Textbook of Uncommon Cancer

To my wife and daughter. *Charles D. Blanke*

To my wife, Beverly, and my daughter, Mary-Michael, to whom I owe everything. *David H. Johnson*

To Dr Mark F. Moots and Fay Moots, to Dr Johns, Dr VandenBerg and Dr Rubinstein, to Dr Posner, to my patients, and to Elizabeth, Hannah, and Skyler; all have been great sources of inspiration. *Paul L. Moots*

To Judy, thanks for tolerating the cold of the northland and the time spent on TUC4, and for being my steadying compass and friend. *Derek Raghavan*

To my wife, Susan, and daughters, Emily and Sarah, for their support and understanding, and to the children and adolescents afflicted by rare cancers and their families who will always be a source of inspiration and motivation. *Gregory H. Reaman*

To my past mentors and current patients and trainees who continue to teach me, and to my family for their continued support. *Peter G. Rose*

To my children, Gabriel, Samantha, and Silas, and to my wife Jennifer, for their love, support, and forbearance in this life I've chosen; to my parents and teachers, I'll always need your guidance; and to my patients, you still inspire me. *Mikkael A. Sekeres*

Textbook of Uncommon Cancer

FOURTH EDITION

Edited by

Derek Raghavan, MD, PhD, FACP, FRACP, FASCO
President, Levine Cancer Institute, Carolinas HealthCare System; Professor/Medicine,
University of North Carolina School of Medicine, Charlotte, NC, USA

Charles D. Blanke, MD, FACP, FRCPC, FASCO
Vice-President, Systemic Therapy, British Columbia Cancer Agency; Professor and Chief,
Medical Oncology, University of British Columbia, Vancouver, BC, Canada

David H. Johnson, MD
Donald W. Seldin Distinguished Chair in Internal Medicine, Professor and Chairman, Department
of Internal Medicine, The University of Texas Southwestern School of Medicine, Dallas, TX, USA

Paul L. Moots, MD
Associate Professor of Neurology and Medicine, Chief, Division of Neuro-Oncology, Vanderbilt-Ingram
Cancer Center, Vanderbilt University Medical Center; Tennessee Valley Healthcare Systems,
Veterans Administration Medical Center, Nashville, TN, USA

Gregory H. Reaman, MD
Professor of Pediatrics and Medicine, The George Washington University School of Medicine
and Health Sciences, Children's National Medical Center, Washington, DC, USA

Peter G. Rose, MD
Head, Section of Gynecologic Oncology, Cleveland Clinic Taussig Cancer Center; Professor of Medicine,
Case Western Reserve University, Cleveland, OH, USA

Mikkael A. Sekeres, MD, MS
Director, Leukemia Program, Associate Professor of Medicine, Department of Hematologic Oncology
and Blood Disorders, Cleveland Clinic Taussig Cancer Institute, Cleveland, OH, USA

WILEY-BLACKWELL

A John Wiley & Sons, Inc., Publication

Published by John Wiley & Sons, Inc., Hoboken, New Jersey
Published simultaneously in Canada

For general information on our other products and services or for technical support, please contact
our Customer Care Department within the United States at (800) 762-2974, outside the United States
at (317) 572-3993 or fax (317) 572-4002.

Wiley also publishes its books in a variety of electronic formats. Some content that appears in print
may not be available in electronic formats. For more information about Wiley products, visit our web
site at www.wiley.com.

Library of Congress Cataloging-in-Publication Data

Textbook of uncommon cancer.
    p. ; cm.
4th ed. / edited by Derek Raghavan ... [et al.].
  Includes bibliographical references and index.
  ISBN 978-1-118-08373-4 (hardback : alk. paper)
  I. Raghavan, Derek. II. Title: 4th ed. / edited by Derek Raghavan ... [et al.].
[DNLM: 1. Neoplasms. 2. Rare Diseases. QZ 200]
616.99′4–dc23

2012021108

Set in 10/11.5pt Times New Roman by SPi Publisher Services, Pondicherry, India

Cover image: Top right-hand image courtesy of Dr Tagawa, bottom right-hand image courtesy of
Dr Rini, top left-hand image courtesy of Dr Raghavan, bottom left-hand image courtesy of Dr Corry
Cover design by Michael Rutkowski

Printed in Singapore
10 9 8 7 6 5 4 3 2

Contents

List of Contributors

Sonia Abuzakhm, MD
Medical Oncology Fellow
Department of Internal Medicine
The Ohio State University
Columbus, OH, USA

Naveed H. Akhtar, MD
Fellow in Medicine
Division of Hematology and Medical Oncology
Department of Medicine
Weill Cornell Medical College of
Cornell University
New York, NY, USA

George A. Alexiou, MD
Chief Resident
Department of Neurosurgery
University Hospital of Ioannina
Ioannina, Greece

Khaled Ali, MD
Department of Solid Tumor Oncology
Cleveland Clinic Taussig Cancer Institute
Glickman Urological Institute
Cleveland, OH, USA

Sonia L. Ali, MD
Medicine Resident and Research Associate
Department of Medicine
Keck School of Medicine at USC
University of Southern California;
Norris Comprehensive Cancer Center and
Hospital
Los Angeles, CA, USA

Michael Alvarado, MD
Assistant Professor
Department of Surgery
University of California San Francisco;
Helen Diller Family Comprehensive
Cancer Center
San Francisco, CA, USA

Deborah K. Armstrong, MD
Associate Professor of Oncology
Department of Medical Oncology
Johns Hopkins Medical Institutions
Baltimore, MD, USA

Rodrigo Arrangoiz, MD, MS
Surgical Oncology Fellow
Fox Chase Cancer Center
Philadelphia, PA, USA

Joseph M. Aulino, MD
Assistant Professor, Neuroradiology

Department of Radiology and
Radiological Sciences
Vanderbilt-Ingram Cancer Center
Vanderbilt University Medical Center
Nashville, TN, USA

Rita Axelrod, MD
Professor, Department of Medical
Oncology
Kimmel Cancer Center
Thomas Jefferson University
Philadelphia, PA, USA

Gildy Babiera, MD
Associate Professor
Department of Surgical Oncology
The University of Texas
MD Anderson Cancer Center
Houston, TX, USA

Sunil Badve, MD, FRCPath
Professor, Pathology and
Laboratory Medicine
Department of Pathology
Indiana University
Indiana, IN, USA

Barbara Bambach, MD
Associate Professor, Oncology
Department of Pediatrics
Roswell Park Cancer Institute;
Associate Professor, Pediatrics
State University of New York at Buffalo
New York, NY, USA

Voichita Bar-Ad, MD
Associate Professor
Department of Radiation Oncology
Kimmel Cancer Center
Thomas Jefferson University
Philadelphia, PA, USA

Richard R. Barakat, MD
Chief, Gynecology Service
Department of Surgery
Memorial Sloan-Kettering
Cancer Center
New York, NY, USA

Gene H. Barnett, MD, FACS
The Rose Ella Burkhardt Chair in
Neurosurgical Oncology
Professor and Director

Rose Ella Burkhardt Brain Tumor and
Neuro-Oncology Center
Cleveland Clinic Neurological Institute;
Department of Neurological Surgery
Cleveland Clinic
Cleveland, OH, USA

Paul M. Barr, MD
Assistant Professor of Medicine and Oncology
Department of Medicine
James P. Wilmot Cancer Center
University of Rochester
Rochester, NY, USA

Rachid Baz, MD
Assistant Member
Department of Malignant Hematology
H. Lee Moffitt Cancer Center and
Research Institute;
Assistant Professor
Department of Oncologic Sciences
and Medicine
University of South Florida
Tampa, FL, USA

Himisha Beltran, MD
Assistant Professor of Medicine and Urology
Division of Hematology and Medical Oncology
Department of Medicine
Weill Cornell Medical College of
Cornell University
New York, NY, USA

Jordan D. Berlin, MD
Professor of Medicine
Department of Medicine
Vanderbilt University Medical Center
Nashville, TN, USA

Charles Biscotti, MD
Staff Pathologist
Department of Anatomic Pathology
Cleveland Clinic
Cleveland, OH, USA

James F. Bishop, AO, MD, MMed, MBBS,
FRACP, FRCPA
Executive Director
Victorian Comprehensive Cancer Centre;
Professor of Cancer Medicine
University of Melbourne;
Professor of Medicine
University of Sydney
Sydney, NSW, Australia

Destin Black, MD
Clinical Assistant Professor/Director
Division of Gynecologic Oncology
Department of Obstetrics and Gynecology
Louisiana State University Health
Sciences Center
New Orleans, LA, USA

Mark Bloomston, MD
Associate Professor of Surgery
Division of Surgical Oncology
The Ohio State University
Columbus, OH, USA

Robert E. Bristow, MD, MBA
Professor and Director
Division of Gynecologic Oncology
Department of Obstetrics and Gynecology
University of California Irvine
Orange, CA, USA

Jubilee Brown, MD
Associate Professor
Department of Gynecologic Oncology and
the Reproductive Sciences
The University of Texas
MD Anderson Cancer Center
Houston, TX, USA

Ronald M. Bukowski, MD
Department of Solid Tumor Oncology
Cleveland Clinic Taussig Cancer Institute
Glickman Urological Institute
Cleveland, OH, USA

Steve Campbell, MD
Professor of Surgery
Department of Urologic Oncology
Cleveland Clinic
Cleveland, OH, USA

Richard D. Carvajal, MD
Assistant Attending Physician
Melanoma/Sarcoma and Developmental
Therapeutics Services
Memorial Sloan-Kettering Cancer Center
New York, NY, USA

Robert C. Castellino, MD
Pediatric Neuro-Oncology Program
Aflac Cancer Center and Blood Disorders Service
Children's Healthcare of Atlanta;
Assistant Professor
Emory University School of Medicine
Emory Children's Center
Atlanta, GA, USA

A. Bapsi Chakravarthy, MD
Assistant Professor
Department of Radiation Oncology
Vanderbilt University School of Medicine
Nashville, TN, USA

Philip R. Chapman, MD
Assistant Professor
Neuroradiology Section

Department of Radiology
University of Alabama
Birmingham, AL, USA

Eunpi Cho, MD
Resident, Department of Internal Medicine
Johns Hopkins University School of Medicine
Baltimore, MD, USA

Maria M. Choudhary, MD
Resident, Department of Internal Medicine
Cleveland Clinic
Cleveland, OH, USA

Christine H. Chung, MD
Associate Professor of Oncology
Department of Medicine
Johns Hopkins Medical Center
Baltimore, MD, USA

Stephen W. Clark, MD, PhD
Assistant Professor
Division of Neuro-Oncology
Department of Neurology
Vanderbilt-Ingram Cancer Center
Vanderbilt University Medical Center
Nashville, TN, USA

Anthony J. Cmelak, MD
Senior Medical Director
Department of Radiation Oncology
Vanderbilt-Ingram Cancer Center
Vanderbilt University Medical Center
Nashville, TN, USA

David Cognetti, MD
Assistant Professor
Department of Otolaryngology-Head and
Neck Surgery
Kimmel Cancer Center
Thomas Jefferson University
Philadelphia, PA, USA

Michael Cooper, MD
Associate Professor
Department of Neurology
Vanderbilt-Ingram Cancer Center
Vanderbilt University Medical Center;
Tennessee Valley Healthcare Systems
Veterans Administration Medical Center
Nashville, TN, USA

Larry J. Copeland, MD
Professor of Obstetrics and Gynecology
James Cancer Hopsital and
Solove Research Institute
The Ohio State University
Columbus, OH, USA

June Corry, MD
Associate Professor
Radiation Oncology Chair
Head and Neck Cancer Service
Peter MacCallum Cancer Centre
Melbourne, VIC, Australia

Bogdan A. Czerniak, MD, PhD
Professor

Department of Anatomic Pathology
The University of Texas
MD Anderson Cancer Center
Houston, TX, USA

Lisa M. DeAngelis, MD
Chairman, Department of Neurology
Memorial Sloan-Kettering Cancer Center;
Professor of Neurology
Department of Neurology and Neuroscience
Weill Cornell Medical College of
Cornell University
New York, NY, USA

Michael Deavers, MD
Professor
Department of Pathology
The University of Texas
MD Anderson Cancer Center
Houston, TX, USA

Louis P. Dehner, MD
Lauren V. Ackerman Department of
Surgical Pathology
Barnes-Jewish Hospital;
Professor, Department of Pathology and
Immunology
St Louis Children's Hospital
Washington University Medical Center
St Louis, MO, USA

John G. Devlin, MD
Attending Physician
Hematology/Oncology Section
Bryn Mawr Medical Specialists Association
Bryn Mawr, PA, USA

Teresa P. Díaz-Montes, MD
Assistant Professor
The Kelly Gynecologic Oncology Service
Department of Gynecology and Obstetrics
Johns Hopkins Medical Institutions
Baltimore, MD, USA

Colin P. Dinney, MD
Chair, Department of Urology
The University of Texas
MD Anderson Cancer Center
Houston, TX, USA

Jeffrey S. Dome, MD, PhD
McKnew Professor of Pediatric Oncology
Chief, Division of Oncology
Children's National Medical Center;
Professor of Pediatrics
George Washington University School of Medicine
Washington, DC, USA

Tanya B. Dorf, MD
Assistant Professor of Medicine
Division of Cancer Medicine
Keck School of Medicine at USC
University of Southern California;
Norris Comprehensive Cancer Center and
Hospital
Los Angeles, CA, USA

Regan M. Duffy, MD, MPH
Fellow in Hematology and Medical Oncology
Division of Hematology and
Medical Oncology
Knight Cancer Institute
Oregon Health and Science University
Portland, OR, USA

Ian O. Ellis, FRCPath
Professor of Cancer Pathology
Department of Histopathology
The University of Nottingham and
Nottingham University Hospitals NHS Trust
Nottingham City Hospital Campus
Nottingham, UK

Kim Ely, MD
Assistant Professor
Department of Pathology
Vanderbilt-Ingram Cancer Center
Vanderbilt University Medical Center
Nashville, TN, USA

Ramez N. Eskander, MD
Clinical Instructor
Division of Gynecologic Oncology
Department of Gynecology and Obstetrics
University of California Irvine
Orange, CA, USA

Mark Faries, MD
Director of Melanoma Research
John Wayne Cancer Institute
Santa Monica, CA, USA

Bonald C. Figueiredo, MD, PhD
Pelé Pequeno Príncipe Research Institute
Faculdades Pequeno Príncipe
Curitiba, PR, Brazil

Jonathan L. Finlay, MB, ChB
Professor of Clinical Pediatrics, Neurology
and Neurological Surgery
Division of Pediatric Hematology/Oncology
Department of Pediatrics
Keck School of Medicine at USC
University of Southern California;
Director, Neuro-oncology Program
Children's Center for Cancer
and Blood Diseases
Children's Hospital Los Angeles
Los Angeles, CA, USA

Douglas B. Flieder, MD
Professor
Department of Pathology
Fox Chase Cancer Center
Philadelphia, PA, USA

Jonathan W. Friedberg, MD, MMSc
Chief, Hematology/Oncology Division
Department of Medicine
James P. Wilmot Cancer Center;
Professor of Medicine and Oncology
University of Rochester
Rochester, NY, USA

Wayne L. Furman, MD
Member, Department of Oncology
St Jude Children's Research Hospital;
Professor, Department of Pediatrics
The University of Tennessee College of
Medicine
Nashville, TN, USA

Giuseppe Giaccone, MD, PhD
Chief, Medical Oncology Branch
National Cancer Institute
Bethesda, MD, USA

Michael Z. Gilcrease, MD, PhD
Professor
Department of Pathology
The University of Texas
MD Anderson Cancer Center
Houston, TX, USA

Bonnie S. Glisson, MD
Professor of Medicine
Department of Thoracic/Head and
Neck Medical Oncology
The University of Texas
MD Anderson Cancer Center
Houston, TX, USA

Helenice Gobbi, MD, PhD
Assistant Professor of Pathology
Department of Pathology
Federal University of Minas Gerais
Belo Horizonte, MG, Brazil

Karyn Goodman, MD
Radiation Oncologist
Department of Radiation Oncology
Department of Medicine
Memorial Sloan-Kettering Cancer Center
New York, NY, USA

Elizabeth G. Grubbs, MD
Assistant Professor
Department of Surgical Oncology
The University of Texas
MD Anderson Cancer Center
Houston, TX, USA

Mouhammed A. Habbra, MD
Assistant Professor
Department of Endocrine Neoplasia and
Hormone Disease
The University of Texas
MD Anderson Cancer Center
Houston, TX, USA

Omid Hamid, MD
Director, Melanoma Center
Chief, Clinical Research
The Angeles Clinic and Research Institute
Santa Monica, CA, USA

Julie E. Hammack, MD
Assistant Professor
Department of Neurology

Mayo Clinic
Rochester, MN, USA

Stephen Hazell, MD
Clinical Anatomic Pathology Unit
Royal Marsden NHS Foundation Trust
London, UK

Bryan T. Hennessy, MD
Consultant Medical Oncologist
Department of Medical Oncology
Beaumont Hospital
Dublin, Ireland

Cynthia E. Herzog, MD
Professor of Pediatrics
Medical Director Pediatric
Clinical Research
Division of Pediatrics
The University of Texas
MD Anderson Cancer Center
Houston, TX, USA

Gabriel N. Hortobagyi, MD
Chair, Breast Medical Oncology
The University of Texas
MD Anderson Cancer Center
Houston, TX, USA

Alan Horwich, MD
Consultant Clinical Oncologist
Academic Unit of Radiotherapy and
Oncology
Institute of Cancer Research and
Royal Marsden NHS Foundation Trust
Sutton, UK

Robert Huddart, MD
Academic Unit of Radiotherapy and
Oncology
Institute of Cancer Research and
Royal Marsden NHS Foundation Trust
Sutton, UK

Winston Huh, MD
Assistant Professor of Pediatrics
Division of Pediatrics
The University of Texas
MD Anderson Cancer Center
Houston, TX, USA

Mohamad A. Hussein, MD
Professor of Medicine and Oncology
Division of Medicine
University of South Florida
Tampa, FL, USA

Arun Jesudian, MD
Clinical Fellow
Division of Gastroenterology and Hepatology
Department of Medicine
Center for Advanced Digestive Care
New York-Presbyterian Hospital
Weill Cornell Medical College of
Cornell University
New York, NY, USA

Anuja Jhingran, MD
Professor
Department of Radiation Oncology
The University of Texas
MD Anderson Cancer Center
Houston, TX, USA

Derek R. Johnson, MD
Instructor in Neurology
Department of Neurology
Mayo Clinic
Rochester, MN, USA

Rima F. Jubran, MD, MPH
Associate Professor of Clinical Pediatrics
Division of Pediatric Hematology/Oncology
Department of Pediatrics
Keck School of Medicine at USC
University of Southern California
Los Angeles, CA, USA

Samer E. Kaba, MD
Vice President
Clinical Research and Medical Management
Scirex Corporation
Horsham, PA, USA

Masako Kasami, MD
Shizuoka Cancer Center
Shizuoka Prefecture
Japan

Matthew H. G. Katz, MD
Assistant Professor
Department of Surgical Oncology
The University of Texas
MD Anderson Cancer Center
Houston, TX, USA

Anna Marie Kenney, PhD
Associate Professor
Departments of Neurological Surgery and
Cell Biology
Vanderbilt-Ingram Cancer Center
Vanderbilt University Medical Center
Nashville, TN, USA

Joshua P. Kesterson, MD
Chief, Division of Gynecologic Oncology
Penn State Milton S. Hershey Medical Center
Hershey, PA USA

Rami Komrokji, MD
Moffitt Cancer Center and Research Institute
Tampa, FL, USA

Michael E. Kupferman, MD
Assistant Professor
Department of Head and Neck Surgery
The University of Texas
MD Anderson Cancer Center
Houston, TX, USA

Athanassios P. Kyritsis, MD
Professor and Chairman
Department of Neurology
University Hospital of Ioannina
Ioannina, Greece

Corey J. Langer, MD, FACP
Professor of Medicine
Abramson Cancer Center
University of Pennsylvania
Philadelphia, PA, USA

Aleksandr Lazaryan, MD
Department of Hematologic Oncology and
Blood Disorders
Taussig Cancer Institute
Cleveland Clinic
Cleveland, OH, USA

Lawrence Leichman, MD
Medical Director
Aptium GI Cancer Consortium
Palm Springs, CA, USA

Shashikant B. Lele, MD
Clinical Chief
Division of Gynecologic Oncology
Roswell Park Cancer Institute
Buffalo, NY, USA

Rong Li, MD, PhD
Fellow
Division of Neuropathology
Department of Pathology
University of Alabama
Birmingham, AL, USA

Patrick J. Loehrer Sr., MD
H. H. Gregg Professor of Medicine
Director
Indiana University Melvin and Bren Simon
Cancer Center;
Associate Dean for Cancer Research
Indiana University School of Medicine
Indianapolis, IN, USA

John S. Macdonald, MD
Chief Medical Officer
Aptium Oncology
Los Angeles, CA, USA

Tobey J. MacDonald, MD
Director, Pediatric Neuro-Oncology Program
Aflac Cancer Center and Blood
Disorders Service
Children's Healthcare of Atlanta;
Associate Professor of Pediatrics
Emory University School of Medicine
Emory Children's Center
Atlanta, GA, USA

Anita Mahajan, MD
Professor
Co-Section Head Pediatric and CNS Radiation
Oncology
Department of Radiation Oncology
The University of Texas
MD Anderson Cancer Center
Houston, TX, USA

Kyle Mannion, MD
Assistant Professor
Department of Otolaryngology
Vanderbilt-Ingram Cancer Center

Vanderbilt University Medical Center
Nashville, TN, USA

Daniela E. Matei, MD
Associate Professor
Department of Medicine, Hematology-Oncology
Indiana University School of Medicine
Indianapolis, IN, USA

Rahel Mathew, MD
Dermatopathology Fellow
Departments of Pathology & Cell Biology and
Dermatology
University of South Florida College of Medicine;
Department of Cutaneous Oncology
H. Lee Moffitt Cancer Center
Tampa, FL, USA

Ingrid A. Mayer, MD, MSCI
Assistant Professor
Division of Hematology Oncology
Department of Medicine
Vanderbilt University School of Medicine
Nashville, TN, USA

Julie Means-Powell, MD
Assistant Professor
Division of Hematology Oncology
Department of Medicine
Vanderbilt University School of Medicine
Nashville, TN, USA

Ruben A. Mesa, MD
Consultant Hematologist
Chair, Division of Hematology and
Medical Oncology
Professor of Medicine
Mayo Clinic
Scottsdale, AZ, USA

Jane L. Messina, MD
Professor
Departments of Pathology & Cell Biology and
Dermatology
University of South Florida College of
Medicine;
Department of Cutaneous Oncology
H. Lee Moffitt Cancer Center
Tampa, FL, USA

Yoav H. Messinger, MD
Director, International PPB Registry
Department of Pediatric Hematology/Oncology
Children's Hospitals and Clinics of Minnesota
Minneapolis, MN, USA

Helen Michael, MD
Professor
Department of Pathology and
Laboratory Medicine
Indiana University School of Medicine
Indianapolis, IN, USA

Kathy D. Miller, MD
Associate Professor of Medicine
Indiana University Melvin and
Bren Simon Cancer Center
Indianapolis, IN, USA

Vincent A. Miller, MD
Consultant, Thoracic Oncology Service
Division of Solid Tumor Oncology
Department of Medicine
Memorial Sloan-Kettering Cancer Center
New York, NY, USA

Randall E. Millikan, MD, PhD
Associate Professor
Department of Genitourinary Medical
Oncology
The University of Texas
MD Anderson Cancer Center
Houston, TX, USA

Brett Mobley, MD
Assistant Professor
Department of Pathology, Microbiology and
Immunology (Neuropathology)
Vanderbilt-Ingram Cancer Center
Vanderbilt University Medical Center
Nashville, TN, USA

Bradley J. Monk, MD, FACS, FACOG
Professor
Division of Gynecologic Oncology
Department of Obstetrics and Gynecology
Creighton University School of
Medicine at St Joseph's Hospital and
Medical Center
Phoenix, AZ, USA

Cesar Moran, MD
Professor
Department of Pathology
The University of Texas
MD Anderson Cancer Center
Houston, TX, USA

David S. Morgan, MD
Associate Professor of Medicine
Division of Hematology Oncology
Department of Medicine
Vanderbilt University School of Medicine
Nashville, TN, USA

Donald L. Morton, MD
Chief, Melanoma Program
Director, Fellowship Program
John Wayne Cancer Institute
Santa Monica, CA, USA

Stacy L. Moulder, MD, MSCI
Associate Professor
Department of Breast Medical Oncology
The University of Texas
MD Anderson Cancer Center
Houston, TX, USA

Barbara A. Murphy, MD
Professor of Medicine
Director, Pain and Symptom Management
Program
Leader, Head and Neck Research Team
Vanderbilt-Ingram Cancer Center
Vanderbilt University Medical Center
Nashville, TN, USA

L. Burt Nabors, MD
Professor
Division of Neuro-Oncology
Department of Neurology
University of Alabama
Birmingham, AL, USA

Govind Nandakumar, MD
Assistant Professor of Surgery
Department of Surgery, Colorectal Surgery
Center for Advanced Digestive Care
New York-Presbyterian Hospital
Weill Cornell Medical College of Cornell University
New York, NY, USA

Herbert B. Newton, MD, FAAN
Professor of Neurology, Neurosurgery
Oncology Director, Division of
Neuro-Oncology
Esther Dardinger Endowed Chair in
Neuro-Oncology
Co-Director, Dardinger Neuro-Oncology
Center
Ohio State University Medical Center and
James Cancer Hospital
Columbus, OH, USA

Kenneth J. Niermann, MD, MSCI
Assistant Professor
Department of Radiation Oncology
Vanderbilt-Ingram Cancer Center
Vanderbilt University School of Medicine
Nashville, TN, USA

Thomas Olencki, MD
Clinical Professor of Medicine
Department of Internal Medicine
The Ohio State University
Columbus, OH, USA

Michael J. Overman, MD
Assistant Professor
Department of Gastrointestinal Medical Oncology
The University of Texas
MD Anderson Cancer Center
Houston, TX, USA

Eric Padron, MD
Moffitt Cancer Center and Research Institute
Tampa, FL, USA

David L. Page, MD
Department of Pathology
Vanderbilt University School of Medicine
Nashville, TN, USA

Paul G. Pagnini, MD
Assistant Professor
Department of Radiation Oncology
Keck School of Medicine at USC
University of Southern California;
Norris Comprehensive Cancer Center and
Hospital
Los Angeles, CA, USA

Kevin T. Palka, MD
Associate Professor
Department of Medicine

Vanderbilt-Ingram Cancer Center
Vanderbilt University Medical Center;
Department of Medicine
Meharry Medical College;
Tennessee Valley Healthcare Systems
Veterans Administration Medical Center
Nashville, TN, USA

Cheryl A. Palmer, MD
Professor
Division of Neuropathology
Department of Pathology
University of Alabama
Birmingham, AL, USA

Alberto S. Pappo, MD
Member, Division of Oncology
Head, Division of Solid Tumors
St Jude Children's Research Hospital
Memphis, TN, USA

John J. Park, MD
Texas Spine and Neurosurgery Center
Methodist Sugar Land Hospital
Sugar Land, TX, USA

Stephanie Perkins, MD
Assistant Professor
Department of Radiation Oncology
Vanderbilt-Ingram Cancer Center
Vanderbilt University Medical Center
Nashville, TN, USA

Sara Peters, MD
Associate Professor of Clinical Pathology
Department of Pathology
The Ohio State University
Columbus, OH, USA

Alexandria T. Phan, MD
Associate Professor
Department of Gastrointestinal Medical
Oncology
The University of Texas
MD Anderson Cancer Center
Houston, TX, USA

M. Catherine Pietanza, MD
Assistant Attending
Thoracic Oncology Service
Department of Medicine
Memorial Sloan-Kettering Cancer Center
New York, NY, USA

Emilia M. Pinto, PhD
Department of Biochemistry and
International Outreach Program
St Jude Children's Research Hospital
Memphis, TN, USA

Hans G. Pohl, MD, FAAP
Associate Professor, Urology and Pediatrics
Director of Pediatric Urology Research
Program Director, Pediatric Urology Fellowship
Division of Urology
Children's National Medical Center;
George Washington University School of
Medicine
Washington, DC, USA

Elizabeta Popa, MD
Assistant Professor
Division of Hematology and Medical Oncology,
Gastrointestinal Oncology
Department of Medicine
Center for Advanced Digestive Care
New York-Presbyterian Hospital
Weill Cornell Medical College of Cornell University
New York, NY, USA

David I. Quinn, MBBS, PhD, FRACP, FACP
Associate Professor of Medicine
Division of Cancer Medicine
Keck School of Medicine at USC
University of Southern California;
Norris Comprehensive Cancer Center and
Hospital
Los Angeles, CA, USA

Kanwal Raghav, MD, MBBS
Fellow, Hematology/Oncology
Division of Cancer Medicine
The University of Texas
MD Anderson Cancer Center
Houston, TX, USA

Gazanfar Rahmathulla, MD
Clinical Scholar
Rose Ella Burkhardt Brain Tumor and
Neuro-Oncology Center
Cleveland Clinic
Cleveland, OH, USA

Arun Rajan, MD
Staff Clinician
Medical Oncology Branch
National Cancer Institute
Bethesda, MD, USA

Emad A. Rakha, FRCPath
Clinical Associate Professor
Department of Histopathology
The University of Nottingham and
Nottingham University Hospitals NHS Trust
Nottingham City Hospital Campus
Nottingham, UK

Nicole M. Randall, MD
Internal Medicine Resident
Department of Oncology
Indiana University School of Medicine
Indianapolis, IN, USA

Chandrajit P. Raut, MD
Assistant Professor of Surgery
Harvard Medical School;
Division of Surgical Oncology
Brigham and Women's Hospital
Center for Sarcoma and Bone Oncology;
Dana-Farber Cancer Institute
Boston, MA, USA

Diane Reidy-Lagunes, MD
Gastrointestinal Oncology Service
Department of Medicine
Memorial Sloan-Kettering Cancer Center;
Assistant Professor of Medicine

Weill Cornell Medical College of Cornell University
New York, NY, USA

Raul C. Ribeiro, MD
Associate Director
Department of Oncology and
International Outreach Program
St Jude Children's Research Hospital
Memphis, TN, USA

John A. Ridge, MD, PhD
Chief, Head and Neck Surgery Section
Professor of Surgical Oncology and
Developmental Therapeutics
Fox Chase Cancer Center
Philadelphia, PA, USA

Gregory J. Riely, MD, PhD
Assistant Attending
Thoracic Oncology Service
Division of Solid Tumor Oncology
Department of Medicine
Memorial Sloan-Kettering Cancer Center;
Assistant Professor
Weill Cornell Medical College of Cornell University
New York, NY, USA

Brian I. Rini, MD, FACP
Associate Professor
Department of Solid Tumor Oncology
Cleveland Clinic Taussig Cancer Institute
Glickman Urological Institute
Cleveland, OH, USA

Brian D. Robinson, MD
Assistant Professor of Pathology and
Laboratory Medicine
Department of Pathology
Weill Cornell Medical College of Cornell University;
Assistant Professor of Pathology in Urology
Weill Cornell Cancer Center
New York, NY, USA

Carlos Rodriguez-Galindo, MD
Department of Pediatric Oncology
Dana-Farber Cancer Institute;
Associate Professor of Pediatrics
Harvard Medical School
Boston, MA, USA

Robert Rosser, MD
Chief of Anatomic Pathology
Desert Regional Medical Center
Palm Springs, CA, USA

Leonard B. Saltz, MD
Chief, Gastrointestinal Oncology Service and
Department of Medicine
Memorial Sloan-Kettering Cancer Center;
Professor of Medicine
Weill Cornell Medical College of
Cornell University
New York, NY, USA

Benjamin Samstein, MD
Assistant Professor of Surgery
Department of Surgery

Columbia University Medical Center
New York, NY, USA

Melinda E. Sanders, MD
Associate Professor
Department of Pathology
Vanderbilt University School of Medicine
Nashville, TN, USA

Alan B. Sandler, MD
Professor of Medicine
Division Chief, Division of Hematology and
Medical Oncology
DeArmond Chair Clinical Cancer Research
Knight Cancer Institute
Oregon Health and Science University
Portland, OR, USA

Inderpal (Netu) S. Sarkaria, MD
Department of Thoracic Surgery
Memorial Sloan-Kettering Cancer Center
New York, NY, USA

Jeanne M. Schilder, MD
Associate Professor
Department of Obstetrics and Gynecology,
Gynecology-Oncology
Indiana University School of Medicine
Indianapolis, IN, USA

Matthew Schniederjan, MD
Department of Pathology
Children's Healthcare of Atlanta
Atlanta, GA, USA

Felice Schnoll-Sussman, MD
Assistant Professor
Division of Gastroenterology and Hepatology
Department of Medicine
Center for Advanced Digestive Care
New York-Presbyterian Hospital
Weill Cornell Medical College of
Cornell University
New York, NY, USA

Kris Ann P. Schultz, MD
Department of Pediatric Hematology/Oncology
Children's Hospitals and Clinics of Minnesota
Minneapolis, MN, USA

Richard A. Scolyer, BMedSci, MBBS, MD,
FRCPA, FRCPath
Consultant Pathologist and Co-Director of
Research
Melanoma Institute Australia;
Senior Staff Specialist
Tissue Pathology and Diagnostic Oncology
Royal Prince Alfred Hospital;
Clinical Professor
The University of Sydney
Sydney, NSW, Australia

Alberto E. Selman, MD
Division of Gynecologic Oncology
Department of Obstetrics and Gynecology
Clinical Hospital
Universidad de Chile
Santiago, Chile

Salyka Sengsayadeth, MD
Clinical Fellow
Department of Medicine
Vanderbilt-Ingram Cancer Center
Vanderbilt University Medical Center
Nashville, TN, USA

Manisha H. Shah, MD
Associate Professor of Internal Medicine
Department of Internal Medicine
The Ohio State University
Columbus, OH, USA

Manish A. Shah, MD
Director, Gastrointestinal Oncology
Division of Hematology and
Medical Oncology, Gastrointestinal
Oncology
Department of Medicine
Center for Advanced Digestive Care
New York-Presbyterian Hospital
Weill Cornell Medical College of
Cornell University
New York, NY, USA

Vladimir Sheynzon, MD
Assistant Professor of Clinical Radiology
Columbia University Medical Center
New York, NY, USA

Chanjuan Shi, MD
Assistant Professor
Department of Pathology, Microbiology and
Immunology
Vanderbilt University Medical Center
Nashville, TN, USA

Arlene O. Siefker-Radtke, MD
Associate Professor
Department of Genitourinary
Medical Oncology
The University of Texas
MD Anderson Cancer Center
Houston, TX, USA

Abby B. Siegel, MD, MS
Assistant Professor of Clinical Medicine
Department of Medicine
Columbia University Medical Center
New York, NY, USA

Allen K. Sills, MD
Associate Professor
Department of Neurosurgery
Vanderbilt-Ingram Cancer Center
Vanderbilt University Medical Center
Nashville, TN, USA

Jean F. Simpson, MD
Professor
Department of Pathology
Vanderbilt University School of Medicine
Nashville, TN, USA

Robert J. Sinard, MD
Associate Professor of Otolaryngology
Department of Otolaryngology

Vanderbilt-Ingram Cancer Center
Vanderbilt University Medical Center
Nashville, TN, USA

Arun D. Singh, MD
Director
Department of Ophthalmic Oncology
Cole Eye Institute
Cleveland Clinic
Cleveland, OH, USA

Gurcharan Singh Khera, MD, FRCR (UK)
Maricopa Integrated Health Trust
Phoenix, AZ, USA

George W. Sledge, Jr., MD
Named Professor of Medicine
Department of Oncology
Indiana University School of Medicine
Indianapolis, IN, USA

B. Douglas Smith, MD
Associate Professor of Oncology
Division of Hematologic Malignancies
Sidney Kimmel Comprehensive Cancer
Center at Johns Hopkins
Baltimore, MD, USA

Vernon K. Sondak, MD
Chair, Department of Cutaneous Oncology
H. Lee Moffitt Cancer Center;
Professor, Departments of Oncologic
Sciences and Surgery
University of South Florida College of Medicine
Tampa, FL, USA

John Sweetenham, MD
Professor
Department of Hematologic Oncology and
Blood Disorders
Taussig Cancer Institute
Cleveland Clinic
Cleveland, OH, USA

Scott T. Tagawa, MD, MS
Assistant Professor of Medicine and Urology
Division of Hematology and
Medical Oncology
Department of Medicine and
Department of Urology
Weill Cornell Medical College of
Cornell University;
Weill Cornell Cancer Center
New York, NY, USA

Shota Tanaka, MD
Neuro-Oncology Fellow
Stephen E. and Catherine Pappas Center
for Neuro-Oncology
Massachusetts General Hospital;
Center For Neuro-Oncology
Dana-Farber Cancer Institute;
Harvard Medical School
Boston, MA, USA

Krishnansu S. Tewari, MD
Associate Professor and Director of Research
Gynecologic Oncology Group at UC Irvine

Division of Gynecologic Oncology
Department of Obstetrics and Gynecology
University of California
Irvine Medical Center
Orange, CA, USA

Anish Thomas, MD
Cinical Fellow
Medical Oncology Branch
National Cancer Institute
Bethesda, MD, USA

John F. Thompson, MD
Executive Director
Melanoma Institute Australia;
Melanoma and Surgical Oncology
Royal Prince Alfred Hospital;
Professor of Melanoma and Surgical Oncology
The University of Sydney
Sydney, NSW, Australia

Raoul Tibes, MD, PhD
Senior Associate Consultant
Associate Director, Acute and Chronic Leukemia
Program
Assistant Professor
Division of Hematology and Medical Oncology
Mayo Clinic
Scottsdale, AZ, USA

Ramon V. Tiu, MD
Assistant Professor of Molecular Medicine
Department of Translational Hematology and
Oncology Research and
Department of Hematologic Oncology and
Blood Disorders
Taussig Cancer Institute
Cleveland Clinic
Cleveland, OH, USA

William D. Travis, MD
Attending Thoracic Pathologist
Department of Pathology
Memorial Sloan-Kettering Cancer Center
New York, NY, USA

Madalina Tuluc, MD
Assistant Professor
Department of Pathology, Anatomy and
Cell Biology
Kimmel Cancer Center
Thomas Jefferson University
Philadelphia, PA, USA

Vicente Valero, MD
Deputy Chairman
Department of Breast Medical Oncology
The University of Texas
MD Anderson Cancer Center
Houston, TX, USA

Russell Vang, MD
Associate Professor
Division of Gynecologic Pathology
Department of Pathology
Johns Hopkins Medical Institutions
Baltimore, MD, USA

Amanda VanSandt, DO
Resident in Pathology
Department of Pathology
Knight Cancer Institute
Oregon Health and Science University
Portland, OR, USA

Valeria Visconte, PhD
Postdoctoral Research Fellow
Department of Translational Hematology and
Oncology Research
Taussig Cancer Institute
Cleveland Clinic
Cleveland, OH, USA

Margaret von Mehren, MD
Professor
Department of Medical Oncology
Director Sarcoma Program
Fox Chase Cancer Center
Philadelphia, PA, USA

Patrick Y. Wen, MD
Director, Center for Neuro-Oncology
Dana-Farber Cancer Institute;
Professor of Neurology
Harvard Medical School
Boston, MA, USA

Mark R. Wick, MD
Professor of Pathology
Associate Director of Surgical Pathology
Department of Pathology
University of Virginia
Charlottesville, VA, USA

Wei Yang, MD
Professor
Department of Diagnostic Radiology
The University of Texas
MD Anderson Cancer Center
Houston, TX, USA

Gerard P. Zambetti, PhD
Department of Biochemistry
St Jude Children's Research Hospital
Memphis, TN, USA

Ming Zhou, MD
Department of Pathology
Cleveland Clinic
Cleveland, OH, USA

Preface

A quarter of a century after the first edition of this textbook, conceived by Chris Williams, John Krikorian, Mark Green and Derek Raghavan, the challenge of "Uncommon Cancers" remains as nearly as daunting as ever. Oncologists still wrestle with these rare malignancies quite often, but few of us have sufficient personal experience to feel confident in the level of evidence governing our management of these conditions. Of importance, we should never forget that, for the individual with an uncommon malignancy, the disease is not only rare but real, and such patients need additional support and care because standard paradigms of care may not exist, and thus the level of clinical uncertainty is much more substantial.

Although there is increasing interest in addressing the problems of our patients with uncommon cancers, the lack of available level 1 (and/or level 2) evidence still confounds the standardization of optimal treatment protocols. As an alternative, we turn to expert collation and interpretation of limited, available information, and thus we continue to believe that our *Textbook of Uncommon Cancer* has a very useful role in providing the basis for the development of management strategies in this setting. As the published case experience and the development of registries have increased in the past 5–6 years, it seems timely to update our book once again. In so doing, we hope that further investigation might be stimulated to develop a strong evidence base for future recommendations.

We have asked our authors to provide a structured overview of the published information and to explain their own approach to management, even in the absence of defined guidelines or level 1–2 data. Our intent is simply to help the clinician inexperienced in treating specific rare tumors, with the intention of improving quality of care, while saving that physician some time.

To keep the book dynamic, we have again evolved changes in the Editorial Board, and we have also modified the structure of the book. Our classic and best received chapters have been updated, but for some topics, new authors have been recruited, who have either completely rewritten, or updated and extended, the contributions from earlier editions. We sincerely thank our past authors for their seminal contributions to past editions and the present work. Some new subjects have also been added.

As always, our families and our support staff have made the sacrifices necessary to facilitate the writing and editing of a large textbook, and we appreciate them greatly, but recognize that it is just not enough to thank them for their support, affection and forbearance.

Derek Raghavan
Charles D. Blanke
David H. Johnson
Paul L. Moots
Gregory H. Reaman
Peter G. Rose
Mikkael A. Sekeres

List of Abbreviations

2-CDA	2-chlorodeoxyadenosine
2HG	2-hydroxyglutarate
3-D	three-dimensional
5-FU	5-fluorouracil
5-HIAA	5-hydroxyindoleacetic acid
17-OHP	17-hydroxyprogesterone
AA	aplastic anemia
AC	atypical carcinoid
ACA	adrenocortical adenoma
ACC	adrenocortical carcinoma/adenoid cystic carcinoma
aCML	atypical chronic myeloid leukemia
ACOSOG	American College of Surgeons Oncology Group
ACT	adrenocortical tumor
ACTH	adrenocorticotropic hormone
ADC	apparent diffusion coefficient
ADCC	antibody-dependent cellular cytotoxicity
ADEM	acute disseminated encephalomyelitis
ADH	antidiuretic hormone
ADOC	adriamycin, cisplatin, cyclophosphamide, vincristine
AFIP	Armed Forces Institute of Pathology
AFP	α-fetoprotein
AFPGC	α-fetoprotein-producing gastric carcinoma
AI	adrenal "incidentaloma"/aromatase inhibitor
AIDS	acquired immunodeficiency syndrome
AJCC	American Joint Commission on Cancer
ALCL	anaplastic large cell lymphoma
ALK	anaplastic lymphoma kinase
ALL	acute lymphoblastic leukemia
allo-SCT	allogeneic stem cell transplantation
AML	angiomyolipoma/acute myelogenous/myeloid leukemia
ANC	absolute neutrophil count
APC	adenomatous polyposis coli
APP	atypical choroid plexus papilloma
APR	abdominoperineal resection
APUD	amine precursor uptake and decarboxylation
AR	androgen receptor
ART	adenocarcinoma of the rete testis
ASC	atypical squamous cells
ASCR	autologous stem cell rescue
ASCT	autologous stem cell transplant

ASCUS	atypical squamous cells of undetermined significance
ASPS	alveolar soft part sarcoma
ATC	anaplastic thyroid carcinomas
ATG	antithymocyte globulin
ATP	adenosine triphosphate
AT/RT	atypical teratoid/rhabdoid tumor
AUC	area under the curve
AV	atrioventricular
BAP1	BRCA1-associated protein-1
BBB	blood–brain barrier
BCC	basal cell carcinoma
BCG	bacillus Calmette–Guérin
BCNU	bis-chloroethylnitrosourea (carmustine)
BCT	breast-conserving treatment
BED	biologically effective dose
BG	Birbeck granules
BHCG	β-human chorionic gonadotropin
BL	Burkitt lymphoma
BMF	bone marrow failure
BML	benign metastasizing leiomyoma
BOT	borderline ovarian tumors
BPH	benign prostatic hyperplasia
BSC	best supportive care
BSCC	basaloid squamous cell carcinoma
BTSG	brain tumor support groups
BTTP	British Testicular Tumour Panel
BWH/DFCI	Brigham and Women's Hospital/Dana-Farber Cancer Institute
BWS	Beckwith–Weidemann syndrome
CAM	cell adhesion molecule
CASR	calcium-sensing receptor
CBC	complete blood count
CBF	core binding factor
CBG	corticosteroid-binding globulin
CCA	clear cell adenocarcinoma
CCAM-PAM	congenital cystic adenomatoid or pulmonary airway malformation
CCG	Children's Cancer Group
CCNU	Lomustine (1-(2-chloroethyl)-3-cyclohexyl-1-nitrosurea)
CCRT	conventional conformal radiotherapy
CCSK	clear cell sarcoma of the kidney

CCyR	complete cytogenetic response	DBA	Diamond–Blackfan anemia
CD	celiac disease	DC	dendritic cell
CDC	collecting duct carcinoma	DCIS	ductal carcinoma in situ
CEA	carcinoembryonic antigen	DEB	drug-eluting bead
CEL-NOS	chronic eosinophilic leukemia-not otherwise specified	DES	diethylstilbestrol
		DFSP	dermatofibrosarcoma protuberans
CgA	chromogranin A	DHEA	dehydroepiandrosterone
CGCL	central giant cell lesion	DHEA-S	dehydroepiandrosterone sulfate
CHG	comparative genomic hybridization	DIA	digital image analysis
CGI	cisplatin, gemcitabine, and ifosfamide	DIC	disseminated intravascular coagulation
CGNP	cerebellar granule neuron precursors	DKC	dyskeratoses congenita
CHOP	cyclophosphamide, doxorubicin, vincristine, and prednisone	DLBCL	diffuse large B cell lymphoma
		DNT	dysembryoplastic neuroepithelial tumor
CHPOR	cyclophosphamide, doxorubicin, vincristine, prednisone, and rituximab	DSRCT	desmoplastic small round cell tumor
		DSS	disease specific survival
CI	confidence interval	DTI	diffusion tensor imaging
CIM	cisplatin, ifosfamide, and mesna	DTPA	diethylene triamine pentaacetic acid
CIN	cervical intraepithelial neoplasia		
CIS	carcinoma in situ	EA	early antigen
CK	cytokeratin	EA-CNR	endoscopically assisted cranioresection
CLL	chronic lymphocytic leukemia	EATL	enteropathy-associated T cell lymphoma
CML	chronic myelocytic leukemia	EBER-1	Epstein–Barr virus early ribonucleic acid-1
CMML	chronic myelomonocytic leukemia	EBNA	Epstein–Barr nuclear antigen
CMN	congenital mesoblastic nephroma	EBRT	external beam radiotherapy
CN	cystic nephroma	EBV	Epstein–Barr virus
CNL	chronic neutrophilic leukemia	ECOG	Eastern Cooperative Oncology Group
CNS	central nervous system	EDR	extreme drug resistance
COG	Children's Oncology Group	EFS	event-free survival
COMS	Collaborative Ocular Melanoma Study	EGB	eosinophilic granular body
CP	craniopharyngioma	EGD	esophagogastroduodenoscopy
CPA	cerebellopontine angle	EGFR	epidermal growth factor receptor
CPC	choroid plexus carcinoma	EGL	external granular layer
CPK	creatine phosphokinase	EIC	endometrial intraepithelial carcinoma
CPP	choroid plexus papilloma	EMA	epithelial membrane antigen/European Medicines Agency
CPT	choroid plexus tumor		
CR	complete remission/response	EMD	endoscopic mucosal dissection
CR1	first complete remission	EMP	extramedullary plasmacytoma
CRC	colorectal carcinoma	EMR	endoscopic mucosal resection
CRF	corticotropin-releasing factor	EMT	epithelial-to-mesenchymal transition
CRH	corticotropin-releasing hormone	ENB	esthesioneuroblastoma
CRPC	castration-resistant prostate cancer	EOC	epithelial ovarian carcinoma
CRS	cytoreductive surgery	EOPPC	extraovarian primary peritoneal carcinoma
CRT	conformal radiotherapy	EORTC	European Organization for Research and Treatment of Cancer
CS	Carney–Stratakis/craniospinal		
CsA	cyclosporine	EP	extramammary Paget disease
CSC	cancer stem cell	EPP	extrapleural pneumonectomy
CSF	cerebrospinal fluid	ER	estrogen receptor
CSI	cranial-spinal irradiation	ERCP	endoscopic retrograde cholangiopancreatography
CSS	cancer-specific survival	ERMS	embryonal rhabdomyosarcoma
CT	computed tomography	ES	Ewing sarcoma
CTL	cytotoxic T lymphocyte	ESS	endometrial stromal sarcoma
CTLA	cytotoxic T lymphocyte antigen	ET	essential thrombocytosis/essential thrombocythemia
CTV	clinical target volume		
CVD	cyclophosphamide, vincristine, and dacarbazine	ETFL	European Task Force on Lymphoma
		EUS	endoscopic ultrasound

FA	Fanconi anemia		HCC	hepatocellular carcinoma
FAC	5-fluorouracil, doxorubicin, and cyclophosphamide		HCC-CC	hepatocellular cholangiocarcinoma
FAM	5-fluorouracil, doxorubicin, and mitomycin-C		HCD	heavy chain disease
FAP	familial adenomatous polyposis		hCG	human chorionic gonadotropin
FC	fibrolamellar carcinoma		HCL	hairy cell leukemia
FDA	Food and Drug Administration		HCT	hematocrit
FDG	fluorodeoxyglucose		HDAC	histone deacetylase
FFS	failure-free survival		HDC	high-dose chemotherapy
FGF	fibroblast growth factor		HDGC	hereditary diffuse gastric cancer
FGFR	fibroblast growth factor receptor		HDR	high-dose rate
FH	(with) favorable histology		H&E	hematoxylin and eosin
FIGO	International Federation of Gynecology and Obstetrics		HES	hypereosinophilic syndrome
			HGF	hepatocyte growth factor/scatter factor
FISH	fluorescent in situ hybridization		HGNEC	high-grade neuroendocrine carcinoma
FLAER	fluorescent labeled aerolysin		HHV	human herpesvirus
FLAIR	fluid-attenuated inversion recovery		HIF	hypoxia-inducible factor
FLIT	fetal lung interstitial tumor		HIPEC	hyperthermic intraperitoneal chemotherapy
FLR	freedom from local recurrence		HIV	human immunodeficiency virus
FMTC	familial medullary thyroid cancer		HL	Hodgkin lymphoma
FNA	fine needle aspiration		HLA	human leukocyte antigen
FNAC	fine needle aspiration cytology		HNPCC	hereditary nonpolyposis colorectal cancer
			HNSCC	head and neck squamous cell carcinoma
GBM	glioblastoma		HPA	hypothalamus-pituitary axis
GC	gemcitabine and cisplatin		HPF	high-power field
GCLS	gastric carcinoma with lymphoid stroma		HPS	hemophagocytic syndrome
GCN	germ cell neoplasm		HPT-JT	hyperparathyroidism–jaw tumor
G-CSF	granulocyte colony-stimulating factor		HPV	human papillomavirus
GCT	platinum, gemcitabine and a taxane/germ cell tumor		HR	hazard ratio
			HSC	hematopoietic stem cells
Gd-DTPA	Gadolinium diethylenetriaminepentacetic acid		HSCT	hematopoietic stem cell transplantation
GE	gastroesophageal		HSTCL	hepatosplenic T cell lymphoma
GEJ	gastroesophageal junction		hTERT	human telomerase reverse transcriptase
GEP	gastroenteropancreatic		HU	Hounsfield unit/hydroxyurea
GETT	Groupe d'Etudes des Tumeurs Thymiques			
GFAP	glial fibrillary acidic protein		IA	intraarterial
GHSG	German Hodgkin Study Group		IARC	International Agency for Research on Cancer
GI	gastrointestinal		IBD	inflammatory bowel disease
GIP	gastric inhibitory polypeptide		ICC	interstitial cells of Cajal
GIST	gastrointestinal stromal tumor		ICP	intracranial pressure
GNB	ganglioneuroblastoma		IDC	invasive ductal carcinoma
G-NET	gastric neuroectodermal tumor		IELSG	International Extranodal Lymphoma Study Group
GnRH	gonadotropin-releasing hormone			
GOG	Gynecologic Oncology Group		IFN	interferon
GPI	glycosylphosphatidylinositol		IFS	infantile fibrosarcoma
GPOH	German Society of Pediatric Oncology and Hematology		Ig	immunoglobulin
			IGF	insulin-like growth factor
GRP	gastrin-releasing peptide		IHC	immunohistochemical
GSC	glioma stem cell		IL	interleukin
GST	gonadal (sex cord) stromal tumor		ILNR	intralobar nephrogenic rest
GTD	gestational trophoblastic disease		IMRT	intensity-modulated radiation therapy
GTR	gross total resection		IMT	inflammatory myofibroblastic tumor
GTV	gross tumor volume		INT	Instituto Nazionale Tumori
			IOM	Institute of Medicine
HAART	highly active antiretroviral therapy		IPACTR	International Pediatric Adrenocortical Tumor Registry
HBV	hepatitis B virus			

IPI	International Prognostic Index	MG	myasthenia gravis/malignant glioma
IPSS	International Prognostic Scoring System	MGA	microglandular adenosis
IRS	Intergroup Rhabdomyosarcoma Study	MGMT	methylguanine methyl transferase
ITP	ifosfamide, taxol, cisplatin	MGUS	monoclonal gammopathy of undetermined
IV	intravenous		significance
IVC	inferior vena cava	MHC	major histocompatibility complex
IVIG	intravenous immune globulin	MIBG	meta-iodobenzylguanidine
IVLBL	intravascular large B cell lymphoma	MIER	minimally invasive endoscopic resection
		MIF	müllerian inhibiting factor
JGCT	juvenile granulosa cell tumor	MKI	multikinase inhibitor
		MM	malignant mesothelioma
KG	ketoglutarate	MMC	mitomycin-C
KPS	Karnofsky performance status	MMMF	man-made mineral fibers
KS	Kaposi sarcoma	MMMT	malignant mixed mesodermal tumor
KTSC	keratinizing thymic squamous carcinoma	MMP	matrix metalloproteinase
		MMR	major molecular response
LAM	lymphangioleiomyomatosis	MMS	Mohs micrographic surgery
LAR	long-acting release/low anterior resection	MMTV	malignant mesothelioma of the tunica vaginalis
LCA	leukocyte common antigen	MOPP	mechlorethamine, vincristine, procarbazine,
LCC	large cell carcinoma		prednosine
LCC-NED	large cell carcinomas with neuroendocrine differentiation	MPE	myxopapillary ependymoma
LCH	Langerhans cell histiocytosis	MPM	malignant pleural mesothelioma
LCNEC	large cell neuroendocrine carcinoma	MPN	myeloproliferative neoplasm
LCNEM	large cell carcinoma with neuroendocrine morphology	MPNST	malignant peripheral nerve sheath tumor
LCT	Leydig cell tumors	MRCP	magnetic resonance cholangiopancreatography
LDH	lactate dehydrogenase	MRI	magnetic resonance imaging
LE	lymphoepitheliomatoid/lymphoepithelioma	MRS	magnetic resonance spectroscopy
LETC	lymphoepithelioma-like thymic carcinoma	MS	mastocytosis
LG	lymphomatoid granulomatosis	MSA	muscle-specific actin
LH	luteinizing hormone	MSD	matched sibling donor
LI	labeling index	MSI-H	microsatellite instability-high phenotype
LMS	leiomyosarcoma	MSKCC	Memorial Sloan-Kettering Cancer Center
LN	lymph node	MTC	medullary thyroid carcinoma
LNI	lymph node involvement	MTD	maximum tolerated dose
LOH	loss of heterozygosity	MTO	C-metomidate
LOI	loss of imprinting	mTOR	mammalian target of rapamycin
LRF	leukemia/lymphoma-related factor	MTP	median time to progression
LVI	lymphovascular invasion	MTSCC	mucinous tubular and spindle cell carcinoma
LVSI	lymph vascular space invasion	MTX	methotrexate
		MVAC	methotrexate, vinblastine, doxorubicin, and cisplatin
MALT	mucosa-associated lymphoid tissue	MVD	microvessel density
MAPK	mitogen-activated protein kinase	MZL	marginal zone lymphoma
MBC	male breast cancer		
MCD	multicentric Castleman disease	NA	not achieved
MCL	mantle cell lymphoma	NADPH	nicotinamide adenine dinucleotide phosphate
MCyR	major cytogenetic response	NB	neuroblastoma
MDACC	MD Anderson Cancer Center	NCB	needle core biopsy
MDNEC	moderately differentiated neuroendocrine carcinoma	NCCN	National Comprehensive Cancer Network
MDS	myelodysplastic syndrome	NCDB	National Cancer Database
MEC	mucoepidermoid carcinoma	NCIC	National Cancer Institute of Canada
MEN	multiple endocrine neoplasia	NDD	neurodegenerative disease
MET	mesenchymal-epithelial transition	NE	neuroendocrine
MFH	malignant fibrous histiocytoma	NEC	neuroendocrine carcinoma
		NED	no evidence of disease
		NEN	neuroendocrine neoplasm

NEPC	neuroendocrine prostate cancer
NET	neuroendocrine tumor
NF	neurofibromatosis
NHL	non-Hodgkin lymphoma
NIH	National Institutes of Health
NLPHL	nodular lymphocyte-predominant Hodgkin lymphoma
NOS	not otherwise specified
NPC	nasopharyngeal cancer
NPCR	National Program of Cancer Registries
NSC	neural stem cell
NSCLC	nonsmall cell lung carcinoma
NSE	neuron-specific enolase
NWTSG	National Wilms Tumor Study Group
OAR	organs at risk
OGCT	ovarian germ cell tumor
OKC	odontogenic keratocyst
ONB	olfactory neuroblastoma
OPC	oligodendrocyte precursor cell
OPG	optic pathway glioma
OR	odds ratio
ORR	overall response rate
OS	overall survival
OSSN	ocular surface squamous neoplasia
PA	pilocytic astrocytoma
PAC	plasma aldosterone concentration
PAP	prostatic acid phosphatase
PARA	paraganglioma
PAS	periodic acid-Schiff
PASH	pseudoangiomatous stroma hyperplasia
PBL	primary breast lymphoma
PBSC	peripheral blood stem cells
PC	prostate cancer
PCL	plasma cell leukemia
PCNA	proliferating cell nuclear antigen
PCNSL	primary central nervous system lymphoma
PCR	polymerase chain reaction
PCV	procarbazine, lomustine, and vincristine
PDGFR	platelet-derived growth factor receptor
PEL	primary effusion lymphoma
PET	positron emission tomography
PFS	progression-free survival
PGE	prostaglandin E
PGS	primary gliosarcoma
PHEO	pheochromocytoma
PHPT	primary hyperparathyroidism
PI3K	phosphoinositide 3´-kinase
PLAP	placenta-like alkaline phosphatase
PLGA	polymorphous low-grade adenocarcinoma
PLL	prolymphocytic leukemia
PLNR	perilobar nephrogenic rest
PMA	pilomyxoid astrocytoma
PMBL	primary mediastinal large B cell lymphoma
PMF	primary myelofibrosis

PNET	primitive neuroectodermal tumor
P-NET	pancreatic neuroectodermal tumor
PNH	paroxysmal nocturnal hemoglobinuria
POG	Pediatric Oncology Group
PPB	pleuropulmonary blastoma
PPI	proton pump inhibitor
PPS	primary pulmonary sarcoma
PPT	pineal parenchymal tumor
PPTID	pineal parenchymal tumor of intermediate differentiation
PR	partial response/progesterone receptor
PRA	plasma renin activity
PRCA	pure red cell aplasia
PRL	primary renal lymphoma
PRRT	peptide receptor radionuclide therapy
PRT	pineal region tumor
PSA	prostate-specific antigen/puromycin-sensitive aminopeptidase
PSBT	peritoneal serous borderline tumor
PSC	primary sclerosing cholangitis
PSCP	papillary serous carcinoma of the peritoneum
PSOC	papillary serous ovarian carcinoma
Ptc	Patched
PTC	papillary thyroid cancer/primary thymic carcinoma
PTH	parathyroid hormone
PTLD	posttransplantation lymphoproliferative disease
PTR	paratesticular rhabdomyosarcoma
PTV	planning target volume
PV	polycythemia vera
PVB	vinblastin, bleomycin and cisplatin
PXA	pleomorphic xanthoastrocytoma
RA	refractory anemia
RAEB	refractory anemia with excess blasts
RARS	refractory anemia with ring sideroblasts
RB	retinoblastoma
RBC	red blood cell
RCC	renal cell carcinoma
RCC Ma	renal cell carcinoma marker
RCMD	refractory cytopenia with multilineage dysplasia
RCUD	refractory cytopenia with unilineage dysplasia
RFA	radiofrequency ablation
RFS	relapse-free survival
RMC	renal medullary carcinoma
RMS	rhabdomyosarcoma
RN	refractory neutropenia
RPLND	retroperitoneal lymph node dissection
RR	response rate
RRSO	risk-reducing salpingo-oophorectomy
RT	radiation therapy/refractory thrombocytopenia
RTK	rhabdoid tumor of the kidney
RTKI	receptor tyrosine kinase inhibitor
RTOG	Radiation Therapy Oncology Group
RT-PCR	reverse transcriptase polymerase chain reaction

SAM	significance analysis of microarray		TDGF	teratocarcinoma-derived growth factor
SBFT	small bowel follow-through		TEC	transient erythroblastopenia of childhood
SBOT	serous borderline ovarian tumor		TGF	transforming growth factor
SBT	serous borderline tumor		TIA	T cell intracellular antigen
SCC	small/squamous cell carcinoma		TIC	tubal intraepithelial carcinoma
SCCRO	squamous cell carcinoma-related oncogene		TKI	tyrosine kinase inhibitor
SCF	stem cell factor		TL	telomere length
SCLC	small cell lung cancer		T-LBL	T cell lymphoblastic lymphoma
SCT	Sertoli cell tumor		T-LGL	T cell large granular lymphocyte leukemia
SCTAT	sex cord tumor with annular tubules		TLN	total lymph nodes
SD	stable disease/standard deviation		t-MDS	therapy-related myelodysplastic syndrome
SDH	succinate dehydrogenase		TMP	taxol, methotrexate, cisplatin
SEER	Surveillance, Epidemiology, and End Results		TNF	tumor necrosis factor
SEGA	subependymal giant cell astrocytoma		TNM	tumor/node/metastasis
SETTLE	spindle cell epithelial tumors of thymic-like epithelium		TRAIL	tumor necrosis factor apoptosis inducing ligand
SFT	solitary fibrous tumor		TRM	tumor-related mortality
SGS	secondary gliosarcoma		TRUS	transrectal ultrasound
SHH	sonic hedgehog		TS	thymidylate synthase
SIADH	syndrome of inappropriate secretion of antidiuretic hormone		TSC	tuberous sclerosis complex
			TSH	thyroid-stimulating hormone
SIB	simultaneous integrated boost		TTF	thyroid transcription factor
SIL	squamous intraepithelial lesion		TTP	time to progression
SIOP	Société Internationale d'Oncologie Pédiatrique		TTT	transpupillary thermotherapy
SLCT	Sertoli–Leydig cell tumor		TUR	transurethal resection
SLL	second-look laparotomy		TURP	transurethral resection of the prostate
SLN	sentinel lymph node			
SLNBx	sentinel lymph node biopsy		UC	urothelial carcinoma
SM	systemic mastocytosis		UFC	urine free cortisol
SMA	smooth muscle actin		UICC	International Union against Cancer
SMN	second malignant neoplasm		UPSC	uterine papillary serous carcinoma
SNP	single nucleotide polymorphism		UM	uveal melanoma
SNUC	sinonasal undifferentiated carcinomas		UV-B	ultraviolet-B
SPB	solitary plasmacytoma of bone			
SPECT	single photon emission computed tomography		VCA	viral capsid antigen
SPTL	subcutaneous panniculitis-like T cell lymphoma		VEGF	vascular endothelial growth factor
SRS	somatostatin receptor scintigraphy/stereotactic radiosurgery		VHL	von Hippel–Lindau
			VMA	vanillylmandelic acid
SSG	Scandinavian Sarcoma Group		VP	ventriculoperitoneal
SSR	somatostatin receptors			
STC	sarcomatoid thymic carcinoma		WAGR	Wilms tumor, aniridia, genitourinary anomalies, mental retardation
STIC	serous tubal intraepithelial carcinoma		WAR	whole-abdominal radiotherapy
STR	subtotal resection		WBC	white blood count
STUMP	stromal tumors of uncertain malignant potential		WBRT	whole-brain radiation therapy
SUV	standardized uptake value		WDTC	well-differentiated thymic carcinmoma
SV40	simian virus 40		WHO	World Health Organization
			WLE	wide local excision
TAE	transhepatic/transcatheter artery embolization		WM	Waldenström macroglobulinemia
T-ALL	T cell acute lymphoblastic leukemia		WT	Wilms tumor
TC	typical carcinoid			
TCC	transitional cell carcinoma		YAP	yes-associated protein
TCCC	thymic clear cell carcinoma			
TCR	T cell receptor		ZES	Zollinger–Ellison syndrome

Section 1: Genitourinary Cancer

1 Uncommon Tumors of the Kidney

Khaled Ali,[1] Ming Zhou,[2] Steve Campbell,[3] Ronald M. Bukowski,[1] and Brian I. Rini[1]

[1] Department of Solid Tumor Oncology, Cleveland Clinic Taussig Cancer Institute, Glickman Urological Institute, Cleveland, OH, USA
[2] Department of Pathology, [3] Department of Urologic Oncology, Cleveland Clinic, Cleveland, OH, USA

Introduction

Tumors of the kidney account for about 3% of adult malignancies.[1] About 64,770 new cases of kidney cancer (40,250 in men and 24,520 in women) were estimated by the American Cancer Society for the year 2012.[2] Renal cell carcinomas (RCC) constitute the bulk of these malignancies and historically they were widely known as *hypernephroma*, a term that was coined by Grawitz in the 19th century, reflecting his belief that they arose from the adrenal gland. RCCs are derived from the epithelial cells of renal tubules and account for more than 80% of primary renal malignant neoplasms. Transitional cell carcinomas, although arising in the renal pelvis, are frequently classified as renal tumors, and account for 7–8%. Other tumors, such as oncocytomas, collecting duct carcinomas (CDCs) of Bellini, and renal sarcomas, are uncommon but are becoming more frequently recognized pathologically. Nephroblastoma (Wilms tumor [WT]) is common in children and accounts for 5–6% of all primary renal tumors.

This chapter focuses on the classification, pathology, genetics, clinical and radiographic manifestations, and surgical and systemic management of the less common malignant and benign tumors of the kidney.

Classification of renal neoplasms

The first classification of renal tumors was proposed by Konig[3] in 1826 based on gross morphological characteristics. Extensive study of renal neoplasms in the last couple of decades has led to a standardized nomenclature by the European and American authorities (Box 1.1).[4] The 2004 World Health Organization (WHO) classification, which includes nearly 50 distinct entities, is based on a combination of immunohistochemistry, histology, and clinical and genetic features that are widely accepted and relatively reproducible.[5] Several large series have shown this classification to have prognostic significance[6] and that it is relevant to diagnosis by fine needle aspiration techniques.[7] It is anticipated that this current classification system will be reassessed in the future.[8]

Molecular diagnostic techniques in renal neoplasms

The application of molecular and cytogenetic techniques has resulted in improved understanding of these tumors. In the forefront among these technologies are comparative genomic hybridization (CGH), fluorescent *in situ* hybridization (FISH), allelic loss analysis, classical cytogenetics, and karyotyping. The von Hippel–Lindau tumor suppressor gene (*VHL*) resides in the short arm of chromosome 3 (3p25.3) and is commonly inactivated by gene mutation or promoter hypermethylation in sporadic clear cell RCC. It is also the causative gene for the von Hippel–Lindau syndrome.[9,10] Papillary RCC, chromophobic RCC, carcinoma of the collecting ducts of Bellini, metanephric adenomas, and renal oncocytomas have also exhibited characteristic chromosomal anomalies.[11–13] RCC associated with chromosomal translocation involving the *TFE3* gene on Xp11.2 has been described as a distinct clinicopathological entity.[14]

Definitive diagnosis of the various histological subtypes based on hematoxylin and eosin (H&E) morphology is possible in the majority of cases. In the minority circumstances where distinction becomes difficult, immunohistochemistry and other molecular techniques are being increasingly relied upon to make the distinction.[15] Renal cell carcinoma marker (RCC Ma) is a monoclonal antibody against the proximal tubular brush border antigen, which is relatively specific for renal neoplasms that originate from the proximal renal tubules, including clear and papillary RCC, despite a rather low sensitivity.[16] The antibody is positive in nearly 80% of clear cell and papillary RCC, is variably expressed in chromophobe RCC, and is absent in oncocytomas and CDCs. CD10 is another marker that helps in the differential diagnosis, by

Box 1.1 WHO histological classification of tumors of the kidney.

Renal cell tumors

- Clear cell renal cell carcinoma
- Multilocular cystic renal cell carcinoma
- Papillary renal cell carcinoma
- Chromophobe renal cell carcinoma
- Carcinoma of the collecting ducts of Bellini
- Renal medullary carcinoma
- Xp11 translocation carcinoma
- Carcinoma associated with neuroblastoma
- Mucinous tubular and spindle cell carcinoma
- Renal cell carcinoma, unclassified
- Papillary adenoma of the kidney
- Oncocytoma

Metanephric tumors

- Metanephric adenoma
- Metanephric adenofibroma
- Metanephric stromal tumor

Nephroblastic tumors

Occurring mainly in children
- Clear cell sarcoma
- Rhabdoid tumor
- Congenital mesoblastic nephroma
- Ossifying renal tumor of infants

Occurring mainly in adults
- Leiomyosarcoma (including renal vein)
- Angiosarcoma
- Rhabdomyosarcoma
- Malignant fibrous histiocytoma
- Hemangiopericytoma
- Osteosarcoma
- Angiomyolipoma
  - Epithelioid angiomyolipoma
- Leiomyoma
- Hemangioma
- Lymphangioma
- Juxtaglomerular cell tumor
- Renomedullary interstitial cell tumor
- Schwannoma
- Solitary fibrous tumor

Mixed epithelial and mesenchymal neoplasms

- Cystic nephroma
- Mixed epithelial and stromal tumor
- Synovial sarcoma

Neuroendocrine tumors

- Carcinoid
- Neuroendocrine carcinoma
- Primitive neuroectodermal tumor

- Neuroblastoma
- Pheochromocytoma

Hematopoietic and lymphoid neoplasms

- Lymphoma
- Plasmacytoma
- Leukemia

Germ cell tumors

- Teratoma
- Choriocarcinoma

Metastatic tumors

Adapted from Eble *et al.*[4] with permission from IARC Press.

being expressed in clear cell and papillary RCC, and absent in chromophobe RCC and oncocytomas.[17] Vimentin is variably expressed in clear cell and papillary RCC and is absent in chromophobe RCC and oncocytomas.[18] Cytokeratins represent a widely used diagnostic immunohistochemical marker in differentiating renal tumors. Cytokeratin 7 (CK7) is strongly positive in most chromophobe RCC, absent in clear cell RCC, and variably expressed in oncocytomas. Routine metaphase cytogenetics, performed on cultured tumor cells, has been used to identify cytogenetic changes associated with each RCC histological subtype. Using specific probe sets, FISH can be used to identify those RCC with characteristic chromosomal alterations.

Papillary adenoma

Background

Historically, adenomas were recognized as lesions smaller than 3 cm based on the work of Bell.[19] This was then modified in 1970 by Murphy and Mostofi who felt that histological differentiation of adenomas from true adenocarcinomas was possible.[20] Renal papillary adenomas are small, discrete, and arise from the renal tubular epithelium. In autopsy studies, they increase in frequency with age (7–40%). At present, the WHO classification system identifies papillary adenomas as epithelial lesions with a tubulopapillary architecture measuring less than 5 mm.[4] An incidence of 7% of papillary adenomas in nephrectomy specimens has been reported. As many papillary adenomas are not easy to identify grossly, the true incidence of renal papillary adenoma may be even higher if broader sampling is achieved in surgical specimens.[21]

Pathology

Papillary adenomas are less than 5 mm in diameter with a low nuclear grade. They appear as pale yellow-gray, well-circumscribed nodules, generally below the renal capsule in the renal cortex. They are usually not encapsulated; however, some have thin pseudocapsules. On microscopic examination, they have tubular, papillary, or tubulopapillary architecture similar to papillary renal cell carcinoma. The cells have scanty cytoplasm with round to oval nuclei and do not have high nuclear grade (Fuhrman nuclear grade 3 or 4). Cytogenetic features include trisomy (chromosome 7 and 17) and loss of the Y chromosome.[22,23] The resemblance of this tumor to renal papillary carcinoma has led to the view that it may represent a precursor lesion of RCC, although this is not firmly established.

Clinical presentation and treatment

Most of these lesions are discovered incidentally. They appear more frequently in patients with underlying kidney disease related to atherosclerosis, scarring, acquired renal cystic disease secondary to hemodialysis, and other malignant conditions of the kidney.[24] With small tumors being increasingly detected incidentally, the current view is to regard all of them as probable early cancers. Renal tumors with diameters 0.5–2 cm often behave in an indolent fashion, although the biological behavior is difficult to ascertain; therefore tumors less than 2 cm are sometimes termed "renal epithelial tumors of uncertain malignant potential" and are observed for progression, while larger tumors may require surgical excision, depending on the clinical scenario. Thus, the primary management of these tumors is surgical, with no established role for chemotherapy or radiation.

Carcinoma of the collecting ducts of Bellini

Background

Collecting duct carcinoma (CDC) is a rare renal tumor derived from the cells of the collecting duct of Bellini, and comprises less than 1% of renal malignancies.[25] Fleming and Lewi described the detailed pathological features of CDC as a distinct entity based on several case reports.[26]

Pathology

This tumor is characterized by a medullary location, with a size ranging from 2 cm to 12 cm, firm whitish-gray appearance, and irregular infiltrative border. It grows radially from the renal hilum to invade into the renal cortex, the renal capsule, and the renal sinus. Histologically, it has an irregular tubulopapillary growth pattern embedded in a desmoplastic stroma (Fig. 1.1a). The tubules are lined with hobnail cells with a scant eosinophilic cytoplasm. The cells display high-grade nuclei with brisk mitotic activity and prominent nucleoli (Fig. 1.1b). Occasionally, sarcomatoid changes or mucin can be seen. Molecular events and cytogenetic changes, which contribute, are poorly characterized and a distinct pattern has not yet emerged. The immunohistochemistry profile is variable, being commonly positive for phytoagglutinins and high molecular weight cytokeratin, with coexpression of vimentin, and negative for CD10 and villin.[27]

Clinical presentation

Collecting duct carcinoma is a highly aggressive tumor, which usually presents in an advanced stage, with gross hematuria, abdominal/back pain, and a flank mass, 40% of the patients being asymptomatic. At diagnosis, it will frequently have distant metastases in the lung, liver, lymph nodes, bone, or adrenal gland. It is more common in males (ratio of about 2:1) with a wide range of age groups (13–83 years with a mean of 55 years). On computed tomography (CT) scan, this tumor appears as a centrally arising infiltrative mass with preservation of the renal contour and minimal enhancement with contrast. Patients can have generalized inflammatory

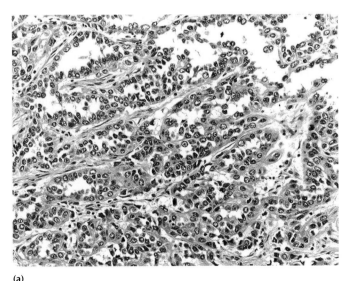

(a)

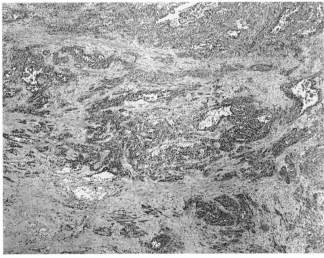

(b)

Figure 1.1 Collecting duct renal cell carcinoma consists of high-grade tumor cells (b) forming complex and angulated tubules or tubulopapillary structures embedded in a remarkably desmoplastic stroma (a).

symptoms secondary to cytokine release from the tumor and the inflammatory reaction associated with the tumor.[26–28]

Treatment and prognosis

The diagnosis of CDC is generally made postoperatively, since radiological distinction from other RCCs is difficult. The prognosis is generally very poor with most patients rapidly developing systemic metastases with a median survival of 22 months.[29] The role of nephrectomy has been debated because of the frequent metastases at presentation and appears to be useful at most for palliation.[30] On the basis of the pathological, immunohistochemical, and cytogenetic similarity to transitional cell carcinomas (TCC) as compared with conventional clear cell RCC, the preferred approach in the treatment of metastatic disease has been with chemotherapy rather than immunotherapy.[31]

In the largest reported series, Dimopoulos et al. reported retrospectively the MD Anderson experience involving 12 patients with CDC treated from 1980 to 1990.[29] Seven of eight patients with metastatic disease were treated with different chemotherapy combinations, with the methotrexate, vinblastine, doxorubicin, and cisplatin (MVAC) regimen being the most common. Only one patient achieved a minor response lasting 5 months. Six patients were treated with a combination of interleukin-2 and interferon (IFN)-α, with a response seen in one patient. Peyromaure et al. reported two complete responses with cisplatin and gemcitabine combination chemotherapy, which lasted 9 and 27 months.[32] Radiotherapy in these series has appeared to have minimal benefit for local recurrence. Chao et al. in a review noted that some patients having regional nodal disease without distant metastasis have had long-term disease-free survival with adjuvant therapy.[33] Cisplatin-gemcitabine has significant activity with a favorable toxicity profile in urothelial cancers. Therefore, a platinum-based regimen is the preferred first-line chemotherapy regimen. There are anecdotal reports of objective responses in CDC patients treated with either sunitinib or sorafenib,[34–36] although other case reports demonstrate no activity of this approach.[37] Therefore, participation in clinical trials of novel therapy is strongly encouraged for these patients given the lack of biological insight and limited therapeutic options.

Renal medullary carcinoma

Background

Renal medullary carcinoma (RMC) was first described by Davis et al.[38] as a sickle cell nephropathy and termed so because of its predominantly medullary location. In a literature review of renal medullary carcinoma by Dimashkieh et al.,[39] hemoglobinopathy was found in 53 of the 55 cases (50 patients had hemoglobin AS, two patients had hemoglobin SC, and one patient had hemoglobin SS disease).

Pathology

Renal medullary carcinoma is a centrally located tumor with an infiltrative growth pattern similar to that of CDC. It is believed to arise from the epithelium of the distal portion of the collecting duct. The right kidney is involved three times more commonly than the left kidney, and the mean tumor size ranges from 4 cm to 12 cm (mean of 7 cm). Renal medullary carcinomas are widely infiltrative, and have variable areas of hemorrhage and necrosis. Histologically, a variety of growth patterns have been described, with reticular growth pattern and compact adenoid cystic morphology being the common features. Most renal medullary carcinomas have areas of poorly differentiated cells with solid sheets of tumor cells. The tumor cells contain vesicular or clear nuclei with prominent nucleoli and amphophilic cytoplasm, which can have a squamoid or rhabdoid quality. The tumor cells are usually high grade and as with CDC, there is often marked desmoplasia and inflammation.[40–43] The immunohistochemical profile is similar to CDC but can be helpful in distinguishing renal medullary carcinoma from other poorly differentiated kidney tumors.

Molecular genetic studies on RMC are rare. Although previously published cases of CDC and RMC reported monosomy of chromosomes 8, 10, and 11, in a series of nine RMCs studied by comparative genomic hybridization, no chromosomal change was observed in eight cases and a loss of chromosome 22 was seen in one case.[42] A more recent series of three RMC patients (one patient with sickle cell disease and two without sickle cell disease) using conventional cytogenetic and single nucleotide polymorphism (SNP) arrays analysis failed to demonstrate a consistent pattern of chromosomal abnormalities between two cases tested. However, all three cases showed increased hypoxia-inducible factor 1α expression. It is thus apparent that no distinct chromosomal numerical or structural defect is constantly observed in renal medullary carcinomas.[44]

Interestingly, two recent case reports demonstrated anaplastic lymphoma kinase (ALK) rearrangement in sickle cell trait-associated renal tumors.[45,46] Further characterization is required but this observation could translate into a therapeutic option (crizotinib, an inhibitor of ALK) in this traditionally treatment-refractory disease.

Clinical presentation

Renal medullary carcinoma is a highly aggressive tumor that occurs almost exclusively in young people (mean age 22 years), predominantly males (male-to-female ratio 2:1) in patients with sickle cell trait. The common presenting symptoms are gross hematuria, abdominal/flank pain or weight loss. Common sites of metastasis at diagnosis include lung, retroperitoneal or mediastinal lymph nodes, bone and liver. Of the patients with adequate staging information available from the two largest case series, 18% had stage III disease and 82% had stage IV disease on presentation.[38,41,42,47–49] Radiological findings in renal medullary carcinoma have been shown to be not specific, although they might provide an indication to the diagnosis given the proper clinical background.[50]

Treatment and prognosis

Renal medullary carcinomas are now widely regarded as a highly aggressive variant of RCC, with an almost uniformly fatal outcome. Early reports of RMC discovered a median survival of 14 weeks after diagnosis. The mean survival after surgery has been about 4 months.[38,51,52] Strouse et al. have reported that only one of the over 80 reported patients is alive at 2 years.[47] This patient had a small tumor (<2 cm) confined to the kidney at the time of resection.

Chemotherapy has been shown to increase survival beyond 4 months in anecdotal reports, but with no reported long-term survivors. In a review of chemotherapy, of the 15 patients assessable for response, there was one complete response, two partial responses, one minor response, one stable disease and 10 patients had progressive disease. Cases from 1995 through 2003 have been reviewed by Simpson et al. who reported on 28 patients. Survival averaged 32 weeks, with notable highest survival in patients on treatment with methotrexate, vinblastine, doxorubicin, and cisplatin – 46 weeks.[52,53]

Numerous current reports suggest limited but some activity (occasional objective responses of limited duration) in patients with RMC.[54–56] A recent case reported by Motzer et al. suggested a complete response to bortezomib (PS-341), a proteasome inhibitor.[57] There are ongoing clinical trials testing the activity of molecular targeted therapy on non-clear cell renal carcinoma but the available data are too preliminary to allow a definitive recommendation and clinical trial participation is encouraged.[58,59] In healthy patients with systemic disease, treatment plans similar to those for urothelial cancers and CDC, with combination cisplatin-based chemotherapy, are a reasonable choice along with inclusion in phase 1 clinical trials. Reports on the role of radiation therapy in the adjuvant setting post surgery and chemotherapy showed no definitive benefit,[41] but reports of palliative radiation for bone metastasis have demonstrated a decline in pain and some reduction in lesion size.[56,60,61]

XP11 translocation neoplasms

Background

Xp11 translocation neoplasms are a subset of RCCs, characterized by various translocations involving chromosome Xp11.2, resulting in fusion of the *TFE3* gene to a variety of recipient genes and overexpression of TFE3 protein. They affect children and young adults predominantly, although some older patients have been reported. Molecular analysis of several different Xp11.2 translocation carcinomas has shown that some bear a translocation that is identical to the breakpoints and *ASPL-TFE3* gene fusion seen in alveolar soft part sarcoma (ASPS).[14] These were recognized as a distinctive subclass in the 2004 WHO renal tumor classification. An unusual renal epithelial neoplasm with a chromosomal translocation involving t(6:11) has been described, which resulted in the overexpression of another transcription factor gene in the same gene family as *TFE3 – TFEB*.[62,63]

Six gene fusion partners of *TFE3* have been reported to date. Five of these six partners have been identified, whereas the identity of the sixth, which is sited on chromosome 3, is still to be determined. The five known gene fusion partners of *TFE3* are *PRCC, ASPL*, polypyrimidine tract-binding protein-

associated splicing factor (*PSF*), non-POU domain-containing octamer-binding (*NONO*; p54[nrb]), and clathrin heavy-chain (*CLTC*) genes, respectively situated on chromosomes 1q21, 17q25, 1p34, Xq12, and 17q23. The t(X;17) (p11.2;q25) or *ASPL-TFE3* translocation RCC and *ASPS* contain the identical *ASPL-TFE3* fusion transcript yet the t(X;17) translocation is always balanced in the Xp11.2 translocation RCC and unbalanced in the *ASPS*.[64]

Pathology

On gross examination, these lesions closely resemble conventional (clear cell) renal carcinomas. They are tan-yellow, and often necrotic and hemorrhagic. The most distinctive histopathological appearance is that of papillary structures lined with clear cells, a finding that is uncommon in other renal carcinomas (Fig. 1.2). They often have a nested architecture, with cells containing clear and granular cytoplasm. The histology of Xp11 translocation carcinomas varies with specific chromosomal translocations. The *ASPL-TFE3* renal carcinomas are notable for cells with voluminous, clear to eosinophilic cytoplasm, discrete cell borders, vesicular nuclear chromatin, and prominent nucleoli. They were previously labeled as the "voluminous cell variant" of pediatric RCC. Hyaline nodules containing psammoma bodies can be seen. In comparison, the *PRCC-TFE3* renal carcinomas ordinarily have less abundant cytoplasm, fewer hyaline nodules with psammoma bodies and a more nested, compact architecture. The immunohistochemistry is positive for TFE3 protein, RCC marker antigen, and CD10. In contrast with traditional RCC, only half of them express epithelial markers such as cytokeratin and epithelial membrane antigen.

Clinical presentation and prognosis

Although RCC is uncommon in children (<5% of all renal tumors), approximately a third of RCC in children and young

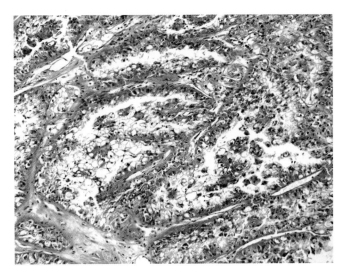

Figure 1.2 Renal cell carcinoma associated with t(X;17) (p11.2; q25) consists of nested to pseudopapillary structures lined with tumor cells with abundant clear, sometimes eosinophilic, cytoplasm.

adults appears to belong to this translocation family of tumors. Some reports have suggested that children who had prior exposure to cytotoxic chemotherapy are at risk for developing Xp11.2 translocation RCC.[65,66]

Even though Xp11.2 translocation RCC has a comparatively good prognosis in childhood, adult-onset Xp11.2 translocation RCC is reported to have a poor prognosis.[67-69] The basis for this is the fact that most patients present with advanced disease at diagnosis and that as yet, there is no effective systemic treatment. Chemotherapy and immunotherapy have not proven to be successful on metastatic lesions.[67,68,70] The clinical behavior of these tumors is still not well characterized. Generally, these carcinomas present at an advanced stage, with lymph node metastases at diagnosis despite their small size in a majority of cases. Even with these advanced stage presentations, the clinical course tends to be variable. This clinical behavior resembles that of ASPS, which has a similar genetic translocation. It can recur 20 or 30 years after the initial diagnosis.

Adequate surgical resection might possibly improve the prognosis. It has been reported that the implication of lymph node dissection in patients with Xp11.2 translocation RCC was greater than that for conventional RCC.[68,71] Only anecdotal reports of the adjuvant use of chemotherapy and immunotherapy in pediatric patients are available and thus adjuvant therapy should not be used outside a clinical trial.[14]

Recently, targeted therapy has demonstrated objective response and prolonged progression-free survival (PFS) in patients with metastatic Xp11.2 translocation RCC. Malouf et al. reported on 21 patients with metastatic Xp11.2 RCC who were treated with vascular endothelial growth factor (VEGF) and mammalian target of rapamycin (mTOR)-targeted therapies.[70] Patients treated with sunitinib were found to have a median PFS of 8.2 months in the first-line setting, while in the setting of second, third or fourth line it showed a median PFS of 11 months. Patients treated with sorafenib had a median PFS of 6 months, whereas patients treated with temsirolimus had a median PFS of 3 months. Seven patients (33%) experienced objective responses. All patients treated with sunitinib and one patient treated with temsirolimus achieved responses. With a median follow-up of 19 months, the median overall survival (OS) was reported to be 27 months. Another retrospective study reported by Choueiri et al. reviewed 15 patients with metastatic Xp11.2 RCC, of whom 10, three, and two received sunitinib, sorafenib, and monoclonal anti-VEGF antibodies, respectively.[72] Five patients had prior systemic treatments. When treated with VEGF-targeted therapy, three patients demonstrated a partial response, seven patients had stable disease, and five patients developed progressive disease. The median PFS and OS of the entire cohort were 7.1 months and 14.3 months, respectively.

Lately mesenchymal-epithelial transition (MET) tyrosine kinase receptor has been studied as a future potential therapeutic target in Xp11.2 RCC. A selective inhibitor of c-Met receptor tyrosine (ARQ-197) kinase has demonstrated safety and tolerability in a phase 1 trial. A phase 2 clinical trial in patients with microphthalmia transcription factor-driven tumors, including translocation-associated RCC, has been completed and is awaiting study results.[70,72,73] Therefore, use of targeted therapeutic agents, preferably in a clinical trial, is favored for this type of tumor, recognizing the relatively limited activity of these agents.

Mucinous tubular and spindle cell carcinoma

Background

These tumors were first described by Farrow et al., who collected a series of eight distinctive tumors that appeared to originate from the collecting tubules.[74] Further studies of this collection of tumors resulted in their classification as "low-grade collecting duct carcinoma,"[75] a term that may not accurately reflect the biology of these tumors. Several other reports also postulated that they represented a low-grade CDC with less biological aggressiveness.[27] However, subsequent characterization and reports of these tumors showed that they had clinical and pathological features quite distinct from CDC. Currently, they are recognized as a separate entity of renal cell tumor in the WHO classification.[4,76-79]

Pathology

Grossly, these tumors are well circumscribed, solid or cystic, large (mean size 6 cm), with a gray or light tan appearance, and a homogeneous, myxoid, and glistening cut surface. Microscopically, they are composed of compressed tubular structures and spindle cells separated by pale mucinous stroma. These can have a configuration simulating leiomyoma or sarcoma.[80] Mitotic activity is minimal with a low Furhman nuclear grade of 1–2. The morphological, immunohistochemical, and ultrastructural features of these lesions indicate an origin from distal nephron segments. They have a complex and variable immunohistochemical profile; with positivity for a wide range of cytokeratins and epithelial membrane antigen. Proximal nephron markers such as CD10 and villin are mostly absent. They also show positivity for Ulex europaeus, peanut, and soya bean agglutinins.[76] On electron microscopy, they have the usual epithelial features resembling the loop of Henle or a distal convoluted tubule. Cytogenetic changes involving chromosome losses of 1, 4, 6, 8, 13 and 14 and gains of chromosomes 7, 11, 16, and 17 have been described.

Clinical presentation

Although more common in middle-aged and elderly women, these tumors can occur in a wide age range (17–82 years with a mean of 53 years) but predominantly in women (female-to-male ratio of 4:1). They usually present as asymptomatic masses on radiological studies. Occasionally, they can present with flank pain or hematuria. Although generally benign in behavior, there are case reports of metastatic disease, presumably due to the sarcomatoid element sometimes found in these tumors.[81,82]

Treatment and prognosis

Previously these mucinous tubular and spindle cell carcinoma (MTSCC)/tumors may have been misdiagnosed as leiomyoma, sarcoma, or CDC. It is crucial to make the diagnosis of these tumors as being distinct from the other tumors in view of the indolent nature of this disease, to prevent undue and excessive treatment. No case series of systemic treatment have been reported to date. There is one case report in the literature of a 61-year-old woman who presented with metastatic MTSCC with a 3 cm right renal mass, a 3 cm left adrenal mass, bulky retroperitoneal adenopathy, a right pulmonary nodule, left hilar adenopathy, and widespread sclerotic bone metastases. Sunitinib was initiated at 50 mg, and symptomatic improvement was noticed a few days after starting treatment. Restaging scans at 12 weeks showed a decrease in size of the retroperitoneal nodal mass and left adrenal lesion whereas other lesions were stable, consistent with a partial response to therapy. At 24 weeks, the patient continued to show clinical benefit from therapy, and a restaging scan showed stable disease.[83]

Therefore, this extraordinarily rare tumor is managed surgically, and, if metastatic, clinical trials should be considered. If trials are unavailable, VEGF-targeted therapy can be considered but based only on the single case report. There are no data supporting the use of chemotherapy in this disease.

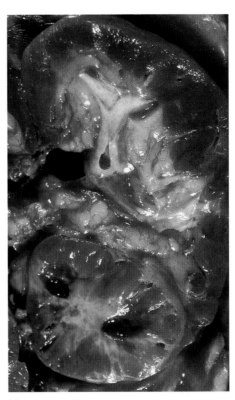

(a)

Oncocytoma

Background

Oncocytomas first came to attention as benign kidney tumors after a case series reported by Klein and Valensi in 1976.[84] They constitute about 3–5% of renal tumors in most large series.[85] However, tumors similar to oncocytomas had been described earlier, by Zippel *et al.* The term *oncocyte* means "swollen cell"; the cells are swollen because of numerous cytoplasmic mitochondria. Similar tumors can occur in the salivary gland, thyroid, parathyroid, and adrenal sites.[86]

Pathology

Oncocytomas are well-circumscribed, nonencapsulated neoplasms with a characteristic central stellate scar, seen in 33%, and most commonly in large tumors (Fig. 1.3a). The median size is about 5 cm but they can be as large as 20 cm. The color is classically mahogany-brown, but can be tan to pale yellow. Hemorrhage can be seen in 20%. They are composed of solid nests and sheets of oncocytes with abundant granular eosinophilic cytoplasm, residing in an edematous, mucopolysaccharide-rich extracellular stromal matrix (Fig. 1.3b). They are thought to arise from the intercalated cells of the collecting duct. The nuclei usually do not exhibit pleomorphism; with an evenly dispersed chromatin, discrete central nucleoli and mitotic activities are rare to absent. Features such as perinephric fat and lymphovascular invasion can be seen and do not appear to confer a worse prognosis.[87,88] However, "atypical features" such as gross involvement of the renal vein, extensive papillary architecture, foci of clear cells, sarcomatoid

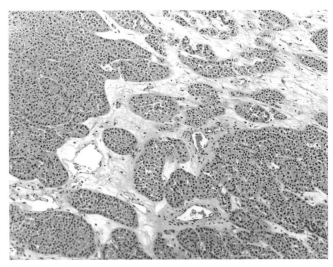

(b)

Figure 1.3 Renal oncocytoma forms a well-circumscribed, nonencapsulated mass with homogeneous cut surface and a central scar (a). The tumor cells (oncocytes) are uniform, round to polygonal with granular eosinophilic cytoplasm and regular round nuclei with evenly dispersed chromatin. They are nested in a loose hypocellular and hyalinized stroma (b).

dedifferentiation, prominent necrosis, and frequent or atypical mitoses carry a different connotation and are inconsistent with a diagnosis of oncocytoma.[89]

The most common differential diagnoses for oncocytomas are chromophobe RCC and clear cell RCC with eosinophilic cells. Making a distinction between these tumors on a cytological aspiration specimen can be difficult.[90] Hale colloidal iron staining, parvalbumin, and vimentin are negative (although focal luminal), as opposed to the diffuse cytoplasmic, colloidal iron staining that can be observed in oncocytoma, and antimitochondrial antibody is positive in oncocytoma and can help in the differential diagnosis.[87] On electron microscopy, they are characterized by numerous normal-appearing mitochondria accounting for the cytoplasmic granularity; leading to the use of the term "mitochondrioma" by some authors.[86,89,91] Microvesicles that are seen in chromophobe RCC are absent in oncocytoma.

Oncocytosis is a condition in which the kidneys contain multifocal oncocytomatous nodules, with oncocytic changes in the renal tubules and cysts in the surrounding regions of the kidney. Multifocality and bilaterality can occur in 5–13% of resected oncocytomas. It behaves in a similar fashion to the solitary tumors. Sometimes, a lesion can contain both oncocytomatous and chromophobe RCC components, a condition referred to as "hybrid oncocytic tumor (HOT tumor)." Therefore, it is crucial to thoroughly examine and adequately sample a lesion that grossly resembles an oncocytoma.[92] The coexistence of oncocytoma with chromophobe RCC and their morphological similarities have sparked a debate as to whether these two entities represent the two extreme ends of the spectrum with a common origin from the intercalated cells of the collecting duct. Recent molecular evidence suggests that renal oncocytoma and chromophobe RCC share not only some morphological similarities, but early cytogenetic alterations also, including loss of chromosomes Y, 1, and 14.

Birt–Hogg–Dube syndrome is a familial, autosomal-dominant syndrome in which the gene, *FLCN* (folliculin), has been localized to the short arm of chromosome 17. This is characterized by dome-shaped skin papules in the facial area, renal tumors (27% of patients), pulmonary cysts, and spontaneous pneumothorax.[93] The most common renal tumor is a hybrid of chromophobe RCC and oncocytoma with multiple tumors in a majority. The possibility of this familial syndrome should be entertained in a diagnosis of renal oncocytosis.[94]

Clinical presentation

Oncocytoma can present anywhere between the ages of 14 and 90 years with no gender predilection. It is detected mostly as an incidental finding on routine imaging studies. Occasionally, patients may have hematuria, flank pain, or a palpable mass. On CT scan, the lesion is usually hypodense, well circumscribed, and peripherally located with a central scar.[95]

Treatment and prognosis

Current literature supports the benign nature of the disease, with surgery being curative.[96] Metachronous lesions have been reported as late as 9 years after initial diagnosis.[97] If the clinical data or preoperative information confirm oncocytoma, it can be treated safely by partial nephrectomy. Therefore, preoperative diagnosis can avoid excessive treatment. However, most patients do undergo nephrectomy because of the inability of current diagnostic methods to reliably distinguish this from renal cell carcinoma, and the occasional coexistence of chromophobe RCC and clear cell RCC with oncocytoma (not readily distinguished on a limited amount of biopsy material). Synchronous and metachronous oncocytoma has been described and surgical management remains the preferred approach. There is no defined role for systemic therapy of renal oncocytoma. The presence of distant disease suggests an alternative histological diagnosis.

Angiomyolipoma

Background

Renal angiomyolipoma is a benign mesenchymal lesion initially described by Grawitz *et al.* in 1900.[98] It accounts for approximately 1% of surgically removed renal tumors. It was also described by Bourneville and Brissaud as part of the tuberous sclerosis complex (TSC) around the same time.[99,100] In 1989 Hartwick *et al.* reported an epithelioid angiomyolipoma with uncommon histological patterns mimicking malignancy, which after further investigation revealed malignant characteristics in some cases. It has recently been classified as a variant of angiomyolipoma with malignant potential.[80]

Pathology

Grossly, renal angiomyolipoma is a large, yellow-gray mass lesion, well demarcated from the kidney but not truly encapsulated. Generally they are solitary but if present in multiple numbers, the picture is that of a dominant tumor with associated smaller lesions. When they grow larger, they usually cause a mass effect rather than infiltrating into surrounding tissue. They are composed of a varying proportion of thick-walled, poorly organized blood vessels, smooth muscle bundles, and mature adipose tissue (Fig. 1.4a), and the varying proportion of each component accounts for the gross appearance of the lesion. Smooth muscle cells are frequently spindle shaped and occasionally rounded epithelioid. Regional lymph node involvement is thought to represent multicentric involvement rather than metastases.[101,102] Infrequently, direct tumor extension into the inferior vena cava and the renal venous system, in the absence of distant metastases, has been described.

The higher prevalence of angiomyolipoma in females has raised the speculation that there may be a sex hormonal potentiation of angiomyolipoma growth. Progesterone and estrogen receptors have been detected in these tumors along with reports of rapid growth during pregnancy.

The immunohistochemical profile is characterized by a coexpression of melanocytic (e.g. HMB-45) (Fig. 1.4b) and smooth muscle (e.g. smooth muscle actin) markers. They can also be positive for CD68, neuron-specific enolase, S-100, desmin, and hormonal receptors whereas the epithelial markers are consistently negative.[4,103–105]

Two genes are known to cause tuberous sclerosis: *TSC gene 1* (*TSC1*) on chromosome 9q34, which encodes hamartin, and *TSC2* on chromosome 16p13, which produces tuberin, a GTPase-activating protein. The biology of these genes has

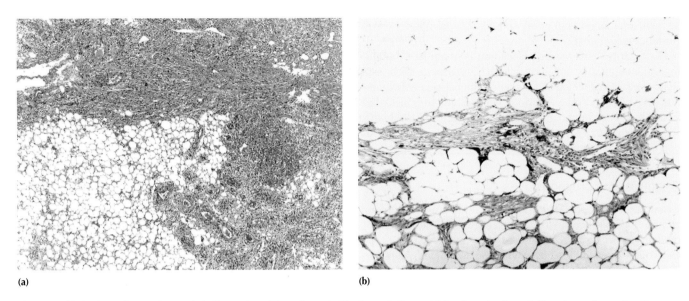

Figure 1.4 (a) Angiomyolipoma characteristically consists of three elements: blood vessels (lower right), adipocytes (lower left), and smooth muscle cells (upper). Melanocytic markers, such as HMB-45, are positive in some tumor cells (b).

been elucidated extensively in recent years. Angiomyolipoma frequently has loss of heterozygosity at one of the two TSC loci in both the sporadic and tuberous sclerosis-associated tumors.[99]

Epithelioid angiomyolipoma is a potentially malignant mesenchymal neoplasm closely related to classic angiomyolipoma. There is a higher association (>50%) with tuberous sclerosis. Patients are frequently symptomatic, both sexes are equally affected, and the mean age of presentation (38 years) is generally younger compared with classic angiomyolipoma. Scarcity of adipose tissue makes radiological diagnosis more difficult. About a third of reported epithelioid angiomyolipoma cases have metastasis to lymph nodes, liver, lungs, or spine.[106–109] Microscopically, there are sheets of epithelioid cells with abundant granular eosinophilic cytoplasm, enlarged vesicular nuclei, and prominent nucleoli. Areas of classic angiomyolipoma can be found interspersed focally. Tumors with necrosis, increased mitotic activity, nuclear atypia, and infiltration into surrounding tissue should be regarded as potentially malignant. The immunohistochemical profile is positive for melanocytic markers such as HMB-45, but not as consistently positive for smooth muscle markers such as actin.[4,80] Although rare, epithelioid angiomyolipoma should be kept in perspective when a diagnosis of angiomyolipoma is made.

Clinical presentation

The prevalence of this tumor in the general population is low.[110,111] Angiomyolipoma can present either sporadically (80%) or in association with the TSC (20%). There is a female preponderance (4:1) in the sporadic form, but not in the tuberous sclerosis-associated tumors. Tuberous sclerosis is an autosomal-dominant disease with incomplete penetrance. It was initially described by Bourneville in 1880, in a girl with mental retardation, epilepsy, and characteristic sclerotic brain lesions

(tubers).[100] Later, in 1900, Bourneville and Brissaud noted the association of the syndrome with renal tumors. Vogt described the classic triad of seizures, mental retardation, and adenoma sebaceum.[112] This triad has been substituted by a constellation of findings that establish the diagnosis. When patients with tuberous sclerosis are followed up, more than half of them show development of angiomyolipoma.

In a pooled analysis by Nelson *et al.*, the authors suggest that tuberous sclerosis-associated angiomyolipoma, in contrast with sporadic cases, is likely to present at an earlier age (mean age 30 versus 52 years), with larger tumors (8.9 versus 5.4 cm), frequent multicentricity (97% versus 13%) and hemorrhage (44% versus 14%).[113] Steiner *et al.* found that tuberous sclerosis-associated tumors were more likely to grow (67% versus 21%) and require surgical intervention (50% versus 28%) during the 4 years of follow-up.[114] De Luca *et al.* reported on 51 patients with sporadic angiomyolipoma who had either immediate surgery or were on observation. Ninety-two percent of the observed patients (mean tumor size 1.5 cm) showed no radiographic growth of angiomyolipoma during the 5-year follow-up. The larger tumors (>4 cm) were more likely to grow (46% versus 27%) or require surgical intervention (54% versus 7%) than smaller tumors.[115]

Angiomyolipoma can present with symptoms such as flank pain, a palpable tender mass, and gross hematuria or as an incidental finding on radiological studies. Morbidities secondary to angiomyolipoma are related to retroperitoneal hemorrhage (Wunderlich syndrome)[116] and renal failure secondary to encroachment of normal renal tissue.[117] Identification of fat in a renal lesion is the key to radiological diagnosis. Some of the lesions contain a minimal amount of fat that may not be detected and may lead to a nephrectomy. There have been reports of fat in RCC tumors, secondary to invasion and entrapment of perirenal fat. Magnetic resonance imaging (MRI) can help in differentiating angiomyolipoma from RCC in select cases and in evaluation during pregnancy. Diagnosis of incidental angiomyolipoma should also prompt a workup for tuberous sclerosis.

Historically there was an association between RCC, angiomyolipoma, and the tuberous sclerosis syndrome. Clear cell RCC appears to develop at a higher rate in patients with tuberous sclerosis syndrome than in general. Eble *et al.* also suggested that some tumors historically diagnosed as RCC in this set of patients may actually have been epithelioid angiomyolipoma, overestimating the association.[118]

Treatment and prognosis

Renal angiomyolipomas are typically slow-growing tumors, and morbidity is secondary to their growth. With the lack of randomized trials, there is considerable controversy as to the exact indication for treating asymptomatic angiomyolipoma, and organ preservation with partial nephrectomy is a preferred approach. Asymptomatic, small, benign-appearing lesions can be observed. Minimal hematuria will usually resolve with hydration and bed rest. In this approach, patients should be cautioned to avoid contact sports and should be followed up closely to evaluate the growth pattern of the lesion.

The primary reasons to intervene should be suspicion of malignancy in a lesion with low fat content, alleviation of symptoms secondary to spontaneous hemorrhage, and risk of rupture or other complications. Surgical removal or core biopsy with immunohistochemical staining should be considered when there is no diagnostic certainty. Symptomatic angiomyolipoma can be managed by either angio-embolization or surgical removal.[113] When clinical risk factors such as childbearing age, large tumor, suspected TSC or anticipated difficulty with periodic reimaging are present, asymptomatic angiomyolipoma can be managed by observation or intervention, according to individual preference.

Retrospective data demonstrate that patients presenting with symptoms or hemorrhage are more likely to have larger tumors. Oesterling *et al.* proposed a 4 cm threshold for the risk of symptoms and intervention in asymptomatic patients.[119] Prospective data from De Luca *et al.*[115] and others suggest that larger lesions may become symptomatic with time, especially in patients with the TSC. These studies have also shown that it is not necessary to treat all large asymptomatic lesions, since they may grow slowly without morbidity. On the basis of available evidence, we suggest that an intervention in an asymptomatic patient should be based on the comprehensive evaluation of the clinical scenario including tumor size, tumor growth pattern, and presence of tuberous sclerosis, patient comorbidities, renal function, pregnancy plans, and compliance.

Surgical intervention for angiomyolipomas is usually reserved for patients with symptoms not responsive to conservative measures, with lesions having renal vein or soft tissue invasion, or with suspicion of malignancy on imaging. Nephron-sparing surgery is the preferred modality because of the benign nature of the tumor. Fazeli-Matin and Novick reported on 27 patients with angiomyolipoma who underwent partial nephrectomy, of whom 21 had a solitary or impaired contralateral kidney.[120] All operated kidneys were functional after surgery, including seven with tumors larger than 12 cm. None of the patients required dialysis postoperatively and none had recurrent angiomyolipoma symptoms at a median follow-up of 39 months.

Pregnancy can complicate the management of young women with angiomyolipoma. While the incidence of hemorrhage during pregnancy is low, the consequences can be catastrophic with potential harm to the mother and fetus. Hormonal links also suggest that these tumors may grow faster secondary to the altered milieu, leading to tumor rupture. Optimal diagnostic methods may be limited by pregnancy, and it may be difficult to distinguish tumor rupture from uterine or placental rupture. This lends greater credence to the belief that women with known angiomyolipoma greater than 4 cm who intend to conceive should be treated prophylactically to avoid the risk of rupture.

Bissler *et al.* reported a 24-month nonrandomized open-label trial, in which all 25 patients were diagnosed with either tuberous sclerosis or sporadic lymphangioleiomyomatosis and least one angiomyolipoma 1 cm in size or more.[121] Sirolimus was administered in the first 12 months and tumor size was reduced to some extent but after stopping treatment, a tendency to increase in tumor size was observed. Of the 25 patients enrolled, 20 completed the 12-month evaluation, and 18 completed the 24-month evaluation. At 24 months, 5 out 18 patients showed a continual reduction in angiomyolipoma volume around 30% or more. Additional data support the role of mTOR in the biology of these neoplasms with case reports of response to mTOR inhibitors.[122] At present, the use of available mTOR inhibitors (temsirolimus, everolimus) is encouraged for metastatic, malignant angiomyolipomas while surgery is the mainstay of therapy for localized, typical angiomyolipomas.

Carcinoids

Background

Primary renal carcinoid is an extremely rare, well-differentiated neuroendocrine tumor with unclear etiology. The origin of this tumor is still unclear, since neuroendocrine cells are not normally present in the renal parenchyma. In 1997, Krishnan *et al.* reported a 20% horseshoe kidney association with the 50 cases of renal carcinoid reported in the literature at that time.[123] The relative risk for a person with horseshoe kidney to develop this tumor is estimated to be 82-fold higher than the general population.[124] It was first reported by Resnick in 1966 in a patient with carcinoid syndrome;[125] however, the majority of the organ-confined tumors do not produce the carcinoid syndrome, which is akin to carcinoids in other organ systems.

Pathology

Grossly, this lesion presents as a solitary, well-circumscribed, moderately firm tumor with a bulging appearance. The color is variable; the appearance is homogeneous with variable focal hemorrhage and calcification.[4] The histopathological features appear to be similar to carcinoid tumors in other organ systems. The cells are uniform in size and arranged in a trabecular pattern. They have small nuclei with "salt and pepper" chromatin and eosinophilic cytoplasm. Immunohistochemical staining is positive for chromogranin, neuron-specific enolase, and keratin. Variable positivity for serotonin, pancreatic polypeptide, prostatic acid phosphatase, and vasoactive intestinal polypeptide has been reported.[126]

Clinical presentation

Most patients present with an asymptomatic mass but they can also present with abdominal pain, mass, or hematuria. Workup for alternate origin is indicated when a lesion is discovered in the kidney, because of the rarity of primary carcinoid of the kidney.[123] Carcinoid symptoms are present in less than 10% of patients on presentation.[4,126,127] The median age at diagnosis is 50 years, with no sex predilection. On CT scan it appears as a circumscribed solid mass with occasional calcification or cystic changes.[127] Some authorities have suggested that an octreotide scan can contribute to accurate staging and diagnosis.[128,129]

Treatment and prognosis

Because of the rarity of the disease, the clinical outcome is difficult to predict. This is also complicated by the fact that a significant proportion of patients with metastatic disease have a prolonged survival. No standard treatment has been approved for locally advanced or metastatic disease.[130] Localized disease has been treated surgically. In one of the largest reviews, with 56 patients, Romero et al. reported that nonmetastatic disease was associated with cure and survival rates of 86% and 96%, respectively, at 48-month follow-up.[131,132]

Carcinoid tumors that arise in horseshoe kidneys tend to have a more indolent course.[123]

Three main prognostic factors have been acknowledged for patients with renal carcinoids.[131]

• Age above 40 years has been associated with a more rapid progression, thus more severe early presentation.
• Tumors measuring less than 4 cm or limited to the renal parenchyma have fewer tendencies to metastasize and hence have a better prognosis.
• Purely solid tumors and those with a mitotic rate higher than 1/10 high-power field (HPF) have also been reported to have a worse prognosis.

Carcinoid crisis secondary to release of vasoactive substances can occur with biopsy or surgical resection of the tumor and can be managed with somatostatin. In patients with a solitary metastasis, especially in the liver, it is appropriate to consider resection of the primary tumor with the metastatic lesions, because of the lack of effective systemic treatment options. Radiation is effective for short-term palliation.

Limited information on the therapy for metastatic renal carcinoid is available. In patients with carcinoid syndrome, symptom control with somatostatin or its analogs such as octreotide is reasonable.[133] For individuals with metastatic disease, systemic treatment options are based on clinical trials in patients with gastrointestinal carcinoids. The need to start systemic therapy is based on tumor anatomy and/or the presence of symptoms and is not indicated immediately for many patients. Interferon produces tumor regression (15%) and biochemical responses in patients with metastatic disease.[134] Combination chemotherapy is of limited value. In an Eastern Cooperative Oncology Group (ECOG) trial, 118 patients with metastatic carcinoid tumor were randomized for treatment with streptozotocin combined with cyclophosphamide or with 5-fluorouracil (5-FU). Objective response rates among the evaluable patients treated with the 5-FU combination were 33% and with the cyclophosphamide combination 26%, with substantial toxicity in both regimens.[135] There are no data supporting other chemotherapy regimens specifically for renal carcinoid and in general the same management approach as for other carcinoid tumors is undertaken.

Advanced neuroendocrine tumor (NET) has demonstrated increased activation of mTOR pathway components plus mTOR inhibitors have shown efficacy in animal models and cell lines and human tumors. This was the rationale for mTOR-targeted therapy for treating advanced NET.[136]

In 2008, Yao et al.[137] published the first phase 2 trial of everolimus in patients with low-grade to intermediate-grade NET. The study enrolled 60 patients with advanced, low-grade to intermediate-grade NET (30 pancreatic NET and 30 lung NET or gastrointestinal NET [carcinoid]). Patients received daily everolimus 5 mg ($n=30$) or 10 mg ($n=30$) orally in combination with octreotide long-acting release (LAR). The overall response rate was 23% in the per-protocol population, in which 13 patients (22%) achieved a partial response (PR), 42 (70%) maintained stable disease, and five (22%) had disease progression. PRs were more frequent in patients with pancreatic NET than in patients with nonpancreatic NET (27% versus 17%). Concerning the different dosages, everolimus 10 mg produced a higher PR rate than 5 mg (30% versus 13%). Median PFS was 60 weeks overall, longer in patients with nonpancreatic NET (63 weeks) than in patients with pancreatic NET (50 weeks). In terms of tumor shrinkage, the majority of patients showed some degree of tumor reduction. This study revealed that everolimus was effective and tolerated in the treatment of low-grade to intermediate-grade NET. Currently there are clinical trials of everolimus ongoing across various types of NET.[136] Even though these studies were not specifically in renal carcinoids, application to these tumors is reasonable.

Lymphoma

Background

Lymphomatous involvement of the kidney occurs in three distinct clinical scenarios. Most commonly, lymphoma of advanced stage involves the kidney secondarily. Posttransplantation lymphoproliferative disease (PTLD) can also involve the kidney secondary to iatrogenic immunosuppression (see Chapters 44 and 48). Primary renal lymphoma (PRL) is the least common. The incidence of PTLD arising in transplant kidneys has been rising in the last couple of decades because of the increasing frequency of transplantations.

Secondary renal involvement tends to be bilateral and is seen with a high incidence (37–47%) in advanced disease. Whether PRL truly exists is still a controversial issue because of its rarity; about 60 cases have been reported and only about 30 cases truly fulfill the diagnostic criteria as PRL.[138,139]

Pathology

Nephrectomy specimens in PRL can have a homogeneous, firm, pale appearance with occasional tumor thrombus or renal vein involvement. The most common pattern is a diffuse involvement with lymphoma cells permeating between the nephrons, a so-called "interstitial pattern." However, nodular involvement with discrete masses and intravascular lymphoma has also been described. Diffuse large B cell is the most common histological type, although Burkitt, lymphoblastic lymphoma, and other histologies have been described. The origin of these tumors is still controversial, since renal parenchyma does not contain any lymphoid tissue. PTLD in transplant kidneys is related to the degree of immunosuppression and Epstein–Barr virus (EBV) infection and can present as a monoclonal or polyclonal process.[4]

Clinical presentation

Due to the silent course of the disease, patients usually present as late manifestations of a systemic disease, although it was found in 34% of autopsies of patients dying of progressive lymphoma or leukemia.[140–142] Patients can present with flank/abdominal pain, fever, cachexia, renal insufficiency, or hematuria. Renal failure was believed to be secondary to general replacement of the functioning parenchyma or bilateral urethral obstruction secondary to enlarged retroperitoneal lymph nodes.[142] However, the diagnosis of renal failure secondary to parenchymal replacement by lymphoma requires exclusion of other causes of renal failure and demonstration of improvement in renal function after starting systemic chemotherapy or radiation therapy.[143,144]

Computed tomography scan is known to be the most sensitive and efficient imaging used for diagnosis and monitoring response to treatment in renal lymphoma.[141,145–147] In a review by Urban et al.,[147] the typical patterns of involvement are single and multiple masses, renal invasion from retroperitoneal disease, perirenal disease, and diffuse renal infiltration. Renal lymphoma should always be kept in mind in patients with immense retroperitoneal lymphadenopathy, splenomegaly, or lymphadenopathy in other parts of the body or uncommon areas within the retroperitoneum.[147,148]

Treatment and prognosis

Patients with PRL are usually treated by nephrectomy, because PRL is regarded clinically as a renal epithelial tumor. Once the renal involvement of lymphoma is confirmed, a thorough search for extrarenal disease and staging studies, such as CT scans and bone marrow biopsy, are warranted to rule out a secondary lymphoma, as the latter is much more common (30 times more common). Stallone et al.[138] have proposed that the diagnosis of PRL be made only when the following criteria are fulfilled:

- lymphomatous renal infiltration
- nonobstructive kidney enlargement
- no extrarenal localization at the time of diagnosis.

If renal lymphoma is expected, consideration should be given to percutaneous biopsy to achieve a pathological diagnosis. Where exploratory surgery is required, intraoperative biopsy and frozen-section analysis will take priority.

Although there have been reports of modest disease-free survival after nephrectomy of PRL, the prognosis is generally poor due to dissemination to secondary sites. Early detection and systemic combination chemotherapy may reverse the renal failure and improve survival by preventing dissemination.[138,148–150] Secondary renal lymphomas are usually seen in the setting of advanced lymphoma and have a dismal prognosis. Nephrectomy is hardly ever indicated for these advanced patients except with severe symptoms, for instance uncontrollable hemorrhage. Patients with advanced lymphoma involving the kidney are treated with conventional therapy (e.g. R-CHOP). PTLD is treated by reducing the immunosuppression if possible; Oertel et al. reported a multicenter phase 2 trial investigating rituximab (anti-CD20 monoclonal antibody) as single agent in 17 patients with PTLD. Transplanted organs were heart ($n=5$), kidney ($n=4$), lung ($n=4$), and liver ($n=4$). Patients were treated with a weekly dose of rituximab for 4 weeks on days 1, 8, 15 and 22. The mean follow-up time is 24.2 months. The mean overall survival period is approximately 3 years with 11 patients that were still alive. In total, nine patients (52.9%) achieved a complete remission, with a mean duration of 17.8 months. Partial remission was observed in one patient, minor remission in two patients, no change in three patients and one patient experienced progressive disease. Two patients relapsed, at intervals 3 and 5 months after obtaining complete remission. Although the kidney was never one of the affected sites in this study, this study proved the feasibility and efficacy of the monoclonal antibody rituximab in the setting of patients with PTLD subsequent to solid organ transplantation.[151]

Renal sarcomas

Background

Primary renal sarcoma in adults is rare, representing approximately 1% of all primary tumors of the kidney.[152–154] Renal sarcomas are less common but more fatal than any other sarcoma in the genitourinary tract, counting the prostate, bladder, and paratesticular area.[155,156] Sarcomatoid components can be seen in approximately 5% of RCC, including clear cell, papillary, chromophobe, and CDCs. It should not be confused with primary renal sarcomas, as the two entities have entirely different biology, pathology, and clinical features.[4,157]

Pathology

Any sarcomas that arise in other parts of the body can occur in the kidney, including leiomyosarcoma, osteosarcoma, malignant fibrous histiocytoma (MFH), angiosarcoma, rhabdomyosarcoma and synovial sarcoma. As in other parts of the body, the diagnosis and classification are traditionally based on H&E histology and immunohistochemistry.[158] However, molecular studies have been increasingly used in the classification of sarcomas. For example, synovial sarcoma of the kidney has a characteristic chromosomal translocation t (X;18) between the *SYT* gene on chromosome 18 and a member of the *SSX* gene family on chromosome X.[159,160]

A wide variety of histological subtypes has been described; as mentioned earlier,leiomyosarcoma is the most common histological subtype of renal sarcoma, representing 50–60% of such tumors.[161,162] Liposarcoma is fairly distinguished from RCC due to the presence of adipose tissue, but it is often confused with angiomyolipoma (AML) or with large, benign renal lipomas.[163] Osteogenic sarcoma is a rare but unique form of renal sarcoma that contains calcium and is usually stony hard.[164,165] Tumor grade, which is recognized as an important prognostic factor in soft tissue sarcomas, is also believed to be prognostic in primary renal sarcomas.

Clinical presentation

The common signs and symptoms that are seen with renal sarcoma in adults include palpable mass, abdominal or flank pain, and hematuria and are like those seen with large, fast-growing RCCs,[166] with a climax incidence in the fifth decade of life.[152,155,163,167] They can spread along tissue spaces and attain a large size before becoming symptomatic, similar to retroperitoneal sarcomas. Systemic symptoms are less commonly reported. Metastasis is generally hematogenous; Saitoh and colleagues reported the common sites of metastases of renal sarcomas where lung was the most common followed by lymph nodes and the liver.[168]

Abdominal CT classically demonstrates a large soft tissue mass connecting or derived from the kidney, a result that is again comparable to that associated with various sarcomatoid RCCs.[152,155,169] Clues that might be indicative of sarcoma rather than of RCC include clear origin from the capsule or perisinuous region, growth to large size, lack of lymphadenopathy, presence of fat or bone suggestive of liposarcoma or osteosarcoma, and hypovascular pattern on angiography, while one notable exception is the hemangiopericytoma, which is highly vascular.[169,170]

Renal liposarcomas in general develop in the fifth and sixth decades of life and frequently grow to enormous size.[166] Preoperative radiographic imaging of the chest should also be performed since this is one of the most common sites of metastatic disease.

Treatment and prognosis

Complete surgical excision is the mainstay of treatment of soft tissue sarcomas at any location with intraoperative screening of margin status. On the basis of case reports in renal sarcomas, complete surgical extirpation of the organ-confined tumor appears to offer patients the only reasonable chance for prolonged survival.[152–154,167] The best outcome is seen with small

tumors (<5 cm) of low histological grade that are confined to the kidneys. Surgical resection of locally recurrent or oligometastatic disease may be beneficial in selected patients as seen with nonrenal metastatic sarcomas.[171] In most case series, leiomyosarcoma has been the most common histological subtype. Karakousis *et al.*[172] reported early disease progression and indicated that most patients die within months regardless of treatment received. However, Vogelzang demonstrated that low-grade sarcomas have a tendency to a more indolent course.[154] In renal liposarcoma, Economou *et al.* reported response to radiation and cisplatin-based chemotherapy in an adjuvant setting.[166] Adjuvant radiation therapy, although commonly used in locally extensive disease, has not been proven to prevent local recurrence or increase survival. Likewise, the use of adjuvant chemotherapy has been described only in case report and case series form for renal sarcoma. Therefore, adjuvant radiation and/or systemic chemotherapy (with sarcoma regimens such as adriamycin and ifosfamide) can be considered for high-risk patients, while appreciating the balance of definite risks and unknown benefits. The benefit of adjuvant chemotherapy in more typical sarcomas is limited, and it is unlikely that the benefit for renal sarcomas is greater.

Metanephric neoplasms

Background

These tumors were first described by Bove *et al.* in1979,[173] and are also known as nephrogenic nephroma.[174] Several reports of similar lesions described under a variety of names then emerged and confirmed them as a distinct entity. They include metanephric adenoma (predominantly epithelial), metanephric adenofibroma, and metanephric stromal tumor (stromal tumor) which is a pediatric tumor identical to the stromal component of metanephric adenofibroma.[175]

Most of the clinical and pathological characteristics of metanephric adenoma were outlined around the mid-1990s in two large series.[176,177] Metanephric adenofibroma was then identified as a biphasic tumor with both epithelial and stromal elements and presented mostly in children and young adults.

Metanephric tumors as a group are highly cellular benign epithelial tumors but in two cases metastasis has been reported. They are also known for their close relationship to WT and are conceptualized by some as being the benign, well-differentiated end of a spectrum of tumors that also includes WT as its malignant counterpart.[175,178–180]

Pathology

These tumors are usually unilateral and seldom multifocal.[181] They tend to grow large, to 0.3–20 cm in their greatest dimension.[182] They are usually unicentric, sharply circumscribed without a capsule (Fig. 1.5a). The cut surface is gray to yellow, with foci of hemorrhage, cystic changes and necrosis being uncommonly present. Histologically, they are composed of tightly packed, small, round acini. Half the tumors contain papillary structures, which resemble primitive glomeruli. Psammoma bodies are frequently present but no blastemal

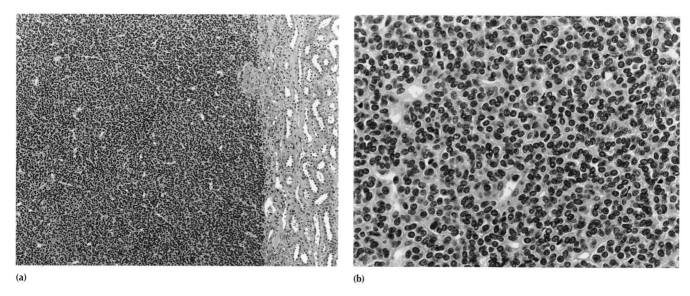

(a)   (b)

Figure 1.5 Metanephric adenoma is sharply demarcated from the adjacent renal parenchyma (a). The tumor cells are closely packed to form tubules with inconspicuous lumens. They have a strikingly uniform appearance with scant cytoplasm and smooth chromatin (b).

elements. The stroma can be inconspicuous or edematous. The cells are generally cuboid with monotonous appearance, scanty cytoplasm, and small, uniform nuclei with inconspicuous nucleoli[4,175–177] (Fig. 1.5b).

Metanephric adenofibroma is composed of nests of epithelial elements similar to metanephric adenoma embedded in bands and sheets of fibroblast-like spindle cells. The proportion of spindle cells and epithelial components in these tumors varies.[183,184] Metanephric stromal tumor, as the name implies, is very similar to the stromal component of metanephric adenofibroma.

Clinical presentation

Metanephric adenoma can occur in children and adults; however, it is predominantly seen in the fifth and sixth decades of life, with a female preponderance (female-to-male ratio 2:1). Metanephric adenofibroma is generally seen in children and young adults from 5 months to 36 years, with a male preponderance. Metanephric stromal tumors are seen mostly in children, with rare adult cases reported. These tumors as a group comprise less than 1% of renal cell neoplasms. Most of these cases are discovered incidentally during radiological studies and workup for incidental hematuria. Radiologically, metanephric adenoma presents as a hypovascular tumor protruding extrarenally. When symptomatic, they can cause abdominal pain and hematuria. Erythrocytosis has also been reported in patients at presentation.[176,185–187]

Yoshioka *et al.*[188] provided evidence that metanephric adenoma cells generate erythropoietin and other cytokines. A number of reports support that the diagnosis of metanephric adenoma can be achieved by percutaneous fine needle aspiration biopsy.[189,190] As using cytological features to make a distinction between metanephric adenoma and Wilms tumor can be challenging, immunocytochemical analysis in this context might be helpful.[189]

Treatment and prognosis

These tumors are benign, with the exception of a few case reports.[179,180] If metanephric adenoma is suspected from the clinical findings, it is important to obtain an intraoperative diagnosis in order to avoid excessive resection. Erythrocytosis associated with these tumors resolve following complete resection. There have been a number of reports supporting partial nephrectomy for metanephric adenoma, mainly in adults.[191–193] A conservative approach to metanephric adenoma, with no surgery, has been described in a few case reports.[6,194] No local recurrence or distant metastasis has been reported for metanephric stromal tumors. Wilms tumor has been reported to have arisen in metanephric adenofibroma and metanephric stromal tumor, pointing to the possible common origin of these entities.[184] Renal angiodysplasia associated with these lesions can cause morbidity secondary to vascular complications. Resection without adjuvant chemotherapy is the preferred modality of treatment. There are no reliable reports of metastatic metanephric adenoma, and therefore no literature supporting any systemic therapy for unresectable disease. Presence of distant metastases should cause one to question the histological diagnosis.

Adult Wilms tumor (nephroblastoma)

Background

Wilms tumor (WT) is the most common malignant renal tumor in children. It affects approximately one in every 8000 children without a significant sex predilection, and about 450 new cases are reported yearly in the United States. Ninety-eight percent of all cases occur in children below the age of 10 years, and less than 300 cases of adult WT have been reported in the literature. It tends to occur with almost the same incidence across the globe, suggesting the absence of an environmental factor. However, the incidence in the United States is highest in

African-Americans and lowest in Asians, indicating a possible genetic predisposition.[4,195] Its true incidence in adults is difficult to ascertain because it is included with renal cell carcinoma in epidemiological reports, and varying diagnostic criteria are utilized in case reports.

Most experts use the following criteria to define adult WT: (i) primary renal neoplasm, (ii) primitive blastematous spindle or round cell component, (iii) formation of abortive or embryonal tubular or glomeruloid structure, (iv) no area of tumor diagnostic of RCC, (v) pictorial confirmation of histology, and (vi) age >15 years.[196,197]

Kilton et al. reported 35 cases of adult Wilms tumor which met the terms of all the above criteria.[198] Approximately 1–2% of pediatric WT cases have a familial origin.

Pathology

In contrast with childhood WTs, which are often multicentric and bilateral, most of the adult WT cases are unicentric, with multicentric and bilateral disease reported in 7% and 5% of patients, respectively. Horseshoe kidneys are associated with a two-fold higher incidence of WT. The gross and microscopic appearance of adult WT otherwise tends to resemble pediatric WT. The gross appearance of WT varies and reflects the proportion of stromal and nonstromal components. Generally WT is pale gray or tan and has a soft consistency; however, tumors with predominant stroma may be white and firm. Cyst formation may be prominent in certain cases.

Wilms tumor contains varying proportions of undifferentiated blastemal cells and differentiated cells of epithelial and stromal lineage. Blastemal cells are undifferentiated, small, mitotically active, rounded or oval, and densely packed with scant cytoplasm. They can occur in several distinctive growth patterns within individual tumors, including diffuse, nodular, serpentine, and basaloid. The epithelial component of WT can manifest as primitive tubules with rosette-like forms and occasionally as glomeruloid structures. Heterologous epithelial differentiation with squamous, mucinous, or ciliated epithelial components can be detected. The stromal component can exhibit significant diversity but is usually composed of spindle cells with a myxoid background. Heterologous elements including skeletal muscle, cartilage, bone, adipose tissue, and neural tissue can be present.

The histological diversity of WT is a hallmark. Characteristically, it has a so-called triphasic pattern with blastemal, epithelial, and stromal components, although monophasic patterns with only one component, and biphasic pattern with two components, are also seen often. Chemotherapy can alter the morphology by inducing maturation of blastemal, epithelial, and stromal elements, leading to a disproportionate reduction of actively proliferating cells as compared to the prechemotherapy specimen. Metastatic WT may comprise a single element or a combination of what is present in the primary tumor. WT-1 antigen is usually identified in the blastemal and epithelial elements, but not in differentiated epithelial or stromal components.[199,200]

Nuclear anaplasia associated with an adverse outcome has been recognized in 5% of pediatric cases and increases in prevalence with age and in certain populations (e.g. African-Americans). Anaplasia requires the presence of multipolar mitotic figures, marked nuclear enlargement (three times that of nonanaplastic nuclei), and nuclear hyperchromasia. The prognostic significance is more profound in diffuse anaplasia compared to focal anaplasia. Extensive blastemal cells have also been identified as an adverse prognostic factor.

Nephrogenic rests are foci of abnormally persistent embryonal renal tissue that are capable of developing into WT. The presence of diffuse or multifocal nephrogenic rests is defined as nephroblastomatosis. There are two variants of nephrogenic rests called perilobar nephrogenic rests (PLNR) and intralobar nephrogenic rests (ILNR). They can be seen in 25–45% of pediatric WT and have also been seen in adult WT patients, as well as in several ectopic sites outside the kidney.

Pediatric WT has been associated with a number of well-known syndromes and genetic mutations. WAGR (Wilms tumor, aniridia, genitourinary anomalies, mental retardation) and Denys–Drash (gonadal dysgenesis, early-onset nephropathy) syndromes are associated with deletion or mutations of the WT1 gene (11p13), a gene critical for renal and gonadal development. Beckwith–Wiedemann syndrome (hemihypertrophy, macroglossia, omphalocele, and visceromegaly) is associated with loss of imprinting on WT2 (11p15). Because of the lack of sufficient cases, the genetics and syndromic associations have not been well elucidated in adults. Recently, a high-resolution genomic analysis of adult WT in a 71-year-old Swedish woman, using a SNP array, displayed a complex genetic profile highly diverse from those observed in pediatrics WT, which indicates that WT in adults may represent a distinct biological entity compared to WT in pediatric patients.[201]

Clinical presentation

The most common clinical presentation of an adult WT is flank pain, hematuria, abdominal mass, or constitutional symptoms. Hypertension, which is commonly presented in pediatric WT, has not been commonly reported in adult WT. While Kilton et al.[198] had described 42% of their patients being symptomatic for more than a year prior to diagnosis, this has not been seen in other adult case series.[196,199,202–205] The tumors are usually fairly large on initial presentation and a varicocele may signal obstruction of the spermatic vein secondary to tumor thrombus in the renal vein or inferior vena cava. Acquired von Willebrand disease has been associated with pediatric WT and testing for this is warranted in adult patients with clinical bleeding tendency. CT findings typically present as a heterogeneous intrarenal mass with a moderately hypovascular outline, but discrimination from RCC can be challenging if not impossible in many cases.[205–207]

Computed tomography scan of the chest and abdomen should be done preoperatively to evaluate for metastases and extrarenal WT. Intravascular extension involving the renal vein and IVC can be seen.

The most common sites for metastasis of WT are the lung, lymph nodes, and the liver. Metastasis to the bone is unusual and a bone scan or skeletal survey is warranted only in the

Table 1.1 Wilms tumor staging system.

Stage	Findings and treatment
I	Tumor limited to the kidney and is resected completely
II	Tumor extends beyond kidney but is resected completely
III	Gross or microscopic residual tumor present and confined to the abdomen
IV	Hematogenous metastasis or lymph node metastasis outside the abdomen and pelvis
V	Bilateral renal involvement at diagnosis; tumor in each kidney should be separately substaged

presence of symptoms. The staging system used by the Children's Oncology Group (COG), Societé Internationale d'Oncologie Pédiatrique (SIOP) (International Society of Pediatric Oncology) and National Wilms Tumor Study Group (NWTSG) has been accepted by most adult WT authorities in the staging of WT (Table 1.1). The staging is based on both radiological and surgical pathology data.

Treatment and prognosis

The prognosis of adults with WT is poor compared to children, who have an 85% chance of cure. This success in pediatric WT represents a paradigm change to multimodality treatment.[208] However, it was also thought that adults are more likely to present with advanced disease and a decline in performance status.[206,209] In the 1980s, most adult case series had reported a long-term survival of about 25%. Even though prior studies have shown comparable results between adult and pediatric WT patient populations when adults are treated on protocols, a recent analysis of the Surveillance, Epidemiology and End Results (SEER) database has demonstrated that adults have a significantly worse overall survival than the pediatric patient populations, which was attributed to inaccurate diagnosis, inadequate staging, and undertreatment.[210]

Prior to the report by Arrigo *et al.* of 27 patients reported to the NWTSG from 1979–87 with a 3-year overall survival of 67%, it was believed that this high rate of cure could not be achieved in adults.[203] This series included six stage I, five stage II, four stage III, 11 stage IV, one stage V patients and four patients with anaplastic histology. In this series, 26 patients underwent nephrectomy, 25 received chemotherapy, and 20 received radiation treatment. This led to the authors' recommendations that patients with stage I disease and favorable histology should be treated with surgery followed by 6 months of postoperative chemotherapy using actinomycin-D and vincristine without postoperative radiation therapy; and for stage II, III, and IV with favourable histology, vincristine, actinomycin-D and doxorubicin for 15 months along with radiation of 2000 cGy to the tumor bed, 1200–1500 cGy to the lungs, 2000 cGy to the liver, and 3000 cGy to other sites as appropriate in patients with metastases at diagnosis.

Kattan *et al.* reported the French experience in 22 adult patients from 1973 to 1992.[204] Their series included four stage I, eight stage II, three stage III and seven stage IV patients. All patients underwent nephrectomy followed by single-modality adjuvant treatment in seven patients (radiotherapy in one and

chemotherapy in six) and combined modality in 15 patients. The chemotherapeutic agents used most often were actinomycin-D, vincristine, and doxorubicin. Two of seven (29%) and 7/15 (47%) patients were disease free after first-line treatment. Salvage chemotherapy had to be given in 13 patients. After a mean follow-up of 100 months, 12/22 patients (55%) were alive, including 10 who were disease free (45%). These authors recommended aggressive treatment including a three-drug regimen (actinomycin-D + vincristine + doxorubicin), regardless of stage, and irradiation starting from stage II.

Terenziani *et al.* reviewed the Italian experience with 17 adult patients between 1983 and 2001 who were treated with an Italian protocol and followed for a median of 131 months.[208] This included eight patients with stage II, four patients with stage III and five patients with stage IV and included one patient with anaplasia. Sixteen patients underwent nephrectomy, 15 received chemotherapy (10 with two drugs and five with three drugs) and seven patients received radiation. The 5-year disease-free survival was 45% with an overall survival of 62%. Reinhard *et al.* reviewed the German experience which included 30 adult patients on the SIOP 93–01 study.[205] Ten patients (33%) had metastatic disease at presentation. There was a predominance of higher stage (stage I, 8; stage II, 7; stage III, 15 patients), with histology revealing intermediate risk in 23 patients and high risk in two patients. Twenty-six patients underwent primary radical nephrectomy and the other four patients received neoadjuvant chemotherapy prior to surgery. Nineteen patients received the intermediate-risk chemotherapy and 11 patients received the high-risk chemotherapy as per protocol. Intermediate-risk chemotherapy included vincristine, actinomycin-D ± doxorubicin for 18–27 weeks, and the high-risk regimen was etoposide, carboplatin, ifosfamide, and doxorubicin for 34 weeks. Fourteen patients received local radiation from 15–35 Gy and three patients received radiation to metastatic sites. Complete remission was obtained in 24 patients (80%) with an event-free survival of 57% and an overall survival of 83% with a median observation time of 4 years.

In an earlier series by Byrd *et al.*, it was noted that adults are at risk for relapse for a greater period of time compared with children.[202] This has not been supported by more recent series.[203,205] Recurrent disease in children has been treated successfully with radiation, multiagent salvage chemotherapy regimens (etoposide, carboplatin, and ifosfamide), or high-dose chemotherapy with stem cell support leading to long-term remissions (30–60%).[211,212]

All existing modern series have lain to rest the skepticism regarding multimodality treatment of WT in adults. A risk-adapted multimodality treatment approach similar to pediatric WT protocols is the current standard of care. In contrast with the pediatric population, where the opinion differs as to whether nephrectomy should be done primarily or after neoadjuvant treatment, there is a consensus opinion that primary surgery is advisable for adult WT because of the difficulty in establishing this rare diagnosis preoperatively. Only in cases of primarily inoperable patients should diagnosis be established by biopsy and neoadjuvant treatment initiated to attempt regression of the tumor and enhance operability. In the absence of bilateral disease, which is rare in adults, the primary surgery should include a radical nephrectomy with lymph node sampling. Although a complete resection of all viable tumor is desirable, surgical effort that may endanger vital organs is not advisable, because local control can be achieved by adjuvant treatment.

Because of the rarity of the disease, there are no established treatment guidelines in adult WT. Treatment should preferably be done in a tertiary center with experience in this disease. Since pathological staging is similar to pediatric Wilms tumor, we propose treating adult patients with similar therapeutic protocols that have been investigated and verified in children.[213] The most recent recommendations available in the literature were based on discussions held with representatives of the renal tumor committees of the SIOP and COG and have been updated with a review of more recently published institutional and trial experiences of adults treated on pediatric protocols as follows.[214]

- Radiation treatment should be given to all patients unless they have a stage I nonanaplastic (favorable histology) WT, when they are treated with a combination chemotherapy regimen such as vincristine and actinomycin-D. Radiation should be used in the adjuvant setting in stage III and IV postoperatively. Pulmonary irradiation is indicated when patients present with lung metastases, regardless of whether complete remission is achieved after chemotherapy or surgery. Abdominal radiotherapy is advised when there is diffuse tumor rupture either before or after surgery.
- Chemotherapy in WT as a general rule needs to be risk adapted based on the histology and should be used in the adjuvant setting in all stages in patients with adequate organ function and performance status. In stage I, chemotherapy based on histology (favorable histology) can be used with a 2–3 drug regimen for 22–25 weeks while unfavorable histology will

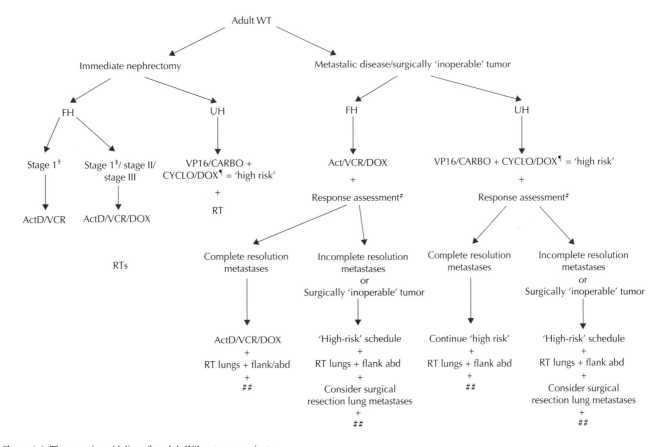

Figure 1.6 Therapeutic guidelines for adult Wilms tumor patients.
[†]Only stage I favorable histology if all four criteria are met, that is:
 1. Stage and histology have been reviewed by a pediatric pathologist experienced in Wilms' tumor;
 2. Histological examination and review has included at least one lymph node;
 3. CT scan of the chest has excluded the presence of lung metastases;
 4. Chemotherapy can be started within 30 days if date of nephrectomy.
[‡]All other stage I Wilms' tumor cases.
[¶]'High risk' chemotherapy schedule.
[#]Response assessment of metastases and operability of the primary tumor after 6 weeks by abdominal/pulmonary CT scan.
[##]Delayed nephrectomy should be considered after 6 weeks of preoperative chemotherapy if a nephrectomy has not been performed at initial diagnosis. If the original diagnosis was made on biopsy only, then in the care of nonresponse or inadequate response to preoperative chemotherapy, the histological diagnosis should be reviewed again and a further biopsy may be warranted if there is any uncertainty. Then in these cases where the Wilms' tumor (histologically confirmed again) remains surgically 'inoperable', we advise to consider changing to the 'high-risk' schedule or go on with this schedule and assess operability again after two to three courses of chemotherapy.
abd, abdominal; ActD, actinomycin D; CARBO, carboplatin; CT, computed tomography; CYCLO, cyclofosfamide; DOX, doxorubicin; FH, favorable histology; VCR, vincristine; VP16, etoposide; RT, radiotherapy; UH, unfavorable histology; WT, Wilms' tumor.

need the four-drug regimen for 25–36 weeks. Chemotherapy for stages II, III and IV (metastatic) is also based on histology and can vary from three- to four-drug regimens for 25–36 weeks. The chemotherapy regimens utilized were based on the existing pediatric experiences. The two-drug regimen was vincristine and actinomycin-D for 22 weeks; the three-drug regimen was vincristine, actinomycin-D, and doxorubicin for 25 weeks; and the four-drug regimen was etoposide, doxorubicin, cyclophosphamide, and carboplatin for 36 weeks. Figure 1.6 describes how to proceed with management.
• Patients with bilateral tumors (stage V disease) should be given primary chemotherapy for about 6–8 weeks followed by nephron-sparing bilateral partial nephrectomy in an attempt to preserve normal renal tissue. Additional chemotherapy and radiation treatment may be needed after the surgery.[215]

Conclusion

Several different tumor types can affect the kidney, ranging from very indolent tumors treated primarily with surgery to more aggressive entities which require multimodal therapy. Close consultation with an expert renal pathologist is critical to ensure a proper diagnosis of these less common entities. More common tumors such as AML and Wilms tumor have established treatment guidelines which should be followed. More rare entities will by definition have only case series and case reports. Such data should be viewed cautiously as low-level evidence when assessing the risk:benefit ratio of a given approach for an individual patient. Future directions include more complete and specific molecular testing of these tumors to identify specific alterations which can be therapeutically targeted.

References

1. Jemal A, *et al.* Cancer statistics, 2005. CA Cancer J Clin 2005; 55(1): 10–30.
2. Siegel R, Naishadham D, Jemal A. Cancer statistics, 2012. CA Cancer J Clin 2012; 62(1): 10–29. Epub ahead of print.
3. Konig G. *Practical Treatment of Diseases of the Kidney as Explained by Case Histories.* Leipzig, Germany: C. Cnobloch, 1826.
4. Eble JN, *et al. Pathology and Genetics of Tumors of the Urinary System and Male Genital Organs.* Lyon, France: IARC Press, 2004.
5. Renshaw AA. Subclassification of renal cell neoplasms: an update for the practising pathologist. Histopathology 2002; 41(4): 283–300.
6. Amin MB, *et al.* Prognostic impact of histologic subtyping of adult renal epithelial neoplasms: an experience of 405 cases. Am J Surg Pathol 2002; 26(3): 281–91.
7. Renshaw AA, Granter SR, Cibas ES. Fine-needle aspiration of the adult kidney. Cancer 1997; 81(2): 71–88.
8. Delahunt B, Eble JN. History of the development of the classification of renal cell neoplasia. Clin Lab Med 2005; 25(2): 231–46.
9. Latif F, *et al.* Identification of the von Hippel–Lindau disease tumor suppressor gene. Science 1993; 260(5112): 1317–20.
10. Cohen D, Zhou M. Molecular genetics of familial renal cell carcinoma syndromes. Clin Lab Med 2005; 25(2): 259–77.
11. Jones TD, Eble JN, Cheng L. Application of molecular diagnostic techniques to renal epithelial neoplasms. Clin Lab Med 2005; 25(2): 279–303.
12. Kovacs G. The value of molecular genetic analysis in the diagnosis and prognosis of renal cell tumours. World J Urol 1994; 12(2): 64–8.
13. Zambrano NR, *et al.* Histopathology and molecular genetics of renal tumors toward unification of a classification system. J Urol 1999; 162(4): 1246–58.
14. Argani P, *et al.* Primary renal neoplasms with the ASPL-TFE3 gene fusion of alveolar soft part sarcoma: a distinctive tumor entity previously included among renal cell carcinomas of children and adolescents. Am J Pathol 2001; 159(1): 179–92.
15. Zhou M, Roma A, Magi-Galluzzi C. The usefulness of immunohistochemical markers in the differential diagnosis of renal neoplasms. Clin Lab Med 2005; 25(2): 247–57.
16. McGregor DK, *et al.* Diagnosing primary and metastatic renal cell carcinoma: the use of the monoclonal antibody 'Renal Cell Carcinoma Marker'. Am J Surg Pathol 2001; 25(12): 1485–92.
17. Avery AK, *et al.* Use of antibodies to RCC and CD10 in the differential diagnosis of renal neoplasms. Am J Surg Pathol 2000; 24(2): 203–10.
18. Kim MK, Kim S. Immunohistochemical profile of common epithelial neoplasms arising in the kidney. Appl Immunohistochem Mol Morphol 2002; 10(4): 332–8.
19. Bell ET. Renal Diseases. Philadelphia, Pennsylvania: Lee and Febiger, 1950.
20. Murphy GP, Mostofi FK. Histologic assessment and clinical prognosis of renal adenoma. J Urol 1970; 103(1): 31–6.
21. Wang KL, *et al.* Renal papillary adenoma – a putative precursor of papillary renal cell carcinoma. Hum Pathol 2007; 38(2): 239–46.
22. Eble JN. Tumors of the kidney. Semin Diagn Pathol 1998; 15: 1–81.
23. Kovacs G, *et al.* The Heidelberg classification of renal cell tumours. J Pathol 1997; 183(2): 131–3.
24. Kipell J. The incidence of benign renal nodules (a clinicopathologic study). J Urol 1971; 106: 503.
25. Mancilla-Jimenez R, Stanley RJ, Blath RA. Papillary renal cell carcinoma: a clinical, radiologic, and pathologic study of 34 cases. Cancer 1976; 38(6): 2469–80.
26. Fleming S, Lewi HJ. Collecting duct carcinoma of the kidney. Histopathology 1986; 10(11): 1131–41.
27. Srigley JR, Eble JN. Collecting duct carcinoma of kidney. Semin Diagn Pathol 1998; 15(1): 54–67.
28. Tokuda N, *et al.* Collecting duct (Bellini duct) renal cell carcinoma: a nationwide survey in Japan. J Urol 2006; 176: 40–3; discussion 43.
29. Dimopoulos MA, *et al.* Collecting duct carcinoma of the kidney. Br J Urol 1993; 71(4): 388–91.
30. Mejean A, *et al.* Is there a place for radical nephrectomy in the presence of metastatic collecting duct (Bellini) carcinoma? J Urol 2003; 169(4): 1287–90.
31. Milowsky MI, *et al.* Active chemotherapy for collecting duct carcinoma of the kidney: a case report and review of the literature. Cancer 2002; 94(1): 111–16.
32. Peyromaure M, *et al.* Collecting duct carcinoma of the kidney: a clinicopathological study of 9 cases. J Urol 2003; 170(4) Pt 1: 1138–40.
33. Chao D, *et al.* Collecting duct renal cell carcinoma: clinical study of a rare tumor. J Urol 2002; 167(1): 71–4.
34. El Tazi M, *et al.* Metastatic collecting duct carcinoma of the kidney treated with sunitinib. World J Surg Oncol 2011; 9: 73.
35. Ansari J, Fatima A, Chaudhri S, Bhatt RI, Wallace M, James ND. Sorafenib induces therapeutic response in a patient with metastatic collecting duct carcinoma of kidney. Onkologie 2009; 32: 44–6.
36. Miyake H, *et al.* Metastatic collecting duct carcinoma of the kidney responded to sunitinib. Int J Clin Oncol 2011; 16: 153–5.
37. Staehler M, *et al.* Carcinoma of the collecting ducts of Bellini of the kidney: adjuvant chemotherapy followed by multikinase inhibition with sunitinib. Clin Genitourinary Cancer 2009; 7(1): 58–61.
38. Davis CJ Jr, Mostofi FK, Sesterhenn IA. Renal medullary carcinoma. The seventh sickle cell nephropathy. Am J Surg Pathol 1995; 19(1): 1–11.
39. Dimashkieh H, Choe J, Mutema G. Renal medullary carcinoma: a report of 2 cases and review of the literature. Arch Pathol Lab Med 2003; 127(3): e135–8.
40. Selby DM, *et al.* Renal medullary carcinoma: can early diagnosis lead to long-term survival? J Urol 2000; 163(4): 1238.

41. Avery RA, *et al*. Renal medullary carcinoma: clinical and therapeutic aspects of a newly described tumor. Cancer 1996; 78(1): 128–32.

42. Swartz MA, *et al*. Renal medullary carcinoma: clinical, pathologic, immunohistochemical, and genetic analysis with pathogenetic implications. Urology 2002; 60(6): 1083–9.

43. Assad L, *et al*. Cytologic features of renal medullary carcinoma. Cancer 2005; 105(1): 28–34.

44. Gatalica Z, Lilleberg S, Monzon F. Renal medullary carcinomas: histopathologic phenotype associated with diverse genotypes. Hum Pathol 2011; 42(12): 1979–88.

45. Debelenko LV, *et al*. Renal cell carcinoma with novel VCL-ALK fusion: new representative of ALK-associated tumor spectrum. Mod Pathol 2010; 24: 430–42.

46. Mariño-Enriquez M, *et al*. ALK rearrangement in sickle cell trait-associated renal medullary carcinoma. Genes, Chromosomes Cancer 2011; 50(3): 146–53.

47. Strouse JJ, *et al*. Significant responses to platinum-based chemotherapy in renal medullary carcinoma. Pediatr Blood Cancer 2005; 44(4): 407–11.

48. Schaeffer EM, *et al*. Renal medullary carcinoma: molecular, pathological and clinical evidence for treatment with topoisomerase-inhibiting therapy. BJU Int 2010; 106: 62–5.

49. Cheng JX, *et al*. Renal medullary carcinoma: rhabdoid features and the absence of INI1 expression as markers of aggressive behavior. Mod Pathol 2008; 21: 647–52.

50. Davidson AJ, *et al*. Renal medullary carcinoma associated with sickle cell trait: radiographic findings. Radiology 1995; 1(95): 83–5.

51. Watanabe IC, *et al*. Renal medullary carcinoma: report of seven cases from Brazil. Mod Pathol 2007; 20: 914–20.

52. Hakimi AA, *et al*. Renal medullary carcinoma: the Bronx experience. Urology 2007; 70: 878–82.

53. Simpson L, *et al*. Renal medullary carcinoma and ABL gene amplification. J Urol 2005; 173: 1883–8.

54. Schaeffer EM, *et al*. Renal medullary carcinoma: molecular, pathological and clinical evidence for treatment with topoisomerase-inhibiting therapy. BJU Int 2010; 106: 62–5.

55. Strouse JJ, *et al*. Significant responses to platinum-based chemotherapy in renal medullary carcinoma. Pediatr Blood Cancer 2005; 44: 407–11.

56. Bell MD. Response to paclitaxel, gemcitabine, and cisplatin in renal medullary carcinoma. Pediatr Blood Cancer 2006; 47: 228.

57. Motzer RJ, *et al*. Treatment outcome and survival associated with metastatic renal cell carcinoma of nonclear-cell histology. J Clin Oncol 2002; 20: 2376–81.

58. Karaman S, *et al*. Renal medullary carcinoma case presenting with abdominal mass. Turk J Cancer 2005; 35: 96–8.

59. Stahlschmidt J, Cullinane C, Roberts P, Picton SV. Renal medullary carcinoma: prolonged remission with chemotherapy, immunohistochemical characterisation and evidence of bcr/abl rearrangement. Med Pediatr Oncol 1999; 33: 551–7.

60. Simpson L, *et al*. Renal medullary carcinoma and ABL gene amplification. J Urol 2005; 173: 1883–8.

61. Rathmell WK, Monk JP. High-dose-intensity MVAC for advanced renal medullary carcinoma: report of three cases and literature review. Urology 2008; 72: 659–63.

62. Argani P, Ladanyi M. Translocation carcinomas of the kidney. Clin Lab Med 2005; 25(2): 363–78.

63. Sidhar SK, *et al*. The t(X;1)(p11.2;q21.2) translocation in papillary renal cell carcinoma fuses a novel gene PRCC to the TFE3 transcription factor gene. Hum Mol Genet 1996; 5(9): 1333–8.

64. Armah H, Parwani A. Xp11.2 translocation renal cell carcinoma. Arch Pathol Lab Med 2010; 134(1): 124–9.

65. Argani P, *et al*. Translocation carcinomas of the kidney after chemotherapy in childhood. J Clin Oncol 2006; 24(10): 1529–34.

66. Ramphal R, Pappo A, Zielenska M, Grant R, Ngan BY. Pediatric renal cell carcinoma: clinical, pathologic, and molecular abnormalities associated with the members of the MIT transcription factor family. Am J Clin Pathol 2006; 126(3): 349–64.

67. Argani P, *et al*. Xp11 translocation renal cell carcinoma in adults: expanded clinical, pathologic, and genetic spectrum. Am J Surg Pathol 2007; 31: 1149–60.

68. Komai Y, *et al*. Adult Xp11 translocation renal cell carcinoma diagnosed by cytogenetics and immunohistochemistry. Clin Cancer Res 2009; 15: 1170–6.

69. Franzini A, *et al*. A case of renal cancer with TFE3 gene fusion in an elderly man: clinical, radiological and surgical findings. Urol Int 2007; 78: 179–81.

70. Malouf GG, *et al*. Targeted agents in metastatic Xp11 translocation/TFE3 gene fusion renal cell carcinoma (RCC): a report from the Juvenile RCC network. Ann Oncol 2010; 21: 1834–8.

71. Geller JI, *et al*. Translocation renal cell carcinoma: lack of negative impact due to lymph node spread. Cancer 2008; 112: 1607–16.

72. Choueiri TK, *et al*. Vascular endothelial growth factor-targeted therapy for the treatment of adult metastatic Xp11.2 translocation renal cell carcinoma. Cancer 2010; 116: 5219–25.

73. Clinical trials phase 2 study in patients with MiT tumors. Available at: http://clinicaltrials.gov/show/NCT00557609. Accessed February 2, 2012.

74. Hennigar R, Epstein J, Farrow GM. Tubular renal cell carcinomas of collecting duct origin. Mod Pathol 1994; 7: 76A.

75. MacLennan GT, Farrow GM, Bostwick DG. Low-grade collecting duct carcinoma of the kidney: report of 13 cases of low-grade mucinous tubulocystic renal carcinoma of possible collecting duct origin. Urology 1997; 50(5): 679–84.

76. Srigley JR. Phenotypic, molecular and ultrastructural studies of a novel low grade renal epithelial neoplasm possibly related to the loop of Henle. Mod Pathol 2002; 15(182A).

77. Amin M. Tubulocystic carcinoma of the kidney. Mod Pathol 2004; 17(137A).

78. Razoky C. Low-grade tubular-mucinous renal neoplasms. Mod Pathol 2002; 15(11): 1162–71.

79. Parwani AV, *et al*. Low-grade myxoid renal epithelial neoplasms with distal nephron differentiation. Hum Pathol 2001; 32(5): 506–12.

80. MacLennan GT, Bostwick DG. Tubulocystic carcinoma, mucinous tubular and spindle cell carcinoma, and other recently described rare renal tumors. Clin Lab Med 2005; 25(2): 393–416.

81. Dhillon J, *et al*. Mucinous tubular and spindle cell carcinoma of the kidney with sarcomatoid change. Am J Surg Pathol 2009; 33: 44–9.

82. Thway K, *et al*. Metastatic renal mucinous tubular and spindle cell carcinoma. Atypical behavior of a rare, morphologically bland tumor. Ann Diag Pathol 2011 Jun 16 [Epub ahead of print].

83. Larkin J, *et al*. Metastatic mucinous tubular and spindle cell carcinoma of the kidney responding to sunitinib. J Clin Oncol 2010; 28: e539–e540.

84. Klein MJ, Valensi QJ. Proximal tubular adenomas of kidney with so-called oncocytic features. A clinicopathologic study of 13 cases of a rarely reported neoplasm. Cancer 1976; 38(2): 906–14.

85. Lieber MM. Renal oncocytoma: prognosis and treatment. Eur Urol 1990; 18(Suppl 2): 17–21.

86. Raghavan D, Brecher M, Johnson D, *et al*. (eds). *Textbook of Uncommon Cancer*, 2nd edn. Chichester: John Wiley & Sons, 1999.

87. Abrahams NA, Tamboli P. Oncocytic renal neoplasms: diagnostic considerations. Clin Lab Med 2005; 25(2): 317–39.

88. Fleming S, O'Donnell M. Surgical pathology of renal epithelial neoplasms: recent advances and current status. Histopathology 2000; 36(3): 195–202.

89. Amin MB, *et al*. Renal oncocytoma: a reappraisal of morphologic features with clinicopathologic findings in 80 cases. Am J Surg Pathol 1997; 21(1): 1–12.

90. Liu J, Fanning CV. Can renal oncocytomas be distinguished from renal cell carcinoma on fine-needle aspiration specimens? A study of conventional smears in conjunction with ancillary studies. Cancer 2001; 93(6): 390–7.

91. Tickoo SK, *et al*. Ultrastructural observations on mitochondria and microvesicles in renal oncocytoma, chromophobe renal cell carcinoma, and eosinophilic variant of conventional (clear cell) renal cell carcinoma. Am J Surg Pathol 2000; 24(9): 1247–56.

92. Tickoo SK, *et al*. Renal oncocytosis: a morphologic study of fourteen cases. Am J Surg Pathol 1999; 23(9): 1094–101.

93. Zbar B, *et al*. Risk of renal and colonic neoplasms and spontaneous pneumothorax in the Birt-Hogg-Dube syndrome. Cancer Epidemiol Biomarkers Prev 2002; 11(4): 393–400.

94. Pavlovich CP, *et al*. Evaluation and management of renal tumors in the Birt-Hogg-Dube syndrome. J Urol 2005; 173(5): 1482–6.

95. Hilton S. Imaging of renal cell carcinoma. Semin Oncol 2000; 27(2): 150–9.

96. Perez-Ordonez B, *et al*. Renal oncocytoma: a clinicopathologic study of 70 cases. Am J Surg Pathol 1997; 21(8): 871–83.

97. Dechet CB, *et al*. Renal oncocytoma: multifocality, bilateralism, metachronous tumor development and coexistent renal cell carcinoma. J Urol 1999; 162(1): 40–2.

98. Grawitz P. Demonstration eines grossen Angio-Myo-Lipoms der Niere. Dtsch Med Wochenschr 1900; 26: 290.

99. Bissler JJ, Kingswood JC. Renal angiomyolipomata. Kidney Int 2004; 66(3): 924–34.

100. Bourneville D-MB. A l'idiotie et epilepsie symptomatique de sclerose tubereuse ou hypertrophique. Arch Neurol 1900; 10: 29–39.

101. Tallarigo C, *et al*. Diagnostic and therapeutic problems in multicentric renal angiomyolipoma. J Urol 1992; 148(6): 1880–4.

102. Abdulla M, *et al*. Renal angiomyolipoma. DNA content and immunohistochemical study of classic and multicentric variants. Arch Pathol Lab Med 1994; 118(7): 735–9.

103. Ashfaq R, Weinberg AG, Albores-Saavedra J. Renal angiomyolipomas and HMB-45 reactivity. Cancer 1993; 71(10): 3091–7.

104. L'Hostis H, *et al*. Renal angiomyolipoma: a clinicopathologic, immunohistochemical, and follow-up study of 46 cases. Am J Surg Pathol 1999; 23(9): 1011–20.

105. Pea M, *et al*. Melanocyte-marker-HMB-45 is regularly expressed in angiomyolipoma of the kidney. Pathology 1991; 23(3): 185–8.

106. Lowe BA, *et al*. Malignant transformation of angiomyolipoma. JUrol 1992; 147(5): 1356–8.

107. Martignoni G, *et al*. Renal angiomyolipoma with epithelioid sarcomatous transformation and metastases: demonstration of the same genetic defects in the primary and metastatic lesions. Am J Surg Pathol 2000; 24(6): 889–94.

108. Mai KT, Perkins DG, Collins JP. Epithelioid cell variant of renal angiomyolipoma. Histopathology 1996; 28(3): 277–80.

109. Eble JN, Amin MB, Young RH. Epithelioid angiomyolipoma of the kidney: a report of five cases with a prominent and diagnostically confusing epithelioid smooth muscle component. Am J Surg Pathol 1997; 21(10): 1123–30.

110. Hajdu SI, Foote FW Jr. Angiomyolipoma of the kidney: report of 27 cases and review of the literature. J Urol 1969; 102(4): 396–401.

111. Fujii Y, *et al*. Benign renal tumors detected among healthy adults by abdominal ultrasonography. Eur Urol 1995; 27(2): 124–7.

112. Vogt H. Zur diagnostik der tuberosen sklerose. Z Erforsch Behandl Jugendl Schwachsinns 1908; 2: 1–12.

113. Nelson CP, Sanda MG. Contemporary diagnosis and management of renal angiomyolipoma. J Urol 2002; 168(4 Pt 1): 1315–25.

114. Steiner MS, *et al*. The natural history of renal angiomyolipoma. J Urol 1993; 150(6): 1782–6.

115. De Luca S, Terrone C, Rossetti SR. Management of renal angiomyolipoma: a report of 53 cases. BJU Int 1999; 83(3): 215–18.

116. Chesa Ponce N, *et al*. Wunderlich's syndrome as the first manifestation of a renal angiomyolipoma. Arch Esp Urol 1995; 48(3): 305–8.

117. Dickinson M, *et al*. Renal angiomyolipoma: optimal treatment based on size and symptoms. Clin Nephrol 1998; 49(5): 281–6.

118. Eble JN. Angiomyolipoma of kidney. Semin Diagn Pathol 1998; 15(1): 21–40.

119. Oesterling JE, *et al*. The management of renal angiomyolipoma. J Urol 1986; 135(6): 1121–4.

120. Fazeli-Matin S, Novick AC. Nephron-sparing surgery for renal angiomyolipoma. Urology 1998; 52(4): 577–83.

121. Bissler JJ, *et al*. Sirolimus for angiomyolipoma in tuberous sclerosis complex or lymphangioleiomyomatosis. N Engl J Med 2008; 358(2): 140–51.

122. Rini BI, Campbell SC, Zhou M. Malignant angiomyolipoma: a rare entity with unusual biology. Oncology 2011; 25: 840–841. [Comment on 'A rare case of metastatic renal epithelioid angiomyolipoma'. Lam ET, *et al*. Oncology 2011; 25(9): 832–8.]

123. Krishnan BT, *et al*. Horseshoe kidney is associated with an increased relative risk of primary renal carcinoid tumor. Clin Urol 1997; 157: 2059–66.

124. Begin LR, *et al*. Renal carcinoid and horseshoe kidney: a frequent association of two rare entities – a case report and review of the literature. J Surg Oncol 1998; 68(2): 113–19.

125. Resnick ME, Unterberger H, McLoughlin PT. Renal carcinoid producing the carcinoid syndrome. Med Times 1966; 94(8): 895–6.

126. Raslan WF, *et al*. Primary carcinoid of the kidney. Immunohistochemical and ultrastructural studies of five patients. Cancer 1993; 72(9): 2660–6.

127. Moulopoulos A, *et al*. Primary renal carcinoid: computed tomography, ultrasound, and angiographic findings. J Comput Assist Tomogr 1991; 15(2): 323–5.

128. McCaffrey JA, *et al*. Carcinoid tumor of the kidney. The use of somatostatin receptor scintigraphy in diagnosis and management. Urol Oncol 2000; 5(3): 108–11.

129. Lamberts SW, *et al*. Somatostatin-receptor imaging in the localization of endocrine tumors. N Engl J Med 1990; 323(18): 1246–9.

130. Kawajiri H, *et al*. Carcinoid tumor of the kidney presenting as a large abdominal mass: report of a case. *Surg Today* 2004; 34: 86–9.

131. Romero FR, *et al*. Primary carcinoid tumors of the kidney. *J Urol* 2006; 176: 2359–66.

132. Konard M, *et al*. Primary renal carcinoid tumour with inferior vena caval tumour. Thrombus Can Urol Assoc J 2009; 3(3): E7–E9.

133. Kulke MH, Mayer RJ. Carcinoid tumors. N Engl J Med 1999; 340(11): 858–68.

134. Oberg K, Eriksson B. The role of interferons in the management of carcinoid tumors. Acta Oncol 1991; 30(4): 519–22.

135. Moertel CG, Hanley JA. Combination chemotherapy trials in metastatic carcinoid tumor and the malignant carcinoid syndrome. Cancer Clin Trials 1979; 2(4): 327–34.

136. Chan H, Grossman AB, Bukowski RM. Everolimus in the treatment of renal cell carcinoma and neuroendocrine tumors. Adv Ther 2010; 27(8): 495–511.

137. Yao JC, *et al*. Efficacy of RAD001 (everolimus) and octreotide LAR in advanced low- to intermediate-grade neuroendocrine tumors: results of a phase II study. J Clin Oncol 2008; 26: 4311–18.

138. Stallone G, *et al*. Primary renal lymphoma does exist: case report and review of the literature. J Nephrol 2000; 13(5): 367–72.

139. Da'as N, *et al*. Kidney involvement and renal manifestations in non-Hodgkin's lymphoma and lymphocytic leukemia: a retrospective study in 700 patients. Eur J Haematol 2001; 67(3): 158–64.

140. Richmond J, *et al*. Renal lesions associated with malignant lymphomas. Am J Med 1962; 32: 184–207.

141. Pollack HM, Banner MP, Amendola MA. Other malignant neoplasms of the renal parenchyma. Semin Roentgenol 1987; 22: 260–74.

142. McVary KT. Lymphoproliferative disease and the genitourinary tract. AUA Update Series 1991; 10: 170–7.

143. Choi JH, *et al*. Bilateral primary renal non-Hodgkin's lymphoma presenting with acute renal failure: successful treatment with systemic chemotherapy. Acta Haematol 1997; 97: 231–5.

144. O'Riordan E, *et al*. Primary bilateral T-cell renal lymphoma presenting with sudden loss of renal function. Nephrol Dial Transplant 2001; 16: 1487–9.

145. Urban BA, Fishman EK. Renal lymphoma: CT patterns with emphasis on helical CT. Radiographics 2000; 20(1): 197–212.

146. Sheeran SR, Sussman SK. Renal lymphoma: spectrum of CT findings and potential mimics. Am J Roentgenol 1998; 171: 1067–72.

147. Jafri SZH, *et al*. CT of renal and perirenal non-Hodgkin lymphoma. Am J Roentgenol 1982; 138: 1101–5.

148. Dimopoulos MA, *et al*. Primary renal lymphoma: a clinical and radiological study. J Urol 1996; 155(6): 1865–7.

149. Yasunaga Y, *et al*. Malignant lymphoma of the kidney. J Surg Oncol 1997; 64(3): 207–11.

150. Okuno SH, et al. Primary renal non-Hodgkin's lymphoma. An unusual extranodal site. Cancer 1995; 75(9): 2258–61.

151. Oertel S, et al. Effect of anti-CD 20 antibody rituximab in patients with post-transplant lymphoproliferative disorder (PTLD). Am J Transplant 2005; 5: 2901–6.

152. Farrow GM, et al. Sarcomas and sarcomatoid and mixed malignant tumors of the kidney in adults. I. Cancer 1968; 22(3): 545–50.

153. Srinivas V, et al. Sarcomas of the kidney. J Urol 1984; 132(1): 13–16.

154. Vogelzang NJ, et al. Primary renal sarcoma in adults. A natural history and management study by the American Cancer Society, Illinois Division. Cancer 1993; 71(3): 804–10.

155. Russo P. Adult genitourinary sarcoma. AUA Update Series 1991; 10: 234–9.

156. Russo P, et al. Adult urological sarcoma. J Urol 1992; 147: 1032–7.

157. Tomera KM, Farrow GM, Lieber MM. Sarcomatoid renal carcinoma. J Urol 1983; 130(4): 657–9.

158. Grignon DJ, et al. Primary sarcomas of the kidney. A clinicopathologic and DNA flow cytometric study of 17 cases. Cancer 1990; 65(7): 1611–18.

159. Argani P, et al. Primary renal synovial sarcoma: molecular and morphologic delineation of an entity previously included among embryonal sarcomas of the kidney. Am J Surg Pathol 2000; 24(8): 1087–96.

160. Ladanyi M, et al. Impact of SYT-SSX fusion type on the clinical behavior of synovial sarcoma: a multi-institutional retrospective study of 243 patients. Cancer Res 2002; 62(1): 135–40.

161. Moudouni SM, et al. Leiomyosarcoma of the renal pelvis. Scand J Urol Nephrol 2001; 35: 425–7.

162. Deyrup AT, Montogomery E, Fisher C. Leiomyosarcoma of the kidney: a clinicopathologic study. Am J Surg Pathol 2004; 28: 178–82.

163. Frank I, Takahashi S, Tsukamoto T, Lieber MM. Genitourinary sarcomas and carcinosarcomas in adults. In: Vogelzang NJ (ed) Comprehensive Textbook of Genitourinary Oncology, 2nd edn. Philadelphia: Lippincott Williams and Wilkins, 2000. pp.1102–19.

164. Micolonghi TS, Liang D, Schwartz S. Primary osteogenic sarcoma of the kidney. J Urol 1984; 133: 1164–6.

165. Leventis AK, et al. Primary osteogenic sarcoma of the kidney – a case report and review of the literature. Acta Oncol 1997; 36: 747–77.

166. Economou JS, Lindner A, deKernion JB. Sarcomas of the genitourinary tract. In: Eilber FR, et al. (eds) The Soft Tissue Sarcomas. Orlando: Grune and Stratton, 1987. p.219.

167. Spellman JE Jr, Driscoll DL, Huben RP. Primary renal sarcoma. Am Surg 1995; 61(5): 456–9.

168. Saitoh H, et al. Metastasis of renal sarcoma. Tokai J Exp Clin Med 1982; 7: 365–9.

169. Shirkhoda A, Lewis E. Renal sarcoma and sarcomatoid renal cell carcinoma: CT and angiographic features. Radiology 1987; 162: 353–7.

170. Smullens SN, Scotti D, Osterholm J, Weiss A. Preoperative embolization of retroperitoneal hemangiopericytomas as an aid in their removal. Cancer 1982; 50: 1870–7.

171. Karakousis CP, et al. Surgery for disseminated abdominal sarcoma. Am J Surg 1992; 163(6): 560–4.

172. Karakousis CP, Gerstenbluth R, Kontzoglou K, Driscoll D. Retroperitoneal sarcomas and their management. Arch Surg 1995; 130: 1104–9.

173. Bove KE, Bhathena D, Wyatt RJ, Lucas BA, Holland NH. Diffuse metanephric adenoma after in utero aspirin intoxication. A unique case of progressive renal failure. Arch Pathol Lab Med 1979; 103: 187–90.

174. Pages A, Granier M. Nephronogenic nephroma (author's transl). Arch Anat Cytol Pathol 1980; 28(2): 99–103.

175. Argani P. Metanephric neoplasms: the hyperdifferentiated, benign end of the Wilms tumor spectrum? Clin Lab Med 2005; 25(2): 379–92.

176. Davis CJ Jr, et al. Metanephric adenoma. Clinicopathological study of fifty patients. Am J Surg Pathol 1995; 19(10): 1101–14.

177. Jones EC, et al. Metanephric adenoma of the kidney. A clinicopathological, immunohistochemical, flow cytometric, cytogenetic, and electron microscopic study of seven cases. Am J Surg Pathol 1995; 19(6): 615–26.

178. Grignon DJ, Eble JN. Papillary and metanephric adenomas of the kidney. Semin Diagn Pathol 1998; 15(1): 41–53.

179. Pins MR, et al. Metanephric adenoma-like tumors of the kidney: report of 3 malignancies with emphasis on discriminating features. Arch Pathol Lab Med 1999; 123(5): 415–20.

180. Renshaw AA, Freyer DR, Hammers YA. Metastatic metanephric adenoma in a child. Am J Surg Pathol 2000; 24(4): 570–4.

181. Hartman DJ, Maclennan GT. Renal metanephric adenoma. J Urol 2007; 178: 1058.

182. Kuroda N, Tol M, Hiroi M, Enzan H. Review of metanephric adenoma of the kidney with focus on clinical and pathobiological aspects. Histol Histopathol 2003; 18 : 253–7.

183. Hennigar RA, Beckwith JB. Nephrogenic adenofibroma. A novel kidney tumor of young people. Am J Surg Pathol 1992; 16(4): 325–34.

184. Arroyo MR, et al. The spectrum of metanephric adenofibroma and related lesions: clinicopathologic study of 25 cases from the National Wilms Tumor Study Group Pathology Center. Am J Surg Pathol 2001; 25(4): 433–44.

185. Netto JMB, et al. Metanephric adenoma: a rare differential diagnosis of renal tumor in children. J Ped Urol 2007; 3: 340–1.

186. Amodio JB, et al. Metanephric adenoma in an 8-year-old child: case report and review of the literature. J Ped Surg 2005; 40: E25–8.

187. Comerci SC, et al. Benign adenomatous kidney neoplasms in children with polycythemia: imaging findings. Radiology 1996; 198: 265–8.

188. Yoshioka K, et al. Production of erythropoietin and multiple cytokines by metanephric adenoma results in erythrocytosis. Pathol Int 2007; 57: 529–36.

189. Khayyata S, Grignon DJ, Aulicino MR, Al-Abbadi MA. Metanephric adenoma vs. Wilms' tumor: a report of 2 cases with diagnosis by fine needle aspiration and cytologic comparisons. Acta Cytol 2007; 51: 464–7.

190. Bosco M, Galliano D, La Saponara F, Pacchioni D, Bussolati G. Cytologic features of metanephric adenoma of the kidney during pregnancy: a case report. Acta Cytol 2007; 51: 468–72.

191. Fielding JR, Visweswaran A, Silverman SG, Granter SR, Renshaw AA. CT and ultrasound features of metanephric adenoma in adults with pathologic correlation. J Comput Assist Tomogr 1999; 23: 441–4.

192. Granter SR, Fletcher JA, Renshaw AA. Cytologic and cytogenetic analysis of metanephric adenoma of the kidney: a report of two cases. Am J Clin Pathol 1997; 108: 544–9.

193. Kosugi M, Nagata H, Nakashima J, Murai M, Hata J. A case of metanephric adenoma treated with partial nephrectomy. Nippon Hinyokika Gakkai Zasshi 2000; 91: 489–92.

194. Hwang SS, Choi YJ. Metanephric adenoma of the kidney: case report. Abdom Imaging 2004; 29(3): 309–11.

195. Breslow N, et al. Age distribution of Wilms' tumor: report from the National Wilms' Tumor Study. Cancer Res 1988; 48(6): 1653–7.

196. Petruzzi MaG D. Adult Wilms tumor. In: Raghavan D, Brecher M, Johnson D, et al. (eds) Textbook of Uncommon Cancer, 2nd edn. Chichester: John Wiley & Sons, 1999.

197. Bozeman G, et al. Adult Wilms' tumor: prognostic and management considerations. Urology 1995; 45(6): 1055–8.

198. Kilton L, Matthews MJ, Cohen MH. Adult Wilms tumor: a report of prolonged survival and review of literature. J Urol 1980; 124(1): 1–5.

199. Huser J, et al. Adult Wilms' tumor: a clinicopathologic study of 11 cases. Mod Pathol 1990; 3(3): 321–6.

200. Khoury JD. Nephroblastic neoplasms. Clin Lab Med 2005; 25(2): 341–61.

201. Karlsson J, et al. High-resolution genomic profiling of an adult Wilms' tumor: evidence for a pathogenesis distinct from corresponding pediatric tumors. Virchows Arch 2011; 459(5): 547–53.

202. Byrd RL, Evans AE, D'Angio GJ. Adult Wilms tumor: effect of combined therapy on survival. J Urol 1982; 127(4): 648–51.

203. Arrigo S, et al. Better survival after combined modality care for adults with Wilms' tumor. A report from the National Wilms' Tumor Study. Cancer 1990; 66(5): 827–30.

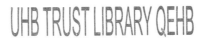

204. Kattan J, *et al*. Adult Wilms' tumour: review of 22 cases. Eur J Cancer 1994; 30A(12): 1778–82.

205. Reinhard H, *et al*. Wilms' tumor in adults: results of the Society of Pediatric Oncology (SIOP) 93–01/Society for Pediatric Oncology and Hematology (GPOH) Study. J Clin Oncol 2004; 22(22): 4500–6.

206. Winter P, *et al*. Wilms' tumor in adults: review of 10 cases. Int Urol Nephrol 1996; 28: 469–75.

207. Orditura M, DeVita F, Catalano G. Adult Wilms' tumor: a case report. Cancer 1997; 15: 1961–5.

208. Terenziani M, *et al*. Adult Wilms' tumor: a monoinstitutional experience and a review of the literature. Cancer 2004; 101(2): 289–93.

209. Akmansu M, Yapici T, Tulay E. Adult Wilms' tumor: a report of two cases and their treatment and prognosis. Int Urol Nephrol 1998; 30: 529–33.

210. Ali A, *et al*. Surveillance, Epidemiology and End Results (SEER) program comparison of adult and pediatric Wilms' tumor. Cancer 2011 Sep 14. doi: 10.1002/cncr.26554 [Epub ahead of print].

211. Abu-Ghosh AM, *et al*. Ifosfamide, carboplatin and etoposide in children with poor-risk relapsed Wilms' tumor: a Children's Cancer Group report. Ann Oncol 2002; 13(3): 460–9.

212. Pein F, *et al*. High-dose melphalan, etoposide, and carboplatin followed by autologous stem-cell rescue in pediatric high-risk recurrent Wilms' tumor: a French Society of Pediatric Oncology study. J Clin Oncol 1998; 16(10): 3295–301.

213. Firoozi F, Kogan BA. Follow-up and management of recurrent Wilms'tumor. Urol Clin North Am 2003; 30: 869–79.

214. Segers H, *et al*., for the SIOP-RTSG and COG Renal Tumour Committee. Management of adults with Wilms' tumor: recommendations based on international consensus. Expert Rev Anticancer Ther 2011; 11(7): 1105–13.

215. Kalapurakal JA, *et al*. Management of Wilms' tumour: current practice and future goals. Lancet Oncol 2004; 5(1): 37–46.

2 Uncommon Cancers of the Bladder

Arlene O. Siefker-Radtke,[1] Bogdan A. Czerniak,[2] Colin P. Dinney,[3] and Randall E. Millikan[1]

[1] Department of Genitourinary Medical Oncology, [2] Department of Anatomic Pathology, [3] Department of Urology, The University of Texas, MD Anderson Cancer Center, Houston, TX, USA

Introduction

The uncommonly encountered tumors arising in the bladder fall naturally into two groups: unusual histologies of urothelial origin and nonurothelial malignancies. While definitive recommendations on the treatment of these variants remain limited, recognition of these variants may have implications regarding the type and timing of chemotherapy, and an impact on surgical planning. Following these lines, we take up the unusual urothelial cancers first, as these are by far the most common and the most clinically important.

About 80% of what is called urothelial carcinoma is of low histological grade, reflecting a primarily hyperplastic process with grossly papillary architecture forming a mass of proliferating but noninvasive cells. Designated "Ta," these lesions tend to recur, and can progress to dysplasia and invasion in 15–20% of patients. However, these neoplasms are, for the most part, more like polyps than true carcinomas. The remaining 20% of urothelial cancer cases display a distinct but often overlapping pattern, with the hallmarks of dysplasia, high histological grade, and invasion.[1] These "nonpapillary" cancers are the source of most of the mortality, and they demonstrate a significant spectrum of histomorphology. At the extreme, they are so unlike transitional cell carcinoma (TCC) that alternative taxonomy is called for. Although quite rare as "pure" variants, it is nevertheless true that about one-third of nonpapillary bladder cancers will exhibit at least focal areas of one of the unusual histologies discussed below. While pure squamous bladder tumors have been classified separately from the more typical urothelial tumors on the basis of gene expression profiling, only a minority of tumors with squamous differentiation were classified with the squamous type.[2] Thus, as a practical matter, there is significant uncertainty about which cases showing minor amounts of variant histology should be considered within the usual spectrum of TCC, and which should be classified as distinct entities.

Diagnosis

The diagnosis of these variant histologies is typically made upon tissue collection at transurethral resection. One exception is in the setting of urachal tumors, in which a midline cystic mass on radiographic imaging is considered pathognomonic for the diagnosis, and should be considered an urachal cancer unless proven otherwise.[3] Pure adenocarcinomas of the bladder are quite rare, and one should always consider the possibility of a metastasis to the bladder with a search for alternate sites based upon clinical suspicion. Radiographic imaging with computed tomography (CT) or magnetic resonance imaging (MRI) of the abdomen and pelvis, and a chest x-ray or CT will help determine the presence of an alternate primary site, and more distant metastases. The utility of positron emission tomography (PET) imaging has been limited by the accumulation of radionuclide in the urine, which may obscure localized disease, or multifocal tumors involving the upper tract and/or bladder. The absence of metastatic disease on PET imaging of small cell urothelial tumors should not lead to the decision to proceed with initial surgery, as PET imaging is unable to detect early microscopic metastases characteristic of small cell tumors. Imaging of the brain may be considered for patients with small cell urothelial cancer, especially for those with stage III or greater disease where the incidence of metastases has been reported to be as high as 50%, or in patients with neurological symptoms.[4]

Sarcomatoid carcinoma of the bladder

Advanced urothelial cancer is generally characterized by more aggressive biological behavior accompanied by phenotypic evolution to patterns that are readily recognized to reflect this more aggressive biology. In this setting, the recognition of areas with spindled histomorphology is fairly common. These biphasic neoplasms with mesenchymal

Textbook of Uncommon Cancer, Fourth Edition. Edited by Derek Raghavan, Charles D. Blanke, David H. Johnson, Paul L. Moots, Gregory H. Reaman, Peter G. Rose and Mikkael A. Sekeres.

spindle cell components seen in combination with epithelial histology are typically described as sarcomatoid carcinomas. When epithelial markers are lost in a significant fraction of tumor cells, the term *carcinosarcoma* is appropriate, but the literature makes no systematic distinction between these two terms. Such cases have been long recognized, and many case series and reviews are available.[5–7] There continue to be several sporadic case reports each year. The typical histological appearance is shown in Figure 2.1.

Almost always, nonspindled areas recognizable as high-grade TCC are also present, suggesting that this pattern results from evolution from a common progenitor. By immunohistochemistry, the spindled areas are generally positive for keratin, epithelial membrane antigen, and vimentin. Analysis of clonality based on loss of heterozygosity (LOH) of microsatellite markers[8,9] and X chromosome inactivation[10] provides strong evidence that although the various components can and do evolve independently once they diverge, they do in fact arise

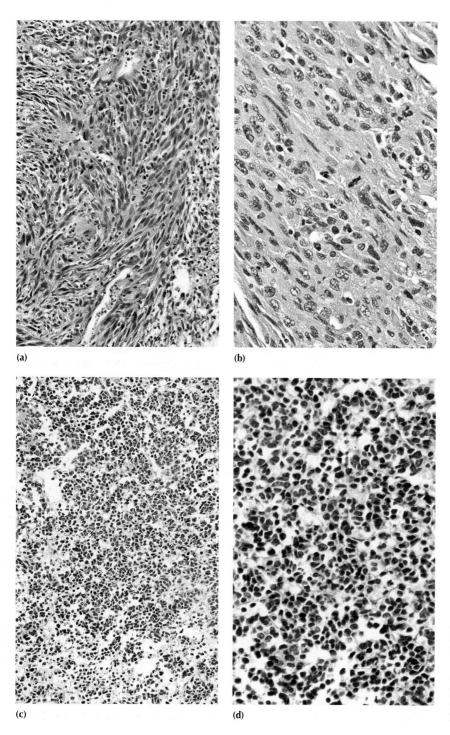

(a)

(b)

(c)

(d)

Figure 2.1 Microscopic features of high-grade urothelial carcinomas with sarcomatoid and small cell phenotype. (a,b) Low- and high-power views of sarcomatoid urothelial carcinoma composed of atypical spindle cells. (c,d) Low- and high-power views of small cell variant of urothelial carcinoma. Note poorly differentiated small cells with inconspicuous cytoplasm and densely packed, hyperchromatic nuclei.

from a common precursor. Emerging evidence implicates the presence of urothelial cancer stem cells in the development of heterogeneous urothelial cancers with mesenchymal phenotype, and that epithelial-to-mesenchymal transition (EMT) may be responsible for sarcomatoid transformation in urothelial cancer.[11]

While it is clear that we can define a subset with a sarcomatoid appearance, it is more important to know what biological significance such morphology portends. Although there do not seem to be particular risk factors, or clinically distinctive features at initial presentation, a recurring theme in the clinical experience with sarcomatoid urothelial cancer is that it has an aggressive natural history and poor outcome relative to that of classic TCC. This is borne out in the MD Anderson registry and in the SEERS database,[12] in both the locally advanced and metastatic settings. In view of this, we consider the presence of a sarcomatoid component in an otherwise minimally invasive bladder cancer to be a strong indication for early cystectomy. We know of no data to recommend any particular therapeutic approach to systemic therapy. Even though we have investigated more intensive chemotherapy in this subset and have seen responses and downstaging with neoadjuvant chemotherapy,[13] we do not have any sense that this is justified by improved outcome, and do not endorse this approach in the absence of a clinical trial.

It is very important to realize that not everything that appears spindled is dangerous.[14] In particular, the postresection sarcomatous nodule and inflammatory pseudotumor must not be confused with the aggressive cancers to which they bear some resemblance. Besides the clinical context, it is reported that the presence of necrosis at the muscle interface and nuclear atypia are the most useful features that distinguish true sarcomas or sarcomatoid carcinomas from these benign conditions.

Although they are extremely uncommon, true sarcomas without an epithelial component do arise in the bladder, and they are taken up in the section on "Sarcoma" below.

Small cell urothelial carcinoma

Like spindled morphology, histological features reminiscent of neuroendocrine carcinomas are commonly encountered in patients with high-grade TCC, especially as it evolves over time. LOH studies of coexisting small cell and TCC suggest descent from a common precursor,[15] just as has been shown for sarcomatoid carcinoma. At present, there is no consensus about the exact diagnostic criteria for declaring a "small cell" or "neuroendocrine" subset. Some authorities place more emphasis on the histomorphology and some on the expression of neuroendocrine markers. At MD Anderson, it has been our sense that the morphology is more predictive of clinical course than any particular pattern of immunohistochemical markers, and thus we continue to prefer the term "small cell carcinoma" and do not require immunohistochemical "confirmation" in order to apply the term. The typical appearance is shown in Figure 2.1.

One occasionally encounters patients with small cell carcinoma found in the prostate and it is not clear if this should be interpreted as being urothelial or prostatic in origin. Unless markedly elevated, prostate-specific antigen (PSA) may not be helpful as elevated levels can be observed when urothelial tumors invade the prostate. Generally, there will be either urothelial dysplasia in the prostatic urethra (favoring an urothelial origin), or signs of dysplasia in the prostatic acini (favoring a prostatic origin). In truth, the distinction matters little, as the foundation of therapy for either primary site is early exposure to systemic chemotherapy with a regimen directed toward the small cell phenotype, followed by local consolidation with either surgery or radiation. Given the frequent presence of other variant histology including sarcomatoid carcinoma, and the presence of carcinoma *in situ* (CIS) which has been reported in up to 76% of patients,[4,16] we would strongly advocate for surgery as the best method for achieving long-term control.

Like its counterpart in the lung, small cell cancer of the bladder is an aggressive, rapidly proliferative tumor characterized by the early development of micrometastases, even in the setting of clinically localized disease. Indeed, it is not uncommon to see patients with very large tumors that had been "completely resected" just 2–3 weeks previously. When small cell is present, it is imperative to efficiently evaluate and stage the patient, and avoid any delays so that chemotherapy can begin quickly, hopefully before metastases become evident on radiographic imaging. In addition to radiographic imaging of the chest, abdomen, and pelvis, a baseline CT or MRI of the brain is recommended in patients with stage III or greater small cell urothelial cancer. A thorough transurethral resection of tumor followed by an exam under anesthesia can help determine the presence of extraorgan extension.

It has long been recognized that cystectomy alone produces markedly inferior results compared to those seen with conventional TCC. Clinical understaging has been the rule, with up to 76% of patients with small cell tumors having metastases at cystectomy.[16] In a recent review of the MD Anderson experience, we found the pathological stage was higher than expected in 56% of patients treated with initial cystectomy.[17] Furthermore, 20% of patients for whom initial cystectomy was planned were found to be surgically unresectable in the operating room, despite a median time from diagnosis to surgery of 24 days.

In view of this experience, many institutions have reported multimodality approaches incorporating systemic therapy with radiation and/or surgery. In a literature review from 1995, Abbas reported that the best disease-free survival was observed when cystectomy was followed by adjuvant chemotherapy, with a median survival of 21.1 months.[18] Of the 19 patients reported by Grignon,[19] four of the five survivors were treated with adjuvant chemotherapy following their cystectomy. Likewise, the University of Southern California Norris Cancer Center reported an improved overall and recurrence-free survival among patients receiving multimodality therapy, the majority of whom received adjuvant chemotherapy.[16] However, the median survival in these patients was only 13 months, with a 5-year survival of 10%.

Neoadjuvant chemotherapy has shown more promising results. Walther[20] reported that 5/7 patients were alive and free of disease at more than 36 months after combined modality treatment; in fact, the five who were alive were treated with preoperative chemotherapy. A retrospective analysis of our own experience in 46 patients who were both candidates for surgery and who had surgically resectable disease found a statistically improved survival for those treated with preoperative chemotherapy.[17] Patients treated with initial cystectomy had median cancer-specific survival (CSS) of 23 months, and a 36% CSS at 5 years. By contrast, for those treated with preoperative chemotherapy, the median CSS has not been reached, and the 5-year CSS was 78%. There were only four cancer-related deaths among the 21 patients treated with initial chemotherapy, and none in the subset "downstaged" to pT2N0M0 or less. It is interesting to note that 7/25 patients treated with initial cystectomy received adjuvant chemotherapy; however, their survival was no better than those treated with cystectomy alone.

As a result of this experience, investigators at the MD Anderson Cancer Center (MDACC) recently completed the first prospective clinical trial in patients with small cell urothelial cancer.[4] Eighteen patients with surgically resectable small cell urothelial cancer (cT2N0M0-cT4aN0M0) were treated with four cycles of neoadjuvant chemotherapy, alternating between ifosfamide with doxorubicin, and etoposide with cisplatin. Pathological downstaging to < pT1N0M0 occurred in 78% of patients, and 72% remain alive and cancer free with a median overall survival of 58 months (Fig. 2.2). The majority of patients with cT3b-4aN0M0 tumors still had viable small cell tumor remaining at surgery, and did more poorly than their lower staged counterparts. It is not yet known whether more cycles of neoadjuvant chemotherapy would affect the outcome in these higher stage patients, or if the outcome is related to adverse biology from higher volume micrometastases.

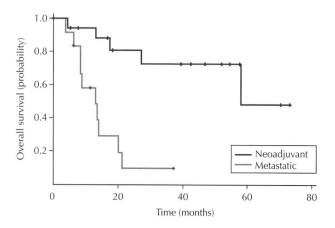

Figure 2.2 Cause-specific survival of patients with resectable and metastatic small cell carcinoma. Kaplan–Meier overall survival (OS) results from a phase 2 clinical trial in small cell urothelial cancer. On the neoadjuvant arm, the median OS time was 58 months (95% confidence interval (CI), 58 months to not achieved (NA)). On the metastatic arm, the median OS time was 13.3 months (95% CI, 8.5 months to NA). Reproduced with permission from Siefker-Radtke A, *et al.*[4] © 2008 American Society of Clinical Oncology. All rights reserved.

Given these results, we take the view that all surgically resectable patients with a small cell component should be treated primarily (and without delay) with four cycles of neoadjuvant chemotherapy incorporating etoposide and cisplatin for those with cT2N0M0 cancer, and two cycles beyond maximal response (usually closer to six cycles) in patients with higher stage, surgically resectable disease. Following chemotherapy, we favor surgical consolidation as the best method for achieving long-term tumor control. This is based on the following observations: most of these patients have widespread dysplasia and CIS, and they often show glandular elements after chemotherapy. Thus, we infer that a significant fraction of patients will not have good long-term control in the bladder by means of radiotherapy. Limited data from radiotherapy retrospective series suggest this is in fact the case, with one series suggesting a lack of long-term control in 60% of patients receiving radiation, with some relapsing in the irradiated field.[21,22]

Unfortunately, given the rapid progression and early metastatic potential of small cell bladder cancer, many patients have metastatic or surgically unresectable disease at presentation. The most frequently reported sites are lymph nodes, liver, bone, lung, and brain.[17,23] With chemotherapy, median survival ranges from 7.5 months to 15 months.[4,17,18] While there are few long-term survivors, a few have been reported in patients undergoing surgical consolidation of initially node-positive disease.[4] Despite the disappointing long-term outcome, small cell urothelial tumors are highly responsive to systemic chemotherapy, and most patients experience marked objective response that is associated with gratifying, albeit temporary, palliation of symptoms.

Unlike the frequency noted in small cell tumors of the lung, brain metastases have only been rarely reported in small cell urothelial cancer. However, when patients were managed on clinical trial, a 50% incidence of brain metastases was noted in patients with stage III or greater small cell urothelial cancer; none were seen in those with lower stage disease.[4] Routine imaging of the brain was not performed on this trial, but was considered only on the basis of clinical suspicion, such as focal neurological findings or unexplained nausea. While it is certainly possible that the close monitoring of patients on clinical trial could account for this finding, an alternative explanation is that use of a small cell-directed chemotherapy regimen may lead to better systemic control in other metastatic sites, allowing the time for clinically evident brain metastases to present. Over 75% of these patients had no progressive tumor elsewhere, suggesting that the issue of prophylactic cranial irradiation will become more relevant in the setting of more effective chemotherapy. Our current recommendations are to consider and discuss prophylactic cranial irradiation with patients with stage III or greater small cell urothelial cancer.

Micropapillary bladder cancer

The histomorphological spectrum of many epithelial cancers is now recognized to include a subset characterized by clusters of high-grade cells nesting in lacunar spaces that have a "micropapillary" architecture. This pattern was first reported in 1982 by Hendrickson *et al.* who described an aggressive variant of endometrial adenocarcinoma with an infiltrative, biologically aggressive pattern of spread, strikingly reminiscent of the behavior of papillary serous carcinoma of the ovary.[24] Subsequently, a micropapillary variant has been recognized in cancers arising from the breast, bladder, thyroid, lung and pancreas, and has thus come to be seen as a general feature of epithelial cancer. It seems likely that this phenotype derives from some fundamental aspect of epithelial carcinogenesis, and the finding of a recognizable "gene signature" that cuts across these different sites would not be surprising.

Investigators from MD Anderson were the first to report a subset of bladder cancers showing such a micropapillary histomorphology, publishing the initial series of 18 patients in 1994.[25] As discussed in the context of sarcomatoid and small cell morphology, it is typical to appreciate a micropapillary component in a context that includes more typical TCC. From this initial series of patients, the micropapillary variant was noted to have a more aggressive clinical course and a particular tendency for prominent lymphovascular invasion. Subsequent case series from around the globe,[26–30] along with many individual case reports, established that micropapillary bladder cancer does have a characteristic morphology (Fig. 2.3) that can be reliably identified. Furthermore, the initially reported propensity for clinical understaging, aggressive behavior and relatively poor response to standard systemic chemotherapy has been fully confirmed.

Ultrastructural studies in the setting of micropapillary breast cancer suggested secretory granules along the basal membrane, where normal cell polarity is lost with secretory activity present at the basal surface, not just at the apical surface.[31] This concept of "inside out" morphology has been reinforced by the demonstration that the mucinous glycoprotein product of the *MUC1* gene is also abnormally localized to the basal surface of micropapillary cancers,[32] including those of bladder origin. Although not yet formally established, it seems likely that a mechanistic connection will be made between this sort of abnormal phenotype and the early submucosal infiltration with early access to lymphatics that characterize the clinical course of these cancers. In our experience, the unusual finding of a bladder cancer that is stage pT1N1 is extremely frequently associated with micropapillary histology.

The clinical management of micropapillary bladder cancer should take into account the very real possibility that it will be clinically understaged and can grow rapidly. Thus, we advocate "early" cystectomy for any tumor that invades the lamina propria, and would certainly urge that any patient with cT1 disease or greater after a trial of intravesical therapy be guided to cystectomy without delay. In one small series of nonmuscle-invasive patients, 67% of patients treated with intravesical bacillus Calmette-Guérin (BCG) progressed to muscle-invasive cancer, with metastases developing in 22% of patients despite close monitoring at an academic institution.[33]

For patients with locally advanced disease, the prognosis is worse than for patients with conventional TCC. In the MD Anderson experience, patients with cT3b or cT4a disease

treated with a combination of systemic chemotherapy and surgery (in any sequence) had an inferior overall cure rate compared to patients with conventional TCC.[34] In the metastatic setting, both the response rate and overall survival of patients with micropapillary cancer are below historical expectation in our hands. Despite aggressive application of combination chemotherapy, patients with micropapillary cancers continue to have a relatively poor outcome. This has been true with methotrexate/vinblastine/doxorubicin/cisplatin (MVAC), with ifosfamide-based combinations,[35] and gemcitabine/cisplatin. It is important to recognize that although the aggregate results are inferior to those obtained for patients with conventional TCC, there are many patients who do well, and thus we continue to offer conventional therapy to patients in this subset.

Adenocarcinoma

Glandular metaplasia is fairly common within the urothelium, and the appearance of cystitis glandularis and cystitis cystica is a familiar consequence of chronic infection, inflammation or irritation as occurs with urolithiasis. In the transformed state, focal areas of glandular differentiation are reasonably common in invasive, nonpapillary TCC. To our knowledge, such focal areas of glandular differentiation do not have any clinical significance with respect to the natural history or response to commonly used systemic agents. Furthermore, it is not unusual to see a remnant of glandular differentiation in a cystectomy specimen following neoadjuvant chemotherapy for a high-grade, nonpapillary TCC, even if no adenocarcinomatous element was appreciated prior to therapy. These relatively common clinical scenarios highlight the morphological repertoire of urothelial histology, and illustrate the difficulty of defining precisely what is meant by "adenocarcinoma of the bladder." In this section, we confine our discussion to cancers that exhibit histology with an adenocarcinoma as the dominant pattern, and without recognizable TCC.

There are many variations of adenocarcinoma encountered within the bladder (see Fig. 2.3). Most authors (including the World Health Organization classification of bladder tumors)[36] include mucinous, signet ring, enteric-type, hepatoid and clear cell (formerly "mesonephric") as recognizable subsets. In addition, an adenoid cystic pattern can also be seen, particularly in the context of transformation of preexisting cystitis cystica. Tumors showing mixtures of these patterns are the rule.[37] Enteric-type histology is especially encountered among cancers arising in an urachal remnant, and these are taken up in a separate section below. Nonetheless, villous adenoma[38] and enteric-type adenocarcinoma do rarely occur in the bladder proper. The immunophenotype of these cancers tends to overlap that seen in colon cancer,[38] and most produce carcinoembryonic antigen (CEA). The diagnostic dilemma for the pathologist is evident, since it could be important to distinguish a colon primary involving the bladder from a primary bladder tumor, and at present, this can only be done by excluding a colon primary by traditional clinical means.

Most adenocarcinomas arising in the bladder proper are of the mucinous or signet ring variety. The male:female ratio is at

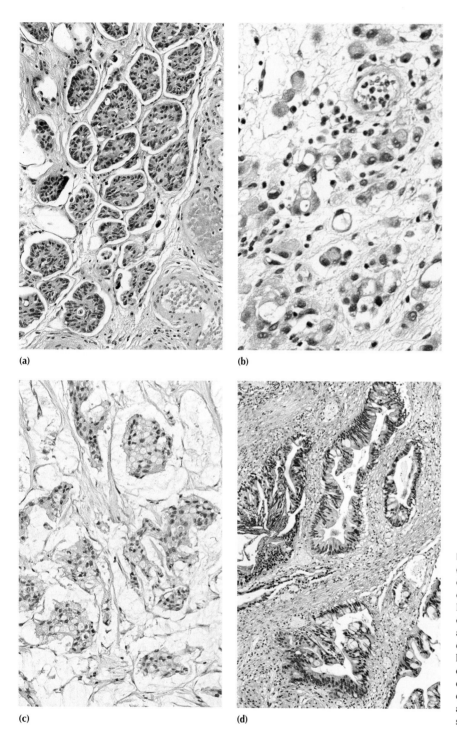

(a)

(b)

(c)

(d)

Figure 2.3 Microscopic features of rare forms of urothelial carcinoma. (a) Micropapillary variant of urothelial carcinoma composed of small nests of atypical epithelial cells arranged in distinct lacunar spaces. (b) Plasmacytoid and signet ring cell variant of urothelial carcinoma. Note loosely arranged oval cancer cells with distinct eosinophilic cytoplasm and eccentric nuclei. Some of the cells have a large mucin-containing cytoplasmic vacuole displacing the nucleus. (c) Mucinous adenocarcinoma composed of nests of cancer cells in lakes of extracellular mucin. (d) Colonic variant of bladder adenocarcinoma composed of large glandular structures with stratified nuclei.

least 2:1, and the age at onset is very similar to that seen in conventional TCC. Bladder exstrophy, a rare developmental anomaly affecting 1 in 50,000 births, is a well-established risk factor,[39] as are other nonphysiological states such as a urinary diversion leaving the bladder in place. Intestinal metaplasia long antedating the appearance of carcinoma is typical in these contexts. Adenocarcinomas also arise in the context of preexisting cystitis cystica (and glandularis), and sometimes in association with schistosomiasis, although squamous histology is more common in the latter context.

It is typical for mucinous adenocarcinomas to be diffusely infiltrative, and to present with irritative symptoms out of proportion to the cystoscopic findings. Cross-sectional imaging typically shows diffusely thickened vesical walls, and frank linitis plastica is well known, especially in the subset with predominantly signet ring histology. We have encountered patients not only with linitis plastica but also with involvement of the seminal vesicles, and even extension down both spermatic cords. Thus, while the cystoscopic appearance may be unimpressive, the examination under anesthesia is typically striking.

The clear cell variant of bladder adenocarcinoma is quite rare, and is also clinically distinct. These cancers usually arise in females (at least 2:1 female predominance), and the median age is younger. More than half of the reported cases appear to arise from the urethra or periurethral glands. They typically express CA-125, and there are other lines of evidence supporting an etiology from müllerian rests.[40] These cancers tend to be quite responsive to taxane-based therapy, such as is used for epithelial ovarian cancer.

The optimal clinical management of adenocarcinoma is of course not settled. Stage is the most important prognostic factor, and unfortunately most patients with adenocarcinoma present with locally advanced disease (cT3 or higher).[41] Thus, for many patients, neoadjuvant systemic therapy is a reasonable consideration, since the historical outcome for surgery only in this setting is poor. Most patients at our center are in fact treated with combination chemotherapy followed by radical surgery. We have seen responses with a variety of chemotherapy regimens in the neoadjuvant and metastatic setting, including those used in the treatment of traditional urothelial cancer, and 5-fluorouracil-based regimens. Nonetheless, the overall response rate is lower than is seen with conventional TCC, and survival exceeding 2 years is uncommon in those with metastases.

Squamous carcinoma

Predominantly squamous carcinoma of the bladder is most commonly encountered in the setting of schistosomiasis in the Middle East, a context which is outside the scope of this chapter since it has a distinct biology, natural history, and treatment as compared to nonbilharzial squamous tumors.

In the West, focal areas of squamous differentiation are commonly encountered among patients with invasive, non-papillary TCC. As is the case for focal glandular differentiation, we know of no clinical significance to this finding. By contrast, pure squamous carcinomas are uncommon, and they show a very distinctive clinical expression. The most common setting for (nonschistosomiasis related) squamous cancer is that of chronic irritation, typically either from urolithiasis (especially stag horn calculi) or from chronic indwelling catheters among patients with paraplegia or with neurogenic bladders from diseases such as multiple sclerosis. It is typical to see keratinizing squamous metaplasia, often with dysplasia, in areas adjacent to these cancers.[42]

Surgery is the mainstay of therapy for squamous cancers.[43] Local control is often a bigger problem than distant progression, in rather marked contrast to the situation with conventional TCC. Sensitivity to chemotherapy is universally reported to be lower for squamous cancers than for conventional TCC, which further reinforces the importance of primary surgical management. Unfortunately, when these cancers are recurrent or metastatic, the expectations of chemotherapy are limited. However, there are certainly patients who enjoy excellent responses, and thus it is difficult to assess the risk:benefit of a trial of chemotherapy. Interestingly, pulmonary metastases from squamous carcinoma of the bladder tend to cavitate

when responding to chemotherapy, behavior not typical of other histologies.

Our experience of trying to deliver chemotherapy in the special context of patients with paraplegia or other diseases causing neurogenic bladder is uniformly unsatisfying, and we cannot endorse use of conventional regimens such as MVAC in this setting. Regimens with some activity include cisplatin, gemcitabine, and ifosfamide (CGI),[43,44] and taxane-cisplatin combinations including taxol, methotrexate, cisplatin (TMP),[45] and ifosfamide, taxol, cisplatin (ITP).[46] Anecdotal experience in our group also suggests benefit with the addition of an epidermal growth factor receptor (EGFR) inhibitor such as cetuximab or panitumumab whenever possible.

Lymphoepithelioma

The descriptive term *lymphoepithelioma* was originally applied to a distinctive tumor occurring in the nasopharynx, composed of a poorly differentiated epithelial component showing syncytial features and a second component consisting of a prominent lymphoid stromal infiltration.[47] In the nasopharynx, these cancers were found to be associated with Epstein–Barr virus, but no such association has been found when this pattern is seen in the bladder.[48] These cancers were also found to be remarkably sensitive to radiotherapy. More recently, morphologically similar cancers have been reported from a great many sites, including thyroid, skin, cervix, lung, and gastrointestinal tract.

There do not seem to be any particularly distinctive features of the clinical presentation of patients with lymphoepithelioma. The clinical importance of recognizing this subset is first to be aware of the potential for misdiagnosing this entity as an extranodal lymphoma, and secondly, to recognize the significantly better prognosis enjoyed by those with this pattern as the predominant (or exclusive) histology. In several series,[49,50] including our own early experience,[47] these cancers have been noted to be more chemosensitive and more radiosensitive than conventional TCC, with many long-term survivors reported when treating "pure" lymphoepithelioma of the bladder with chemotherapy alone.[47,49]

Strikingly, however, patients with only "focal" expression of a lymphoepithelioma pattern have a poor prognosis.[47,49,50] When more typical urothelial histology is present, our current practice is to treat as a typical urothelial tumor, with surgery and neoadjuvant or adjuvant chemotherapy as determined by tumor stage. Only in those with a pure lymphoepithelioma would we recommend treatment with chemotherapy alone.

Plasmacytoid

Plasmacytoid tumors of the bladder derive their name from their morphological appearance of a small to medium-sized cell with an eccentric nucleus and abundant amphophilic to eosinophilic cytoplasm characteristically seen in plasma cells. The presence of cytokeratin markers and lack of staining for lymphoma markers, vimentin, and mucin production can aid in differentiating these tumors from plasmacytomas, lymphomas, signet ring cell tumors, and rhabodmyosarcomas.[51] CD138, a plasma cell marker, has been found to be positive in plasmacytoid urothelial tumors, and cannot be relied upon to reliably differentiate between these and plasmacytomas.[51-53]

Although fewer than 75 cases have been reported in the literature, plasmacytoid tumors are high grade and aggressive, typically presenting with higher stage disease.[52,53] Few long-term survivors have been reported when plasmacytoid was the predominant histology. This is borne out in the experience at MDACC, even in the setting of neoadjuvant chemotherapy. There is a marked predilection for this tumor to present or eventually metastasize to the peritoneum. A characteristic clinical picture is for patients to develop peritoneal carcinomatosis approximately 6 months after chemotherapy, even in cases downstaged to pT0N0 with neoadjuvant chemotherapy. Chemotherapy regimens used in the treatment of traditional urothelial cancer, including dose-dense MVAC, and gemcitabine with cisplatin, display activity in these tumors.

Urachal cancer

The urachus is a vestigial structure which, while important in some species, has no role in the development of humans. The precursor of the urachal ligament initially arises from the cloaca at the terminal end of the hindgut. During embryogenesis, the cloaca divides, forming the urogenital sinus, which develops into the bladder and sex organs, and the anorectal canal, which becomes the rectum. The bladder is formed from the medial portion of the urogenital sinus. Superior to this, the lumen of the allantois is obliterated to form the urachus. By adulthood, the urachus coalesces with the obliterated umbilical arteries to form the ligamentum commune. While the urachal ligament most frequently connects with the dome of the bladder, it can also attach to the posterior or anterior bladder wall, usually in the midline.[54] A remnant lumen may persist in the wall of the bladder as a tiny tubular or cystic structure, and can communicate with the lumen of the bladder in up to one-third of adults.[55,56] Columnar cells, glandular islands, and transitional cell epithelium may be present in such an urachal remnant.[57] When malignancy is found to arise in such a remnant, the histology is overwhelming enteric-type adenocarcinoma.

Two theories have been proposed for the development of urachal tumors. One is that these adenocarcinomas originate from enteric rests left behind from the cloaca during embryological development. This would explain the histological resemblance to adenocarcinomas of the rectum. An alternate hypothesis is that these tumors arise from metaplasia. Supportive evidence includes the occurrence of adenocarcinomas in exstrophic bladders despite transitional epithelium at birth, the occasional development of other enteric-type tumors in the ureter and renal pelvis which are not of cloacal origin, and the observation of adenocarcinoma arising from cystitis glandularis.

Whatever the details of their origin, it is clear that these cancers have a clinical expression that is quite distinct from typical urothelial cancer. No risk factors have been identified and in particular, smoking and other environmental factors which figure so prominently in typical TCC seem not to be relevant. Patients with urachal cancer are typically much younger, with a reported median age at diagnosis of 47–57 years, with many cases reported in the third and fourth decades.[58,59] In addition, these cancers occur equally in men and women (TCC is about 3:1 male to female), and they display markedly less susceptibility to cisplatin-based chemotherapy.

The majority of urachal tumors display enteric-type histology, resembling adenocarcinomas of the colon and rectum. These tumors often have glandular structures with mucin production; colloid and/or signet ring cell histology may be present. More rarely, sarcomatoid, squamous, and transitional cell histology have been reported.[57,59] Remnants of normal or focally ulcerative surface epithelium may overlie the tumor. Normal epithelium overlying the tumor strongly supports the diagnosis of urachal carcinoma. However, the destruction of this layer by tumor can make the distinction between urachal and nonurachal bladder adenocarcinoma difficult. The presence of cystitis cystica or cystitis glandularis transitioning to malignancy favors a diagnosis of an adenocarcinoma of the bladder proper, as opposed to an urachal origin.

Most patients have locally advanced disease at diagnosis, usually presenting with gross hematuria and irritative voiding symptoms, but often presenting with no urinary complaints at all. Patients may report voiding mucoid material, a feature consistent with the typical histology. Erythema and umbilical discharge have also been reported, and we have seen patients initially diagnosed with an "umbilical infection." The presence of a cystic midline mass with calcifications at the bladder dome on radiographic imaging is nearly pathognomonic (Fig. 2.4). As a practical matter, all patients with enteric-type adenocarcinoma involving the bladder dome should be regarded as having urachal cancer until proven otherwise.

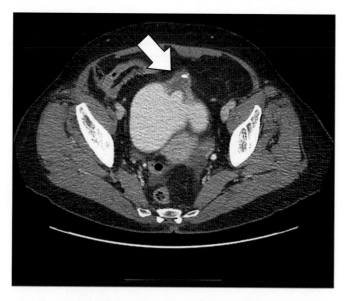

Figure 2.4 Radiographic features of urachal cancer. The appearance of a midline, cystic, bladder mass with microcalcifications is nearly pathognomonic for the diagnosis of urachal cancer.

Nonetheless, it is important to recognize that these tumors can occur all along the urachal ligament, and may produce a palpable mass anywhere from the umbilicus to the symphysis. While involvement of the bladder is frequently present, it is not a requirement for the diagnosis.

The majority of patients present with locally advanced disease, with tumor that invades the bladder wall. The diagnosis is typically made by cystoscopy and biopsy. In addition to the location in the bladder dome and the unusual histology, an important clue to the recognition of an urachal origin is the typical finding of tumor in the muscularis propria with unremarkable urothelium overlying the cancer. By contrast, adenocarcinomas arising from the urothelium grow from "the inside to the outside" and are frequently associated with the presence of urothelial dysplasia or even focal areas of recognizable transitional cell cancer. The only other important differential consideration in the differential diagnosis is "drop metastasis" from an ovarian or upper gastrointestinal (or pancreatic) primary tumor, although these tend to involve the cul-de-sac and not the bladder dome. Invasion from an urachal primary into the large or small bowel is fairly common, and we have seen several cases of "multifocal colon cancer" or "bladder cancer metastatic to the colon" that turned out to be urachal cancers eroding into the gut at one or more locations.

As with colon cancer, evaluation of serum tumor markers may be helpful, especially in the context of evaluating response to therapy. As with other tumor types, an elevation of CA-125 should raise suspicion for the presence of peritoneal carcinomatosis which is an extremely common finding in patients with urachal cancers. Elevations in CEA and CA-19-9 may also be useful in monitoring response to chemotherapy, especially when peritoneal disease cannot be easily measured on CT imaging.

Appropriate surgical management of urachal carcinoma requires that the diagnosis be made preoperatively, based on recognition of this possibility in the appropriate clinical setting. Cross-sectional imaging is the key to recognizing the diagnosis. On CT, urachal carcinoma often appears as a low-attenuation mass at the dome of the bladder, typically in the midline or slightly to one side (see Fig. 2.4). Because of the relatively high recurrence rate following the treatment of this disease, en bloc resection of the umbilicus, urachus, overlying peritoneum and posterior rectus fascia lateral to the medial umbilical ligament, bladder, and pelvic lymph nodes is now the standard operation. The recognition that urachal tumors are predominantly extravesical and not associated with a field effect suggested to surgeons that in most cases even bulky tumors could be completely resected with adequate margins by an en bloc dissection with only a partial cystectomy.[59,60] Contemporary series report that neither local recurrence nor outcome is threatened by this approach. Rather, survival is more tightly linked to the stage at presentation, the presence of lymph node metastasis, and the ability to achieve a negative surgical margin than with the performance of a partial or total cystectomy.[58,61,62] A radical cystectomy is indicated during salvage surgery to treat a positive surgical margin or to remove an inadequately controlled urachal ligament, which occurs when the diagnosis was not made preoperatively. In a series of patients referred to MD Anderson,[58] it was remarkable that only 19 of 35 patients undergoing primary surgical management had en bloc resection of the urachal ligament and umbilicus. The importance of proper surgical management was reinforced by the finding that 13 of the 16 long-term survivors reported in this series were treated with en bloc resection including umbilectomy.

Unfortunately, patients with nodal or peritoneal involvement discovered at surgery have a median survival of about 25 months, and demonstrate a clinical course that is virtually indistinguishable from that of patients with clinically apparent metastases at diagnosis.[58] In view of this finding, and the demonstrated benefit of perioperative chemotherapy for colorectal cancer, the use of adjuvant or neoadjuvant chemotherapy for urachal cancer would seem to be a reasonable consideration. Unfortunately there are essentially no data bearing on this point directly, so we are left to extrapolate from our experience with other enteric adenocarcinomas. Since we do have some systemic therapies with clinically relevant response rates (see below), it seems appropriate to discuss adjuvant therapy with patients at particularly high risk of recurrence, including those with tumor in the lymph nodes, on the peritoneal surface, or in the setting of inadequate surgery, including either the presence of positive margins, or where the urachal ligament was not controlled.[58]

Not surprisingly, few long-term survivors have been observed once metastases develop. The most frequently involved sites include bone, lung, liver, lymph nodes and brain. Peritoneal carcinomatosis is common, especially in the setting of positive surgical margins and the presence of peritoneal implants at cystectomy. Lack of en bloc resection of the umbilicus with the urachal ligament and bladder dome may also increase this risk. We have seen several operative notes indicating a spillage of cystic contents into the peritoneal cavity when the ligament was resected below the umbilicus, leaving the umbilicus in place.

Historically, chemotherapy has had little impact in the treatment of urachal cancer. This is particularly so in the context of chemotherapy regimens traditionally employed for transitional cell carcinoma.[62] More recently, responses have been reported in the setting of 5-fluorouracil-based chemotherapy regimens.[58,63] Currently, we are enrolling patients on a phase 2 trial using combination chemotherapy with 5-fluorouracil, leucovorin, gemcitabine, and cisplatin. Results in the first 20 patients show objective response in just over one-third of patients.[3] In keeping with the clinical manifestations of this disease being so closely related to colorectal cancer, we have observed anecdotal responses in patients treated with capecitabine and irinotecan-based regimens, and to the antiepidermal growth factor antibody cetuximab.

Sarcoma

Sarcomas are quite uncommon in the urinary tract. Many patients referred to our institution with tumors diagnosed as sarcomas turn out to have epithelial components on review, and thus are best classified as carcinosarcomas, as described above. Nonetheless, sarcomas that appear to arise within the bladder without a detectable epithelial component do occur. Prior radiotherapy is a recognized risk factor and the typical delay of two or three decades from radiation exposure to secondary cancer seems to apply. Urinary sarcomas have also been reported in the setting of prior exposure to cyclophosphamide[64,65] and in some children with neurofibromatosis type 1.[66]

In adults, the most commonly reported histological subtype is leiomyosarcoma,[67,68] and rhabdomyosarcoma is the most common malignant bladder tumor in children.[69] Of course, many tumors display areas with more than one pattern of differentiation.

Clinical management follows the principles of sarcoma management in other sites. In general, surgery is the mainstay of therapy.[68] If the primary tumor is quite large and it shows a histology for which a reasonable response to chemotherapy can be anticipated, such as osteogenic sarcoma, then neoadjuvant chemotherapy is given. Outcome is primarily driven by stage. The presence of lymphovascular invasion and positive margins has also been associated with a higher risk of relapse.[68] It is our impression that patients with sarcoma are more susceptible to tumor implants in the urethra after a transurethal resection (TUR) but this has not been formally studied, nor has it been reported by other centers.

References

1. Dinney CPN, McConkey DJ, Millikan RE, et al. Focus on bladder cancer. Cancer Cell 2004; 6: 111–16.

2. Blaveri E, Simko JP, Korkola JE, et al. Bladder cancer outcome and subtype classification by gene expression. Clinical Cancer Res 2005; 11:4044–55.

3. Siefker-Radtke A. Urachal carcinoma: surgical and chemotherapeutic options. Expert Rev Anticancer Ther 2006; 6: 1715–21.

4. Siefker-Radtke AO, Kamat AM, Grossman HB, et al. Phase II clinical trial of neoadjuvant alternating doublet chemotherapy with ifosfamide/doxorubicin and etoposide/cisplatin in small-cell urothelial cancer. J Clin Oncol 2009; 27: 2592–7.

5. Baschinsky DY, Chen JH, Vadmal MS, et al. Carcinosarcoma of the urinary bladder – an aggressive tumor with diverse histogenesis. A clinicopathologic study of 4 cases and review of the literature. Arch Pathol Lab Med 2000; 124: 1172–8.

6. Lopez-Beltran A, Pacelli A, Rothenberg HJ, et al. Carcinosarcoma and sarcomatoid carcinoma of the bladder: clinicopathological study of 41 cases. J Urol 1998; 159: 1497–503.

7. Perret L, Chaubert P, Hessler D, et al. Primary heterologous carcinosarcoma (metaplastic carcinoma) of the urinary bladder: a clinicopathologic, immunohistochemical, and ultrastructural analysis of eight cases and a review of the literature. Cancer 1998; 82:1535–49.

8. Gronau S, Menz CK, Melzner I, et al. Immunohistomorphologic and molecular cytogenetic analysis of a carcinosarcoma of the urinary bladder. Virchows Arch 2002; 440:436–40.

9. Halachmi S, DeMarzo AM, Chow NH, et al. Genetic alterations in urinary bladder carcinosarcoma: evidence of a common clonal origin. Eur Urol 2000; 37: 350–7.

10. Sung MT, Wang M, MacLennan GT, et al. Histogenesis of sarcomatoid urothelial carcinoma of the urinary bladder: evidence for a common clonal origin with divergent differentiation. J Pathol 2007; 211: 420–30.

11. McConkey DJ, Lee S, Choi W, et al. Molecular genetics of bladder cancer: emerging mechanisms of tumor initiation and progression. Urol Oncol 2010; 28: 429–40.

12. Wright JL, Black PC, Brown GA, et al. Differences in survival among patients with sarcomatoid carcinoma, carcinosarcoma and urothelial carcinoma of the bladder. J Urol 2007; 178: 2302–6; discussion 2307.

13. Black PC, Brown GA, Dinney CP. The impact of variant histology on the outcome of bladder cancer treated with curative intent. Urol Oncol 2009; 27: 3–7.

14. Iczkowski KA, Shanks JH, Gadaleanu V, et al. Inflammatory pseudotumor and sarcoma of urinary bladder: differential diagnosis and outcome in thirty-eight spindle cell neoplasms. Mod Pathol 2001; 14: 1043–51.

15. Cheng L, Jones TD, McCarthy RP, et al. Molecular genetic evidence for a common clonal origin of urinary bladder small cell carcinoma and coexisting urothelial carcinoma. Am J Pathol 2005; 166: 1533–9.

16. Quek ML, Nichols PW, Yamzon J, et al. Radical cystectomy for primary neuroendocrine tumors of the bladder: the University of Southern California experience. J Urol 2005; 174: 93–6.

17. Siefker-Radtke AO, Dinney CP, Abrahams NA, et al. Evidence supporting preoperative chemotherapy for small cell carcinoma of the bladder: a retrospective review of the M. D. Anderson cancer experience. J Urol 2004; 172: 481–4.

18. Abbas F, Civantos F, Benedetto P, et al. Small cell carcinoma of the bladder and prostate. Urology 1995; 46(5): 617–30.

19. Grignon DJ, Ro JY, Ayala AG, et al. Small cell carcinoma of the urinary bladder. A clinicopathologic analysis of 22 cases. Cancer 1992; 69(2):527–36.

20. Walther PJ. Adjuvant/neo-adjuvant etoposide/cisplatin and cystectomy for management of invasive small cell carcinoma of the bladder. J Urol 2002; 167: 285.

21. Lohrisch C, Murray N, Pickles T, et al. Small cell carcinoma of the bladder: long term outcome with integrated chemoradiation. Cancer 1999; 86(11): 2346–52.

22. Sejima T, Miyagawa I: 'Successful' chemo- and radiotherapy prior to radical cystectomy does not necessarily correlate with clinical course in small cell carcinoma of the bladder. Urol Int 2005; 74: 286–8.

23. Sved P, Gomez P, Manoharan M, et al. Small cell carcinoma of the bladder. BJU Int 2004; 94: 12–17.

24. Hendrickson M, Ross J, Eifel P, et al. Uterine papillary serous carcinoma: a highly malignant form of endometrial adenocarcinoma. Am J Surg Pathol 1982; 6: 93–108.

25. Amin MB, Ro JY, el-Sharkawy T, et al. Micropapillary variant of transitional cell carcinoma of the urinary bladder. Histologic pattern resembling ovarian papillary serous carcinoma. Am J Surg Pathol 1994; 18: 1224–32.

26. Johansson SL, Borghede G, Holmang S. Micropapillary bladder carcinoma: a clinicopathological study of 20 cases. J Urol 1999; 161: 1798–802.

27. Maranchie JK, Bouyounes BT, Zhang PL, et al. Clinical and pathological characteristics of micropapillary transitional cell carcinoma: a highly aggressive variant. J Urol 2000; 163: 748–51.

28. Samaratunga H, Khoo K. Micropapillary variant of urothelial carcinoma of the urinary bladder: a clinicopathological and immunohistochemical study. Histopathology 2004; 45: 55–64.

29. Nassar H. Carcinomas with micropapillary morphology: clinical significance and current concepts. Adv Anat Pathol 2004; 11:297–303.

30. Alvarado-Cabrero I, Sierra-Santiesteban FI, Mantilla-Morales A, et al. Micropapillary carcinoma of the urothelial tract. A clinicopathologic study of 38 cases. Ann Diagn Pathol 2005; 9:1–5.

31. Luna-More S, Gonzalez B, Acedo C, et al. Invasive micropapillary carcinoma of the breast. A new special type of invasive mammary carcinoma. Pathol Res Pract 1994; 190:668–74.

32. Nassar H, Pansare V, Zhang H, et al. Pathogenesis of invasive micropapillary carcinoma: role of MUC1 glycoprotein. Mod Pathol 2004; 17: 1045–50.

33. Kamat AM, Gee JR, Dinney CPN, et al. The case for early cystectomy in the treatment of nonmuscle invasive micropapillary bladder carcinoma. J Urol 2006; 175: 881–5.

34. Kamat AM, Dinney CP, Gee JR, et al. Micropapillary bladder cancer: a review of the University of Texas M. D. Anderson Cancer Center experience with 100 consecutive patients. Cancer 2007; 110: 62–7.

35. Siefker-Radtke A, Millikan RE, Kamat AM, et al. A phase II trial of sequential neoadjuvant chemotherapy with ifosfamide, doxorubicin, and gemcitabine (IAG), followed by cisplatin, gemcitabine, and ifosfamide

(CGI) in locally advanced urothelial cancer: final results from the M. D. Anderson Cancer Center. J Clin Oncol 2008; 26: 269s.

36. Eble J, *et al. World Health Organization Classification of Tumours. Pathology and Genetics of Tumours of the Urinary Systatem and Male Genital Organs.* Lyon, France: IARC Press, 2004.

37. Grignon DJ, Ro JY, Ayala AG, *et al.* Primary adenocarcinoma of the urinary bladder. A clinicopathologic analysis of 72 cases. Cancer 1991; 67: 2165–72.

38. Tamboli P, Mohsin SK, Hailemariam S, *et al.* Colonic adenocarcinoma metastatic to the urinary tract versus primary tumors of the urinary tract with glandular differentiation: a report of 7 cases and investigation using a limited immunohistochemical panel. Arch Pathol Lab Med 2002; 126: 1057–63.

39. Nielsen K, Nielsen KK. Adenocarcinoma in exstrophy of the bladder – the last case in Scandinavia? A case report and review of literature. J Urol 1983; 130: 1180–2.

40. Mai KT, Yazdi HM, Perkins DG, *et al.* Multicentric clear cell adenocarcinoma in the urinary bladder and the urethral diverticulum: evidence of origin of clear cell adenocarcinoma of the female lower urinary tract from Mullerian duct remnants. Histopathology 2000; 36: 380–2.

41. Lughezzani G, Sun M, Jeldres C, *et al.* Adenocarcinoma versus urothelial carcinoma of the urinary bladder: comparison between pathologic stage at radical cystectomy and cancer-specific mortality. Urology 2010; 75: 376–81.

42. Lagwinski N, Thomas A, Stephenson AJ, *et al.* Squamous cell carcinoma of the bladder: a clinicopathologic analysis of 45 cases. Am J Surg Pathol 2007; 31: 1777–87.

43. Kassouf W, Spiess PE, Siefker-Radtke A, *et al.* Outcome and patterns of recurrence of nonbilharzial pure squamous cell carcinoma of the bladder: a contemporary review of The University of Texas M D Anderson Cancer Center experience. Cancer 2007; 110: 764–9.

44. Pagliaro LC, Millikan RE, Tu SM, *et al.* Cisplatin, gemcitabine, and ifosfamide as weekly therapy: a feasibility and phase II study of salvage treatment for advanced transitional-cell carcinoma. J Clin Oncol 2002; 20: 2965–70.

45. Tu SM, Hossan E, Amato R, *et al.* Paclitaxel, cisplatin and methotrexate combination chemotherapy is active in the treatment of refractory urothelial malignancies. J Urol 1995; 154: 1719–22.

46. Galsky MD, Iasonos A, Mironov S, *et al.* Prospective trial of ifosfamide, paclitaxel, and cisplatin in patients with advanced non-transitional cell carcinoma of the urothelial tract. Urology 2007; 69: 255–9.

47. Amin MB, Ro JY, Lee KM, *et al.* Lymphoepithelioma-like carcinoma of the urinary bladder. Am J Surg Pathol 1994; 18: 466–73.

48. Gulley ML, Amin MB, Nicholls JM, *et al.* Epstein–Barr virus is detected in undifferentiated nasopharyngeal carcinoma but not in lymphoepithelioma-like carcinoma of the urinary bladder. Human Pathol 1995; 26: 1207–14.

49. Williamson SR, Zhang S, Lopez-Beltran A, *et al.* Lymphoepithelioma-like carcinoma of the urinary bladder: clinicopathologic, immunohistochemical, and molecular features. Am J Surg Pathol 2011; 35: 474–83.

50. Tamas EF, Nielsen ME, Schoenberg MP, *et al.* Lymphoepithelioma-like carcinoma of the urinary tract: a clinicopathological study of 30 pure and mixed cases. Mod Pathol 2007; 20: 828–34.

51. Ro JY, Shen SS, Lee HI, *et al.* Plasmacytoid transitional cell carcinoma of urinary bladder: a clinicopathologic study of 9 cases. Am J Surg Pathol 2008; 32: 752–7.

52. Nigwekar P, Tamboli P, Amin MB, *et al.* Plasmacytoid urothelial carcinoma: detailed analysis of morphology with clinicopathologic correlation in 17 cases. Am J Surg Pathol 2009; 33: 417–24.

53. Keck B, Stoehr R, Wach S, *et al.* The plasmacytoid carcinoma of the bladder – rare variant of aggressive urothelial carcinoma. Int J Cancer 2011; 129: 346–54.

54. Schubert GE, Pavkovic MB, Bethke-Bedurftig BA. Tubular urachal remnants in adult bladders. J Urol 1982; 127: 40–2.

55. Begg RC. The urachus: its anatomy, histology and development. J Anat 1930; 64: 170–83.

56. Hammond G, Yglesias L, Davis J. Urachus, its anatomy and associated fasciae. Anat Rec 1941; 80: 271.

57. Sheldon CA, Clayman RV, Gonzalez R, *et al.* Malignant urachal lesions. J Urol 1984; 131: 1–8.

58. Siefker-Radtke AO, Gee J, Shen Y, *et al.* Multimodality management of urachal carcinoma: the M. D. Anderson Cancer Center experience. J Urol 2003; 169: 1295–8.

59. Henly DR, Farrow GM, Zincke H. Urachal cancer: role of conservative surgery. Urology 1993; 42: 635–9.

60. Herr HW. Urachal carcinoma: the case for extended partial cystectomy. J Urol 1994; 151: 365–6.

61. Herr HW, Bochner BH, Sharp D, *et al.* Urachal carcinoma: contemporary surgical outcomes. J Urol 2007; 178: 74–8; discussion 78.

62. Molina JR, Quevedo JF, Furth AF, *et al.* Predictors of survival from urachal cancer: a Mayo Clinic study of 49 cases. Cancer 2007; 110: 2434–40.

63. Logothetis CJ, Samuels ML, Ogden S. Chemotherapy for adenocarcinomas of bladder and urachal origin: 5-fluorouracil, doxorubicin, and mitomycin-C. Urology 1985; 26: 252–5.

64. Pedersen-Bjergaard J, Jonsson V, Pedersen M, *et al.* Leiomyosarcoma of the urinary bladder after cyclophosphamide. J Clin Oncol 1995; 13: 532–3.

65. Tanguay C, Harvey I, Houde M, *et al.* Leiomyosarcoma of urinary bladder following cyclophosphamide therapy: report of two cases. Mod Pathol 2003; 16: 512–14.

66. Sung L, Anderson JR, Arndt C, *et al.* Neurofibromatosis in children with rhabdomyosarcoma: a report from the Intergroup Rhabdomyosarcoma study IV. J Pediatr 2004; 144: 666–8.

67. Mills SE, Bova GS, Wick MR, *et al.* Leiomyosarcoma of the urinary bladder. A clinicopathologic and immunohistochemical study of 15 cases. Am J Surg Pathol 1989; 13: 480–9.

68. Spiess PE, Kassouf W, Steinberg JR, *et al.* Review of the M.D. Anderson experience in the treatment of bladder sarcoma. Urol Oncol 2007; 25: 38–45.

69. Leuschner I, Harms D, Mattke A, *et al.* Rhabdomyosarcoma of the urinary bladder and vagina: a clinicopathologic study with emphasis on recurrent disease: a report from the Kiel Pediatric Tumor Registry and the German CWS Study. Am J Surg Pathol 2001; 25: 856–64.

Section 1: Genitourinary Cancer

3 Urethral Cancer

Sonia L. Ali,[1] **Tanya B. Dorf,**[2] **Paul G. Pagnini,**[3] and **David I. Quinn**[2]

[1] Department of Medicine, [2] Division of Cancer Medicine, [3] Department of Radiation Oncology, Keck School of Medicine at USC, University of Southern California; Norris Comprehensive Cancer Center and Hospital, Los Angeles, CA, USA

Introduction

Primary carcinoma of the urethra is rare, representing less than 0.1% of all genitourinary neoplasms,[1,2] or less than 80 patients each year up to the 1998 American Cancer Society estimates, the last year in which cancers considered of rare incidence were routinely reported.[3] In a review of the National Cancer Institute Surveillance, Epidemiology, and End Results (SEER) database covering approximately 10% of the United States population for the period 1973–2002, 1075 men and 540 women were diagnosed with urethral cancer, with an annual age-adjusted incidence rate of 4.3 per million and 1.5 per million, respectively.[4] Due to its low incidence, no institution has been able to amass enough patients to evaluate different therapeutic options and develop consistent treatment strategies. Management decisions are therefore based on retrospective reports. The following discussion will review the important aspects of natural history, epidemiology, prognosis, and clinical management in men and women.

Anatomy

The anatomy and histology of the urethra differ greatly between males and females, which leads to differences in pathological presentations. In the female the urethra is a 4 cm-long tubular conduit that courses obliquely anteroinferiorly from the internal urethral meatus through the urogenital diaphragm to the external uretral meatus. Multiple paraurethral glands of Skene (derivatives of the urogenital sinus and homologous to the prostate in males) secrete mucous material that provides urethral lubrication during sexual intercourse.[5] By convention, in the female, the distal third of the urethra is called the anterior urethra, while the proximal two-thirds is called the posterior urethra.[6–8] The proximal third of the female urethra is lined with transitional cell epithelium with the distal two-thirds lined with stratified squamous epithelium.[6,9] The male urethra, on the other hand, is divided into prostatic, membranous, and penile segments.[6,10] The prostatic urethra is surrounded by the prostate, where the posterior wall of the urethra forms an elevation, the verumontanum (colliculus seminales). The midline of the male urethra has an opening, the utriculus prostaticus, which is the rudimentary male homolog of the uterus.[11]

The urethra is located within the urogenital triangle and pierces the superficial and deep perineal spaces of the pelvic floor. Cancers of the anterior urethra preferentially drain into superficial inguinal lymph nodes. The posterior urethra (prostatic, membranous, and bulbar segments in the male and the proximal two-thirds of the urethra in the female) generally drains into pelvic lymphatic channels.[6] Lymphatic drainage of the posterior urethra in the female is to the pelvic lymph nodes while the anterior urethra drains into the superficial and deep inguinal lymph nodes.[7] Lymphatic drainage of the bulbomembranous urethra in the male is to the pelvic lymph nodes, while the penis drains to the superficial and deep inguinal nodes.[7]

Epidemiology

Unique among the urological neoplasms, cancer of the urethra is more common in women than men, with a ratio of between 2:1 and 4:1[4,12] (Table 3.1). Cases have been reported in all age groups, but most present in the sixth decade of life or later with a peak in incidence in the 75–84-year range.[4] The relative incidence of urethral cancer in African-Americans exceeds that of the white population in the United States. The incidence of transitional cell carcinoma is similar between the two groups but squamous cell cancer predominates in African-American men and adenocarcinoma in African-American women.[4,13]

Because of the small number of cases reported, it is difficult to ascertain significant etiological agents. Even so, chronic inflammation due to either infection or irritation seems to play some role in the development of squamous cancers. A history of venereal disease, urethritis, multiple urethral instrumentation, and strictures is a common finding in men.[14,15] Human papillomaviruses (HPV) of genotype 16 and 18 are associated

Textbook of Uncommon Cancer, Fourth Edition. Edited by Derek Raghavan, Charles D. Blanke, David H. Johnson, Paul L. Moots, Gregory H. Reaman, Peter G. Rose and Mikkael A. Sekeres.
© 2012 John Wiley & Sons, Inc. Published 2012 by John Wiley & Sons, Inc.

Table 3.1 Summary of several contemporary series of urethral carcinoma.

Center	CHHRI Manchester[183] 1936–1964	U of TN + MVAH Memphis[155] 1961–1980	MDACC Houston[184] 1979–1990	MSKCC New York[185] 1958–1996	BAKCC Detroit[22] 1980–1996	NCKUH Taiwan[24] 1988–2001	TMH, Mumbai, India[186] 1991–2000	MDACC Houston[187] 1955–1989	WUSM, St. Louis[188] 1959–1995	MSKCC New York[189] 1958–1994	PMH, Toronto, Canada[190] 1961–1990	Mayo Clinic, Rochester[191] 1948–1999
Predominant primary local therapy	RT	Surgery	Surgery	Surgery	Neoadjuvant RT + CT then Surgery	Surgery	Surgery, CT, RT	RT	RT with or without surgery	Surgery or RT	RT	Surgery
Characteristic												
Number	132	16	23	46	21	21	18	97	44	72	34	53
Gender: M:F	132 female only	16 male only	23 male only	46 male only	11:10	14:7	36:18 only female data reported	97 female only	44 female only	72 female only	34 female only	53 female only
Age, years												
Median	NR	62.5	61	59.5	NR	53	NR	63	NR	60	67	63
Mean	62.2	63	NR	59.2	59.2	52.6	58	NR	67	59	NR	63
Range	38–86	38–84	23–78	36–92	32–80	28–72	45–72	36–89	37–89	21–84	30–80	36–92
Follow-up, months												
Mean	NR	43.7	50	NR	NR	55.6	NR	NR	NR	NR	NR	NR
Median	–	18.5	NR	125	42.1	36	NR	105	99	85	84	174
Range	–	2–160	5–156	1–336	5–96	5–160	18–70	20–337	30–282	0–384	21–325	19–337
Histological type												
Adenocarcinoma	4 (3)	1 (6)	0	1 (2)	8 (38)	6 (43)	9 (50)	34 (35)	23	25 (35)	6 (18)	14
Squamous	64 (49)	8 (50)	19 (83)	29 (63)	11 (52)	5 (36)	5 (28)	40 (41)	13	28 (39)	15 (44)	21
Transitional	19 (14)	2 (13)	3 (13)	15 (33)	1 (5)	3 (21)	4 (22)	21 (22)	5	11 (15)	13 (38)	15
Other	5 (4)	5 (31) (SCC + TCC)	1 (4)	1 (2)	1 (5)	0	0	2 (3)	3	8 (11)	0	0
Tumor location												
Distal	–	5 (31)	15 (65)	18 (39)	7 (64)	5 (35)	9 (50)	34 (35)	20 (47)	25 (35)	14 (41)	29 (55)
Proximal or entire (bulbomembranous/ prostatic)	–	11 (69)	8 (35)	28 (61)	4 (36)	9 (65)	9 (50)	63 (65)	23 (53)	40 (56)	20 (59)	24 (45)
Stage												
I–II	86 (65)	8 (50)	6 (26)	21 (49)	9 (43)	6 (43)	9 (50)	40 (41)	13 (30)	19 (31)	8 (24)	27 (51)
III–IV	46 (35)	8 (50)	17 (74)	22 (51)	12 (57)	8 (57)	9 (50)	57 (59)	31 (70)	42 (69)	26 (76)	26 (49)
5-year overall survival (%)	42	–	41	42	–	–	33	41	42	32	58	51
5-year overall survival – Stage I–II (%)	–	–	83	83	–	–	50	–	–	78	–	59
5 year overall survival – Stage III–IV (%)	–	37.5	31	36	–	–	0	–	–	22	–	42

BAKCC, Barbara A. Karmanos Cancer Center; CHHRI, Christie Hospital and Holt Radium Institute; CT, chemotherapy; MDA, University of Texas MD Anderson Cancer Center; MSKCC, Memorial Sloan Kettering Cancer Center; MVAH, Memphis Veterans Administration Hospital; NCKUH, National Cheng Kung University Hospital; NR, not reported; PMH, Princess Margaret Hospital; RT, Radiation therapy; TMH, Tata Memorial Hospital; WUSM, Washington University School of Medicine; U of TN, University of Tennessee.

with human urogenital tumors.[16–20] Although proliferative lesions such as papillomas, adenomas, and leukoplakia may also be important, especially in women, few associations have been substantiated.[21] Heavy metal exposure, especially with arsenic, and the presence of urethral diverticulae appear to be important predisposing factors to adenocarcinoma of the bulbomembranous urethra in selected female populations.[22–25]

Pathology

Benign lesions

In older surgical literature, before the widespread use of estrogen replacement therapy in postmenopausal women, 90% of the reported urethral masses in females were caruncles.[26] Though these lesions are often asymptomatic, they can produce pain or hematuria in estrogen-deficient women. Caruncles histologically exhibit hyperplastic squamous epithelium with underlying submucosal vascularity, fibrosis, and inflammation.[27] There are very few reports in the literature of benign tumors of the urethra. They include nephrogenic adenomas, papillomas, paragangliomas, amyloidosis, hemangiomas,[28] fibromas, leiomyomas,[29–31] and sarcoidosis.

Nephrogenic adenomas of the urinary tract are the most reported benign tumors of the urethra[32,33] and are more common in renal transplant recipients where the derivation of cells from the renal tubular epithelium has recently been documented.[34] Most nephrogenic adenomas occur in the urinary bladder (55%), second most often in the urethra (41%), followed by 4% in the ureters. The remaining nephrogenic adenomas occur in the prostate, but stain negatively for prostate-specific antigen (PSA) but positively for PAX-2.[35,36] These lesions represent benign metaplastic proliferation of urothelium, occurring mostly in males.[37,38] Usually there is some associated trauma.[39] In females, it can occur in a urethral diverticulum..[40–44] The most common microscopic pattern is tubular, with the cystic pattern seen in 72% of cases. Eosinophilic secretions are found in 75% of cases and basophilic secretions in 25%.[45] These lesions do not transform into a malignancy but can recur after transurethral resection.[37]

Papillomas of the urethra are rare, occurring mainly in men.[46–48] Paragangliomas outside the adrenals occur in only 10%, rarely in the urinary tract. The bladder is the most common site, the ureter less frequently and rarely in the urethra.[49] The cases are usually in elderly men and often discovered as an incidental finding. Grossly they are polypoid or pedunculated lesions. Most occur at or proximal to the verumontanum and measure up to 15 mm in maximum dimension. There is no immunoreactivity for PSA or prostatic acid phosphatase. Neuroendocrine cells are normal cellular constituents in the bladder, prostate and prostatic urethra, including von Brunn's nests and glandular metaplasia.[50,51] Another benign lesion is amyloidosis of the urethra.[52,53] When found, a workup for systemic amyloidosis and myeloma should be performed since it is such a rare lesion, with less than 30 reported cases.[54] If localized, these lesions can spontaneously regress.[55]

Urethral capillary hemangioma has been reported rarely in the world literature, with less than 20 cases.[56] It has the tendency to recur locally, though its histology of vascular sinuses and hemorrhages is clearly benign. Sex hormone cycles influence the clinical manifestations of this tumor in the female urethra in 7% of patients.[57] There are only two reports of urethral leiomyoma presenting in pregnancy with measurable estrogen receptors (ER)[58,59] but leiomyomas can occur without pregnancy in women.[60] Grossly, it appears as a fleshy tumor, at times pedunculated. Microscopically, abundant muscle fibers are seen and the cells have elongated nuclei with mitosis. Estrogen receptors have been found in the male urethra in asymptomatic and symptomatic patients undergoing transurethral resection of the prostate (TURP) due to symptomatic infravesical obstruction, as well as in patients with bladder cancer using the Abbott ER-ICA monoclonal assay for immunohistochemical demonstration of ERs,[61] while it is not demonstrated in the bladder. Bodker et al. note that the difference between ER expression in the bladder and the prostatic urethra cannot be explained embryologically, since both the bladder and urethra are derived from the urogenital sinus.[61] They proposed instead that the periurethral glands may have contributions from the müllerian ducts, which in the female give rise to the ER-positive uterine tissue. Out of 21 reported patients with leiomyoma of the urethra, there is only one detailed case of ER-positive staining occurring in a male.[62]

Solitary urethral sarcoidosis is a rare occurrence,[63] requiring workup for systemic sarcoidosis. An infection often seen in the urethra is condyloma acuminata. [64–71] It often is associated with bladder or penis involvement.[68,69,72–75] It is an important entity, because it may be a premalignant lesion.[76,77]

Malignant lesions

Carcinoma of the urethra is a rare tumor, with 1200 cases reported in women and 600 reported in men. In females, most are squamous cell carcinomas (55%), 18% adenocarcinoma, 16% transitional cell carcinomas, and the remaining 11% a mixture of rare tumors.[11] In males, 80% of the tumors are squamous cell carcinomas, 15% transitional cell carcinomas and the remainder are adenocarcinomas. Most urethral cancers in the male are located in the bulbomembranous urethra (60%), 30% in the penile urethra, and the remainder in the prostatic urethra.[7]

Gross appearance

The gross appearance of urethral cancers may appear as papillomatous, mucosal thickening or induration, or as a small spreading or superficial ulcer. As the lesion becomes more advanced, it will appear as indurated, annular constricting, or fungating.[11]

Microscopic appearance

Squamous cell carcinoma of the urethra usually has an area of focal keratinization that identifies it as squamous cell carcinoma (Figs 3.1–3.3). Transitional cell carcinoma (TCC) of the urethra is indistinguishable from the appearance seen in TCC of the bladder (Fig. 3.4). Thus, one may see a papillary

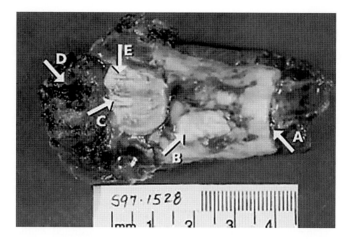

Figure 3.1 Gross pathological specimen (longitudinal) of a squamous cell carcinoma of the proximal urethra (segmental resection). (A) The distal margin of the tumor. (B) The polypoid-appearing squamous cell carcinoma. (C) The proximal margin of the tumor. (D) Periurethral soft tisssue. (E) Squamous metaplasia.

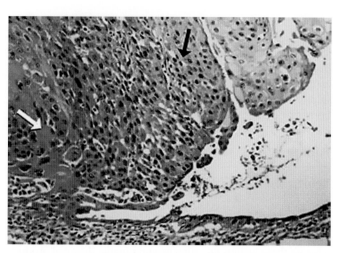

Figure 3.3 Micrograph of Figure 3.2, polypoid squamous cell carcinoma of the urethra. The white arrow represents the area of keratinization. The black arrow represents the polypoid portion of the tumor. Running along the bottom of the micrograph is a tongue of squamous metaplasia.

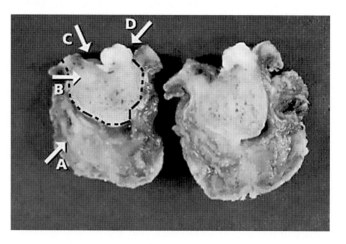

Figure 3.2 Cross-sections of the pathological specimen of the squamous cell carcinoma of the proximal urethra seen in Figure 3.1. (A) The periurethral soft tissue. (B) Cavities of the corpus cavernosum and corpus spongiosum. (C) The urethral opening. (D) The polypoid-shaped squamous cell carcinoma. The unlabeled specimen on the right represents the tumor at the level of the bulbomembranous urethra.

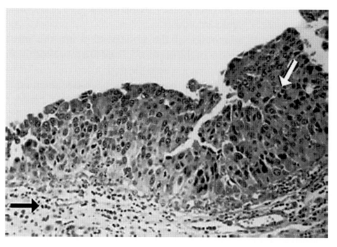

Figure 3.4 Micrograph of a high-grade transitional cell carcinoma of the urethra. The black arrow represents the lamina propria layer. The white arrow represents the TCC.

appearance, *in situ*, papillary and infiltrating, or infiltrating carcinoma of any grade. A thorough examination of the urothelium must be performed for sites of concurrent malignancy, especially in the case of previous cystectomy for bladder carcinoma.

Adenocarcinoma of the urethra requires careful workup of possible extraurethral sources. There is a frequently reported clear cell variant of adenocarcinoma, exhibiting glycogen-rich cells (Fig. 3.5). The clear cell variant can stain positive with antibodies to PSA and prostatic acid phosphatase.[23,78–87] Adenocarcinoma of the female urethra accounts for 10% of all urethral cancers,[87] with the derivation of adenocarcinoma either from Skene's glands and producing PSA or from urethritis transiting through intestinal metaplasia and producing mucin and not PSA. Dodson *et al.* evaluated 13 primary adenocarcinomas of the female urethra and found two histological groups:

columnar/mucinous (11 cases) and clear cell (two cases). The conclusion was that female urethral adenocarcinoma has more than one tissue of origin, with a minority arising from the Skene's glands, accounting for less than 0.003% of all genital tract malignancies in females.[86,87] Another case series supporting more than one tissue of origin of female urethral adenocarcinoma was reported by Murphy *et al.* who stained 12 formalin-fixed archival tissue cases of primary female urethral adenocarcinoma, using an antibody against a unique colonic epithelial epitope and reactive in areas of intestinal metaplasia called Das1. Of the 12 cases, nine were columnar/mucinous adenocarcinoma, two clear cell adenocarcinoma and one a cribriform pattern resembling adenocarcinoma of the prostate. All columnar/mucinous adenocarcinomas reacted positively with the Das1 antibody but did not react with the PSA antibody. The tumor with a cribriform pattern reacted strongly with PSA but

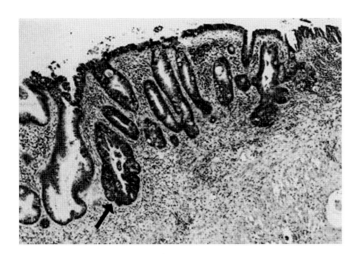

Figure 3.5 Micrograph of an adenocarcinoma of the urethra. The arrow is pointing to infiltrating colonic-type glands.

not with Das1 antibody. The two clear cell adenocarcinomas did not react with either antibody. Benign urethral specimens demonstrated strong reactivity to the antibody used in areas of urethritis glandularis while normal, inflamed urethral mucosa and transitional cell carcinoma did not react.[88] More recent research has focused on derivation of clear cell cancers from nephrogenic adenomas and metaplasia.[89–91]

Rare histologies

Rare tumors of the urethra include non-Hodgkin lymphoma, reported in less than 25 well-documented cases, mainly in females. The lesion appears as a firm meatal epithelium mass that may resemble a caruncle.[92–94] Even rarer are extramedullary plasmacytomas of the urethra, reported in less than 15 patients.[95–101] In these cases, patients do not necessarily develop multiple myeloma as seen in solitary plasmacytomas of the bone.

There are less than 15 cases of primary carcinoid tumor of the urethra in the medical literature.[102–107] In the original case report, the lesion grossly appeared as a ventral palpable mass in the midpenile urethra and at the fossa navicularis. It was thought to be a TCC of the urethra. After 15 months with several intervening procedures, the patient developed facial flushing, sweating, diarrhea, loss of weight, and weakness. On examination, he was found to have an enlarged liver which when palpated triggered waves of pain, flushing, and sweating. Liver biopsy confirmed a carcinoid malignancy that prompted review of all previous pathology from the segmental resection, recurrence treated by penile urethrectomy, bladder papilloma recurrence, and palpable lymph nodes. The original urethral pathology was reviewed again with argentaffin stains and electron microscopy, and it was determined that it was consistent with a carcinoid primary.[102] Subsequent experience with urethral carcinoid suggests a good prognosis for primary lesions treated with local therapy but the potential for symptomatic recurrence many years later.[104–107]

There are also many reports of melanoma of the urethra in the literature. It is the most common nonurothelial malignancy in this location.[108–128] The general pattern with urethra melanoma is that it can be difficult to distinguish from benign lesions such as caruncles, from condylomata and from urothelial derived tumors.[120,122,129] Lesions are typically polypoid and involve the distal urethra, possibly being more common in women with around 20% being amelanotic.[124,125,130,131] Melanoma of the urethra has a high rate of locoregional recurrence and mortality rates of 60–70% by 3 years, but with reported cases living many years after multimodal therapy.[125,132,133]

Paget's disease of the urethra usually occurs as an extension from vulvar, penile, or bladder cancer.[134–138] There is only one case of primary Paget's disease of the urethra which occurred in a 58-year-old African-American male seen at the Medical College of Virginia. The man presented with a history of urinary incontinence, overflow, dysuria, and hematuria. In 19 g of prostatic tissue obtained from a transurethral resection, there was a variety of morphologies. The specimen contained squamous metaplasia and poorly differentiated carcinoma, which had clear cells, suggesting glandular pattern. Paget cells were seen in the basal portion of the prostatic urethra.[139]

Investigations

Symptoms and findings on physical examination

The female patient usually presents with hemorrhagic spotting, dyspareunia, and on pelvic exam a palpable urethral mass. Most tumors arise in the anterior urethra. The rest are in the proximal two-thirds or posterior urethra.[7] The male patient usually presents with difficulty voiding and/or a bloody urethral discharge. On examination, a palpable nodule is felt in the urethra on examination of the penis and provides a rough estimate of the extent of the disease.[7,11,140–142] Approximately 20% of patients present with palpably enlarged inguinal lymph nodes, representing metastases. There is only one documented report of a patient presenting with sudden-onset urinary retention and acute renal failure, who was later found to have a leiomyoma of the urethra.[143]

Staging

The American Joint Commission on Cancer (AJCC) staging system (Box 3.1) is uniform with the International Union against Cancer (UICC), which makes reporting of treatment and survival more consistent in the worldwide literature.[144]

Endoscopic examination

Most diagnoses are made initially by cystourethroscopy and biopsy. One must be careful not to confuse a mucin-producing tumor with the anesthetic jelly used in endoscopy.[145]

Radiological studies

The gold standard for identifying the urethral defect is still retrograde urethrography.[7,11,140–142] Pelvic computed tomography (CT) is useful in identifying enlarged pelvic or retroperitoneal nodes. Multicoil magnetic resonance imaging (MRI) has enhanced the ability to visualize abnormalities of the female

Box 3.1 Clinico-pathological staging for urethral cancer.

Primary tumor (T) (men and women)

Tx	Primary tumor cannot be assessed
T0	No evidence of primary tumor
Ta	Noninvasive papillary, polypoid, or verrucous carcinoma
Tis	Carcinoma *in situ*
T1	Tumor invades subepithelial connective tissue
T2	Tumor invades any of the following: corpus spongiosum, prostate, periurethral muscle
T3	Tumor invades any of the following: corpus cavernosum, beyond prostate capsule, anterior vagina, bladder neck
T4	Tumor invades other adjacent organs

Urothelial (transitional cell) carcinoma of the prostate

Tis pu	Carcinoma *in situ*, involvement of the prostatic urethra
Tis pd	Carcinoma *in situ*, involvement of the prostatic ducts
T1	Tumor invades subepithelial connective tissue
T2	Tumor invades any of the following: prostatic stroma, corpus spongiosum, periurethral muscle
T3	Tumor invades any of the following: corpus cavernosum, beyond prostatic capsule, bladder neck (extraprostatic extension)
T4	Tumor invades other adjacent organs (invasion of the bladder)

Regional lymph nodes (N)

Nx	Regional lymph nodes cannot be assessed
N0	No regional lymph node metastasis
N1	Metastasis in a single lymph node, 2 cm or less in greatest dimension
N2	Metastasis in a single lymph node more than 2 cm in greatest dimension, or in multiple lymph nodes

Distant metastasis (M)

Mx	Distant metastasis cannot be assessed
M0	No distant metastasis
M1	Distant metastasis

Stage grouping

Stage 0a	Ta	N0	M0
Stage 0is	Tis	N0	M0
	Tis pu	N0	M0
	Tis pd	N0	M0
Stage I	T1	N0	M0
Stage II	T2	N0	M0
Stage III	T1	N1	M0
	T2	N1	M0
	T3	N0	M0
	T3	N1	M0
Stage IV	T4	N0	M0
	T4	N1	M0
	Any T	N2	M0
	Any T	Any N	M1

Reproduced from Edge and Byrd.[182] Used with the permission of the American Joint Committee on Cancer (AJCC), Chicago, Illinois. The original source for this material is the AJCC Cancer Staging Manual, Seventh Edition (2010) published by Springer Science and Business Media LLC, www.springer.com

urethra and periurethral tissues, contributing to surgical planning.[5] Endovaginal ultrasound or MRI coil may further define anatomical structures in selected cases.[146,147] Positron emission tomography (PET) scan has been used to evaluate biological activity in pelvic or retroperitoneal nodes. A PET scan also obviates the need for a bone scan, since uptake will be seen in the cortex or medullary cavity of bones in advanced disease.

Prognosis and natural history

The 5-year overall survival after a diagnosis of urethral carcinoma ranges from 32% to 51% (see Table 3.1) with 10-year overall survival of 29% in a recent report on male urethral cancer using the population-based SEER database.[148] In the SEER database, advanced age, higher grade, higher T stage, lymph node involvement, systemic metastases, other histology versus TCC, and no surgery versus radical resection were predictors of death and death from disease.[148] Clinical and pathological stages predict the prognosis of the patient: patients with stage I or II disease at diagnosis have a 50–83% 5-year overall survival compared to 0–42% for those with stage III or IV disease (see Table 3.1). The presence of local invasion and/or lymph node metastases has consistently been associated with a poorer outcome. In addition, involvement of the bulbomembranous (proximal) urethra or the entire length of urethra has a poorer prognosis than involvement limited to the distal segment. Adenocarcinoma has a poorer survival compared to either transitional or squamous cell carcinoma in many series but not all.[148] In contrast, tumor grade, while it may have predictive significance as a single variable in some series, is often not significant when other factors such as stage are incorporated.[148]

Squamous cell and TCC tend to progress by spread to local lymph node groups, typically the inguinal groups, then paraaortic lymph nodes and subsequently the lungs and other visceral organs. Adenocarcinoma tends to have a slightly different pattern of spread, with early involvement of the peritoneum and associated ascites even in the absence of lymph node involvement. Subsequently patients may develop lung (pleural), liver, and bone metastases.

Treatment

Surgery

Surgery in the female patient

Anatomical presentation of the tumor determines the treatment approach. In the more common anterior urethral lesions (distal one-third) where the goal is curative, the cure rate of 75% at 5 years can be obtained by either surgery or radiation.[7,142] Laser resection and fulguration can treat urethral tumors that are restricted to the mucosa and that are very superficial.[12,149] The advantage of the laser over local excision is the absence of bleeding, faster healing, and the possible avoidance of hypertrophic scar associated with deeper penetration seen in surgery. However, there is a higher chance of recurrence, but the laser resection can be repeated.[150] For anterior urethral tumors of low clinical stage that are small and visible, local excision is all that should be necessary, with transurethral resection reserved for lesions in the submucosa (Tis or T1 tumors). Partial urethrectomy, based on clinical situation, can be performed on Tis, T1, and T2 lesions of the anterior urethra.[12] Total urethrectomy is used with T2/T3 lesions where bladder preservation is possible.[12,151]

For tumors of the posterior urethra, the overall survival rate is only 10–17% at 5 years. Patients presenting with involvement of both posterior and anterior urethra also have a poor prognosis. Surgery involves an anterior pelvic exenteration, urinary diversion, and ilioinguinal dissection.[7,142] For defects that are too large for primary closure, the gracilis musculocutaneous flap provides healthy tissue with its own blood and nerve supply to close the wound.[152]

If the tumor is a Skene's (periurethral) gland carcinoma, and preoperatively the PSA is elevated, postoperative levels of PSA titers should decrease after surgical removal.[86]

Surgery in the male patient

As in the female, anatomical presentation of the tumor determines the treatment approach; overall survival rates are 22% at 5 years for penile urethra tumors and only 10% at 5 years for bulbomembranous urethral tumors.[7,142,153] Surgery for penile urethra tumors involve local excision, partial or total penectomy. Local excision can provide long-term disease control in distal tumors when followed by adjuvant radiation therapy.[154–158] A more established procedure for distal tumors is partial penectomy. The advantage of this procedure is a 2 cm proximal margin while preserving sufficient penile length to allow urination in a standing position with excellent disease control.[153]

The ideal patient for radical penectomy is one with T2 disease (involvement of corpus spongiosum) whose tumor does not extend proximal to the midbulb or a patient with a distal neoplasm. If there is evidence of T3 disease, *en bloc* resection with cystoprostatectomy is the best surgical option.[153] *En bloc* resection of the penis, bilateral ilioinguinal node dissection, cystoprostatectomy and urinary diversion should be performed if surgery is the treatment option for carcinoma of the bulbomembranous urethra.

Radiotherapy

Radiotherapy in the female patient

Early lesions can be treated with interstitial irradiation with excellent results (75% 5-year rates), with surgery used for failures or persistent tumors. The technique employs afterloading brachytherapy catheters utilizing iridium-192 (Ir-192) to form a volume implant in a circular pattern around the urethral orifice, with placement based on tumor volume, with the use of MRI for pretreatment planning.[159] The treatment is carried out using a disposable Syed-Neblett template with blind-end stainless steel (17-gauge) or Flex-guide catheters. After verification, simulation films are taken with dummy seeds, a low-dose Ir-192 treatment is delivered between 60 and 70 Gy at a rate of 60–120 cGy per hour to the periphery of the implant when used alone.

For patients with bulky disease, the whole pelvis is treated with external beam irradiation for control of subclinical disease to a total of 45–50 Gy in 5–5½ weeks. The portals cover the inguinal, external, and internal iliac lymph nodes. If the inguinal nodes are involved, they are boosted to 60 or 65 Gy with separate electron beams. There is debate on whether the legs should be frog-legged to flatten the dose to the perineum or closed, and the choice is left to the treating radiation oncologist's experience. Confluent moist desquamation is inevitable, which may require a treatment break of 1 or 2 weeks, with topical care with Domeboro's solution and Silvadene 1% cream. Bolus or tissue compensators can reduce this complication. An additional 20–35 Gy is delivered by afterloading the interstitial implant using a modified disposable Syed-Neblett template for a total dose of 70–80 Gy.[159] Follow-up consists of physical examination and cystoscopy every 3 months, with biopsy at the first visit to be sure there is no residual disease.[160]

For tumors of the anterior meatus, the 5-year survival rates are reported to be 100%.[158,161] In a study of 62 patients with primary carcinoma of the female urethra treated with combined radiation therapy, 42 patients (67.7%) had tumors of the anterior urethra; 20 women (32.3%) had involvement of the posterior urethra. The overall survival rate was 64.5%, with anterior urethral carcinomas having a higher 5-year survival rate (71.4%). Patients with posterior carcinoma have a 5-year survival of only 50%.[162] Follow-up consists of physical examination and cystoscopy every 3 months, with biopsy at the 3-month point to check for residual disease.

For patients with urethral carcinoma who are medically inoperable, treatment can be delivered with external beam radiation therapy and high-dose intracavitary brachytherapy.[140] Georgetown University reported on four women with locally advanced urethral cancer who received whole-pelvis external beam radiotherapy to a planned dose of 45 Gy in 1.8 Gy fractions using AP-PA fields. The anterior field included the inguinal nodes and was not opposed by the posterior field. The inguinal fields were boosted separately with electron fields. A high-dose rate (HDR) afterloader with a 10 Ci Ir-192 source was used to boost therapy. The treatment was carried out by running the source down a modified 20 Fr Foley catheter in a vaginal cylinder to displace the mucosa of the posterior wall. A shield was placed posteriorly within the cylinder to provide further protection to the posterior vaginal wall and rectum. Patients received three or four HDR intracavitary implants, with a 7 Gy isodose cloud encompassing the tumor with margin. The total dose is 66–70 Gy. All three patients had a functioning urethra afterwards. Two died of complications of metastatic disease at 22 and 25 months, with one dying of an unrelated medical problem 12 months later. The remaining patient was disease free at 55 months with only urethral meatal telangiectasia and occasional urinary urgency.

Radiotherapy in the male patient

Radiation therapy in distal urethral lesions provides organ preservation. Early lesions, as in females, can be treated with intracavitary radiation with or without interstitial needles implanted around the urethral meatus. For more advanced lesions, a technique uses parallel-opposed fields with the penis suspended vertically by a urethral catheter[163] or by using a tissue-equivalent mold. This technique is not useful to treat inguinal nodes, however. It can be combined with an intracavitary boost using a modified 20 Fr Foley catheter. All patients develop a brisk skin reaction and swelling, which should subside in 2–4 weeks. In the long term, patients can develop urethral meatal strictures.

Radiation therapy for primary non-Hodgkin lymphoma of the urethra can be the primary mode of treatment for early-stage disease.[93] Plasmacytoma of the urethra can be treated with a low dose of pelvic irradiation (41.4 Gy), with a long-term disease-free survival (more than 12 years).[95]

Cytotoxic chemotherapy

Chemotherapy was previously only considered for urethral cancers with inguinal or pelvic node involvement where the survival rates at 5 years are 10% to 30% or for patients presenting with metastatic disease. The drugs most commonly used have been cisplatin (CDDP), bleomycin, and methotrexate (MTX).[7] Single agents can provide a useful palliative response for some patients.[164] The overall approach to locally advanced disease (T3 or greater) and patients with posterior urethral tumors has evolved because of data showing extremely poor outcomes for patients treated with single-modality local treatments. Patients commonly relapse in a pattern where loss of local disease control and development of distant metastases are contemporaneous or only separated by a few months. This better understanding of the disease has led to the use of chemotherapy with or without radiation in the neoadjuvant setting for patients having surgery or as primary therapy for those with distant spread who need local disease control for quality of life and morbidity benefit.

Urethral carcinomas are generally very responsive to platinum-based cytoxic regimens. Neoadjuvant strategies in this disease show very high complete response rates to chemotherapy either alone or in combination with radiation therapy.[22] As with surgery and radiation therapy, there are no prospective evaluations of response and outcome nor clinical trials of cytotoxic therapy in urethral carcinoma because of the rarity of the disease. On this basis, chemotherapeutic strategies are derived either from experience in urethral cancer or from paradigm extrapolation from more common cancers occurring in the pelvis with similar histologies.

Based on this, some oncologists model therapy for squamous cell urethral carcinoma on cervical, vulvar and anal carcinoma therapies, urethral transitional carcinoma on that used for urothelial TCC and adenocarcinoma with rectal carcinoma.

• Current standard therapy for squamous cell carcinoma (SCC) of cervix or vulva involves cisplatin (with or without 5-fluorouracil) given concurrently with radiation therapy while that for anal SCC is either 5-fluorouracil and mitomycin-C or cisplatin and mitomycin-C given concurrently with radiation.[165–167]

• In urothelial cancer, methotrexate, vinblastine, adriamycin (doxorubicin), and cisplatin (MVAC) is a long-term standard for adjuvant or neoadjuvant treatment.[168] A randomized phase 3 trial run by the European Organization for Research and Treatment of Cancer (EORTC) compared MVAC with gemcitabine and cisplatin (GC) in patients with metastatic TCC and found response and survival to be virtually identical but with less toxicity in the GC arm.[169] In patients with localized bladder cancer, concurrent single-agent cisplatin and radiation therapy (RT) results in good local disease control and bladder preservation in up to 70% of patients, with surgical salvage for the remaining 30%.[170] In addition, the activity of three drug regimens incorporating platinum, gemcitabine and a taxane (GCT) has produced impressive response rates in advanced bladder cancer, including cases with uncommon histological types such as squamous cell or adenocarcinoma.[171,172] Whether GCT is superior to GC in advanced TCC awaits the outcome of a phase 3 trial completed by the EORTC with assistance from the Southwest Oncology Group.[173]

• Rectal adenocarcinoma is routinely treated with radiation therapy and 5-fluorouracil before surgery.[174,175] Several trials are testing whether the addition of new platinums such as oxaliplatin or biological agents targeted at angiogenesis or the epidermal growth factor receptor might further improve outcomes.[176,177]

Combined chemoradiotherapy

Chemoradiotherapy has been explored in patients with tumors that are locally advanced or involve the proximal urethra.[178–181] The radiation therapy dose is a minimum of 30 Gy with a maximum dose of 55 Gy. The use of concurrent cytoxic agents in this setting is commonplace but selection of drugs used varies. Use of weekly cisplatin, infusional 5-fluorouracil and/or mitomycin-C every 6 weeks as single agents or in combination, dependent upon the oncologist's familiarity with each regimen, is reasonable. Our approach at the University of Southern California has been to use weekly cisplatin at a dose of 20 mg/m² of body surface area in combination with 5-fluorouracil 350–450 mg/m² per day infused over 4 days every third week. This regimen is used, dependent upon patient tolerance, for 6 weeks concurrently with radiation therapy. The common side-effects of this approach include inflation of the skin, bladder, urethra, vagina and rectum, dehydration from diarrhea and electrolyte imbalance from cisplatin. These are all manageable if the clinicians providing treatment are diligent in assessing for these effects. Once radiation therapy is complete, we normally give another 6 weeks of chemotherapy with cisplatin and 5-fluorouracil to complete the therapeutic program.

Chemotherapy for metastatic disease

Cisplatin and 5-fluorouracil have been considered a standard in this disease for many years. Recently we have utilized a regimen combining cisplatin or carboplatin with gemcitabine and a taxane. We have found this combination tolerable and in a purely historical and anecdotal sense more efficacious than cisplatin and 5-fluorouracil. While significant disease shrinkage and clinical improvement are common, complete response of all disease amounting to remission is rare and all patients relapse and eventually die, usually from their cancer. In this setting, newer biological agents typically targeting tyrosine receptor kinases or ligands activating the vascular endothelial or epidermal growth factor pathways are theoretically attractive. Until we have some indication of response of these patients in phase 1 trials or are able to better profile patients to determine their response, advice on and indeed indiscriminate use of these agents in patients with urethral cancer remains unwise.

Conclusion

Although embryologically the urethra comes from the same urogenital sinus as the bladder, tumors are more variable, though rare. Treatment also is more variable, based on anatomical location of the tumor and histology, which determines overall survival. Urethral cancers are usually reported in small case reports and therefore there is no clear standard of care. When possible, if the possibility of cure is not compromised, organ preservation should be the primary goal.

Acknowledgment

The authors wish to acknowledge contributors to prior editions including Oscar Streeter, Jocelyn Speight, Garth Green and Peter Nichols.

References

1. Srinivas V, Khan SA. Female urethral cancer – an overview. Int Urol Nephrol 1987; 19: 423–7.
2. Srinivas V, Khan SA. Male urethral cancer. A review. Int Urol Nephrol 1988; 20: 61–5.
3. Landis SH, Murray T, Bolden S, et al. Cancer statistics, 1999. CA Cancer J Clin 1999; 49: 8–31.
4. Swartz MA, Porter MP, Lin DW, et al. Incidence of primary urethral carcinoma in the United States. Urology 2006; 68: 1164–8.
5. Prasad SR, Menias CO, Narra VR, et al. Cross-sectional imaging of the female urethra. technique and results. Radiographics 2005; 25: 749–61.
6. Carroll PR, Dixon CM. Surgical anatomy of the male and female urethra. Urol Clin North Am 1992; 19: 339–46.
7. Terry PJ, Cookson MS, Sarosdy MF. Carcinoma of the urethra and scrotum. In: Raghavan D, Scher HI, Leibel SA, et al. (eds) *Principles and Practice of Genitourinary Oncology.* Philadelphia: Lippincott–Raven, 1997. pp 347–54.
8. Krieg R, Hoffman R. Current management of unusual genitourinary cancers. Part 2. Urethral cancer. Oncology (Williston Park) 1999; 13: 1511–7, 1520; discussion 1523–4.
9. Sullivan MP, Yalla SV. Physiology of female micturition. Urol Clin North Am 2002; 29: 499–514, vii.
10. Yiee JH, Baskin LS. Penile embryology and anatomy. Scient World J 2010; 10: 1174–9.
11. Mostofi FK, Davis CJ Jr, Sesterhenn IA. Carcinoma of the male and female urethra. Urol Clin North Am 1992; 19: 347–58.
12. Narayan P, Konety B. Surgical treatment of female urethral carcinoma. Urol Clin North Am 1992; 19: 373–82.
13. Meis JM, Ayala AG, Johnson DE. Adenocarcinoma of the urethra in women. A clinicopathologic study. Cancer 1987; 60: 1038–52.
14. Kaplan GW, Bulkey GJ, Grayhack JT. Carcinoma of the male urethra. J Urol 1967; 98: 365–71.
15. Bostwick DG, Lo R, Stamey TA. Papillary adenocarcinoma of the male urethra. Case report and review of the literature. Cancer 1984; 54: 2556–63.
16. Wiener JS, Liu ET, Walther PJ. Oncogenic human papillomavirus type 16 is associated with squamous cell cancer of the male urethra. Cancer Res 1992; 52: 5018–23.
17. Wiener JS, Walther PJ. A high association of oncogenic human papillomaviruses with carcinomas of the female urethra. Polymerase chain reaction-based analysis of multiple histological types. J Urol 1994; 151: 49–53.
18. Li N, Yang L, Zhang Y, et al. Human papillomavirus infection and bladder cancer risk. a meta-analysis. J Infect Dis 2011; 204: 217–23.
19. Moonen PM, Bakkers JM, Kiemeney LA, et al. Human papilloma virus DNA and p53 mutation analysis on bladder washes in relation to clinical outcome of bladder cancer. Eur Urol 2007; 52: 464–8.
20. Shigehara K, Sasagawa T, Kawaguchi S, et al. Etiologic role of human papillomavirus infection in bladder carcinoma. Cancer 2011; 117: 2067–76.
21. Vesa Llanes J, Domingo Ferrerons R, Muntane Hombrados MJ, et al. Inverted papilloma of the prostatic urethra. Histopathogenetic considerations. Arch Esp Urol 1994; 47: 1022–4.
22. Gheiler EL, Tefilli MV, Tiguert R, et al. Management of primary urethral cancer. Urology 1998; 52: 487–93.
23. Oliva E, Young RH. Clear cell adenocarcinoma of the urethra. A clinicopathologic analysis of 19 cases. Mod Pathol 1996; 9: 513–20.
24. Tsai YS, Yang WH, Tong YC, et al. Experience with primary urethral carcinoma from the blackfoot disease-endemic area of South Taiwan. Increased frequency of bulbomembranous adenocarcinoma? Urol Int 2005; 74: 229–34.
25. Thomas AA, Rackley RR, Lee U, et al. Urethral diverticula in 90 female patients. A study with emphasis on neoplastic alterations. J Urol 2008; 180: 2463–7.
26. Marshall PC, Uson AC, Melicow MM. Neoplasms and caruncles of the female urethra. Surg Gynecol Obstet 1960; 110: 723–33.
27. Dmochowski RR, Ganabathi K, Zimmern PE, et al. Benign female periurethral masses. J Urol 1994; 152: 1943–51.
28. Hayashi T, Igarashi K, Sekine H. Urethral hemangioma. Case report. J Urol 1997; 158: 539–40.
29. Scholl AJ, Braasch WF. Primary tumors of the urethra. Ann Surg 1922; 76.
30. Pacik D, Dolezel J, Skoumal R, et al. Very rare angioleiomyoma of the male urethra. Int Urol Nephrol 1993; 25: 479–84.
31. Costantini E, Cochetti G, Porena M. Vaginal para-urethral myxoid leiomyoma. Case report and review of the literature. Int Urogynecol J Pelvic Floor Dysfunct 2008; 19: 1183–5.
32. Ford TF, Watson GM, Cameron KM. Adenomatous metaplasia (nephrogenic adenoma) of urothelium. An analysis of 70 cases. Br J Urol 1985; 57: 427–33.
33. Rahemtullah A, Oliva E. Nephrogenic adenoma. An update on an innocuous but troublesome entity. Adv Anat Pathol 2006; 13: 247–55.
34. Mazal PR, Schaufler R, Altenhuber-Muller R, et al. Derivation of nephrogenic adenomas from renal tubular cells in kidney-transplant recipients. N Engl J Med 2002; 347: 653–9.
35. Young RH. Nephrogenic adenomas of the urethra involving the prostate gland. A report of two cases of a lesion that may be confused with prostatic adenocarcinoma. Mod Pathol 1992; 5: 617–20.
36. Tong GX, Melamed J, Mansukhani M, et al. PAX2. A reliable marker for nephrogenic adenoma. Mod Pathol 2006; 19: 356–63.
37. Berger BW, Bhagavan SB, Reiner W, et al. Nephrogenic adenoma. Clinical features and therapeutic considerations. J Urol 1981; 126: 824–6.
38. Bhagavan BS, Tiamson EM, Wenk RE, et al. Nephrogenic adenoma of the urinary bladder and urethra. Hum Pathol 1981; 12: 907–16.
39. Carcamo Valor PI, San Millan Arruti JP, Cozar Olmo JM, et al. Nephrogenic adenoma of the upper and lower urinary tract. Apropos of 22 cases. Arch Esp Urol 1992; 45: 423–7.
40. Peterson LJ, Matsumoto LM. Nephrogenic adenoma in urethral diverticulum. Urology 1978; 11: 193–5.
41. Klutke CG, Akdman EI, Brown JJ. Nephrogenic adenoma arising from a urethral diverticulum. Magnetic resonance features. Urology 1995; 45: 323–5.

42. Medeiros LJ, Young RH. Nephrogenic adenoma arising in urethral diverticula. A report of five cases. Arch Pathol Lab Med 1989; 113: 125–8.

43. Miyake O, Hara T, Matsumiya K, *et al.* A case of nephrogenic adenoma in the female urethral diverticulum. Hinyokika Kiyo 1990; 36: 1189–92.

44. Pamplona M, Paniagua P, Gimeno F, *et al.* Nephrogenic adenoma in urethral diverticulum in women. Actas Urol Esp 1990; 14: 277–8.

45. Oliva E, Young RH. Nephrogenic adenoma of the urinary tract. A review of the microscopic appearance of 80 cases with emphasis on unusual features. Mod Pathol 1995; 8: 722–30.

46. Cheng CW, Chan LW, Chan CK, *et al.* Is surveillance necessary for inverted papilloma in the urinary bladder and urethra? Aust NZ J Surg 2005; 75: 213–17.

47. Fine SW, Chan TY, Epstein JI. Inverted papillomas of the prostatic urethra. Am J Surg Pathol 2006; 30: 975–9.

48. Sung MT, Maclennan GT, Lopez-Beltran A, *et al.* Natural history of urothelial inverted papilloma. Cancer 2006; 107: 2622–7.

49. Boyle M, Gaffney EF, Thurston A. Paraganglioma of the prostatic urethra. A report of three cases and a review of the literature. Br J Urol 1996; 77: 445–8.

50. Freedman SR, Goldman RL. Normal paraganglia in the human prostate. J Urol 1975; 113: 874–5.

51. Kiernan M, Gaffney EF. The endocrine-paracrine cells of von Brunn's nests and glandular metaplasia in the supramontanal prostatic urethra. Histopathology 1990; 16: 365–9.

52. Branson AD, Kiser WS, Gifford RW Jr, *et al.* Localized amyloidosis of the urethra. Report of a case. J Urol 1969; 101: 68–70.

53. Ichioka K, Utsunomiya N, Ueda N, *et al.* Primary localized amyloidosis of urethra. Magnetic resonance imaging findings. Urology 2004; 64: 376–8.

54. Provet JA, Mennen J, Sabatini M, *et al.* Primary amyloidosis of urethra. Urology 1989; 34: 106–8.

55. Brown RD, Mulhollan JA, Childers JH, *et al.* Localized amyloidosis of the urethra. Diagnostic implications and management. J Urol 1988; 140: 1536–8.

56. Roberts TW, Melicow MM. Pathology and natural history of urethral tumors in females. Review of 65 cases. Urology 1977; 10: 583–9.

57. Fry M, Wheeler JS Jr, Mata JA, *et al.* Leiomyoma of the female urethra. J Urol 1988; 140: 613–14.

58. Kato T, Kobayashi T, Ikeda R, *et al.* Urethral leiomyoma expressing estrogen receptors. Int J Urol 2004; 11: 573–5.

59. Kesari D, Gemer O, Segal S, *et al.* Estrogen receptors in a urethral leiomyoma presenting in pregnancy. Int J Gynaecol Obstet 1994; 47: 59–60.

60. Dasan JC, Rao K, Nalini V. Leiomyoma of the female urethra – a clinical curiosity. Int J Gynaecol Obstet 1989; 28: 381–3.

61. Bodker A, Balslev E, Juul BR, *et al.* Estrogen receptors in the human male bladder, prostatic urethra, and prostate. An immunohistochemical and biochemical study. Scand J Urol Nephrol 1995; 29: 161–5.

62. Ohtani M, Yanagizawa R, Shoji F, *et al.* Leiomyoma of the male urethra. Eur Urol 1982; 8: 372–3.

63. Ho KL, Hayden MT. Sarcoidosis of urethra simulating carcinoma. Urology 1979; 13: 197–9.

64. Cetti NE. Condyloma acuminatum of the urethra. Problems in eradication. Br J Surg 1984; 71: 57.

65. Kesner KM. Extensive condylomata acuminata of male urethra. Management by ventral urethrotomy. Br J Urol 1993; 71: 204–7.

66. Lindner HJ, Pasquier CM Jr. Condylomata acuminata of the urethra. J Urol 1954; 72: 875–9.

67. Redman JF, Meacham KR. Condyloma acuminata of the urethral meatus in children. J Pediatr Surg 1973; 8: 939–41.

68. Bissada NK, Cole AT, Fried FA. Extensive condylomas acuminata of the entire male urethra and the bladder. J Urol 1974; 112: 201–3.

69. Bissada NK, Redman JF, Sulieman JS. Condyloma acuminatum of male urethra. Successful management with 5-fluorouracil. Urology 1974; 3: 499–501.

70. Mininberg DT, Rudick DH. Urethral condyloma acuminata in male children. Pediatrics 1976; 57: 571–3.

71. Cardamakis E, Kotoulas IG, Metalinos K, *et al.* Treatment of urethral condylomata acuminata or flat condylomata with interferon-alpha 2a. J Urol 1994; 152: 2011–13.

72. Benoit G, Orth G, Vieillefond A, *et al.* Presence of papilloma virus type 11 in condyloma acuminatum of bladder in female renal transplant recipient. Urology 1988; 32: 343–4.

73. Asvesti C, Delmas V, Dauge-Geffroy MC, *et al.* Multiple condylomata of the urethra and bladder disclosing HIV infection. Ann Urol (Paris) 1991; 25: 146–9.

74. Pompeius R, Ekroth R. A successfully treated case of condyloma acuminatum of the urethra and urinary bladder. Eur Urol 1976; 2: 298–9.

75. Wallin J. 5-Fluorouracil in the treatment of penile and urethral condylomata acuminata. Br J Vener Dis 1977; 53: 240–3.

76. Libby JM, Frankel JM, Scardino PT. Condyloma acuminatum of the bladder and associated urothelial malignancy. J Urol 1985; 134: 134–6.

77. Noronha RF, Sundaram M. Are intraurethral condylomata premalignant? Br J Urol 1984; 56: 546–7.

78. Tanabe ET, Mazur MT, Schaeffer AJ. Clear cell adenocarcinoma of the female urethra. Clinical and ultrastructural study suggesting a unique neoplasm. Cancer 1982; 49: 372–8.

79. Assimos DG, O'Conor VJ. Clear cell adenocarcinoma of the urethra. J Urol 1984; 131: 540–1.

80. Young RH, Scully RE. Nephrogenic adenoma. A report of 15 cases, review of the literature, and comparison with clear cell adenocarcinoma of the urinary tract. Am J Surg Pathol 1986; 10: 268–75.

81. Hull MT, Eglen DE, Davis T, *et al.* Glycogen-rich clear cell carcinoma of the urethr. An ultrastructural studya. Ultrastruct Pathol 1987; 11: 421–7.

82. Kusuyama Y, Yoshida M, Uekado Y, *et al.* Clear cell adenocarcinoma of the female urethra. A case report. Acta Pathol Jpn 1988; 38: 217–23.

83. Ebisuno S, Miyai M, Nagareda T. Clear cell adenocarcinoma of the female urethra showing positive staining with antibodies to prostate-specific antigen and prostatic acid phosphatase. Urology 1995; 45: 682–5.

84. Seballos RM, Rich RR. Clear cell adenocarcinoma arising from a urethral diverticulum. J Urol 1995; 153: 1914–15.

85. Drew PA, Murphy WM, Civantos F, *et al.* The histogenesis of clear cell adenocarcinoma of the lower urinary tract. Case series and review of the literature. Hum Pathol 1996; 27: 248–52.

86. Dodson MK, Cliby WA, Keeney GL, *et al.* Skene's gland adenocarcinoma with increased serum level of prostate-specific antigen. Gynecol Oncol 1994; 55: 304–7.

87. Dodson MK, Cliby WA, Pettavel PP, *et al.* Female urethral adenocarcinoma. Evidence for more than one tissue of origin? Gynecol Oncol 1995; 59: 352–7.

88. Murphy DP, Pantuck AJ, Amenta PS, *et al.* Female urethral adenocarcinoma. Immunohistochemical evidence of more than 1 tissue of origin. J Urol 1999; 161: 1881–4.

89. Hartmann A, Junker K, Dietmaier W, *et al.* Molecular evidence for progression of nephrogenic metaplasia of the urinary bladder to clear cell adenocarcinoma. Hum Pathol 2006; 37: 117–20.

90. Tong GX, Weeden EM, Hamele-Bena D, *et al.* Expression of PAX8 in nephrogenic adenoma and clear cell adenocarcinoma of the lower urinary tract. Evidence of related histogenesis? Am J Surg Pathol 2008; 32: 1380–7.

91. Herawi M, Drew PA, Pan CC, *et al.* Clear cell adenocarcinoma of the bladder and urethra. Cases diffusely mimicking nephrogenic adenoma. Hum Pathol 2010; 41: 594–601.

92. Kahn DG, Rothman PJ, Weisman JD. Urethral T-cell lymphoma as the initial manifestation of the acquired immune deficiency syndrome. Arch Pathol Lab Med 1991; 115: 1169–70.

93. Selch MT, Mark RJ, Fu YS, *et al.* Primary lymphoma of female urethra. Long-term control by radiation therapy. Urology 1993; 42: 343–6.

94. Inuzuka S, Koga S, Imanishi D, *et al.* Primary malignant lymphoma of the female urethra. Anticancer Res 2003; 23: 2925–7.

95. Mordkin RM, Skinner DG, Levine AM. Long-term disease-free survival after plasmacytoma of the urethra. A case report and review of the literature. Urology 1996; 48: 149–50.

96. Campbell CM, Smith JA Jr, Middleton RG. Plasmacytoma of the urethra. J Urol 1982; 127: 986.

97. Mark JA, Pais VM, Chong FK. Plasmacytoma of the urethra treated with transurethral resection and radiotherapy. J Urol 1990; 143: 1010–1.

98. Witjes JA, de Vries JD, Schaafsma HE, et al. Extramedullary plasmacytoma of the urethra. A case report. J Urol 1991; 145: 826–8.

99. Lemos N, Melo CR, Soares IC, et al. Plasmacytoma of the urethra treated by excisional biopsy. Scand J Urol Nephrol 2000; 34: 75–6.

100. Kraus-Tiefenbacher U, Gutwein S, Hopner U, et al. Plasmocytoma of the urethra. Onkologie 2004; 27: 166–8.

101. Gokce O, Acar O, Tunc M, et al. Primary urethral plasmacytoma. A case report and literature review. Kaohsiung J Med Sci 2008; 24: 274–7.

102. Sylora HO, Diamond HM, Kaufman M, et al. Primary carcinoid tumor of the urethra. J Urol 1975; 114: 150–3.

103. Katayama M, Hara A, Hirose Y, et al. Carcinoid tumor in the female urethral orifice. Rare case report and a review of the literature. Pathol Int 2003; 53: 102–5.

104. Chen KT. Primary carcinoid tumor of the urethra. J Urol 2001; 166: 1831–2.

105. Murali R, Kneale K, Lalak N, et al. Carcinoid tumors of the urinary tract and prostate. Arch Pathol Lab Med 2006; 130: 1693–706.

106. Smith M, Lucia MS, Werahera PN, et al. Carcinoid tumor of the verumontanum (colliculus seminalis) of the prostatic urethra with a coexisting prostatic adenocarcinoma. a case report. J Med Case Reports 2010; 4: 16.

107. Chen YB, Epstein JI. Primary carcinoid tumors of the urinary bladder and prostatic urethra. A clinicopathologic study of 6 cases. Am J Surg Pathol 2011; 35: 442–6.

108. Buckle AE. Primary malignant melanoma of the female urethra. Br J Surg 1969; 56: 548–50.

109. Guinn GA, Ayala AG. Male urethral cancer. Report of 15 cases including a primary melanoma. J Urol 1970; 103: 176–9.

110. Geelhoed GW, Myers GH Jr. Primary melanoma of the male urethra. J Urol 1973; 109: 634–7.

111. Iyer KM, Shah AL, Bapat RD, et al. Primary malignant melanoma of the male urethra. Indian J Cancer 1974; 11: 213–14.

112. Morrow CP, DiSaia PJ. Malignant melanoma of the female genitalia. A clinical analysis. Obstet Gynecol Surv 1976; 31: 233–71.

113. Iversen K, Robins RE. Mucosal malignant melanomas. Am J Surg 1980; 139: 660–4.

114. Ariel IM. Malignant melanoma of the female genital system. A report of 48 patients and review of the literature. J Surg Oncol 1981; 16: 371–83.

115. Begun FP, Grossman HB, Diokno AC, et al. Malignant melanoma of the penis and male urethra. J Urol 1984; 132: 123–5.

116. Stein BS, Kendall AR. Malignant melanoma of the genitourinary tract. J Urol 1984; 132: 859–68.

117. Manivel JC, Fraley EE. Malignant melanoma of the penis and male urethra. 4 case reports and literature review. J Urol 1988; 139: 813–16.

118. Pow-Sang JM, Klimberg IW, Hackett RL, et al. Primary malignant melanoma of the male urethra. J Urol 1988; 139: 1304–6.

119. Kim CJ, Pak K, Hamaguchi A, et al. Primary malignant melanoma of the female urethra. Cancer 1993; 71: 448–51.

120. Rashid AM, Williams RM, Horton LW. Malignant melanoma of penis and male urethra. Is it a difficult tumor to diagnose? Urology 1993; 41: 470–1.

121. Aragona F, Maio G, Piazza R, et al. Primary malignant melanoma of the female urethra. A case report. Int Urol Nephrol 1995; 27: 107–11.

122. Radhi JM. Urethral malignant melanoma closely mimicking urothelial carcinoma. J Clin Pathol 1997; 50: 250–2.

123. Pandey M, Mathew A, Abraham EK, et al. Primary malignant melanoma of the mucous membranes. Eur J Surg Oncol 1998; 24: 303–7.

124. Oliva E, Quinn TR, Amin MB, et al. Primary malignant melanoma of the urethra. A clinicopathologic analysis of 15 cases. Am J Surg Pathol 2000; 24: 785–96.

125. DiMarco DS, DiMarco CS, Zincke H, et al. Outcome of surgical treatment for primary malignant melanoma of the female urethra. J Urol 2004; 171: 765–7.

126. Katz EE, Suzue K, Wille MA, et al. Primary malignant melanoma of the urethra. Urology 2005; 65: 389.

127. Sanchez-Ortiz R, Huang SF, Tamboli P, et al. Melanoma of the penis, scrotum and male urethra. A 40-year single institution experience. J Urol 2005; 173: 1958–65.

128. Van Geel AN, den Bakker MA, Kirkels W, et al. Prognosis of primary mucosal penile melanoma. A series of 19 Dutch patients and 47 patients from the literature. Urology 2007; 70: 143–7.

129. Lopez JI, Angulo JC, Ibanez T. Primary malignant melanoma mimicking urethral caruncle. Case report. Scand J Urol Nephrol 1993; 27: 125–6.

130. Nakamoto T, Inoue Y, Ueki T, et al. Primary amelanotic malignant melanoma of the female urethra. Int J Urol 2007; 14: 153–5.

131. Sugaya K, Yazaki T, Ishikawa S, et al. A case of amelanotic malignant melanoma of the female urethra. Jpn J Clin Oncol 1983; 13: 435–9.

132. Comploj E, Palermo S, Trenti E, et al. Unexpected long survival in primary malignant melanoma of the male urethra. Case Rep Dermatol 2009; 1: 93–9.

133. Altarac S, Papes D. Primary malignant melanoma of the female urethra. 10-year survival. Med Oncol 2011 Sep 3 [Epub ahead of print].

134. Lee RA, Dahlin DC. Paget's disease of the vulva with extension into the urethra, bladder, and ureters. A case report. Am J Obstet Gynecol 1981; 140: 834–6.

135. Begin LR, Deschenes J, Mitmaker B. Pagetoid carcinomatous involvement of the penile urethra in association with high-grade transitional cell carcinoma of the urinary bladder. Arch Pathol Lab Med 1991; 115: 632–5.

136. Damotte D, Chretien Y, Dufour B, et al. Paget's disease of the prostatic urethra revealing a bladder carcinoma. Histopathology 1998; 33: 492–4.

137. Tomaszewski JE, Korat OC, LiVolsi VA, et al. Paget's disease of the urethral meatus following transitional cell carcinoma of the bladder. J Urol 1986; 135: 368–70.

138. Fujisawa Y, Nakamura Y, Takahashi T, et al. Penile preservation surgery in a case of extramammary Paget's disease involving the glans penis and distal urethra. Dermatol Surg 2008; 34: 823–30; discussion 830–1.

139. Salazar G, Frable WJ. Extramammary Paget's disease. A case involving the prostatic urethra. Am J Clin Pathol 1969; 52: 607–12.

140. Kuettel MR, Parda DS, Harter KW, et al. Treatment of female urethral carcinoma in medically inoperable patients using external beam irradiation and high dose rate intracavitary brachytherapy. J Urol 1997; 157: 1669–71.

141. Cohen MS, Triaca V, Billmeyer B, et al. Coordinated chemoradiation therapy with genital preservation for the treatment of primary invasive carcinoma of the male urethra. J Urol 2008; 179: 536–41; discussion 541.

142. Karnes RJ, Breau RH, Lightner DJ. Surgery for urethral cancer. Urol Clin North Am 2010; 37: 445–57.

143. Leung YL, Lee F, Tam PC. Leiomyoma of female urethra causing acute urinary retention and acute renal failure. J Urol 1997; 158: 1911–12.

144. Greene FL, Page DL, Fleming ID, et al. Urethra, 6th edn. New York: Springer-Verlag, 2002.

145. Yachia D, Turani H. Colonic-type adenocarcinoma of male urethra. Urology 1991; 37: 568–70.

146. Elsayes KM, Mukundan G, Narra VR, et al. Endovaginal magnetic resonance imaging of the female urethra. J Comput Assist Tomogr 2006; 30: 1–6.

147. Wieczorek AP, Wozniak MM, Stankiewicz A, et al. 3-D high-frequency endovaginal ultrasound of female urethral complex and assessment of inter-observer reliability. Eur J Radiol 2010; 81: e7–e12.

148. Rabbani F. Prognostic factors in male urethral cancer. Cancer 2010; Dec 14 [Epub ahead of print].

149. Dann T, Schuller J, Schmeller NT, et al. Treatment of distal urethral cancer by laser coagulation. Urologe A 1989; 28: 296–9.

150. Staehler G, Chaussy C, Jocham D, et al. The use of neodymium-YAG lasers in urology. Indications, technique and critical assessment. J Urol 1985; 134: 1155–60.

151. Desgrandchamps F, Sergent B, Alamanis C, et al. Total extended ++urethrectomy and transureteral continent cystostomy in the treatment of urethral melanoma in women. Report of a case. Prog Urol 1995; 5: 720–3.

152. Larson DL, Bracken RB. Use of gracilis musculocutaneous flap in urologic cancer surgery. Urology 1982; 19: 148–51.

153. Zeidman EJ, Desmond P, Thompson IM. Surgical treatment of carcinoma of the male urethra. Urol Clin North Am 1992; 19: 359–72.

154. Bracken RB, Henry R, Ordonez N. Primary carcinoma of the male urethra. South Med J 1980; 73: 1003–5.

155. Hopkins SC, Nag SK, Soloway MS. Primary carcinoma of male urethra. Urology 1984; 23: 128–33.

156. Mandler JI, Pool TL. Primary carcinoma of the male urethra. J Urol 1966; 96: 67–72.

157. Ray B, Canto AR, Whitmore WF Jr. Experience with primary carcinoma of the male urethra. J Urol 1977; 117: 591–4.

158. Prempree T, Amornmarn R, Patanaphan V. Radiation therapy in primary carcinoma of the female urethra. II. An update on results. Cancer 1984; 54: 729–33.

159. Micaily B, Dzeda MF, Miyamoto CT, et al. Brachytherapy for cancer of the female urethra. Semin Surg Oncol 1997; 13: 208–14.

160. Klein FA, Ali MM, Kersh R. Carcinoma of the female urethra. Combined iridium Ir 192 interstitial and external beam radiotherapy. South Med J 1987; 80: 1129–32.

161. Antoniades J. Radiation therapy in carcinoma of the female urethra. Cancer 1969; 24: 70–6.

162. Weghaupt K, Gerstner GJ, Kucera H. Radiation therapy for primary carcinoma of the female urethra. A survey over 25 years. Gynecol Oncol 1984; 17: 58–63.

163. Heysek RV, Parsons JT, Drylie DM, et al. Carcinoma of the male urethra. J Urol 1985; 134: 753–5.

164. Eisenberger MA. Chemotherapy for carcinomas of the penis and urethra. Urol Clin North Am 1992; 19: 333–8.

165. Flam M, John M, Pajak TF, et al. Role of mitomycin in combination with fluorouracil and radiotherapy, and of salvage chemoradiation in the definitive nonsurgical treatment of epidermoid carcinoma of the anal canal. results of a phase III randomized intergroup study. J Clin Oncol 1996; 14: 2527–39.

166. Green JA, Kirwan JM, Tierney JF, et al. Survival and recurrence after concomitant chemotherapy and radiotherapy for cancer of the uterine cervix. A systematic review and meta-analysis. Lancet 2001; 358: 781–6.

167. Ryan DP, Compton CC, Mayer RJ. Carcinoma of the anal canal. N Engl J Med 2000; 342: 792–800.

168. Sternberg CN, Yagoda A, Scher HI, et al. M-VAC (methotrexate, vinblastine, doxorubicin and cisplatin) for advanced transitional cell carcinoma of the urothelium. J Urol 1988; 139: 461–9.

169. Von der Maase H, Hansen SW, Roberts JT, et al. Gemcitabine and cisplatin versus methotrexate, vinblastine, doxorubicin, and cisplatin in advanced or metastatic bladder cancer. Results of a large, randomized, multinational, multicenter, phase III study. J Clin Oncol 2000; 18: 3068–77.

170. Kachnic LA, Kaufman DS, Heney NM, et al. Bladder preservation by combined modality therapy for invasive bladder cancer. J Clin Oncol 1997; 15: 1022–9.

171. Hussain M, Vaishampayan U, Du W, et al. Combination paclitaxel, carboplatin, and gemcitabine is an active treatment for advanced urothelial cancer. J Clin Oncol 2001; 19: 2527–33.

172. Hussain M, Vaishampayan U, Smith DC. Novel gemcitabine-containing triplets in the management of urothelial cancer. Semin Oncol 2002; 29: 20–4.

173. De Wit R. Overview of bladder cancer trials in the European Organization for Research and Treatment. Cancer 2003; 97: 2120–6.

174. Bosset JF, Calais G, Mineur L, et al. Enhanced tumorocidal effect of chemotherapy with preoperative radiotherapy for rectal cancer. Preliminary results – EORTC 22921. J Clin Oncol 2005; 23: 5620–7.

175. Sauer R, Becker H, Hohenberger W, et al. Preoperative versus Postoperative chemoradiotherapy for rectal cancer. N Engl J Med 2004; 351: 1731–40.

176. Cunningham D, Humblet Y, Siena S, et al. Cetuximab monotherapy and cetuximab plus irinotecan in irinotecan-refractory metastatic colorectal cancer. N Engl J Med 2004; 351: 337–45.

177. Hurwitz H, Fehrenbacher L, Novotny W, et al. Bevacizumab plus irinotecan, fluorouracil, and leucovorin for metastatic colorectal cancer. N Engl J Med 2004; 350: 2335–42.

178. Lutz ST, Huang DT. Combined chemoradiotherapy for locally advanced squamous cell carcinoma of the bulbomembranous urethra. A case report. J Urol 1995; 153: 1616–18.

179. Tran LN, Krieg RM, Szabo RJ. Combination chemotherapy and radiotherapy for a locally advanced squamous cell carcinoma of the urethra. A case report. J Urol 1995; 153: 422–3.

180. Hussein AM, Benedetto P, Sridhar KS. Chemotherapy with cisplatin and 5-fluorouracil for penile and urethral squamous cell carcinomas. Cancer 1990; 65: 433–8.

181. Lee KC. Carcinoma of the female urethra responsive to moderate dose chemoradiotherapy. J Urol 2000; 163: 905–6.

182. Edge SB, Byrd DR. *AJCC Cancer Staging Manual*, 7th edn. New York: Springer, 2010.

183. Pointon RC, Poole-Wilson DS. Primary carcinoma of the urethra. Br J Urol 1968; 40: 682–93.

184. Dinney CP, Johnson DE, Swanson DA, et al. Therapy and prognosis for male anterior urethral carcinoma. An update. Urology 1994; 43: 506–14.

185. Dalbagni G, Zhang ZF, Lacombe L, et al. Male urethral carcinoma. Analysis of treatment outcome. Urology 1999; 53: 1126–32.

186. Thyavihally YB, Wuntkal R, Bakshi G, et al. Primary carcinoma of the female urethra. Single center experience of 18 cases. Jpn J Clin Oncol 2005; 35: 84–7.

187. Garden AS, Zagars GK, Delclos L. Primary carcinoma of the female urethra. Results of radiation therapy. Cancer 1993; 71: 3102–8.

188. Grigsby PW. Carcinoma of the urethra in women. Int J Radiat Oncol Biol Phys 1998; 41: 535–41.

189. Dalbagni G, Zhang ZF, Lacombe L, et al. Female urethral carcinoma. An analysis of treatment outcome and a plea for a standardized management strategy. Br J Urol 1998; 82: 835–41.

190. Milosevic MF, Warde PR, Banerjee D, et al. Urethral carcinoma in women. Results of treatment with primary radiotherapy. Radiother Oncol 2000; 56: 29–35.

191. Dimarco DS, Dimarco CS, Zincke H, et al. Surgical treatment for local control of female urethral carcinoma. Urol Oncol 2004; 22: 404–9.

4 Uncommon Cancers of the Prostate

Scott T. Tagawa,[1,2,4] Naveed H. Akhtar,[1] Brian D. Robinson,[3,4] and Himisha Beltran[1]

[1] Division of Hematology and Medical Oncology, Department of Medicine, [2] Department of Urology, [3] Department of Pathology, Weill Cornell Medical College of Cornell University, New York, NY, USA
[4] Weill Cornell Cancer Center, New York, NY, USA

Introduction

The prostate is an exocrine organ present in all mammals, normally weighing 20–25 g in an adult male.[1,2] It is derived from the urogenital sinus, with growth directed by dihydrotestosterone during the third month of fetal growth. Epithelial buds invade the mesenchyme to develop into the prostate, forming the various zones. There are three predominant cell types making up prostatic tissue: luminal epithelial cells, basal cells, and neuroendocrine (NE) cells. Stromal cells and prostatic tissue matrix are also important parts of the prostatic milieu for normal development and function, as well as malignant processes.

Unlike some of the other accessory sexual glands in men, the prostate is frequently involved with hyperplasia and malignancy.[1] The most common malignancy of the prostate, by far, is adenocarcinoma. This cancer, the most common in men other than basal cell and squamous carcinomas of the skin, is also a leading cause of cancer death, resulting in over 28,170 deaths in the United States in 2012.[3] However, there are other malignancies affecting this organ that are less uncommon.

This chapter reviews four major uncommon primary cancers of the prostate: neuroendocrine prostate cancer (NEPC), sarcoma, urothelial carcinoma (UC), and lymphoma. In each section, we will review the pathology of the disease, discuss the clinical presentation and diagnostic points, review prognosis and treatment options, and conclude with our recommendations.

Neuroendocrine prostate cancer

The epithelial compartment of the normal prostate gland is composed of basal cells, secretory (luminal) epithelial cells, and NE cells. Prostate adenocarcinoma or prostate cancer (PC) shows features of secretory cells. Basal cells are androgen insensitive and have recently been shown to display stem cell features. The physiological role of NE cells in the normal prostate is not well established, but they are thought to be involved in regulation of epithelial cell growth and differentiation. NE cells contain dense-core cytoplasmic granules that store peptide hormones and prohormones, including chromogranin A (CgA), neuron-specific enolase (NSE), chromogranin B, somatostatin, bombesin, and calcitonin gene family peptides (calcitonin, katacalcin, and calcitonin gene-related peptide).[4,5] Normal prostatic NE cells lack the proliferation-associated Ki-67 antigen, are considered differentiated postmitotic cells, and do not express p63 or prostate-specific antigen (PSA). They lack androgen receptor (AR) expression, and are thus androgen insensitive.

Neuroendocrine prostate cancer, sometimes termed anaplastic PC, is an aggressive subtype of PC characterized by a morphology composed of small blue round cells, similar to small cell carcinomas of other primary sites. These tumors frequently do not express AR,[6] have modest elevation of PSA, markers of NE differentiation (i.e. NSE and chromogranin A) and metastasize frequently. *De novo* NEPC is considered uncommon, representing <1% of newly diagnosed PCs. However, secondary NEPC arising after therapy of prostate adenocarcinoma is more common and may represent a significant proportion of late-stage PCs. Primary and secondary NEPC can look and act similarly, and molecular analyses suggest that they have similar molecular profiles. Focal NE differentiation can be seen in 5–10% of localized PCs, and this proportion rises with disease progression.[7] The amount of NE differentiation in prostate tumors correlates with the rate of tumor progression, adverse outcome, and with surrogate markers of adverse outcome (such as tumor grade and stage).[8,9] NE cells may also contribute to a significant percentage of PCs developing resistance to hormonal therapy. Elevated serum chromogranin A levels are associated with worse survival in men with metastatic PC, adding prognostic information to clinical stage and Gleason grade.[10] These tumors are highly aggressive, with nearly all patients dying within 1 year of diagnosis.

Textbook of Uncommon Cancer, Fourth Edition. Edited by Derek Raghavan, Charles D. Blanke, David H. Johnson, Paul L. Moots, Gregory H. Reaman, Peter G. Rose and Mikkael A. Sekeres.

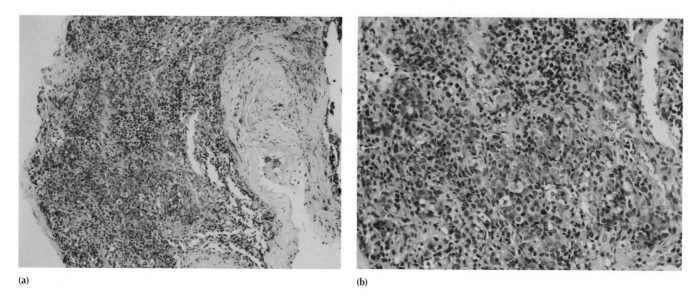

(a)   (b)

Figure 4.1 Neuroendocrine prostate cancer. Low- (a) and high-power (b) views of NEPC showing sheets of densely packed cells with nuclear molding, increased nucleus:cytoplasm (N:C) ratio, coarse chromatin, and irregular nuclear membranes.

Pathology

As initially reported in the literature, NEPC was associated with clinical syndromes suggesting ectopic hormone production, thus focusing histopathological study on particular morphological and functional features consistent with NE differentiation. For more than 60 years, it has been recognized that endocrine-paracrine cells (argentaffin or argyrophil staining) are present in the normal and hyperplastic prostate gland.[11–13]

The amount of NE differentiation increases during progression of prostate adenocarcinoma, and can progress to a predominantly neuroendocrine phenotype that may sometimes become indistinguishable from *de novo* NEPC.

Pathologically, NEPC is characterized by sheets and nests of uniform cells almost devoid of specific cell-to-cell orientation. At best, there is some focal suggestion of perivascular or peripheral palisading along the epithelial–stromal interfaces but more typically, no such arrangement is apparent. Microscopic or larger foci of tumor necrosis are prominent, as is the "streaming effect" of hematoxyphilic debris. The tumor infiltrates widely and diffusely in a lymphoma-like fashion with poorly circumscribed margins at the advancing edge. Lymphatic and blood vessel permeation is usually evident, and small tumor emboli may be seen at a distance from the infiltrating edge of the carcinoma. The stroma between the tumor islands is immature and fibroblastic. Remnants of normal prostatic tissue may be seen, entrapped or encircled by the carcinoma. Figure 4.1 demonstrates the pathological representation of NEPC.

Cytologically, the small uniform cells have rounded hyperchromatic nuclei, coarse chromatin, and usually absent or inconspicuous nucleoli. Mitotic figures are numerous, occurring at a rate of 5–10 per high-power field in most regions. The cytoplasm is scanty and, in many areas, the nuclei appear "naked." Mucin stains are negative, while argyrophil granules (Grimelius technique) are variably present. Argentaffin

granules are usually not observed (Fontana–Masson method). The electron microscopic features of NEPC are similar to those of small cell carcinomas occurring at other sites, and include typical small (140–250 nm), roughly circular neurosecretory dense-core granules.[14,15] Small, well-formed desmosomes have been described in at least one clinical study[16] and this observation has been confirmed in xenograft studies.

Immunohistochemical (IHC) staining is often positive for NE elements (NSE, synaptophysin, and chromogranin) and sometimes other various polypeptide hormones (including adrenocorticotropic hormone [ACTH], antidiuretic hormone [ADH], and corticotropin-releasing factor [CRF]). IHC is often negative for classic markers of prostatic glandular differentiation (PSA and prostatic acid phosphatase [PAP]). In tumors that are progressing from prostate adenocarcinoma to NEPC, mixed histologies and IHC profiles can be seen even within the same tumor focus. In those tumors with a mixed pattern, the adenocarcinoma is of the moderately to poorly differentiated microacinar or cribriform type, with intermingling of tumor elements and transitional areas.

We regard identification of an adenocarcinoma component as an important confirmation that the tumor has arisen in the prostate, although it is not an absolute requirement for the diagnosis of NEPC. If not present, NEPC can be confirmed as prostatic in origin by performing fluorescent *in situ* hybridization (FISH) breakapart assay to evaluate for the *TMPRSS2-ERG* gene fusion. However, if FISH is negative, this does not rule out prostatic origin since fusion is present in only half of NEPC. Even when fusion is positive, IHC staining for Erg is often negative (since Erg expression is driven by AR and NEPC is not). Therefore, FISH is preferred over IHC to evaluate for *TMPRSS2-ERG* gene fusion in NEPC.

Just as small cell carcinoma of the lung was thought to arise from the so-called bronchial K cells,[17] the histologically similar NEPC was initially considered to arise from this type of cell.[18] However, recent studies have shown that there is likely a similar cell of origin of NEPC and prostate adenocarcinoma. The PC-specific *TMPRSS2-ERG* gene fusion is present in approximately 50% of NEPC as well as prostate adenocarcinoma, and there is concordance of fusion in mixed tumors. This distinguishes NEPC from small cell carcinomas from other primary sites, and suggests that the pathogenesis may be different. Since the upstream genes commonly involved in *ERG* gene rearrangements are androgen regulated (e.g. TMPRSS2), the downstream Erg protein expression is limited only to the adenocarcinoma component of mixed tumors. Thus, *ERG* fusion-positive NEPC is AR negative and Erg protein negative.

It has also been suggested that the neuropeptides released by NE cells in the prostate may facilitate the development of androgen independence, acting as autocrine and paracrine growth factors for malignant cells. In PC cells, neuropeptides have been shown to promote cell growth, migration and protease expression.[19] For instance, the neuropeptides bombesin and gastrin-releasing peptide (GRP) transmit their signals through G protein-coupled receptors, which are often overexpressed in PC and can aberrantly activate androgen receptor (AR) in the absence of androgen.[20]

Expression of tumor markers

Polypeptide hormones constitute the major biochemical markers of NEPC, exhibiting features characteristic of the endocrine-paracrine cells described above (so-called amine precursor uptake and decarboxylation [APUD] cells). The production of these hormones is associated morphologically with argyrophil staining or, at an ultrastructural level, with the presence of the neurosecretory granules. A range of peptide hormones is produced, including the chromogranins, calcitonin, an immunoreactive parathyroid hormone (PTH)-like substance, and a thyroid-stimulating hormone (TSH)-like substance. However, even in classic adenocarcinoma of the prostate, hypercalcemia has been reported, which may be due to the production of an immunoreactive PTH-like substance.[21] Further evidence for the overlap between classic adenocarcinoma and NEPC has been provided by Pruneri *et al.*,[22] who immunohistochemically documented the production of chromogranin A, chromogranin B, and secretogranin II in more than half of a series of 64 patients with classic adenocarcinoma of the prostate. They identified a correlation between these neurocrine hormones and the areas of poor differentiation, although in this small series they did not find obvious correlations between the expression of these peptides and the ultimate prognosis.

To date, ACTH appears to be the most common ectopic hormone in NEPC, usually identified only on the basis of biochemical, immunohistochemical, or endocrinological tests,[14,23–25] although occasionally presenting with a variant of Cushing syndrome. ADH production has also been described in association with NEPC,[26,27] and there has been a case report of metastatic NEPC that elaborated corticotropin.[28] A xenografted NEPC cell line from Raghavan *et al.* has been shown to produce low levels of bombesin-like immunoreactivity and of somatostatin.[29]

Neuron-specific enolase, an enzyme of anaerobic glycolysis that is present in NE cells, has been extensively reported as a marker of small cell carcinoma of the lung. Its expression has been found to vary with both the proliferative state and the level of oxygenation of bronchogenic NE cancer.[30] There tends to be discordance of expression between NSE and the classic prostate markers. For example, Ghandur-Mnaymneh *et al.*[26] reported that NSE was expressed in pure NEPC, none of which stained for PSA or PAP, an observation confirmed by Ro *et al.*[15] Conversely, Ro *et al.* have described one case of NEPC that stained for PSA and PAP but did not express NSE.[15] In mixed tumors, the adenocarcinoma components do not stain for NSE whereas approximately 50% of tumors express this antigen in regions of NE differentiation.[26]

Other tumor markers have been reported in cases of NEPC, although their clinical utility appears limited. For example, carcinoembryonic antigen (CEA) has been demonstrated in up to 25% of classic PCs,[31,32] but is not a specific marker. Its expression has been correlated with decreasing differentiation of the adenocarcinoma cells.[31,33] In a detailed xenograft study, the authors of the previous chapter have shown marked heterogeneity of expression of CEA (representing about 25% of cells), in contrast to nearly uniform immunohistochemical staining of cells for NSE and epithelial membrane antigen (EMA).[29,34] This further illustrates the limitations of CEA as a potential marker of NEPC.

Another marker, calcitonin, was evaluated retrospectively in 16 patients with widely metastatic small cell carcinoma of the prostate (five pure NEPC and 11 combined with adenocarcinoma). Nine of 16 (56%) had elevated serum calcitonin level (range 42–2654 pg mL^{-1}), which chemically supported the diagnosis of NEPC. Survival analysis by log-rank test did not show a statistically significant prognostic value of serum calcitonin. However, patients with extremely high serum calcitonin level tended to have poor survival.[35]

Epithelial membrane antigen is expressed in normal prostate cells[36] and is seen focally in up to 80% of prostate adenocarcinomas, although its presence does not correlate with histological grade.[31,32] It is not found on cells of normal endocrine tissue or in classic NE tumors, but has been reported to be expressed by certain NE cancers of the lung.[36]

As noted previously, although PSA and PAP are not usually expressed in foci of NEPC, they may be detected immunohistochemically in coexistent regions of adenocarcinoma. By contrast, these markers have been reported in both the adenocarcinoma and carcinoid components of prostatic carcinoid tumors.[37–39] However, it is also possible that this distribution may be inaccurate, reflecting the artifacts of the immunohistochemical techniques used in the early 1980s, before the availability of monoclonal antibodies and some of the sophisticated controls that are routinely applied today.

Cases of NEPC have been described in which no ectopic hormone production has been detected.[16,40,41] Furthermore, in several cases in which ectopic hormone production is thought to have occurred, the diagnosis has merely been presumptive, on the basis of biochemical changes (e.g. hypokalemic alkalosis) or autopsy data (adrenal hyperplasia).[42–44]

Clinical application of tumor markers

In clinical practice, the role of neuroendocrine markers in the serum and in tissue has been restricted predominantly to diagnosis, and in particular to the more detailed characterization of undifferentiated tumors. The demonstration of increased serum levels of NSE or chromogranin may suggest the presence of occult elements of NE differentiation in a patient thought to suffer from a classic high-grade adenocarcinoma of the prostate. Because early recognition of this clinical entity seems important (see below), one should have a low threshold for checking levels of these better-defined markers, which may indicate the presence of clinically important NE components. However, in contrast to the serial measurement of blood levels of α-fetoprotein and human chorionic gonadotropin in the management of germ cell and trophoblastic tumors, CEA and NSE appear to have little role in monitoring the clinical course of NEPC as they often correlate poorly with the changing level of tumor burden.

Angelsen *et al.*[45] have studied the serum and tissue expression of NE markers in a series of 22 cases of PC, with tissue specimens obtained by transurethral resection (and thus subject to some geographical selection bias). They correlated tissue and blood levels of PSA, NSE, chromogranin A, and chromogranin B, and found significant discordance of expression. In their study, none of the patients had elevated blood levels of NSE, despite the presence of NSE-positive tumor cells in 77% of the tumors. However, a positive correlation was identified between the number of chromogranin A staining cells and the serum values of chromogranin A, although the number of cases was relatively small.[45] Other investigators have suggested that chromogranin A and/or NSE may be markers of prognosis in patients with adenocarcinoma of the prostate.[46–49] However, clearly more prospective data are needed before clinical decisions can be made on this basis alone.

The potential role of monitoring ectopic hormone levels has not yet been defined in this context. It is not clear whether their presence (or their corresponding clinical syndromes) acts as an adverse prognostic determinant *per se*, although several cases of NEPC with ectopic hormone production have been characterized by short survival. However, this may simply be a function of tumor volume, with larger tumors producing sufficient quantities of these hormones to allow detection in the circulation.

Molecular alterations in neuroendocrine prostate cancer

Gene expression profiling and assessment of DNA copy number alterations comparing prostate adenocarcinoma and NEPC has revealed dramatic gene expression and copy number differences.[50,51] Neural developmental genes and G2/M phase cell cycle genes are significantly upregulated in NEPC, and AR signaling and luminal epithelial genes are decreased.[50,51] *EZH2*, a polycomb gene associated with tumor aggressiveness in several tumor types including prostate,[52] is also upregulated in NEPC. The *TMPRSS2-ERG* prostate cancer-specific gene fusion is present in approximately 50% of NEPC,[53–56] similar to the frequency in prostate adenocarcinoma,[55] suggesting a

similar cell of origin and distinguishing NEPC from small cell carcinoma of other primary sites. The frequency of less common PC gene fusions in NEPC is unknown. The genes encoding Aurora kinase A (*AURKA*) and N-myc (*MYCN*) have also been shown to be overexpressed and coamplified in 40% of NEPC and 5% of prostate adenocarcinomas and have been shown to cooperate to promote the NE phenotype in preclinical models.[50]

Neuroendocrine prostate cancer models

The NCI-H660 cell line was derived from a lymph node metastasis of a patient with pure NEPC, initially thought to be small cell lung cancer but later classified as prostate. It is also one of few PC cells lines that harbor the *TMPRSS2-ERG* gene fusion. The PC3 cell line, derived from an androgen-independent bone metastasis, has also recently been characterized as NEPC, lacking PSA and AR and expressing NE and stem cell markers. Prostate adenocarcinoma LNCaP cells can transdifferentiate into NE-like cells in response to androgen deprivation or other cytokine exposure *in vitro*.[57] This line has been used to study the relationship between hormone suppression and outgrowth of NE cells, and appears to suggest that the change in histology reflects an induction of NE differentiation by hormonal deprivation.[58]

Patient-derived and serially passaged NEPC xenograft models such as UCRU-PR-2,[59] MDA 146.10 and MDA 155.2,[51] LTL-352[60] and others are valuable tools for exploring genomic mutations as well as testing new drugs *in vivo*. These xenografts have all been described as morphologically consistent with NEPC with NE marker expression and lack of PSA and androgen receptor. In addition, the transgenic TRAMP mouse model of PC may lend itself to the detailed characterization of the progression towards NEPC.[61,62]

Flow cytometry has shown UCRU-PR-2 to be consistently diploid.[63] The karyotype was hypodiploid with nonrandom losses of chromosomes 6, 7, 10, and 13, and with structural rearrangements of chromosomes 1 and 2,[64] demonstrating the characteristics of prostatic adenocarcinoma (deletion of chromosome 10) and a similarity of the 1p+ chromosome that has been reported in some samples of bronchogenic small cell lung cancer. The Australian team of investigators postulated that this line might exhibit stem cell function with variable differentiation, which could be elicited by implantation of tumors at different physical sites, but were unable to demonstrate any such changes in differentiation in tumors growing at different sites.[34]

Histogenesis

To date, the histogenesis of NEPC has been controversial and several different theories exist. NE cells are scattered throughout the prostate gland and prostatic epithelium, including ducts and acini.[65] Although NE cells are a constant feature of the prostatic ducts and periurethral region, they seem to disappear from normal peripheral prostate tissue during childhood and return at puberty, although the basis of this fluctuation is not known.[66] It was suggested that NEPC is derived from the neural crest line/APUD cell system.[67] This

Table 4.1 Neuroendocrine prostate cancer clinical summary.*

Series	Median age (range)	Presence of AdCa (%)	Ectopic hormone production	Liver metastases	Bone metastases	Initial transient response to hormonal therapy	Comments
Historical*	66 (49–89)	62%	9 of 14 case reports	41%	52%	60%	References 14–16, 23, 26, 40, 43, 44, 63, 75, 76, 82, 378
WCMC 2011[†]	74 (50–89)	100%[†]	NR	48%	93%	100%	Median survival 17 months

AdCa, adenocarcinoma; NR, not reported.

* Adapted from Tagawa ST *et al.* Uncommon cancers of the prostate. In: Raghavan D *et al.* (eds) *Textbook of Uncommon Cancer*, 3rd edn. New York: Wiley & Sons, 2006.

[†] Series of patients with metastatic PC treated with hormonal therapy with subsequent clinical diagnosis of NEPC

was not confirmed by the embryological studies that showed an endodermal origin.[68] Another common theory is the progression of typical adenocarcinoma to NEPC as a product of final dedifferentiation according to the model of divergent differentiation.[69] A third theory presents a direct stem cell origin for NEPC based on the lack of immunohistological staining for PSA, lack of androgen receptor positivity, and high MIB-1 labeling.[70]

In the majority of reported cases, the identification of NE elements is preceded by adenocarcinoma, often involving an interval of several years. Whether the production of polypeptide hormones is attributed to an endodermal or neuroectodermal origin, this index of functional differentiation is most easily explained by origin from a pluripotential stem cell. Whatever the histogenesis, it is clear that NEPC is often intimately associated with elements of adenocarcinoma. Thus, the formulation of a plan of management, both diagnostic and therapeutic, should take into account the presence of tumor cells with a wide range of potential functional characteristics. Furthermore, the paradigms of management of classic adenocarcinoma of the prostate may require modification, as it appears likely that NEPC has previously been underdiagnosed, and may well account for a proportion of "resistant" prostatic adenocarcinomas.

Clinical presentation

Extrapulmonary small cell carcinomas (SCC) have presented a diagnostic and therapeutic challenge to oncologists since their first description by Duguid and Kennedy in 1930.[71] Although sometimes misdiagnosed as metastatic small cell lung carcinoma, small cell anaplastic carcinomas and NEPC share many of the same characteristics; they are extremely aggressive, metastasize early and often, and do not respond to many traditional chemotherapeutic regimens. Estimated to comprise only 0.1–0.4% of all common forms of cancer and 2–4% of all small cell carcinomas,[72] rarity adds to difficulties in their diagnosis and treatment.

The malignant capacity of NEPC leads to metastasis more often to soft tissues, lung, and liver than to bone. Dauge and Delmas found the degree of aggressive behavior to be directly proportional to the extent of NE differentiation.[73] Metastasis to rare sites such as the pericardium has also been reported.

In contrast to adenocarcinoma of the prostate, NEPC can present with metastatic disease to the bone that is purely lytic. Patients with NEPC more frequently present with metastatic disease, tend to have a greater proportion of brain metastases, and are younger than patients with prostatic adenocarcinoma. The aggressive nature of SCC is evident by a median survival of 5.2 months after primary diagnosis. Concomitant adenocarcinoma can be present elsewhere in the prostate gland of patients with NEPC, and serum PSA and PAP levels may be elevated in this disease.

In the past, the prospective clinical diagnosis of NEPC was rarely made, with the majority of cases diagnosed either late in the course of the disease or at autopsy. More recently, there has been an increasing level of prospective histological recognition of this entity, thus presenting the cases for management at a point at which treatment decisions can affect outcome. As shown in Table 4.1, there are many similarities to the presentation of classic adenocarcinoma of prostate, whether antecedent or concomitant adenocarcinoma is present.

The population of patients consists of males, predominantly in the age range 60–80 years, often with features of local and distant involvement.[14,15,74–81] The presenting symptoms include urinary outflow obstruction, frequency, perineal pain or discomfort, nocturia, hematuria, and occasionally, rectal symptoms due to the effects of the enlarged prostate. A common feature that distinguishes NEPC from classic adenocarcinoma clinically may be the relative paucity of osseous involvement. Although bone metastases may occur with NEPC, it is more common for this entity to demonstrate a predominance of lymph node, pulmonary, hepatic, brain, and soft tissue involvement. We have recently reviewed our cases at Weill Cornell Medical College of clinically and/or pathologically diagnosed cases of NEPC arising from prior adenocarcinoma after hormonal therapy. As seen in Table 4.1, this population may be slightly older and with a higher proportion of bone metastases as might be suspected for a population presenting with metastatic PC treated with hormonal therapy. Nevertheless, liver involvement is common and median survival may be as short as 7.7 months from the time of NEPC diagnosis for some subsets.

Many patients present with neurological symptoms in association with unrecognized brain metastasis, rarely seen in adenocarcinoma of the prostate.[82] McCutcheon *et al.* reviewed

38 patients with antemortem intracerebral metastasis found on a review of 7994 PC patients treated over an 18-year period, noting that SCC comprised 0.5% of the patient cohort but 26% of patients with brain metastasis.[83] All patients with NEPC originally presented with stage D disease in comparison to only half of the adenocarcinoma patients; they tended to have greater numbers of brain metastases and were younger than patients with adenocarcinoma. Surprisingly, patients with brain metastases of pure adenocarcinoma had lower mean survival even though they originally presented at a lower stage of disease than those with NEPC.

Paraneoplastic syndromes occur in 10% of patients with SCC of the prostate. These syndromes include thyrotoxicosis, inappropriate ADH production, hypercalcemia, and adrenal hyperfunction. Ectopic production of thyroxine causing thyrotoxicosis and ultimately death has been reported.[78] In these instances, biochemical disturbances such as hypokalemic alkalosis or hyponatremia have required treatment if recognized in time. In one case, the presenting feature of hypokalemic alkalosis was an acute psychosis,[44] although the usual metabolic abnormalities are more classically associated with clouding of consciousness, constipation, anorexia, and malaise.

Diagnosis

Perhaps the most important prerequisite for the correct diagnosis of NEPC is initial awareness of the entity. In the patient with an unusual presentation of PC or the presence of an apparent paraneoplastic syndrome, the appropriate physical examination and biochemical tests, such as measurement of NSE, chromogranin A, calcitonin, or ACTH, may help establish the diagnosis. Electrolyte abnormalities, including hyponatremia, and the presence of hypercalcemia may suggest the diagnosis. It should be noted that patients with ectopic ACTH production may not show classic Cushing syndrome, and may appear cachexic and pigmented.

The diagnosis of NEPC is primarily based on morphology, though immunohistochemistry can support or confirm the diagnosis. Typically, one or more of NE markers, chromogranin A, synaptophysin, NSE, and CD56 are positive by immunohistochemistry. In a minority of cases (10%), NE markers are all negative but the morphology still supports the diagnosis. Again, immunohistochemistry is typically negative for AR, PSA, and PAP, distinguishing NEPC from conventional prostate adenocarcinoma. The presence of the prostate-specific *ERG* gene fusion by FISH breakapart occurs in approximately 50% of NEPC, which rules out small cell carcinoma from other primary sites.[84,85]

Prostate-specific antigen level should also be measured in the blood as it may reflect the presence of a component of adenocarcinoma. In fact, from xenograft studies, it appears likely that NEPC itself may release low levels of PAP.[63] The demonstration of modest elevations of PSA level, in the presence of a large tumor load with extensive metastases, should raise the suspicion of NEPC as the diagnosis. In recent times, we have tended not to routinely measure PAP level, although occasionally its presence will increase the diagnostic suspicion of prostatic origin of an undifferentiated tumor.

Complete staging of this tumor is required, along with a bone scan and computed tomography (CT) scan of the chest, abdomen, and pelvis with intravenous and oral contrast. The presence of lytic bone metastases will increase suspicion of the presence of metastatic NE elements. Magnetic resonance imaging (MRI) scan may increase the level of definition of the prostatic primary tumor and local extension, but has no clear advantage over CT scan. The usefulness of positron emission tomography (PET) has been described for small cell lung cancer,[86,87] but has not been evaluated in NEPC. However, based upon limited information available in small cell carcinoma of other sites,[88,89] as well as proven uptake in small cell lung cancer (SCLC), PET may be of use in the staging of NEPC, particularly in suspected limited stage disease. If definitive local therapy is planned, or in the presence of neurological symptoms, an MRI scan of the brain and occasionally a bone marrow aspiration and biopsy should also be considered before defining the plan of management.

Treatment

Untreated NEPC may be rapidly progressive and fatal. However, despite its aggressiveness and grave prognosis, NEPC is sensitive to cytotoxic chemotherapy and radiation. Early introduction of chemotherapy may afford a survival advantage. Effective palliation can be achieved, and in some series treatment has achieved a 2-year survival of 20% of patients.[78] Considered rare, transient remissions have been seen in patients who have received multimodality therapy with chemotherapy, surgery, and radiation.

In view of the infrequent early diagnosis of this condition, it is not possible to define the single "optimal" approach to the management of localized NEPC.[78,79] However, in small cell cancers of other sites, including the lung and urinary bladder, primary surgery as monotherapy has had very poor results and has largely been abandoned. Integral to any approach is the early diagnosis of NEPC and the definition of the extent of disease, as outlined above.

Patients with NEPC that appears to be localized to the prostate are highly likely to have occult metastatic disease. Thus a multimodal approach to a patient who is otherwise healthy is logical. Such an approach may include both systemic therapy with cytotoxic chemotherapy (with or without hormone therapy) and possibly local therapy with external beam radiation or radical prostatectomy. Possible approaches include:
• radical radiotherapy, in an attempt to achieve local control and perhaps cure
• radical prostatectomy, to control the adenocarcinomatous elements and to reduce the bulk of the primary tumor (less relevant if the patient has previously presented with adenocarcinoma of the prostate, with the current syndrome representing NEPC)
• concurrent or sequential combination cytotoxic chemotherapy, administered to control both local disease and systemic micrometastases in a fashion analogous to that employed for bronchogenic NE carcinoma.[90]

Local therapy is generally reserved for the healthy patient with apparently localized disease, and should usually be preceded by systemic chemotherapy. Clinical studies in bladder SCC have suggested the superiority of this approach to one beginning with surgery.[91] Median cancer-specific survival (CSS) for resectable patients treated with initial cystectomy was 23 months, with 36% disease free at 5 years, which is similar to poor survival in patients treated with primary surgery reported by Quek *et al*.[92] Patients receiving neoadjuvant chemotherapy did not reach the median CSS ($p = 0.026$) with CSS at 5 years of 78%. No cancer-related deaths were observed beyond 2 years, though no similar comparison has been made for NEPC. Unfortunately, many cases of NEPC are not recognized on biopsy or clinical presentation, but are rather diagnosed on the radical prostatectomy specimen. In such cases adjuvant chemotherapy will generally be offered, based on the experience in SCC of the lung.

With regard to the optimal dose of radical radiotherapy, there is controversy as to whether a lower dose (40–50 Gy over 4–5 weeks) is appropriate (based on the marked radiosensitivity of NE cancer at other sites), or whether a more conventional, higher dose (75.6+ Gy at 1.8 Gy per fraction) should be applied, analogous to prostatic adenocarcinoma. Just as in the treatment of adenocarcinoma of the prostate, definitive conformal radiation therapy using either three-dimensional (3-D) conformal radiotherapy (CRT) or intensity modulated radiation therapy (IMRT) should be used to limit toxicity to surrounding critical organs (i.e. rectum and bladder). We believe that the latter approach should be used in view of the potential for admixture of elements of NE and adenocarcinoma in these tumors.

No controlled studies of adjuvant cytotoxic chemotherapy have been carried out in cases of localized NEPC, and it is not possible to make any specific recommendations at present. In view of the rarity of the disease, it is unlikely that the appropriate randomized studies will be completed. Thus, any decision regarding the use of adjuvant cytotoxic chemotherapy should be influenced substantially by considerations such as the age and general fitness of the patient, geographical accessibility, available facilities, and patient preferences.

There is only a relatively scanty literature regarding the management of extensive NEPC with chemotherapy. The cytotoxic agents that are active against bronchogenic NE cancer, including cyclophosphamide, vincristine, doxorubicin, cisplatin, carboplatin, etoposide, and paclitaxel,[93] produce objective responses in metastatic NEPC, although specific objective response rates have not been defined clearly for single agents.[26,78,79] The use of three- or four-drug combination regimens yields objective response rates of 60–75% in NE cancer of the lung.[93,94] The available literature suggests that the response to chemotherapy for NEPC may be lower than that for bronchogenic tumors, perhaps in view of the heterogeneity of NEPC with the admixture of elements of adenocarcinoma.

Galanis *et al*. retrospectively reviewed 81 cases of extrapulmonary small cell carcinoma treated between 1974 and 1994 at a single institution.[95] Tumor sites included the head and neck, genitourinary, gastrointestinal, and gynecological systems. Among patients treated initially with surgical resection, 75%

(30/40) relapsed with a median disease-free survival of 6 months despite adjuvant chemotherapy and/or radiotherapy. The majority of recurrences (80%) occurred in distant sites with median survival of 18 months. Five-year overall survival was reported in 13%. The best predictor of long-term disease-free survival after local therapy was disease localized to primary organ at presentation. For patients with localized disease, chemotherapy with radiotherapy showed equal efficacy to surgery. Metastatic disease had a response rate of 73% to platinum-based therapies with a medium duration of response of 8.5 months. The authors concluded that surgery can be curative in organ-confined disease but due to the high rate of systemic recurrence and the chemoresponsiveness of the tumor, platinum-based adjuvant regimens must be considered.

In a single-institution phase 2 trial of combination therapy consisting of doxorubicin, etoposide, and cisplatin in patients with NEPC, Papandreou questioned the belief in three- or four-drug regimens. When 38 patients were treated with this regimen, a 61% response rate was seen with no complete responses. While toxicity was substantially greater than historical cisplatin-etoposide regimens, notwithstanding the serious problems of historical controls, median time to progression of 5.8 months and median survival of 10.5 months failed to improve upon the historical outcome.[96]

Similarly, in another study by Flechon *et al*. carboplatin and etoposide were given to patients with anaplastic progressive metastatic castration-resistant prostate cancer (CRPC) with or without NE differentiation. In the 60 patients included, the objective response rate was 8.9% in the 46 patients with measurable disease. A NE response was observed in 31% of cases for NSE and 7% for CgA. The PSA response rate was 8%. The median overall survival was 9.6 months (95% confidence interval (CI) 8.7–12.7). Due to poor response and high toxicity (i.e. neutropenia, thrombocytopenia and anemia), the benefit:risk ratio of the study was poor.[97]

Although there is no specific evidence to support improved survival, chemotherapy can provide palliation, and complete responses have been reported.[40] We have usually treated such cases with etoposide and carboplatin or cisplatin, using relatively conventional doses,[90,94] and anticipate a response rate of 50–60%. A common approach has been to use etoposide at a dose of 360–500 mg m², delivered over 3–5 days per cycle, with cisplatin at a total dose of 60–100 mg m² or carboplatin at an area under the curve (AUC) dose of 5–6, each cycle being repeated every 21–28 days. Although newer agents, such as gemcitabine, taxanes, and irinotecan, appear to have a role in the management of bronchogenic NE, their role has not yet been defined for NEPC. There are no clinical data for the use of targeted biological agents.

Much more complex and controversial is the decision regarding the role of initial hormonal therapy. Where the patient has a histological diagnosis of concurrent adenocarcinoma and NEPC or high circulating blood level of PSA, it is worth considering the role of castration as part of initial treatment. We usually use the gonadotropin-releasing hormone (GnRH) agonists in this situation, as they are potentially reversible if there is no evidence of hormone response by the tumor.

The role of hormonal manipulation should not be trivialized. In several cases summarized in Table 4.1, sustained objective initial remission was achieved by bilateral orchiectomy or by the use of systemic estrogens (without cytotoxic chemotherapy). As many of these cases of NEPC were diagnosed *post hoc*, it is not clear whether the impact of hormonal manipulation at initial presentation was directed toward pure elements of adenocarcinoma or whether NEPC itself truly responded to the hormonal therapy.

It should also be emphasized that patients treated initially by hormonal manipulation alone for NEPC should be monitored very closely. Some of the available case reports describe rapid deterioration and death within a few weeks after the institution of hormonal treatment. If a patient with NEPC fails to respond to hormonal manipulation, cytotoxic chemotherapy should be applied. In the management of prostatic adenocarcinoma, we usually allow a minimum of 2 months before assessing the response to hormonal manipulation (unless the patient is rapidly deteriorating). By contrast, the patient with NEPC should be reviewed within 2–4 weeks, depending upon the extent and severity of the disease. On an empirical basis, we will often begin treatment with cytotoxic chemotherapy simultaneously with initiation of hormonal therapy or without it at all if there is a high index of suspicion (or histological confirmation) of NEPC. It is again emphasized that these principles are derived from our clinical practice and explicit empiricism, rather than representing the results of structured, randomized trials.

As more extensive molecular analyses of NEPC are generated, it is likely that more effective drug targets will be identified and will lead to the clinical development of targeted therapies. For instance, based on extensive genomic studies and preclinical evaluation, targeting Aurora kinase A inhibition may be an effective treatment strategy[50] but has yet to undergo clinical evaluation.

The specific implication of the diagnosis of "carcinoid" of the prostate is not completely clear, although there is a general consensus that classic prostate carcinoids are less aggressive in their natural history than NEPC.[75,81] If the diagnostic distinction can be made between prostatic carcinoid and NEPC, analogous to the situation that applies to tumors of the thorax, there is a greater tendency to apply localized treatment (in particular, surgical resection) for prostatic carcinoids. In carcinoids at other sites, cytotoxic chemotherapy appears to have a substantially lesser role than for NE cancer, and thus we have been less inclined to use systemic chemotherapy for prostatic carcinoids without evidence of spread. In the workup of such tumors of the prostate, octreotide scanning can elucidate sites of metastatic disease. Somatostatin analogs may be useful in controlling systemic carcinoid symptoms and have shown antiproliferative actions on human PC cell line LNCaP.[98] Therapy with somatostatin analogs has been shown to inhibit tumor growth *in vitro* with evaluable responses seen in patients.[99]

Prognosis

Traditionally, the prognosis for NEPC has been dismal. Although the majority of patients in the literature have survived less than 6 months from the time of documentation of NEPC, it should be noted that most of them did not receive cytotoxic therapy and were diagnosed with advanced disease. More recently, with the earlier recognition of NEPC, we have seen prolonged survival among patients who have been treated aggressively with definitive local treatment combined with systemic chemotherapy.[78,79]

In a retrospective review of 180 patients with genitourinary small cell carcinoma,[100] primary surgical therapy was the only parameter that predicted survival in NEPC. Median survival was 7 months in the 60 patients reviewed. The NE component of these carcinomas was resistant to antiandrogen therapy, possibly because of lack of estrogen and testosterone receptors. Hormonal manipulation and systemic chemotherapy did not have a significant impact on the natural history of this disease. Patient and tumor characteristics were not survival determinants on subgroup analysis. No further conclusions could be made because of the nature of the study.

Given the rarity of NEPC, it is unclear whether the late diagnosis of this disease is ultimately responsible for the poor outcome of its patients or whether the presence of NE elements *per se* confers a worse survival, with conflicting data from different series.[82,101] The definition of median survival is complicated by the fact that several of the reported cases have apparently had biphasic tumors with elements of adenocarcinoma and NE carcinoma. Thus some cases with prolonged survival may have reflected the sustained initial responses to hormonal manipulation because of an initial dominance of adenocarcinoma. The rapid decline after documentation of NEPC may have reflected a selection process because of (i) the outgrowth of NE carcinoma after initial treatment, (ii) failure to apply the most appropriate treatment for a NE carcinoma, or (iii) an altered biological state of the tumor, consequent upon initial hormonal therapy.

Recommendations

The biology of NEPC is still incompletely understood, although our evolving recognition of the mechanisms of cell cycle regulation and gene control is providing insights into the disease. Morphologically and functionally, it bears a closer resemblance to bronchogenic NE carcinoma than to classic prostatic adenocarcinoma. However, in many patients, there is also a substantial overlap with the characteristics of adenocarcinoma, either due to the presence of concurrent elements of this histological subtype or as an inherent biological function of the NE cell. The use of multimodality therapy is considered to be standard although no clear consensus exists on the ideal approach for localized or locally advanced disease. The abundance of case reports, heterogeneity of data, and failure of clinical diagnosis of this entity have led to difficulty in determining its optimal treatment. There is a clear consensus only on the belief that the prognosis is poor with this histology.

Although rare, one of the most important aspects of clinical management is the need to consider this entity early in the differential diagnosis of a poorly differentiated prostatic neoplasm as it appears that early recognition, with the concomitant use of cytotoxic chemotherapy, is associated with the potential for long-term survival and even with the possibility of ultimate cure. Given the above information, strong consideration should be given to a referral to an experienced center with multidisciplinary care. Even in the setting of localized disease, systemic therapy should be considered. In all cases, if available, participation in a clinical trial is suggested.

Sarcomas of the prostate

When compared with other malignancies, sarcomas are uncommon. In the United States, an estimated 11,280 new cases of soft tissue sarcoma will be diagnosed in 2012 with 3900 expected deaths.[3] Since soft tissue sarcomas may occur in almost any anatomical site, specific numbers for sarcomas are unknown. However, based on extrapolation of estimates from several countries, the worldwide incidence is approximately 30 cases per million in the population (International Agency for Research on Cancer [IARC] data).[102]

Primary prostatic occurrences of this relatively uncommon cancer are even more rare, and only case reports and small retrospective series exist. Although cancer of the prostate is one of the most common malignancies, the fraction of these that are sarcomas is exceedingly rare. During a period in which 31,882 deaths from prostatic malignancy occurred, 35 cases of prostatic sarcoma were identified.[103] Schmidt presented a single institution's experience over the 40-year period from 1933 to 1973 in which 12 cases of prostatic sarcoma were identified among over 5000 cases of adenocarcinoma of the prostate (0.24%).[104] Investigators from Memorial Sloan-Kettering Cancer Center reported that 16% of genitourinary sarcomas seen over a 25-year period arose from the prostate.[105]

This section will review the pathology of prostatic sarcomas, provide information relevant to clinical situations, and review treatment options.

Pathology

Sarcomas may be classified on the basis of their biological behavior, tissue of origin, site of occurrence, histological appearance and/or grade, immunohistochemical profile, molecular profile, and/or microarray analysis. Therefore within the rare entity of sarcoma of the prostate, there may be many more subclassifications. Amongst sarcomas of the adult prostate, leiomyosarcoma appears to be the most common followed by rhabdomyosarcomas (RMS).[104,106,107] In contrast, malignant fibrous histiocytoma and liposarcoma are historically the two most common subtypes of soft tissue sarcoma overall. Another rare variant are tumors of specialized prostatic stroma, which have occasionally shown overt malignant (sarcomatous) behavior.[108,109]

The difficulty and importance of sarcoma classification should not be overlooked. Several studies have demonstrated that pathologists with specific sarcoma experience at specialized centers will have different interpretations from local pathologists.[110–113] These differences in interpretations may have prognostic implications, and may be especially important in the context of clinical trials.[112,113]

Historical case reports and series describing the frequency of sarcoma subtypes should be viewed critically, as many were based on the use of light microscopy alone. The use of immunohistochemical techniques, and to a lesser degree electron microscopy, has permitted a more accurate identification of sarcoma subtypes. For example, equivocal diagnoses of the most common sarcomas of the prostate, RMS and leiomyosarcoma, can often be confirmed by the demonstration on electron microscopy of the presence of thick and thin filaments or Z-band material[114,115] or immunohistochemical positivity for antigens highly specific to muscle tissue, such as desmin, myoglobin, the M subunit of creatine phosphokinase (CPK), skeletal muscle myosin, or muscle-specific actin.[114] Furthermore, some of the sarcoma subtypes have been found to be highly associated with individual cytogenetic abnormalities, thereby providing another potential means to arrive at a more definitive diagnosis.[116,117] For example, t(l2;16)(ql3;pl1) has been identified in myxoid liposarcoma. The presence of this translocation would support this diagnosis over that of the myxoid variants of malignant fibrous histiocytoma, a distinction that is often difficult to make. Other associations include t(X;18)(pll.2;qll.2) with synovial sarcoma, and t(2;13) (q37;ql4) with alveolar RMS.

The use of microarray analysis has been developed to characterize tumors by gene expression patterns.[118,119] This technology permits simultaneous analysis (profiling) of multiple gene expression markers. Alveolar RMS, Ewing sarcoma, gastrointestinal stromal tumors, and synovial sarcoma have all been characterized.[120–123] This technology also reveals the drawback of less precise histological subtyping of sarcomas, such as malignant fibrous histiocytoma, which has variable gene expression profiles.[119] Recently, the diagnostic gene expression profiles linking signaling pathways to different sarcoma subtypes were demonstrated and a hypoxia-induced metastatic profile was identified in the pleomorphic, high-grade sarcomas. These findings suggest the diagnostic utility and application of expression data for improved selection of high-risk patients.[124] In addition, potential therapeutic molecular targets may be discovered.[122]

With the above caveats in mind when reading the historical literature of sarcoma, and in particular, rare sarcomas such as primary sarcoma of the prostate, several subtypes have been described. Many of the histological subtypes of sarcoma that are more commonly found at other locations in the body have also been described in the prostate.[104,106,107,125–132] In this review, we will limit our specific discussions to the more common sarcomas of the adult prostate (leiomyosarcoma and RMS), tumors of specialized prostatic stroma (i.e. prostatic stromal sarcoma), and some other interesting tumors (e.g. carcinosarcoma, postradiotherapy prostatic sarcoma, Ewing sarcoma and inflammatory myofibroblastic tumor) before discussing the broader clinical aspects of sarcoma of the prostate.

Leiomyosarcoma

Prostatic leiomyosarcoma is an extremely rare neoplasm that accounts for less than 0.1% of primary prostate malignancies.[133] It is the most common primary sarcoma of the prostate in adults and comprises 38–52% of primary prostatic sarcomas (Fig. 4.2a).[107] Vandoros et al. presented an analysis of 54 cases of leiomyosarcoma of the prostate from 1988 to 2008. The

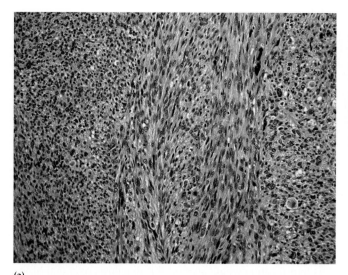
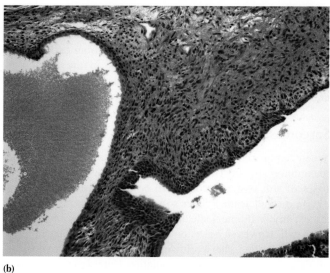

(a)   (b)

Figure 4.2 Prostatic sarcoma. (a) Pathological appearance of leiomyosarcoma of the prostate. H&E section shows intersecting fascicles of atypical spindled cells with eosinophilic cytoplasm, marked nuclear pleomorphism, and hyperchromasia. (b) Pathological appearance of stromal sarcoma of the prostate. Hypercellular stroma is composed of atypical spindled cells and interspersed benign glands. The stromal cells show loosely fascicular growth pattern, nuclear pleomorphism, and hyperchromasia, and tend to show condensation beneath the glandular component.

median age of the cohort was 63.8 years (range 40–80). Among 38 patients for whom clinical data regarding presenting symptoms were available, 89.4% had obstructive urinary symptoms and 25.6% had perineal or rectal pain. Less frequent manifestations were burning on ejaculation and hematuria, both presented as initial symptoms in only 5.2% of the patients. Median survival was estimated at 17 months (95% CI 20.7–43.7 months) and the 1-, 3-, and 5-year survival rates were 68%, 34%, and 26%, respectively. The only factors predictive of long-term survival were negative surgical margins and absence of metastatic disease at presentation.[134] This report is consistent with previous investigators reporting median survival of 16–49 months.[104,106,107]

Rhabdomyosarcoma

Although adult RMS is infrequently described in the literature, it is probably even less common than the literature would suggest.[135–139] In a Finnish study involving 880 cases of soft tissue sarcoma among adults older than 40 years, 25 of these were originally identified as RMSs. However, when these 25 cases were retrospectively evaluated by histology, immuno-chemistry, and electron microscopy, with strict criteria for the diagnosis of striated muscle differentiation, only two of the 25 cases were convincingly demonstrated to be RMS. Both tumors arose in the urogenital region, one in the prostate and the other in the bladder, and both patients died within 3 months of diagnosis. Of interest, 30 pleomorphic sarcomas in this series were also evaluated to determine whether any case of RMS was misdiagnosed, but none of the latter was found.[140]

Smith and Dehner reviewed the records of the Armed Forces Institute of Pathology and found 55 primary sarcomas of the prostate (including pediatric patients).[106] Twenty-three of the 55 patients (42%) were classified as having RMS. Of these, 17 were embryonal RMS (median age 16), four alveolar, and two other. Waring *et al.* published a case series of adult prostatic

embryonal RMS. Six cases from the post-1958 literature (after reclassification of RMS) met criteria of patients at least 18 years of age, having prostate as the origin of disease, and adequate clinical information. The median age was 31 years (mean = 39) and median survival was 8 months from the diagnosis.[141]

Inflammatory myofibroblastic tumors

These tumors are rare lesions with uncertain pathogenesis and can also be termed pseudosarcomatous fibromyxoid tumors, inflammatory pseudotumors, pseudosarcomatous myofibroblastic tumors, fibromyxoid pseudotumors, pseudomalignant spindle cell proliferation, and nodular fasciitis.[142] The pathogenesis of inflammatory myofibroblastic tumor (IMT) is unknown. Positive cytokeratin reactivity is considered by some to be a requirement for the diagnosis of sarcomatoid carcinoma; however, many IMTs may also show at least focal cytokeratin reactivity.[143] Recently, *ALK* gene rearrangements have been reported in approximately 75% of IMTs, and immunohistochemical detection of ALK expression or FISH detection of *ALK* gene rearrangements can be a useful diagnostic adjunct.[144,145] The distinction of IMT from malignant sarcoma of prostate is paramount, as IMTs are benign lesions that require only conservative surgical management.

Prostatic stromal sarcoma

Tumors of specialized prostatic stroma may be purely stromal or, more commonly, contain admixed benign epithelial components.[146–148] This category of tumor encompasses the cystic-epithelial stromal tumor classically referred to as cystosarcoma phyllodes. Overall, these lesions are extremely rare. They exhibit a spectrum of histological features similar to malignant phyllodes tumors of the breast. Although a benign clinical course has been emphasized in some reports, cumulative evidence in literature indicates that these lesions should be considered neoplasms rather than atypical hyperplasia due to the frequent early recurrences with possible dedifferentiation, infiltrative growth, and potential for extraprostatic spread in some cases. Prostatic stromal sarcomas are rare, with 82 cases reported in the literature. These cases have been published under a variety of diagnoses, including phyllodes tumor and prostatic stromal tumors of uncertain malignant potential (STUMP).[149–163] Prostatic stromal sarcomas have occasionally been shown to be capable of aggressive behavior and cause rapid death.[154,155,163]

Histologically, most of these tumors are biphasic, consisting of stromal and epithelial components arranged to form cysts lined by hyperplastic epithelium. The proliferating stroma is of variable cellularity and sometimes shows subepithelial condensation (Fig. 4.2b). The lining epithelium is benign, with basal cell and secretory layers that show immunoreactivity typical of benign prostatic epithelium, but the epithelial components may show various metaplastic and proliferative changes such as basal cell hyperplasia or squamous metaplasia.[151] There is wide variability in the stromal-to-epithelial ratio, stromal cellularity, cytologic atypia, and mitotic activity. These variable features, as well as the presence or absence of necrosis, have been quantified and used to assign a tumor grade. The mean age of patients who present with prostatic stromal sarcomas is about 55 years (range: 22–86 years) and 40% of the patients are younger than 50 years.[164]

The use of the term "stromal tumor of uncertain malignant potential" (STUMP) is generally reserved for lesions diagnosed on needle core biopsy, where limited tissue is available for evaluation and overt malignant features are not identified. In these cases, final classification as stromal hyperplasia with atypia, low-grade stromal sarcoma, or high-grade stromal sarcoma (e.g. cystosarcoma phyllodes) may be performed on the fully excised tumor if surgical resection is recommended as a means of therapy. These lesions differ from one another histologically and immunohistochemically, and each requires its own clinical management strategy.[165] Investigations of gene amplifications indicate that epidermal growth factor receptor (EGFR) and AR are frequently and strongly expressed in both epithelial and stromal components of prostatic stromal sarcomas.[165]

Carcinosarcoma

Another unusual histology found in the prostate, but less exclusive to it than adult RMS and cystosarcoma phyllodes, is carcinosarcoma. This mixture of malignant epithelial and malignant mesenchymal elements has been described in less than 100 cases.[104,166–180] Carcinosarcoma is a difficult lesion to diagnose. It must be distinguished from (i) a primary carcinoma that has become anaplastic and spindle shaped, (ii) a primary carcinoma that has produced nonmalignant sarcomatous changes in the stroma, and (iii) the "collision" of a separately occurring carcinoma and a sarcoma.[104]

Mostofi and Price have defined carcinosarcoma as a malignant mixed tumor with carcinomatous and sarcomatous components, the latter consisting of neoplastic cartilage or bone.[181] Indeed, in the absence of malignant heterologous elements, such as bone, cartilage, or striated muscle, it may be difficult to ascertain mesenchymal differentiation of cells that do not have an epithelial appearance.[172]

Many theories have been proposed to explain the origin of carcinosarcoma. Chung et al. inoculated specific epithelial and fibroblast cell lines into either adult male syngeneic rats or athymic nude mice and induced the development of tumors that resembled carcinosarcoma.[182] In this model, the investigators were able to establish that the fibroblasts influenced the epithelial cells. Recently, data by Elo et al. demonstrated that disruption of fibroblast growth factor (FGF) signaling pathways by increased epithelial production of FGF-8b leads to strongly activated and atypical stroma, which precedes development of prostate cancer with mixed features of adenocarcinoma and sarcoma in the prostates of transgenic mice.[183] The symptoms and signs experienced by a patient with carcinosarcoma are not distinctive from those experienced by a patient with either adenocarcinoma or sarcoma of the prostate. The largest study entails study of pathology specimens from 42 patients. Clinical information was available on 32 patients; 21 patients had prior history of adenocarcinoma of prostate. The percentage of sarcomatoid growth ranged from 5% to 99%. The sarcomatoid component did not show immunoreactivity for PSA in eight cases. Of patients with meaningful follow-up, 6/7 died in the first year of diagnosis of carcinosarcoma. Survival had no association with morphology.[180]

Radiation-associated sarcoma

Sarcomas may develop in a prostate in a previous therapeutic radiation field. The impact of radiation exposure on the development of a subsequent malignancy has been described historically, and therapeutic radiation also carries with it a risk of secondary malignancy, with an incidence of sarcoma in 0.8% of described women receiving adjuvant radiotherapy for breast cancer.[184] The specific risk of radiation-associated sarcoma in the prostate is unknown. A retrospective single-institution study estimated the risk with long-term follow-up to be 0.03–0.8% with a multitude of sites and reasons for the radiotherapy.[185] In a review of patients treated surgically at a single institution for radiation-induced soft tissue sarcomas, 14% of the cases developed after radiotherapy for prostate cancer (third most frequently after breast cancer 29% and lymphoma 15%).[186]

The histology of these sarcomas has been reported as variable (with the caveats described at the beginning of this section even more important), with malignant fibrous histiocytomas and osteosarcomas among the most frequent.[187] The majority of the cases reported in the literature tend to be high grade and often associated with a poor prognosis.[186–188] Postradiation sarcomas of the prostate do not appear to behave differently from similar sarcomas in other sites when stratified for grade, based on the more than 20 cases that have been reported.[186,189–195] Canfield et al. reported a case of sarcoma developing after brachytherapy for adenocarcinoma of the prostate.[195] They concluded from their review of the literature that many of the cases, especially those with short latency periods, may in fact be carcinosarcoma or dedifferentiation of adenocarcinoma. The clinical presentation of radiation-associated prostatic sarcomas does not appear to be significantly different from that of other prostatic sarcomas, although pain may be a more prominent symptom after radiation than in de novo cases.

Ewing sarcoma/primitive neuroectodermal tumor of prostate

Based on immunohistochemical and molecular studies, Ewing sarcoma (ES) and primitive neuroectodermal tumor (PNET) are now considered a single entity with different clinical manifestations/disease phenotype. ES/PNET is reported to occur in various organs but it rarely occurs in the prostate, with only two reported cases in the literature.[196,197] Both reports show variable immunohistochemical staining. Kumar *et al.* showed that viable neoplastic cells show diffuse, intense cell surface immunoreactivity for CD99. The tumor cells were positive for vimentin, S-100, NSE and synaptophysin (the latter focally) and negative for cytokeratin, desmin and CD45.[196] Funahashi *et al.* showed that the neoplastic cells exhibit diffuse, immunoreactivity for CD99, as well as for NSE, CD56, MIB-1, and p53. The tumor cells were negative for AE1/AE3, chromogranin A, S-100, EMA, αSMA, CD34, and bcl-2. FISH analysis revealed a characteristic chromosomal translocation t(11; 22) (q24; q12) for ES/PNET.[197]

Although primary ES/PNET of the prostate is an extremely rare soft tissue sarcoma, it should be considered in the differential diagnosis of a prostate tumor. Several approaches, including cytogenetic methods, are important for an early, accurate diagnosis of ES/PNET.

Clinical characteristics

Obstructive symptoms are the most common complaints in men presenting with sarcoma of the prostate. These obstructive symptoms may range from mild to acute urinary obstruction and its consequences. Other relatively common symptoms include hematuria, pyuria, and dysuria. Other reported clinical signs and symptoms include urinary incontinence, changes in bowel habits, weight loss, fever, edema, and pain.

The most common sites of metastatic disease include lymph nodes, lungs, and bones. In their review of adult embryonal RMS, Waring *et al.* reported clinical characteristics of the disease differentiating it from adenocarcinoma of the prostate, including a younger age at diagnosis, higher frequency of a suprapubic mass, more lymph nodal metastases, presence of osteolytic bone metastases, and rapid clinical course.[141] However, since any space-occupying lesion of the prostate can cause similar subjective and objective evidence of disease, none of these is distinctive to prostatic sarcoma.

It has been suggested that there may be differences found by digital rectal exam. Sarcoma may be smooth, tense, and symmetrical; soft and balloon like, or smooth and firm. These consistencies can be distinguished from the fixed, hard, and irregular consistency that is usually characteristic of the gland in adenocarcinoma.[104,105,129] Nonetheless, the consistency of prostatic sarcoma mimics that of prostatic adenocarcinoma in the majority of cases; only approximately 20% of sarcomas have these unique features at palpation.[107]

An important point is that it is unusual for children or young adults to have an abnormal prostate or to present with symptoms of urinary obstruction, and this clinical picture should alert the examiner to the possibility of sarcoma. The differential diagnosis of an abnormal prostate examination finding in the older patient includes benign prostatic hypertrophy, cysts or abscesses of the prostate, cysts or neoplasms of the seminal vesicles and müllerian duct remnants, tuberculous prostatitis, sarcomas or UC of the bladder invading the prostate, or metastatic lesions to the prostate. Tissue diagnosis is usually achieved by conventional means; that is, by transrectal biopsy under ultrasound guidance.

In general, there are few radiological characteristics of prostatic malignancies that may be diagnostic in differentiating an adenocarcinoma from another malignancy.[198] However, the characteristics of sarcomas may give some clues. Sarcomas are often associated with marked prostatic enlargement in comparison to other prostatic malignancies. Apart from this general difference, imaging may play a larger clinical role in staging and treatment response than in diagnosis of the primary lesion. There have been several reports of a few cases of different imaging modalities of prostatic sarcoma. Figure 4.3 demonstrates the CT appearance of a prostatic sarcoma. The most common and probably the most clinically useful modalities in the right context are ultrasonography, CT, and MRI. Both pelvic and transrectal ultrasonography results have been described in prostatic sarcomas. Pelvic ultrasonography has proved to be useful in pediatric pelvic RMSs, but is probably not as useful as other imaging modalities in adults.[199,200] Computed tomography has demonstrated utility in pelvic malignancies, but is rarely diagnostic of a prostatic sarcoma, with the exception of the unique appearance of prostatic stromal sarcomas, particularly the phyllodes variant.[151]

Bartolozzi *et al.* have described the MR findings of prostatic sarcoma. Of interest, in three of four cases MR images showed the site of origin to be the central area of the prostate, with compression of a clearly recognizable peripheral zone, which may be relevant in differentiating sarcomas from carcinomas.[201] In a recent study, the correlation of imaging features of prostate sarcoma with clinical findings was analyzed. Prostate sarcoma was characteristically shown to be a large and heterogeneous mass with hypervascular, heterogeneous, and rapid enhancement on CT and MRI. The main MR feature was a marked increase in the choline:citrate ratio. The clinical manifestations corresponded mainly to local mass effects and tumor invasion.[202]

Prognostic factors

Prognosis of individual categories of sarcoma of the prostate has been described above. Since there have been no formal prospective studies validating prognostic factors in prostatic sarcoma, we can only extrapolate based on historical cases and relevant factors from sarcoma in other anatomical sites. However, the same limitations described above regarding difficulties in classifying sarcomas apply even to some prospective studies of sarcoma, particularly when it comes to analysis by histological type. The site of origin of sarcomas has been described as a prognostic factor in soft tissue sarcomas overall, with nonextremity sites of origin having higher risk of death.[203,204] This fact alone implies that prostatic sarcomas will have a poorer prognosis than the same counterpart found on an extremity. Recently Janet *et al.* showed that the histological subtype of

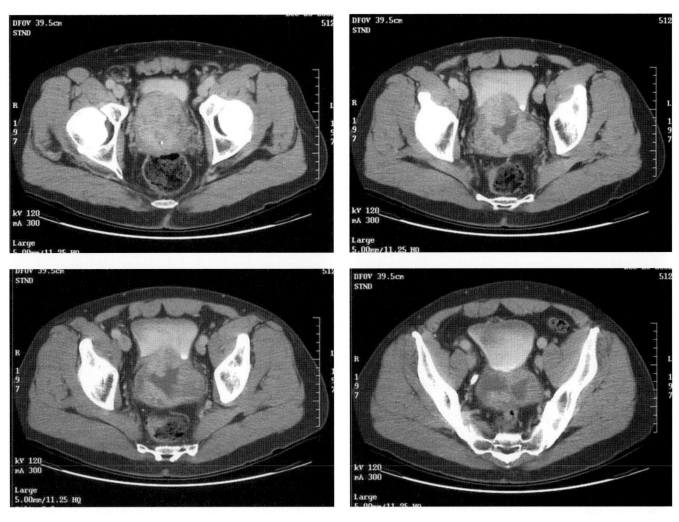

Figure 4.3 Computed tomography image of malignant fibrous tumor of the prostate. Notice the enlarged heterogenous prostate with areas of central necrosis. The seminal vesicles are pushed posteriorly with the mass pushing into the bladder base without invasion. The trigone is elevated and the rectum spared, with tumor extending into the pouch of Douglas, consistent with a prostatic sarcoma. Reproduced with permission from Tagawa ST *et al.* Uncommon cancers of the prostate. In: Raghavan D *et al.* (eds) *Textbook of Uncommon Cancer*, 3rd edn. New York: Wiley & Sons, 2006.

prostate sarcoma has prognostic significance; however, no differences in survival outcomes with respect to tumor size or grade have been noted. Presence of metastasis at the time of diagnosis was a poor predictor of outcome.[205] Kattan's postoperative nomogram may be clinically useful in soft tissue sarcoma overall, but is of unproven utility in sarcoma of prostatic origin.[203]

The prognosis of sarcoma of the prostate is variable. Patients presenting with metastatic disease or large high-grade lesions may have a rapidly progressive course and a short survival. Other patients may have an indolent course, with or without aggressive therapy. The factors mentioned above, in addition to other patient characteristics and preferences, must be kept in mind when developing a treatment plan. Young patients with high-grade prostatic sarcomas tend to have a poor prognosis in spite of aggressive treatment.

Treatment

Surgery continues to be the primary modality of therapy for localized soft tissue sarcomas. However, there are reports of treatment with primary radiotherapy. Multimodality therapy has also been used (and advocated) for localized disease. Systemic chemotherapy has been used for metastatic disease. We will discuss the available data and give our recommendations, particularly with reference to specific clinical circumstances.

The largest amount of data about prospective treatment comes from soft tissue sarcomas of the extremities. For this disease, complete surgical excision with clean margins has produced the best long-term results, particularly with regard to recurrence-free survival.[206,207] Postoperative radiotherapy has been added to surgery and appears to decrease local recurrence rates, particularly with high-grade lesions.[208] Preoperative radiotherapy has also been studied, although there are no published prospective randomized controlled trials looking at survival in this setting. Retrospective multivariate analysis has found no significant difference in outcome between preoperative and postoperative radiotherapy.[209]

In a study of 176 adults with primary soft tissue sarcomas of the head and neck, patients with negative margins had 85% survival at 5 years versus a 28% survival among those whose margins were positive.[210] In another study of 57 patients with head and neck, breast, and trunk sarcomas, completely resected disease resulted in a 77% 3-year survival (median follow-up, 35 months).[211] Among 50 patients with primary colorectal sarcomas, complete resections led to a median survival of 174 months, whereas a less than complete resection achieved a median survival of only 12 months.[212]

In another study among patients with soft tissue sarcomas at all locations except the viscera, 66 of 107 patients with an initial recurrence were rendered disease free by surgery.[213] Their actuarial survival at 3 years was 51% compared to a median survival of 7.4 months among patients not rendered disease free. Thirty (45%) of the 66 remained disease free at the time of the report (median follow-up 28 months), but the other 36 had recurrence. Sixteen (44%) of these 36 were again rendered disease free; their survival was 18 months, compared to 6 months for those whose disease could not be completely resected. However, only four of these 16 remained disease free at follow-up.

The use of radiotherapy as an adjunctive treatment following complete resection, because of the common presence of microscopic residual disease and local recurrence, is often considered. There are limited data in nonextremity sarcoma to support this practice, but sarcomas are known to be moderately radiosensitive. As in the case of extremity sarcomas, we do not recommend adjuvant radiotherapy for "low-grade" lesions that have been resected with negative surgical margins. In cases of "high-grade" sarcomas, we recommend consideration of conformal radiation therapy (either 3-D CRT or IMRT) to either 60 Gy (with negative margins of resection) or at least 66–70 Gy (with positive margins of resection) at 2 Gy per fraction. In addition, for low-grade sarcomas with positive surgical margins, adjuvant CRT should be considered. In general, RMSs require significantly lower doses of radiation depending upon the response to initial chemotherapy (40 Gy with a complete response to chemotherapy, or at least 50 Gy if less than a complete response is achieved) and margin status after resection (40 Gy with negative margins, or at least 50–55 Gy with positive margins). Case reports suggest that radiotherapy has a useful palliative role for the prostatic sarcoma that cannot be completely resected. However, its curative potential without the use of surgery is anecdotal. Surgery alone seems acceptable for low-grade lesions (e.g. low-grade prostatic stromal sarcoma), if clear margins can be obtained, although metastatic stromal sarcoma has been treated successfully with chemotherapy in an anecdotal report.[160] The role of chemotherapy will be discussed in further detail below.

The reader must be aware, however, that the foundation from which these recommendations are built is not firm. Data on nonextremity sarcomas have been collected retrospectively, often over several years. Different studies may generate dissimilar results for several reasons. Factors that vary between studies include the skills of the participating surgeons, surgical practices and supportive care over time, staging techniques, histopathological classification, adjunctive therapies to surgery, the differing mix of prognostic factors, and follow-up intervals. Even within studies, attempts to dissect some of these influences through the use of multivariate analyses have

been limited. In addition, for the determination of the effect of surgery on recurrent disease, the influential role of lead-time bias needs to be considered. Even if these interpretive difficulties could somehow be obviated, it remains clear that there is significant room for therapeutic improvement and innovation, and a continuing need for well-structured clinical trial design in this context.

From a therapeutic perspective, the prostatic sarcoma that has been most critically examined is RMS, although the majority of cases happen in the pediatric age range. There have been many contributors to the development and evaluation of therapeutic strategies in RMS, but the Intergroup Rhabdomyosarcoma Study (IRS) Committee, which receives patient data from centers around the world and has coordinated trials since 1972, has been the most instrumental. As adult prostatic RMS is an uncommon manifestation of an uncommon problem, we will only briefly review the salient therapeutic findings.

The first Intergroup Rhabdomyosarcoma Study (IRS-I) approached bladder–prostate sarcomas with a primary extirpative surgery, if feasible, followed by radiotherapy (50–60 Gy) and chemotherapy (vincristine, dactinomycin, and cyclophosphamide).[214] On the basis of the data suggesting that the bladder salvage rate was higher if chemotherapy and radiotherapy were applied initially, followed by surgery only if malignancy remained, one of the major objectives of IRS-II, III, and IV was to continue to improve disease control and survival with increased bladder preservation. Bladder preservation rates improved from 25% in IRS-II to 60% in IRS-III.[215–217] In IRS-IV, 82% of patients with nonmetastatic RMS survived for 6 years and 55 of 88 patients retained their bladder without relapse.[217,218] Unfortunately, the favorable results in the pediatric age group have not carried over to patients diagnosed with RMS or other prostatic sarcomas beyond puberty, who have a poor prognosis in spite of multimodal therapy.

The role of chemotherapy for soft tissue sarcomas in the setting of both adjuvant therapy and metastatic disease has been extensively reviewed and is only briefly discussed here.[219] A broad range of traditional cytotoxic agents, including doxorubicin, ifosfamide and cyclophosphamide, methotrexate, cisplatin and carboplatin, dacarbazine, actinomycin-D, and etoposide, have demonstrable activity against soft tissue sarcomas, with reported objective response rates for advanced disease in the wide range of 0–40%. No optimal agent has been defined, although there is a practical current consensus that doxorubicin and ifosfamide should be regarded as the anchors of treatment.

Although there is no consensus regarding the respective merits of single-agent and combination chemotherapy, it is generally agreed that combination chemotherapy regimens yield higher objective response rates (60–70% versus 0–40%), but without clear evidence of survival benefit. In current practice, the CYVADIC and MAID regimens, incorporating cyclophosphamide or ifosfamide in combination with doxorubicin and dacarbazine, are widely used for advanced soft tissue sarcomas, although there is considerable controversy as to whether the toxicity of these regimens is justified by the modest reported outcomes. Outside a clinical trial, our practice has been to administer combination chemotherapy with doxorubicin and ifosfamide with mesna prophylaxis (AIM) without dacarbazine to reduce toxicity while attempting to maintain the efficacy of combination chemotherapy. Gemcitabine and docetaxel are often used for patients unable to receive an anthracycline or ifosfamide due to cardiac or renal impairment.[220]

With respect to adjuvant therapy, controversy persists regarding its role, even in the treatment of more common extremity sarcomas. Prostatic sarcomas should be regarded as "deep" tumors, irrespective of stage and grade, when considering the role of adjuvant chemotherapy.[221] The literature on adjuvant chemotherapy of sarcomas is dominated by series including extremity sarcomas, although these reports have often included nonextremity tumors as well, making it more difficult to give specific recommendations regarding prostatic sarcomas. An updated metaanalysis by Pervaiz et al. confirms the marginal efficacy of chemotherapy in localized resectable soft tissue sarcoma with respect to local recurrence, distant recurrence, overall recurrence, and overall survival. These benefits are further improved with the addition of ifosfamide to doxorubicin-based regimens, but must be weighed against associated toxicities.[222–224] When nonextremity sarcomas have been treated exclusively in adjuvant trials, there has been no clear demonstration of prolonged survival, although one trial did show an improvement in disease-free survival.[225] However, each of these studies was conducted with such small numbers of patients, possibly used suboptimal chemotherapy, and/or suffered from such low statistical power that the issue of adjuvant therapy for nonextremity sarcoma should more properly be considered unresolved.

Given the limitations of conventional cytotoxic single-agent and combination regimens, newer agents and approaches have been applied in both the adjuvant and metastatic settings. Alternative anthracyclines have been investigated in addition to nonanthracycline combinations such as taxanes and gemcitabine.[226] Hyperthermia and intraoperative photodynamic therapy are being combined with other modalities in an attempt to improve response. Preoperative chemotherapy has also been studied, but remains unproven in this context. In theory, the attractions of this strategy include (i) the reduction of requisite surgery or conversion of a nonresectable mass to an operable lesion, (ii) sparing of nonresponders from further ineffective chemotherapy in the adjuvant setting, (iii) identification of patients with a poor prognosis, thereby stimulating a change in approach, (iv) possible radiosensitization of tumor tissues, and (v) possible effect on occult metastatic deposits before completion of definitive local therapy. In addition, regimens of high-dose chemotherapy are being evaluated in soft tissue sarcomas, although we are unaware of specific protocols for patients with prostatic sarcomas. As we move towards a molecular basis of diagnosis, targeted therapies may come into play.[207] Thus far, the only targeted therapies to have proven clinical benefit are imatinib and newer derivatives for gastrointestinal stromal tumors.

Recommendations

As with all cases of rare tumors, consideration should be given to referral to an experienced center with multidisciplinary care.

Pathological review of the available tissue by an experienced, specialized pathologist is important in guiding further therapy. In general, for soft tissue sarcoma of the prostate, based on the data for other nonextremity sarcomas, it appears reasonable to approach resectable prostatic sarcomas with initial aggressive surgery. Complete resection of all gross disease should be the primary goal, as lesser resections do not appear to prolong survival. This usually includes cystoprostatectomy and, often, total pelvic exenteration. On the basis of the data for high-grade extremity sarcoma demonstrating the equivalence of limb-sparing surgery followed by radiation therapy to amputation, it is not unreasonable to adopt a similar approach in high-grade prostatic sarcomas; that is, resection of all gross disease with an attempt at "clear" margins followed by radiation therapy. We recommend CRT (either 3-D CRT or IMRT) to deliver high doses of adjuvant irradiation (60–70 Gy depending upon the margin status and grade of sarcoma). Significant doses of radiation therapy can be delivered to the prostate bed often with a tolerable degree of side-effects. For low-grade tumors, such as low-grade leiomyosarcomas or stromal sarcomas, surgical resection is probably all that is warranted, but local recurrences are very common. For recurrences, complete resection of disease should be considered, whether the recurrence is local or distant. Given the morbidity associated with these procedures, resection should be attempted only if the surgeon believes that all gross disease can be successfully removed.

Adjuvant chemotherapy programs for sarcomas have occasionally been associated with a prolonged disease-free interval and rarely with a longer survival. Although the prolongation of disease-free status is not an unreasonable goal, the inconsistency of this result, especially in the setting of nonextremity sarcoma, suggests that the role of adjuvant chemotherapy for prostatic sarcoma should be confined to the investigational setting. Patients with good performance status and locally advanced or metastatic prostatic sarcoma are candidates for chemotherapy, although its benefits, if any, are likely to be modest. Despite increases in toxicity without clear survival benefit, in patients in whom control of metastatic disease followed by resection is a possibility, combination chemotherapy is recommended. Until new agents are found, anthracyclines and ifosfamide, with or without dacarbazine, remain the drugs of choice. These limitations emphasize the importance of continued innovative approaches and the entry of eligible patients into well-structured clinical trials.

Urothelial carcinoma of the prostate

Primary urothelial carcinoma (UC) most commonly arises in the bladder, but may arise from the urothelium of the renal pelvis, ureter, posterior urethra, or distal excretory prostatic ducts. Solitary UC of the prostate is a rare entity, much less common than the approximate 73,510 cases and 14,880 deaths from bladder cancer expected in the United States in 2012[3] (or the 386 cases per 100,000 people worldwide).[227] Much more commonly, the prostate is involved either as a synchronous or a metachronous lesion to one in the urinary bladder. Certain aspects of UC of the prostate continue to be confusing, namely, staging and pathogenesis. Some of this confusion is derived from the historically imprecise nomenclature for this tumor.

Melicow and Hollowell are generally given credit for the first description of urothelial cancer involving the prostate in 1952, although earlier authors may have examined prostates with evidence of UC.[228–230] Bowen's disease was used to describe 30 cases of UC in situ (CIS). Three patients with CIS of the prostate were found incidentally after open prostatectomy. Ortega et al. used the term Paget's disease for in situ UC of the prostate.[231] The association of CIS of the urinary bladder and that of the prostatic urethra was also noted.[232] Franks and Chesterman presented a case similar to the previous ones and stressed the use of the term "cancer in situ" rather than the eponymous titles Bowen or Paget.[233] Ende et al. hypothesized the origin of these cancers from the prostatic ducts as they enter the prostatic urethra, later confirmed by others.[234–236] In 1972, Johnson et al. demonstrated the first cases of noncontiguous UC of the bladder and the prostate.[237] Seemayer et al. raised concern about patients with CIS of the bladder and the subsequent development of prostatic ductal UC, which according to them may occur quickly and silently.[238] Many of the early case reports note the presence of infection or cystitis without frank bladder tumors in association with UC of the prostate. Grabstald theorized that some of these lesions actually represented unappreciated CIS of the bladder.[239]

In this section we will review primary UC of the prostate. Primary UC is defined as carcinoma arising from the transitional cell epithelium of the prostatic structures without upper tract or bladder cancer.[240] Much more commonly, the epithelium of the prostatic urethra or ducts is involved secondary to a bladder cancer.[237] Any review of the literature is confounded by the admixture of primary and secondary UCs. In many cases of primary UC, the extent of histological investigation of the bladder is uncertain.[241] Also confusing the situation are some early reviews, which considered UC of the prostate to be more closely related to adenocarcinoma of the prostate than to a UC elsewhere in the urinary system.[242] Adley et al. have described a rare high-grade urothelial-type adenocarcinoma arising in the prostate. This primary prostatic tumor mimicked metastatic colorectal adenocarcinoma due to its striking morphological resemblance as well as overlapping immunohistochemical phenotype.[243] It is common for these reports to include a history of hormonal therapy without response.

Incidence

The true incidence of this rare disease is difficult to determine. As noted above, the diagnosis of this entity in some historical reports is doubtful. There may be an increasing frequency of the finding of UC of the prostatic structures, although this may instead reflect an increased pathological awareness or an emphasis on urothelial mapping with inclusion of prostatic sampling.[244–246] A 9-year pathological experience of 2724 cases of prostatic cancers revealed 122 cases (4.5%) of UC of the prostate.[247] Of these, 46 (1.7%) were thought to be solitary lesions without UCs of the urinary bladder. Other studies report that primary UC of the prostate comprises 1–5% of all primary prostatic neoplasms.[234,242,248–250]

As discussed previously, UC of the prostate occurs in strong association with that of the urinary bladder. In an effort to determine the incidence of bladder UC-derived involvement of the prostate, a number of authors have performed pathological evaluation of the prostate in specimens removed for treatment of bladder cancer. Pagano et al. reported on 72 of 562 (13%) patients with pathologically staged prostatic involvement after cystectomy for T1 to T4 disease.[251] Others have found an incidence of 12–43%.[252–255]

A retrospective pathological review by Kirk et al. reported a 55% incidence of UC invasive to the prostate, dysplasia, or CIS of the prostatic ducts in cystoprostatectomy specimens.[256] These authors conclude that the high incidence of these malignant or premalignant abnormalities portends a poor prognosis for nonoperative therapy. A retrospective review of a 20-year experience at the Mayo Clinic notes that 23% of prostatic UC were true primary lesions without disease elsewhere in the urinary tract.[248]

Pathogenesis and etiology

It is likely that the risk factors for the development of UC of the prostate are the same as those for UC elsewhere in the urinary system. These presumptive carcinogenic agents include tobacco smoke, aromatic amines (β-naphthylamine, benzidine), analgesics (especially phenacetin-containing analgesics), cyclophosphamide, radiation, and chronic inflammation or infection.[257]

Several less established associations have been proposed. Intact RNA of human papillomavirus type 6 has been detected in grade 1 UCs of the distal urethra; investigators have postulated a role of this virus as an agent for the development of UCs arising from transitional cell epithelium as analogous to condylomata arising from squamous epithelium.[258] A role for chronic irritation from cystitis or urethritis has been proposed but not proven.[214] Asbestos has been reported as a risk factor in a case report.[259] CIS is the putative precursor lesion, but other changes have been identified. Ullmann and Ross presented nine cases with abnormal epithelial changes of the periurethral prostatic glands of patients with benign bladders.[260] These abnormalities included hyperplasia, hyperplasia with atypia, and CIS. Although they were not able to show temporal progression of these lesions to frank invasive UC, they have been proposed as potential precursor lesions.

Johnson et al. identified three mechanisms of development: (i) direct extension from an invasive bladder lesion, (ii) prostatic urethral implantation from a lesion elsewhere in the urinary tract, and (iii) de novo development from the prostatic urothelium.[237] Other patterns of involvement include contiguous intraepithelial spread and metastatic spread. Supporting evidence for intraepithelial spread of transitional carcinoma is provided by prostate mapping studies of cystoprostatectomy specimens.[261] The authors of the chapter in the previous edition and colleagues examined eight cases of transitional cell CIS of the seminal vesicles.[262] The finding of CIS of the seminal vesicles is very highly associated with carcinoma of the bladder and prostate, and it is always found with UC of the prostatic ducts. As the seminal vesicles contain columnar and no urothelium, this is most consistent with mucosal spread via the prostatic ducts (in the absence of evidence of transmural penetration from the bladder).[262]

Pathology

The vast majority of primary prostatic carcinomas are adenocarcinomas, with several variants (acinar, ductal, mucinous, sarcomatoid, neuroendocrine, and signet ring).[263–265] Grossly, adenocarcinoma and UC of the prostate are indistinguishable.[242,266] The gland may be firm, irregular, fixed, and enlarged.[266,267] UC involving the prostatic urethra, ducts, and acini is generally easily distinguishable from adenocarcinoma, and follows the same pathological criteria of urothelial cancer elsewhere.[265] UC is typically moderately to poorly differentiated and often found with significant chronic inflammation but not particularly associated with squamous metaplasia.[266,268] Prostatic urethral dysplasia has been associated with UC of the bladder.[269]

There is a strong association of UC of the prostate and CIS of the bladder. The study by Wishnow and Ro noted that 100% (25 of 25 cases) of their patients with UC of the prostate had multifocal CIS of the bladder.[270] Johnson noted a substantial but lesser association (70%).[237] Prout et al. evaluated the significance of urothelial CIS of the urinary bladder with and without invasive cancer.[271] In their patients who underwent cystectomy for CIS of the bladder, 66% had carcinoma of the prostatic urethra, ducts, or stroma. A more recent study by Cheville et al. found a 76% concordance with historical or contemporaneous CIS of the urinary bladder.[272] Although secondary involvement of the prostate with invasive UC of the bladder is not the subject of this chapter, we refer the reader to studies documenting the significant risk of urethral recurrence, which may be mistaken for prostatic UC.[272–274]

As may be expected by the high incidence of prostatic adenocarcinoma in the population most at risk for UC, there are a number of cases of concomitant prostatic UC and incidental adenocarcinoma. In the large retrospective review by Cheville et al., four of 50 (8%) patients had prostate adenocarcinoma.[272] Other studies note a larger coincidence of 20–50%, which is comparable to the rates of incidental adenocarcinoma in the general population.[237,275–277]

High-grade UCs may be difficult to distinguish from poorly differentiated adenocarcinoma.[247] Nuclear characteristics are often useful; urothelial cancer cells tend to have larger, more pleomorphic nuclei with more irregularly distributed and coarsely granular chromatin.[268] The determination may also be facilitated by the use of immunohistochemical stains for PSA and PAP; however, these may be false negative in a poorly differentiated adenocarcinoma.[278] Squamous cell carcinoma occurs rarely in the prostate and may be indistinguishable from high-grade UC. Focal keratinization and lack of urothelial differentiation are suggestive and stains for keratin may support this differentiation.[268]

Urothelial carcinoma involving the prostate tends to be of high grade.[247,279] In a series of 110 cases of UC of the prostate examined by Goebbels et al. there were no specimens with grade 1 histology, 24 with grade 2, and 86 prostates with grade 3 UC. Fifty percent of cases have prominent tumor-associated inflammation. This is in contradistinction to prostatic adenocarcinoma, which usually lacks an inflammatory response.[247]

When the prostate is involved with UC, there exists a substantial risk of distant metastasis. In one study, 20% of patients had metastases to bone and lung at presentation.[275] The presence of invasive (into prostatic stroma) UC has been associated with a 100% risk of also having metastatic disease in one study.[270] Curtis et al. have reported two cases of adenocarcinoma arising from prostatic urethra and/or proximal prostatic ducts, and distinguishing primary urethral adenocarcinoma from secondary colonic adenocarcinoma based on H&E morphology alone may be impossible, especially on prostate needle biopsies.[280]

Clinical features

The diagnosis of UC of the prostate has been made in males from age 7 years to the very elderly, with a mean age at diagnosis in the eighth decade.[281,282] Many patients complain of irritative voiding symptoms such as urgency, frequency, dysuria, or hematuria.[237] In those patients with concomitant bladder cancer, these symptoms may be referable to the vesical disease.[275,283] A number of studies report patient presentations with obstructive voiding complaints.[234,237,284] However, concomitant benign prostatic hyperplasia (BPH) is common in this age group, and the etiology of symptoms may be difficult to distinguish. Because the age at presentation tends to be similar to that of prostatic adenocarcinoma, there is a significant coincidence of prostate cancer. Occasionally, UC is diagnosed in younger patients.[240,285] Primary presentation with nasal skin metastasis from suspected primary UC of the prostate has been described.[286] Prior to the advent of serum PSA testing and immunohistochemical staining for PSA, UC occasionally presented as a castration-resistant "adenocarcinoma."[242,284,287] Signs of prostate involvement with UC may include prostate nodularity and firmness.[237]

Diagnosis

Cytology is currently a cornerstone for diagnosis and surveillance of UCs but voided cytology alone will not distinguish bladder from prostate origin. Epstein reported prostate UC in a patient with a history of bladder cancer diagnosed by prostatic cytological aspirate.[288] Transrectal ultrasound (TRUS) results of 221 patients with carcinoma of the prostate were reviewed retrospectively, including two cases of confirmed UC involving the prostate.[289] These two patients had identifiable hypoechoic lesions involving both the anterior and posterior regions, which were indistinguishable from those found on TRUS of the adenocarcinomatous prostate. In another study, TRUS was unable to identify UC invasive to the prostatic urethra.[290] This same study identified hypoechoic lesions in five of seven patients with stromal invasion and in 100% of patients with involvement of the ejaculatory ducts. UC of the prostate from bladder cancer may also be identified using CT scan.[291]

Algaba et al. reviewed their cystoscopic findings of five patients with UC involving the prostate.[275] Four of these had no abnormalities; one had findings related to the concomitant bladder cancer but a negative prostatic urethra. A prospective review by Montie *et al.* noted that only one of 10 patients with UC of the prostate had cystoscopic evidence of the cancer.[244] This patient had a visible papillary lesion of the prostatic urethra. Incidental prostatic UC has been identified by needle biopsy for presumed adenocarcinoma, as well as by transurethral or open prostatectomy for benign prostatic hypertrophy.[246,292] Albert *et al.* described a diagnosis made after transperineal needle biopsy performed for evaluation of an abnormal digital rectal examination.[246]

As there is considerable coincidence of prostatic and bladder involvement with UC and the preoperative identification of the malignancy in the prostate could potentially alter management, adequate biopsy of the prostate is a necessary component for staging of primary bladder cancer.[293–295] This is especially true for high-risk patients such as those with CIS or with cancer near the bladder neck. Rikken *et al.* performed endoscopic cold cup prostatic urethral biopsies prior to mitomycin-C therapy for bladder carcinoma.[296] They noted a CIS or superficial cancer incidence of 27%. Complete pathology was not obtained. This is within the range of incidence from several studies, but slightly lower than the frequency of UC of the prostate reported by some authors.[253,297]

A prospective evaluation of three biopsy techniques – transperineal needle core biopsy, transrectal fine needle aspiration of the prostate, and transurethral resection biopsy – was performed prior to radical cystoprostatectomy and whole-mount 4–5 mm step-section pathological evaluation.[297] The results indicate a 20% diagnostic accuracy with perineal needle biopsy and a 40% accuracy with transrectal aspiration. Transurethral resection biopsy correctly identified prostatic involvement in 90% of cases, was 83% correct in defining ductal involvement, and was 40% accurate for prostatic stromal invasion. The authors' recommended technique was to perform deep resectoscope biopsy of the prostate at the 5 and 7 o'clock urethral positions. Sakamoto *et al.*, who performed prostatic mapping of cystoprostatectomy specimens,[298] confirmed this technique to be the most accurate. They noted that the finding of carcinoma in the prostatic ducts at the 5 and 7 o'clock positions at the level of the verumontanum should raise suspicion of a deeper involvement. Although there exists a theoretical risk of implantation after resection of a bladder tumor and prostate biopsy, Laor *et al.* found no increased risk of subsequent development of a new prostatic UC implant.[299]

Controversy exists over the best staging system for UC of the prostate. Some authors have used traditional staging systems for adenocarcinoma of the prostate, while others have used similar ones from UC of the bladder. To be practical, the staging system must predict prognosis. Much of the argument over staging has revolved around secondary involvement of the prostate rather than the primary prostatic UC.[249,251,255]

Prognosis

The discussion of prognosis is often made difficult by the reporting of cases in which prostatic involvement may have been shown to be truly secondary by today's diagnostic standards.

The literature has been confounded with discussions of UC with additional prostatic involvement rather than true primary prostatic UC. The prognosis of patients diagnosed with UC of the prostate has traditionally been very poor; they commonly have metastatic disease at diagnosis.[267,275,292,300–303] Laplante and Brice note that "if invasion into the prostate gland is proved, the prognosis is so poor that radical cystectomy for cure appears unreasonable."[293] This may reflect the overall historically poor prognosis of patients with advanced-stage bladder cancer.

Recent studies indicate more optimistic survival after aggressive therapy of the associated primary bladder cancer, although these reports often describe bladder UC with prostatic involvement.[304] Cheville *et al.* reviewed 50 cases of primary prostatic UC, including CIS of the prostatic urethra and prostatic ducts (bladder CIS was included, but current or historical invasive bladder UC was excluded).[272] All patients were treated with radical cystoprostatectomy. Overall 5-year survival was 40%. Patients were broken into four categories of disease with different survival: CIS only (62% 5-year survival), prostatic stromal invasion (35% 5-year survival), extraprostatic extension (0% 5-year survival), and lymph node metastases (30% 5-year survival). Only CIS survival (38% of the patients reported) was statistically significant from the others.

Management

For many years the treatment of UC with hormone ablation was reported, always with unsuccessful results, and numerous studies have documented this inefficacy.[249,267] The value of intravesical bacillus Calmette-Guérin (BCG) for the treatment of UC of the prostate remains controversial. Several authors have investigated the use of BCG as initial or as definitive therapy for CIS of the prostatic urethra.[305–309] Orihuela *et al.* used BCG intravesical therapy as treatment for 15 patients who had superficial UC of the bladder and mucosal involvement of the prostate.[308] They noted successful treatment in 87% of patients after a mean follow-up of 37 months. They considered the presence of prostatic urethritis and granulomas after the treatment to be a sign of prostatic exposure to the BCG and indicative of adequate therapeutic effect. Lamm considered intravesical BCG therapy to be the treatment of choice for superficial UC of the prostatic urethra.[310] The question remains as to how adequately the prostatic urothelium is exposed to therapeutic BCG. Transurethral resection (TUR), particularly of the bladder neck, has been recommended to facilitate exposure of the lesion to the bacillus; however, some authors do not recommend TUR prior to intravesical treatment.[305,309,311,312] Intravesical chemotherapy for primary prostatic UC has not been reported to our knowledge. A report by Lockhart and colleagues noted a 36% recurrence rate in the prostatic urothelium after intravesical mitomycin-C therapy for superficial bladder UC.[313] However, the prostates were not sampled prior to therapy and this may in fact represent untreated lesions rather than recurrent lesions. Droller and Walsh reported progression to prostatic involvement in three patients undergoing intravesical chemotherapy.[314]

Transurethral resection of UC lesions of the prostate has been used; early reports noted reasonable survival rates with this method for urothelial and mixed cancers.[234,300] Shenasky and Gillenwater recommended transurethral resection with repeat surveillance cystourethroscopy as a definitive therapy for superficial low-grade urothelial cancer of the prostate.[315] These authors recommended aggressive therapy for high-grade lesions or those invasive into the parenchyma.

Some authors have reported results of radiation therapy for UC of the prostate. On the basis of the aggressiveness of this tumor, Kopelson *et al.* suggested that radiotherapy is the treatment of choice.[316] Schellhammer *et al.* noted 20% 5-year survival of patients with stromal invasion who underwent preoperative radiotherapy followed by radical cystoprostatectomy.[317] Frazier and colleagues found no difference in the local recurrence rate or survival of patients with and without preoperative radiation treatment.[318]

Occasional reports of success with primary systemic chemotherapy have been published.[267,300,301,319–321] On the basis of historical data, it is likely that the most efficacious regimens for unresectable UC of the prostate would be methotrexate, vinblastine, doxorubicin, and cisplatin (MVAC), delivered in the classic way or in dose-dense fashion,[245,322] or gemcitabine and cisplatin.[323] Recently, intraarterial delivery of MVAC for prostatic UC has been reported with favorable short-term results.[324]

Recommendations

Urothelial cancer of the prostate is almost always associated with UC elsewhere in the urinary system and is rarely primary. It may be an incidental finding in suspected prostatic adenocarcinoma and tends to be high grade. The diagnostic method of choice is deep transurethral resections through the prostatic urethra. The incidental finding or suspicion of solitary prostatic UC necessitates evaluation of the entire urothelium, including mapping biopsy of the urinary bladder under anesthesia and upper tract evaluation with CT urogram.

If UC of the bladder is discovered to be associated with prostatic urethral mucosal or stromal invasion, the treatment is largely driven by the bladder cancer. The treatment of choice is neoadjuvant cisplatin-based chemotherapy followed by cystoprostatectomy. Urethrectomy is generally reserved for patients with stromal involvement, a positive apical margin at surgery, or those for whom a cutaneous diversion is planned (as opposed to a neobladder reconstruction). Patients not undergoing primary urethrectomy must be followed up by life-long periodic voided or urethral washing cytology to detect recurrence in the remnant urethra. A full discussion of the management of this more common disease is outside the scope of this chapter.

As this is a rare disease, consideration may be given for referral to an experienced center and enrollment on a clinical trial, if available. For the patient with primary UC of the prostate in the absence of bladder involvement, treatment should take into consideration the stage of the disease and the patient's general condition. Superficial mucosal involvement or CIS can be effectively treated with TURP and intravesical BCG. Patients with stromal invasion or recurrence after BCG require surgical excision, with radical prostatectomy or cystoprostatectomy depending on the extent of disease, and full bilateral pelvic node dissection. We would consider adjuvant radiotherapy to a dose of at least 66 Gy at 2 Gy per fraction for patients with positive surgical margins. For patients with locally advanced disease, systemic chemotherapy may be employed in the hope of downstaging the patient and allowing surgical excision. Patients with metastatic disease who are candidates for therapy should receive systemic chemotherapy. The combination of gemcitabine and cisplatin is a reasonable option with consideration of dose-dense MVAC in select individuals for patients with metastatic disease, although the preferred option is participating in a clinical trial. (Editorial note: the use of dose-dense MVAC regimen remains highly controversial for urothelial malignancy, and there is no level 1 evidence to support its use, in preference to the standard MVAC regimen, in urothelial cancer of the prostate.)

Primary lymphoma of the prostate

In 2012, there will be an expected 79,190 new cases of lymphoma with 20,130 deaths (18,940 non-Hodgkin lymphoma [NHL], 1190 Hodgkin lymphoma) and 47,150 new cases of leukemia in the United States.[3] Worldwide, the WHO reports via Globocan 2008 that there are approximately 424,350 (356,431 NHL, 67,919 Hodgkin lymphoma) and 350,434 new cases of leukemia per year.[227] Only a small fraction of these will involve the prostate, and even fewer will be of primary prostatic origin, with less than 70 reported cases of primary lymphoma of prostate. This section reviews this uncommon disease.

Prostatic involvement with systemic hematological malignancy

Although tumors secondarily involving the prostate are not the subject of this chapter, we will briefly review prostatic involvement by hematological malignancies. Cases of both systemic leukemia and lymphoma have been reported to involve the prostate. In 1937, Jacobi *et al.* reported leukemic involvement of the prostate.[325] Several other case reports and reviews of the literature have been published since then.[326–331] Butler *et al.* reported on a large retrospective review of 4862 prostatectomies with six cases of leukemic infiltration identified.[332] It appears that the predominant type of leukemia involving the prostate is chronic lymphocytic leukemia (CLL), with only a few reported cases of acute myeloid leukemia and even fewer with chronic myeloid leukemia. One interesting case of acute myelogenous leukemia affecting the prostate was reported by Thalhammer *et al.*, the case of a 68-year-old man who developed granulocytic sarcoma (extramedullary leukemia) of the prostate as the initial site of relapse 9 years after complete remission.[333] The predominance of CLL is not entirely unexpected because of the prevalence of this chronic disease compared to other leukemic subtypes. The exact subtypes of leukemia (and lymphoma) are difficult to attribute because of different pathological interpretation and classification schemes over the years.

Systemic lymphoma has also been described to involve the prostate. The largest series of prostatic lymphoma by Bostwick *et al.* describes 62 cases. In that series, secondary prostatic involvement was more common than primary prostatic lymphoma.[334] Weimar *et al.* described a large retrospective series of 1068 patients with lymphoma and described genitourinary involvement.[335] The genitourinary tract was involved in 6.7% of cases (49 cases of NHL, 23 cases of Hodgkin lymphoma), but prostatic involvement was not explicitly described in any case. A review of 6000 male autopsies revealed an incidence of 0.82% (49 patients) of prostatic lymphomatous involvement.[336] In a review of extranodal lymphomas, only three of 1467 (0.2%) cases had documented prostatic involvement.[337] Rosenberg reviewed 1269 cases of lymphosarcoma and only identified two (0.16%) with prostatic involvement.[338] A series from the MD Anderson Cancer Center reviewed 2928 untreated patients with lymphoma presenting to their center from 1980 through 1991 and found three cases (0.1%) of primary lymphoma of the prostate.[339] Of 3446 cases of prostatic malignancies treated during that time, these three cases represented 0.09% of prostatic malignancies.

Nearly all reported cases of prostatic lymphoma are of non-Hodgkin type, with only a few reported cases of Hodgkin disease involving the prostate. One such interesting case described by Klotz *et al.* reported a case of stage IV nodular sclerosing Hodgkin lymphoma with an initial response to surgery, chemotherapy, and radiation.[340] A subsequent presentation with acute urinary retention revealed recurrence in the prostate, with subsequent long-term response to radiotherapy.

The clinical presentation of secondary involvement of the prostate by hematological malignancies is difficult to interpret. In a large surgical series all patients were symptomatic, although it is interesting to note that while there were six cases of leukemic infiltration into the prostate, eight other cases with systemic leukemia and prostatic obstructive symptoms were found to have leukemia-free prostates.[332] Since the common types of leukemia with prostatic involvement are rare in people younger than 50 years old, it stands to reason that many patients with leukemia will have prostatic symptoms, even though on the basis of reported data only a minority of these will have leukemic involvement. Primary presentation of leukemia with prostatic symptoms has been reported.[330] However, in modern times with the majority of patients with CLL (the most common type of leukemia with prostatic involvement by far) presenting with either peripheral lymphadenopathy and/or laboratory abnormalities, we expect this to be an even more uncommon phenomenon. In a recent study by Verma *et al.*, records of 1445 patients with CML/myeloproliferative neoplasm (MPN) or other hematological malignancies treated with tyrosine kinase inhibitors were reviewed to investigate the frequency and characteristics of second malignancies (other than AML, acute lymphocytic leukemia or myelodysplastic syndrome). After a median follow-up of 107 (range 13–362) months after CML/MPN diagnosis, 66 (4.6%) patients developed second malignancies, including 10 (0.7%) prostate cancer cases.[341]

Primary lymphoma of the prostate

In 1877, Coupland reported the first case of prostatic lymphoma.[342] Since then, more cases and small series have been reported. In Bostwick's original series[343] of prostatic lym-

phoma, a modification of criteria described by King and Cox[344] was used to define primary lymphoma of the prostate. The criteria are simply: (i) presenting symptoms attributable to prostatic enlargement, (ii) involvement of the prostate predominantly, with or without adjacent tissue, and (iii) absence of involvement of liver, spleen, or lymph nodes within 1 month of diagnosis of prostatic involvement.[334,343] As these criteria have been used in the literature since then (sometimes referred to as the Bostwick and Mann criteria), we will follow the classification. It should be noted, however, that these criteria would exclude patients who on autopsy or biopsy are found to have lymphoma present only in their prostate if they did not present with symptoms of prostatic enlargement.

Bostwick's 1998 series of 62 patients includes 22 patients with primary lymphoma of the prostate.[334] The most common histology amongst patients with primary prostatic lymphoma was diffuse large B cell lymphoma in 55%, followed by small lymphocytic lymphoma (CLL) in 18%. There were two cases of high-grade, Burkitt-like lymphoma. Several other cases or smaller series have also been reported in the last decade, fulfilling the same criteria as those for primary lymphoma of the prostate.[339,345–367] The majority of these cases was also large B cell lymphoma, with some small cell or mixed types with two additional cases of small noncleaved NHL, although the specific subtypes of NHL are not well described in all cases. There are emerging data regarding viruses and NHL, specifically human immunodeficiency virus (HIV), Epstein–Barr virus (EBV), and hepatitis C, but there are no studies in this regard for primary lymphoma of the prostate.

Recently, Koga *et al.* reported a patient who was diagnosed with primary mucosa-associated lymphoid tissue (MALT) lymphoma of the prostate. The patient was staged as extranodal marginal zone B cell MALT-type lymphoma of the prostate, low grade and stage I and had a good response to radiation therapy.[368] In another report a patient was diagnosed with primary MALT of prostate concurrent with adenocarcinoma of the prostate.[369] Chin *et al.* also reported a case of diffuse large B cell malignant lymphoma of prostate which subsequently developed features of moderately differentiated adenocarcinoma.[363] These two case reports have opened a new debate that chronic inflammation may trigger the malignant transformation in the prostatic tissue. Furthermore, the expression of leukemia/lymphoma-related factor (LRF), also known as Pokemon factor, has been studied in BPH and prostate cancer tissue sections.[370] Semi-quantitative reverse transcriptase polymerase chain reaction (RT-PCR) and western immunoblot analyses demonstrated significantly higher messenger RNA transcripts and protein expression in cancer compared to BPH. High expression of LRF suggests that it may have a potential role in the pathogenesis of both BPH and prostate cancer.[367]

Clinical presentation

In the more recent Bostwick series, 91% (43 of 47) of all patients (including secondary prostatic lymphomatous involvement and unknown cases) presented with symptoms of prostatic enlargement.[334] Nine patients (19%) had hematuria at presentation. Only three patients (6%) had B symptoms. Cystoscopically, there were no reported pathognomonic findings, with urethral luminal narrowing and bladder trabeculation as in nodular hyperplasia. PSA was known in 10 patients, and elevated above 4 ng mL^{-1} in two. In the 22 patients meeting the criteria for primary prostatic lymphoma, 16 (73%) developed extraprostatic sites of disease more than 1 month after diagnosis. Since symptoms need to be present to fulfill the criteria put forth for primary lymphoma of the prostate, all of the other recent case reports have presented with symptoms, again the most common being obstructive symptoms, with hematuria described not uncommonly. There are few data on PSAs of all these reported cases. In one of the cases of small cell lymphoma, PSA was found to be 4.8 ng/mL with a prostatic nodule and a well-circumscribed hypoechoic lesion on ultrasound.[352] In another patient with follicular NHL of the prostate, laboratory data showed a significantly elevated PSA level.[356] Chin et al. reported a patient with PSA of 13 ng/mL.[363] While several of the case reports have described the ultrasonic appearance of the involved prostate, one case from the Mayo Clinic describes the ultrasound characteristics in detail.[371] The prostate in a 39-year-old man appeared enlarged, but normal landmarks could be identified. Several areas of hypoechogenicity were identified, including the area of extraprostatic extension felt on digital rectal examination.

More recently, F-18 fluorodeoxyglucose positron emission tomography/computed tomography (FDG PET/CT) has been used to evaluate and stage primary and secondary prostate lymphoma. Hodgson et al. reported that in a patient who was incidentally diagnosed with prostate lymphoma on biopsy, FDG PET/CT revealed markedly increased uptake of FDG in prostate and after combination chemotherapy showed complete metabolic response.[372] Cimarelli and Li have reported two different cases where FDG PET/CT was successfully employed to assess the response of a CD 20+ NHL involving prostate and a large B cell NHL of prostate to chemotherapy.[373,374] As there is no prospective evaluation of the utility of FDG PET/CT in prostate lymphoma, it is reasonable to extrapolate its use in other lymphoma subsets for evaluation of extent of disease, treatment response, and prognosis.[375]

Prognosis

In Bostwick's original series, the median survival was 8 months overall (mean survival 2 months) and only 4 months (mean 8 months) for the primary prostatic lymphoma patients.[343] In the follow-up series, 13 of 22 patients with primary prostatic lymphoma were known to have died, with nine of them having lymphoma as their cause of death (median survival in these patients was 23 months). Most of the other case reports and series have quoted relatively short survival statistics, with several notable exceptions. There have been a few cases with long-term survival after local therapy (surgery and/or radiotherapy) as well as with chemotherapy and/or multimodality therapy, which will be discussed below.

Treatment

Primary lymphoma of the prostate is, by definition, a local or regional disease (at least at the time of clinical presentation) and therefore, attempts at local therapy alone have been reported historically. Many of the cases and series reported are surgical series, with the diagnosis of lymphoma only becoming known after prostatectomy. Several case reports after prostatectomy have reported poor outcomes but at least one case of a large cell lymphoma removed by radical retropubic prostatectomy and no further treatment resulted in a disease-free survival of 13 years at the time of reporting.[346] Likewise, there have been a few cases of patients treated with radiotherapy alone. Two cases resulted in rapid progression and death (5- and 11-month survival from diagnosis),[342,349] but another case treated with radiotherapy alone resulted in 24-month disease-free survival at the time of reporting.[345] Fukutani et al. presented a review of treatment of 23 reported cases of malignant prostate lymphoma in 2003. The majority of the patients were older than 60 years and their histopathology was mostly intermediate NHL according to the Working Formulation Classification. Nineteen out of 23 cases (83%) were divided into localized stage, i.e. stage I or II. In these reports, three of five cases treated with either radical prostatectomy or radiotherapy alone resulted in death or progressive disease. On the other hand, 11 out of 16 cases (69%) who received chemotherapy alone or with other therapy obtained complete response.[376] Care should be taken to examine each case on an individual basis.

Several important points should be noted when considering local therapy for primary lymphoma of the prostate. The pathological subtype of lymphoma has often been overlooked in the historical literature when outcome has been reported. This may be illustrated by a case reported by Braslis et al. of a 65-year-old man with recurrent urinary tract infections found to have an abnormal result on digital rectal examination and a mildly elevated PSA level.[352] A transrectal biopsy revealed small cell lymphoma. The patient received no treatment for this usually indolent lymphoma and was alive and well with no change on rectal examination, in the PSA level or the clinical symptoms at the time of reporting. As reported historically in the literature, indolent lymphomas such as this may have a 70% 10-year survival without impact by early aggressive therapy.[377]

Another important point to note is the natural history of lymphoma in general. While several cases of subtypes of true stage IE lymphoma may result in long-term survival with localized therapy alone, it is noteworthy that in the largest series, 16 of 22 patients (73%) developed extraprostatic sites of disease between 1 and 59 months after diagnosis.[334] Only seven of 22 patients (32%) received systemic therapy. In a series from the MD Anderson Cancer Center, all three patients were treated with systemic chemotherapy: two with specific therapies for aggressive small noncleaved lymphoma and one with cyclophosphamide, doxorubicin, vincristine, and prednisone (CHOP) combination chemotherapy.[339] It is noteworthy that historical reports on systemic therapy for NHL of the prostate were prior to the introduction of rituximab.[361] It is likely that the addition of rituximab to standard chemotherapy (e.g. R-CHOP) would lead to improvement in outcome in this subset of patients as well.

Recommendations

For patients discovered to have a hematological malignancy affecting their prostate, we recommend evaluation at a center with expertise in several areas, including hematology/ oncology, urology, radiation oncology, and pathology. If available, enrollment in a clinical trial should be considered. After thorough review of the pathology, extensive workup for other sites of disease should be performed, including complete history and physical, laboratory evaluation, CT of the body, functional imaging with PET (in particular for higher grades of lymphoma), and a bone marrow biopsy. If indicated, tests for infectious etiologies, such as HIV and/or hepatitis C should be considered. After workup, multidisciplinary evaluation should be performed. Taking into consideration the pathology (type and grade), stage, clinical status and symptoms, comorbidities, and patient preferences, a treatment plan should be rendered. For those patients presenting with an incidental diagnosis of low-grade lymphoma of the prostate (i.e. asymptomatic), consideration may be given to surveillance. Systemic combination chemotherapy for intermediate to high-grade tumors should be strongly considered, regardless of a negative staging workup. Outside a clinical trial, the most common regimen recommended for diffuse large B cell lymphoma would be R-CHOP. For patients with bulky local disease, a discussion about the risks and benefits of radiotherapy in addition to chemotherapy is reasonable on a case-by-case basis, extrapolating from results in bulky lymphomas of other sites.

In any patient presenting in an unusual fashion, in particular younger men with obstructive prostatic symptoms and/or hematuria, the diagnosis of lymphoma of the prostate should be considered. A transrectal ultrasound with biopsy may be diagnostic, prompting the workup as stated above. For the small subset of patients discovered to have lymphoma of the prostate only after prostatectomy, we recommend extensive workup (as above) to evaluate other sites of disease. It is not known whether "adjuvant" therapy for this subset of patients will affect outcome. However, given the historically poor prognosis for this subset of patients, especially those men with intermediate to high-grade lesions, referral to an experienced center is warranted and combination chemotherapy should be considered.

References

1. Partin AW, Rodriguez R. The molecular biology, endocrinology, and physiology of the prostate and seminal vesicles. In: Walsh PC, *et al.* (eds) *Campbell's Urology*, 8th edn. Philadelphia: Saunders, 2002. pp.1237–96.
2. Scher HI. Cancer of the prostate. In: Devita VT Jr, Hellman S, Rosenberg SA (eds) *Cancer Principles and Practice of Oncology*, 7th edn. Philadelphia: Lippincott Williams and Wilkins, 2005. pp.1192–259.
3. Siegel R, Naishadham D, Jemal A. Cancer statistics, 2012. CA Cancer J Clin 2012; 62(1): 10–29.
4. Di Sant'Agnese PA. Neuroendocrine differentiation in human prostatic carcinoma. Hum Pathol 1992; 23: 287–96.
5. Abrahamsson PA. Neuroendocrine cells in tumour growth of the prostate. Endocr Relat Cancer 1999; 6: 503–19.
6. Nakada SY, di Sant'Agnese PA, Moynes RA. The androgen receptor status of neuroendocrine cells in human benign and malignant prostatic tissue. Cancer Res 1993; 53: 1967–70.
7. Mucci NR, Akdas G, Manely S, Rubin MA. Neuroendocrine expression in metastatic prostate cancer: evaluation of high throughput tissue microarrays to detect heterogeneous protein expression. Hum Pathol 2000; 31: 406–14.
8. Weinstein MH, Partin AW, Veltri RW, Epstein JI. Neuroendocrine differentiation in prostate cancer: enhanced prediction of progression after radical prostatectomy. Hum Pathol 1996; 27: 683–7.
9. Berruti A, Bollito E, Cracco CM, *et al.* The prognostic role of immunohistochemical chromogranin a expression in prostate cancer patients is significantly modified by androgen deprivation therapy. Prostate 2010; 70: 718–26.
10. Berruti A, Mosca A, Tucci M, *et al.* Independent prognostic role of circulating chromogranin A in prostate cancer patients with hormone-refractory disease. Endocr Relat Cancer 2005; 12: 109–17.
11. Pretl K. Zur Frage der Endokrinie der menschlichen Vorsfeherdruse. Virchows Arch A Pathol Anat 1944; 312: 392–404.
12. Feyrter F. Uber das urogenitale Helle-Zelien System des Menschen. Z Mikrosk Anat Forsch 1951; 57: 324–44.
13. di Sant'Agnese PA, de Mesy Jensen KL, Churukian CJ, Agarwal MM. Human prostatic endocrine–paracrine (APUD) cells. Arch Pathol Lab Med 1985; 109: 607–12.
14. Wenk RE, Bhagavan BS, Levy R, Miller D, Weisburger W. Ectopic ACTH, prostatic oat cell carcinoma and marked hypernatremia. Cancer 1977; 40: 773–8.
15. Ro JY, Têtu B, Ayala AG, Ordóñez NG. Small cell carcinoma of the prostate. II. Immunohistochemical and electron microscopic studies of 18 cases. Cancer 1987; 59: 977–82.
16. Schron DS, Gipson T, Mendelsohn G. The histogenesis of small cell carcinoma of theprostate. An immunohistochemical study. Cancer. 1984; 53: 2478–80.
17. Bonikos DS, Bensch KG. Endocrine cells of bronchial and bronchiolar epithelium. Am J Med 1977; 63: 765–71.
18. Azzopardi JG, Evans DJ. Argentaffin cells in carcinoma: differentiation from lipofuscin and melanin in prostatic epithelium. J Pathol 1971; 104: 247–51.
19. Vashchenko N, Abrahamsson PA. Neuroendocrine differentiation in prostate cancer: implications for new treatment modalities. Eur Urol 2005; 47: 147–55
20. Yang JC, Ok JH, Busby JE, Borowsky AD, Kung HJ, Evans CP. Aberrant activation of androgen receptor in a new neuropeptide-autocrine model of androgen-insensitive prostate cancer. Cancer Res 2009; 69: 151–60.
21. Barkin J, Crassweller PO, Roncari DA, Onrot J. Hypercalcemia associated with cancer of prostate without bony metastases. Urology 1984; 24: 368–71.
22. Pruneri G, Galli S, Rossi RS, *et al.* Chromogranin A and B and secretogranin II in prostatic adenocarcinomas: neuroendocrine expression in patients untreated and treated with androgen deprivation therapy. Prostate 1998; 34: 113–20.
23. Newmark SR, Dlhuh RG, Bennett AH. Ectopic adrenocorticotropin syndrome with prostatic carcinoma. Urology 1973; 2: 666–8.
24. Vuitch MF, Mendelsohn G. Relationship of ectopic ACTH production to tumor differentiation. A morphologic and immunohistochemical study of prostatic carcinoma with Cushing's syndrome. Cancer 1982; 47: 296–9.
25. Slater D. Carcinoid tumour of the prostate associated with inappropriate ACTH secretion. Br J Urol 1985; 57: 591–2.
26. Ghandur-Mnaymneh L, Satterfield S, Block NL. Small cell carcinoma of the prostate gland with inappropriate antidiuretic hormone secretion: morphological, immunohistochemical and clinical expressions. J Urol 1986; 135: 1263–6.
27. Sellwood RA, Spencer J, Azzopardi JG, Wapnick S, Welbourn RB, Kulatilake AE. Inappropriate secretion of antidiuretic hormone by carcinoma of the prostate. Br J Surg 1969; 56: 933–5.
28. Carey RM, Varma SK, Drake CR Jr, *et al.* Ectopic secretion of corticotropin-releasing factor as a cause of Cushing's syndrome. A clinical, morphologic and biochemical study. N Engl J Med 1984; 311: 13–20.
29. Jelbart ME, Russell PJ, Fullerton M, Russell P, Funder J, Raghavan D. Ectopic hormone production by a prostatic small cell carcinoma xenograft line. Mol Cell Endocrinol 1988; 55: 167–72.
30. Reeve JG, Stewart J, Watson JV, Wulfrank D, Twentyman PR, Bleehen NM. Neuron specific enolase expression in carcinoma of the lung. Br J Cancer 1986; 53: 519–28.

31. Ellis DW, Leffers S, Davies JS, Ng AB. Multiple immunoperoxidase markers in benign hyperplasia and adenocarcinoma of the prostate. Am J Clin Pathol 1984; 81: 279–84.

32. Heyderman E, Brown BM, Richardson TC. Epithelial markers in prostatic, bladder and colorectal cancer. An immunoperoxidase study of epithelial membrane antigen, carcino-embryonic antigen, and prostatic acid phosphatase. J Clin Pathol 1984; 37: 1363–9.

33. Ghazizadeh M. Immunohistochemical detection of CEA in benign hyperplasia and adenocarcinoma of the prostate with monoclonal antibody. J Urol 1984; 131: 501–4.

34. Jelbart ME, Russell PJ, Russell P, et al. Site-specific growth of the prostate xenograft line UCRU-PR-2. Prostate 1989; 14: 163–75.

35. Sim SJ, Glassman AB, Ro JY, Lee JJ, Logothetis CJ, Liu FJ. Serum calcitonin in small cell carcinoma of the prostate. Ann Clin Lab Sci 1996; 26: 487–95.

36. Sloane JP, Ormerod MG. Distribution of epithelial membrane antigen in normal and neoplastic tissues and its value in diagnostic tumor pathology. Cancer 1981; 47: 1786–95.

37. Ansari MA, Pintozzi RL, Choi YS, Ladove RF. Diagnosis of carcinoid-line metastatic prostatic carcinoma by an immunoperoxidase method. Am J Clin Pathol 1981; 76: 94–8.

38. Ghali VS, Garcia RL. Prostatic adenocarcinoma with carcinoidal features producing adrenocorticotropic syndrome. Cancer 1984; 54: 1043–8.

39. Almagro UA. Argyrophilic prostatic carcinoma. Case report with literature review on prostatic carcinoid and 'carcinoid-like' prostatic carcinoma. Cancer 1985; 55: 608–14.

40. Hindson DA, Knight LL, Ocker JM. Small-cell carcinoma of prostate. Transient complete remission with chemotherapy. Urology 1985; 26: 182–4.

41. Smith CS. Small cell carcinoma of the prostate. J Urol 1985; 133: 371A (abstract 1029).

42. Sommers SC. Endocrine changes with prostatic carcinoma. Cancer 1957; 10: 345–58.

43. Wise HM Jr, Pohl HL, Gazzaniga A, Harrison JH. Hyperadrenocorticism associated with 'reactivated' prostatic carcinoma. Surgery 1965; 57: 655–64.

44. Hall TC. Symptomatic hypokalaemic alkalosis in hyperadrenocorticism secondary to carcinoma of the prostate. Cancer 1968; 21: 190–2.

45. Angelsen A, Syversen U, Haugen OA, Stridsberg M, Mjølnerød OK, Waldum HL. Neuroendocrine differentiation in carcinomas of the prostate: do neuroendocrine serum markers reflect immunohistochemical findings? Prostate 1997; 30: 1–6.

46. Wu JT, Astill ME, Liu GH, Stephenson RA. Serum chromogranin A: early detection of hormonal resistance in prostate cancer patients. J Clin Lab Anal 1998; 12: 20–5.

47. Berruti A, Dogliotti L, Mosca A, et al. Potential clinical value of circulating chromogranin A in patients with prostate carcinoma. Ann Oncol 2001; 12(Suppl 2): S153–7.

48. Isshiki S, Akakura K, Komiya A, Suzuki H, Kamiya N, Ito H. Chromogranin a concentration as a serum marker to predict prognosis after endocrine therapy for prostate cancer. J Urol 2002; 167: 512–15.

49. Kamiya N, Akakura K, Suzuki H, et al. Pretreatment serum level of neuron specific enolase (NSE) as a prognostic factor in metastatic prostate cancer patients treated with endocrine therapy. Eur Urol 2003; 44: 309–14.

50. Beltran H, Rickman DS, Park K, et al. Molecular characterization of neuroendocrine prostate cancer and identification of new drug targets. Cancer Discovery 2011; 1(6): 487–95.

51. Aparicio A, Tzelepi V, Araujo JC, et al. Neuroendocrine prostate cancer xenografts with large-cell and small-cell features derived from a single patient's tumor: morphological, immunohistochemical, and gene expression profiles. Prostate 2011; 71(8): 846–56.

52. Sreekumar A, Poisson LM, Rajendiran TM, et al. Metabolomic profiles delineate potential role for sarcosine in prostate cancer progression. Nature 2000; 457(7231): 910–14.

53. Lotan TL, Gupta NS, Wang W, et al. ERG gene rearrangements are common in prostatic small cell carcinomas. Mod Pathol 2011; 24(6): 820–8.

54. Williamson SR, Zhang S, Yao JL, et al. ERG–TMPRSS2 rearrangement is shared by concurrent prostatic adenocarcinoma and prostatic small cell carcinoma and absent in small cell carcinoma of the urinary bladder: evidence supporting monoclonal origin. Mod Pathol 2011; 24(8): 1120–7.

55. Mosquera JM, Mehra R, Regan MM, et al. Prevalence of TMPRSS2-ERG fusion prostate cancer among men undergoing prostate biopsy in the United States. Clin Cancer Res 2009; 15(14): 4706–11.

56. Tai S, Sun Y, Squires JM, et al. PC3 is a cell line characteristic of prostatic small cell carcinoma. Prostate 2011; 71(15): 1668–79.

57. Yuan TC, Veeramani S, Lin MF. Neuroendocrine-like prostate cancer cells: neuroendocrine transdifferentiation of prostate adenocarcinoma cells. Endocr Relat Cancer 2007; 14(3): 531–47.

58. Noordzij MA, van Weerden WM, de Ridder CM, van der Kwast TH, Schröder FH, van Steenbrugge GJ. Neuroendocrine differentiation in human prostatic tumor models. Am J Pathol 1996; 149(3): 859–71.

59. Van Haaften-Day C, Raghavan D, Russell P, et al. Xenografted small cell undifferentiated cancer of prostate: possible common origin with prostatic adenocarcinoma. Prostate 1987; 11(3): 271–9.

60. Tung WL, Wang Y, Gout PW, Liu DM, Gleave M, Wang Y. Use of irinotecan for treatment of small cell carcinoma of the prostate. Prostate 2011; 71(7): 675–81.

61. Chiaverotti T, Couto SS, Donjacour A, et al. Dissociation of epithelial and neuroendocrine carcinoma lineages in the transgenic adenocarcinoma of mouse prostate model of prostate cancer. Am J Pathol 2008; 172(1): 236–46.

62. Perez-Stable C, Altman NH, Mehta PP, Deftos LJ, Roos BA. Prostate cancer progression, metastasis, and gene expression in transgenic mice. Cancer Res 1997; 57: 900–6.

63. Van Haaften–Day C, Russell P, Carr S, Wright L. Xenografted small cell undifferentiated cancer of prostate: possible common origin with prostatic adenocarcinoma. Prostate 1988; 11: 271–9.

64. Pittman S, Russell PJ, Jelbart ME, Wass J, Raghavan D. Flow cytometric and karyotypic analysis of a primary small cell carcinoma of the prostate: a xenografted cell line. Cancer Genet Cytogenet 1987; 26: 165–9.

65. Cohen RJ, Glezerson G, Taylor LF, Grundle HA, Naudé JH. The neuroendocrine cell population of the human prostate gland. J Urol 1993; 150: 365–8.

66. Pearse AGE, Pollak JM. Neural crest origin of the endocrine polypeptide (APUD) cell of the gastrointestinal cell and pancreas. Gut 1971; 12: 783–8.

67. Pearse AG, Takor T. Embryology of the diffuse neuroendocrine system and its relationship to the common peptides. Fed Proc 1979; 38: 2288–94.

68. LeDouarin N, Tellet MA. The migration of neural crest cells to the wall of the digestive tract in the avian embryo. J Embryol Exp Morphol 1972; 30: 31–48.

69. Schron DS, Gipson T, Mendelsohn G. The histogenesis of small cell carcinoma of the pancreas: an immunohistological study. Cancer 1984; 53: 2478–80.

70. Helpap BB, Kollerman J, Ochler U. Neuroendocrine differentiation in prostatic carcinoma: histogenesis, biology, clinical relevance, and future therapeutic perspectives. Urol Int 1999; 62: 133–8.

71. Duguid JB, Kennedy AM. Oat cell tumors of mediastinal glands. J Pathol Bacteriol 1930; 33: 93–9.

72. Brown JR, Wieczorek TJ, Shaffer K, Salgia R. Small-cell cancers, an unusual reaction to chemotherapy. J Clin Oncol 2003; 21: 2437–43.

73. Dauge MC, Delmas V. APUD type endocrine tumor of the prostate. Incidence and prognosis in association with adenocarcinoma. Prog Clin Biol Res 1987; 243A: 529.

74. Newmark SR, Dluhy RG, Bennett AH. Ectopic adrenocorticotropin syndrome with prostatic carcinoma. Urology 1973; 2: 666–8.

75. Lovern WJ, Fariss BL, Wettlaufer JN, Hane S. Ectopic ACTH production in disseminated prostatic adenocarcinoma. Urology 1975; 5: 817–20.

76. Holland EA. Prostatic adenocarcinoma with ectopic ACTH production. Br J Urol 1978; 50: 538–41.

77. Hindson DA, Knight LL, Ocker JM. Small-cell carcinoma of prostate. Transient complete remission with chemotherapy. Urology 1985; 26: 182–4.

78. Osterling JE, Hauzeur CG, Farrow GM. Small cell anaplastic carcinoma of the prostate: a clinical, pathologic and immunohistochemical study of 27 patients. J Urol 1992; 147: 804–7.

79. Amato RJ, Logothetis CJ, Hallinan R, Ro JY, Sella A, Dexeus FH. Chemotherapy for small cell carcinoma of prostatic origin. J Urol 1992; 147: 935–7.

80. Montasser AY, Ong MG, Mehta VT. Carcinoid tumor of the prostate associated with adenocarcinoma. Cancer 1979; 44: 307–10.

81. Wasserstein PW, Goldman RL. Diffuse carcinoid of prostate. Urology 1981; 18: 407–9.

82. Têtu B, Ro JY, Ayala AG, Ordóñez NG, Johnson DE. Small cell carcinoma of the prostate, Part 1: A clinicopathologic study of 20 cases. Cancer 1987; 59: 1803–9.

83. McCutcheon IE, Eng DY, Logothetis CJ. Brain metastases from prostate carcinoma. Antemortem recognition and outcome after treatment. Cancer 1999; 86: 2301–11.

84. Scheble VJ, Braun M, Wilbertz T, et al. ERG rearrangement in small cell prostatic and lung cancer. Histopathology 2010; 56: 937–43.

85. Scheble VJ, Braun M, Beroukhim R, et al. ERG rearrangement is specific to prostate cancer and does not occur in any other common tumor. Mod Pathol 2010; 23: 1061–7.

86. Bradley JD, Dehdashti F, Mintun MA, Govindan R, Trinkaus K, Siegel BA. Positron emission tomography in limited-stage small-cell lung cancer: a prospective study. J Clin Oncol 2004; 22: 3248–54.

87. Brink I, Schumacher T, Mix M, Ruhland S, et al. Impact of [18F]FDG-PET on the primary staging of small-cell lung cancer. Eur J Nucl Med Mol Imaging 2004; 31: 1614–20.

88. Torii K, Kawabe J, Hayashi T, et al. A case of small cell carcinoma of the esophagus detected incidentally by FDG–PET. Ann Nucl Med 2004; 18: 699–702.

89. Chander S, Ergün EL, Westphal S, Powell W, Zerin JM, Nandkumar U. Small cell carcinoma of the parotid gland: evaluation with FDG PET imaging. Clin Nucl Med 2004; 29: 502–3.

90. Bishop JF, Raghavan D, Stuart-Harris R, et al. Carboplatin (CBDCA, JM-8) and VP-16–213 in previously untreated patients with small cell lung cancer. J Clin Oncol 1987; 5: 1574–9.

91. Siefker-Radtke AO, Dinney CP, Abrahams NA, et al. Evidence supporting preoperative chemotherapy for small cell carcinoma of the bladder: a retrospective review of the MD Anderson cancer experience. J Urol 2004; 172: 481–4.

92. Quek ML, Nichols PW, Yamzon J, et al. Radical cystectomy for primary neuroendocrine tumors of the bladder: the University of Southern California experience. J Urol 2005; 174: 93–6.

93. Murren JR, Turrisi AT, Pass HI. Small cell lung cancer. In: Devita VT Jr, Hellman S, Rosenberg SA (eds) Cancer Principles and Practice of Oncology, 7th edn. Philadelphia: Lippincott Williams and Wilkins, 2005. pp. 810–43.

94. Creaven PJ, Raghavan D, Pendyala L, Loewen G, Kindler HL, Berghorn EJ Jr. Paclitaxel and carboplatin in early phase studies: Roswell Park Cancer Institute experience in the subset of patients with lung cancer. Semin Oncol 1997; 24(Suppl 12): 138–43.

95. Galanis E, Frytak S, Lloyd RV. Extrapulmonary small cell carcinoma. Cancer 1997; 79: 1729–36.

96. Papandreou CN, Daliani DD, Thall PF, et al. Results of a phase II study with doxorubicin, etoposide, and cisplatin in patients with small-cell carcinoma of the prostate. J Clin Oncol 2002; 20: 3072–80.

97. Fléchon A, Pouessel D, Ferlay C, et al. Phase II study of carboplatin and etoposide in patients with anaplastic progressive metastatic castration-resistant prostate cancer (mCRPC) with or without neuroendocrine differentiation: results of the French Genito-Urinary Tumor Group (GETUG) P01 trial. Ann Oncol 2011; 22(11): 2476–81.

98. Brevini TA, Bianchi R, Motta M. Direct inhibitory effect of somatostatin on the growth of the human prostate cancer cell line LNCaP: possible mechanisms of action. J Clin Endocrinol Metab 1993; 77: 626.

99. Spieth ME, Lin G, Nguyen TT. Diagnosis and treating small-cell carcinomas of prostatic origin. Clin Nucl Med 2002; 27: 11–17.

100. Mackey JR, Au HJ, Hugh J, Venner P. Genitourinary small cell carcinoma: determination of clinical and therapeutic factors associated with survival. J Urol 1998; 159: 1624–9.

101. Weinstein MH, Partin AW, Veltri RW, Epstein JI. Neuroendocrine differentiation in prostate cancer: enhanced prediction of progression after radical prostatectomy. Hum Pathol 1996; 27: 683–7.

102. www.iarc.fr/en/publications/pdfs-online/pat-gen/

103. Stirling WC, Ash JE. Sarcoma of the prostate. J Urol 1939; 41: 515–33.

104. Schmidt JD, Welch MJ. Sarcoma of the prostate. Cancer 1976; 37: 1908–12.

105. Dotan ZA, Tal R, Golijanin D. Adult genitourinary sarcoma: the 25-year Memorial Sloan-Kettering experience. J Urol 2006; 176(5): 2033–8.

106. Smith BH, Dehner JP. Sarcoma of the prostate gland. Am J Clin Pathol 1972; 58: 43–50.

107. Sexton WJ, Lance RE, Reyes AO, Pisters PW, Tu SM, Pisters LL. Adult prostate sarcoma: the MD Anderson Cancer Center experience. J Urol 2001; 166: 521–5.

108. Laturnus JM, Gebhard M, Sommerauer M, Jocham D, Doehn C. Stromal tumour of uncertain malignant potential of the prostate (STUMP) – a case report. Akt Urol 2010; 41(3): 197–9.

109. Fukuhara S, Matsuoka Y, Hanafusa T, Nakayama M, Takayama H, Tsujihata M. A case report of prostatic stromal tumor of uncertain malignant potential (STUMP). Hinyokika Kiyo 2008; 54(5): 377–81.

110. Coindre JM, Trojani M, Contesso G, David M, Rouesse J, Bui NB. Reproducibility of a histopathologic grading system for adult soft tissue sarcoma. Cancer 1986; 58: 306–9.

111. Shiraki M, Enterline HT, Brooks JJ, et al. Pathologic analysis of advanced adult soft tissue sarcomas, bone sarcomas, and mesotheliomas. The Eastern Cooperative Oncology Group (ECOG) experience. Cancer 1989; 64: 484–90.

112. Alvegard TA, Berg NO. Histopathology peer review of high-grade soft tissue sarcoma: the Scandinavian Sarcoma Group experience. J Clin Oncol 1989; 7: 1845–51.

113. Fletcher CD, Gustafson P, Rydholm A, Willén H, Akerman M. Clinicopathologic re-evaluation of 100 malignant fibrous histiocytomas: prognostic relevance of subclassification. J Clin Oncol 2001; 19: 3045–50.

114. Enzinger FM, Weiss SW. General considerations. In: Enzinger FM, Weiss SW (eds) Soft Tissue Sarcomas. St. Louis, Missouri: CV Mosby, 1988. pp. 1–17.

115. Reddick RL, Michellitch H, Triche TJ. Malignant soft tissue tumors (malignant fibrous histiocytoma, pleomorphic liposarcoma, and pleomorphic rhabdomyosarcoma): an electron microscope study. Hum Pathol 1979; 10: 327–43.

116. Sandberg AA, Turc-Carel C, Gemmill RM. Chromosomes in solid tumors and beyond. Cancer Res 1988; 48: 1049–59.

117. Mitelman F, Kaneko Y, Trent JM. Report of the committee on chromosome changes in neoplasia. Cytogenet Cell Genet 1990; 55: 358–86.

118. Khan J, Wei JS, Ringnér M, et al. Classification and diagnostic prediction of cancers using gene expression profiling and artificial neural networks. Nat Med 2001; 7: 673–9.

119. Nielsen TO, West RB, Linn SC, et al. Molecular characterization of soft tissue tumors: a gene expression study. Lancet 2002; 359: 1301–7.

120. Khan J, Saal LH, Bittner ML, Chen Y, Trent JM, Meltzer PS. CDNA microarrays detect activation of a myogenic transcription program by the PAC3-FKHR fusion oncogene. Proc Natl Acad Sci USA 1999; 96: 13264–9.

121. Lessnick SL, Dacwag CS, Golub TR. The Ewing's sarcoma oncoprotein EWS/FLI induces a p53-dependent growth arrest in primary human fibroblasts. Cancer Cell 2002; 1: 393–401.

122. Allander SV, Nupponen NN, Ringnér M, et al. Gastrointestinal stromal tumors with KIT mutations exhibit a remarkably homogeneous gene expression profile. Cancer Res 2001; 61: 8624–8.

123. Allander SV, Ehrenborg E, Luthman H, Powell DR. Expression of synovial sarcoma by cDNA microarrays: association of ERBB2, IGHBP2, and ELF3 with epithelial differentiation. Am J Pathol 2002; 161: 1587–95.

124. Francis P, Namløs HM, Müller C. Diagnostic and prognostic gene expression signatures in 177 soft tissue sarcomas: hypoxia-induced transcription profile signifies metastatic potential. BMC Genom 2007; 8: 73.

125. Bain GO, Danyluk JM, Shnitka TK, Jewell LD, Manickavel V. Malignant fibrous histiocytoma of prostate gland. Urology 1985; 26: 89–91.

126. Hulbert JC, Rodriguez PN, Cummings KB. Perineal liposarcoma: diagnosis and management. J Urol 1984; 131: 1185–7.

127. Smith DM, Manivel C, Kapps D, Uecker J. Angiosarcoma of the prostate: report of 2 cases and review of the literature. J Urol 1986; 135: 382–4.

128. Cea PC, Ward JN. Sarcoma of the prostate 13 years after suprapubic prostatectomy. J Urol 1977; 117: 129–30.

129. Mottola A, Selli C, Carini M, Natali A, Gambacorta G. Leiomyosarcoma of the prostate. Eur Urol 1985; 11: 131–3.

130. Cheville JC, Dundore PA, Nascimento AG, et al. Leiomyosarcoma of the prostate. Report of 23 cases. Cancer 1995; 76: 1422–7.

131. Iwasaki H, Ishiguro M, Ohjimi Y, et al. Synovial sarcoma of the prostate with t(x; 18) (p11.2; q11.2). Am J Surg Pathol 1999; 23: 220–6.

132. Williams DH, Hua VN, Chowdhry AA, Laskin WB, Kalapurakal JA, Dumanian GA. Synovial sarcoma of the prostate. J Urol 2004; 171: 2376.

133. Miedler JD, MacLennan GT. Leiomyosarcoma of the prostate. J Urol 2007; 178: 668.

134. Vandoros GP, Manolidis T, Karamouzis MV, et al. Leiomyosarcoma of the prostate: case report and review of 54 previously published cases. Sarcoma 2008; 2008: 458709.

135. Peterson LJ, Paulson DF. Rhabdomyosarcoma in adult prostate. Urology 1974; 3: 689–92.

136. Dupree WB, Fisher C. Rhabdomyosarcoma of prostate in adult. Long-term survival and problem of histologic diagnosis. Urology 1982; 19: 80–2.

137. Keenan DJM, Graham WH. Embryonal rhabdomyosarcoma of the prostatic-urethral region in an adult. Br J Urol 1985; 57: 241.

138. Palmer MA, Viswanath S, Desmond AD. Adult prostatic rhabdomyosarcoma. Br J Urol 1993; 71: 489–90.

139. Wang KF, Wu B, Zhang Y. Adult prostate sarcoma: a report of 6 cases with clinical analysis. Zhonghua Nan Ke Xue 2007l; 13(7): 617–19.

140. Miettinen M. Rhabdomyosarcoma in patients older than 40 years of age. Cancer 1988; 62: 2060–5.

141. Waring PM, Newland RC. Prostatic embryonal rhabdomyosarcoma in adults. A clinicopathologic review. Cancer 1992; 69: 755–62.

142. Harik LR, Merino C, Coindre JM, Amin MB, Pedeutour F, Weiss SW. Pseudosarcomatous myofibroblastic proliferations of the bladder: a clinicopathologic study of 42 cases. Am J Surg Pathol 2006; 30(7): 787–94.

143. Iczkowski KA, Shanks JH, Gadaleanu V, et al. Inflammatory pseudotumor and sarcoma of urinary bladder: differential diagnosis and outcome in thirty-eight spindle cellneoplasms. Mod Pathol 2001; 14(10): 1043–51.

144. Montgomery EA, Shuster DD, Burkart AL, et al. Inflammatory myofibroblastic tumors of the urinary tract: a clinicopathologic study of 46 cases, including a malignant example inflammatory fibrosarcoma and a subset associated with high-grade urothelial carcinoma. Am J Surg Pathol 2006; 30(12): 1502–12.

145. Tsuzuki T, Magi-Galluzzi C, Epstein JI. ALK-1 expression in inflammatory myofibroblastic tumor of the urinary bladder. Am J Surg Pathol 2004; 28(12): 1609–14.

146. Herawi M, Epstein JI. Specialized stromal tumors of the prostate: a clinicopathologic study of 50 cases. Am J Surg Pathol 2006; 30(6): 694–704.

147. Nagar M, Epstein JI. Epithelial proliferations in prostatic stromal tumors of uncertain malignant potential (STUMP). Am J Surg Pathol 2011; 35(6): 898–903.

148. Bostwick DG, Hossain D, Qian J, et al. Phyllodes tumor of the prostate: long-term followup study of 23 cases. J Urol 2004; 172(3): 894–9.

149. López-Beltran A, Gaeta JF, Huben R, Croghan GA. Malignant phyllodes tumor of prostate. Urology 1990; 35: 164–7.

150. Manivel C, Shenoy BV, Wick MR, Dehner LP. Cystosarcoma phyllodes of the prostate. Arch Pathol Lab Med 1986; 110: 534–8.

151. Reese JH, Lombard CM, Krone K, Stamey TA. Phyllodes type of atypical prostatic hyperplasia: a report of 3 new cases. J Urol 1987; 138: 623–6.

152. Yokota T, Yamashita Y, Okuzono Y, et al. Malignant cystosarcoma phyllodes of prostate. Acta Pathol Jpn 1984; 34: 663–8.

153. Gueft B, Walsh MA. Malignant prostatic cystosarcoma phyllodes. NY State J Med 1975; 75: 2226–8.

154. Yum M, Miller JC, Agrawal BL. Leiomyosarcoma arising in atypical fibromuscular hyperplasia (phyllodes tumor) of the prostate with distant metastasis. Cancer 1991; 68: 910–15.

155. Têtu B, Ro JY, Ayala AG, Srigley JR, Bégin LR, Bostwick DG. Atypical spindle cell lesions of the prostate. Semin Diagn Pathol 1988; 5: 284–93.

156. Gaudin PB, Rosai J, Epstein JI. Sarcomas and related proliferative lesions of specialized prostatic stroma: a clinicopathologic study of 22 cases. Am J Surg Pathol 1998; 22: 148–62.

157. Watanabe M, Yamada Y, Kato H, et al. Malignant phyllodes tumor of the prostate: retrospective review of specimens obtained by sequential transurethral resection. Pathol Int 2002; 52: 777–83.

158. Kim HS, Lee JH, Nam JH, et al. Malignant phyllodes tumor of prostate. Pathol Int 1999; 49: 1105–8.

159. Schapmans S, van Leuven L, Cortvriend J, Beelaerts W, van Erps P.Phyllodes tumor of the prostate. A case report and review of the literature. Eur Urol 2000; 38: 649–53.

160. Lam KC, Yeo W. Chemotherapy induced complete remission in malignant phyllodes tumor of the prostate metastasizing to the lung. J Urol 2002; 168: 1104–5.

161. Tijare JR, Shrikhande AV, Shrikhande VV. Phyllodes type of atypical prostatic hyperplasia. J Urol 1999; 162: 803–4.

162. Yamamoto S, Ito T, Miki M, Serizawa H, Maekawa S, Furusato M. Malignant phyllodes tumor of the prostate. Int J Urol 2000; 7: 378–81.

163. Young JF, Jensen PE, Wiley CA. Malignant phyllodes tumor of prostate. A case report with immunohistochemical and ultrastructural studies. Arch Pathol Lab Med 1992; 116: 296–9.

164. Bostwick DG, Hossain D, Qian J, et al. Phyllodes tumor of the prostate: long-term follow up study of 23 cases. J Urol 2004; 172: 894–9.

165. Wang X, Jones TD, Zhang S, et al. Amplifications of EGFR gene and protein expression of EGFR, Her-2/neu, c-kit, and androgen receptor in phyllodes tumor of the prostate.Mod Pathol 2007; 20: 175–82.

166. Zenklusen HR, Weymuth G, Rist M, Mihatsch MJ. Carcinosarcoma of the prostate in combination with adenocarcinoma of the prostate and adenocarcinoma of the seminal vesicles. A case report with immunocytochemical analysis and review of the literature. Cancer 1990; 66: 998–1001.

167. Wick MR, Young RH, Malvesta R, Beebe DS, Hansen JJ, Dehner LP. Prostatic carcinosarcomas. Clinical, histologic, and immunohistochemical data on two cases, with a review of the literature. Am J Clin Pathol 1989; 92: 131–9.

168. Ginesin Y, Bolkier M, Moskovitz B, Lichtig C, Levin DR. Carcinosarcoma of the prostate. Eur Urol 1986; 12: 441–2.

169. Krastanova LJ, Addonizio JC. Carcinosarcoma of prostate. Urology 1981; 18: 85–8.

170. Tannenbaum M. Carcinoma with sarcomatoid changes or carcinosarcoma of prostate. Urology 1975; 6: 91–3.

171. Quay SC, Proppe KH. Carcinosarcoma of the prostate: case report and review of the literature. J Urol 1981; 125: 436–8.

172. Martin SA, Fowler M, Catalona WJ, Boyarsky S. Carcinosarcoma of the prostate: report of a case with ultrastructural observations. J Urol 1979; 122: 709–11.

173. Hokamura K, Kurozumi T, Tanaka K, Yamaguchi A. Carcinosarcoma of the prostate. Acta Pathol Jpn 1985; 35: 481–7.

174. Lindboe CF, Mjones J. Carcinosarcoma of prostate. Immunohistochemical and ultrastructural observations. Urology 1992; 40: 376–80.

175. Nazeer T, Barada JH, Fisher HA, Ross JS. Prostatic carcinosarcoma: case report and review of literature. J Urol 1991; 146: 1370–3.

176. Kubosawa H, Matsuzaki O, Kondo Y, Takao M, Sato N. Carcinosarcoma of the prostate. Acta Pathol Jpn 1993; 43: 209–14.

177. Shannon RL, Ro JY, Grignon DJ, *et al.* Sarcomatoid carcinoma of the prostate. A clinicopathologic study of 12 patients. Cancer 1992; 69: 2676–82.

178. Fukawa T, Numata K, Yamanaka M, *et al.* Prostatic carcinosarcoma: a case report and review of literature. Int J Urol 2003; 10: 108–13.

179. Dundore PA, Cheville JC, Nascimento AG, Farrow GM, Bostwick DG. Carcinosarcoma of the prostate: report of 21 cases. Cancer 1995; 76: 1035–42.

180. Hansel DE, Epstein JI. Sarcomatoid carcinoma of the prostate: a study of 42 cases. Am J Surg Pathol 2006; 30(10): 1316–21.

181. Mostofi FK, Price EB. Malignant tumors of the prostate. In: *Atlas of Tumor Pathology: Tumors of Male Genital System,* series 2, part8. Washington, DC: Armed Forces Institute of Pathology, 1973. pp. 257–8.

182. Chung LW, Chang SM, Bell C, Zhau HE, Ro JY, von Eschenbach AC. Co-inoculation of tumorigenic rat prostate mesenchymal cells with non-tumorigenic epithelial cells results in the development of carcinosarcoma in syngeneic and athymic animals. Int J Cancer 1989; 43: 1179–87.

183. Elo TD, Valve EM, Seppänen JA, *et al.* Stromal activation associated with development of prostate cancer in prostate-targeted fibroblast growth factor 8b transgenic mice. Neoplasia 2010; 12(11): 915–27.

184. Pierce SM, Recht A, Lingos TI, *et al.* Long-term radiation complications following conservative surgery (CS) and radiation therapy (RT) in patients with early stage breast cancer. Int J Radiat Oncol Biol Phys 1992; 23: 915–23.

185. Mark RJ, Poen J, Tran LM, Fu YS, Selch MT, Parker RG. Postirradiation sarcomas. A single-institution study and review of the literature. Cancer 1994; 73: 2653–62.

186. Cha C, Antonescu CR, Quan ML, Maru S, Brennan MF. Long-term results with resection of radiation-induced soft tissue sarcomas. Ann Surg 2004; 239: 903–10.

187. Laskin WB, Silverman TA, Enzinger FM. Postradiation soft tissue sarcomas. An analysis of 53 cases. Cancer 1988; 62: 2330–40.

188. Huvos AG, Woodard HQ, Cahan WG, Higinbotham NL, Stewart FW, Butler A, Bretsky SS. Postradiation osteogenic sarcoma of bone and soft tissues. A clinicopathologic study of 66 patients. Cancer 1985; 55: 1244–55.

189. Scully JM, Uno JM, McIntyre M, Mosely S. Radiation-induced prostatic sarcoma: a case report. J Urol 1999; 144: 746–8.

190. McKenzie M, MacLennan I, Kostashuk E, Bainbridge T. Postirradiation sarcoma after external beam radiation for localized adenocarcinoma of the prostate: report of three cases. Urology 1999; 53: 1228.

191. Prevost JB, Bossi A, Sciot R, Debiec-Rychter M. Post irradiation sarcoma after external bean radiation therapy for localized adenocarcinoma of the prostate. Tumori 2004; 90: 618–21.

192. Terris MK. Transrectal ultrasound appearance of radiation-induced prostatic sarcoma. Prostate 1998; 37: 182–6.

193. Joerger M, Oehlschlegel C, Cerny T, Gillessen S. Postradiation high-grade myofibroblastic sarcoma of the prostate – a rare entity of prostatic tumors – responding to liposomal doxorubicin. Onkologie 2002; 25(6): 558–61.

194. Nishiyama T, Ikarashi T, Terunuma M, Ishizaki S. Osteogenic sarcoma of the prostate. Int J Urol 2001; 8(4): 199–201.

195. Canfield SE, Gans TH, Unger P, Hall SJ. Postradiation prostatic sarcoma: de novo carcinogenesis or dedifferentiation of prostatic adenocarcinoma. Tech Urol 2001; 7(4): 294–5.

196. Kumar V, Khurana N, Rathi AK, *et al.* Primitive neuroectodermal tumor of prostate. Indian J Pathol Microbiol 2008; 51(3): 386–8.

197. Funahashi Y, Yoshino Y, Hattori R. Ewing's sarcoma/primitive neuroectodermal tumor of the prostate. Int J Urol 2009; 16(9): 769.

198. Varghese SL, Grossfeld GD. The prostatic gland: malignancies other than adenocarcinomas. Radiol Clin North Am 2000; 38(1): 179–202.

199. Geoffray A, Couanet D, Montagne JP, Leclere J, Flamant F. Ultrasonography and computed tomography for diagnosis and follow-up of pelvic rhabdomyosarcomas in children. Pediatr Radiol 1987; 17(2): 132–4.

200. Bahnson RR, Zaontz MR, Maizels M, Shkolnik AA, Firlit CF. Ultrasonography and diagnosis of pediatric genitourinary rhabdomyosarcoma. Urology 1989; 33(1): 64–8.

201. Bartolozzi C, Selli C, Olmastroni M, Menchi I, di Candio G. Rhabdomyosarcoma of the prostate: MR findings. Am J Roentgenol 1988; 150(6): 1333–4.

202. Ren FY, Lu JP, Wang J, Ye JJ, Shao CW, Wang MJ. Adult prostate sarcoma: radiological-clinical correlation. Clin Radiol 2009; 64(2): 171–7.

203. Kattan MW, Leung DH, Brennan MF. Postoperative nomogram for 12-year sarcoma-specific death. J Clin Oncol 2002; 20(3): 791–6.

204. Borden EC, Baker LH, Bell RS, *et al.* Soft tissue sarcomas of adults: state of the translational science. Clin Cancer Res 2003; 9(6): 1941–56.

205. Janet NL, May AW, Akins RS. Sarcoma of the prostate: a single institutional review. Am J Clin Oncol 2009; 32(1): 27–9.

206. Markhede G, Angervall L, Stener B. A multivariate analysis of the prognosis after surgical treatment of malignant soft-tissue tumors. Cancer 1982; 49(8): 1721–33.

207. Pisters PW, Leung DH, Woodruff J, Shi W, Brennan MF. Analysis of prognostic factors in 1,041 patients with localized soft tissue sarcomas of the extremities. J Clin Oncol 1996; 14(5): 1679–89.

208. Yang JC, Chang AE, Baker AR, *et al.* Randomized prospective study of the benefit of adjuvant radiation therapy in the treatment of soft tissue sarcomas of the extremity. J Clin Oncol 1998; 16(1): 197–203.

209. Zagars GK, Ballo MT, Pisters PW, Pollock RE, Patel SR, Benjamin RS. Preoperative vs. postoperative radiation therapy for soft tissue sarcoma: a retrospective comparative evaluation of disease outcome. Int J Radiat Oncol Biol Phys 2003; 56(2): 482–8.

210. Farhood AI, Hajdu SI, Shiu MH, Strong EW. Soft tissue sarcomas of the head and neck in adults. Am J Surg 1990; 160(4): 365–9.

211. Glenn J, Kinsella T, Glatstein E, *et al.* Results of multimodality therapy of resectable soft-tissue sarcomas of the retroperitoneum. Surgery 1985; 97: 316–25.

212. Meijer S, Peretz T, Gaynor JJ, Tan C, Hajdu SI, Brennan MF. Primary colorectal sarcoma. A retrospective review and prognostic factor study of 50 consecutive patients. Arch Surg 1990; 125(9): 1163–8.

213. Potter DA, Glenn J, Kinsella T, *et al.* Patterns of recurrence in patients with high-grade soft-tissue sarcomas. J Clin Oncol 1985; 3(3): 353–66.

214. Maurer HM, Beltangady M, Gehan EA, *et al.* The Intergroup Rhabdomyosarcoma Study–I. A final report. Cancer 1988; 61(2): 209–20.

215. Maurer HM, Gehan EA, Beltangady M, *et al.* The Intergroup Rhabdomyosarcoma Study–II. Cancer 1993; 71(5): 1904–22.

216. Crist W, Gehan EA, Ragab AH, *et al.* The Third Intergroup Rhabdomyosarcoma Study. J Clin Oncol 1995; 13: 610–30.

217. Crist WM, Anderson JR, Meza JL, *et al.* Intergroup Rhabdomyosarcoma Study–IV: results for patients with nonmetastatic disease. J Clin Oncol 2001; 19(12): 3091–102.

218. Arndt C, Rodeberg D, Breitfeld PP, Raney RB, Ullrich F, Donaldson S. Does bladder preservation (as a surgical principle) lead to retaining bladder function in bladder/prostate rhabdomyosarcoma? Results from Intergroup Rhabdomyosarcoma Study IV. J Urol 2004; 171(6 Pt 1): 2396–403.

219. Brennan MF. Soft tissue sarcoma: advances in understanding and management. Surgeon 2005; 3(3): 216–23.

220. Maki RG. Gemcitabine and docetaxel in metastatic sarcoma: past, present, and future. Oncologist 2007; 12(8): 999–1006.

221. American Joint Committee on Cancer. Soft tissue sarcoma. In: *AJCC Cancer Staging Manual,* 6th edn. Philadelphia: Lippincott-Raven, 2002. pp. 221–8.

222. Pervaiz N, Colterjohn N, Farrokhyar F, Tozer R, Figueredo A, Ghert M. A systematic meta-analysis of randomized controlled trials of adjuvant chemotherapy for localized resectable soft-tissue sarcoma. Cancer 2008; 113(3): 573–81.

223. Frustaci S, Gherlinzoni F, de Paoli A, *et al.* Adjuvant chemotherapy for adult soft tissue sarcomas of the extremities and girdles: results of the Italian Randomized Cooperative Trial. J Clin Oncol 2001; 19(5): 1238–47.

224. Petrioli R, Coratti A, Correale P, *et al.* Adjuvant epirubicin with or without ifosfamide for adult soft-tissue sarcoma. Am J Clin Oncol 2002; 25(5): 468–73.

225. Glenn J, Kinsella T, Glatstein E, *et al*. A randomized, prospective trial of adjuvant chemotherapy in adults with soft tissue sarcomas of the head and neck, breast, and trunk. Cancer 1985; 55(6): 1206–14.

226. Verma S, Younus J, Stys-Norman D, Haynes AE, Blackstein M. Ifosfamide-based combination chemotherapy in advanced soft-tissue sarcoma: a practice guideline. Curr Oncol 2007; 14(4): 144–8.

227. Ferlay J, Shin HR, Bray F. Estimates of worldwide burden of cancer in 2008: GLOBOCAN 2008. Int J Cancer 2010; 127(12): 2893–917.

228. Melicow MM, Hollowell JW. Intra-urothelial cancer: carcinoma in situ, Bowen's disease of the urinary system: discussion of thirty cases. J Urol 1952; 68: 763–72.

229. Kahler JE. Carcinoma of the prostate gland: a pathologic study. J Urol 1939; 41: 557.

230. Thompson GJ. Transurethral resection of malignant lesions of the prostate gland. JAMA 1942; 120: 1105.

231. Ortega LG, Whitmore WF, Murphy AI. In situ carcinoma of the prostate with intraepithelial extension into the urethra and bladder. Cancer 1953; 6: 898.

232. Salazar G, Frable WJ. Extramammary Paget's disease: a case involving the prostatic urethra. Am J Clin Pathol 1969; 52: 607–12.

233. Chesterman FC, Franks LM. Intra-epithelial carcinoma of prostatic urethra, peri-urethral glands, and prostatic ducts (Bowen's disease of urinary epithelium). Br J Cancer 1956; 10: 223–5.

234. Ende N, Woods LP, Shelley HS. Carcinoma originating in ducts surrounding the prostatic urethra. Am J Clin Pathol 1963; 40: 183–9.

235. Karpas CM, Moumgis B. Primary transitional cell carcinoma of prostate gland: possible pathogenesis and relationship to reserve cell hyperplasia of prostatic periurethral ducts. J Urol 1969; 101: 201–5.

236. Bates HR. Transitional cell carcinoma of the prostate. J Urol 1969; 101: 206–7.

237. Johnson DE, Hogan JM, Ayala AG. Transitional cell carcinoma of the prostate. A clinical morphological study. Cancer 1972; 29: 287–93.

238. Seemayer TA, Knaack J, Thelmo WL, Wang NS, Ahmed MN. Further observations on carcinoma in situ of the urinary bladder: silent but extensive intraprostatic involvement. Cancer 1975; 36: 514–20.

239. Grabstald H. Prostatic biopsy in selected patients with carcinoma in situ of the bladder: preliminary report. J Urol 1984; 132: 1117–18.

240. Rhamy RK, Buchanan RD, Spalding MJ. Intraductal carcinoma of the prostate gland. J Urol 1973; 109: 457–60.

241. Montie JE, Wood DP Jr, Mendendorp SV, Levin HS, Pontes JE. The significance and management of transitional cell carcinoma of the prostate. Semin Urol 1990; 8: 262–8.

242. Rubenstein AB, Rubnitz ME. Transitional cell carcinoma of the prostate. Cancern1969; 24: 543–6.

243. Adley BP, Maxwell K, Dalton DP, Yang XJ. Urothelial-type adenocarcinoma of the prostate mimicking metastatic colorectal adenocarcinoma. Int Braz J Urol 2006; 32(6): 681–7.

244. Montie JE, Mirsky H, Levin H. Transitional cell carcinoma of the prostate in a series of cystectomies: incidence and staging problems. J Urol 1986; 135: 243A (abstract 557).

245. Matzkin H, Soloway MS, Hardeman S. Transitional cell carcinoma of the prostate. J Urol 1991; 146: 1207–12.

246. Albert PS, Mallouh C, Nagamatsu GR. Transitional-cell carcinoma of prostate: an enigma. Urology 1973; 2: 128–30.

247. Goebbels R, Amberger L, Wernert N, Dhom G. Urothelial carcinoma of the prostate. Appl Pathol 1985; 3: 242–54.

248. Zincke H, Utz DC, Farrow GM. Review of the Mayo Clinic experience with carcinoma in situ. Urology 1985; 26(4 Suppl): 39–46.

249. Tannenbaum M. Transitional cell carcinoma of prostate.Urology 1975; 5: 674–8.

250. Dhom G, Mohr G. Urothel-Carcinome in der Prostata. Urologe A 1977; 16: 70–2.

251. Pagano F, Bassi P, Ferrante GL, *et al*. Is stage pT4a (D1) reliable in assessing transitional cell carcinoma involvement of the prostate in patients with a concurrent bladder cancer? A necessary distinction for contiguous or noncontiguous involvement. J Urol 1996; 155: 244–7.

252. Schellhammer PF, Bean MA, Whitmore WF. Prostatic involvement by transitional cell carcinoma: pathogenesis, patterns and prognosis. J Urol1977; 118: 399–403.

253. Wood DP Jr, Montie JE, Pontes JE, VanderBrug Medendorp S, Levin HS. Transitional cell carcinoma of the prostate in cystoprostatectomy specimens removed for bladder cancer. J Urol 1989; 141: 346–9.

254. Honda N, Yamada Y, Okada M, *et al*. Clinical study of transitional cell carcinoma of the prostate associated with bladder transitional cell carcinoma. Int J Urol 2001; 8: 662–8.

255. Esrig D, Freeman JA, Elmajian DA, *et al*. Transitional cell carcinoma involving the prostate with a proposed staging classification for stromal invasion. J Urol 1996; 156: 1071–6.

256. Kirk D, Savage A, Makepeace AR, Gostelow BE. Transitional cell carcinoma involving the prostate – an unfavorable prognostic sign in the management of bladder cancer?. Br J Urol 1981; 53: 610.

257. Hudson MA, Catalona WJ. Urothelial tumors of the bladder, upper tracts, and prostate. In: Gillenwater JY *et al*. (eds) *Adult and Pediatric Urology*. St Louis, Missouri: Mosby-Year Book, 1996.

258. Mevorach RA.. Human papillomavirus type 6 in grade I transitional cell carcinoma of the urethra. J Urol 1990; 143: 126.

259. Monseur J, Leguéné B, Lebouffant L, Tichoux G. Asbestose du col vésical et de la prostate. J Urol 1986; 92: 17.

260. Ullmann AS, Ross OA. Hyperplasia, atypism, and carcinoma in situ in prostatic periurethral glands. Am J Clin Pathol 1967; 47: 497.

261. Mahadevia PS, Koss LG, Tar IJ. Prostatic involvement in bladder cancer: prostate mapping in 20 cystoprostatectomy specimens. Cancer 1986; 58: 2096.

262. Montie JE, Wojno K, Klein E, Pearsall C, Levin H. Transitional cell carcinoma in situ of the seminal vesicles: 8 cases with discussion of pathogenesis, and clinical and biological implications. J Urol 1997; 158: 1895.

263. Dube VE, Farrow GM, Greene LF. Prostatic adenocarcinoma of ductal origin. Cancer 1973; 32: 402.

264. Aydin F. Endometrioid adenocarcinoma of prostatic urethra presenting with anterior urethral implantation. Urology 1993; 41: 91.

265. Bostwick DG. Neoplasms of the prostate. In: Bostwick DG, Eble JN (eds) *Urologic Surgical Pathology*. St. Louis, Missouri: Mosby-Year Book, 1997.

266. Sawczuk I, Tannenbaum M, Olsson CA, deVere White R. Primary transitional cell carcinoma of prostatic periurethral ducts. Urology 1985; 25: 339.

267. Greene LF, O'Dea MJ, Dockerty MB. Primary transitional cell carcinoma of the prostate. J Urol 1976; 116: 761.

268. Murphy WM, Gaeta JF. Diseases of the prostate gland and seminal vesicals. In: Murphy WM (ed) *Urological Pathology*. Philadelphia: WB Saunders, 1989.

269. Bryan RL, Newman J, Suarez V, Kadow C, O'Brien JM. The significance of prostatic urothelial dysplasia. Histopathology 1993; 22: 501.

270. Wishnow KI, Ro JY. Importance of early treatment of transitional cell carcinoma of prostatic ducts. Urology 1988; 32: 11.

271. Prout GR Jr, Griffin PP, Daly JJ, Heney NM. Carcinoma in situ of the urinary bladder with and without associated vesical neoplasms. Cancer 1983; 52: 524.

272. Cheville JC, Dundore PA, Bostwick DG, *et al*. Transitional cell carcinoma of the prostate: clinicopathologic study of 50 cases. Cancer 1998; 82: 703.

273. Freeman JA, Esrig D, Stein JP, Skinner DG. Management of the patient with bladder cancer: urethral recurrence. Urol Clin North Am 1994; 21: 645.

274. Freeman JA, Tarter TA, Esrig D, *et al*. Urethral recurrence in patients with orthotopic ileal neobladders. J Urol 1996; 156: 1615.

275. Algaba F, Santaularia JM, Lamas M, Ayala G. Transitional cell carcinoma of the prostate. Eur Urol 1985; 11: 87–90.

276. Winfield HN, Reddy PK, Lange PH. Coexisting adenocarcinoma of prostate in patients undergoing cystoprostatectomy for bladder cancer. Urology 1987; 30: 100.

277. Pritchett TR, Moreno J, Warner NE, *et al*. Unsuspected prostatic adenocarcinoma in patients who have undergone radical cystoprostatectomy for transitional cell carcinoma of the bladder. J Urol 1988; 139: 1214.

278. Dhom G. Histopathology of prostate carcinoma: diagnosis and differential diagnosis. Pathol Res Pract 1985; 179: 277.

279. Marshall VF. The relation of the preoperative estimate to the pathologic demonstration of the extent of vesical neoplasms. J Urol 1952; 68: 714.

280. Curtis MW, Evans AJ, Srigley JR. Mucin-producing urothelial type adenocarcinoma of prostate: report of two cases of a rare and diagnostically challengingentity. Mod Pathol 2005; 18(4): 585–90.

281. Samsonov VA, Kolomoitsev SV. Dimorphic (transitional-anaplastic) ductal cancer of the prostate. Arkh Patol 1984; 46: 71.

282. Lemberger RJ, Bishop MC, Bates CP, Blundell W, Ansell ID. Carcinoma of the prostate of ductal origin. Br J Urol 1984; 56: 706.

283. Zincke H, Utz DC, Farrow GM. Review of the Mayo Clinic experience with carcinoma in situ. Urology 1985; 26: 39.

284. Nicolaisen GS, Williams RD. Primary transitional cell carcinoma of the prostate. Urology 1984; 24: 544.

285. Wolfe JHN, Lloyd-Davies RW. The management of transitional cell carcinoma of the prostate. Br J Urol 1981; 53: 253.

286. Razvi M, Firfer R, Berkson B. Occult transitional cell carcinoma of the prostate presenting as skin metastasis. J Urol 1975; 113: 734.

287. Wendelken JR, Schellhammer PF, Ladaga LE, El-Mahdi AM. Transitional cell carcinoma: cause of refractory cancer of the prostate. Urology 1979; 13: 557.

288. Epstein NA. The cytologic appearance of metastatic transitional cell carcinoma. Acta Cytol 1977; 21: 723.

289. Griffiths GJ, Clements R, Jones DR, Roberts EE, Peeling WB, Evans KT. The ultrasound appearances of prostatic cancer with histological correlation. Clin Radiol 1987; 38: 219.

290. Terris MK, Villers A, Freiha FS. Transrectal ultrasound appearance of transitional cell carcinoma involving the prostate. J Urol 1990; 143: 953.

291. Beer M, Schmidt H, Riedl R. Klinische Wertigkeit des präoperativen Stagings von Blasen– und Prostatakarzinomen mit NMR und Computertomographie. Urologe A 1989; 28: 65.

292. Bates HR, Thornton JL. Carcinoma of prostatic ducts. Am J Clin Pathol 1966; 45: 96.

293. Laplante M, Brice M. The upper limits of hopeful application of radical cystectomy for vesical carcinoma: does nodal metastasis always indicate incurability? J Urol 1973; 109: 261.

294. Thelmo WL, Seemayer TA, Madarnas P, Mount BM, Mackinnon KJ. Carcinoma in situ of the bladder with associated prostatic involvement. J Urol 1974; 111: 491.

295. Greene LF, Mulcahy JJ, Warren MM, Dockerty MB. Primary transitional cell carcinoma of the prostate. J Urol 1973; 110: 235.

296. Rikken CHM, van Helsdingen PJRO, Kazzaz BA. Are biopsies from the prostatic urethra useful in patients with superficial bladder carcinoma? Br J Urol 1987; 59: 145.

297. Wood DP Jr, Montie JE, Pontes JE, Levin HS. Identification of transitional cell carcinoma of the prostate in bladder cancer patients: a prospective study. J Urol 1989; 141: 83–5.

298. Sakamoto N, Tsuneyoshi M, Naito S, Kumazawa J. An adequate sampling of the prostate to identify prostatic involvement by urothelial carcinoma in bladder cancer patients. J Urol 1993; 149: 318.

299. Laor E, Grabstald H, Whitmore WF. The influence of simultaneous resection of bladder tumors and prostate on the occurrence of prostatic urethral tumors. J Urol 1981; 126: 171.

300. Chibber PJ, McIntyre MA, Hindmarsh JR, Hargreave TB, Newsam JE, Chisholm GD. Transitional cell carcinoma involving the prostate. Br J Urol 1981; 53: 605–9.

301. Kirk D, Hinton CE, Shaldon C. Transitional cell carcinoma of the prostate. Br J Urol 1979; 51: 575–8.

302. Raz S, Mclorie G, Johnson S, Skinner DG. Management of the urethra in patients undergoing radical cystectomy for bladder carcinoma. J Urol 1978; 120: 298.

303. Solsona E, Iborra I, Ricós JV, Monrós JL, Casanova JL, Almenar S. The prostate involvement as prognostic factor in patients with superficial bladder tumors. J Urol 1995; 154: 1710.

304. Reese JH, Freiha FS, Gelb AB, Lum BL, Torti FM. Transitional cell carcinoma of the prostate in patients undergoing radical cystoprostatectomy. J Urol 1992; 147: 92.

305. Palou J, Xavier B, Laguna P, Montlleó M, Vicente J. In situ transitional cell carcinoma involvement of prostatic urethra: bacillus Calmette–Guerin therapy without previous transurethral resection of the prostate. Urology 1996; 47: 482.

306. Bretton PR, Herr HW, Whitmore WF Jr, et al Intravesical bacillus Calmette–Guerin therapy for in situ transitional cell carcinoma involving the prostatic urethra. J Urol 1989; 141: 853.

307. Hillyard RW, Ladaga L, Schellhammer PF. Superficial transitional cell carcinoma of the bladder associated with mucosal involvement of the prostatic urethra: results of treatment with intravesical bacillus Calmette–Guerin. J Urol 1988; 139: 290.

308. Orihuela E, Herr HW, Whitmore WF. Conservative treatment of superficial transitional cell carcinoma of prostatic urethra with intravesical BCG. Urology 1989; 34: 231.

309. Schellhammer PF, Ladaga LE, Moriarty RP. Intravesical bacillus Calmette–Guerin for treatment of superficial transitional cell carcinoma of the prostatic urethra in association with carcinoma of the bladder. J Urol 1995; 153: 53.

310. Lamm D. Re: Transitional cell carcinoma of the prostate, editorial. J Urol 1991; 146: 1630.

311. Droller MJ. Bacillus Calmette–Guerin in the management of bladder cancer. J Urol 1986; 135: 331.

312. Siami P, Chinn S, Clayton M, Ray V, Rubenstein M, Guinan P. BCG in management of transitional cell carcinoma invasive to prostate. Urology 1989; 34: 381.

313. Lockhart JL, Chaikin L, Bondhus MJ, Politano VA. Prostatic recurrences in the management of superficial bladder tumors. J Urol 1983; 130: 256.

314. Droller MJ, Walsh PC. Intensive intravesical chemotherapy in the treatment of flat carcinoma in situ: is it safe? J Urol 1985; 134: 1115.

315. Shenasky JH, Gillenwater JY. Management of transitional cell carcinoma of the prostate. J Urol 1972; 108: 462.

316. Kopelson G, Harisiadis L, Romas NA, Veenema RJ, Tannenbaum M. Periurethral prostatic duct carcinoma: clinical features and treatment results. Cancer 1978; 42: 2894.

317. Schellhammer PF, Bean MA, Whitmore WF Jr. Prostatic involvement by transitional cell carcinoma: pathogenesis, patterns and prognosis. J Urol 1977; 118(3): 399–403.

318. Frazier HA, Robertson JE, Dodge RK, Paulson DF. The value of pathologic factors in predicting cancer-specific survival among patients treated with radical cystectomy for transitional cell carcinoma of the bladder and prostate. Cancer 1993; 71: 3993.

319. Taylor HG, Blom J. Transitional cell carcinoma of the prostate: response to treatment with adriamycin and cis-platinum. Cancer 1983; 51: 1800.

320. Alexander SJ, Lee SS, Bekhrad A. Transitional cell carcinoma of the prostate: response to treatment with cisplatinum and cyclophosphamide. J Urol 1984; 131: 975.

321. Dexeus FH, Logothetis CJ, Samuels ML, Ayala AG, Hossan E. Complete responses in metastatic transitional cell carcinoma of the prostate with cisplatin regimens. J Urol 1987; 137: 122.

322. Takashi M, Sakata T, Nagai T, et al. Primary transitional cell carcinoma of prostate: case with lymph node metastasis eradicated by neoadjuvant methotrexate, vinblastine, doxorubicin, and cisplatin (M-VAC) therapy. Urology 1990; 36: 96.

323. Von der Maase H, Andersen L, Crinò L, Weinknecht S, Dogliotti L. Weekly gemcitabine and cisplatin combination therapy in patients with transitional cell carcinoma of the urothelium: a phase II clinical trial. Ann Oncol 1999; 10(12): 1461–5.

324. Maruyama T, Yamada Y, Ueda Y. A case of primary urothelial carcinoma of the prostate responsive to MVAC intra-arterial chemotherapy: a case report. Hinyokika Kiyo 2011; 57(5): 255–9.

325. Jacobi M, Panoff CE, Herzlich J. Leukemic infiltration of the prostate. J Urol 1937; 38: 494–9.

326. Johnson MA, Gundersen A. Infiltration of the prostate bland by chronic lymphatic leukemia. J Urol 1953; 69: 681–5.

327. Tighe JR. Leukaemic infiltration of the prostate. Br J Surg 1960; 47: 658–60.

328. Vinnicombe J. Leukaemic infiltration of the prostate. Br J Urol 1963; 35: 297–8.

329. Waddington RT. Leukaemic infiltration of the prostate in a patient with chronic lymphatic leukaemia – a case report. Br J Urol 1973; 45: 184–6.

330. Dajani YF, Burke M. Leukemic infiltration of the prostate: a case study and clinicopathological review. Cancer 1976; 38: 2442–6.

331. Gunlusoy B, Cicekl S, Selek E, Sayhan S, Minareci S, Arslan M. A case report: leukaemic infiltration and hyperplasia of the prostate. Int Urol Nephrol 2004; 36(1): 55–6.

332. Butler MR, O'Flynn JD. Prostatic disease in the leukaemic patient – with particular reference to leukaemic infiltration of the prostate – a retrospective clinical study. Br J Urol 1973; 45: 179–83.

333. Thalhammer F, Gisslinger H, Chott A, et al. Granulocytic sarcoma of the prostate as the first manifestation of a late relapse of acute myelogenous leukaemia. Ann Hematol 1994; 68: 97–9.

334. Bostwick DG, Iczkowski KA, Amin MB, Discigil G, Osborne B. Malignant lymphoma involving the prostate: report of 62 cases. Cancer 1998; 83: 732–8.

335. Weimar G, Culp DA, Loening S, Narayana A. Urogenital involvement by malignant lymphomas. J Urol 1980; 125: 230–1.

336. Zein TA, Huben R, Lane W, Pontes JE, Englander LS. Secondary tumors of the prostate. J Urol 1985; 133: 615–16.

337. Freeman C, Berg JW, Cutler SJ. Occurrence and prognosis of extranodal lymphomas. Cancer 1972; 29: 252–60.

338. Rosenberg SA, Diamond SD, Jaslowitz B, Craver LF. Lymphosarcoma: a review of 1269 cases. Medicine 1961; 40: 31–84.

339. Sarris A, Dimopoulos M, Pugh W, Cabanillas F. Primary lymphoma of the prostate: good outcome with doxorubicin-based combination chemotherapy. J Urol 1995; 153: 1852–4.

340. Klotz LH, Herr HW. Hodgkin's disease of the prostate: a detailed case report. J Urol 1986; 135: 1261–2.

341. Verma D, Kantarjian H, Strom SS, et al. Malignancies occurring during therapy with tyrosine kinase inhibitors (TKIs) for chronic myeloid leukemia (CML) and other hematologic malignancies. Blood 2011; 118(16): 4353–8.

342. Coupland S. Lymphoma of the prostate. Trans Pathol Soc Lond 1877; 28: 179.

343. Bostwick DG, Mann RB. Malignant lymphomas involving the prostate. Cancer 1985; 56: 2932–8.

344. King LS, Cox TR. Lymphosarcoma of the prostate. Am J Pathol 1951; 27: 801–23.

345. Fell P, O'connor M, Smith JM. Primary lymphoma of prostate presenting as bladder outflow obstruction. Urology 1987; 29: 555–6.

346. Patel DR, Gomez GA, Henderson ES, Gamarra M. Primary prostatic involvement in non-Hodgkin lymphoma. Urology 1988; 32: 96–8.

347. Kerbl K, Pauer W. Primary non-Hodgkin lymphoma of prostate. Urology 1988; 32: 347–9.

348. Suzuki H, Nakada T, Iijima Y, et al Malignant lymphoma of the prostate. Report of a case. Urol Int 1991; 47: 172–5.

349. Sarlis NJ, Knight RA, Sarlis I, Papadimitriou K, Kehayas P. Primary non-Hodgkin lymphoma of the prostate gland. Int Urol Nephrol 1993; 25: 163–8.

350. Morozumi M, Takasu H, Watanabe T, Okada M. Primary non-Hodgkin lymphoma of the prostate: a case report. Nippon Hinyokika Gakkai Zasshi 1993; 84: 2023–63.

351. Mounedji-Boudiaf L, Culine S, Devoldère G, et al. Primary, highly malignant B-cell lymphoma of the prostate. Apropos of a case and review of the literature. Bull Cancer 1994; 81: 334–7.

352. Braslis KG, Lee N, Machet D, Peters J. Primary prostatic lymphoma: a rare prostatic malignancy. Aust N Z J Surg 1994; 64: 58–9.

353. Parks RW, Henry PG, Abram WP, Best BG. Primary non-Hodgkin's lymphoma of the prostate mimicking acute prostatitis. Br J Urol 1995; 76: 409.

354. Ghose A, Baxter-Smith DC, Eeles H, Udeshi U, Priestman TJ. Lymphoma of the prostate treated with radiotherapy. Clin Oncol (R Coll Radiol) 1995; 7: ar134.

355. Bell CR, Napier MP, Morgan RJ, Dick R, Jarmulowicz M, Jones AL. Primary non-Hodgkin's lymphoma of the prostate gland: case report and review of the literature. Clin Oncol (R Coll Radiol) 1995; 7: 409–10.

356. Miyahara T, Oyabul Y, Hayashi T, Shimizu S, Tanaka H, Matsuoka K. A case of malignant lymphoma of the prostate. Nihon Hinyokika Gakkai Zasshi 2005; 96(6): 644–6.

357. Solis V, Rosenberg RJ, Spencer RP. B cell lymphoma: a case with localized involvement of the prostate on F-18-FDG examination. Clin Nucl Med 2005; 30(4): 236–7.

358. Alvarez CA, Rodriguez BI, Perez LA. Primary diffuse large B-cell lymphoma of the prostate in a young patient. Int Braz J Urol 2006; 32(1): 64–5.

359. Shen XJ, Zheng XG, Zhou XJ, Zhou HB. [Non-hodgkin's lymphoma of the prostate: a report of 2 cases and review of the literature]. Zhonghua Nan Ke Xue 2007; 13(10): 895–8.

360. Oosterheert JJ, Budel LM, Vos P, Wittebol S. High levels of serum prostate-specific antigen due to PSA producing follicular non-hodgkin's lymphoma. Eur J Haematol 2007; 79(2): 155–8.

361. Taleb A, Ismaili N, Belbaraka R, et al. Primary lymphoma of the prostate treated with rituximab based chemotherapy: a case report and review of the literature. Cases J 2009; 2: 8875.

362. Fehr M, Templeton A, Cogliatti S, Aebersold F, Egli F, Gillessen S, Cathomas R. Primary manifestation of small lymphocytic lymphoma in the prostate. Onkologie 2009; 32(10): 586–8.

363. Chin K, Fujimura M, Sekit N, et al. [Case of malignant lymphoma of the prostate complicated with prostate adenocarcinoma]. Nihon Hinyokika Gakkai Zasshi 2009; 100(7): 698–702.

364. Kini JR, Kini H, Pai MR, Naik R. Primary diffuse large B-cell lymphoma of the prostate presenting as urinary retention. Indian J Pathol Microbiol 2010; 53(1): 194–5.

365. Wang GW, Chen DB, Shen DH. [Diffuse large B-cell lymphoma of prostate: report of a case]. Zhonghua Bing Li Xue Za Zhi 2011; 40(6): 412–13.

366. Steuter J, Weisenburger DD, Bociek RG, et al. Non-hodgkin lymphoma of the prostate. Am J Hematol 2011; 86(11): 952–4.

367. Kishimoto N, Takao T, Yamamoto K, et al. [A case of primary malignant lymphoma of the prostate]. Hinyokika Kiyo 2011; 57(8): 445–9.

368. Koga N, Noguchi M, Moriya F, Ohshima K, Yoshitake N, Matsuoka K. A case of primary mucosa-associated lymphoid tissue lymphoma of the prostate. Rare Tumors 2009; 1(2): e55.

369. Kang JJ, Eaton MS, Ma Y, Streeter O, Kumar P. Mucosa-associated lymphoid tissue lymphoma and concurrent adenocarcinoma of the prostate. Rare Tumors 2010; 2(3): e54.

370. Aggarwal H, Aggarwal A, Hunter WJ 3rd, Yohannes P, Khan AU, Agrawal DK. Expression of leukemialymphoma related factor (LRFPokemon) in human benign prostate hyperplasia and prostate cancer. Exp Mol Pathol 2011; 90(2): 226–30.

371. Rainwater LM, Barrett DM. Primary lymphoma of the prostate: transrectal ultrasonic appearance. Urology 1990; 36: 522–5.

372. Hodgson R, Huang YT, Steinke K, Ravi Kumar AS. FDG-PETCT in evaluation and prognostication of primary prostate lymphoma. Clin Nucl Med 2010; 35(6): 418–20.

373. Cimarelli S, Lachenal F, Ricard F, et al. A case of advanced non-hodgkin's lymphoma involving the prostate: staging and treatment monitoring using F-18 FDG PETCT imaging. Clin Nucl Med 2010; 35(6): 425–7.

374. Li G, Dhawan M, Takalkar AM, Lilien DL. FDG PETCT imaging suggests lymphoma involving prostate may be more resistant to treatment. Clin Nucl Med 2011; 36(3): 255–7.

375. Cronin CG, Swords R, Truong MT, et al. Clinical utility of PET/CT in lymphoma. Am J Roentgenol 2010; 194(1): W91–W103.

376. Fukutani K, Koyama Y, Fujimori M, Ishida T. [Primary malignant lymphoma of the prostate: report of a case achieving complete response to combination chemotherapy and review of 22 Japanese cases]. Nihon Hinyokika Gakkai Zasshi 2003; 94(6): 621–5.

377. Horning SJ, Rosenberg SA. The natural history of initially untreated low-grade non-Hodgkin's lymphomas. N Engl J Med 1984; 311: 1471–5.

378. Bleichner JC, Chun B, Klappenbach RS. Pure small cell carcinoma of the prostate with fatal liver metastasis. Arch Pathol Lab Med 1986; 110: 1041–4.

Section 1: Genitourinary Cancer

5 Rare Tumors of the Testis and Paratesticular Tissues

Robert Huddart,[1] Stephen Hazell,[2] and Alan Horwich[1]

[1] Academic Unit of Radiotherapy and Oncology, Institute of Cancer Research and Royal Marsden NHS Foundation Trust, Sutton, UK

[2] Clinical Anatomic Pathology Unit, Royal Marsden NHS Foundation Trust, London, UK

Introduction

The testes originate embryologically from the retroperitoneum. They have both endocrine and reproductive functions, and tumors of the testes and their adnexae (Fig. 5.1) reflect this diversity both of origin and function. The majority of testicular cancers arise from germinal epithelium.[1] Rarely tumors of lymphoid, interstitial, or ductal origin arise in the testes and this chapter describes these together with tumors of paratesticular, mesothelial, and connective tissues. The main sections of this chapter cover the following areas:

- non-Hodgkin lymphoma of the testis
- gonadal (sex cord) stromal tumors
- malignant mesothelioma of the tunica vaginalis
- adenocarcinoma of the rete testis
- paratesticular rhabdomyosarcoma.

Non-Hodgkin lymphoma of the testis

History

The first description of malignant lymphoma of the testis in 1877 is credited to the French worker Malassez.[2] In a case report published by Hutchinson,[3] many of the notable features of this disease were illustrated in that the patient was elderly, had bilateral tumors, and the disease disseminated widely to involve bone and subcutaneous tissues (a feature also of Malassez's original case). Gowing[4] reported on 128 cases. Seventy-eight percent of patients were over 50 years of age, 20% had bilateral testicular involvement, and 62% had died of disseminated disease within 2 years. However, 15 of 124 patients treated by orchidectomy survived disease free for 5 or more years, supporting the conclusion that testicular lymphoma occurs as a primary manifestation of non-Hodgkin lymphoma (NHL) as well as in the context of disseminated disease.

The prognosis has been considered poor, in keeping with the aggressive histology (see Fig. 5.1). However, the importance both of stage, emphasized by Kiely et al.,[5] and the exact histological type[6] is now recognized, as is the high systemic relapse rate even in patients with early-stage disease, leading to the investigation of systemic therapy in patients with stage I presentation.

A retrospective outcomes study on behalf of the International Extranodal Lymphoma Study Group (IELSG) has been reported by Zucca et al., based on 373 patients from 23 institutions worldwide.[7] This provided a tool for defining the clinical features and outcome of this subset of lymphoma which differs from its nodal counterpart in several respects.

Epidemiology and etiology

Testicular tumors are rare, affecting from <1 to 4.5 patients per 1,000,000 men per year, and there are marked racial and geographic variations.[8] The reported incidence is increasing[9] and the vast majority of these tumors arise from germinal epithelium. NHL accounts for approximately 5% of all testicular neoplasms. The relative incidence increases with age (Fig. 5.2). In patients over 50 years old, lymphomas account for 25–50% of all testicular neoplasms.[10] Nearly 80% of the cases reported by the British Testicular Tumour Panel (BTTP) were over 50, contrasting with just three children reported in the same series.[4]

The testis is an uncommon site of presentation for NHL.[11,12] The Princess Margaret Hospital, Toronto, serving a population of 4 million, saw 1934 new patients with NHL between 1967 and 1978, of whom 16 (0.83%) had a primary testicular presentation.[10] Wahal et al.[13] reported on NHL in north India, and of 1283 cases, 264 (21%) were extranodal, of which 20 (1.5%) presented with a testicular lesion.

Pathology

Testicular lymphoma may present with a very large testicular mass. Kiely et al.[5] recorded one case measuring 16 cm × 9 cm and weighing 750 g. In the BTTP series,[4] the largest tumor

Textbook of Uncommon Cancer, Fourth Edition. Edited by Derek Raghavan, Charles D. Blanke, David H. Johnson, Paul L. Moots, Gregory H. Reaman, Peter G. Rose and Mikkael A. Sekeres.
© 2012 John Wiley & Sons, Inc. Published 2012 by John Wiley & Sons, Inc.

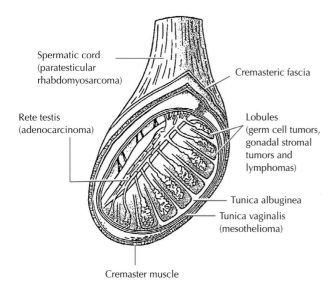

Figure 5.1 Diagram of testis and spermatic cord indicating sites of tumor origin. Paratesticular rhabdomyosarcoma may arise from connective tissue of the cord or of adjacent structures.

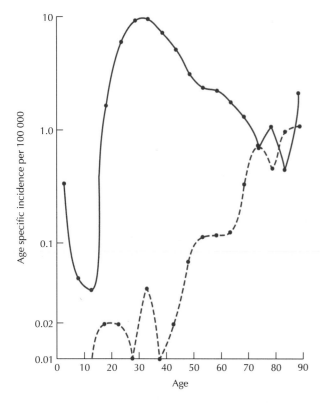

Figure 5.2 Incidence of germ cell tumous and of lymphomas of the testis by age of presentation. Data from Thames Cancer Registry.

measured 13 cm × 10 cm × 8 cm and weighed 380 g. The cut surface may appear homogeneous or have yellowish areas of necrosis present and the color has been variously described as cream, pink, gray or buff. No capsule is present and the lesions have ill-defined edges. Local extension is common.

Table 5.1 Prognosis of testicular lymphoma.

Author	Stage*	Number	% disease-free survival at 5 years
Zucca[7]	I	214	54
	II	80	48
	III–IV	79	30
	I–IV	373	48
Gowing[4]	I–IV	128	12
Mazloom[52]	I–IV	75	>2000 59%
			<2000 52%
Jackson[17]	I–IV	194	14.5
Read[225] †	I/IIA	24	40
	IIB/IV	27	0
	I–IV	51	20
Crellin[226]	I–IV	34	33
Zietman[227]	I	26	61

* Staging according to the Ann Arbor classification.
† I + IIA – no palpable metastases; IIB–IV – clinically overt metastases.

Gowing[4] gave a full histological description of these tumors and the morphological features that help to distinguish them from seminoma. In this series all the tumors were composed of either poorly differentiated cells of the lymphocytic series or of lymphomas of larger undifferentiated cell type.

The classification most widely applied to testicular lymphoma in the past has been that of Rappaport[14] and using this, virtually all reported cases are of diffuse histiocytic or diffuse poorly differentiated lymphocytic type. Turner et al.[6] reported on 35 cases of malignant lymphoma of the testis classified by both the Rappaport criteria and the International Working Formulation of non-Hodgkin's lymphoma.[15] All the tumors showed a diffuse pattern of growth and 29 were diffuse histiocytic lymphomas. In the Working Formulation, 22 of these were of intermediate grade (large cell cleaved, large cell non-cleaved) and seven high grade (immunoblastic lymphoma). In subsequent studies the majority of testicular lymphomas have been found to be of intermediate grade.[16,17] Immunohistological studies have suggested that the majority are tumors of B lymphocytes.[18] The majority of the tumors are classified in the recent WHO classification as diffuse large B cell lymphoma[19] of nongerminal center type.[20] It has been suggested that rapid dissemination associated with this tumor may be due to the lack of expression of adhesion molecules.[21] The tumors usually have BCL-2 protein, but not the t(14;18) translocation typical of follicular lymphomas.[22] They are not generally associated with Epstein–Barr virus (EBV) or human herpesvirus (HHV)8 viruses.[23]

Prognosis and patterns of relapse

The prognosis of testicular NHL is unsatisfactory (Table 5.1), with early reports showing particularly poor results. In the BTTP series,[4] 62% had died of disseminated lymphoma within 2 years of presentation and only 15 of the 124 patients treated by orchidectomy survived 5 or more years postoperatively. Jackson and Montessori[17] confirmed this low 5-year survival

Table 5.2 Testicular lymphoma: stage distribution.

	Number of cases				
Author	IE	IIE	IIIE	IV	Stage IV major sites involved (n)
Zucca[7]	214	80	79		Bone marrow (18), CNS (11), adrenal glands (9), skin (9), bone (8), kidney (7)
Duncan[43]	10	8	2	4	Skin (3), lung (1)
Read[225]	28		6	17	Bone (4), skin (4), lung (3), CNS (3), upper airways (4), bone marrow (2), liver (1)
Baldetorp[16]	8	8	3	5	Bone (2), liver (1), skin (1)
Crellin[226]	13	10	3	8	Bone (2), marrow (3), pelvis (3), kidney (3)

Table 5.3 Testicular lymphoma: sites of relapse.

Author	Number of cases	Number relapsing	Major sites of relapse
Zucca[7]	Stage I (214)	102	Contralateral testis plus other nodal and extranodal sites (Stage I: 19, II: 5, III/IV: 7, total:31) All CNS relapse (Stage I: 27, II: 12, III/IV: 17, total: 56) Isolated CNS relapse (Stage I: 17, II: 6, III/IV: 11, total: 34)
	Stage II (80)	44	
	Stage III–IV (79)	49	
	Total (373)	195	
Duncan[43]	24	13	Upper airways (5), bone (5), nodal (4), CNS (2)
Read[225]	51	32	Liver (11), skin (9), CNS (5), lung (5), bone (2)
Baldetorp[16]	24	13	Nodal (6), upper airways (2), other testes (3)
Crellin[226]	34	23	CNS (6), testis (2), lung (3), heart (2), marrow (2), thyroid (1), and nodal sites

rate by tabulating reported series up to 1977 and found only 28 out of 194 (14.5%) patients surviving disease free for more than 5 years. However, more recent reports of aggressive multimodality treatment using a combination of systemic and intrathecal chemotherapy and scrotal and lymphatic radiotherapy have demonstrated improved survivals, depending upon the prognostic factors present.[24,25] The IELSG multicenter review[7] revealed a median survival of 4.8 years and a 5-year and 10-year overall survival (OS) of 48% and 27% respectively for the whole group. A majority of these patients were, however, stage I. In keeping with the aggressive nature of the disease, most patients who succumb to lymphoma do so within the first 2–3 years, but there are a proportion of deaths that occur later. Sussman et al.[26] noted that of 37 patients, 24 (65%) died of disseminated disease; 71% of these died within the first year post orchidectomy, 17% within the second, 4% within the third, none in the fourth, and 8% within the fifth year of follow-up. In the IELSG report, lymphoma-related deaths were seen up to 14 years from diagnosis.[7] Gundrum et al.[27] reported a population-based study from the USA of 769 patients with similar outcomes. The overall pattern of this lymphoma also seems similar in China.[28]

In the IELSG report, the factors significantly associated with a favorable prognosis on univariate analysis were good performance status, limited stage, absence of a bulky mass, normal serum lactate dehydrogenase (LDH) and β2-microglobulin, and absence of additional extranodal involvement, absence of B symptoms, favourable International Prognostic Index, anthracycline-based chemotherapy, and prophylactic scrotal irradiation. However, on multivariate analysis only the latter four remained significant. Among stage I patients, the group of those with normal LDH, age less than 60 years, and a performance status 1 had a significantly better outcome, with a 5-year OS of 81% and progression-free survival (PFS) of 68%. This small subset of patients has a prognosis approaching that of their nodal lymphoma counterparts.[7]

These tumors usually present with early-stage disease but can disseminate widely on recurrence (Tables 5.2, 5.3). In the BTTP series,[4] 13 patients (10%) had clinical evidence of disseminated disease at the time of orchidectomy. In the recent SEER series,[27] 76% were in stage I or II. The sites of possible metastatic involvement are numerous and reflect both lymphatic and hematogenous spread. In the IELSG study, the sites of extranodal involvement at presentation were bone marrow (5%), central nervous system (CNS) (3%), adrenal glands and skin (2.5% each), bone and kidney (2% each) and soft tissue, gastrointestinal tract and liver (1% each).[7]

Sites of involvement at relapse are varied (see Table 5.3). There appears to be a particular risk of relapse in the CNS.[29–35] In a multicenter Rare Cancer Network study of 36 patients, CNS was found to be the principal site of relapse (8/14 relapses).[36] This has led to intrathecal chemotherapy prophylaxis as part of routine management of these patients and recurrence after this seems to be less common.[30,32,37] Relapse in the contralateral testis is a particular problem and affects survival,[7] but is preventable by prophylactic radiotherapy.[7,38]

Clinical features

Enlargement of the testicle is the usual presenting feature. The duration of symptoms in Talerman's series[39] varied from a few weeks to 3 years but was usually less than 6 months. Pain is present in 8–25% of cases and in the 402 cases reported up to 1985, there was a right-sided preponderance of 1.3:1. The clinical features that may help to differentiate lymphoma from the more common germ cell tumors and seminoma are the patient's greater age, the tendency to bilateral involvement, lack of association with maldescent, the different pattern of metastatic spread, and a lack of gynecomastia. Many other authors have commented on this striking difference in age distribution from the more usual testicular tumors. In the series of Eckert and Smith,[40] the mean age for lymphoma was 59.8 years compared to 33 years for teratoma and 42.3 years for seminoma.

In the IELSG report, the median age at presentation was 66 years (range 19–91 years). Overall, 79% had stage I–II disease, 90% had no B symptoms, 5% had bulky disease (defined as >10 cm diameter) and 47% had a raised LDH.[7] Bilateral synchronous primaries occur in about 2–5% of cases.[4,41,42] Duncan

Author	Stage	Number of patients	Radiotherapy prescription	Disease-free survival	
Duncan[43]	IE	9	30–40 Gy in 20–24# in 34 days	45%	
	IIE	7	Daily fractionation	30%	at 5 years
Read[225]*	I/IIA	24	30 Gy in 20# over 4 weeks	40%	
	IIB	4		0%	at 5 years
Tepperman[10]	IE	4	25 Gy in 20# over 4 weeks	75%	
	IIE	6		17%	at 2 years
Buskirk[228]	IE	8	25–40 Gy in 20# over 4 weeks	50%	
	IIE	3		33%	at 2 years

Table 5.4 Testicular lymphoma: radiotherapy results.

*Manchester staging system.
Gy, gray.
#, Fraction.

et al.[43] commented that patients presenting with bilateral testicular lymphoma usually have advanced disease, with only one of 11 patients then reported in the medical literature surviving more than 2 years following locoregional therapy.

In childhood, testicular lymphoma is rarely localized[44,45] and Burkitt lymphoma is the most common type,[46] although it has also been reported in the elderly[47] (see also Chapters 44 and 48).

Investigation and staging

Patients should be staged according to the Ann Arbor classification.[48] Important areas of clinical assessment include the contralateral testis, regional and other lymph node areas, the skin, and the central nervous system.

The following investigations are recommended: full blood count and differential count, erythrocyte sedimentation rate, bone marrow aspirate and trephine biopsy, renal and liver function tests, α-fetoprotein and β-human chorionic gonadotropin (BHCG) estimation, chest x-ray, computed tomography (CT) of the chest and abdomen, and cerebrospinal fluid cytology.

Management and outcome

Important considerations for appropriate management include the patient's age and general condition, the histological subtype, and the stage of the disease.

Surgery

A radical inguinal orchidectomy is the recommended procedure. Historically, this was the only method of treatment and can result in cure of a minority of patients.[4] In the IESLG study,[7] 41 patients had orchidectomy as the sole treatment. Their PFS was significantly shorter than those of patients receiving additional chemotherapy and/or radiotherapy (median PFS, 1.0 versus 5.4 years). The OS was also shorter, but the difference did not reach statistical significance (median OS, 2.1 versus 6.4 years; $p = 0.07$).

Radiotherapy

Abdominal and pelvic lymph node irradiation, e.g. by an inverted-Y field, has been employed either as an adjuvant following orchidectomy or to treat overt disease, and either alone or in combination with chemotherapy. The radiotherapy prescription as shown in Table 5.4 has varied in different institutions, with a midplane dose recommendation of between 30 and 40 Gy in 20 fractions over 4 weeks using megavoltage equipment. With orchidectomy and adjuvant radiotherapy, approximately 50% of stage I patients and 20% of stage II patients can be expected to be long-term survivors. In view of the high systemic relapse rate, consideration should be given to the use of adjuvant chemotherapy in early-stage disease as in early-stage lymphoma at other sites.[45,49] For patients with bulky localized NHL, there may be an advantage to the addition of involved field radiotherapy (RT) after CT. This would be a consideration in those presenting with abdominal node metastases, or who have an involved unresected contralateral testis.

Adjuvant irradiation of the scrotal sac along with the contralateral remaining testicle has been shown to improve outcome. In the IELSG report, a continuous risk of recurrence in the contralateral testis (15% at 3 years, 42% at 15 years) was present in patients not receiving radiotherapy to the contralateral testis ($p=0.003$). Prophylactic radiotherapy to the contralateral testis was also associated with better PFS (5-year PFS, 36% versus 70%; $p<0.001$) and OS (5-year OS, 38% versus 66%; $p<0.001$) rates. Among patients receiving radiotherapy to the primary testicular site of involvement, the OS was longer for those receiving an irradiation dose of at least 30 Gy ($p=0.02$),[7] and this prevented relapse in the testis in the prospective study reported by Vitolo.[50]

Chemotherapy

Treatment results are improved by the use of combination chemotherapy regimens. In the IELSG study,[7] combination chemotherapy with anthracycline-containing regimens significantly improved the outcome in all patients (5-year PFS, 35% versus 55%; $p <0.001$, and 5-year OS, 39% versus 52%; $p=0.02$). Even when the analysis was limited to stage I–II patients, the benefit was statistically significant for PFS and OS. Patients receiving six or more cycles of chemotherapy had a better long-term outcome than those treated for a shorter period (10-year OS, 44% versus 19%; $p=0.03$). Cyclophosphamide, doxorubicin, vincristine, and prednisone (CHOP) was the standard until reports of improved survival with the addition of rituximab to the CHOP chemotherapy[51] and though individual studies appear to show improved prognosis recently,[50,52] the population-based US study did not demonstrate better survival in those treated in the rituximab era.[27]

Recommendations

In view of the high systemic relapse rate even for patients with early-stage disease, we would recommend systemic chemotherapy in all patients. The management of patients with advanced disease should be as for advanced lymphoma at other sites. The choice of chemotherapy would depend on the age and health of the patient and preference of the treating institution. At least six cycles of CHOP with rituximab should be considered appropriate for advanced disease although fewer courses, three or four, may be sufficient in stage I–II disease. Adult patients with stage II disease should be considered for adjuvant involved-field nodal RT to a dose of 30–40 Gy, possibly depending on positron emission tomography (PET) assessment of response. Irradiation of the contralateral scrotal sac is also recommended to a dose of 30 Gy using a technique which delivers this dose to the entire testis, such as with high energy electrons. All patients should be considered for CNS staging and prophylaxis with intrathecal chemotherapy.

Gonadal (sex cord) stromal tumors

Introduction

Mostofi et al.[53] referred to Sertoli and Leydig cell tumors as "tumors of the specialized gonadal stroma" and suggested a common origin for these cell types. The term sex cord stromal tumors, which is used for analogous ovarian tumors, may be more appropriate.[54] They are uncommon, accounting for approximately 4% of all testicular neoplasms, have a broad age distribution at presentation and may be hormonally active. Expression of the S-100 protein has been reported.[55]

Testicular stromal cells include Leydig and Sertoli cells. Leydig cells are named after Franz von Leydig (1821–1908), the German anatomist who first described them. They arise embryologically from the posterior urogenital ridge, secreting primarily testosterone but also lesser amounts of estrogens. They are capable of producing testosterone from cholesterol and can secrete just under 10 mg of testosterone per day.[56]

Sertoli cells are named after the Milan physiologist Enrico Sertoli (1842–1910). They form the supporting cells of the seminiferous tubules lying between the germinal cells, often with clumps of spermatids buried in their cytoplasm. Sertoli cells have certain features characteristic of hormone-producing cells, and although apparently unable to generate steroids, they may be able to promote their interconversion.

The majority of gonadal (sex cord) stromal tumors (GSTs) are Leydig cell tumors (LCT), with smaller numbers of Sertoli cell tumors and occasional rarities such as granulosa cell tumors. Mixed GSTs have been described, and one example revealed the germ cell cytogenetic marker isochromosome i(12p) in an inguinal node metastasis.[57] Most GSTs are benign but about 10% metastasize. It is difficult to predict the malignant phenotype from the presenting characteristics. Surgery remains the mainstay of treatment.

Leydig cell tumors

Epidemiology and etiology

In the BTTP series of 2739 testicular tumors, 43 (1.6%) were LCTs.[58] Mostofi[59] recorded a 3% and Ward et al.[60] a 2% incidence. The diagnosis and incidence of these and other sex cord tumours may have increased with the increased detection of impalpable testicular lesions by ultrasound. Leonhartsburger et al.[61] reported that in the period 1999–2008 LCTs made up 14.7% of 197 tumors seen. This apparent increase may be due to increased detection of an impalpable lesion. In an overview of impalpable lesions sex cord tumours (predominantly Leydig cell) accounted for 35% of lesions.[62]

Most published cases of LCTs have occurred in adult life but they can rarely occur in childhood.[63] The age of the patients in the BTTP series ranged from 21 to 81 and similar results have been seen in more recent series, with a mean age at onset of around 35–45.[64–68]

Leydig cell hyperplasia may occur with testicular atrophy and LCTs may be associated with maldescent, atrophy, and infertility.[58,62,64,67] Carmignani et al.[62] noted that infertility was a risk factor (relative risk 9.6) for diagnosis of a sex cord tumor in impalpable testicular lesions. Constant luteinizing hormone stimulation of the testis in experimental animals can induce both Leydig cell hyperplasia and LCT. Malignant Leydig cell tumors are rare and are thought to account for approximately 10% of cases; by 1985, only 37 cases of malignant LCT had been described; the average age was nearly 63 years.[69] The precise proportion of LCTs which are malignant tumors is highly variable, with some series reporting rates much less than 10%. For instance, Suardi et al.[70] had no relapses in 37 patients treated between 1990 and 2006, whilst Giannarini et al.[64] and Loeser et al.[67] also reported no metastatic recurrences in 17 and 16 patients respectively treated conservatively. This variability may in part depend on the rate of clinical versus incidentally detected tumors and the size of tumor detected.

Pathology and biology

These tumors, which are rarely bilateral, arise within the substance of the testis and are usually well demarcated with a striking yellow-brown color. Necrosis and hemorrhage may be seen. They can vary widely in size, the range in the BTTP series being 0.7–10 cm,[58] and sometimes involve the rete testis and spermatic cord.

The tumor cells may be polygonal or fusiform in shape with prominent nucleoli and abundant eosinophilic or granular cytoplasm. Characteristic crystalloids of Reinke are seen in about a third of cases, and these have been used to aid in cytological diagnosis.[71] Mitotic figures can be frequent and do not necessarily imply malignancy.[58] The absence of seminiferous tubules within the tumor helps to differentiate LCT from Leydig cell hyperplasia (Figs 5.3, 5.4).

Features of the primary lesion that should arouse suspicion of malignancy include large size (>5 cm), lack of encapsulation, presence of satellite nodules, areas of necrosis, and on microscopy, a high mitotic rate (>3/10 high-power field [HPF]) and blood vessel or lymphatic invasion.[58] In the review by

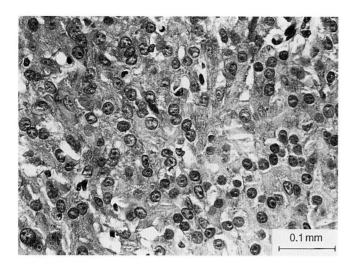

Figure 5.3 Leydig cell tumor composed of relatively uniform cells with rounded nuclei and abundant cytoplasm (H&E, 310×).

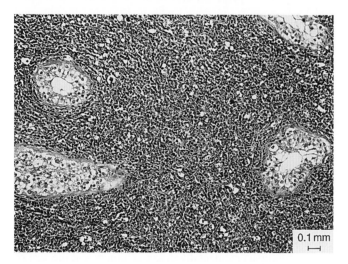

Figure 5.4 Diffuse B cell lymphoma involving testis. The infiltrate is interstitial and widely separates seminiferous tubules which contain only Sertoli cells (H&E, 62×).

Kim et al.,[69] 84% of the malignant LCTs were 5 cm or greater in diameter, 74% had an infiltrative margin, and 72% lymphatic or vascular invasion. A recent multivariate analysis of histological factors performed at the Royal Marsden/Charing Cross Hospitals studied 23 patients with stromal tumors (18 LCTs, four Sertoli cell and one granulosa cell). Moderate/marked nuclear atypia, mitoses per 10 HPF and presence of prominent nucleoli predicted for malignant phenotype.[68] However, histological prediction is not entirely reliable and the occurrence of metastasis is the only definite proof of malignancy.[72] Cheville et al.[73] reported 30 cases of LCT of the testis (23 tumors were localized and seven had metastasized). Patients with LCTs that metastasized were diagnosed at a mean age of 62 years (range, 39–70 years) compared with 48 years (range, 9–79 years) in patients with nonmetastasizing tumors ($p = 0.25$). Leydig cell tumors that metastasized were significantly larger than nonmetastasizing tumors (mean, 4.7 versus 2.6 cm, respectively; $p = 0.008$). In this study, the presence of

cytological atypia, necrosis, angiolymphatic invasion, increased mitotic activity, atypical mitotic figures, infiltrative margins, extension beyond the testicular parenchyma, DNA aneuploidy, and increased MIB-1 activity was significantly associated with metastatic behavior in Leydig cell tumors.

Inhibin was reported to be the most sensitive marker, with positive staining in 100% LCTs and a very useful marker to differentiate testicular sex cord-stromal tumors from germ cell tumors.[74,75] Melan A and calretinin are also frequently expressed, as is CD99 in approximately two-thirds.

Metastases are present at diagnosis in about 25% of malignant cases and develop in the remainder when they occur, usually within 3 years. Recurrence after 5 years is uncommon.[76] The most common sites of metastases include the regional lymph nodes (68%), liver (45%), lung (45%), and bone (27%).

Clinical features

Although stromal tumors may present in childhood, these usually do not metastasize.[76–78] Most LCTs present with a testicular mass or, increasingly, as an impalpable hypoechoic lesion on ultrasound. A proportion of patients (~10–25%) can present with gynecomastia or, in children, with precocious puberty.[64,67,79] Malignant LCT tumors generally occur in adults with a testicular mass.[73] Though the age range is similar to benign LCTs, the median age tends to be older,[80] ranging from 20–82 years with the median age being 58 years. Painless testicular enlargement was present in 81%. All patients in this series by definition had metastases, 72% with regional node involvement, 43% with pulmonary metastases, 38% with hepatic metastases, and 28% with lung involvement.[80] Gynecomastia was present in 19%. Metastases were present in 22% at presentation and developed within 1 year in a further 19%.

Investigations

A full endocrinological assessment of the pituitary/gonadal axis is advised, with particular attention to androgen, estrogen, and progesterone production.[59,78,81] The value of these data is that if elevated titers are noted, they can act as a tumor marker. A case report has indicated that spermatic venous blood from the tumor-bearing testis had high concentrations of testosterone and androstenedione.[82] Elevations of urinary ketosteroids were seen in 14 of 22 patients (64%), of serum and/or urinary androgens in 12 of 22 patients (54%), and of serum of urinary estrogens in 11 of 22 patients (50%) with metastatic LCT.[82] Increased 17-hydroxyprogesterone (17-OHP) in a child may suggest congenital adrenal hyperplasia; however, in Leydig cell tumors plasma cortisol levels are normal and the 17-OHP does not suppress with dexamethasone.[83] CT scanning of the chest and abdomen should also be performed.

Management and prognosis
Surgery

Inguinal orchidectomy has traditionally been the treatment of choice for LCT and will cure the majority of patients. Over recent years, several groups have treated small tumors by partial orchidectomy and reported high levels of local control. Malignancy is often defined in terms of the presence of metastatic disease and surgery has been used to resect

Table 5.5 Outcome of patients undergoing retroperitoneal lymph node dissection for sex cord tumors.

Author	Region	Year	Tumor types	n	Metastatic lymph nodes	Clinical mets	Mean FU	Deaths
Di Tonno[224]	NE Italy	2009	Leydig	5	0	1	81	1
Mosharafa[83]	Indiana	2003	Leydig 6 Sertoli 4 Mixed 5 Granulosa 1 Undifferentiated 1	17	9	6	40	6
Peschel[168]	Austria	2003	Leydig	6	0	0	12	0
			Leydig 18 Sertoli 4 Granulosa 1	23	5			

FU, follow up; mets, metastases.

established regional nodal disease in the retroperitoneum[84,85] and solitary pulmonary metastases with long-term benefit.[86] As established metastatic disease is generally incurable, this has raised the question as to whether prophylactic retroperitoneal lymph node dissection (RPLND) should be undertaken, and this has been addressed in a number of recent studies summarized in Table 5.5. Laparoscopic RPLND may be a less invasive approach.[87] Most patients have multiple sites of metastases and surgery can offer useful palliation in some circumstances.[88]

Radiotherapy

Radiotherapy was prescribed for 11 of 32 patients with malignant LCT reviewed by Grem et al.[80] No objective responses were seen but two patients (one with bone metastases and one with a retroperitoneal mass) noted reduction in pain. Total radiation dose varied but no response was recorded in patients receiving 48 Gy[89] or 50 Gy[90] as well as in those receiving lower doses.

Chemotherapy

Systemic chemotherapy has been presented only in the setting of advanced metastatic disease. Two out of seven patients treated with the agent o,p′-DDD (see also Chapter 10) responded, one with a reduction in liver size and falling urinary 17-ketosteroids and another with resolution of pulmonary nodules.[82,91]

Standard chemotherapy regimens have had no major benefit[92] and more experimental therapy with lonidamine, which can impair spermatogenesis, probably via changes induced in Sertoli cells, although producing symptomatic improvement in one of two patients, produced no objective responses.[82]

Prognosis of those with metastasis is variable, with a median survival of 2 years (range 2 months to 17 years).

Recommendations

Inguinal orchidectomy is recommended both to establish the diagnosis and to remove the primary lesion. In those patients whose tumors appear benign and whose hormone profile returns to normal post orchidectomy, no further treatment is recommended beyond surveillance, reserving lymphadenectomy for those who relapse either solely in regional nodes or with limited resectable pulmonary disease. Those patients with histological features suggestive of malignancy should be fully investigated and considered for template retroperitoneal node dissection. Radiotherapy and chemotherapy appear to be ineffective but may be considered for palliation of patients with widespread or unresectable disease.

Sertoli cell tumors

Epidemiology and etiology

In the BTTP series there were 32 Sertoli cell tumors (SCTs) (1.2%).[58] At least seven exhibited malignancy. This figure is in keeping with other large reported series.[69] The age of patients ranged from 2 months to 80 years, with seven patients presenting in the first decade of life. Godec[93] reported the 11th case of malignant SCT (excluding the BTTP series patients) and noted only two cases in children. SCT may be found either as pure tumors or in combination with germ cell tumors or other gonadal stromal tumors; the etiology remains obscure. The variable clinical course of these tumors has been reviewed by Giglio et al.[94] Sertoli cell tumor may occur in association with Peutz–Jeghers syndrome when feminization has been reported to be due to increased transcription of the aromatase P450 gene.[95,96]

Pathology and biology

A full description of these tumors is provided by Symington and Cameron.[58] SCTs arise within the testis and in the BTTP series showed considerable variation in size (1–30 cm).[58] They were well demarcated, and creamy white or tan in color, with occasional foci of hemorrhage or necrosis. Histologically, SCTs usually show solid or gland-like tubule formation, forming nests and cords separated by fibrous tissue (Fig. 5.5) with considerable variation in pattern both within individual tumors and between different tumors. The tumor cells may appear clear because of intracytoplasmic lipid, and Call–Exner-like bodies or focal calcifications are sometimes noted within larger aggregations of cells. Immunohistochemical evidence of vimentin (100%), frequent cytokeratin (60–80%), S-100 (30–60%), focal calretinin (50%) and inhibin (30–90%) is seen in both neoplastic and normal Sertoli cells. Epithelial membrane antigen (EMA) is usually negative but has been noted to show increased expression in malignant cases.[97]

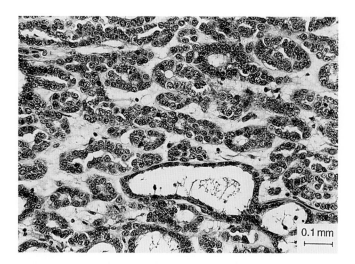

Figure 5.5 Sertoli cell tumor with a pattern of variably sized tubules in a loose fibrous stroma (H&E, 155×).

In the BTTP series, seven cases were malignant. The sites of metastatic involvement included regional nodes, liver, lung, bone, and brain. In four of seven cases the tumor invaded the rete testis, epididymis, or spermatic cord, and in all cases lymphatic and/or vascular invasion was seen. In the Boston series of 60 Sertoli cell tumors,[98] the pathological features that best correlated with a clinically malignant course were as follows: a tumor diameter of 5.0 cm or greater, necrosis, moderate-to-severe nuclear atypia, vascular invasion and a mitotic rate of more than 5 mitoses per 10 HPF. Only one of nine benign tumors for which follow-up data of 5 years or more were available had more than one of these features, whereas five of seven malignant tumors had at least three. As with Leydig tumors, staining for inhibin is common, but lack of staining may be a marker of malignant potential.[99]

The distinction of Sertoli cell tumors from seminoma may be difficult. Henley et al. highlighted 13 malignant Sertoli cell tumors of the testis with light microscopic features that mimicked seminoma with a nested growth pattern, prominence of clear cells, lymphoid infiltrate, cytoplasmic glycogen and prominent nucleoli.[100] However, a panel including inhibin-α, EMA and OCT3/4 would help to resolve this.

The time from presentation to detection of metastases in a review[101] was generally short, with eight of 11 malignant cases developing metastases within 1 year, although long disease-free intervals are occasionally noted.

Clinical features

Sertoli cell tumors usually present with testicular swelling: 29 of 32 cases in the BTTP series did so in this manner.[58] They may also be discovered on routine examinations or as an incidental finding either at autopsy or at operation for maldescent.[59]

Gabrilove et al.[102] reported on 72 cases of SCT, of which 60 were benign. Seventeen cases presented at less than 1 year of age, and 28 between 20 and 45 years. Malignancy was noted in only one child less than 10 years of age and was predominantly seen in patients over 25 years of age. Gynecomastia was

recorded in 17 of the 72 cases and was associated with malignancy in seven. Hormone studies have been infrequent but elevation of serum and urinary estrogens and testosterone has been reported. Young et al.[98] described 60 Sertoli cell tumors of the testis, with an age range from 15 to 80 years (mean, 45 years). In 14 cases a testicular mass had been enlarging slowly, the longest period being 14 years (mean 3.7 years). Only five patients had testicular pain. Four patients had metastatic disease at the time of presentation. All the tumors were unilateral and ranged from 0.3 cm to 15 cm (mean 3.6 cm) in size.

Investigations

A full endocrinological assessment of the pituitary/gonadal axis is advised with particular attention being paid to androgen, estrogen, and progesterone production.[59] CT scanning of the chest, abdomen and pelvis should be performed, particularly when the primary tumor exhibits features of malignancy. BHCG, α-fetoprotein, and placental alkaline phosphatase should also be measured to exclude germ cell tumor.

Management and prognosis
Surgery

In general, the management and issues are similar as for Leydig cell tumors. Inguinal orchidectomy has been the treatment of choice for SCT and will cure the majority of patients but partial orchidectomy/local excision has grown in popularity and for small tumors achieves good long-term control rates.

Like Leydig tumors, RPLND has been performed both as a staging/adjuvant[103] procedure and to resect established metastatic disease. The value of the former procedure, although not tested in a trial setting, is apparent in case reports in which long-term survivors are reported following resection of both microscopic and macroscopic nodal disease.[104,105] In Godec's series reviewing 11 cases with malignant SCT, four had retroperitoneal lymph node dissection for nodal disease and three remained disease free at 5 years, 7 months, and 6 months respectively.[101] Mosharafa et al.[85] reviewed 17 patients with malignant sex cord stromal tumors who underwent retroperitoneal lymph node dissection. All patients with stage I disease were alive without disease at last follow-up (mean 4.5 years). Six of eight patients with stage II–III tumors died of disease within 9 months to 6 years after surgery (median 1.2 years).

Radiotherapy

Radiotherapy has also been prescribed as adjuvant treatment to the inguinal nodes and to treat recurrent disease. In a review of metastasizing Sertoli cell tumors, Madson and Hultberg reported that irradiation of para-aortic lymph nodes may provide effective local treatment. None of 13 patients they reviewed developed para-aortic lymph node recurrences.[106] In general, high radiation doses (40 Gy) have been recommended.

Chemotherapy

Chemotherapy has been infrequently prescribed for this rare tumor, which does not appear to be chemosensitive, except possibly in childhood.[105]

Recommendations

Inguinal orchidectomy is recommended both to establish the diagnosis and to remove the primary lesion. In small tumors partial orchidectomy is an alternative in experienced centers. In those patients whose tumors appear benign and whose hormone profile returns to normal after orchidectomy, no further treatment is recommended. Patients with histological features suspicious of malignancy should be fully investigated and if no evidence of spread of disease is found, it is reasonable to consider either retroperitoneal node dissection or close surveillance. Patients who have disease limited to the regional nodes at presentation should have initially a retroperitoneal lymphadenectomy performed. Addition of radiotherapy is of uncertain benefit and radiotherapy should be reserved for palliation of patients with widespread or unresectable disease.

The prognosis is variable. In the BTTP series,[58] six of seven patients with malignant SCT died within 18 months, and one after 18 years (histologically confirmed). In the series of Godec,[93] four of 11 remain alive, deaths occurring within 2 years in five of seven who died.

Large cell calcifying Sertoli cell tumor

A rare subtype of Sertoli cell tumor is the large cell calcifying Sertoli cell tumor.[107–111] Only 48 cases have been reported in the literature as reviewed recently by Giglio et al.[94] It is generally seen in childhood and adolescence and is sometimes associated with other abnormalities, including Leydig cell and pituitary tumors,[112] and may form part of the autosomal dominantly inherited Carney complex.[113,114] It presents as a slowly enlarging testicular mass, but may be bilateral or multifocal. Grossly, the tumor is well circumscribed, and microscopically it has fibrous septa, with calcification, which separate sheets, cords, and solid nests of cells with abundant eosinophilic cytoplasm. Ultrastructurally,[115,116] they resemble Sertoli cells, and characteristic Charcot–Böttcher crystalloids have been demonstrated in one case.[112] Testosterone and estradiol have been demonstrated in the neoplastic cells by immunohistochemistry,[113] along with a different immunoreactivity with greater expression of inhibin, S-100 and vimentin than conventional SCTs.[117]

Kratzer et al.[118] reported six malignant and six benign large cell calcifying Sertoli cell tumors of the testis and reviewed the literature. Malignant tumors were unilateral and solitary and occurred at a mean age of 39 years (range 28–51 years), whereas the benign neoplasms were bilateral and multifocal in 28% of cases and occurred at a mean age of 17 years (range 2–38 years). Only one malignant tumor occurred in a patient with evidence of a genetic syndrome (Carney syndrome), whereas 36% of benign tumors had various genetic syndromes or endocrine abnormalities. Most of the tumors in the latter cases were bilateral and multifocal. There were strong associations of malignant behavior with size >4 cm, extratesticular growth, gross or microscopic necrosis, high-grade cytological atypia, vascular space invasion, and mitotic rate greater than three mitoses per 10 HPF.[118] Management guidelines are as for other Sertoli cell tumors.

Adenocarcinoma of the rete testis

History

This tumor was first described by Curling.[119] Feek and Hunter[120] outlined the histological criteria for diagnosis and Schoen and Rush[121] emphasized its aggressive nature. Sarma and Weillbaecher[122] reviewed the literature, indicating that long-term survival post orchidectomy was possible.

Epidemiology and etiology

This is a very rare tumor with only about 45 cases reported in the English literature.[123] The age at presentation ranges from 30 to 91 years with a median of 47 and mean of 50 years.[122,124,125] The etiology is unknown although some patients have had a history of undescended testis,[126] chronic epididymitis[127] or trauma.

Pathology and biology

The rete testis forms part of the collecting system of the testis and tumors arising in the region tend to be located at the hilum. A full description of these tumors is given by Mostofi and Price,[128] who described the tendency for this tumor to form papillary structures, although solid and tubular patterns are also seen. There is usually moderate nuclear pleomorphism and mitotic activity.

Immunohistochemistry shows positivity for cytokeratins (CAM5.2 and CK7), EMA and less often CEA.[117] There is also evidence of expression of the cell lineage specific transcription factors for wolffian duct development, PAX2 and PAX8, in both normal and neoplastic rete epithelium.[129]

The differential diagnosis includes germ cell tumor invading the rete testis, adenocarcinoma arising from embryonic remnants, and, particularly, mesothelioma. Also, in cryptorchidism the relative increase or even hyperplasia of the cells of the collecting system can be misinterpreted as adenocarcinoma of the rete testis (ART). Criteria for diagnosis[54] include a predominant location in the rete, a pattern consistent with origin from rete epithelium, continuity between tumor and normal rete epithelium, and absence of a primary carcinoma elsewhere. The differential diagnosis includes malignant mesothelioma, certain ovarian-type tumors, metastatic adenocarcinoma, epididymal carcinoma, and malignant Sertoli cell tumor.[130]

Adenocarcinoma of the rete testis is an aggressive tumor by virtue of both local extension and local recurrence after excision, and wide dissemination. In 17 cases reviewed by Sarma with adequate follow-up data, 10 patients developed metastases within 1 year of presentation.[122] Sites of metastatic involvement included regional nodes, lung, and liver. In a literature review by Sanchez-Chapado et al.,[131] information about disease-free survival was collected in 38 patients. As many as 40% of them died within the first year of diagnosis. Three- and 5-year disease-free survivals were 49% and 13%, respectively. Tumors that were organ confined and small (testicular mass <5 cm in maximum diameter) behave better than those disseminated at diagnosis or of a bigger size.

Clinical features

The tumor may arise in either testis. The most common presenting feature is an enlarging scrotal mass which may be tender and can have an associated hydrocele in about a quarter of patients.[130] About 20% present ART with symptoms due to either nodal or metastatic disease and about an additional 30% will be found to have metastasis on staging.[132]

Investigation and staging

The authors recommend CT scanning of the thorax and abdomen to assess extent of disease at diagnosis.[133] Chest x-ray and routine hematological and biochemical tests should also be performed as well as serum estimations of α-fetoprotein and BHCG, and placental alkaline phosphatase in order to help in the differential diagnosis.

Management and prognosis

Surgery

Complete surgical excision is the mainstay of treatment. A radical inguinal orchidectomy is recommended because local recurrence has been recorded after scrotal interference.[134] Local recurrence has also been reported when the tumor is adherent to the scrotum[132] and hemi-scrotectomy may be considered in these circumstances.

As ART has a high metastatic rate and is resistant to nonsurgical therapies, a few case reports have reported using adjuvant retroperitoneal lymph node dissection.[135–137] There is limited information on the success of this approach. Patients with negative lymph nodes may have better prognosis[122,136,138] and at least one patient reported to have had resected involved lymph nodes has remained disease free at 3.5 years.[139]

Radiotherapy

This has been prescribed to treat extensive local disease at the primary site, following orchidectomy as an adjuvant to the regional lymph nodes, and to treat metastatic disease.

The one patient presenting with extensive local disease and treated with radiotherapy alone (dose not stated) died 40 days from presentation, having had no apparent response.[132,140] In the five patients receiving adjuvant radiotherapy, one died at 2 months with metastases involving the skin and inguinal nodes. Follow-up times were less than 1 year in the remainder, the impact of radiotherapy in an adjuvant setting remaining unclear.[122] Of 14 patients presenting with or developing metastases, radiotherapy was prescribed in seven. In only one case was comment made about a beneficial response to radiotherapy, the patient remaining symptom free at 5 months from presentation. Dose–response data and information on local control with radiotherapy could not be ascertained[122] although in the report by Whitehead et al.,[141] no regression was seen despite an applied dose of 76 Gy using cobalt-60.

Chemotherapy

This has been infrequently used and only in the setting of overt metastatic disease. No responses have been seen to combinations of cyclophosphamide, 5-fluorouracil, and actinomycin-D[142] or to single-agent methotrexate.[122]

Recommendations

Patients should have a radical inguinal orchidectomy and a hemi-scrotectomy if scrotal violation has occurred. This establishes the diagnosis and should control the primary site. If no evidence of metastases is present on staging then consideration should be given to retroperitoneal lymph node dissection, based on isolated reports of benefit. An alternative policy is one of surveillance, with particular attention being paid to the regional lymph nodes, reserving surgery for patients relapsing in the site alone.

Patients with metastatic disease limited to the regional nodes should be managed by surgery. Patients with distant metastases should be treated with palliative intent, reserving radiotherapy and chemotherapy for specific symptoms. More information is required on the chemotherapy responsiveness of these tumors, perhaps with newer chemotherapy agents.

The prognosis overall is poor, with a 5-year survival of only 13%. Prompt diagnosis and resection of a small-sized tumor appear to offer the best chance for cure.

Malignant mesothelioma of the tunica vaginalis

Introduction

The tunica vaginalis surrounds the testis, having been formed from the processus vaginalis, which is part of the peritoneum that is carried down to the scrotum during the descent of the testis. Malignant mesothelioma of the tunica vaginalis (MMTV) is extremely rare and was first described in 1957.[143] Its association with prior asbestos exposure has been emphasized.[144] Surgery represents the only potentially curative treatment and must be meticulously performed in view of the tendency for local recurrence. Careful appraisal of regional nodes is important as this represents a major pathway of dissemination. In the presence of metastatic disease, radiotherapy and chemotherapy are used palliatively, with optimal treatment yet to be defined.

Epidemiology and etiology

Malignant mesotheliomas can arise from any part of the body where a mesothelial membrane exists[145]; tumors of the tunica vaginalis, however, are very rare, accounting for less than 5% of all mesotheliomas.[146,147] A literature review in 1998 found only 80 cases.[148] The age range of these patients was 7–87 years with a median age of 60 years.

Although there are several mechanisms hypothesized for the development of tunical mesothelioma, the exposure to asbestos or asbestos-containing materials remains the only established risk factor. In the literature review by Plas,[148] asbestos exposure was documented in 34.2% of the patients. Even this may be an underestimate as detailed case notes were available in only half of the patients. Even a family history of asbestos exposure has been associated with development of MMTV.[149] Other suggested associations include chronic immunosuppression,[150] chromosomal abnormalities such as losses on 1p, 3p, 6q, 9q, and monosomy 22,[151] radiation exposure,[152] simian virus 40 (SV40) exposure,[153] trauma and previous hernia repair.[130,144]

Pathology and biology

The tumor usually presents as a hydrocele associated with a scrotal mass. The hydrocele fluid is often clear but can be bloodstained and the tumor is seen as a papillary structure or nodules[154,155] standing out from the clear smooth lining of the sac. Great variation in histological appearance occurs but, like pleural mesothelioma, solid, papillary-glandular, and occasionally biphasic patterns are seen. In general, mesothelial cells may produce hyaluronic acid but, unlike many adenocarcinomas, do not produce periodic acid-Schiff (PAS)-positive mucin.[156] Analysis of 20 cases showed a similar picture to that found in mesotheliomas elsewhere, with all staining positive for caretinin and EMA, 90% for thrombomodulin, 83% for CK7 and 72% for CK5-6, but were negative for CK20 and CEA.[157] Mesothelial cells also have distinct ultrastructural features, including abundant, elongated microvilli, and electron microscopy can be helpful in diagnosis.[158]

Regional lymph node involvement has been reported in three of eight cases undergoing laparotomy, and diffuse visceral nodules were seen in a further two cases.[144] Distant metastases at presentation are rare but are seen on relapse, with pulmonary involvement being the most readily apparent. MMTV also tends to recur locally and in the regional lymph nodes.[144,159] Time from initial therapy to relapse can vary considerably, from months to many years. In a series of 24 patients there were nine recurrences, three by 1 year, five by 2 years and seven by 3 years from presentation.[144]

Additionally, there is a rare variant with a well-differentiated papillary pattern which can be regarded as having "uncertain malignant potential."[160,161]

Clinical features and prognosis

Malignant mesothelioma of the tunica vaginalis presents with a scrotal mass in association with a hydrocele and there may be a history of prior asbestos exposure. The diagnosis may be helped by Doppler as well as scrotal ultrasound.[162] The tumor can produce multiple nodules[154,163] and occasionally malignant mesothelioma of the peritoneum can spread to involve the tunica vaginalis and vice versa.[164] The presence of a bilateral MMTV was reported in only two patients (3.8%) in the review by Plas.[148] Primary metastatic presentation was seen in 15% of the cases. Lymphatic spread was most common followed by spread to lung, liver, and pleura. Rare cases of cerebral metastasis have also been reported.[165] Interestingly, the review also highlighted the difficulty of diagnosing the disease preoperatively. In only two of the 74 published cases (2.7%) was an accurate preoperative diagnosis made of the malignant disease.

The clinical course is variable although prognostic information may be derived from details of presentation and histology.[166] Plas et al.[148] reported that age over 60 years and presence of metastatic disease were significant factors for a poorer outcome on univariate analysis. Patients with a positive history of asbestos exposure also did worse, with a shorter disease-free interval.

Investigations and staging

Ultrasound of the testis is a useful initial diagnostic test and the features on ultrasound have been summarized in a recent report.[167] In view of the propensity to spread to involve abdominal lymph nodes and lung, lymphangiography and CT scanning of the thorax and abdomen are recommended along with routine hematological and biochemical investigations. Data from pleural mesothelioma suggest a role for fluorodeoxyglucose (FDG) PET scanning to help staging.[168]

Management

Surgery

Surgery is the mainstay of treatment for MMTV and a radical inguinal orchidectomy is the optimal surgical procedure for localized tumor.[164] Transscrotal procedures are associated with local recurrence and where scrotal violation has occurred, hemi-scrotectomy should be considered. After primary surgery, complete remission has been reported in 47.5% patients with a median follow-up of 12 months. Most patients with recurrent tumor went on to develop disseminated disease (83.9%). The median time to tumor recurrence was 10.5 months (range, 2–180 months). More than 60% of recurrences developed within the first 2 postoperative years.[148]

Patients who have radiological evidence of regional lymph node involvement with no evidence of distant metastases require lymph node dissection, which can be curative. One such patient with histologically confirmed regional node involvement survived 15 years disease free following this procedure.[169]

Retroperitoneal lymph node dissection as an adjuvant therapy is more controversial. As no other therapy except surgery is curative in MMTV, an argument for a RPLND at presentation can be made in a patient with good general health; however, benefit from this treatment depends on the abdominal nodes being the only site of metastases. Of eight patients undergoing laparotomy, three were found to have lymph node involvement, of whom only one survived disease free. Three patients had negative laparotomies, of whom one relapsed with groin nodes, one at the primary site, and one remained disease free. The two remaining patients were discovered to have multiple visceral nodules of disease at laparotomy. Sixteen patients did not undergo laparotomy and of these, only two relapsed with abdominal disease at 5 and 19 years respectively.[144] A reasonable alternative approach would therefore be to monitor patients radiologically, reserving lymphadenectomy for those who relapse only in nodes.

Radiotherapy

Radiotherapy alone has been prescribed as part of the primary management of MMTV in 10 of 74 cases reported in the literature.[148,170–172] The total doses prescribed varied from 25 to 60 Gy, and fractionation and overall time were not specified. A complete remission was reported in five (50%) of 10 cases with a maximum follow-up of 12 months. Follow-up times ranged from 1.5 to 36 months and the impact of radiotherapy on survival is not clear.

Radiotherapy has also been used for those patients who develop local recurrence following surgery.[144] Of three patients with such a complication, one received radiotherapy (45 Gy total dose over approximately 1 month) following resection of the recurrence and, although he subsequently died from pulmonary metastases, he suffered no further local recurrences.

Chemotherapy

A number of agents have been used to treat recurrent or metastatic MMTV. In the review by Plas, partial remission, defined as stable disease or reduction of tumor volume, was reported in two of 10 cases receiving chemotherapy (20%). No improvement in symptoms or tumor size was seen in six patients (60%), and none of the patients experienced complete remission. Combined chemotherapy and radiotherapy was given to six patients with disseminated disease and partial remission was seen in three patients, including one who had had stable disease for 16 years.[148]

The similarity between MMTV and malignant mesothelium at other sites would suggest that chemotherapy is not curative.[163,173] The combination of cisplatin with either pemetrexed or raltitrexed can prolong survival.[174,175]

Recommendations

Radical inguinal orchidectomy and hemi-scrotectomy lead to a high local control rate. PET scanning may improve sensitivity of staging. Patients with no evidence of metastatic disease should be followed clinically with special attention being paid to the primary site, peritoneum, and regional lymph nodes. Patients relapsing in these sites with no evidence of other disease should undergo further surgery, and if resection margins are in doubt, consideration may be given to high-dose local radiotherapy. Similarly, patients presenting with metastatic disease solely involving the regional nodes should undergo radical surgery in an attempt to cure.

Patients relapsing with disseminated disease or who have unresectable disease should be managed with palliative intent. The efficacy of current chemotherapy makes this a reasonable palliative option in fitter patients.

Paratesticular rhabdomyosarcoma

History

Rokitansky is credited with the first reported case of rhabdomyosarcoma affecting the spermatic cord[176] and in 1934, a review by Hirsch[177] pointed out that the majority of cases occurred in childhood. Tanimura and Furata[178] reviewed the literature and noted that the majority of patients died with disseminated disease within 1 year and that the overall prognosis was poor. The value of chemotherapy in rhabdomyosarcoma was clearly demonstrated in the 1970s.[179] At present, attempts are being made to reduce toxicity from chemotherapy in early-stage disease and improve results for bad-risk patients, and overall cure rates have improved to over 80%.[180]

Epidemiology and etiology

Rhabdomyosarcoma is the most frequently encountered malignant tumor affecting the soft tissues in childhood. Between 1954 and 1973, 2048 cases of malignancy in childhood were recorded by the Manchester Children's Tumour Registry (CTR), and of these, 85 cases (4%) were rhabdomyosarcoma. The overall incidence in the UK is approximately four cases per year per million of the population under 15 years of age[181] and this figure is in keeping with the United States experience reported by Young and Miller.[182] Paratesticular rhabdomyosarcoma represents 4–8% of rhabdomyosarcoma at all sites.

An association with genetically transmitted disease exists, rhabdomyosarcoma occurring more frequently in particular with von Recklinghausen disease.[183] Interestingly, in von Recklinghausen disease, compound tumors consisting of schwannian elements and rhabdomyosarcoma are seen.[184] These are sometimes called "triton" tumors after the experiments of Locatelli,[185] in which implantation of the cut end of the sciatic nerve into tritons (a small salamander) induced the growth of supernumerary limbs, leading to the supposition that endoneural cells may be able to differentiate into muscle. There may also be a higher incidence of breast cancer in relatives,[183] a pattern consistent with the Li–Fraumeni cancer syndrome.[186]

The age incidence of rhabdomysarcoma shows two peaks, an early one around 5 years of age and one later on during adolescence. This bimodal distribution in age of presentation is also seen in paratesticular rhabdomyosarcoma which represents about 40% of all paratesticular malignancies.[187]

Pathology and biology

Paratesticular rhabdomyosarcoma (PTR) usually arises in the spermatic cord but it can compress or invade neighboring structures such as the epididymis or testes, and may be very extensive.

The histologicl subtype of PTR is most commonly embryonal rather than pleomorphic or alveolar and, as indicated by Willis,[188] resembles primitive embryonic tissue. In an Italian and German Cooperative Group study, 84% of the 198 patients with PTR had embryonal histology while only 8% had alveolar histology, a proportion significantly smaller than in the rhabdomyosarcoma population as a whole (20–30%).[189] The embryonal and alveolar histologies have distinctive molecular characteristics which assist diagnostic confirmation. Unique translocations between the *FKHR* gene on chromosome 13 and either the *PAX3* gene on chromosome 2 or the *PAX7* gene on chromosome 1 are characteristic of alveolar rhabdomyosarcoma.[190,191] Genomic amplification is rare in embryonal rhabdomyosarcoma, although gains of whole chromosomes occur commonly while gene amplification commonly occurs in alveolar rhabdomyosarcoma.[192]

Table 5.6 Classification of rhabdomyosarcoma.

The Rhabdomyosarcoma Group of the International Society of Paediatric Oncology (SIOP) Classification[196]	
1. Embryonal type (293 cases)	
1.1 Dense	
1.1.1 Poorly differentiated	37%
1.1.2 Well differentiated	14%
1.2 Loose	
1.2.1 Botryoid	11%
1.2.2 Nonbotryoid	15%
1.3 Alveolar	
2. Adult type (1 case)	
Intergroup Rhabdomyosarcoma Classification (IRS) system (581 cases)[197]	
1. Embryonal	57%
2. Alveolar	19%
3. Botryoid	6%
4. Pleomorphic	1%
5. Special undifferentiated type 1	4%
6. Special undifferentiated type 2	3%
7. Undifferentiated mesenchymal sarcoma	10%

Research on myocyte development shows that cross-striations do not become apparent until the 14th week of embryonic life and the absence of such striations does not therefore preclude the diagnosis of rhabdomyosarcoma.[193,194] The usual histological appearance is of a myxoid stroma in association with small dark ovoid or spindle cells with varying degrees of myoblastic differentiation.[195] These ovoid cells may show enlargement around an eccentrically placed nucleus, producing the so-called "tadpole" or "tennis racket" cells. Two histopathological classifications are shown in Table 5.6.[196,197] The prognostic significance of such groupings is not yet clear.

Although electron microscopy can help to establish the diagnosis by showing actin and myosin filaments and Z-bands, immunohistochemistry is much more sensitive.[198] Antibodies to myogenin and MyoD1, as well as desmin and smooth muscle actin (SMA), help to differentiate rhabdomyosarcoma from other small round cell tumors of childhood such as neuroblastoma, Ewing sarcoma, or lymphoma, and from other paratesticular sarcomas in adults. It is only nuclear staining of both myogenin and MyoD1 that is diagnostic.[199]

In rhabdomyosarcoma, site, stage, and histological type are important prognostic factors,[200–204] paratesticular and orbital primaries being favorable. Both the Intergroup Rhabdomyosarcoma Study Group (IRS)[202] and an Italian cooperative study[205] have confirmed the better prognosis of embryonal compared to alveolar or pleomorphic histology. LaQuaglia et al.[206] identified the importance of completeness of surgical resection in a multivariate analysis of mortality in 28 patients with PTR. Other important and statistically significant factors from large studies are tumor resectability, local invasiveness, nodal involvement, patient's age at diagnosis (>10 years) and tumor size (>5 cm).[189,207] Patients with either local invasiveness or tumor size more than 5 cm represented the worst-risk group. In those with metastatic disease, the number of involved sites is important.[208]

The majority of the patients with PTR have localized disease. In a European study,[189] retroperitoneal lymph node assessment was done with CT scan in all 216 patients and retroperitoneal lymph node involvement was detected in 21 (10%). The disease was localized in 92% of the cases as compared to 25% for rhabdomyosarcomas at other sites. Hematogenous metastases are uncommon at presentation, occurring in less than 5% of patients, mainly in liver, bone marrow, and lung. The most common sites of recurrence after treatment for early-stage disease include the groin, retroperitoneal lymph nodes, lung, bone, and bone marrow.[209]

Clinical features

The most common presenting feature is an enlarging painless scrotal mass.[187] Less commonly, symptoms are due to metastatic disease, especially in the regional lymph nodes. The presence of a scrotal mass in a child, especially if separate from the testis, should suggest the possibility of rhabdomyosarcoma.

Investigation

The following investigations are recommended: full blood count, α-fetoprotein and BHCG estimation (to differentiate germ cell cancer), renal and liver function tests, CT scanning of the thorax and abdomen, isotope bone scan, and bone marrow aspirate and biopsy. Also the primary tumor should be imaged clearly in view of the adverse significance of local extension.[210]

The International Union against Cancer (UICC) published a TNM classification in 1982[211] for rhabdomyosarcoma which has been widely accepted. In Table 5.7 the IRS classification,[212] which has been compared with the UICC TNM classification,[202] is also shown.

Management and prognosis

Surgery

Radical inguinal orchidectomy both confirms the diagnosis and usually completely removes the primary tumor. Resection of the scrotal skin is usually performed when there is scrotal tissue involvement or for primary reexcision after a prior transscrotal approach. In patients with residual disease after primary surgery that is not amenable to reexcision, a second surgery after chemotherapy is recommended.[213]

With orchidectomy alone, information from collected surgical series suggests an approximately 50% 2-year relapse-free survival rate, this figure being higher in those under 7 years of age compared to those over 7 years of age. For example, of seven cases of PTR reported by Malek et al.,[214] essentially treated by orchidectomy, three patients remained disease free (follow-up of 1, 3, and 39 years) and four patients subsequently developed metastases (all older children). Arlen et al.[169] also correlated risk of recurrence with older age.[215]

Surgery has been used diagnostically to sample retroperitoneal nodes and also as a therapeutic measure. However, the use of RPLND in paratesticular rhabdomyosarcoma is controversial, with conflicting data emerging from the European and

Table 5.7 Staging of rhabdomyosarcoma.

TNM	Summary	pTNM	
T1	Confined to organ/tissue	Limited to organ	pT1
T1a	<5 cm	Excision complete	
T1b	=5 cm		
T2	Involving other organs/tissues	Invasion beyond organ	pT2
	Effusion	Excision incomplete	
T2a	<5 cm	Microscopic residual tumor	pT3a
T2b	=5 cm	Macroscopic residual tumor	pT3b
T3/4	(Not applicable)	Nonresectable tumor	PT3c
N1	Regional involvement	Nodes completely resected	pN1a
		Nodes incompletely resected	pN1b
M0	No distant metastasis		
M1	Metastasis present		

Intergroup Rhabdomyosarcoma Study (IRS)[212]

Group I	Localized disease, completely removed, regional nodes not involved
	I.1 Confined to muscle or organ of origin
	I.2 Contiguous involvement with infiltration outside the muscle organs of origin, as through fascial planes
	Inclusion in this group includes both gross impression of complete removal and microscopic confirmation of complete removal
Group II	II.1 Grossly removed tumor with microscopic residual disease; no evidence of gross residual tumor; no evidence of regional node involvement
	II.2 Regional disease, completely removed (no microscopic residual disease)
	II.3 Regional disease with involved nodes, grossly removed, but with evidence of microscopic residual disease
Group III	Incomplete resection or biopsy with gross residual disease
Group IV	Distant metastatic disease present at onset

Reproduced with permission from Buskirk SJ, *et al.*[228]

IRS studies. In the Italian and German Cooperative Group study,[189] surgical assessment of the retroperitoneal lymph nodes was recommended as a staging procedure for all patients in the earlier studies. Thereafter, it was avoided in patients with clearly negative nodes on imaging and reserved for patients with doubtful retroperitoneal involvement. No significant difference was observed in the rate of positive node detection between the two periods.

Surgery also has a role in the management of patients who relapse and, when combined with chemotherapy and radiotherapy, has led to prolonged survival.[179]

Radiotherapy

The IRS series examined the role of local radiotherapy in 13 patients with completely excised primaries and no evidence of nodal metastases, randomizing patients to receive or not to receive local radiotherapy, in addition to adjuvant chemotherapy. No patient in either arm developed local recurrence, suggesting that radiotherapy to the primary site is not usually indicated but could be considered if scrotal contamination has occurred[209] or there is residual disease after surgery.

Radiotherapy to the regional nodes has also been recommended as an adjuvant in stage I PRT and also to treat known abdominal or pelvic nodal disease, often in conjunction with chemotherapy and surgery. However, radiotherapy to the para-aortic and pelvic lymph nodes in young children will produce growth impairment. Tefft *et al.*[216] addressed the question of regional lymph node irradiation in rhabdomyosarcoma of the genitourinary tract in childhood, reporting on 58 cases. Thirty-eight patients had lymph node sampling of which 15 were

positive; 11 out of the 15 patients with positive lymph nodes and six out of 23 with negative lymph node sampling received radiotherapy, as did 10 patients with no node sampling. The radiation prescription varied up to a maximum of 45 Gy in 5–6 weeks. In the entire series, only one patient (who received 45 Gy to the regional nodes) failed in regional nodes. Radiotherapy in combination with surgery and chemotherapy can result in prolonged survival in patients relapsing in regional lymph nodes.[179]

In nonmetastatic rhabdomyosarcoma, the European approach has been to pursue less aggressive local therapies, to reduce the long-term toxicity risks[217] so that radiotherapy was avoided in patients who achieve complete response with surgery and chemotherapy. The US group protocols place more emphasis on maintaining a high disease-free rate.[218]

Chemotherapy

The adjuvant value of chemotherapy in rhabdomyosarcoma in which all disease has been apparently surgically resected was demonstrated by Heyn *et al.*,[219] where eight of 15 patients (53%) treated by surgery and local radiotherapy developed recurrence of metastases versus three of 17 (17.6%) receiving adjuvant chemotherapy (actinomycin-D and vincristine). This achieved statistical significance ($p = 0.03$). The study by Olive *et al.*[179] on 19 children with complete tumor removal and negative lymphangiograms confirms the effectiveness of combination chemotherapy as an adjuvant. All but one of the 19 received adjuvant chemotherapy alone with combinations of vincristine, adriamycin, actinomycin-D, and cyclophosphamide, and of these 18, only one relapsed with spermatic cord

Table 5.8 Rhabdomyosarcoma: results of treatment.

Series	Stage	Number of patients	Treatment	% disease-free survival	Median duration of observation
Ferrari[189]*	Gp I	164	C	91	9 years
	Gp II	21	S,R,C	95	
	Gp III	13	S,R,C	76	
SIOP MMT 84[207]	I–III	27	C	93	7 years
SIOP MMT 89[207]	I–III	69	C	78	7 years
Olive[179]†	I	19	C	89	>3 years
	II–IV	13	–	46	–
Hamilton[201]‡	All	17	S,R,C	88	5 years
	I	12	R,C	90	5 years
Loughlin[203]	All	12	S, CT	74	
Blyth[229]	All	18	S,R,C	89	4 years
Raney[209]*	Gp I	57	S,R,C	93	
	Gp II	20	S,R,C	90	3 years
	Gp III	4	R,C	67	
	Gp IV	14	R,C	67	
LaQuaglia[206]	All	28	S,R,C	57	

* IRS staging system (see Table 5.7).
† SIOP staging system.
‡ RMH/Barts staging system.
S, abdominal surgery; R, radiotherapy; C, chemotherapy.

and iliac lymph node involvement, and he was successfully salvaged with combined modality treatment and was considered cured 56 months later.

Multiagent chemotherapy is an important component of the multidisciplinary approach in treatment of these tumors. Various combinations and dose schedules have been used in different protocols in Europe and North America. Overall, regimens have been progressively reduced in intensity and duration over the years. The active agents include vincristine, dactinomycin, cyclophosphamide, ifosfamide and doxorubicin.

In the Italian and German Cooperative Group study, 106 patients with low-risk disease, i.e. favorable histology, T1N0M0, and complete resection at diagnosis (IRS group I), received chemotherapy alone. The 5-year survival of this subset was 99.1%.[189] The International Society of Pediatric Oncology (SIOP) studies (MMT 84 and MMT 89) systematically studied the role of combination chemotherapy in PTR.[207] The standard first-line chemotherapy for all patients in MMT 84 was combination therapy with ifosfamide, vincristine, and dactinomycin. In the MMT 89 study, an attempt was made to avoid alkylating agents for those patients in whom tumors had been completely resected at primary surgery (stage I pT1). These patients received only vincristine and dactinomycin. Important prognostic factors influencing survival were large tumors (>5 cm) and males aged >10 years.[217]

Due to the low frequency of metastatic PTR, inferences regarding the role of chemotherapy in metastatic PTR may be drawn from studies of rhabdomyosarcoma at other sites. Using vincristine and actinomycin-D in conjunction with appropriate surgery and radiotherapy, Heyn et al.[220] achieved a 20% 5-year survival in 14 patients with metastatic disease at presentation. In the Italian and German Cooperative Group study, the 5-year survival rate for the PTR patients with metastases was 22.2%.[189] The IRS[212,221] tested vincristine and actinomycin-D against those two agents plus cyclophosphamide (VAC) and found no

survival difference between the two regimens in patients with microscopic residual disease and/or nodal involvement, with approximately a 70% relapse-free survival at 5 years. They also compared VAC and VAC plus adriamycin in patients with more advanced disease (gross residual disease/systemic metastases), achieving a response rate of over 80% in each arm with no differences in duration of response or survival being noted. In the report of Maurer et al.,[212] 423 children had been entered on the IRS series, 85 of whom had microscopic or regional nodal disease and 151 had gross residual or metastatic disease. Less than 10% of patients with metastatic disease at presentation were alive at 2 years compared to over 60% with gross residual disease post surgery at presentation. Of 14 patients with PTR treated with VAC ± adriamycin ± radiotherapy, there were 12 complete remissions, of whom three relapsed, leading to a 3-year survival estimate of 64%.[202]

In the Children's Solid Tumour Group study,[172] the 5-year predicted actuarial survival rate for children with rhabdomyosarcoma confined to the tissue of origin and no evidence of nodal or metastatic spread was 86% compared to 21% for those with extension outside the tissue of origin. Of the 73 children reported, 14 had distant metastases at presentation and were treated with VAC chemotherapy, surgery being usually confined to biopsy only and radiotherapy being prescribed for bulky disease. Approximately 15% survived for 2 years. The results of treatment are shown in Table 5.8. There is a suggestion that ifosfamide be used in place of cyclophosphamide.[222] A detailed discussion of modern chemotherapy approaches can be found in the review by Sultan and Ferrari.[223]

Recommendations

Primary surgery consists of a high inguinal orchidectomy. RPLND is not routinely recommended for staging. Adjuvant treatment is indicated following primary surgery for clinical stage I PTR and the most extensive experience has been with VAC chemotherapy. Cure rates are high (approximately 90%) and less toxic chemotherapy, such as deletion of the alkylating agent, can be employed in those with negative surgical staging. The need for postchemotherapy irradiation is not established in good prognosis patients.

Patients presenting with abdominal lymph node involvement should be managed by combined modalities. It is beneficial to use chemotherapy post orchidectomy and use nodal disease as a marker of response. In patients with a complete radiological response, an argument for continued chemotherapy alone can be made but an alternative is to recommend surgical confirmation of response. In those presenting prior to their growth spurt with residual disease post chemotherapy, the authors would recommend a surgical approach to the control of intraabdominal disease. In older teenagers with residual postchemotherapy disease, radiotherapy may be considered guided by detail of excision and pathology.

Disseminated PTR should be managed as rhabdomyosarcoma at other sites, and although high response rates are seen using combinations of vincristine, cyclophosphamide, and adriamycin,[214] overall survival is poor at approximately 25%.

Acknowledgments

This work was undertaken at the Royal Marsden NHS Foundation Trust which received a proportion of its funding from the NHS Executive; we acknowledge NHS funding to the NIHR Biomedical Research Centre. The views expressed in this publication are those of the authors and not necessarily those of the NHS Executive. This work was supported by the Institute of Cancer Research (ICR), and Cancer Research UK (CUK) grant number C46/A10588 to the ICR Section of Radiotherapy.

References

1. Woodward P, *et al*. Germ cell tumours. In: Eble JN, *et al*. (eds) *Pathology and Genetics of Tumours of the Urinary System and Male Genital Organs*. Lyon, France: IARC Press, 2004. pp.221–49.
2. Malassez M. Lymphadenome du testicule. Bull Soc Anat Paris 1877; 52: 176.
3. Hutchinson J. Lymphosarcoma of both testes with considerable interval of time. BMJ 1889; 1: 413.
4. Gowing NFC. Malignant lymphoma of the testis. In Pugh RCB (ed) *Pathology of the Testis*. London, England: Blackwell Scientific Publications, 1976. pp.334–55.
5. Kiely JM, *et al*. Lymphoma of the testis. Cancer 1970; 26: 847–52.
6. Turner RR, Colby TV, MacKintosh FR. Testicular lymphomas: a clinico-pathologic study of 35 cases. Cancer 1981; 48: 2095–102.
7. Zucca E, *et al*. Patterns of outcome and prognostic factors in primary large-cell lymphoma of the testis in a survey by the International Extranodal Lymphoma Study Group. J Clin Oncol 2003; 21: 20–7.
8. Whelan SL, *et al*. *Patterns of Cancer in Five Continents*. IARC Scientific Publications No 102. Lyon, France: IARC Press, 1990.
9. Waterhouse JAH. Epidemiology of testicular tumours. J R Soc Med 1985; 78: 3–7.
10. Tepperman BS, *et al*. Non-Hodgkin's lymphoma of the testis. Radiology 1982; 142: 203–8.
11. Economopoulos T, *et al*. Primary extranodal non-Hodgkin's lymphoma in adults: clinicopathological and survival characteristics. Leuk Lymphoma 1996; 21: 131–6.
12. Freilone R, *et al*. Combined modality treatment with a weekly brief chemotherapy (ACOP-B) followed by locoregional radiotherapy in localized-stage intermediate- to high-grade non-Hodgkin's lymphoma. Ann Oncol 1996; 7: 919–24.
13. Wahal KM, Mehrotra R, Agarwal PK. Extranodal lymphomas in North India. J Indian Med Assoc 1983; 80: 130–2.
14. Rappaport H. Tumors of the hematopoietic system. In: *Atlas of Tumor Pathology*. Washington, DC: Armed Forces Institute of Pathology, 1966. pp.91–161.
15. Non-Hodgkin's Lymphoma Pathologic Classification Project. National Cancer Institute sponsored study of classifications of non-Hodgkin's lymphomas. Cancer 1982; 49: 2112–35.
16. Baldetorp LA, *et al*. Malignant lymphoma of the testis. Br J Urol 1984; 56: 525–30.
17. Jackson SM, Montessori GA. Malignant lymphoma of the testis: review of 17 cases in British Columbia with survival related to pathological subclassification. J Urol 1980; 123: 881–3.
18. Nonomura N, *et al*. Malignant lymphoma of the testis: histological and immunohistological study of 28 cases. J Urol 1989; 141: 1368–71.
19. World Health Organization. *Pathology and Genetics of Tumours of Hematopoietic and Lymphoid Tissues*. Lyon, France: IARC Press, 2001.
20. Al-Abbadi MA, Hattab EM, Tarawneh MS, Amr SS, Orazi A, Ulbright TM. Primary testicular diffuse large B-cell lymphoma belongs to the non-germinal center B-cell-like subgroup: a study of 18 cases. Mod Pathol 2006; 19(12): 1521–7.
21. Horstmann WG, Timens W. Lack of adhesion molecules in testicular diffuse centroblastic and immunoblastic B cell lymphomas as a contributory factor in malignant behaviour. Virchows Arch 1996; 429: 83–90.
22. Lambrechts AC, *et al*. Lymphomas with testicular localisation show a consistent BCL-2 expression without a translocation (14;18): a molecular and immunohistochemical study. Br J Cancer 1995; 71: 73–7.
23. Hyland J, Lasota J, Jasinski M, Petersen RO, Nordling S, Miettinen M. Molecular pathological analysis of testicular diffuse large cell lymphomas. Hum Pathol 1998; 29(11): 1231–9.
24. Linassier C, *et al*. Stage I-IIE primary non-Hodgkin's lymphoma of the testis: results of a prospective trial by the GOELAMS Study Group. Clin Lymphoma 2002; 3: 167–72.
25. Visco C, *et al*. Non-Hodgkin's lymphoma affecting the testis: is it curable with doxorubicin-based therapy? Clin Lymphoma 2001; 2: 40–6.
26. Sussman EB, *et al*. Malignant lymphoma of the testis. A clinicopathologic study of 37 cases. J Urol 1977; 118: 1004–7.
27. Gundrum JD, Mathiason MA, Moore DB, Go RS. 2009 Primary testicular diffuse large B-cell lymphoma: a population-based study on the incidence, natural history, and survival comparison with primary nodal counterpart before and after the introduction of rituximab. J Clin Oncol 2009; 27(31): 5227–32.
28. Cao B, *et al*. A clinical analysis of primary testicular diffuse large B-cell lymphoma in China. Hematology 2011; 16(5): 291–7.
29. Björkholm M, *et al*. Central nervous system occurrence in elderly patients with aggressive lymphoma and a long-term follow-up. Ann Oncol 2007; 18(6): 1085–9.
30. Park BB, *et al*. Consideration of aggressive therapeutic strategies for primary testicular lymphoma. Am J Hematol 2007; 82(9): 840–5.
31. Fonseca R, *et al*. Testicular lymphoma is associated with a high incidence of extranodal recurrence. Cancer 2000; 88: 154–61.
32. Hasselblom S, Ridell B, Wedel H, Norrby K, Sender Baum M, Ekman T. Testicular lymphoma – a retrospective, population-based, clinical and immunohistochemical study. Acta Oncol 2004; 43: 758–65.
33. Keldsen N, Michalski W, Bentzen SM, Hansen KB, Thorling K. Risk factors for central nervous system involvement in non-Hodgkins lymphoma – a multivariate analysis. Acta Oncol 1996; 35: 703–8.
34. Ostronoff M, *et al*. Localized stage non-Hodgkin's lymphoma of the testis: a retrospective study of 16 cases. Nouv Rev Fr Hematol 1995; 37: 267–72.
35. Sasai K, *et al*. Primary testicular non-Hodgkin's lymphoma: a clinical study and review of the literature. Am J Clin Oncol 1997; 20: 59–62.

36. Zouhair A, *et al.* Outcome and patterns of failure in testicular lymphoma: a multicenter Rare Cancer Network study. Int J Radiat Oncol Biol Phys 2002; 52: 652–6.

37. Arkenau HT, *et al.* The role of intrathecal chemotherapy prophylaxis in patients with diffuse large B-cell lymphoma. Ann Oncol 2007; 18(3): 541–5.

38. Vitolo U, *et al.* for the Gruppo Italiano Multiregionale Linfomi e Leucemie (GIMURELL). Dose-dense and high-dose chemotherapy plus rituximab with autologous stem cell transplantation for primary treatment of diffuse large B-cell lymphoma with a poor prognosis: a phase II multicenter study. Haematologica 2009; 94(9): 1250–8.

39. Talerman, A. A Primary malignant lymphoma of the testis. J Urol 1977; 118: 783–6.

40. Eckert H, Smith JP. Malignant lymphoma of the testis. BMJ 1963; 2(5362): 891–4.

41. Hurley LJ, Burke CR, Shetty SK, Previte SR, Sakr OE, Libertino JA. Bilateral primary non-Hodgkin's lymphoma of the testis. Urology 1996; 47: 596–8.

42. Kupfer H, von der Beek K. Recurrence in the other testicle of a non-Hodgkin's lymphoma with no other manifestations. Br J Urol 1995; 76: 516.

43. Duncan PR, Checa F, Gowing NFC, McElwain TJ, Peckham MJ. Extranodal non-Hodgkin's lymphoma presenting in the testicle: a clinical and pathologic study of 24 cases. Cancer 1980; 45: 1578–84.

44. Haddy TB, Sandlund JT, Magrath IT. Testicular involvement in young patients with non-Hodgkin's lymphoma. Am J Pediatr Hematol Oncol 1988; 10: 224–9.

45. Kellie SJ, Pui CH, Murphy SB. Childhood non Hodgkin's lymphoma involving the testis: clinical features and treatment outcome. J Clin Oncol 1989; 7: 1066–70.

46. Doll DC, Weiss RB. Malignant lymphoma of the testis. Am J Med 1986; 81(3): 515–24.

47. Leonard MP, Schlegel PN, Crovatto A, Gearhart JP. Burkitt's lymphoma of the testis: an unusual scrotal mass in childhood. J Urol 1990; 143: 104–6.

48. Carbone PP, Kaplan HS, Musshoff K, Smithers DW, Tubiana T. Report of the committee on Hodgkin's disease staging classification. Cancer Res 1971; 31: 1860–1.

49. Roche H, *et al.* Stage IE non Hodgkin's lymphoma of the testis: a need for a brief aggressive chemotherapy. J Urol 1989; 141: 554–6.

50. Vitolo U, *et al.* First-line treatment for primary testicular diffuse large B-cell lymphoma with rituximab-CHOP, CNS prophylaxis, and contralateral testis irradiation: final results of an international phase II trial. J Clin Oncol 2011; 29(20): 2766–72.

51. Coiffier B, *et al.* CHOP chemotherapy plus rituximab compared with CHOP alone in elderly patients with diffuse large-B-cell lymphoma. N Engl J Med 2002; 346: 235–42.

52. Mazloom A, Fowler N, Medeiros LJ, Iyengar P, Horace P, Dabaja BS. Outcome of patients with diffuse large B-cell lymphoma of the testis by era of treatment: the M. D. Anderson Cancer Center experience. Leuk Lymphoma 2010; 51(7): 1217–24.

53. Mostofi FK, Theiss EA, Ashley DJ. Tumors of specialized gonadal stroma in human male patients. Cancer 1959; 12: 944–57.

54. Young RH, Talerman A. Testicular tumors other than germ cell tumors. Semin Diagn Pathol 1987; 4: 342–60.

55. McLaren K, Thomson D. Localisation of S-100 protein in a Leydig and sertoli cell tumour of testis. Histopathology 1989; 15: 649–52.

56. Campbell EJ, Dickinson CJ, Slater JD, Edwards CR, Sikora EK. Sex and reproduction. In: Campbell EJ, Dickinson CJ, Slater JD, Edwards CR, Sikora EK (eds) *Clinical Physiology.* London: Blackwell Scientific Publications, 1984. pp.651–708.

57. Oosterhuis JW, *et al.* A malignant mixed gonadal stromal tumor of the testis with heterologous components and I(12P) in one of its metastases. Cancer Genet Cytogenet 1989; 41: 105–14.

58. Symington T, Cameron KM. Testicular diseases. In: Pugh RC (ed) *Pathology of the Testis.* London: Blackwell Scientific Publications 1976. pp.259–303.

59. Mostofi FK. Testicular tumours. Cancer 1973; 32: 1186–201.

60. Ward JA, Krantz S, Mendeloff J, Haltiwanger E. Interstitial cell tumour of the testis: report of two cases. J Clin Endocrinol Metab 1960; 20: 1622–32.

61. Leonhartsberger N, *et al.* Increased incidence of Leydig cell tumours of the testis in the era of improved imaging techniques. BJU Int 2011; 108(10): 1603–7.

62. Carmignani L, Morabito A, Gadda F, Bozzini G, Rocco F, Colpi GM. Prognostic parameters in adult impalpable ultrasonographic lesions of the testicle. J Urol 2005; 174(3): 1035–8.

63. Johnstone G. Pre-pubertal gynaecomastia in association with an interstitial cell tumour of the testis. Br J Urol 1967; 39: 211–20.

64. Giannarini G, *et al.* Long-term followup after elective testis sparing surgery for Leydig cell tumors: a single center experience. J Urol 2007; 178(3 Pt 1): 872–6.

65. Al-Agha OM, Axiotis CA. An in-depth look at Leydig cell tumor of the testis. Arch Pathol Lab Med 2007; 131(2): 311–17.

66. Carmignani L, *et al.* Conservative surgical therapy for leydig cell tumor. J Urol 2007; 178(2): 507–11.

67. Loeser A, *et al.* Testis-sparing surgery versus radical orchiectomy in patients with Leydig cell tumors. Urology 2009; 74(2): 370–2.

68. Dudderidge TJ, *et al.* Diagnosis of prostate cancer by detection of minichromosome maintenance 5 protein in urine sediments. Br J Cancer 2010; 103(5): 701–7.

69. Kim I, Young RH, Scully RE. Leydig cell tumours of the testis. Am J Surg Pathol 1985; 9: 177–92.

70. Suardi N, *et al.* Leydig cell tumour of the testis: presentation, therapy, long-term follow-up and the role of organ-sparing surgery in a single-institution experience. BJU Int 2009; 103(2): 197–200.

71. Assi A, Sironi M, Bacchioni AM, Declich P, Cozzi L, Pasquinelli G. Leydig cell tumor of the testis: a cytohistological, immunohistochemical, and ultrastructural case study. Diagn Cytopathol 1997; 16: 262–6.

72. Goswitz JJ, Pettinato G, Manivel JC. Testicular sex cord-stromal tumors in children: clinicopathologic study of sixteen children with review of the literature. Pediatr Pathol Lab Med 1996; 16: 451–70.

73. Cheville JC, Sebo TJ, Lager DJ, Bostwick DG, Farrow GM. Leydig cell tumor of the testis: a clinicopathologic, DNA content, and MIB-1 comparison of nonmetastasizing and metastasizing tumors. Am J Surg Pathol 1998; 22: 1361–7.

74. Iczkowski KA, Bostwick DG, Roche PC, Cheville JC. Inhibin A is a sensitive and specific marker for testicular sex cord-stromal tumors. Mod Pathol 1998; 11: 774–9.

75. Young RH. Sex cord-stromal tumors of the ovary and testis: their similarities and differences with consideration of selected problems. Mod Pathol 2005; 18(Suppl 2): S81–98.

76. Harms D, Kock LR. Testicular juvenile granulosa cell and Sertoli cell tumours: a clinicopathological study of 29 cases from the Kiel Paediatric Tumour Registry. Virchows Arch 1997; 430: 301–9.

77. Thomas JC, Ross JH, Kay R. Stromal testis tumors in children: a report from the prepubertal testis tumor registry. J Urol 2001; 166: 2338–40.

78. Valensi P, Coussieu C, Kemeny JL, Attali JR, Amouroux J, Sebaoun J. Endocrine investigations in two cases of feminizing Leydig cell tumour. Acta Endocrinol (Copenh) 1987; 115: 365–72.

79. Carmignani L, *et al.* Conservative surgical therapy for leydig cell tumor. J Urol 2007; 178(2): 507–11.

80. Grem JL, Robins I, Wilson KS, Gilchrist K, Trump DL. Metastatic Leydig cell tumor of the testis. Cancer 1986; 58: 2116–19.

81. Mineur P, de Cooman S, Hustin J, Verhoeven G, de Hertogh R. Feminizing testicular Leydig cell tumor: hormonal profile before and after unilateral orchidectomy. J Clin Endocrinol Metab 1987; 64: 686–91.

82. Sasano H, Maehara I, Ueno J, Orikasa S, Nagura H. Leydig cell tumor of the testis: analysis of testosterone production and secretin by three-dimensional histoculture. Endocr J 1996; 43: 73–8.

83. Solish SB, Goldsmith MA, Voutilainen R, Miller WL. Molecular characterization of a Leydig cell tumor presenting as congenital adrenal hyperplasia. J Clin Endocrinol Metab 1989; 69: 1148–52.

84. Lockhart JL, Dalton DL, Vollmer RT, Glenn JF. Non functioning interstitial cell carcinoma of testes. Urology 1976; 8: 392–4.

85. Mosharafa AA, *et al*. Does retroperitoneal lymph node dissection have a curative role for patients with sex cord-stromal testicular tumors? Cancer 2003; 98: 753–7.

86. Parker RG. Treatment of apparent solitary pulmonary metastases. J Thorac Cardiovasc Surg 1958; 36: 81–7.

87. Peschel R, Gettman MT, Steiner H, Neururer R, Bartsch G. Management of adult Leydig-cell testicular tumors: assessing the role of laparoscopic retroperitoneal lymph node dissection. J Endourol 2003; 17: 777–80.

88. Sawin PD, van Gilder JC. Spinal cord compression from metastatic Leydig's cell tumor of the testis: case report. Neurosurgery 1996; 38: 407–11.

89. Feldman PS, Kovacs K, Horvath E, Adelson GL. Malignant Leydig cell tumor: clinical, histologic and electron microscopic features. Cancer 1982; 49: 714–21.

90. Davies JM. Testicular cancer in England and Wales: some epidemiological aspects. Lancet 1981; 1: 928–32.

91. Azer PC, Braunstein GD. Malignant Leydig cell tumour: objective tumor response to o,p'-DDD. Cancer 1981; 47: 1251–5.

92. Farkas LM, Székely JG, Pusztai C, Baki M. High frequency of metastatic Leydig cell testicular tumours. Oncology 2000; 59: 118–21.

93. Godec CJ. Malignant Sertoli cell tumour of the testicle. Urology 1985; 26: 185–8.

94. Giglio M, Medica M, de Rose AF, Germinale F, Ravetti JL, Carmignani G. Testicular sertoli cell tumours and relative sub-types. Analysis of clinical and prognostic features. Urol Int 2003; 70: 205–10.

95. Ceccamea A, *et al*. Feminizing Sertoli cell tumour associated with Peutz–Jeghers syndrome (histologic and ultrastructural study). Tumori 1985; 71: 379–85.

96. Young S, Gooneratne S, Straus FH 2nd, Zeller WP, Bulun SE, Rosenthal IM. Feminizing Sertoli cell tumors in boys with Peutz–Jeghers syndrome. Am J Surg Pathol 1995; 19: 50–8.

97. Bostwick DG, Cheng L. *Urologic Surgical Pathology*, 2nd edn. Edinburgh: Mosby Elsevier Inc, 2008.

98. Young RH, Koelliker DD, Scully RE. Sertoli cell tumors of the testis, not otherwise specified: a clinicopathologic analysis of 60 cases. Am J Surg Pathol 1998; 22: 709–21.

99. Compérat E, Tissier F, Boyé K, De Pinieux G, Vieillefond A. Non-Leydig sex-cord tumors of the testis. The place of immunohistochemistry in diagnosis and prognosis. A study of twenty cases. Virchows Arch 2004; 444: 567–71.

100. Henley JD, Young RH, Ulbright TM. Malignant Sertoli cell tumors of the testis: a study of 13 examples of a neoplasm frequently misinterpreted as seminoma. Am J Surg Pathol 2002; 26: 541–50.

101. Nielsen K, Jacobsen GK. Malignant sertoli cell tumour of the testis, an immunohistochemical study and a review of the literature. APMIS 1988; 96: 755–60.

102. Gabrilove JL, Freiberg EK, Leiter E, Nicolis GL. Feminising and non-feminising Sertoli cell tumours. J Urol 1980; 124: 757–67.

103. Weitzner S, Addridge JE, Lamar Weems W. Stertoli cell tumour of the testis. J Urol 1979; 13: 87–9.

104. Herera LO, Wilks H, Wills JS, Loper GE. Malignant (androblastoma) Sertoli cell tumor of testis. J Urol 1981; 18: 287–90.

105. Sharma S, Seam RK, Kapoor HL. Malignant sertoli cell tumour of the testis in a child. J Surg Oncol 1990; 44: 129–31.

106. Madson E, Hultberg B. Metastasizing Sertoli cell tumors of the human testis – a report of two cases and a review of the literature. Acta Oncol 1990; 29: 946–9.

107. Buchino JJ, Buchino JJ, Uhlenhuth ER. Large-cell calcifying Sertoli cell tumour. J Urol 1989; 141: 953–4.

108. Perez-Atayde AR, *et al*. Large-cell calcifying Sertoli cell tumour of the testis. An ultrastructural immunocytochemical and biochemical study. Cancer 1983; 51: 2287–92.

109. Plata C, *et al*. Large cell calcifying Sertoli cell tumour of the testis. Histopathology 1995; 26: 255–9.

110. Proppe KH, Scully RE. Large cell calcifying Sertoli cell tumor of the testis. Am J Clin Pathol 1980; 74: 607–19.

111. Waxman M, Damjanov I, Khapra, A, Landau SJ. Large cell calcifying Sertoli tumor of the testis. Light microscopic and ultrastructural study. Cancer 1984; 54: 1574–81.

112. Carney JA, Gordon H, Carpenter PC, Shenoy BV, Go LV. The complex of myxomas, spotty pigmentation and endocrine overactivity. Medicine (Baltimore) 1985; 64: 270–83.

113. Carney JA. The Carney complex (myxomas, spotty pigmentation, endocrine overactivity, and schwannomas). Dermatol Clin 1995; 13: 19–26.

114. Noszian IM, Balon R, Eitelberger FG, Schmid N. Bilateral testicular large-cell calcifying sertoli cell tumor and recurrent cardiac myxoma in a patient with Carney's complex. Pediatr Radiol 1995; 25: S236–7.

115. Horn T, Jao W, Keh PC. Large-cell calcifying Sertoli cell tumor of the testis: a case report with ultrastructural study. Ultrastruct Pathol 1983; 4: 359–64.

116. Proppe KH, Dickersin GR. Large cell calcifying Sertoli cell tumour of the testis. Light microscopic and ultrastructural study. Hum Pathol 1982; 13: 1109–14.

117. Emerson RE, Ulbright TM. Morphological approach to tumours of the testis and paratestis. J Clin Pathol 2007; 60(8): 866–80.

118. Kratzer SS, *et al*. Large cell calcifying Sertoli cell tumor of the testis: contrasting features of six malignant and six benign tumors and a review of the literature. Am J Surg Pathol 1997; 21: 1271–80.

119. Curling TB. Observations on cystic disease of the testicle. Medic Chir Trans 1853; 36; 449.

120. Feek JD, Hunter WC. Papillary carcinoma arising from rete testis. Arch Pathol 1945; 30; 399.

121. Schoen SS, Rush BF. Adenocarcinoma of the rete testis. J Urol 1959; 82: 356–63.

122. Sarma DP, Weillbaecher TG. Adenocarcinoma of the rete testis. J Surg Oncol 1985; 30: 67–71.

123. Menon PK, Vasudevarao, Sabhiki A, Kudesia S, Joshi DP, Mathur UB. A case of carcinoma rete testis: histomorphological, immunohistochemical and ultrastructural findings and review of literature. Indian J Cancer 2002; 39: 106–11.

124. Crisp-Lindgren N, Travers H, Wells MM, Cawley LP. Papillary adenocarcinoma of rete testis. Autopsy findings, histochemistry, immunohistochemistry, ultrastructure and clinical correlations. Am J Surg Pathol 1988; 12: 492–501.

125. Mrak RE, Husain MM, Schaefer RF. Ultrastructure of metastatic rete testis adenocarcinoma. Arch Pathol Lab Med 1990; 114: 84–8.

126. Dundon C. Carcinoma of the rete testis occurring ten years after orchidopexy. Br J Urol 1952; 24: 58–63.

127. Desberg T, Tanno V. Adenocarcinoma of the rete testis. J Urol 1964; 91: 87–9.

128. Mostofi FK, Price EB. *Tumors of the Male Genital System*. Washington DC: AFIP, 1973. pp.170–3.

129. Tong GX, *et al*. PAX8 and PAX2 immunostaining facilitates the diagnosis of primary epithelial neoplasms of the male genital tract. Am J Surg Pathol 2011; 35(10): 1473–83.

130. Amin MB. Selected other problematic testicular and paratesticular lesions: rete testis neoplasms and pseudotumors, mesothelial lesions and secondary tumors. Mod Pathol 2005; 18(Suppl 2): S131–45.

131. Sanchez-Chapado M, Angulo JC, Haas GP. Adenocarcinoma of the rete testis. Urology 1995; 46: 468–75.

132. Skailes GE, Menasce L, Banerjee SS, Shanks JH, Logue JP. Adenocarcinoma of the rete testis. Clin Oncol (R Coll Radiol) 1998; 10(6): 401–3.

133. Musser JE, Ernest AJ, Thibault GP, McMann LP. Primary adenocarcinoma of the rete testis: improved staging accuracy with CT-PET. Urology 2011; 77(2): 334.

134. Schapira HE, Engel M. Adenocarcinoma of rete testis. NY State J Med 1972; 72: 1283–5.

135. Stein JP, Freeman JA, Esrig D, Chandrasoma PT, Skinner DG. Papillary adenocarcinoma of the rete testis: a case report and review of the literature. Urology 1994; 44(4): 588–94.

136. Burns MW, Chandler WL, Krieger JN. Adenocarcinoma of rete testis. Role of inguinal orchiectomy plus retroperitoneal lymph node dissection. Urology 1991; 37(6): 571–3.

137. Farhat F, Culine S, Terrier-Lacombe MJ, Droz JP. [Adenocarcinoma of rete testis. Apropos of a case and review of the literature]. Bull Cancer 1995; 82(2): 167–72.

138. Orozco RE, Murphy WM. Carcinoma of the rete testis: case report and review of the literature. J Urol 1993; 150: 974–7.

139. Winter CC, Puente E, Lai DY, Sharma HM. Papillary carcinoma of rete testis. Urology 1981; 18(2): 168–70.

140. Roy JB, Boumann WE, Lewis TM, Fahmy A, Pitha, J. Adenocarcinoma of rete testis. J Urol 1979; 14: 270–2.

141. Whitehead ED, Valensi QJ, Brown JS. Adenocarcinoma of the rete testis. J Urol 1972; 107: 992–99.

142. Smith JJ, Malone MJ, Geffin J, Silverman ML, Libertino JA. Retroperitoneal lymph node dissection in malignant mesothelioma of tunica vaginalis testis. J Urol 1990; 144: 1242–3.

143. Barbera V, Rubino M. Papillary mesothelioma of the tunica vaginalis. Cancer 1957; 10: 183–9.

144. Antman K, Cohen S, Dimitrov NV, Green M, Muggia F. Malignant mesothelioma of the tunica vaginalis testis. J Clin Oncol 1984; 2: 447–51.

145. Antman KH, Osteen R, Sugarbaker DJ, Herman T, Weissman L, Corson J. Mesothelioma cancer. Princ Pract Oncol Updates 1989; 3: 1–16.

146. Serio G, Ceppi M, Fonte A, Martinazzi M. Malignant mesothelioma of the testicular tunica vaginalis. Eur Urol 1992; 21: 174–6.

147. Tischoff I, Neid M, Neumann V, Tannapfel A. Pathohistological diagnosis and differential diagnosis. Recent Results Cancer Res 2011; 189: 57–78.

148. Plas E, Riedl CR, Pfluger H. Malignant mesothelioma of the tunica vaginalis testis: review of the literature and assessment of prognostic parameters. Cancer 1998; 83: 2437–46.

149. Vianna NJ, Polan AK. Non-occupational exposure to asbestos and malignant mesothelioma in females. Lancet 1978; 1: 1061–3.

150. Lew F, Tsang P, Holland JF, Warner N, Selikoff IJ, Bekesi JG. High frequency of immune dysfunctions in asbestos workers and in patients with malignant mesothelioma. J Clin Immunol 1986; 6: 225–33.

151. Taguchi T, Jhanwar SC, Siegfried JM, Keller SM, Testa JR. Recurrent deletions of specific chromosomal sites in 1p, 3p, 6q, and 9p in human malignant mesothelioma. Cancer Res 1993; 53: 4349–55.

152. Cavazza A, et al. Post-irradiation malignant mesothelioma. Cancer 1996; 77: 1379–85.

153. Stenton SC. Asbestos, Simian virus 40 and malignant mesothelioma. Thorax 1997; 52(Suppl 3): S52–7.

154. Tyagi G, Munn CS, Kiser LC, Wetzner SM, Tarabulcy E. Malignant mesothelioma of tunica vaginalis testis. Urology 1989; 34: 102–4.

155. Bisceglia M, Dor DB, Carosi I, Vairo M, Pasquinelli G. Paratesticular mesothelioma. Report of a case with comprehensive review of literature. Adv Anat Pathol 2010; 17(1): 53–70.

156. Kannerstien M, Churg J. Histochemistry in the diagnosis of malignant mesothelioma. Ann Clin Lab Sci 1973; 3: 207–11.

157. Winstanley AM, Landon G, Berney D, Minhas S, Fisher C, Parkinson MC. The immunohistochemical profile of malignant mesotheliomas of the tunica vaginalis: a study of 20 cases. Am J Surg Pathol 2006; 30(1): 1–6.

158. Ehya H. Cytology of mesothelioma of the tunica vaginalis metastasis to the lung. Acta Cytol 1985; 29: 79–84.

159. Hai B, Yang Y, Xiao Y, Li B, Chen C. Diagnosis and prognosis of malignant mesothelioma of the tunica vaginalis testis. Can Urol Assoc J 2011; 8: 1–4.

160. Brimo F, Illei PB, Epstein JI. Mesothelioma of the tunica vaginalis: a series of eight cases with uncertain malignant potential. Mod Pathol 2010; 23(8): 1165–72.

161. Trpkov K, Barr R, Kulaga A, Yilmaz A. Mesothelioma of tunica vaginalis of "uncertain malignant potential" – an evolving concept: case report and review of the literature. Diagn Pathol 2011; 6: 78.

162. Aggarwal P, Sidana A, Mustafa S, Rodriguez R. Preoperative diagnosis of malignant mesothelioma of the tunica vaginalis using Doppler ultrasound. Urology 2010; 75(2): 251–2.

163. Prescott S, Taylor RE, Sclare G, Busuttil A. Malignant mesothelioma of the tunica vaginalis testis: a case report. J Urol 1988; 140: 623–4.

164. Schure PJ, van Dalen KC, Ruitenberg HM, van Dalen T. Mesothelioma of the tunica vaginalis testis: a rare malignancy mimicking more common inguino-scrotal masses. J Surg Oncol 2006; 94(2): 162–4.

165. Mah E, Bittar RG, Davis GA. Cerebral metastases in malignant mesothelioma: case report and literature review. J Clin Neurosci 2004; 11: 917–18.

166. Grove A, Jensen ML, Donna A. Mesotheliomas of the tunica vaginalis testis and hernial scs. Virchows Arch 1989; 415: 283–92.

167. Mak CW, Cheng TC, Chuang SS, Wu RH, Chou CK, Chang JM. Malignant mesothelioma of the tunica vaginalis testis. Br J Radiol 2004; 77: 780–1.

168. Gerbaudo VH, Mamede M, Trotman-Dickenson B, Hatabu H, Sugarbaker DJ. FDG PET/CT patterns of treatment failure of malignant pleural mesothelioma: relationship to histologic type, treatment algorithm, and survival. Eur J Nucl Med Mol Imaging 2011; 38(5): 810–21.

169. Arlen M, Grabstald H, Whitemore WF Jr. Malignant tumours of the spermatic cord. Cancer 1969; 23: 525–32.

170. Eimoto T, Inoue I. Malignant fibrous mesothelioma of the tunica vaginalis: a histologic and ultrastructural study. Cancer 1977; 39: 2059–66.

171. Kasdon EJ. Malignant mesothelioma of the tunica vaginalis propria testis: report of two cases. Cancer 1969; 23: 1144–50.

172. Kingston JE, McElwain TJ, Malpas JS. Childhood rhabdomyosarcoma: experience of the Children's Solid Tumour Group. Br J Cancer 1983; 48: 195–207.

173. Aisner J, Wiernik PH. Chemotherapy in the treatment of malignant mesothelioma. Semin Oncol 1981; 8: 335–43.

174. Van Meerbeeck JP, et al. Randomized phase III study of cisplatin with or without raltitrexed in patients with malignant pleural mesothelioma: an intergroup study of the European Organisation for Research and Treatment of Cancer Lung Cancer Group and the National Cancer Institute of Canada. J Clin Oncol 2005; 23(28): 6881–9.

175. Vogelzang NJ, et al. Phase III study of pemetrexed in combination with cisplatin versus cisplatin alone in patients with malignant pleural mesothelioma. J Clin Oncol 2003; 21(14): 2636–44.

176. Gowing NF. Paratesticular tumours of connective tissue and muscle. In: Pathology of the Testis. London: Blackwell Scientific Publications, 1976. p.36

177. Hirsch EF. Rhabdomyosarcoma of the spermatic cord. Am J Cancer 1934; 20: 398–403.

178. Tanimura H, Furata M. Rhabdomyosarcoma of the spermatic cord. Cancer 1968; 22: 1215–20.

179. Olive D, et al. Para-aortic lymphadenectomy is not necessary in the treatment of localised paratesticular rhabdomyosarcoma. Cancer 1984; 54: 1283–7.

180. Pappo AS, Shapiro DN, Crist WM. Rhabdomyosarcoma. Biology and treatment. Pediatr Clin North Am 1997; 44: 953–72.

181. Draper GJ, et al. Childhood Cancer in Britian 1953–1975: Incidence, Mortality and Survival. Studies in Medical and Population Subjects, Vol. 37. London: HMSO, 1982.

182. Young JL, Miller RW. Incidence of malignant tumours in US children. J Pediatr 1975; 86: 254–8.

183. Alexander F. Pure testicular rhabdomyosarcoma. Br J Cancer 1968; 22: 498–501.

184. Woodruss JM, Chernik NL, Smith MC, Millett WB, Foote FW Jr. Peripheral nerve tumors with rhabdomyosarcomatous differentiation (malignant Triton tumors). Cancer 1973; 32: 426.

185. Locatelli P. Formation de Membres Surnuméraires. CR Assoc 20e réunion Turin 1925; 279–82.

186. Birch JM, et al. Cancer in the families of children with soft tissue sarcoma. Cancer 1990; 66: 2239–48.

187. Ahmed HU, Arya M, Muneer A, Mustaq I, Sebire NJ. Testicular and paratesticular tumors in the prepubertal population. Lancet Oncol 2010; 11: 476–83.

188. Willis RA. *Pathology of Tumours*. London: Butterworth, 1948.

189. Ferrari A, *et al*. Paratesticular rhabdomyosarcoma: report from the Italian and German Cooperative Group. J Clin Oncol 2002; 20: 449–55.

190. Barr FG. Molecular genetics and pathogenesis of rhabdomyosarcoma. J Pediatr Hematol Oncol 1997; 19: 483–91.

191. Merlino G, Helman LJ. Rhabdomyosarcoma – working out the pathways. Oncogene 1999; 18: 5340–8.

192. Weber-Hall S, *et al*. Gains, losses, and amplification of genomic material in rhabdomyosarcoma analyzed by comparative genomic hybridization. Cancer Res 1996; 56: 3220–4.

193. Patton RB, Horn RC Jr. Rhabdomyosarcoma: clinical and pathological features and comparison with human fetal and embryonal skeletal muscle. Surgery 1962; 52: 572–84.

194. Porterfield JF, Zimmermann LE. Rhabdomyosarcoma of the orbit. A clinico pathological study of 55 cases. Virchows Arch [A] 1962; 335: 329–44.

195. Marsden HB. The pathology of soft-tissue sarcomas with emphasis on childhood tumours. In: D'Angio GJ, Evans AE (eds) *Bone Tumours and Soft Tissue Sarcomas*. London: Edward Arnold, 1985. pp.14–25.

196. Flamant F, Rodary CH, Voute PR, Otten J. Primary chemotherapy in the treatment of rhabdomyosarcoma in children: trial of the International Society of Paediatric Oncology SIOP preliminary results. Radiother Oncol 1985; 3: 187–293.

197. Gaiger AM, Soule EH, Newton WA. Pathology of rhabdomyosarcoma. Experience of the intergroup rhabdomyosarcoma study 1972-8. Natl Cancer Inst Monogr 1981; 56: 19–27.

198. Fisher C. The value of electron microscopy and immunohistochemistry in the diagnosis of soft tissue sarcomas: a study of 200 cases. Histopathology 1990; 16: 441–55.

199. Fisher C. *Diagnostic Pathology of Soft Tissue*. Salt Lake City, UT: Amirsys Publishing Inc, 2011.

200. Ghavimi F, Mandell L, Heller G, LaQuaglia M, Exelby P. Genitourinary rhabdomyosarcoma (RMS) in children: Memorial Sloan–Kettering Cancer Experience (Meeting Abstract). Med Pediatr Oncol 1989; 17: 308.

201. Hamilton CR, Pinkerton R, Horwich A. The management of paratesticular rhabdomyosarcoma. Clin Radiol 1989; 40: 314–17.

202. Lawrence WJ, *et al*. Lymphatic metastases with childhood rhabdomyosarcoma. A report from the Intergroup Rhabdomyosarcoma Study. Cancer 1987; 60: 910–15.

203. Loughlin KR, *et al*. Genitourinary rhabdomyosarcoma in children. Cancer 1989; 63: 1600–6.

204. Rodary C, *et al*. Prognostic factors in 281 children with non metastatic rhabdomyosarcoma (RMS) at disgnosis. Med Pediatr Oncol 1988; 16: 71–7.

205. Carli M, Grotto P, Cavazzana A, Perilongo G, Ninfo V. Prognostic significance of histology in childhood rhabdomyosarcoma (RMS): improved survival with a new histologic 'leiomyomatous' subtype (Meeting abstract). Proc Am Soc Clin Oncol 1990; 9: 1153.

206. LaQuaglia MP, *et al*. Mortality in pediatric paratesticular rhabdomyosarcoma: a multivariate analysis. J Urol 1989; 142: 473–8.

207. Stewart RJ, *et al*. Treatment of children with nonmetastatic paratesticular rhabdomyosarcoma: results of the Malignant Mesenchymal Tumors studies (MMT 84 and MMT 89) of the International Society of Pediatric Oncology. J Clin Oncol 2003; 21: 793–8.

208. Breneman JC, *et al*. Prognostic factors and clinical outcomes in children and adolescents with metastatic rhabdomyosarcoma – a report from the Intergroup Rhabdomyosarcoma Study IV. J Clin Oncol 2003; 21(1): 78–84.

209. Raney RB, *et al*. Paratesticular sarcoma in childhood and adolescence. A report from the intergroup rhabdomyosarcoma studies I and II, 1973–1983. Cancer 1987; 60: 2337–43.

210. Rodary C, *et al*. Prognostic factors in 951 nonmetastatic rhabdomyosarcoma in children: a report from the international rhabdomyosarcoma workshop. Med Pediatr Oncol 1991; 19: 85–95.

211. Spiesse B, Hermanek P, Scheibe O, Wagner G. pTNM classification of malignant tumours. In: Spiesse B, Hermanek P, Scheibe O, Wagner G (eds) *INM Atlas: Illustrated Guide to the TNM*. Berlin: Springer, 1982.

212. Maurer HM. The Intergroup Rhabdomyosarcoma Study: update, November 1978. Natl Cancer Inst Monogr 1981; 56: 61–8.

213. Dall'Igna P, *et al*. Primary transcrotal excision for paratesticular rhabdomyosarcoma: is hemiscrotectomy really mandatory? Cancer 2003; 97: 1981–4.

214. Malek RS, Utz DC, Farrow GM. Malignant tumours of the spermatic cord. Cancer 1972; 29: 1108–13.

215. Bisogno G, *et al*. Rhabdomyosarcoma in adolescents: a report from the AIEOP Soft Tissue Sarcoma Committee. Cancer 2012; 118: 821–7.

216. Tefft M, *et al*. Radiation to regional nodes for rhabdomyosarcoma of the genitourinary tract in children: is it necessary? Cancer 1980; 45: 3065–8.

217. Stevens MC, *et al*. Treatment of nonmetastatic rhabdomyosarcoma in childhood and adolescence: third study of the International Society of Paediatric Oncology – SIOP Malignant Mesenchymal Tumor 89. J Clin Oncol 2005; 23(12): 2618–28.

218. Donaldson SS, Anderson JR. Rhabdomyosarcoma: many similarities, a few philosophical differences. J Clin Oncol 2005; 23(12): 2586–7.

219. Heyn RM, Holland R, Newton WA, Tefft M, Breslow N, Hartmann JR. The role of combined chemotherapy in the treatment of rhabdomyosarcoma in children. Cancer 1974; 34: 2128–42.

220. Heyn RM. Late effects of therapy in rhabdomyosarcoma. Clin Oncol 1985; 4: 287–97.

221. Maurer HM, Moon T, Donaldson M. The Intergroup Rhabdomyosarcoma Study: a preliminary report. Cancer 1977; 40: 2015–26.

222. Crist WM, *et al*. Prognosis in children with rhabdomyosarcoma: a report of the intergroup rhabdomyosarcoma studies I and II. Intergroup Rhabdomyosarcoma Committee [see comments]. J Clin Oncol 1990; 8: 443–52.

223. Sultan I, Ferrari A. Selecting multimodal therapy for rhabdomyosarcoma. Expert Rev Anticancer Ther 2010; 10(8): 1285–301.

224. Di Tonno F, *et al*. Lessons from 52 patients with Leydig cell tumor of the testis: the GUONE (North-Eastern Uro-Oncological Group, Italy) experience. Urol Int 2009; 82(2): 152–7.

225. Read, G. Lymphomas of the testis – results of treatment 1960–1977. Clin Radiol 1981; 32: 687–92.

226. Crellin AM, Hudson BV, Bennett MH, Harland S, Hudson GV. Non-Hodgkin's lymphoma of the testis. Radiother Oncol 1993; 27: 99–106.

227. Zietman AL, Coen JJ, Ferry JA, Scully RE, Kaufman DS, McGovern FG. The management and outcome of stage IA(E) nonHodgkin's lymphoma of the testis. J Urol 1996; 155: 943–6.

228. Buskirk SJ, Evans RG, Banks PM, O'Connell MJ, Earle JD. Primary lymphoma of the testis. Int J Radiat Oncol Biol Phys 1982; 8: 1699–703.

229. Lawrence W Jr, Anderson JR, Gehan EA, Maurer H. Pretreatment TNM staging of childhood rhabdomyosarcoma: a report of the Intergroup Rhabdomyosarcoma Study Group. Children's Cancer Study Group. Pediatric Oncology Group. Cancer 1997; 80: 1165–70.

Section 2: Head and Neck Cancer

6 Uncommon Tumors of the Oral Cavity and Adjacent Structures

Voichita Bar-Ad,[1] **Madalina Tuluc,**[2] **David Cognetti,**[3] **and Rita Axelrod**[4]

[1] Department of Radiation Oncology, [2] Department of Pathology, Anatomy and Cell Biology, [3] Department of Otolaryngology-Head and Neck Surgery, [4] Department of Medical Oncology, Kimmel Cancer Center, Thomas Jefferson University, Philadelphia, PA, USA

Introduction

Head and neck cancer is the sixth most common malignancy worldwide.[1,2] Oral cavity cancer represents approximately 30% of head and neck region tumors and 3% of all cancers in the United States.[3] In the United States, oral cavity cancer is most commonly associated with tobacco and alcohol use.[1,4] However, recent data have demonstrated an increased incidence of oral tongue carcinoma in younger nonsmokers and nondrinkers.[1] The vast majority (about 95%) of oral cavity tumors is represented by squamous cell carcinomas[5,6] but a multitude of other pathological types may be diagnosed and are discussed in this chapter (Box 6.1).

Tumors involving the oral cavity mucosa

Verrucous carcinoma, an uncommon variant of squamous cell carcinoma

Verrucous carcinoma is a rare and distinct pathological and clinical variant of well-differentiated squamous cell carcinoma. It is commonly associated with the chronic use of tobacco or with the practice of chewing betel nut.[7] However, recent studies have revealed a potential role of human papillomavirus (HPV) in the development and progression of verrucous carcinoma.[8,9] Patients often present with extensive, slow-growing, white, warty lesions, resembling a cauliflower. Common sites of mucosal involvement are the buccal mucosa, mandibular alveolar ridge, gingiva, and tongue. The distinction of verrucous carcinoma from classic squamous cell carcinomas is made difficult by the extensive nature of these tumors, mimicking an invasive cancer.[10] Diagnosis can be difficult, at times requiring repeated biopsies. Cell kinetics of verrucous carcinoma may be more similar to those of normal epithelium than to those of classic squamous cell carcinoma. Mitotic figures are confined to the basal layer, unlike in invasive squamous cell carcinoma (Fig. 6.1).[11] Proliferative verrucous leukoplakia is considered to be a precursor of verrucous carcinoma.[12] Oral lesions that progress to verrucous carcinoma reveal DNA-aneuploidy on flow cytometry examination and maintain an abnormal aneuploid cell line during disease progression.[13]

Verrucous carcinoma tends to be locally aggressive. It has the potential to involve large surface areas of the oral cavity, but is unlikely to metastasize.[14] The complicated management of verrucous carcinoma is related to the persistent nature of this tumor and high risk of recurrence. Surgery has classically been the treatment of choice for these lesions. Neck dissection is typically not necessary for verrucous carcinoma given the rarity of nodal metastasis. The role of radiotherapy and chemotherapy remains controversial.[7,15]

Malignant melanoma

Malignant melanoma originates from the proliferation of melanocytes, which represent cells derived from the neural crest and constitute the melanin pigment in the basal layer of the epithelium. While most melanomas arise in the skin, they may also arise from mucosal membranes or other sites where neural crest cells migrate.[16] Although their function is not completely understood, the presence of melanocytes in the mucous membranes has been well established.[16,17]

Malignant melanoma of the oral cavity is a very uncommon tumor and accounts for only about 2% of all melanomas. The risk factors for mucosal malignant melanoma are not well defined.[17,18] Melanocytic nevi are thought to be precursors of oral cavity mucosal melanoma in only a small minority of cases.[17] When oral nevi occur, they are most frequently diagnosed on the palate; this is also the most common site of oral cavity mucosal melanoma.[17] The peak age for diagnosis of mucosal melanoma is between 65 and 79 years of age, on average two decades later than cutaneous melanomas.[17] These tumors may occur at any location in the oral cavity, but

Box 6.1 Uncommon tumors of the oral cavity and adjacent structures.

Tumors involving the oral cavity mucosa

- Verrucous carcinoma, an uncommon variant of squamous cell carcinoma
- Malignant melanoma

Tumors of the minor salivary glands

- Pleomorphic adenoma
- Mucoepidermoid carcinoma
- Adenoid cystic carcinoma
- Acinic cell carcinoma
- Carcinoma ex-pleomorphic adenoma
- Polymorphous low-grade adenocarcinoma
- Adenocarcinoma, not otherwise specified
- Undifferentiated carcinoma

Soft tissue sarcomas

- Malignant fibrous histiocytoma
- Angiosarcoma
- Synovial sarcoma
- Leiomyosarcoma
- Rhabdomyosarcoma

Tumors of the bone

- Central giant cell lesions of the jaw
- Chondrosarcoma
- Osteosarcoma
- Histiocytosis X

Odontogenic tumors

- Ameloblastoma
- Malignant ameloblastoma and ameloblastic carcinoma
- Odontogenic keratocyst
- Cementoblastoma

Other neoplasms

- Burkitt lymphoma
- Kaposi sarcoma

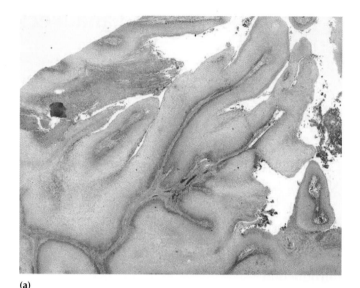

(a)

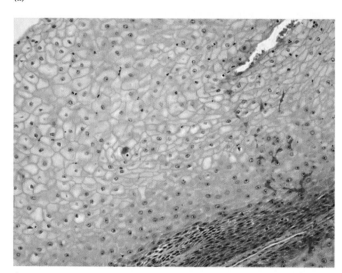

(b)

Figure 6.1 (a) Verrucous carcinoma (H&E, 40×). (b) Verrucous carcinoma (H&E, 200×).

they more commonly affect the hard palate and the maxillary alveolar mucosa.[16,17] The majority of mucosal malignant melanomas of the oral cavity appear as new lesions from apparently normal mucosa, whereas about one-third to half of the tumors are preceded by oral pigmentations for several months or years.[17]

Oral cavity malignant melanomas must be differentiated from other pigmented oral lesions, including physiological or racial pigmentation, amalgam tattoo, oral melanotic macule, melanocytic nevus, melanoacanthoma, Kaposi sarcoma, Peutz–Jeghers syndrome, Addison disease, and drug- or smoking-associated melanosis.[17,19] Oral amelanotic

melanoma is very rare, representing only about 10% of oral cavity mucosal melanomas.[17] The prognosis of amelanotic melanomas of the oral cavity is poorer than that of pigmented melanomas, in part due to delays in establishing the correct diagnosis and initiating treatment. Moreover, amelanotic forms are considered to be biologically more aggressive than pigmented melanomas. Histological examination together with immunostaining with S-100 antigen and more specific markers (HMB-45, Melan-A, antityrosinase) are the keys in the diagnosis of amelanotic melanoma (Fig. 6.2).[17,20,21]

Oral cavity malignant melanomas frequently remain asymptomatic as brown, dark blue or black macules and are usually diagnosed only when mucosal ulceration or bleeding is present.[17] The lack of early symptoms and the unusual locations in which they occur may explain the fact that the majority of primary mucosal melanomas are diagnosed at advanced stages.[17]

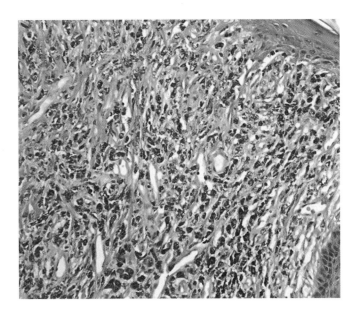

Figure 6.2 Malignant melanoma (H&E, 200×).

In contrast to cutaneous melanomas, the classification of mucosal melanoma in subtypes is controversial, and no correlation has been found between depth of invasion and outcome.[17,22] Mucosal melanomas may be histologically similar to cutaneous lentigo malignant melanoma in its radial growth phase. Once invasion occurs, however, oral cavity mucosal melanomas are very aggressive and can metastasize with vertical growth similar to superficial spreading cutaneous melanoma.[17] The American Joint Committee on Cancer (AJCC) has not published guidelines for the staging of oral malignant melanomas.[17]

The main treatment of localized, nonmetastatic mucosal malignant melanoma of the oral cavity is wide surgical excision.[22] Advances in surgical technique may allow more extensive resection and reconstruction.[23] However, the likelihood of local recurrence after resection is about 50%.[24] Postoperative radiotherapy has been used in patient with high-risk disease and has been shown to be associated with a reduced risk of locoregional failure. Postoperative radiotherapy probably does not improve overall survival, however. Disease-specific mortality is increased for advanced primary lesions and when regional lymph node metastases are present at the time of diagnosis.[22,24] Moreover, despite effective locoregional treatment, including surgical resection and postoperative radiotherapy, most patients with mucosal malignant melanoma die of distant metastases.[22] It remains unclear at the present time if chemotherapy and/or immunotherapy might help prevent distant metastases for these patients.[22,25,26] Mucosal malignant melanoma of the oral cavity is associated with a poorer prognosis than the cutaneous malignant melanomas.[17] Reported 5-year survival rates for primary mucosal melanomas range from approximately 15% to 50%.[17,23,24]

Early diagnosis and treatment are essential to improving the prognosis of oral cavity malignant melanoma.[23] The dental clinician must therefore thoroughly examine the oral cavity and any pigmented lesion that exhibits growth must be biopsied.

Moreover, the development of new, more effective systemic treatment to prevent distant metastases is urgently needed.

Tumors of the minor salivary glands

The salivary glands consist of three large, paired, major salivary glands (parotid, submandibular, and sublingual) and hundreds of minor salivary glands.[27] The minor salivary glands are widely distributed in the upper aerodigestive tract, palate, buccal mucosa, base of tongue, floor of mouth, gingiva, lips, paranasal sinuses, nasal cavity, pharynx, and trachea.[27] Salivary gland tumors represent less than 5% of head and neck malignancies and only 0.4% of all cancers in the United States.[27,28] The majority (88%) of minor salivary gland tumors are malignant, compared to only 25% of parotid tumors.[29,30]

Etiological factors associated with salivary gland tumors have not been defined clearly; cigarette smoking and exposure to irradiation have been described as potential risk factors.[31–34] Patients typically present with a painless lump. Local invasion is the initial route of spread of malignant salivary gland tumors, depending on the location and histological type. The incidence of nodal involvement depends on the stage of the primary tumor, tumor location, and histological type. Squamous cell carcinoma, undifferentiated cancer, and salivary duct cancer are associated with the greatest risk of nodal spread. An intermediate risk is associated with mucoepidermoid tumors. Acinic cell carcinoma, adenoid cystic carcinoma, and carcinoma ex-pleomorphic adenoma rarely spread to lymph nodes.[35,36] Distant metastases are found at presentation in about 3% of cases, and develop within 10 years of follow-up in 33% of cases. The most common sites of distant spread are the lung and bone.[37] Distant metastases are more frequently seen with adenoid cystic, salivary duct, squamous cell, and undifferentiated carcinomas.[29,38–41] A formal staging system has not been developed for minor salivary gland tumors.

In general, the management of malignant salivary gland tumors includes surgical resection followed by postoperative radiation therapy for unfavorable prognostic factors (locally advanced tumors with involvement of adjacent organs, close or positive surgical margins, bone involvement, perineural invasion, high-grade tumors, and recurrent disease).[37,42] The role of radiosensitizing chemotherapy remains controversial and is currently under study by cooperative groups (RTOG 1008/ NCT01220583) and others.[43] For patients at high risk of recurrence in this setting, we would consider radiosensitizing chemotherapy with cisplatin either as high dose 100 mg/m² every 3 weeks or as weekly therapy at a lower dose of 40 mg/m²/week, each for nonadenoid cystic carcinomas.

A number of molecular abnormalities have been identified in salivary gland cancers that may lead to more specific therapies in the future. In adenoid cystic cancer, a specific translocation, t(6:9)(q22–23;p23–24) has been identified.[44] The fusion product of the *myb* oncogene and transcription factor NF1B results in dysregulation of *myb* and downstream pathways involved in cell cycle control, angiogenesis and other pathways.[44] In mucoepidermoid cancer, a CRTC-MAML2 translocation has been identified. Interestingly, wild-type *CRTC* gene members are activators of cyclic AMP response proteins, linked to the regulation of glucose and fatty acid metabolism.[45–47] In adenocarcinomas and salivary duct tumors, a proportion of tumors may show presence of androgen and/or estrogen receptors.[48] Her 2 neu has been identified in a minority of cases. These receptors, when present, may be exploited for therapy, but there is no standard for this now. A recent study of lapatinib in salivary gland tumors for tumors expressing EGFR or erb b2 (Her 2 neu) did not show response, but did show tumor stabilization.[49]

In general, for salivary gland malignancies, chemotherapy can result in symptom improvement or response in metastatic disease, but does not lead to cure. Further, responses are not durable. Therefore, treatment is generally reserved for patients who have symptomatic and/or rapidly progressive disease. Patients with asymptomatic slowly growing lung metastases, for example, are best treated with observation and, in selected cases, resection. Locally recurrent disease is generally treated with re-resection where possible. Other agents used for squamous cell cancers of the head and neck, such as cisplatin, fluorouracil, vinorelbine and others, have shown activity.[50,51] Taxanes have demonstrated efficacy in mucoepidermoid or adenocarcinoma, but not in adenoid cystic cancers in a cooperative group series.[52] Despite the identification of new targets, treatment with small molecules has largely been disappointing, with stable disease and few minor responses seen.

Molecularly targeted therapies are intuitively promising, but clinical trials have not shown major responses. Improvements in progression-free survival have been noted.

Pleomorphic adenoma

Pleomorphic adenomas are the most common tumors of the major and minor salivary glands.[53,54] About 90% of the cases occur in the parotid gland, with only 10% of cases developing from the minor salivary glands (most commonly from the minor salivary glands of the palate, lips, and buccal mucosa).[54,55] Pleomorphic adenoma is diagnosed more frequently in women than in men, with a median age at the time of diagnosis of 43–46 years.[55,56] Pleomorphic adenoma usually presents as a region of slow-growing, painless, firm swelling, without ulceration or bleeding of the overlying mucosa.[55] Microscopically, the tumor does not have a true capsule, and the tumor has finger-like projections into the normal surrounding tissues, called pseudopodia.[29,57,58] Pleomorphic adenoma comprises both /epithelial and mesenchymal structures (Fig. 6.3).[55] It appears that there is no difference in clinical behavior of the tumor based on the proportion of these elements.[59] Recent studies have suggested that both epithelial and mesenchymal (myxoid, hyaline, chondroid, osseous) elements arise from the same cell clone, which may be a myoepithelial or ductal reserve cell.[59] A monoclonal cell pattern has been described in the stromal and epithelial elements in most cases.[59]

The mainstay of therapy for pleomorphic adenoma is surgical resection. Although classified as a benign tumor, pleomorphic adenoma carries a risk of local recurrence after initial surgery, that varies largely with surgical technique.[29] Changes in surgical approaches, with abandonment of enucleation,

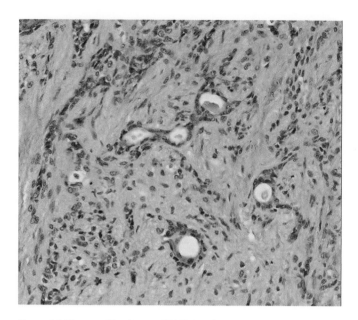

Figure 6.3 Pleomorphic adenoma (H&E, 200×).

have significantly reduced the recurrence rate from 20–40% to less than 4% in the last few decades.[60] Adequate resection typically involves wide local excision of the tumor and its surrounding pseudocapsule, along with the adjacent mucosa to achieve clear margins.[55,60] Recent studies have shown that cell proliferation activity, expression of progesterone and estrogen receptors, and MUC1/DF3 mucin glycoprotein may correlate with risk of tumor recurrence.[61,62] Furthermore, the potential for malignant transformation to carcinoma ex-pleomorphic adenoma has been reported in the literature.[29,54,63] Radiotherapy is generally not recommended, due to the typical patient's young age, benign histology, and the remote possibility of subsequent radiation-induced malignancy.[64]

Mucoepidermoid carcinoma

Mucoepidermoid carcinoma is the most common malignant tumor of the salivary glands.[65,66] When the tumor arises from the minor salivary glands, it is most commonly located on the palate, retromolar trigone, floor of mouth, buccal mucosa, lips and tongue.[65] Mucoepidermoid carcinoma is diagnosed more frequently in women than in men. The greatest incidence is between the third and the sixth decades of life, but it may be diagnosed at any age.[65,66] Mucoepidermoid carcinoma represents the most common malignant salivary gland tumor diagnosed in children and adolescents.[65–68]

The histopathological grading criteria for mucoepidermoid carcinoma remain controversial. Low-grade mucoepidermoid carcinomas, especially those arising in minor salivary glands, contain a prominent mucin-secreting component composed of columnar cells lining cystic spaces. The low-grade tumors are usually less than 4 cm in diameter, well circumscribed, and predominantly cystic. On microscopy, the majority of tumor cells are represented by well-differentiated epidermoid and mucus-producing cells with few mitoses (<3 mitoses per 10 high-power fields [HPF]) and minimal nuclear polymorphism (Fig. 6.4a). Intermediate-grade tumors are less cystic and show a predilection to form large, irregular nests or sheets of malignant cells (Fig. 6.4b). High-grade tumors, which are frequently larger than 4 cm in diameter, typically display an increased degree of atypia, areas of hemorrhage and necrosis, ill-defined margins, and numerous mitoses (>4 mitoses per 10 HPF)[65,69] (Fig. 6.4c). The proportion of proliferating tumor cells progressively increases with tumor grade, as demonstrated by the immunoreactivity of proliferating cell nuclear antigen (PCNA) and Ki-67 proliferation antigen.[65,67,70]

Surgical excision is the treatment of choice for all mucoepidermoid carcinomas.[68] Adequate tumor resection is essential in all grades of tumor. Recurrence rates of 50% have been reported in cases of positive surgical margins for low- and intermediate-risk tumors. This may increase to 80% for high-grade lesions that are resected with positive margins.[65,71] Postoperative radiotherapy is generally indicated for high-grade tumors and in cases with positive surgical margins in order to improve local control and possibly long-term survival.[66,72,73] Prognosis is related to histological grade, adequacy of surgical resection, and clinical staging. Low-grade mucoepidermoid carcinoma is associated with a high 5-year survival rate of 90–100%.[65,69] Intermediate- and high-risk mucoepidermoid carcinomas have a greater tendency to recur and metastasize and are associated with 10- and 15-year survival rates of about 40% and 33%, respectively.[65,656,74] Recent studies have demonstrated that the mucoepidermoid tumors positive for *p27* expression and CRTC1-MAML2 fusion are associated with favorable clinical and pathological features and long-term outcome.[41]

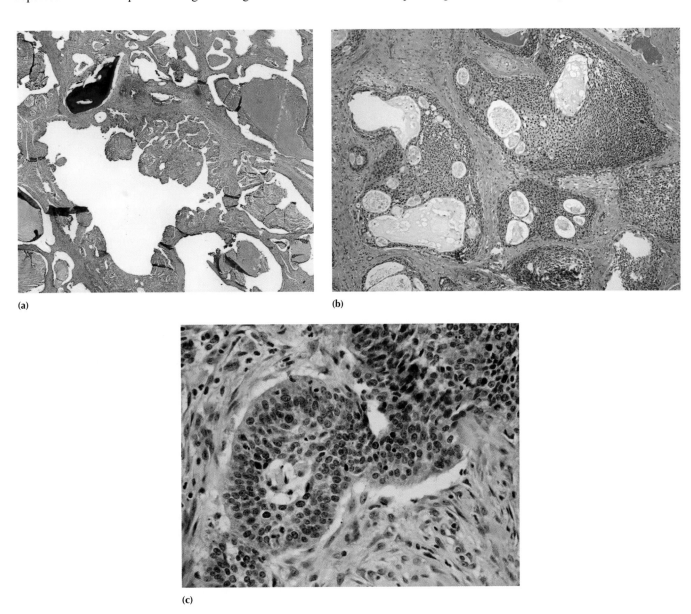

(a)

(b)

(c)

Figure 6.4 (a) Mucoepidermoid carcinoma, low grade (H&E, 40×). (b) Mucoepidermoid carcinoma, intermediate grade (H&E, 40×). (c) Mucoepidermoid carcinoma, high grade (H&E, 400×).

Adenoid cystic carcinoma

Adenoid cystic carcinoma is the most frequent minor salivary gland tumor, and it most commonly involves the palate.[30,37,40] A relatively equal gender distribution has been described.[75] This tumor occurs in adults in the fifth, sixth, and seventh decades[65] and is characterized by slow growth and a tendency to recur locally as well as to disseminate systemically, sometimes at very late stages in the course of disease.[29,37,40] Adenoid cystic carcinoma has a strong neurotropism, which represents a major route of tumor dissemination.[76] Perineural invasion of adenoid cystic carcinoma may be evaluated by computed tomography (CT), showing foramenal enlargement, as well as by magnetic resonance imaging (MRI).[77]

Growth pattern is characterized as cribriform, tubular, and solid[76] (Fig. 6.5). Recent studies have demonstrated a high incidence of loss of heterozygosity (LOH) at chromosome 6q23–35, which correlates with clinical and histological parameters in salivary gland adenoid cystic carcinoma.[78] Although several studies reported a favorable prognosis for the tubular and cribriform subtypes of adenoid cystic carcinoma compared with the solid variant, many authors question the prognostic significance of tumor grade and express the need for standardization using classification systems[79] (see Fig. 6.5). Perineural invasion has been identified as an unfavorable prognostic factor.[80–82]

Distant metastases are more frequent than regional lymph node involvement for adenoid cystic carcinoma.[76] Lung metastases prevail while other sites of distant spread may include bones, liver and brain.[83,84] Distant metastases seem to occur irrespective of the control of the primary tumor.[85,86] Sung *et al.* reported that half of the patients who developed distant metastases did not show evidence of locoregional failure.[86] Metastases from adenoid cystic carcinoma may remain asymptomatic for a long period of time. This is particularly true for pulmonary

metastases, which tend to progress very slowly.[84,86–88] Recent data show that expression of cysteine-rich protein 61 (Cyr61) appears to be significantly correlated with tumor angiogenesis and metastases in adenoid cystic carcinoma and may be an important target in antiangiogenetic therapy.[89]

Adenoid cystic carcinoma should be managed with a multidisciplinary approach. Surgical resection alone may be associated with high risk of local recurrence, and postoperative radiotherapy is often indicated.[76] When a named branch of a cranial nerve is involved by adenoid cystic carcinoma, the nerve pathways to the base of skull should be electively treated. When only focal perineural invasion of small unnamed nerves is present, the need for irradiation of the base of skull depends on the location of the primary tumor; for tumors of the palate or paranasal sinuses, the base of skull is included into the radiotherapy fields due to its proximity to the tumor bed.[90] Chemotherapy is not indicated in the initial local management of disease. The role of systemic chemotherapy for adenoid cystic carcinoma remains unclear.

The role of chemotherapy for metastatic adenoid cystic cancer overall remains controversial and clinical trial enrollment, where feasible, is preferred. Molecular and immunohistochemistry from the tumor may help to guide therapy, but this has not been validated in controlled trials.[91] Chemotherapy is reserved for patients with rapidly progressive systemic disease not amenable to local palliative radiation therapy or surgery. Tumors that overexpress ERCCI are less likely to respond to cisplatin-containing agents; tumors that overexpress RRM1 are less likely to respond to gemcitabine, and tumors with low levels of expression of TS are more likely to respond to agents such as fluorouracil or pemetrexed.[92–96] Regimens for otherwise unspecified salivary gland cancers often parallel those for other head and neck squamous cell cancers. Given cooperative group data, we would avoid taxanes for adenoid cystic cancers.[52] A regimen of cisplatin (50 mg/m^2) adriamycin (50 mg/m^2) and cyclophosphamide (500 mg/m^2) every 3 weeks has been used for metastatic salivary gland cancers[50] with responses in the range of 50% of patients and we have used this when clinical trials are not available. Other reasonable regimens may include cisplatin and vinorelbine.[51]

Acinic cell carcinoma

Acinic cell carcinoma is an uncommon malignant neoplasm of the salivary glands. The tumor commonly presents in the fifth decade of life and demonstrates bilateral involvement in approximately 3% of cases.[97] Acinic cell carcinoma represents the second most frequent salivary gland tumor diagnosed in children, after mucoepidermoid carcinoma.[98] The tumor is composed primarily of serous acinar cells (Fig. 6.6). A capsule may be present, and the tumor may have a multinodular appearance.[99] Cytogenetic alterations have been described in acinic cell carcinomas, including chromosome 6q rearrangement, loss of chromosome Y, and gains of chromosome 7 and 8.[100,101] The general management includes surgical resection followed by postoperative radiation therapy for unfavorable prognostic factors (locally advanced tumors with involvement of adjacent organs or close or positive surgical margins).[37,42]

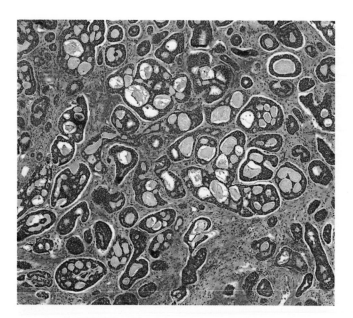

Figure 6.5 Adenoid cystic carcinoma, predominantly cribriform pattern (H&E, 40×).

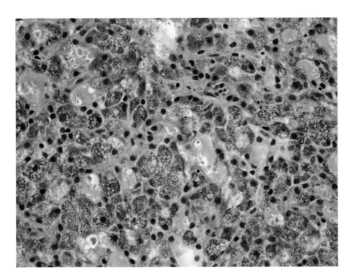

Figure 6.6 Acinic cell carcinoma (H&E, 200×).

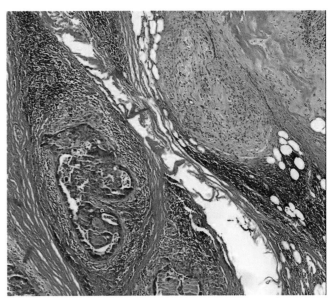

Figure 6.7 Carcinoma ex pleomorphic adenoma (H&E, 40×).

Carcinoma ex-pleomorphic adenoma

Carcinoma ex-pleomorphic adenoma is defined as a carcinoma arising from a benign pleomorphic adenoma. The disease is uncommon, representing only about 12% of all malignant salivary gland neoplasms.[102] The tumor is diagnosed most commonly in the sixth to eighth decades of life and is slightly more frequent in women.[102] Carcinoma ex-pleomorphic adenoma is considered a malignant transformation within a primary or recurrent pleomorphic adenoma.[103] In published series, 20–25% of the patients diagnosed with carcinoma ex-pleomorphic adenoma have a previously treated pleomorphic adenoma.[104,105]

The development of carcinoma ex-pleomorphic adenoma seems to follow a multistep model. Based on the presence and extent of invasion of the carcinomatous component outside the capsule, carcinoma ex-pleomorphic adenoma can be subdivided into three categories: noninvasive (known as intracapsular carcinoma ex-pleomorphic adenoma), minimally invasive (<1.5 mm penetration into the extracapsular tissue) and invasive (greater than 1.5 mm invasion by the malignant component from the tumor capsule into the adjacent organs)[106,107] (Fig. 6.7). Patients with noninvasive or minimally invasive tumors have a better prognosis than patients with invasive carcinoma ex-pleomorphic adenoma. Furthermore, tumor size, tumor grade, and completeness of tumor resection have been shown to be prognostic indicators in patients diagnosed with carcinoma ex-pleomorphic adenoma.[107]

Treatment of carcinoma ex-pleomorphic adenoma involves surgical resection and neck dissection (in cases of cervical nodal involvement).[102] Postoperative radiotherapy is used for patients with high-grade disease, positive surgical margins, perineural invasion, or lymph node involvement.[108] Patients may also be offered the option of postoperative combined chemoradiotherapy, although there are limited published data on the effectiveness of chemotherapy in the management of this lesion.[104,108]

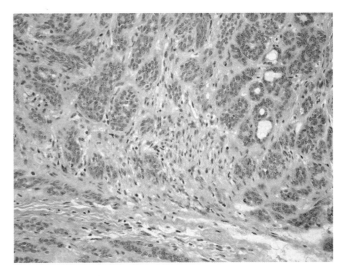

Figure 6.8 Polymorphous low-grade adenocarcinoma (H&E, 200×).

Polymorphous low-grade adenocarcinoma

Polymorphous low-grade adenocarcinoma (PLGA) is a generally slow-growing neoplasm with low metastatic potential that almost always arises in the minor salivary glands of the palate and buccal mucosa.[109,110] A typical finding is the presence of concentric whorls, creating target-like (onion skin-like) patterns, reminiscent of lobular carcinoma of the breast. The histological appearance varies and can include solid, trabecular, tubular, papillary, and cribriform patterns.[101] Invasion of adjacent organs and perineural and vascular invasion are common.[109,110] Although the heterogeneous morphological features of PLGA are somewhat distinct, difficulty with diagnosis may arise due to morphological overlap with other primary salivary neoplasms, especially adenoid cystic carcinoma; shared histological features include ill-defined borders, solid and cribriform growth patterns, and neurotropism[111] (Fig. 6.8).

Immunohistochemical markers may be helpful in differentiating PLGA from adenoid cystic carcinoma, particularly carcinoembryonic antigen (CEA), vimentin, smooth muscle actin (SMA), c-kit and Ki-67.[75,111,112] The distinction between PLGA and adenoid cystic carcinoma is essential for appropriate management and follow-up. Despite its infiltrative growth pattern and neurotropism, the overall prognosis of PLGA remains favorable, with low recurrence rates and excellent prognosis following complete tumor excision.[111]

Soft tissue sarcomas

Soft tissue sarcomas represent only 1% of all malignancies and 1% of all head and neck malignant tumors.[113] There is a variable male predominance with a median age at the time of diagnosis of 50–55 years.[114] A small proportion of head and neck soft tissue sarcoma (3%) occurs in areas that have been previously irradiated.[114,115] Most patients present with a painless mass.[116,117] The head and neck soft tissue sarcomas occur most frequently in the scalp, face and neck areas and very uncommonly in the oral cavity, larynx or pharynx.[114] The histologies of head and neck soft tissue sarcomas are represented by malignant fibrous histiocytoma, angiosarcoma, rhabdomyosarcoma, malignant schwannoma and malignant peripheral nerve sheath tumors, dermatofibrosarcoma protuberans, fibrosarcoma, leiomyosarcoma, synovial sarcoma, liposarcoma, and desmoid tumors.[114] Desmoid tumors, also called aggressive fibromatosis, are locally aggressive benign tumors with a favorable prognosis.[118] Dermatofibrosarcoma protuberans is a low-grade cutaneous lesion with a favorable prognosis, although it rarely may metastasize.[119] However, most head and neck soft tissue sarcomas are high-grade tumors.[114] The rate of lymph node metastasis is generally very low, and the risk of distant metastases is related to histological type, tumor grade, and tumor size.[114,118,120] The most common site of distant metastases is the lung.[114]

Management of sarcomas of the head and neck area is similar to that of other areas. Radical resection is the optimal treatment. However, it is usually not feasible to achieve a complete compartmental resection for head and neck soft tissue sarcomas. Therefore, recurrence rates after wide local excision for high-grade head and neck soft tissue sarcomas may be as high as 50%.[114,121] Postoperative radiation therapy is indicated for patients with low-grade soft tissue sarcomas with close (<1 cm) or positive margins and patients with high-grade tumors.[114] The reported local control rates after surgery alone or surgery combined with postoperative radiotherapy are between 60% and 70% and are influenced by the tumor grade, tumor size, and margins status.[114] Distant metastases develop in 10–30% of head and neck soft tissue sarcoma patients.[114] Five-year overall survival rates are between 60% and 70% and vary with age, histological grade, invasion of deep structures, and adequacy of surgical resection.[114]

The role of adjuvant chemotherapy is not clearly defined. Taxanes have been shown to be uniquely effective in angiosarcomas.[122] For marginally resectable disease, neoadjuvant therapy can be used appropriate to the tumor type. The body of experience in head and neck sarcomas is not as large as

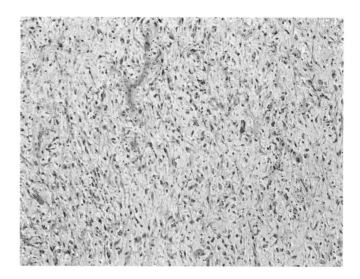

Figure 6.9 Malignant fibrous hystiocytoma (H&E, 40×).

with extremity sarcomas. However, positron emission tomography-computed tomography (PET-CT) has been used in some series to gauge response to chemotherapy.[123]

Malignant fibrous histiocytoma

Malignant fibrous histiocytoma represents the most common soft tissue sarcoma of the head and neck region[124] and seems to be the most frequent sarcoma diagnosed in patients with prior radiation exposure in the head and neck areas.[125,126] Radiation-induced malignant fibrous histiocytoma of the head and neck region appears to be associated with a particularly poor prognosis.[127] Most malignant fibrous histiocytomas are considered high grade (Fig. 6.9). Nodal metastases are extremely rare, but distant metastases are common.[125] Surgical resection is the primary therapy for head and neck malignant fibrous histiocytoma. However, given the high rates of local recurrence (86% after marginal resection, 66% after wide local excision, and 27% after radical resection), adjuvant radiation therapy should be considered.[125,128] The role of adjuvant chemotherapy for head and neck malignant fibrous histiocytoma remains undefined. The 5-year overall survival for patients with head and neck malignant fibrous histiocytoma (48%) has been reported to be much lower than for patients with malignant fibrous histiocytoma arising in the trunk or extremities (77%).[128]

Angiosarcoma

Head and neck angiosarcoma most commonly presents as a purple scalp lesion in elderly white men.[129] Angiosarcoma of the oral cavity is extremely rare[130] (Fig. 6.10). Angiosarcoma has a significantly worse prognosis when compared to other soft tissue sarcomas.[131,132] These tumors are aggressive and tend to recur locally and to metastasize early despite multimodality treatment, including surgery and postoperative radiation therapy. Complete resection is often challenging due to multifocal disease involvement.[129] Results with surgery alone

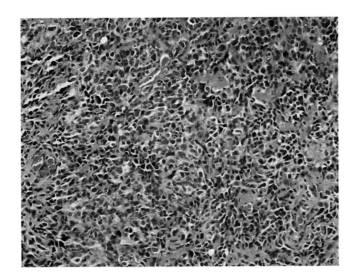

Figure 6.10 Angiosarcoma (H&E, 200×).

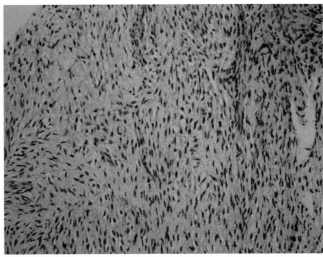

Figure 6.11 Synovial sarcoma, monophasic type (H&E, 200×).

have been disappointing due to a high rate of local recurrence.[129] Some series have suggested that combined modality treatment offers the best prognosis; extensive surgery followed by postoperative radiation therapy is considered optimal, but the effect of chemotherapy is uncertain.[129,133,134] The 5-year overall survival reported in the literature is very poor, ranging between 10% and 20%.[129,130,133]

Synovial sarcoma

Synovial sarcoma is a high-grade histological variant of sarcoma. The tumor is rarely found in the head and neck area (the most common sites being hypopharynx and parapharyngeal spaces).[135–137] Synovial sarcoma is the fourth most frequent variety of sarcoma following malignant fibrous histiocytoma, liposarcoma, and rhabdomyosarcoma.[138] Two subtypes of synovial sarcoma have been described in the literature: monophasic (containing only spindle cells) and biphasic (containing spindle and epithelioid cells). The biphasic subtype appears to be more common and is generally considered more aggressive than the monophasic subtype[135,139] (Fig. 6.11). The characteristic translocation present in 99% of the cases is represented by t(X;18). Finding this translocation is important for confirming the diagnosis of synovial sarcoma, especially for the monophasic subtype, where the differential diagnosis includes other spindle cell tumors such as hemangiopericytoma, fibrosarcoma, leiomyosarcoma, malignant schwannoma, and malignant peripheral nerve sheath tumors.[135,140] Overall and disease-free survival rates reported in the recent literature for head and neck synovial sarcoma vary from approximately 45% to 50%.[141]

Treatment for synovial sarcomas follows a multimodality approach including surgical resection, postoperative radiotherapy and systemic treatment.[135] Postoperative radiation therapy has been shown to improve prognosis for head and neck synovial sarcoma.[135,141,142] Ifosfamide-based chemotherapy has been investigated, especially for tumors in the hypopharynx and larynx sites, where a complete surgical resection is

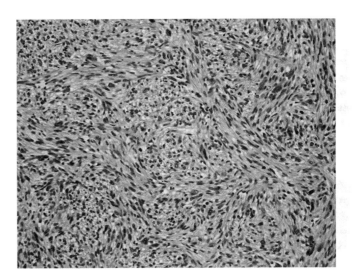

Figure 6.12 Leiomyosarcoma (H&E, 200×).

sometimes not feasible.[135,137,143] Recent data have suggested the likely role of epidermal growth factor receptor (EGFR) and human epithelial growth factor receptor 2 (Her 2 neu) in the carcinogenesis of synovial sarcoma, thus suggesting that the anti-EGFR monoclonal antibody may play a therapeutic role in the treatment of synovial sarcomas.[135,144,145]

Leiomyosarcoma

Leiomyosarcoma of the oral cavity is very rare, representing only 3–10% of leiomyosaromas arising in the head and neck region.[146,147] They represent mesenchymal tumors that exhibit smooth muscle differentiation[146] (Fig. 6.12). The peak incidence occurs between the fifth and seventh decades of life. The patients present with a slowly growing nodule that infiltrates adjacent tissues.[146] Nodal metastases rate was reported in 15% of the cases. Distant metastases occur in 39% of the cases, most frequently in the lung.[148]

The main treatment of oral cavity leiomyosarcoma is wide surgical resection with histologically proven negative surgical margins. However, complete surgical removal of oral leiomyosarcoma may be difficult and the recurrence rate reported in some series is 36%.[148] The reported disease-free survival at 5 years is only 23%.[148] Postoperative radiation therapy may be used[136] although some authors question its utility.[146] The role of chemotherapy is not yet defined.[146]

Rhabdomyosarcoma

Rhabdomyosarcoma is a rare tumor in adults, accounting for only 2–5% of tumors in the head and neck region. On the other hand, it represents approximately 60% of head and neck tumors in children.[149] The most frequent site of rhabdomyosarcoma is in fact the head and neck region, with the orbit being the single most common site. Rhabdomyosarcoma of the oral cavity is very uncommon, representing only 10–12% of all head and neck cases.[149] Oral cavity rhabdomyosarcoma is a nonparameningeal rhabdomyosarcoma. The most common subsites of involvement for the oral cavity rhabdomyosarcoma are tongue, soft palate, hard palate, and buccal mucosa.[149,150] Four subtypes have been described based on histological findings: embryonal rhabdomyosarcoma, alveolar rhabdomyosarcoma, botryoid and spindle cell rhabdomyosarcoma, and undifferentiated botryoid and spindle cell rhabdomyosarcoma[149,151,152] (Fig. 6.13).

Surgical resection is generally difficult for head and neck rhabdomyosarcomas due to the location of parameningeal rhabdomyosarcoma and involvement of adjacent critical structures.[149] A multimodality treatment approach, including chemotherapy, surgery, and radiotherapy, has been shown to improve survival rates for rhabdomyosarcoma over the last few decades.[149,153–155]

Tumors of the bone

Central giant cell lesions of the jaw

The term "giant cell lesion" is currently used to describe the entire spectrum of lesions formerly known as "giant cell reparative granuloma." "Giant cell reparative granuloma" comprises lesions with similar histological features, rich in giant cells but with a wide variety of clinical behavior.[156] At one end of the spectrum, there are small lesions, discovered incidentally, with no aggressive features. At the other end, there are large, multilocular lesions with evidence of aggressive behavior, including rapid growth, root resorption, pain, paresthesia, and increased recurrence rate. The indolent type of central giant cell lesion (CGCL) may be "reactive" (some of them are associated with tooth extraction or implants), but in aggressive lesions, a genetic abnormality is likely to play a role. Whether the two ends of this spectrum represent two different disease entities, one reactive and one neoplastic,[156] is currently not clear. The noncommittal term "central giant cell lesion" is therefore favored.

The nonaggressive and the aggressive lesions show similar histology, with a variable osteoclastic giant cell population embedded in a richly vascularized stroma, spindle-shaped mesenchymal cells, and round monocyte-macrophages. Giant cells vary in number from very few to many and they may be aggregated focally or present diffusely throughout the lesion. Mitoses are common but they are not atypical (Fig. 6.14). Correlation of histological features with clinical behavior is debatable; aggressiveness is clinical and radiographically determined. CGCL is histologically identical to the brown tumor of hyperparathyroidism. Therefore, in all patients with CGCL, especially patients with multiple giant cell lesions, evaluation of serum calcium and parathyroid hormone levels is necessary.

Central giant cell lesions may arise sporadically or in association with cherubism, Noonan syndrome, Jaffe–Campanacci syndrome, neurofibromatosis type 1 or Ramon syndrome. In most cases of cherubism, the lesions tend to regress after puberty with resolution of the facial deformities. In some patients, varying degrees of facial alterations can persist. Given the natural history of the disease with involution after puberty, there is no right answer to the question of whether to treat or simply observe patients; the optimal therapy for cherubism has not been determined.

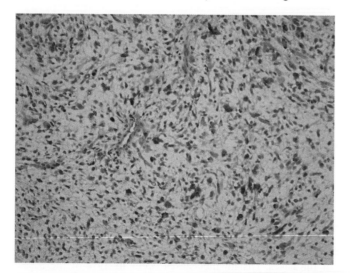

Figure 6.13 Rhabdomyosarcoma, botryoid type (H&E, 200×).

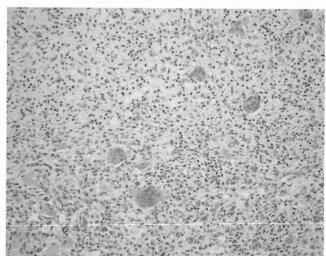

Figure 6.14 Central giant cell lesion (H&E, 200×).

Sporadic CGCL occurs in young patients, twice as often in the mandible as in the maxilla. Women are affected more frequently than men, especially in high estrogen states such as pregnancy. Most CGCL are asymptomatic and are discovered incidentally during dental radiological examination. A small number of cases manifest clinically with pain, paresthesia, or perforation of the cortical bone plate. Radiographically, CGCL presents as a well-delineated radiolucent lesion. While most small lesions are unilocular, the majority of the large lesions are multilocular and expansile, with a radiographical appearance resembling ameloblastoma. Root resorption and displacement of the teeth may be observed.

Central giant cell lesions are treated by curettage, and the recurrence rate varies from 11% to 50% or more. Alternative therapeutic options in patients with aggressive tumors are represented by calcitonin, corticosteroids and interferon-α2. All three therapeutic options have been proven effective in controlling recurrences, but they require months before regression is seen. Radiation therapy and chemotherapeutic agents such as methotrexate, doxorubicin, and cyclophosphamide have also been employed.

Chondrosarcoma

Chondrosarcoma of the jaw and facial bones is very uncommon, comprising only 0.1% of all head and neck malignancies.[156] Because of similar histological features, chondroblastic osteosarcoma may be misdiagnosed as chondrosarcoma, especially considering that chondroid differentiation in osteosarcoma of the jaw is more common than in osteosarcoma of long bones. The most common location in the craniofacial bones is the maxilla; less common locations include the mandible, nasal septum, and paranasal sinuses. A significant proportion of head and neck chondrosarcomas arise from the cartilaginous components of the larynx. Patients with gnathic chondrosarcomas, especially the mesenchymal variant, are usually younger than those with extragnathic involvement, and no sex or race predilection has been identified. The most common clinical symptom is bony expansion with secondary malocclusion and loosening of the teeth. Pain tends to be an unusual complaint. Chondrosarcomas arising in the nasal cavity or maxillary sinus present with nasal obstruction, congestion, and epistaxis.

Radiographically, chondrosarcomas present as radiolucent lesions with poorly defined borders. Spotty calcifications with a ring-like pattern are specific for chondrosarcomas but are present only in tumors that exhibit significant calcifications. Frequently chondrosarcomas permeate bony trabeculae of the preexisting bone, making it difficult to determine the exact extent of the tumor. When teeth are involved, root resorption or symmetrical widening of the periodontal ligament is also noted.

Histologically, chondrosarcomas are tumors composed of cartilage with various degrees of cellularity and maturation. There are three histological grades of chondrosarcoma that correlate well with the prognosis. The great majority of gnathic tumors are grade 1 chondrosarcomas. They are composed of chondroid matrix with increased cellularity and

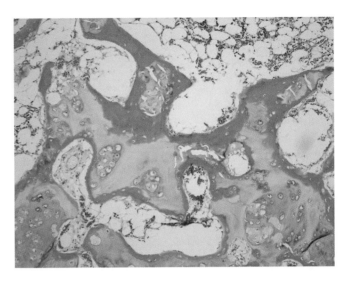

Figure 6.15 Chondrosarcoma, low grade (H&E, 200×).

scattered atypical nuclei or binucleated cells (Fig. 6.15). Grade 2 tumors show increased cellularity, especially at the periphery of the lobules, greater nuclear atypia, and low mitotic rate. Prominent myxoid areas are present in the cartilaginous matrix. Grade 3 tumors are highly cellular, pleomorphic, demonstrate increased mitotic activity, and may show spindle cell transformation. There is minimal cartilaginous matrix, and liquefaction necrosis may be present.[156,157]

One of the unusual variants of chondrosarcoma, the mesenchymal chondrosarcoma, deserves special discussion because it involves predominantly the jaw bones. This tumor occurs in a younger patient population, during the second and third decades of life, and histologically it presents as a bimorphic tumor composed of islands of well-differentiated cartilage juxtaposed with small, round cell undifferentiated malignancy with a hemangiopericytoma-like arrangement. Surgical treatment with *en bloc* resection with 2–3 cm margins is the recommended treatment for chondrosarcoma. Because wide and clear surgical margins can be difficult to achieve in the head and neck area, the location of the tumor becomes one of the most important prognostic factors. Tumor grade has also prognostic value; the risk of distant metastases increases with grade. Grade 1 tumors rarely, if ever, metastasize, while the metastatic rate for grade 3 tumors reaches 70%. Mesenchymal chondrosarcoma has a worse prognosis, with lower 5- and 10-year survival compared to conventional chondrosarcomas. Radiation and chemotherapy are less effective and are used primarily for unresectable tumors.[156]

Osteosarcoma

Gnathic osteosarcoma is a malignant mesenchymal neoplasm in which the cellular stroma of the tumor directly produces osteoid and may also produce variable amounts of cartilaginous matrix. The etiology is unknown, but most osteosarcomas contain clonal chromosomal aberrations. While most osteosarcomas arise *de novo*, some arise post

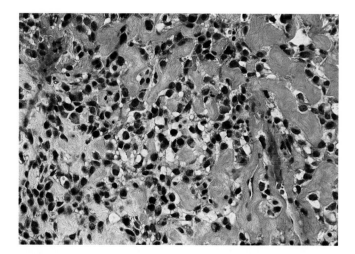

Figure 6.16 Osteosarcoma, osteoblastic type (H&E, 200×).

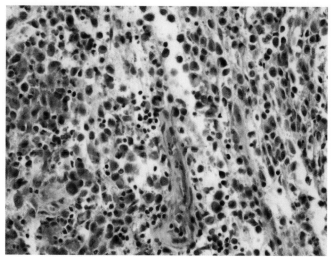

Figure 6.17 Langerhans cell histiocytosis (H&E, 200×).

radiation therapy, in Paget disease, or in preexisting benign osseous tumors.[158] Gnathic osteosarcomas have a slight male predominance, and most patients are in the third and fourth decades of life at the time of diagnosis. The maxilla and mandible are affected with equal frequency, and patients usually present with swelling and pain.

Radiographically, osteosarcomas vary from a dense, sclerotic lesion to mixed sclerotic to radiolucent lesion. Tumors involving teeth may cause root resorption and symmetrical widening of the periodontal ligament that results from tumor infiltration along the periodontal space. CT scans are invaluable in evaluating tumor extent, tumoral calcifications, and soft tissue involvement.[159] Histologically, the hallmark of osteosarcoma is production of osteoid by malignant tumor cells. There is a great deal of variability in respect to stromal cellularity, degree of cytological atypia, mitotic activity, and the amount of matrix material produced in the tumor. Several histological subtypes have been described, based mainly on the type and amount of stroma produced in the tumor (osteoblastic, chondroblastic, fibroblastic)[156] (Fig. 6.16). These subtypes, however, do not have any prognostic or therapeutic significance.

Most gnathic osteosarcomas are low-grade tumors so prognosis in patients with jaw osteosarcoma is better than in patients with tumors of the long bones. Treatment consists of wide surgical excision with neoadjuvant or postsurgical chemotherapy with a variety of agents. Most protocols involve neoadjuvant chemotherapy, followed by surgical excision with pathological examination of the resected specimen to appreciate the effect of chemotherapy on the tumor. One of the most important prognostic factors is the ability to achieve complete surgical excision. Local recurrence with uncontrolled local disease more often causes death than distant metastases for head and neck osteosarcomas. Therefore, postoperative radiation therapy has been employed in order to reduce local recurrence rates.[160,161] Distant metastases are less common in gnathic osteosarcoma than in osteosarcoma of the long bones. The most commonly affected sites are the lungs and the brain.

Langerhans cell histiocytosis

Langerhans cell histiocytosis (LCH) includes a group of diseases of unknown etiology that have in common abnormal proliferation of bone marrow-derived histiocytes (Langerhans cells). The spectrum of Langerhans cell histiocytosis includes three classic entities: eosinophilic granuloma (localized chronic form), Hand–Schuller–Christian disease (disseminated chronic form) and Letterer–Siwe disease (disseminated acute form).[157] Due to overlapping clinical features, it is often difficult to categorize patients into one of these three subtypes.

The pathogenesis of Langerhans cell histiocytosis is unknown and proposed hypotheses include dysfunction of the immune system with hypersensitivity reaction to an unknown antigen with stimulation of the histiocytic-macrophage system, deficiency of T suppressor cells, and altered immunoglobulins. An inflammatory origin is suspected due to the microscopic characteristics and clinical evolution of the disease but so far, none of the proposed pathogenic mechanisms has been proven.

The disease can be localized or disseminated with multiorgan involvement. Children are affected more often than the adults; more than 50% of cases occur in patients younger than 15 years old. The head and neck are frequently involved in LCH, usually with bone involvement (skull, jaws). Patients present clinically with pain and tenderness secondary to bone involvement accompanied by ulcerative or proliferative mucosal lesions, if the lesion breaks out of bone. Patients can present with otitis media in cases with temporal bone involvement. In rare cases, ulcerated oral mucosal lesions can occur in the absence of bone lesions. Mucosal lesions can be associated with cervical lymphadenopathy, which is a reflection of histiocytic infiltration. Lesions in the body of maxilla or mandible can mimic a periapical inflammatory condition.

Radiographically, osseous involvement by Langerhans cell histiocytosis produces sharply punched-out, radiolucent lesions. Confirmation of diagnosis requires microscopic examination and identification of the lesional Langerhans cells. These are enlarged, pale-staining mononuclear cells with indented, lobated, or folded ("coffee bean") nuclei. Langerhans cells demonstrate reactivity with CD1a and CD207 antibodies. An increased number of eosinophils is present in the background (Fig. 6.17).

Localized disease to the head and neck area requires conservative surgical treatment. Low doses of radiation therapy are used for less accessible bone lesions. For chronic disseminated disease, the ideal treatment has yet to be established. Good response is usually achieved with single-agent chemotherapy using prednisolone, etoposide, vincristine or cyclosporine.[145] A combination of prednisone and vincristine seems to reduce the risk of recurrence. Visceral involvement and very young age at diagnosis have a negative effect on survival.

Odontogenic tumors

Ameloblastoma

With an incidence that equals the combined frequency of all other odontogenic tumors, ameloblastoma is the most common clinically significant gnathic tumor. It is a benign, slow-growing, and locally aggressive tumor with a significant risk of local recurrence. Ameloblastoma arises from the enamel organ or its progenitor cell lines, from the epithelial lining of an odontogenic cyst, from the basal cells of the oral mucosa, or from rests of dental lamina.[156,157] Eighty percent of ameloblastomas are located in the mandible (two-thirds in the posterior mandible), where they usually develop at the site of an impacted tooth. In 20% of patients, ameloblastomas develop in the maxilla. Maxillary ameloblastomas can invade the maxillary sinus and present clinically as sinonasal tumors. Conventional (multicystic) ameloblastoma is prevalent during the third to the seventh decades of life, with no gender or racial predilection. Unicystic ameloblastoma occurs in a younger population, with 50% of tumors diagnosed in the second decade of life. Peripheral ameloblastoma is the least common of the three and probably arises from dental lamina rests. It is located in the gingival or alveolar soft tissue.

Ameloblastomas usually present as variably sized painless jaw swellings or, in cases of peripheral tumors, as a painless sessile or pedunculated gingival lesion. Most small ameloblastomas are asymptomatic, and they are detected during dental radiological examination. The most typical radiographic feature is a uni- or multilocular radiolucent lesion with scalloped borders ("honeycomb" or "soap bubble" appearance). Frequently, there is associated cortical bone expansion, resorption of the adjacent teeth roots, and an unerupted tooth. Although in the multicystic type, the radiological characteristics are highly suggestive of ameloblastoma, numerous other odontogenic and nonodontogenic lesions may show similar features and should be included in the differential diagnosis (odontogenic keratocyst, central giant cell granuloma, ameloblastic fibroma, calcifying epithelial odontogenic tumor, intraosseous mucoepidermoid carcinoma). Maxillary tumors may show less distinct radiological borders and often fill the maxillary sinus.

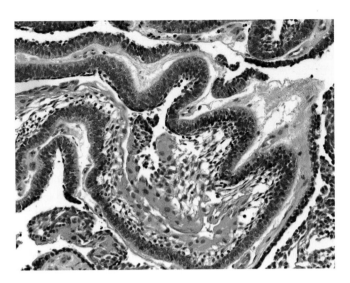

Figure 6.18 Ameloblastoma (H&E, 200×).

The classic histological features are represented by islands of proliferating epithelium resembling the enamel organ. Several histological subtypes have been described but all have in common epithelial islands of edematous epithelium resembling stellate reticulum surrounded by tall, columnar basophilic odontogenic cells exhibiting reverse polarity. The cell cytology is bland with little pleomorphism and mitotic activity[157,162] (Fig. 6.18). Recent studies have shown that p53 and metallothionein expression in ameloblastoma is significantly higher than other benign odontogenic tumors, which may explain the more aggressive nature of this tumor.[163,164]

Patients with conventional ameloblastomas are treated by surgical resection. Because the conventional ameloblastoma infiltrates between intact cancellous bone trabeculae at the periphery of the lesion, it is recommended that the margin of resection should be at least 1.0–1.5 cm beyond the radiological margins of the lesion. Recurrence rates of up to 15% have been reported after marginal or *en bloc* resection, and delayed recurrence after many years has been reported. Unicystic ameloblastomas can be treated by simple enucleation. Recurrence rates of 10–20% have been described after enucleation and curettage of unicystic ameloblastomas. Due to risk of local recurrence, patients should remain under long-term follow-up. Peripheral ameloblastoma shows a lower recurrence rate, after local surgical excision.

Radiation therapy has seldom been used as adjuvant treatment because of the intraosseous location of the tumor and the potential for a secondary, radiation-induced malignancy. The most promising results with potential therapeutic implications come from studies focused on sonic hedgehog (SHH) and Pi3K/Akt/mTOR signaling.[165] The expression of SHH signaling molecules in ameloblastomas at the mRNA and protein levels has suggested that these molecules may play a role in cell proliferation.

Immunohistochemistry studies have also revealed aberrant signaling in the Pi3K, Akt and mTOR pathways. Involvement of the two pathways in ameloblastoma survival/growth opens the door for nonsurgical therapy, with SHH-specific inhibitors together with Pi3K, Akt or mTOR blocking agents that could potentially be used locally, minimizing major systemic effects.[163,166–168]

Malignant ameloblastoma and ameloblastic carcinoma

Malignant variants of ameloblastoma include metastasizing ameloblastoma and ameloblastic carcinoma. Metastasizing ameloblastoma is an ameloblastoma that metastasizes despite a benign histological appearance, making this a purely retrospective diagnosis. It occurs over a wide age range (4–75 years), and the interval between the initial diagnosis of ameloblastoma and first metastasis varies from 1 to 30 years. Patients with metastasizing ameloblastoma have a poor prognosis. About 50% of patients with documented metastases have died of their disease.

Ameloblastic carcinoma occurs in older patients (during the sixth and seventh decades of life) and is composed of cells that, although mimicking the architectural pattern of ameloblastoma, exhibit profound cytological atypia, increased mitotic activity, and necrosis (Fig. 6.19). Possible involvement of CpG island hypermethylation of the *p16* gene in the malignant transformation in a case of ameloblastic carcinoma ex ameloblastoma has been described in the recent literature.[169] Patients present with swelling and pain, located most commonly in the posterior mandible. Radiographical findings are consistent with an aggressive tumor, with ill-defined margins, cortical destruction, and foci of calcification.[145] Ameloblastic carcinoma commonly metastasizes to lungs and cervical lymph nodes.[170,171] Spread to viscera and other bones has also been described.

Ameloblastic carcinoma caries a poor prognosis. Because of the rarity of large clinical series with long-term follow-up, there is no consensus on treatment guidelines. Treatment consists of radical surgical excision. The efficacy of adjuvant radiation or chemotherapy as a postsurgical treatment is not

clear. However, radiotherapy and chemotherapy should be considered for locally advanced disease and metastatic lesions not amenable to surgical excision.[170,172]

Odontogenic keratocyst

Odontogenic keratocyst (OKC) is a distinctive form of developmental odontogenic cyst that arises from rests of the dental lamina. Because OKCs demonstrate a neoplastic-like growth potential, with a high rate of local recurrence, in the latest World Health Organization classification of odontogenic tumors these lesions have been classified as "keratocystic odontogenic tumor."[157] OKC demonstrates predilection for involvement of the posterior mandible, in the region of the third molar. It is most common between 10 and 40 years of age, and males are affected more commonly than females. Most OKCs are discovered incidentally during dental radiological examination. In rare cases, patients present with swelling and pain.

Radiologically, OKC presents as a well-defined radiolucent unilocular lesion with smooth borders that is associated with an unerupted tooth in 25–40% of cases.[157] Larger lesions may appear multilocular. Multifocal OKCs and cases diagnosed in children should raise the possibility of Gorlin syndrome (nevoid basal cell carcinoma syndrome) which is an autosomal dominant disorder characterized by a mutation of *PTCH* (patched tumor suppressor gene) located on chromosome 9q22. Signs and symptoms of this syndrome include multiple cutaneous basal cell carcinomas, multiple OKCs, calcification of falx cerebri, skeletal abnormalities involving ribs and vertebrae, and increased frequency of certain neoplasms.

The diagnosis of OKC is based on characteristic histopathological features represented by a uniformly thin epithelial lining (6–8 cells thick) lacking rete ridges and covered by a corrugated parakeratotic layer (Fig. 6.20). OKCs may show satellite cysts and islands of odontogenic epithelium, more common in patients with Gorlin syndrome. Treatment of OKCs consists of enucleation and curettage. OKCs tend to recur after treatment, with recurrence rates in large series of approximately 30%. Multiple recurrences are not unusual, and sometimes recurrences occur after 10 years or more following the initial surgery. In very rare circumstances, a locally aggressive OKC requires local resection and bone grafting.[157]

Cementoblastoma

Cementoblastoma is a rare benign odontogenic tumor that accounts for less than 1% of all odontogenic tumors. It affects young adults, with most cases diagnosed before 30 years of age. There is no gender predilection. More than 75% of cases arise in the mandible, usually in the premolar and molar regions. Although benign, cementoblastoma may exhibit locally aggressive behavior, including cortical erosion, displacement of adjacent teeth, maxillary sinus involvement, and infiltration into the pulp chamber and root canals.[173,174] Clinically, cementoblastoma presents with swelling and pain due to bony expansion of the alveolar ridge. Radiographically,

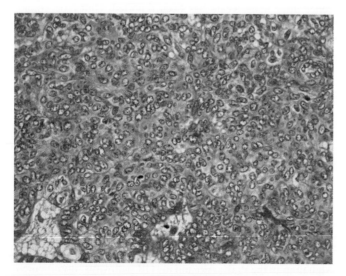

Figure 6.19 Ameloblastic carcinoma (H&E, 400×).

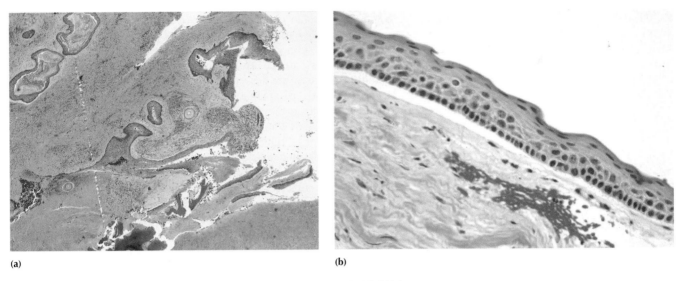

(a)   (b)

Figure 6.20 (a) Odontogenic keratocyst (H&E, 40×). (b) Odontogenic keratocyst (H&E, 200×).

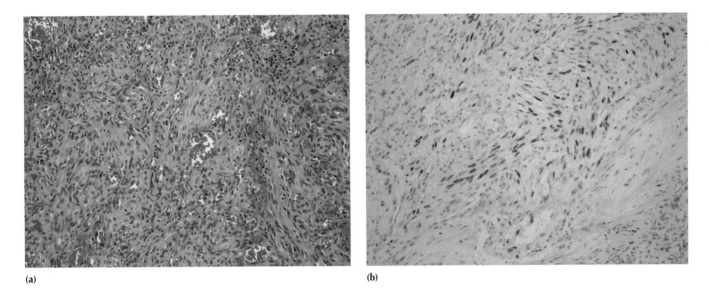

(a)   (b)

Figure 6.21 (a) Kaposi sarcoma (H&E, 200×). (b) Kaposi sarcoma (HHV8 stain, 200×).

the tumor appears as a well-circumscribed opaque mass attached to the root of the involved tooth with a surrounding thin radiolucent zone. The attachment to the root of involved tooth is a pathognomonic radiographical finding. Histologically, cementoblastoma is characterized by masses of hypocellular cementum embedded in a fibrovascular stroma. Multinucleated giant cells are often seen. Prominent cementoblastic rimming and formation of basophilic reversal lines with a pagetoid appearance are also present.[157]

Differential diagnosis of cementoblastoma includes osteoblastoma and osteosarcoma.[173,175] Osteoblastoma and cementoblastoma are essentially identical histologically and the only distinguishing feature is the attachment of cementoblastoma to the root of a tooth. Differentiation of the osteosarcoma from cementoblastoma requires correlation with the clinical and radiological findings.

The treatment of choice for cementoblastoma is complete surgical excision of the mass with removal of the affected tooth. Incomplete removal raises the risk of recurrence and some authors advocate curettage after extraction to decrease the overall rate of recurrence.

Other neoplasms

Kaposi sarcoma

Kaposi sarcoma is an angioproliferative disorder characterized by proliferation of spindle cells, neoangiogenesis, inflammation and edema[176–178] (Fig. 6.21). The major forms of Kaposi sarcoma consist of classic, African endemic, immunosuppression-associated or transplant-associated, and AIDS-associated Kaposi sarcoma.[176,179] Head and neck region involvement is frequent in AIDS-associated Kaposi sarcoma, but it is uncommon in other Kaposi sarcoma variants.[176,178,180] A decrease in AIDS-associated Kaposi sarcoma has been seen in Europe and North America since the introduction of highly active antiretroviral therapy (HAART), but a dramatic increase in Kaposi sarcoma has been noticed in Africa.[176,181–183] Human herpesvirus type 8 (HHV-8) has been demonstrated universally in Kaposi sarcoma lesions.[176–178,184]

Oral cavity involvement is very frequent in AIDS-associated Kaposi sarcoma. Oral lesions represent the first presentation of Kaposi sarcoma in 22% of HIV-positive individuals, and 71% of the HIV-positive individuals developing Kaposi sarcoma will develop oral Kaposi sarcoma lesions at some point.[176,178,180] Patients present with deep red to blue-purplish macular, plaque, and nodular lesions, particularly on the palate. The tumor may also involve the tongue, gingiva, buccal mucosa, pharynx, major salivary glands, and jaw bones.[176,177,180]

Patients with AIDS-associated Kaposi sarcoma should be treated with HAART, particularly in early stages of disease.[176,185] Systemic treatment is indicated for rapidly progressive, extensive oral Kaposi sarcoma.[176,186] Liposomal anthracyclines (pegylated liposomal doxorubicin) are chemotherapeutic agents commonly used for disseminated Kaposi sarcoma. Pegylated liposomal doxorubicin with HAART provides complete or partial response rates in more than 70% of cases with disseminated disease.[176,186,187] Local approaches include intralesional chemotherapy, radiotherapy, laser therapy, and cryotherapy.[176,185–188] Intralesional vinblastine is widely used for oral Kaposi sarcoma.[188]

Burkitt lymphoma

Burkitt lymphoma is a small, noncleaved B cell lymphoma, first described as a malignancy occurring in the jaws of African children.[189] The African form of the disease commonly affects children aged 5–7 years and is characterized by jaw tumors in 60–80% of cases. Epstein–Barr virus (EBV) titers are positive in more than 90% of cases; abdominal masses are less frequent, occurring only in about half of cases; paraplegia indicating central nervous system involvement is the presenting symptom in about one-third of the cases.[190] Patients diagnosed with the American, nonendemic form of Burkitt lymphoma most frequently present with an abdominal mass. Head and neck involvement is less common than in the African variant and usually presents with cervical adenopathy. Involvement of the facial bones, jaw, and other extranodal sites in the head and neck is diagnosed in fewer than 10% of nonendemic Burkitt lymphoma patients. Central nervous system involvement is also a rare presenting symptom, but it eventually occurs in nearly half of cases during the course of disease. Unlike in African Burkitt lymphoma, less than 20% of American variant cases have positive titers for EBV.[191–193]

Histological features of American Burkitt lymphoma are similar to the African variant, with a "starry sky" pattern of undifferentiated, small lymphocytes interspaced with large histiocytes. Multiple mitotic figures are usually present and represent rapidly enlarging tumor mass[190] (Fig. 6.22). Burkitt lymphoma is associated with unique cytogenetic translocations involving the *c-MYC* oncogene on chromosome 8, which appears to be involved in the pathogenesis of this type of lymphoma.[193]

Burkitt lymphoma is one of the fastest-growing tumors in humans, and rapid diagnosis and treatment are essential. Treatment of Burkitt lymphoma includes aggressive multi-agent chemotherapy with central nervous system prophylaxis.[193,194] The use of autologous stem cell transplantation appears to benefit patients with chemotherapy-sensitive relapsed Burkitt lymphoma. The role of allogeneic stem cell transplantation remains to be determined.[194]

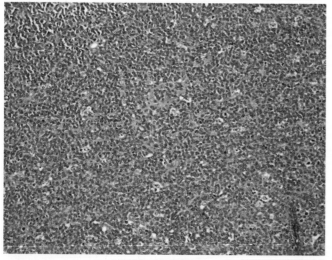

(a)

(b)

Figure 6.22 (a) Burkitt lymphoma (H&E, 40×). (b) Burkitt lymphoma (Ki67 stain, 40×).

References

1. Halperin EC, Perez CA, Brady LW, Wazer DE, Freeman C, Prosnitz LR. *Perez and Brady's Principles and Practice of Radiation Oncology*, 5th edition. Philadelphia: Wolters Kluwer/Lippincott Williams & Wilkins, 2007. p. 891.

2. American Cancer Society. Cancer Facts and Figures 2006. www.cancer.org.

3. Greenle RT, Murray T, Bolden S, *et al.* Cancer statistics 2000. CA Cancer J Clin 2000; 50: 7–33.

4. Dobrossy L. Epidemiology of head and neck cancer: magnitude of the problem. Cancer Metastases Rev 2005; 24: 9–17.

5. Million RCN, Mancuso A. *Oral Cavity*. Philadelphia: J.B. Lippincott, 1994.

6. Patel, Snehal G, Archer, Daniel J, Henk, J Michael. Tumours of the Oral Cavity. In *Principles and Practice of Head and Neck Oncology*. Rhys-Evans PH, Montgomery PQ, Gullane PJ (eds). London: Martin Dunitz, 2003. p. 166.

7. Santoro A, Pannone G, Contaldo M, *et al.* A troubling diagnosis of verrucous squamous cell carcinoma ("the bad kind" of keratosis) and the need of clinical and pathological correlations: a review of the literature with a case report. J Skin Cancer 2011; 2011; 370605.

8. Eversole LR. Pappilary lesions of the oral cavity: relationship to human papillomaviruses. J Calif Assoc 2000; 28: 922–7.

9. Miller CS, White DK. Human papillomavirus expression in oral mucosa, premalignant conditions, and squamous cell carcinoma: a retrospective review of the literature. Oral Surg Oral Med Oral Pathol Oral Radiol Endod 1996; 82: 57–68.

10. Woolgar JA, Triantafyllou A. Pitfalls and procedures in the histopathological diagnosis of oral and oropharyngeal squamous cell carcinoma and a review of the role of pathology in prognosis. Oral Oncol 2009; 45: 361–85.

11. Ferlito A, Antonutto A, Silvestri F. Histological appearances and nuclear DNA content of verrucous squamous cell carcinoma of the larynx. J Oto-Rhino-Laryngol Relat Special 1976; 38: 65–85.

12. Maraki D, Boecking A, Pomjanski N, Megahed M, Becker J. Verrucous carcinoma of the buccal mucosa: histopathological, cytological and DNA-cytometric features. J Oral Pathol Med 2006; 35: 633–5.

13. Hemmer J, Kraft K. High-resolution DNA flow cytometry in oral verrucous carcinoma. Oncol Rep 2000; 7: 433–5.

14. Jordan RC. Verrucous carcinoma of the mouth. J Can Dent Assoc 1995; 61: 797–801.

15. Yoshimura Y, Mishima K, Obara S, Nariaib Y, Yoshimura H, Mikami T. Treatment modalities for oral verrucous carcinomas and their outcome: contribution of radiotherapy and chemotherapy. Int J Clin Oncol 2001; 6: 192–200.

16. Boulaadas M, Benazzou S, Mourtada F, *et al.* Primary oral malignant melanoma. J Craniofac Surg 2007; 18: 1059–561.

17. Ferniano F, Lanza A, Bounaiuto C, Gombos F, DiSoirito F, Cirillo N. Oral malignant melanoma: a review of the literature. J Oral Pathol Med 2008; 37(7): 383–8.

18. Freedman DM, Sigurdson A, Doody MM, Rao RS, Linet MS. Risk of melanoma in relation to smoking, alcohol intake, and other factors in a large occupational cohort. Cancer Causes Control 2003; 14: 847–57.

19. Hatch CL. Pigmented lesions of the oral cavity. Dent Clin North Am 2005; 49: 185–201.

20. Rapini RP. Oral melanoma. Diagnosis and treatment. Semin Cutan Med Surg 1997; 16: 320–2.

21. Notani K, Shindoh M, Yamazaki Y, *et al.* Amelanotic malignant melanomas of the oral mucosa. Br J Oral Maxillofac Surg 2002; 40: 195–200.

22. Tanaka N, Mimura M, Ogi K, Amagasa T. Primary malignant melanoma of the oral cavity: assessment of outcome from the clinical records of 35 patients. Int J Oral Maxillofac Surg 2004; 33: 761–5.

23. Ebenezer J. Malignant melanoma of the oral cavity. Indian J Dent Res 2006; 17(2): 94–6.

24. Mendenhall WM, Amdur RJ, Hinerman RW, Werning JW, Villaret DB, Mendenhall NP. Head and neck mucosal melanoma. Am J Clin Oncol 2005; 28: 626–30.

25. Eggermont AM, Robert C. New drugs in melanoma: it's a whole new world. Eur J Cancer 2011; 47(14): 2150–7.

26. Eggermont AM, Testori A, Maio M, Robert C. Anti-CTLA-4 antibody adjuvant therapy in melanoma. Semin Oncol 2010; 37(5): 455–9.

27. Halperin EC, Perez CA, Brady LW, Wazer DE, Freeman C, Prosnitz LR. *Perez and Brady's Principles and Practice of Radiation Oncology*, 5th edition. Philadelphia: Wolters Kluwer/Lippincott Williams & Wilkins, 2007. p. 874.

28. Sun BC, Curtis R, Melbye M, *et al.* Salivary gland cancer in the United States. Cancer Epidemiol Biomarkers Prev 1999; 8: 1095–100.

29. Spiro RH. Salivary neoplasms: overview of 35-year experience with 2,807 patients. Head Neck Surg 1986; 8: 177–84.

30. Jones AS, Beasley NJP, Houghton DJ, *et al.* Tumors of the minor salivary glands. Clin Otolaryngol 1998; 23: 27–33.

31. Swanson GM, Burns PB. Cancers of the salivary gland: workplace risks among women and men. Ann Epidemiol 1997; 7: 369–74.

32. Modan B, Alfandary E, Tamir A, *et al.* Increased risk of salivary gland tumors after low-dose irradiation. Laryngoscope 1998; 108: 1095–7.

33. Saku T, Hayashi Y, Takahara O, *et al.* Salivary gland tumors among atomic bomb survivors, 1950–1987. Cancer 1997; 79: 1465–575.

34. Whatley WS, Thompson JW, Rao B. Salivary gland tumors in survivors of childhood cancer. Otolaryngol Head Neck Surg 2006; 134: 385–8.

35. Regis de Brito Santos I, Kowalski LP, Cavalcante de Araujo V, *et al.* Multivariate analysis of risk factors for neck metastases in surgically treated parotid carcinoma. Arch Otolayngol Head neck Surg 2001; 127: 46–60.

36. Terhaard CHJ, Lubsen H, Rasch CRN, *et al.* The role of radiotherapy in the treatment of malignant salivary gland tumors. Int J Radiat Oncol Biol Phys 2006; 61: 103–11.

37. Terhaard CHJ, Lubsen H, van der Tweel I, *et al.* Salivary gland carcinoma: independent prognostic factors for locoregional control, distant metastases, and overall survival. Results of the Dutch Head and Neck Oncology Cooperative Group. Head Neck 2004; 26(8): 681–93.

38. Guzzo M, di Palma S, Grandi C, *et al.* Salivary duct carcinoma. Clinical characteristics and treatment strategies. Head Neck 1997; 19: 126–33.

39. Jaehne M, Roeser K, Jaekel T, *et al.* Clinical and immunohistologic typing of salivary duct carcinoma. A report of 50 cases. Cancer 2005; 103: 2526–33.

40. Parsons JT, Mendenhall WM, Stringer P, *et al.* Management of minor salivary gland carcinomas. Int J Radiat Oncol Biol Phys 1996; 35: 443–54.

41. Miyabe S, Okabe M, Nagatsuka H, *et al.* Prognostic significance of p27Kip1, Ki-67, and CRTC1-MAML2 fusion transcript in mucoepidermoid carcinoma: a molecular and clinicopathologic study of 101 cases. J Oral Maxillofac Surg 2009; 67(7): 1432–41.

42. Beckhardt RN, Weber RS, Zane R, *et al.* Minor salivary gland tumors of the palate: clinical and pathologic correlates of outcome. Laryngoscope 1995; 105: 1155–60.

43. Schoenfeld JD, Sher DJ, Norris CM Jr, *et al.* Salivary gland tumors treated with adjuvant intensity-modulated radiotherapy with or without concurrent chemotherapy. Int J Radiat Oncol Biol Phys 2012; 82(1): 308–14.

44. Persson M, Andren Y, Mark J, Horlings HM, Persson F, Stenman G. Recurrent fusion of MYB and NFIB transcription factor genes in carcinomas of the breast and head and neck. Proc Natl Acad Sci USA 2009; 106(44): 18740–4.

45. Conkright MD, Canelttieri G, Screaton R, *et al.* TORCs: transducers of regulated CREB activity. Mol Cell 2003; 12: 413–23.

46. Iourgenko V, Zhang W, Mickanin C, *et al.* Identification of a family of cAMP response element-binding protein coactivators by genome-scale functional analysis in mammalian cells. Proc Natl Acad Sci USA 2003; 100: 12147–52.

47. Coxon A, Rozenblum E, Park YS, *et al.* Mect1-Maml2 fusion oncogene linked to the aberrant activation of cyclic AMP/CREB regulated genes. Cancer Res 2005; 65: 7137–44.

48. Williams MD, Roberts D, Blumenschein GR, *et al.* Differential expression of hormonal and growth factor receptors in salivary duct carcinomas:

biologic significance and potential role in therapeutic stratification of patients. Am J Surg Pathol 2007; 31: 1645–52.

49. Aqulnik M, Cohen EW, Cohen RB, *et al.* Phase II study of lapatinib in recurrent or metastatic epidermal growth factor receptor and/or erbB2 expressing adenoid cystic carcinoma and non adenoid cystic carcinoma malignant tumors of the salivary glands. J Clin Oncol 2007; 25(25): 3978–84.

50. Creagan ET, Woods JE, Schutt AJ, *et al.* Cyclophosphamide, adriamycin and cisdiaminodichloroplatinum in the treatment of advanced nonsquamous cell head and neck cancer. Cancer 1983; 52: 2007–10.

51. Airoldi M, Pedani F, Succo G, *et al.* Phase II randomized trial comparing vinorelbine versus vinorebine plus cisplatin in patients with recurrent salivary gland malignancies. Cancer 2001; 91(3): 541–7.

52. Gilbert J, Li Y, Pinto H, *et al.* Phase II trial of taxol in salivary gland malignancies (E1394): a trial of the Eastern Cooperative Oncology Group. Head Neck 2006; 28(3): 197–204.

53. Garcia Berrocal JR, Ramirez Camacho R, Trinidad A, Salas C. Mixed tumor (pleomorphic adenoma) of head and neck. Typical and atypical patterns. An Otorrinolaringol Ibero Am 2000; 27: 333–40.

54. Clauser L, Mandrioli S, Dallera V, Sarti E, Galie M, Cavazzini L. Pleomorphic adenoma of the palate. J Craniofac Surg 2004; 15(6): 1206–9.

55. Dalati T, Hussein MR. Juvenile pleomorphic adenoma of the cheek: a case report and review of literature. Diagn Pathol 2009; 4: 32.

56. Wang D, Li Y, He H, Liu L, Wu L, He Z. Intraoral minor salivary gland tumors in a Chinese population: a retrospective study of 737 cases. Oral Surg Oral Med Oral Pathol Oral Radiol Endod 2007; 104: 94–100.

57. Stennert E, Wittekindt C, Klussmann JP, *et al.* Recurrent pleomorphic adenoma of the parotid gland: a prospective histopathological and immunohistochemical study. Laryngoscope 2004; 114: 158–63.

58. Wittekindt C, Streubel K, Arnold G, *et al.* Recurrent pleomorphic adenoma of the parotid gland: analysis of 108 consecutive patients. Head Neck 2007; 29: 822–8.

59. Lee PS, Sabbath-Solitare M, Redondo TC, Ongcapin EH. Molecular evidence that the stromal and epithelial cells in pleomorphic adenomas of salivary gland arise from the same origin: clonal analysis using human androgen receptor gene (HUMARA) assay. Hum Pathol 2000; 31: 498–503.

60. Redaelli de Zinis LO, Piccioni M, Antonelli AR, *et al.* Management and prognostic factors of recurrent pleomorphic adenoma of the parotid gland: personal experience and review of the literature. Eur Arch Otorhinolaryngol 2008; 265: 447–52.

61. DeRoche TC, Hoschar AP, Hunt JL. Immunohistochemical evaluation of androgen receptor, HER-2/neu, and p53 in benign pleomorphic adenomas. Arch Pathol Lab Med 2008; 132: 1907–11.

62. Hamada T, Matsukita S, Goto M, *et al.* Mucin expression in pleomorphic adenoma of salivary gland: a potential role of MUC1 as a marker to predict recurrence. J Clin Pathol 2004; 57: 813–21.

63. Lewis JE, Olsen KD, Sebo TJ. Carcinoma ex pleomorphic adenoma: pathologic analysis of 73 cases. Hum Pathol 2001; 32: 596–604.

64. Halperin EC, Perez CA, Brady LW, Wazer DE, Freeman C, Prosnitz LR. *Perez and Brady's Principles and Practice of Radiation Oncology*, 5th edition. Philadelphia: Wolters Kluwer/Lippincott Williams & Wilkins, 2007. p. 882.

65. Triantafillidou K, Dimitrakopoulos J, Iordanidis F, Koufogiannis D. Mucoepidermoid carcinoma of minor salivary glands: a clinical study of 16 cases and review of the literature. Oral Diseases 2006; 12: 364–70.

66. Brandwein MS, Ivanov K, Wallace DI, *et al.* Mucoepidermoid carcinoma: a clinicopathologic study of 80 patients with special reference to histological grading. Am J Surg Pathol 2001; 25: 835–45.

67. Hicks J, Flaitz C. Mucoepidermoid carcinoma of salivary glands in children and adolescents: assessment of proliferation markers. Oral Oncol 2000; 36: 454–60.

68. Caccamese JF, Ord RA. Paediatric mucoepidermoid carcinoma of the palate. Int J Oral Maxillofac Surg 2002; 31: 136–9.

69. Goode RK, Auclair PL, Ellis GL. Mucoepidermoid carcinoma of the major salivary glands: clinical and histopathologic analysis of 234 cases with evaluation of grading criteria. Cancer 1998; 82: 1217–24.

70. Okabe M, Inagaki H, Murase T, Inoue M, Nagai N, Eimoto T. Prognostic significance of p27 and Ki-67 expression in mucoepidermoid carcinoma of the intraoral minor salivary gland. Mod Pathol 2001; 14: 1008–14.

71. Healey WV, Perzin KH, Smith L. Mucoepidermoid carcinoma of salivary gland origin. Classification, clinicalpathologic correlation, and results of treatment. Cancer 1970; 26: 368–88.

72. North CA, Lee DJ, Piantadosi S, Zahurak M, Johns ME. Carcinoma of the major salivary glands treated by surgery or surgery plus postoperative radiotherapy. Int J Radiat Oncol Biol Phys 1990; 18: 1319–26.

73. Hosokawa Y, Shirato H, Kagei K, *et al.* Role of radiotherapy for mucoepidermoid carcinoma of salivary gland. Oral Oncol 1999; 35: 105–11.

74. Guzzo m, Andreola S, Sirizzotti G, Cantu G. Mucoepidermoid carcinoma of the salivary glands: clinicopathologic review of 108 patients treated at the National Cancer Institute on Milan. Ann Surg Oncol 2002; 9: 688–95.

75. Darling MR, Schneider JW, Phillips VM. Polymorphous low-grade adenocarcinoma and adenoid cystic carcinoma: a review and comparison of immunohistochemical markers. Oral Oncol 2002; 38(7): 641–5.

76. Martinez-Rodriguez N, Leco-Berrocal I, Rubio-Alonso L, Arias-Irimia O, Martinez-Gonzalez JM. Epidemiology and treatment of adenoid cystic carcinoma of the minor salivary glands: a meta-analysis study. Med Oral Pathol Oral Cir Buccal. 2011; 16(7): e884–9.

77. Caldeneyer KS, Matthews VP, Righi PD, *et al.* Imaging features and clinical significance of perineural spread or extension of head and neck tumors. Radiographics 1998; 18: 87–100.

78. Stallmach I, Zenklusen P, Komminoth P, *et al.* Loss of heterogeneity at chromosome 6q23-35 correlates with clinical and histologic parameters in salivary glands adenoid cystic carcinoma. Virchows Arch 2002; 440: 77–84.

79. Kokemueller H, Eckardt A, Brachvogel P, Hausamen JE. Adenoid cystic carcinoma of the head and neck: a 20 years experience. Int J Oral Maxillofac Surg 2004; 33: 25–31.

80. Huang M, Ma D, Sun K, Yu G, Guo C, Gao F. Factors influencing survival rate in adenoid cystic carcinoma of the salivary glands. Int J Oral Maxillofac Surg 1997; 26: 435–9.

81. Khan AJ, di Giovanna MP, Ross DA, *et al.* Adenoid cystic carcinoma: a retrospective clinical review. Int J Cancer 2001; 96: 149–58.

82. Garden AS, Weber RS, Morrison WH, Ang KK, Peters LJ. The influence of positive margins and nerve invasion in adenoid cystic carcinoma of the head and neck treated with surgery and radiation. Int J Radiat Oncol Biol Phys 1995; 32: 619–26.

83. Simpson JR, Thawley SE, Matsuba HM. Adenoid cystic salivary gland carcinoma: treatment with irradiation and surgery. Radiology 1984; 151(2): 509–12.

84. Umeda M, Nishimatsu N, Masago H, *et al.* Tumour-doubling time and onset of pulmonary metastases from adenoid cystic carcinoma of the salivary gland. Oral Surg 1999; 88: 473–8.

85. Matsuba HM, Spector GJ, Thawley SE, Simpson JR. Mauney FJ, Pikul FJ. Adenoid cystic salivary gland carcinoma. A histopathologic review of treatment failure patterns. Cancer 1986; 57: 519–24.

86. Sung MW, Kim KH, Kim JW, *et al.* Clinicopathologic predictors and impact of distant metastases from adenoid cystic carcinoma of the head and neck. Arch Otolaryngol Head Neck Surg 2003; 129: 1193–7.

87. Van der Waal JE, Becking AG, Snow GB, van der Waal I. Distant metastases of adenoid cystic carcinoma of the salivary glands and the value of diagnostic examination during follow up. Head Neck 2003; 24: 779–83.

88. Spiro RH. Distant metastases in adenoid cystic carcinoma of the salivary origin. Am J Surg 1997; 174: 495–8.

89. Tang QL, Chen WL, Tan XY, *et al.* Expression and significance of Cyr61 in distant metastasis cells of human primary salivary adenoid cystic carcinoma. Oral Surg Oral Med Oral Pathol Oral Radiol Endod 2011; 112(2): 228–36.

90. Halperin EC, Perez CA, Brady LW, Wazer DE, Freeman C, Prosnitz LR. *Perez and Brady's Principles and Practice of Radiation Oncology*, 5th edition. Philadelphia: Wolters Kluwer/Lippincott Williams & Wilkins, 2007. p. 883.

91. Von Hoff DD, Stephenson Jr JJ, Rosen P, *et al*. Pilot study using molecular profiling of patients' tumors to find potential targets and select treatments for their refractory cancers. J Clin Oncol 2010; 28: 4877–83.

92. Rosell R, Crino L, Danenberg K, *et al*. Targeted therapy in combination with gemcitabine in non-small cell lung cancer. Semin Oncol 2003; 30(4 Suppl. 10): 19–25.

93. Righi L, Papotti MG, Ceppi P, *et al*. Thymidylate synthase but not excision repair cross-complementation group 1 tumor expression predicts outcome in patients with malignant pleural mesothelioma treated with pemetrexed-based chemotherapy. J Clin Oncol 2010; 28: 1534–9.

94. Edler D, Glimelius B, Hallstrom M, *et al*.Thymidylate synthase expression in colorectal cancer: a prognostic and predictive marker of benefit from adjuvant fluorouracil-based chemotherapy. J Clin Oncol 2002; 20: 1721–8.

95. Quintela-Fandino M, Hitt R, Medina P, *et al*. DNA-repair gene polymorphisms predict favorable clinical outcome among patients with advanced squamous cell carcinoma of the head and neck treated with cisplatin-based induction chemotherapy. J Clin Oncol 2006; 24: 4333–9.

96. Lord RVN, Brabender J, Gandara D, *et al*. Low ERCC1 expression correlates with prolonged survival after cisplatin plus gemcitabine chemotherapy in non-small cell lung cancer. Clin Cancer Res 2002; 8: 2286–91.

97. Levin JM, Robinson DW, Lin F. Acinic cell carcinoma: collective review, including bilateral cases. Arch Surg 1975; 11: 64–8.

98. Krolls SO, Trodahl JN, Boyers RC. Salivary gland lesions in children: a review of 430 cases. Cancer 1972; 30: 459–69.

99. Depowski PL, Setzen G, Chui A, Koltai PJ, Dollar J, Ross JS. Familial occurrence of acinic cell carcinoma of the parotid gland. Arch Pathol Lab Med 1999; 123: 1118–20.

100. Jin Y, Mertens F, Limon J, Mandahl N, Wennerberg M. Characteristics of karyotype features in lacrimal and salivary gland carcinomas. Br J Cancer 1994; 70: 42–7.

101. El-Naggar AK, Abdul-Karim FW, Hurr K, Callender D, Luna MA, Batsakis JG. Genetic alterations in acinic cell carcinoma of the parotid gland as determined by microsatellite analysis. Cancer Genet Cytogenet 1998; 102: 19–24.

102. Anthony J, Gopalan V, Smith RA. Carcinoma ex pleomorphic adenoma: a comprehensive review of clinical, pathological and molecular data. Head Neck 2011; Jul 9 [Epub ahead of print].

103. Gnepp DR. Malignant mixed tumours of the salivary glands: a review. Pathol Annu 1993; 28: 279–328.

104. Nouraei SA, Hope KL, Kelly CG, *et al*. Carcinoma ex benign pleomorphic adenoma of the parotid gland. Plast Reconstr Surg 2005; 116: 1206–13.

105. Zbaren P, Zbaren S, Caversaccio MD, Stauffer E. Carcinoma ex pleomorphic adenoma: diagnostic difficulty and outcome. Otolaryngol Head Neck Surg 2008; 138: 601–5.

106. LiVolsi VA, Perzin KH. Malignant mixed tumours: a clinico-pathological study. Cancer 1977; 39: 2209–30.

107. Barnes L, Eveson JW, Reichart P, Sidransky D (eds). *World Health Organization Classification of Tumours. Pathology and Genetics of Head and Neck Tumours*. Lyon: IARC Press. 2005.

108. Luers JC, Wittekindt C, Streppel M, *et al*. Carcinoma ex-pleomorphic adenoma of the parotid gland. Study and implications for diagnostics and therapy. Acta Oncol 2009; 48: 132–6.

109. Skalova A, Sima R, Kaspirkova-Nemcova J, *et al*. Cribriform adenocarcinoma of minor salivary gland origin principally affecting the tongue: characterization of new entity. Am J Surg Pathol 2011; 35: 1168–76.

110. Luna MA, Wenig BM. Polymorphous low-grade adenocarcinoma. In: Barnes EL, Eveson JW, Reichart P, Sidransky D (eds) *World Health Organization Classification of Tumours. Pathology and Genetics of Head and Neck Tumours*. Lyon: IARC Press, 2005. pp.223–4.

111. Beltran D, Faquin WC, Gallagher G, August M. Comparison of polymorphous low-grade adenocarcinoma and adenoid cystic carcinoma. J Oral Maxillofac Surg 2006; 64: 415–23.

112. Saghravanian N, Mohtasham N, Jafarzadeh H. Comparison of immunohistochemical markers between adenoid cystic carcinoma and polymorphous low-grade adenocarcinoma. J Oral Sc 2009; 51(4): 509–14.

113. Sturgis EM, Potter BO. Sarcomas of the head and neck region. Curr Opin Oncol 2003; 15: 239–52.

114. Mendenhall WM, Mendenhall CM, Werning JW, Riggs CE, Mendenhall NP. Adult head and neck soft tissue sarcomas. Head Neck 2005; 27: 916–22.

115. Balm AJ, van Coevoorden F, Boske, *et al*. Report of a symposium on diagnosis and treatment of adult soft tissue sarcomas in the head and neck. Eur J Surg Oncol 1995; 21: 287–9.

116. Krauss DH, Dubner S, Harrison LB, *et al*. Prognostic factors for recurrence and survival in head and neck soft tissue sarcomas. Cancer 1994; 74: 697–702.

117. Dijkstra MD, Balm AJM, van Coevoorden F, *et al*. Survival of adult patients with head and neck soft tissue sarcomas. Clin Otolaryngol 1996; 21: 66–71.

118. Mendenhall WM, Zlotecki RA, Morris CG, Hochwald SN, Scarborough MT. Aggressive fibromatosis. Am J Clin Oncol 2005; 28: 211–15.

119. Mendenhall WM, Zlotecki RA, Scarborough MT. Dermatofibrosarcoma protuberans. Cancer 2004; 101: 2503–8.

120. Brant TA, Parsons JT, Marcus RB, *et al*. Preoperative irradiation for soft tissue sarcomas of the trunk and extremities in adults. Int J Radiat Oncol Biol Phys 1990; 19: 899–906.

121. Parsons JT, Zlotecki RA, Reddy KA, Mitchell TP, Marcus RB Jr, Scarborough MT. The role of radiotherapy and limb-conserving surgery in the management of soft-tissue sarcomas in adults. Hematol Oncol Clin North Am 2001; 15: 377–88.

122. Penel N, Bui BN, Bay JO, *et al*. Phase II trial of weekly paclitaxel for unresectable angiosarcoma: the ANGIOTAX study. J Clin Oncol 2008; 26(32): 5269–74.

123. Benz MR, Czernin J, Allen-Auerbach MS, *et al*. FDG PET imaging predicts histologic treatment responses after the initial cycle of chemotherapy in high grade soft tissue sarcomas. Clin Cancer Res 2009; 15(8): 2856–63.

124. Sturgis EM, Potter BO. Sarcomas of the head and neck region. Curr Opin Oncol 2003; 15: 239–52.

125. Clark DW, Moore BA, Patel SR, *et al*. Malignant fibrous histiocytoma of the head and neck region. Head Neck 2011; 33(3): 303–8.

126. Ko JY, Chen CL, Lui LT, Hsu MM. Radiation-induced malignant fibrous histiocytoma in patients with nasopharyngeal carcinoma. Arch Otolaryngol Head Neck Surg 1996; 122: 535–8.

127. Wang CP, Chang YL, Ting LL, Yang TL, Ko JY, Lou PJ. Malignant fibrous histiocytoma of the sinonasal tract. Head Neck 2009; 31: 85–93.

128. Sabesan T, Xuexi W, Yongfa Q, Pingzhang T, Ilankovan V. Malignant fibrous histiocytoma. Outcome of tumours in the head and neck compared with those in the trunk and extremities. Br J Oral Maxillofac Surg 2006; 44(3): 209–12.

129. Mark RJ, Tran LM, Sercarz J, Fu YS, Calcaterra TC, Juillard GF. Angiosarcoma of the head and neck. The UCLA experience 1955 through 1990. Arch Otolaryngol Head neck Surg 1993; 119: 973–8.

130. Maddox JC, Evans HL. Angiosarcoma of skin and soft tissue: a study of forty-five cases. Cancer 1981; 48: 1907–21.

131. Ward JR, Feigenberg SJ, Mendenhall NP, Marcus RB Jr, Mendenhall WM. Radiation therapy for angiosarcoma. Head Neck 2003; 25: 873–8.

132. Willers H, Hug EB, Spiro IJ, Efird JT, Rosenberg AE, Wang CC. Adult soft tissue sarcomas of the head and neck treated by radiation and surgery or radiation alone: pattern of failure and prognostic factors. Int J Radiat Oncol Biol Phys 1995; 33: 585–93.

133. Holden CA, Spittle MF, Jones EW. Angiosarcoma of the face and scalp, prognosis and treatment. Cancer 1987; 59: 1046–57.

134. Morales PH, Lindberg RD, Barkley HT. Soft tissue angiosarcomas. Int J Radiat Oncol Biol Phys 1981; 7: 1655–9.

135. Rigante M, Visocchi G, Petrone G, Mule A, Bussu F. Synovial sarcoma of the parotid gland: a case report and review of the literature. Acta Otorhinolaryngol Ital 2011; 31: 43–6.

136. Carillo R, Rodriguez-Peralto JL, Bastakis JG. Synovial sarcoma of the head and neck. Ann Otol Rhinol Laryngol 1992; 101:367–370.

137. Dei Tos AP, Dal Cin P, Sciot R, *et al*. Synovial sarcoma of the larynx and hypopharynx. Ann Otol Rhinol Laryngol 1998; 107: 1080–5.

138. Sachse F, August C, Alberty J. *Malignant fibrous histiocytoma in the parotid gland. Case series and literature review.* HNO 2006; 54: 116–20.

139. Spillane AJ, A'Hern R, Judson IR, et al. Synovial sarcoma: a clinico-pathologic, staging, and prognostic assessment. J Clin Oncol 2000; 18: 3794–803.

140. Ihak RA, Lydiatt WM, Lydiatt DD, et al. Synovial sarcoma of the head and neck: chromosomal translocation (X;18) as a diagnostic aid. Head Neck 1997; 19: 549–53.

141. Wang H, Zhang J, He X, et al. Synovial sarcoma in the oral and maxillofacial region: report of 4 cases and review of the literature. J Oral Maxillofac Surg 2008; 66: 161–7.

142. Bukachevsky RP, Pincus RL, Shechtman FG, et al. Synovial sarcoma of the head and neck. Head Neck 1992; 14: 44–8.

143. Bilgic B, Mete O, Ozturk AS, et al. Synovial sarcoma: a rare tumor of the larynx. Pathol Oncol Res 2003; 9: 242–5.

144. Olsen RJ, Lydiatt WM, Koepsell SA, et al. C-erb-B2 (HER2/neu) expression in synovial sarcoma of the head and neck. Head Neck 2005; 27: 883–92.

145. Thomas DG, Giordano TJ, Sanders D, et al. Expression of receptor tyrosine kinases epidermal growth factor receptor and HER-2/neu in synovial sarcoma. Cancer 2005; 103: 830–8.

146. Muzio LL, Favia G, Mignogna MD, Piattelli A, Maiorano E. Primary intraoral leiomyosarcoma of the tongue: an immunohistochemical study and review of the literature. Oral Oncol 2000; 36: 519–24.

147. Piattelli A, Artese L. Leiomyosarcoma of the tongue: a case report. J Oral Maxillofac Surg 1995; 53: 698–701.

148. Schenberg ME, Slootweg PJ, Koole R. Leiomyosarcomas of the oral cavity. Report of four cases and review of the literature. J Craniomaxillofac Surg 1993; 21: 342–7.

149. Miloglu O, Altas SS, Buyukkurt MC, Erdemci B, Altun O. Rhabdomyosarcoma of the oral cavity: a case report. Eur J Dent 2011; 5(3): 340–3.

150. Peters E, Cohen M, Altini M, Murray J. Rhabdomyosarcoma of the oral and paraoral region. Cancer 1989; 63: 963–6.

151. Franca CM, Caran EM, Alves MT, Barreto AD, Lopes NN. Rhabdomyosarcoma of the oral tissues – two new cases and literature review. Med Oral Patol Oral Cir Bucal 2006; 11: 136–40.

152. Gordon-Nunez MA, Piva MR, Dos Anjos ED, Freitas RA. Orofacial rhabdomyosarcoma: report of a case and review of the literature. Med Oral Patol Oral Cir Bucal 2008; 13: 765–9.

153. Sekhar MS, Desai S, Kumar GS. Alveolar rhabdomyosarcoma involving the jaws: a case report. J Oral Maxillofac Surg 2000; 58: 1062–5.

154. Wiener ES. Head and neck rhabdomyosarcoma. Semin Pediatric Surg 1994; 3(3): 203–6.

155. Raney RB, Meza J, Anderson JR, et al. Treatment of children and adolescents with localized parameningeal sarcoma: experience of the Intergroup Rhabdomyosarcoma Study Group protocols IRS-II through -IV, 1978–1997. Med Pediatr Oncol 2002; 38(1): 22–32.

156. Thompson LDR. *Head and Neck Pathology.* New York: Churchill Livingstone, 2006.

157. Neville B, Damm DD, Allen CM, Bouquot J. *Oral and Maxillofacial Pathology.* Philadelphia: Saunders, 2009.

158. De S, Ghosh S, Mondal D, Sur PK. Osteosarcoma of the mandible – second cancer in a case of Hodgkin's lymphoma post-chemotherapy. J Cancer Res Ther 2010; 6: 336–8.

159. Padilla RJ, Murrah VA. The spectrum of gnathic osteosarcoma: caveats for the clinician and the pathologist. Head Neck Pathol 2011; 5: 92–9.

160. Fayda M, Aksu G, Yaman Agaoglu F, et al. The role of surgery and radiotherapy in treatment of soft tissue sarcomas of the head and neck region: review of 30 cases. J Craniomaxillofac Surg 2009; 37: 42–8.

161. Jaffe N. Osteosarcoma: review of the past, impact on the future. The American experience. Cancer Treat Res 2009; 152: 239–62.

162. Slater LJ. Diagnostic criteria for unicystic ameloblastoma: ameloblastic versus ameloblastomatous epithelium. Oral Surg Oral Med Oral Pathol Oral Radiol Endod 2011; 111: 536–8.

163. Gadbail AR, Patil R, Chaudhary M. Co-expression of Ki-67 and p53 protein in ameloblastoma and keratocystic odontogenic tumor. Acta Odontol Scand 2011; Jul 25 [Epub ahead of print].

164. Ribeiro AL, Nobre RM, Rocha GC, et al. Expression of metallothionein in ameloblastoma. A regulatory molecule? J Oral Pathol Med 2011; 40: 516–19.

165. Salehinejad J, Zare-Mahmoodabadi R, Saghafi S, et al. Immuno-histochemical detection of p53 and PCNA in ameloblastoma and adenomatoid odontogenic tumor. J Oral Sci 2011; 53: 213–17.

166. Muraki E, Nakano K, Maeda H, et al. Immunohistochemical localization of Notch signaling molecules in ameloblastomas. Eur J Med Res 2011; 16: 253–7.

167. Borkosky SS, Gunduz M, Beder L, et al. Allelic loss of the ING gene family loci is a frequent event in ameloblastoma. Oncol Res 2010; 18: 509–18.

168. Kumamoto H, Ohki K. Detection of Notch signaling molecules in ameloblastomas. J Oral Pathol Med. 2008; 37: 228–34.

169. Karakida K, Aoki T, Sakamoto H, et al. Ameloblastic carcinoma, secondary type: a case report. Oral Surg Oral Med Oral Pathol Oral Radiol Endod 2010; 110: e33–7.

170. Yoon HJ, Hong SP, Lee JI, Lee SS, Hong SD. Ameloblastic carcinoma: an analysis of 6 cases with review of the literature. Oral Surg Oral Med Oral Pathol Oral Radiol Endod 2009; 108: 904–13.

171. Devenney-Cakir B, Dunfee B, Subramaniam R, et al. Ameloblastic carcinoma of the mandible with metastasis to the skull and lung: advanced imaging appearance including computed tomography, magnetic resonance imaging and positron emission tomography computed tomography. Dentomaxillofac Radiol 2010; 39: 449–53.

172. Lucca M, d'Innocenzo R, Kraus JA, Gagari E, Hall J, Shastri K. Ameloblastic carcinoma of the maxilla: a report of 2 cases. J Oral Maxillofac Surg 2010; 68: 2564–9.

173. Bilodeau E, Collins B, Costello B, Potluri A. Case report: a pediatric case of cementoblastoma with histologic and radiographic features of an osteoblastoma and osteosarcoma. Head Neck Pathol 2010; 4: 324–8.

174. Huber AR, Folk GS. Cementoblastoma. Head Neck Pathol 2009; 3: 133–5.

175. Brannon RB, Fowler CB, Carpenter WM, Corio RL. Cementoblastoma: an innocuous neoplasm? A clinicopathologic study of 44 cases and review of the literature with special emphasis on recurrence. Oral Surg Oral Med Oral Pathol Oral Radiol Endod 2002; 93: 311–20.

176. Ramirez-Amador V, Martinez-Mata G, Gonzalez-Ramirez I, Anaya-Saavedra G, de Almeida OP. Clinical, histological and immunohisto-chemical findings in oral Kaposi's sarcoma in a series of Mexican AIDS patients. Comparative study. J Oral Pathol Med 2009; 38(4): 328–33.

177. Feller L, Wood NH, Lemmer J. HIV-associated Kaposi sarcoma: pathogenic mechanisms. Oral Surg Oral Med Oral Pathol Oral Radiol Endod 2007; 104(4): 521–9.

178. Szajerka T, Jablecki J. Kaposi's sarcoma revisited. AIDS Rev 2007; 9(4): 230–6.

179. Sissolak G, Mayaud P. AIDS-related Kaposi's sarcoma: epidemiological, diagnostic, treatment and control aspects in sub-Saharan Africa. Trop Med Int Health 2005; 10(10): 981–92.

180. Chokunonga E, Levy LM, Bassett MT, Mauchaza BG, Thomas DB, Parkin DM. Cancer incidence in the African population of Harare, Zimbabwe: second results from the cancer registry 1993-1995. Int J Cancer 2000; 85(1): 54–9.

181. Eltom M, Jemal A, Mbulaiteye SM, Devesa SS, Biggar RJ. Trends in Kaposi's sarcoma and non-Hodgkin's lymphoma incidence in the Unites States from 1973 through 1998. J Natl Cancer Inst 2002; 94(16): 1204–10.

182. Jones JL, Hanson DL, Dworkin MS, Jaffe HW. Incidence and trends in Kaposi's sarcoma in the era of effective antiretroviral therapy. J Acquir Immune Defic Syndr 2000; 24(3): 270–4.

183. Ganem D. KSHV infection and the pathogenesis of Kaposi's sarcoma. Annu Rev Pathol 2006; 1: 273–86.

184. Bower M, Weir J, Francis N, *et al.* The effect of HAART in 254 consecutive patients with AIDS-related Kaposi's sarcoma. AIDS 2009; 23(13): 1701–6.

185. Di Lorenzo G, Konstantinopoulos PA, Pantanowitz L, Li Trolo R, de Placido S, Dezube BJ. Management of AIDS-related Kaposi's sarcoma. Lancet Oncol 2007; 8(2): 167–76.

186. Martin-Carbonero L, Palacios R, Valencia E, *et al.* Kaposi Sarcoma Spanish Group. Long-term prognosis of HIV-infected patients with Kaposi sarcoma treated with pegylated liposomal doxorubicin. Clin Infect Dis 2008; 47(3): 410–17.

187. Ramirez-Amador V, Esquivel-Pedraza L, Lozada-Nur F, *et al.* Intralesional vinblastine vs sodium tetradecyl sulfate for the treatment of oral Kaposi's sarcoma. A double blind, randomized clinical trial. Oral Oncol 2002; 38(5): 460—7.

188. Caccialanza M, Marca S, Piccinno R, Eulisse G. Radiotherapy of classic and human immunodeficiency virus-related Kaposi's sarcoma: results in 1482 lesions. J Eur Acad Dermatol Venerol 2008; 22(3): 297–302.

189. Burkitt D. A Sarcoma involving the jaws in African children. Br J Surg 1958; 46: 218–23.

190. Wang MB, Strasnick B, Zimmerman MC. Extranodal American Burkitt's lymphoma of the head and neck. Arch Otolaryngol Head Neck Surg 1992; 118: 193–9.

191. Levine AM, Pavlova Z, Pockros AW, *et al.* Small noncleaved follicular center cell lymphoma: Burkitt and non-Burkitt variants in the United States, I: clinical features. Cancer 1983; 52: 1073–9.

192. Ziegler JL. Burkitt's lymphoma. N Engl J Med 1981; 305: 735–45.

193. Bociek RG. Adult Burkitt's lymphoma. Clin Lymphoma 2005; 6(1): 11–20.

194. Feinberg SM, Ou SH, Gu M, Shibuya TY. Burkitt's lymphoma of the base of tongue: a case report and review of literature. Ear Nose Throat J 2007; 86(6): 356–60.

Section 2: Head and Neck Cancer

7 Rare Tumors of the Larynx

Kyle Mannion,[1] Kenneth J. Niermann,[2] Joseph M. Aulino,[3] and Barbara A. Murphy[4]

[1] Department of Otolaryngology, [2] Department of Radiation Oncology, [3] Department of Radiology and Radiological Sciences, [4] Department of Medicine, Vanderbilt-Ingram Cancer Center, Vanderbilt University Medical Center, Nashville, TN, USA

Introduction

The larynx is a specialized organ that plays a critical role in vocalization, deglutition, and airway protection. Thus, cancers arising from this site have a profound impact on functionality and quality of life. There were an estimated 12,740 new cases of laryngeal cancer and 3560 deaths related to laryngeal cancer in United States in 2011.[1] Over 90% of cases are squamous cell carcinoma (SCC), with smoking and alcohol reported as the primary risk factors. Nonsquamous histopathology subtypes represent an uncommon and heterogeneous group of malignancies. This chapter aims to characterize uncommon malignancies that occur in the larynx, discuss current therapeutic considerations, and provide prognostic information.

Anatomy, presentation, and staging

The larynx is divided into three anatomical subsites based on embryological development: the *supraglottis*, which include the epiglottis, aryepiglottic folds, false vocal cords, and portions of the arytenoid cartilages, the *glottis*, which is composed of the true vocal cords, and the *subglottis*, which extends from the glottis inferiorly to the bottom of the cricoid cartilage. These subdivisions each drain to different nodal basins. See Figures 7.1–7.3.

The presenting symptoms of laryngeal cancers reflect the unique functionality of this organ. Patients commonly present with respiratory symptoms of wheezing or shortness of breath due to airway impingement by tumor. Impending airway obstruction, which is characterized by stridor and use of the accessory muscles of respiration, is not uncommon and must be treated with urgent tracheotomy. Patients may also present with cough or respiratory infections secondary to aspiration resulting from the inability to provide adequate airway protection while swallowing. Involvement of the vocal cord may result in hoarseness or changes in voice quality. Additional presenting symptoms may include dysphagia with or without weight loss, sore throat, and a neck mass. Since many of these symptoms are seen with upper respiratory tract infections or allergies, delay in diagnosis is common.

Laryngeal cancers are staged based on the TNM system. Due to the unique anatomical structures of the three laryngeal subsites, each subsite has a specific T-stage system (Table 7.1). Of note, for all three subsites, loss of vocal cord mobility corresponds to a T stage of 3. The nodal staging and overall staging system for all three subsites are the same (Tables 7.2, 7.3).

An appropriate staging workup begins with a physical examination, including careful palpation of the neck to identify nodal metastases and endoscopic visualization of the primary tumor. Most patients will undergo a direct laryngoscopy under anesthesia in order to clearly define the extent of the disease and to assess airway patency. Supplemental imaging with a computed tomography (CT) scan, magnetic resonance imaging (MRI) and/or positron emission tomography (PET)/CT scan to assess local and regional spread is considered standard for patients with locally advanced disease. In addition, a chest x-ray or chest CT is usually obtained to help exclude metastatic disease.

Imaging of the larynx

The vast majority of laryngeal tumors (SCC) arise from epithelium, and can be readily identified by the endoscopist. Most of the uncommon tumors of the larynx present primarily as a *submucosal* mass lesion, and are seen by the endoscopist as an area of fullness or asymmetry deep to the intact mucosa.[2] Cross-sectional imaging of the neck, with CT and/or MR, is used to define the submucosal extent of known epithelial tumors, for characterization of primarily submucosal lesions (tumors with an intact overlying mucosa), and for identification of regional metastatic involvement. Imaging shows the relationship of the tumor to the surrounding structures identifies cartilage involvement and aids the endoscopist in directing biopsy.

Textbook of Uncommon Cancer, Fourth Edition. Edited by Derek Raghavan, Charles D. Blanke, David H. Johnson, Paul L. Moots, Gregory H. Reaman, Peter G. Rose and Mikkael A. Sekeres.
© 2012 John Wiley & Sons, Inc. Published 2012 by John Wiley & Sons, Inc.

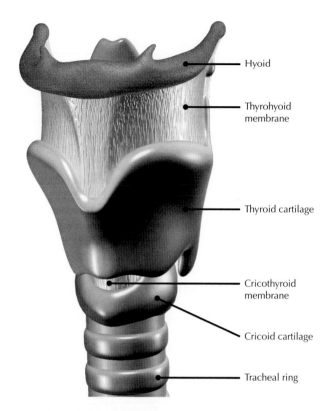

Figure 7.1 External laryngeal skeleton. Courtesy of Mark Sabo.

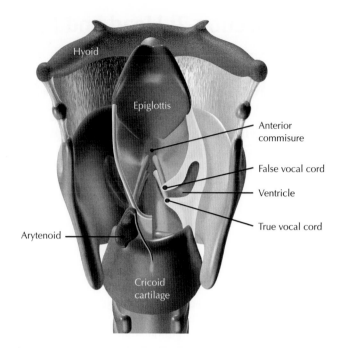

Figure 7.3 Posterior view of endolaryngeal structure. Courtesy of Mark Sabo.

Laryngeal *epithelial* tumors (SCC, spindle cell carcinoma) have a similar, nonspecific imaging appearance. Laryngeal *submucosal* tumors may display imaging characteristics that suggest a particular diagnosis, such as calcification or hypervascularity.[2] Chondrosarcoma and chondroma arise from hyaline cartilage, and 80% of tumors contain calcifications, which may be stippled or in the form of "rings and arcs,"[3] well characterized by CT imaging. These lesions are indistinguishable from each other by imaging, and may coexist within the same tumor mass. These submucosal lesions are centered in and destroy cartilage, most commonly arising in the cricoid cartilage posterior lamina.[4] These lesions usually display T2-hyperintense signal on MR images because of the high water content of hyaline cartilage.

The submucosal minor salivary gland tumors and neuroendocrine cancers mimic the appeance of epithelial neoplasm with cross-sectional imaging, without specific imaging findings to suggest a histological diagnosis.

There are a number of histology-specific behaviors that merit comments. Patients with laryngeal adenoid cystic carcinoma, most commonly arising in the subglottis, often present with locally advanced disease, and the typical imaging findings of vocal cord paralysis may be evident. Patients with adenoid cystic carcinoma chondrosarcoma and chondroma frequently recur late, so more extended surveillance may be indicated. Using CT, precise determination of the size and extent of a laryngeal chondrosarcoma can be made. MRI can aid in determining the soft tissue extent of the lesion when appropriate.[5] For mucoepidermoid cancer, careful assessment of regional nodes is critical. For patients with adenoid cystic carcinoma, screening the chest for metastatic disease with CT is advisable. There is variable uptake by adenoid cystic cancers on PET, thus their role in this tumor has yet to be defined.

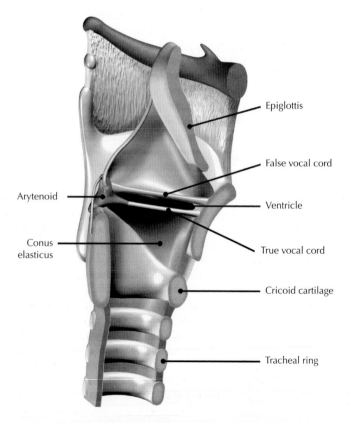

Figure 7.2 Midsagittal section of larynx. Courtesy of Mark Sabo.

Table 7.1 Primary tumor (T).

	T1	T1a	T1b	T2	T3	T4a	T4b
Supraglottis	Tumor limited to one subsite of supraglottis with normal vocal cord mobility			Tumor invades mucosa of more than one adjacent subsite of supraglottis or glottis region without fixation of the larynx.	Tumor limited to larynx with vocal cord fixation and/or invades any of the following: postcricoid area, preepiglottic space, paraglottic space, and/or inner cortex of thyroid cartilage. Moderately advanced local disease	Tumor invades through the thyroid cartilage and/or invades tissue beyond larynx (e.g. tracheo-esophagus). Very advanced local disease	Tumor invades prevertebral space, encases carotid artery, or invades mediastinal structures
Glottis	Tumor limited to the vocal cord(s) (may involve anterior or prosterior commissure) with normal vocal cord mobility	Tumor limited to one vocal cord	Tumor involves both vocal cords	Tumor extends to supraglottis and/or subglottis, and/or with impaired vocal cord mobility	Tumor limited to the larynx with vocal cord fixation and/or invasion of paraglottic space. Moderately advanced local disease	Tumor invades through the outer cortex of the thyroid cartilage and/or invades tissues beyond thyroid, or esophagus. Very advanced local disease	Tumor invades prevertebral space, encases carotid artery, or invades mediastinal structures
Subglottis	Tumor limited to the subglottis			Tumor extends to vocal cord(s) with normal or impaired mobility	Tumor limited to the larynx with vocal cord fixation	Moderately advanced local disease. Tumor invades cricoid or thyroid cartilage and/or invades tissue beyond the larynx (e.g. esophagus)	Tumor invades prevertebral fascia, encases carotid artery, or invades mediastinal structures

Table 7.2 Regional lymph nodes (N).

NX	N0	N1	N2	N2a	N2b	N2c	N3
Regional lymph nodes cannot be assessed	No regional lymph node metastasis	Metastasis in a single ipsilateral lymph node, 3 cm or less in greatest dimension	Metastasis in a single ipsilateral lymph node, more than 3 cm but not more than 6 cm in greatest bilateral or contralateral lymph nodes, none more than 6 cm in greatest dimension	Metastasis in a single ipsilateral lymph node, more than 3 cm but not more than 6 cm in greatest dimension	Metastasis in multiple ipsilateral lymph nodes, none more than 6 cm in greatest dimension	Metastasis in bilateral or contralateral lymph nodes, none more than 6 cm in greatest dimension	Metastasis in a lymph node, more than 6 cm in greatest dimension	*Note: Metastases at level VII are considered regional lymph node metastases

Pathological subtypes

Tumors of epithelial origin

Verrucous carcinoma
Epidemiology and biology
First described in 1948 by Lauren V. Ackerman,[6] verrucous carcinoma is an exophytic lesion with a papillary micronodular appearance.[7] It is a variant of SCC with specific clinical and morphological features and is felt to exist within the continuum between benign squamous hyperplasia and frank SCC. Verrucous carcinoma makes up only 1–2% of laryngeal carcinomas. The larynx is the second most common site of occurrence in the head and neck after the oral cavity.[8,9] It has been suggested that verrucous carcinomas may develop from a benign precursor.[10] A clear association has been established between the use of tobacco products and verrucous carcinoma.[11,12] Some investigators have implicated the human papillomavirus (HPV) in the pathogenesis of these tumors but the data are mixed; thus the role of HPV in verrucous carcinomas remains unclear.[13–15] Frank invasive SCC can develop from highly proliferative lesions.

Pathology
Grossly, verrucous carcinoma appears as a fungating, papillomatous, shaggy, grayish-white neoplasm (Fig. 7.4). Microscopically, it appears as a well-differentiated SCC with minimal cytological atypia. The surface of the lesion is densely keratinized with a well-circumscribed deep margin. The borders are often described

Table 7.3 Overall stage groupings.

Group	T	N	M
0	Tis	N0	M0
I	T1	N0	M0
II	T2	N0	M0
III	T3	N0	M0
	T1	N1	M0
	T2	N1	M0
	T3	N1	M0
	T4a	N0	M0
IVA	T4a	N1	M0
	T1	N2	M0
	T2	N2	M0
	T3	N2	M0
	T4a	N2	M0
	T4b	Any N	M0
IVB	Any T	N3	M0
IVC	Any T	Any N	M1

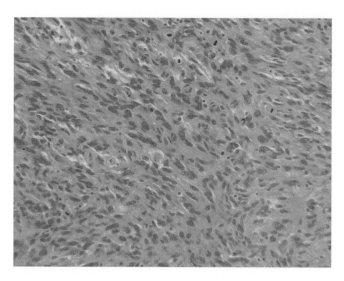

Figure 7.5 Spindle cell carcinoma of the larynx (H&E, 200×). Courtesy of Richard Prayson.

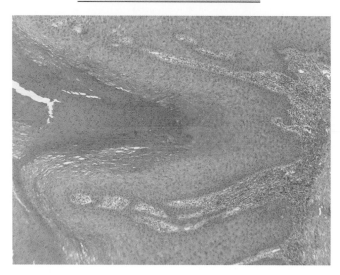

Figure 7.4 Verrucous carcinoma of the larynx (H&E, 50×). Courtesy of Richard Prayson.

as "pushing" rather than infiltrative and are usually surrounded by an inflammatory infiltrate. Mitoses are rare and the usual cytological criteria of malignancy are lacking.[8,12,15] Hybrid tumors which contain elements of both verrucous carcinoma and SCC are noted occasionally and should be treated as SCC. Failure to identify elements of SCC may occur when biopsy samples of large lesions do not contain both elements.

Clinical presentation and behavior

Most tumors present as stage I lesions.[9] Despite occasional local destruction, disease is locally contained in greater than 90% of cases.[9] Regional and distant spread of verrucous carcinoma is exceedingly rare.[16,17] Overall 5-year survival for laryngeal verrucous lesions is 86.9%. Mortality is most commonly associated with anaplastic transformation. In the past, it has been hypothesized that radiotherapy may lead to transformation to a more aggressive histopathological variant[15] but this hypothesis has been disputed.[18,19] Regardless, the primary treatment modality for resectable tumors is surgery, with radiation therapy being reserved for lesions that are

unresectable or recurrent. Five-year survival rates for patients treated with surgery was 94% versus 66% 5-year survival in patients treated with radiation alone.[9]

Spindle cell (sarcomatoid) carcinoma
Biology and epidemiology

Spindle cell (sarcomatoid) carcinomas of the larynx (Fig. 7.5) make up 1.3–2.7% of head and neck cancers.[20,21] Spindle cell carcinoma has a male-to-female ratio of 13:1, is associated with a history of tobacco use (87%) and heavy alcohol consumption (65%), and occurs most commonly in the seventh decade of life.[21] The tumor is composed of spindle and epithelial components. Theories regarding the histogenesis of this tumor include:
• originating from two synchronous tumors, a carcinoma and a sarcoma from nearby sites (collision tumor)
• originating from an undifferentiated pluripotential cell which differentiates toward both squamous epithelium and stroma (carcinosarcoma)
• the spindle cells may be a nonneoplastic reaction of the stroma to the presence of the carcinoma (pseudosarcoma)
• the spindle cells may be modified malignant epithelial cells (spindle cell carcinoma).[22]
The latter theory is currently most widely accepted. Numerous terms have been used in the literature to describe this entity: *carcinosarcoma, pseudosarcoma, pseudocarcinoma, pseudocarcinosarcoma, pseudosarcomatous carcinoma, spindle cell carcinoma, spindle cell variant of squamous carcinoma, SCC with pseudosarcoma, pleomorphic carcinoma, metaplastic carcinoma*, and *polypoid SCC*.

Pathology

Grossly, the majority of these tumors appear polypoid and rarely sessile or ulcerated. Most of these lesions are carcinomas with spindle-shaped cells. Spindle cell (sarcomatoid) carcinoma appears as a biphasic tumor composed of two components: one which is SCC (invasive or *in situ*), another composed of a bland or pleomorphic spindle cell stroma. When present, the squamous portion makes the diagnosis fairly routine. Unfortunately, this portion is often elusive. When both are clearly present, the sarcomatoid and carcinomatous components commonly abut each other with minimal areas of blending.

The sarcomatoid portion can vary in appearance such that the tumor will imitate malignant fibrous histiocytoma, leiomyosarcoma, fibrosarcoma, or fibromatosis. Immunophenotypical analysis of these tumors produces variable results. Thompson et al. noted variable staining with smooth muscle actin (32.5%), muscle-specific actin (15.4%), S-100 (4.9%), and desmin (1.6%). Epithelial markers were also variably reactive.[21] Two recent case reports have demonstrated deviation from this pattern.[23,24] These studies demonstrate that the combination of a variable microscopic appearance and variable immunostaining leads to difficulties in making this diagnosis.

Clinical presentation and behavior

In general, these tumors behave similarly to SCC and are treated in the same way. Based on staging T1–T4, 22.5%, 36.0%, 56.5%, and 66.7% of patients died, respectively.[21] These data support a worsening progress with larger lesions. Tumors occurring in patients with a history of radiation treatment appear to be more aggressive. Overall 5-year survival irrespective of tumor/node/metastasis (TNM) classification was recently found to be 58.8%.[21] 19.3% of patients developed metastatic disease: the rate varied based on laryngeal subsite (glottis 12.1%, supraglottis 35.7%, subglottis 100%).[21]

Basaloid squamous cell carcinoma
Biology and epidemiology

First described in 1928 by Montgomery[25] and characterized by Wain et al.,[26] basaloid SCC of the upper aerodigestive tract is thought to arise from the pluripotential basal cell layer of the epithelium. The typical patient is an elderly male with a history of tobacco and/or alcohol abuse. Epstein–Barr virus has been detected in three cases of nasopharyngeal basaloid squamous carcinoma, but a causative role has not yet been established.[27] Alternative terms existing in the literature include *basosquamous carcinoma* and *metatypical carcinoma*. Within the larynx, the most common subsite is the supraglottis.

Pathology

Grossly, basaloid squamous carcinoma appears as an exophytic lesion, which is sometimes ulcerated. Microscopically, the tumor is described as being composed of two portions, basaloid and squamous. The basaloid component consists of growths of small, crowded cells in a lobular arrangement, close to the mucosa. These cells have scant cytoplasm and round-to-oval nuclei with small basophilic nucleoli. Small cystic spaces containing mucinous-like material are interspersed within these lobules. Mitoses are common. The squamous component is either frank invasive SCC or foci of squamous differentiation, squamous dysplasia, or carcinoma *in situ*.[26] The tumors commonly stain for p53 with variable focal S-100 positivity. Basaloid squamous carcinoma can be confused with adenoid cystic carcinoma (particularly the solid subtype) or small cell undifferentiated (neuroendocrine)

carcinoma if not carefully examined. The identification of mitoses, nuclear pleomorphism, and necrosis points toward a diagnosis of basaloid squamous carcinoma.[28]

Clinical presentation and behavior

Basaloid squamous carcinoma is an aggressive subtype of SCC with a high incidence of nodal and distant metastases at the time of presentation.[29–31] In a study of 20 head and neck cancer patients with basaloid tumors, five patients had died of the disease and four patients were alive with the disease.[27] Recently, several reports have challenged this assertion, suggesting that this tumor behaves similarly to SCC.[32–34] In general, treatment should be administered based on principles that guide the treatment of SCC; that is, multimodality treatment should always be considered for advanced lesions.

Tumors derived from salivary glands

Adenoid cystic carcinoma
Biology and epidemiology

Adenoid cystic carcinoma is the most common malignant tumor of the minor salivary glands. There are approximately 120 cases of laryngeal adenoid cystic carcinoma reported in the literature. Males and females are equally affected. The etiology of minor salivary gland tumors is unclear but several factors have been postulated to play a role. These include lead, asbestos, alcohol, and ionizing radiation.[35,36] The subglottis is the most common subsite.[29] For laryngeal adenoid cystic cancers, the survival rates vary. Alavi reported 2-year and 5-year survival rates of 100% and 75%, respectively.[37] In contrast, Mahlstedt reported a 5-year survival rate of 33%.[38] These variations are likely due to small sample sizes of this rare lesion.

Pathology

Grossly, the lesions usually appear as exophytic masses with intact mucosal coverage. Batsakis initially defined four histopathological patterns: cribiform, tubular (glandular), solid, and hyaline (cylindromatous).[39] These patterns were refined by the creation of a grading system for adenoid cystic carcinoma. Grade I is predominantly tubular, grade II is cribiform, and grade III is solid.[4,39] The usual microscopic pattern is described as cribiform with nests and columns of bland cells arranged concentrically around gland-like spaces filled with periodic acid-Schiff (PAS)-positive material. True glands may also be seen (Fig. 7.6).

Clinical presentation and behavior

Adenoid cystic carcinomas have a distinct behavior pattern. This tends to be a very slow growing tumor and survival is often measured in decades rather than years. Perineural invasion with skip lesions and a submucosal growth pattern are hallmarks of this tumor. Thus, this tumor is often diagnosed when it is locally advanced and local recurrences are common.[40] Unlike most epidermoid cancers, nodal spread to regional lymph nodes is uncommon and is most common in tumors with a solid pattern.[40,41] Neck dissections are therefore reserved for patients with clinically abnormal nodes or pathologically proven nodal metastases.[42] Over time, adenoid cystic

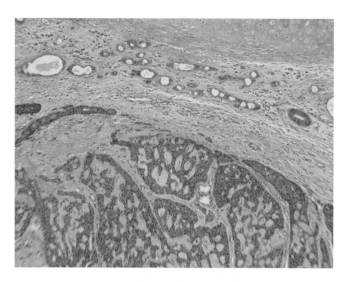

Figure 7.6 Adenoid cystic carcinoma of the larynx (H&E, 100×). Courtesy of Richard Prayson.

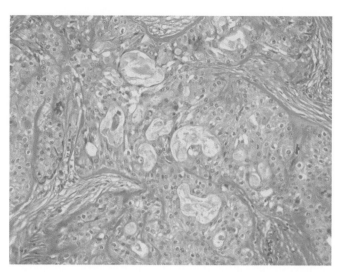

Figure 7.7 Mucoepidermoid carcinoma of the larynx (H&E, 200×). Courtesy of Richard Prayson.

carcinomas frequently develop distant metastases. Common sites include the lungs (most common), bone, and liver.

Mucoepidermoid carcinoma
Biology and epidemiology

These tumors are believed to develop from ductal components of the submucosal salivary glands.[37] The most common sites include the floor of the laryngeal ventricle, the false vocal folds, and the anterior commissure. The true vocal cords are rarely involved.[38] Males and patients aged 40–80 years are more commonly affected.[43]

Pathology

Mucoepidermoid carcinomas are composed of several different cell types, which include clear cells, mucoid cells, columnar cells, epidermoid cells, and intermediate cells (Fig. 7.7). The classification and grading of the tumor depend on the relative presence of each cell type.[39] Mucoepidermoid carcinomas have been divided into three different grades: low, intermediate, and high. Low-grade mucoepidermoid carcinoma is composed of well-formed glandular or cystic spaces lined by a single layer of mucin-producing cells and flattened epidermoid cells. Low-grade tumors do not feature pleomorphism or mitoses. Intermediate-grade tumors have a greater tendency to form solid nests of cells. They are more cellular and pleomorphic with greater numbers of intermediate cells and occasional mitoses. High-grade mucoepidermoid tumors exhibit depletion of mucoid elements. There are numerous mitoses and solid nests of intermediate or epidermoid cells.[44] This lesion is often difficult to distinguish from SCC.[41]

Behavior and treatment

Laryngeal mucoepidermoid carcinoma occurs most commonly in the supraglottis where the density of minor salivary glands is highest. The behavior of mucoepidermoid cancers is highly variable depending on the histological grade. Low-grade lesions are less likely to spread to regional lymph nodes or distant sites. Patients with intermediate- or high-grade mucoepidermoid

carcinoma frequently present with cervical metastases. Thus, the diagnostic workup needs to be tailored to fit the individual patient. Patients with high-grade lesions have a propensity for the development of metastatic disease. Five-year survival has been reported as 100% for low-grade tumors but only 53% at 3 years for patients with high-grade mucoepidermoid carcinoma.[40]

Lesions of mesenchymal origin
Chondrosarcoma
Biology and epidemiology

Chondrosarcoma is the most common nonepithelial tumor of the larynx (Fig. 7.8), comprising 0.1–1% of all laryngeal neoplasms.[42,45–47] The etiology of chondrosarcoma is unclear. Its occurrence has been described following Teflon injections and radiation therapy.[48–51] Smoking is not considered to be an etiological factor.[46] The occurrence of chondrosarcoma is associated with ossification of the laryngeal cartilages. Because ossification commences at sites of muscle insertion (the posterior cricoid ring and the posterior thyroid lamina), chondrosarcomas occur more commonly in these areas.[45,46,52,53] The timing of cartilaginous ossification also determines the age range for this tumor. Ossification begins in the third decade of life and increases with old age.[54] As a result, patients between ages 50 and 80 years are most commonly affected but tumors have been reported in patients as young as 33 and as old as 91.[55–57]

It has been suggested that the majority of chondrosarcomas are juxtaposed with benign chondromas that have been exposed to a degree of ischemia. Thompson and Gannon noted that the ischemic areas were usually found directly abutting chondrosarcoma.[46] This occurred in 62% of the tumors in their study.

Pathology

Grossly, both chondroma and chondrosarcoma appear as smooth, firm lesions.[45,52] The distinction between chondroma and chondrosarcoma is a difficult one to make. This often comes down to personal interpretation.[46] Chondromas of the laryngeal

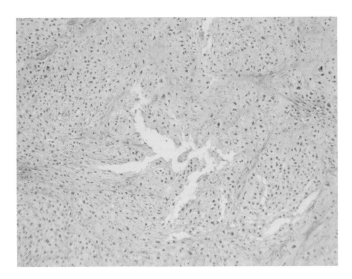

Figure 7.8 Chondrosarcoma of the larynx (H&E, 100×). Courtesy of Richard Prayson.

cartilages will resemble normal cartilage, but the nuclei are often larger.[58–60] Low-grade chondrosarcomas often contain chondroma patterns within them. Therefore, a single biopsy of a cartilaginous tumor may not provide adequate tumor sampling. Evans described cells with plump nuclei, more than one cell with two such nuclei, giant cartilage cells with large single or multiple nuclei, or cells with clumps of chromatin. They grouped chondrosarcoma into grades I (well differentiated), II (moderately differentiated), and III (poorly differentiated).[61] The subdivisions are based on mitotic rate, cellularity, and nuclear size. Well-differentiated lesions often show only focal areas that meet criteria for malignancy. In contrast, malignant features are present in a greater area of moderate and high-grade tumors.

Additional subtypes of chondrosarcoma are dedifferentiated chondrosarcoma, clear cell chondrosarcoma, and myxoid chondrosarcoma. Dedifferentiated chondrosarcoma is also known as chondrosarcoma with additional malignant mesenchymal component (CAMMC). It is considered a grade III lesion. These lesions demonstrate an abrupt transition into a malignant, highly cellular proliferation with a high mitotic count. Clear cell chondrosarcoma is extremely rare in the larynx with only three cases reported. It is characterized by rounded cells with a predominantly clear cytoplasm with a sparse intervening matrix. Two of the described cases involved recurrences but no distant metastases have been described.[48,62,63] Myxoid chondrosarcoma features a myxoid background matrix production with the neoplastic chondrocytes arranged in a "string of pearls" distribution while including other required features of chondrosarcoma. It is required that >10% of the lesion demonstrate this pattern to be considered a myxoid chondrosarcoma.[46] These lesions are designated as grade II tumors. Thompson and Gannon note that this designation did significantly affect patient outcome.[46]

Clinical presentation and behavior

Within the larynx, chondrosarcoma most commonly occurs in the cricoid cartilage, followed by the thyroid cartilage.

Chondrosarcomas of the arytenoid cartilages and epiglottis are rare.[46,53] Because chondroma and chondrosarcoma are slow-growing lesions, symptoms develop slowly over time. These tumors most commonly demonstrate local growth and destruction. Regional and distant metastases are rare, but have been reported.[46] Survival following treatment of laryngeal chondrosarcoma is generally quite good. Rinaldo reported a 5-year survival rate of 90%.[52] A larger study noted overall survival of 96.3% at an average follow-up of 10.9 years. In this study, 5-year and 10-year disease-free survival rates were 78.9% and 47.8%, respectively.[46] Interestingly, 5-year survival rates for grade I, II, and III tumors were reported as 78%, 79% and 100%, respectively. Increasing tumor grade is associated with a higher risk of recurrence but does not seem to affect overall survival.

Lesions of neuroendocrine origin

Neuroendocrine carcinoma
Biology and epidemiology

Currently, neuroendocrine tumors are divided into the following subgroups: *well-differentiated neuroendocrine carcinoma (NEC) (true carcinoid), moderately differentiated NEC (MDNEC) (atypical carcinoid), and poorly differentiated NEC (small cell carcinoma)*. Moderately differentiated tumors, which are intermediate between the other (less common) extremes of NEC, make up the bulk of laryngeal NEC. Indeed, 90% of laryngeal NEC is moderately differentiated. The well-differentiated subtype is the least common.[49] The histogenesis of laryngeal NEC is unknown. The only well-documented neuroendocrine structure present in the larynx is the paraganglion. However, paragangliomas are much less common when compared to NEC.[49] A recent study aimed at identifying additional neuroendocrine cells in the larynx was successful but these cells do not appear to be the precursors of NEC.[50] NEC most commonly occurs in the sixth or seventh decade with a predilection for males. Within the larynx, the supraglottis is most commonly affected. Affected patients commonly have a history of tobacco use.

Pathology

The microscopic appearance of NEC varies based on the level of differentiation. In many cases, diagnosis is aided by the use of immunohistochemistry with both neuroendocrine and epithelial markers. Well-differentiated NEC of the larynx is characterized by cell nests composed of uniform cells separated by a fibrovascular or hyalinized connective tissue stroma. The nuclei are round or oval with a vesicular or stippled chromatin pattern and eosinophilic cytoplasm. These tumors demonstrate epithelial mucin staining and argyrophilia in addition to cytokeratin, chromogranin, and neuron-specific enolase positivity. On ultrastructural definition, abundant neurosecretory granules, cellular junctional complexes, and inter- and intracellular lumina are seen.

Moderately differentiated NEC is polypoid or nodular, displaying varying degrees of surface ulceration. The tumor is submucosal and growth characteristics including glandular, organoid, trabecular, acinar, solid, and nesting patterns are present. Light microscopic features of this tumor may be nonspecific. Combinations of patterns are frequently reported within the same specimen. Delicate fibrovascular or hyaline stroma separates nests of tumor. The tumor cells are large, round, or polyhedral, containing eosinophilic cytoplasm with a round-to-oval pleomorphic, eccentrically placed nucleus with a stippled chromatin pattern. Nucleoli may be present. Perineural, perivascular, and perilymphatic involvement is common. However, vascular or lymphatic invasion is rare. Histochemical, immunocytochemical, and ultrastructural examination of MDNEC demonstrates both epithelial and neuroendocrine differentiation. Neurosecretory granules are common but not abundant.[51,64,65]

Calcitonin is a useful immunohistochemical marker in moderately differentiated lesions. Calcitonin expression is reported to be as high as 80% in this subtype.[66] In cases where calcitonin expression is present, the tumor may appear similar to medullary thyroid carcinoma.

Poorly differentiated NEC lesions are characterized by sheets of undifferentiated small cells with minimal cytoplasm and pleomorphic, hyperchromatic nuclei with delicate chromatin and absent or inconspicuous nucleoli. Mitoses and individual cell necrosis are common. Vascular and perineural invasion are also quite common. Compared to the better differentiated neuroendocrine tumors, the special histochemical, immunochemical, and ultrastructural investigations are less uniform due to the undifferentiated nature of this tumor type; nevertheless, evidence of both epithelial and neuroendocrine differentiation is clear.[64] Scant neurosecretory granules are present.

Clinical presentation and behavior

The pattern of behavior of laryngeal NEC with regard to local recurrence and distant metastases varies based on tumor differentiation. Well-differentiated tumors generally have an indolent course and are treated with surgery.[67,68] Moderately differentiated tumors have a greater tendency toward local recurrence and metastatic disease. These tumors, like the well-differentiated subtype, are considered chemo- and radio-resistant. Surgery is the primary form of therapy and total laryngectomy is often necessary for all but small lesions.[69] Poorly differentiated tumors are much more aggressive and commonly metastasize to the bone, liver, lungs, brain, and adrenal glands.[70] Transient response is seen after treatment with several cytotoxic agents, including the platinum complexes, etoposide, the taxanes, gemcitabine, and ifosfamide. A specific role for neoadjuvant or adjuvant chemotherapy, while attractive in principle, has not been defined. Mean survival for patients with poorly differentiated NEC is less than 1 year.[70]

An unusual feature of laryngeal NEC is the predilection for cutaneous and subcutaneous metastases.[71,72] This type of metastasis can occur regardless of tumor grade. It has been suggested that the occurrence of cutaneous metastases is related to dedifferentiation of a portion of the primary tumor. Prognosis for these patients is poor.[71] It is important to differentiate these metastases from primary Merkel cell carcinoma and metastatic visceral undifferentiated small cell carcinoma.

Treatment considerations

Overview

Preservation of function is of great importance in patients with laryngeal cancers, so the critical treatment question for any histological subtype is to determine whether a function preservation approach is feasible. In order to make this determination, it must be established whether the tumor is radiation sensitive or not. If it is not, then primary surgery is the only curative treatment option. Earlier stages of disease may be amenable to a function-sparing surgical approach. If the tumor is advanced, the only curative option may be total laryngectomy with or without radiation-based adjuvant therapy.

Decision making for radiation-sensitive tumors is more complex. Early-stage disease may be amenable to curative, function-sparing treatment with either surgery or radiation. Under these circumstances, the long-term effects of therapy will help guide the patient's decision making. For those patients with locally advanced disease, two options may be considered: surgery followed by adjuvant radiation (with or without chemotherapy) or chemoradiation. Chemoradiation is often the choice for function preservation but in selected patients, function-sparing surgery may be an option. When both radiation and surgical function preservation approaches are options, the choice of therapy is once again based on anticipated side-effects. General prejudice is that surgical approaches are associated with increased toxicity but this is not always the case. Chemoradiation therapy in the treatment of squamous cell carcinoma of the larynx has been proven to carry a 43% rate of severe late toxicity[73] and the radiation dose delivered to structures in the upper aerodigestive tract has been shown to have a significant adverse impact on long-term function. Specifically, increased dose to the aryepiglottic folds, false vocal folds, and lateral pharyngeal walls correlates with increased weight loss and worse quality of life scores.[74] Surgery should be considered if functional debility can be limited by avoiding high-dose radiation to the pharynx. Finally, if surgery and radiation therapy are both expected to be part of the patient's treatment, surgery should be performed first to avoid increased risk of healing problems.

Surgical considerations

Once the decision has been made to undertake a surgical treatment approach, the anatomical extent of a given tumor dictates which surgical options are available, and consequently the functional impact of surgery. The primary surgical options are transoral partial laryngectomy, open partial laryngectomy, and total laryngectomy.

The key questions that the head and neck surgeon can answer are: is the tumor amenable to laryngeal preservation surgery (partial laryngectomy), and if so, will the extent of partial laryngectomy provide a lesser functional impact on the patient than total laryngectomy? The intuitive answer to the second question is that partial laryngectomy will always be better for the patient than total laryngectomy, but this is often not the case. There are specific patient-related and tumor-related factors that predict better outcome with a total laryngectomy, even when surgical laryngeal preservation is possible. Specifically, glottic tumor involvement and particularly arytenoid involvement should temper the consideration of partial laryngetomy. True vocal cord resection always produces a negative impact on the voice and often on swallowing as well. If the supraglottic structures and both arytenoids can be preserved, aspiration is rarely a problem and the patient can be taught to phonate with the false vocal folds with acceptable voice quality.

Many surgeons have performed partial laryngectomy with resection of one arytenoid, but very careful patient selection is necessary. While arytenoid involvement doesn't preclude partial laryngectomy, the impact on speech and swallowing can be significant. Similarly, a patient with limited pulmonary reserve has a limited ability to cope with a partial laryngectomy as virtually every partial resection carries some risk of aspiration. Partial laryngectomy should be undertaken in these patients only with careful patient selection and extensive counseling. In all cases, the patient must know that total laryngectomy may become the only option based on surgical findings and intraoperative frozen section analysis. They must also know of the potential for aspiration and/or a nonfunctional laryngeal remnant, which could lead to total laryngectomy at a later date.

Functional outcome with surgical intervention

It is important to discuss functional outcome after total laryngectomy with patients. Gadepalli et al.[75] recently showed that 95% of patients undergoing total laryngectomy rated their voice as good postoperatively versus 5% whose voice was poor or absent. Similarly, 3–5% were limited to a liquid diet (either by mouth or gastrostomy tube) while the other 95–97% tolerated a soft or regular diet by mouth. These authors showed an obvious decrease in functional outcomes when total pharyngectomy was also required in addition to a total laryngectomy.

Differing partial laryngectomy techniques carry different functional outcomes. Advancement of both technology and surgical technique over the past two decades has led to a significant transition from open partial laryngectomy to transoral approaches (with laser, robotic, or traditional instruments) for tumors amenable to laryngeal preservation. The difference between these techniques and their applications is beyond the scope of this discussion, as they are, at their most basic level, different tools to accomplish the same end. What is important to know is that as transoral techniques have evolved, they have produced better functional outcomes than open partial laryngectomy.[76]

Generally, supraglottic tumors should be considered good candidates for primary surgery in patients without significant comorbidities, particularly pulmonary disease. Voice outcomes are generally excellent, but swallowing may be impaired. While most supraglottic laryngectomees aspirate, the rate of aspiration pneumonia after transoral supraglottic resection is low at 0–11.5%.[77–79] Supracricoid laryngectomy is a very oncologically sound procedure that resects both vocal cords, most of the thyroid cartilage, and the whole supraglottis if necessary. Patients achieve a significantly altered but functional voice and, like supraglottic laryngectomy, a moderate risk of

aspiration. In an analysis of over 450 patients undergoing supracricoid laryngectomy, Benito et al.[80] found an 11.6% risk of aspiration pneumonia. Thirty-four percent had a temporary gastrostomy tube (for a mean duration of 8 months), 1.6% of patients required a permanent gastrostomy tube, and 3.7% required total laryngectomy. The resection of one arytenoid was significantly associated with both permanent feeding tube use and conversion to total laryngectomy. Many other variations of partial laryngectomy exist that are tailored to the particular location of a given tumor.

Special considerations for histological subtypes

The specific tumor types often guide the treating physicians to surgical or nonsurgical therapy. Many of these issues have been addressed above.

In general, low-grade tumors that carry high cure rates with surgical resection should always be considered for surgical management. Verrucous carcinoma tends to be exophytic and carries a low rate of metastasis, and should be treated with primary transoral resection when possible. Even if total laryngectomy is necessary, this can often be a single modality treatment. Similarly, low-grade mucoepidermoid carcinoma should be treated in the same fashion. This tumor's propensity to occur in the supraglottis typically makes it amenable to transoral resection techniques. Low-grade chondrosarcomas pose a somewhat unique surgical disease. These tumors tend to grow slowly and carry very low rates of metastasis. If only the anterior cricoid is involved, cricotracheal resection may be curative but when the posterior cricoid is involved, total larygectomy is typically the treatment of choice. The indolent nature of the disease allows for at least temporary and often permanent avoidance of total laryngectomy by debulking the tumor transorally with narrow margins.[81] This carries a relatively high rate of local recurrence (20%).[82] These recurrences can often be treated with repeat debulking. Eventually, the airway compromise can no longer be relieved in this fashion, or the cricoarytenoid joints become involved and total laryngectomy becomes the only option.

High-grade tumors or those that tend to be locally invasive require more aggressive surgical management that mimics the management of squamous cell carcinoma of the larynx. Finally, tumors that carry a high risk of regional metastases should undergo neck dissection. In the N0 neck, a 20% risk of occult metastases is a good rule of thumb as an indication for neck dissection. In most of these cases, the risk of bilateral neck disease must be considered in treatment planning.

Radiation considerations

The principles in planning radiation therapy for squamous cell carcinoma of the hypopharynx and larynx are also applicable to the treatment of the rarer malignancies that involve this region. The coverage volumes and techniques that are applied for squamous cell cancers, including conventional three-dimensional radiation therapy and intensity-modulated radiation therapy, may also be applied to other less common histologies, with some important distinctions.

Dose considerations for radiation therapy

As is the case for squamous cell carcinoma, radiation doses are prescribed based on the specifications of a given tumor. When gross, unresected disease is present, whether at the primary site or at a site of nodal spread, the target dose for therapy is 70 gray. For sites that have been resected but where there is still residual disease, or if there are features suggesting a high risk of recurrence, 60 gray is administered. At-risk nodal regions without evidence of active disease are treated with a prophylactic dose of 50 gray.

Lymph node volumes at risk according to anatomical subsite

With cancers of the laryngeal region, it is very important to consider the rich network of lymphatic structures that provide drainage and are therefore at risk for regional spread. Given the lack of any large clinical studies detailing the nodal drainage pattern of laryngeal cancers of rare histologies, many clinicians extrapolate the nodal drainage patterns from squamous cell carcinoma to determine which nodal regions are at risk for the rarer histologies. For tumors involving the supraglottis, the lymphatic channels at risk include the bilateral jugular chain. The supraglottis is a midline structure and has significant risk of neoplastic spread bilaterally. The cervical nodes that are most frequently involved are those at leves II, II, and IV. Levels IA, IB, and V are seldom involved.[83–85] Tumors involving the subglottis have a less, but still significant risk for lymph node involvement. Here, the regions at highest risk include the prelaryngeal, pretracheal, and supraclavicular nodal regions.[86] Unlike the regions of the supraglottis and subglottis, the true vocal cords are nearly devoid of lymphatic capillaries. T1 and T2 lesions have a less than 2% risk for node metastases, while the risk approaches 20% for T3 lesions and 30% for T4 lesions, especially when the tumor spreads into the lymphatic-rich regions of the subglottis or supraglottis.[87]

Special considerations for histological subtypes

Verrucous carcinoma

The most common variant of squamous cell carcinoma involving the larynx, verrucous carcinoma is considered to have a relatively low metastatic potential. Radiation therapy is usually reserved for larger tumors, including T3 and T4 lesions. In these cases, only the primary tumor is covered with radiation therapy, with little need for prophylactic radiation coverage of regional lymph nodes. When radiation is used as primary treatment, about a third of the patients have local relapse; in these cases nearly all patients can be salvaged surgically, with a 97% 5-year disease-specific survival.[88]

Spindle cell (sarcomatoid) carcinoma

These tumors are typically small and may be treated with radiation alone. For larger lesions which require total laryngectomy, postoperative radiation therapy to the primary site is frequently indicated.[89]

Basaloid squamous cell carcinoma

These tumors should be regarded as a subtype of squamous cell cancers with a highly aggressive behavior pattern. Thus, the radiation treatment approach to these tumors is practically the same as that for squamous cell carcinoma, namely multimodal chemoradiation, with radiation covering the primary tumor site, as well as cervical lymph nodes at risk.[90,91]

Adenoid cystic carcinoma

There is a strong role for postoperative radiation therapy in these tumors, owing to their high potential for perineural invasion. Standard radiation fields are modified to cover areas of local extension, as well as perineural spread, as these tumors can track along cranial nerves to the base of the skull. Specifically, if a named cranial nerve is involved in these tumors, this must be encapsulated within the radiation portal. In these cases, brachytherapy may be employed to replace or augment external beam radiotherapy to minimize normal tissue morbidity.[92]

Mucoepidermoid carcinoma

This typically low-grade, slow-growing, and well-circumscribed cancer can usually be effectively treated by surgery alone. In the high-grade variants, there is an increased risk of lymph node spread and it is appropriate to administer adjuvant radiation therapy to the primary tumor site and nodal volumes at risk.[93,94]

Chondrosarcoma

Radiation treatment for this histology is considered less effective than surgery and is thus reserved for patients who are not candidates for surgical resection. There is generally low malignant potential for nodal spread; thus, when radiation therapy is indicated, radiotherapy volumes are limited to the area of primary disease, without prophylactic radiation to regional lymph nodes. To effectively reach local control, radiation doses should be 60 gray or higher.[95]

Neuroendocrine carcinoma

For well-differentiated neuroendocrine tumors involving the larynx, radiation therapy is usually only indicated when a complete resection is not possible. Prophylactic regional lymph nodes are not typically included in the radiation treatment volume. For the moderately or poorly differentiated tumors of this subtype, radiation therapy may be used for locally advanced disease with or without the addition of chemotherapy.

Chemotherapy considerations

Studies evaluating the role of chemotherapy in laryngeal cancer with nonsquamous histologies are lacking. Clearly, systemic chemotherapy is the treatment of choice for patients with metastatic or recurrent noncurable disease. The role of chemotherapy becomes more unclear in patients with locally advanced disease. In general, one extrapolates from data from other disease sites where the specific histological subtype is most commonly found. For example, verrucous carcinoma, spindle cell carcinoma and basaloid squamous carcinomas behave in a manner which is most similar to squamous cell carcinoma of the head and neck. Thus, in patients with locally advanced disease who are treated with radiation therapy for curative intent, induction and/or concurrent chemotherapy may be considered using agents such as cisplatin, carboplatin, paclitaxel, docetaxel, and 5-fluorouracil (5-FU). For patients with locally advanced, poorly differentiated neuroendocrine tumors, treatment with cisplatin and etoposide may be considered as adjunctive to radiation therapy. When making a decision to add chemotherapy to either primary or adjunctive radiation, the potential for treatment benefit must be carefully weighed against the established increase in acute and late toxicities.

Conclusion

The rare tumors of the larynx discussed in this chapter are a diverse group of malignancies with unique characteristics. Careful consideration of the relevant differential diagnoses generally helps determine the correct diagnosis. Because these tumors are uncommon, treatment parameters are less well defined. When possible, conservation surgery or a radiation-based approach should be attempted to spare function. Still, treatment of the more aggressive, radiation-resistant tumors may require laryngectomy in order to eradicate disease.

References

1. Siegel R, Ward E, Brawley O, Jermal A. The impact of eliminating socioeconomic and racial disparities on premature cancer deaths. CA Cancer J 2011; 61: 212–36.
2. Becker M, Burkhardt K, Dulguerov P, Allal A. Imaging of the larynx and hypopharynx. Eur J Radiol 2008, 66: 460–79.
3. Burggraaff BA, Weinstein GA. Chondrosarcoma of the larynx. Ann Otol Rhinol Laryngol 1992; 101: 183–4.
4. Thompson LDR, Gannon FH. Chondrosarcoma of the larynx: a clinico-pathologic study of 111 cases with a review of the literature. Am J Surg Pathol 2002; 26: 836–51.
5. Mishell JH, Schild JA, Mafee MF. Chondrosarcoma of the larynx. Diagnosis with magnetic resonance imaging and computed tomography. Arch Otolaryngol Head Neck Surg 1990; 116: 1338–41.
6. Ackerman LV. Verrucous carcinoma of the oral cavity. Surgery 1948; 23: 670–8.
7. Lawson W, Biller HF, Suen JY. Cancer of the larynx. In: Myers EN, Suen JY (eds) Cancer of the Head and Neck. New York: Churchil Livingstone, 1989. pp. 533–93.
8. Batsakis JG. Tumors of the Head and Neck. Clinical and Pathological Considerations, 2nd edn. Baltimore, MD: Williams and Wilkins, 1979.
9. Koch BB, et al. Commission on cancer, American College of Surgeons. American Cancer Society. National survey of head and neck verrucous carcinoma: patterns of presentation, care, and outcome. Cancer 2001; 92(1): 110–20.
10. Ishiyama A, et al. Papillary squamous neoplasms of the head and neck. Laryngoscope 1994; 104: 1446–52.
11. Spiro R. Verrucous carcinoma, then and now. Am J Surg 1998; 175: 393–7.
12. Ferlito A, Recher G. Ackerman's tumor (verrucous carcinoma) of the larynx: a clinicopathologic study of 77 cases. Cancer 1980; 7(46): 1617–30.
13. Miyamoto T, et al. Association of cutaneous verrucous carcinoma with human papillomavirus type 16. Br J Dermatol 1999; 140(1): 168–9.
14. Lubbe J, et al. HPV-11 and HPV-16-associated oral verrucous carcinoma. Dermatology 1996; 192: 217–21.
15. Fliss DM, et al. Laryngeal verrucous carcinoma: a clinicopathologic study and detection of human papillomavirus using polymerase chain reaction. Laryngoscope 1994; 104: 146–52.
16. McCaffrey TV, Witte M, Ferguson MT. Verrucous carcinoma of the larynx. Ann Otol Rhinol Laryngol 1998; 107: 391–5.
17. Orvidas LJ, et al. Verrucous carcinoma of the larynx: a review of 53 patients. Head Neck 1998; 20: 197–203.
18. Ferlito A, Rinaldo A, Mannara GM. Is primary radiotherapy an appropriate option for the treatment of verrucous carcinoma of the head and neck? J Laryngol Otol 1998; 112: 132–9.
19. Tharp ME, Shidnia H. Radiotherapy in the treatment of verrucous carcinoma of the head and neck. Laryngoscope 1995; 104: 391–6.
20. Howell JH, Hyams VJ, Sprinkle PM. Spindle cell carcinomas of the nose and paranasal sinuses. Surg Forum 1978; 29: 565–8.
21. Thompson LDR, et al. Spindle cell (sarcomatoid) carcinomas of the larynx. Am J Surg Pathol 2002; 26: 153–70.
22. Friedmann I, Pyris J. The larynx in systemic pathology. In: Symmers WS, Symmers C (eds) Nose, Throat and Ears, 3rd edn. Edinburgh: Churchill Livingstone, 1986.
23. Miyahara H, et al. Spindle cell carcinoma of the larynx. Auris Nasus Larynx 2004; 31: 177–82.
24. Marioni G, et al. Spindle-cell tumors of the larynx: diagnostic pitfalls. A case report and review of the literature. Acta Otolaryngol 2003; 123: 86–90.
25. Montgomery H. Dermatopathology. New York: Harper and Row, 1967.
26. Wain SL, et al. Basaloid squamous carcinoma of the tongue, hypopharynx, and larynx. Hum Pathol 1986; 17: 1158–66.
27. Paulino AFG, et al. Basaloid squamous cell carcinoma of the head and neck. Laryngoscope 2000; 110: 1479–82.
28. Eryilmaz A, et al. Basaloid squamous cell carcinoma of the larynx. J Laryngol Otol 2002; 116: 52–3.
29. Ferlito A, et al. Basaloid squamous cell carcinoma of the larynx and hypopharynx. Ann Otol Rhinol Laryngol 1997; 106: 1024–35.
30. Raslan WF, et al. Basaloid squamous cell carcinoma of the head and neck: a clinicopathological and flow cytometric study of 10 new cases with review of the English literature. Am J Otolaryngol 1994; 15: 204–11.
31. Bahar G, et al. Basaloid squamous carcinoma of the larynx. Am J Otolaryngol 2003; 24: 204–8.
32. Bracero F, et al. Hypopharynx and larynx basaloid squamous carcinoma: our experience with 6 cases. Acta Otorrinolaringol Esp 2001; 52: 229–36.
33. Luna MA, et al. Basaloid squamous carcinoma of the upper aero-digestive tract: clinicopathologic and DNA flow cytometric analysis. Cancer 1990; 66: 537–42.
34. Erisen LM, et al. Basaloid squamous cell carcinoma of the larynx: a report of four new cases. Laryngoscope 2004; 114: 1179–83.
35. Ellis GL, Auclair PL, Gnepp DR. Surgical Pathology of the Salivary Glands. Philadelphia: WB Saunders, 1991.
36. Spitz MR, et al. Salivary gland cancer. A case-controlled investigation of risk factors. Arch Otolaryngol Head Neck Surg 1990; 116: 1163–6.
37. Alavi S, et al. Glandular carcinoma of the larynx: the UCLA experience. Ann Otol Rhinol Laryngol 1999; 108: 485–9.
38. Mahlstedt K, Ussmuller J, Donath K. Malignant sialogenic tumours of the larynx. J Laryngol Otol 2002; 116: 119–22.
39. Batsakis JG, Luna MA, El-Naggar A. Histopathologic grading of salivary gland neoplasms: III. Adenoid cystic carcinoma. Ann Otol Rhinol Laryngol 1990; 99: 1007–9.
40. Damiani JM, et al. Mucoepidermoid-adenosquamous carcinoma of the larynx and hypopharynx: a report of 21 cases and review of the literature. Otolaryngol Head Neck Surg 1981; 89: 235–43.
41. Cumberworth VL, et al. Mucoepidermoid carcinoma of the larynx. J Laryngol Otol 1989; 103: 420–3.
42. Saleh HM, et al. Laryngeal chondrosarcoma: a report of five cases. Eur Arch Otorhinolaryngol 2002; 259: 211–16.
43. Shonai T, et al. Mucoepidermoid carcinoma of the larynx: a case which responded completely to radiotherapy and a review of the literature. Jap J Clin Oncol 1998; 28: 339–42.
44. Healy WV, Persin KH, Smith L. Mucoepidermoid carcinoma of salivary gland origin. Classification, clinicopathologic correlations, and results of treatment. Cancer 1970; 26: 368–88.
45. Uygur K, et al. Chondrosarcoma of the thyroid cartilage. J Laryngol Otol 2001; 115: 507–9.

46. Thompson LDR, Gannon FH. Chondrosarcoma of the larynx: a clinicopathologic study of 111 cases with a review of the literature. Am J Surg Pathol 2002; 26: 836–51.

47. Wang SJ, et al. Chondroid tumors of the larynx: computed tomographic findings. Am J Otolaryngol 1999; 20: 379–82.

48. Said S, et al. Clear cell chondrosarcoma of the larynx. Otolaryngol Head Neck Surg 2001; 125: 107–8.

49. Ferlito A, Shaha AR, Rinaldo A. Neuroendocrine neoplasms of the larynx: diagnosis, treatment and prognosis. ORL 2002; 64: 108–13.

50. Chung JH, et al. Neuroendocrine carcinomas of the larynx and an examination of non-neoplastic larynx tissue for neuroendocrine tissue for neuroendocrine cells. Laryngoscope 2004; 114: 1264–70.

51. El-Naggar AK. Laryngeal neuroendocrine carcinoma: victims of semantics. Arch Pathol Lab Med 1992; 116: 237–8.

52. Rinaldo A, Howard DJ, Ferlito A. Laryngeal chondrosarcoma: a 24-year experience at the Royal National Throat, Nose and Ear Hospital. Acta Otolaryngol 2000; 120: 680–8.

53. Thome R, Thome DC, de la Cortina RA. Long-term follow-up of cartilaginous tumors of the larynx. Otolaryngol Head Neck Surg 2001; 124: 634–40.

54. Baatenburg de Jong RJ, van Lent S, Hogendoorn PCW. Chondroma and chondrosarcoma of the larynx. Curr Opin Otolaryngol Head Neck Surg 2004; 12: 98–105.

55. Nicolai P, et al. Laryngeal chondrosarcoma: incidence, pathology, biological behavior and treatment. Ann Otol Rhinol Laryngol 1990; 99: 515–23.

56. Lavertu P, Tucker HM. Chondrosarcoma of the larynx: case report and management philosophy. Ann Otol Rhinol Laryngol 1984; 93: 452–6.

57. Cantrell RW, et al. Conservative surgical treatment of chondrosarcoma of the larynx. Ann Otol Rhinol Laryngol 1980; 89: 567–71.

58. Batsakis JG, Raymond AK. Cartilage tumors of the larynx. South Med J 1988; 81: 481–4.

59. Chiu LD, Rasgon BM. Laryngeal chondroma: a benign process with long-term implications. Ear Nose Throat J 1996; 75: 540–9.

60. Devaney KO, Ferlito A, Silver CE. Cartilaginous tumors of the larynx. Ann Otol Rhinol Laryngol 1995; 104: 251–5.

61. Evans HL, Ayala AG, Romsdahl MM. Prognostic factors in chondrosarcoma of bone: a clinicopathologic analysis with emphasis on histologic grading. Cancer 1977; 40: 818–31.

62. Kleist B, et al. Clear cell chondrosarcoma of the larynx: a case report of a rare histologic variant in an uncommon localization. Am J Surg Pathol 2002; 26: 386–92.

63. Obenauer S, et al. Unusual chondrosarcoma of the larynx: CT findings. Eur Radiol 1999; 9: 1625–8.

64. Millroy CM, Ferlito A. Immunohistochemical markers in the diagnosis of neuroendocrine neoplasms of the head and neck. Ann Otol Rhinol Laryngol 1995; 104: 413–18.

65. Batsakis JG, El-Naggar AK, Luna MA. Neuroendocrine tumors of the larynx. Ann Otol Rhinol Laryngol 1992; 101: 710–14.

66. Wenig BM, Hyams VJ, Heffner DK. Moderately differentiated neuroendocrine carcinoma of the larynx. Cancer 1988; 62: 2658–76.

67. Baugh RF, et al. Carcinoid (neuroendocrine carcinoma) of the larynx. Ann Otol Rhinol Laryngol 1987; 96: 315–21.

68. Patterson SD, Yarington CT. Carcinoid tumor of the larynx: the role of conservative therapy. Ann Otol Rhinol Laryngol 1987; 96: 12–14.

69. Gripp FM, et al. Neuroendocrine neoplasms of the larynx. Importance of the correct diagnosis and differences between atypical carcinoid tumors and small-cell neuroendocrine carcinoma. Eur Arch Otorhinolaryngol 1995; 252: 280–6.

70. Machens A, Holzhausen JH, Dralle H. Minimally invasive surgery for recurrent neuroendocrine carcinoma of the supraglottic larynx. Eur Arch Otorhinolaryngol 1999; 256: 242–6.

71. Schmidt U, et al. Well-differentiated (oncocytoid) neuroendocrine carcinoma of the larynx with multiple skin metastases: a brief report. J Laryngol Otol 1994; 108: 272.

72. Ottinetti A, et al. Cutaneous metastasis of the neuroendocrine carcinoma of the larynx: report of a case. J Cutan Pathol 2003; 30: 512–15.

73. Machtay M, et al. Factors Associated with severe late toxicity after chemoradiation for locally advanced head and neck cancer: an RTOG analysis. J Clinical Oncology 2008; 21: 3582.

74. Dornfeld K, et al. Radiation doses to structures within and adjacent to the larynx are correlated with long-term diet- and speech-related quality of life. Int J Rad Oncol Biol Phys 2007; 68: 750.

75. Gadepalli C, et al. Functional results of pharyngo-laryngectomy and total laryngectomy: a comparison. J Laryngol Otol 2012; 126(1): 52–7.

76. Rodrigo JP, et al. Transoral laser surgery for supraglottic cancer. Head and Neck 2008; 30(5): 658.

77. Killisch M, et al. Functional results following partial supraglottic resection. Comparison of conventional surgery vs transoral laser microsurgery. Adv Otorhinolaryngol 1995; 49: 237.

78. Cabanillas R, et al. Functional outcomes of transoral laser surgery of supraglottic carcinoma compared with a trancervical approach. Head and Neck 2004; 26: 653.

79. Peretti G, et al. Comparison of functional outcomes after endoscopic versus open-neck supraglottic laryngectomies. Ann Otol Rhinol Laryngol 2006; 115: 827.

80. Benito J, et al. Aspiration after supracricoid partial laryngectomy: incidence, risk factors, management, and outcomes. Head and Neck 2010; 32: 679.

81. Bathala S, et al. Chondrosarcoma of the larynx: review of the literature and clinical experience. J Laryngol Otol 2008; 122: 1127.

82. Thompson LD. Chondrosarcoma of the larynx. ENT J 2004; 83(9): 609.

83. Lindberg R. Distribution of cervical lymph node metastases from squamous cell carcinoma of the upper respiratory and digestive tracts. Cancer 1972; 29(6): 1446–9.

84. Byers RM, Wolf PF, Ballantyne AJ. Rationale for elective modified neck dissection. Head Neck Surg 1988; 10(3): 160–7.

85. Shah JP. Patterns of cervical lymph node metastasis from squamous carcinomas of the upper aerodigestive tract. Am J Surg 1990; 160(4): 405–9.

86. Letterman M. Cancer of the larynx. I: natural history in relation to treatment. Br J Radiol 1971; 44: 569.

87. Kaplan MJ, et al. Glottic carcinoma. The roles of surgery and irradiation. Cancer 1984; 53(12): 2641–8.

88. Strojan P, et al. Verrucous carcinoma of the larynx: determining the best treatment option. Eur J Surg Oncol 2006; 32(9): 984–8.

89. Olsen KD, Lewis JE, Suman VJ. Spindle cell carcinomas of the larynx and hypopharynx. Otolaryngol Head Neck Surg 1997; 116: 47–52.

90. Banks ER, Frierson HF Jr, Mills SE, George E, Zarbo RJ, Swanson PE. Basaloid squamous cell carcinoma of the head and neck: a clinicopathologic and immunohistochemical study of 40 cases. Am J Surg Pathol 1992; 16(10): 939–46.

91. Ferlito A, Rinaldo A, Altavilla G, Doglioni C. Basaloid squamous cell carcinoma of the larynx and hypopharynx. Ann Otol Rhinol Laryngol 1997; 106(12): 1024–35.

92. Spiro JD, Spiro RH. Salivary tumors. In: Shah J (ed) Cancer of the Head and Neck. Hamilton, ON: BC Decker, 2001. p. 240.

93. Armstrong JG, et al. The indications of elective treatment of the neck in cancer of the major salivary glands. Cancer 1992; 69: 615–19.

94. Frankenthaler RA, et al. Predicting occult lymph node metastasis in parotid cancer. Arch Otolaryngol Head Neck Surg 1993; 119: 517–20.

95. Rich TA, et al. Clinical and pathologic review of 48 cases of chordoma. Cancer 1985; 56: 182–7.

8 Nasopharyngeal Carcinoma in Nonendemic Populations

June Corry[1] and Bonnie S. Glisson[2]

[1] Head and Neck Cancer Service, Peter MacCallum Cancer Centre, Melbourne, VIC, Australia

[2] Department of Thoracic/Head and Neck Medical Oncology, The University of Texas MD Anderson Cancer Center, Houston, TX, USA

Introduction

The first histologically confirmed case of cancer of the nasopharynx was probably that reported by Michaux[1] who, in 1845, described a 45-year-old male with carcinoma of the base of the skull. There is anthropological evidence, however, that the disease has existed for many centuries. For example, Strouhal[2] described an ancient Egyptian skull from the cemetery at Naga-ed-Der in Upper Egypt with features consistent with extensive destruction by a nasopharyngeal cancer. The first English language review of the disease is contained in the textbook *A Treatise on Disease of the Nose and Throat* by Bosworth in 1889.[3] Further details of the history of this fascinating disease may be found in the article by Muir.[4]

Cancer of the nasopharynx, in the generic sense, includes carcinomas, sarcomas, and lymphomas. Throughout the world, however, "nasopharyngeal cancer" pragmatically refers to carcinoma and to a specific category of carcinoma, abbreviated as NPC. Potentially a source of confusion, NPC designates nonglandular malignancies arising from the epithelium lining the surface and crypts of the nasopharynx. On the basis of ultrastructural features, all types of NPC may be regarded as variants of squamous cell carcinoma (Fig. 8.1) and are subclassifiable as groups based on their predominant pattern as viewed by the light microscope.[5–9] NPC represents a nearly unique model in human neoplasia because of its etiopathogenic relationships with viral infection, neoplastic transformation, and immune response of the host.[10] Its clinicopathological aspects, histology, clinical staging systems, and genetic as well as environmental variables have further positioned NPC in a stalking-horse role in oncological research.

Anatomy of the nasopharynx

Gross anatomy

The roof of the nasopharynx begins behind the posterior nasal choanae and slopes downward where it becomes continuous with the posterior wall. The bony roof and posterior wall are formed serially by the basisphenoid, basiocciput, and anterior arch of the atlas. The lateral and posterior walls are, in part, upward extensions of the boundaries of the oropharynx. In the lower part of the lateral wall, the superior constrictor muscle sends its fibers posteriorly to attach to the basisphenoid. Between the upper border of the superior constrictor and the skull base is stretched the pharyngobasilar fascia with the eustachian tube lodged between the medial pterygoid plate and the superior constrictor. The tubal ampulla's inward bulge creates a slit-like space between it and the posterior wall – the pharyngeal recess or fossa of Rosenmüller, filled, in part, by the levator palati muscle that lies between the pharyngobasilar fascia and the mucous membrane.[11]

The nasopharyngeal lymphoid tissue or adenoid is concentrated at the junction of the roof and the posterior wall of the postnasal space. There are other lymphoid aggregates about the tubal openings. The sensory nerve supply to the postnasal space is provided by the glossopharyngeal and maxillary nerves. Beneath the mucous membrane of the roof is the vestigial pharyngeal hypophysis. Lying in the mid-ine near the vomerosphenoidal articulation, its presence is a reminder of the embryological origin of the anterior pituitary from Rathke's pouch. The hypophyseal vestige may be partly or completely surrounded by the basisphenoid. Also in the midline but dorsal along the roof and separated from the pharyngeal hypophysis by adenoidal tissue is an epithelial recess, sometimes called the pharyngeal bursa, an occasional locus of inflammation or cyst formation. Believed to be formed by a tethering of pharyngeal endoderm to the tip of the embryonic notochord, the recess has no relationship with Rathke's pouch.[11]

Microscopic anatomy

Batsakis *et al.*[5] have summarized our current knowledge of the histology of the mucosa of the nasopharynx. It is composed of three basic cell types: pseudostratified columnar (respiratory)

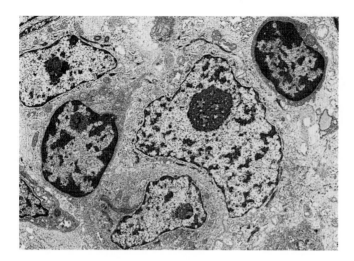

Figure 8.1 Electron micrograph of undifferentiated carcinoma of nasopharynx showing epidermoid characteristics, for example, cell junctions and tonofilaments. Original magnification: ×9000.

Table 8.1 Age-adjusted incidence rates by ethnic grouping.

Incidence	Rate*	Ethnic grouping
Very high	>25	Indigenous southern Chinese
High	15–25	Emigrant southern Chinese (Singapore, USA)
Intermediate	5–15	Non-Chinese South-east Asians, Arabs, Eskimos
Moderate to low	1–5	Northern Chinese, Polynesians, central Africans, Maltese
Rare	<1	Caucasians, people of Indian subcontinent, Japanese, Koreans

* Per 100,000 in males.

cells, squamous cells, and intermediate (pseudostratified) cuboidal cells. All three types are found during fetal development, with the respiratory type being the first to evolve. There is an increase in squamous epithelium until, in the adult nasopharynx, the dominance of respiratory over squamous epithelium is reversed. A commensurate increase in the intermediate type of epithelium is not seen, but it persists at junctions between respiratory and squamous epithelia with its greatest density at the junction of the oropharynx and nasopharynx. In the adult, squamous epithelium covers approximately 60% of the entire nasopharyngeal surface. The intermediate epithelium is aptly named since it is intermediate in a topographic as well as cytological sense. Investigations in nonhuman species have indicated a change of some of the intermediate cells to either ciliated respiratory or squamous cells.[5] Resembling the intermediate cell layers in both respiratory and squamous epithelia, the intermediate epithelium's greatest density is in the sites of predilection for NPC and it is also the closest normal histological homolog of the nonkeratinizing or undifferentiated carcinomas of the nasopharynx.[5]

Epidemiology and etiology of nasopharyngeal carcinoma

The etiology of NPC is very likely multifactorial: genetic, environmental, and viral. There are at least three major risk factors: (i) a genetically determined predisposition allowing an Epstein–Barr virus (EBV) infection of the type that permits (ii) integration of the genome of the virus into the chromosomes of some nasopharyngeal epithelial cells, thereby priming them for (iii) neoplastic transformation by some environmental cofactor. Alternatively, the environmental agent(s) may trigger the viral genome in the cells to oncogenic activity.

Although environmental factors appear to be essential, the high frequency in disparate ethnic groups points to different operative agents for each group.[5,7,10] As judged by age-specific incidences, Scandinavians and American blacks and whites appear to have a different etiological origin for NPC from that

of Chinese Americans, or Hong Kong or Singapore Chinese. In the Chinese, the incidence curves rise sharply after the third decade; those for non-Chinese show a rise after the fourth or fifth decade. Native Alaskans have a curve pattern similar to that of Chinese, but Tunisians have a bimodal curve, with an early peak in the second decade. In all ethnic groups, the incidence in males is two to three times greater than that in females.

On the basis of data published in the latest edition of *Cancer Incidence in Five Continents*,[12] the world's highest incidence rates are found in Hong Kong (particularly among the boat people). With its population primarily derived from Guandong Province in south-eastern China, Hong Kong has consistently reported very high rates of about 25–30 per 100,000 in males and 10–15 per 100,000 in females. Cantonese Chinese who have migrated to other parts of the world retain a high predisposition to the disease, although at a lesser rate than those living in China.[13] Intermediate rates (5–15 per 100,000 in males) are reported in other peoples of South-east Asia (Malays, Indonesians, Filipinos, Thais, and Vietnamese), Eskimos, and North African Arabs. A relatively low-to-moderate incidence (1–5 per 100,000) occurs in northern Chinese, Polynesians, Maltese, and central Africans. The disease is rare, <1 per 100,000, in Caucasians, Japanese, Koreans, and the population of the Indian subcontinent (Table 8.1).

In Europe, the populations of the southern countries (Spain, Italy, France, Balkan states) are at a relatively higher risk than those from northern countries. In the past, the increased risk was linked to populations living on the Mediterranean Sea coast. The recent data do not seem to confirm this finding. In fact, only Malta and Israel (Jews born in Africa or Asia) show higher incidence rates, whereas the coastal populations of Spain, Italy, and the Balkan states have a lower incidence than those living in the interior parts of those countries.

Levine and others[14] have studied demographic patterns for NPC in the United States. These were obtained from the Third National Cancer Survey, the Surveillance Epidemiology and End Results (SEER) program, and the Connecticut Tumor Registry. Approximately seven of every eight malignant tumors of the nasopharynx (1202 patients) were classified as NPC. While 84% of white patients with cancer of the nasopharynx had NPC, more than 90% of nonwhite patients had NPC. The preponderance of NPC in the case material held for all but the younger patients; sarcomas were more frequent among whites under 10 years of age. White patients had the highest frequency of squamous cell carcinomas. Undifferentiated carcinomas were more common in black and Chinese-American patients and were relatively frequent in young patients of all races. Chinese-Americans have a greater risk of developing NPC than any other racial/ethnic group in the United States. Whites and blacks have similar risks, except in younger age groups where there is a minor postadolescent age peak in NPC risk that is more pronounced for blacks than for whites in the United States.[15] A similar young age peak has been observed in other parts of the world such as India, Tunisia, and Sudan, but remains unexplained. The apparent high risk in the young black population in the United States has been considered to be related to rural residence and low socioeconomic status.[16]

The morbidity data from the United States do not show outstanding geographic or temporal variation in the NPC risk for whites.[14,16] Only the relatively high mortality rate in Alaska stands out as a significant factor in mortality studies of the states and counties.

Epstein–Barr virus and biological implications

Epstein–Barr virus (EBV) is ubiquitous in humans, and antibodies to polypeptides of the virus are present in over 80% of human serum samples from the USA, and in higher percentages from Asian and African populations.[10,17] Practically no one escapes infection from this herpes group virus. Primary infections often remain clinically inapparent or not recognized as being due to EBV, particularly in subjects under the age of 5 years.

The consequences of EBV infection vary in different populations: it is associated predominantly with infectious mononucleosis in the western hemisphere, Burkitt lymphoma in Africa, and NPC in Asia. Occurrence of these three EBV-associated diseases is unusual outside their normally associated populations, strongly suggesting the role of additional factors in the populations at risk. The apparent differences in geographic distribution of the three main EBV-associated diseases have also prompted suggestions that different strains of EBV are prevalent in different areas, but this has not been verified and likely is not a factor.[10]

Whether clinically manifest or not, primary EBV infections establish a permanent EBV carrier state in the lymphatic system and also in the major salivary glands.[18] This is reflected in the life-long persistence of EBV-specific antibodies, at almost constant titers, and an intermittent excursion of EBV into the oropharynx.[10,18,19]

The association between EBV and NPC was initially discovered in 1966 by Old et al.,[20] who showed that patients with undifferentiated carcinoma of the nasopharynx had elevated IgG and IgA antibody titers against EBV early and viral capsid antigens (VCA). Since then a large number of studies have shown that essentially all cases of undifferentiated carcinoma of the nasopharyngeal type throughout the world contain the EBV genome regardless of the local incidence of the tumor or the ethnicity of the patients. Epstein–Barr nuclear antigen (EBNA 1) is expressed in practically all NPCs. Evidence

strengthening the causal association of EBV with NPC in genetically predisposed groups was provided by the demonstration that preinvasive dysplastic lesions of the nasopharynx contain monoclonal copies of the EBV genome (using the criterion of terminal repeat reiteration frequency), indicating that EBV infection is likely to be an early initiating event in the development of NPC.[21] Reports on the association between EBV and keratinizing (WHO type 1) NPC are contradictory. Although some studies have been unable to demonstrate the presence of EBV in keratinizing NPC, others have shown positive hybridization signals although expression of viral encoded transcripts appears to be downregulated, once tumor cells differentiate and produce keratin.[22] Recent data indicate that a subset of keratinizing NPC cases in the US are associated with human papillomavirus.[23]

Although EBV infection is clearly an important factor in the pathogenesis of NPC, its ubiquitous distribution contrasted with the distinct geographical epidemiology of NPC implicates a multistep process. Genetic predisposition is obviously a factor.[24] It would also appear that in high-risk groups, environmental carcinogens such as salted fish may play a role. Genetic polymorphisms in cytochrome p450 enzymes, such as the c2 allele of *CYP2E*, which metabolically activates nitrosamines, may be responsible for this association with salted fish exposure.[25] In geographic areas of sporadic incidence, tobacco and ethanol exposure increase the risk for development of keratinizing (WHO type 1) but not nonkeratinizing NPC (type 2 or 3).[26] A population-based case–control study in the United States showed an odds ratio of 1.9 for NPC when the glutathione *S*-transferase M1 gene (*GSTM1*) is absent.[27] Interestingly, although this enzyme is involved in the metabolism of tobacco carcinogens, the relationship between *GSTM1* absence and risk was not modified by tobacco exposure and the risk was similar among Caucasians, African-Americans, and Asians, and across histological types.

Genetics

Several genetic systems have been investigated in patients with NPC. In southern Chinese populations, a strong association with human leukocyte antigen (HLA) alleles A2, B14, and B46 has been observed. This susceptibility may be due to a gene closely linked to HLA loci as suggested by Lu et al.[28] However, data from other races are inconclusive. Burt et al.[29] investigated associations between NPC and HLA antigens at the HLA-A, -B, -C, and -DQ loci and alleles at the DRB1 locus in a population-based multicenter study in the United States. Data from 82 cases and 140 controls were presented, making this the largest study yet performed in an area of sporadic incidence of NPC. An analysis was undertaken to compare their results with previously published findings. This found a significant protective association with A2 antigen in non-Chinese, a protective association with A11 across all races, and increased risk associated with B5 in Caucasians. Associations were found to be more pronounced in younger patients.

Familial segregation of NPC is noted in areas of endemic incidence and, more rarely, in Caucasians. However, no specific inherited gene in familial NPC has been identified and the possibility that shared exposure to an environmental carcinogen contributes to familial clustering cannot be excluded.

Early karyotyping analyses of primary tumors and cell lines showed nonrandom structural or numerical abnormalities in defined regions of chromosomes 1, 3p, 3q, 5q, 9p, 11q, 12, 13q, 14q, and X.[30–33] More recent studies utilizing comparative genomic hybridization in primary NPC have shown numerous genetic events, both gains and losses, suggesting the involvement of both oncogenes and tumor suppressor genes.[30] The most critical of these in NPC appear to be inactivation of tumor suppressor genes on 3p (*RASSF1A, FHIT, RARβ2*), 9p (*p15INK4B, p16/INK4A*), 11q (*TSLC1*), 13q (*EDNRB*), 14q, and 16 q and increased copy number and expression of c-*myc* at 8q24 and *EGFR* at 7p12.

On the basis of the accumulating evidence of genetic and epigenetic alterations, a theoretical model for the molecular pathogenesis of NPC has been proposed.[30] In endemic NPC, it can be hypothesized that germline genotypes for HLA and polymorphic genes for carcinogen metabolism, detoxification, and DNA repair predispose to persistence of DNA damage in the nasopharyngeal epithelium. Chronic exposure to environmental carcinogens with associated DNA damage may then lead to evolution of tumorigenic clones. Interaction of these with the cellular mechanisms induced by latent EBV infection then cooperate in the initiation of carcinogenesis. Because this model derives from studies in the endemic population, relevance to NPC in areas of sporadic incidence, even if EBV associated, is not clear. Continued investigation in this area is critical not only to further the understanding of pathogenesis but also for strategies in prevention and early diagnosis, and to identify potential targets for biologic-based therapy.

Pathology

Classification and histology of nasopharyngeal carcinoma

Regardless of geographic distributions, the nonglandular, nonlymphomatous, and nonsarcomatous malignancies are the most common neoplasms of the nasopharynx[5] (Box 8.1). In high-risk regions, these carcinomas dominate cancer statistics for the head and neck.

Over the years, diversity of diagnostic nomenclature and an absence of a uniform histological reporting system have bedeviled correlation with results of therapy and prognosis.[5] In consequence, in 1978 the World Health Organization (WHO) divided NPC into three histological types: squamous (type 1), nonkeratinizing (type 2), and undifferentiated (type 3).[5,7,9] Type 1 histology is uncommon in areas of endemic incidence while it represents approximately 25% of cases in North America.[31] Type 3 tumors represent the vast majority of cases in southern China (90–95%) and both types 2 and 3 are associated with elevated EBV serology at diagnosis.[32] The latter association with EBV and the finding that NPC tissue sometimes shows a mixed pattern of types 2 and 3 led to a revised WHO classification in 1991.[33] This defined NPC as either keratinizing squamous cell carcinomas (WHO type 1) or nonkeratinizing carcinomas. The second group was subdivided into

Box 8.1 Carcinomas of the nasopharynx.

Nasopharyngeal carcinoma (NPC)

- Keratinizing squamous cell carcinoma (WHO type 1)
- Nonkeratinizing carcinoma
  - Differentiated nonkeratinizing carcinoma (WHO type 2)
  - Undifferentiated carcinoma (WHO type 3)

Basaloid squamous cell carcinoma

Adenocarcinomas

- Salivary type
- Nonsalivary type

Neuroendocrine carcinoma

Teratocarcinoma

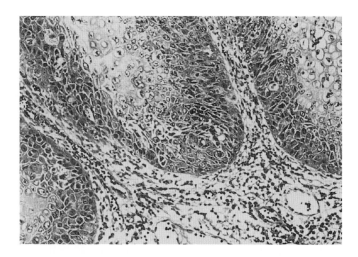

Figure 8.2 Keratinizing squamous cell carcinoma of the nasopharynx, WHO type 1 (H&E, original magnification: 400×).

differentiated (WHO type 2) and undifferentiated (WHO type 3) carcinomas. In 2005, the classification was revised to add basaloid histology, a rarely identified fourth subtype.[34]

Squamous cell carcinoma of the nasopharynx is similar to squamous cell carcinoma in other anatomical sites of the upper aerodigestive tract mucosa. The carcinomas manifest obvious and readily identifiable keratin products, and their growth pattern is typical of that found in any other squamous cell carcinomas (Fig. 8.2). In general, the carcinoma is moderately differentiated and is accompanied by a desmoplastic host response. Since it is preponderantly a surface growth, endoscopic examination of the nasopharynx usually identifies the carcinoma. The average age of patients with squamous cell carcinoma of the nasopharynx is somewhat higher than that of all NPC patients. It is rarely found in patients younger than 40 years.[9]

Like the squamous cell carcinomas, differentiated nonkeratinizing carcinomas exhibit variable degrees of differentiation within the limits of their definition. The cells have a maturation

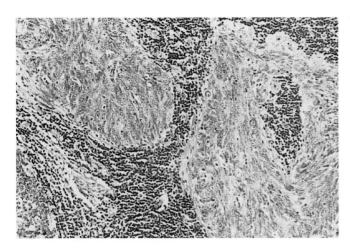

Figure 8.3 Nonkeratinizing carcinoma of the nasopharynx, WHO type 2. Note the sharp delimitation from surrounding lymphoid tissue and in this example, a spindle character to the neoplastic cells (H&E, original magnification: 360×).

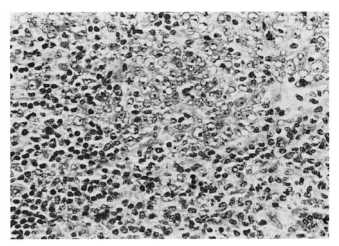

Figure 8.5 WHO type 3 NPC or undifferentiated carcinoma. Vesicular nuclei, prominent nucleoli, indistinct cell membranes, and a lymphoid-like character are manifested. Note intimate relationship with nonneoplastic lymphocytes (H&E, original magnification: 420×).

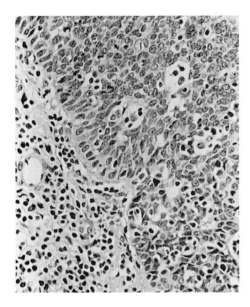

Figure 8.4 Differentiated nonkeratinizing carcinoma, WHO type 2. This example manifests, in addition to neoplasm, stroma demarcation, clear cells and "intermediate type" cells (H&E, original magnification: 400×).

sequence that ends without evidence of squamous differentiation at the light microscopic level (Figs 8.3, 8.4). Growth may be papillary and/or plexiform. The cells have fairly well-defined cell margins and the neoplastic islands are usually quite well delineated from the adjacent stroma. In some of the carcinomas, there is a pseudostratified arrangement of cells, not unlike that noted for the intermediate epithelium of the nasopharynx. While histological differences between squamous cell carcinoma and nonkeratinizing carcinomas are sharp, those between nonkeratinizing and undifferentiated carcinomas are sometimes vague and may be arbitrary, thus their shared group in the most recent WHO classification.

Undifferentiated carcinoma of the nasopharynx is composed of primitive cells whose most consistent feature is a single, prominent nucleolus, and a nucleus with distinct membrane and, in many cases, nuclear vesiculation (Fig. 8.5). In contrast with the other NPC types, the cell margins of this carcinoma are often indistinct and the tumor often has a syncytial appearance. The cellular arrangement, however, is variable, with masses, strands, or individual cells lying in a lymphoid stroma. The variety of cytoplasmic forms and growth patterns has given rise to descriptive terms such as anaplastic, clear cell, spindle cell, simplex, and lymphoepithelioma. Undifferentiated NPC has a striking invasive and metastasizing capability, and tissue reactions to the infiltrating tumor are usually limited. Fibrosis and desmoplasia, for example, are never prominent unless there has been prior radiation therapy.[9] Usually, there is no discernible reaction and the carcinoma maintains an intimate relationship with lymphoid tissues.

The presence or absence of lymphocytes in NPC is not a factor while making the diagnosis. It is now firmly established that the lymphocytes are not neoplastic or integral to the carcinomas. They can be found in all three of the WHO types, but are most often associated with undifferentiated carcinomas. Approximately 98% of undifferentiated, 70% of nonkeratinizing, and 37% of squamous cell carcinomas of the nasopharynx are associated with lymphocytes.[9] The lymphoid "stroma" is not entirely passive. Metastases of undifferentiated NPC to nonlymphoid tissues may also have an accompaniment of lymphoid cells.

Several histological findings of a host response to NPC merit mention. Some may have as yet an unknown prognostic value; others, in the presence of undifferentiated NPC, may mislead the surgical pathologist to a diagnosis of lymphoid neoplasm. A mixture of lymphoid cells and plasma cells, sometimes associated with polymorphonuclear leukocytes, is found in nearly all forms of NPC. A mild-to-moderate stromal eosinophilia is evident in about one-fourth of the carcinomas, most often with the undifferentiated types, where it may be a conspicuous feature. Some authors have also reported an amyloid-like material in the stroma and also sometimes in the cytoplasm of the carcinoma cells.[35] The amyloid, unlikely to be of a secondary type, is found most often in association with nonkeratinizing NPC. In the lymphoid tissue immediately adjacent to undifferentiated NPC, there may be a predominance of T lymphocytes, a finding of possible significance because of the inherently B cell nature of the lymphoid tissue of the nasopharynx. T zone histiocytes (Langerhans cells and precursors) at primary carcinoma sites may also play a role in an immune reaction.[36] In lymph nodes with or without metastases from NPC and, on occasion, in the nasopharynx itself, tuberculoid granulomas are found. Usually around the neoplasm, the epithelioid granulomas may be accompanied by large numbers of eosinophils, fibrosis, and caseous necrosis. Infective granulomas or Hodgkin disease may be simulated.

Despite the variations in histological appearance of the WHO types, their proposed mode of histogenesis, the lability and maturational tendencies of the nasopharyngeal epithelium, and clinicopathological findings suggest all three types may be histologically homogeneous. The tendency for an epidermoid differentiation and the light optic findings of a mixed cell or intermediate population in otherwise prototypic histologic classes support this homogeneity, as does ultrastructure. Shanmugaratnam et al.[7] have indicated that features of more than one histological type were present in 25% of all NPCs studied in a Singapore population. In such instances, classification is based on the predominant type found in the primary lesion.

Carcinomas histologically similar or indistinguishable from NPC types 2 and 3 have been found elsewhere in the epithelium of Waldeyer's ring,[37] the larynx,[38] the thymus,[39] major salivary glands,[18] and cervix.[40] The role of EBV in some of these carcinomas is strongly suggested by serological profiles, by the presence of EBV-associated nuclear antigen in the carcinoma cells, and by high levels of viral genomes in the DNA. A histomorphological feature common to all carcinomas is an intimacy between epithelium and lymphoid cells, not unlike that of the nasopharyngeal mucosa. This "lymphoepithelium" is found in the base of the tongue, tonsillar and adenoidal crypts, in association with salivary ducts, laryngeal "tonsil" and obviously in the thymus. These "lymphoepithelial carcinomas" are infrequent, for example, less than 5% of the base of the tongue and tonsil carcinomas, but their biological behavior and response to treatment further qualify them as *carcinomas of nasopharyngeal type*.

Immunological aspects of nasopharyngeal carcinoma

In the 1980s, a collaborative prospective study of North American patients with different histopathological types of NPC identified certain biological characteristics of EBV that have clinical importance for diagnosis and possibly for the management of the disease.[10,41] Immunovirological tests having diagnostic significance include antibody titers to VCA and early antigen (EA). The VCA (IgA) is more specific, while the EA is more sensitive. These tests may help resolve the diagnosis in patients who present with metastatic carcinoma in a neck node from an unknown primary. In addition, antibody-dependent cellular cytotoxicity (ADCC) assays titrating EBV-induced

membrane antigen complex appear to be predictive of clinical outcome and prognosis in patients with NPC types 2 and 3. High ADCC titers at diagnosis are associated with a more favorable prognosis, regardless of the disease stage. The incidence of positive titers in NPC appears to be the same regardless of tumor size and hence can complement the diagnostic evaluation of patients. In southern China, positive titers for IgA to VCA have been used in screening programs, with predominantly early-stage NPC diagnosed.[42]

Anti-EBV serological findings distinguish WHO type 1 from types 2 and 3 carcinomas. Types 2 and 3 carcinomas manifest characteristic anti-EBV profiles and are more often small and submucosal, and may be clinically occult.[9] They are more radiosensitive than WHO type 1 carcinomas. WHO types 2 and 3 carcinomas appear to occur at an earlier age, manifest longer disease-free periods after treatment, and have a better survival even though early and advanced metastases to the neck are more common, as is the risk of distant metastasis.[9,16]

Early results of NPC screening in high-risk populations using a transoral brush biopsy appear promising. The brush provides nasopharyngeal cell DNA, which is tested for EBV genomic sequences using polymerase chain reaction (PCR). In a sample population of 178 (21 with NPC and 157 without), a sensitivity of 90% and a specificity of 99% were found for detecting NPC using this technique.[43] EBV DNA can also be quantified in plasma with PCR, which has been shown to identify NPC with high sensitivity and specificity in the endemic population.[44] A large prospective trial is ongoing to assess the value of plasma screening for NPC in an endemic area. There have also been interesting results using plasma EBV DNA before and after treatment as a prognostic factor. Due to the lack of consensus on cut points in EBV DNA levels, and thus far, the lack of a clear impact on management, this has not been routinely integrated into care.[45]

Clinical presentation and diagnosis of nasopharyngeal carcinoma

Nasopharyngeal carcinoma, especially of WHO types 2 and 3, usually arises in the region of the fossa of Rosenmüller. The early symptoms of the disease are neither pathognomonic nor specific. The clinical presentation of NPC in the North American population has been documented in a collaborative prospective study.[46]

Over a third of patients will notice a mass in the neck as their first symptom and approximately an equal number will have a sensation of unilateral ear fullness or plugging and hearing loss. A persistent serous otitis media, especially if unilateral in an otherwise healthy adult, should arouse suspicion of a carcinoma of the nasopharynx. A cancer of the nasopharynx will seldom produce choanal or nasal obstruction but initial bleeding or bloody nasal drainage will be noticed by approximately one-fifth of the patients. The triad of a mass in the neck, a conductive hearing loss, and nasal obstruction with blood-tinged drainage will frequently be present by the time the diagnosis of NPC is made.

The proximity of the foramen lacerum and thus the floor of the middle cranial fossa allows for direct tumor extension into

Table 8.2 Frequency of cranial nerve involvement in cancer of the nasopharynx.*

	Cranial nerves											
	I	II	III	IV	V	VI	VII	VIII	IX	X	XI	XII
Number of patients	13	114	236	207	521	600	133	49	264	233	154	358
Frequency (%)	0.5	4.0	8.2	7.2	18.1	20.9	4.6	1.7	9.2	8.1	5.4	12.5

* Based on 2871 patients of whom 641 (22.3%) manifested cranial nerve involvement.
Adapted from Sawaki et al.[47] with permission.

the cranium and involvement of adjacent nerves. One-fifth of patients will have symptoms of cranial nerve involvement at diagnosis. Facial pain and paresthesias suggest tumor infiltration of the trigeminal nerve branches, and diplopia from paralysis of the lateral rectus muscle is a sign of involvement of the abducens nerve. Involvement of cranial nerves III and IV indicates more advanced disease along the cavernous sinus. Tumor extension may occur laterally into the parapharyngeal space and involve cranial nerves IX, X, and XI, producing a jugular foramen syndrome. A persistent occipitotemporal headache, especially unilateral, is reported by one of every six patients. Only very occasionally will NPC invade the parotid gland and cause facial nerve paralysis. Proptosis will occur when cancer invades through the posterior portion of the orbit. Trismus is an indication of pterygoid muscle invasion and cancer extension into this space.

At diagnosis, nine of every 10 patients will have palpable lymph node metastases with bilateral involvement in half of them. The lymph nodes most frequently involved are in the subdigastric area and in the chain along the spinal accessory nerve in the posterior triangle. The sentinel lymph node for NPC is located underneath the upper insertion of the sternocleidomastoid muscle. Frequently the neck mass is large and painless, and it can enlarge quite rapidly because of necrosis or hemorrhage. Retropharyngeal lymph node metastasis, when extensive, produces a characteristic syndrome of pain referred to the ipsilateral neck, ear, head, forehead, and orbit. It may be associated with a stiff neck or pain when cervical dorsiflexion is attempted.

Physical examination includes inspection of the nasopharynx, either indirectly with a mirror or preferably by direct visualization through a fiberoptic endoscope. The tumor usually appears as an asymmetrical mass with telangiectasia on its friable surface and centered in the fossa of Rosenmüller. Depending on the size of the primary tumor, distortion of the soft palate can occur. Straw-colored serous otitis media is usually unilateral. Evaluation of the cranial nerves may show subtle signs of tumor infiltration. The earliest signs are usually extraocular muscle dysfunction, especially lateral rectus palsy, and signs of trigeminal nerve involvement such as hyperesthesia and atrophy of masticatory muscles. The relative frequency of involvement of each cranial nerve is indicated in Table 8.2.[47]

Biopsy of the tumor in the nasopharynx can be done under topical anesthetic by cocaine applications through the nasal cavity. Palpation of the neck, especially in the upper third, will frequently reveal lymph node metastases that are often of large size, multiple, and sometimes fixed to the surrounding structures. Keratinizing carcinomas (WHO type 1) produce fewer lymph node metastases than the nonkeratinizing carcinomas (WHO types 2 and 3).

Radiological evaluation of the nasopharynx, the base of the skull, paranasal sinuses, and the neck is mandatory for appropriate staging and treatment. Computed tomography (CT) allows for the definition of the extent of primary tumor and the amount of invasion and infiltration of surrounding structures. Bone destruction at the floor of the sphenoid sinus, the adjacent middle cranial fossa, the clivus, and the pterygoid plates can be documented, as well as the extension of tumor through the foramen lacerum into the middle cranial fossa, laterally into the parapharyngeal space, anteriorly into the nasal cavity, and anterolaterally into the orbit. It is important to demonstrate invasion into the posterior ethmoid cells and adjacent portion of the maxillary antrum. Magnetic resonance imaging (MRI) further improves radiological staging of the disease, particularly for detecting base of skull invasion and intracranial extension. Ng et al. reported on 67 patients who had both staging CT and MRI scans. They found that staging MRI demonstrated skull base invasion and intracranial extension in a further 20% patients compared with their staging CT.[48] Poon et al. reported similar results.[49] They compared results of 48 patients who had both staging CT and MRI and found that MRI demonstrated increased volume of disease and upstaged disease in 16 patients (33%), of whom eight (25%) had their T stage upgraded. Consequently MRI is now considered the optimal standard diagnostic staging tool in NPC (Fig. 8.6).

Computed tomography and MRI scans may also reveal metastatic spread to lymph nodes that is undetectable clinically. For example, Figure 8.7 shows a patient in whom obviously involved retropharyngeal lymph nodes were demonstrated radiographically. Accurate delineation of disease is a *sine qua non* for optimal radiation dose delivery to the entire gross tumor volume. It is presumably the explanation for the fascinating finding of a prognostic impact of MRI in NPC. This was first demonstrated by Lee et al.[50] In their series of 2687 patients, 860 (32%) were staged by MRI, which resulted in significantly better outcomes than in those staged by CT. Despite a significantly higher stage in the MRI group (T3–4 46 versus 27%, N2–3 37 versus 27%), their 5-year local failure-free rate and overall survival rate were significantly better than those of the CT-staged patients: 91% versus 87% and 80% versus 74%. Using

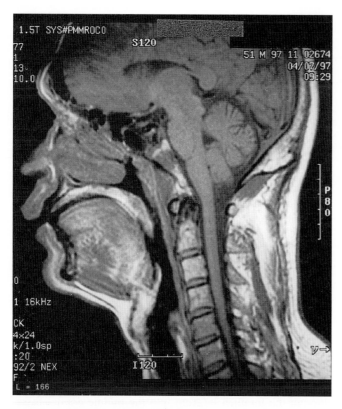

Figure 8.6 Sagittal T1-weighted MRI image of a patient with clinically localized NPC showing invasion of the clivus by tumor. The tumor appears as a dark area within the bright signal of normal marrow.

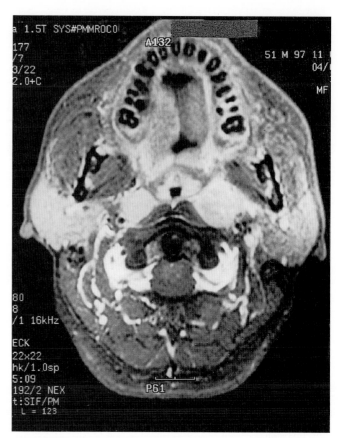

Figure 8.7 Axial T1-weighted fat-saturated contrast-enhanced MRI image showing bilaterally enlarged retropharyngeal lymph nodes harboring metastases from NPC.

multifactorial analysis, Corry *et al*. have also demonstrated a significant independent impact of staging MRI on local control and overall survival in Asian and non-Asian patients.[51]

The majority of patients with NPC present with locoregionally advanced disease, and at least one-fifth of patients can be reckoned to have had occult distant metastases at presentation on the basis of relapse patterns following treatment.[52,53] Sites of predilection for metastatic spread are presented in Table 8.3.[54] Kumar *et al*. prospectively evaluated 139 patients with WHO type 3 NPC with chest x-ray, liver ultrasonography, and bone scan.[55] The incidence of occult metastatic disease increased with higher overall stage and N status, with less than 5% yield for patients with N0–2 disease compared to a 14.3% yield for patients with N3 disease. The current US National Comprehensive Cancer Network guidelines recommend imaging of chest, liver, and bone, and/or a PET-CT scan for patients with WHO types 2 and 3 NPC associated with N2–3 disease.[56] We, and others, have found PET-CT to have high sensitivity in the detection of distant metastatic disease in regionally advanced NPC, and use it as the screening tool of choice over a combination of chest x-ray/CT, liver ultrasound, and bone scintigraphy. [57–60]

Staging

For many years three separate staging systems had been used for NPC. Among Caucasians, the American Joint Commission for Cancer (AJCC) system was most commonly used in the

Table 8.3 Distant metastatic sites of nasopharyngeal carcinoma: a study of 2637 patients.

Metastatic site	Number of patients (%)
Bones	342 (41)
Lungs	256 (30)
Liver	121 (14)
Distant lymph nodes	101 (12)
Brain	18 (2)

Modified with permission from Huang and Chu.[54]

United States and the similar International Union Against Cancer (UICC) system elsewhere in the western world. By contrast, in South-eastern Asia the Ho system[61] was used. The UICC and AJCC criteria were merged into a joint classification with international consensus in 1997. The combined criteria embrace many features of the Ho system and its derivatives, providing a staging system for NPC that is quite different from cancers in other mucosal primary sites of the head and neck. The most recent revision of the combined system (*AJCC Cancer Staging Manual*, 7th edition) is detailed in Box 8.2 and the stage groupings presented in Table 8.4.[62]

Central to the staging system is the use of cross-sectional imaging with CT and/or MRI to demonstrate the extent of

Box 8.2 Unified TNM staging system.

Primary tumor (T)

TX   Primary tumor cannot be assessed
T0   No evidence of primary tumor
Tis   Carcinoma *in situ*
T1   Confined to the nasopharynx, or extends to oropharynx and/or nasal cavity, no parapharyngeal extension
T2   With parapharyngeal extension
T3   Skull base and/or paranasal sinuses
T4   Intracranial extension and/or cranial nerves, infratemporal fossa/masticator space, hypopharynx, or orbit

Regional lymph nodes (N)

NX   Cannot be assessed
N0   No regional lymph node metastasis
N1   Unilateral metastasis in lymph node(s), 6 cm or less in greatest dimension, above the supraclavicular fossa or unilateral/bilateral retropharyngeal
N2   Bilateral metastasis in lymph node(s), 6 cm or less in greatest dimension, above the supraclavicular fossa
N3   Metastasis in a lymph node(s)
      N3a greater than 6 cm in dimension
      N3b extension to the supraclavicular fossa

Table 8.4 Stage grouping: nasopharynx.

Stage	T	N	M
Stage 0	Tis	N0	M0
Stage I	T1	N0	M0
Stage II	T2	N0	M0
	T1	N1	M0
	T2	N0	M0
	T2	N1	M0
Stage III	T1	N2	M0
	T2	N2	M0
	T3	N0	M0
	T3	N1	M0
	T3	N2	M0
Stage IVA	T4	N0	M0
	T4	N1	M0
	T4	N2	M0
Stage IVB	Any T	N3	M0
Stage IVC	Any T	Any N	M1

primary tumor and nodal involvement. The principle adopted was that data guiding the staging revision should be based on tumors whose extent was assessed using cross-sectional imaging since outcomes based on previous clinical and radiological findings would likely be invalid. The main differences between the previous UICC/AJCC staging system from the sixth edition in 2002 and the new classification are as follows.

T categories
• T1: includes tumors confined to the nasopharynx and those extending to the oropharynx or nasal cavity. Previously, extension to those sites was classified as T2a.

• T2: parapharyngeal space extension (previously T2b) is the only criterion for T2. This is defined as posterolateral infiltration beyond the pharyngobasilar fascia.
• T3 and T4 criteria are not altered.

N categories
The critical prognostic significance of level of lymph node involvement in the neck, as well as size and laterality, has been recognized. Multiplicity and clinical fixity of nodes are not criteria for staging.
• N1: the N1 category includes nodes up to 6 cm in greatest dimension, provided they are unilateral and above the supraclavicular fossa. Bilateral retropharyngeal node involvement is also classified as N1 in the 7th edition revision of the AJCC staging.[62]
• N2: includes bilateral lymph nodes above the supraclavicular fossa of the neck up to 6 cm in size.
• N3: presence of nodes greater than 6 cm in diameter or any involvement of or extension to the supraclavicular fossa, delimited by medial and lateral margins of the clavicle and the point where the shoulder meets the neck, constitutes N3.

Management and prognosis

While there is good evidence that addition of concurrent chemotherapy to radiotherapy improves locoregional control and overall survival in patients with locally advanced disease, radiotherapy remains the backbone of treatment in NPC.

Radiotherapy

Because of the rarity of NPC in nonendemic areas, most published series are relatively small and span long periods over which both diagnostic and therapeutic technologies have undergone a revolution. In the first edition of this textbook, a tabulation of all Caucasian series published between 1980 and 1986 was provided. Mostly these included patients diagnosed between the 1950s and 1970s, that is, in the era preceding cross-sectional imaging. Reported overall 5-year survivals averaged around 40%.

The largest reported radiotherapy series from a nonendemic area remains that from the MD Anderson Cancer Center (MDACC) detailing the outcome of patients treated with radiation alone at that institution between 1954 and 1992.[63] There were 378 patients; 85% were Caucasian or Hispanic, the remainder being Asian (8%), African-American (5%), and Arabic (2%). Three-fourths of the patients presented with AJCC (1992) stage IV disease. The histology was 51% squamous carcinoma (including poorly differentiated tumors), 41% lymphoepitheliomas, and 8% unclassified. WHO type 2 cases are not discernible from this series as they are mixed with the squamous carcinomas and the lymphoepitheliomas (Dr Fady Geara, Beirut, personal communication). The overall 5-, 10-, and 20-year actuarial rates of survival were 48%, 34%, and 18%, respectively, and the corresponding disease-specific survival rates were 53%, 45%, and 39%.
• *Primary site control*: 5- and 10-year actuarial local control rates were 71% and 66%, the falloff between 5 and 10 years reflecting the propensity of this disease for late recurrence.

A total of 100 patients experienced local tumor failure, of whom 17 had concurrent regional recurrence, five had distant metastases, and nine had both regional and distant failure. Multivariate analysis revealed T stage, tumor differentiation, and cranial nerve palsies as independent prognostic determinants of local control. The 10-year local control rate was 79% for lymphoepithelioma compared to 54% for squamous carcinoma. As reflected in the revised staging system, patients with skull base involvement had a much better 10-year local control rate (50%) than those with cranial nerve palsies (26%).

• *Neck control*: the 5-, 10-, and 20-year regional control rates were 84%, 83%, and 83%, respectively. The great majority of patients with regional failure had concurrent local and/or distant failure with isolated regional recurrence in only nine (2.4%) cases.

• *Distant metastases*: the 5-, 10-, and 20-year rates of distant metastasis were 30%, 32%, and 32%, respectively. Multivariate analysis showed that the combination of nodal stage and level in the neck was the most potent determinant of distant metastasis, ranging from 10% for those with nodes less than 3 cm in size in the upper two-thirds of the neck to 65% for those with larger nodes involving the lower third of the neck. This is consistent with the current staging system.

Although a large series, only patients in the last decade of that four-decade study period were CT staged, and the 1992 AJCC system was used. Additionally, this retrospective series did not classify patients by WHO type, given that many were diagnosed before this classification came into common use. There are now several large non-Caucasian series, staged by CT and the AJCC/UICC 1997 classification, detailing current results of treatment with radiotherapy. The largest is the Hong Kong experience reported by Lee *et al.*[50] This series detailed 2687 CT-staged patients, the vast majority with WHO type 3 histology. There were 7% stage I, 41% stage II, 25% stage III, and 28% stage IVA–IVB patients. Radiotherapy alone to a median dose of 66 Gy was used to treat 77% of patients. The 5-year local, nodal, and distant failure-free survival (FFS) rates for all patients were 85%, 94%, and 81%, respectively. The progression-free survival and overall survival rates for patients in stages I, II, III, and IV were 85% and 90%, 73% and 84%, 62% and 75%, and 44% and 58%, respectively.

These two series demonstrate significantly different results and typify the inherent difficulties in comparing series over very different time frames. The differences in staging investigations, staging systems, pathological classification, and treatment techniques are all relevant to the differing outcomes. However, another very relevant and interesting point is the different histologies in the two series. There is general agreement that, stage for stage, patients with WHO types 2 and 3 NPC do better than patients with WHO type 1 tumors, especially with regard to local control with radiation.[64] Historically, however, WHO types 2 and 3 have been associated with greater risk for distant recurrence. It has also been assumed that better outcomes from endemic areas are at least in part due to the very low incidence of WHO type 1 in those series. It is not clear whether there is a difference in treatment outcome between stage- and histology-matched Asian and non-Asian NPC patients.

A retrospective analysis of North American NPC patients with Chinese ancestry (parents born in China, Hong Kong, or Taiwan) compared to non-Chinese was performed by Su and Wang.[65] The series included 131 non-Chinese and 41 Chinese patients treated at one institution with definitive radiation between 1979 and 1996. Only 20% of patients received any form of chemotherapy. Patients were staged according to the AJCC/UICC 1997 classification with data from their examination and CT imaging. Chinese patients were younger, more likely to have stage IV disease and WHO type 3 histology, and less likely to have ongoing tobacco exposure than non-Asians. In a multivariate analysis that controlled for stage, age, WHO type, and treatment, Chinese patients had a fourfold increased risk of distant metastases. Race did not predict overall survival or local control, though there was a trend to worse disease-specific and overall survival in the Chinese patients. Independent of race, WHO type 3 histology was associated with better local control and survival.

In a series from the Peter MacCallum Cancer Centre, Australia, treatment outcomes of Caucasian (born in Europe, Australia, Middle East, and Pacific Islands) and Asian (born in southern China or south-east Asia) NPC patients were compared.[51] All patients had WHO types 2 or 3 disease and were staged using the 1997 UICC/AJCC criteria. The mean potential follow-up time was 9.6 years (range 1.0–18.5 years). There were 158 patients: 86 Asian and 72 Caucasians. Stage groupings were: I 12 patients; II 32 patients; III 59 patients; and IV 55 patients. Ninety-nine percent of patients had staging CT and/or MRI. Female sex, age <45 years, and performance status of zero were more commonly observed in Asian patients. Other putative prognostic factors were not significantly different between the groups. Treatment consisted of radiotherapy alone in 30% (early-stage disease), and chemotherapy and radiotherapy combinations in the remainder (locoregionally advanced disease), the majority receiving neoadjuvant chemotherapy and concurrent chemoradiation. There were no significant differences in treatment between the two groups (although this may have reflected small case numbers). The 5-year rates for freedom from local recurrence (FLR), FFS, and overall survival (OS) for Asian and Caucasian patients were 74% versus 82%, 61% versus 55%, and 75% versus 63%, respectively. Corresponding 10-year figures were 62% versus 82%, 43% versus 48%, and 58% versus 49%. There were no significant differences in FFS or OS between Asian and Caucasian patients, perhaps again reflecting the case numbers. However, the FLR interval was significantly worse in the Asian group (hazard ratio (HR) 2.37; 95% confidence interval (CI) 1.11–5.06), while duration of freedom from distant metastasis tended to be better (HR 0.71; 95% CI 0.33–1.53). While this study provides no evidence that race is an independent prognostic factor for overall survival in patients with WHO types 2 and 3 NPC, it does suggest that relapse patterns may vary, with a higher rate of late primary failures (offset by a lower rate of distant failure) in the Asian population. Further confirmatory studies with larger patient cohorts are indicated.

Comparison of the impact of race in patients with WHO type 1 NPC has been difficult given the rarity of this histological subtype in Asian patients. Marks *et al.* analyzed cases from the National Cancer Data Base (USA) diagnosed between

1985 and 1994.[66] Their data showed the expected predominance of type 1 histology in non-Asians, and better survival for patients with type 2 and 3 tumors. However, no independent association of survival with race, independent of the histological type, was identified. Using the SEER database from the US, a retrospective matched analysis of Caucasian and Asian patients with NPC was performed by Bhattacharyya.[67] Pairs were matched for age, gender, AJCC stage, WHO type, and treatment modality. Of 171 matched pairs studied, 45% (77 in each group) of patients were WHO type 1 with 47% and 8% WHO types 2 and 3, respectively. The majority (82%) were stage III or IV. While overall survival was higher in those of Chinese ethnicity, no differences in disease-specific survival, overall and stratified by stage, were identified.

Given the differences in racial definitions, it is perhaps not surprising that the data discussed above are contradictory in many aspects. Overall, they do not support an independent effect of race on survival of patients with NPC. Further investigations will be necessary to determine if race influences relapse patterns in a consistent manner independent of stage, WHO type, and treatment.

Philosophy and technique

The propensity of cancer of the nasopharynx to metastasize and spread locally beyond the confines of the nasopharynx mandates large treatment volumes for all stages of disease. The primary tumor may extend anteriorly into the nasal cavity, superiorly into the floor of the sphenoid sinus or through the foramen lacerum into the cavernous sinus, anterosuperiorly into the posterior ethmoid air cells and orbits, laterally into the parapharyngeal space and sphenopalatine fossa, and inferiorly into the oropharynx (Fig. 8.8). Lymphatic spread most commonly involves the jugular chain of lymphatics and the posterior cervical chain. In addition, retropharyngeal nodes may be involved (see Fig. 8.7). These lymphatic pathways are included in the planning target volumes for all stages of disease. Delineation of the primary target volume is based on the extent of disease determined by clinical and radiological evaluation.

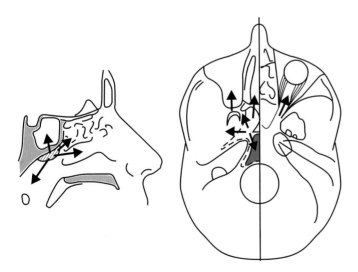

Figure 8.8 Potential routes of spread of primary tumor.

The latter should include both transverse and coronal CT cuts. As in all radiotherapy, the objective of treatment is to deliver a dose to the target volume tailored to the extent of disease present while respecting the tolerance of the normal tissues irradiated. Achieving this objective is technically difficult. The use of intensity-modulated radiotherapy (IMRT) has been a very exciting development in radiotherapy in general, and in the treatment of NPC in particular.

Treatment plan

Radiotherapy techniques for NPC have evolved enormously since the original techniques of parallel opposed photon fields reducing off spinal cord and junctioned with either posterior electron fields or an oblique bilateral photon field with central shielding (Ho technique).[68] These techniques provided good coverage of the planning target volume (PTV) for early-stage disease, but produced unnecessary morbidity associated with irradiation of the major salivary glands, and the gross tumor volume (GTV) coverage is generally poor in locally advanced disease. Conventional conformal radiotherapy (CCRT) techniques provided significant improvement in GTV coverage and parotid sparing in locally advanced disease. A good example of CCRT is the "boomerang technique" which utilizes two asymmetrical arcs to rotate around the spinal cord/brainstem, typically from 340° to 80° and 280° to 20.[69] This generates a dosimetry that nicely approximates the extent of disease commonly seen in locally advanced NPC, whilst respecting the tolerance of the spinal cord/brainstem and sparing the parotid glands. This technique is further improved by dividing the two arcs into three minor arcs of 30–35° ("Tri-arc" technique), which then also enables a reduction of radiation dose to the inner ears. Nevertheless, the falloff in dose, particularly superiorly for disease close to the optic nerve/chiasm, is not as fast as with IMRT. A diagram detailing the evolution of RT techniques is given for historical context (Fig. 8.9), as the standard radiotherapy technique for NPC is now IMRT.

Intensity-modulated radiotherapy

Intensity-modulated radiotherapy is a novel approach in the planning and delivery of radiation therapy. Unlike conventional radiotherapy, IMRT usually involves inverse planning, whereby dose/volume constraints for targets and normal tissues are defined *a priori*, then optimized with the use of a computer algorithm. Treatment is typically delivered with the help of multileaf collimators that move in and out of the beam's path during treatment, modulating the beam's intensity.

Patients are immobilized supine in a cast, in a hard palate vertical position, and 2 mm CT slices, with intravenous contrast, are taken from the skull vertex to well below the sternal notch. These upper and lower levels need to be well beyond the treated area if noncoplanar fields are to be used. Fusion of the CT images with MRI images is used to further improve the delineation of disease, particularly in T4 disease. It is important for the radiation oncologist to review the diagnostic imaging with a head and neck specialist radiologist. On the axial slices, the gross tumor in both the primary site (GTVp) and nodes (GTVn) disease, and areas at risk of subclinical disease, particularly the draining regional lymph nodes, are contoured.

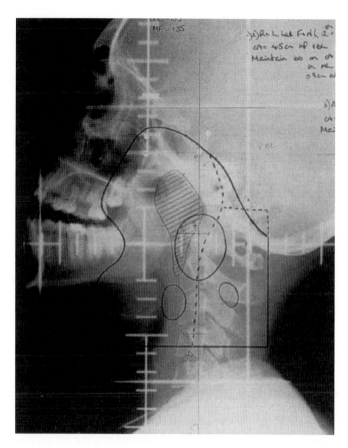

Figure 8.9 Simulation film for the previous standard plan of treatment of a patient with NPC stage T2aN1 included as historical reference (see text).

All relevant organs at risk (OAR) are delineated – optic nerves/chiasm, temporal lobes, lens, brainstem, spinal cord, inner ears, parotid glands, pharyngeal constrictor muscles, and brachial plexus – and avoidance structures such as the oral cavity and glottic larynx are also contoured.

Our current standard is for delivery of dose using a simultaneous integrated boost (SIB) technique, where the GTV is treated to 70 Gy over 7 weeks and lower risk regions receive 63 Gy (high-risk subclinical disease) or 56 Gy (low-risk subclinical disease) over 7 weeks. The PTV63 and PTV56 over 7 weeks equates to 60 Gy and 50 Gy over 6 and 5 weeks, respectively, using a correction factor of 0.6 Gy per extra treatment day to compensate for the potential for accelerated repopulation. The PTV 70 Gy is delineated by expansion from the GTV primary, using a minimum margin of 10 mm. These margins usually need to be constricted when the gross disease is in close proximity to the brainstem and/or optic nerve/chiasm.

The rapid falloff in dose with IMRT can be advantageous, but it also means that frequently there needs to be judicious use of PTV63 and/or PTV56 to ensure dose is delivered with appropriate margins. In this regard, it is important for the PTV63 to cover the entire anatomical boundaries of the nasopharynx, the anterior half of the clivus (whole clivus if involved), skull base (foramen ovale and rotundum bilaterally), pterygoid fossa, parapharyngeal space, inferior sphenoid sinus (in T3–4 disease the entire sphenoid sinus), and the posterior fourth of the nasal cavity and maxillary sinuses (to ensure coverage of the pterygopalatine fossae). The cavernous sinus should also be included in patients with T3–4 disease that involves the roof of the nasopharynx. The PTV63 volume should be at least 15 mm from the GPVp. It is acceptable in patients with early-stage disease (T1–2,N0) for these structures mentioned above to be covered by the PTV56 volume.

Nodal coverage in NPC is comprehensive. The involved nodes are usually treated to 70 Gy, but 63–68 Gy over 7 weeks is acceptable for nodes less than 2 cm in size. The high-risk subclinical disease nodal regions to be treated to 63 Gy include the bilateral retropharyngeal nodes and the upper jugulodigastic nodes (level 2a) bilaterally. The nodes with low risk of subclinical disease to be covered with PTV56 include the bilateral mid and low jugular nodes, the posterior cervical, and supraclavicular nodes. The submandibular nodes (level 1b) are included when in close proximity to involved level 2a nodes. Once all these structures are contoured, an optimal plan is then developed using IMRT software, usually involving 7–10 fields (Fig. 8.10). Whilst the entire treatment volume can be treated with IMRT fields, better sparing of the midline structures (mucosa, pharyngeal constrictors, and glottic larynx) can be achieved by junctioning with a bilateral anterior neck field with a 2 cm central lead shield. It is important to realize the complexities of junctioning an IMRT plan with an anterior lower neck field and the subsequent dose uncertainties at that junction. We minimize this by placing the isocenter at or near that junction, with a 1 cm overlap contributed to by 50% of each of the IMRT and anterior neck fields.

The radiation oncologist needs to review the dose volume histograms of the GTVp, GTVn, PTVs and OAR as well as reviewing the dosimetry on each axial slice. The aim is to deliver 100% of the prescribed dose to the GTV and at least 95% to the PTVs, whilst ensuring that the dose tolerances of critical organs at risk are respected, that dose to noncritical OAR is as low as feasible, and that any high-dose areas are not in structures like the mandible, and are small, e.g. more than 77 Gy <5% and more than 80 Gy <1% of the PTV70 volume.

In more advanced primaries, some compromise in margin (and/or dose) may be required to respect the brainstem and optic nerve/chiasm dose tolerance of 54 Gy in 2 Gy fractions. Nevertheless, when gross disease is closely applied to these structures, we increase the tolerance dose constraint to 59 Gy when given in 1.7 Gy fractions over 7 weeks (i.e. biologically equivalent dose to 54 Gy in 2 Gy fractions using an $\alpha{:}\beta$ ratio of 2). This is supported by the QANTEC data.[70]

An important consideration when large nodal disease extends into the lower neck/supraclavicular fossa is the brachial plexus. We demarcate this structure from the level of the junction of C4–5 vertebral bodies, contoured from the exit foramina at the transverse spinous process towards the direction of the external jugular vein. but not extending beyond the prevertebral muscles/fascia. We limit the maximum brachial plexus dose to 66 Gy.

Results with intensity-modulated radiotherapy
The largest series of NPC patients treated with IMRT from nonendemic areas are from North America. Lee *et al.* reported

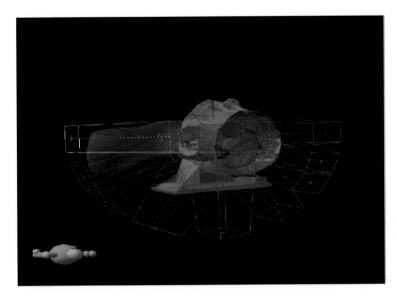

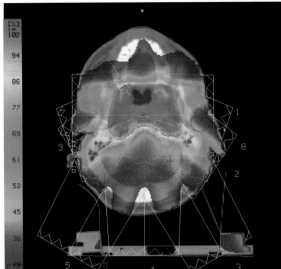

Figure 8.10 IMRT beam arrangement and dose cloud.

on 67 patients, 55 (82%) of whom were Chinese, treated at the University of California at San Francisco.[71] WHO types 2 and 3 histology were evenly distributed with no WHO type 1 patients in the series. Concurrent and adjuvant chemotherapy was given to 75% of patients. The prescribed dose was 65–70 Gy to the GTV, 60 Gy to the clinical target volume (CTV, i.e. GTV plus a margin of potential microscopic spread), and 50–60 Gy to the clinically negative neck. Twenty-six patients were treated with a brachytherapy boost and one with gamma-knife radiosurgery following external beam treatment. The disease was in AJCC/UICC 1997 stage I in eight, stage II in 12, stage III in 33, and stage IV in 25 patients. T3 and T4 disease was identified in 15 and 14 patients, respectively (43%). Median follow-up was relatively short at 31 months, but the 4-year locoregional control was excellent at 98%; the 4-year overall survival was 88%. The median parotid dose was 34 Gy, but this still resulted in only grades 0–1 xerostomia at 24 months in 98% of the 41 evaluable patients.

A second North American series from the Memorial Sloan Kettering Cancer Center reports on 74 patients: 43% were Asian; 5% had WHO type 1, 30% WHO type 2, and 65% WHO type 3 histology; 6% stage I, 16% stage II, 30% stage III, 47% stage IV, and 43% T3–4.[72] Concurrent and adjuvant chemotherapy was given to 93% of patients. IMRT was given with accelerated fractionation, either concomitant boost or dose painting to 70 Gy. Median follow-up was again relatively short at 35 months. The 3-year rates of local and regional control are 91% and 93%, respectively. The rate of local control was not significantly different from the historical control of 79% at this institution for patients treated before 1998 with 3-D planning. Local control was 100% for T1–2 and 83% for T3–4, with 5/6 local recurrences in the target volume. Progression-free and overall survival were 67% and 83%, respectively.[72]

Larger IMRT series from endemic areas show impressive early results regarding disease control. Tham *et al.* reviewed 195 patients with undifferentiated NPC, 63% with stage III–IV disease, including 26% with T4 disease. The 3-year local

relapse-free survival was 93% and the disease-free survival was 82%.[73] Similar excellent results were reported by Ng *et al.* where 193 patients, 93% with stage III–IV disease, had a 2-year local progression-free survival of 95%, distant metastatic disease-free survival was 90% and overall survival was 92%.[74] The RTOG 0225 study demonstrated the transportability of IMRT in the treatment of NPC. Seventeen North American centers enrolled 68 patients, 94% WHO 2–3 and 93% stage III–IV, with 19% T4. The 2-year loco-regional progression-free survival was 89%, the distant metastates-free survival was 85%, the PFS was 73% and the OS was 80%.[75]

These studies all consistently demonstrate high locoregional control rates using IMRT for locally advanced NPC. Although the follow-up for all these IMRT series is relatively short, the disease control rates will still be impressive even if there were to be a 10% degradation in results with longer follow-up. The prescribed dose of 70 Gy is not a significant escalation of dose *per se* compared to historical series. It is the ability of IMRT to deliver the entire prescribed radiation dose to the entire GTV, whilst respecting the dose constraints of surrounding critical tissues, that constitutes relative dose escalation. Previously, the posteromedial aspects of gross disease received up to 30% less of the prescribed dose due to the technical limitations of the radiotherapy techniques used.[69]

There are no randomized trials comparing IMRT and CCRT in NPC. It seems unlikely that such studies will be performed in the future given the general availability, clear dosimetric advantages, and current clinical results demonstrated by the use of IMRT.

The acute toxicities seen with IMRT are similar to those with all RT techniques; it is the late treatment toxicities that are expected to be reduced by using IMRT. There are two randomized studies comparing IMRT with parallel opposed RT in early-stage NPC.[76,77] Both of these studies showed significant reduction in the severity of xerostomia and improved quality of life in patients treated with IMRT.

Radiation dose and fractionation

There are no randomized trials specifically addressing the question of optimal radiation dose in NPC. As mentioned above, the standard recommended doses (derived empirically) are 70 Gy in 2 Gy fractions to areas of gross disease, and 50 Gy in 2 Gy fractions to uninvolved nodal regions. Given the tight margins that are required around gross disease, we recommend a "buffer zone" of 60 Gy transitioning into the 50 Gy volume. When IMRT is used, it is very labor intensive to use a shrinking field technique. We, and others, treat all volumes in 35 fractions over 7 weeks using differential dose per fraction to provide biologically equivalent doses, that is, 63 Gy and 56 Gy at 1.8 and 1.6 Gy per fraction respectively. With the increased availability of IMRT, it is an opportune time for a randomized trial to establish the optimal radiation dose required in the context of defined WHO histology, a common staging system, and use of concurrent chemotherapy.

The question of whether altered dose fractionation is of benefit in treating NPC is unclear. Teo *et al.* randomized 159 patients with WHO type 3 NPC to receive either conventional radiotherapy (60 Gy in 2.5 Gy fractions over 30 days) or conventional/accelerated radiotherapy (20 Gy in 2.5 Gy fractions, a further 51.2 Gy using 1.6 Gy twice daily, total 71.2 Gy in 40 fractions over 31 days).[78] This study did not show improved locoregional control or overall survival in the higher dose arm. However, only half the planned accrual was achieved before the study was terminated because of unacceptable neurological toxicity in the high-dose arm.

Both retrospective and prospective studies by Lee *et al.*[79] suggested improved local control in patients with stage IV(A-B) disease treated with accelerated fractionation (66 Gy in 2 Gy fractions, delivered 6 days per week) compared to a historical control group treated with conventional fractionation. The prospective phase II study included induction chemotherapy with cisplatin and 5-fluorouracil and concurrent chemoradiation with intermittent cisplatin. At 3 years, locoregional and distant failure-free rates were 77% and 75% respectively, and overall survival was 71%. On the basis of these promising results, a subsequent 2 × 2 randomized study comparing conventional radiotherapy (CF), accelerated radiotherapy (AF), each with or without concurrent and adjuvant chemotherapy (+C), was begun.[80] A major eligibility criterion for this study was T3–4 N0–1 staging. This restrictive eligibility contributed to poor accrual and the study was closed prematurely at 189 patients instead of the planned 464. The results suggest that patients treated with AF + C have significantly better locoregional control, but with only a trend to improved overall survival. Although the study is underpowered due to premature closure, the potential significance of trends should not be ignored in developing hypotheses for future trials.

Role of chemotherapy

The current standard of care for locoregionally advanced NPC in North America was established by the Intergroup 0099 trial, a randomized comparison of radiation alone (70 Gy) versus concurrent chemoradiation with intermittent high-dose cisplatin for three cycles followed by adjuvant chemotherapy with cisplatin and 5-FU for three cycles.[81] Patient eligibility included those with stage III–IV disease by the AJCC 1992 classification. Accrual to this trial was stopped prematurely when an interim analysis indicated significant benefit for survival in the chemotherapy arm. This trial was criticized for a high rate of ineligibility, a relatively poor outcome with radiation alone, and early closure leading to only 69 and 78 eligible patients in control and experimental arms, respectively. Additionally, 30% of patients in this study had WHO type 1 histology, and there was substantial doubt that this approach would be beneficial in endemic NPC, which typically is composed of more than 95% WHO types 2 and 3, and thus, in general, is more radiosensitive.

Since the results of the Intergroup 0099 were published, more than 10 randomized trials of chemoradiation versus radiation have been completed in patients with endemic NPC. The majority of these have been included in one or both of two metaanalyses which have confirmed the survival impact of the addition of chemotherapy to radiation for advanced NPC.[82] In the first of these by Baujat *et al.*, individual patient data from eight trials were analyzed, from both endemic and sporadic incidence areas, and including chemotherapy as induction, concurrent, and/or adjuvant settings.[82] The relative risk of death was reduced by 18% with the addition of chemotherapy in all settings (HR 0.82, $p = 0.006$); however, for trials with concurrent chemoradiation the risk of death was reduced by 40% (HR 0.60) as opposed to only induction or adjuvant chemotherapy which were associated with a HR of 0.97 and 0.99, respectively. Chemotherapy was associated with reduction in both locoregional (HR 0.76) and distant failure (HR 0.72) and overall resulted in a 10% improvement in event-free (tumor recurrence or death) survival at 5 years. Notably, the impact of chemotherapy on both overall and event-free survival was strongest in patients with WHO type 1 NPC, but was significant in those with type 2 and 3 as well.

In the most recent metaanalysis, Zhang *et al.* included only trials from the endemic incidence areas, and only those with concurrent chemoradiation, with or without adjuvant chemotherapy.[83] Individual patient data from the seven trials included were not analyzed. Nevertheless, their findings in general recapitulate those of Baujat *et al.*[82] The risk of death at 5 years was reduced by 26% in favor of the chemotherapy-treated patients (HR 0.74); given the predominance of the radiosensitive WHO types 2 and 3 (99.7% of patients), the impact of chemotherapy was most prominent in reducing distant failure, though locoregional control was also improved.

Departing from the findings of most randomized trials including patients with head and neck squamous cell carcinoma (HNSCC) of other common mucosal primary sites, patients with NPC in the endemic areas appear to benefit from reduced distant failure whether chemotherapy is given concurrently with radiation or as induction/adjuvant to chemoradiation. This is being further studied in several ongoing trials from the endemic area in which induction chemotherapy followed by chemoradiation is compared to chemoradiation alone (NCT01245959, NCT00997906, NCT00201396, NCT00379262). GORTEC-NPC2006 (NCT00828386) is investigating this question in patients with NPC from areas of sporadic incidence.

Prior to the era of chemoradiation brought about by the results of Intergroup 0099, neoadjuvant and adjuvant chemotherapy had been studied in seven randomized trials. These were all negative for a survival impact, though one neoadjuvant trial showed improved progression-free survival for the chemotherapy arm.[84] An older metaanalysis published in 2004 included these and three concurrent chemoradiation trials with a total of 10 studies and 2450 patients.[85] Both neoadjuvant chemotherapy and concurrent chemoradiation resulted in significant improvements in locoregional and distant control, while adjuvant chemotherapy did not. The HR for death in all studies was 0.82 ($p = 0.01$), corresponding to an absolute survival benefit of 4% after 3 years. The use of chemoradiation was associated with a HR of 0.48 ($p = 0.004$) and a survival improvement of 20% after 3 years. Neoadjuvant and/or adjuvant chemotherapy did not affect overall survival. Despite these negative findings, treatment with adjunctive full-dose chemotherapy, especially for high-risk patients (advanced N or T stage), continues to be actively studied as reflected in the trials listed above. This is in part driven by the observation that distant recurrence is the predominant mode of failure in the IMRT era, even with concurrent chemotherapy.

The difficulties in identifying a benefit from adjuvant chemotherapy, whether given sequentially following radiation or after concurrent chemoradiation, may lie to some extent in the poor tolerance and thus inadequate drug exposure in that setting. Treatment in the induction setting is much better tolerated and thus more consistently given. Further, it offers the advantage of cytoreduction that can facilitate radiation for very advanced T stage disease that encroaches on critical neighboring structures such as brain, brainstem, and optic tracts. New induction regimens integrating taxanes and/or gemcitabine with platins, with and without fluoropyrimidines are being studied, as discussed above. Results of a randomized phase 2 trial of docetaxel/cisplatin followed by chemoradiation with weekly cisplatin, compared to chemoradiation alone reported by Hui *et al.*, lend support to the potential value of this paradigm.[86] Importantly, cisplatin dose intensity during chemoradiation was not altered in the patients on the induction arm. Further, there was a trend to improved 3-year progression-free survival (88% versus 60%, $p = 0.12$) and a significant increase in overall survival at 3 years (94% versus 68%) with sequential therapy.

A major effort in ongoing trials for patients with locoregionally advanced disease is improving tolerance for both induction and concurrent chemoradiation. In that regard, regimens devoid of infusional 5-FU and its attendant toxicity and logistical difficulty are being studied, such as docetaxel,or gemcitabine, and cisplatin.[86] Many ongoing trials have also opted for a weekly cisplatin schedule during radiation as opposed to the every 3 week schedule given in Intergroup 0099.[81] Although these two schedules have not been directly compared, efficacy outcomes with the weekly schedule with regard to disease control and survival appear equivalent and many oncologists prefer it based on the perception of improved tolerance and dosing flexibility.[86–88]

Carboplatin is generally better tolerated than cisplatin and is the preferred platinating agent in the elderly, for those with renal insufficiency, preexistent neuropathy or hearing loss, and reduced functional status. It has been directly compared to cisplatin in a randomized phase 3 trial of 206 patients with advanced NPC in Thailand treated with both concurrent and adjuvant chemotherapy based on Intergroup 0099.[89] Estimated efficacy outcomes at 3 years appeared equivalent (disease-free and overall survival 63% versus 61% and 78% versus 79% for cisplatin and carboplatin arms, respectively). Cisplatin was clearly more toxic than carboplatin and fewer patients received the intended drug exposure on the cisplatin arm. Although these data are of interest, confirmatory trials are necessary before accepting carboplatin as equivalent to cisplatin in curative-intent treatment.

Pretreatment evaluation and follow-up

Every patient should have an audiogram and a careful dental evaluation before treatment. Teeth that show signs of decay or periodontal disease need to be either restored or ablated. Every patient is submitted to a thorough prophylactic program.[90] For patients with advanced disease in whom the pituitary and hypothalamus will be in the primary radiation beam, baseline endocrine assessments of hypophyseal function should be done prior to commencement of radiotherapy. This permits early identification of hormonal deficiencies and initiation of appropriate replacement therapy.[91]

After completion of therapy, patients should be examined at regular intervals, every 3 months for the first 2 years, every 4 months for the third year, and every 6 months through the fifth year after treatment. A follow-up evaluation is done every year thereafter. During follow-up, the disease status is evaluated for recurrence at the primary site or the neck nodes and for clinical signs of distant metastases. Attention should also be directed to possible sequelae of treatment and prevention of infectious complications in the head and neck area. The external auditory canals will be deficient in normal cerumen production and all patients should be instructed about prevention of external otitis. The auditory canal will be dry and the normal migration of the epithelium within the auditory canal is impaired. As a result, debris tends to collect and may impact. Patients should be advised to avoid manipulation of the ear canal and to seek medical advice promptly if irritation develops. Patients with carcinoma of the nasopharynx often present with serous otitis media. After treatment, this may subside but may persist in a chronic form. If this sequela causes bothersome symptoms, it can be managed with indwelling tympanic membrane ventilation tubes, although this has to be weighed against the subsequent high risk of chronic otitis media. The incidence of chronic hearing loss following treatment of NPC has generally been underappreciated, as there have been few prospective studies. The need for permanent hearing aids must be assessed and they must be recommended as required in the follow-up of these patients.

Dental and oral cavity care should be meticulous and the application of fluoride solutions in the form of stannous fluoride or sodium fluoride by custom-fitted carriers should be done routinely. There are products now available, such as toothpastes with high fluoride levels (e.g. Neutrofluor 5000™ and Dentacal™; casein phosphate peptide amorphous calcium phosphate), that protect against the deleterious effects of xerostomia on dentition and should be recommended prophylactically. Dental extractions after radiation therapy should be avoided whenever possible. If extractions are unavoidable, extreme precautions are necessary to minimize the risk of osteoradionecrosis.[50]

Radiation to the temporomandibular joints and masticatory muscles, especially in patients who receive systemic chemotherapy, may cause trismus. This usually does not set in before 3–6 months after treatment, but is progressive. Patients, especially teenagers and young adults, need to be instructed about its prevention and encouraged to do active jaw exercises. The effect of irradiation on the mucosa of the sinonasal tract is a metaplastic transformation of the epithelium from ciliary columnar respiratory epithelium to cuboidal or squamous stratified epithelium with loss of ciliary function and very often loss of the mucus-secreting elements. In spite of these changes, it is rare that patients experience sinonasal infections. Nevertheless, if they do occur they should be treated promptly and aggressively to avoid undesirable necrosis of soft tissue and osteoradionecrosis of facial bones.

Irradiation of part or the entire pituitary hypothalamic axis is unavoidable when there is cancerous bony invasion of the base of the skull. In such patients, an annual evaluation of the pituitary function and of the thyroid and pituitary adrenal axis is therefore recommended. Proper replacement therapy should be tailored to identified deficiencies.[91]

Management of recurrent or metastatic nasopharyngeal carcinoma

Radiotherapy

Locally recurrent NPC, especially if limited to the primary site, without intracranial extension, should be considered for retreatment with radiotherapy. Pryzant et al.[92] reported the results of retreatment of 53 patients with megavoltage irradiation at the MDACC between 1954 and 1989. Overall 5-year actuarial local control was 35%. Much better results were achieved in a subset of nine patients with recurrent disease confined to the nasopharynx in whom treatment with an intracavitary brachytherapy boost was possible: seven of these patients achieved durable local control. In this series, eight of 53 patients sustained severe complications of retreatment, which were fatal in five. The most significant factor predicting for severe complications was a total cumulative dose of external beam therapy greater than 100 Gy. Similar results were reported by Fu et al.[93] in a series of 74 patients retreated at the University of California at San Francisco between 1957 and 1995. Overall locoregional progression-free survival was 40%. Significant factors predicting for locoregional control were histological type (WHO type 1 worse), time to diagnose a recurrence (longer than 5 years best), and use of brachytherapy in patients with disease confined to the nasopharynx. Complications were significantly increased in patients who received cumulative doses greater than 120 Gy.

The definitive study of risk factors for complications of retreatment is from Hong Kong, where Lee et al.[94] reported on a series of 654 patients retreated between 1976 and 1992. Of these, 539 received external beam therapy alone. The biologically effective dose (BED) of the initial treatment and to a lesser extent the retreatment BED were significant determinants of risk; interestingly, there was no evidence that the time between treatments influenced residual tolerance. In all series, there is clearly less morbidity when a component of brachytherapy is used, reflecting the smaller volume of tissue receiving a high retreatment dose. This was again demonstrated in a recent series by Koutcher et al.[95] who reviewed 29 patients: 16 were retreated with external beam RT (EBRT), using IMRT in the majority, and 13 also received brachytherapy (CMT). The 5-year actuarial local control rates were the same in both groups (52%) but severe complications (temporal lobe necrosis and cranial neuropathies) were higher in the EBRT group. The limitation of brachytherapy in treating disease that extends beyond the nasopharynx can be partially overcome by using modern stereotactic conformal techniques or heavy particle therapy.[96–99]

Several centers have published results of IMRT for treating recurrent NPC. Chua et al. retreated 31 patients with locally recurrent NPC (45% with recurrent T4 disease).[100] Patients received induction chemotherapy and median 54 Gy, with a radiosurgical boost (approximately 10 Gy) in 10 patients. The 1-year locoregional control rate was 56%, but for rT1–3 disease it was 100% compared to 35% for rT4 disease. Severe late toxicity at 1 year was 25% (including 10% cranial neuropathies and 7% brain necrosis). Lu et al. demonstrated a 9-month locoregional control rate of 100% for 49 patients (including 51% rT4) retreated with 70 Gy using IMRT.[101] No subsequent late complication data have been published for either of these series. No results of retreatment with proton beam therapy have yet been published, although theoretically dose to OAR could be reduced using this technology.[102]

Overall it is apparent that there is clinical value in retreatment with RT in selected patients with recurrent NPC disease. Paradoxically, the benefits of IMRT as the current standard for initial treatment of NPC, with its ability to consistently deliver 63 Gy to the posterior aspect of the clivus which is in close proximity to the brainstem, will limit the "available dose" for future use of RT in retreatment of recurrent disease.

Radiotherapy also has a role in the palliative treatment of regional or distant metastatic sites in patients with incurable disease. The most common indication is for painful bony or liver metastases.

Surgery

Technical advances in skull base surgery along with better imaging to define the extent of recurrent disease make salvage surgery also an option for patients with localized recurrence. A variety of approaches have been described but fall into three main groups: inferior/inferolateral,[103–105] lateral,[106,107] and anterolateral.[108] Long-term control rates averaging 38% have been reported,[105,108] a figure that compares favorably with retreatment by radiotherapy. However, it is likely that a greater degree of selection is applied to patients being considered for surgical resection than those for re-irradiation. In a highly selected group from Hong Kong (22 patients over a 10-year period), the anterolateral (maxillary swing) approach provided local control in 82% at 3 years.[109]

Isolated neck recurrences after treatment of NPC are rare (especially for WHO types 2 and 3). However, for patients who do relapse regionally, and in whom no distant disease can be demonstrated, neck dissection is indicated and can be curative. For example, Wei *et al.* reported on 51 patients who underwent radical neck dissection for persistent or recurrent neck disease following radiotherapy.[110] Actuarial 5-year survival and neck control rates were 38% and 66%, respectively. More recently, Yen *et al.*[111] published outcome data on 31 patients undergoing salvage neck surgery in Taiwan over a 14-year period (emphasizing the rarity of the condition). In this series, overall 5-year survival after neck dissection was 67%.

Systemic therapy for recurrent disease

For recurrence in the neck and distant metastatic sites, with or without failure at the primary site, systemic chemotherapy is generally indicated unless functional status is quite poor. Active single agents include the platinating agents, fluoropyrimidines, taxoids, gemcitabine, methotrexate, anthracyclines, bleomycin, and ifosfamide. Platin-based doublets have been studied most commonly and appear most effective in producing complete responses. Overall median survival for patients with incurable recurrent NPC and palliative chemotherapy ranges from 12 to 15 months in most trials. Aggressive triplet or quadruplet combinations may produce higher overall response rates than doublets, but are generally associated with substantial toxicity, including treatment-related death, without a clear impact on survival (reviewed by Guo and Glisson[112]).

Although chemotherapy for most patients with recurrent disease is of palliative benefit only, in the experience of the group at the Institut Gustave Roussy, a small subset of patients (approximately 10%) were long-term survivors (disease free for 82+ to 190+ months) and appear to have been cured.[113] Seventy-five percent of the long-term survivors had isolated bone metastases and many of them were treated with consolidative radiation after a complete response to chemotherapy.

Because the prognosis for most patients with recurrence, especially distant metastases, is quite poor, the investigation of molecular-targeted agents is attractive. Two series have shown that expression of the epidermal growth factor receptor (EGFR) is observed in >80% of endemic NPC, though prognostic import to expression was not consistent.[114,115] A trial with cetuximab, a monoclonal antibody to EGFR, in combination with carboplatin in patients with recurrent disease previously treated with cisplatin demonstrated a partial response rate of 12%.[116] This is nearly identical to response rates seen with cetuximab as a single agent, or combined with cisplatin or carboplatin in platin-refractory patients with squamous cancers of other head and neck sites.[117] Based on these results, cetuximab and nimotuzumab, another antibody to EGFR, are being studied in combination with chemotherapy and/or chemoradiation in patients with locally advanced disease.

Another obvious target for biological therapy of NPC is the association with EBV. In a series of 23 patients, Louis *et al.* have reported on the feasibility of developing *ex vivo* expanded EBV-specific cytotoxic T lymphocytes (CTL) from previously treated patients.[118] These patients were infused with autologous CTL following chemotherapy for recurrence. Of the eight patients who were infused in remission, five remained free of progression 17–75 months from treatment, at the time of publication. Objective regression was observed in 7/15 (48%) patients with progressive disease at the time of treatment. Efficacy appeared most promising for patients with locoregional disease. This approach has also been studied by Comoli *et al.* in a smaller series of 10 patients with similar findings.[119]

Vaccination with dendritic cells primed with viral antigens and peptides with viral vectors integrated have also been studied and demonstrate EBV-specific immune response.[120] Both adoptive immunotherapy and vaccines strategies are being further investigated in patients at high risk for recurrence or in combination with chemotherapy for recurrent disease.

Conclusion

Although nasopharyngeal cancer is a rare disease in Caucasians and other nonendemic populations, there is strong evidence that the results of treatment are significantly influenced by the quality of medical care rendered. Results have improved dramatically over the past three decades and can confidently be predicted to improve further as a result of continuing progress in medical imaging, radiotherapy technical capability, and improved efficacy and tolerance for systemic therapy. In the next decade it is hoped that personalizing therapy based on molecular profiling, in addition to the clinical parameters of T and N stage, will further refine decision making with regard to radiotherapy and systemic therapy.

To ensure that patients with NPC receive optimum treatment, they should ideally be managed in a major cancer center where the experience and expertise to handle the complexities of the disease are available. Furthermore, they should, wherever possible, be enrolled in clinical trials designed to resolve unanswered questions surrounding the disease and its management. As the medical resources available to countries with high endemic rates of NPC increase, opportunities for international collaboration to test new treatment strategies in a timely way should not be lost.

References

1. Michaux L. Carcinoma de base du crâne. In: Godfredsen E (ed) Ophthalmologic and neurologic symptoms of malignant nasopharyngeal tumours. Acta Psychiat Scand 1944; 34(Suppl. 1): 323.
2. Strouhal E. Ancient Egyptian case of carcinoma. Bull N Y Acad Med 1978; 54: 290.
3. Bosworth FH. *A Treatise on Disease of the Nose and Throat*, vol. 1. New York: Wood, 1889.
4. Muir CS. Nasopharyngeal cancer – a historical vignette. CA Cancer J Clin 1983; 33: 180.
5. Batsakis JG, Solomon AR, Rice DH. The pathology of head and neck tumors: carcinoma of the nasopharynx, part II. Head Neck Surg 1981; 3: 511.

6. Michaels L, Hyams VJ. Undifferentiated carcinoma of the nasopharynx. A light and electron microscopical study. Clin Otolaryngol 1977; 2: 105.

7. Shanmugaratnam K, *et al*. Histopathology of nasopharyngeal carcinoma. Correlations with epidemiology, survival rates and other biological characteristics. Cancer 1979; 44: 1029.

8. Taxy JB, Hidvegi DF, Battifora H. Nasopharyngeal carcinoma: antikeratin immunohistochemistry and electron microscopy. Am J Clin Pathol 1985; 83: 320.

9. Weiland LH, Neel HB, Pearson GR. Nasopharyngeal carcinoma. Curr Hematol Oncol 1986; 4: 379.

10. Henle W, Henle G. Epidemiologic aspects of Epstein–Barr Virus (EBV-associated) diseases. Ann NY Acad Sci 1980; 354: 326.

11. Watson CRR. The anatomy of the post-nasal space: its significance in local malignant invasion. Australas Radiol 1972; 16: 118.

12. Parkin DM , Whelan SL , Ferley J , Raymond L , Young J (eds). Cancer Incidence in Five Continents, vol. VII, no. 143. Lyon: IARC, 1997.

13. Lee HP, *et al*. Recent trends in cancer incidence among Singapore Chinese. Int J Cancer 1988; 42: 159.

14. Levine PH, Connelly RR, Easton JM. Demographic patterns for nasopharyngeal carcinoma in the United States. Int J Cancer 1980; 26: 741.

15. Greene MH, Fraumeni JF, Hoover R. Nasopharyngeal cancer among young people in the United States: radical variations by cell type. J Natl Cancer Inst 1977; 58: 1267.

16. Easton JM, Levine PH, Hyams VJ. Nasopharyngeal carcinoma in the United States. A pathologic study of 177 US and 30 foreign cases . Arch Otolaryngol 1980; 106: 88.

17. Neel HB. A prospective evaluation of patients with nasopharyngeal carcinoma: a overview. J Otolaryngol 1986; 15: 137.

18. Wolf H, Haus M, Wilmes E. Persistence of Epstein–Barr virus in the parotid gland. J Virol 1984; 51: 795.

19. Lung ML, *et al*. Evidence that respiratory tract is a major reservoir for Epstein–Barr virus. Lancet 1985; 1: 389.

20. Old LJ, *et al*. Precipitating antibodies in human serum to an antigen present in cultured Burkitt's lymphoma cells. Proc Natl Acad Sci USA 1966; 56: 1699.

21. Pathmanathan R, *et al*. Clonal proliferation of cells infected with Epstein–Barr virus in preneoplastic lesions related to nasopharyngeal carcinoma. N Engl J Med 1995; 333: 693.

22. Rajadurai P, *et al*. Undifferentiated, nonkeratinizing and squamous cell carcinoma of the nasopharynx: variants of EBV infected neoplasia. Am J Pathol 1995; 146(6): 1355.

23. Lo EJ, *et al*. Human papillomavirus and WHO type I nasopharyngeal carcinoma. Laryngoscope 2010; 120(10):1990.

24. Choi PHK, *et al*. Nasopharyngeal carcinoma: genetic changes, Epstein–Barr virus infection, or both. A clinical and molecular study of 36 patients. Cancer 1993; 72: 2873.

25. Hildesheim A, *et al*. CYP2E1 genetic pleomorphisms and risk of nasopharyngeal carcinoma in Taiwan. J Natl Cancer Inst 1997; 89: 12207–12.

26. Vaughan TL, *et al*. Nasopharyngeal carcinoma in a low-risk population: defining risk factors by histological type. Cancer Epidemiol Biomarkers Prev 1996; 5: 587–93.

27. Goldsmith DB, West TM, Morton R. HLA association with nasopharyngeal carcinoma in Southern Chinese: a meta-analysis. Clin Otolaryngol 2002; 27: 61–7.

28. Lu SJ, *et al*. Linkage of a nasopharyngeal carcinoma susceptibility locus to the HLA region. Nature 1990; 346: 470–1.

29. Burt RD, *et al*. Associations between human leukocyte antigen type and nasopharyngeal carcinoma in Caucasians in the United States. Cancer Epidemiol Biomarkers Prev 1996; 5(11): 879.

30. Lo KW, *et al*. Focus on nasopharyngeal carcinoma Cancer Cell 2004; 5: 423.

31. Nicholls JM. Nasopharyngeal carcinoma: classification and histological appearances. Adv Anat Pathol 1997; 4: 71–84.

32. Krueger GRF, *et al*. Histological types of nasopharyngeal carcinoma as compared to EBV serology. Anticancer Res 1981; 8: 27.

33. Shanmugaratnam K, Sobin LH. Histological typing of tumours of the upper respiratory tract and ear. In: Shanmugaratnam K, Sobin LH (eds) *International Histological Classification of Tumours*, 2nd edn. Genevea: WHO, 1991. pp.32–3.

34. Chan JKC, Pilch BZ, Kuo TT, *et al*. Nasopharyngeal carcinoma. In: Barnes L, Eveson JW, Reichart P, Sidransky D (eds) *World Health Organization Classification of Tumours. Pathology and genetics. Head and neck tumors*. Lyon: IARC Press, 2005. pp. 83–97.

35. Prathap K, Looi LM, Prasad U. Localized amyloidosis in nasopharyngeal carcinoma. Histopathology 1984; 8: 27.

36. Nomori H, *et al*. Histiocytes in nasopharyngeal carcinoma in relation to prognosis. Cancer 1986; 57: 100.

37. Moller P, *et al*. Lymphoepithelial carcinoma (Schmincke type) as a derivate of the tonsillar crypt epithelium. Virchows Arch A Pathol Anat Histopathol 1984; 405: 83.

38. Micheau C, *et al*. Lymphoepitheliomas of the larynx (undifferentiated carcinomas of nasopharyngeal type). Clin Otolaryngol 1979; 4: 43.

39. Rosai J. 'Lymphoepithelioma-like' thymic carcinoma. Another tumor related to Epstein–Barr virus? N Engl J Med 1985; 312: 1320.

40. Mills SE, Austin MB, Randall ME. Lymphoepithelioma-like carcinoma of the uterine cervix with inflammatory stroma. Am J Surg Pathol 1985; 9: 883.

41. Neel HB, *et al*. Applications of Epstein–Barr virus serology to the diagnosis and staging of North American patients with nasopharyngeal carcinoma. Otolaryngol Head Neck Surg 1983; 91: 225.

42. Zong YS, *et al*. Immunoglobulin A against viral capsid antigen of Esptein–Barr virus and indirect mirror examination of the nasopharynx in the detection of asymptomatic nasopharyngeal carcinoma. Cancer 1992; 69: 3–7.

43. Tune CE, *et al*. Nasopharyngeal brush biopsies and detection of nasopharyngeal cancer in a high-risk population. J Natl Cancer Inst 1999; 91(9): 796–800.

44. Chan KC, Lo YM. Circulating EBV DNA as a tumor marker for nasopharyngeal carcinoma. Semin Cancer Biol 2002; 12: 489.

45. Chan AT, *et al*. Phase II study of neoadjuvant carboplatin and paclitaxel followed by radiotherapy and concurrent cisplatin in patients with locoregionally advanced nasopharyngeal carcinoma: therapeutic monitoring with plasma EBV DNA. J Clin Oncol 2004; 22: 3053–60.

46. Neel HB. Nasopharyngeal carcinoma: clinical presentation, diagnosis, treatment and prognosis. Otolaryngol Clin North Am 1985; 18: 479.

47. Sawaki S, Sugano H, Hirayama T. Analytical aspects of symptoms of nasopharyngeal malignancies. In: de-The G, Ito Y (eds) *Nasopharyngeal Carcinoma: Etiology and Control*, vol. 147, no. 20. Lyon: IARC, 1978. p. 63.

48. Ng SH, *et al*. Nasopharyngeal carcinoma: MRI and CT assessment. Neuroradiology 1997; 39: 741–6.

49. Poon PY, Tsang VH, Munk PL. Tumour extent and T stage of NPC: a comparison of MRI and CT findings. Can Assoc Radiol J 2000; 51(5): 287–95.

50. Lee AW, *et al*. Treatment results for nasopharyngeal carcinoma in the modern era: the Hong Kong experience. Int J Radiat Oncol Biol Phys 2005; 61: 1107–16.

51. Corry J, *et al*. Relapse patterns in WHO 2/3 nasopharyngeal cancer: is there a difference between ethnic Asian versus non-Asian patients? Int J Radiat Oncol Biol Phys 2006; 64: 63–71.

52. Vikram B, *et al*. Patterns of failure in carcinoma of the nasopharynx. Failure at distant sites. Head Neck Surg 1986; 8: 276.

53. Geara FB, *et al*. Carcinoma of the nasopharynx treated by radiotherapy alone: determinants of distant metastasis and survival. Radiother Oncol 1997; 43: 53.

54. Huang SC, Chu GL. Nasopharyngeal cancer: study 11. Int J Radiat Oncol Biol Phys 1981; 7: 713.

55. Kumar MB, *et al*. Tailoring distant metastatic imaging for patients with clinically localized undifferentiated nasopharyngeal carcinoma. Int J Radiat Oncol Biol Phys 2004; 58: 688–93.

56. Pfister DG, *et al*. Head and neck cancers. J Natl Compr Canc Netw 2011; 9: 597–650.

57. Liu FY, *et al*. 18-FDG PET can replace conventional work-up in primary M staging of nonkeratinizing nasopharyngeal carcinoma. J Nucl Med 2007; 48(10): 1614.

58. Ng SH, *et al*. Staging of untreated nasopharyngeal carcinoma with PET/CT: comparison with conventional imaging work-up. Eur J Nucl Med Mol Imaging 2009; 36(1): 12.

59. Law A, *et al*. The utility of PET/CT in staging and assessment of treatment response of nasopharyngeal cancer. J Med Imaging Radiat Oncol 2011; 55(2): 199.

60. Chua ML, *et al*. Comparison of 4 modalities for distant metastasis staging in endemic nasopharyngeal carcinoma. Head Neck 2009; 31(3): 346.

61. Ho JH. Stage classification of nasopharyngeal carcinoma: a review. IARC Sci Publ 1978; 20: 99.

62. Edge SB, Byrd DR, Compton CC, Fritz AG, Greene FL, Trotti A (eds). *AJCC Cancer Staging Manual*, 7th edn. New York: Springer, 2011.

63. Sanguinetti G, *et al*. Carcinoma of the nasopharynx treated by radiotherapy alone: determinants of local and regional control. Int J Radiat Oncol Biol Phys 1997; 37(5): 985.

64. Reddy SP, *et al*. Prognostic significance of keratinization in nasopharyngeal carcinoma. Am J Otolaryngol 1995; 16: 103–8.

65. Su CK, Wang CC. Prognostic value of Chinese race in nasopharyngeal cancer. Int J Radiat Oncol Biol Phys 2002; 54: 752–8.

66. Marks JE, Phillips JL, Menck HR. The National Cancer Data Base report on the relationship of race and national origin to the histology of nasopharyngeal carcinoma. Cancer 1998; 83: 582–8.

67. Bhattacharyya N. The impact of race on survival in nasopharyngeal carcinoma: a matched analysis. Am J Otolaryngol 2004; 25: 94–7.

68. Ho JH. An epidemiologic and clinical study of nasopharyngeal carcinoma. Int J Radiat Oncol Biol Phys 1978 4: 181–98.

69. Corry J, *et al*. The "boomerang" technique: an improved method for conformal treatment of locally advanced nasopharyngeal cancer. Australas Radiol 2004; 8: 170–80.

70. Mayo C, *et al*. Radiation associated brainstem injury. Int J Radiat Oncol Biol Phys 2010; 76(3): S36–410.

71. Lee N, *et al*. Intensity-modulated radiotherapy in the treatment of nasopharyngeal carcinoma: an update of the UCSF experience. Int J Radiat Oncol Biol Phys 2002; 53: 12–22.

72. Wolden SL, *et al*. Intensity modulated radiation therapy (IMRT) for nasopharynx cancer: update of the Memorial Sloan-Kettering experience. Int J Radiat Oncol Biol Phys 2006; 64: 57–62.

73. Tham IW, *et al*. Treatment of nasopharyngeal carcinoma using intensity-modulated radiotherapy: the National Cancer Center Singapore experience. Int J Radiat Oncol Biol Phys 2009; 75(5): 1481.

74. Ng WT, *et al*. Clinical outcomes and patterns of failure after intensity-modulated radiotherapy for nasopharyngeal carcinoma. Int J Radiat Oncol Biol Phys 2011; 179(2): 420.

75. Lee N, *et al*. Intensity-modulated radiation therapy with or without chemotherapy for nasopharyngeal carcinoma: radiation therapy oncology group phase II trial 0225. J Clin Oncol 2009; 27(22): 3684.

76. Kam MK, *et al*. Prospective randomized study of intensity-modulated radiotherapy on salivary gland function in early-stage nasopharyngeal carcinoma patients. J Clin Oncol 2007; 25(31): 4873.

77. Pow EH, *et al*. Xerostomia and quality of life after intensity-modulated radiotherapy vs. conventional radiotherapy for early-stage nasopharyngeal carcinoma: initial report on a randomized controlled clinical trial. Int J Radiat Oncol Biol Phys 2006; 66(4): 981.

78. Teo PM, *et al*. Final report of a randomized trial on altered-fractionated radiotherapy in nasopharyngeal carcinoma prematurely terminated by significant increase in neurologic complications. Int J Radiat Oncol Biol Phys 2000; 48: 1311–22.

79. Lee AW, *et al*. Treatment of stage IV (A-B) nasopharyngeal carcinoma by induction-concurrent chemoradiotherapy and accelerated fractionation. Int J Radiat Oncol Biol Phys 2005; 63: 1331–8.

80. Lee AW, *et al*. A randomized trial on addition of concurrent-adjuvant chemotherapy and/or accelerated fractionation for locally-advanced nasopharyngeal carcinoma. Radiother Oncol 2011; 98(1): 15.

81. Al-Sarraf MML, *et al*. Chemo-radiotherapy vs radiotherapy in patients with locally advanced nasopharyngeal cancer: phase III randomized Intergroup study (0099) (SWOG 8892, RTOG 8817, ECOG 2388). J Clin Oncol 1998; 16: 1310.

82. Baujat B, *et al*. Chemotherpay in locally advanced nasopharyngeal carcinoma: an individual patient data meta-analysis of eight randomized trials and 1753 patients. Int J Radiat Oncol Biol Phys 2006; 64(1): 47.

83. Zhang L, *et al*. The role of concurrent chemoradiotherpay in the treatment of locoregionally advanced nasopharyngeal carcinoma among endemic population: a meta-analysis of the phase III randomized trials. BMC Cancer 2010; 10: 558.

84. International Nasopharynx Cancer Study Group. Preliminary results of a randomized trial comparing neoadjuvant chemotherapy (cisplatin, epirubicin, bleomycin) plus radiotherapy vs. radiotherapy alone in stage IV undifferentiated nasopharyngeal carcinoma: a positive effect on progression-free survival. Int J Radiat Oncol Biol Phys 1996; 35: 463–9.

85. Langendijk JA, *et al*. The additional value of chemotherapy to radiotherapy in locally advanced nasopharyngeal carcinoma: a meta-analysis of the published literature. J Clin Oncol 2004; 22: 4604–12.

86. Hui EP, *et al*. Randomized phase ii trial of concurrent cisplatin-radiotherapy with or without neoadjuvant docetaxel and cisplatin in advanced nasopharyngeal carcinoma. J Clin Oncol 2009; 27(2): 242.

87. Chen Y, *et al*. Preliminary results of a prospective randomized trial comparing concurrent chemoradiotherapy plus adjuvant chemotherapy with radiotherapy alone in patients with locoregionally advanced nasopharyngeal carcinoma in endemic regions of China. Int J Radiat Oncol Biol Phys 2008; 71(5): 1356.

88. Chan AT, *et al*. Overall survival after concurrent cisplatin-radiotherapy compared with radiotherapy alone in locoregionally advanced nasopharyngeal carcinoma. J Natl Cancer Inst 2005; 97(7): 536.

89. Chitapanarux I, *et al*. Chemoradiation comparing cisplatin versus carboplatin in locally advanced nasopharyngeal cancer: a randomized, non-inferiority, open trial. Eur J Cancer 2007; 43: 1399.

90. Daly T. Dental care in the irradiated patients. In: Fletcher GH (ed) *Textbook of Radiotherapy*, 3rd edn. Philadelphia: Lea and Febiger, 1980. p. 229.

91. Samaan NA, *et al*. Hypothalamic, pituitary and thyroid dysfunction after radiotherapy of the head and neck. Int J Radiat Oncol Biol Phys 1982; 8: 1857.

92. Pryzant RM, *et al*. Re-treatment of nasopharyngeal carcinoma in 53 patients. Int J Radiat Oncol Biol Phys 1992; 22: 941.

93. Fu KK, Hwang JM, Phillips T. Re-irradiation of locally recurrent nasopharyngeal carcinoma. In@ Proceedings of the UICC Workshop on Nasopharyngeal Cancer, Singapore, February 11–14 1998. pp. 173–87.

94. Lee AW, *et al*. Reirradiation for recurrent nasopharyngeal carcinoma: factors affecting therapeutic ratio and ways for improvement. Int J Radiat Oncol Biol Phys 1997; 34: 43.

95. Koutcher L, *et al*. Reirradiation of locally recurrent nasopharynx cancer with external beam radiotherapy with or without brachytherapy. Int J Radiat Oncol Biol Phys 2010; 76(1): 130.

96. Buatti JM, *et al*. Linac radiosurgery for locally recurrent nasopharyngeal carcinoma: rationale and technique. Head Neck 1995; 17: 14.

97. Cmelak AJ, *et al*. Radiosurgery for skull base malignancies and nasopharyngeal carcinoma. Int J Radiat Oncol Biol Phys 1997; 37: 997.

98. Feehan PE, *et al*. Recurrent locally advanced nasopharyngeal carcinoma treated with heavy charged particle irradiation. Int J Radiat Oncol Biol Phys 1992; 23: 881.

99. Leung TW, *et al*. Sterotactic radiotherapy for locally recurrent nasopharyngeal carcinoma. Int J Radiat Oncol Biol Phys 2009; 75(3): 734.

100. Chua DT, *et al*. Reirradiation of nasopharyngeal carcinoma with intensity-modulated radiotherapy. Radiother Oncol 2005; 77(3): 290.

101. Lu TX, *et al*. [Intensity-modulated radiation therapy for 49 patients with recurrent nasopharyngeal carcinoma.] Zhonghua Zhong Liu Za Zhi 2003; 25(4): 386.

102. Liu SW, *et al*. A treatment planning comparison between proton beam therapy and intensity-modulated x-ray therapy for recurrent nasopharyngeal carcinoma. J Xray Sci Technol 2010; 18(4): 443.

103. Fee WE, Robertson JR, Goffinet DR. Long-term survival after surgical resection for recurrent nasopharyngeal cancer after radiotherapy failure. Arch Otolaryngol Head Neck Surg 1991; 117: 1233.

104. Tu G-Y, *et al*. Salvage surgery for nasopharyngeal carcinoma. Arch Otolaryngol Head Neck Surg 1988; 114: 328.

105. Morton RP, *et al*. Transcervico-mandibulo-palatal approach for surgical salvage of recurrent nasopharyngeal cancer. Head Neck 1996; 18: 352.

106. Panje WR, Gross CE. Treatment of tumours of the nasopharynx: surgical therapy. In: Thawley SE, Panje WR (eds) *Comprehensive Management of Head and Neck Tumors*, vol. 1. Philadelphia: WB Saunders, 1987. p. 662.

107. Fisch U. The infratemporal approach for nasopharyngeal tumours. Laryngoscope 1983; 93: 36–43.

108. Wei WI, *et al*. Maxillary swing approach for resection of tumours in and around the nasopharynx. Arch Otolaryngol Head Neck Surg 1995; 121: 638.

109. Chan JY, *et al*. Nasopharyngectomy for locally advanced recurrent nasopharynx carcinoma: exploring the limits. Head Neck 2011 Aug 4 [Epub ahead of print].

110. Wei WI, *et al*. Efficacy of radical neck dissection for the control of cervical metastasis after radiotherapy for nasopharyngeal carcinoma. Am J Surg 1990; 160: 439–42.

111. Yen KL, *et al*. Salvage neck dissection for cervical recurrence of nasopharyngeal carcinoma. Head Neck Surg 1997; 123: 725–9.

112. Guo Y, Glisson B. Systemic treatment for incurable recurrent and/or metastatic nasopharyngeal carcinoma. In: Lu JJ, Cooper JS, Lee AWM (eds) *Nasopharyngeal Cancer: Multidisciplinary Management*. Berlin: Springer Verlag, 2009. pp. 267–74.

113. Fandi A, *et al*. Long-term disease-free survivors in metastatic undifferentiated carcinoma of nasopharyngeal type. J Clin Oncol 2000; 18: 1324–30.

114. Chua DT, *et al*. Prognostic value of epidermal growth factor receptor expression in patients with advanced stage nasopharyngeal carcinoma treated with induction chemotherapy and radiotherapy. Int J Radiat Oncol Biol Phys 2004; 59: 11–20.

115. Leong JL, *et al*. Epidermal growth factor receptor expression in undifferentiated carcinoma of the nasopharynx. Laryngoscope 2004; 114: 153–7.

116. Chan ATC, *et al*. Multicenter, phase II study of cetuximab in combination with carboplatin in patients with recurrent or metastatic nasopharyngeal carcinoma. J Clin Oncol 2005; 23: 3568–76.

117. Trigo J, *et al*. Cetuximab monotherapy is active in patients with platinum-refractory recurrent/metastatic squamous cell carcinoma of the head and neck: results of a phase II study (Meeting proceedings) (Abstract 5502). J Clin Oncol 2004; 22(14s): 488.

118. Louis CU, *et al*. Adoptive transfer of EBV-specific T cells results in sustained clinical response in patients with locoregional nasopharyngeal carcinoma. J Immunother 2010; 33: 983.

119. Comoli P, *et al*. Cell therapy of stage IV nasopharyngeal carcinoma with autologous Epstein–Barr virus-targeted cytotoxic T-lymphocytes. J Clin Oncol 2005; 23: 8942.

120. Lin CL, *et al*. Immunization with Epstein–Barr virus peptide-pulsed dendritic cells induces functional CD8v+T-cell immunity and may lead to tumor regression in patients with EBV-positive nasopharyngeal carcinoma. Cancer Res 2002; 62: 6952.

Section 2: Head and Neck Cancer

9 Esthesioneuroblastoma

Barbara A. Murphy,[1] Salyka Sengsayadeth,[1] Joseph M. Aulino,[2] Christine H. Chung,[3] Kim Ely,[4] Robert J. Sinard,[5] and Anthony J. Cmelak[6]

[1] Department of Medicine, [2] Department of Radiology and Radiological Sciences, [4] Department of Pathology, [5] Department of Otolaryngology, [6] Department of Radiation Oncology, Vanderbilt-Ingram Cancer Center, Vanderbilt University Medical Center, Nashville, TN, USA
[3] Department of Medicine, Johns Hopkins Medical Center, Baltimore, MD, USA

Introduction

Esthesioneuroblastoma (ENB), also termed olfactory neuroblastoma (ONB), is a rare malignancy of neural crest origin, which comprises about 6% of nasal cavity and paranasal sinuses tumors.[1,2] First described by Berger and Luc[3] in 1924, more than 1400 cases have since been reported in the literature.[4] The neoplasm develops from the olfactory epithelium of the cribriform plate, the superior upper one-third of the nasal septum, and the upper surface of the superior turbinate, and has a propensity to invade the skull base and intracranial space.[5] ENB has been known by many names including esthesioneurocytoma, olfactory intranasal neuroblastoma, esthesioneuroepithelioma, olfactory esthesioneuroma, tumor of olfactory placode, and neuroolfactory tumor.[6] The rarity of this tumor has led to the slow progress in our understanding of its pathobiology and the lack of consensus regarding treatment.

Currently, there are no clearly established risk factors or causal agents. ENB occurs across the age spectrum from toddlers to the elderly, and previous studies have shown a bimodal age distribution with an early peak in the teen years and a later peak in the fifth decade of life. More recent studies are showing a more unimodal age distribution, with the highest incidence in the fifth decade.[7] No racial or gender predilection has been noted.[8] The most common presenting symptoms include nasal congestion, anosmia, recurrent epistaxis, pain, headache, and diplopia.[2] Rare cases have also presented with paraneoplastic manifestations such as Cushing syndrome due to ectopic adrenocorticotropic hormone (ACTH) secretion or hyponatremia due to syndrome of inappropriate secretion of antidiuretic hormone (SIADH). Because many of these symptoms are nonspecific and can be attributed to chronic sinusitis, diagnosis can be delayed for prolonged periods of time, and hence patients often present with locally advanced disease.

Since ENB is a rare tumor, individual investigators see and treat only a handful of cases. Thus, pooling of cases is critical.

A number of reviews published over the years have provided insight into the natural history of ENB and have helped in the development of treatment paradigms.[9–16] More recently, two large metaanalyses have been conducted by Broich (1997)[6] and Dulguerov (2001).[2] Broich provides a detailed listing of 208 documented reports between 1924 and 1994 totaling 970 cases of ENB. Dulguerov reported on 26 selected studies that include 390 patients, the majority of which have 5-year survival data. Together, these reports have provided important insights into this uncommon disease.

In general, ENB is considered to be a slow-growing tumor with a prolonged disease course. In the metaanalysis conducted by Broich et al.,[6] the 5-year overall survival of 234 patients was as follows: 68% alive without disease, 13% alive with disease, and 19% dead. When compared to other nonsquamous cell neoplasms of the nasal cavity and paranasal sinuses, 5- and 10-year survival rates are relatively high (Fig. 9.1).[17] There is a subset of patients with poorly differentiated tumors, whose disease course is characterized by rapid progression with high rates of metastatic disease. However, some feel that these rapidly growing tumors represent a different pathological entity, in particular, the clinically aggressive sinonasal undifferentiated carcinomas (SNUC).[15] Miyamoto argues that the designation of high-grade tumors as SNUCs instead of ENB explains the high survival rates reported in some series.[18] Advances in molecular biology will hopefully answer this question in due time.

Staging

Esthesioneuroblastoma usually involves the ethmoid sinuses, and commonly involves the maxillary sinuses, sphenoid sinuses, frontal sinuses, orbits, anterior cranial fossa dura, cavernous sinus, and frontal lobes. The primary tumor more commonly extends inferiorly into the nasal cavity and paranasal sinuses than superiorly to involve the brain.[19] Involvement of

Textbook of Uncommon Cancer, Fourth Edition. Edited by Derek Raghavan, Charles D. Blanke, David H. Johnson, Paul L. Moots, Gregory H. Reaman, Peter G. Rose and Mikkael A. Sekeres.
© 2012 John Wiley & Sons, Inc. Published 2012 by John Wiley & Sons, Inc.

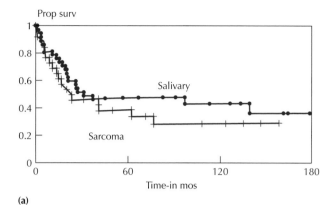

(a)

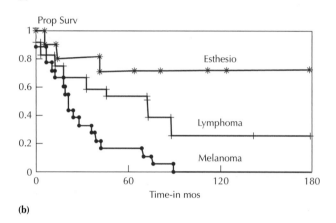

(b)

Figure 9.1 Comparative survival for ENB and other tumors involving the base of skull.[17] (a) Actuarial survival for patients with salivary-type cancer and sarcoma. (b) Actuarial survival for patients with melanoma, lymphoma, and ENB. Reproduced from Spiro *et al.*[17] with permission from John Wiley & Sons, Inc.

these critical structures by tumor has profound implications for staging, treatment, and functional outcome.

There is no uniform staging system, but the most commonly used are the Kadish and Dulguerov classifications. The original staging system for ENB was proposed by Kadish *et al.* in 1976[11] (Table 9.1). Tumors were categorized into three stages: A, confined to the nasal cavity, B, confined to the nasal and paranasal cavities, and C, tumors extending beyond the nasal and paranasal cavities. Only 5% of patients presented with clinically evident nodal disease; however, with time, it has become evident that this cohort of patients has a significantly worse survival (29% for node-positive versus 64% for node-negative disease).[2] Thus, in 1993, Morita recommended the addition of stage D, presence of metastases, to accommodate this cohort of patients.[13] Biller *et al.* proposed the first staging system using the TNM classification in 1990.[20] T3 tumors extended to include the brain and were distinguished from T4 tumors by operability. Finally, in 1992, Dulguerov proposed a staging system that could be based on computed tomography (CT) or magnetic resonance imaging (MRI) findings, thus allowing nonoperative staging.[21]

Because of the nonspecific nature of the presenting symptoms, patients may be symptomatic for prolonged periods of time prior to diagnosis. Therefore, the majority of patients pre-

Table 9.1 Staging systems.

Stage	Extension
Kadish	
A	Limited to the nasal cavity
B	Involving the nasal and paranasal cavities
C	Extending beyond the nasal and paranasal cavities
Morita	
A	Limited to the nasal cavity
B	Involving the nasal and paranasal cavities
C	Extending beyond the nasal and paranasal cavities
D	Presence of metastases
Biller	
T1	Limited to the nasal and paranasal cavities
T2	Extension to periorbital tissue and cranial cavity
T3	Extending to the brain with good operability
T4	Nonoperable extension to the brain
Dulguerov	
T1	Nasal and paranasal cavities excluding the sphenoid
T2	T1 plus extension to the sphenoid
T3	Extending to the orbit and anterior fossa
T4	Extension to the brain

sent with locally advanced disease. In a metaanalysis conducted by Dulguerov, studies using the Kadish staging system reported the following stages at presentation: stage A, 12%, stage B, 27%, and stage C, 61%. Studies using the Dulguerov staging system reported the following T stages at presentation: T1, 25%, T2, 25%, T3, 33%, and T4, 17%.[2] Patients uncommonly present with distant metastases; disseminated disease is usually a feature of recurrence.[19,22,23] Hematogenous spread to the lung, bone, liver, pancreas, skin, mediastinum, and brain has been described.[19,22–24]

Unfortunately, other than the presence or absence of nodal disease, current staging systems fail to consistently predict outcome. In the metaanalysis conducted by Dulguerov, 5-year survival based on stage was as follows: Kadish stage A, 72% (standard deviation [SD] 41), stage B, 59% (SD 44), and stage C, 47% (SD16); Dulguerov stage T1, 81% (SD 17), T2, 93% (SD 14), T3, 33% (SD 33), and T4, 48% (SD 41).

Pathology

Morphological characteristics

Esthesioneuroblastomas are polypoid, red-gray to tan lesions that are composed of discrete lobules of monotonous cells set in a delicate neurofibrillary background (Fig. 9.2). Less commonly, these nodules may coalesce to produce a sheet-like growth pattern with minimal intervening connective tissue. The eosinophilic fibrillary stroma is present in variable amounts in approximately 86% of cases and has been shown ultrastructurally to represent neuronal cell processes. When this fibrillary material is prominent, Homer–Wright rosettes are typically found, with about 28% of instances containing well-developed pseudorosettes. True or Flexner–Wintersteiner rosettes may also be seen, being identified in about 5% or less of tumors. In rare examples, admixed ganglion cells,[25] rhabdomyoblasts,[26]

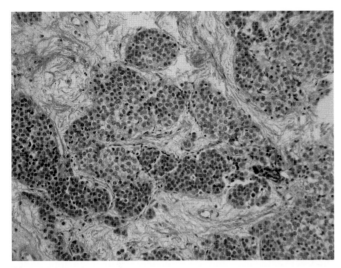

(a)

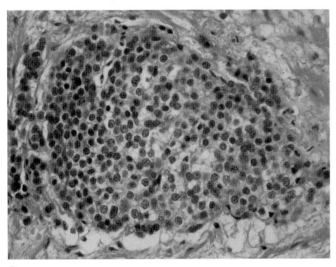

(b)

Figure 9.2 (a) Low magnification: ENB is composed of clustered nests of cells in fibrillary matrix; (b) high magnification: the uniform "small blue cells" have indistinct nucleoli. Cell borders are difficult to appreciate.

and melanin pigment[27] are evident. Cytologically, the neoplastic cells possess small, hyperchromatic, round to oval nuclei with a stippled or "salt and pepper" chromatin possessing inconspicuous nucleoli. The cytoplasm is usually sparse with indistinct cell membranes; however, occasional ENBs may have more abundant eosinophilic cytoplasm. Most cases display a mild-to-moderate degree of nuclear atypia and a low mitotic rate. Necrosis, dystrophic calcification, and lymphovascular invasion are unusual findings. When pleomorphism is pronounced and the proliferation index high, the possibility of another neoplasm should be entertained.

Microscopic grading

In 1988, Hyams and associates[28] proposed a system for grading ENB, which takes into account the following morphological features: lobular architecture, neurofibrillary background,

formation of rosettes, nuclear pleomorphism, mitotic activity, necrosis, and dystrophic calcification. On the basis of these criteria, a numerical grade was assigned from I to IV, with grade I corresponding to the most differentiated lesions and grade IV the least differentiated tumors. Some have found this classification to be an accurate indicator of local recurrence and survival,[2,13,14,18] while others have found it to be of limited value in predicting outcome.[29–31]

Immunohistochemistry

The typical immunohistochemical profile of ENB includes reactivity for markers of neuroendocrine differentiation, with 64–94% labeling with synaptophysin[32–34] and up to 100% with neuron-specific enolase (NSE).[33,34] Chromogranin is less consistent, with only occasional studies reporting variable expression.[33,35] Other neuroendocrine/neural markers such as CD56 and CD57 (Leu-7) are also often positive.[3] Between 73%[33] and 88%[32,34] of cases demonstrate a distinctive peripheral staining pattern with antibodies to S-100 protein. This distribution of S-100-positive cells corresponds to the Schwann cells at the tumor/stroma interface ultrastructurally. Frierson[33] observed that nearly all ENBs in his series were labeled with one or more antibodies that detected neuronal cytoskeletal proteins (class III β-tubulin isotype 82%, microtubule-associated protein 73%, neurofilament 200 kD 73%). These results are in agreement with those in other analyses.[25,34] Recently, a few authors have noted that some ENBs have been found to stain for keratin. Approximately 19–36% of cases have been positive for low molecular weight keratin (CAM5.2).[33,34] They are, however, usually negative or at most focal and sporadically positive for AE1/AE3.[33,34] Immunoreactivity for epithelial membrane antigen (EMA) and carcinoembryonic antigen (CEA) is typically absent.[33,35]

Electron microscopy

On ultrastructural examination, ENB is consistently characterized by numerous intracytoplasmic, neurosecretory, dense-core granules, and cell processes.[32] The neurosecretory, dense-core granules range in size from 80 to 230 nm (mean 140 nm, most granules measuring 100–180 nm) and contain electron-dense cores of relatively uniform shape. Longitudinally arranged neural tubules and an occasional synaptic junction are present within neuronal processes.[36,37] In addition to these structures, sustentacular-like cells can be seen at the periphery of cell nests. These cells are usually devoid of dense-core granules and microtubules.[32]

Differential diagnosis

Esthesioneuroblastoma is a member of the family of "small round cell tumors" and bears histological resemblance to embryonal rhabdomyosarcoma, lymphoma, and Ewing sarcoma/peripheral neuroectodermal tumor (ES/PNET). Usually, it can be distinguished by close attention to morphological, immunohistochemical, and anatomical detail. Specifically, its neurofibrillary stroma, immunophenotype (NSE+, synaptophysin+, leukocyte common antigen [LCA]−, desmin−, and 013−), and confinement to the olfactory epithelium are defining features. In addition, the presence of characteristic S-100-reactive dendritic cells around lobules of tumor cells in ENB is a finding not shared by these other small round cell neoplasms and contrasts with the diffuse, strong staining seen in malignant melanoma.

Molecular biology

Because of the limitations of histological diagnosis by light microscopy, various molecular techniques have been applied to look for characteristic cytogenetic and molecular features of ENBs. With the recent development of molecular technologies such as comparative genomic hybridization (CGH), genomics, and proteomics, the identification of ENB tumors and pathological classification systems will become more sophisticated. The additional biological information will also greatly facilitate clinical management.

Initial evidence indicated that ENB was related to PNET and ES due to the presence of the characteristic translocation found in PNET and ES, t(11 : 22)(q24;q12), causing a gene fusion EWS/FLI1, in ENB cell lines established from metastatic lesions.[38–40] However, emerging molecular evidence indicates that ENB is a distinct entity. Further studies of ENB demonstrated that tumors lack the characteristic EWS gene rearrangement (measured by fluorescent *in situ* hybridization, FISH), reverse transcriptase polymerase chain reaction (RT-PCR) and southern blot analyses), and immunohistochemical analyses indicate that ENB tumors also lack the ES-associated MIC2 antigen.[34,41,42] Furthermore, in one study, expression levels of the human achaete-scute homolog (hASH1) gene, which is critical in olfactory neuronal differentiation and expressed in immature olfactory cells, appeared useful as a diagnostic marker.[43] All four ENB were positive, and 19 poorly differentiated tumors of sinonasal region were negative. In addition, there was an inverse relationship between hASH1 level and grade of the tumor.

Comparative genomic hybridization was performed in a study of 12 ENB patients, including 12 primary tumors and their 10 metastatic/recurrent lesions.[44] This study showed numerous individual chromosomal abnormalities and also a characteristic pattern of chromosomal imbalance consisting of deletions on chromosomal 3p12-p14 and overrepresentations on 17q12 and 17q25 in almost all cases. A more recent study by Guled *et al.* used array comparative genomic hybridization, and the study demonstrated that the most frequent changes included additions at 7q, 9p, 20 p/q, and X p/q as well as deletions at 2q, 6q, 22q, and Xp/q. This study also demonstrated, not surprisingly, that high-grade ENBs had more cytogenetic abnormalities than low-grade ENBs.[45]

Thus, ENB may be separated from other small round cell tumor types through its distinct cytogenetic pattern. In a comparison between the primary tumor, a metachronous lymph node, and two intraspinal metastatic lesions, a high number of shared overlapping alterations were found. This result supports the hypothesis of an underlying clonal process. However, metastatic/recurrent lesions had a higher mean number of chromosomal aberrations per tumor (16 versus 23). Specific patterns of alteration associated with metastatic/recurrent disease could also be determined (deletions in chromosome 5, 6q, 7q, 11, and 15q21, and amplifications of 1p32-p34, 1q12, 2p22-p24). More importantly, these patterns had clinical implications and were associated with a worse prognosis.

Imaging

General imaging considerations

Although ENB is an uncommon tumor, the imaging appearance has been well documented (Figs 9.3, 9.4).[24,46–49] The determination of tumor extent is essential for staging and appropriate therapy. The differential diagnosis of sinonasal tumors is extensive, and unfortunately the imaging appearance of ENB is relatively nonspecific. The imaging differential diagnosis of a mass centered in the superior nasal cavity includes squamous cell carcinoma, minor salivary gland tumor (adenoid cystic carcinoma, mucoepidermoid carcinoma, undifferentiated carcinoma, adenocarcinoma), melanoma, ENB, sarcoma (especially rhabdomyosarcoma), neuroma, lymphoma, and meningioma.[49,50] However, the diagnosis of ENB should be entertained prior to biopsy if certain clinical and imaging findings are identified.

Given that ENB arises from the basal cells of the olfactory epithelium,[51,52] the location of the tumor centered in the superior nasal cavity within the olfactory recess is predictable. However, the olfactory epithelium extends inferiorly to the middle turbinates and can be found in the paranasal sinuses, explaining the occasional *atypical* locations of these tumors[12,48] including the sphenoid sinus, sellar and parasellar region, the nasopharynx, or the petrous apex.[53–60]

Computed tomography imaging of local disease

Facial CT images are most useful to identify bony changes of erosion and remodeling,[49] and to identify calcifications. Images in the axial and coronal planes generated using a bone contrast setting should be obtained and carefully inspected for subtle erosions of the cribriform plate, lamina papyracea, and other facial bone structures. With multidetector CT scanner hardware, high-resolution coronally reformatted images can be generated from axial source data, limiting radiation and patient discomfort. Calcifications have been identified within ENB[11,24,46,47,61] and are better seen on CT than MR images. However, the imaging appearance of residual, partially destroyed bone could be confused with tumor calcifications.[62,63] Rarely, ENB tumors may cause a hyperostotic reaction in adjacent bone.[64] If MR imaging cannot be performed, enhanced CT imaging of the anterior skull base is required to help identify intracranial extension. The use of CT to determine the extent of tumor is limited by retained sinus secretions, which may be of the same density as the tumor, and enhancing, thickened mucosa may also mimic tumor. Enhanced CT (or MR) imaging of the neck is used to identify regional nodal involvement.

Figure 9.3 Esthesioneuroblastoma with intracranial extension. (a) Axial T1-weighted image shows tumor within the superior left nasal cavity and left ethmoid air cells (*asterisks*). Mildly T1-hyperintense signal within the left sphenoid and posterior left ethmoid air cells reflects retained secretions (*arrows*). (b) Coronal T1-weighted postcontrast image reveals cyst formation adjacent to the intracranial component, characteristic of esthesioneuroblastoma. (c) Coronal T1-weighted postcontrast image, obtained 7 years after clinical presentation, shows bilateral convexity dural-based enhancing recurrent tumors. Classic adjacent cyst formation (C).

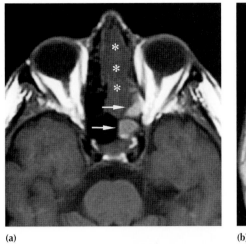

(a)

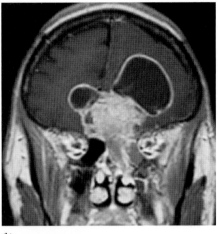

(b)

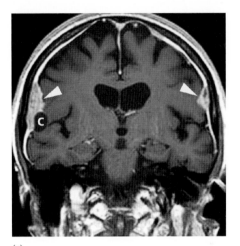

(c)

Magnetic resonance imaging of local disease

The MR imaging appearance of ENB is not specific for this tumor.[48,49] On T1-weighted images the tumor is hypo- to isointense, and on T2-weighted images the signal is iso- to hyperintense, compared with the brain. Contrast enhancement of the tumor is variable but always present. MR imaging is useful to distinguish tumor from retained paranasal sinus secretions, usually displaying different signal characteristics. T2-weighted images are most useful to differentiate tumor from sinus secretions,[49,65,66] although precontrast T1-weighted images occasionally contribute information to make the distinction.[49,66] Enhanced images may also be useful to separate secretions from tumor.[47,49,61,67] Although epistaxis is a frequent presenting symptom for ENB, no hemorrhage is seen within these tumors by imaging, unless a recent biopsy has been performed.[48,49,61,65] Face MR imaging is superior to CT for assessment of intracranial extension of tumor through the cribriform plate to involve the dura, leptomeninges, and brain.[47,68–72] Cystic changes adjacent to areas of intracranial extension of a sinonasal mass have been described as specific for the diagnosis of ENB.[48,62] Although tumor involvement of the olfactory nerves has been reported,[73] frank perineural tumor spread is not characteristic of this malignancy.

The face MR imaging protocol of sinonasal tumors should include postcontrast coronal fat-suppressed T1-weighted images for evaluation of intracranial, dural, and leptomeningeal involvement, and for determining orbit invasion. Dedicated, small field-of-view imaging through the orbits and anterior skull base allows improved resolution compared with routine neck MR imaging, which typically includes lower resolution images through the face. If CT images through the neck have not been obtained, it would be appropriate to perform MR imaging of the neck at the time of the face MRI, to help identify involved cervical nodes.

Computed tomography versus magnetic resonance imaging for local disease

Computed tomography is superior to MRI for evaluation of bone detail, including bony anterior skull base destruction,[69,71] paranasal sinus and facial bone erosion,[69] and tumor calcifications. MRI outperforms CT for determining dural and leptomeningeal involvement[49,71] as well as differentiating sinus secretions from tumor.[47,49,66]

Magnetic resonance and CT imaging of the face and orbits for evaluation of local disease are complementary, and should

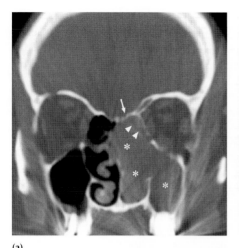

(a)

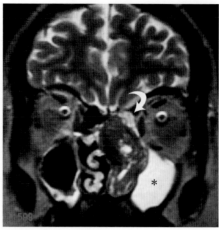

(b)

Figure 9.4 Coronal images through left nasal cavity esthesioneuroblastoma with cribriform plate involvement. (a) CT image in a bone window setting shows opacification of the left nasal cavity and left maxillary sinus (*white asterisks*). Left ethmoid air cells appear opacified as well (*arrowheads*). The bony left cribriform plate is slightly attenuated (*arrow*). (b) T2-weighted image (slightly anterior to (a) shows the retained secretions within the left maxillary sinus (*black asterisk*). The left ethmoid air cells are not completely replaced by tumor (*curved arrow*), as suggested on the CT exam. (c) Postcontrast T1-weighted image shows tumor extension across the cribriform plate (*double arrows*), without nodular dural enhancement. Retained left maxillary sinus secretions (*large arrow*).

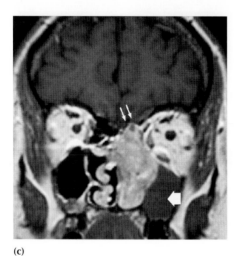

(c)

both be performed for accurate staging and surgical planning.[69,73] The CT and MR images should be carefully inspected for lamina papyracea destruction, orbit periosteum involvement and displacement, extraocular muscle involvement and displacement, and orbit fat involvement. Unfortunately, both CT and MR imaging underestimate orbit involvement by sinonasal tumors when compared with intraoperative assessment.[73,74] Therefore, intraoperative assessment remains the gold standard for the determination of the extent of local disease.[73,75]

Regional and distant disease

Computed tomography has been shown to perform slightly better than MR imaging for the detection of nodes involved by metastatic squamous cell carcinoma,[76] and this would seem to be the case for other metastatic tumors as well. CT imaging is also more sensitive than physical examination for detecting involved nodes,[77–79] and should complement the clinical evaluation routinely. Nodal metastases from ENB usually arise in level II, and retropharyngeal nodes are commonly involved.[80] Nuclear medicine bone scan has been used to characterize osseous involvement at distant sites,[22] and CT scanning of the

chest, abdomen, and pelvis may be useful to detect solid organ involvement. Nuclear medicine whole-body fluorodeoxyglucose positron emission tomography (FDG-PET) scanning appears sensitive to the detection of widespread disease. Although this newer technology remains to be explored, a relative lack of specificity may limit utility.[81] Despite this limitation, FDG-PET shows promise in evaluating for both regional and distant metastatic disease, and will likely become a routine diagnostic method for ENB staging.

Molecular imaging

Despite the theorized neural crest cell origin of the tumor, ENB does not reliably display increased uptake of radioiodinated metaiodobenzylguanidine (^{131}I-MIBG) by nuclear medicine imaging, although cases have been reported.[82,83] Prado *et al.* presented a case of absent ^{131}I-MIBG uptake, possibly related to the histologically undifferentiated nature of the tumor.[84] In that same patient, increased radiotracer accumulation of technetium-99 methylcysteinate dimer (^{99m}Tc-ECD) was identified during evaluation of cerebral blood flow related to the activity of the enzyme esterase within the tumor tissue. Similarly, strong uptake of [111]indium-labeled octreotide, a somatostatin analog, has been shown in primary and metastatic ENB, suggesting a future role for somatostatin receptor-directed radionuclide therapy.[81,85]

The role of FDG PET/CT molecular imaging for staging and restaging (and surveillance) has not yet been determined. Although most nodal metastases are moderate to strongly FDG avid,[80] the low specificity of PET/CT is a concern for some oncologists (Murphy BA, personal communication). An early report has shown that the degree of FDG uptake (SUV) has been correlated with histologic grade of ENB.[86] FDG-PET shows promise in evaluating for both regional and distant metastatic disease, and will likely become a routine diagnostic method for ENB staging, complementing MR and CT.

Recurrence and surveillance imaging

Because of the low incidence of ENB, there are no prospective studies of imaging surveillance. Since a third of patients with regional recurrence are salvageable,[2] aggressive imaging screening as an adjunct to physical examination for the detection of cervical lymphadenopathy is recommended.[76–79] Late recurrences have been reported[11,30] and lifetime surveillance has been proposed.[87,88] Lund *et al.* found that more than half of recurrences occurred adjacent to or within the orbit, suggesting dedicated orbit MR imaging for surveillance.[89] Unfortunately, postoperative and postradiation granulation tissue can be indistinguishable from tumor in the paranasal sinuses,[49,66] often requiring biopsy or serial MR imaging to detect an interval change. Cerebral radiation necrosis may mimic recurrence intracranially.[90] Dural recurrence of ENB is thought to arise after violation of the dura by tumor or surgery,[91] and may be confused with a hematogenous metastatic deposit (see Fig. 9.3). FDG-PET/CT imaging may play a future role in the distinction of postoperative and postradiation changes from recurrent tumor. We suggest baseline face and brain MR imaging 8–16 weeks after surgery and radiation, then every 4–6 months for 5–8 years, with consideration of annual imaging surveillance thereafter.

Although the survival rate of patients with disseminated disease is dismal,[2] radiochemotherapy and bone marrow transplantation have been used successfully to treat metastatic disease.[87] Koka *et al.* reported a 40% rate of distant metastases in their series, of which the most common site was bone (82% of patients with metastases).[22] They therefore proposed that nuclear medicine bone scans be used for routine screening of metastases. However, the metastatic rate to bone is substantially lower in most series, and the cost-effectiveness of this approach is questionable.

Treatment

Historical perspective

Historically, ENB was treated with either surgery or radiation therapy. A case review of 104 patients with ENB was reported by Skolnick in 1966.[92] Five-year survival was 64% for patients treated with surgery and 38% for patients treated with radiation therapy. Early reports documented a high rate of local recurrence with a significant percentage of patients experiencing multiple recurrences over extended periods of time.[10,12] Although recurrence rates were high, some investigators reported high rates of salvage. Although there is no Class I evidence or consensus for treatment, two advances in treatment have made a dramatic impact on outcome: the use of craniofacial resections and the use of combined modality therapy. Because of the two aforementioned metaanalyses, craniofacial resection followed by radiotherapy tends to be considered the gold standard.[2] Craniofacial resection, which allows the *en bloc* removal of tumor, is described below under surgical considerations.

Treatment of early-stage disease

Early-stage lesions below the cribriform plate that exhibit no bony erosion or cranial nerve involvement can be treated with definitive irradiation with good tumor control and preservation of function. However, the vast majority of these tumors will be resected with negative margins and without compromising olfaction or vision. Therefore, the standard practice is to observe or, more commonly, to irradiate postoperatively using moderate doses of 50–60 Gy with conformal treatment planning (3D or intensity-modulated radiation therapy – IMRT) to minimize dose to the optic apparatus, pituitary, and the brain.[93] Elective nodal irradiation is generally not indicated in this setting if imaging (CT, MR, PET) is normal due to the low risk (less than 15%) of subclinical metastases.[94]

Treatment of locally advanced resectable disease

Patients with more advanced local disease benefit from a multimodality approach incorporating surgery, radiation, and chemotherapy. In this setting, the risk of regional nodal and distant metastases becomes a factor in decision making for the clinician. In addition, functional impairment from radical resection increases and the ability to resect all gross disease with clear margins becomes more difficult. Anatomically, ENBs typically arise against the cribriform plate, so both the olfactory epithelium and the overlying dura must be removed to ensure complete resection of the tumor. Anterior craniofacial resection, combining neurosurgical and otolaryngotological expertise, has been the favored surgical approach to allow *en bloc* resection of tumor while minimizing risk to local structures. While this approach has not been evaluated in randomized fashion, most analyses demonstrate a survival advantage compared to the previously used transfacial approach.[19,95]

Local control of 65–100% has been reported, with larger retrospective studies favoring the use of postoperative irradiation even in patients with negative surgical margins. In the Broich metaanalysis,[6] combined modality therapy demonstrated a clear superiority to single modality therapy (72.5% for surgery and radiation therapy versus 62.5% for surgery alone and 53.9% for radiation alone). Similar results were reported in the Dulguerov metaanalysis[2] (65% for surgery and radiation therapy versus 48% for surgery alone versus 37% for radiation alone). Although death rates were highest with radiation alone, this may represent a cohort with a high percentage of patients with advanced nonresectable disease. Foote and colleagues[14] from the Mayo Clinic reported results in 49 patients, 32 of whom had advanced local disease, who underwent surgery with or without postoperative irradiation. The 5-year local control, disease-free survival, and overall survival rates were 65.3%, 54.8%, and 69.1%, respectively. Postoperative irradiation (mean 55.5 Gy) improved local tumor control even in patients with gross total resection.

Some have argued against the combined approach, citing a high rate of complications.[96] In addition, an analysis done by Kane et al. recently reported on 956 patients with median follow-up of 3 years that showed no difference in overall survival between patients who underwent surgery compared to those who underwent surgery plus adjuvant radiation therapy at 5 years (78% versus 75%) or 10 years (67% versus 61%) ($p=0.3$).[97] More recent reports using updated craniofacial surgical techniques and 3D conformal RT or IMRT do not corroborate these concerns and strongly advocate postoperative irradiation with modern techniques in essentially all cases.[16,98]

Unresectable and marginally resectable disease

Unfortunately, some patients will present with unresectable disease. Although criteria vary, patients with invasion of the optic chiasm, the cavernous sinus, and middle fossa are generally considered unresectable.[99] In addition, patients with extensive or bilateral frontal lobe involvement are considered poor surgical candidates. In patients with tumors that are unresectable or marginally resectable, preoperative radiotherapy with or without chemotherapy has been attempted for tumor downsizing with some success.

Because of the histological similarity to small cell carcinomas, investigators have utilized cisplatin-based chemotherapy regimens to treat ENB. Some reports indicate that systemic chemotherapy may be highly effective in previously untreated ENB. In a report by Kim et al., nine of 11 patients had an objective response to a combination of cisplatin, ifosfamide, and etoposide.[100] In a report by Mishima,[101] nine of 12 previously untreated patients who received cyclophosphamide, doxorubicin, and vincristine with continuous infusion cisplatin and etoposide had at least a partial response after two cycles of therapy. Conversely, of three patients treated with induction therapy by investigators at the Johns Hopkins, none had a response.[23] Koka[22] reported the results of 40 patients with ENB treated at the Institut Gustave Roussy. Sixteen patients received induction chemotherapy. Only five (31%) patients had a complete response to induction chemotherapy; however, response to chemotherapy predicted survival in those patients who were treated with definitive radiation therapy. More recently, Porter et al. reported a series of 12 patients with advanced disease treated at the Mayo Clinic with adjuvant chemotherapy with variable combinations of cisplatin, etoposide, ifosfamide, bleomycin, and cyclophosphamide. There was an improved median survival of 83 months versus 78 months and improved median progression-free survival of 2.9 years versus 0.9 years in the adjuvant chemotherapy group versus no adjuvant chemotherapy.[102]

Investigators at the University of Virginia have been strong advocates for the use of preoperative radiation therapy or chemoradiation for patients with Kadish stage B and C disease. Preoperative doses of 45–50 Gy were utilized to remain within optic nerve tolerance. Polin et al. reported that two-thirds of patients experienced a significant reduction in tumor burden.[103] Responding patients experienced an improved disease-free survival. Overall 5- and 10-year survival for the entire patient cohort was 81% and 54.5%, respectively. Others have used radiation with chemotherapy after tumor debulking in order to minimize surgical morbidity. Wieden et al. reported using this approach with postoperative radiation (55.8 Gy), cisplatin and 5-fluorouracil with good survival.[104]

Radiotherapy with chemotherapy has also been used as definitive treatment in locally advanced tumors as well. Fitzek et al. reported 5-year local control of 88% and 5-year survival of 74% in 19 patients treated with etoposide and cisplatin with concomitant-boost radiation.[105] Bhattacharyya[106] utilized a similar approach using daily radiation to 68 Gy, utilizing resection only for incomplete tumor response. Eight of nine patients were able to forego surgery and complications were low. No patients had experienced recurrent tumor with short follow-up.

In a recent case series, Sohrabi et al. report two cases of advanced ENB treated with neoadjuvant chemotherapy, in similar fashion to treatment of small cell lung cancer. The preoperative regimen included cisplatin 60 mg/m² on days 1 and 23 for two cycles and etoposide 120 mg/m² on days 1 through 3 and 23 through 25 given concurrently with 50 Gy of radiation in 25 fractions. While there were complications in both cases, surgery was not delayed, and both patients achieved complete pathological responses and were disease free at 24 and 30 months of follow-up.[107]

Despite the mixed results, chemotherapy is being incorporated more frequently into a combined modality approach for patients with advanced disease. Its role in the treatment armamentarium still needs definition but these results do indicate that in selected cases, particularly in advanced disease, platinum-based chemotherapy can offer additional therapeutic benefit.

Nodal disease

Approximately 5% of patients present with cervical node metastases.[2] However, cervical metastases eventually occur in 20–25% of patients.[108] The presence of involved cervical lymph nodes at diagnosis is an important prognostic factor.[2,19,22,23,109,110] In a study by Koka et al., the 2-year survival of patients with palpable lymph nodes at presentation was 0% compared with 78% for patients presenting with N0 disease.[22] They also noted no correlation of advanced clinical stage (tumor size) with cervical nodal metastases, suggesting aggressive nodal evaluation even with small primary lesions. Treatment options include resection, radiation therapy, or a combination of both. The survival rate in this cohort of patients is poor.

In the Dulguerov metaanalysis, there is reported 5% presence of cervical metastases at diagnosis. This metaanalysis also showed survival data of 29% in initially N+ patients compared with 64% in N0 patients. Thus, this decreased survival had led the authors to recommend aggressive therapy with neck dissection and postoperative radiotherapy. This stance has also been adopted by most centers in treatment of patients with cervical nodal disease. There are no data to guide the extent of the neck dissection in this patient population, and most centers would advocate selective dissection. Usually, the contralateral neck is not dissected, barring any suspicious nodes or nodes crossing the midline.[2]

Because of the poor prognosis of patients with nodal disease, the question has arisen as to how to deal with the clinically negative neck. In a literature review evaluating neck recurrences, Beitler[111] reported that 19% (21 of 110 patients) developed a neck recurrence. Thus, neck recurrence is relatively frequent. Similar results have been reported by others. In a review of 320 patients from 15 reports, Rinaldo[112] reported that 23.4% of patients developed nodal disease. Neck recurrences can be delayed; 10 of 21 patients in Beitler's study developed a recurrence within 24 months of diagnosis, and 18 of 21 had recurred within 60 months. Contralateral neck recurrence is common; hence, some authors have advocated bilateral neck treatment when nodal disease develops. In a metaanalysis of 678 patients by Gore and Zanation, 79 (12.4%) developed late cervical metastases, and analysis indicated a survival advantage in patients who received combined surgery and radiotherapy (odds ratio (OR) of 8.6, $p < 0.003$) versus those who received surgery or radiation alone. There was no statistical difference in analysis of surgery alone versus radiation alone. This led authors to recommend a combined salvage modality of surgery and radiotherapy for late neck metastasis given this survival advantage (59%–14%).[94]

Despite aggressive salvage therapy, a third of patients who develop neck recurrence will die of the disease. This has led some investigators to ask whether prophylactic treatment of the neck with either surgery or radiation would be beneficial.[112] Koka[22] reported a neck failure rate of 0% (0 of 12) in patients receiving elective neck radiation versus 19% (4 of 21) in patients who did not. This area remains controversial with no clear evidence that prophylactic neck irradiation changes the natural history of the disease or increases overall survival, although some institutions advocate treating prophylactically in the immediate postoperative period.[113] Confirmatory data are limited so some advocate treating the neck only when it is found to be clinically involved.[110]

Patterns of recurrence after primary treatment

The median time to first recurrence is generally less than 2 years but late recurrences are common. In one study, the longest time from presentation to recurrence was 13.3 years.[15] Thus, follow-up must be protracted. The most common site of recurrence is local. Local recurrence rates have dropped significantly with the use of combined modality therapy and now occur in approximately 15–30% of patients.[6,13,14,61,87,111] Salvage rates after local recurrence are approximately 30–50%.[2] The second most common site of recurrence is in regional lymph nodes at 15–29%. The salvage rate for patients with nodal disease is about 30%. Although patients seldom present with

distant metastases, 8–17% of patients will develop disseminated disease at some point during their disease process.[19,22,23,61,87] Long-term survivors have been reported with high-dose chemotherapy and stem cell transplantation.

Chemotherapy for recurrent disease

As expected, response rates in previously treated patients were substantially lower. In a report by investigators at Mayo clinic,[114] 10 patients with Kadish stage C disease were treated with platinum-based chemotherapy. Nine of 10 patients had recurrent disease. Two of four patients with high-grade tumors responded to chemotherapy. None of the low-grade tumors responded. Stewart *et al.* reported the results of eight patients with recurrent ENB or poorly differentiated sinonasal tumors, treated with high-dose chemotherapy and autologous bone marrow transplant. At the time of reporting, three patients were alive and another patient had survived 5 years, but relapsed and died after a second transplant. Treatment with high-dose therapy remains experimental.[115]

Surgical considerations

The surgical management of ENB consists of an *en bloc* resection of the tumor, the olfactory epithelium from which it arises, the cribriform plate and its adjacent dural covering, and any other involved structures. This type of resection is best accomplished through what is called a *craniofacial resection*. There are several surgical approaches available to achieve this *en bloc* removal, and the choice of which one to use depends on the anatomical extent of tumor, the individual surgeon's preference, and certain patient factors.

Transfacial approaches to the anterior skull base can be viewed as a progression of increased exposure with extension of incisions that sequentially allow retraction of "modules" of the facial structure. These approaches are combined with a bifrontal craniotomy to gain superior exposure while protecting the frontal lobes of the brain. The lateral rhinotomy is the most basic unilateral approach to tumors of the anterior skull base. The incision begins under the medial aspect of the brow, curves medially and inferiorly between the nasal root and medial canthus, and then courses inferiorly between the nasal and medial cheek subunits, and then curves around the nasal ala. Superiorly, the incision is carried down to the underlying nasal bone and nasal process of the maxilla, while inferiorly the incision connects to the pyriform aperture. This allows removal of the medial maxilla for exposure, and the removed segment of bone can be replaced at the end of the case.

This basic approach allows exposure for tumors involving the maxillary and ethmoid sinus and the anterior portion of the sphenoid sinus, with limited extension into the nasopharynx and clivus. When tumors spread posterolaterally into the infratemporal fossa, the incision can be extended under the eye out to the lateral canthus, providing improved lateral exposure at the price of potential ocular complications.

Tumors with contralateral extension beyond the pterygoid plates require a more bilateral exposure such as that achieved with a midfacial degloving. This approach was designed to expose the maxilla without using facial incisions, primarily for repair of facial fractures. The approach begins with incisions in the nose and under the upper lip that separate the nasal pyramid and facial soft tissues from the underlying bone. Bone cuts are then made, as dictated by the extent of the tumor.

The bicoronal flap is a critical step in the exposure of the anterior cranial fossa from above. It begins with an incision extending from one helical root of the ear to the other, just posterior to the hairline. The pericranial tissues are then elevated forward to the supraorbital vessels and glabella medially and to the lateral orbital rims laterally. The craniotomy is then designed as dictated by the location of the tumor. Generally, a low craniotomy facilitates exposure by minimizing the amount of frontal lobe retraction needed to visualize the anterior cranial fossa. Tumor extension superiorly into the frontal sinus may preclude a low craniotomy, depending on the degree of pneumatization of the sinus. Preoperative imaging provides the information necessary for designing the craniotomy.

Resection of the tumor at this point connects the cranial and facial approaches. After tumor removal, dural defects are repaired with grafts of fascia lata to make the closure watertight. The frontonasal bone segment is replaced and secured into position with miniplates. The frontal sinus is then "cranialized" by removal of the posterior wall and the frontal bone plate is returned to its anatomical position and secured with miniplates or sutures through small drill holes.

The list of complications that can occur with anterior skull base surgery includes those common to surgical procedures in general (such as infection, hemorrhage) and those specific to the anterior skull base (including cerebrospinal fluid (CSF) leak and pneumocephalus). As experience with the procedure and its modifications has grown over the decades, craniofacial resection is no longer considered a procedure of last resort. It is a viable, relatively safe procedure as long as careful attention is paid to the basic surgical principles of careful handling of tissues and accurate closure of dura to obtain anatomical separation of the sterile intracranial environment from the contaminants of the sinonasal cavities.

In recent years, treatment of ENB has involved increasing use of endoscopically assisted cranioresection (EA-CNR) or minimally invasive endoscopic resection (MIER) in selected cases to reduce postoperative morbidity. Several case series have shown good survival and fewer complications associated with these techniques.[116–121] Devaiah *et al.* reviewed published outcomes in a metaanalysis of surgical techniques (open, endoscopic, and endoscopic assisted) for treatment of ENB. In this 16-year analysis, 361 patients were identified, and results indicated that endoscopic/endoscopic-assisted surgery produced better survival rates ($p = 0.0019$, hazard ratio (HR) = 2.39, 95% confidence interval (CI) = 1.20–5.76) than open surgery after adjusting for publication year. However, the limitations of this metaanalysis include small sample sizes, individual skill variations, and the fact that most of the open surgeries were performed on Kadish stages C and D while the endoscopic technique was more commonly used in Kadish Stage A and B. This may be reflecting that the role of endoscopic surgery may still be reserved for less advanced tumors. However, this does indicate that endoscopic surgery is a promising modality that

minimizes invasiveness without compromising oncological principles in carefully selected patients.[117]

Radiation therapy considerations

Radiotherapy should be delivered in fractions of 1.8–2.0 Gy to minimize risk of late normal tissue complications. Three-dimensional or intensity-modulated techniques should be utilized to limit dose to surrounding sensitive structures. Tissue homogeneity corrections are important in this group of patients, particularly after surgical resection where large air spaces may be present. Homogeneity within the high-dose region should be kept within 10% of the prescribed dose, if possible. This is more important when treating to doses over 60 Gy, when areas receiving greater than 110% dose will be at risk for radiation necrosis. Tolerance doses for brain, optic nerves, chiasm, retina, and pituitary need to be maintained to avoid catastrophic complications. In order to improve the therapeutic ratio, some have used conformal irradiation in combination with proton beam or radiosurgery.[105] Zabel and colleagues showed that this technique could simultaneously improve target coverage and lower doses to adjacent critical structures significantly.[122]

References

1. Svane-Knudsen V, *et al.* Cancer of the nasal cavity and paranasal sinuses: a series of 115 patients. Rhinology 1998; 36: 12–14.
2. Dulguerov P, Allal AS, Calcaterra TC. Esthesioneuroblastoma: a meta-analysis and review. Lancet Oncol 2001; 2: 683–90.
3. Berger L, Luc G, Richard D. L'esthesioneuroepitheliome olfactif. Bull Cancer 1924; 13: 410–21.
4. Christmas DA, Mirante JP, Yanagisawa E. Endoscopic view of an esthesioneuroblastoma that resembles a benign polyp. Ear Nose Throat J 2004; 83: 668–70.
5. Mishima Y, *et al.* Combination chemotherapy and radiotherapy with stem cell support can be beneficial for adolescents and adults with esthesioneuroblastoma. Cancer 2004; 101: 1437–44.
6. Broich G, Pagliari A, Ottaviani F. Esthesioneuroblastoma: a general review of the cases published since the discovery of the tumour in 1924. Anticancer Res 1997; 17: 2683–706.
7. Arnesen MA, Scheithauer BW, Freeman S. Cushing syndrome secondary to olfactory neuroblastoma. Ultrastruct Pathol 1994; 18: 61–8.
8. Al Ahawal M, *et al.* Olfactory neuroblastoma: report of a case associated with inappropriate antidiuretic hormone secretion. Ultrastruct Pathol 1993; 18: 437–9.
9. Lewis JS, *et al.* Nasal tumors of olfactory origin. Arch Otolaryngol 1965; 81: 169–74.
10. Elkon D, *et al.* Esthesioneuroblastoma. Cancer 1979; 44: 1087–94.
11. Kadish S, Goodman S, Wang CC, Olfactory neuroblastoma, a clinical analysis of 17 cases. Cancer 1976; 37: 1571–6.
12. Shah JP, Feghali J. Esthesioneuroblastoma. Am J Surg 1981; 142: 456–8.
13. Morita A, Ebersold MJ, Olsen KD. Esthesioneuroblastoma prognosis and management. Neurosurgery 1993; 32: 706–14.
14. Foote RL, *et al.* Esthesioneuroblastoma: the role of adjuvant radiation therapy. Int J Radiat Biol Phys 1993; 27: 835–42.
15. Levine PA, Gallagher R, Cantrell R. Esthesioneuroblastoma: reflections of a 21-year experience. Laryngoscope 1999; 109: 1539–43.
16. Spaulding CA, *et al.* Esthesioneuroblastoma: a comparison of two treatment eras. Int J Radiat Biol Phys 1988; 15: 581–90.
17. Spiro JD, Soo KC, Spiro RH. Nonsquamous cell malignant neoplasms of the nasal cavity and paranasal sinuses. Head Neck 1995; 17: 114–18.

18. Miyamoto RC, *et al*. Esthesioneuroblastoma and sinonasal undifferentiated carcinoma: impact of histologic grading and clinical staging on survival and prognosis. Laryngoscope 2000; 110: 1262–5.

19. Dias FL, *et al*. Patterns of failure and outcome in esthesioneuroblastoma. Arch Otolaryngol Head Neck Surg 2003; 129: 1186–92.

20. Biller HF, *et al*. Esthesioneuroblastoma: surgical treatment without radiation. Laryngoscope 1990; 100: 1199–201.

21. Dulguerov P, Calcaterra T, Esthesioneuroblastoma: the UCLA experience 1970–1992. Laryngoscope 1992; 102: 843–9.

22. Koka VT, *et al*. Aesthesioneuroblastoma. J Laryngol Otol 1998; 112: 628–33.

23. Resto VA, *et al*. Esthesioneuroblastoma: the Johns Hopkins experience. Head Neck 2000; 22: 550–8.

24. Manelfe C, *et al*. Computer tomography in olfactory neuroblastoma: one case of esthesioneuroepithelioma and four cases of esthesioneuroblastoma. J Comput Assist Tomogr 1978; 2: 412–20.

25. Mills SE, Frierson HF. Olfactory neuroblastoma – a clinicopathologic study of 21 cases. Am J Surg Pathol 1985; 9: 317–27.

26. Slootweg PJ, Lubsen H. Rhabdomyoblasts in olfactory neuroblastoma. Histopathology 1991; 19: 182–4.

27. Curtis JL, Rubinstein LJ. Pigmented olfactory neuroblastoma. Cancer 1982; 49: 2136–43.

28. Hyams VJ, Batsakis VJ, Michaels L (eds). Tumors of the upper respiratory tract and ear. Atlas of Tumor Pathology, Fascicle 25. Washington, DC: Armed Forces Institute of Pathology, 1988. pp. 240–8.

29. Papadaki H, *et al*. Relationship of p53 gene alterations with tumor progression and recurrence in olfactory neuroblastoma. Am J Surg Pathol 1986; 20: 715–21.

30. Diaz EM, *et al*. Olfactory neuroblastoma: the 22-year experience at one comprehensive cancer center. Head Neck 2005; 27: 138–49.

31. Ingeholm P, *et al*. Esthesioneuroblastoma: a Danish clinicopathological study of 40 consecutive cases. APMIS 2002; 110: 639–45.

32. Hirose T, *et al*. Olfactory neuroblastoma. An immunohistological, ultrastructural, and flow cytometric study. Cancer 1995; 76: 4–19.

33. Frierson HF, *et al*. Olfactory neuroblastoma. Additional immunohistochemical characterization. Am J Surg Pathol 1990; 94: 547–53.

34. Argani P, *et al*. Olfactory neuroblastoma is not related to the Ewing family of tumors: absence of EWS/FLI1 gene fusion and MIC2 expression. Am J Surg Pathol 1987; 22: 391–8.

35. Axe S, Kuhajda FP. Esthesioneuroblastoma. Intermediate filaments, neuroendocrine, and tissue-specific antigens. Am J Clin Pathol 1987; 88: 139–45.

36. Min K. Usefulness of electron microscopy in the diagnosis of "small" round cell tumors of the sinonasal region. Ultrastruct Pathol 1995; 19: 347–63.

37. Taxy JB, *et al*. The spectrum of olfactory neural tumors – a light microscopic immunohistochemical and ultrastructural analysis. Am J Surg Pathol 1986; 10: 687–95.

38. Whang-Peng J, *et al*. Translocation t(11;22) in esthesioneuroblastoma and their metastases. Cancer Genet Cytogenet 1987; 29: 155–7.

39. Cavazzana AO, *et al*. Olfactory neuroblastoma is not a neuroblastoma but is related to primitive neuroectodermal tumor (PNET). Prog Clin Biol Res 1988; 271: 463–73.

40. Sorensen PH, *et al*. Olfactory neuroblastoma is a peripheral primitive neuroectodermal tumor related to Ewing's sarcoma. Proc Natl Acad Sci USA 1996; 93: 1038–43.

41. Mezzelani A, *et al*. Esthesioneuroblastoma is not a member of the primitive peripheral neuroectodermal tumour-Ewing's group. Br J Cancer 1999; 81: 586–91.

42. Kumar S, *et al*. Absence of EWS/FLI1 fusion in olfactory neuroblastomas indicates these tumors do not belong to the Ewing's sarcoma family. Hum Pathol 1999; 30: 1356–60.

43. Mhawawech P, *et al*. Human achaete-scute homologue (hASH1) mRNA level as a diagnostic marker to distinguish esthesioneuroblastoma from poorly differentiated tumors arising in the sinonasal tract. Am J Clin Pathol 2004; 122: 100–5.

44. Bockmuhl U, *et al*. CGH pattern of esthesioneuroblastoma and their metastases. Brain Pathol 2004; 14: 158–63.

45. Guled M, Myllykangas S, Frierson HF Jr, Mills SE, Knuutila S, Stelow EB. Array comparative genomic hybridization analysis of olfactory neuroblastoma. Mod Pathol 2008; 21(6): 770–8.

46. Hurst RW, *et al*. Computer tomographic features of esthesioneuroblastoma. Neuroradiology 1989; 31: 253–7.

47. Li C, *et al*. Olfactory neuroblastoma: MR evaluation. Am J Neuroradiol 1993; 14: 1167–71.

48. Derdeyn CP, *et al*. MRI of esthesioneuroblastoma. J Comput Assist Tomogr 1994; 18: 16–21.

49. Schuster JJ, Phillips CD, Levine PA. MR of esthesioneuroblastoma (olfactory neuroblastoma) and appearance after craniofacial resection. Am J Neuroradiol 1994; 15: 1169–77.

50. Loevner LA, Sonners AI. Imaging of neoplasms of the paranasal sinuses. Magn Reson Imaging Clin North Am 2002; 10: 467–93.

51. Michaeu C. A new histological approach to olfactory esthesioneuroma. Cancer 1977; 40: 314–18.

52. Cantrell RW, Ghorayeb BY, Fitz-Hugh GS, Esthesioneuroblastoma: diagnosis and treatment. Ann Otol Rhinol Laryngol 1977; 86: 760–5.

53. Castro L, de la Pava S, Webster JH. Esthesioneuroblastoma: a report of 7 cases. Am J Roentgenol Rad Ther Nucl Med 1969; 105: 7–13.

54. Mashberg A, Thoma KH, Wasilewski EJ. Olfactory neuroblastoma (esthesioneuroblastoma) of the maxillary sinus. Oral Surg Oral Med Oral Pathol 1960; 13: 908–12.

55. Sawar M. Primary sellar-parasellar esthesioneuroblastoma. Am J Roentgenol 1979; 133: 140–1.

56. Chacko G, Chandi Chandy MJ. Primary sphenoid and petrous apex esthesioneuroblastoma: case report. Br J Neurosurg 1998; 12: 264–6.

57. Roy A, *et al*. Correspondence: aesthesioneuroblastoma arising in pituitary gland. Neuropathol Appl Neurobiol 2000; 26: 177–9.

58. Sharma SC, *et al*. Isolated esthesioneuroblastoma of sphenoid sinus. Am J Otolaryngol 2002; 23: 287–9.

59. Chirico G, *et al*. Primary sphenoid esthesioneuroblastoma studied with MR. J Clin Imag 2003; 27: 38–40.

60. Mariani L, *et al*. Esthesioneuroblastoma of the pituitary gland: a clinico-pathological entity? J Neurosurg 2004; 101: 1049–52.

61. Pickuth D, Heywang-Kobrunner SH. Imaging of recurrent esthesioneuroblastoma. Br J Radiol 1999; 72: 1052–7.

62. Som PM, *et al*. Sinonasal esthesioneuroblastoma with intracranial extension: marginal tumor cysts as a diagnostic MR finding. Am J Neuroradiol 1994; 15: 1259–62.

63. Som PM, Lidov M. The significance of sinonasal radiodensities: ossification, calcification, or residual bone? Am J Neuroradiol 1994; 15: 917–22.

64. Roegenbogen VS, *et al*. Hyperostotic esthesioneuroblastoma: CT and MR findings. J Comput Assist Tomogr 1988; 12: 52–6.

65. Schroth G, *et al*. MR imaging of esthesioneuroblastoma. J Comput Assist Tomogr 1986; 10: 316–19.

66. Som PM, *et al*. Sinonasal tumors and inflammatory tissues: differentiation with MR imaging. Radiology 1988; 167: 803–9.

67. Lanzieri CF, *et al*. Use of gadolinium-enhancing MR imaging for differentiating mucoceles from neoplasms in the paranasal sinuses. Radiology 1991; 178: 425–8.

68. Sze G, *et al*. MR imaging of the cranial meninges with emphasis on contrast enhanced and meningeal carcinomatosis. Am J Neuroradiol 1989; 10: 965–75.

69. Kraus DH, *et al*. Complementary use of computer tomography and magnetic imaging in assessing skull base lesions. Laryngoscope 1992; 102: 623–9.

70. Eisen MD, *et al*. Use of pre-operative MR to predict dural, perineural, and venous sinus invasion of skull base tumors. Am J Neuroradiol 1996; 17: 1937–45.

71. Ishida H, Mohri M, Amatsu M. Invasion of the skull base by carcinomas: histopathologically evidenced findings with CT and MRI. Eur Arch Otorhinolaryngol 2002; 259: 535–9.

72. Maroldi R, Ambrosi C, Farina D. Metastatic disease of the brain: extra-axial metastases. Eur Radiol 2005; 15: 617–26.

73. Eisen MD, *et al.* Preoperative imaging to predict orbital invasion by tumor. Head Neck 2000; 22: 456–62.

74. Maroldi R, *et al.* MR of malignant nasosinusal neoplasm. Frequently asked questions. Eur Radiol 1997; 24: 181–90.

75. Som PM, *et al.* Ethmoid sinus disease: CT evaluation in 400 cases. Part III. Radiology 1986; 159: 605–9.

76. Curtin HD, *et al.* Comparison of CT and MR imaging in staging neck metastases. Radiology 1998; 207: 123–30.

77. Shingaki S, *et al.* Computer tomographic evaluation of lymph node metastases in head and neck carcinomas. J Craniomaxillofac Surg 1995; 23: 233–7.

78. Merritt RM, *et al.* Detection of cervical metastasis: a meta-analysis comparing computer tomography with physical exam. Arch Otolaryngol Head Neck Surg 1997; 123: 149–52.

79. Atula TS, *et al.* Assessment of cervical lymph node status in head and neck cancer patients: palpation, computer tomography and low field magnetic resonance imaging compared with ultra-sound-guided fine-needle aspiration cytology. Eur Radiol 1997; 25: 152–61.

80. Howell MC, Branstetter BF 4th, Snyderman CH. Patterns of regional spread for esthesioneuroblastoma. Am J Neuroradiol 2011; 32: 929–33.

81. Yu J, *et al.* Ectopic Cushing's syndrome caused by an esthesioneuroblastoma. Endocr Pract 2004; 10: 119–24.

82. Kairemo KJA, *et al.* Imaging of olfactory neuroblastoma – an analysis of 17 cases. Auris Nasus Larynx 1998; 25: 173–9.

83. Sasajima T, *et al.* High uptake of 123I-metaiodobenzylguanidine related to olfactory neuroblastoma revealed by single-photon emission CT. Am J Neuroradiol 2000; 21: 717–20.

84. Prado GLM, *et al.* Olfactory neuroblastoma visualized by technetium-99m-ECD SPECT. Radiat Med 2001; 19: 267–70.

85. Ramsey HA, Kairemo KJ, Jekunen AP. Somatostatin receptor imaging of olfactory neuroblastoma. J Laryngol Otol 1996; 110: 1161–3.

86. Mahmood Y, *et al.* 18F-Fluorodeoxyglucose (FDG) PET/CT-based evaluation of esthesioneuroblastoma: correlating standardized uptake value with histological tumor grade. Poster presentation. J Nucl Med 2007; 48 (Suppl 2): 365P.

87. Eden BV, *et al.* Esthesioneuroblastoma: long-term outcome and patterns of failure – the University of Virginia experience. Cancer 1994; 73: 2556–62.

88. Girod D, Hanna E, Marentette L. Esthesioneuroblastoma. Head Neck 2001; 23: 500–5.

89. Lund VJ, *et al.* Olfactory neuroblastoma: past, present, and future? Laryngoscope 2003; 11: 502–7.

90. Tran TA, *et al.* Delayed cerebral radiation necrosis. Am J Roentgenol 2003; 180: 70.

91. Valenzuela R, Hanna E, Loevner LA, Shatzkes DR, Michel MA, Ginsberg LE. Dural metastases: a form of recurrence of uncommon sinonasal malignancies [oral abstract]. Program and Abstracts of the Forty-fourth Annual Meeting of the American Society of Head & Neck Radiology, Houston, Texas, October 6–10, 2010. p. 177.

92. Skolnick EM, Massari FM, Tenta LT, Olfactory neuroepithelioma. Arch Otolaryngol 1966; 84: 644–53.

93. Chao KS, *et al.* Esthesioneuroblastoma: the impact of treatment modality. Head Neck 2001; 23: 749–57.

94. Gore MR, Zanation AM. Salvage treatment of late neck metastasis in esthesioneuroblastoma: a meta-analysis. Arch Otolaryngol Head Neck Surg 2009; 135: 1030–4.

95. Ketcham AS, *et al.* The ethmoid sinuses: a re-evaluation of surgical resection. Am J Surg 1973; 126: 469–76.

96. Olsen KD, de Santo L. Olfactory neuroblastoma. Acta Otolaryngol 1983; 109: 797–802.

97. Kane AJ, *et al.* Posttreatment prognosis of patients with esthesioneuroblastoma. J Neurosurg 2010; 113: 340–51.

98. O'Connor TA, *et al.* Olfactory neuroblastoma. Cancer 1989; 63: 2426–8.

99. Levine PA, McLean WC, Cantrell RW. Esthesioneuroblastoma: the University of Virginia experience 1960–1985. Laryngoscope 1986; 96: 742–6.

100. Kim DW, *et al.* Neoadjuvant etoposide, ifosfamide, and cisplatin for the treatment of olfactory neuroblastoma. Cancer 2004; 101: 2257–60.

101. Mishima Y, *et al.* Combination chemotherapy (cyclophosphamide, doxorubicin, and vincristine with continuous-infusion cisplatin and etoposide) and radiotherapy with stem cell support can be beneficial for adolescents and adults with esthesioneuroblastoma. Cancer 2004; 101: 1437–44.

102. Porter AB, *et al.* Retrospective review of adjuvant chemotherapy for esthesioneuroblastoma. J Neurooncol 2008; 90: 201–4.

103. Polin RS, *et al.* The role of pre-operative adjuvant treatment in the management of esthesioneuroblastoma: the University of Virginia Experience. Neurosurgery 1998; 42: 1029–37.

104. Wieden PL, Yarington CT Jr, Richardson RG. Olfactory neuroblastoma. Chemotherapy and radiotherapy for extensive disease. Arch Otolaryngol 1984; 110: 759–60.

105. Fitzek MM, *et al.* Neuroendocrine tumors of the sinonasal tract. Results of a prospective study incorporating chemotherapy, surgery, and combined proton-photon radiotherapy. Cancer 2002; 94: 2623–34.

106. Bhattacharyya N, *et al.* Successful treatment of esthesioneuroblastoma and neuroendocrine carcinoma with combined chemotherapy and proton radiation: results in 9 cases. Arch Otolaryngol Head Neck Surg 1997; 123: 34–40.

107. Sohrabi S, *et al.* Neoadjuvant concurrent chemoradiation for advanced esthesioneuroblastoma: a case series and review of the literature. J Clin Oncol 2011; 29: e358–61.

108. Zanation AM, *et al.* When, how and why to treat the neck in patients with esthesioneuroblastoma: a review. Eur Arch Otorhinolaryngol 2010; 267: 1667–71.

109. Homzie MJ, Elkon D. Olfactory esthesioneuroblastoma. Cancer 1980; 46: 2509–13.

110. Rinaldo A, *et al.* Esthesioneuroblastoma and cervical lymph node metastases: clinical and therapeutic implications. Acta Otolaryngol 2002; 122: 215–21.

111. Beitler JJ, *et al.* Esthesioneuroblastoma: is there a role for elective neck treatment? Head Neck 1991; 13: 321–6.

112. Ferlito A, Rinaldo A, Rhys-Evans PH. Contemporary clinical commentary: esthesioneuroblastoma: an update on management of the neck. Laryngoscope 2003; 113: 1935–8.

113. Monroe AT, *et al.* Radiation therapy for esthesioneuroblastoma: rationale for elective neck irradiation. Head Neck 2003; 25: 529–34.

114. McElroy E, Buckner JC, Lewis JE. Chemotherapy for advanced esthesioneuroblastoma: the Mayo clinic experience. Neurosurgery 1998; 42: 1023–7.

115. Stewart FM, *et al.* High-dose chemotherapy and autologous marrow transplant for esthesioneuroblastoma and sinonasal undifferentiated carcinoma. Am J Clin Oncol 1989; 12: 217–21.

116. Batra PS, *et al.* Outcomes of minimally invasive endoscopic resection of anterior skull base neoplasms. Laryngoscope 2010; 120: 9–16.

117. Devaiah AK, Andreoli MT. Treatment of esthesioneuroblastoma: a 16-year meta-analysis of 361 patients. Laryngoscope 2009; 119: 1412–16.

118. Suriano M, *et al.* Endoscopic treatment of esthesioneuroblastoma: a minimally invasive approach combined with radiation therapy. Otolaryngol Head Neck Surg 2007; 136: 104–7.

119. Yuen AP, *et al.* Endoscopic-assisted cranionasal resection of olfactory neuroblastoma. Head Neck 2005; 27: 488–93.

120. Liu JK, *et al.* Endoscopic-assisted craniofacial resection of esthesioneuroblastoma: minimizing facial incisions – technical note and report of 3 cases. Minim Invasive Neurosurg 2003; 46: 310–15.

121. Casiano RR, Numa WA, Falquez AM. Endoscopic resection of esthesioneuroblastoma. Am J Rhinol 2001; 15: 271–9.

122. Zabel A, *et al.* The role of stereotactically guided conformal radiotherapy for local tumor control of esthesioneuroblastoma. Strahlenther Onkol 2002; 178: 187–91.

Section 3: Endocrine Tumors

10 Adrenal Neoplasms

Alexandria T. Phan,[1] Mouhammed A. Habbra,[2] Elizabeth G. Grubbs,[3] and Cesar Moran[4]

[1] Department of Gastrointestinal Medical Oncology, [2] Department of Endocrine Neoplasia and Hormone Disease,
[3] Department of Surgical Oncology, [4] Department of Pathology, The University of Texas MD Anderson Cancer Center, Houston, TX, USA

Introduction

The adrenal glands are chiefly responsible for releasing hormones in response to stress through the synthesis of corticosteroids such as cortisol and catecholamines such as epinephrine, and in response to plasma osmolarity changes through the secretion of aldosterone. The adrenal cortex is divided into functional zones, including zona glomerulosa, zona fasciculata, and zona reticularis. The outermost layer, the zona glomerulosa, is the main site for production of mineralocorticoids, mainly aldosterone, which is largely responsible for the long-term regulation of blood pressure by affecting the functions of the kidneys. The innermost cortical layer, the zona reticularis, produces androgens, mainly dehydroepiandrosterone (DHEA) and DHEA sulfate (DHEA-S). Situated between the glomerulosa and reticularis, the zona fasciculata is responsible for producing glucocorticoids, chiefly cortisol. Whereas the zona glomerulosa is primarily regulated by angiotensin II, both the zona fasciculata and the zona reticularis are regulated by corticotropin or adrenocorticotropic hormone (ACTH).[1] Both these zones become hypofunctional and atrophic when ACTH is deficient; on the other hand, they become hypertrophic and hyperplastic when ACTH is secreted in excess.

Neoplasms of the adrenal glands can be primary, secondary, or incidental. Primary adrenal neoplasms are further divided into benign or malignant originating from the cortex or the medulla. Within the adrenal cortex, there are benign adrenocortical adenomas (ACAs) and malignant adrenocortical carcinomas (ACCs). On the other hand, benign and malignant pheochromocytomas (PHEO) make up the neoplasms of the adrenal medulla. Secondary adrenal gland neoplasms refer to malignant metastatic disease from other primary sites. Among the common malignancies with secondary metastatic involvement of the adrenal glands are melanoma, lymphoma, and carcinomas of the lung, breast, colon, and rectum.[2] With the advent of more sectional body computed tomography (CT)/magnetic resonance imaging (MRI) scans performed for abdominal symptoms, incidental findings of adrenal masses are discovered.[2] These are referred to as adrenal "incidentalomas" (AIs).

Clinical manifestations of adrenal neoplasms are typified by the hormones being oversecreted or symptoms relating to mass effects from cancerous infiltration or metastasis. Understanding of the physiological functions of the adrenal glands will help to decipher the primary site of pathology, cortex or medulla. Clinical behaviors such as distant metastases or disease recurrences are often used to distinguish malign from benign pathology. Fortunately, benign neoplasms of the adrenal glands are more common than malignant diseases. Radiological and laboratory evaluations help to determine the extend of diseases and hormonal functionality of the neoplasms. Major modalities of radiological assessments include CT and MRI scans. Pathological assessment of adrenal glands, especially with regard to any malignant potential, is difficult, mainly because of the lack of published large series and the clinical and biological heterogeneity of the disease.

Both ACC and malignant PHEO are rare primary malignancies of the adrenal glands, occurring with an approximate annual incidence of 0.6–1.67 per 100,000[3] and 0.0005–0.0011 per 100,000[4] respectively. Patients presenting with localized neoplasm of the adrenal glands should undergo surgical resection, and most benign conditions are curable. However, malignant adrenal neoplasms such as ACCs rarely have durable survival because of their high frequency of recurrence and/or metastases at the time of diagnosis. Antineoplastic therapeutic options are limited and there is none with clear documentation of survival benefits over placebo alone. Standard of care therapy for malignant adrenal neoplasms is based on consensus recommendations, not on level 1 evidence.[5] Pharmaceutical interest in drug development for these rare diseases is nonexistent, because of the lack of commercial potential, and effective treatment options are limited. Additionally, clinical heterogeneity and rarity of diseases make formal clinical research and drug development programs very difficult without international collaborative efforts.

However, the fast accrual rate and early completion of an international randomized phase 3 placebo-controlled study in advanced ACCs has recently demonstrated that meaningful clinical research for these orphan malignancies is feasible.[6] Continued scientific advancement, clinical research, and collaborations will further personalize drug development and improve prognosis in malignancies of the adrenal glands.

Neoplasms of the adrenal cortex

Clinical presentation

As in most endocrine neoplasms, clinical presentations reflect the neoplastic burden or are the result of hormonal oversecretion. While it is possible for a neoplasm producing hormones (functional) to have symptoms from both the hormones and the disease burden, the reverse is not true for a neoplastic process without hormonal overproduction (nonfunctional). Both malignant and benign neoplasms of the adrenal cortex can be either functional or nonfunctional (Fig. 10.1). Patients can present with constitutional symptoms such as fever, night sweats, cachexia, anorexia, weight loss, malaise and fatigue. Certain symptoms such as abdominal discomfort, pain, and fullness can be associated with nausea, vomiting, early satiety, and dyspepsia. Specific to the location of the adrenal glands in proximity to the kidneys, liver, and inferior vena cava (IVC), nonfunctional symptoms may include flank pain, dysuria, urinary frequency or hesitancy resulting from obstructive hydronephrosis, and lower extremity edema associated with tumor thrombosis of the IVC.

Whether adrenal masses appear unilateral or bilateral, evaluation for malignancy necessitates good understanding of the epidemiology of secondary and primary malignancies that typically involve the adrenal glands. The knowledge that metastatic spread of other primary malignancies is more common than primary adrenal cancer, along with a healthy appreciation that unilateral adrenal involvement frequently correlates with benign adrenal pathology, will go a long way to contributing to the correct diagnosis.

Clinical parameters important for differentiating malignant from benign adrenal tumors include size and imaging characteristics of the adrenal mass. As demonstrated in a retrospective analysis of a large database from the National Italian Study Group on Adrenal Tumors, the maximum diameter of the adrenal mass is predictive of malignancy.[7] ACC were significantly associated with mass size, with 90% being more than 4 cm in diameter when discovered. Angeli *et al.* had suggested that a 4 cm maximal adrenal diameter cutoff has 93% sensitivity and 76% specificity for detecting ACC.[7] Additionally, the smaller the ACC at the time of diagnosis, the more favorable the overall prognosis.

The complex of symptoms is variable, based on what is affected by neoplastic infiltration or malignant spread. Hormone overproducing adrenal tumors are found, respectively, in 40% to 60% of ACC cases, and approximately 20% to 80% of ACA cases.[8-10] Functional neoplasms of the adrenal glands, more than those that are nonfunctional, are diagnosed at earlier cancer stages. Possible explanations for this include that the size of neoplastic growth is not the criterion for hormonal overproduction or possibly that the clinical manifestations of the hormones lead to earlier diagnosis. The effects of neoplastic growth typically imply that the burden of disease is bulky, with significantly more local infiltration, and ultimately increased likelihood of advanced stage at diagnosis. Because the adrenal cortex can produce pure glucocorticoids, minerocorticoids, sex steroids or combinations, clinical manifestations attributable to functional adrenocortical neoplasms are the effects of isolated or combined oversecretion of hormones. Disorders from the excess productions of cortisol, aldosterone, or androgen are respectively referred to as Cushing syndrome, Conn syndrome, and adrenogenital syndrome. Signs and symptoms of these hormonal syndromes associated with functional tumors of the adrenal cortex are listed in Table 10.1.

Cushing syndrome

Cushing syndrome is defined as a pathological condition caused by high levels of plasma cortisol, which can be caused by neoplastic growth that produces cortisol or ACTH. The paraventricular nucleus (PVN) of the hypothalamus releases corticotropin-releasing hormone (CRH), which stimulates the pituitary gland to release ACTH, causing the adrenal glands to release cortisol from the zona fasciculata of the adrenal cortex. Elevated levels of cortisol exert negative feedback on the pituitary, which decreases the amount of ACTH released from the pituitary gland.

The most common etiology of Cushing syndrome is from a pituitary adenoma overproducing ACTH, which in turn elevates cortisol via its stimulation of the adrenal glands; this specific condition, called Cushing disease (pituitary Cushing syndrome), is responsible for 70% of Cushing syndrome

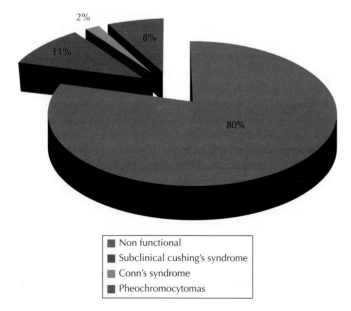

2%

8%

11%

80%

■ Non functional
■ Subclinical cushing's syndrome
■ Conn's syndrome
■ Pheochromocytomas

Figure 10.1 Prevalence of endocrine activity in adrenal incidentalomas.

Table 10.1 Clinical manifestations of hormonal syndromes associated with adrenal neoplasm.

Clinical conditions	Characteristic signs and symptoms
Cushing syndrome (hyperadrenocorticism)	Rapid weight gain, central obesity, buffalo hump, and moon face Dryness, easy bruising, purple/red striae, telangiectasia, acanthosis nigricans, facial acne, impaired wound healing, hyperhidrosis, baldness, and hirsutism Decreased libido, impotence, amenorrhea, oligomenorrhea, infertility, diabetes (hyperglycemia), polyuria, polydipsia, hypertension and hypokalemia Proximal muscle weakness, myalgia, arthralgia, osteopenia or osteoporosis Bowel ileus, abdominal fullness, flatulence, nausea with or without vomiting Insomia, euphoria to depression, and anxiety to psychosis
Conn syndrome (hyperaldosteronism)	Chronic headache Hypertension, hypokalemia, hypernatremia, hypocalcemia, and metabolic alkalosis Bowel ileus, abdominal fullness, flatulence, nausea with or without vomiting Myalgias, muscle weakness and cramps
Adrenogenital syndrome (hyperandrogenism)	*Virilization syndrome* – clitoromegaly, deepening of the voice, increased muscle mass, decreased breast size and amenorrhea *Feminization syndrome* – gynecomastia and testicular atrophy Hirsutism, acne, and androgenic alopecia Decreased libido, impotence, amenorrhea, oligomenorrhea, and infertility
Pheochromocytoma	*Classic triad* – episodic headache, sweating, and tachycardia *Common* – sustained or paroxysmal hypertension, headache variable, generalized sweating, palpitations, dyspnea, generalized weakness, and panic attack-type symptoms *Less common* – pallor, orthostatic hypotension, visual blurring, papilledema, weight loss, polyuria, polydipsia, constipation, increased erythrocyte sedimentation rate, hyperglycemia, leukocytosis, psychiatric disorders, secondary erythrocytosis

cases.[11] The other causes of Cushing syndrome include prolonged use of glucocorticoid drugs as well as ACAs and functional ACC. Hyperadrenocorticism is the most frequent hormonal syndrome in ACCs, accounting for approximately 30–40% of functional cases or 20–30% of all cases.[12] On the other hand, Cushing syndrome is found in less than 1% of all ACAs.[13]

Neoplastic growth of the adrenal cortex, such as ACA or ACC causing *adrenal* Cushing syndrome, produces elevated cortisol levels leading to negative feedback on the pituitary, resulting in a very low ACTH level. On the other hand, *pituitary* Cushing syndrome (Cushing disease) results in both elevated ACTH and cortisol levels; the ACTH level remains high because the neoplastic process in the pituitary (pituitary adenoma) dampens its responsiveness to the negative feedback of the circulating high cortisol level. *Paraneoplastic* Cushing syndrome is caused by ectopic overproduction of ACTH from malignancies not in the hypothalamus-pituitary-adrenal axis (HPA), such as small cell lung cancer[14] or pancreatic neuroendocrine carcinoma.[15] Another differential diagnosis of Cushing syndrome is *pseudo*-Cushing syndrome, commonly found in patients taking oral contraceptives, especially those with estrogen. Exogenous estrogen will increase cortisol-binding globulin and thereby cause the total cortisol level to be elevated.[16] Generally, however, patients with this pseudo-Cushing syndrome do not have typical clinical manifestations of Cushing syndrome because their free 24-h urine cortisol level is normal.

The most frequent symptoms include rapid weight gain, particularly isolated weight gain in trunk and face with sparing of the limbs (central obesity), development of fat pads along the clavicle and back of neck (buffalo hump) and face (moon face). Striking skin changes are also common, which include thinning of the skin leading to dryness, easy bruising, as well as formation of purple or red striae on the trunk, buttocks, arms, legs or breasts.[17,18] Other symptoms include facial acne, hirsutism, baldness, and proximal muscle weakness. Hyperadrenocorticism can also affect other endocrine systems leading to reduced libido, impotence, amenorrhea or oligomenorrhea and infertility. Both diabetes and hypertension are secondary disorders of Cushing syndrome. By enhancing epinephrine's vasoconstrictive effect as well as exhibiting its mineralocorticoid activity, cortisol excess can lead to persistent hypertension, which can be difficult to control, and hypokalemia.[19] Hyperglycemia in Cushing syndrome results from insulin resistance. Patients frequently suffer from various psychological disturbances, ranging from euphoria to depression as well as anxiety and psychosis.[20]

Conn syndrome

Conn syndrome (primary hyperaldosteronism) results from excess production of aldosterone produced only by the zona glomerulosa, the outermost functional layer of the adrenal cortex. Again both ACCs and ACAs can cause oversecretion of aldosterone but unlike Cushing syndrome, Conn syndrome is usually found among patients with ACAs, with an estimated prevalence of 7%[21,22] of all ACA cases compared to 1.5%[23] of all ACC cases. Among the several known etiologies of Conn syndrome, the most common include bilateral idiopathic hyperplasia (70%), unilateral idiopathic hyperplasia (20%), and aldosterone-producing ACA (<5%).[24] Having nothing to do with neoplastic or hyperplastic processes of the adrenal cortex, secondary hyperaldosteronism is related to decreased cardiac output which is associated with elevated renin levels.

Aldosterone augments renal sodium-potassium exchange, resulting in concurrent hypernatremia and hypokalemia as the principal sign of hyperaldosteronism. A state of significant hypokalemia activates the sodium-hydrogen pumps in the nephron to increase excretion of hydrogen ions, further exacerbating hypernatremia.[25] The hydrogen ions that are exchanged for sodium are generated by carbonic anhydrase in the renal tubule, causing increased production of bicarbonate. The increased bicarbonate and excreted hydrogen combine to generate metabolic alkalosis. The high pH associated with alkalosis reduces the availability of calcium to tissue, often resulting in symptoms of hypocalcemia. The sodium retention triggers plasma volume expansion and elevated blood pressure. Increased glomerular filtration rate and decreased renin release from the granular cells of the juxtaglomerular apparatus are the consequences of elevated blood pressure.[26]

Aside from persistent elevation of blood pressure, other manifesting problems of Conn syndrome include myalgias, weakness, and chronic headaches. The muscle cramps are due to neuron hyperexcitability seen in the setting of hypocalcemia, muscle weakness is secondary to hypoexcitability of skeletal muscles in the setting of hypokalemia, and headaches are thought to be due to both electrolyte imbalance and hypertension.[27]

Adrenogenital syndrome

The adrenal cortex also produces a minor portion of the body's sex steroids; androgens are the predominant sex steroids. Pathological overproduction of adrenal androgens can lead to hyperandrogenism in women. The most common androgen is testosterone and the most common female sex steroid being produced is estrogen. Neoplasms of the adrenal cortex affecting the functional zona reticularis are very rare, and the resulting diagnostic signs of hyperandrogenism include hirsutism, acne, androgenic alopecia, and virilization. Hirsutism, defined as excessive growth of terminal hair in a masculine pattern in women, is the most commonly used clinical diagnostic criterion of excess androgens in women.[28] The presence of hirsutism is usually determined by using a standardized scoring system of hair growth. Depending on the definition, hirsutism is present in up to 80% of patients with hyperandrogenism.[29] Acne and androgenic alopecia are other common androgenic skin changes, and might be observed without hirsutism in some hyperandrogenic women. However, the isolated presence of any of these manifestations is not used as a diagnostic criterion for hyperandrogenism. Virilization is a relatively uncommon feature of hyperandrogenism and its presence often suggests androgen-producing neoplasms.[30] On the other hand, the extremely rare estrogen-secreting adrenocortical neoplasms usually induce gynecomastia and testicular atrophy in men.

The adrenal androgens, normally secreted by the fetal adrenal zone or the zona reticularis of the adrenal cortex, are steroid hormones with weak androgenic activity. Although adrenal androgens do not appear to play a major role in the fully androgenized adult man, they seem to play a role in the adult woman and in both sexes before puberty. Girls, women,

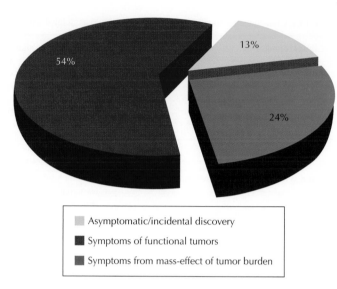

Figure 10.2 Presenting symptoms at diagnosis of ACC.

and prepubertal boys may be negatively affected by adrenal androgen oversecretion, in contrast to adult men.

In practice, clinical presentations of functional adrenocortical neoplasms (ACAs and ACCs) are often due to oversecretions of more than one hormone (Fig. 10.2). Rapidly progressing Cushing syndrome with or without virilization is the most common endocrine syndrome associated with ACC in adults.[31] Rarely, ACCs may also secrete mineralocorticoids causing hypertension and pronounced hypokalemia; even more rarely, cosecretion of aldosterone and cortisol has been reported.[32] The extremely rare estrogen-secreting tumors may induce gynecomastia and testicular atrophy in men. Patients who have oversecretion of multiple hormones causing mixed hormonal syndromes almost always have malignant disease or ACC.[33] Cushing syndrome is the most common condition among cases of functional ACA, followed by sex steroid- and rarely adosterone-secreting ACAs. Approximately 80% of adrenal incidentalomas are hormonally inactive, while less than 20% produce hormones – Conn syndrome (40–50%), PHEO (40–50%) and Cushing syndrome (<10%).[34]

Laboratory evaluation

Laboratory workup is important as part of diagnosis as well as management of neoplasms of the adrenal cortex. Hormonal production is characteristic of functional sections of the adrenal gland, cortex versus medulla and cortical functional zones. However, in clinical practice, physical signs and symptoms are typically overlapping or vague and not hormonally specific; most patients will have overproduction of more than one hormone. Therefore, laboratory workup will need to be inclusive of all the usual hormones associated with the adrenal cortex, evaluating for overproduction of glucocorticosteroids (cortisol), mineralcorticosteroid (aldosterone), and sex steroids (androgens). Fortunately, there is a limited number of laboratory values considered to be important or diagnostic.

Table 10.2 Laboratory workup for hormonal syndromes associated with functional adrenal neoplasm.

Clinical conditions	Diagnostic laboratory tests	Results
Cushing syndrome (hyperadrenocorticism)	24-h urine free cortisol	↑
	Plasma cortisol concentration	↑
	Plasma ACTH concentration	↓
	Plasma cortisol concentration, after dexamethasone suppression test	↑
Conn syndrome (hyperaldosteronism)	Plasma aldosterone concentration (PAC)	↑
	Plasma renin activity (PRA)	↓
	Aldo:renin ratio (PAC:PRA)	>20–30
Adrenogenital syndrome (hyperandrogenism)	Plasma concentrations of DHEA and/or DHEA-S	↑
	Plasma concentration of testosterone	↑/wnl
	Plasma concentration of cortisol	↑/wnl
	24-h urine 17-ketosteroids	↑
	24-h urine cortisol	↑/wnl
Pheochromocytoma	24-h urine fractionated catecholamines and metanephrines	
	Norepinephrine	↑2×ULN (>170 µg)
	Epinephrine	↑2×ULN (>35 µg)
	Dopamine	↑2×ULN (>700 µg)
	Normetanephrine	↑2×ULN (>900 µg)
	Metanephrine	↑2×ULN (>400 µg)

ACTH, adrenocorticotropic hormone; DHEA, dehydroepiandrosterone; DHEA-S, dehydroepiandrosterone sulfate; wnl, within normal limits.

While there are many differential diagnoses for each hormone pathologically being overproduced, the rest of this section will mainly concentrate on the laboratory workup for hormonal syndromes associated with neoplasms of the adrenal cortex. Table 10.2 summarizes these diagnostic laboratory tests.

Hypercortisolism: Cushing syndrome

Cortisol (hydrocortisone) functions mainly to increase blood sugar through stimulation of gluconeogenesis, as well as to suppress the immune system and aid in fat, protein and carbohydrate metabolism.[31] Cortisol, a glucocorticoid, is produced within the zona fasciculata of the adrenal cortex, and its secretion/release is regulated by the HPA axis. Specifically, the secretion of CRH by the hypothalamus triggers the anterior pituitary secretion of ACTH, which is carried by the blood to the adrenal cortex, where it triggers glucocorticoids to be released into the circulation. Like most serum levels, serum cortisol level denotes blood plasma concentration.

Cortisol concentration in the serum undergoes diurnal variation where the level peaks in the early morning and reaches its lowest level around 3–5 h after the onset of sleep.[35] This pattern can be easily altered by many foods/drinks, drugs, and common conditions, such as depression, stress, fever, surgery, fear, pain and temperature extremes. Additionally, most serum cortisol is bound to proteins such as corticosteroid-binding globulin (CBG) and serum albumin.[36] Therefore changes in nutritional status or protein homeostasis can further affect the true amount of cortisol in the body, or total free cortisol. A more accurate and reliable assessment of total free cortisol is a 24-h urine free cortisol.[37,38] In patients suspected of having primary hypercortisolism (adrenal Cushing syndrome), plasma concentration of cortisol can be variable but elevated 24-h urine cortisol and reactive suppressed plasma concentration of ACTH levels are accurate and reproducible as diagnostic criteria.

Another important diagnostic tool in Cushing syndrome is the dexamethasone suppression test, which is used to evaluate the status of the HPA axis and determine the etiology of hypercortisolism. Serving as an exogenous glucocorticoid that is 30–40 times more potent than cortisol, dexamethasone is orally administered at low (1–2 mg) or high (8 mg) doses at 11pm to midnight and levels of serum dexamethasone and cortisol are drawn at 8am (for overnight test) or serum ACTH and dexamethasone and 24-h urine cortisol, and 17-hydroxycorticosteroids (17-OHCS) (for standard 2-day test).[39,40] The premise behind the low-dose dexamethasone test is that if the HPA axis is normal, any supraphysiological dose dexamethasone is sufficient to suppress pituitary ACTH, leading to reductions in cortisol secretion and its plasma concentration in serum as well as in 24-h urine excretion. The basis for high-dose tests is the fact that ACTH secretion in pituitary Cushing syndrome is only relatively resistant to glucocorticoid negative feedback inhibition and will not suppress normally with either the overnight or the 2-day low-dose test.[41] By increasing the dose of dexamethasone, ACTH secretion can be suppressed in most patients with pituitary Cushing syndrome, while most nonpituitary malignant tumors that produce ectopic ACTH are not responsive to glucocorticoid negative feedback. The overnight test at low dose is a quick screening test for nonsuppressible cortisol production and subclinical or clinical Cushing syndrome, while the 2-day test is used to evaluate suppressibility in patients with an equivocal overnight test or in patients who have not had an overnight test.[42]

Hyperaldosteronism: Conn syndrome

Adrenal aldosterone synthesis is regulated by the renin-angiotensin system, along with plasma concentration of potassium and ACTH.[43] In addition to angiotensin (A) III, the production of aldosterone is also stimulated by the elevation of plasma concentrations of AII, ACTH or potassium which are responses to reduce plasma sodium concentration. The level of AII is regulated by AI, which is in turn regulated by the renal hormone renin. The end-organs affected by aldosterone are the distal tubules and collecting ducts within the nephron of the kidney, promoting sodium and water retention while lowering plasma potassium.[43] By definition, in Conn syndrome (primary hyperaldosteronism), there is an elevation of the plasma aldosterone concentration (PAC). Elevation of aldosterone results in reabsorption of sodium into the blood and secretion of potassium into urine. Decrease and increase in plasma concentrations of potassium and sodium, respectively, will result in downregulation of AII and, in turn, reduction in plasma renin activity (PRA). Neither AII nor renin is able to downregulate the constitutively formed aldosterone.[44] Hence, an elevated PAC:PRA ratio resulting from increased PAC and decreased PRA makes this assay a useful diagnostic tool in patients suspected of having Conn syndrome.

Hyperandrogenism: adrenogenital syndrome

Androgens are byproducts of the synthesis of cortisol in the adrenal glands and thus ACTH is the major regulator for production and secretion.[45] The primary adrenal androgens are DHEA and DHEA-S, which are also produced by the testes or ovaries (which only contribute less than 10% of the total body DHEA and DHEA-S).[45] Both of these adrenal androgens have only minor endogenous androgenic effects. However, a small percentage of DHEA/DHEA-S is converted to androstenedione, and then to testosterone and estrogen by the tissues of the adrenal glands, the peripheral tissues of the integumentary system, the prostate, external genitalia and adipose tissue.[46] In men, less than 5% of testosterone comes from the adrenal glands; on the other hand, in women, adrenally secreted testosterone and androstenedione (and those that are peripherally converted from DHEA and DHEA-S) contribute substantially to total androgen production.[47]

While oversecretion of DHEA and DHEA-S defines adrenogenital syndromes, particularly adrenal hyperandrogenism, the clinical manifestations of hirsutism and virilization (or feminization) are caused by the more potent sex steroids, androstenedione and testosterone (or estrogen). Serum levels of DHEA and DHEA-S do not vary diurnally but chronologically, meaning that concentrations rise throughout puberty, reaching a peak in the third decade, and then progressively decline.[48] Hence, the time of day when blood is drawn for testing is irrelevant in determining plasma concentrations of DHEA and DHEA-S.

Androgen-secreting adrenal cortical neoplasms are typically malignant ACCs.[49] Primary adrenal androgen-secreting neoplasms can be diagnosed by demonstrating elevated plasma concentration of DHEA or DHEA-S or testosterone that does not fall in response to dexamethasone. Unlike ACAs, ACCs will produce excesses of not only DHEA, DHEA-S, testosterone infrequently and estrogen rarely, but also cortisol and many steroid intermediates. In fact, the most common diagnostic laboratory findings of ACCs producing androgens are elevated plasma concentration of DHEA and DHEA-S, urinary 17-ketosteroid excretion, along with elevation of cortisol in

both serum and urine.[32] Urinary 17-ketosteroids are excreted metabolites of DHEA and DHEA-S.

Radiological evaluation

The two most common modalities used for radiological workup of adrenal cortical neoplasms are CT and MRI scans. Aside from evaluating the anatomy of adrenal cortex, which is important for any surgical planning, other important objectives include the delineation of characteristics denoting carcinoma from those of adenoma or hyperplasia, and the determination of extent of cancer staging. While size plays an important role in evaluation for malignancy, equally crucial are the radiological characteristics of the adrenal mass. Specific descriptions about lipid content, consistency and border, rate and quantity of contrast washout are used to distinguish benign from malignant adrenal tumor and distant adrenal metastasis originating from other primary sites.[50,51] Evaluation of lipid content, through assessment of mass density, may be even more informative than the size of the mass in determining whether a lesion is a primary or secondary adrenal malignancy.[51]

On CT scans, the density of the image is attributed to x-ray attenuation. The intracytoplasmic fat in adenomas results in low attenuation while nonadenomas have higher attenuation on nonenhanced CT images. The Hounsfield scale is a semi-quantitative method of measuring x-ray attenuation. Attenuation on CT scans, as expressed in Hounsfield units (HU) on an unenhanced scan, is equivalent to the density of fat. Typical precontrast HU values indicating adipose tissue are between -20 to -150 HU, and kidney has 20–150 HU. Therefore, an adrenal mass measuring less than 10 HU on a nonenhanced CT scan has a nearly 100% likelihood of being a benign adenoma. In a retrospective analysis of 151 patients with adrenal masses at the Cleveland Clinic, Hamrahian and colleagues[52] were able to demonstrate that HU on nonenhanced CT scans can usually distinguish benign from malignant pathology. Mean HU (+ standard deviation (SD)) for ACA, ACC, metastases from other sites, and PHEO were $16+14$, $37+4$ and $39+15$, and $39+8$, respectively. In this series, a nonenhanced CT HU <10 or a combination of tumor size <4 and HU <20 excluded nonadenomas in 100% of cases.[52] However, the lipid-rich nature of the adenomas is commonly found in only 70% of cases; 30% of adenomas do not contain large amounts of lipid and thus become indistinguishable from nonadenomas on nonenhanced CT scans. Adding adrenal consistency and border to lipid nature quantified by values of HU will further improve the predictive potential of imaging characteristics. For example, a homogeneous adrenal mass with a smooth border and attenuation value <10 HU on nonenhanced CT is more likely to be a benign adrenal adenoma.[53] Degree and rate of contrast washout on delayed enhanced CT scans can also help to differentiate malignant from benign adrenal masses. Adenomas typically exhibit rapid contrast washout, whereas nonadenomas have delayed washout. Ten minutes after administration of contrast, an absolute contrast medium washout of >50% was reported to be 100% sensitive and specific for adenomas.[54,55] Additional radiological features suggestive of ACC include inhomogeneity, irregular borders, calcifications, invasion of surrounding structures, and regional lymph node enlargement.[56]

Important phenotypes on CT scan include lipid nature, border, rate and percentage of contrast washout, while MRI scan has other benefits not available to CT. One important advantage of MRI is its ability to better display local invasion from ACC.[57] Additionally, differences between T1- and T2-weighted images from conventional spin-echo MRI can distinguish benign adenomas from ACC and PHEO. On gadolinium-DPTA-enhanced MRI, adenomas demonstrate mild enhancement and a rapid washout of contrast, while malignant lesions show rapid and marked enhancement and slower washout pattern. ACAs lose signal on out-of-phase images but appear relatively bright on in-phase images, on chemical shift imaging (CSI) MRI which is a form of lipid-sensitive imaging. Important radiological phenotypes of adrenal masses that are useful in the evaluation of malignancy are summarized in Table 10.3.

Other radiological modalities had been used to delineate malignant from benign adrenal tumors. Attempting to improve radiological specificity or sensitivity correlating to tumor biology, radiolabeled nuclear scans such as iodine-131-meta-iodo-benzylguanidine (MIBG) scan and indium-111-pentetreotide (OctreoScan™) have been used to evaluate adrenal masses. The MIBG scan takes advantage of the fact that cells, particularly tumor cells of the neuroectodermal origin, specifically take up and incorporate iodine into their vital cell cycle. Therefore, MIBG is particularly useful for evaluating thyroid pathology, PHEO, and other neuroendocrine tumors. On the other hand, OctreoScan™ is used for the identification and localization of neuroendocrine tumors. The success of OctreoScan™ is based upon the physiology of somatostatin receptors (SSR). SSRs are found in the cells of neuroectodermal origin, particularly those that produce hormones in response to autonomic nervous system activity. Hence, this imaging technique is helpful in the workup of adrenal tumor where the differential diagnoses include PHEO.

Recent additions to radiological modalities targeting tumor proliferation or biology include positron emission tomography (PET) with either 18-fluoro-2-deoxy-D-glucose (FDG-PET)[58] or 11C-metomidate (MTO-PET).[59] FDG-PET coregistration with CT (PET/CT) scan has recently become popular in the radiological workup of neoplasms arising from the adrenal cortex. Retrospective reports have suggested that PET/CT scans are useful tools to distinguish ACC from ACA. The applications of PET/CT scans in other solid malignancies would suggest that theoretically they can be used similarly in ACCs to determine early metabolic response to antineoplastic therapy, and to evaluate for occult metastatic foci not otherwise visualized with traditional CT or MRI.[60] Due to inconsistency of tumor signal and lack of outcomes from long-term follow-up in patients with adrenal masses, PET/CT scans currently have limited usage in patients without documented malignant cancer. Despite its popularity, indications and applications for PET/CT scan are relatively uncharted, awaiting validating prospective evidence. For now, PET/CT scans can be most helpful in patients with confirmed diagnosis or prior history of malignancy.

Pathological evaluation

Primary adrenocortical neoplasms are either benign adenoma, ACA or malignant, where ACC is the most frequent. Infrequently primary adrenal lymphomas and soft tissue

Table 10.3 Adrenal incidentalomas: radiological characteristics in evaluation of malignancy.

Clinical diagnoses		Characteristics		
		General	**On CT scan**	**On MRI scan**
Benign	**ACA**	Round, homogeneous Smooth border Sharp margination Diameter <4 cm Unilateral	Unenhanced CT attenuation <10 HU Rapid contrast washout (at 10 min after contrast administration >50% washout)	Same intensity with liver on both T1- and T2-weighted MRI Lost signal on out-of-phase images on chemical shift MRI (=increased lipid content)
Malignant	**Pheo**	Increased vascularity Cystic and hemorrhagic changes Variable diameter size Maybe bilateral	Unenhanced CT attenuation >20 HU Delay contrast washout (at 10 min after contrast administration <50% washout)	High signal intensity compared to the liver on T2-weighted MRI
	ACC	Irregular shape, heterogeneous Calcification Diameter >4 cm Unilateral Evidence of local invasion or metastases	Unenhanced CT attenuation >20 HU Heterogeneous contrast enhancement on CT with IV contrast Delay contrast washout (at 10 min after contrast administration <50% washout)	Low signal intensity compared to the liver on T1-weighted MRI High-intermediate signal intensity compared to the liver on T2-weighted MRI (=increased water intensity)
	Metastases	Irregular shape, heterogeneous bilateral	Unenhanced CT attenuation >20 HU Heterogeneous contrast enhancement on CT with IV contrast Delay contrast washout (at 10 min after contrast administration <50% washout)	Same-low signal intensity compared to the liver on T1-weighted MRI High-intermediate signal intensity compared to the liver on T2-weighted MRI (=increased water intensity)

ACA, adrenocortical adenoma; ACC, adrenocortical carcinoma; CT, computed tomography; HU, Hounsfield unit; IV, intravenous; MRI, magnetic resonance imaging; Pheo, pheochromocytoma.

sarcomas of the adrenal cortex have been reported.[61] Additionally, rare variants of ACC include oncocytic, myxoid, carcinosarcoma, adenosquamous, and clear cell.

However, unlike most other solid tumors, the delineating line between malignant and benign is blurred when the diagnosis relies solely on pathological features. Uniquely in adrenal tumors, other features such as radiological and clinical are used to assist with separating malignant from benign. In the absence of local invasion or distant metastasis, the pathological diagnosis of ACC based on gross and microscopic data can be very difficult. Macroscopic features indicative of malignancy are tumor weight, hemorrhage, breached tumor capsule and necrosis, while the most widely used microscopic diagnostic tool remains the Weiss score.

In a study of metastasizing and nonmetastasizing adrenocortical neoplasms, among 43 patients followed for a median of 11 years, Weiss[62] demonstrated the utility of nine histomorphological criteria in predicting the biology of adrenocortical neoplasms. A Weiss score is obtained by summing the values of these nine different parameters; three parameters are structural (low percentage of clear cells, diffuse architecture, necrosis), three are cytological (atypia, atypical mitoses, high mitotic rate >1 of 10 high-power fields), and three are related to invasion (vein invasion, sinusoidal invasion, and capsular invasion). A Weiss score of >3 is consistent with a malignant adrenal tumor with a sensitivity of 100% and specificity of 96%.[63] No single criterion could distinguish benign from malignant tumor biology; all but one of the benign adrenocortical tumors had two or fewer criteria, where ACCs have been found in tumors with a score of <2.[64] In a later study, Weiss[63] modified the diagnostic criteria for benign and malignant adrenocortical neoplasms; tumors exhibiting >3 adverse histological features were considered malignant. In a more recent study, Stojadinovic et al.[65] identified six morphological prognostic factors that correlated significantly with disease-specific survival in ACC: venous, capsular, and adjacent organ invasion; tumor necrosis and mitotic rate; and atypical mitosis. Both studies identified mitotic activity as the single most important determinant of tumor-related mortality from ACC.[63,65]

As an alternative to the morphological approach, a wide array of immunohistochemical (IMHC), chromosomal, genetic, and molecular markers have been tested in ACC to identify reliable diagnostic and prognostic factors. Tumor staining with Ki-67 has been utilized to help differentiate benign from malignant adrenal tumors. A cutoff value between ACAs and ACCs has been found to vary from 1.5% to 4%,[66] whereas high expression of Ki-67 (>10%) has been associated with poor survival.[67] Other markers, such as zinc finger transcription factor Snail, cyclin E, E-cadherin, topoisomerase IIα, HER-neu, and N-cadherin assessed by IMHC, have been used for the diagnosis of ACC, as well as for predicting biological behavior in adrenocortical neoplasms.[64] Additionally, IMHC evaluation of adrenal 4 binding protein (Ad4BP) or SF-1 has been reported to aid in the differentiation of ACC from metastatic malignancies,[68] although with limited results.

Despite significant advancements in molecular genetics and genetic signatures of many diseases and conditions, the only reliable method to establish a pathological diagnosis remains the Weiss score. Therefore, thorough understanding of clinical features, biological behaviors, underlying oncological history, and differential diagnoses of other pathological processes will go further than relying solely on pathology to distinguish malignant from benign. Differential diagnoses of adrenal mass, both unilateral and bilateral, are summarized in Table 10.4, while a summary of the Weiss score system is presented in Table 10.5.

Adrenal incidentaloma/adrenocortical adenoma

Epidemiology

Adrenocortical adenoma is a benign neoplasm that can be hormonally silent or hormone secreting. Functional adenomas produce steroids independently from both ACTH and renin-angiotensin systems. They can produce symptoms of hypercortisolism,

Table 10.4 Differential diagnoses of adrenal mass(es).

Unilateral mass (90%)	Bilateral masses (10%)
Adrenocortical adenoma	Bilateral adrenocortical adenomas
Adrenocortical carcinoma	
Pheochromocytoma	Bilateral pheochomocytoma
Metastatic disease	Metastatic disease
Congenital adrenal hyperplasia	Bilateral congenital adrenal hyperplasia
Cyst	Bilateral macronodular adrenal disease
Massive macronodular adrenal disease	
Nodular variant of adrenocortical adenoma	ACTH-dependent Cushing (pituitary/ectopic)
Myolipoma	
Neuroblastoma	Lymphoma
Ganglioneuroma	
Amyloidosis	Amyloidosis
Granuloma/tnfection (TB, fungal)	Granuloma/infection (TB, fungal)
Hemorrhage	Hemorrhage
Infiltrative disease to adrenal	Infiltrative disease to bilateral adrenals

ACTH, adrenocorticotropic hormone; TB, tuberculosis.

Table 10.5 Pathological determinants of adrenal neoplasms.

Features associated with malignancy	
Low % of clear cells	
Diffuse architecture	
Tumor necrosis	***Weiss Score >3***
Cell atypia	**≈ Malignant**
Atypical mitoses	**Adrenal Tumor**
High mitotic rate (>1/10 HPF)	*[sensitivity 100%,*
Venous/vascular invasion	*specificity 96%]*
Sinusoidal invasion	
Adrenal capsular invasion	
Features associated with adverse survival outcomes	
Tumor necrosis	***Stojadinovic***
High mitotic rate (>1/10 HPF)	***Adverse Criteria***
Venous/vascular invasion	**≈ Disease-Specific**
Adrenal capsular invasion	**Survival of**
Adjacent organ invasion	**Adrenocortical**
	Carcinoma

HPF, high-power field.

hyperaldosteronism, and rarely produce virilization or feminization. While a minority present with symptoms of hormonal excess, many are discovered incidentally on abdominal imaging studies and are then referred to as AIs.

An incidentaloma is an adrenal mass lesion greater than 1 cm in diameter. CT scans and ultrasonography have markedly increased the clinical dilemma of differentiation and diagnosis among a wide variety of radiologically recognized asymptomatic adrenal lesions. In the modern era when usage of radiological imaging is a common and primary method of working up symptoms, it is no wonder that the incidence of AI is increased. Adrenal tumors are most often discovered as an incidental finding, in over 4% of high-resolution abdominal imaging studies.[69] Most AIs are nonfunctional, but as many as 15% of them are functional, most commonly secreting cortisol and causing subclinical Cushing syndrome. In a series of 1004 AIs, 85% were nonfunctional, 9% were defined as subclinical Cushing syndrome, 4% were PHEOs, and 1.6% were aldosteronomas.[51]

Discovery of an adrenal mass necessitates two simultaneous workup pathways: (1) to determine if it is malignant and (2) to determine if it is functional. In a Mayo Clinic series of 61,054 abdominal CT scans performed from 1985 to 1990, adrenal masses were seen in 2006 patients (3%) with less than 1% of them being greater than 1 cm, referred to as AIs.[70] In a more recent report, utilizing higher resolution CT scanners, Bovio et al.[71] reported a 4% prevalence of AI on abdominal CT scan. The prevalence rate of AI is approximately 1–5% of abdominal imaging studies[72] and 5–15% of autopsies.[73]

A common presentation of ACA or AI is as a unilateral adrenal mass, while less frequently bilateral involvement occurs in approximately 10–15% of cases.[7,74] It is also important to remember that, although bilateral ACA or AI can occur, metastatic spread of other primary cancers is more prevalent. Other differential diagnosis of bilateral incidentally discovered adrenal masses includes congenital adrenal hyperplasia, lymphoma, granulomatous infection, hemorrhage, ACTH-dependent Cushing, PHEO, amyloidosis, infiltrative disease of the adrenal glands, and ACTH-independent bilateral macronodular adrenal hyperplasia.

Tumorigenesis

Better understanding of the molecular pathogenesis of adrenal tumors, benign or malignant, has suggested two mechanisms. Accumulation of activated protooncogenes and inactivated tumor suppressor genes will ultimately lead to monoclonal population of adrenal tumor cells. While the majority of adrenal tumors are sporadic, a small minority are associated with a hereditary syndrome, suggesting some specific possible gene abnormalities that may have contributed to the generation of primary adrenal tumors. These syndromes include Li–Fraumeni[75,76] and Beckwith–Wiedemann.[77] Activating mutation of the CTNNB1 gene has also been linked to the development of adrenal carcinoma, where many of these are the result of point mutations altering the Ser45 gene in exon 3.[78–80] Primary tumors of the adrenal glands are also believed to result from expression of aberrant receptors that are responsive to agonists leading to growth

and malignant transformation. Evidence has suggested that cortisol-secreting adenomas arise from aberrant expressions and activation of non-ACTH receptors in the adrenal cortical tissues. These aberrant receptors include gastric inhibitory polypeptide (GIP), β-adrenergic agonists, V1-vasopressin, serotonin, and luteinizing hormone/human chorionic gonadotropin.[81] A suggested schema for hormonal evaluation in patients with AI is presented in Figure 10.3.

Management

Discovery of AI necessitates evaluation for malignancy and hormonal production. A review of the available data suggests that the incidence rate of malignancy is small (<0.03%) in all adrenal AIs that are 1.5–6 cm. However, this rate increases considerably with tumors larger than 6 cm (up to 15%).[82] These incidentalomas become clinically relevant only when they become functional tumors with hormonal secretions or if they display features consistent with malignant change. The objective in the management of patients with functional tumor is mainly to control hormonal overproduction. Depending on cancer stage, cure and/or disease control should be the objectives for patients with malignant adrenal tumors.

All patients with documented PHEO and primary aldosteronism should undergo definitive surgery. Unilateral adrenalectomy is the treatment of choice for most patients with hormone-secreting unilateral ACAs, and many with incidentally discovered adrenal masses. Laparoscopic adrenal surgery is a safe, effective, and less expensive procedure than open adrenalectomy for patients with AI, adosterone- or cortisol-secreting ACA, and PHEO.[83] A review of 308 articles on laparascopic adrenal surgery suggested that it is safe and less expensive than open adrenalectomy for these patients.[84] Additionally, laparoscopic surgery may require a longer operative time but it is associated with less postoperative pain and shorter hospital stays, where the average length of hospital stay ranged from 1.5 to 4 days with laparoscopic adrenalectomy compared with 5.3–10 days with open surgery.[85,86] Hence laparoscopic adrenal surgery is recognized as a standard surgical approach for patients with smaller adenomas (<6 cm in diameter).[87,88] However, for patients with documented ACC, indications for laparascopic adrenal surgery are still controversial and no standard of care surgical approach is universally accepted.

In the majority of patients with hormone-secreting ACAs or incidentalomas, terminating hormonal excess and cure can be achieved with complete surgical resection. Postoperative and possibly chronic glucocorticoid therapy may be necessary for many of the patients post adrenalectomy. Rare instances of AI or ACA, such as documented subclinical Cushing syndrome, can be monitored and treated as indicated by symptoms and clinical manifestations. However, younger patients and those who have metabolic disorders attributable or possibly related to autonomous glucocorticoid secretion should be considered for surgical resection.[89] Adrenal masses with either suspicious imaging phenotype or size larger than 4 cm should be considered for resection as the probability of having ACC increases.[53]

The management of bilateral adrenal masses is different from that for unilateral masses. In patients carrying a diagnosis

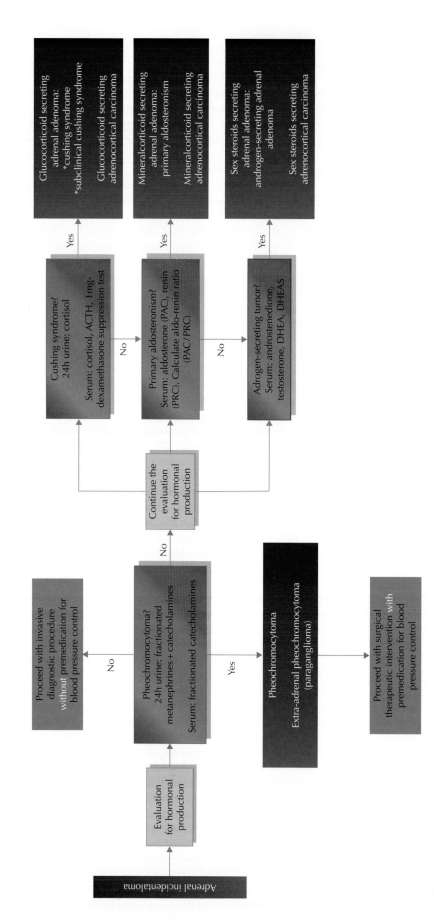

Figure 10.3 Adrenal incidentalomas: evaluation for hormonal production.

of subclinical ACTH-independent bilateral macronodular adrenal hyperplasia, size is not an indication for surgery, as some can be as large as 5–10 cm with insufficient hormone production or low potential for malignant transformation to necessitate surgery. Additionally, in patients with known history of other malignancy, metastatic involvement should be included among the differential diagnoses of bilateral adrenal masses.

Along with all clinical and radiological parameters used to differentiate benign from malignant disease, the patient's access to care, history of therapeutic compliance and own wishes should be considered and weighed when close surveillance of nonfunctioning AI is selected. Time and duration of follow-up evaluations should be personalized for each patient. Concrete and evidence-based recommendations are lacking because of nonexistent prospective data. In the absence of prospective studies, it is reasonable to repeat imaging at intervals of 6–12 months. A refined protocol defining type of radiological studies, frequency and duration of surveillance should be guided by each person's clinical circumstances, imaging phenotype, and the clinical judgment of the treating physician. Furthermore, there is no evidence to suggest that close surveillance will improve overall survival duration or rates in patients with AI. Adrenal masses reaching 4 cm in diameter, enlarging more than 1 cm during a follow-up interval, and associated with new-onset hormonal syndromes should be resected as definitive treatment.

Adrenocortical carcinomas

Epidemiology

Other malignant primary cancers of the adrenal cortex exist but they are extremely rare and their management is generally decided case by case and treatment can be with chemotherapy or palliative radiation or surgery. The rest of this section will focus on malignant ACCs, which are also extremely rare, representing approximately 1–2 new cases per million of the population per year,[90] respectively. This is probably a gross underdiagnosis. The estimated incidence is approximately 8–10 times higher in children in southern Brazil, where a number of environmental and genetic risk factors have been identified.[91] ACC can develop at any age but typically has a bimodal age distribution with disease peaks before the age of five and in the fourth and fifth decades.[92] ACC is a heterogeneous disease with wide variation in cancer aggressiveness, and neither age of presentation nor associated hormonal syndromes typically can predict the course of disease or survival outcomes. Detection before metastases become overt is difficult. Reports have suggested that functional ACCs occur more frequently in women, while men are more likely to present with nonfunctional ACCs.[93]

Tumorigenesis

Although most cases of ACC appear to be sporadic, some have been described as a component of several hereditary syndromes. Some insight into the tumorigenesis of ACC is gleaned by analysis of these hereditary syndromes, such as Li–Fraumeni syndrome (*p53* gene on 17p13), multiple endocrine neoplasia type 1 (MEN 1, *menin* gene on 11q13), and Beckwith–Wiedemann syndrome (insulin-like growth factor [IGF] 2 from 11p15.5).[94,95] Hereditary syndromes with a predisposition for ACC are summarized in Table 10.6.

The exact etiology of sporadic ACC remains elusive. Loss of heterozygosity (LOH) has also been found in loci related to von Hippel–Lindau (*3p*) and retinoblastoma genes (*13q*).[96] Overexpression of IGF genes is related strongly to

Table 10.6 Adrenocortical carcinoma: associated hereditary cancer syndromes.

Syndromes	Associated neoplastic conditions	Genetic pathology	Molecular mechanisms
Li–Fraumeni Syndrome with predisposition to variable and wide range of tumor development	Breast cancer Soft tissue and bone sarcomas Brain tumors **Adrenocortical carcinoma**	*TP53* gene (chromosome 17p13)	Inactivation of tumor suppressor gene, *TP53* by predominantly missense mutation
Beckwith–Wiedemann Pediatric overgrowth disorder with predisposition to tumor development	Wilms tumor Neuroblastoma Hepatoplastoma **Adrenocortical carcinoma**	Key genes: *IGF2, H19, CDKIC, KCNQ1* and *KCNQ1OT1* genes (chromosome 11p15)	Microduplication of 11p15, potentially from parental imprinting
Multiple endocrine neoplasia 1 (MEN 1) Syndrome with predisposition to development of several endocrine tumors	Parathyroid adenoma Anterior pituitary adenoma Thymic/bronchial/pancreatic/duodenal/ neuroendocrine tumor/gastrinomas Lipomas/angiolipomas/angiomyolipomas/ spinal cord ependymomas **Adrenal adenoma** **Adrenocortical carcinoma**	*MEN 1* gene Other rare genes: CDK inhibitor genes such as *CDKN1B* (p27), *CDKN2B* (p15), *CDKN2C* (p18), *CDKN1A* (p21) genes (chromosome 11q13)	Mainly inactivating mutations of the *MEN1* gene causing dysfunction of the the protein product menin
Sarcoma breast lung adrenal (SBLA)	Sarcoma Breast cancer Brain tumors Lung and laryngeal cancers Leukemia and lymphoma **Adrenocortical carcinoma**	*SBLA* gene – to be determined (not yet localized to a chromosome or genetic loci)	Not yet defined

the tumorigenesis of ACC. Both IGF-1 and IGF-2 are involved in differentiation of the adrenal cortex. High levels of these factors may play a role in tumorigenesis and dedifferentiation.[97–99] Specifically molecular studies of ACC cells show *in situ* mutations of the *TP53* and *TP57* genes (both antioncogenes) and increased production of IGF-2.[97,99,100] The *P53* gene mutations are the most common in human cancer. A potential role for this in sporadic ACC is suggested by the frequent finding of LOH at the 17p13 locus in cases of sporadic ACC.[99] Definite germline mutations of the *P53* gene have also been demonstrated in more than 90% of children with ACC from southern Brazil, which has the highest prevalence of sporadic ACC in the world.[101] Amplification of steroidogenic factor-1 (SF-1) expression has also been described in this population.[101] Another genetic locus of interest is the 11-p region that may also harbor a tumor suppressor gene and has been implicated in linkage studies in subjects with the Beckwith–Wiedemann syndrome. LOH at band 11p15 and overexpression of IGF-2, whose gene is carried on this genetic locus, have been described in cases of sporadic ACC.[99,102] Other studies demonstrate that some of these tumor cells express menin, the aberrant gene product in patients with type I (MEN-1).[102] In other studies, the hybrid gene is associated with glucocorticoid-responsive aldosteronism (GRA).[103] Several reports suggest that while benign adrenal tumors retain expression of the type 2 MHC antigens, these are lost in adrenocortical carcinoma cells. Furthermore, while adrenal adenomas can be monoclonal (43%), polyclonal (28%), or mixed (28%), virtually all ACCs are monoclonal.[104]

The squamous cell carcinoma-related oncogene (SCCRO) is a novel gene involved in the hedgehog-signaling pathway of mammalian development, including the adrenal cortex. SCCRO is one of the newly described "oncodevelopmental" genes, important in normal cellular function in the regulated state and carcinogenesis in the dysregulated state. In a recent study of murine ACC,[105] high levels of SCCRO were observed in 94% of benign adrenal adenomas, while loss of SCCRO was related to over 65% of ACC. Loss of expression was related to a worse outcome and may represent a marker of dedifferentiation.

Beuschlein *et al.*[106] describe some newly discovered roles of proteins and peptides in the tumorigenesis of ACC in both the murine and human models. Inhibin and activin are dimeric glycoproteins in the transforming growth factor (TGF)-β family of ligands. Activin is a ubiquitous protein, while inhibin is expressed mostly in the gonads, adrenal cortex, and pituitary gland. They are known to play important roles as paracrine and autocrine factors regulating growth and differentiation. Archival ACC immunostaining has shown strong inhibin and activin receptor presence. Activin has been shown to inhibit proliferation, induce apoptosis and modulate ACTH-induced cortisol secretion. *In vitro*, activin treatment of ACC cultured cells inhibits steroidogenesis in a dose-dependent manner.

Luteinizing hormone (LH) may also regulate cortisol secretion by the adrenal cortex, while human chorionic gonadotropin (hCG) and gonadotropin-releasing hormone (GnRH) have been shown to stimulate DHEA-S, and pure androgen-secreting tumors. The existence of an LH/hCG receptor found in some ACC tumors has lead researchers to postulate that hormone-stimulated LH receptor expression could act as a tumor promoter when expressed ectopically in the adrenal cortex. Other oncogenetic events, however, may be necessary to induce frank carcinogenesis.[6]

A recent Bulgarian study analyzed serum levels of circulating vascular endothelial growth factor (VEGF) and prostaglandin E (PGE) in 75 patients with functional adrenal masses, such as aldosteronoma, pheochromocytoma, cortisol-secreting adenoma, ACC, and normal subjects. Researchers found that all patients with adrenal masses had elevated circulating serum levels of VEGF as compared with normal subjects, while patients with ACC had statistically significant higher levels of VEGF than patients with benign tumors. There was no difference in PGE levels across groups. VEGF and PGE are markers for angiogenesis. Overexpression of VEGF has been correlated in the past with functional activity of tumors as well as malignancy.[107] Some studies have correlated the serum levels of VEGF with tumor aggressiveness and patient outcome.[108] In the Bulgarian study, patients with cortisol-secreting tumors and ACC had the highest levels of circulating VEGF. All patients with ACC had cortisol hypersecretion; therefore, the authors postulated that while specific angiogenesis in cortisol-producing tumors is higher than other adrenal tumors, this assay alone might not be able to differentiate adenomas from carcinoma.[107]

A definitive proof for a hyperplasia-to-adenoma-to-carcinoma sequence, which occurs with colon cancer, is lacking, although a multistep tumor progression model has been suggested as a possible etiological basis for sporadic ACC. A possible unifying hypothesis might include alterations in intercellular communication, paracrine and autocrine effects of various growth factors, cytokines elaborated by the tumor cells, and promiscuous expression of various ligand receptors on the cell membranes of the cells that causes them to be in a state of perpetual hyperstimulation. These combined mechanisms could lead to clonal adrenal cellular hyperplasia, autonomous proliferation, tumor formation, and hormone elaboration.[99] The fact that the normal adrenal cortex has multiple areas of adrenomedullary cells (often forming large cell nests) and that adrenocortical cells also are scattered in the adrenal medulla suggests a close interaction between the two groups of cells, despite their distinct phylogenetic and embryonic origins. The relevance of the paracrine interactions of these cells in the pathogenesis of adrenal cortex and adrenal tumors as a whole is still being actively investigated.

Cancer diagnostic evaluation and staging

Cancer staging is a common concept in oncology, which entails radiological evaluation and determination of neoplastic spread, which, by definition, is a malignant process. Once a pathological diagnosis of ACC is made, staging workup is done to assess disease spread. Imaging with CT, MRI and FDG-PET/CT scans is the foundation for staging. Bone scan or bone survey is indicated if there are relevant clinical signs and symptoms of bony involvement. In recent years, the FDG-PET/CT scan has been used by clinicians to distinguish between benign and malignant lesions as well as for staging of asymptomatic metastatic sites.[60] However, the use of FDG-PET/CT scan in diagnosis and staging of ACC is yet to be validated. A new method of adrenal imagining is 11C-metomidate-PET. Metomidate binds to adrenal 11-β-hydroxylase and is therefore an excellent tool to distinguish lesions of adrenocortical origin from other lesions.[109] This is still mostly available in research centers and more so in those centers in Europe.

Staging can be based on clinical information, mainly radiological features describing size, characteristics of the tumor (T), involvement of locoregional lymph nodes (N), and existence of distant metastasis (M). Stage grouping can also be based on pathological information obtained during primary surgical resection. Most investigators use a surgical staging system based upon tumor size, nodal involvement and the presence or absence of metastases that was developed initially by MacFarlane in 1958[110] and subsequently modified by Sullivan et al. in 1978.[111] Since then, many revised staging systems have been proposed by different investigators.[112]

Until recently, the variability in the staging systems used in individual studies complicated the comparison of reported results. The TNM clinical cancer staging system for malignancy of the adrenal cortex was introduced for the first time in the current 7th edition of the American Joint Cancer Committee (AJCC) cancer staging manual published in 2010.[113] It remains unclear if total number of lymph nodes resected or number of lymph nodes positive for metastastic involvement, tumor grade and differentiation, weight of resected tumor, as well as lymphovascular or perineural invasion are independent prognostic determinants in ACC. Vascular invasion is still considered a prognostic determinant

of survival for ACC but it has not yet been incorporated into this first version of the TNM classification because of inconsistencies in the available data.[113] Table 10.7 represents the AJCC TNM cancer staging system for the adrenal cortex.

Natural history of disease and prognosis

The majority of patients will present with advanced-stage disease. Approximately 70% of ACCs will have spread beyond the adrenal gland at the time of diagnosis. Stages I and II will comprise about 32% of the population, while 68% will have stages III and IV at presentation.[114] The 5-year overall survival (OS) rate is 35–58%.[115] It is apparent that the more advanced stage of disease correlates with the less durable survival outcome. Complete resection (curative, definitive, or negative margins without microscopic residual [R0]) results in the best chance for cure among patients who present with locally advanced and resectable disease. An estimated 70% of ACC patients will have local recurrence or metastatic disease,after radical resection. Published data on cohorts with adult ACCs have suggested that risk of recurrence is increased among patients with capsular extension, vascular invasion, and incomplete resection. However, the rarity of the disease limits adequate study population size to correlate or validate any prognostic factor (molecular or clinical). It remains controversial whether or not patients with functional ACC and size of tumor mass have a different prognosis from those without hormonal functionality.

In recent years, with the advances in study of the human genome, tissue microarray has enabled multimolecular profiling. Investigators from the Memorial Sloan-Kettering Cancer Center analyzed the molecular profile of 124 patients with

Table 10.7 American Joint Cancer Committee TNM cancer staging for adrenal cortex.

Groupings	T	N	M	5-Year overall survival (%)
Stage I	T1	N0	M0	
Stage II	T2	N0	M0	
Stage III	T1	N1	M0	
	T2	N1	M0	
	T3	N0	M0	
Stage IV	T3	N1	M0	
	T4	N0	M0	
	T4	N1	M0	
	Any T	Any N	M1	
Primary tumor (T)	**Definitions**			
TX	Primary tumor cannot be assessed			
T0	No evidence of primary tumor			
T1	Tumor <5 cm in greatest diameter, no extraadrenal invasion			
T2	Tumor >5 cm in greatest diameter, no extraadrenal invasion			
T3	Tumor of any size with local invasion, but not invading adjacent organs (kidney, diaphragm, great vessels, pancreas, spleen and liver)			
T4	Tumor of any size with invasion of adjacent organs (kidney, diaphragm, great vessels, pancreas, spleen and liver)			
Regional lymph nodes (N)	**Definitions**			
NX	Regional (paraaortic, periaortic, retroperitoneal) lymph nodes cannot be assessed			
N0	No regional (paraaortic, periaortic, retroperitoneal) lymph node metastasis			
N1	Metastasis in regional (paraaortic, periaortic, retroperitoneal) lymph node(s)			
Distant metastasis (M)	**Definitions**			
M0	No distant metastasis			
M1	Distant metastasis			

ACC or adrenal adenomas, correlating with disease outcome, particularly the disease-specific survival. These investigators discovered that there was a significant variation in cell cycle regulatory protein expression among ACCs and between tumor and normal tissue. Furthermore, the presence of distant metastases, older age (>45 years), and incomplete resection (R1) were determinants of poor survival.[65]

Management and therapeutic options
Treatment for localized/resectable disease

Complete oncological surgical resection resulting in surgical margins without carcinoma invasion (R0) remains the only chance for durable remission and thus cure. All ACC patients with localized disease should be considered for surgery. Despite operative intervention, most patients with ACCs have a poor prognosis for several reasons. Cancer recurrence has been reported to be as high as 50–80%[8] because of a potential for micrometastasis that is undefined. Adrenalectomy can be performed with open laparotomy or be assisted with laparoscopy. Retrospective data analyses have been underpowered and results have been controversial as to which technique is associated with optimal survival outcomes for patients with resectable disease.[116] While it is technically feasible, laparoscopic adrenalectomy is still considered suboptimal as a definitive surgery and inadequate as curative treatment for patients with large ACC, particularly those with IVC infiltration. It has been recommended that a transabdominal approach through a subcostal incision be used for any suspected or proven ACC, facilitating maximal exposure for complete surgical resection and minimizing tumor spillage.[117] The presence of IVC invasion should not be considered as metastatic disease, but rather as tumor extension. In such cases, the surgical procedure should be more aggressive, attempting to remove completely the intravascular extension.[117]

Recurrent local and metastatic disease is common and reoperation should be attempted when feasible and clinically appropriate. Metastases occur most often in the lymph nodes, liver, lung, and bone.[118] Prospective and consistent retrospective data identifying clinical parameters of resectable ACC are lacking. It has been proposed that size of primary tumor and vascular invasion are predictive of those patients who may benefit most from primary cancer resection.[118] Unfortunately, many of the proposed clinical parameters are derived from retrospective series which have lacked the power to detect differential significance adequate for use as either predictive or prognostic criteria.

For other solid cancers, such as pancreatic, thoracic and head and neck cancers, published data suggested that surgical resection performed at centers of excellence results in improved outcomes compared to those performed elsewhere.[119] In a single-institution retrospective analysis of cases of ACC operated with curative intent, Grubbs et al.[120] demonstrated that survival outcomes were significantly improved compared to those cases operated elsewhere. The consistently reported parameters predictive of durable survival outcomes following curative resection include the volume of surgeries performed in the hospital, experience of surgeons and low perioperative morbidity.[119] While it is more difficult to quantify, patient selection

for resection is the most important confounder in all of these reports. In our center, we rely on a multidisciplinary clinical team and discuss such cases at a tumor board when making management decisions because of the complexity of the decision process for this disease.

Adjunctive treatments given before (neoadjuvant/preoperative), after (adjuvant/postoperative) or sandwiching (perioperative) definitive surgery have been reported to show improved survival outcomes compared to definitive surgery alone in several solid cancers, although the data for ACC are less definitive.

Attempts at local control with radiotherapy of the resected bed have been evaluated in small case series of ACC patients with R0 resection. Fassnacht et al.[121] reported that, among 14 patients with resected ACC, adjuvant radiotherapy to the resected tumor bed was effective in reducing the local recurrence, where the probability of freedom from local recurrence significantly increased compared to no adjuvant radiotherapy (79% versus 12%, $p < 0.01$). The investigators also reported that there was no significant improvement of disease-free survival (DFS) or OS with adjuvant radiotherapy. Aside from this small study, the role of adjuvant radiotherapy is not clearly defined as very little information about its efficacy has been reported in ACC cases.

There is no proven role for adjuvant systemic therapy, although there have been case reports[122] of patients who were treated with adjuvant mitotane and other agents after completion of surgical resection.

Treatment for advanced/metastatic/unresectable disease

For those patients who present with resectable disease, approximately 50–80% will eventually have recurrent or metastatic disease, after curative resection. The majority of ACC patients will present with unresectable disease or metastatic disease, requiring medical therapy with either hormonal therapy if the disease is functional and/or cytotoxic therapy with combination chemotherapy or mitotane alone.

Hypersecretion of hormonal steroids in ACC frequently contributes to the disease burden and can severely affect quality of life. Clinical manifestations of primary adrenal cortical tumors with hormonal secretion should be treated. Therapy for endocrine syndromes of ACC can be either via surgical removal of all hormone-producing neoplastic tissues or with medical treatment. The goals are to control and reverse, if possible, the clinical manifestations by normalizing hormonal overproduction, while avoiding permanent dependence upon medications or hormonal deficiency. Specifically in the many patients with ACC, medical management of hormonal overproduction is crucial to the success of antineoplastic therapy and should be concurrent and part of the overall objective of cancer control and/or treatment. Cushing syndrome from hypercortisolism is the most common symptom complex found in functional ACCs, while much less frequent functional conditions in ACC are the symptom complexes of adrenogenital syndrome and hyperaldosteronism.

In addition to dietary sodium restriction (<100 mEq/day), maintenance of ideal bodyweight, alcohol avoidance, and regular aerobic exercise to control hypertension in patients with hyperaldosteronism, mineralocorticoid receptor antagonists such as spironolactone or eplerenone and potassium-sparing diuretics such as amiloride or triamterene can be effective alternatives to control the aldosterone level.[123] Spironolactone competes with aldosterone for receptor sites in the distal renal tubule, increasing sodium chloride and water excretion while conserving potassium and hydrogen ions. Its current indications include edema associated with excessive aldosterone excretion, hypertension, primary hyperaldosteronism, hyperkalemia, cirrhosis of the liver accompanied by edema or ascites, nephrotic syndrome, and severe heart failure but it has even been used rarely to treat female acne, hirsutism, hypertension and as a diuretic. Commonly observed side-effects of spironolactone include gynecomastia, hyperkalemia, amenorrhea, abdominal cramps, nausea, vomiting, diarrhea, headache, and urticaria. Compared to spironolactone, eplerenone is a highly selective mineralocorticoid receptor antagonist, having 0.1% of the binding affinity to androgen receptors and <1% of the binding affinity to progresterone receptors.[124,125] Because of its selectivity, eplerenone is associated with a lower incidence of endocrine side-effects. On the other hand, potassium-sparing diuretics that block the aldosterone-sensitive sodium channel in the collecting tubules, such as amiloride[126] or triamterene,[127] can also block the renal effects of aldosterone, lowering the blood pressure and raising the serum potassium concentration. Frontline medical therapy for hyperaldosteronism remains aldosterone antagonist agents.

Antiandrogen therapy is the medical treatment of choice for androgen-secreting ACCs. Women can be treated with spironolactone or flutamide to block the action of androgens. In addition to being an antagonist to the aldosterone receptor, spironolactone also acts as a progesterone agonist and androgen receptor antagonist. Flutamide is an oral nonsteroidal antiandrogen capable of inhibiting androgen uptake and binding of androgen in target tissues. It is used to treat prostate cancer, but has also been reported to be effective against female hirsutism.[128] Common side-effects of flutamide include galactorrhea, nausea/vomiting, and hot flashes in women taking flutamide. The most relevant to ACC patients with hepatic metastases is that both spironolactone and flutamide can rarely cause hepatotoxicity. Therefore frequent monitoring of liver functions is indicated when using either of these drugs in metastatic ACC, especially in patients with significant hepatic tumor burden.

Typically, hypercortisolism from an ACTH-pituitary tumor, ectopic ACTH secretion, or cortisol secretion from ACA or ACC is treated primarily with surgical resection. However, when surgery is contraindicated or unsuccessful or not indicated because of metastatic/widespread ACC, medical therapy is often required. Commonly used agents include glucocorticoid receptor antagonists, adrenal enzyme inhibitors, and adrenolytic agents. Mifepristone (RU-486) is no longer available in the United States where its major indication had been to terminate pregnancy, but it has been used in Europe with some efficacy for patients with hypercortisolism. This is a synthetic steroid that acts as a competitive antagonist of the glucocorticoid and progesterone receptors. Therefore, mifepristone does not inhibit steroidogenesis, but instead it antagonizes the peripheral actions of glucocorticoids and progestogens. Common side-effects of mifepristone include vaginal bleeding

and uterine cramping as well as headaches, dizziness, abdominal cramping, nausea, vomiting, and diarrhea.

Aminoglutethimide (which is also no longer commercially available), ketoconazole, metyrapone, trilostane, fluconazole, and etomidate inhibit one or more enzymes in cortisol synthesis. These agents are commonly used for patients with Cushing disease or ACTH-producing pituitary tumors and rarely used in those with primary functional ACA or ACC. Among these, the most commonly used inhibitors of cortisol synthesis are ketoconazole and metyrapone. Ketoconazole inhibits the first step in cortisol biosynthesis and, to a lesser extent, the conversion of 11-deoxycortisol to cortisol. Its side-effects include headache, sedation, nausea/vomiting, gynecomastia, decreased libido, and impotence, although these effects are dose dependent. Though rare, ketoconazole can cause reversible hepatotoxicity and should be used cautiously in patients with hepatic metastases with already elevated liver enzymes. Metyrapone is an 11-β-hydroxylase inhibitor that blocks the final step in cortisol biosynthesis as well as increasing adrenal androgen production which can cause an increase in hirsutism in women. Its drug-related side-effects include salt retention and hypertension along with nausea and vomiting. Currently the availability of metyrapone is limited to registered prescribers on a compassionate need basis directly from the manufacturer, Novartis Pharmaceuticals Corporation.

Mitotane is the only drug approved by the FDA for the treatment of ACC. It was developed in 1960 as an insecticide (DDT) and is taken up by the adrenal cortex, causing necrosis. Mitotane is an adrenocorticolytic drug that is used primarily for the treatment of ACC, and rarely used to achieve medical adrenalectomy during or after pituitary irradiation in patients with Cushing disease or as an adjunctive medication in patients with ectopic ACTH secretion. Uniquely, mitotane is used to both block hormonal production in functional ACC and cause cytotoxic effects on malignant cells in ACC. It acts on adrenocortical cell mitochondria to inhibit 11-β-hydroxylase and cholesterol side-chain cleavage enzymes. While most of the zonal tissues in the adrenal cortex are affected by mitotane, the zona glomerulosa is relatively spared during initial exposure, suggesting that mineralocorticoid replacement may not be necessary until prolonged mitotane exposure has occurred. Additionally, it alters the metabolism of cortisol by decreasing the production of 17-hydroxycorticosteroids by converting cortisol instead into 6-β-hydrocortisol. Additionally, mitotane has several important extraadrenal actions. In addition to its actions in the adrenocortical tissues, mitotane can also:

- inhibit cholesterol oxidase leading to new-onset or worsening hypercholesterolemia
- accelerate the metabolism of halogenated synthetic glucocorticoids such as dexamethasone and fludrocortisone, indicating that patients on mitotane should be getting cortisol or prednisolone instead of their halogenated counterparts as exogeneous glucocorticoids replacement
- increase serum concentrations of other binding globulins including sex hormone-binding globulin and thyroid-binding globulin, leading to artificial decreases in serum concentrations of both free testosterone and FT4.

This drug has a cytotoxic effect on human adrenal tissue, both normal adrenals and ACC. Specifically, mitotane is metabolized into an acyl chloride that binds to important macromolecules in the mitochondria, causing mitochondrial destruction and necrosis of the adrencortical cells. Furthermore, mitotane leads to focal degeneration of the fascicular and particularly the reticular zone whereas changes of the zona glomerulosa are relatively slight. It also reverses gene-expressed chemotherapy resistance (multi-drug resistance, MDR) by reducing cellular drug efflux.

Mitotane is a difficult drug to manage as it has a narrow therapeutic index, where antitumor activity occurred at a level >14 mg/L but toxic side-effects occurred at a level >22 mg/L. Aside from adrenal suppression/insufficiency, the side-effects of mitotane are many, but most frequently gastrointestinal or involving the central nervous system.[129] In general, adverse effects are reversible after cessation of mitotane. However, since mitotane accumulates in adipose tissue, the half-life is long, and blood levels and adverse effects usually increase over time even if the dose remains unchanged. Patients on mitotane should be monitored for side-effects and have close surveillance of blood levels of mitotane, adrenal function and clinical evidence of side-effects. Due to its adrenolytic activity and increased metabolic clearance of glucocorticoids, adrenal replacement with long-acting glucocorticoids such as decadron and prednisone is necessary. Because the clinical manifestations of mitotane side-effects and those of mitotane-induced adrenal insufficiency are the same, high awareness of both will allow for better compliance.

Typical practice is to start with a low dose (1.5–2 g per day) of mitotane and titrate 0.5 g weekly, to reach the desired therapeutic serological level. Concurrent administration of glucocorticoids is also recommended. Blood levels of mitotane can be evaluated 2 weeks after starting therapy, and serum ACTH, renin, 24-h urine free cortisol (UFC) or 17-OH cortisol are used to monitor for adequate adrenal function. Patients on mitotane are also advised to discontinue the drug in the event of trauma, surgery, shock or other medical insult (e.g. sepsis) and aggressive adrenal replacement therapy should then be instituted by the medical team (a warning bracelet will often assist in alerting the medical team to this need).

Mitotane is used in several clinical contexts, including recurrent, metastatic or unresectable disease, alone or in combination with other cytotoxic agents.[129] Though still controversial, mitotane has been used in the setting of adjuvant therapy after curative or complete surgical resection. It controls endocrine hypersecretion in 70–75% of patients with functional ACC.[114] As a single agent, the average objective tumor response rate of mitotane is seen in up to 20–30% of patients.[114] Hormonal amelioration can be observed independent of tumor response. Mitotane control of endocrine hypersecretion usually occurs with serum concentrations >7 mg/L, and objective antitumor response and long-term survival benefits are observed only when serum mitotane concentrations are consistently >14 mg/L.[130]

Having both antihormonal and antitumor effects, mitotane is theoretically an ideal agent for the management of ACC. However, as it is slow to reach the therapeutic level and has dose-limiting toxicity, mitotane alone is frequently insufficient to rapidly control hypersecretion or tumor growth in all patients.

Experience with cytotoxic chemotherapy in ACC is limited, partly due to the rarity of the disease, and there are very few well-designed studies assessing the efficacy of therapy. Several combinations of cytotoxic agents have been used and the available evidence suggests that cisplatin-based chemotherapy has activity in ACC. Various chemotherapy regimens have been combined with mitotane, which was theoretically added to the efficacy of the cytotoxic agent by blocking cellular efflux via MDR suppression. Berruti et al. reported an objective response rate with mitotane-etoposide-adriamycin-cisplatin (M-EAP) combination chemotherapy of 49% among 28 patients with advanced ACC.[131] This success comes at the cost of significant toxicity. Subsequent studies have not been able to reproduce the same tumor efficacy, and response rate with cisplatin-based chemotherapy is more generally thought to be 20–30%.[132] Another regimen proposed because of a lower side-effect profile is a combination of mitotane and streptozotocin (M-S), for which Khan et al. reported an objective response rate of 36% among eight patients with advanced ACC.[133] Review of selected published data using combination chemotherapy in advanced ACC resulted in a tumor response rate of about 32%.[114] Without randomized controlled trials via large international efforts, the optimal frontline chemotherapy regimen cannot be determined. The same large cooperative effort will also be required to assess whether or not the addition of mitotane to a chemotherapy regimen will increase tumor response rate. Currently international cooperation has led to an ongoing trial, FIRM-ACT, in which patients with advanced ACC are randomized between M-EAP and M-S as frontline therapy.[134]

Systemic therapy for ACC continues to be disappointing, with significant toxicity profile and low tumor efficacy and no survival benefits. The only FDA-approved choice for unresectable, advanced, or metastatic ACC is mitotane, alone or in combination with chemotherapy. Preclinical data, mainly from case series protein expression profiles of ACC tissues, have identified several targets for drug development in ACC: VEGF and its receptor (VEGFR),[135,136] epidermal growth factor receptor (EGFR),[137,138] insulin receptor,[139] or IGF-1 receptor (IGF-1R).[140,141] Clinical studies of inhibitors of EGFR, such as small molecule tyrosine kinase inhibitors (gefitinib, erlotinib) alone or in combination with cytotoxic chemotherapy, have been disappointing. No objective responses were observed with gefitinib 250 mg daily in a phase 2 study conducted via Darthmouth-Hitchcock Norris Cotton Cancer Center NCT00215202.[142] In another phase 2 study, 10 ACC patients were treated with oral erlotinib 100 mg daily and intravenous gemcitabine 800 mg/m^2/2 weeks. Quinkler et al.[143] reported only one patient who experienced a minor response, while nine of 10 patients had died after a median of 5.5 months after treatment initiation. Experience with anti-VEGF/VEGFR therapy has not been much different. No objective responses were reported with bevacizumab, a monoclonal antibody against VEGF-A ligand. In this study, bevacizumab was administered at 5 mg/kg intravenously in combination with oral capecitabine at 950 mg/m^2 twice daily for

14 days, every 3 weeks to 10 patients with refractory advanced/metastatic ACC.[144]

Perhaps the most promising and advanced drug development program is along the pathway of the insulin-like growth factor. Approximately 90% of ACCs overexpress IGF-2, and preclinical studies have suggested that IGF-2 functions in an autocrine fashion to stimulate proliferation of ACC cells.[145] Inhibitors of IGF-R1 reduced proliferation and cell viability in cultures.[141,146] Figitumumab, a human monoclonal antibody against IGF-R1, was given to patients with ACC at an intravenous dose of 20 mg/kg every 21 days with or without mitotane. However, only data regarding safety, tolerability, and pharamcokinetics of the arm where patients were treated with figitumumab were reported. Haluska et al.[147] reported one episode of grade 4 toxicity (hyperuricemia, proteinuria and elevated γ-glutamyltransferase; while no objective response was observed, eight of 14 patients in this study achieved stable disease.

In a phase 1 study of intermittent dosing of OSI-906, a dual tyrosine kinase inhibitor of IGF-1R and insulin receptor (IR) in patients with advanced solid tumors, 61 patients were treated. Among 11 patients with advanced and refractory ACC, one had a durable partial response (73% reduction by the standard NCI Response Evaluation Criteria in Solid Tumors, "RECIST", criteria) of 16 months' duration, and four had stable disease at 3 months' duration.[148] Results from the phase 1 study among ACC patients have led to the international registration phase 3 randomized placebo-controlled study of OSI-906 in patients with locally advanced or metastatic ACC (GALACCTIC), NCT00924989, conducted by Astellas Pharma Inc., at more than 200 sites. The primary endpoint was overall survival. The study was opened in 2009 and had completed its planned accrual of 135 patients early in 2011; the completion of this study represents a monumental achievement of international collaboration, as well as being the first ever phase 3 study in ACC. Interim efficacy analysis is due in the summer of 2012, and results are anxiously anticipated by many physicians and patients.

Neoplasms of the adrenal medulla

The most frequent adult primary malignancy of the adrenal medulla is PHEO and its extraadrenal variant, paraganglioma (PARA). Catecholamine-secreting tumors are rare neoplasms, probably occurring in less than 0.2% of patients with hypertension.[149] Specifically, PHEO occurs less frequently than ACC; estimated incidence for PHEO is 2–8 in 1 million people and approximately 1000 cases (benign and malignant) diagnosed in the United States yearly.[149] PHEO is commonly diagnosed among young or middle-aged adults, and can occur earlier in hereditary cases.[150] Similar to ACC, the treatment modality offering the best chance for durable remission or cure is complete surgical resection. The prognosis of patients with PHEO presenting with unresectable, metastatic or metastatic recurrent disease is poor and options are predominantly limited to palliative therapy.

Approximately 10% of PHEOs are bilateral,[151] while 20% occur in children.[152] Furthermore, approximately 15%[153] are located outside the adrenal gland, and of these, 95%[154] are in the abdomen. Frequently, PHEO is a catecholamine-producing benign neoplasm but in about 10–26% cases it is malignant.[155,156] Differentiating features between benign and malignant neoplasms are based predominantly on clinical aggressiveness and clinical/radiological documentation of metastatic involvement outside the adrenal glands.

Clinical presentations

Pheochromocytoma is usually suggested by the history in a symptomatic patient, discovery of an incidental adrenal mass, or the family history in a patient with familial disease (Table 10.8). In one report of 107 patients, the average age at diagnosis was 47 years, and the average tumor size was 4.9 cm.[150] Occurring very rarely is the the classic triad of symptoms consisting of episodic headache, sweating, and tachycardia,[157] while the most common presentation is hypertension. Frequently, hypertension can be either paroxysmal or sustained[157] but approximately 5–15% of patients present with normal blood pressure.[158] Headache, which may be mild or severe, and variable in duration, occurs in up to 90% of symptomatic patients.[158] Generalized sweating occurs in about 60% of symptomatic patients. Less common symptoms and signs include pallor, orthostatic hypotension, visual blurring, papilledema, weight loss, polyuria, polydipsia, constipation, hyperglycemia, leukocytosis, psychiatric disorders, and rarely, clinical features associated with secondary erythrocytosis due to overproduction of erythropoietin.[159] The symptoms of PHEOs may also be caused by neoplastic oversecretion of norepinephrine (NE), epinephrine (E), and dopamine (DOPA).

With the more widespread use of computerized imaging, an increasing number of asymptomatic patients are diagnosed with PHEO in the course of investigation of an AI or in the workup of one of the genetic forms of the disease. In a case series of 150 PHEO patients treated at the Mayo Clinic, 15 (10%) patients had their diagnoses made by incidental finding on abdominal CT scans performed for other indications.[160]

Most catecholamine-secreting tumors are sporadic. However, some patients have the disease as part of a familial disorder. In these patients the catecholamine-secreting tumors are more likely to be bilateral adrenal PHEOs or paragangliomas. Hereditary PHEOs typically present at a younger age than sporadic cases.[161] Additionally, sporadic PHEO is usually diagnosed on the basis of symptoms or an incidental discovery on CT/MRI scans. Several familial syndromes are associated with predisposition for PHEO, including von Hippel–Lindau (VHL), MEN-2, and neurofibromatosis (NF)-1; all have autosomal dominant inheritance, with associated frequencies of developing PHEO of 10–20%, 50%, and 0.1–5.7% respectively.[162,163] When PHEO is associated with MEN 2 syndrome, symptoms are present in only about 50% of patients and only 30% have hypertension.[164] It is not known whether this difference is due to screening or is a real difference in the clinical expression of the disease. A similar finding has been observed with PHEO associated with VHL disease, as 35% of patients have no symptoms, a normal blood pressure, and normal laboratory values for fractionated catecholamines.[165]

Table 10.8 Pheochromocytoma/paraganglioma: associated hereditary cancer syndromes.

Syndromes	Associated neoplastic conditions	Genetic pathology	Molecular mechanisms
Von Hippel–Lindau (VHL)	Renal clear cell carcinoma Pancreatic neuroendocrine carcinoma ***Pheochromocytoma and paraganglioma*** Pancreatic/epididymal serous cystadenomas Hemangioblastoma Retinal angiomas	*VHL* (chromosome 3p25)	Missense or *de novo* mutation of *VHL* gene, which functions as a tumor suppressor. VHL protein has many functions and interactions, including angiogenesis, cycle regulation, renal gatekeeper
Multiple endocrine neoplasm 2 (MEN 2)	Medullary thryoid carcinoma ***Pheochromocytoma*** Cutaneous lichen amyloidosis Mucocutaneous/intestinal neuromas Papillary thyroid carcinoma	*RET* (chromosome 10q11)	Missense activating mutation of *RE*, which functions as a protooncogene
Neurofibromatosis 1 (NF 1)	Neurofibroma Central nervous system gliomas ***Pheochromocytoma and paraganglioma*** Pancreatic neuroendocrine carcinoma	*NF1* (chromosome 17q11)	Deletion and translocation leading to deactivating mutations in the *NF1* gene, which functions as a tumor suppressor
Familial paraganglioma	***Paraganglioma*** Renal cell carcinoma	*SDH-B* (subunit B, an iron-sulfur protein, chromosome 1p36) *SDH-C* (subunit C, integral membrane protein, chromosome 1q21) *SDH-D* (subunit D, integral membrane protein, chromosome 11q23) *SDH-AF2* (assembly factor 2, chromosome 11q12) *SDH-A* (subunit A, flavaprotein, chromosome 5p15)	Mutations in the *SDH* gene which compose portions of the mictochondrial complex II, a tumor suppressor gene involve in the electron transport chain and the tricarboxylic acid cycle

RET, rearranged during transfection; SDH, succinate dehydrogenase subunit genes.

Laboratory evaluation and diagnosis

The diagnosis is typically confirmed by measurements of urinary and plasma fractionated metanephrines and catecholamines. There is still no consensus as to the most specific and optimal methods for diagnosing catecholamine-producing neoplasms. Many experts still agree that a 24-h urine collection for fractionated catecholamines and metanephrines remains the most reliable case detection method, with 98% sensitivity and 98% specificity.[160,166] This should also include measurement of urinary creatinine to verify an adequate collection. The diagnostic cutoffs for most 24-h urinary fractionated metanephrine assays are based on normal ranges derived from a normotensive volunteer reference group, and this can result in excessive false-positive testing. A positive test is considered to be a two-fold elevation above the upper limit of normal in urine catecholamines or metanephrines (see Table 10.2). Proponents of plasma fractionated metanephrines have suggested that plasma testing should be a first-line diagnostic test for PHEO, where the sensitivity and specificity are reported to be 96–100% and 85–89%,[166,167] respectively. Tricyclic antidepressants interfere most frequently with the interpretation of 24-h urinary catecholamines and metabolites. Furthermore, catecholamine secretion may be appropriately increased in situations of physical stress or illness (e.g. stroke, myocardial infarction, congestive heart failure, obstructive sleep apnea). Therefore, the clinical circumstances under which catecholamines and metanephrines are measured must be assessed in each case.

Other ancillary tests used to confirm the diagnosis of PHEO include clonidine suppression test, plasma chromogranin-A (CGA) and neuropeptide-Y, 24-h urinary vanillylmandelic acid (VMA) excretion as well as provocative testing and suppression testing such as histamine and glucagon stimulation tests. For any of the biochemical tests, sensitivity will be lower and specificity higher for hereditary compared to sporadic PHEO because tumors detected in patients with a familial disposition tend to be small masses that release catecholamines in amounts that are often too low to be detected. In contrast, sporadic PHEOs tend to be larger and present with typical signs and symptoms of catecholamine excess.

In one multicenter cohort study that included 214 patients with confirmed PHEO and 644 patients who were determined not to have the tumor (both groups being tested for either sporadic or familial PHEO), investigators reported that sensitivity was highest for plasma fractionated metanephrines (99%) followed by urinary fractionated metanephrines (97%) and specificity was highest for urinary VMA (96%) followed by urinary total metanephrines (93%).[167] In another analysis, the diagnostic efficacy of plasma fractionated metanephrines and 24-h urinary total metanephrines (sum of metanephrine + normetanephrine) in combination with fractionated catecholamines was compared in 349 outpatients tested for PHEO.[166] The sensitivities of plasma fractionated metanephrines compared to urinary total metanephrines in combination with urinary fractionated catecholamines were 97% versus 90%, while the specificities were 85% versus 96%.[166] Based on another systematic review and metaanalysis of plasma fractionated metanephrines, including three studies of 56 patients with and 445 subjects without PHEO, the posttest probabilities with positive plasma fractionated metanephrine values would be 2.8% and 23.7% in the patient with hypertension or AI, respectively.[168] Thus, plasma fractionated metanephrines are very sensitive (97–100%), but not very specific (85–89%) for PHEO, so measurement of plasma fractionated metanephrines is useful to rule out PHEO, but a positive test only slightly increases suspicion of disease when screening for sporadic PHEO.

Pathological evaluation

Image-guided needle biopsy of PHEO should be avoided due to a high rate of biopsy-related complications. This was illustrated in a report of 20 patients who were diagnosed at the time of needle biopsy, of whom 14 (70%) developed biopsy-related complications.[169] Complications included low frequency (41%) of having a R0 resection, delay in going to R0 resection (15%), labile hypertension (15%), hematoma (30%), nondiagnostic biopsy (25%), and pain (25%).[169] Interventional radiologists commonly use narrow gauge biopsy needles to obtain adrenal samples, which yield scant diagnostic tissue and further complicate pathological evaluation.

Differentiation between various adrenal neoplasms can be challenging, so the histological diagnosis of PHEO relies heavily on pathological expertise, and various immunohistochemical antibody panels, consisting of combinations of antibodies against various markers such as chromogranin, SF-1, MART, calretinin or inhibin.[170] Many different panels had been proposed to be effective in distinguishing adrenal cortical lesions from PHEOs, but none are pathognomonic. While it is common to expect pathological tissue to be the most important in making a diagnosis in oncological practice, PHEOs are typically diagnosed based on clinical probabilities and confirmed with laboratory results.

Cancer diagnostic evaluation and staging

Among patients suspected to have a PHEO, the diagnosis is rarely confirmed. Biochemical confirmation of the diagnosis should be followed by radiological evaluation to locate the tumor, not the other way around. The most common extraadrenal locations are the superior and inferior abdominal paraaortic areas (75%), the urinary bladder (10%), the thorax (10%), and the head, neck, and pelvis (5%).[153] The most commonly used radiological modalities for evaluation of PHEOs are CT and MRI scans. With CT, there is some exposure to radiation but no risk of exacerbation of hypertension if current radiographic contrast agents are given. CT with low-osmolar contrast is safe for patients with PHEO, even without α- or β-blocker pretreatment, as illustrated in a report of 22 such patients.[171] With MRI,

there is neither radiation nor dye. This more expensive test can distinguish PHEOs from other adrenal masses; on T2-weighted images PHEOs appear hyperintense and other adrenal tumors isointense, as compared with the liver.[172] MRI lacks the superior spatial resolution of CT. In patients with the MEN 2 syndrome, CT imaging may miss about one-quarter of the tumors.[172] In a selected group of patients with a 40% incidence of PHEOs, the respective positive and negative predictive values of CT were 69% and 98%.[173]

If abdominal and pelvic CT or MRI is negative in the presence of clinical and biochemical evidence of PHEOs, one ought first to reconsider the diagnosis. If it is still considered likely, then MIBG scintigraphy may be done. A MIBG scan can detect tumors not detected by CT or MRI or multiple tumors when CT or MRI is positive.[173] However, this radioactive scintigraphy is indicated in patients with large (>10 cm) adrenal PHEOs (increased risk of malignancy).[153] MIBG findings should always be corroborated by findings on computed imaging. Other radiological modalities include OctreoScan™ and FDG- or ^{11}C-metomidate (MTO)-PET/CT scan, none of which has very high sensitivity or specificity for PHEOs.

Natural history of disease and prognosis

Pheochromocytoma is a rare neuroendocrine tumor, occurring in <0.2% of patients with hypertension. In at least 10% of patients, the tumor is discovered incidentally during CT or MRI of the abdomen for unrelated symptoms. Additionally, no formal TNM staging system exists for PHEO. So prognosis of patients with newly diagnosed PHEO relies on clinical features such as size of the tumor, extraadrenal involvement or distant metastatic foci. The risk of malignancy is higher for PARA than for PHEO, especially if the patient has a mutation in succinate dehydrogenase subunit B (SDH-B),[174] and is also higher in some forms of variant VHL.[175] The only reliable clue to the presence of a malignant PHEO is local invasion or distant metastases, which may occur as long as 20 years after resection.

Surgical removal of a PHEO does not always lead to long-term cure of PHEO or even control of hypertension, even in patients with a benign tumor. In one series of 176 patients, PHEO recurred in 29 (16%) and the recurrence was malignant in 15 (52%).[176] Recurrence was more likely in patients with familial PHEO/PARA, right adrenal tumors, and extraadrenal tumors. Thus, long-term monitoring is indicated in all patients, even those apparently cured. Most patients should have annual biochemical screening and anatomical evaluation with CT or MRI scans can be done on routine schedule, typically every 4 months for the first 2–3 years after definitive surgery followed by every 6 months thereafter until 5–10 years out from surgery.

Management and therapeutic options

Preoperative medical management

When AI is suspected to be catecholamine producing or after a diagnosis of PHEO is made, definitive surgery should only be performed after appropriate medical preparation.

Cardiovascular and hemodynamic variables must be monitored closely. Continuous measurement of intraarterial pressure and heart rhythm is required. Objectives of preoperative medical therapy include hypertensive control and volume expansion. Combined α- and β-adrenergic blockade, calcium channel blockers, and metyrosine have all been used successfully to achieve goals for preoperative management. Combined α- and β-adrenergic blockade blockade is one approach to control blood pressure and prevent intraoperative hypertensive crises.

An α-adrenergic blocker is given 10–14 days preoperatively to normalize blood pressure and expand the contracted blood volume. A longer duration of preoperative α-adrenergic blockade is indicated in patients with recent myocardial infarction, catecholamine cardiomyopathy, refractory hypertension, and catecholamine-induced vasculitis. Phenoxybenzamine is the preferred drug for preoperative preparation to control blood pressure and arrhythmia in most centers in the United States. It is an irreversible, long-acting, nonspecific α-adrenergic blocking agent. The initial dose is 10 mg once or twice daily, and the dose is increased by 10–20 mg in divided doses every 2–3 days as needed to control blood pressure and clinical episodes of hypertension-related symptoms. The final dose of phenoxybenzamine is typically between 20 and 100 mg daily. Typical side-effects of phenoxybenzamine include orthostasis, nasal stuffiness, fatigue, and retrograde ejaculation for men. With their more favorable side-effect profiles, selective α1-adrenergic blocking agents (e.g. prazosin, terazosin, or doxazosin) are preferable to phenoxybenzamine when long-term pharmacological treatment is indicated (e.g. for metastatic PHEO). However, treatment with these agents is not routinely used preoperatively because of incomplete α-adrenergic blockade.

After adequate α-adrenergic blockade has been achieved, β-adrenergic blockade is initiated, which typically occurs 2–3 days preoperatively. The β-adrenergic blocker should never be started first because blockade of vasodilatory peripheral β-adrenergic receptors with unopposed α-adrenergic receptor stimulation can lead to a further elevation in blood pressure. β-Adrenergic blockers should be started slowly and at lower doses. For example, propranolol 10 mg is administered orally every 6 h on the first day of β-adrenergic blockade and β-adrenergic blockade is converted to a single long-acting dose starting the second day. The dose can be increased as necessary to control the tachycardia, where the goal heart rate is 60–80 beats per minute. In general, the patient is ready for surgery in 10–14 days after initiation of α-adrenergic blockade.

Although preoperative α-adrenergic blockade is widely recommended, a second regimen that has been effectively utilized involves the administration of a calcium channel blocker.[177] Nicardipine is the most commonly used calcium channel blocker in this setting; the starting dose is 30 mg twice daily of the sustained-release preparation. It is given orally to control blood pressure preoperatively and as an intravenous infusion intraoperatively. The main role for this class of drugs may be either to supplement the combined α- and β-adrenergic blockade protocol when blood pressure control is inadequate

or to replace the adrenergic blockade protocol in patients with intolerable side-effects.

Another approach involves the administration of metyrosine (α-methyl-para-tyrosine), which inhibits catecholamine synthesis. In one report, the patients given metyrosine had a smoother perioperative course than those given phenoxybenzamine alone.[178] Metyrosine should be used with caution and only when other agents have been ineffective or in patients in whom tumor manipulation or destruction will be significant.[178] With appropriate indications, metyrosine can be initiated at 250 mg every 6 h on day 1, 500 mg every 6 h on day 2, 750 mg every 6 h on day 3, and 1000 mg every 6 h on the day before the procedure, with the last dose (1000 mg) on the morning of the procedure.[178] With this short-course metyrosine therapy, the main side-effect is hypersomnolence. The side-effects of metyrosine can be disabling and with long-term therapy they include sedation, depression, diarrhea, anxiety, nightmares, crystalluria and urolithiasis, galactorrhea, and extrapyramidal signs. Metyrosine may be added to α- and β-adrenergic blockade when the resection will be difficult or if destructive therapy is planned. The extrapyramidal effects of phenothiazines or haloperidol may be potentiated and their use concomitantly with metyrosine should be avoided. High fluid intake to avoid crystalluria is suggested for any patient taking more than 2 g daily.

Blood pressure should be monitored twice daily in the outpatient setting with the patient in the seated and standing positions. Target blood pressure is less than 120/80 mmHg (seated), with systolic blood pressure greater than 90 mmHg (standing); both targets should be modified on the basis of the patient's age and comorbid disease. On the second or third day of α-adrenergic blockade, patients are encouraged to start a diet high in sodium content (>5000 mg daily) because of the catecholamine-induced volume contraction and the orthostasis associated with α-adrenergic blockade. This degree of volume expansion may be contraindicated in patients with congestive heart failure or renal insufficiency.

Treatment of localized/resectable disease

The laparoscopic approach to the adrenal gland is the procedure of choice for patients with solitary intraadrenal PHEO, <8 cm in diameter and without malignant radiological features. Both the laparoscopic transabdominal and retroperitoneal approaches have been used successfully, although there is some evidence that the retroperitoneal approach is preferable.[179] A retrospective review reported better operative outcomes with the retroperitoneal approach compared with the transabdominal approach, with decreased operative time (84 versus 117 min), decreased intraoperative blood loss (200 mL versus 340 mL), shorter hospital stay (5 versus 8 days), and lower complication rates (7% versus 12%).[180]

Laparoscopic adrenalectomy is safe and effective and hence the preferred surgical option as definitive therapy in PHEO. Because approximately 30% of PHEO cases associated with MEN 2 will be bilateral,[151] complete bilateral adrenalectomy is recommended for MEN 2 patients. Patients with VHL have less diffuse medullary disease and cortical-sparing bilateral adrenalectomy is an option for these patients when bilateral disease is evident on imaging.[181] If a bilateral adrenalectomy is planned preoperatively, the patient should receive glucocorticoid stress coverage while awaiting transfer to the operating room. Glucocorticoid coverage should be initiated in the operating room if unexpected bilateral adrenalectomy is necessary. Postoperative hypotension can be avoided by adequate fluid replacement and hypoglycemia. After tumor removal, catecholamine secretion should fall to normal in approximately 1 week.

Treatment for advanced/metastatic/unresectable disease

There are no curative treatments for malignant PHEO unless the sites of disease are surgically resectable. However, individual cases of malignant PHEO can be evaluated for palliative adrenalectomy to improve symptom control and quality of life. Painful skeletal metastatic lesions can be treated with external radiation therapy. In initial studies, tumor irradiation with 131I-MIBG has proven to be of some therapeutic value in selected patients.[182]

There are few data addressing the benefit of systemic antineoplastic therapy in these patients. A chemotherapy program consisting of cyclophosphamide, vincristine, and dacarbazine (CVD) is sometimes used initially, based on an early trial that reported high response rates and symptomatic improvement with this regimen.[183] Overall, objective response rate was noted in 55%, while biochemical responses were seen in 72%,[183] with 20 months' median duration of response and 3.3 years' median OS duration.[183] Effective cytoreduction and blood pressure control were observed in 33% of the 54 patients with PHEO and paragangliomas treated with CVD containing chemotherapy at the University of Texas MD Anderson Cancer Center.[184] Additionally, the use of tyrosine kinase inhibitors, such as sunitinib, in four patients with malignant PHEO/PARA appeared promising in normalizing blood pressure and improving quality of life.[185]

Conclusion

Neoplasms of the adrenal gland can be primary or secondary; secondary neoplasms are malignancies from another primary site metastasizing to the adrenal glands. Primary adrenal neoplasms are rare malignancies where the majority are fortunately benign tumors capable of oversecreting hormones that can manifest as clinical or subclinical symptoms. The foundation of management of adenomas of the adrenal cortex and adrenal incidentalomas is diagnostic workup requiring both laboratory and radiological evaluations. Fortunately, imaging features on CT and MRI can be helpful in distinguishing malignant from benign tumors. Diagnostic evaluation of all adrenal masses needs to exclude the possibility of catecholamine-secreting tumors of the adrenal medulla such as pheochromocytoma and paragangliomas. Prevalence of malignant pheochromocytoma is variably reported as 10–20%. Adrencortical carcinoma is the rare malignant primary tumor of the adrenal cortex, where the majority of patients will have advanced and unresectable disease. Cancer recurrence occurred in >50% of patients with adrenocortical carcinoma after curative resection. Curative therapy does not exist for advanced, unresectable or metastatic adrenocrtical carcinoma and pheochromocytoma.

Hereditary syndromes associated with these deadly malignancies have provided directions for identifying therapeutic targets in drug development; OSI-906 is a small molecule tyrosine kinase inhibitor of IGF-1R and IR that has led the way by completing its accrual ahead of projected schedule in a registration phase 3 randomized placebo-controlled study for patients with refractory advanced adrenocortical carcinoma.

While the prognoses for primary adrenal malignancies are grim, the commercial interest in drug development for orphan diseases and improved molecular understanding of these rare malignancies will hopefully result in the introduction of more effective and less toxic therapy for patients afflicted with either adrenocortical carcinoma or malignant pheochromocytoma.

References

1. Astwood EB, Greep RO, Geiger SR. *Endocrinology: Adrenal Gland.* American Physiological Society, 1975, Bethesda, pp. 1–742.
2. Brunt LM, Moley JF. Adrenal incidentaloma. World J Surg 2001; 25(7): 905–13.
3. Zografos GC, Driscoll DL, Karakousis CP, Huben RP. Adrenal adenocarcinoma: a review of 53 cases. J Surg Oncol 1994; 55(3): 160–4.
4. McNeil AR, Blok BH, Koelmeyer TD, Burke MP, Hilton JM. Phaeochromocytomas discovered during coronial autopsies in Sydney, Melbourne and Auckland. Aust N Z J Med 2000; 30(6): 648–52.
5. Kopf D, Goretzki PE, Lehnert H. Clinical management of malignant adrenal tumors. J Cancer Res Clin Oncol 2001; 127(3): 143–55.
6. Wy LA, Carlson HE, Kane P, Li X, Lei ZM, Rao CV. Pregnancy-associated Cushing's syndrome secondary to a luteinizing hormone/human chorionic gonadotropin receptor-positive adrenal carcinoma. Gynecol Endocrinol 2002; 16(5): 413–17.
7. Angeli A, Osella G, Ali A, Terzolo M. Adrenal incidentaloma: an overview of clinical and epidemiological data from the National Italian Study Group. Horm Res 1997; 47(4–6): 279–83.
8. Abiven G, *et al.* Clinical and biological features in the prognosis of adrenocortical cancer: poor outcome of cortisol-secreting tumors in a series of 202 consecutive patients. J Clin Endocrinol Metab 2006; 91(7): 2650–5.
9. Libè R, Fratticci A, Bertherat J. Adrenocortical cancer: pathophysiology and clinical management. Endocr Rel Cancer 2007; 14(1): 13–28.
10. Koschker AC, Fassnacht M, Hahner S, Weismann D, Allolio B. Adrenocortical carcinoma – improving patient care by establishing new structures. Exp Clin Endocrinol Diabetes 2006; 114(02): 45–51.
11. Fehm HL, Voigt KH. Pathophysiology of Cushing's disease. Pathobiol Annu 1979; 9: 225–55.
12. Latronico AC, Chrousos GP. Adrenocortical tumors. J Clin Endocrinol Metab 1997; 82(5): 1317–24.
13. Orth DN. Cushing's syndrome. N Engl J Med 1995; 332(12): 791–803.
14. Garrido M, Ponce C, Escalante S, Sanz V, Mena A. Cushing's paraneoplastic syndrome as first manifestation of an adenocarcinoma of unknown origin. Clin Translat Oncol 2006; 8(8): 621–3.
15. Bertani H, *et al.* Unusual paraneoplastic syndrome accompanies neuroendocrine tumours of the pancreas. Case Rep Med 2011; May 10 [Epub ahead of print].
16. Newell-Price J, Trainer P, Besser M, Grossman A. The diagnosis and differential diagnosis of Cushing's syndrome and pseudo-Cushing's states. Endocr Rev 1998; 19(5): 647–72.
17. Ross EJ, Marshall-Jones P, Friedman M. Cushing's syndrome: diagnostic criteria. QJM 1966; 35(2): 149–92.
18. Ross E, Linch D. Cushing's syndrome – killing disease: discriminatory value of signs and symptoms aiding early diagnosis. Lancet 1982; 320(8299): 646–9.

19. Arai K, Chrousos GP. Syndromes of glucocorticoid and mineralocorticoid resistance. Steroids 1995; 60(1): 173–9.

20. Kelly WF, Checkley SA, Bender DA. Cushing's syndrome, tryptophan and depression. Br J Psychiatry 1980; 136(2): 125–32.

21. Lim Jr RC, Nakayama DK, Biglieri EG, Schambelan M, Hunt TK. Primary aldosteronism: changing concepts in diagnosis and management. Am J Surg 1986; 152(1): 116–21.

22. Conn JW, Knopf RF, Nesbit RM. Clinical characteristics of primary aldosteronism from an analysis of 145 cases. Am J Surg 1964; 107(1): 159–72.

23. Vallotton MB. Primary aldosteronism. Part I Diagnosis of primary hyperaldosteronism. Clin Endocrinol 1996; 45(1): 47–52.

24. Lingam RK, et al. Diagnostic performance of CT versus MR in detecting aldosterone-producing adenoma in primary hyperaldosteronism (Conn's syndrome). Eur Radiol 2004; 14(10): 1787–92.

25. Telner AH. Adrenal cortical carcinoma: an unusual cause of hyperaldosteronism. Can Med Assoc J 1983; 129(7): 731–2.

26. Thanavaro JL. Diagnosis and management of primary aldosteronism. Nurse Pract 2011; 36(4): 12–21; quiz –2.

27. Seccia TM, Fassina A, Nussdorfer GG, Pessina AC, Rossi GP. Aldosterone-producing adrenocortical carcinoma: an unusual cause of Conn's syndrome with an ominous clinical course. Endocr Relat Cancer 2005; 12(1): 149–59.

28. Onselen JV. Hirsutism: causes and treatment for women. Br J Nurs 2011; 20(16): 985–6.

29. Yildiz BO. Diagnosis of hyperandrogenism: clinical criteria. Best Pract Res Clin Endocrinol Metab 2006; 20(2): 167–76.

30. Patel SS, Carrick KS, Carr BR. Virilization persists in a woman with an androgen-secreting granulosa cell tumor. Fertil Steril 2009; 91(3): 933.

31. Scott HW Jr, Abumrad NN, Orth DN. Tumors of the adrenal cortex and Cushing's syndrome. Ann Surg 1985; 201(5): 586–94.

32. Allolio B, Fassnacht M. Adrenocortical carcinoma: clinical update. J Clin Endocrinol Metab 2006; 91(6): 2027–37.

33. Wajchenberg BL, et al. Adrenocortical carcinoma. Cancer 2000; 88(4): 711–36.

34. Gopan T, Remer E, Hamrahian AH. Evaluating and managing adrenal incidentalomas. Cleveland Clin J Med 2006; 73(6): 561–8.

35. Edwards S, Evans P, Hucklebridge F, Clow A. Association between time of awakening and diurnal cortisol secretory activity. Psychoneuroendocrinology 2001; 26(6): 613–22.

36. Lentjes EGWM, Romijn FHTPM. Temperature-dependent cortisol distribution among the blood compartments in man. J Clin Endocrinol Metab 1999; 84(2): 682–7.

37. Flack MR, et al. Urine free cortisol in the high-dose dexamethasone suppression test for the differential diagnosis of the Cushing syndrome. Ann Intern Med 1992; 116(3): 211–17.

38. Hamrahian AH, Oseni TS, Arafah BM. Measurements of serum free cortisol in critically ill patients. N Engl J Med 2004; 350(16): 1629–38.

39. Ness-Abramof R, et al. Overnight dexamethasone suppression test: a reliable screen for Cushing's syndrome in the obese. Obesity 2002; 10(12): 1217–21.

40. Nugent C, Nichols T, Tyler F. Diagnosis of Cushing's syndrome: single dose dexamethasone suppression test. Arch Intern Med 1965; 116(2): 172–6.

41. Tyrrell JB, Findling JW, Aron DC, Fitzgerald PA, Forsham PH. An overnight high-dose dexamethasone suppression test for rapid differential diagnosis of Cushing's syndrome. Ann Intern Med 1986; 104(2): 180–6.

42. Kirk LF Jr, Hash RB, Katner HP, Jones T. Cushing's disease: clinical manifestations and diagnostic evaluation. Am Fam Physician 2000; 62(5): 1119–27, 33–4.

43. Nakamaru M, Misono K, Naruse M, Workman R, Inagami T. A role for the adrenal renin–angiotensin system in the regulation of potassium-stimulated aldosterone production. Endocrinology 1985; 117(5): 1772–8.

44. Seccia TM, Fassina A, Nussdorfer GG, Pessina AC, Rossi GP. Aldosterone-producing adrenocortical carcinoma: an unusual cause of Conn's syndrome with an ominous clinical course. Endocr Rel Cancer 2005; 12(1): 149–59.

45. Odell WD, Parker LN. Control of adrenal androgen production. Endocr Res 1984; 10(3–4): 617–30.

46. Grover PK, Odell WD. Correlation of in vivo and in vitro activities of some naturally occurring androgens using a radioreceptor assay for 5alpha-dihydrotestosterone with rat prostate cytosol receptor protein. J Steroid Biochem 1975; 6(10): 1373–9.

47. Henry GB. Androgen production in women. Fertil Steril 2002; 77(Suppl 4): 3–5.

48. Šulcová J, Hill M, Hampl R, Stárka L. Age and sex related differences in serum levels of unconjugated dehydroepiandrosterone and its sulphate in normal subjects. J Endocrinol 997; 154(1): 57–62.

49. Wolthers OD, et al. Androgen secreting adrenocortical tumours. Arch Dis Child 1999; 80(1): 46–50.

50. Young WF. The incidentally discovered adrenal mass. N Engl J Med 2007; 356(6): 601–10.

51. Mantero F, Arnaldi G. Management approaches to adrenal incidentalomas. A view from Ancona, Italy. Endocrinol Metab Clin North Am 2000; 29(1): 107–25, ix.

52. Hamrahian AH, et al. Clinical utility of noncontrast computed tomography attenuation value (Hounsfield units) to differentiate adrenal adenomas/hyperplasias from nonadenomas: Cleveland Clinic experience. J Clin Endocrinol Metab 2005; 90(2): 871–7.

53. Grumbach MM, et al. Management of the clinically inapparent adrenal mass ("incidentaloma"). Ann Intern Med 2003; 138(5): 424–9.

54. Szolar DH, et al. Adrenocortical carcinomas and adrenal pheochromocytomas: mass and enhancement loss evaluation at delayed contrast-enhanced CT. Radiology 2005; 234(2): 479–85.

55. Pena CS, Boland GW, Hahn PF, Lee MJ, Mueller PR. Characterization of indeterminate (lipid-poor) adrenal masses: use of washout characteristics at contrast-enhanced CT. Radiology 2000; 217(3): 798–802.

56. Bharwani N, et al. Adrenocortical carcinoma: the range of appearances on CT and MRI. Am J Roentgenol 2011; 196(6): W706–W14.

57. Bharwani N, et al. Adrenocortical carcinoma: the range of appearances on CT and MRI. Am J Roentgenol 2011; 196(6): W706–14.

58. Groussin L, et al. 18F-Fluorodeoxyglucose positron emission tomography for the diagnosis of adrenocortical tumors: a prospective study in 77 operated patients. J Clin Endocrinol Metab 2009; 94(5): 1713–22.

59. Hennings J, Hellman P, Ahlstrom H, Sundin A. Computed tomography, magnetic resonance imaging and 11C-metomidate positron emission tomography for evaluation of adrenal incidentalomas. Eur J Radiol 2009; 69(2): 314–23.

60. Nunes M, et al. 18F-FDG PET for the identification of adrenocortical carcinomas among indeterminate adrenal tumors at computed tomography scanning. World J Surg 2010; 34(7): 1506–10.

61. Moreira SG Jr, Pow-Sang JM. Evaluation and management of adrenal masses. Cancer Control 2002; 9(4): 326–34.

62. Weiss LM. Comparative histologic study of 43 metastasizing and nonmetastasizing adrenocortical tumors. Am J Surg Pathol 1984; 8(3): 163–9.

63. Weiss LM, Medeiros LJ, Vickery AL Jr. Pathologic features of prognostic significance in adrenocortical carcinoma. Am J Surg Pathol 1989; 13(3): 202–6.

64. Stojadinovic A, et al. Adrenocortical adenoma and carcinoma: histopathological and molecular comparative analysis. Mod Pathol 2003; 16(8): 742–51.

65. Stojadinovic A, et al. Adrenocortical carcinoma: clinical, morphologic, and molecular characterization. J Clin Oncol 2002; 20(4): 941–50.

66. Arola J, Salmenkivi K, Liu J, Kahri AI, Heikkila P. p53 and Ki67 in adrenocortical tumors. Endocr Res 2000; 26(4): 861–5.

67. Terzolo M, et al. Immunohistochemical assessment of Ki-67 in the differential diagnosis of adrenocortical tumors. Urology 2001; 57(1): 176–82.

68. Sbiera S, et al. High diagnostic and prognostic value of steroidogenic factor-1 expression in adrenal tumors. J Clin Endocrinol Metab 2010; 95(10): E161–71.

69. Davenport C, et al. The prevalence of adrenal incidentaloma in routine clinical practice. Endocrine, 2011; 40 (1): 80–83.

70. Herrera MF, Grant CS, van Heerden JA, Sheedy PF, Ilstrup DM. Incidentally discovered adrenal tumors: an institutional perspective. Surgery 1991; 110(6): 1014–21.

71. Bovio S, et al. Prevalence of adrenal incidentaloma in a contemporary computerized tomography series. J Endocrinol Invest 2006; 29(4): 298–302.

72. Kloos RT, Gross MD, Francis IR, Korobkin M, Shapiro B. Incidentally discovered adrenal masses. Endocr Rev 1995; 16(4): 460–84.

73. Mansmann G, Lau J, Balk E, Rothberg M, Miyachi Y, Bornstein SR. The clinically inapparent adrenal mass: update in diagnosis and management. Endocr Rev 2004; 25(2): 309–40.

74. Barzon L, et al. Incidentally discovered adrenal tumors: endocrine and scintigraphic correlates. J Clin Endocrinol Metab 1998; 83(1): 55–62.

75. Figueiredo BC, et al. Penetrance of adrenocortical tumours associated with the germline TP53 R337H mutation. J Med Genet 2006; 43(1): 91–6.

76. Sidhu S, et al. Mutation and methylation analysis of TP53 in adrenal carcinogenesis. Eur J Surg Oncol 2005; 31(5): 549–54.

77. Gicquel C, et al. Structural and functional abnormalities at 11p15 are associated with the malignant phenotype in sporadic adrenocortical tumors: study on a series of 82 tumors. J Clin Endocrinol Metab 1997; 82(8): 2559–65.

78. Tissier F, et al. Mutations of beta-catenin in adrenocortical tumors: activation of the Wnt signaling pathway is a frequent event in both benign and malignant adrenocortical tumors. Cancer Res 2005; 65(17): 7622–7.

79. Tadjine M, Lampron A, Ouadi L, Horvath A, Stratakis CA, Bourdeau I. Detection of somatic beta-catenin mutations in primary pigmented nodular adrenocortical disease (PPNAD). Clin Endocrinol (Oxf) 2008; 69(3): 367–73.

80. Gaujoux S, et al. Wnt/beta-catenin and 3′,5′-cyclic adenosine 5′-monophosphate/protein kinase A signaling pathways alterations and somatic beta-catenin gene mutations in the progression of adrenocortical tumors. J Clin Endocrinol Metab 2008; 93(10): 4135–40.

81. Lacroix A, Ndiaye N, Tremblay J, Hamet P. Ectopic and abnormal hormone receptors in adrenal Cushing's syndrome. Endocr Rev 2001; 22(1): 75–110.

82. Grumbach MM, et al. Management of the clinically inapparent adrenal mass ("incidentaloma"). Ann Intern Med 2003; 138(5): 424–9.

83. Liao CH, Lai MK, Li HY, Chen SC, Chueh SC. Laparoscopic adrenalectomy using needlescopic instruments for adrenal tumors less than 5 cm in 112 cases. Eur Urol 2008; 54(3): 640–6.

84. Gill IS, Meraney AM, Thomas JC, Sung GT, Novick AC, Lieberman I. Thoracoscopic transdiaphragmatic adrenalectomy: the initial experience. J Urol 2001; 165(6 Pt 1): 1875–81.

85. Linos DA, Stylopoulos N, Boukis M, Souvatzoglou A, Raptis S, Papadimitriou J. Anterior, posterior, or laparoscopic approach for the management of adrenal diseases? Am J Surg 1997; 173(2): 120–5.

86. Hansen P, Bax T, Swanstrom L. Laparoscopic adrenalectomy: history, indications, and current techniques for a minimally invasive approach to adrenal pathology. Endoscopy 1997; 29(4): 309–14.

87. Duh QY, et al. Laparoscopic adrenalectomy. Comparison of the lateral and posterior approaches. Arch Surg 1996; 131(8): 870–5; discussion 5–6.

88. Wells SA, Merke DP, Cutler GB Jr, Norton JA, Lacroix A. Therapeutic controversy: the role of laparoscopic surgery in adrenal disease. J Clin Endocrinol Metab 1998; 83(9): 3041–9.

89. Toniato A, Merante-Boschin I, Opocher G, Pelizzo MR, Schiavi F, Ballotta E. Surgical versus conservative management for subclinical Cushing syndrome in adrenal incidentalomas: a prospective randomized study. Ann Surg 2009; 249(3): 388–91.

90. Schteingart DE, et al. Management of patients with adrenal cancer: recommendations of an international consensus conference. Endocr Relat Cancer 2005; 12(3): 667–80.

91. Ribeiro RC, et al. Adrenocortical tumors in children. Braz J Med Biol Res 2000; 33(10): 1225–34.

92. Golden SH, Robinson KA, Saldanha I, Anton B, Ladenson PW. Clinical review: prevalence and incidence of endocrine and metabolic disorders in the United States: a comprehensive review. J Clin Endocrinol Metab 2009; 94(6): 1853–78.

93. Grubbs Ee Lee JE. Limited prognostic value of the 2004 International Union Against Cancer staging classification for adrenocortical carcinoma: proposal for a revised TNM classification. Cancer 2009; 115(24): 5847; author reply 8.

94. Steenman M, Westerveld A, Mannens M. Genetics of Beckwith–Wiedemann syndrome-associated tumors: common genetic pathways. Genes Chromosomes Cancer 2000; 28(1): 1–13.

95. Hatada I, et al. An imprinted gene p57KIP2 is mutated in Beckwith–Wiedemann syndrome. Nat Genet 1996; 14(2): 171–3.

96. Suh I, Guerrero MA, Kebebew E. Gene-expression profiling of adrenocortical carcinoma. Expert Rev Mol Diagn 2009; 9(4): 343–51.

97. Trezzi R, Poli F, Fellegara G. "Dedifferentiated" adrenal cortical neoplasm. Int J Surg Pathol 2009; 17(4): 343–4.

98. De Krijger R, Papathomas T. Adrenocortical neoplasia: evolving concepts in tumorigenesis with an emphasis on adrenal cortical carcinoma variants. Virchows Archiv 2010; 460(1): 9–18.

99. Bernard MH, et al. A case report in favor of a multistep adrenocortical tumorigenesis. J Clin Endocrinol Metab 2003; 88(3): 998–1001.

100. Schmitt A, et al. IGFII and MIB1 immunohistochemistry is helpful for the differentiation of benign from malignant adrenocortical tumours. Histopathology 2006; 49(3): 298–307.

101. Ribeiro RC, et al. An inherited p53 mutation that contributes in a tissue-specific manner to pediatric adrenal cortical carcinoma. Proc Natl Acad Sci U S A 2001; 98(16): 9330–5.

102. Soon PS, et al. Loss of heterozygosity of 17p13, with possible involvement of ACADVL and ALOX15B, in the pathogenesis of adrenocortical tumors. Ann Surg 2008; 247(1): 157–64.

103. Dluhy RG, Lifton RP. Glucocorticoid-remediable aldosteronism (GRA): diagnosis, variability of phenotype and regulation of potassium homeostasis. Steroids 1995; 60(1): 48–51.

104. Soon PSH, McDonald KL, Robinson BG, Sidhu SB. Molecular markers and the pathogenesis of adrenocortical cancer. Oncologist 2008; 13(5): 548–61.

105. Sarkaria IS, et al. Squamous cell carcinoma-related oncogene is highly expressed in developing, normal, and adenomatous adrenal tissue but not in aggressive adrenocortical carcinomas. Surgery 2004; 136(6): 1122–8.

106. Beuschlein F, Galac S, Wilson DB. Animal models of adrenocortical tumorigenesis. Mol Cell Endocrinol 2011; Nov 11 [Epub ahead of print].

107. Hoeben A, Landuyt B, Highley MS, Wildiers H, van Oosterom AT, de Bruijn EA. Vascular endothelial growth factor and angiogenesis. Pharmacol Rev 2004; 56(4): 549–80.

108. Bernini GP, et al. Angiogenesis in human normal and pathologic adrenal cortex. J Clin Endocrinol Metab 2002; 87(11): 4961–5.

109. Fitzgerald PA, et al. Malignant pheochromocytomas and paragangliomas: a phase II study of therapy with high-dose 131I-metaiodobenzylguanidine (131I-MIBG). Ann N Y Acad Sci 2006; 1073: 465–90.

110. Macfarlane DA. Cancer of the adrenal cortex; the natural history, prognosis and treatment in a study of fifty-five cases. Ann R Coll Surg Engl 1958; 23(3): 155–86.

111. Sullivan M, Boileau M, Hodges CV. Adrenal cortical carcinoma. J Urol 1978; 120(6): 660–5.

112. Lee JE, et al. Surgical management, DNA content, and patient survival in adrenal cortical carcinoma. Surgery 1995; 118(6): 1090–8.

113. Edge SB, Compton CC. The American Joint Committee on Cancer: the 7th edition of the AJCC cancer staging manual and the future of TNM. Ann Surg Oncol 2010; 17(6): 1471–4.

114. Phan A. Adrenal cortical carcinoma – review of current knowledge and treatment practices. Hematol Oncol Clin North Am 2007; 21(3): 489–507.

115. Alexandria TP. Adrenal cortical carcinoma—review of current knowledge and treatment practices. Hematol Oncol Clin North Am 2007; 21(3): 489–507.

116. Gonzalez RJ, et al. Laparoscopic resection of adrenal cortical carcinoma: a cautionary note. Surgery 2005; 138(6): 1078–86.

117. Tauchmanova L, et al. Andrenocortical carcinomas: twelve-year prospective experience. World J Surg 2004; 28(9): 896–903.

118. Porpiglia F, *et al*. Retrospective evaluation of the outcome of open versus laparoscopic adrenalectomy for stage I and II adrenocortical cancer. Eur Urol 2010; 57(5): 873–8.

119. Birkmeyer NJ, Goodney PP, Stukel TA, Hillner BE, Birkmeyer JD. Do cancer centers designated by the National Cancer Institute have better surgical outcomes? Cancer 2005; 103(3): 435–41.

120. Grubbs EG, *et al*. Recurrence of adrenal cortical carcinoma following resection: surgery alone can achieve results equal to surgery plus mitotane. Ann Surg Oncol 2009; 17(1): 263–70.

121. Fassnacht M, *et al*. Efficacy of adjuvant radiotherapy of the tumor bed on local recurrence of adrenocortical carcinoma. J Clin Endocrinol Metab 2006; 91(11): 4501–4.

122. Terzolo M, *et al*. Adjuvant mitotane treatment for adrenocortical carcinoma. N Engl J Med 2007; 356(23): 2372–80.

123. Ghose RP, Hall PM, Bravo EL. Medical management of aldosterone-producing adenomas. Ann Intern Med 1999; 131(2): 105–8.

124. Pitt B, *et al*. Aggressive lipid-lowering therapy compared with angioplasty in stable coronary artery disease. Atorvastatin versus Revascularization Treatment Investigators. N Engl J Med 1999; 341(2): 70–6.

125. Zannad F, *et al*. Eplerenone in patients with systolic heart failure and mild symptoms. N Engl J Med; 364(1): 11–21.

126. Griffing GT, Cole AG, Aurecchia SA, Sindler BH, Komanicky P, Melby JC. Amiloride in primary hyperaldosteronism. Clin Pharmacol Ther 1982; 31(1): 56–61.

127. Ganguly A, Weinberger MH. Triamterene-thiazide combination: alternative therapy for primary aldosteronism. Clin Pharmacol Ther 1981; 30(2): 246–50.

128. Loszio FA, Toth S, Kocsis J, Pavo, Szecsi M. Testosterone-secreting gonadotropin-responsive adrenal adenoma and its treatment with the antiandrogen flutamide. J Endocrinol Invest 2001; 24(8): 622–7.

129. Hahner S, Fassnacht M. Mitotane for adrenocortical carcinoma treatment. Curr Opin Invest Drugs 2005; 6(4): 386–94.

130. Hermsen IG, *et al*. Plasma concentrations of o,p'DDD, o,p'DDA, and o,p'DDE as predictors of tumor response to mitotane in adrenocortical carcinoma: results of a retrospective ENS@T multicenter study. J Clin Endocrinol Metab 2011; 96(6): 1844–51.

131. Berruti A, Terzolo M, Pia A, Angeli A, Dogliotti L. Mitotane associated with etoposide, doxorubicin, and cisplatin in the treatment of advanced adrenocortical carcinoma. Italian Group for the Study of Adrenal Cancer. Cancer 1998; 83(10): 2194–200.

132. Ahlman H, *et al*. Cytotoxic treatment of adrenocortical carcinoma. World J Surg 2001; 25(7): 927–33.

133. Khan TS, *et al*. Streptozocin and o,p'DDD in the treatment of adrenocortical cancer patients: long-term survival in its adjuvant use. Ann Oncol 2000; 11(10): 1281–7.

134. Allolio B, Fassnacht M. Clinical review: adrenocortical carcinoma: clinical update. J Clin Endocrinol Metab 2006; 91(6): 2027–37.

135. Britvin TA, Kazantseva IA, Kalinin AP, Kushlinskii NE. Vascular endothelium growth factor in the sera of patients with adrenal tumors. Bull Exp Biol Med 2005; 140(2): 228–30.

136. Pawlikowski M, Winczyk K, Sledz B. Immunohistochemical detection of angiotensin receptors AT1 and AT2 in adrenal tumors. Folia Histochem Cytobiol 2008; 46(1): 51–5.

137. Sasano H, Suzuki T, Shizawa S, Kato K, Nagura H. Transforming growth factor alpha, epidermal growth factor, and epidermal growth factor receptor expression in normal and diseased human adrenal cortex by immunohistochemistry and in situ hybridization. Mod Pathol 1994; 7(7): 741–6.

138. Nakamura M, *et al*. An analysis of potential surrogate markers of target-specific therapy in archival materials of adrenocortical carcinoma. Endocr Pathol 2009; 20(1): 17–23.

139. Chang Q, Li Y, White MF, Fletcher JA, Xiao S. Constitutive activation of insulin receptor substrate 1 is a frequent event in human tumors: therapeutic implications. Cancer Res 2002; 62(21): 6035–8.

140. Backlin C, Rastad J, Skogseid B, Hellman P, Akerstrom G, Juhlin C. Immunohistochemical expression of insulin-like growth factor 1 and its receptor in normal and neoplastic human adrenal cortex. Anticancer Res 1995; 15(6B): 2453–9.

141. Barlaskar FM, *et al*. Preclinical targeting of the type I insulin-like growth factor receptor in adrenocortical carcinoma. J Clin Endocrinol Metab 2009; 94(1): 204–12.

142. Samnotra V. Phase II trial of ZD1839 (IRESSA) in patients with non-resectable adrenocortical carcinoma (ACC). Invest New Drugs 2003; 21(3): 341–5.

143. Quinkler M, *et al*. Treatment of advanced adrenocortical carcinoma with erlotinib plus gemcitabine. J Clin Endocrinol Metab 2008; 93(6): 2057–62.

144. Wortmann S, *et al*. Bevacizumab plus capecitabine as a salvage therapy in advanced adrenocortical carcinoma. Eur J Endocrinol 2010; 162(2): 349–56.

145. Libe R, Fratticci A, Bertherat J. Adrenocortical cancer: pathophysiology and clinical management. Endocr Relat Cancer 2007; 14(1): 13–28.

146. Almeida MQ, *et al*. Expression of insulin-like growth factor-II and its receptor in pediatric and adult adrenocortical tumors. J Clin Endocrinol Metab 2008; 93(9): 3524–31.

147. Haluska P, *et al*. Safety, tolerability, and pharmacokinetics of the anti-IGF-1R monoclonal antibody figitumumab in patients with refractory adrenocortical carcinoma. Cancer Chemother Pharmacol 2010; 65(4): 765–73.

148. Carden CP, *et al*. Phase I study of intermittent dosing of OSI-906, a dual tyrosine kinase inhibitor of insulin-like growth factor-1 receptor (IGF-1R) and insulin receptor (IR) in patients with advanced solid tumors. J Clin Oncol 2010; 28(15s): Abstr 2530.

149. Donckier JE, Michel L. Phaeochromocytoma: state of the art. Acta Chir Belg 2010; 110(2): 140–8.

150. Guerrero MA, *et al*. Clinical spectrum of pheochromocytoma. J Am Coll Surg 2009; 209(6): 727–32.

151. Pacak K, Eisenhofer G, Ilias I. Diagnosis of pheochromocytoma with special emphasis on MEN2 syndrome. Hormones (Athens) 2009; 8(2): 111–16.

152. Waguespack SG, *et al*. A current review of the etiology, diagnosis, and treatment of pediatric pheochromocytoma and paraganglioma. J Clin Endocrinol Metab 2010; 95(5): 2023–37.

153. Whalen RK, Althausen AF, Daniels GH. Extra-adrenal pheochromocytoma. J Urol 1992; 147(1): 1–10.

154. Bravo EL. Pheochromocytoma: new concepts and future trends. Kidney Int 1991; 40(3): 544–56.

155. Eisenhofer G, *et al*. Malignant pheochromocytoma: current status and initiatives for future progress. Endocr Relat Cancer 2004; 11(3): 423–36.

156. Gimenez-Roqueplo AP, *et al*. Mutations in the SDHB gene are associated with extra-adrenal and/or malignant phaeochromocytomas. Cancer Res 2003; 63(17): 5615–21.

157. Stein PP, Black HR. A simplified diagnostic approach to pheochromocytoma. A review of the literature and report of one institution's experience. Medicine (Baltimore) 1991; 70(1): 46–66.

158. Manger WM, Gifford RW. Pheochromocytoma. J Clin Hypertens (Greenwich) 2002; 4(1): 62–72.

159. Bravo EL, Gifford RW Jr. Pheochromocytoma. Endocrinol Metab Clin North Am 1993; 22(2): 329–41.

160. Kudva YC, Sawka AM, Young WF Jr. Clinical review 164: the laboratory diagnosis of adrenal pheochromocytoma: the Mayo Clinic experience. J Clin Endocrinol Metab 2003; 88(10): 4533–9.

161. Neumann HP, *et al*. Germ-line mutations in nonsyndromic pheochromocytoma. N Engl J Med 2002; 346(19): 1459–66.

162. Walther MM, Herring J, Enquist E, Keiser HR, Linehan WM. von Recklinghausen's disease and pheochromocytomas. J Urol 1999; 162(5): 1582–6.

163. Dluhy RG. Pheochromocytoma – death of an axiom. N Engl J Med 2002; 346(19): 1486–8.

164. Pomares FJ, Canas R, Rodriguez JM, Hernandez AM, Parrilla P, Tebar FJ. Differences between sporadic and multiple endocrine neoplasia type 2A phaeochromocytoma. Clin Endocrinol (Oxf) 1998; 48(2): 195–200.

165. Walther MM, *et al.* Clinical and genetic characterization of pheochromocytoma in von Hippel–Lindau families: comparison with sporadic pheochromocytoma gives insight into natural history of pheochromocytoma. J Urol 1999; 162(3 Pt 1): 659–64.

166. Sawka AM, Jaeschke R, Singh RJ, Young WF Jr. A comparison of biochemical tests for pheochromocytoma: measurement of fractionated plasma metanephrines compared with the combination of 24-hour urinary metanephrines and catecholamines. J Clin Endocrinol Metab 2003; 88(2): 553–8.

167. Lenders JW, *et al.* Biochemical diagnosis of pheochromocytoma: which test is best? JAMA 2002; 287(11): 1427–34.

168. Sawka AM, Prebtani AP, Thabane L, Gafni A, Levine M, Young WF Jr. A systematic review of the literature examining the diagnostic efficacy of measurement of fractionated plasma free metanephrines in the biochemical diagnosis of pheochromocytoma. BMC Endocr Disord 2004; 4(1): 2.

169. Vanderveen KA, *et al.* Biopsy of pheochromocytomas and paragangliomas: potential for disaster. Surgery 2009; 146(6): 1158–66.

170. Sangoi AR, McKenney JK. A tissue microarray-based comparative analysis of novel and traditional immunohistochemical markers in the distinction between adrenal cortical lesions and pheochromocytoma. Am J Surg Pathol 2010; 34(3): 423–32.

171. Baid SK, *et al.* Brief communication: radiographic contrast infusion and catecholamine release in patients with pheochromocytoma. Ann Intern Med 2009; 150(1): 27–32.

172. Bravo EL. Evolving concepts in the pathophysiology, diagnosis, and treatment of pheochromocytoma. Endocr Rev 1994; 15(3): 356–68.

173. Bravo EL. Diagnosis of pheochromocytoma. Reflections on a controversy. Hypertension 1991; 17(6 Pt 1): 742–4.

174. Neumann HP, *et al.* Distinct clinical features of paraganglioma syndromes associated with SDHB and SDHD gene mutations. JAMA 2004; 292(8): 943–51.

175. Nielsen SM, *et al.* Genotype-phenotype correlations of pheochromocytoma in two large von Hippel–Lindau (VHL) type 2A kindreds with different missense mutations. Am J Med Genet A 2010; 155A(1): 168–73.

176. Amar L, Servais A, Gimenez-Roqueplo AP, Zinzindohoue F, Chatellier G, Plouin PF. Year of diagnosis, features at presentation, and risk of recurrence in patients with pheochromocytoma or secreting paraganglioma. J Clin Endocrinol Metab 2005; 90(4): 2110–16.

177. Ulchaker JC, Goldfarb DA, Bravo EL, Novick AC. Successful outcomes in pheochromocytoma surgery in the modern era. J Urol 1999; 161(3): 764–7.

178. Steinsapir J, Carr AA, Prisant LM, Bransome ED Jr. Metyrosine and pheochromocytoma. Arch Intern Med 1997; 157(8): 901–6.

179. Nehs MA, Ruan DT. Minimally invasive adrenal surgery: an update. Curr Opin Endocrinol Diabetes Obes 2010; 18(3): 193–7.

180. Li H, *et al.* Experience of retroperitoneal laparoscopic treatment on pheochromocytoma. Urology 2010; 77(1): 131–5.

181. Baghai M, Thompson GB, Young WF Jr, Grant CS, Michels VV, van Heerden JA. Pheochromocytomas and paragangliomas in von Hippel–Lindau disease: a role for laparoscopic and cortical-sparing surgery. Arch Surg 2002; 137(6): 682–8; discussion 8–9.

182. Rose B, *et al.* High-dose 131I-metaiodobenzylguanidine therapy for 12 patients with malignant pheochromocytoma. Cancer 2003; 98(2): 239–48.

183. Averbuch SD, *et al.* Malignant pheochromocytoma: effective treatment with a combination of cyclophosphamide, vincristine, and dacarbazine. Ann Intern Med 1988; 109(4): 267–73.

184. Ayala-Ramirez M, *et al.* Clinical benefits of systemic chemotherapy for patients with metastatic pheochromocytomas or sympathetic extra-adrenal paragangliomas: insights from the largest single-institutional experience. Cancer 2011; Oct 17 [Epub ahead of print].

185. Jimenez C, *et al.* Use of the tyrosine kinase inhibitor sunitinib in a patient with von Hippel–Lindau disease: targeting angiogenic factors in pheochromocytoma and other von Hippel–Lindau disease-related tumors. J Clin Endocrinol Metab 2009; 94(2): 386–91.

11 Uncommon Cancers of the Thyroid

Sonia Abuzakhm,[1] **Mark Bloomston,**[2] **and Manisha H. Shah**[1]

[1] Department of Internal Medicine, [2] Division of Surgical Oncology, The Ohio State University, Columbus, OH, USA

Introduction

Thyroid cancers are relatively uncommon, with 44,670 new cases and 1690 deaths estimated in the United States for 2010.[1] This accounts for 2.9% of all new cancer diagnoses and 0.3% of cancer-related deaths. Thyroid cancer is by far the most common endocrine malignancy, representing 95% of all new endocrine cancer cases, and is more common in women than men by a ratio of 3:1.[1] However, thyroid cancer accounts for only 64% of endocrine cancer-related deaths, indicating the rather indolent nature of the disease relative to other cancers.

Thyroid cancers are traditionally classified by histology into differentiated, medullary, and anaplastic thyroid cancer, accounting for 90%, 5%, and 1–2% of thyroid cancers, respectively. Differentiated thyroid cancers are further categorized into papillary (80–85%), follicular (10–15%), and the less common Hürthle cell carcinoma (3–5%). These tumors tend to arise from follicular cells which line the colloid follicles within the thyroid and are involved in the concentration of iodine and the production of thyroid hormone. These same cells likely also give rise to anaplastic thyroid carcinomas (ATC). Medullary thyroid carcinoma (MTC) develops from the parafollicular cells, sometimes called calcitonin-producing C-cells, which are found in the upper and middle thirds of the thyroid gland and are embryologically derived from the neural crest. Immune cells are commonly found within the substance of the thyroid and give rise to lymphomas which represent 1–3% of thyroid malignancies. More rare tumors account for less than 1% of thyroid malignancies and include sarcoma, insular carcinoma, primary squamous carcinoma, malignant teratoma, mucoepidermoid carcinoma, and hemangioendothelioma.

This chapter will focus on the diagnosis and management of medullary thyroid cancer (both sporadic and familial), Hürthle cell carcinoma, anaplastic cancer, lymphoma, and these other rare tumors.

Medullary thyroid carcinoma

First described in 1959 as a solid thyroid neoplasm without follicular histology and a marked propensity for lymph node metastasis, the origin of MTC would not be known until the late 1960s when the parafollicular C-cell was described.[2,3] The correlation between C-cells and MTC was further strengthened in the 1970s when it became obvious that calcitonin would become one of the most sensitive and specific tumor markers in oncology.[4] Investigators quickly began developing an understanding of the familial associations of MTC which has led to the defining of genetic changes in the *RET* protooncogene important for both the heritable and sporadic forms of the disease.[5] MTC is now one of the best characterized solid tumor malignancies given our understanding of its genetic, molecular, pathological, biochemical, and clinical features.

Hereditary features of medullary thyroid carcinoma

Medullary thyroid carcinoma accounts for approximately 3–5% of all thyroid cancers and is associated with familial syndromes in 25–30% of cases. It is a principal component of multiple endocrine neoplasia (MEN) type 2A (MTC, pheochromocytoma, hyperparathyroidism) and 2B (MTC, pheochromocytoma, mucosal ganglioneuromatosis, marfanoid body habitus) as well as being part of its own syndrome of familial medullary thyroid cancer (FMTC). These syndromes show an autosomal dominant pattern of inheritance with MEN 2 variants being caused by mutations in the *RET* protooncogene.[5] MEN 2A is caused by mutations in extracellular cysteine residues such as mutation at codon 634 while MEN 2B results from a methionine to threonine mutation at codon 918 in the tyrosine kinase catalytic domain. Familial MTC is caused by the same mutation as MEN 2A as well as, less commonly, mutations in the intracellular portion of the protein.[6]

These distinct, well-defined mutations coupled with effective treatment options make genetic screening for the associated familial syndromes not only possible but mandatory in patients diagnosed with MTC. Referral of such patients to a cancer geneticist for evaluation and genetic counseling is essential. As well, the prominence of pheochromocytoma in MEN 2 emphasizes the importance of ruling out MEN 2 by genetic screening for pheochromocytoma by plasma metanephrines/normetanephrines in patients presenting with MTC.

Medullary thyroid carcinoma in the setting of MEN 2 is characterized by 100% penetrance with invasive carcinoma present by the first year of life in MEN 2B and lymph node metastases reported by age 2.[7] MTC in patients with MEN 2A, albeit less aggressive than in MEN 2B, is often present by age 2 with lymph node metastases by age 5.[8] FMTC, the least aggressive of the three familial MTC syndromes, is characterized by MTC presenting in the second or third decade of life. These differences in presentation affect the recommendations regarding timing of prophylactic thyroidectomy in children with the associated mutations. Early thyroidectomy in patients with biochemical evidence of MTC by provocative (with calcium and pentagastrin stimulation) calcitonin screening of at-risk family members or without biochemical evidence of MTC in patients with germline mutations can be curative or preventive in all patients with MEN 2.[9,10]

The current recommendations for the management of the thyroid based upon the 2001 consensus guidelines for MEN 2 emphasize the use of *RET* mutation testing rather than calcitonin testing in at-risk individuals.[11] This is based upon several points:

- early thyroidectomy can significantly alter the course of MTC in MEN 2
- thyroidectomy is relatively well tolerated and safe
- waiting for biochemical evidence of MTC may leave patients with residual disease following thyroidectomy
- genetic testing is a more sensitive screening method than stimulated calcitonin testing.

Based upon this, patients with MEN 2B genotype (codon 883, 918, and 922 mutations) are at the highest risk and it is recommended that they undergo thyroidectomy and central node dissection by 6 months of age, preferably within the first month of life. Mutations at codons 634, 620, 618, and 611 are also at relatively high risk and patients with these mutations are recommended to undergo thyroidectomy with or without central node dissection by 5 years of age. The recommendations for patients at lowest risk (codon 609, 768, 790, 791, 804, and 891 mutations) are less rigid, with some advocating thyroidectomy by age 5, by age 10, or on the basis of provocative calcitonin testing.

Clinical presentation and diagnosis

Most MTCs present with sporadic disease as an asymptomatic thyroid mass. Patients with heavy tumor burden and very high calcitonin levels may present with secretory diarrhea as their primary symptom. At the time of presentation, up to 75% of patients will have lymph node metastases with distant metastases being common. Thus, MTC is typically a systemic disease with distant metastasis to the lungs, liver, and/or bones. Serum calcitonin is a sensitive and specific

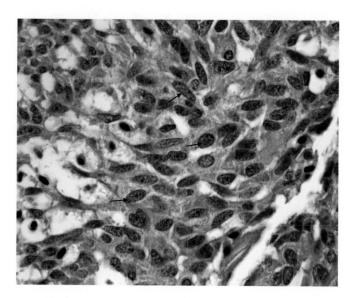

Figure 11.1 Medullary thyroid carcinoma. Note finely stippled "salt-and-pepper" chromatin (*arrows*).

tumor marker in MTC that has diagnostic and prognostic value. In addition, serum carcinoembryonic antigen (CEA) has been used to assess the degree of dedifferentiation of the tumors in these patients. Since MTC derives from C-cells and not follicular cells, they do not concentrate iodine, thus rendering radioactive iodine scan ineffective for workup.[12] Conventional computed tomography (CT) or magnetic resonance imaging (MRI) scans, and nuclear imaging techniques such as ^{131}I metaiodobenzylguanidine (MIBG), somatostatin receptor scintigraphy, and radiolabeled CEA antibody or anticalcitonin antibody, have been utilized to survey for metastatic disease, each with suboptimal sensitivity.[13–16] All patients with apparent sporadic MTC should undergo genetic testing as up to 6% of such patients have been found to carry germline *RET* mutation.[11]

The diagnosis of MTC can be confirmed by fine needle aspiration (FNA). Histologically, MTC is a type of neuroendocrine carcinoma demonstrating several patterns: glandular, solid, spindle cell, oncocytic, clear cell, papillary, small cell, and giant cell. The nuclei of MTC cells are round with stippled "salt-and-pepper" chromatin, similar to other neuroendocrine tumors found elsewhere in the body (Fig. 11.1). Features associated with poor outcome include necrosis, squamous pattern, presence of oxyphilic cells in the tumor and absence of cells with intermediate cytoplasm, and less than 50% calcitonin reactivity.[17]

Treatment

Surgical

As systemic chemotherapy and radiation are ineffective against MTC, surgical resection is the mainstay of treatment.[18] Total thyroidectomy is recommended for familial and sporadic cases given the multifocal nature of the MTC in 90% and 20% of patients, respectively. Total thyroidectomy also enhances the ability to utilize calcitonin levels to assess for adequacy of resection and monitor for recurrence. Since

MTC has a propensity for early lymph node metastasis, thyroidectomy should be accompanied by central node dissection, clearing all tissue from the hyoid down to the innominate vessels inferiorly and the internal jugular veins laterally. Thorough removal of all tissue in these central compartments by an experienced surgeon reduces local recurrence and improves overall survival.[19] Clinically suspicious nodes in the lateral neck should be sampled and, if positive, lateral neck dissection undertaken. Routine removal of nodes in levels II through V bilaterally or ipsilateral modified radical neck dissection should also be considered in larger palpable thyroid tumors (i.e. greater than 2 cm) since occult metastases can occur in 75% of ipsilateral and 47% of contralateral jugular nodes.[20,21]

Controversy exists regarding the ideal management of the parathyroid glands at the time of prophylactic or curative thyroidectomy. Some experts advocate total parathyroidectomy with reimplantation to ensure complete removal of all thyroid tissue and all central nodal tissue. This may also prevent future hyperparathyroidism in patients with MEN 2A.[6] Others believe this is unnecessary to achieve adequate thyroid resection and the risk of postoperative hyperparathyroidism, even in the face of MEN 2A, is uncommon.[22]

Management of persistent or recurrent calcitonin elevation

While thyroidectomy is often curative in children with MEN 2A and FMTC diagnosed by genetic testing, more than 50% of patients presenting with palpable disease will fail to achieve a "biochemical cure" following resection of all known gross disease.[23] The course of these patients is rather indolent, with only 35% progressing to demonstrable disease, as shown by van Heerden *et al.* in 1990.[23] In this study of 31 patients, 11 patients recurred during the 12-year follow-up period. These patients all went on to resection and none had normalization of their calcitonin levels. Still, 5- and 10-year survival for all patients was 90% and 86%, respectively. Based upon these findings, patients with persistently elevated calcitonin levels without obvious disease should be followed with interval CT scanning of the neck, chest, and abdomen and surgery reserved for those patients with appearance of measurable disease. However, if a patient has not had adequate clearance of all nodal tissue at risk as described above at the time of thyroidectomy, central neck dissection with or without lateral neck dissection should be considered. If adequate neck dissection has been completed, then blind neck reexploration is discouraged.[6]

Distant metastases are present at the time of diagnosis in 12% of patients with sporadic MTC compared to 20% in MEN 2B. Only 3% of patients with MEN 2A and 2% with FMTC will present with synchronous metastases.[24] The liver is a common site of distant disease, but metastatic deposits are often small and therefore difficult to detect with radiographic imaging techniques. This has led some to propose staging laparoscopy in patients being considered for clearance of persistent or recurrent neck disease with occult liver metastases identified in 20%.[25] Resection of recurrent MTC offers the best chance of long-term survival and symptom palliation with median survival of over 8 years reported.[26]

Nonoperative treatment

Radioactive iodine treatment is ineffective in MTC since thyroid C-cells do not concentrate iodine. Also, the results of external beam radiation therapy (EBRT) have been disappointing. Analysis of Surveillance, Epidemiology and End Results (SEER) data by a univariate analysis showed that EBRT was not associated with a significant improvement in overall survival.[27] EBRT is beneficial in improving local control of disease for high-risk patients, as shown by retrospective studies.[28,29] Similarly, various chemotherapeutic regimens consisting of doxorubicin, dacarbazine, streptozotocin, and 5-fluorouracil administered as single agents or in combination consistently produce short-lived response rates of 15–30%.[30,31]

This has led investigators to seek novel therapeutic strategies targeting genetic and molecular defects in MTC. Multikinase inhibitors (MKIs) targeting *RET* and other critical growth factor receptors, including vascular endothelial growth factor receptors (VEGFR), have been the focus of early-phase clinical trials in patients with sporadic and hereditary MTC. Data from trials using imatinib, motesanib, vandetanib, sorafenib, sunitinib, and XL184 (cabozantinib) are summarized in Table 11.1.[32–39] The median age of patients on these trials was 45–60 years. Treatment with oral MKIs was generally well tolerated, with common toxicities including diarrhea, hand foot syndrome, fatigue, rash, and hypertension. Many of these side-effects may be chronic in nature and therefore can be disabling even when severity is mild or moderate. Patient education, early recognition, and treatment of MKI-associated side-effects are essential. In addition to symptomatic treatment, dose reductions or drug holidays from MKI may be necessary. Furthermore, rare but life-threatening side-effects are also associated with MKIs, including thrombosis, bleeding, and bowel perforation.

Vandetanib, an oral inhibitor of *RET*, VEGFR, and EGFR signaling pathways, is the first MKI to be approved by the Food and Drug Administration (FDA) for the treatment of symptomatic or progressive MTC in patients with unresectable, locally advanced, or metastatic disease. This approval was based on the results of a multicenter international randomized, double-blind, placebo-controlled phase 3 trial of vandetanib in patients with locally advanced or metastatic MTC (see Table 11.1).[39] In the study, 331 patients (90% sporadic MTC, 10% hereditary MTC) were randomized 2:1 to vandetanib 300 mg daily ($n=231$) or placebo ($n=191100$). Cross-over from placebo to vandetanib was allowed. The primary endpoint was progression-free survival (PFS) and secondary endpoints included objective response rate, disease control, biochemical response and overall survival. After a median follow-up of 24 months, PFS was significantly improved in the vandetanib arm (hazard ratio (HR) 0.45, 95% confidence interval (CI) 0.30–0.69, $p=0.0001$). Median PFS was 19.8 months in the placebo arm and not reached in the vandetanib arm. Statistically significant outcomes were also observed in favor of vandetanib with respect to secondary endpoints, except for overall survival. Common adverse events for vandetanib were similar to those reported with other MKIs as described above.

Table 11.1 Summary of clinical trials of multikinase inhibitors in locally advanced and metastatic MTC.

Drug	Dose	Key targets	Number of patients (sporadic, hereditary, unknown)	PR n (%)	SD n (%)	SD >6 months n (%)	Duration of PR, months	Median PFS, months	Comments
Phase 1–2 trials of multikinase inhibitors in patients with MTC									
Imatinib[32]	600–800 mg PO daily	PDGFR, KIT, RET	15 (11,4,0)	0	4 (27)	4 (27)	NA	NR	Lack of objective response, considerable toxicity
Motesanib[33]	125 mg PO daily	VEGFR 1–3, PDGFR, KIT, RET	91 (76,13,2)	2 (2)	74 (81)	44 (48)	5 and 8	12	37% of patients had reduction >50% from baseline in calcitonin, 76% had reduction of tumor measurement from baseline
Vandetanib[34]	300 mg PO daily	VEGFR, EGFR, RET	30 (0,30,0)	6 (20)	22 (73)	16 (53)	10 (median)	28	80% and 53% of patients respectively had reduction >50% from baseline in calcitonin and CEA, 83% of patients had a reduction in tumor measurement from baseline
Vandetanib[35]	100 mg PO daily	VEGFR, EGFR, RET	19 (0,19,0)	3 (16)	12 (63)	10 (53)	6 (median)	NR	16% and 5% of patients respectively had reduction >50% from baseline in calcitonin and CEA
Sorafenib[36]	400 mg PO twice daily	VEGFR 1–3, PDGFR, RET, BRAF	16 (16,0,0)	1 (6)	14 (87)	10 (62)	21	18	69% of patients had reduction from baseline of calcitonin and CEA but this did not correlate with degree or duration of RECIST response
Sunitinib[37]	50 mg PO daily	VEGFR2, PDGFR, RET, KIT	23 (NR)	8 (35)	13 (57)	13 (57)	9 (median)	7	44% of patients had reduction >30% from baseline in calcitonin, evidence of PR or SD >6 months was observed in 7 of 9 patients with a M918T RET mutation
XL-184[38]	MTD 175mg PO daily (0.08–11.52 mg/kg PO daily, or 175–265 mg PO daily)	c-MET, VEGFR2, RET	37 (22,3,6)	10 (29)*	15 (41)	15 (41)	4 – 35+ Median duration not yet reached	NR	48% of patients had reduction of tumor size by 30% or more from baseline
Phase 3 trial of vandetanib versus placebo in patients with MTC									
Vandetanib[39]	300 mg orally daily	VEGFR, RET, EGFR	331 (298,3,0)	NR	NR	NR	NR	Not reached	Statistically significant PFS was observed for vandetanib versus placebo (HR 0.45, 95% CI 0.30–0.69, $p = 0.0001$)

* Based on $n = 35$, number of patients with measurable disease.

BRAF, V-raf murine sarcoma viral oncogene B1; CEA, carcinoembryonic antigen; CI, confidence interval; EGFR, epidermal growth factor receptor; HR, hazard ratio; MTC, medullary thyroid carcinoma; MTD, maximum tolerated dose; NA, not applicable; NR, not reported; PDGFR, platelet-derived growth factor receptor; PFS, progression-free survival; PO, per os; PR, partial response; SD, stable disease; VEGFR, vascular endothelial growth factor receptor. c-MET, RET, and KIT are protooncogenes.

In the setting of metastatic MTC, several treatment options are available and they are summarized here, per the NCCN guidelines[40]:

• clinical trial
• external beam radiotherapy for localized symptoms
• vandetanib
• consideration of other MKIs, such as sorafenib or sunitinib, if clinical trials or vandetanib are not available or appropriate for the patient, or if the patient progresses on vandetanib
• systemic chemotherapy using dacarbazine or combinations including dacarbazine.

In the clinic, we individualize therapy based on several factors, including degree of tumor burden, pace of progression, presence of associated comorbid conditions, and patient's willingness to accept treatment-associated risks. Due to the fact that novel MKI therapies at best improve PFS and have not been shown to prolong overall survival, we currently do not recommend vandetanib or other MKI therapies if a patient has low tumor burden or slowly progressive or asymptomatic disease. Clinicians and patients must be aware of risks involved with MKIs, including chronic side-effects that range from mild to severe intensity and can adversely impact quality of life. There is also a risk of about 1% of life-threatening adverse events, such as pulmonary embolism, bowel perforation or bleeding. In the setting of symptomatic or significantly progressive MTC in patients with locally advanced or metastatic disease, we recommend treatment on clinical trial (preferred) or vandetanib 300 mg orally once daily. For patients with progressive disease on vandetanib, our next preferred treatment is clinical trial if available, or consideration of other commercially available MKIs, specifically sorafenib 400 mg orally twice daily or sunitinib 50 mg once daily.

Hürthle cell carcinoma

Hürthle cell carcinomas are oxyphilic tumors that arise from follicular cells, not from the parafollicular C-cells attributed to the 19th-century pathologist after whom these tumors were mistakenly named by Ewing in 1919.[41] This uncommon variant of follicular carcinoma is referred to as oxyphil tumor, oncocytoma, mitochondrioma, or Askanazy cell tumor. The natural history and optimal treatment of Hürthle cell tumors are not completely agreed upon. Their histological features and thyroglobulin production suggest that they arise from follicular cells, but they do not appear to be variants of follicular carcinoma.[42]

Clinical presentation and diagnosis

Hürthle cell carcinoma presents in the fifth to seventh decades of life with a 3:1 female preponderance. The typical presentation is that of a slow-growing thyroid nodule with lymphadenopathy, vocal cord paralysis, and distant metastasis being uncommon. Approximately only 10% of metastasis from Hürthle cell carcinomas concentrate iodine, compared with 75% of metastases from follicular carcinoma.

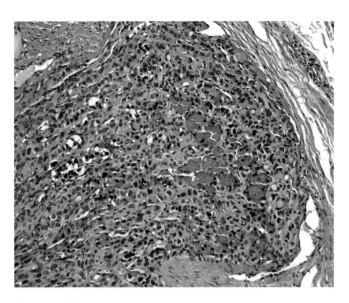

Figure 11.2 Hürthle cell carcinoma.

Diagnosis of Hürthle cell neoplasm is confirmed by FNA though the determination of invasive carcinoma cannot be made by cytological examination alone.[43] Hürthle cells show characteristic abundant granular acidophilic cytoplasm filled with mitochondria and nuclei that are usually vesicular and uniform (Fig. 11.2). The determination of invasive malignancy is based upon demonstration of capsular invasion or angioinvasion which can only be assessed in the resected specimen.[44] Clearly, local invasion, lymph node spread, and distant metastasis also classify Hürthle cell neoplasms as malignant. Grossly, these tumors have a distinct tan-brown color and are typically well encapsulated. Approximately 20% of Hürthle cell tumors will turn out to be cancers. Thyroid scanning typically demonstrates a "cold" nodule but is not reliable in distinguishing between benign and malignant tumors.

Treatment

The debate about the optimal resection for Hürthle cell carcinoma (total thyroidectomy versus lobectomy) follows the discussion of the optimal management of differentiated thyroid cancers. Though lobectomy may be adequate for smaller (less than 1 cm) tumors, total thyroidectomy offers several advantages:

• though local recurrence rates are low following lobectomy, they are fatal in over one-third of patients
• multifocal disease is found in up to 35%
• removal of all thyroid tissue facilitates radioactive iodine uptake in persistent or recurrent disease for surveillance and ablative purposes (though these tumors tend not to concentrate iodine)
• thyroglobulin assays are more sensitive for recurrent disease in the absence of normal thyroid tissue.[45,46] Any remaining normal thyroid tissue should be ablated with radioactive iodine postoperatively.

Surveillance consists of serum thyroglobulin measurement in the hypothyroid state. When serum thyroglobulin levels are still detectable after total thyroidectomy and ablation or if they begin to rise, recurrence should be sought. Radioiodine scanning is a reasonable early test to detect the few Hürthle cell carcinomas that take up iodine.[47] Recurrences occur in 23–29% of patients after a median of 4 years from resection.[46] Most recurrences are in the neck, with the lung being the most common site of distant metastasis. Surgical resection is the mainstay of treatment for recurrent disease as chemotherapy and external beam radiation are of little benefit. Median survival after recurrence is 34 months.[48]

The optimal management of patients with distant metastases is controversial. There are anecdotal reports that radioactive iodine therapy may be effective in this setting[49] but in general it is believed that metastatic Hürthle cell thyroid carcinomas do not accumulate radioactive iodine (contrary to follicular thyroid cancer) and that radioactive iodine therapy is unlikely to be beneficial. In accordance with the current NCCN guidelines[40] for the treatment of clinically progressive or symptomatic metastatic disease, we recommend:
• treatment with clinical trials for nonradioiodine-responsive tumors
• consideration of MKIs, specifically pazopanib, sorafenib, or sunitinib, if clinical trials are not available or appropriate
• systemic therapy if a clinical trial is not available
• best supportive care.
In the next section, we describe the evidence for treatment of metastatic and progressive Hürthle cell thyroid cancers with MKIs.

Experimental treatment

Since there is no effective systemic treatment currently for iodine-refractory metastatic differentiated thyroid cancers, early-phase clinical trials are investigating the use of MKIs in this setting. While the majority of patients on these trials have papillary thyroid histology, there are patients with follicular and Hürthle cell subtypes who are also enrolled. Here we describe results of phase 2 clinical trials of MKIs that enrolled 10 or more patients with Hürthle cell cancer and efficacy results are reported separately for this group of patients. In a phase 2 trial of sorafenib in iodine-refractory metastatic thyroid cancer, patients with papillary thyroid cancer were enrolled into Arm A and patients with follicular, Hürthle cell, anaplastic or mixed thyroid carcinoma were enrolled into Arm B.[50] The primary endpoint was objective response rate after administration of sorafenib 400 mg twice daily until disease progression, illness preventing therapy, or unacceptable toxicity. For the combined group of Hürthle cell patients ($n=9$) and follicular ($n=2$) thyroid cancer patients, stable disease was achieved in nine patients (82%) and in six patients (54%), stable disease was durable for greater than 6 months. There were no complete or partial responses in this group and one patient had progressive disease. Median PFS was estimated to be 4.5 months with 30% PFS rate at 1 year. Median OS was 24 months with 64% alive at 1 year. Sorafenib was generally well tolerated, but did require dose reduction in most patients

in this subset (73%), secondary to hand foot skin rashes, diarrhea, arthralgia and hypertension.

The efficacy of pazopanib, a small molecule inhibitor of VEGFR–1, –2, and –3, PDGFR, and *KIT*, was also studied in a phase 2 trial of 37 patients with metastatic, rapidly progressive, and iodine-refractory differentiated thyroid cancers.[51] The histological subtypes included in the study were follicular ($n=11$), Hürthle cell ($n=11$), and papillary ($n=15$). All patients received pazopanib 800 mg daily, administered in 4-week cycles, until disease progression or unacceptable toxicity. There were no complete responses and 18 out of 37 total patients (49%) had a radiographic partial response by RECIST criteria. Partial responses were observed in five out of 11 patients (45%) with Hürthle cell tumors. The study's reported median PFS for all patients was 11.7 months and PFS at 1 year was 47%. Median OS was not reached and OS for all patients was 81% at 1 year. Of significance, the partial responses induced by pazopanib were found to be durable, with a 66% likelihood of a response lasting more than 1 year. The most common adverse effects included fatigue, skin hypopigmentation, diarrhea and nausea, and adverse effects led to dose reduction in 16 (43%) patients.

Anaplastic thyroid carcinoma

The marked aggressive nature of anaplastic thyroid carcinoma clearly distinguishes it from its well-differentiated counterparts where long-term survival is expected. With a median survival of only 5 months and less than 20% of patients surviving 1 year from diagnosis, anaplastic carcinoma is one of the most rapidly growing and deadly cancers.[52] The incidence of anaplastic carcinoma is declining.[53] This decline may be related to previous overestimates of the incidence of disease due to misclassification of lymphomas, medullary carcinomas, and "insular" variants of follicular carcinoma.[54] Some reports do suggest that the true incidence of ATC is indeed declining, likely related to the decrease in endemic goiter associated with dietary iodine supplementation.[55]

Anaplastic thyroid carcinoma commonly coexists with differentiated thyroid cancer, leading many investigators to surmise that the former may represent dedifferentiation of the more indolent well-differentiated neoplasms.[56,57] Several genetic alterations have been implicated in pathogenesis of ATC. Discovery of activating mutations in the B-type RAF kinase (*BRAF*) gene in papillary thyroid cancer (PTC)[58] has advanced our understanding of progression of differentiated thyroid tumors to ATC. Frequency of *BRAF* mutation in PTC is 45% (28–69%) while in ATC it is 24% (0–100%).[59] However, *BRAF* mutation has been consistently present in both differentiated and undifferentiated components of ATC, suggesting a possible role of *BRAF* in dedifferentiation. Furthermore, frequent mutations in *p53* (83%),[60] *β-catenin* (61%),[61] and *RAS* (52%)[62] have been described in ATC. While activating mutations in *RAS* and *BRAF* oncogenes are implicated in differentiated thyroid carcinoma, inactivating mutations in *p53* tumor suppressor gene are exclusively present in poorly differentiated thyroid tumors. Finally, upregulation of minichromosome maintenance proteins (MCM) is reported in 65% of ATC.[63]

Clinical presentation and diagnosis

Unlike well-differentiated thyroid cancers, ATC tends to be a disease of the elderly, presenting in the seventh decade of life with a mean age at diagnosis of approximately 71 years.[64] Like other thyroid cancers, there is a female preponderance of disease, though less drastic (1.5–2:1). Patients almost uniformly present with a rapidly enlarging mass with evidence of local invasion, with symptoms of dysphagia, hoarseness, and stridor being common. At diagnosis, the primary is typically large with an average tumor size of 6.4 cm (range, 1–15 cm), 38% have extrathyroidal tumors and/or lymph node invasion, and 43% have distant metastasis.[64] The most common sites of metastases are the lungs and pleura, present in up to 90% of patients with distant metastases, and less commonly bone, brain, skin, and liver.

Anaplastic thyroid carcinoma are divided into three histological subtypes: large cell, spindle cell, and squamoid. Each subtype is named for cell patterns to which they are similar, with squamoid resembling nonkeratinizing squamous cell carcinoma, spindle cell being "sarcoma-like," and large cell demonstrating more pleomorphism than the other patterns. All subtypes are characterized by high mitotic activity, foci of necrosis, and both intra- and extrathyroidal extensive invasion.

Treatment

Anaplastic thyroid carcinoma is associated with an extremely rapid course and despite aggressive treatment is almost always fatal. There are no prospective randomized well-designed trials conducted to guide therapy for such rare cancer. In general, a multimodality regimen with surgery, radiation and chemotherapy is recommended for this aggressive cancer in patients who have a good performance status, preserved organ function, and those who desire an intensive approach.

Most patients present with extensive local disease and this ultimately causes death secondary to airway compromise. For this reason, local disease control, whether palliative or curative, is of the utmost importance. When possible, total thyroidectomy with or without neck dissection should be sought as the mainstay of treatment. Survival in resected patients is significantly longer in patients not amenable to resection, though still very poor.[65] Debulking operations to control local disease combined with adjuvant external beam radiation in hyperfractionated doses has shown significant improvements in survival (7–8 months with clearing of neck disease versus 1 month with residual neck disease) even when distant disease was present.[66] Further, adjuvant radiation in standard or hyperfractionated doses in combination with chemotherapy, specifically doxorubicin, platinum or taxanes, and surgery when feasible has been shown to be an effective treatment in anaplastic thyroid cancer.[67,68] Still, survival beyond 1 year is rare.

A recent review of a single-institution experience with aggressive multimodal therapy suggested improved survival outcomes with use of intensity-modulated radiation therapy (IMRT) combined with radiosensitizing plus adjuvant chemotherapy, as compared to historical outcomes in patients with stage IVA and IVB ATC.[52] In this review, 25 newly diagnosed ATC patients were evaluated and 10 out of 25 patients had regionally confined disease and selected aggressive therapy with surgery if feasible, and IMRT plus radiosensitizing and adjuvant chemotherapy. Out of the 10 patients, seven received multiagent chemotherapy (including combinations of doxorubicin, docetaxel, cisplatin, paclitaxel, and carboplatin) with five of the 10 receiving combination doxorubicin and docetaxel. At the time of publication, five out of 10 patients (50%) were alive and cancer free, all were followed greater than 32 months, with a median overall survival of 5 years. Overall survival at 1 and 2 years was 70% and 60% respectively, compared to 1-year survival of 20% in the historical group of similar patients at the same institution treated with surgery and postoperative radiation. It is important to note that out of 25 initial patients, only 10 chose to proceed with the described multimodality treatment, demonstrating bias toward a selected group of patients. The results are encouraging and suggest that IMRT in combination with adjuvant and radiosensitizing chemotherapy may have a significant impact on survival in locoregionally confined ATC.

Given the lack of any durable benefits from radiotherapy or chemotherapy in this aggressive disease, targeted therapies are currently being studied in clinical trials. One targeted therapy, CA4P or fosbretabulin tromethamine (a vascular disrupting agent), was studied in the largest prospective randomized clinical trial in ATC to date, and demonstrated a tripling of 1-year overall survival when combined with carboplatin and paclitaxel.[69] In this multicenter trial, 80 patients with ATC who may have received prior surgery, radiotherapy or chemotherapy were randomized 2:1 to receive up to six cycles of carboplatin and paclitaxel with CA4P (CA4P arm) or without CA4P (control arm). Following 6 months of therapy on the CA4P arm, patients without progression could continue treatment with CA4P until disease progression. The median overall survival time for the CA4P arm was 5.2 months compared to 4.0 months for the control arm. One-year survival was 27% for the CA4P arm and 9% for the control arm. Adverse effects, including hypertension and neutropenia, were more common in the CA4P arm. Further clinical trials are needed to define the optimal role of targeted therapies in anaplastic thyroid cancer.

Insular carcinoma

First described in 1907 by Langhans and named in 1984 by Carcangiu,[70] insular carcinoma represents a follicular cell-derived, poorly differentiated variant of thyroid cancer. Though generally considered as having a better outcome than anaplastic carcinoma, prognosis is still poor. With only a few series reported, insular carcinomas appear to represent less than 5% of thyroid cancers.[71]

Clinical presentation and diagnosis

Insular carcinoma typically presents as a rapidly enlarging mass in patients over the age of 50 with a female predilection but has also been reported in the very young.[72] Local invasion evidenced by hoarseness, dyspnea, and dysphagia is common. Cervical lymph node involvement at the time of presentation is common with distant metastasis typically occurring in the lungs and bone.

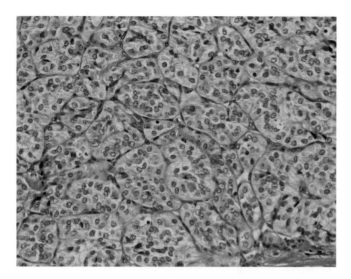

Figure 11.3 Insular carcinoma, characterized by well-defined solid clusters of small, uniform tumor cells that are associated with small, thyroglobulin-containing follicles.

Definitive diagnosis is made histologically with demonstration of solid clusters of tumor cells with small follicles within the clusters (Fig. 11.3). Foci of necrosis, vascular invasion, and frequent mitotic figures are commonplace along with extrathyroidal extension of disease.[73] Definitive cytological characteristics are lacking, making FNA ineffective for diagnosis.

Treatment

Total thyroidectomy has been the mainstay of therapy in the only three large reports.[70,71] Neck dissection is added to thyroidectomy given the high incidence of lymph node metastasis. Radioactive iodine has been utilized with variable response rates.[71] External beam radiation is largely ineffective, as is chemotherapy. Even with early aggressive surgical therapy with or without radioiodine treatment, prognosis in these patients is poor, with 10-year survival less than 50%.[71,74] Clinical behavior of such disease is more consistent with poorly differentiated or anaplastic thyroid carcinoma than differentiated thyroid carcinomas. The role of novel therapies such as MKIs in this type of thyroid cancer remains unclear. Given the aggressive nature of insular carcinoma and its propensity for local recurrence and distant metastases, we recommend aggressive management, including total thyroidectomy followed by radioactive iodine ablation, and in selected individuals the addition of chemotherapy.

Primary thyroid lymphoma

Primary thyroid lymphoma accounts for 1% of all lymphomas and are almost all non-Hodgkin lymphomas.[75] Since the thyroid does not inherently contain lymphoid tissue, primary thyroid lymphomas may arise in the context of acquired lymphoid aggregation, such as in autoimmune thyroid disease (e.g. Hashimoto thyroiditis).[76] The majority (70–90%) are intermediate-grade diffuse large B cell lymphomas or, less commonly, mucosa-associated lymphoid tissue lymphomas or MALTomas.

Clinical presentation and diagnosis

Primary thyroid lymphomas tend to present in the seventh decade of life and have at least a 3:1 female preponderance. These tumors typically present as a slow-growing thyroid mass, with invasive symptoms of hoarseness, stridor, or dysphagia being less common. "B-type" symptoms of fever, night sweats, and weight loss are only seen in about 20% of patients.[75]

The key to diagnosing and planning therapy for primary thyroid lymphoma, like other lymphomas, rests on accurate histological subtyping. This generally requires core or open surgical biopsy to obtain enough tissue for immunophenotypic and cytogenetic analysis, though FNA is sometimes sufficient. Next, accurate staging is accomplished by imaging with either CT or MRI. Though MRI has been shown to be more accurate than CT in evaluating the extent of local disease in the neck, advancements in CT technology make both imaging modalities equally effective in preoperative planning.[77] Radioactive iodine and technetium uptake scans are generally not helpful due to variable uptake patterns.

Treatment

The role of surgery in the management of primary thyroid lymphoma outside the context of obtaining adequate tissue for diagnosis is debatable. Many believe that diffuse large B cell lymphomas should be considered a systemic disease with no role for thyroidectomy. These patients have been managed with chemoradiation with 5-year survivals of 70% reported using doxorubicin-based regimens (see Chapters 44 and 48).[78] The more indolent MALT lymphomas when localized to the thyroid (stage IE) respond well to total thyroidectomy, with 5-year survivals up to 90% when complete resection is possible.[79]

Sarcoma

Often confused with spindle cell variant of anaplastic carcinoma, sarcoma of the thyroid includes liposarcoma, angiosarcoma, leiomyosarcoma, and dendritic cell types.[80,81] The management of these entities is similar to other sarcomas and consists of aggressive surgical resection including total thyroidectomy with removal of any involved lymph nodes or adjacent structures. Patients harboring tumors with pathological features suggestive of advanced disease, including extracapsular spread, high mitotic rate, abundant nuclear pleomorphism, or unresectable disease, warrant postoperative radiotherapy with adjuvant chemotherapy recommended for more aggressive subtypes (e.g. dendritic cell sarcoma).[80]

Squamous cell carcinoma

Primary squamous cell carcinoma (SCC) of the thyroid is extremely uncommon, accounting for less than 1% of all thyroid malignancies. Several theories exist as to the origin of this rare cancer. Some have suggested that it arises from remnants of the thyroglossal duct with cystic formation within the field of cancer cells being seen.[82] Chronic inflammation of the thyroid such as that seen in Hashimoto disease may lead to squamous metaplasia and, ultimately, SCC.[83] Finally SCC may arise as a direct transition from papillary or follicular carcinoma.[84]

Clinical presentation and diagnosis

Patients with primary SCC of the thyroid present in the fifth or sixth decade of life with a rapidly enlarging thyroid mass. There is a female preponderance (2–3:1) with many patients having a long-standing history of goiter with sudden enlargement. Evidence of local invasion as well as lymph node metastasis are common at the time of diagnosis. Distant metastasis is uncommon.

The diagnosis of primary SCC of the thyroid requires exclusion of an alternative source of SCC that has involved the thyroid by hematogenous or contiguous spread. These may arise from the aerodigestive tract most commonly, though spread from breast, gastrointestinal and renal sources should be considered. Workup therefore consists of FNA of the thyroid mass to confirm the diagnosis of SCC along with upper endoscopy and CT of the neck, chest, and abdomen. Histological findings of primary thyroid SCC are like those of other primaries and not unique to the thyroid, emphasizing the importance of thorough workup.

Treatment

Radical resection, when possible, including total thyroidectomy with resection of adjacent involved structures and neck dissection, yields the best chance for local control and long-term survival.[85] This is often not possible due to extensive esophageal and/or tracheal involvement. External beam radiation may be beneficial as adjuvant therapy when complete resection has been achieved but is otherwise not helpful.[84] These characteristics render SCC of the thyroid highly lethal, similar to anaplastic carcinoma, with survival rates generally less than 1 year.

Malignant teratoma

Extragonadal germ cell tumors are very uncommon in adults and are always malignant. They even less commonly arise in the thyroid with the mediastinum and retroperitoneum being more common sites.[86] Early descriptions reported poor survival though more recent reports suggest improved outcomes with the addition of chemotherapy.[87]

The median age at presentation is 28 years with a thyroid mass being the most common finding. Current treatment recommendations are total thyroidectomy followed by chemotherapy using a bleomycin, etoposide, and cisplatin (BEP) regimen and external beam radiation.[88] These recommendations are based upon anecdotal reports with no large experiences reported.

Malignant hemangioendothelioma

These heterogeneous vascular tumors are exceedingly rare, with few cases reported in the literature. Histologically intermediate between a benign hemangioma and a conventional angiosarcoma, these tumors have been classified into four categories including epithelioid, spindle cell, kaposiform, and endovascular papillary. Malignant hemangioendotheliomas were first described by Weiss and Enzinger in 1982 and have similar morphology to other tumors reported in the skin, bone, lung, pleura, liver, peritoneum, and anterior mediastinum.[89] They can be distinguished from anaplastic carcinomas by immunohistochemistry and their endothelial origin confirmed by staining for factor VIII-related antigen, *Ulex europaeus*, and CD31.[90]

Clinical presentation and diagnosis

Patients tend to present in the seventh decade of life with men more commonly diagnosed than women (2:1). The typical presentation is that of an enlarging neck mass, often with local compressive effects. Metastases to lymph nodes and lung are common at the time of presentation.

Histologically, hemangioendotheliomas are often unencapsulated and ill defined. The cells are eosinophilic and pleomorphic with uniform nuclei. Cytoplasmic vacuolization is remarkable and distinctive, suggesting a failed attempt at lumen formation.[90] Epithelioid cells predominate and are arranged in nests and short cords embedded in an abundant matrix.

Treatment

Hemangioendotheliomas are aggressive tumors. As such, radical resection is the mainstay of therapy.[91] External beam radiation as adjuvant therapy for patients with extensive disease or with positive margins has been applied. Radiation may also play a role in palliation for patients with advanced disease. Chemotherapy has been applied in the setting of metastatic or recurrent disease, utilizing more typical sarcoma regimens. Extensive experience with this management scheme is lacking. Median survivals range from 2 to 14 months with few long-term survivors reported.[91,92]

Mucoepidermoid carcinoma

These tumors are most commonly found in salivary glands, particularly the parotid, but have been described rarely in the thyroid.[93] The origin of these tumors is debated, with early reports hypothesizing that they arose from thyroglossal duct remnants and ectopic salivary gland tissue.[94,95] This has given way to the two more modern theories that continue to be debated, of an ultimobranchial origin based purely upon histological evidence[96] and a follicular epithelial origin using both histological and molecular evidence.[97] Though they typically are reported as low-grade malignancies, aggressive tumors with rapid patient demise have been reported.

Clinical presentation and treatment

Patients present with a neck mass in the fifth to eighth decades of life. More often present in women (2–3:1), lymph node metastasis at the time of diagnosis is common. Distant metastases to lungs and bone are rare.[97] While lobectomy or subtotal thyroidectomy is often adequate, Steele *et al.*

advocate more aggressive surgery until we understand more about the natural history of the disease.[98] Chemotherapy, external beam radiation, and radioactive iodine have all been used in different combinations but limited experience prevents definitive recommendations regarding metastatic or recurrent disease.

Secondary thyroid malignancies

The thyroid gland is an unusual site for clinically evident metastasis, representing 1–2% of thyroid malignancies, though autopsy studies report incidences as high as 24% in patients dying from metastatic disease.[99] These lesions are usually multifocal and rarely the only site of metastasis but may present prior to the primary lesion being found. Renal cell carcinoma is the most common primary with esophagus, breast, stomach, colon, skin, lung, pancreas, and melanoma also reported.[100] The latency period between initial therapy for the primary malignancy and the development of thyroid metastasis varies by tumor type, with very long delays of 7–9 years commonly seen in renal cell carcinoma metastases.[100]

Patients typically present with a thyroid nodule. Diagnosis is made by FNA or thyroidectomy. Cytological evaluation is most helpful in patients with known malignancies or poor surgical risk. Distinguishing between primary anaplastic carcinoma of the thyroid and poorly differentiated adenocarcinoma metastasis can prove difficult, though positive immunostaining for thyroglobulin suggests a primary thyroid malignancy. Currently, FNA cytology is recommended prior to thyroidectomy, particularly in the face of previous cancer.

The management of metastases to the thyroid is individualized. Since it is a harbinger of systemic disease, it is often not curable. Thus treatment and, ultimately, survival are predicated on the presence of other sites of metastasis and the natural history of the primary. When appropriate, thyroidectomy can result in long-term survival when the thyroid represents the only site of metastasis. Patients with renal cell carcinoma fare better following metastasectomy, with 56% 4-year survival reported.[100] Palliative thyroidectomy is an option for local symptoms but, as expected, few patients survive beyond 2 years.[101] Systemic therapy is tailored to the site of origin and is beyond the scope of this chapter.

Conclusion

The thyroid gland is a complex organ composed of several cell types, making it fertile ground for many unusual malignancies. While on the whole the thyroid is the most commonly affected endocrine organ, the cancers described above are fairly uncommon. As such, few endocrinologists or surgeons have amassed a great experience with each type. Still, thorough workup, early diagnosis, and aggressive surgical therapy are the common threads among these rare thyroid cancers, recognizing the potential of advanced and often incurable disease.

References

1. Jemal A, Siegel R, Xu J, et al. Cancer statistics, 2010. CA Cancer J Clin 2010; 60: 277–300.
2. Hazard JB, Hawk WA, Crile G Jr. Medullary (solid) carcinoma of the thyroid: a clinicopathologic entity. J Clin Endocrinol Metab 1959; 19: 152–61.
3. Williams ED. Histogenesis of medullary carcinoma of the thyroid. J Clin Pathol 1966; 19: 114–18.
4. Wells SA Jr, Baylin SB, Linehan WM, et al. Provocative agents and the diagnosis of medullary carcinoma of the thyroid gland. Ann Surg 1978; 188: 139–41.
5. Komminoth P. The RET proto-oncogene in medullary and papillary thyroid carcinoma. Molecular features, pathophysiology and clinical implications. Virchows Arch 1997; 431: 1–9.
6. Quayle FJ, Moley JF. Medullary thyroid carcinoma: including MEN 2A and MEN 2B syndromes. J Surg Oncol 2005; 89: 122–9.
7. Skinner MA, DeBenedetti MK, Moley JF, et al. Medullary thyroid carcinoma in children with multiple endocrine neoplasia types 2A and 2B. J Pediatr Surg 1996; 31: 177–81; discussion 181–2.
8. Modigliani E, Cohen R, Campos JM, et al. Prognostic factors for survival and for biochemical cure in medullary thyroid carcinoma: results in 899 patients. The GETC Study Group. Groupe d'etude des tumeurs a calcitonine. Clin Endocrinol (Oxf) 1998; 48: 265–73.
9. Wells SA Jr, Dilley WG, Farndon JA, et al. Early diagnosis and treatment of medullary thyroid carcinoma. Arch Intern Med 1985; 145: 1248–52.
10. Rodriguez GJ, Balsalobre MD, Pomares F, et al. Prophylactic thyroidectomy in MEN 2A syndrome: experience in a single center. J Am Coll Surg 2002; 195: 159–66.
11. Brandi ML, Gagel RF, Angeli A, et al. Guidelines for diagnosis and therapy of MEN type 1 and type 2. J Clin Endocrinol Metab 2001; 86: 5658–71.
12. Sone T, Fukunaga M, Otsuka N, et al. Metastatic medullary thyroid cancer: localization with iodine-131 metaiodobenzylguanidine. J Nucl Med 1985; 26: 604–8.
13. Thomas CC, Cowan RJ, Albertson DA, et al. Detection of medullary carcinoma of the thyroid with I-131 MIBG. Clin Nucl Med 1994; 19: 1066–8.
14. Edington HD, Watson CG, Levine G, et al. Radioimmunoimaging of metastatic medullary carcinoma of the thyroid gland using an indium-111-labeled monoclonal antibody to CEA. Surgery 1988; 104: 1004–10.
15. Frank-Raue K, Bihl H, Dorr U, et al. Somatostatin receptor imaging in persistent medullary thyroid carcinoma. Clin Endocrinol (Oxf) 1995; 42: 31–7.
16. Krausz Y, Rosler A, Guttmann H, et al. Somatostatin receptor scintigraphy for early detection of regional and distant metastases of medullary carcinoma of the thyroid. Clin Nucl Med 1999; 24: 256–60.
17. Franc B, Rosenberg-Bourgin M, Caillou B, et al. Medullary thyroid carcinoma: search for histological predictors of survival (109 proband cases analysis). Hum Pathol 1998; 29: 1078–84.
18. Evans DB, Fleming JB, Lee JE, et al. The surgical treatment of medullary thyroid carcinoma. Semin Surg Oncol 1999; 16: 50–63.
19. Dralle H, Damm I, Scheumann GF, et al. Compartment-oriented microdissection of regional lymph nodes in medullary thyroid carcinoma. Surg Today 1994; 24: 112–21.
20. Duh QY, Sancho JJ, Greenspan FS, et al. Medullary thyroid carcinoma. The need for early diagnosis and total thyroidectomy. Arch Surg 1989; 124: 1206–10.
21. Moley JF, DeBenedetti MK. Patterns of nodal metastases in palpable medullary thyroid carcinoma: recommendations for extent of node dissection. Ann Surg 1999; 229: 880–7; discussion 887–8.
22. Decker RA, Geiger JD, Cox CE, et al. Prophylactic surgery for multiple endocrine neoplasia type IIa after genetic diagnosis: is parathyroid transplantation indicated? World J Surg 1996; 20: 814–20; discussion 820–1.
23. Van Heerden JA, Grant CS, Gharib H, et al. Long-term course of patients with persistent hypercalcitoninemia after apparent curative primary

surgery for medullary thyroid carcinoma. Ann Surg 1990; 212: 395–400; discussion 400–1.

24. Kouvaraki MA, Shapiro SE, Lee JE, *et al.* Surgical management of thyroid carcinoma. J Natl Compr Canc Netw 2005; 3: 458–66.

25. Moley JF, Debenedetti MK, Dilley WG, *et al.* Surgical management of patients with persistent or recurrent medullary thyroid cancer. J Intern Med 1998; 243: 521–6.

26. Chen H, Roberts JR, Ball DW, *et al.* Effective long-term palliation of symptomatic, incurable metastatic medullary thyroid cancer by operative resection. Ann Surg 1998; 227: 887–95.

27. Martinez SR, Beal SH, Chen A, *et al.* Adjuvant external beam radiation for medullary thyroid carcinoma. J Surg Oncol 2010; 102: 175–8.

28. Brierley J, Tsang R, Simpson WJ, *et al.* Medullary thyroid cancer: analyses of survival and prognostic factors and the role of radiation therapy in local control. Thyroid 1996; 6: 305–10.

29. Fife KM, Bower M, Harmer CL. Medullary thyroid cancer: the role of radiotherapy in local control. Eur J Surg Oncol 1996; 22: 588–91.

30. Orlandi F, Caraci P, Berruti A, *et al.* Chemotherapy with dacarbazine and 5-fluorouracil in advanced medullary thyroid cancer. Ann Oncol 1994; 5: 763–5.

31. Schlumberger M, Abdelmoumene N, Delisle MJ, *et al.* Treatment of advanced medullary thyroid cancer with an alternating combination of 5 FU-streptozocin and 5 FU-dacarbazine. The Groupe d'Etude des Tumeurs a Calcitonine (GETC). Br J Cancer 1995; 71: 363–5.

32. De Groot JW, Zonnenberg BA, van Ufford-Mannesse PQ, *et al.* A phase II trial of imatinib therapy for metastatic medullary thyroid carcinoma. J Clin Endocrinol Metab 2007; 92: 3466–9.

33. Schlumberger MJ, Elisei R, Bastholt L, *et al.* Phase II study of safety and efficacy of motesanib in patients with progressive or symptomatic, advanced or metastatic medullary thyroid cancer. J Clin Oncol 2009; 27: 3794–801.

34. Wells SA Jr, Gosnell JE, Gagel RF, *et al.* Vandetanib for the treatment of patients with locally advanced or metastatic hereditary medullary thyroid cancer. J Clin Oncol 2010; 28: 767–72.

35. Robinson BG, Paz-Ares L, Krebs A, *et al.* Vandetanib (100 mg) in patients with locally advanced or metastatic hereditary medullary thyroid cancer. J Clin Endocrinol Metab 2010; 95: 2664–71.

36. Lam ET, Ringel MD, Kloos RT, *et al.* Phase II clinical trial of sorafenib in metastatic medullary thyroid cancer. J Clin Oncol 2010; 28: 2323–30.

37. De Souza JA, Busaidy N, Zimrin A, *et al.* Phase II trial of sunitinib in medullary thyroid cancer (MTC). J Clin Oncol 2010; 28: 15s (suppl; abstr 5504).

38. Kurzrock R, Sherman SI, Ball DW, *et al.* Activity of XL184 (Cabozantinib), an oral tyrosine kinase inhibitor, in patients with medullary thyroid cancer. J Clin Oncol 2011; 29: 2660–6.

39. Wells SA Jr. RB, Gagel R, *et al.* Vandetanib (VAN) in locally advanced or metastatic medullary thyroid cancer (MTC): A randomized, double-blind phase III trial (ZETA). J Clin Oncol 2010; 28: 15s (suppl; abstr 5503).

40. National Comprehensive Cancer Network (NCCN) www.nccn.org/professionals/physician_gls/pdf/thyroid.pdf.

41. Ewing J. *Neoplastic Disease*, 3rd edn. Philadelphia: WB Saunders, 1928.

42. Masood S, Auguste LJ, Westerband A, *et al.* Differential oncogenic expression in thyroid follicular and Hurthle cell carcinomas. Am J Surg 1993; 166: 366–8.

43. Tyler DS, Winchester DJ, Caraway NP, *et al.* Indeterminate fine-needle aspiration biopsy of the thyroid: identification of subgroups at high risk for invasive carcinoma. Surgery 1994; 116: 1054–60.

44. Massidda B, Nicolosi A, Mura E, *et al.* [Hurthle-cell tumors of the thyroid]. Minerva Chir 1992; 47: 913–17.

45. Ditkoff BA, Chabot J, Jin S, *et al.* Hurthle cell cancer of the thyroid: the incidence of multifocal and bilateral disease. Thyroidol Clin Exp 1995; 7: 49–53.

46. McDonald MP, Sanders LE, Silverman ML, *et al.* Hurthle cell carcinoma of the thyroid gland: prognostic factors and results of surgical treatment. Surgery 1996; 120: 1000–4; discussion 1004–5.

47. Caplan RH, Abellera RM, Kisken WA. Hurthle cell neoplasms of the thyroid gland: reassessment of functional capacity. Thyroid 1994; 4: 243–8.

48. Grossman RF, Clark OH. Hurthle Cell Carcinoma. Cancer Control 1997; 4: 13–17.

49. Besic N, Vidergar-Kralj B, Frkovic-Grazio S, *et al.* The role of radioactive iodine in the treatment of Hurthle cell carcinoma of the thyroid. Thyroid 2003; 13: 577–84.

50. Kloos RT, Ringel MD, Knopp MV, *et al.* Phase II trial of sorafenib in metastatic thyroid cancer. J Clin Oncol 2009; 27: 1675–84.

51. Bible KC, Suman VJ, Molina JR, *et al.* Efficacy of pazopanib in progressive, radioiodine-refractory, metastatic differentiated thyroid cancers: results of a phase 2 consortium study. Lancet Oncol 2010; 11: 962–72.

52. Foote RL, Molina JR, Kasperbauer JL, *et al.* Enhanced survival in locoregionally confined anaplastic thyroid carcinoma: a single-institution experience using aggressive multimodal therapy. Thyroid 2011; 21: 25–30.

53. Are C, Shaha A. Anaplastic thyroid carcinoma: biology, pathogenesis, prognostic factors, and treatment approaches. Ann Surg Oncol 2006; 13: 453–64.

54. Samaan NA, Ordonez NG. Uncommon types of thyroid cancer. Endocrinol Metab Clin North Am 1990; 19: 637–48.

55. Agrawal S, Rao RS, Parikh DM, *et al.* Histologic trends in thyroid cancer 1969–1993: a clinico-pathologic analysis of the relative proportion of anaplastic carcinoma of the thyroid. J Surg Oncol 1996; 63: 251–5.

56. Hadar T, Mor C, Shvero J, *et al.* Anaplastic carcinoma of the thyroid. Eur J Surg Oncol 1993; 19: 511–16.

57. Venkatesh YS, Ordonez NG, Schultz PN, *et al.* Anaplastic carcinoma of the thyroid. A clinicopathologic study of 121 cases. Cancer 1990; 66: 321–30.

58. Cohen Y, Xing M, Mambo E, *et al.* BRAF mutation in papillary thyroid carcinoma. J Natl Cancer Inst 2003; 95: 625–7.

59. Xing M. BRAF mutation in thyroid cancer. Endocr Relat Cancer 2005; 12: 245–62.

60. Fagin JA, Matsuo K, Karmakar A, *et al.* High prevalence of mutations of the p53 gene in poorly differentiated human thyroid carcinomas. J Clin Invest 1993; 91: 179–84.

61. Garcia-Rostan G, Tallini G, Herrero A, *et al.* Frequent mutation and nuclear localization of beta-catenin in anaplastic thyroid carcinoma. Cancer Res 1999; 59: 1811–15.

62. Garcia-Rostan G, Zhao H, Camp RL, *et al.* Ras mutations are associated with aggressive tumor phenotypes and poor prognosis in thyroid cancer. J Clin Oncol 2003; 21: 3226–35.

63. Guida T, Salvatore G, Faviana P, *et al.* Mitogenic effects of the up-regulation of minichromosome maintenance proteins in anaplastic thyroid carcinoma. J Clin Endocrinol Metab 2005; 90: 4703–9.

64. Kebebew E, Greenspan FS, Clark OH, *et al.* Anaplastic thyroid carcinoma. Treatment outcome and prognostic factors. Cancer 2005; 103: 1330–5.

65. McIver B, Hay ID, Giuffrida DF, *et al.* Anaplastic thyroid carcinoma: a 50-year experience at a single institution. Surgery 2001; 130: 1028–34.

66. Levendag PC, de Porre PM, van Putten WL. Anaplastic carcinoma of the thyroid gland treated by radiation therapy. Int J Radiat Oncol Biol Phys 1993; 26: 125–8.

67. Tennvall J, Lundell G, Wahlberg P, *et al.* Anaplastic thyroid carcinoma: three protocols combining doxorubicin, hyperfractionated radiotherapy and surgery. Br J Cancer 2002; 86: 1848–53.

68. Troch M, Koperek O, Scheuba C, *et al.* High efficacy of concomitant treatment of undifferentiated (anaplastic) thyroid cancer with radiation and docetaxel. J Clin Endocrinol Metab 2010; 95: E54–7.

69. Sosa JA, Elisei R, Jarzab Bea. A randomized phase II/III trial of a tumor vascular disrupting agent fosbretabulin tromethamine (CA4P) with carboplatin (C) and paclitaxel (P) in anaplastic thyroid cancer (ATC): final survival analysis of the FACT trial. J Clin Oncol 2011; 29 (suppl; abstr 5502).

70. Carcangiu ML, Zampi G, Rosai J. Poorly differentiated ("insular") thyroid carcinoma. A reinterpretation of Langhans' "wucherde Struma". Am J Surg Pathol 1984; 8: 655–68.

71. Ashfaq R, Vuitch F, Delgado R, *et al.* Papillary and follicular thyroid carcinomas with an insular component. Cancer 1994; 73: 416–23.

72. Rijhwani A, Satish GN. Insular carcinoma of the thyroid in a 10-year-old child. J Pediatr Surg 2003; 38: 1083–5.

73. Sobrinho-Simoes MS, Fonesca E. Recently described tumors of the thyroid. In: Anthony PP, Macsween RNM (eds) *Recent Advances in Histopathology*. Edinburgh: Churchill Livingstone, 1994. pp.213–29.

74. Flynn SD, Forman BH, Stewart AF, *et al*. Poorly differentiated ("insular") carcinoma of the thyroid gland: an aggressive subset of differentiated thyroid neoplasms. Surgery 1988; 104: 963–70.

75. Glass AG, Karnell LH, Menck HR. The National Cancer Data Base report on non-Hodgkin's lymphoma. Cancer 1997; 80: 2311–20.

76. Thieblemont C, Mayer A, Dumontet C, *et al*. Primary thyroid lymphoma is a heterogeneous disease. J Clin Endocrinol Metab 2002; 87: 105–11.

77. Takashima S, Nomura N, Noguchi Y, *et al*. Primary thyroid lymphoma: evaluation with US, CT, and MRI. J Comput Assist Tomogr 1995; 19: 282–8.

78. Skarsgard ED, Connors JM, Robins RE. A current analysis of primary lymphoma of the thyroid. Arch Surg 1991; 126: 1199–203; discussion 1203–4.

79. Widder S, Pasieka JL. Primary thyroid lymphomas. Curr Treat Options Oncol 2004; 5: 307–13.

80. Galati LT, Barnes EL, Myers EN. Dendritic cell sarcoma of the thyroid. Head Neck 1999; 21: 273–5.

81. Merimsky O, Issakov J, Kollender Y, *et al*. Sarcoma and thyroid disorders: a common etiology? Oncol Rep 2002; 9: 863–9.

82. Akbari Y, Richter RM, Papadakis LE. Thyroid carcinoma arising in thyroglossal duct remnants. Report of a case and review of the literature. Arch Surg 1967; 94: 235–9.

83. LiVolsi VA, Merino MJ. Squamous cells in the human thyroid gland. Am J Surg Pathol 1978; 2: 133–40.

84. Harada T, Shimaoka K, Yakumaru K, *et al*. Squamous cell carcinoma of the thyroid gland – transition from adenocarcinoma. J Surg Oncol 1982; 19: 36–43.

85. Sarda AK, Bal S, Arunabh, *et al*. Squamous cell carcinoma of the thyroid. J Surg Oncol 1988; 39: 175–8.

86. Buckley NJ, Burch WM, Leight GS. Malignant teratoma in the thyroid gland of an adult: a case report and a review of the literature. Surgery 1986; 100: 932–7.

87. Ueno NT, Amato RJ, Ro JJ, *et al*. Primary malignant teratoma of the thyroid gland: report and discussion of two cases. Head Neck 1998; 20: 649–53.

88. Tsang RW, Brierley JD, Asa SL, *et al*. Malignant teratoma of the thyroid: aggressive chemoradiation therapy is required after surgery. Thyroid 2003; 13: 401–4.

89. Suster S, Moran CA, Koss MN. Epithelioid hemangioendothelioma of the anterior mediastinum. Clinicopathologic, immunohistochemical, and ultrastructural analysis of 12 cases. Am J Surg Pathol 1994; 18: 871–81.

90. Siddiqui MT, Evans HL, Ro JY, *et al*. Epithelioid haemangioendothelioma of the thyroid gland: a case report and review of literature. Histopathology 1998; 32: 473–6.

91. Rhomberg W, Boehler F, Eiter H, *et al*. Treatment options for malignant hemangioendotheliomas of the thyroid. Int J Radiat Oncol Biol Phys 2004; 60: 401–5.

92. Ladurner D, Totsch M, Luze T, *et al*. [Malignant hemangioendothelioma of the thyroid gland. Pathology, clinical aspects and prognosis]. Wien Klin Wochenschr 1990; 102: 256–9.

93. Bhandarkar ND, Chan J, Strome M. A rare case of mucoepidermoid carcinoma of the thyroid. Am J Otolaryngol 2005; 26: 138–41.

94. Diaz-Perez R, Quiroz H, Nishiyama RH, Primary mucinous adenocarcinoma of thyroid gland. Cancer 1976; 38: 1323–5.

95. Rhatigan RM, Roque JL, Bucher RL. Mucoepidermoid carcinoma of the thyroid gland. Cancer 1977; 39: 210–14.

96. Harach HR. A study on the relationship between solid cell nests and mucoepidermoid carcinoma of the thyroid. Histopathology 1985; 9: 195–207.

97. Wenig BM, Adair CF, Heffess CS. Primary mucoepidermoid carcinoma of the thyroid gland: a report of six cases and a review of the literature of a follicular epithelial-derived tumor. Hum Pathol 1995; 26: 1099–108.

98. Steele SR, Royer M, Brown TA, *et al*. Mucoepidermoid carcinoma of the thyroid gland: a case report and suggested surgical approach. Am Surg 2001; 67: 979–83.

99. Berge T, Lundberg S. Cancer in Malmo 1958–1969. An autopsy study. Acta Pathol Microbiol Scand 1977; 260(Suppl): 1–235.

100. Mirallie E, Rigaud J, Mathonnet M, *et al*. Management and prognosis of metastases to the thyroid gland. J Am Coll Surg 2005; 200: 203–7.

101. Rosen IB, Walfish PG, Bain J, *et al*. Secondary malignancy of the thyroid gland and its management. Ann Surg Oncol 1995; 2: 252–6.

Section 3: Endocrine Tumors

12 Parathyroid Carcinoma

Rodrigo Arrangoiz and John A. Ridge

Fox Chase Cancer Center, Philadelphia, PA, USA

Introduction

Parathyroid carcinoma is certainly a rare malignancy. Based on the Surveillance, Epidemiology, and End Results (SEER) database, the reported incidence of parathyroid cancer is less than one per million population per year over a 16-year period from 1988 to 2003.[1] It is an uncommon cause of primary hyperparathyroidism (PHPT), accounting for less than 5% of PHPT cases.[2–4] This chapter reviews the incidence, pathophysiology, clinical presentation, diagnosis, treatment, and prognosis of this disease.

Embryology, anatomy and physiology

The parathyroid glands develop as epithelial thickenings of the dorsal endoderm of the third and fourth branchial pouches. As a consequence of their migration, the derivatives of the third branchial pouch become the inferior parathyroid glands, while those of the fourth branchial pouch become the superior parathyroid glands. The inferior parathyroid glands are closely related to the thymus gland, which is derived from the ventral portion of the third branchial pouch. This intimate relationship usually ends during the 8th week of gestation, leaving the parathyroid gland near the level of the lower border of the thyroid gland. Sometimes the inferior parathyroid glands can become encapsulated within the thymus or thyrothimic tract and may be carried into the anterior mediastinum.[5] The superior parathyroid glands descend into the neck to associate with the posterior border of the upper pole of the thyroid. They may be found within the gland parenchyma, but infrequently the superior glands continue their migration caudally, and they may be found anywhere along the course of the tracheoesophageal groove into the posterior mediastinum.[6,7]

The parathyroid glands are usually found on the posterior surface of the thyroid gland, each with its own capsule of connective tissue. They are occasionally within the thyroid capsule, but may even follow a blood vessel deep into a sulcus of the thyroid.[5] Typically, four parathyroid glands are present, two superior and two inferior, with an average size and weight of approximately $5 \times 3 \times 2$ mm and 40–60 mg each.[6,7] It is not uncommon to have more or fewer glands. When fewer than four glands are found, the possibility of an ectopic gland is difficult to exclude.[5] Two parathyroid glands may be fused to one another; such a pair can be differentiated from a bilobate gland only by the presence of a cleavage plane between them.[8] Hooghe et al., in a study of 416 parathyroidectomies, found parathyroid glands in ectopic locations in 19% of the cases (distant to the thyroid lobes, along the esophagus, or in the upper anterior mediastinum within thymic remnants). Among these patients, 5% had supernumerary parathyroids.[9]

In a study of 354 autopsy specimens, Alveryd observed that both the superior and inferior parathyroid glands are usually supplied by the inferior thyroid artery: 86% on the right side, 77% on the left. When the inferior thyroid artery is absent, both the superior and inferior parathyroid glands are supplied by the superior thyroid artery in the majority of cases.[10]

The chief (or "principal") cells form a major portion of the parathyroid parenchyma and oxyphilic cells form a minor part. The parathyroid cells participate in the secretion of the parathyroid hormone, parathormone (PTH), and thus in the regulation of calcium and phosphate metabolism. The *PTH* gene is located on chromosome 11. By sensing extracellular calcium levels, the parathyroid gland cells rely on a G-protein-coupled membrane receptor, designated the calcium-sensing receptor (CASR), to regulate PTH secretion.[11] Low levels of 1,25-dihydroxy vitamin D, catecholamines, and hypomagnesemia can also stimulate PTH secretion. PTH is synthesized through a precursor hormone, preproPTH, which is cleaved first to pro-PTH and then to the final 84-amino acid PTH. The half-life of PTH is some 2–6 min.[12,13] In the liver, PTH is metabolized into the active N-terminal component and the relatively inactive C-terminal fraction. The C-terminal component is excreted by the kidneys and accumulates in chronic renal failure.[14]

Textbook of Uncommon Cancer, Fourth Edition. Edited by Derek Raghavan, Charles D. Blanke, David H. Johnson, Paul L. Moots, Gregory H. Reaman, Peter G. Rose and Mikkael A. Sekeres.
© 2012 John Wiley & Sons, Inc. Published 2012 by John Wiley & Sons, Inc.

The function of PTH is to regulate calcium levels through its actions on three organs: the bone, kidney, and gut. It increases the resorption of bone by stimulating osteoclasts and promotes the release of calcium and phosphate into the circulation. At the level of the kidney, calcium is primarily absorbed in conjunction with sodium in the proximal convoluted tubule, but adjustments can occur more distally (via an active transport mechanism, PTH acts to limit calcium excretion at the distal convoluted tubule). PTH also inhibits phosphate reabsorption (at the proximal convoluted tubule) and bicarbonate reabsorption and inhibits the Na^+/H^+ antiporter, which results in a mild metabolic acidosis in hyperparathyroid states. Both hypophosphatemia and PTH enhance 1-hydroxylation of 25-hydroxyvitamin D, which is responsible for its indirect effect of increasing intestinal calcium absorption. Adenomatous, hyperplastic, or malignant changes in the parathyroid glands result in the loss of feedback inhibition, increased secretion of parathyroid hormone, and subsequent hypercalcemia.

Epidemiology

Parathyroid carcinoma is rare, with a reported incidence from less than 1% to as high as 5% among cases of PHPT. These statistics are similar worldwide, except for Japan, where a significantly higher proportion of patients with PHPT are found to have parathyroid cancer.[15] In earlier series published in the United States, the incidence ranged from 1% (by Cope) in 1966 to as high as 4% (by Schantz and Castleman) in 1973.[3,16,17] In series from Italy and Japan, it has been reported as nearly 5%.[15,18,19] Obara and Fujimoto, in a collective review, found an incidence of 2.1% among more than 4000 cases of PHPT.[2] More recently, two cancer registry reports of parathyroid cancer have been published. The largest of these describes 286 patients with parathyroid carcinoma registered in the US National Cancer Database (NCDB) between 1985 and 1995.[9] The second was reported by Lee et al. from the SEER database over a 16-year period.[1] They reported an incidence of parathyroid cancer of less than one per million population per year. They noted that during the study time period, the incidence of parathyroid carcinomas increased by 60%, from 3.58 per 10 million population during the 1988–1991 period to 5.73 per 10 million population during 2000–2003. The increase in incidence was attributed to the increase in the frequency of operations performed for PHPT because routine calcium screening has become more common, and surgical guidelines for PHPT were liberalized after 2002.[20]

In contrast to PHPT, which predominantly affects women, there is no gender predilection with parathyroid carcinoma. The NCDB found a nearly even ratio of 51% men to 49% women,[9] which was recently confirmed by Lee et al. in their review of SEER database.[1] Parathyroid carcinoma tends to present at a younger age than benign hyperparathyroidism (by a mean of 10 years), often in the fifth decade of life compared with PHPT, which frequently presents in the sixth decade.[21]

Etiology

The etiology of parathyroid carcinoma is poorly understood. One risk factor seems to be previous radiation therapy to the head and neck: five cases in the literature report parathyroid carcinoma in the setting of distant radiation exposure.[22] There is a well-described genetic predisposition: about 2% of parathyroid carcinoma cases have been reported to have a family history of PHPT.[23] Multiple endocrine neoplasia (MEN) type 1 (Wermer syndrome) and MEN 2A (Sipple syndrome) have been associated with an increased risk of developing parathyroid cancer.[24] However, the association between family history and parathyroid cancer appears to be more common than parathyroid cancer and MEN.

Hyperparathyroidism–jaw tumor (HPT-JT) is a rare autosomal dominant inherited disorder that is characterized by having hyperparathyroidism (90%) and ossifying fibromas of the maxilla and mandible (30%). Less commonly, renal cysts (10%), harmartomas, and Wilms tumors have also been reported with this syndrome. The most common finding in this syndrome is PHPT but in about 10–15% of the cases parathyroid carcinoma is identified.[24–26] HPT-JT syndrome results from germline mutations in the tumor suppressor gene *CDC73* (formerly *HRPT2*) located on chromosome 1.[27]

Another risk factor that has been implicated in the development of parathyroid carcinoma is secondary and tertiary hyperparathyroidism.[28] Khan et al. reported on 18 cases of parathyroid carcinoma developing in this setting, which occurred approximately 6 years after the start of hemodialysis.[28]

Genetics

No specific gene has been implicated as a cause of parathyroid carcinoma; however, several genes may be involved in the pathogenesis of this malignancy. The *CDC73* (formerly *HRPT2*) gene is a tumor suppressor gene that may contribute to the pathogenesis of parathyroid carcinoma when mutated.[27,29] Somatic mutations of the *CDC73* gene are present in 66–100% of sporadic parathyroid carcinomas.[30,31]

The normal *CDC73* gene encodes the protein parafibromin.[26,27] Parafibromin has been shown to be a tumor suppressor by transfection studies in which wild-type parafibromin inhibited tumor cell growth, but transfection with missense parafibromin mutants had no impact on cell growth.[25] The vast majority of the mutations reported are nonsense mutations that result in loss of parafibromin expression, although mutations in noncoding regulatory regions or gene inactivation by promoter methylation have also been part of the pathogenesis.[32] Less than 1% of benign sporadic parathyroid adenomas harbor mutations in the *CDC73* gene.[33] As discussed above, *CDC73* gene mutations have been identified in patients with the HPT-JT syndrome. Parathyroid carcinoma is overrepresented among HPT-JT patients with a frequency of 10–15% (in contrast to less than 1–5% among all patients with hyperparathyroidism).[24] In 15 patients with sporadic parathyroid carcinomas, 10 had *CDC73* mutations and 30% of these mutations were germline in origin. Each of these mutations resulted in failure of parafibromin production, thereby implicating *CDC73* and its product, parafibromin, as tumor suppressors of parathyroid cancer.[29]

Parafibromin has an inhibitory effect on cyclin D1 activity; its loss leads to neoplastic transformation. Cyclin D1, an oncogene located at chromosome band 11q13, is overexpressed in parathyroid adenomas and carcinomas.[24,33,34] The level of cyclin D1 is significantly higher in parathyroid carcinomas than adenomas.[25] Transfection of NIH3T3 mouse cells and HEK-293 human cells with wild-type parafibromin inhibited expression of cyclin D1. Transfection with mutant parafibromin had no impact on cyclin D1 expression. These findings suggest that *CDC73* mutations with loss of parafibromin expression may result in increases in cyclin D1 expression and contribute to neoplasia. However, parafibromin is present in other tissues without neoplastic transformation associated with mutations.[25]

Other oncogenes and tumor suppressor genes have been implicated in the pathogenesis of parathyroid carcinoma. Loss of heterozygosity in chromosome 13q, a region containing two tumor suppressor genes, *RB1* (retinoblastoma, 13q14.3) and *BRCA2* (13q12.3), has been linked to parathyroid carcinomas.[33] Cryns *et al.* reported that loss of heterozygosity at the *RB1* locus was found in 100% carcinomas (11/11 samples), but in only 5% of adenomas (1/19 samples). Near-complete or total absence of *RB1* expression was identified in immunohistochemical studies in 88% of the carcinomas, whereas the adenomas demonstrated normal *RB1* staining patterns.[35] These genes have not been linked to the pathogenesis of parathyroid carcinoma by all reports, suggesting that the gene expression may be epigenetically regulated or that other tumor suppressors in this region may be important in parathyroid carcinogenesis.[36] Other genes associated with loss of heterozygosity that have linked to parathyroid cancer include *PTEN*, *MET*, *TP53*, and *HRAS*.[33,37]

The *APC* (adenomatous polyposis coli) gene was recently implicated in the pathogenesis of parathyroid carcinoma; loss of its expression via hypermethylation of its promoter region was found in five of five parathyroid carcinomas.[38] This mutation was associated with the accumulation of nonphosphorylated β-catenin, suggesting aberrant activation of the WNT/β-catenin signaling pathway.

In more than 90% of parathyroid carcinomas the *CCND1* gene (formerly *PRAD1*) is overexpressed.[37] This oncogene was identified during the molecular characterization of several large sporadic parathyroid adenomas harboring DNA rearrangements that involved the *PTH* gene (chromosome 11). The exact role of this gene in the pathogenesis of parathyroid carcinomas remains to be ascertained.

Pathology

Schantz and Castleman established the classic histological criteria for parathyroid cancers.[3] They distinguished parathyroid carcinoma as a separate entity and found that there was no evidence that cancer developed from adenomas or hyperplasia of the parathyroid glands. They described that parathyroid carcinomas are characterized by chief cells (which are almost always the predominant cell type) arranged in a trabecular, solid, or acinar pattern with the loss of the typical lobular pattern (Fig. 12.1). In diagnosing parathyroid cancer, they found fibrous trabeculae in 90%, mitotic figures in 81%, capsular invasion in 67%, and blood vessel invasion in 12% of the cases.[3] As evidenced by their frequency, such findings are not consistent. These classic features are seldom present as frequently as initially reported. One recent study noted fibrous bands, mitosis,

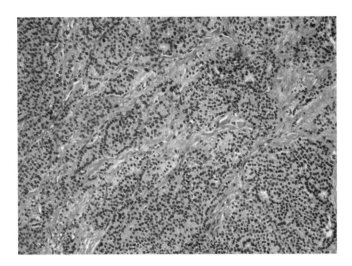

Figure 12.1 The classic features of parathyroid carcinoma.

and vascular invasion in only 37% of the patients.[39] Another review of 27 cases of parathyroid cancer reported fibrous bands in 44%, mitotic figures in 40%, vascular invasion in 37%, capsular invasion in 26%, trabeculae in 11%, and lymphatic invasion in 11% of the cases.[40] An additional study compared histopathological features found in 16 parathyroid carcinomas with those found in 45 typical adenomas and eight atypical adenomas. The qualities that were found to be most specific for parathyroid carcinoma, and not present in typical or atypical adenomas, were capsular invasion (94%), adjacent soft tissue invasion (69%), and vascular invasion (81%).[41]

Many of the features used to diagnose parathyroid carcinoma, including adherence to surrounding structures, fibrous bands, trabecular growth pattern, and mitosis, can also be found in benign lesions.[42,43] Some authors consider vascular invasion, defined as the presence of affected vessels within the tumor capsule or surrounding soft tissues, pathognomonic of carcinoma[44] but the overall diagnostic value of both vascular and capsular invasion remain subject to debate.[45]

A series of 95 cases of parathyroid carcinoma from the Swedish Cancer Registry reported on reevaluations of histopathology by pathologists unaware of the initial diagnosis. At the first surgical procedure, only 74% of cases were correctly diagnosed as parathyroid carcinoma, and in 19% of cases a benign initial diagnosis was rendered. On reevaluation, 43% were diagnosed unequivocally as malignant, while 57% were read as histologically equivocal, that is, displaying varying combinations of suspicious findings.[18] These results highlight the difficulty of assigning a conclusive pathological diagnosis of this rare cancer.

The utility of immunohistochemical staining for cell cycle-associated antigens (such as Ki-67 and cyclin D1) in distinguishing parathyroid carcinomas from parathyroid adenomas at this time is limited because of its significant overlap.[33] Efforts to evaluate loss of the parafibromin protein by immunohistochemical studies, loss of heterozygosity, or mutations in the *CCND1* gene may be useful as adjuncts to the diagnosis of this condition.[46]

Intraoperative findings that might help distinguish a parathyroid carcinoma from a benign condition include a firm, gray-white, spherical tumor with a thick capsule adherent to adjacent structures (in contrast to benign adenomas that are red-brown and soft). The structures typically invaded are the thyroid (89%), the strap muscles (71%), the recurrent laryngeal nerve (26%), the esophagus (18%), and the trachea (17%).[22] These cancers usually weigh between 2 g and 10 g. Clinical findings in the operating room are not invariably suspicious for carcinoma and frozen sections are not reliable enough to assure real-time diagnosis.[47] Local invasion seems to be the most highly suggestive feature indicating cancer.[22]

Staging

There is no standard staging system for parathyroid cancer. A TNM (tumor, nodes, and metastasis) staging system has proven difficult to develop for parathyroid carcinoma because of the rarity of the condition. The tumor size and lymph node status at presentation have not been strong predictors of survival.[20] However, Shaha and Shah proposed a TNM-based staging system focused upon tumor size greater or less than 3 cm, the presence of regional lymph node metastases, and the presence of distant metastases.[48]

One potentially useful means of characterizing the extent of disease is whether it is limited to the parathyroid gland, locally invasive, or having metastases. A histological classification system may give an indication of prognosis. In one proposed system, where capsular and vascular invasion identifies parathyroid carcinoma, tumors with limited local infiltration were classified as low grade and those with widespread infiltration as high grade. Low-grade lesions with limited local invasion correlated with cure, while high-grade tumors with widespread infiltration correlated with metastases.[49]

Clinical presentation

The clinical presentation of patients with parathyroid carcinoma almost invariably results from hypercalcemia due to the parathyroid hormone produced by the tumor. Symptoms include the classic "bones, stones, groans, and psychic moans" associated with hypercalcemia of hyperparathyroidism; however, in patients with parathyroid carcinoma, they occur more frequently and in more severe forms.

Less than 5% of patients with parathyroid carcinoma will be asymptomatic and in contrast to benign PHPT, the frequency of a palpable neck mass, renal disease, or bone disease is estimated to be greater than 35–40%.[22] Paralysis of the recurrent laryngeal nerve is also a relatively common finding. Parathyroid hormone levels are usually higher in carcinoma than in hyperparathyroidism. Alkaline phosphatase levels are also elevated.[21]

The clinical manifestations at presentation of hypercalcemia from parathyroid carcinoma in several reported series are shown in Table 12.1. The organ systems most commonly affected are skeletal and renal. Skeletal complications, including diffuse osteopenia, osteoporosis, osteitis fibrosa cystica, bone pain, or pathological fractures, are reported in 30–91% of cases.[2,19,21,40,50] Renal complications including nephrolithiasis, nephrocalcinosis, and impaired renal function are seen in 21–60% of cases. [2,19,21,40,50]

Neuromuscular and neuropsychiatric manifestations are frequently vague in presentation but can often be elicited through a thorough review of systems. In a series reported by Busaidy et al., symptoms of fatigue were reported in 33%, arthralgia in 22%, and headaches in 26% of the cases.[40] Loss of concentration, malaise, polydipsia, polyuria, and depression may also be present. Recurrent severe pancreatitis and peptic ulcer disease may be seen.[33]

The physical finding most associated with parathyroid carcinoma is a palpable cervical lymph node but this represents a distinct minority of cases. Cervical lymphadenopathy is present on examination of patients with parathyroid carcinoma with reported frequencies of 15–75%.[2,3,40,41,50,52] However, it is exceedingly rare in patients with benign causes of primary hyperparathyroidism. Stojadinovic et al. studied a series of 73 patients with parathyroid adenomas, atypical adenomas, and carcinomas. They reported the incidence of a palpable neck

	Busaidy et al.[40]	Iacobone et al.[19]	Wynne et al.[50]	Obara and Fujimoto[15]	Shane and Bilezikian[51]	Schantz and Castleman[3]
No. of patients	27	19	40	163	62	61
Skeletal	30%	63%	91% (20/22)	39%	70%	62%
Renal	44%	53%	56% (14/25)* 38%†	48%	60%	30%* 21%†
Neuromuscular	33%‡	37%	27%§	–	–	8%‡
	22%§	–	–	–	–	–
	26%¶	–	–	–	–	–
Pancreatitis	4%	–	–	5%	10%	10%
Gastrointestinal	15%	16%	–	–	–	13%
Asymptomatic	30%	21%	7%	2%	2%	–

Table 12.1 Frequency of clinical manifestations of hypercalcemia with parathyroid carcinoma.

* Calculi.
† Intrinsic.
‡ Weakness, lethargy.
§ Myalgia, arthralgia.
¶ Headaches.

mass in carcinoma of 75% (16/20), versus atypical adenoma of 25% (2/8), and adenoma 0% (0/45).[41] Hoarseness resulting from recurrent laryngeal nerve palsy may provide a clue to the presence of a carcinoma. Hypercalcemic crisis may develop in patients with marked hyperparathyroidism. This condition presents with nausea, vomiting, anorexia, constipation, acute pancreatitis, shortened QT interval, apathy, drowsiness, and coma, and if left untreated, it can lead to death.[33]

A serum calcium level greater than 14–15 mg/dL[-1] should raise suspicion of parathyroid carcinoma.[33] Average calcium levels measured in patients with parathyroid cancer in multiple published series range from 13.4 to 15.9 mg/dL[-1].[2,3,18,20,40,41,50,53] In a published series comparing parathyroid carcinoma to atypical adenomas and typical adenomas, the average serum calcium levels were 14, 12, and 11 mg/dL[-1] respectively.[41] Alkaline phosphatase levels are usually higher in patients with carcinoma compared with those found in benign parathyroid disease. Increased serum and urinary human chorionic gonadotropin levels (the hyperglycosylated isoform) have also been reported in patients with parathyroid carcinomas and may have value as diagnostic and prognostic adjuncts.[54] A subset of parathyroid cancers also overproduces the N-terminal form of parathyroid hormone; the clinical implications of this are still unknown.[55]

Patients with parathyroid carcinoma frequently show markedly elevated parathyroid hormone levels. PHPT is usually associated with parathyroid hormone levels less than twice the upper limit of normal values. Patients with parathyroid carcinoma often have parathyroid hormone levels five times greater than the upper limit of normal values.[2,18,50] Table 12.2 shows average calcium levels and the magnitudes of parathyroid hormone elevations from published series in which both values were reported.

Imaging studies

Imaging studies are typically those that have been employed in PHPTs. The sestamibi nuclear medicine scan is the most sensitive test for identifying parathyroid tumors. Sestamibi with single photon emission computed tomography (SPECT) adds three-dimensional imaging. Ultrasound is increasingly employed for imaging the neck. It can identify tumor invasion of local structures. Computed tomography (CT) scan and magnetic resonance imaging (MRI) are useful for imaging the mediastinum and sites of distant metastases, but are seldom

Table 12.2 Serum calcium and parathyroid hormone levels in patients with parathyroid carcinoma.

Author	Serum calcium (No. of patients)	Magnitude of parathyroid hormone level elevation* (No. of patients)
Wynne et al.[50]	14.6 mg/dL[-1] (43)	10.2× (21)
Sandelin et al.[18]	14.4 mg/dL[-1] (95)	1.3–75× (24)
Obara and Fujimoto[2]	15.0 mg/dL[-1] (163)	>5× (53)

*Elevation is the multiple of the upper limit of normal values.

performed because preoperative recognition of parathyroid cancer is not common.

Positron emission tomography (PET) has also shown utility for the detection of metastatic parathyroid cancers.[56] An important caution in this scenario is that brown tumors can be fluorodeoxyglucose avid on this imaging modality and may be mistaken for metastases.[57]

Needle biopsy of suspected parathyroid carcinoma should not be performed because of the risk of tumor seeding.[2,58]

Operative findings

Clinical diagnosis of parathyroid carcinoma at operation is important so that the appropriate resection can be performed. The surgeon should be prepared to perform the necessary operation on clinical grounds alone. Tumor appearance, size, and local invasion are important. The cancer often differs markedly from a typical parathyroid adenoma. Instead, the surgeon encounters a gray-white, lobulated, firm tumor, which may exceed 2.5 cm in diameter, weighing more than 4 g, and invading or adherent to adjacent structures.

The average diameter of parathyroid carcinoma tumors in published series ranges from 2.5 to 3.3 cm.[3,18,40] The largest published series of parathyroid carcinomas, from the US NCDB, reported an average tumor diameter of 3.3 cm in 174 measurable cases.[20] Schantz and Castleman reported a weight range of 0.8–42.4 g in 24 cases.[3] The weight range reported in a published series from the Swedish Cancer Registry was 1.05–40 g in 35 cases.[18]

Parathyroid carcinoma tends to arise in inferior parathyroid glands. In a study of 16 cases, six had cancers in the left inferior gland, nine were in the right inferior gland, and one was in a mediastinal fifth gland, while no cases involved superior glands.[4] In another series, out of 19 cases with tumor locations reported, 15 involved inferior glands, three involved superior glands, and one involved a mediastinal gland.[40]

An important distinguishing feature of parathyroid carcinoma at operation is tumor invasion of local tissue and adjacent structures. Invasion may occur into local adipose tissue or into adjacent structures such as thyroid, esophagus, and recurrent laryngeal nerve. The incidence of local invasion is 44–70% in reported series, with invasion of fat most common.[18,40] Invasion of adjacent structures has been reported as 23–37%.[18,40] Structures most frequently invaded are the thyroid, the strap muscles, the recurrent laryngeal nerve, the esophagus, and the trachea.[22] In a series of 163 patients with parathyroid carcinoma, 38 had invasion of local structures, with the thyroid[50] and recurrent laryngeal nerve[6] most frequently involved.[2]

Cervical lymph node management is controversial. The incidence of occult cervical lymph node metastasis has been reported to be as high as 32%, which resulted in recommendations for formal lymph node dissection at the initial operation.[53] However, several reported series cite an incidence of cervical lymph node involvement at less than 5%.[2,4,18] Hence, there has been no standard surgical approach to clinically uninvolved cervical lymph nodes.

The lack of a standard regarding lymph node dissection/sampling is likely a confounding factor in the reporting of the incidence of lymph node metastases at presentation. The Swedish Cancer Registry found only three lymph node metastases in 95 cases; however, 84 of them (88%) did not undergo lymphadenectomy.[18] In published series in which lymph node dissections were regularly performed, the incidence of lymph node metastasis at initial operation was 11–15%.[3,20,40] In the US NCDB review of 286 cases, only 105 had cervical lymph node status reported, of which 15% showed lymph node involvement at initial operation.[20]

Treatment

The only curative treatment for parathyroid carcinoma is surgical resection. If parathyroid cancer is suspected preoperatively, obtaining anatomical imaging such as CT will be useful in defining the extent of disease and will help plan the operation. However, not uncommonly, the diagnosis will be made intraoperatively and in some occasions postoperatively. The resection should be performed without disruption of the tumor capsule, as this can result in "seeding" of the surgical bed. Similarly, disruption of adhesions between tumor and local structures can result in tumor implants. In addition, local cervical lymph nodes may harbor metastases.

No prospective data guide recommendations for resection. However, the suggested operation for parathyroid carcinoma is *en bloc* resection including tumor, adherent tissues, the ipsilateral thyroid, with ipsilateral lymphadenectomy of levels IV, VI, and the tracheoesophageal groove.[2,21,48,58] The recurrent laryngeal nerve should be sacrificed if involvement is recognized preoperatively (by a paralyzed vocal cord) or if invasion is identified at operation. If cervical lymph nodes are clinically involved at operation, then a comprehensive cervical lymphadenectomy should be performed.[48]

The majority of patients with parathyroid carcinoma undergo an inadequate initial operation. This may be due to lack of recognition of parathyroid carcinoma at operation in the majority of cases[20] but surgeons may be reluctant to pursue the recommended resection as well. For instance, few surgeons are willing to sacrifice the recurrent laryngeal nerve or to pursue a formal node dissection in the absence of documented malignancy. In addition, many patients are not identified until recurrence ensues. As many as 19% of cases are initially interpreted as benign by pathologists.[18] Analysis of the US NCDB results found that only 13% of operations performed for parathyroid carcinoma were the recommended *en bloc* resection of tumor with adjacent structures and lymphatic tissue, while 60% underwent resection of parathyroid glands only, and 6% had excisional biopsies performed. The inadequacy of resection is further exemplified by the finding that 39% of cases did not report tumor size, suggesting that the cancer was disrupted or incompletely resected, which could result in seeding of the surgical bed.[20]

Analysis of results from the Swedish Cancer Registry found that only 44% of cases received the recommended operation for parathyroid carcinoma (tumor resection with partial or total thyroidectomy, with or without neck dissection).

Resection of tumor alone or multiple parathyroid glands occurred in 51% of cases. Multivariate analysis showed that patients treated with more extensive, *en bloc* operations had a longer relapse-free period and longer survival.[18] Analysis of the SEER database by Lee *et al.*[1] revealed that 79% of parathyroid cancers were resected by simple parathyroidectomy, whereas only 13% of patients underwent *en bloc* resection. These data highlight the difficulty both in differentiating benign from malignant disease intraoperatively, and in undertaking the appropriate resection.

A published series of seven cases suggests the importance of a complete initial operation. Two patients underwent *en bloc* resection of tumor and ipsilateral thyroid with adherent structures as well as ipsilateral central compartment lymph node dissection and ipsilateral thymectomy, with no adjuvant therapy. They were cured. The other five patients underwent lesser operations; three developed lung metastases and two died from recurrent or metastatic parathyroid carcinoma. Of note is that one of those five patients had a tumor resection alone that was read as complete, but local recurrence and lung metastases ensued and led to death from disease.[52] Patients with local recurrence or distant metastasis may be submitted to reoperation and metastasectomy, with the goal of reducing parathyroid hormone levels and hypercalcemia.[19,59] Parathyroid cancers metastasize via the lymphatic and hematogenous routes, with lung, bone, and liver being the most common distant metastatic sites. Multiple operations may be required.

In situations where the parathyroid carcinoma is identified during the final pathological examination, reoperation with excision of the ipsilateral thyroid lobe, contiguous structures, and lymph nodes (level IV, VI) may be considered if the patient remains hypercalcemic or pathological findings confirm extensive vascular or capsular invasion.[33]

The role of adjuvant radiation therapy in the management of parathyroid carcinoma remains undefined. The evidence available is limited because of small sample sizes and retrospective nature of the studies. Several small series studying radiation therapy in the adjuvant setting have seemed promising in prevention of local relapse in patients with locally advanced disease.[40,59] The results in patients with bulky recurrence have not been as favorable.[60] In a series from the MD Anderson Cancer Center,[40] six of 18 patients with the diagnosis of locally invasive disease received adjuvant radiation therapy (dosage between 50 to 63 Gy) within 2 months after surgery. Only one of six patients treated with adjuvant radiation developed recurrent disease compared with five of 12 patients who did not receive radiation treatment. The authors noted that five of eight patients with tumors whose invasive character was unrecognized had recurrence, compared with six of 18 with locally invasive disease, suggesting that radiation may decrease local relapse rates.

Chemotherapy has not been an effective treatment option for parathyroid carcinoma. Regimens including nitrogen mustard, adriamycin, dacarbazine, methotrexate, lomustine, cyclophosphamide, 5-fluorouracil, and others have been unsuccessful.[21,24,33,61–64] Further studies are required to evaluate newer treatment options including antiparathyroid hormone immunotherapy,[65] octreotide therapy to reduce parathyroid hormone secretion,[66] and telomerase inhibitors.[67–69] Despite the

Table 12.3 Recurrence and survival rates for parathyroid carcinoma.

Author	Number of patients	Recurrence incidence (%)	5-year survival (%)	10-year survival (%)
Kleinpeter et al.[52]	23	22	86	69
Busaidy et al.[40]	26	42	85	77
Hundahl et al.[20]	286	N/A	86	49
Sandelin et al.[18]	95	42	85	70

introduction of several new cytotoxic agents since our previous review, including the taxanes, gemcitabine, novel platinum complexes and a series of novel tyrosine kinase inhibitors and vascular inhibitors, there are no published series (or even case reports) that indicate their utility in the treatment of parathyroid carcinoma.

Calcium-reducing agents, including bisphosphonates, plicamycin, and calcitonin, have been utilized in the treatment of hypercalcemia secondary to parathyroid carcinoma with varying success and without durable effect.[2,21] Calcimimetics work by modulating the calcium receptor. They are molecules that allosterically modulate the calcium receptor selectively by increasing receptor sensitivity to ionized calcium levels, affecting the negative feedback loop and decreasing parathyroid hormone secretion from parathyroid cells.[70] This treatment has been successful in primary and secondary hyperparathyroidism and may have potential in treating hypercalcemia secondary to parathyroid carcinoma.[21,70]

Prognosis

Most parathyroid carcinomas are characterized by their slow, progressive, indolent course. Patient surveillance is important as most of these tumors recur. Reported rates range from 22% to 100%, perhaps owing in part to the fact that many cases are not appreciated until review at the time of recurrence.[18,40,51,52] This frequently occurs years after the initial presentation, so the recommended follow-up interval is not well established. Some authors recommend follow-up every 4–6 months.[33] The diagnosis is often assigned on the basis of recurrent hypercalcemia (often debilitating) and hyperparathyroidism. Metastases may occur through either lymphatic or hematogenous routes. The most common sites of recurrence are the cervical lymph nodes and the tumor bed (50–75%), followed by lung (22–40%), liver (10–28%), and bone (5–28%).[3,18,48] Other sites, such as brain, are reported, but rare.[71] Tumor can be detected by means of sestamibi, CT, and MRI.[52,58]

Schantz and Castleman reported a recurrence rate of 30% in 59 cases with a clear relationship between early recurrence and death from the disease. Ten patients had recurrence within 2 years of initial diagnosis and nine (90%) died from recurrent tumor. Eight patients had a recurrence more than 2 years after presentation and only three of the eight (38%) died of recurrent disease.[3] In a large series reporting on disease recurrence in 95 parathyroid carcinoma patients, the Swedish Cancer Registry found that the incidence of recurrence was 42% with an average time to recurrence of 33 months (range: 1–228 months). A significant advantage for *en bloc* resection was demonstrated

with a recurrence incidence of 21% after *en bloc* resection, versus 58% after tumor resection alone ($p=0.0002$ for recurrence, $p=0.003$ for survival).[18] This study is particularly important as it demonstrated that the initial type of operation, *en bloc* resection, has a statistically significant impact on recurrence and survival, a benefit that could not be established by smaller studies.[18,40,52]

Multivariate analysis of the Swedish Cancer Registry demonstrated that the type of operation (*en bloc* versus tumor resection) and histopathology (invasive versus atypical) were statistically significant factors correlating with both increased disease-free and overall survival.[18] Evaluation of the US NCDB found that tumor size and lymph node status had no significant impact on survival.[20]

Favorable long-term survival rates are sometimes seen in patients with parathyroid carcinoma. Five-year survival rates were reported as 85% from the US NCDB and Swedish Cancer Registry, and 50–90% in other series.[18,20,41,52] Ten-year survival of 49–77% has been reported.[18,20,52] A more recent review of cases from the SEER database reported overall 10-year survival rates of 68%.[1] The cause of death is hypercalcemia in the overwhelming majority of cases.[2,3,40,41] Table 12.3 shows recurrence and survival rates for parathyroid carcinoma.

Conclusion

Parathyroid carcinoma is an uncommon cause of primary hyperparathyroidism. The morbidity and mortality are related to hypercalcemia resulting from tumor production of parathyroid hormone. The initial goals of therapy for this cancer are complete removal of the tumor and prevention of recurrence.

It is important to be aware of preoperative findings that might suggest the diagnosis of parathyroid carcinoma. These include skeletal and renal complications from hypercalcemia, the presence of a palpable neck mass, and markedly elevated serum calcium and parathyroid hormone levels. Sestamibi scanning is the most sensitive noninvasive study for localization, while the addition of ultrasound can be helpful for identifying tumor invasion of surrounding structures. At operation for benign disease, it is essential to recognize findings indicative of parathyroid carcinoma, such as tumor invasion or adherence to surrounding structures. Otherwise, the best opportunity for cure will be lost.

The first-line treatment is adequate resection at the initial operation. This consists of *en bloc* resection of tumor, ipsilateral thyroid, adherent tissues, and regional lymphadenectomy (including the ipsilateral central compartment and lower cervical chain). Despite the morbidity of such an operation, surgeons who see a

Box 12.1 Summary of diagnosis and treatment of parathyroid carcinoma.

Presentation

- Skeletal and renal complications are common

Physical examination

- Palpable cervical mass

Laboratory values

- Calcium >14 mg/dL^{-1}
- Parathyroid hormone level increased >5×

Radiology

- Sestamibi, ultrasound

Operative findings

- *Gross*: gray-white tumor (>3 cm) adherent to or invading local tissue and structures
- *Micro*: invasion through gland capsule into surrounding tissue, lymphatics, and vessels

Treatment

- *En bloc* resection of tumor, adherent tissue and structures, ipsilateral thyroid, and ipsilateral lymphadenectomy of the central compartment and lower cervical chain
- For recurrence: reoperation and metastasectomy. Radiation has no established role. Chemotherapy has been ineffective

substantial number of patients with hyperparathyroidism should be prepared to undertake the curative procedure on clinical grounds. This represents a challenge for the profession.

The frequency of recurrence in parathyroid carcinoma is high but good long-term survival rates can be achieved. Operation is the most effective treatment for recurrence or metastasis. Second-line treatment options with calcium-reducing medications may serve a future role in reducing morbidity as advances are made. A summary of diagnosis and treatment of parathyroid carcinoma is given in Box 12.1.

References

1. Lee PK, *et al*. Trends in the incidence and treatment of parathyroid cancer in the United States. Cancer 2007; 109(9): 1736–41.
2. Obara T, Fujimoto Y. Diagnosis and treatment of patients with parathyroid carcinoma: an update and review. World J Surg 1991: 15(6): 738–44.
3. Schantz A, Castleman B. Parathyroid carcinoma. A study of 70 cases. Cancer 1973; 31(3): 600–5.
4. Favia G, *et al*. Parathyroid carcinoma: sixteen new cases and suggestions for correct management. World J Surg 1998; 22(12): 1225–30.
5. Skandalakis JE, *et al. Skandalakis' Surgical Anatomy: The Embryologic and Anatomic Basis of Modern Surgery*, vol. 1. New York: McGraw-Hill, 2004.
6. Doherty GM, Wells SA. Parathyroid glands. In: Greenfield LJ, Mulholland MW, Oldham KT, Zelenock GB, Lillemoe KD (eds). *Essentials of Surgery - Scientific Principles and Practice*. Philadelphia: Lippincott Williams and Wilkins, 1997. pp. 419–425.
7. Van Heerden JA, Smith SL. *Parathyroidectomy for Primary Hyperparathyroidism (Adenoma and Carcinoma)*, 3rd edn. Boston, Massachusetts: Little, Brown and Co, 1997.
8. Wang C. The anatomic basis of parathyroid surgery. Ann Surg 1976: 183(3): 271–5.
9. Hooghe L, Kinnaert P, van Geertruyden J. Surgical anatomy of hyperparathyroidism. Acta Chirurg Belg 1992; 92(1): 1–9.
10. Alveryd A. Parathyroid glands in thyroid surgeryI. Anatomy of parathyroid glands. II. Postoperative hypoparathyroidism – identification and autotransplantation of parathyroid glands. Acta Chirurg Scand 1968; 389: 1–120.
11. Raue F, *et al*. The role of the extracellular calcium-sensing receptor in health and disease. Exper Clin Endocrinol Diabetes 2006; 114(8): 397–405.
12. Mace AD, *et al*. Intra-operative parathyroid hormone monitoring using a laboratory based multichannel analyser. Clin Otolaryngol 2008; 33(2): 134–7.
13. Mandell DL, *et al*. The influence of intraoperative parathyroid hormone monitoring on the surgical management of hyperparathyroidism. Arch Otolaryngol Head Neck Surg 2001; 127(7): 821–7.
14. Carling T. Molecular pathology of parathyroid tumors. Trends Endocrinol Metab 2001; 12(2): 53–8.
15. Fujimoto Y, *et al*. Surgical treatment of ten cases of parathyroid carcinoma: importance of an initial en bloc tumor resection. World J Surg 1984; 8(3): 392–400.
16. Cope O. The study of hyperparathyroidism at the Massachusetts General Hospital. N Engl J Med 1966; 274(21): 1174–82.
17. Cope O, Nardi GL, Castleman B. Carcinoma of the parathyroid glands: 4 cases among 148 patients with hyperparathyroidism. Ann Surg 1953; 138(4): 661–71.
18. Sandelin K, *et al*. Prognostic factors in parathyroid cancer: a review of 95 cases. World J Surg 1992; 16(4): 724–31.
19. Iacobone M, Lumachi F, Favia G. Up-to-date on parathyroid carcinoma: analysis of an experience of 19 cases. J Surg Oncol 2004; 88(4): 223–8.
20. Hundahl SA, *et al*. Two hundred eighty-six cases of parathyroid carcinoma treated in the U.S. between 1985–1995: a National Cancer Data Base Report. The American College of Surgeons Commission on Cancer and the American Cancer Society. Cancer 1999; 86(3): 538–44.
21. Shane E. Clinical review 122: Parathyroid carcinoma. J Clin Endocrinol Metab 2001; 86(2): 485–93.
22. Koea JB, Shaw JH. Parathyroid cancer: biology and management. Surg Oncol 1999; 8(3): 155–65.
23. Harrison LB, Sessions RB, Hong WK (eds). *Head and Neck Cancer - A Multidisciplinary Approach*, 3rd edition. Philadelphia: Lippincott, Williams and Wilkins, 2009.
24. Mittendorf EA, McHenry CR. Parathyroid carcinoma. J Surg Oncol 2005; 89(3): 136–42.
25. Woodard GE, *et al*. Parafibromin, product of the hyperparathyroidism–jaw tumor syndrome gene HRPT2, regulates cyclin D1/PRAD1 expression. Oncogene 2005; 24(7): 1272–6.
26. Szabo J, *et al*. Hereditary hyperparathyroidism–jaw tumor syndrome: the endocrine tumor gene HRPT2 maps to chromosome 1q21–q31. Am J Hum Genet 1995; 56(4): 944–50.
27. Carpten JD, *et al*. HRPT2, encoding parafibromin, is mutated in hyperparathyroidism–jaw tumor syndrome. Nat Genet 2002; 32(4): 676–80.
28. Khan MW, *et al*. Parathyroid carcinoma in secondary and tertiary hyperparathyroidism. J Am Coll Surg 2004; 199(2): 312–19.
29. Shattuck TM, *et al*. Somatic and germ-line mutations of the HRPT2 gene in sporadic parathyroid carcinoma. N Engl J Med 2003; 349(18): 1722–9.
30. Howell VM, *et al*. HRPT2 mutations are associated with malignancy in sporadic parathyroid tumours. J Med Genet 2003; 40(9): 657–63.
31. Cetani F, *et al*. Genetic analyses of the HRPT2 gene in primary hyperparathyroidism: germline and somatic mutations in familial and sporadic parathyroid tumors. J Clin Endocrinol Metab 2004; 89(11): 5583–91.

32. Hewitt KM, *et al*. Aberrant methylation of the HRPT2 gene in parathyroid carcinoma. Ann Otol Rhinol Laryngol 2007; 116(12): 928–33.

33. Fang SH, Lal G. Parathyroid cancer. Endocr Pract 2011; 17(Suppl 1): 36–43.

34. Zhang C, *et al*. Parafibromin inhibits cancer cell growth and causes G1 phase arrest. Biochem Biophys Res Commun 2006; 350(1): 17–24.

35. Cryns VL, *et al*. Loss of the retinoblastoma tumor-suppressor gene in parathyroid carcinoma. N Engl J Med 1994; 330(11): 757–61.

36. Shattuck TM, *et al*. Mutational analyses of RB and BRCA2 as candidate tumour suppressor genes in parathyroid carcinoma. Clin Endocrinol 2003; 59(2): 180–9.

37. Hunt JL, *et al*. Allelic loss in parathyroid neoplasia can help characterize malignancy. Am J Surg Pathol 2005; 29(8): 1049–55.

38. Svedlund J, *et al*. Aberrant WNT/beta-catenin signaling in parathyroid carcinoma. Mol Cancer 2010; 9: 294.

39. Clayman GL, *et al*. Parathyroid carcinoma: evaluation and interdisciplinary management. Cancer 2004; 100(5): 900–5.

40. Busaidy NL, *et al*. Parathyroid carcinoma: a 22-year experience. Head Neck 2004; 26(8): 716–26.

41. Stojadinovic A, *et al*. Parathyroid neoplasms: clinical, histopathological, and tissue microarray-based molecular analysis. Hum Pathol 2003; 34(1): 54–64.

42. McKeown PP, McGarity WC, Sewell CW. Carcinoma of the parathyroid gland: is it overdiagnosed? A report of three cases. Am J Surg 1984; 147(2): 292–8.

43. Bondeson AG, Bondeson L, Thompson NW. Clinicopathological peculiarities in parathyroid disease with hypercalcaemic crisis. Eur J Surg 1993; 159(11–12): 613–17.

44. Delellis RA. Challenging lesions in the differential diagnosis of endocrine tumors: parathyroid carcinoma. Endocr Pathol 2008; 19(4): 221–5.

45. Marcocci C, *et al*. Parathyroid carcinoma. J Bone Mineral Res 2008; 23(12): 1869–80.

46. Gill AJ, *et al*. Loss of nuclear expression of parafibromin distinguishes parathyroid carcinomas and hyperparathyroidism–jaw tumor (HPT-JT) syndrome-related adenomas from sporadic parathyroid adenomas and hyperplasias. Am J Surg Pathol 2006: 30(9): 1140–9.

47. Thompson SD, Prichard AJ. The management of parathyroid carcinoma. Curr Opin Otolaryngol Head Neck Surg 2004; 12(2): 93–7.

48. Shaha AR, Shah JP. Parathyroid carcinoma: a diagnostic and therapeutic challenge. Cancer 1999; 86(3): 378–80.

49. Kameyama K, Takami H. Proposal for the histological classification of parathyroid carcinoma. Endocr Pathol 2005; 16(1): 49–52.

50. Wynne AG, *et al*. Parathyroid carcinoma: clinical and pathologic features in 43 patients. Medicine 1992; 71(4): 197–205.

51. Shane E, Bilezikian JP. Parathyroid carcinoma: a review of 62 patients. Endocr Rev 1982; 3(2): 218–26.

52. Kleinpeter KP, *et al*. Is parathyroid carcinoma indeed a lethal disease? Ann Surg Oncol 2005; 12(3): 260–6.

53. Holmes EC, Morton DL, Ketcham AS. Parathyroid carcinoma: a collective review. Ann Surg 1969; 169(4): 631–40.

54. Rubin MR, *et al*. Human chorionic gonadotropin measurements in parathyroid carcinoma. Eur J Endocrinol 2008; 159(4): 469–74.

55. Rubin MR, *et al*. An N-terminal molecular form of parathyroid hormone (PTH) distinct from hPTH(1 84) is overproduced in parathyroid carcinoma. Clin Chem 2007; 53(8): 1470–6.

56. Arslan N, Rydzewski B. Detection of a recurrent parathyroid carcinoma with FDG positron emission tomography. Clin Nucl Med 2002; 27(3): 221–2.

57. Kemps B, *et al*. Brown tumors simulating metastases on FDG PET in a patient with parathyroid carcinoma. Eur J Nucl Med Mol Imaging 2008; 35(4): 850.

58. Fraker DL. Update on the management of parathyroid tumors. Curr Opin Oncol 2000; 12(1): 41–8.

59. Munson ND, *et al*. Parathyroid carcinoma: is there a role for adjuvant radiation therapy? Cancer 2003; 98(11): 2378–84.

60. Kirkby-Bott J, *et al*. One stage treatment of parathyroid cancer. Eur J Surg Oncol 2005: 31(1): 78–83.

61. Chahinian AP, *et al*. Metastatic nonfunctioning parathyroid carcinoma: ultrastructural evidence of secretory granules and response to chemotherapy. Am J Med Sci 1981; 282(2): 80–4.

62. Chahinian AP. Chemotherapy for metastatic parathyroid carcinoma. Arch Intern Med 1984; 144(9): 1889.

63. Bukowski RM, *et al*. Successful combination chemotherapy for metastatic parathyroid carcinoma. Arch Intern Med 1984; 144(2): 399–400.

64. Calandra DB, *et al*. Parathyroid carcinoma: biochemical and pathologic response to DTIC. Surgery 1984. 96(6): 1132–7.

65. Betea D, *et al*. Hormonal and biochemical normalization and tumor shrinkage induced by anti-parathyroid hormone immunotherapy in a patient with metastatic parathyroid carcinoma. J Clin Endocrinol Metab 2004; 89(7): 3413–20.

66. Denney AM, Watts NB. The effect of octreotide on parathyroid carcinoma. J Clin Endocrinol Metab 2004; 89(2): 1016.

67. Pacini F, *et al*. Telomerase and the endocrine system. Nat Rev Endocrinol 2011; 7(7): 420–30.

68. Falchetti A, *et al*. Azidothymidine induces apoptosis and inhibits cell growth and telomerase activity of human parathyroid cancer cells in culture. J Bone Mineral Res 2005; 20(3): 410–18.

69. Kouniavsky G, Zeiger MA. The role of telomeres and telomerase in endocrine tumors. Discovery Med 2010; 10(53): 340–7.

70. Weigel RJ. Nonoperative management of hyperparathyroidism: present and future. Curr Opin Oncol 2001; 13(1): 33–8.

71. Kern M, *et al*. Intracranial metastatic parathyroid carcinoma. Case report and review of the literature. J Neurosurg 2004; 101(6): 1065–9.

13 Metaplastic Breast Carcinoma

Ingrid A. Mayer,[1] Helenice Gobbi,[3] and A. Bapsi Chakravarthy[2]

[1] Department of Medicine, [2] Department of Radiation Oncology, Vanderbilt University School of Medicine, Nashville, TN, USA
[3] Department of Pathology, Federal University of Minas Gerais, Belo Horizonte, MG, Brazil

Introduction

Metaplastic carcinoma represents less than 5% of all breast carcinomas and is a very heterogeneous disease. It is characterized by tumors containing both epithelial and mesenchymal cell types. The pathological phenotype is the best predictor of the clinical behaviour of metaplastic carcinoma. Due to its rarity, treatment decisions are made based on limited retrospective data. Following histological confirmation, surgical options should be discussed with the patient. However, the optimal adjuvant systemic therapy is unclear.

Historical background

The term metaplastic carcinoma is used for a heterogeneous group of tumors containing cells of both epithelial and mesenchymal phenotype. The metaplastic changes include epithelial (squamous) and sarcomatous elements (osseous, chondroid, loose spindle and fibromyxoid stroma, dense spindle and fibrosarcomatoid stroma).[1] Various synonyms have been used for similar lesions but the large number of terms has not helped to better understand the biology and prognosis of these tumors.[2] In the new WHO classification of breast tumors, metaplastic carcinomas were grouped as pure epithelial metaplastic carcinomas (including squamous cell carcinoma, adenocarcinoma with spindle cell metaplasia, adenosquamous carcinoma, and mucoepidermoid carcinoma) and mixed epithelial/mesenchymal metaplastic carcinomas.[3] The WHO classification is difficult to follow because spindle cell metaplastic carcinomas without admixed adenocarcinoma, heterologous elements or squamous differentiation are included in neither the "purely epithelial" nor the "mixed epithelial and mesenchymal" category.[4] The classification of metaplastic carcinomas into two main categories of monophasic ("sarcomatoid" or spindle cell carcinomas) and biphasic "sarcomatoid" carcinomas ("carcinosarcomas" or "malignant mixed tumors") would be more appropriate from a diagnostic point of view.[2]

Biology and epidemiology

Metaplastic carcinoma is a rare disease with heterogeneous pathological features. The incidence of metaplastic carcinoma represents less than 5% of breast malignancies. Due to its rarity, treatment decisions are made primarily based on retrospective data. The prognosis is variable depending on the degree of mesenchymal component in the tumor. Five-year survival rates range from 40% to 65%.

An accurate assessment of the incidence of metaplastic breast cancers is difficult because these tumors have been designated under a variety of names, and authors tend to report incidence based on specific subtypes. There are many examples in the literature of initial "misdiagnosis." High-grade monophasic tumors have been classified as pure sarcomas and low-grade spindle cell metaplastic tumors are often misinterpreted as fibromatosis.[5-7] Metaplastic carcinomas may arise within fibrosclerotic breast lesions such as papillomas, complex sclerosing lesions, and nipple adenomas.[8,9] Two main variants of low-grade metaplastic tumors are described in association with fibrosclerotic lesions: fibromatosis-like tumors[5] and adenosquamous carcinoma.[8] The neoplastic nature of such low-grade tumors is sometimes difficult to distinguish from reactive myofibroblastic proliferation that can occur within complex sclerosing lesions and papillomas.[10]

A recent report by Hennessy *et al.*[11] compared 28 metaplastic carcinomas of the breast with common breast cancers using comparative genomic hybridization, transcriptional profiling, and reverse-phase protein arrays and by sequencing for common breast cancer mutations. Their findings suggest that metaplastic carcinomas showed unique DNA copy number aberrations compared with common breast cancers. A statistically significantly higher proportion of *PIK3CA* mutations were detected in metaplastic carcinomas, compared to the other subsets of breast cancers. By transcriptional profiling, metaplastic breast cancers are characterized by low expression of GATA3-regulated genes and of genes responsible for cell–cell adhesion with enrichment for markers linked to stem cell function and epithelial-to-mesenchymal transition (EMT). In contrast to other breast cancers, most metaplastic carcinomas showed a significant similarity to a "tumorigenic" signature defined using CD44[+]/CD24[-] breast tumor-initiating stem cell-like cells. These data suggest that metaplastic carcinomas may arise from an earlier, more chemoresistant breast epithelial precursor than other types of breast cancers.

Another small series analyzed a variety of tumor markers in archived, paraffin-embedded blocks from six primary metaplastic carcinomas, and found a high frequency of p53 overexpression/mutation, high levels of e-cadherin, and high frequency of the angiogenesis markers vascular endothelial growth factor (VEGF) and hypoxia-inducible factor (HIF)-1α expression.[12]

Pathology

Gross pathology

Metaplastic tumors show no specific macroscopic features, but the majority of cases have been reported to be circumscribed, hard, and rubbery. Tumors range in size from 0.5 to 21 cm, with an average size of 3–5 cm. Heterologous elements, especially bone and cartilage, may be evident on gross examination. Tumors which are predominantly squamous may have cystic degeneration.[7,13–15] Although spindle cell carcinomas are often grossly spiculated or well circumscribed, microscopically they show a more infiltrative border.[5,7]

Microscopic appearances

Because the microscopic pathology of metaplastic breast tumors is so varied, multiple histological sections are necessary for an accurate diagnosis of these lesions and to determine whether the tumor is monophasic of pure spindle cell pattern or of biphasic epithelial and mesenchymal morphology.[2] Although in most cases two patterns, dominant and minor, are recognized, often more are intermixed. The most common pattern of metaplastic tumors is the spindle cell pattern, which can be pure or in combination with squamous, glandular or sarcomatous elements, such as bone, cartilage, and osteoclastic-like giant cells.

Spindle cell metaplastic carcinoma

Tumors composed of dominant spindle cells frequently associated with an invasive squamous or glandular component are referred to as *monophasic* sarcomatous carcinoma or spindle cell metaplastic carcinomas. The spindle cells in these tumors can vary from a relatively bland appearance to aggressive patterns resembling high-grade sarcomas.[7] The lowest-grade spindle cell metaplastic tumors show low cellularity intermixed with more fibromyxoid stroma, with only sparse recognizable squamous or glandular elements closely mimicking fibromatosis (Fig. 13.1). We chose the term "fibromatosis-like metaplastic tumors" for such lesions to avoid the word carcinomas because neither the phenotype nor the behavior is that of a carcinoma.[5,16]

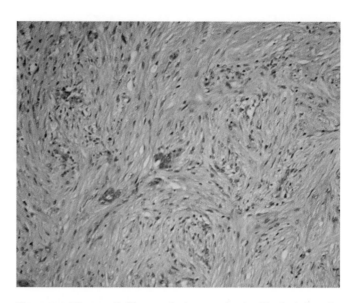

Figure 13.1 Fibromatosis-like metaplastic tumor showing bland spindle cell proliferation with few glandular elements (*center and left*) (H&E, 200×).

In tumors that are almost entirely composed of spindle cells, the epithelial elements may be difficult to recognize.[7,17,18] The spindle cells coexpress myoepithelial (actins, p63, CD10, maspin, P-cadherin) and mesenchymal markers such as vimentin. The consistent expression of myoepithelial markers in spindle cell metaplastic carcinomas is helpful in the diagnosis and indicates myoepithelial differentiation of such tumors.[4,5,19,20] The spindle cells of metaplastic carcinomas are usually negative for estrogen receptor (ER) and progesterone receptor (PR) and HER2/neu. Positivity, when present in these tumors, is confined to the adenocarcinomatous component.[21]

Adenosquamous carcinoma

Adenosquamous carcinoma is a variant of metaplastic carcinoma composed of small glandular structures intimately admixed with variable amounts of solid nests of squamous differentiation in a collagenous stroma (Fig. 13.2).[13,22] Squamous metaplasia varies from syringoma-like differentiation, well-differentiated keratinizing areas to poorly differentiated nonkeratinizing foci. Although benign squamous metaplasia has been described in different types of benign lesions and invasive mammary carcinomas (representing less than 5–10% of the tumor), the term "metaplastic carcinoma" is reserved for tumors that show metaplasia as a dominant pattern.[10,13] The squamous component is negative for ER, PR, and HER2/neu while the positivity of the glandular component is dependent on its degree of differentiation.[21]

Primary squamous carcinoma of the breast denotes a carcinoma entirely composed of metaplastic squamous cells with no connection to the skin or continuity with the nipple. Tumors with less squamous differentiation are referred to as adenocarcinomas with extensive squamous differentiation or adenosquamous carcinomas. Squamous cell carcinomas assume several phenotypes including keratinizing, nonkeratinizing or spindled.[3,23]

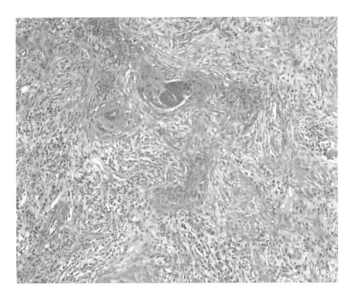

Figure 13.2 Low-grade adenosquamous metaplastic carcinoma showing islands of squamous cells merging with the spindle cells (H&E, 200×).

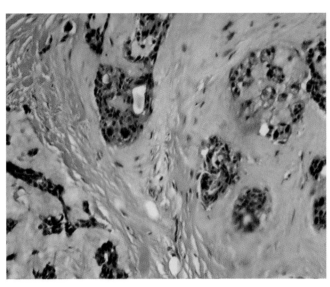

Figure 13.3 Matrix-producing metaplastic carcinoma presenting groups of epithelial cells within condromyxoid stroma (H&E, 200×).

Metaplastic carcinoma with sarcomatous metaplasia

A broad range of patterns is seen in this wide variety of tumors, including those designated as "matrix producing carcinomas" (Fig. 13.3) and carcinosarcomas.[3] These tumors are composed of infiltrating carcinoma mixed with spindle cells and heterologous elements ranging from bland chondroid and osseous differentiation to high-grade sarcomas including fibrosarcoma, malignant fibrous histiocytoma, osteosarcoma, chondrosarcoma, liposarcoma, rhabdomyosarcoma, and leiomyosarcoma. The epithelial component of the sarcomatous metaplastic carcinomas may have squamous features, but it is more commonly of ductal nonspecial type and usually of grade 2 or 3 morphology.[3] When the mesenchymal component is malignant, the designation of carcinosarcoma has been used.[3,14] Some authors use the term "pseudosarcomatous" to describe these lesions.[24] Although heterologous elements, such as bone and cartilage, may be associated with metaplastic carcinoma, foci of benign heterologous elements may also be present in other mammary carcinomas without known adverse clinical implications.[25]

The majority of biphasic sarcomatous carcinomas are negative for ER, PR, and HER2/neu in both the adenocarcinoma and the mesenchymal elements. The spindle cells may show focal positivity for cytokeratin and p63.[19,21,25]

Grade

The proportion and grading of epithelial and sarcomatous elements present in metaplastic tumors of the breast would be expected to have potential clinical relevance.[5,16] However, in most published series a correlation of histological grade and prognosis has not been considered, despite the accepted clinical utility of histological grading in both soft tissue sarcoma and mammary carcinoma.[7] Similarly, grading of sarcomatous elements in metaplastic carcinomas would be expected to have

potential clinical relevance. It is also important to grade the carcinomatous component when it is significant in extent. In general, most cases with predominant squamous and glandular lesions are intermediate- to high-grade adenocarcinomas with areas of squamous metaplasia of similar grade. It is recommended that squamous carcinomas should be graded based mainly on nuclear features and, to a lesser degree, cytoplasmic differentiation.[3]

Clinical aspects: presentation, diagnostic considerations, and techniques

As these tumors can contain both carcinomatous and mesenchymal elements, it is likely that the clinical behavior will also be a combination of these two elements. The average ages at diagnosis and clinical presentation of metaplastic carcinomas are similar to those for the more common invasive mammary carcinomas. In spite of the variety of histological patterns of metaplastic breast carcinomas, most patients present with a solitary, nontender palpable mass or a mammographic density.

Metaplastic carcinomas may present as a density on mammography and a microlobulated mass on ultrasonography. Although microcalcifications are usually absent, large coarse calcifications have been associated with metaplastic tumors with osteosarcomatous elements. Complex echogenicity with solid and cystic components may be seen sonographically and high signal intensity on T2-weighted MRI. These image features are related to necrosis and cystic degeneration found histopathologically.[26–28]

Due to its heterogeneous histopathological pattern, the use of fine needle aspiration to diagnose metaplastic carcinoma has been considered limited with a relatively high false-negative rate.[29] The accuracy of preoperative diagnosis by this method is reported to be approximately 50%.

The final diagnoses of cases initially misdiagnosed as metaplastic carcinomas using cytology have included both benign and malignant conditions. The carcinomatous components are usually easily identified, but the squamous and/or sarcomatous components are generally less obvious.[30] The use of core needle biopsy and mammatome is also limited in the diagnosis of metaplastic carcinomas, and the final diagnosis should be made after complete excision and adequate histopathological examination of the entire tumor.[31]

Treatment

Metaplastic carcinoma is a very rare and heterogeneous disease. Although there are several series describing the pathological findings of this disease, these consist of generally less than 25 patients accrued over many years and treated with many different modalities.

Locoregional treatment: surgery and radiation

Retrospective series generally describe mastectomy as the surgery most commonly performed for these patients. Although some of these small retrospective studies have remarked on the use of radiation, they have not distinguished between radiation used as a component of breast conservation and postmastectomy radiation.[32] In a retrospective analysis from the MD Anderson Cancer Center (MDACC), 100 sarcomatoid breast cancer patients have been identified. All but one had surgery and 54% have had radiation as a component of treatment. Although 50% of first recurrences were local, the abstract does not report whether this was more common in patients who did not receive postoperative radiation.[33]

A retrospective analysis of patients with metaplastic breast carcinoma diagnosed from 1988 to 2006 was performed, utilizing the Surveillance, Epidemiology, and End Results (SEER) database.[34] Among 1501 patients, radiation was given to 580 (38.6%). Almost half of the patients had tumors between 2 and 5 cm, and 70% had high-grade tumors. About half of the patients underwent mastectomy as their definitive surgery; the other half had lumpectomies. Ten-year overall survival and disease-specific survival rates were 53.2% and 68.3%, respectively. In the overall analysis, patients receiving radiation therapy demonstrated 36% and 26% decreases in death from any cause and breast-related mortality, respectively. Roughly 25% of mastectomy patients received radiation therapy (RT), due to tumors ≥5 cm or greater than four metastatic axillary lymph nodes. Mastectomy patients who received RT demonstrated a 33% decreased risk of death from all-cause mortality. These findings seem to support the use of adjuvant radiation for patients with metaplastic breast carcinoma.

Systemic treatment: chemotherapy

Adjuvant systemic therapy has not been routinely administered for metaplastic carcinoma. The few reported series in which chemotherapy, radiation therapy, or the combination was administered in the adjuvant setting cover an admixture of tumors, including those with both predominant epithelial and mesenchymal components.[7,23,24,35,36] In a review of the Mayo Clinic experience of 28 patients with pathology-reviewed

primary metaplastic carcinoma, 13 of them received adjuvant systemic therapy.[37] These mostly consisted of "standard" regimens containing anthracycline and tamoxifen for women with ER- and/or PR-positive tumors. Since no difference was observed in the rate or recurrence between patients who did and did not receive adjuvant therapy, the authors suggest that the use of "standard" regimens for adenocarcinoma of the breast may be relatively ineffective for metaplastic breast cancer.

Conversely, in an MDACC review series,[32] in the 50 patients identified with metaplastic cancer of the breast, the addition of systemic chemotherapy with anthracycline-containing regimens to mastectomy (but not to wide local excision) yielded statistically significant better recurrence rates, particularly in stage II disease. In a more recent retrospective review of 100 patients from MDACC with sarcomatoid/ metaplastic carcinoma of the breast,[33] no differences were observed in the 5-year relapse-free survival between patients who did and did not receive adjuvant chemotherapy, although a total of three patients treated with an anthracycline/ifosfamide-based regimen did remain recurrence free.

Once distant disease develops, patients uniformly do poorly. The vast majority of patients die from their disease. A small retrospective single-institution series from Japan observed a modest response rate to taxane-containing regimens in the metastatic treatment of metaplastic carcinomas.[38]

Metaplastic carcinomas are rarely estrogen and/or progesterone positive.[7] Nevertheless, in those patients who are hormone positive, we would recommend the use of hormonal therapy using the same guidelines as those used for the more common infiltrating ductal carcinomas, despite the seeming lack of efficacy in this setting. Although metaplastic carcinomas are rarely HER2/neu amplified, they often express HER1. This raises the intriguing possibility of exploring treatments with EFGR tyrosine kinase inhibitors in selected patients in the context of clinical trials.[39]

In view of reports of the high frequency of the angiogenesis markers VEGF and HIF-1α[12] and higher proportion of *PIK3CA* mutations in metaplastic breast carcinomas,[11] Moulder et al. initiated a single-institution phase 1 trial where patients with metastatic metaplastic carcinoma were treated with a combination of liposomal doxorubicin, bevacizumab (a monoclonal antibody against VEGF) and temsirolimus (an mTOR inhibitor).[40] The first five patients in the study had metastatic high-grade sarcomatoid metaplastic carcinoma, and all had been previously treated with docetaxel in the adjuvant or metastatic setting. The first two patients in the trial achieved a complete response and partial response, respectively. Neither of them had previous exposure to anthracyclines. One patient had stable disease for approximately 6 months, despite previous anthracycline exposure. The two patients that were heavily pretreated with several lines of chemotherapeutics, including anthracyclines and taxanes, developed disease progression.

Prognosis

Metaplastic carcinomas represent a heterogeneous and rare group of tumors whose prognosis is unclear since much of the data are derived from small cases series.[2,6,8,27] The best predictor for the clinical behavior of metaplastic carcinoma is the phenotype. This approach is helpful in tumors with pure mesenchymal appearance. However, metaplastic carcinoma may contain significant components of both invasive mammary carcinoma and mesenchymal neoplasm. In this setting, one might predict the tumor to behave with the combined potential of each of the components taken separately.[1] The clinical behavior of the low-grade fibromatosis-like metaplastic tumors appears to be that of fibromatosis with a tendency for local recurrence and low or no metastatic potential.[5,9] Low-grade adenosquamous carcinomas also have an excellent prognosis, but a small number of cases can behave in a locally aggressive manner. Recurrence appears to be related to the adequacy of local excision.[13] Lymph node metastases in these tumors are extremely rare. The higher grade biphasic sarcomatous carcinomas tend to behave more like sarcomas, with a potential for both local recurrence and distant metastases, especially via hematogenous spread to the lung.[41]

In general, the incidence of lymph node metastases in metaplastic carcinoma is much lower when compared to invasive ductal carcinoma of similar size, ranging between 5% and 26%. The likelihood of lymph node involvement with metaplastic carcinoma may be a reflection of the amount and grade of epithelial elements.[3] Low-grade lesions such as matrix-producing metaplastic carcinoma and low-grade adenosquamous carcinoma appear to have an extremely low incidence of metastases to regional lymph nodes.[3,22] Tumors which consist predominantly of epithelial elements tend to behave similarly to carcinomas and may have lymph node involvement by the epithelial elements. In contrast, the mesenchymal elements of sarcomatous metaplasia of the breast typically do not metastasize to regional lymph. Tumors which consist predominantly of high-grade mesenchymal elements tend to behave like pure sarcomas and spread hematogenously to distant sites.[16] Although some series have found no correlation between lymph node involvement and prognosis, this is likely due to the small number of patients involved in these studies.

The pattern of progression is usually that of local recurrence followed by metastases to the lungs followed by spread to other anatomical sites. However, patients with low-grade tumors, such as fibromatosis-like and adenosquamous, usually present with local recurrences but no distant metastases.[9,22,42] Recurrence appears to be related to the extent of initial surgery. Patients undergoing excisional biopsy had higher rates of local recurrence than patients undergoing mastectomy. The increased recurrence rate after excisional biopsy alone for the low-grade tumors did not translate into increased mortality.[5,42] Some authors reported a correlation between size of the primary metaplastic tumor in the breast and recurrence rates as well as survival. Tumors that are larger in size are more likely to recur and patients are more likely to die of disease.[3]

In general, 5-year survival rates of metaplastic carcinoma made up predominantly of epithelial elements are reported around 65%, comparable to ductal carcinoma of similar size.[2,3] The presence of squamous metaplasia appears to have no effect on the clinical behavior of the breast lesion with which it is associated. Patients with biphasic sarcomatoid carcinomas appear to have a very poor prognosis and lower survival rate, with 5-year survival around 40%.[2] However, Wargotz and Norris reported a 5-year survival of 64% for patients with the "matrix-producing" subtype of metaplastic carcinoma.[15]

Recommendations

Following histological confirmation of the diagnosis, surgical options should be discussed with the patient. Breast conservation should be offered to patients who can obtain a margin-negative excision. Adjuvant systemic therapy with anthracycline-containing regimens should be discussed with patients who have a component of adenocarcinoma or when lymph nodes are involved. Tamoxifen or aromatase inhibitors should be considered in patients with ER- and/or PR-positive tumors. There is a paucity of data on metastatic management of this disease, but it seems reasonable to use those agents found to be most active in ductal carcinoma if the largest component is adenocarcinoma or agents used in sarcomas if the sarcomatoid features are most prevalent in the metastatic lesion. Clinical trial participation should be encouraged.

Given the lack of prospective data on the role of radiation in the treatment of metaplastic carcinomas, we have generally applied the same criteria as used in the treatment of soft tissue sarcomas in other sites. If a lumpectomy with negative margins (at least 2 mm) can be achieved then postlumpectomy radiation to a total dose of 6000 cGy is utilized. Radiation therapy is used to maximize local control without sacrificing cosmetic results. If the tumor size or breast:tumor ratio precludes breast conservation, mastectomy would be recommended. If the tumor can be removed with wide surgical margins (≥2 cm), postmastectomy radiation would not be recommended. If the margins are close, postmastectomy radiation to a total dose of 6000 cGy should be considered. We would treat the regional nodes only if four or more lymph nodes were involved at the time of axillary dissection.

References

1. Page DLA, Anderson TJ. Uncommon types of invasive carcinoma. In: Page DLA, Anderson TJ (eds) *Diagnostic Histopathology of the Breast*. Edinburgh: Churchill Livingstone, 1987. pp.236–52.

2. Pinder SE, Elston CW, Ellis IO. Invasive carcinoma – unusual histological types. In: Elston CW, Ellis IO (eds) *The Breast*. Edinburgh: Churchill Livingstone, 1998. pp.283–337.

3. Ellis IO SS, *et al*. Invasive breast carcinoma. In: Tavassoli F DP (ed) *WHO Classification of Tumours: Pathology and Genetics of Tumours of the Breast and Female Genital Organs*. Lyon, France: IARC Press, 2003. pp.13–59.

4. Leibl S, Gogg-Kammerer M, Sommersacher A, Denk H, Moinfar F. Metaplastic breast carcinomas: are they of myoepithelial differentiation? Immunohistochemical profile of the sarcomatoid subtype using novel myoepithelial markers. Am J Surg Pathol 2005; 29: 347–53.

5. Gobbi H, Simpson JF, Borowsky A, Jensen RA, Page DL. Metaplastic breast tumors with a dominant fibromatosis-like phenotype have a high risk of local recurrence. Cancer 1999; 85: 2170–82.

6. Gersell DJ, Katzenstein AL. Spindle cell carcinoma of the breast. A clinicopathologic and ultrastructural study. Hum Pathol 1981; 12: 550–61.

7. Wargotz ES, Deos PH, Norris HJ. Metaplastic carcinomas of the breast. II. Spindle cell carcinoma. Hum Pathol 1989; 20: 732–40.

8. Denley H, *et al*. Metaplastic carcinoma of the breast arising within complex sclerosing lesion: a report of five cases. Histopathology 2000; 36: 203–9.

9. Gobbi H, Simpson JF, Jensen RA, Olson SJ, Page DL. Metaplastic spindle cell breast tumors arising within papillomas, complex sclerosing lesions, and nipple adenomas. Mod Pathol 2003; 16: 893–901.

10. Gobbi H, Tse G, Page DL, Olson SJ, Jensen RA, Simpson JF. Reactive spindle cell nodules of the breast after core biopsy or fine-needle aspiration. Am J Clin Pathol 2000; 113: 288–94.

11. Hennessy BT, *et al*. Characterization of a naturally occurring breast cancer subset enriched in epithelial-to-mesenchymal transition and stem cell characteristics. Cancer Res 2009; 69: 4116–24.

12. Kochhar R, Howard EM, Umbreit JN, Lau SK. Metaplastic breast carcinoma with squamous differentiation: molecular and clinical analysis of six cases. Breast J 2005; 11: 367–9.

13. Rosen PP, Oberman HA. Invasive carcinoma. In: *Tumors of the Mammary Gland*. Washington, DC: Armed Forces Institute of Pathology, 1993. pp.157–257.

14. Wargotz ES, Norris HJ. Metaplastic carcinomas of the breast. III. Carcinosarcoma. Cancer 1989; 64: 1490–9.

15. Wargotz ES, Norris HJ. Metaplastic carcinomas of the breast. I. Matrix-producing carcinoma. Hum Pathol 1989; 20: 628–35.

16. Borowsky A, Gobbi H. Metaplastic carcinoma of the breast: grading and behavior of predominantly spindle cell tumors. Pathol Case Rev 1999; 4: 208–13.

17. Adem C, Reynolds C, Adlakha H, Roche PC, Nascimento AG. Wide spectrum screening keratin as a marker of metaplastic spindle cell carcinoma of the breast: an immunohistochemical study of 24 patients. Histopathology 2002; 40: 556–62.

18. Kurian KM, Al-Nafussi A. Sarcomatoid/metaplastic carcinoma of the breast: a clinicopathological study of 12 cases. Histopathology 2002; 40: 58–64.

19. Reis-Filho JS, *et al*. Novel and classic myoepithelial/stem cell markers in metaplastic carcinomas of the breast. Appl Immunohistochem Mol Morphol 2003; 11: 1–8.

20. Koker MM, Kleer CG. p63 expression in breast cancer: a highly sensitive and specific marker of metaplastic carcinoma. Am J Surg Pathol 2004; 28: 1506–12.

21. Barnes PJ, Boutilier R, Chiasson D, Rayson D. Metaplastic breast carcinoma: clinical-pathologic characteristics and HER2/neu expression. Breast Cancer Res Treat 2005; 91: 173–8.

22. Rosen PP, Ernsberger D. Low-grade adenosquamous carcinoma. A variant of metaplastic mammary carcinoma. Am J Surg Pathol 1987; 11: 351–8.

23. Wargotz ES, Norris HJ. Metaplastic carcinomas of the breast. IV. Squamous cell carcinoma of ductal origin. Cancer 1990; 65: 272–6.

24. Kaufman MW, Marti JR, Gallager HS, Hoehn JL. Carcinoma of the breast with pseudosarcomatous metaplasia. Cancer 1984; 53: 1908–17.

25. Popnikolov NK, Ayala AG, Graves K, Gatalica Z. Benign myoepithelial tumors of the breast have immunophenotypic characteristics similar to metaplastic matrix-producing and spindle cell carcinomas. Am J Clin Pathol 2003; 120: 161–7.

26. Chang YW, *et al*. Magnetic resonance imaging of metaplastic carcinoma of the breast: sonographic and pathologic correlation. Acta Radiol 2004; 45: 18–22.

27. Gunhan-Bilgen I, Memis A, Ustun EE, Zekioglu O, Ozdemir N. Metaplastic carcinoma of the breast: clinical, mammographic, and sonographic findings with histopathologic correlation. Am J Roentgenol 2002; 178: 1421–5.

28. Velasco M, *et al*. MRI of metaplastic carcinoma of the breast. Am J Roentgenol 2005; 184: 1274–8.

29. Ribeiro-Silva A, Luzzatto F, Chang D, Zucoloto S. Limitations of fine-needle aspiration cytology to diagnose metaplastic carcinoma of the breast. Pathol Oncol Res 2001; 7: 298–300.

30. Johnson TL, Kini SR. Metaplastic breast carcinoma: a cytohistologic and clinical study of 10 cases. Diagn Cytopathol 1996; 14: 226–32.

31. Hoda SA, Rosen PP. Observations on the pathologic diagnosis of selected unusual lesions in needle core biopsies of breast. Breast J 2004; 10: 522–7.

32. Gutman H, Pollock RE, Janjan NA, Johnston DA. Biologic distinctions and therapeutic implications of sarcomatoid metaplasia of epithelial carcinoma of the breast. J Am Coll Surg 1995; 180: 193–9.

33. Hennessy B, Giordano S, Broglio K, Hortobagyi GN, Valero V. Sarcomatoid (metaplastic) carcinoma of the breast: the U.T. M. D. Anderson Cancer Center (MDACC) and SEER database experience. Proceedings of the American Society of Clinical Oncology, 2005, Orlando, FL. J Clin Oncol 2005; 23(16 S Pt 1): 614.

34. Tseng W, Martinez S. Metaplastic breast cancer: to radiate or not to radiate? Ann Surg Oncol 2011; 18: 94–103.

35. Lazarevic B, Katatikarn V, Marks RA. Primary squamous-cell carcinoma of the breast. Diagnosis by fine needle aspiration cytology. Acta Cytol 1984; 28: 321–4.

36. Toikkanen S. Primary squamous cell carcinoma of the breast. Cancer 1981; 48: 1629–32.

37. Rayson D, Adjei AA, Suman VJ, Wold LE, Ingle JN. Metaplastic breast cancer: prognosis and response to systemic therapy. Ann Oncol 1999; 10: 413–19.

38. Chen IC, *et al*. Lack of efficacy to systemic chemotherapy for treatment of metaplastic carcinoma of the breast in the modern era. Breast Cancer Res Treat 2011; 130(1): 345–51.

39. Leibl S, Moinfar F. Metaplastic breast carcinomas are negative for Her-2 but frequently express EGFR (Her-1): potential relevance to adjuvant treatment with EGFR tyrosine kinase inhibitors? J Clin Pathol 2005; 58: 700–4.

40. Moulder S, *et al*. Responses to liposomal doxorubicin, bevacizumab, and temsirolimus in metaplastic carcinoma of the breast: biologic rationale and implications for stem-cell research in breast cancer. J Clin Oncol 2011; 29: e572–5.

41. Pitts WC, *et al*. Carcinomas with metaplasia and sarcomas of the breast. Am J Clin Pathol 1991; 95: 623–32.

42. Sneige N, *et al*. Low-grade (fibromatosis-like) spindle cell carcinoma of the breast. Am J Surg Pathol 2001; 25: 1009–16.

14 Adenoid Cystic Carcinoma of the Breast

Melinda E. Sanders,[1] Masako Kasami,[3] Julie Means-Powell,[2] and David L. Page[1]

[1] Department of Pathology, [2] Department of Medicine, Vanderbilt University School of Medicine, Nashville, TN, USA
[3] Shizuoka Cancer Center, Shizuoka Prefecture, Japan

Introduction and historical background

Adenoid cystic carcinoma (ACC) of the breast, when properly and rigidly defined, accounts for about 0.1% of all invasive breast malignancies. Strict criteria were identified by the 1970s, aided by the use of electron microscopic features and histochemistry that recognized the orderly arrangement of dichotomous features.[1] Carcinomas of this type and of similar histopathology have been described in the literature by a variety of terms, including carcinoma adenoides cysticum, adenocystic carcinoma, pseudoadenomatous basal cell carcinoma, adenocystic basal cell cancer, basaloma, adenomyoepithelioma, cylindromatous carcinoma, and adenocystic basaloid carcinoma.[1,2] Unfortunately, there is no guarantee that these related terms will identify cases we now diagnose as ACC based on strictly defined histological features. "Adenocystic" has been used generically for tumors of similar patterns, probably including what we now call "invasive cribriform carcinoma."[1]

Adenoid cystic carcinoma was initially described by Billroth in 1856.[3] However, the term ACC of the breast, which is first credited to Spies in 1930[4] and later Geschicter in 1945,[5] is the appropriate specific term for this special tumor type.

Biology and epidemiology

Carcinomas termed "ACC" occur in many sites, including the major and minor salivary glands, lacrimal glands, maxillary sinuses, nasopharynx, external ear, esophagus, skin, tongue, trachea, bronchi, uterus, cervix, and Bartholin's glands.[2,6–8] ACC of the breast is so named because of its microscopic similarity to these tumors of the same name. Despite its rarity in the breast, it is important to be aware of the unique, defining elements of ACC because of its excellent prognosis at this site. This starkly contrasts with its behavior elsewhere, as well as the behavior of similarly appearing cancers of the breast. An important observation associates the origin of some ACC with

examples of microglandular adenosis (MGA)[9] and ACC *in situ* involving intraductal papillomas.[10]

Adenoid cystic carcinoma of the breast accounts for about 0.1% of all invasive breast malignancies.[1] Age at diagnosis is varied, with a range from 31 to 90 years. Incidence rates increase prominently at age 35–44 years, with a less marked rise in older ages and an apparent plateau beginning at 55–64 years.[11] ACC is more common in whites than in African-American women.[11]

In sharp contrast to similar tumors in other organs, ACC presenting in the breast is much less aggressive. In most instances, the tumor grows slowly[1,2–14] and has a low malignant potential.[14] It is unusual for patients to have metastases at the time of diagnosis; however, these tumors can recur both locally, likely as a result of inadequate excision, and rarely with limited patterns of metastatic disease many years after initial presentation. In fact, ACC of the breast has been reported to recur more than 20 years after diagnosis.[13] Nevertheless, patients may live for many years following documented distant metastases[15,16] and most of the few reported deaths from mammary ACC are aberrant high-grade examples or lack clear case definition and histological verification.[17–25] Most recent studies report 10-year survival rates of 95%.[11,26]

Molecular biology and genetics

Recurrent translocations in epithelial tumors are uncommon and in the breast have been previously reported only in secretory carcinomas.[27] Persson *et al.*[28] recently reported a t(6;9)(q22-23;p23-24) translocation in ACC of the breast and head and neck. This translocation results in fusions encoding "gain-of-function" chimeric transcripts predominantly consisting of MYB exon 14 linked to the last coding exon(s) of NFIB. These fusions all result in deletion of micro-RNA target sites in MYB exon 15 which are responsible for negative regulation of MYB expression. Deletion of these sites likely results in disruption of

MYB repression, leading to activation of critical MYB targets, including genes associated with apoptosis, cell cycle control, cell growth/angiogenesis, and cell–cell adhesion.

Mutations in genes encoding members of the phosphoinositide-3-kinase (PIK3CA) pathway have been recently reported in approximately 30% of breast cancers.[29–31] The PIK3CA pathway is one of the most important pathways in cancer metabolism and growth.[29] Vranic *et al.*[32] report the coexistence of mutations in both PIK3CA (Ex1 + 169 A>C) and PTEN (IVS4-3 C>T) in a putative mammary ACC and a subsequent renal metastasis. These specific mutations have not been previously reported. Until a larger number of well-characterized cases can be tested, the significance of these mutations is unclear. However, their presence raises the possibility that mTOR inhibitors may be useful in rare patients with metastatic disease.[33]

Although ACC of the breast is uniformly negative for estrogen receptor as typically tested by antibodies against the full-length estrogen receptor α (ER-α66), a recent study including 11 cases of pure ACC of the breast demonstrated strong positivity for ER-α36, a novel isoform of ER-α66 which localizes to the cytoplasm on the cell membrane, in eight cases.[34] ER-α36 mediates nonclassic nongenomic estrogen signaling, which includes activation of the mitogen-activated protein kinase (MAPK/ERK) signaling pathway.[35,36] The significance of this expression is unclear in ACC but it is certainly consistent with the reported lack of utility of antiestrogen therapy in ACC.[18]

Pathology

Breast cancer classification

Among the several carefully defined special types of breast cancer, ACC is a prime example of the necessity of strictly defining a set of pathological features that guarantee a unique, usually excellent clinical behavior and prognosis.[37–39] Unlike other special types of invasive breast cancer,[40,41] ACC does not appear to be enriched in screening settings, although this phenomenon may not be discernible because of the rarity of ACC. In general, the special types of breast cancer, including ACC, are associated with a very good to excellent overall survival, as is readily identified by their greatly increased representation in 20-year survivors of invasive breast cancer.[42]

Histopathology of adenoid cystic carcinoma of the breast

Breast ACC was first proposed as an entity because of its histopathological similarity to the tumors of the same name in the salivary glands. A dual cell population composed of cytokeratin-positive epithelial cells and vimentin-positive myoepithelial cells present in well-formed islands of cohesive cells forming small, sharply defined cystic spaces within these islands are the hallmarks of this tumor (Figs 14.1, 14.2). Nodular and diffusely infiltrating smaller, usually rounded collections of infiltrating tumor may coexist, but maintenance of the same cytology and intercellular arrangements is a defining feature.

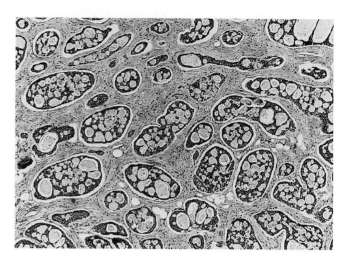

Figure 14.1 Low-power view of adenoid cystic carcinoma. Notice the sharp borders of the tumor islands within the surrounding stroma and the crisp definition of rounded spaces in each infiltrating island.

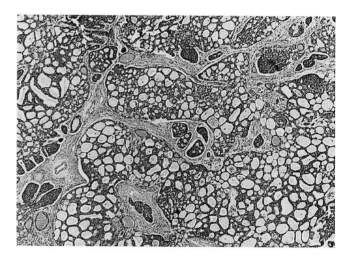

Figure 14.2 Low-power view of infiltrating adenoid cystic carcinoma with larger island pattern than in Figure 14.1 and some stromal reaction.

The typical cribriform morphology consists of glandular and pseudoglandular structures (Fig. 14.3), with true glands filled with brightly eosinophilic mucin and pseudolumens filled with more basophilic basement membrane-like material. In some cases, the basement membrane-like material predominates, forming irregular islands (Fig. 14.4). On a periodic acid-Schiff stain, the contents of the "true" lumens stain pink as is typical of epithelial mucins, which are of near neutral pH, whereas the basement membrane material or "stromal mucin" in the "pseudolumens" is more acidic and stains pale pink or blue (Fig. 14.5).[1,43] The main proliferating element is a population of modified myoepithelial cells as demonstrated by positive staining for smooth muscle actins, vimentin,[44] p63,[45] CK 5/6, CK14, and CK 17 (Fig. 14.6). These cells are grouped in nests outlining the "pseudolumens" or more irregular islands of basement membrane-like material. The true epithelial lumens, also referred to as the "glandular" or "adenoid" component, are lined by cytokeratin and epithelial membrane

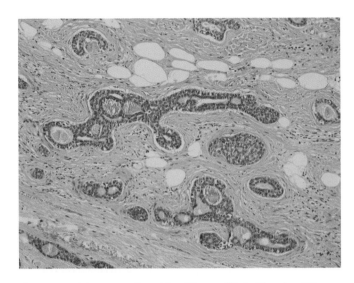

Figure 14.3 Higher power view of "true" lumens filled with eosinophilic mucin and "pseudolumens" filled with basement membrane-like material.

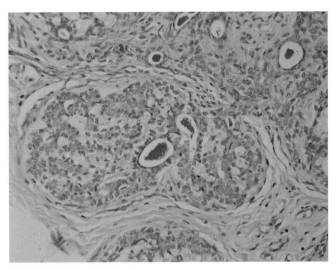

Figure 14.5 Periodic acid-Schiff stain of adenoid cystic carcinoma stains the mucin in the few "true" lumena bright pink while the predominating basement membrane-like material stains pale pink.

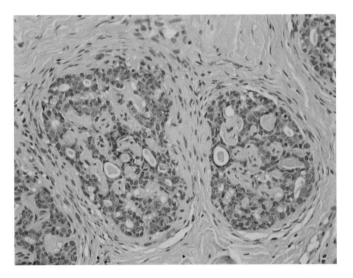

Figure 14.4 Example of adenoid cystic carcinoma with basement membrane-like material predominating and surrounded by largely myoepithelial cells.

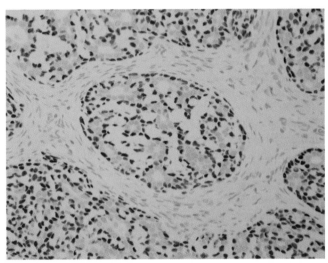

Figure 14.6 The myoepithelial stain p63 highlights the predominantly myoepithelial population in this adenoid cystic carcinoma while the epithelial cells forming the true lumena remain unstained.

antigen-positive cells and demonstrate conserved basolateral markers of normal epithelial polarity including fodrin, E-cadherin, and β-catenin.[44] Electron microscopy can also be used to demonstrate these two defining patterns.[2,43,46]

All strictly defined ACCs reported in the literature are estrogen receptor (ER) and progesterone receptor (PR) negative.[23,47–50] However, these findings should not be used as an indicator of poor outcome. In fact, the detailed study of markers of epithelial polarity in ACC by Kasami *et al.*,[44] demonstrating a status of advanced normal differentiation despite the capacity for local invasion, is consistent with the usual lack of distant metastasis.

Approximately 65% of cases also show strong membranous staining for EGFR and c-kit.[45,51,52] However, overexpression of both as demonstrated by immunohistochemistry is not the result of gene amplification.[53] Furthermore, patients with advanced ACC of the head and neck did not show benefit from

imatinib mesylate (Gleevec®).[54] Thus, while useful diagnostically, it does not appear that either of these markers plays a significant role in the pathogenesis of ACC.

Although not often mentioned in the literature, *in situ* patterns may occasionally be present in conjunction with areas of invasive tumor,[10,44] although there is no recognized adenoid cystic form of *in situ* carcinoma without attendant invasion. We have identified several cases of ACC with *in situ*-like areas involving papillomas but also with classic ACC present in the surrounding soft tissue. Single case reports of ACC arising in a fibroadenoma[10,55] and adenomyoepithelioma[56] have been described; however, the ACC-like areas were apparently focal and confined to these otherwise benign lesions without evidence of classic ACC in the surrounding breast tissue.

Shin and Rosen[10] have described a solid variant of ACC that exhibits a >90% solid growth pattern composed of basaloid

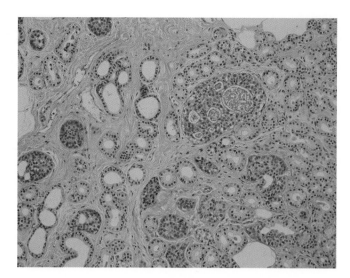

Figure 14.7 Example of microglandular adenosis with coexistent adenoid cystic carcinoma showing an admixture of the simplified glands of microglandular adenosis lined by a single layer of epithelial cells with small nuclei and eosinophilic cytoplasm, more complex epithelial-lined glands with cribriform spaces or solid growth consistent with atypical MGA as well as glands expanded by myoepithelial cells and pseudolumena with basophilic basement membrane-like material.

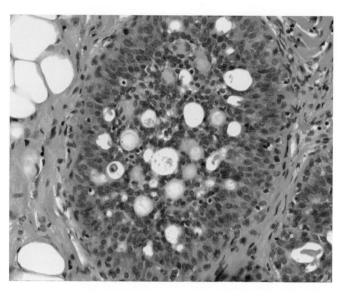

Figure 14.8 Example of collagenous spherulosis showing regular, round spaces within an island of benign proliferating epithelium containing rigid, spherular deposits of eosinophilic hyaline material composed of laminin and type IV collagen.

cells with moderate to occasionally marked nuclear atypia and rare to brisk mitotic activity. Ductules reminiscent of the intercalated ducts in salivary gland tumors identifiable by the presence of larger cells with eosinophilic cytoplasm and normochromatic nuclei arranged around the lumen were also present in tumor islands. These tumors show the same immunohistochemical profile of a typical ACC. Despite the presence of a single lymph node metastasis in two of the nine described patients, no patient developed recurrent or distant disease after initial treatment.[10]

Rarely, ACC may be intermixed with or appear to arise from a benign but infiltrative and equally rare condition, microglandular adenosis (MGA).[9] Altered myoepithelial cells appear to be the major neoplastic element in both ACC and "atypical MGA," which shows recognizable features of typical MGA but with glandular proliferations of greater architectural complexity and cytological atypia. In such cases, the single layer of lining epithelium typical of MGA is replaced by stratified cells with intraluminal bridging.[57–59] In cases of MGA with coexistent ACC (Fig. 14.7), many of the haphazardly spaced glands of MGA contain the typical dual cell population and architectural features of ACC.[9]

There is an important mimicker of mammary ACC, usually easily recognized as bounded by the basement membrane of lobular units, consisting of aggregates of well-circumscribed eosinophilic spherules termed "collagenous spherulosis" (Fig. 14.8). Although relatively uncommon, it is an extremely important pattern to recognize and is usually confined to a single lobular unit or a clustering of lobular units in an otherwise benign breast. The spaces are lined by basement membrane material as originally defined by Clement and colleagues[60] using an antibody to type IV collagen (a basement membrane-related collagen).

Similarities between adenoid cystic and invasive cribriform carcinoma

Superficially, the histological pattern characteristic of ACC is similar to that of invasive cribriform carcinoma.[61–63] Both of these special types of breast carcinoma are characterized by small, sharply defined, rounded spaces within islands of epithelial cells. The first difference is that invasive cribriform carcinoma is named because it mimics quite precisely the pattern of noninvasive cribriform ductal carcinoma *in situ*.[61–63] This pattern is only superficially similar to ACC and does not include the dual cell population with attendant special histochemical and immunohistochemical findings described above. Their differences have also been described by electron microscopy.[64] However, both invasive cribriform carcinoma and ACC show increased representation in prevalence screening mammography, presumably because of their slow growth and lack of significant metastatic activity.[40,41,65,66]

Clinical aspects: presentation, diagnostic considerations, and techniques

Average age at diagnosis of ACC in the breast is varied but most cases occur in the fifth and sixth decades (range 31–90 years). Similar to those with other slower-growing mammary carcinomas, patients present with a mobile breast mass, which may be present for years before diagnosis.[7,8] The size of these tumors at diagnosis may be large but the range is similar to invasive breast cancers in general. Current cases are diagnosed by mammographic imaging, diagnostic ultrasound or magnetic resonance imaging (MRI) at an average size of 2 cm.[11] However, in circumstances in which the breast mass was neglected, tumors as large as 10 cm have been reported.[6,46] Unlike typical mammary carcinoma, the breast mass may be painful or tender.[7,8,67,68] A significant feature, particularly with regard to complete excision, is the relatively frequent presence of a diffuse pattern of infiltration peripherally that is not apparent on gross examination, associated with a dominant, more compact centrally located tumor mass.

There is no predilection for either the left or the right breast[7,69] and no bilateral lesions have been reported. Most cases occur in the upper outer quadrant and most commonly in the region of the nipple or areola.[2,6,70] Fixation to skin, nipple, or pectoral muscles[7,12,68] is uncommon and bloody discharge is rare.[67] As with typical mammary carcinoma, ACC in males is rare[12,20,25,71,72] but when present, it generally presents and behaves similarly to ACC in females.

As with other special types of breast cancer, it is mandatory to identify the unique histological features of ACC that predict an excellent prognosis before rendering this diagnosis; dual differentiation in the majority of the neoplasm. Ro and colleagues have presented a few cases attempting to further refine the prognostic ability of the histological features.[23] These investigators devised a grading system for breast ACC, dividing cases into three categories: grade I tumors were completely glandular and cystic, lacking a solid component; grade II tumors contained solid areas constituting less than 30% of the mass; and grade III tumors were those in which the solid component made up more than 30% of the mass. Unfortunately, this effort was hampered by the paucity of cases and lack of strict adherence to the dimorphic criteria. Indeed, the single grade III case in this study was not the dimorphic "special type" of breast cancer and should be regarded as a generic, high-grade breast cancer. This is very important because this woman, who presented with positive axillary nodes at the time of diagnosis and died 2 years later with liver and brain metastases, is often cited as evidence that ACC of the breast can act badly. In fact, this tumor was twice as large as any other tumor in the study (6.0 cm) and was >90% solid. Although demonstrated to be of myoepithelial origin by electron microscopy and positivity for S-100, the photomicrographs show a tumor composed of very large, solid neoplastic islands containing cells of significantly higher grade than the usual ACC. This approach has also been specifically denied by the later important works of Shin and Kleer, which described solid variants of ACC that have few of the lumina but the same dual cell population and excellent prognosis.[10,73] Kleer additionally found that nuclear grade and proliferative activity did not predict capacity for local recurrence or distant metastasis.[10,73]

In contrast to the usual breast cancer histologies, in breast ACC the routine sampling of axillary lymph nodes at the time of initial surgery has not been considered useful in providing prognostic information nor has this procedure contributed to local control. In fact, regional lymph node involvement is quite rare. After a review of over 200 cases in the literature, we were only able to find six histologically confirmed cases of breast ACC involving axillary lymph nodes.[10,23,25,46,47] Controversy surrounds the diagnosis of one of these cases[25] because of the presence of psammoma bodies and necrosis. These features are not typical of breast ACC, calling into question the accuracy of the diagnosis.[24,74,75] At least one group suggests that this case in fact represents a variant of papillary and cribriform carcinoma.[69] Of the remaining five accepted cases, the tumors were

large, ranging from 5 to 15 cm.[10,23,46,47] Two of these patients had clinically positive lymph nodes at presentation[23,46,47] and two were from patients with solid variant tumors described by Shin but did not show evidence of local or distant recurrence on follow-up.[10]

A more recently published study utilizing California Cancer Registry data reports that 5% of 144 women with ACC had lymph node involvement. Despite the lack of central pathology review and a precise case definition, the 10-year relative cumulative survival was 100% in patients with negative lymph nodes, while that for patients with positive lymph nodes was 32.7%,[26] consistent with previous conclusions that knowledge of lymph node status does not contribute to local control. A similar population-based study using Surveillance, Epidemiology and End Results (SEER) data reported 2.5% lymph node involvement among 338 women with mammary ACC; however, it also reported that 20% of tumors were ER positive, calling into question the significance of these data.[11]

Local recurrence and metastatic potential

Local recurrence after primary surgical therapy is an infrequent occurrence. We were able to confirm 10 cases of local recurrence from ACC,[2,7,16,23,74,76–78] nine of which had undergone local excision. The remaining patient had a simple mastectomy. The margins from the initial resection of these tumors were not well documented. Therefore, considering that local recurrence is such an infrequent occurrence, it may be that inadequate attention was given to the margins at the time of initial resection in cases of local recurrence. Furthermore, two cases of local recurrence were reported as grade II tumors by Ro et al. and are not consistent with pure ACC.[23] These two tumors are described as behaving more aggressively, which may account for the development of local recurrence in these cases.

Similar to local recurrence, metastasis from ACC is rare. In fact, we were able to confirm only seven cases in the literature since 1970.[15,16,23,46,49,76] Peters and Wolff[69] presented one additional case of a patient who developed lung and liver metastases found on radiological studies, but no biopsy was performed to confirm the presence of metastases from ACC. When metastasis does occur, the lung[15,16,46,76] is the most frequently observed site. In fact, there are no accepted cases of distant metastases in which pulmonary metastasis did not occur. Other sites of metastases include bone,[23,49] kidney,[15,49] and brain.[16] Most recently, studies by Khanfir and Coates report the occurrence of metastatic disease in four patients in each series (6.5% and 1%, respectively).[79,80] However, these studies acknowledge up to 29.5% of cases demonstrating ER positivity and 63% of cases demonstrating unknown ER status. Furthermore, the ER status and tumor grade of the cases with metastatic disease cannot be determined from the presented data.

Although data on distant metastases from breast ACC are appropriately sparse, the pattern of mestastatic spread appears to be very different from that of carcinoma of no special type. Patients typically developed a solitary distant metastasis several years from initial presentation. In one reported case, a patient with a 10 cm mass present for 10–20 years had evidence of disease metastatic to the lung at the time of presentation.[46] In a series of 12 patients with ACC reported by Ro *et al.*, only one patient had died of disease at the time of follow-up after developing distant metastases.[23] However, this particular patient did not have classic histology for breast ACC, which probably accounts for the tumor's uncharacteristically aggressive behavior.

Treatment

Management of primary tumors

Historically, surgical treatment of the primary tumor has varied from excisional biopsy to radical mastectomy. In the literature, simple mastectomy is frequently proffered as the treatment of choice unless the tumors are large or there are clinically enlarged axillary lymph nodes.[2,7,24,50,69] However, we believe the preferred initial treatment of breast ACC is local excision to negative margins (4–5 mm is typically adequate) since this is a relatively indolent disease. Furthermore, although the incidence of local recurrence increases with more conservative surgery (similar to other breast cancer histologies), distant metastasis following local failure is exceedingly rare. In addition, patients who experience local failures can be salvaged with more extensive surgical procedures. In the existing literature, only one patient initially treated with local excision who developed local recurrence subsequently died from distant metastases.[22] An additional patient for whom the type of initial treatment was unknown, but axillary nodes were negative, developed a metastasis to the clavicle at 3 years, metastases to the lung, kidney, scalp, and eye at 5 years and subsequently died at 6 years following her initial diagnosis.[49]

When excisional biopsy is performed as the primary initial surgical procedure, special attention must be given to the surgical margins because these tumors grow in an infiltrative pattern. In the series presented by Ro *et al.*, all 12 tumors showed focal infiltration at the border, with tumor extension into adipose tissue.[23] Also, Peters and Wolff noted insidious extensions around a grossly obvious lesion, which would be impossible to detect clinically.[69] We believe that the primary reason why these tumors recur locally is inadequate resection of the tumor with histologically positive margins. Because axillary lymph node metastasis is unusual with breast ACC and of questionable prognostic significance, we agree with others who advocate performing axillary node dissection only in patients with large tumors or clinically involved axillary lymph nodes.[6,7,26]

There are few reliable data regarding adjuvant hormonal or radiation therapy and its effects on local recurrence and survival in this disease. In addition, there does not appear to be a proven means of predicting patients who may benefit from adjuvant systemic therapy,[68] and chemotherapy is not advocated. Seven recent studies purporting to examine outcome in ACC[17–20,79] are all flawed by limited or absent central pathological review and no mention of pathological criteria for accepting a case as ACC. Cases included were diagnosed from 1960 to 2007,[17–20,79,80] during which time criteria for ACC were refined considerably. In addition, three of these studies report

46%,[17] 29%,[19] and 20% of cases as ER positive, a finding that argues that these tumors were not actually ACC but rather invasive cribriform carcinoma or other low-to-intermediate grade cancers with focal cribriform features. In the first,[17] all women given hormonal therapy had ER-positive tumors. Of 11 women with ER- and PR-negative tumors, six received no adjuvant therapy, three had an unknown adjuvant therapy status but all were alive and well with no evidence of disease at 1, 5, and 11 years after initial surgery, and two women received radiotherapy, one of whom was alive and well without evidence of recurrence at 5 years while the other experienced distant metastasis to an unspecified site 6 years following diagnosis but was alive and well 2 years later. In fact, the only reported death in this study[17,79] was a woman with an ER-positive tumor associated with distant metastatic disease at the time of diagnosis.

A recent study suggesting that adjuvant radiotherapy improves survival admittedly reports a statistically significant difference in stage between the radiotherapy versus no radiotherapy groups, with the lower stage lesions predominating in the radiation therapy group.[79] This finding, in combination with the lack of central pathology review and the fact that more than 50% of cases in each group were either ER positive or of unknown ER status, makes the authors' conclusions tenuous. In the second study,[19] it is not mentioned whether adjuvant therapy was given following surgery and its effect on outcome.

Until these reports, there was only one report of an ER-positive ACC of the breast[1] and even this case has been questioned because there has not been any reported confirmation of this histological diagnosis.[24] Based on our review of the literature, there are no definitively diagnosed cases of ACC in which hormone therapy in the adjuvant setting was administered. In one report, tamoxifen was given in the setting of metastatic ACC; however, the tumor failed to respond.[18] Accordingly, we do not believe antiestrogen hormone therapy has a therapeutic role in this malignancy.

Management of local recurrence

Local recurrence is commonly treated by repeat surgical excision. A variety of surgical approaches have been used, including wide local excision, simple mastectomy, modified radical mastectomy, radical mastectomy, and *en bloc* resection of the pectoralis muscle and axilla. The median time from initial diagnosis to local recurrence was 5 years but recurrence occurred as early as 6 months[25] and as late as 22 years.[13] Only one patient who developed local recurrence subsequently died with distant metastases.[22] Of interest, this patient did not have a pure ACC tumor by pathological description.

These admittedly limited data suggest that local recurrence with typical ACC histology is not a harbinger of systemic disease.

Management of distant recurrence

Several modalities have been used for the management of distant metastases, including surgical resection, chemotherapy, radiation therapy, and hormone therapy. However, the effectiveness of these modalities is difficult to determine because of the paucity of patients involved. The presence of solitary, large distant metastases may respond best to surgical excision.[15,16] This is exemplified by a woman who had a pulmonary metastasis successfully surgically resected 6 years after mastectomy and a subsequent renal metastasis successfully resected 12 years after mastectomy.

Recommendations

We believe the preferred initial treatment of breast ACC is local excision to negative margins (at least 4–5 mm) since this is a relatively indolent disease. Although the incidence of local recurrence increases with more conservative surgery (similar to other breast cancer histologies), distant metastasis following local failure is exceedingly rare. Patients who experience local recurrences can be salvaged with more extensive surgical procedures. We advocate performing axillary node dissection only in patients with large tumors or clinically involved axillary lymph nodes. Adjuvant chemotherapy or radiotherapy is not advocated. Antiestrogen hormone therapy does not appear to have a role in this malignancy.

It is difficult to comment on the effectiveness of surgical resection, chemotherapy, radiation therapy, and hormone therapy in the management of distant metastases because of the paucity of patients in the literature and imprecise case definition in some reports. Hormonal therapy and chemotherapy have a limited role, if any, in the management of distant disease. A surgical approach to solitary metastases seems defensible given the fact that patients may live for many years following resection of documented distant metastases. Finally, the recent report of a PIK3CA and PTEN mutation in ACC raises the possibility that mTOR inhibitors may be useful in rare patients with metastatic disease and progression.[33]

References

1. Azzopardi JG, Ahmed A, Millis RR. Problems in breast pathology. Major Probl Pathol 1979; 11: i–xvi, 1–466.
2. Qizilbash AH, Patterson MC, Oliveira KF. Adenoid cystic carcinoma of the breast. Light and electron microscopy and a brief review of the literature. Arch Pathol Lab Med 1977; 101: 302–6.
3. Billroth T. Die cylindergeschwalst. Berlin: G Reimer, 1856.
4. Spies J. Adenoid cystic carcinoma: generalized metastases in three cases of basal cell type. Arch Surg 1930; 21: 365–404.
5. Geschickter CF. Diseases of the Breast: Diagnosis, Pathology, and Treatment. Philadelphia: J.B. Lippincott, 1945.
6. Anthony PP, James PD. Adenoid cystic carcinoma of the breast: prevalence, diagnostic criteria, and histogenesis. J Clin Pathol 1975; 28: 647–55.
7. Cavanzo FJ, Taylor HB. Adenoid cystic carcinoma of the breast. An analysis of 21 cases. Cancer 1969; 24: 740–5.
8. Galloway JR, Woolner LB, Clagett OT. Adenoid cystic carcinoma of the breast. Surg Gynecol Obstet 1966; 122: 1289–94.
9. Acs G, Simpson JF, Bleiweiss IJ, et al. Microglandular adenosis with transition into adenoid cystic carcinoma of the breast. Am J Surg Pathol 2003; 27: 1052–60.
10. Shin SJ, Rosen PP. Solid variant of mammary adenoid cystic carcinoma with basaloid features: a study of nine cases. Am J Surg Pathol 2002; 26: 413–20.
11. Ghabach B, Anderson WF, Curtis RE, Huycke MM, Lavigne JA, Dores GM. Adenoid cystic carcinoma of the breast in the United States (1977 to 2006): a population-based cohort study. Breast Cancer Res 2010; 12: R54.
12. Hjorth S, Magnusson PH, Blomquist P. Adenoid cystic carcinoma of the breast. Report of a case in a male and review of the literature. Acta Chir Scand 1977; 143: 155–8.
13. Lusted D. Structural and growth patterns of adenoid cystic carcinoma of breast. Am J Clin Pathol 1970; 54: 419–25.
14. Prioleau PG, Santa Cruz DJ, Buettner JB, Bauer WC. Sweat gland differentiation in mammary adenoid cystic carcinoma. Cancer 1979; 43: 1752–60.
15. Herzberg AJ, Bossen EH, Walther PJ. Adenoid cystic carcinoma of the breast metastatic to the kidney. A clinically symptomatic lesion requiring surgical management. Cancer 1991; 68: 1015–20.
16. Koller M, Ram Z, Findler G, Lipshitz M. Brain metastasis: a rare manifestation of adenoid cystic carcinoma of the breast. Surg Neurol 1986; 26: 470–2.
17. Arpino G, Clark GM, Mohsin S, Bardou VJ, Elledge RM. Adenoid cystic carcinoma of the breast: molecular markers, treatment, and clinical outcome. Cancer 2002; 94: 2119–27.
18. Kontos M, Fentiman IS. Adenoid cystic carcinoma of the breast. Int J Clin Pract 2003; 57: 669–72.
19. McClenathan JH, de la Roza G. Adenoid cystic breast cancer. Am J Surg 2002; 183: 646–9.
20. Millar BA, Kerba M, Youngson B, Lockwood GA, Liu FF. The potential role of breast conservation surgery and adjuvant breast radiation for adenoid cystic carcinoma of the breast. Breast Cancer Res Treat 2004; 87: 225–32.
21. Nayer HR. Case report section; cylindroma of the breast with pulmonary metastases. Dis Chest 1957; 31: 324–7.
22. O'Kell RT. Adenoid cystic carcinoma of the breast. Mo Med 1964; 61: 855–8.
23. Ro JY, Silva EG, Gallager HS. Adenoid cystic carcinoma of the breast. Hum Pathol 1987; 18: 1276–81.
24. Sumpio BE, Jennings TA, Merino MJ, Sullivan PD. Adenoid cystic carcinoma of the breast. Data from the Connecticut Tumor Registry and a review of the literature. Ann Surg 1987; 205: 295–301.
25. Verani RR, van der Bel-Kahn J. Mammary adenoid cystic carcinoma with unusual features. Am J Clin Pathol 1973; 59: 653–8.
26. Thompson K, Grabowski J, Saltzstein SL, Sadler GR, Blair SL. Adenoid cystic breast carcinoma: is axillary staging necessary in all cases? Results from the California Cancer Registry. Breast J 2011; 17: 485–9.
27. Tognon C, Knezevich SR, Huntsman D, et al. Expression of the ETV6-NTRK3 gene fusion as a primary event in human secretory breast carcinoma. Cancer Cell 2002; 2: 367–76.
28. Persson M, Andren Y, Mark J, Horlings HM, Persson F, Stenman G. Recurrent fusion of MYB and NFIB transcription factor genes in carcinomas of the breast and head and neck. Proc Natl Acad Sci U S A 2009; 106: 18740–4.
29. Baselga J. Targeting the phosphoinositide-3 (PI3) kinase pathway in breast cancer. Oncologist 2011; 16(Suppl 1): 12–19.
30. Castaneda CA, Cortes-Funes H, Gomez HL, Ciruelos EM. The phosphatidyl inositol 3-kinase/AKT signaling pathway in breast cancer. Cancer Metastasis Rev 2010; 29: 751–9.
31. Dupont Jensen J, Laenkholm AV, Knoop A, et al. PIK3CA mutations may be discordant between primary and corresponding metastatic disease in breast cancer. Clin Cancer Res 2011; 17: 667–77.
32. Vranic S, Bilalovic N, Lee LM, Kruslin B, Lilleberg SL, Gatalica Z. PIK3CA and PTEN mutations in adenoid cystic carcinoma of the breast metastatic to kidney. Hum Pathol 2007; 38: 1425–31.
33. Dancey JE. Therapeutic targets: MTOR and related pathways. Cancer Biol Ther 2006; 5: 1065–73.
34. Vranic S, Gatalica Z, Deng H, et al. ER-alpha36, a novel isoform of ER-alpha66, is commonly over-expressed in apocrine and adenoid cystic carcinomas of the breast. J Clin Pathol 2011; 64: 54–7.
35. Wang Z, Zhang X, Shen P, Loggie BW, Chang Y, Deuel TF. Identification, cloning, and expression of human estrogen receptor-alpha36, a novel variant of human estrogen receptor-alpha66. Biochem Biophys Res Commun 2005; 336: 1023–7.
36. Wang Z, Zhang X, Shen P, Loggie BW, Chang Y, Deuel TF. A variant of estrogen receptor-{alpha}, hER-{alpha}36: transduction of estrogen- and antiestrogen-dependent membrane-initiated mitogenic signaling. Proc Natl Acad Sci U S A 2006; 103: 9063–8.

37. Page DL, Anderson TJ. How should we categorize breast cancer? Breast 1993; 2: 217–19.

38. Pereira H, Pinder SE, Sibbering DM, *et al.* Pathological prognostic factors in breast cancer. IV: Should you be a typer or a grader? A comparative study of two histological prognostic features in operable breast carcinoma. Histopathology 1995; 27: 219–26.

39. Simpson JF, Page DL. Prognostic value of histopathology in the breast. Semin Oncol 1992; 19: 254–62.

40. Anderson TJ, Lamb J, Donnan P, *et al.* Comparative pathology of breast cancer in a randomised trial of screening. Br J Cancer 1991; 64: 108–13.

41. Cowan WK, Kelly P, Sawan A, *et al.* The pathological and biological nature of screen-detected breast carcinomas: a morphological and immunohistochemical study. J Pathol 1997; 182: 29–35.

42. Dixon JM, Page DL, Anderson TJ, *et al.* Long-term survivors after breast cancer. Br J Surg 1985; 72: 445–8.

43. Koss LG, Brannan CD, Ashikari R. Histologic and ultrastructural features of adenoid cystic carcinoma of the breast. Cancer 1970; 26: 1271–9.

44. Kasami M, Olson SJ, Simpson JF, Page DL. Maintenance of polarity and a dual cell population in adenoid cystic carcinoma of the breast: an immunohistochemical study. Histopathology 1998; 32: 232–8.

45. Mastropasqua MG, Maiorano E, Pruneri G, *et al.* Immunoreactivity for c-kit and p63 as an adjunct in the diagnosis of adenoid cystic carcinoma of the breast. Mod Pathol 2005; 18(10); 1277–82.

46. Wells CA, Nicoll S, Ferguson DJ. Adenoid cystic carcinoma of the breast: a case with axillary lymph node metastasis. Histopathology 1986; 10: 415–24.

47. Pastolero G, Hanna W, Zbieranowski I, Kahn HJ. Proliferative activity and p53 expression in adenoid cystic carcinoma of the breast. Mod Pathol 1996; 9: 215–19.

48. Sheen-Chen SM, Eng HL, Chen WJ, Cheng YF, Ko SF. Adenoid cystic carcinoma of the breast: truly uncommon or easily overlooked? Anticancer Res 2005; 25: 455–8.

49. Trendell-Smith NJ, Peston D, Shousha S. Adenoid cystic carcinoma of the breast: a tumour commonly devoid of oestrogen receptors and related proteins. Histopathology 1999; 35: 241–8.

50. Zaloudek C, Oertel YC, Orenstein JM. Adenoid cystic carcinoma of the breast. Am J Clin Pathol 1984; 81: 297–307.

51. Azoulay S, Lae M, Freneaux P, *et al.* KIT is highly expressed in adenoid cystic carcinoma of the breast, a basal-like carcinoma associated with a favorable outcome. Mod Pathol 2005; 18: 1623–31.

52. Page DL. Adenoid cystic carcinoma of breast, a special histopathologic type with excellent prognosis. Breast Cancer Res Treat 2005; 93: 189–90.

53. Vranic S, Frkovic-Grazio S, Lamovec J, *et al.* Adenoid cystic carcinomas of the breast have low Topo IIalpha expression but frequently overexpress EGFR protein without EGFR gene amplification. Hum Pathol 2010; 41: 1617–23.

54. Hotte SJ, Winquist EW, Lamont E, *et al.* Imatinib mesylate in patients with adenoid cystic cancers of the salivary glands expressing c-kit: a Princess Margaret Hospital phase II consortium study. J Clin Oncol 2005; 23: 585–90.

55. Blanco M, Egozi L, Lubin D, Poppiti R. Adenoid cystic carcinoma arising in a fibroadenoma. Ann Diagn Pathol 2005; 9: 157–9.

56. Van Dorpe J, de Pauw A, Moerman P. Adenoid cystic carcinoma arising in an adenomyoepithelioma of the breast. Virchows Arch 1998; 432: 119–22.

57. James BA, Cranor ML, Rosen PP. Carcinoma of the breast arising in microglandular adenosis. Am J Clin Pathol 1993; 100: 507–13.

58. Kay S. Microglandular adenosis of the female mammary gland: study of a case with ultrastructural observations. Hum Pathol 1985; 16: 637–41.

59. Rosenblum MK, Purrazzella R, Rosen PP. Is microglandular adenosis a precancerous disease? A study of carcinoma arising therein. Am J Surg Pathol 1986; 10: 237–45.

60. Clement PB, Young RH, Azzopardi JG. Collagenous spherulosis of the breast. Am J Surg Pathol 1987; 11: 411–17.

61. Page DL, Dixon JM, Anderson TJ, Lee D, Stewart HJ. Invasive cribriform carcinoma of the breast. Histopathology 1983; 7: 525–36.

62. Simpson JF, Page DL. Status of breast cancer prognostication based on histopathologic data. Am J Clin Pathol 1994; 102: S3–8.

63. Venable JG, Schwartz AM, Silverberg SG. Infiltrating cribriform carcinoma of the breast: a distinctive clinicopathologic entity. Hum Pathol 1990; 21: 333–8.

64. Wells CA, Ferguson DJ. Ultrastructural and immunocytochemical study of a case of invasive cribriform breast carcinoma. J Clin Pathol 1988; 41: 17–20.

65. Page DL. Prognosis and breast cancer. Recognition of lethal and favorable prognostic types. Am J Surg Pathol 1991; 15: 334–49.

66. Stutz JA, Evans AJ, Pinder S, *et al.* The radiological appearances of invasive cribriform carcinoma of the breast. Nottingham Breast Team. Clin Radiol 1994; 49: 693–5.

67. Jaworski RC, Kneale KL, Smith RC. Adenoid cystic carcinoma of the breast. Postgrad Med J 1983; 59: 48–51.

68. Leeming R, Jenkins M, Mendelsohn G. Adenoid cystic carcinoma of the breast. Arch Surg 1992; 127: 233–5.

69. Peters GN, Wolff M. Adenoid cystic carcinoma of the breast. Report of 11 new cases: review of the literature and discussion of biological behavior. Cancer 1983; 52: 680–6.

70. Friedman BA, Oberman HA. Adenoid cystic carcinoma of the breast. Am J Clin Pathol 1970; 54: 1–14.

71. Ferlito A, di Bonito L. Adenoid cystic carcinoma of the male breast: report of a case. Am Surg 1974; 40: 72–6.

72. Miliauskas JR, Leong AS. Adenoid cystic carcinoma in a juvenile male breast. Pathology 1991; 23: 298–301.

73. Kleer CG, Oberman HA. Adenoid cystic carcinoma of the breast: value of histologic grading and proliferative activity. Am J Surg Pathol 1998; 22: 569–75.

74. Peters GN, Wolff M, Haagensen CD. Tubular carcinoma of the breast. Clinical pathologic correlations based on 100 cases. Ann Surg 1981; 193: 138–49.

75. Steinman A, Pepus M, McSwain G. Adenoid cystic carcinoma of the breast. South Med J 1978; 71: 851–4.

76. Lim SK, Kovi J, Warner OG. Adenoid cystic carcinoma of breast with metastasis: a case report and review of the literature. J Natl Med Assoc 1979; 71: 329–30.

77. Wilson WB, Spell JP. Adenoid cystic carcinoma of breast: a case with recurrence and regional metastasis. Ann Surg 1967; 166: 861–4.

78. Woyke S, Domagala W, Olszewski W. Fine structure of mammary adenoid cystic carcinoma. Pol Med J 1970; 9: 1140–8.

79. Coates JM, Martinez SR, Bold RJ, Chen SL. Adjuvant radiation therapy is associated with improved survival for adenoid cystic carcinoma of the breast. J Surg Oncol 2010; 102: 342–7.

80. Khanfir K, Kallel A, Villette S, *et al.* Management of adenoid cystic carcinoma of the breast: a Rare Cancer Network study. Int J Radiat Oncol Biol Phys 2011; May 11 [Epub ahead of print].

15 Non-Hodgkin Lymphoma of the Breast

David S. Morgan[1] and Jean F. Simpson[2]

[1]Department of Medicine, [2]Department of Pathology, Vanderbilt University School of Medicine, Nashville, TN, USA

Introduction

Non-Hodgkin lymphoma (NHL) localized to the breast is an uncommon disease. Most series and cases reported in the literature use a case definition devised by Wiseman and Liao[1] and modified by Hugh *et al.*,[2] which describes cases of "primary" breast lymphoma (PBL) as having the following characteristics: both mammary tissue and lymphomatous infiltrate present in close association in an adequate histological specimen, and no evidence of widespread lymphoma by standard staging techniques or preceding extramammary lymphoma, although ipsilateral axillary node involvement is allowed if both lesions present simultaneously.

Considerably more common is "secondary" NHL of the breast, that is, NHL which involves the breast as one of several sites of nodal and/or extranodal involvement at the first diagnosis or as a site of relapse. "Secondary" breast lymphoma is perhaps twice as common as primary breast lymphoma.[3] Hodgkin disease involving the breast[4–9] is very rare and will not be discussed here.

The traditional case definition for primary breast lymphoma is somewhat at odds with the modern understanding that NHL is a disseminated disease in almost all cases.[10,11] It is not now customary to define most lymphomas as "primary" or "secondary." However, because of the specific diagnostic and therapeutic challenges it presents to clinicians, radiologists, and pathologists, this review will focus on localized, "primary" NHL of the breast. Specifically, a breast mass may often initiate a diagnostic and treatment algorithm optimized for adenocarcinoma of the breast, which may include mammogram, ultrasound, and even excisional biopsy before the true diagnosis of NHL is recognized. The diagnosis and management of so-called "secondary" cases are similar to those of other cases of NHL with one or more extranodal foci of involvement, and are not discussed here.

Historical background

The nomenclature, classification, and treatment of the diseases we now call NHLs have changed radically since they were first recognized in the 19th century, and therefore it is difficult to assess data from reports in the older literature. Lymphoid neoplasms of the breast have been recognized at least since 1880 when Gross removed an upper outer quadrant breast mass from a 22-year-old woman which was said to show "lymphadenoid sarcoma."[12] A handful of cases was reported in the late 19th and early 20th centuries.[13–15] In 1944, Adair and Hermann reported five cases of breast lymphosarcoma among 3033 cases of malignant breast tumors (0.16%) seen over a period of 20 years at Memorial Hospital.[16] Since then, numerous reports, mostly case reports and small case series as well as a few larger series, have described the clinical and pathological features and discussed the management of this disease.[2,3,5,17–40] Many older reports are of limited utility to the modern clinician for two reasons: first, they focus on comparing and differentiating NHL of the breast and carcinoma of the breast, and second, there is little focus on the pathological subtypes of lymphoma seen in the breast. Newer reports approach this entity in its most straightforward form, that is, as an extranodal NHL. As such, the focus is on the special clinicopathological aspects of PBL in distinction to other NHLs.[5,38,39]

Etiology and epidemiology

Extranodal involvement in advanced-stage lymphoma is quite common and its incidence varies by histological subtype, the most common sites being the gastrointestinal tract, the paranasal sinuses, and the respiratory tract. Breast involvement is not uncommon, and is said to be particularly common in Burkitt or other high-grade lymphomas.[20,21]

The discovery of NHL in an extranodal site as the sole (Ann Arbor stage IE[41]) focus of involvement is also common in clinical practice, found in perhaps one-third of NHL cases. Some extranodal lymphomas arise in mucosa-associated lymphoid tissue (MALT)[42] which is found in a variety of sites, most notably the gastrointestinal tract but also occasionally in the breast.[43] MALT lymphomas are reported to have a distinctive morphology, immunohistochemical phenotype, and natural history (see below). Other histological subtypes seen in breast lymphoma recapitulate the range of subtypes seen in nodal disease, including reports of follicle center cell lymphoma, diffuse large B cell lymphoma,[5,38,39,44,45] mantle cell lymphoma,[46] anaplastic large cell lymphoma,[47–49] and Burkitt lymphoma.[50] A report from Chanan-Khan et al.[51] details three cases of HIV-positive patients with PBL, although it is not known if immunocompromised patients are particularly prone to this localization.

The incidence of NHL with breast localization only (with or without clinically apparent involvement of the associated axillary lymph nodes) is quite low. Reflecting the clinical problem of distinguishing this entity from carcinoma of the breast, many authors have reported its rate of occurrence as a percentage of all operable breast malignancies seen in single-institution series. These historical reviews have placed the relative incidence at 0.05–0.18% of breast neoplasms,[2,26,29,33,52–55] although a few series put this figure as high as 1.1%.[1,56,57] PBL is said to make up about 2.2% of all extranodal lymphomas[58] and 0.7% of all NHLs in population-based studies.[2]

Most cases have been reported in women; fewer than 10 cases have been reported in men.[27,29,59–61] Although most reported cases have been in persons of European or Asian descent,[27,61,62] it is unclear whether this represents a higher incidence in those groups or reflects reporting bias. The reported age at diagnosis varies widely, from 9 years to 95 years,[27,33,60,63] with the greatest frequency in the sixth decade.[2,5,24,26,29,33,64] Many investigators have reported a bimodal age distribution,[16,27,33,65] with distinct clinical characteristics and outcomes in the two groups (see below).

Pathology

Recent advances may improve our understanding of the clinicopathological features of primary breast lymphoma. Acceptance of clinically relevant classification systems and the standard practice of immunophenotyping lymphoid neoplasms may result in more accurate comparison of published series of lymphomas. In the past, some studies of breast lymphomas may not have been carefully defined, and have included pseudolymphomas,[3,52] granulocytic sarcomas,[5] or even poorly differentiated carcinomas.[5] Adopting more precise diagnostic approaches, as well as use of defining criteria for primary breast lymphoma,[1,2] should result in greater understanding of these unusual neoplasms. The following review of histopathology of primary breast lymphoma is based on studies that have adhered to these tenets.

Primary breast lymphoma is a heterogeneous disease, even when limited to the defining criteria stated above.[1,2] It does seem that there are two distinct clinicopathological groups of patients, however. Women in the first group are younger and

Table 15.1 Reported incidence of primary breast lymphoma presenting as MALT-type lymphoma.

Study	Number of cases	Number (%) of MALT lymphomas
Bobrow et al.[70]	9	0
Prevot et al.[71]	14	0
Mattia et al.[3]	9	4 (44%)
Ariad et al.[36]	6	0
Lin et al.[5]	21	0
Hugh et al.[2]	20	7 (35%)
Tan et al.[73]	14	0
Jeon et al.[27]	7	0
Arber et al.[37]	41	2 (5%)
Kuper-Hommel et al.[67]	38	8 (20%)
Farinha et al.[31]	14	9 (64%)

often have a bilateral presentation, often associated with pregnancy or recent childbirth, and the disease behaves aggressively. Classically, the histological correlate of this type of primary breast lymphoma is high-grade, small noncleaved cell, Burkitt-type lymphoma,[66] although diffuse large cell or immunoblastic lymphoma is also described[5,37] in this setting. The second group of patients has an age range that overlaps that of primary breast carcinoma, and the presenting symptom is usually a unilateral breast mass. This group demonstrates the broad morphological spectrum of malignant lymphoma, with the preponderance of cases being intermediate to high grade (see below).[5] The same histological subtypes found in node-based lymphomas are also present in breast lymphoma, and there does not appear to be any unique subtype occurring exclusively in the breast, although diffuse large cell lymphoma is commonly reported.[5,37,67,68]

Some authors have suggested that primary breast lymphomas are often MALT type.[3] MALT lymphoma is a low-grade lymphoma characterized by a proliferation of follicle marginal zone-type cells (centrocyte-like cells or monocytoid B cells), often with surrounding reactive germinal centers, plasmacytic differentiation, Dutcher bodies, follicular colonization, and lymphoepithelial lesions. These lymphomas typically express pan-B cell markers. Although mammary tissue is not considered a normal site of MALT, it is possible that low-grade lymphomas similar to MALT lymphoma could arise in the breast in "acquired MALT," as in the setting of infection or autoimmune disease.[42]

In support of the concept of MALT-type lymphomas of the breast, Mattia et al.[3] have presented clinical and pathological findings from nine cases of primary breast lymphoma. Of these, eight were of low grade (Working Formulation and Kiel classification) and four were classified as MALT-type lymphomas (Table 15.1). No lymphoepithelial lesions, typically found in MALT-type lymphomas of more usual sites, were identified. In their cases, MALT-type lymphomas constituted a distinct subset with a markedly increased potential for prolonged disease-free survival after local therapy (see below). Hugh et al.[2] presented the clinical and pathological features of 20 cases of PBL and found seven (35%) to be monocytoid B cell lymphomas, histologically identical to lymphomas arising in MALT.

One histopathological feature of lymphomas of MALT origin is the presence of lymphoepithelial lesions, characterized by malignant lymphoid infiltrates involving glandular epithelium.[42] These lymphoepithelial lesions may be seen in PBL not otherwise characteristic of MALT lymphoma, however. In contrast, lymphoepithelial lesions were not identified in MALT-like lymphomas of the breast in the series presented by Mattia et al.[3] Burke stresses site-specific differences about MALT lymphomas, including those involving the breast.[69]

Other studies (see Table 15.1) have not found MALT-type lymphomas to be characteristic of primary breast lymphomas,[70,71] including the largest reported series[37] of primary breast lymphoma (41 cases). In this study, derived largely from consultative cases, as well as others,[27,36,71–73] intermediate- and high-grade lymphomas predominate.

In summary, the histopathology of primary breast lymphoma is heterogeneous. Although the Burkitt-type PBL that affects younger women does appear to be a distinctive clinicopathological entity, the majority of PBL have histopathological characteristics that overlap with lymphomas in other sites, with both aggressive and relatively indolent forms represented.

The rarity of PBL has been attributed to the paucity of normal lymphocytes in this location.[43] Some investigators have suggested that PBL occurs in the setting of a preexisting breast lymphocytic lobulitis.[72,74] The immunophenotype of the lymphocytes in lobulitis is predominantly B cells, with increased expression of HLA-DR by the lobular epithelium.[75–77] In contrast, however, the lymphocytic infiltrate in PBL has been shown to be of T cell origin.[70,71,78] And although lobular atrophy was a frequent finding in the study by Arber et al.,[37] lobulitis in surrounding benign breast epithelium was not identified, nor was it seen in the series by Mattia et al.[3]

Immunohistochemical analysis of primary breast lymphoma

A detailed comparison of the immunophenotype of reported primary breast lymphomas is difficult, because reported series vary widely in reagents and methodology used. In spite of these inconsistencies, the vast majority (>90%) of primary breast lymphomas are of B cell lineage by immunophenotyping studies.[2,3,5,27,36,37,70–73] A few studies have also explored immunoglobulin (Ig) heavy chain expression, with documentation of monoclonal Ig.[2,3,52]

Immunohistochemical evidence supporting MALT-type differentiation in PBL has not been studied in great detail. In the series presented by Mattia et al.[3] that described four PBL as being MALT-like (see above), one case was further characterized as being CD5, CD10, and CD23 negative, an immunophenotype reported for MALT lymphoma.[79] Arber et al.[37] studied frozen sections of seven PBL with antibodies to mantle (UCL3D3) and marginal cells (UCL4D12). One of the seven cases, a monocytoid B cell lymphoma, was positive for both, while the remaining six cases representing other types of lymphomas were negative. Farinha et al. reported nine of 14 PBL as MALTomas, and stress the importance of immunohistochemistry in assessing the MALT characteristics of PBL.[31] Thus, in the few examples reported, the immunophenotype of

MALT-type lymphomas involving the breast is consistent with that histopathological diagnosis.

Molecular and cytogenetic studies

Reports of cytogenetic and molecular analysis of primary breast lymphomas are infrequent. In a karyotypic study of MALT-type lymphomas, Ott et al.[79] described the t(11;18)(q21;q21) chromosome translocation as a frequent and specific aberration in low-grade MALT-type lymphomas. The single breast low-grade lymphoma included in this series did not contain clonal aberration, however. Bobrow et al.[70] used polymerase chain reaction (PCR) to screen their cases of PBL for t(14;18), but none was positive for this translocation. This finding was not unexpected since less than 5% of extranodal lymphomas show this finding.[80] Others have used the lack of Ig heavy chain gene rearrangement as supportive evidence of T cell lineage in a case of PBL.[81]

Clinical presentation

Breast lymphoma is rarely suspected clinically. The demographic profile, presenting symptoms, and initial evaluation of patients generally point to a diagnosis of carcinoma of the breast or occasionally to a benign lesion, both of which are much more common than NHL of the breast. Therefore, the rate of clinical misdiagnosis is quite high, and the potential for inappropriate treatment is likewise high.

The most common presentation is a painless, palpable mass which is often reported to have enlarged very rapidly, or a new lesion seen on screening mammogram.[3,82] Reported sizes range from 1 cm to 19 cm and multiple lesions may be seen. Less common is a presentation reminiscent of inflammatory breast cancer, with diffuse thickening or hardening of the breast, sometimes with an overlying violaceous skin color. Skin retraction, nipple retraction, and nipple discharge are not usually seen; Liberman et al. report that these findings were absent in all 32 patients in their series.[83] The constitutional ("B") symptoms of NHL (fever, night sweats, and weight loss) are unusual but occasionally seen with high-grade histologies.

Many investigators have reported that involvement of the right breast is more common,[17,24,29,38,84,85] although others have found no lateralization.[3,5] Up to 25% are reported to be bilateral at presentation,[2] with additional patients (9% in one series[20]) developing involvement of the contralateral breast later or as a relapse site.[35,86] Involvement of the upper outer quadrant appears to be more common than involvement of other parts of the breast.[53,60,87] The right predominance and the upper outer quadrant localization are unexplained, but neither seems to have prognostic or management implications.

A number of groups have reported the occurrence of lymphoma in proximity to the capsule of silicone breast implants.[48,49,88–92] The histological subtype in the majority of cases is anaplastic large cell lymphoma (ALCL), without ALK expression. In all, less than 30 cases of ALCL associated with breast implants have been reported. Causality has not been proven but a Dutch population-based, case–control study reports that the hazard ratio for the ALCL histology was 18.2

in the presence of silicone breast implants.[49] As ALCL of the breast is exceedingly rare, however, this still represents an incidence of only 00.1–0.3 per 100,000 women with breast implants in The Netherlands.

In summary, the clinical presentation is very similar to breast carcinoma, although bilaterality, rapid breast enlargement, absence of nipple discharge and skin retraction, multiple lesions, violaceous skin changes over the lesion, and soft and mobile axillary lymph nodes (as opposed to the harder lymph nodes typical of metastatic carcinoma) have been reported as features suggestive of breast lymphoma.[5]

Similarly, the radiographic findings are not characteristic; the mammogram and ultrasound findings are similar to those in other breast diseases, both malignant and benign.[83] The most common mammogram finding is one or multiple focal masses, sometimes with a thin rim of radiolucency (a finding usually associated with nonmalignant lesions). Less common is diffusely increased breast density with skin thickening, which may be interpreted as consistent with inflammatory breast cancer.[83,93] Spiculated masses and miliary densities have been described infrequently.[94,95] Liberman reviewed 32 cases of breast NHL, 21 of them primary, and correlated mammogram and histological findings. The majority of mammograms, 69%, showed a solitary uncalcified mass, 9% showed multiple uncalcified masses, 9% diffuse increased opacity, and 13% no abnormal findings. In the cases with mammographically detected masses, 28% were well circumscribed, while the remainder were incompletely circumscribed. None of the masses was spiculated. The findings did not correlate with histological subtypes.[83] Thus, no mammographic finding is specific for breast lymphoma. A small series by Schouten, which reported the prospective interpretation of mammograms, is perhaps illustrative: of seven mammograms, all were read as "abnormal," two as "suggesting lymphoma," and three as "malignancy."[20]

The ultrasonographic findings are even less well described and are reported as showing a wide spectrum of findings. In one retrospective series, eight patients had sonograms; seven of the studies showed a mass. All the masses were hypoechoic, with homogeneous echotexture in six.[83]

Magnetic resonance (MR) imaging of breast NHL has been described.[96–98] The findings on MR are not pathognomonic and are similar to other breast neoplasms.

Investigation and staging

As for all breast masses, there is a low threshold for biopsy. The most reliable diagnosis requires an incisional or excisional biopsy, and some authors have warned that diagnoses made by frozen section examination may be inaccurate at distinguishing lymphoma from breast carcinoma.[57] While some authors have also cautioned against core needle biopsies,[33] others have pointed out that immunoperoxidase studies performed on core samples or fine needle aspiration samples may facilitate making a diagnosis of breast lymphoma.[94]

Once a diagnosis of breast lymphoma is made, the investigation should proceed as for the staging of any other extranodal lymphoma, and should include the following:

- a detailed history with attention to systemic symptoms of lymphoma (unexplained fever greater than 101°F, loss of more than 10% of bodyweight, and unexplained night sweats)
- computed tomography scans of the chest, abdomen and pelvis
- bone marrow biopsy
- blood studies, including a complete blood count with differential and platelets, chemistries including lactate dehydrogenase, and perhaps β2-microglobulin
- consideration of lumbar puncture with cytology.

Fluorodeoxyglucose-positron emission tomography (FDG-PET) has become a common staging modality, especially for intermediate- and high-grade lymphoma. As expected, FDG avidity of breast lymphoma has been reported.[99] PET may aid in distinguishing PBL from disseminated NHL, or conversely, it may identify previously unknown breast involvement in a systemic NHL. It is likely to be a useful tool for staging and follow-up of aggressive breast lymphoma.[99]

Treatment and outcome

Determining definitive treatment recommendations for breast lymphoma from the reported case series is difficult. There are no clinical trials, the case series are small and typically describe nonuniform treatments. The classification system for NHLs has evolved and the concept of MALT lymphoma has been explored. In general, during the time period covered by the older case series, common treatments for NHL have evolved from surgery to adjuvant radiotherapy to combination chemotherapy and chemoimmunotherapy.

In the past, physicians used and reported the results of the treatments they had available, so early investigators favored surgical treatment,[16] while later authors have advocated radiotherapy, chemotherapy, or both after excisional biopsy.[20,24,26,33,36,53,55] Lamovec and Jancar, for example, advocated radiotherapy after excisional biopsy based on their small series, in which those receiving radiotherapy after excisional biopsy had fewer recurrences than those who had excisional biopsy alone.[26] Schouten et al. advocated aggressive chemotherapy based on their small series,[20] and other authors began to advocate chemotherapy when such factors as high-grade histology, high lactate dehydrogenase level, axillary node involvement, and bulky disease are present.[24]

It is perhaps more instructive, however, to follow the paradigms now elucidated for systemic NHLs. Specifically, the histological subtype, as well as the staging and risk factor data, predict the natural history and should guide the optimal therapy in NHL whether with a localized nodal, localized extranodal, or systemic presentation.[17,18,22,23,25,28,35,38,39,44,51]

In the absence of clear data to the contrary from the literature, it seems reasonable to base the treatment of primary breast lymphoma on the generally accepted recommendations for other extranodal lymphomas. Primary breast lymphomas, as defined for the purposes of this discussion (see above), are stage IE or IIE in the Ann Arbor staging system.[41] Histological subtypes are defined according to the 2008 WHO classification of lymphoma or may be grouped as low, intermediate or high grade according to the Working Formulation classification of lymphoma.[100]

The standard therapy for apparently localized low-grade lymphoma is radiotherapy alone,[101] with the caveat that dissemination of low-grade lymphoma is the rule and that many patients with apparently localized disease have occult disease elsewhere. For this reason, some clinicians would advocate the anti-CD20 antibody rituximab, single agent alkylator therapy such as chlorambucil or cyclophosphamide, a fludarabine-based combination, or a nonanthracycline-based alkylator combination such as cyclophosphamide, vincristine, and prednisone, rather than radiotherapy alone. A period of observation without treatment may be appropriate for selected patients with indolent histology and clinical behavior.

Low-grade lymphomas of MALT in the gastrointestinal tract or salivary gland, where they are most common and best characterized, behave indolently.[102–104] Although relatively few reports[2,3,26] have addressed the question of whether breast low-grade MALT lymphomas are similarly indolent, there is evidence that this histological subtype may represent a special case in which excision alone is adequate for some patients. For example, Mattia et al., among nine cases of primary breast lymphoma, observed four patients with low-grade lymphoma of MALT who were treated with excision alone. Three were alive with no evidence of disease at 10, 12, and 48 months' follow-up.[3] In reviewing the literature, they identified 17 patients in whom this diagnosis is relatively secure, 10 of whom had a durable complete remission "most after local treatment only." They concluded that there is a recognizable subset of patients with this histological subtype in the older literature who had an indolent course with minimal treatment.[3]

Ample data now support the treatment of localized intermediate-grade lymphomas, including extranodal presentations, with abbreviated chemotherapy (for example, three cycles of cyclophosphamide, doxorubicin, vincristine, prednisone, and rituximab (CHOPR), or the equivalent) followed by involved field radiotherapy.[105,106] For those patients with bulky disease or other adverse prognostic features, some clinicians might consider longer courses of chemotherapy followed by radiotherapy. For some cases, some clinicians would choose to omit the radiotherapy (for example, if the fields would involve the ventricle) and would give chemotherapy alone.

Of particular concern are reports that central nervous system (CNS) relapse is particularly common with diffuse large B cell lymphoma of the breast,[17,22,30,35,38,45] raising the question of CNS prophylaxis. Because of the small numbers of patients, no risk factors for CNS progression or relapse have been identified. Reported CNS relapse rates range from 0% to 29%,[5,45] although some reports include patients with high-grade histologies.

The optimal treatment regimen for extranodal Burkitt or other high-grade lymphoma has not been well described; however, it should be seen as a potentially curable disease requiring aggressive chemotherapy and CNS prophylaxis similar to the treatment of nodal high-grade lymphomas.

Like much of the data on primary breast lymphoma, the reported results of treatment in the older literature vary widely. Five-year survival rates ranging from 9%[107] to 85%[33] are reported, likely reflecting the heterogeneous histological subtypes, variations in staging, and nonstandardized treatment of patients in the various small series. In general, early reports described an aggressive, rapid course with early relapse: Lattes, for example, reported 17 of 33 patients dead in the first year.[107] It has been suggested that these poor outcome data reflect understaging of patients and thus inadequate treatment.[20] Undoubtedly some of these patients had Burkitt or other high-grade lymphoma.

As noted above, many authors have distinguished two patterns of clinical behavior of primary breast lymphoma. The first affects younger women, many of them pregnant or recently post partum, and many of African or Italian descent, who have a bilateral presentation, Burkitt-like histological subtype and a very rapid and aggressive clinical course.[2,16,27,108–113] CNS relapses are reportedly common in this group.[2] The other pattern is of older women with unilateral breast involvement. A variety of histological subtypes is seen, and the clinical course is in general more indolent.[2,114] Age, which probably discriminates these two groups, has been reported to be a significant prognostic factor. One series reported median survival times of 10.3 months in patients under 45 years old and 25.5 months in those older than 45,[27] and similarly, Hugh et al., extracting data on 235 patients described in the literature, reported median survival of 9.5 and 47 months for those younger than and older than 40, respectively.[2] It is very likely that age is a surrogate marker for the true determinant of clinical behavior, which is histology, Burkitt and other high-grade lymphomas being more common in younger patients and indolent lymphomas being more common in older patients.

In the more recent series, histological subtype is reported as a major prognostic factor, as it is in other lymphomas.[3,27,29,36,38,39,44,55] It is likely that the outcomes for patients with breast lymphoma are generally similar to other extranodal NHL patients, with long survival times. Low-grade lymphomas of MALT tend to have favorable outcomes with a variety of treatments, including radiotherapy, surgery, chemotherapy or antibody therapy with rituximab.[3,5,17,26] Localized radiotherapy may be particularly useful in this group. A report by Ganjoo et al. reported four of five low-grade (four marginal zone lymphomas/MALT and one follicle center cell lymphoma), localized patients treated with radiotherapy in remission at a median follow-up of 5.8 years.[39] Follicle center cell lymphomas of the breast can be treated similarly, with the caveat that, like follicle center cell lymphomas elsewhere, they tend to relapse in disseminated sites and therefore systemic treatment may be more appropriate than radiotherapy.

The reported survival times for intermediate- and high-grade histological subtypes of primary breast lymphoma (e.g. diffuse large B cell lymphoma, anaplastic large cell lymphoma, Burkitt lymphoma) diagnosed with current techniques and treated with modern chemotherapy or combined modality therapy are fairly consistent. With combination chemotherapy (for example, cyclophosphamide, doxorubicin, vincristine, prednisone – CHOP) or chemoimmunotherapy (CHOPR), intermediate-grade breast lymphoma is probably curable.[28,38,39,44,45] For example, in a retrospective analysis the International, Extranodal Lymphoma Study Group reported 204 patients with diffuse large B cell lymphoma. In the 143 who received an anthracycline-containing chemotherapy regimen, the 5-year overall survival was 73% (progression-free survival data not given).[38] Ganjoo *et al.* estimated the progression-free survival of their patients with diffuse large B cell lymphoma as 61% at a median follow-up of 3.8 years.[39] While some reports indicate that patients with localized diffuse large B cell lymphoma of the breast have approximately the same cure rate as their counterparts with nodal presentations of the same stage, Validire *et al.* reported 68 patients in their series who had a markedly worse progression-free survival and overall survival when compared to historical controls.[45] The International Prognostic Index[115] (negative features of elevated lactate dehydrogenase (LDH), age greater than 60, stage III or IV, more than one extranodal site, and Eastern Cooperative Oncology Group (ECOG) performance status greater than 2) has been validated in this group of patients.[39,45] One report notes that those presenting with bilateral disease (5% of their group, *n*=11) fare much worse, with early progression and poorer survival (progression-free survival 1.3 years), and they suggest that those patients be regarded as having stage IV disease.[38]

The pattern of relapse of PBL is worthy of special note. CNS relapse of aggressive disease is reported throughout the literature on PBL, although its rarity makes it difficult to estimate the frequency of this occurrence or to determine whether it is more frequent than in other extranodal lymphomas. Validire *et al.* reported three CNS relapses among 38 patients with diffuse large B cell lymphoma, for a rate of 8%,[45] while Ryan *et al.* reported 11 CNS relapses among 204 diffuse large B cell lymphoma patients (5%).[38] Relapse in the ipsilateral or contralateral breast is common, although the use of radiotherapy seems to decrease that risk in the ipsilateral breast, while anthracycline-containing chemotherapy reduces the risk in the contralateral breast, at least among patients with diffuse large B cell lymphoma.[38]

Recommendations

In summary, the rational treatment of localized breast lymphoma should be similar to that of other extranodal lymphomas. MALT lymphoma has a lower potential for dissemination and may be particularly suited to treatment with local irradiation or even resection alone. Other low-grade lymphomas such as follicle center cell lymphoma may be treated with any of the low-grade lymphoma regimens such as rituximab alone or chemoimmunotherapy combinations. Diffuse large B cell lymphoma should be treated with chemotherapy containing anthracycline and rituximab (such as CHOPR) either alone for "full course" or with an abbreviated course followed by local irradiation. Consideration should be given to administering prophylactic intrathecal chemotherapy to those with diffuse large B cell lymphoma. Burkitt lymphoma can be treated with a regimen appropriate for that histological subtype with CNS prophylaxis.

References

1. Wiseman C, Liao KT. Primary lymphoma of the breast. Cancer 1972; 29(6): 1705–12.
2. Hugh JC, *et al.* Primary breast lymphoma. An immunohistologic study of 20 new cases. Cancer 1990; 66(12): 2602–11.
3. Mattia AR, Ferry JA, Harris NL. Breast lymphoma. A B-cell spectrum including the low grade B-cell lymphoma of mucosa associated lymphoid tissue. Am J Surg Pathol 1993; 17(6): 574–87.
4. Eufemio G. Case report. Primary malignant lymphoma of the breast. Acta Med Philipp 1966; 2(4): 201–5.
5. Lin Y, Govindan R, Hess JL. Malignant hematopoietic breast tumors. Am J Clin Pathol 1997; 107(2): 177–86.
6. Kuechkens H. Ein lokales lymphogranulom der brust in form eines mammatumors. Beitr pathol Anat Allge Pathol 1928; 80: 135–7.
7. Raju GC, Jankey N, Delpech K. Localized primary extranodal Hodgkin's disease (Hodgkin's lymphoma) of the breast. J R Soc Med 1987; 80(4): 247–9.
8. Abuin JC, Gonzalez R. [Mammary localization of Hodgkin's disease]. Rev Sanid Milit Argent 1968; 67(1): 45–8.
9. Lawler MR Jr, Riddell DH. Hodgkin's disease of the breast. Arch Surg 1966; 93(2): 331–4.
10. Horning SJ, *et al.* Detection of non-Hodgkin's lymphoma in the peripheral blood by analysis of antigen receptor gene rearrangements: results of a prospective study. Blood 1990; 75(5): 1139–45.
11. Stetlet-Stevenson M, *et al.* Detection of occult follicular lymphoma by specific DNA amplification. Blood 1988; 72(5): 1822–5.
12. Gross S. *Tumors of the Mammary Gland.* New York: Appleton and Co, 1880.
13. Halsam W. Birmingh M Rev 1889; 25: 286.
14. Geist SH, Wilensky AO. Sarcoma of the breast. Ann Surg 1915; 62(1): 11–21.
15. Bilroth I. *Handbuch der Frauenkrankheiten.* Stuttgart: F. Enke, 1880.
16. Adair F, Hermann J. Primary lymphosarcoma of the breast. Surgery 1944; 16: 836.
17. Wong WW, *et al.* Primary non-Hodgkin lymphoma of the breast: the Mayo Clinic experience. J Surg Oncol 2002; 80(1): 19–25; discussion 26.
18. Vigliotti ML, *et al.* Primary breast lymphoma: outcome of 7 patients and a review of the literature. Leuk Lymphoma 2005; 46(9): 1321–7.
19. Smith MR, Brustein S, Straus DJ. Localized non-Hodgkin's lymphoma of the breast. Cancer 1987; 59(2): 351–4.
20. Schouten JT, Weese JL, Carbone PP. Lymphoma of the breast. Ann Surg 1981; 194(6): 749–53.
21. Sabate JM, *et al.* Lymphoma of the breast: clinical and radiologic features with pathologic correlation in 28 patients. Breast J 2002; 8(5): 294–304.
22. Ribrag V, *et al.* Primary breast lymphoma: a report of 20 cases. Br J Haematol 2001; 115(2): 253–6.
23. Park YH, *et al.* Primary malignant lymphoma of the breast: clinicopathological study of nine cases. Leuk Lymphoma 2004; 45(2): 327–30.
24. Misra A, Kapur BM, Rath GK. Primary breast lymphoma. J Surg Oncol 1991; 47(4): 265–70.
25. Lyons JA, *et al.* Treatment of prognosis of primary breast lymphoma: a review of 13 cases. Am J Clin Oncol 2000; 23(4): 334–6.
26. Lamovec J, Jancar J. Primary malignant lymphoma of the breast. Lymphoma of the mucosa-associated lymphoid tissue. Cancer 1987; 60(12): 3033–41.
27. Jeon HJ, *et al.* Primary non-Hodgkin malignant lymphoma of the breast. An immunohistochemical study of seven patients and literature review of 152 patients with breast lymphoma in Japan. Cancer 1992; 70(10): 2451–9.
28. Ha CS, *et al.* Localized primary non-Hodgkin lymphoma of the breast. Am J Clin Oncol 1998; 21(4): 376–80.
29. Giardini R, Piccolo C, Rilke F. Primary non-Hodgkin's lymphomas of the female breast. Cancer 1992; 69(3): 725–35.
30. Gholam D, *et al.* Primary breast lymphoma. Leuk Lymphoma 2003; 44(7): 1173–8.
31. Farinha P, *et al.* High frequency of MALT lymphoma in a series of 14 cases of primary breast lymphoma. Appl Immunohistochem Mol Morphol 2002; 10(2): 115–20.
32. Domchek SM, *et al.* Lymphomas of the breast: primary and secondary involvement. Cancer 2002; 94(1): 6–13.
33. Dixon JM, *et al.* Primary lymphoma of the breast. Br J Surg 1987; 74(3): 214–16.

34. Cohen PL, Brooks JJ. Lymphomas of the breast. A clinicopathologic and immunohistochemical study of primary and secondary cases. Cancer 1991; 67(5): 1359–69.

35. Au WY, et al. Lymphoma of the breast in Hong Kong Chinese. Hematol Oncol 1997; 15(1): 33–8.

36. Ariad S, et al. Breast lymphoma. A clinical and pathological review and 10-year treatment results. S Afr Med J 1995; 85(2): 85–9.

37. Arber DA, et al. Non-Hodgkin's lymphoma involving the breast. Am J Surg Pathol 1994; 18(3): 288–95.

38. Ryan G, et al. Primary diffuse large B-cell lymphoma of the breast: prognostic factors and outcomes of a study by the International Extranodal Lymphoma Study Group. Ann Oncol 2008; 19(2): 233–41.

39. Ganjoo K, et al. Non-Hodgkin lymphoma of the breast. Cancer 2007; 110(1): 25–30.

40. Lin YC, et al. Clinicopathologic features and treatment outcome of non-Hodgkin lymphoma of the breast – a review of 42 primary and secondary cases in Taiwanese patients. Leuk Lymphoma 2009; 50(6): 918–24.

41. Carbone PP, et al. Report of the Committee on Hodgkin's Disease Staging Classification. Cancer Res 1971; 31(11): 1860–1.

42. Isaacson P, Wright DH. Extranodal malignant lymphoma arising from mucosa-associated lymphoid tissue. Cancer 1984; 53(11): 2515–24.

43. Ferguson DJ. Intraepithelial lymphocytes and macrophages in the normal breast. Virchows Arch A Pathol Anat Histopathol 1985; 407(4): 369–78.

44. Ogawa T, et al. Primary non-Hodgkin's lymphoma of the breast treated nonsurgically: report of three cases. Breast Cancer 2011; 18(1): 68–72.

45. Validire P, et al. Primary breast non-Hodgkin's lymphoma: a large single center study of initial characteristics, natural history, and prognostic factors. Am J Hematol 2009; 84(3): 133–9.

46. Windrum P, et al. Mantle cell lymphoma presenting as a breast mass. J Clin Pathol 2001; 54(11): 883–6.

47. Lazzeri, D, et al. ALK-1-negative anaplastic large cell lymphoma associated with breast implants: a new clinical entity. Clin Breast Cancer 2011; 11(5): 283–96.

48. Jewell M, et al. Anaplastic large T-cell lymphoma and breast implants: a review of the literature. Plast Reconstr Surg 2011; 128(3): 651–61.

49. de Jong D, et al. Anaplastic large-cell lymphoma in women with breast implants. JAMA 2008; 300(17): 2030–5.

50. Lingohr P, Eidt S, Rheinwalt KP. A 12-year-old girl presenting with bilateral gigantic Burkitt's lymphoma of the breast. Arch Gynecol Obstet 2009; 279(5): 743–6.

51. Chanan-Khan A, et al. Non-Hodgkin's lymphoma presenting as a breast mass in patients with HIV infection: a report of three cases. Leuk Lymphoma 2005; 46(8): 1189–93.

52. Akbari CM, Welch JP, Pastuszak W. Primary lymphoproliferative disorders of the breast. Conn Med 1995; 59(11): 651–5.

53. Decosse JJ, et al. Primary lymphosarcoma of the breast. A review of 14 cases. Cancer 1962; 15: 1264–8.

54. Jernstrom P, Sether J. Primary lymphosarcoma of the mamary gland. JAMA 1967; 201: 506.

55. Mambo NC, Burke JS, Butler JJ. Primary malignant lymphomas of the breast. Cancer 1977; 39(5): 2033–40.

56. Dao AH, Adkins RB Jr, Glick AD. Malignant lymphoma of the breast: a review of 13 cases. Am Surg 1992; 58(12): 792–6.

57. Telesinghe PU, Anthony PP. Primary lymphoma of the breast. Histopathology 1985; 9(3): 297–307.

58. Freeman C, Berg JW, Cutler SJ. Occurrence and prognosis of extranodal lymphomas. Cancer 1972; 29(1): 252–60.

59. De Souza LJ, Talvalkar GV, Morjaria JH. Primary malignant lymphoma of the breast. Indian J Cancer 1978; 15(4): 30–5.

60. Lawler MR Jr, Richie RE. Reticulum cell sarcoma of the breast. Cancer 1967; 20(9): 1438–46.

61. Murata T, et al. Primary non-Hodgkin malignant lymphoma of the male breast. Jpn J Clin Oncol 1996; 26(4): 243–7.

62. Tanaka T, et al. Primary malignant lymphoma of the breast. With a review of 73 cases among Japanese subjects. Acta Pathol Jpn 1984; 34(2): 361–73.

63. Pullen CM, Cass AJ. Bilateral primary lymphoma of the breast. Aust N Z J Surg 1996; 66(12): 845–7.

64. Cohen Y, et al. [Primary breast lymphoma]. Harefuah 1993; 125(1–2): 24–6, 63.

65. Latteri MA, et al. Primary extranodal non-Hodgkin lymphomas of the uterus and the breast: report of three cases. Eur J Surg Oncol 1995; 21(4): 432–4.

66. Poulsen LO, et al. Immunologic observations in close relatives of two sisters with mammary Burkitt's lymphoma. Mammary Burkitt's lymphoma in sisters. Cancer 1991; 68(5): 1031–4.

67. Kuper-Hommel MJ, et al. Treatment and survival of 38 female breast lymphomas: a population-based study with clinical and pathological reviews. Ann Hematol 2003; 82(7): 397–404.

68. Vignot S, et al. Non-Hodgkin's lymphoma of the breast: a report of 19 cases and a review of the literature. Clin Lymphoma 2005; 6(1): 37–42.

69. Burke JS. Are there site-specific differences among the MALT lymphomas – morphologic, clinical? Am J Clin Pathol 1999; 111(1 Suppl 1): S133–43.

70. Bobrow LG, et al. Breast lymphomas: a clinicopathologic review. Hum Pathol 1993; 24(3): 274–8.

71. Prevot S, et al. [Primary non-Hodgkin's malignant lymphoma of the breast. Anatomopathologic diagnosis of 14 cases]. Bull Cancer 1990; 77(2): 123–36.

72. Aozasa K, et al. Malignant lymphoma of the breast. Immunologic type and association with lymphocytic mastopathy. Am J Clin Pathol 1992; 97(5): 699–704.

73. Tan PH, Sng IT. Breast lymphoma – a pathologic study of 14 cases. Ann Acad Med Singapore 1996; 25(6): 783–90.

74. Rooney N, et al. Primary breast lymphoma with skin involvement arising in lymphocytic lobulitis. Histopathology 1994; 24(1): 81–4.

75. Lammie GA, et al. Sclerosing lymphocytic lobulitis of the breast – evidence for an autoimmune pathogenesis. Histopathology 1991; 19(1): 13–20.

76. Schwartz IS, Strauchen JA. Lymphocytic mastopathy. An autoimmune disease of the breast? Am J Clin Pathol 1990; 93(6): 725–30.

77. Tomaszewski JE, et al. Diabetic mastopathy: a distinctive clinicopathologic entity. Hum Pathol 1992; 23(7): 780–6.

78. Giedsing Hansen T, et al. Primary non-Hodgkin's lymphoma of the breast (PLB): a clinicopathological study of seven cases. APMIS 1992; 100(12): 1089–96.

79. Ott G, et al. The t(11;18)(q21;q21) chromosome translocation is a frequent and specific aberration in low-grade but not high-grade malignant non-Hodgkin's lymphomas of the mucosa-associated lymphoid tissue (MALT-) type. Cancer Res 1997; 57(18): 3944–8.

80. Raghoebier S, et al. Essential differences in oncogene involvement between primary nodal and extranodal large cell lymphoma. Blood 1991; 78(10): 2680–5.

81. Anania G, et al. Primary non-Hodgkin's T-cell lymphoma of the breast. Eur J Surg 1997; 163(8): 633–5.

82. Slanetz PJ, Whitman GJ. Non-Hodgkin's lymphoma of the breast causing multiple vague densities on mammography. Am J Roentgenol 1996; 167(2): 537–8.

83. Liberman L, et al. Non-Hodgkin lymphoma of the breast: imaging characteristics and correlation with histopathologic findings. Radiology 1994; 192(1): 157–60.

84. El-Ghazawy IM, Singletary SE. Surgical management of primary lymphoma of the breast. Ann Surg 1991; 214(6): 724–6.

85. Eskelinen M, et al. Lymphoma of the breast. Ann Chir Gynaecol 1989; 78(2): 149–52.

86. Zinzani PL, et al. Bilateral primary breast lymphoma: a case of local recurrence. Leuk Lymphoma 2003; 44(4): 737–8.

87. Andre JM, et al. [Malignant lymphomas and other hematosarcomas with initial breast localization. Retrospective study of 20 cases]. Bull Cancer 1983; 70(5): 401–9.

88. Cook PD, et al. Follicular lymphoma adjacent to foreign body granulomatous inflammation and fibrosis surrounding silicone breast prosthesis. Am J Surg Pathol 1995; 19(6): 712–17.

89. Gaudet G, et al. Breast lymphoma associated with breast implants: two case-reports and a review of the literature. Leuk Lymphoma 2002; 43(1): 115–19.

90. Sahoo S, et al. Anaplastic large cell lymphoma arising in a silicone breast implant capsule: a case report and review of the literature. Arch Pathol Lab Med 2003; 127(3): e115–18.

91. Duvic M, *et al.* Cutaneous T-cell lymphoma in association with silicone breast implants. J Am Acad Dermatol 1995; 32(6): 939–42.

92. Keech JA Jr, Creech BJ. Anaplastic T-cell lymphoma in proximity to a saline-filled breast implant. Plast Reconstr Surg 1997; 100(2): 554–5.

93. Meyer JE, Kopans DB, Long JC. Mammographic appearance of malignant lymphoma of the breast. Radiology 1980; 135(3): 623–6.

94. Meyer JE, *et al.* Large-core breast biopsy to obtain tissue for tumor markers in breast lymphoma. AJR Am J Roentgenol 1994; 162(6): 1500.

95. Pameijer FA, *et al.* Non-Hodgkin's lymphoma of the breast causing miliary densities on mammography. Am J Roentgenol 1995; 164(3): 609–10.

96. Demirkazik FB. MR imaging features of breast lymphoma. Eur J Radiol 2002; 42(1): 62–4.

97. Naganawa S, *et al.* MR Imaging of the primary breast lymphoma: a case report. Breast Cancer 1996; 3(3): 209–13.

98. Darnell A, *et al.* Primary lymphoma of the breast: MR imaging features. A case report. Magn Reson Imaging 1999; 17(3): 479–82.

99. Bakheet SM, *et al.* F-18 FDG positron emission tomography in primary breast non-Hodgkin's lymphoma. Clin Nucl Med 2001; 26(4): 299–301.

100. National Cancer Institute sponsored study of classifications of non-Hodgkin's lymphomas: summary and description of a working formulation for clinical usage. The Non-Hodgkin's Lymphoma Pathologic Classification Project. Cancer 1982; 49(10): 2112–35.

101. Shipp M, Mauch P, Harris N. Non-Hodgkin's lymphomas. In: DeVita V, Hellman S, Rosenberg S (eds) *Cancer: Principles and Practice of Oncology*. Philadelphia: Lippincott-Raven, 1997. pp.2165–220.

102. Isaacson PG. Gastrointestinal lymphoma. Hum Pathol 1994; 25(10): 1020–9.

103. Radaszkiewicz T, Dragosics B, Bauer P. Gastrointestinal malignant lymphomas of the mucosa-associated lymphoid tissue: factors relevant to prognosis. Gastroenterology 1992; 102(5): 1628–38.

104. Wotherspoon AC, *et al.* Helicobacter pylori-associated gastritis and primary B-cell gastric lymphoma. Lancet 1991; 338(8776): 1175–6.

105. Miller TP, *et al.* Chemotherapy alone compared with chemotherapy plus radiotherapy for localized intermediate- and high-grade non-Hodgkin's lymphoma. N Engl J Med 1998; 339(1): 21–6.

106. Persky DO, *et al.* Phase II study of rituximab plus three cycles of CHOP and involved-field radiotherapy for patients with limited-stage aggressive B-cell lymphoma: Southwest Oncology Group study 0014. J Clin Oncol 2008; 26(14): 2258–63.

107. Lattes R. Sarcomas of the breast. Int J Radiat Oncol Biol Phys 1978; 4(7–8): 705–8.

108. Carbone A, *et al.* Primary lymphoblastic lymphoma of the breast. Clin Oncol 1982; 8(4): 367–73.

109. Durodola JI. Burkitt's lymphoma presenting during lactation. Int J Gynaecol Obstet 1976; 14(3): 225–31.

110. Jones DE, *et al.* Burkitt's lymphoma: obstetric and gynecologic aspects. Obstet Gynecol 1980; 56(4): 533–6.

111. Kay S. Lymphosarcoma of the female mammary gland. AMA Arch Pathol 1955; 60(5): 575–9.

112. Shepherd JJ, Wright DH. Burkitt's tumour presenting as bilateral swelling of the breast in women of child-bearing age. Br J Surg 1967; 54(9): 776–80.

113. Tweeddale DN, Mahr MM. Secondary lymphosarcoma of the breast in pregnancy. Report of a case. Obstet Gynecol 1964; 24: 584–6.

114. Brustein S, *et al.* Malignant lymphoma of the breast. A study of 53 patients. Ann Surg 1987; 205(2): 144–50.

115. International Non-Hodgkin's Lymphoma Prognostic Factors Project. A predictive model for aggressive non-Hodgkin's lymphoma. N Engl J Med 1993; 329(14): 987–94.

16 Male Breast Cancer

Nicole M. Randall,[1] Kathy D. Miller,[2] and George W. Sledge Jr.[1]

[1] Department of Oncology, Indiana University School of Medicine, Indianapolis, IN, USA
[2] Indiana University Melvin and Bren Simon Cancer Center, Indianapolis, IN, USA

Introduction

Although breast cancer is an uncommon malignancy in men, it has been recognized since antiquity. The earliest mention of breast cancer appears in the Edwin Smith Surgical Papyrus dating from 3000 to 2500 BC and refers to a man.[1] The first clinical description is attributed to the 14th-century English surgeon John of Aderne who warned a priest with a large breast mass that treatment by a barber "would bring him to death."[2] The subsequent scattered case reports were compiled by Williams in the late 19th century[3] but an exhaustive and detailed review of the basic characteristics of the disease did not appear until 1927.[4]

Knowledge of many of the relevant aspects of the disease and appropriate therapy remains limited. Large series of male breast cancer (MBC) are rare, retrospective, and cover extended time periods, generally at single institutions, during which methods of diagnosis, staging, and treatment may have changed dramatically. Prospective, randomized trials are not available. Treatment for men has therefore been based on the known biology of MBC and the knowledge gained from controlled clinical studies performed in women.

Biology and epidemiology

The American Cancer Society estimated that in 2010 approximately 1970 men would be diagnosed with breast cancer in the United States, and that 390 patients would die from the disease.[5] This accounts for 0.9% of all breast cancer cases, and only 0.25% of all malignancies in men. In the United States, breast cancer is responsible for 0.13% of all cancer deaths in men. The incidence of MBC, once thought to be relatively stable, now seems to be increasing. Incidence of MBC increased significantly from 0.86 to 1.06 per 100,000 population over the last 26 years.[6] Rates of *in situ* tumors increased most rapidly, up by 123% among men. Invasive localized disease rates were found to have increased by a more modest 37%. Conversely, the

disease rates of invasive regional and distant breast carcinoma declined for men and women during the 1980s and 1990s. For example, the distant disease rate was found to have decreased 41% among men from 0.09 per 100,000 man-years during 1975–1980 to 0.05 per 100,000 man-years during 1997–2001.[7] Advances in screening mammography could not account for the dramatic increases noted in early-stage breast carcinoma among men, given that men are not routinely screened for breast carcinoma. However, a heightened awareness of male breast carcinoma might result in the earlier detection of "symptomatic" *in situ* and invasive localized tumors because of the easier detection of lesions in men with a small breast volume.[7]

The prevalence of MBC increases with age, from 0.1 cases per 100,000 at 30–34 years to 6.5 cases per 100,000 at 85 years and older.[8] The disease is extremely rare before the age of 30, although two children have been reported with the disease.[9] The mean age at diagnosis is approximately 63–71 years, nearly 10 years older than the corresponding mean age for women.[8,10–12] The reason for this age difference is not known.

As with female breast cancer, the incidence of MBC varies with geographic location, with higher rates in North America and Europe and lower rates in Asia. The lowest rates are reported in Finland and Japan,[13] and the highest incidence occurs in several African nations.[14] In Zambia, nearly 15% of patients diagnosed with breast cancer are men.[15] Regions with the highest incidence of MBC coincide with areas of increased incidence of liver disease, suggesting a possible association with higher estrogen levels.

The cause of MBC remains elusive. Many etiological factors have been proposed but supporting evidence is generally thin and based on small numbers of patients (Box 16.1). One commonly reported factor is a hormonal imbalance between estrogen and androgens. The association between estrogen levels and breast cancer in men is of interest because estrogen-related risk factors have been strongly implicated in female breast cancer. The imbalance between estrogen and

Box 16.1 Factors implicated in the etiology of male breast cancer.

- Estrogen – androgen imbalance
  - Exogenous estrogen
  - Klinefelter syndrome
  - Treatment for prostate cancer
  - Chronic liver disease
  - Obesity
- Testicular abnormalities
  - Orchiectomy
  - Mumps orchitis
  - Cryptorchidism
  - Excess heat exposure
- Increased prolactin
  - Drugs
  - Head trauma
- Ionizing radiation
- Family history
- Genetic syndromes: *BRCA2*

androgen may be the result of either estrogen excess or androgen deficiency. Conditions associated with MBC that increase levels of circulating estrogens in the body include chronic liver disease,[7,16] obesity early in life,[17,18] and pharmacological estrogen therapy, particularly in prostate cancer.[19] In obese men, estrogen production, metabolism, and bioavailability are enhanced. Levels of circulating estrogens may be increased with conversion of androgens to estradiol and estrone in peripheral adipose tissue.[20] The treatment required for male to female transsexuality has been implicated in MBC. Surgical and chemical castration and prolonged administration of large doses of female hormones produce the estrogen–androgen imbalance.[21,22] Similarly, estrogen therapy used in prostate cancer could lead to hormonal imbalance. Kanhai et al. demonstrated that after chemical castration for prostate cancer, there was moderate acinar and lobular formation of breast tissue.[19]

Disorders of testicular function result in hormonal imbalance by decreasing androgen production. A number of conditions have been implicated, including mumps orchitis, orchiectomy, undescended testes, and testicular injury.[23] Several case series have found an unusually high association with Klinefelter syndrome, where patients display a eunuchoid habitus, gynecomastia, and small, firm testes. Patients have high levels of gonadotropins and low levels of androgens.[24] Klinefelter syndrome has been documented by karyotype in up to 7% of MBC patients.[25,26] Occupational environmental exposure to high temperatures has been associated with increased risk of breast cancer in men. The increased temperature presumably results in testicular damage with altered androgen and estrogen levels. Among the affected are men working in steel and rolling mills, those involved in machinery repair and motor vehicle manufacturing, and blast furnace workers.[27,28] Exposure to carcinogens such as polycyclic aromatic hydrocarbons, nitrosamines, and metal fumes may also play a role.[29] Hyperprolactinemia, whether precipitated by drugs, brain trauma, or skull fractures, may increase the risk of developing breast cancer.[30] Radiation-induced breast cancers have also been reported.[31,32]

The relationship between gynecomastia, a proliferation of normal breast tissue under estrogenic stimulation, and MBC remains controversial. Microscopic evidence of ductal hyperplasia has been found in 40% of men with breast cancer.[33] In addition, autopsy studies have shown gynecomastia to be prevalent in as many as 50% of all MBC patients.[34] However, reviews of healthy men have found clinical gynecomastia to be present in 35–40%,[35] and therefore the rates of gynecomastia in MBC patients may be similar to those in the general population.[36]

Molecular biology and genetics

A possible familial association has been recognized for many years, with increased risk for close male and female relatives of MBC patients.[37] Data from the Surveillance, Epidemiology, and End Results (SEER) program showed that men with a positive family history have an odds ratio of 3.98 for developing breast cancer.[38] Advances in molecular analysis over the last decade have allowed the identification of breast cancer susceptibility genes, *BRCA1* and *BRCA2*. Although most studies of *BRCA1* carriers do not seem to be associated with an increased risk of MBC,[39] one study demonstrated a 10.5% (8 of 76) incidence of *BRCA1* mutations in Ashkenazi Jewish men with breast cancer.[40] The lifetime risk for breast cancer in a male with *BRCA1* mutation carrier is just over 1%.[41] *BRCA2* mutations, on the contrary, are the strongest risk factor for male breast cancer.[41] The lifetime risk for breast cancer in a male *BRCA2* mutation carrier is approximately 7%, which is 80–100 times greater than the general population.[41] Wooster et al. localized the gene to chromosome 13q12-13 and described multiple cases of MBC linked to this area.[42]

The prevalence of *BRCA2* mutations in men with breast cancer remains unclear. In a study of 237 families affected by breast cancer including at least one affected male, 76% were because of *BRCA2*.[43] The frequency of *BRCA* mutations in a population-based series of 54 male patients without a strong family history found only two (4%) with *BRCA2* mutations.[44]

PTEN tumor suppressor gene and *CHEK2* kinase are two genes associated with female breast cancer that have also been associated with MBC. In addition, there are 25 genes, including the *AR* gene and *CYP17* gene, that have also been suspected in MBC but have no definite role in female patients.[24]

Clinical presentation and diagnostic considerations

The clinical manifestations of MBC have been well described by several authors.[10,28,45] The most common presentation, a painless, firm subareolar mass, is seen in 75–85% of patients. There is a slight predilection for the left breast (1.07:1) in most collective series, with bilateral disease being quite unusual.[10,13,36,46] Other presenting symptoms include nipple discharge, ulceration or bleeding of the nipple, pain or swelling of the breast, or symptoms related to metastatic disease.[47]

In addition to the palpable mass, common physical examination findings include nipple retraction, inversion or fixation, nipple discharge, and mastitis. The rate of nipple involvement has been reported to be as high as 40–50% because of the sparsity of breast tissue and the central location of tumors.[36] Signs of Paget disease occur in approximately 3–5% of patients.[10,48] Paget disease in men is nearly always associated with an underlying invasive cancer.[49] Clinically involved axillary nodes occur in 40–55% of patients at presentation.[49,50] Palpable axillary adenopathy with an occult breast tumor, however, is uncommon in men.[9] The frequency of locally advanced disease with skin ulceration has declined as the delay in diagnosis has decreased from 18 months in older series to less than 6 months in some series after 1981.[9,51,52]

The main differential diagnosis is between gynecomastia and breast cancer. Other benign tumors of the male breast include lipoma, inclusion cyst, lymph node, fat necrosis, and leiomyoma, but are exceedingly rare.[53] In men suspected of having breast cancer, the diagnostic evaluation should parallel that recommended for women. The distinction on physical examination may be difficult but a bloody nipple discharge strongly favors carcinoma.[54,55] Several studies have demonstrated that mammography can reasonably differentiate gynecomastia and breast cancer.[52,56,57] One study of 100 male patients demonstrated 90% accuracy in differentiating the two pathologies.[56] An uncalcified mass is most commonly seen; microcalcifications are less frequent and tend to be more scattered with a coarse appearance.[55,57] Ultrasonography has proven helpful in imaging lesions in the male breast, with 80% of breast cancers having irregular margins.[57] Complex cystic lesions, heterogeneous hypoechoic lesions, and increased vascularity are other ultrasonographic signs concerning malignancy.[58] Fine needle aspiration biopsy with conventional cytological examination has been demonstrated to be very accurate, with high sensitivity and specificity.[59] If cytology is inconclusive (5%) or the specimen is insufficient (22%), an open biopsy is required and should be performed if any question remains following diagnostic imaging. Additional evaluation following cytological diagnosis should include biochemical evaluation of renal and liver function, and a plain chest radiograph. Bone scans, abdominal computed tomography, and brain imaging should be reserved for patients with symptoms, laboratory abnormalities, or advanced disease. The values of serum tumor markers such as CEA, CA15-3, and CA 27-29 have not been evaluated in MBC.

Pathology

Virtually all known histological types of breast cancer have been reported in men. As in women, infiltrating ductal carcinoma, with or without an intraductal component, predominates and accounts for 85–90% of cases.[59] Ductal carcinoma in situ (DCIS) is the most common type of in situ (noninvasive) tumor in men.[59] Given the absence of screening mammography in men, the striking rise in DCIS seen in women is unlikely to be paralleled in men. Medullary, tubular, papillary, mucinous, and inflammatory variants have been reported in a minority of patients. Conventional wisdom suggested that lobular carcinoma did not occur in men because of the lack of terminal differentiation in the rudimentary male breast. Both invasive and in situ forms of lobular carcinoma, however, have been reported extremely rarely.[60,61] Benign and malignant sarcomas have been well described and may account for up to 8% of male breast tumors.[62] The breast is not often considered a site of metastatic disease; however, prostate cancer is the most common tumor to metastasize to the breast.[63]

Estrogen and progesterone receptors are more commonly positive in MBC than in the female counterpart. A study using data from the SEER database demonstrated 90% positivity in 680 MBC patients with known estrogen receptor status.[6] Similarly, progesterone receptors were found to be positive in over 81% in those with known receptor status. Consistently high levels of estrogen (81%) and progesterone (74%) receptors are found in the largest literature review of studies of 1301 MBC patients.[36] Approximately 65–90% of MBC tumors are both estrogen and progesterone receptor positive.[59] These rates approximate those seen in older women, possibly because of the similarities in physiological estrogen status. In contrast with female breast cancer, there is no correlation between age and receptor positivity.

The prognostic utility of estrogen and progesterone receptors in men has not been established. The number of studies looking at the prognostic impact of hormone receptors in men is limited. Data from the SEER database demonstrated similar 5-year survival rates in both the hormone receptor-positive and -negative groups.[6] In addition, two large studies demonstrate contrasting results. A study of 229 patients from the Princess Margaret Hospital did not find any significant difference in overall survival after adjustment for key factors such as size of tumor, lymph node status, and type of treatment.[64] A study of 215 patients from Wisconsin, however, did find an improved overall survival after adjustment for tumor stage and lymph node status.[46] One recent study found expression of androgen receptor in tumor tissue to be an independently adverse factor for both disease-free and overall survival.[65]

The role of Her-2/neu expression in MBC is also not well defined, but MBC tumors are less likely than female breast cancers to express Her-2/neu. A recent review of Her-2/neu by immunohistochemistry in pooled data of 511 male patients demonstrated 37% overexpression.[36] However, the antibody preparations and definitions for positive staining varied significantly among the studies. More contemporary studies suggest that older studies may have overestimated the rate of Her-2/neu overexpression.[66]

Recently, 65 patients were studied by immunohistochemistry. Scoring was performed according to currently established guidelines and 9% (6/65) demonstrated 2+ or 3+ overexpression.[67] Another study of 99 patients found that 15.1% (15/99) demonstrated 2+ or 3+ overexpression.[68] These cases were then tested for Her-2/neu gene amplification by fluorescence in situ hybridization (FISH). Seven of seven 3+ staining samples demonstrated gene amplification, as well as four of eight 2+ staining samples. Her-2/neu gene amplification/protein overexpression did not correlate with tumor state, histological grade, estrogen/progesterone receptor status, or the axillary lymph node status. In addition, in recent studies Her-2/neu positivity is lower in males (2–15%) than in female breast cancer patients (18–20%).[68] In two studies, MBC tumors were around three times less likely to be Her-2 positive than FBC tumors (5% versus 15%).[59] It is unknown if Her-2/neu overexpression in males has the same prognostic implications as in females; however, one study found decreased disease-free survival with Her-2/neu overexpression.[67]

Treatment

Localized disease

The traditional approach most often used in series prior to 1960 was the Halstedian radical mastectomy. The pattern of surgical treatment has been based on the extent of disease at presentation and the standard of care for contemporary women. While randomized trials have proven the safety and efficacy of less aggressive surgical procedures in women with breast cancer, similar data do not exist for men. The finding that modified radical mastectomy is equivalent to radical mastectomy in prospective randomized trials in women has led to the use of modified radical mastectomy in men. Studies that have compared radical mastectomy and modified radical mastectomy in men have found no difference in local recurrence rates and in overall survival rates.[51,69,70] Most modern series use modified radical mastectomy as the standard local therapy for men.[36] Breast cosmesis is not a primary consideration for most men. Therefore, there has been little enthusiasm for investigating breast-conserving treatments. Successful breast conservation with lumpectomy and radiation therapy, however, has been described in a small series of patients with small breast cancers.[71]

The use of the sentinel node procedure has replaced axillary node dissection in women with a clinically negative axilla, and is now accepted as a reliable method to establish axillary node status for invasive MBC. There are many large reviews demonstrating its efficacy and accuracy in women. It is also the subject of three large prospective, randomized trials which demonstrated equivalent overall survival, disease-free survival, and regional control between sentinel lymph node resection compared with conventional axillary lymph node dissection, and with fewer complications.[72–74] In men, however, there have been a very limited number of patients evaluated with the sentinel node procedure. One trial of 18 patients using only colloid human albumin labeled with ,[99]Tc demonstrated successful identification of the node in all patients. Six of 18 patients (33%) had positive sentinel nodes.[75] Two other series used the combination of blue dye and ^{99m}Tc-radiolabeled colloidal albumin. All patients in the two series had successful identification of sentinel nodes (nine and seven patients).[76,77] Five of nine patients (56%) and one of seven patients (14%) had positive sentinel nodes, respectively. Routine axillary dissections were not performed in either trial and therefore false-negative rates could not be determined. On the basis of these limited data, it appears that the sentinel node procedure in MBC patients is successful in the hands of experienced

surgeons, avoids unnecessary removal of uninvolved lymph nodes, and reduces length of hospital stay.[49]

The role of adjuvant radiotherapy to the chest wall and axilla is poorly defined. The use of radiotherapy has varied widely, with some institutions recommending radiation only to those patients with inoperable tumors,[78] while others recommend radiation to nearly all patients.[50] Several retrospective reviews have found that postmastectomy radiation does reduce the risk of local recurrence but does not improve overall survival.[10,46,79] Given the lack of definitive data, it seems reasonable to consider local radiation in patients with risk factors similar to those described in women, i.e. those with large primary tumors, chest wall invasion, or multiple positive lymph nodes. Radiation to the axilla can be reduced especially after complete axillary lymph node dissection, when the risk of axillary recurrence is less than 1%.[80] Although uncommon, when breast conservation is chosen in men, adjuvant radiation therapy is indicated, as in women.

The significant benefit of adjuvant hormonal therapy in women combined with the high frequency of estrogen receptor expression in MBC has sparked interest in the use of adjuvant hormonal therapy to prevent systemic recurrence. Ribeiro and Swindell reported the results of an unselected series of patients with stage II and III disease treated with adjuvant tamoxifen for 1 to 2 years.[81] After a median follow-up of 49 months, the 39 treated patients had a 5-year actuarial survival of 61%, compared with 44% in a historical control group. Two other series have found an improved survival after treatment with tamoxifen.[45,64] Although these patients reported few serious side-effects, the experience at the Memorial Sloan-Kettering Cancer Center is quite different. Between 1990 and 1993, 24 patients received tamoxifen as adjuvant therapy for MBC. More than half the patients reported at least one side-effect, most commonly decreased libido, weight gain, hot flushes, and mood alterations or depression. Five patients (20.8%) discontinued therapy within 1 year.[82] Although the side-effects reported by Anelli et al. should not be taken lightly, they are hardly life-threatening in severity and should not discourage the use of adjuvant tamoxifen in men. Further, while the standard duration of therapy with tamoxifen in women is 5 years, most reviews in men have been for less than 2 years of tamoxifen. Therefore, the benefit may be underestimated if proportional benefit parallels duration of treatment as in women.

The finding of increased disease-free survival in postmenopausal women with anastrozole has not yet resulted in significant reports of the adjuvant use of third-generation aromatase inhibitors in men.[83] Harlan et al. studied the patterns of care for men with breast cancer diagnosed between 2003 and 2004 in a population-based sample who were treated in communities throughout the United States, and found that the use of tamoxifen decreased the risk of death from cancer; however, there was no decrease in mortality among men who received aromatase inhibitors.[84] The authors summarize that their data support the use of tamoxifen as the hormone agent of choice for men with breast cancer, and that aromatase inhibitors should not be used for treatment of men with breast cancer outside the context of a clinical trial.[84] In congruence, based on their review of the literature, Gomez-Raposo *et al.* conclude that tamoxifen is the gold standard of adjuvant hormone therapy, and aromatase inhibitors should not be used in the adjuvant setting because data on their effectiveness in men are scarce.[85]

Doyen *et al.* reported on the largest experience of the efficacy of aromatase inhibitors (AIs) in MBC patients; they administered AIs to 15 metastatic patients, and showed acceptable activity, with two complete responses, four partial responses, and two cases of disease stabilization.[86] A case series of two metastatic male breast cancer patients with clinical conditions of pulmonary thromboembolism and detached retina, for which tamoxifen might not be safe, were started on anastrozole after adjuvant chemotherapy, and demonstrated high suppression of estrogen synthesis after 6 weeks (near 80%), comparable with that observed in postmenopausal women treated with letrozole.[87] However, additional research into the role and effect of aromatase inhibitors in men with breast cancer is needed. Furthermore, the improved disease-free survival in women switching to exemestane or letrozole after 2–3 years or 5 years, respectively, of treatment with tamoxifen has also not been reported in men.[88,89]

Recommendations for adjuvant chemotherapy have been largely based on studies performed in women. The National Cancer Institute (NCI) completed a phase 2 study of 24 men with stage II disease and histologically proven nodal involvement. All patients received cyclophosphamide, methotrexate, and 5-fluorouracil (CMF) for a total of 12 months, beginning within 4 weeks of definitive surgery. None of the patients received adjuvant radiation therapy. After a median follow-up of 46 months, the projected 5-year survival of 80% compares well with historical controls in females. Two of the four patients with recurrent disease were disease free for more than 60 months, raising the question as to whether adjuvant therapy prevents or merely delays recurrence.[90] In a similar study of stage II and III patients using doxorubicin-based chemotherapy, Patel *et al.* found a 5-year survival of over 85%, with 64% of patients remaining disease free.[91]

Other authors have found improved outcomes with adjuvant chemotherapy.[36] Preferred adjuvant chemotherapy combinations include drugs such as doxorubicin, cyclophosphamide, paclitaxel, trastuzumab, methotrexate, fluorouracil, etc.[92] The rarity of MBC precludes randomized trials of adjuvant therapy in this population. The limited data available suggest that adjuvant hormonal or chemotherapy may improve disease-free and overall survival in patients with node-positive disease compared to that achieved with local therapies alone. Furthermore, adjuvant therapy should be considered in patients with tumors larger than 1 cm.

The treatment of men with pure DCIS requires special mention. Cutuli *et al.* reviewed 31 men treated at 19 French regional cancer centers over a 22-year period.[93] All patients were treated with surgical excision: six underwent lumpectomy and 25 underwent mastectomy. Axillary dissection in 19 patients found no evidence of nodal involvement. After a median follow-up of 83 months, four patients had a local recurrence, including three of those initially treated with lumpectomy and negative surgical margins. One patient's disease remained *in situ*; three had developed invasive disease but were salvaged with radical surgical excision. One patient developed contralateral DCIS. One patient developed metastasis and died 30 months after local recurrence.[93] As in women, DCIS is primarily a local disease with an excellent prognosis. Simple mastectomy without axillary node dissection is the treatment of choice.

Prognosis

The same tumor-node-metastasis (TNM) system is used to stage both male and female breast cancer. Older series demonstrated higher rates of presentation with regional disease and correspondingly low 5-year survival rates.[94] Scheike found an increase in patients presenting with stage I disease, from 20% in 1943–1957 to 44% in 1958–1972.[48] There was a similar decrease in patients with stage IV disease, although the percentage of patients with stage II disease remained constant. In comparison, recent NCI SEER data demonstrate that 41% of male patients present with disease localized to the breast. In addition, 37% present with regional node involvement.[7] According to the American Joint Committee on Cancer (AJCC) staging, these patients presented as stage 0–10%, stage I–29%, stage II–38%, stage III–7%, and stage IV–8%.

Despite increases in the number of patients diagnosed with localized disease, the number of patients presenting with distant metastasis has not changed greatly. In the past, approximately 10% of both male and female patients presented with overt metastasis but more recently this number was approximately 7–8%.[7] The risk of contralateral second breast cancer in men with a diagnosis of carcinoma of the breast was greatly increased in 1788 men in the SEER database. This risk was greater in men diagnosed with the first breast cancer before the age of 50 and was not associated with the type of treatment.[95]

Stage and axillary nodal status continue to be the most important prognostic indicators in MBC (Table 16.1). One report correlated survival with the number of pathologically involved nodes; Guinee *et al.* found 5-year survivals of 90%, 73%, and 55% for patients with 0, 1–3, and four or more positive nodes, respectively.[50] Similarly, Lartigau *et al.* reported 10-year survivals of 84%, 44%, and 14% for patients with 0, 1–3, and four or more involved lymph nodes.[78] Tumor size appears to be an important prognostic factor with 5-year survival of 74% for T1, 53% for T2, and 37% for T3 lesions. Histological grade also correlates well with survival; 5-year survival decreased from 74% for grade I tumors to 53% for those with grade III histological features.[6] The prognostic significance of ancillary studies used in female breast cancer has been poorly evaluated in men. DNA ploidy, percentage of cells in S-phase, Ki-67, cathepsin D, and p53 have not demonstrated a reproducible correlation with prognosis.

The relative prognosis of men and women with breast cancer has been the subject of much debate. Early reports suggested a much worse survival for men compared with women. In studies in which male and female patients were matched for age and stage, however, survivals were similar.[50,98,99] A recent large population-based registry study in Sweden demonstrated that there is no evidence to support the hypothesis that sex is a

Author	Years	Total patients	Five-year overall survival (%)		
			All	LN negative	LN positive
Ramantanis et al.[94]	1937–1974	138	32.5	56.5	30.8
Yap et al.[96]	1945–1975	87	42	77	37
Heller et al.[33]*	1949–1976	97	40	79	11
Donegan et al.[46]	1953–1995	156	50	73.6[†]	64.7[†]
Cutuli et al.[10,93]	1960–1986	397	65	82	61
Guinee et al.[50‡]	1965–1986	335	NR	90	65
Erlichman et al.[47]	1967–1981	89	NR	77	37
Borgen et al.[52,97]	1975–1990	104	85	100	60

Table 16.1 Overall survival based on pathological axillary nodal status.

LN, lymph node; NR, not reported.
*10-year survival rate.
[†]Survival calculated for operable patients only.
[‡]Disease-specific survival.

prognostic factor for breast cancer, as both female and male breast cancer patients had similar survival rates.[99] The previously observed differences in prognosis were thought to result from delays in diagnosis rather than a different biology or tumor aggressiveness. Comparisons that further stratify for the number of axillary nodes involved confirm similar survival.[50] Thus, while stage for stage the prognosis is equivalent in men and women, the tendency for more advanced disease at presentation and older median age seen in men may result in a lower overall survival. These differences are most likely because of the older age of male patients, death from other causes, and the lower life expectancy of men in the general population.[6,69] The 5-year survival rates for men with stages I–IV breast tumors are 96%, 84%, 52%, and 24%, respectively; the rates do not differ significantly from 5-year survival rates for female breast cancer.[6,59]

Metastatic disease

The median survival from the time of presentation with metastatic disease is about 26.5 months,[70] although the range is large and long-term survivors have been reported.[100] Since approximately 8% of men present with metastatic disease and many of those treated locally will recur at some point during the course of their illness, the need for effective treatment cannot be overemphasized. Strategies for treatment of men with disseminated disease have mirrored those developed for women. Hormonal therapy, either ablative or additive, and systemic chemotherapy have both been used with some success; however, controlled studies are lacking.

Hormonal therapy has been the mainstay of treatment since Farrow and Adair first reported healing of skeletal metastasis after orchiectomy in 1942.[101] In a review of 70 men treated with orchiectomy, Meyskens et al. found a collective response rate of 67% with a median duration of response of 22 months.[102] In addition, one review found that patients who responded to orchiectomy were more likely to respond to second-line ablative therapies, and responding patients had improved survival.[103] Jaiyesimi et al. reviewed ablative therapies in 447 patients and found response rates of 55% for orchiectomy,

80% for adrenalectomy, and 56% for hypophysectomy.[104] Investigators at the Roswell Park Memorial Institute confirm the effectiveness of adrenal ablation. Eight of 10 patients responded with a median duration of response of 15 months. Of these eight patients, five had previously responded to orchiectomy and three had had no prior response.[105]

Despite excellent response rates to hormonal ablation, these treatments have rarely been used as first-line therapy since the advent of effective additive hormonal treatments. Additive hormonal therapies eliminate the psychological opposition to orchiectomy and the substantial surgical morbidity and side-effect risk associated with adrenalectomy and hypophysectomy while preserving response. The overall response rates of additive therapies have been reported as 75% for androgens, 57% for antiandrogens, 40% for aminoglutethimide, and 49% for tamoxifen.[36] The efficacy of tamoxifen in metastatic MBC has been documented in sporadic case reports and small series. Patterson et al. found 31 patients in 16 collected reports with a cumulative response rate of 48%.[106] Lopez et al. treated 24 patients with advanced disease and reported a response rate of 38%.[107] Median duration of response was 21 months with a range of 8–60 months. While these response rates are somewhat lower than those reported with orchiectomy, the percentage of patients with estrogen receptor-positive tumors in each study is not known. The relationship between steroid receptor status and response to tamoxifen is clear. In both reports, more than 80% of known receptor-positive patients responded while there were no documented responses in those patients known to be receptor negative.

The widespread use of aromatase inhibitors in postmenopausal women has not yet been exported to men with breast cancer. Success with the early aromatase inhibitor aminoglutethimide has been limited in men. In women, the third-generation aromatase inhibitors anastrozole, letrozole, and exemestane have shown good results compared with tamoxifen as first-line agents. In the only reported series (in men) to date, three out of five men responded to nastrozole, with a mean duration of response of 8 months.[108] A recent case reported an ongoing clinical complete response of 12 months with the use of letrozole.[109] Other hormonal manipulations have also documented effectiveness in small studies. Medroxyprogesterone, cyproterone acetate, the combination of the gonadotropin-releasing hormone agonist analog buserelin and the antiandrogen flutamide have had variable success. Other agents that have produced temporary regressions include estrogens, prednisone, and androgens.

Systemic chemotherapy has not been rigorously studied in MBC. As many patients benefit from hormonal manipulations, chemotherapy is generally reserved as second-line therapy for those patients whose disease has become refractory to hormonal agents. Lopez *et al.* directly compared hormonal therapy and chemotherapy in a small series of 14 patients, and higher response rates were observed after hormonal therapy.[107] At least two studies have suggested that though the response to chemotherapy is often faster in men than in women with metastatic breast cancer, the duration of response is shorter.[12,110] Reported response rates for the various regimens include 67% for 5-fluorouracil, doxorubicin, cyclophosphamide, 55% for other doxorubicin-containing regimens, and 33% for CMF-like regimens.[36] Preferred single agents for recurrent and metastatic cases are doxorubicin, epirubicin, paclitaxel, docetaxel, capecitabine, vinorelbine, gemcitabine, etc.[92]

Recommendations

Carcinoma of the male breast is uncommon but not rare. The limited numbers of patients and the inability to conduct cooperative studies have prevented careful research. Accordingly, conclusions must be based on the available literature. The following recommendations find some support in the available data but cannot and should not be regarded as definitively proven.

• Carcinoma of the male breast is analogous to carcinoma of the female breast. The lone exception is the higher rate of estrogen receptor positivity and response to hormonal therapy seen in men.
• Genetic factors such as *BRCA2* increase the risk of developing MBC but overall account for a minority of patients.
• A modified radical mastectomy is the surgical procedure of choice for most patients. Total mastectomy and sentinel node biopsy can be considered by experienced surgeons.
• Radiation therapy may reduce the risk of local recurrence in patients with large tumors and/or multiple positive lymph nodes but has no impact on survival.
• Adjuvant hormonal therapy with tamoxifen and adjuvant chemotherapy may improve survival in patients with axillary nodal involvement. Treatment decisions need to be individualized.
• Metastatic disease is highly responsive to hormonal therapy; this should be the initial mode of treatment in men with hormone receptor-positive cancers. Ablative therapies may have a higher response rate but are generally much less acceptable to patients than tamoxifen. Many patients will respond to sequential hormonal therapies.
• Response rates to cytotoxic chemotherapy are similar to those seen in women and may provide palliation to patients in whom hormonal therapy is no longer effective.

References

1. Breasted JH. The Edwin Smith Surgical Papyrus. Chicago: University of Chicago Press, 1930. pp.403–6.
2. Holleb AI, Freeman HP, Farrow JH. Cancer of male breast. I. N Y State J Med 1968; 68: 544–53.
3. Williams W. Cancer of the male breast, based on records of 100 cases; with remarks. Lancet 1889; 2: 261–3.
4. Wainwright J. Carcinoma of the male breast. Arch Surg 1927; 14: 846–52.
5. American Cancer Society. *Cancer Facts and Figures 2010*. Atlanta, Georgia: American Cancer Society, 2010.
6. Giordano SH, *et al.* Breast carcinoma in men: a population-based study. Cancer 2004; 101(1): 51–7.
7. Anderson WF, Devesa SS. Breast carcinoma in men. Cancer 2005; 103(2): 432–3; author reply 433.
8. Donegan W. Cancer of the male breast. In: Donegan W (ed) *Cancer of the Breast*, 3 rd edn. Philadelphia: WB Saunders, 1988. pp.716–27.
9. Crichlow RW. Carcinoma of the male breast. Surg Gynecol Obstet 1972; 134(6): 1011–19.
10. Cutuli B, *et al.* Male breast cancer: results of the treatments and prognostic factors in 397 cases. Eur J Cancer 1995; 31A(12): 1960–4.
11. Anderson WF, *et al.* Is male breast cancer similar or different than female breast cancer? Breast Cancer Res Treat 2004; 83(1): 77–86.
12. Ribeiro G. Male breast carcinoma – a review of 301 cases from the Christie Hospital & Holt Radium Institute, Manchester. Br J Cancer 1985; 51(1): 115–19.
13. Ewertz M, *et al.* Incidence of male breast cancer in Scandinavia, 1943–1982. Int J Cancer 1989; 43(1): 27–31.
14. El-Gazayerli M, Abdel-Aziz A. On bilharziasis and male breast cancer in Egypt. Br J Cancer 1963; 17: 556–71.
15. Bhagwandeen SB. Carcinoma of the male breast in Zambia. East Afr Med J 1972; 49(2): 89–93.
16. Sorensen HT, *et al.* Risk of breast cancer in men with liver cirrhosis. Am J Gastroenterol 1998; 93(2): 231–3.
17. Ballerini P, *et al.* Hormones in male breast cancer. Tumori 1990; 76(1): 26–8.
18. Ewertz M, *et al.* Risk factors for male breast cancer – a case-control study from Scandinavia. Acta Oncol 2001; 40(4): 467–71.
19. Thellenberg C, *et al.* Second primary cancers in men with prostate cancer: an increased risk of male breast cancer. J Urol 2003; 169(4): 1345–8.
20. Hsing AW, *et al.* Risk factors for male breast cancer (United States). Cancer Causes Control 1998; 9(3): 269–75.
21. Symmers WS. Carcinoma of breast in trans-sexual individuals after surgical and hormonal interference with the primary and secondary sex characteristics. BMJ 1968; 2(597): 82–5.
22. Kanhai RC, *et al.* Short-term and long-term histologic effects of castration and estrogen treatment on breast tissue of 14 male-to-female transsexuals in comparison with two chemically castrated men. Am J Surg Pathol 2000; 24(1): 74–80.
23. Thomas DB, *et al.* Breast cancer in men: risk factors with hormonal implications. Am J Epidemiol 1992; 135(7): 734–48.
24. Weiss JR, Moysich KB, Swede H. Epidemiology of male breast cancer. Cancer Epidemiol Biomarkers Prev 2005; 14(1): 20–6.
25. Evans DB, Crichlow RW. Carcinoma of the male breast and Klinefelter's syndrome: is there an association? CA Cancer J Clin 1987; 37(4): 246–51.
26. Hultborn R, *et al.* Prevalence of Klinefelter's syndrome in male breast cancer patients. Anticancer Res 1997; 17(6D): 4293–7.
27. Rosenbaum PF, *et al.* Occupational exposures associated with male breast cancer. Am J Epidemiol 1994; 139(1): 30–6.
28. Pollan M, Gustavsson P, Floderus B. Breast cancer, occupation, and exposure to electromagnetic fields among Swedish men. Am J Ind Med 2001; 39(3): 276–85.
29. Cocco P, *et al.* Case-control study of occupational exposures and male breast cancer. Occup Environ Med 1998; 55(9): 599–604.
30. Olsson H, Ranstam J. Head trauma and exposure to prolactin-elevating drugs as risk factors for male breast cancer. J Natl Cancer Inst 1988; 80(9): 679–83.

31. Eldar S, Nash E, Abrahamson J. Radiation carcinogenesis in the male breast. Eur J Surg Oncol 1989; 15(3): 274–8.

32. Ron E, *et al*. Male breast cancer incidence among atomic bomb survivors. J Natl Cancer Inst 2005; 97(8): 603–5.

33. Heller KS, *et al*. Male breast cancer: a clinicopathologic study of 97 cases. Ann Surg 1978; 188(1): 60–5.

34. Andersen JA, Gram JB. Male breast at autopsy. Acta Pathol Microbiol Immunol Scand A 1982; 90(3): 191–7.

35. Braunstein GD. Gynecomastia. N Engl J Med 1993; 328(7): 490–5.

36. Giordano SH, Buzdar AU, Hortobagyi GN. Breast cancer in men. Ann Intern Med 2002; 137(8): 678–87.

37. Olsson H, *et al*. Population-based cohort investigations of the risk for malignant tumors in first-degree relatives and wives of men with breast cancer. Cancer 1993; 71(4): 1273–8.

38. Rosenblatt KA, *et al*. Breast cancer in men: aspects of familial aggregation. J Natl Cancer Inst 1991; 83(12): 849–54.

39. Hall JM, *et al*. Linkage of early-onset familial breast cancer to chromosome 17q21. Science 1990; 250(4988): 1684–9.

40. Frank TS, *et al*. Clinical characteristics of individuals with germline mutations in BRCA1 and BRCA2: analysis of 10,000 individuals. J Clin Oncol 2002; 20(6): 1480–90.

41. Johansen Taber KA. Male breast cancer: risk factors, diagnosis, and management (review). Oncol Rep 2010; 24(5): 1115–20.

42. Wooster R, *et al*. Localization of a breast cancer susceptibility gene, BRCA2, to chromosome 13q12-13. Science 1994; 265(5181): 2088–90.

43. Ford D, *et al*. Genetic heterogeneity and penetrance analysis of the BRCA1 and BRCA2 genes in breast cancer families. The Breast Cancer Linkage Consortium. Am J Hum Genet 1998; 62(3): 676–89.

44. Friedman LS, *et al*. Mutation analysis of BRCA1 and BRCA2 in a male breast cancer population. Am J Hum Genet 1997; 60(2): 313–19.

45. Ribeiro G, *et al*. A review of the management of the male breast carcinoma based on an analysis of 420 treated cases. Breast 1996; 5: 141–6.

46. Donegan WL, *et al*. Carcinoma of the breast in males: a multiinstitutional survey. Cancer 1998; 83(3): 498–509.

47. Erlichman C, Murphy KC, Elhakim T. Male breast cancer: a 13-year review of 89 patients. J Clin Oncol 1984; 2(8): 903–9.

48. Scheike O. Male breast cancer. 5. Clinical manifestations in 257 cases in Denmark. Br J Cancer 1973; 28(6): 552–61.

49. Gennari R, *et al*. Male breast cancer: a special therapeutic problem. Anything new? Int J Oncol 2004; 24(3): 663–70.

50. Guinee VF, *et al*. The prognosis of breast cancer in males. A report of 335 cases. Cancer 1993; 71(1): 154–61.

51. Gough DB, *et al*. A 50-year experience of male breast cancer: is outcome changing? Surg Oncol 1993; 2(6): 325–33.

52. Borgen PI, *et al*. Current management of male breast cancer. A review of 104 cases. Ann Surg 1992; 215(5): 451–7; discussion 457–9.

53. Appelbaum AH, *et al*. Mammographic appearances of male breast disease. Radiographics 1999; 19(3): 559–68.

54. Amoroso WL, Robbins GF, Treves N. Serous and serosanguinous discharge from the male nipple. Arch Surg 1956; 73(2): 319–29.

55. Dershaw DD, *et al*. Mammographic findings in men with breast cancer. Am J Roentgenol 1993; 160(2): 267–70.

56. Evans GF, *et al*. The diagnostic accuracy of mammography in the evaluation of male breast disease. Am J Surg 2001; 181(2): 96–100.

57. Gunhan-Bilgen I, *et al*. Male breast disease: clinical, mammographic, and ultrasonographic features. Eur J Radiol 2002; 43(3): 246–55.

58. Yang WT, *et al*. Sonographic features of primary breast cancer in men. Am J Roentgenol 2001; 176(2): 413–16.

59. Joshi A, Kapila K, Verma K. Fine needle aspiration cytology in the management of male breast masses. Nineteen years of experience. Acta Cytol 1999; 43(3): 334–8.

60. Sanchez AG, Villanueva AG, Redondo C. Lobular carcinoma of the breast in a patient with Klinefelter's syndrome. A case with bilateral, synchronous, histologically different breast tumors. Cancer 1986; 57(6): 1181–3.

61. Nance KV, Reddick RL. In situ and infiltrating lobular carcinoma of the male breast. Hum Pathol 1989; 20(12): 1220–2.

62. Visfeldt J, Scheike O. Male breast cancer. I. Histologic typing and grading of 187 Danish cases. Cancer 1973; 32(4): 985–90.

63. Green LK, Klima M. The use of immunohistochemistry in metastatic prostatic adenocarcinoma to the breast. Hum Pathol 1991; 22(3): 242–6.

64. Goss PE, *et al*. Male breast carcinoma: a review of 229 patients who presented to the Princess Margaret Hospital during 40 years: 1955–1996. Cancer 1999; 85(3): 629–39.

65. Kwiatkowska E, *et al*. BRCA2 mutations and androgen receptor expression as independent predictors of outcome of male breast cancer patients. Clin Cancer Res 2003; 9(12): 4452–9.

66. Bloom K, *et al*. Male breast carcinomas do not show amplification of the her-2/neu gene (Abstract). Breast Cancer Res Treat 2000; 64(1): 127.

67. Wang-Rodriguez J, *et al*. Male breast carcinoma: correlation of ER, PR, Ki-67, Her2-Neu, and p53 with treatment and survival, a study of 65 cases. Mod Pathol 2002; 15(8): 853–61.

68. Rudlowski C, *et al*. Her-2/neu gene amplification and protein expression in primary male breast cancer. Breast Cancer Res Treat 2004; 84(3): 215–23.

69. Ouriel K, Lotze MT, Hinshaw JR. Prognostic factors of carcinoma of the male breast. Surg Gynecol Obstet 1984; 159(4): 373–6.

70. Digenis AG, *et al*. Carcinoma of the male breast: a review of 41 cases. South Med J 1990; 83(10): 1162–7.

71. Vetto J, *et al*. Stages at presentation, prognostic factors, and outcome of breast cancer in males. Am J Surg 1999; 177(5): 379–83.

72. Krag DN, *et al*. Sentinal-lymph-node resection compared with conventional axillary-lymph-node dissection in clinically node-negative patients with breast cancer: overall survival findings from the NSABP B-32 randomized phase 3 trial. Lancet Oncol 2010; 11(10): 927–33.

73. Lucci A, *et al*. Surgical complications associated with sentinel lymph node dissection (SLND) plus axillary lymph node dissection compared with SLND alone in the American College of Surgeons Oncology Group Trial Z0011. J Clin Oncol 2007; 25(24): 3657–63.

74. Wilke LG, *et al*. Surgical complications associated with sentinel lymph node biopsy: results from a prospective international cooperative group trial. Ann Surg Oncol 2006; 13(4): 491–500.

75. De Cicco C, *et al*. Sentinel node biopsy in male breast cancer. Nucl Med Commun 2004; 25(2): 139–43.

76. Goyal A *et al*. ALMANAC Trialists Group. Sentinel lymph node biopsy in male breast cancer patients. Eur J Surg Oncol 2004; 30(5): 480–3.

77. Albo D, *et al*. Evaluation of lymph node status in male breast cancer patients: a role for sentinel lymph node biopsy. Breast Cancer Res Treat 2003; 77(1): 9–14.

78. Lartigau E, *et al*. Male breast carcinoma: a single centre report of clinical parameters. Clin Oncol (R Coll Radiol) 1994; 6(3): 162–6.

79. Zabel A, *et al*. External beam radiotherapy in the treatment of male breast carcinoma: patterns of failure in a single institute experience. Tumori 2005; 91(2): 151–5.

80. Cutuli B. The impact of loco-regional radiotherapy on the survival of breast cancer patients. Proc Eur J Cancer 2000; 36(15): 1895–902.

81. Ribeiro G, Swindell R. Adjuvant tamoxifen for male breast cancer (MBC). Br J Cancer 1992; 65(2): 252–4.

82. Anelli TF, *et al*. Tamoxifen administration is associated with a high rate of treatment-limiting symptoms in male breast cancer patients. Cancer 1994; 74(1): 74–7.

83. Howell A, *et al*. ATAC Trialists' Group. Results of the ATAC (Arimidex, Tamoxifen, Alone or in Combination) trial after completion of 5 years' adjuvant treatment for breast cancer. Lancet 2005; 365(9453): 60–2.

84. Harlan LC, *et al*. Breast cancer in men in the United States: a population-based study of diagnosis, treatment and survival. Cancer 2010; 116(15): 3558–68.

85. Gomez-Raposo C, *et al*. Male breast cancer. Cancer Treat Rev 2010; 36(6): 451–7.

86. Doyen J, *et al*. Aromatase inhibition in male breast cancer patients: biological and clinical implications. Ann Oncol 2010; 21(6):1243–45.

87. Bighin C, *et al*. Estrone sulphate, FSH, and testosterone levels in two male breast cancer patients treated with aromatase inhibitors. Oncologist 2010; 15(12): 1270–2.

88. Coombes RC, *et al.* Intergroup Exemestane Study. A randomized trial of exemestane after two to three years of tamoxifen therapy in postmenopausal women with primary breast cancer. N Engl J Med 2004; 350(11): 1081–92.

89. Goss PE, *et al.* A randomized trial of letrozole in postmenopausal women after five years of tamoxifen therapy for early-stage breast cancer. N Engl J Med 2003; 349(19): 1793–802.

90. Bagley CS, *et al.* Adjuvant chemotherapy in males with cancer of the breast. Am J Clin Oncol 1987; 10(1): 55–60.

91. Patel HZ II, Buzdar AU, Hortobagyi GN. Role of adjuvant chemotherapy in male breast cancer. Cancer 1989; 64(8): 1583–5.

92. Barh D. Biomarkers, critical disease pathways, drug targets, and alternative medicine in male breast cancer. Curr Drug Targets 2009; 10(1): 1–8.

93. Cutuli B, *et al.* Ductal carcinoma in situ of the male breast. Analysis of 31 cases. Eur J Cancer 1997; 33(1): 35–8.

94. Ramantanis G, Besbeas S, Garas JG. Breast cancer in the male: a report of 138 cases. World J Surg 1980; 4(5): 621–3.

95. Auvinen A, Curtis RE, Ron E. Risk of subsequent cancer following breast cancer in men. J Natl Cancer Inst 2002; 94(17): 1330–2.

96. Yap HY, *et al.* Male breast cancer: a natural history study. Cancer 1979; 44(2): 748–54.

97. Borgen PI, *et al.* Carcinoma of the male breast: analysis of prognosis compared with matched female patients. Ann Surg Oncol 1997; 4(5): 385–8.

98. El-Tamer MB, *et al.* Men with breast cancer have better disease-specific survival than women. Arch Surg 2004; 139(10): 1079–82.

99. Thalib L, Hall P. Survival of male breast cancer patients: population-based cohort study. Cancer Sci 2009; 100(2): 292–5.

100. Siddiqui T, *et al.* Cancer of the male breast with prolonged survival. Cancer 1988; 62(8): 1632–6.

101. Farrow J, Adair F. Effect of orchiectomy on skeletal metastases from cancer of the male breast. Science 1942; 95: 654.

102. Meyskens FL Jr, Tormey DC, Neifeld JP. Male breast cancer: a review. Cancer Treat Rev 1976; 3(2): 83–93.

103. Kantarjian H, *et al.* Hormonal therapy for metastatic male breast cancer. Arch Intern Med 1983; 143(2): 237–40.

104. Jaiyesimi IA, *et al.* Carcinoma of the male breast. Ann Intern Med 1992; 117(9): 771–7.

105. Kennedy BJ, Kiang DT. Hypophysectomy in the treatment of advanced cancer of the male breast. Cancer 1972; 29(6): 1606–12.

106. Patterson JS, Battersby LA, Bach BK. Use of tamoxifen in advanced male breast cancer. Cancer Treat Rep 1980; 64(6–7): 801–4.

107. Lopez M, *et al.* Hormonal treatment of disseminated male breast cancer. Oncology 1985; 42(6): 345–9.

108. Giordano SH, *et al.* Efficacy of anastrozole in male breast cancer. Am J Clin Oncol 2002; 25(3): 235–7.

109. Zabolotny BP, Zalai CV, Meterissian SH. Successful use of letrozole in male breast cancer: a case report and review of hormonal therapy for male breast cancer. J Surg Oncol 2005; 90(1): 26–30.

110. Lopez M, *et al.* Chemotherapy in metastatic male breast cancer. Oncology 1985; 42(4): 205–9.

Section 4: Breast Cancer

17 Phyllodes Tumor of the Breast

Emad A. Rakha and Ian O. Ellis

Department of Histopathology, The University of Nottingham and Nottingham University Hospitals NHS Trust, Nottingham City Hospital Campus, Nottingham, UK

Introduction and historical background

Phyllodes tumor of the breast is a rare biphasic fibroepithelial neoplasm that has the potential for recurrence and metastases. Although phyllodes tumor may have been described as early as the 1770s, it was first fully characterized in 1838 by Johannes Müller, who used the term cystosarcoma phyllodes. The term phyllode, which is derived from the Greek word *phullon* or leaf, was chosen to describe the leaf-like projection of the stroma into cystic spaces while sarcoma was used to describe the "fleshy" consistency of the tumor. However, the term cystosarcoma is a misleading description, as the tumors are rarely cystic and the majority follow a benign clinical course. In fact, the use of cystosarcoma to describe this lesion was not intended to connote malignancy as a benign nature was implied in the original account. In total, more than 60 synonyms have been reported [1] but the preferred term used by most authorities and by the World Health Organization is "phyllodes tumor." Although the term periductal stromal tumor was used in the past to describe phyllodes tumor, some authors prefer to maintain this term to describe rare biphasic breast tumors with stromal proliferation of variable cellularity and atypia around open tubules and ducts lacking a phyllodes architecture, to distinguish these from the typical phyllodes tumors.[2]

Epidemiology and biology

Epidemiology

Phyllodes tumors are rare and account for <1% (0.2–0.9%) of all mammary neoplasms and 2.5% of fibroepithelial lesions in the breast,[1] in contrast to fibroadenomas, which are the most common benign breast lesion. Although it has been reported that in the United States the average annual age-adjusted incidence rate of malignant cystosarcoma phyllodes is 2.1 per 1 million women, approximately 500 cases annually,[3,4] in a large population-based study collected from the Surveillance, Epidemiology, and End Results Program (SEER) during a period of 20 years (1983–2002), only 821 cases were identified, indicating a lower incidence.[5] In Nottingham, we identified 32 cases over a 15-year period (1975–1990).[6] There seems to be an ethnic difference, with greater incidence occurring in Asians.[7] In the United States, Latin-American whites have a higher risk of phyllodes tumor than other racial-ethnic groups.[4] Not only the incidence but also the size of phyllodes tumors and patient age may be associated with ethnic origin; it was reported that the mean size was larger in African-Americans than in whites and the age tends to be younger in Latina and Asian patients.[8] In a study of 124 phyllodes tumors diagnosed in American patients, Pimiento et al.[9] found that 42% of the patients were Caucasian, 43% were Hispanic, and 12% were black, with a higher percentage of borderline and malignant tumors in Hispanic patients who also tended to have larger tumors and higher mitotic rates.

The peak incidence occurs between 37 and 50 years of age (10–20 years later than the peak incidence of fibroadenomas). Although very rare, phyllodes tumors can also occur in young women. Younger women, however, had a significantly higher chance of having a benign phyllodes tumor or a tumor of small size.[10,11] Phyllodes tumors are thought not to occur in the male breast because of the absence of a lobuloalveolar structure; however, there have been reports of fibroadenomas and phyllodes tumors arising in men usually in association with gynecomastia.[12–14]

Phyllodes tumors are usually unilateral and solitary but rare cases presenting as multifocal or bilateral have been reported.[15,16] Phyllodes tumors are predominantly breast neoplasms but similar lesions can occur in the prostate gland[17] and in supernumerary breast tissue in the vulva and axilla.[18,19]

Biology

No etiological or predisposing factors have been associated with phyllodes tumors, with the exception of Li–Fraumeni syndrome, a rare autosomal dominant condition characterized by the development of multiple tumors. There is a reported association between malignant phyllodes tumors and nulliparity.[20] Although the etiological relationship between fibroadenomas and phyllodes tumors remains unclear, some authors believe that phyllodes tumors arise from fibroadenomas due to their close histological resemblance, frequent coexistence, and molecular similarities. Many patients develop both lesions either synchronously or metachronously, and histological features of both fibroadenomas and phyllodes tumors have been identified in some tumors.[21,22] Coexisting fibroadenoma is found histologically in up to 40% of cases but is not always apparent clinically. In a previous study of 293 patients with phyllodes tumors, 37% (109 patients) reported a history of fibroadenoma diagnosed before identification of their phyllodes tumors.[23] It has also been suggested that, in a proportion of fibroadenomas, a somatic mutation can result in a monoclonal proliferation, histologically indistinguishable from the polyclonal element but with a propensity for local recurrence and progression to a phyllodes tumor. Molecular studies suggested that phyllodes tumors can progress from fibroadenomas.[24–26] Clonal analysis of the stroma, using X-chromosome inactivation studies, from patients who sequentially developed fibroadenomas and phyllodes tumors at the same site showed that both lesions were monoclonal and expressed the same inactivated allele, appearing to support this hypothesis.[27] However, it is important to note that monoclonality is not a feature of fibroadenomas and some authors demonstrated that the fibroadenoma with stromal monoclonality show mixed features with a phyllodes component,[26] an observation that suggests that these cases are fibroadenoma-like areas in heterogeneous phyllodes tumors.

Displaying a broad range of clinical and pathological behavior, phyllodes tumors should be regarded as a spectrum of fibroepithelial neoplasms rather than a single disease entity. At the extreme end of the spectrum, malignant phyllodes tumors resemble a soft tissue sarcoma and if inadequately treated, have a propensity for rapid growth and metastatic spread. At the other extreme, benign phyllodes are often indistinguishable from cellular fibroadenomas and can be cured by local surgery. However, with the nonoperative management of fibroadenomas widely adopted, the importance of phyllodes tumors lies in the need to differentiate them from other benign breast lesions and to adopt a considered approach to management.

Like fibroadenomas, phyllodes tumors arise from the stroma and epithelium of the terminal duct lobular units; however, only the stromal elements comprise the neoplastic component of these tumors. These stromal elements, which are derived from the periductal rather than intralobular stromal cells of the breast,[28,29] are a key component in the differentiation of phyllodes tumors from fibroadenomas and in determining histological classification (benign, borderline, and malignant subtypes). It is generally the stromal component that becomes malignant and has the ability to metastasize, resembling sarcoma. Although clonality studies have also demonstrated that only the stroma of phyllodes tumors is monoclonal (neoplastic) while the epithelium is polyclonal,[24,25] stromal induction by the epithelial component has also been postulated.

This is supported by observations which show that density of stromal mitotic figures correlates with proximity to the epithelium in phyllodes tumors.[30] In fact, current evidence supports a model where initiation of phyllodes tumor involves interactions between the epithelium and stroma and these interactions are lost with the progression to malignancy such that growth of the stroma becomes independent of the epithelium. Loss of the stromal–epithelial interdependency, increased stromal proliferation, angiogenesis, and matrix alterations appear to be involved in the progression to malignancy.[31] Epithelial component may be present in recurrent phyllodes tumors in the breast or chest wall; however, metastatic deposits are composed of stromal components only, apart from two case reports that claimed epithelial component in the lung metastasis.[32,33]

It has been postulated that in benign tumors, stromal proliferation to a certain extent is under the control of the epithelium. Although the epithelium promotes stromal growth, it may also limit it in benign tumors, because any excessive stromal growth alters the epithelium:stroma ratio. Epithelial growth, sometimes manifest as hyperplasia, may in turn be promoted by the stroma. Once the stroma of the tumor acquires specific, as yet unknown mutations and becomes malignant, the stromal proliferation becomes autonomous and no longer requires a mitogenic stimulus from the epithelium. This results in a reduction in the epithelium:stroma ratio, as is typically seen in malignant phyllodes tumors, in which the epithelium may be very hard to find or is present only as a single layer of luminal epithelial cells, in contradistinction to the hyperplasia seen in many benign phyllodes tumors.

Traditionally phyllodes tumors are graded based on a set of histological features into benign, borderline, and malignant subtypes. The incidence of each subtype varies widely in different series (Table 17.1). One of the reasons for this variation is the lack of standard interpretation of the histological features used to define benign and malignant phyllodes tumors. In a review of 36 published studies that included histological classification of tumors, we found that 63% were reported as benign (1527/2413 cases), 17% (399/2413 cases) borderline, and 20% (487/2413 cases) malignant (see Table 17.1[1,11,34]). Local recurrence is reported in 10% (163/1616) of benign, 20% (87/431) of borderline, and 19% (89/471) of malignant phyllodes tumors. Collectively, we found that 13% (339/2518) of all phyllodes tumors recurred, results similar to those reported in phyllodes tumors without histological subtyping (13%,[8] 15% (8–22%)[1]). However, local recurrence per se is not an indicator of malignancy because it has been described in benign, borderline, and malignant phyllodes tumors.

Repeated local recurrence has also been reported without the development of distant metastases or reduced survival.[11] Recurrence of phyllodes tumors is thought to relate more to inadequate excision rather than histological subtype.[35] Surgical margins <1 cm are associated with the highest risk of local recurrence. Other factors reported to be associated with local recurrence include patient age, surgical approach, mitotic activity, and the presence of tumor necrosis.[23,36] Hajdu et al.[37] showed that recurrence is due to intracanalicular or intracystic extension in 50% of recurrent phyllodes tumors and recommended that phyllodes should be excised with a generous

Table 17.1 Distribution of benign, borderline, and malignant tumors in different published series and the number of local recurrences and distant metastases in each histological group.

Series	Year of publication	Size of series	Tumor classification			Number of recurrences			Number of metastases		
			Benign	Borderline	Malignant	Benign	Borderline	Malignant	Benign	Borderline	Malignant
Treves and Sunderland[22]	1951	77	41 (54%)	18 (23%)	18 (23%)	4 (10%)	4 (22%)	10 (54%)	0	0	9 (50%)
Lester and Stout[97]	1953	58	28 (48%)	10 (17%)	20 (35%)	1 (4%)	1 (10%)	1 (5%)	1 (4%)	1 (10%)	2 (10%)
Pietruszka and Barnes[35]	1978	42	18 (43%)	5 (12%)	19 (45%)	4 (22%)	1 (20%)	1 (5%)	0	1 (20%)	4 (21%)
Murad et al.[98]	1988	25	15 (60%)	—*	10 (40%)	4 (27%)	—	6 (60%)	0	—	4 (40%)
Salvadori et al.[99]	1989	81	28 (35%)	32 (39%)	21 (26%)	1 (4%)	10 (31%)	3 (14%)	0	1 (3%)	1 (5%)
Bartoli et al.[100]	1990	106	92 (87%)	12 (11%)	2 (2%)	6 (6%)	0	0	0	0	0
Cohn-Cedermark et al.[73]	1991	77	42 (55%)	—*	35 (45%)	†	†	†	4 (10%)	3 (14%)	12 (34%)
Grimes MM[101]	1992	100	51 (51%)	22 (22%)	27 (27%)	14 (27%)	7 (32%)	7 (26%)	0	0	6 (22%)
Zurrida et al.[85]	1992	216	140 (64%)	46 (21%)	30 (14%)	11 (8%)	9 (20%)	7 (23%)	—	0	
Moffat et al.[6]	1995	32	23 (72%)	4 (13%)	5 (17%)	6 (26%)		1 (20%)	0	0	0
Stebbing and Nash[102]	1995	33	24 (73%)	6 (18%)	3 (9%)	5 (21%)	3 (50%)	0	0	0	0
Reinfuss et al.[103]	1996	170	92 (54%)	19 (11%)	59 (35%)	4 (4%)	3 (16%)	7 (12%)	4 (4%)	2 (11%)	19 (32%)
Yamada et al.[104]	1997	118	110 (94%)	4 (3%)	4 (3%)	6 (5%)	0	2 (50%)	0	0	1 (25%)
Rajan et al.[10]	1998	45	34 (75%)	8 (18%)	3 (7%)	4 (12%)	0	2 (67%)	0	0	1 (33%)
Mokbel et al.[105]	1999	30	21 (70%)	2 (7%)	7 (23%)	2 (10%)	0	3 (43%)	0	0	1 (14%)
Chaney et al.[40]	2000	101	58 (56%)	12 (12%)	30 (29%)	3 (5%)	0	1 (33%)	1 (2%)	0	7 (23%)
Chen et al.[36]	2005	172	131 (76%)	12 (7%)	29 (17%)	19 (15%)	0	7 (23%)	0	1 (8%)	2 (7%)
Tan et al.[38]	2005	335	250 (75%)	54 (16%)	31 (9%)	25 (10%)	11 (20%)	7 (23%)	0	0	2 (6%)
Abdalla et al.[96]	2006	79	31 (39%)	27 (34%)	21 (27%)	3 (10%)	7 (26%)	6 (29%)	1 (3%)	3 (11%)	6 (28%)
Taira et al.[39]	2007	45	31 (69%)	5 (11%)	9 (20%)	3 (10%)	0	3 (33%)	0	0	1 (11%)
Pezner et al.[84]‡	2008	376	—	376	—	—	51 (14%)	—	—	37 (10%)	—
Belkacemi et al.[34]	2008	443	284 (64%)	80 (18%)	79 (18%)	31 (11%)	23 (29%)	22 (28%)	0	0	15 (19%)
Barth et al.[3]	2009	46	0	16 (35%)	30 (65%)	0	0	0	0	0	2 (7%)
Guillot et al.[11]	2011	165	114 (69%)	37 (22%)	14 (9%)	7 (6%)	8 (22%)	0	0	0	2 (14%)

* These studies did not use a borderline category.
† This data not available from the publication.
‡ Population based study with no histological grading.

margin. Most recurrent tumors are histologically similar to the primary neoplasms but frequently are more cellular, with focally atypical periductal areas. Upgrading to the next category is observed in approximately 25% of the cases.[38]

The incidence of metastases varies among the reported series. From Table 17.1, it can be seen that 0–50% of the malignant tumors in the quoted series have developed metastases, with an average of 22% (97/441). It is also interesting to note that occasional benign or borderline tumors can become metastatic, and metastases have been reported to occur up to 12 years after initial diagnosis. Table 17.1 shows that 3% (12/285) of borderline and 1% (11/1476) of benign phyllodes tumors develop distant metastasis. Collectively, 5% (120/2308) of phyllodes tumors, regardless of their histological subtype, develop distant metastasis. Unlike local recurrence, distant metastasis is related to tumor size and histological features such as stromal cellularity, stromal overgrowth, stromal atypia, and the presence of heterologous stromal elements. Metastatic spread is, as for sarcomas of other sites, via the hematogenous route. The sites most commonly involved are the lung, pleura, and bone; axillary lymph nodes are rarely involved.[39,40]

Molecular biology

Most recent studies of phyllodes tumors have concentrated on the genetic changes detected in the tumors. Comparative genomic hybridization (CGH) and array CGH have been used to delineate the cytogenetic abnormalities of phyllodes tumors, and it has been reported that histologically malignant phyllodes tumors tend to show more chromosomal changes than the benign and borderline counterparts. In a study conducted by Sawyer *et al.*, the molecular analysis of phyllodes tumors reveals distinct changes in the epithelial and stromal components.[41] In another recent study, genetic alterations were identified by application of array CGH in 91% (10 of 11) of cases of phyllodes tumors. In this study, the mean number of chromosomal events was 5.5 (range 0–16) per case, and a mean of two gains (range 0–10) and three losses (range 0–9) was seen per case. Recurrent copy number gain was seen on chromosome 1q, 2p, 3q, 7p, 8q, 16q, and 20 and recurrent loss on chromosome 1q, 4p, 10, 13q, 15q, 16, 17p, 19 and X, with gain of 1q and loss of 3p being the most frequent chromosomal changes. On the other hand, no copy number changes were detected in fibroadenomas. Hence, genomic instability may be an early event in the genesis of phyllodes tumors.[42]

The genetic changes that cause a phyllodes tumor to become malignant are yet to be defined. Gain of 1q material was significantly associated with histologically defined stromal overgrowth and was associated with recurrence.[43] Studies looking at ploidy show that diploid phyllodes tumors tend to be biologically indolent whereas most aneuploid tumors are associated with a poor clinical outcome.[44] On the basis of patterns of chromosomal changes, some authors have reported more similarity between benign and borderline phyllodes tumors compared with malignant tumors,[45] whereas other authors reported more similarity between borderline and malignant phyllodes tumors compared with benign tumors.[46]

Based on methylation profiles, Kim *et al.*[47] have suggested that phyllodes tumors segregate into only two groups: the benign group and the combined borderline and malignant group. Ang *et al.*[48] have carried out microarray gene expression profiling of 21 phyllodes tumors (six benign, 10 borderline, five malignant). They identified a list of 29 genes that were able to classify them according to their histological grade. Among these 29 genes are those responsible for matrix formation, cell adhesion, epidermis formation, and cell proliferation. In this study comparative genomic microarray analysis showed an increasing number of chromosomal changes with increasing histological grade.

A number of pathways and markers have been implicated in the pathogenesis of phyllodes tumor including hormone receptors, members of the Wnt pathway, cell cycle proteins, factors involved in angiogenesis, tyrosine kinase receptors, and matrix metalloproteases. Molecular markers have also attracted attention as diagnostic and prognostic markers to complement the conventional clinicopathological factors that show limited power in the outcome prediction. Although many show a correlation with the grading of phyllodes tumors, none of the available molecular markers to date have shown the ability to consistently predict the outcome or recurrence.

Phyllodes tumors are associated with Li–Fraumeni syndrome, caused by germline *TP*p53 mutations. Although breast carcinoma and sarcomas are numerically most frequent in this syndrome, Birch found that the greatest increases relative to the general population rates were in adrenocortical carcinoma and phyllodes tumor.[49] Studies of *TP*p53 expression have shown that abnormal expression does occur in some borderline and malignant phyllodes tumors and is associated with known negative prognostic factors. The staining pattern of *TP*p53 in malignant phyllodes tumors, and very occasionally in borderline tumors, is characteristically diffuse strong nuclear staining, particularly in the high cellularity stromal area and in the subepithelial location. Most studies, however, were unable to demonstrate the ability of *TP*p53 to predict outcome or recurrence in phyllodes tumors and its overall prognostic utility remains uncertain.[50–53]

Several studies have investigated the role of proliferation markers such as Ki-67 (MIB1) in phyllodes tumors. MIB1 expression shows a positive correlation with tumor grade.[52–55] The reported incidence of MIB1 expression in phyllodes tumors ranged from 5% to 25% in benign cases and from 15% to 100% in malignant cases. The utility of Ki-67 in predicting outcome is variable, with some studies suggesting MIB1 to be useful in predicting outcome[52,53,55] and others suggesting that it may also be associated with likelihood of recurrence.[53] It was also reported that both MIB1 index and p53 stromal expression are associated with outcome and can provide significant prognostic information in patients with phyllodes tumors.[45,53] Other proliferation and cell cycle-associated markers assessed in phyllodes tumors include C-myc, p16, cyclin D1, and pRb.[55–57] C-myc overexpression has been found to be associated with malignant phyllodes tumors.[56] Ploidy studies have demonstrated that benign phyllodes tumor is diploid whilst aneuploidy is identified in some borderline to malignant phyllodes tumors. S-phase fraction also shows a progressive increase from benign to borderline to malignant phyllodes.[44]

The expression of c-kit (CD117) shows progressive increase from benign to malignant phyllodes, ranging from 0–46% in benign lesions to 0–100% in malignant lesions, by immunohistochemistry.[50,56,58,59] Interestingly, some authors reported that high stromal expression of c-kit was related to recurrence.[50] The underlying mechanism of c-kit expression remains uncertain, because known activation mutations in gastrointestinal stromal tumor have not been demonstrated in the majority of c-kit overexpressed phyllodes tumors.[56,58] The potential of tyrosine kinase inhibitor (imatinib mesylate; Glivec™) for treatment of malignant phyllodes tumors remains to be explored.

CD10 (CALLA) has been reported to be significantly increased from low (0–6%) expression in benign phyllodes tumors to high (32–50%) in borderline to frankly malignant phyllodes tumors.[60,61] CD10 expression has also been reported in some high-grade spindle cell and pleomorphic sarcomas of the breast; however, these sarcomas lack the typical fibroepithelial pattern of phyllodes tumors and they often coexpress myoepithelial markers and epidermal growth factor receptor (EGFR). Features may be associated with myoepithelial neoplasms or some forms of metaplastic carcinoma. Morphology, associated *in situ* lesions and other immunohistochemical markers such as epithelial markers (i.e. high molecular weight and broad-spectrum cytokeratins) may help differentiation in such situations. Unlike c-kit and CD10, the expression of CD34 and bcl2 is most common in benign phyllodes and decreases gradually in borderline and malignant phyllodes.[62,63]

In phyllodes tumors, estrogen receptor (ER)-α and progesterone receptor (PR) are detected mainly within the epithelium, with PR expression being common and ER expression less common. ER and PR expression has been shown in 43% and 84% of the epithelium respectively, and less than 5% of the stromal cells.[64] Androgen receptor is reported to be expressed in the epithelium of 70% of cases.[59] However, stromal cells express ER-β.[65] EGFR protein expression and gene amplification are detected in 35% of phyllodes tumors.[59] In phyllodes tumors there is increased expression with increasing malignancy, ranging from 12–16% in benign phyllodes tumors to 56–63% in malignant phyllodes tumors.[59,66,67] In addition to tumor grade, EGFR expression is associated with stromal cellularity, mitosis, stromal nuclear pleomorphism, and stromal overgrowth.[66] None of the phyllodes tumors is reported to be positive for Her-2/neu.[53,59]

discoloration and dilated veins, and pressure necrosis can occur in larger lesions. While certain clinical features may raise the index of suspicion, phyllodes tumor is not clinically distinguishable from fibroadenoma and other benign breast lesions. The diagnosis of phyllodes tumor should be considered and ruled out in the diagnostic pathway of larger fibroadenoma.

Of the 40 patients reviewed by Mangi *et al.*,[86] 37 presented with a palpable mass, seven complained of pain, and three were detected on mammographic screening. Similar to this study, many other series reflect the majority of patients presenting with a palpable mass. On examination, phyllodes tumors are smooth, mobile, and well circumscribed (often diagnosed as a fibroadenoma). A clue to it being a phyllodes tumor is if there is a recent history of rapid increase in size. This feature of rapid growth may lead to stretched or even ulcerated overlying skin. It is important to note that such "suspicious" presenting signs do not necessarily predict the behavior of the tumor. Nonetheless, as is the case with all breast lumps, they should undergo a triple assessment to rule out malignant change. Phyllodes tumors are found more commonly in the upper outer quadrant with an equal propensity to occur in either breast. Fixation to the skin or the pectoralis muscles has been reported but ulceration is uncommon, even in patients with histologically malignant tumors. A proportion of patients have previously had a fibroadenoma and in a minority these have been multiple. Occasionally, fibroadenomas present simultaneously with a phyllodes tumor and synchronous bilateral phyllodes tumors have been reported. The diagnosis of a phyllodes tumor should be considered in all women, particularly over the age of 35, who present with a rapidly growing but clinically benign breast lump.

Malignant phyllodes tumor is not known to metastasize to lymph nodes but rather hematogenously. Thus, unlike carcinomas, evaluation of the axilla beyond clinical examination is not necessary. Palpable lymph nodes may be elicited on presentation in up to 20% of patients but this is thought to be a feature of tumor necrosis. Carcinoma arising within a phyllodes tumor has been reported and in one case report there was metastasis of the lymph node but it was from the carcinomatous component.[69] Even though the male breast lacks the lobuloalveolar complex, there have been isolated case reports of phyllodes tumor arising within the male breast. The literature is scant, with such data limited to isolated case reports; thus it is difficult for us to draw definitive conclusions on its natural history in males.

Clinical presentation and diagnosis

Presentation

Phyllodes tumors occur over a wide age range (median age 45). These lesions (both benign and malignant) typically present as a symptomatic breast (or rarely axillary) lump. Presentation may be precipitated by a sudden increase in size in a long-standing breast lesion. Size at presentation is often larger than for fibroadenoma, although increased breast awareness and the impact of screening have resulted in a trend towards presentation at smaller tumor sizes.[68] Overlying skin may show bluish

Pathology

Macroscopic appearances

Phyllodes tumors, by their very nature, grow radially, compressing the adjacent breast parenchyma and creating a pseudocapsule through which tongues of phyllodes stroma may protrude and grow into adjacent breast tissue. Macroscopically, phyllodes tumors typically form a firm, bulging lobulated single or multinodular mass. They vary in size from less than 2 cm to more than 10 cm in diameter, with an average size of 5 cm.[6,35] However, tumors of more than 20 cm

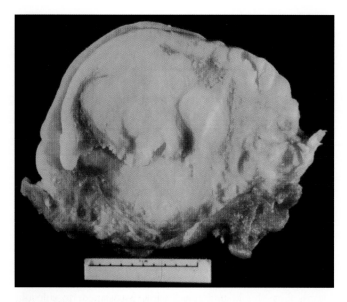

Figure 17.1 The cut surface appearance of a phyllodes tumor showing the characteristic cleft leaf bud-like appearance.

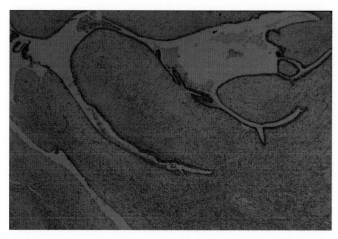

Figure 17.2 The histological appearance of a benign phyllodes tumor showing the combination of clefted epithelial-lined spaces and hypercellular stroma.

are recorded in many series. They are usually well circumscribed, often with a bosselated contour. The cut surface has a characteristic whorled pattern, resembling a compressed leaf bud (Fig. 17.1), with visible clefts. Larger tumors frequently exhibit cystic spaces and foci of hemorrhage, degeneration and necrosis may be present, particularly in malignant tumors.

Histological appearances

The histological hallmark of phyllodes tumor is the coexistence of proliferating stromal elements admixed with epithelial elements that are typically lining elongated clefts, ducts, and sparse lobular elements. The stroma of phyllodes tumor exhibits a considerable degree of heterogeneity within the same lesion and varies from case to case. Foci indistinguishable from fibroadenoma may be seen adjacent to highly cellular areas with stromal expansion. Stromal cellularity is often more dense adjacent to epithelial elements, the so-called periductal stroma, and these areas usually display the highest mitotic activity. When this pattern of periductal stromal condensation is exaggerated, particularly in association with a predominant pericanalicular growth pattern and lack of clefts, some authors call these lesions periductal stroma tumor/sarcoma.[2,70] Pseudoangiomatous stroma hyperplasia (PASH) may occur in phyllodes tumors and in some cases it may be a prominent feature. Lipomatous and osseous metaplasia can occur in the stroma. Myxoid changes may occur in phyllodes tumors as in fibroadenoma but it tends to be patchy. The epithelial element consists of the usual two layers of basal myoepithelial and luminal epithelial cells. Focal epithelial hyperplasia is not uncommon and observed in approximately a third of cases and this may occasionally be florid. There is usually a positive correlation between epithelial hyperplasia and stromal cellularity and stromal mitotic activity. In rare cases, florid epithelial hyperplasia may be extensive and atypical, giving the impres-

sion of ductal carcinoma *in situ*, but the significance of these cases remains uncertain. Case reports of lobular neoplasia and ductal carcinoma *in situ* occurring in phyllodes tumors have been recorded; associated invasive carcinoma is an even greater rarity. Epithelial metaplasia such as squamous or apocrine metaplasia, areas of adenosis, and sclerosing adenosis may be seen in phyllodes tumors.

As no single histological criterion is of determinate significance in the diagnosis of phyllodes tumors, several histological characteristics are assessed. Furthermore, grading into benign, borderline, and malignant categories is rather based on a constellation of histological characteristics. Histological features of borderline and malignant phyllodes tumors were first defined by Pietruszka and Barnes,[35] [35], modified by Azzopardi,[71] and adopted by the World Health Organization.[72] These histological features include:
• degree of stromal hypercellularity which is best assessed on thin sections in the periductal areas or between ducts
• stromal expansion/overgrowth (defined as the absence of epithelial element in the expanded stroma or increased stroma:epithelium ratio)
• stromal cell atypia and mitotic activity including the presence of atypical mitoses
• tumor margins
• presence of necrosis and malignant heterologous (i.e. osteosarcomatous or chondrosarcomatous) elements.
However, it important to note that none of these histological factors alone or in combination is useful in predicting local recurrence, which is strongly related to completeness of local excision. Histological features of malignancy, however, may be associated with the development of distant metastasis.
• Benign phyllodes tumors: the stroma is characteristically more cellular than in a fibroadenoma (Fig. 17.2), the spindle cells exhibit no or mild degree of pleomorphism and mitoses are infrequent (0–4 mitoses/10 high-power field [HPF]). There is a minimal stromal overgrowth and the margin is pushing with no evidence of

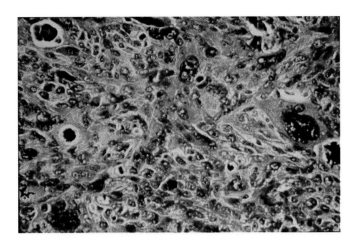

Figure 17.3 A malignant phyllodes tumor showing stromal overgrowth with stromal cell atypia and increased mitotic frequency.

invasion of the surrounding tissue. The presence of occasional bizarre stromal giant cells does not indicate malignant change.

• *Malignant phyllodes tumors*: at the other end of the spectrum, a minority of tumors will show frankly sarcomatous change, characterized by marked stromal overgrowth and hypercellularity (Fig. 17.3), significant nuclear atypia, and an increased mitotic count (≥10 mitoses /10 HPF). In particular, specific patterns such as rhabdomyosarcoma, angiosarcoma, chondrosarcoma, and osteosarcoma are clear indicators of malignancy. In fact, the presence of frank malignant stroma combined with the fibroepithelial pattern is sufficient for a diagnosis of malignant phyllodes tumor though these lesions often show other features of malignancy such as infiltrative margin.

• *Borderline phyllodes tumors*: there remains an intermediate group of tumors with appearances that pose problems for the pathologist and clinician in predicting the likelihood of local recurrence and metastatic malignant potential. A number of studies[7,35,37,38,72,73] have addressed this question since Norris and Taylor[74] first suggested that an infiltrative rather than a pushing margin, cellular atypia, increased mitotic count, and large size all favored malignancy. Using semi-quantitative criteria derived from those proposed by Pietruszka and Barnes[35] and by Ward and Evans,[75] Moffat et al.[6] have divided phyllodes tumors into three groups: benign, borderline, and malignant. The histological characteristics used included its margin (pushing or infiltrating), stromal cellularity (mild, moderate, or severe), stromal overgrowth (mild, moderate, or severe), tumor necrosis (present or absent), cellular atypia (mild, moderate, or severe), and the number of mitoses per high-power field. Cases with intermediate features are classified as borderline tumors. These may include all features but in the moderate degree category or some of the features but with moderate to severe degrees, such as infiltrative margins, moderate to marked stromal cellularity and overgrowth and moderately high mitotic counts (4–9 mitoses/10 HPF). It is our policy in Nottingham to classify phyllodes tumors showing intermediate features as borderline rather than low-grade malignant phyllodes; we do not subclassify malignant phyllodes into low grade and high grade. We classify tumors showing all features of malignancy, such as high mitotic counts

(>10/10 HPF) and infiltrative margins, or those showing frank sarcomatous stroma (i.e. fibrosarcoma, chondrosarcoma or angiosarcoma), regardless of other features, as malignant phyllodes. Tumors showing one or two features of malignancy such as infiltrative margin, moderate to significant stromal atypia and/or a high mitotic count with occasional atypical mitotic figure but lacking other features are classified as borderline tumors.

Sarcomatous overgrowth

Sarcomatous differentiation is a rare but important event in phyllodes tumors. Guerrero has reviewed the literature back to 1979 and identified a total of 30 documented cases.[76] The most common histological type is liposarcoma, accounting for a total of 23 cases (adipose differentiation ranged from mature fat to liposarcoma). Malignant fibrous histiocytoma (MFH) was identified in three cases, rhabdomyosarcoma and chondrosarcoma in one case each, and by multiple histological types. Powell et al.[77] studied 14 patients with adipose differentiation and concluded that malignant phyllodes tumor with adipose differentiation can be graded histologically on the basis of this component and that despite the high-grade histology in some instances, the patients had an excellent prognosis when the tumors were completely excised.

Because of the rarity of this event, little is known about the clinical behavior, treatment, and prognosis of such tumors. However, others have observed that most clinically malignant phyllodes tumors reported in the literature that have metastasized have had overgrowth of an obvious sarcomatous element on histological examination.[78] This malignant element has often been something other than low-grade fibrosarcoma (e.g. high-grade sarcoma, liposarcoma, rhabdomyosarcoma). It is also reported that among the various subtypes of stromal sarcomas, angiosarcoma is characterized by a high risk of occurrence in irradiated fields and by a poor prognosis with a high risk of lung metastases. Therefore, close examination of the stroma with multiple sections is mandatory. The truly malignant phyllodes tumor may be present only in a portion of the phyllodes tumor.

Use of biological markers

Benign phyllodes tumors show low levels of proliferation with low MIB1 index and negative/weak staining for p53, c-kit and CD10 but they exhibit strong expression of CD34 and bcl2. Malignant phyllodes tumors show high MIB1 index, positive staining for p53, c-kit and CD10 but negative/weak patchy staining for CD34. Borderline tumors show a profile of intermediate features. Cytokeratins (CK), CD34 and bcl2 are useful in cases lacking the typical fibroepithelial pattern to exclude metaplastic carcinomas, which is CK positive and CD34 and bcl2 negative.[79] ER, PR and Her-2 are of little diagnostic or prognostic value in phyllodes tumors. Although many markers assessed in phyllodes tumors are correlated with histological grade, none of them has been able to independently predict patient outcome. At present, strict histological assessment and generous sampling of these tumors provide the most clinically useful information.

Differential diagnosis

In most cases, the distinction from fibroadenoma is straightforward, but difficulties may be encountered with small lesions. A leaf-like pattern and hypercellular stroma favor a diagnosis of phyllodes tumor, but size alone cannot be used as a distinguishing feature. Stromal heterogeneity is a feature of phyllodes tumor while the stroma is usually homogeneous in fibroadenoma though it may be variable from one fibroadenoma to another. Some phyllodes tumors may show fibroadenoma-like stroma which may have diagnostic implications, particularly in a limited sample such as a core biopsy. Mitotic figures are extremely unusual in the stroma of a fibroadenoma and when occasional mitosis is seen, such as in younger women or in the juvenile variant, it is usually associated with epithelial proliferative activity and mitotic figures in the epithelium. Stromal fat and heterologous elements (i.e. osteochondroid areas) are features of phyllodes tumors and rarely seen in a fibroadenoma. Most fibroepithelial lesions with adipose differentiation are phyllodes tumors.

Although CD34 immunohistochemistry shows strong positivity in the stroma of fibroadenoma and its expression decreases in borderline and becomes weak or focally negative in malignant phyllodes, we do not find it useful in differentiating fibroadenoma from benign phyllodes. Proliferation markers such as Ki-67 may be helpful in this regard.

Fibromatosis, primary sarcoma, and metaplastic carcinoma of the breast, although very rare, must be distinguished from malignant phyllodes tumors. Again, the mixture of elements, with the leaf-like epithelial clefts, is a feature of phyllodes tumor not seen in the other lesions. Metaplastic carcinoma may be distinguished by positive immunostaining of the spindle cells with epithelial markers such as broad-spectrum cytokeratins, as mentioned above.

Diagnosis

The major challenge in making a preoperative imaging diagnosis is that neither mammography nor ultrasonography can reliably distinguish phyllodes tumors from fibroadenomas.[1] In mammography, both will appear as well-defined oval or lobulated masses with rounded borders. Coarse microcalcifications may be present. A radiolucent "halo" may be seen around the lesion, due to compression of the surrounding breast stroma. Such features can even mimic a well-circumscribed carcinoma. No mammographic indicators have been identified that allow differentiation between benign and malignant tumors. Preoperative diagnosis using ultrasonography is also known to be disappointing. Phyllodes tumors often show smooth contours with low-level homogeneous internal echoes, intramural cysts, and the absence of posterior acoustic enhancement. Certain features could raise suspicion of the mass being a phyllodes tumor, such as smooth walls, low-level internal echoes and echo-free margins. Identification of a cyst within a solid lesion by ultrasound is highly suggestive of phyllodes tumor.

Recently, modalities such as magnetic resonance imaging (MRI), color flow Doppler and even vascular embolization have been employed with varying degrees of success. The role of MRI has not been fully elucidated. Although some authors reported that MRI cannot precisely differentiate phyllodes tumors from fibroadenomas,[80] others have indicated that several MRI findings can be used to help determine the histological grade of phyllodes tumors and that dynamic enhancement patterns may be helpful for the diagnosis of larger tumors (>3 cm).[81] Other experimental approaches include proton magnetic resonance spectroscopy and scintimammography. Current evidence, however, indicates that many phyllodes tumors cannot be distinguished from fibroadenomas on radiological grounds, nor can benign and malignant variants be reliably differentiated.

Preoperative diagnosis of phyllodes tumors

The recurring theme in phyllodes tumor is one of underdiagnosis by pathologists. Accurate preoperative diagnosis allows correct surgical planning and avoidance of reoperation, either to achieve wider excision or for subsequent tumor recurrence. Many studies have employed fine needle aspiration cytology (FNAC) as part of their triple assessment. However, in the assessment of phyllodes tumors, FNAC has significant limitations with an overall accuracy of 63%. Cytologically, it is often easier to differentiate benign from malignant phyllodes tumors than to separate benign phyllodes tumors from fibroadenomas as both tumors share a dimorphic pattern with both epithelial and stromal components. The key diagnostic features relate to the stroma, including the presence of hypercellular stromal fragments, well-delineated borders to stromal fragments, stromal nuclear atypia, isolated stromal cells with bare nuclei, and blood vessels crossing the stroma. The value of FNAC in the diagnosis of phyllodes tumor remains controversial.

The use of core biopsy invariably provides a superior result for tissue diagnosis.[82–84] It should be borne in mind that the histological characteristics of a phyllodes tumor can vary in different regions and a core biopsy sample, which is of limited size, may not include all parts of the lesion. Phyllodes tumor usually shows increased stromal cellularity and mitotic activity; however, juvenile fibroadenoma may also have cellular stroma, presenting a source of increased diagnostic difficulty.

Diagnosis relies on recognition of one or preferably a combination of features. In a previous study,[83] we found that four features were significantly more common in cores from phyllodes tumors and had a κ statistic of >0.6 in a reproducibility study: stromal cellularity increased in at least 50% compared with typical fibroadenoma; stromal overgrowth (×10 field with no epithelium); fragmentation; and adipose tissue within stroma. In this study, tumor heterogeneity was the main cause for false-negative results. Komenaka et al.[68] have reported a 93% negative predictive value and an 83% positive predictive value for phyllodes in a needle core biopsy (NCB) diagnosis. In this study nine cases were equivocal on core biopsies and the histological outcome was fibroadenoma in five and phyllodes tumor in four cases. In a previous study of 54 phyllodes tumors, 70% were diagnosed as phyllodes/cellular fibroepithelial lesion on NCB.[11] Stromal proliferation in juvenile fibroadenoma tends to be relatively uniform, whereas in phyllodes tumor it is often (though not always) more prominent in the periductal areas. Some authors also suggested that proliferation markers (i.e. Ki-67) may be helpful in this context.[54]

The guidelines recommend that phyllodes tumor should be designated lesions of uncertain malignant potential (B3) on needle core biopsy reporting and in the cases where it cannot be differentiated from fibroadenoma it should be called a "cellular fibroepithelial lesion" to avoid underdiagnosis of phyllodes tumor, with correlation to clinical and imaging findings. If there is clinical suspicion of a phyllodes tumor, formal excision is recommended to allow comprehensive assessment of its characteristics. This should ideally occur in the context of a multidisciplinary meeting. Malignant phyllodes tumors with malignant stroma are coded as malignant (B5).

Treatment

Surgery

Margin of excision, especially incomplete excision, is the principal cause of local recurrence. For benign lesions, surgery should be guided by the size of the lesion and the breast. Small lesions can safely undergo wide local excision with a 1–2 cm margin. As some of these patients are young, cosmesis should be an important aspect of the surgical decision-making process. Oncoplastic procedures such as partial mastectomy and latissimus dorsi flaps and envelope mastectomy with reconstruction have shown excellent results. Mastectomy should be reserved for larger lesions, where the breast is too small or achieving an acceptable clearance margin provides a poor cosmetic outcome (i.e. size of lesion versus size of breast).

In older series, the frequency of mastectomy ranged from 52% to 87% of patients; however, studies including recent series have shown that increasing numbers of patients are treated by breast-preserving lumpectomy procedures.[5,8] In a study of 165 patients presenting with phyllodes tumor between 1994 and 2008, Guillot et al.[11] reported that 97% of patients underwent breast-conserving treatment, of whom three had oncoplastic surgery. Only five patients (3%) had a mastectomy, of whom three (two malignant and one borderline) had very large tumors (≥100 mm). In a population-based study of 821 phyllodes diagnosed from 1983 to 2002, a significant increase in the use of wide excision or breast conservation compared with mastectomy was observed in recent years.[5] There is at present no role for axillary staging sampling or clearance, and we do not envisage a role for sentinel node biopsy.

Because excision of the tumor and not surrounding breast tissue is the goal, this provides an opportunity, even in large tumors, for extensive skin and nipple sparing. If breast-conserving surgery is used and an adequate margin is not achieved, some authors argue against immediate reexcision.[85] Timely reexcision of breast recurrences is more appropriate in that situation, requiring close clinical surveillance. However, overwhelmingly, the published data clearly show that achieving a tumor-free margin is imperative to achieving the best local regional control. Moffat et al. showed that in 32 women with a median follow-up of 135 months, five had local recurrence and all possessed involved margins.[6] Mangi et al.[86] reported on

40 patients and again showed a significant correlation between local recurrence and involved margins ($p < 0.05$).

The average interval between the diagnosis of primary benign and recurrent benign phyllodes tumors is 2 years but several years may elapse between apparent recurrences. Pezner et al.[8] have demonstrated a correlation between type of surgery and local recurrence; 5-year local control rates were 79% for 169 lumpectomy patients and 91% for 207 mastectomy patients treated by surgery alone. They found a correlation between size of tumor and recurrence rate; 5-year local control rates were 91% for 0–2 cm tumors, 85% for 2–5 cm tumors, and 59% for 5–10 cm tumors treated by lumpectomy alone. For mastectomy patients, 5-year local control rates were 100% for 0–2 cm tumors, 95% for 2–5 cm tumors, 88% for 5–10 cm tumors, and 85% for 10–20 cm tumors.[8] Incompletely treated multiplicity is a likely cause of so-called recurrence in some settings, as it is for fibroadenoma. In the advent of local recurrence for benign phyllodes, a reexcision with wider margins is recommended.

Malignant phyllodes tumors show a propensity to recur or metastasize if margins are involved. Kapiris et al.[87] studied 45 women with phyllodes tumor. Of 24 patients treated conservatively, local recurrence occurred in 40% and distant metastasis in 27%. Both events were related to margin status. Although the trend for so-called malignant phyllodes tumor has been to obtain mastectomy, in Barth's review[88] there was no difference in survival for women with histologically malignant phyllodes tumor based on type of surgical treatment. He concluded that survival was not impaired by breast-conserving surgery.

In summary, clear margin status is associated with a low local recurrence rate regardless of histological features of the lesion. We recommend ensuring wide local excision with clear margins (≥10 mm) even if this means mastectomy, especially in cases of malignant phyllodes tumor.

Radiotherapy

Akin to soft tissue sarcoma, adjuvant radiotherapy (RT) has been recommended for malignant phyllodes tumor patients to reduce the risk of local recurrence. RT has been recommended for patients with adverse pathological findings such as close or positive surgical margins or tumor size greater than 5 cm.[89,90] Other authors have concluded that the value of RT has not been established or that RT should not be routinely used.[5,36,78,91] In a population-based study of 821 phyllodes tumors, it was even reported that adjuvant radiotherapy predicted for worse cause specific survival when implemented compared with surgery alone.[5] Unfortunately, the value of adjuvant RT has not been extensively studied for malignant phyllodes tumors mainly because of the rarity of the tumor and the limited number of patients who have received adjuvant RT. McGowan et al. used RT in 10 of 32 (31%) patients but did not provide a separate analysis of local control.[92] Soumarova et al. used adjuvant RT for 17 of 25 (68%) malignant phyllodes tumor patients and local recurrence was noted in two of 17 (12%) who received RT and two of eight (25%) who did not.[89]

In 2009, Barth et al.[3] published the results of a clinical trial which enrolled 46 women who presented with borderline

($n = 16$) or malignant ($n = 30$) phyllodes tumors that were treated with a margin-negative breast-conserving resection and adjuvant RT. The primary endpoint was local recurrence. During a median follow-up of 56 months (range, 12–129 months), none of the 46 patients developed a local recurrence (local recurrence rate 0%; 95% confidence interval 0–8). These authors therefore concluded that margin-negative resection combined with adjuvant radiotherapy is very effective therapy for local control of borderline and malignant phyllodes tumors.[3] In 2010, another clinical trial (Phyllodes Tumor Partial Breast Radiation Study) was commenced to determine the efficacy of partial breast radiation therapy after a lumpectomy for phyllodes tumor. This study aims to recruit 50 patients (≥18 years old) with a histological diagnosis of borderline or malignant tumors. Results of this trial are awaited.

Following wide local excision, postoperative RT is currently not recommended routinely in Nottingham but it may have a role in preventing local recurrence if negative margins cannot be achieved. We would therefore recommend offering adjuvant RT to those patients with borderline or malignant tumors where clear margins cannot be achieved surgically, as these patients are at high risk of local recurrence. For patients with malignant, inoperable local recurrence or metastatic tumors, RT may offer some palliation and occasional complete responses are documented.[93]

Chemotherapy

As in more conventional sarcomas, the efficacy of chemotherapy in these tumors is limited but it can be useful for treating symptomatic metastases. Chemotherapy is based on the guidelines for the treatment of sarcomas rather than breast carcinomas. The most commonly used drugs are those used for the treatment of soft tissue sarcomas outside the breast – doxorubicin and ifosfamide.[94] The role of routine postoperative chemotherapy in malignant phyllodes tumors remains uncertain. Because of the rarity of the disease, no large randomized controlled trials have been performed. The only randomized study looking at this question randomized 28 patients with malignant phyllodes tumors to receive adjuvant doxorubicin and dacarbazine or observation. Adjuvant chemotherapy did not impact on survival.[95] On the basis of these data, we at present do not recommend adjuvant chemotherapy for malignant phyllodes tumors.

Hormonal and biological therapy

In the past, when biochemical assays were performed to assess estrogen and progesterone receptor status, it was thought that phyllodes tumors were progesterone receptor positive. This led to the suggestion that hormonal therapy may be useful in the treatment of advanced, malignant phyllodes tumors. However, immunohistochemical studies have all shown that estrogen and progesterone receptors are expressed only in glandular elements of phyllodes tumors and not in the stroma. It is therefore unlikely that these types of drugs will be useful in the treatment of malignant phyllodes tumors.

Recent increased understanding of the molecular biology of phyllodes tumors brings the potential for use of targeted biological therapy. c-kit (CD117) is expressed in phyllodes tumors. The success of the therapeutic agent imatinib (Glivec™) targeted at this receptor for gastrointestinal stromal tumor has led the authors to speculate that imatinib may be a potentially useful drug for its management.

Characteristics and management of recurrent disease

Parker and Harries have reviewed the characteristics associated with local recurrence.[1] Local recurrence rates range from 10% to 40%, with an average of 15%; local recurrence appears to be related to the extent of the initial surgery and should be regarded as a failure of primary surgical treatment. Whether malignant tumors have an increased risk of recurrence is unclear but when it does occur, it is invariably seen earlier than with benign tumors; local recurrence usually occurs within the first few years of surgery and histologically resembles the original tumor. Of great importance is that local recurrences are less likely to evolve into malignancy if this feature was not present in the primary tumor.[6,78] Occasionally, recurrent tumors show increased cellularity and more aggressive histological features than the original lesion. Hajdu et al. found malignant transformation in two out of 28 recurrent benign phyllodes tumors and they showed some evidence that any large or second recurrence may be life threatening.[37]

In most patients, local recurrence is isolated and is not associated with the development of distant metastases; in a minority of patients repeated local recurrence occurs over a prolonged period with no survival disadvantage and this is often seen irrespective of the histological type of the tumor.[73] It was therefore concluded that local recurrence can usually be controlled by further wide excision and mastectomy is not invariably required but should be considered for local recurrence after local surgery for borderline or malignant tumors. However, in a study of 478 patients with malignant phyllodes tumors, Pezner et al.[8] found that in multivariate survival analysis, survival was adversely affected by local recurrence. Kapiris et al.[87] have reported that local recurrence with subsequent metastatic spread and survival following treatment of malignant phyllodes tumors are related to excision margins and tumor size. Occasionally, aggressive local recurrence can result in widespread chest wall disease with direct invasion of the underlying lung parenchyma, and isolated reports of good palliation in this situation with radiotherapy have been published.

Characteristics and management of metastatic disease

Parker and Harries have also recently reviewed the characteristics associated with metastatic disease.[1] Overall, less than 10% of patients with phyllodes tumors develop distant metastases and this phenomenon is more common (approximately 20%) in patients with histologically malignant tumors. Most distant metastases develop without evidence of local recurrence. The most common sites for distant metastases are the lung, bone, and abdominal viscera. These often occur in the absence of lymph node metastases and histologically contain only the stromal element. The risk of metastatic disease does not appear to be influenced by the extent of the initial surgery and appears to be predetermined by tumor biology. Few reports have been published about distant metastases after excision of a benign phyllodes tumor, except when histologically malignant local recurrence occurs. Metastatic phyllodes tumors have a poor prognosis and no long-term survival has been reported. Isolated reports have been published about palliation of metastatic disease with single-agent or combination chemotherapy, but the exact role of chemotherapy in metastatic phyllodes tumors remains to be defined.

Prognosis

Most malignant phyllodes tumors do not recur or metastasize while some histologically benign tumors can show an aggressive clinical course. Consequently, it has been suggested that all phyllodes tumors should be regarded as having malignant potential. In view of this relatively indolent behavior of the majority, radical surgery for all phyllodes tumors is unnecessary and attempts have been made to identify clinical and histopathological prognostic factors. Overall survival for malignant phyllodes tumors has been reported to be in the range of 42–95%, depending on length of follow-up. A retrospective pooled study of 821 malignant phyllodes patients reported cause-specific survival rates of 91% at 5 years and 89% at 10 years.[5] In a study of 443 phyllodes tumors, Belkacemi et al.[34] have reported overall survival rates of 97% and 96% at 5- and 10-year follow-up respectively. However, lower figures have also been reported; for instance Chaney et al.,[40] using 101 phyllodes tumors, have reported overall survival rates of 88% and 79%, and 62% at 5 and 10 years, respectively.

Little consensus exists regarding the relative importance of the clinicopathological and molecular features, and different factors appear to be important in predicting local recurrence and metastatic spread. No reliable clinical prognostic factors other than incompleteness of excision have been identified that predict local recurrence. Patient age does not appear to be important but tumors presenting in adolescence do seem to be less aggressive irrespective of their histological type. The risk of local recurrence is increased in incompletely excised lesions. McGowan et al.[92] found that the 5-year local recurrence failure rate increased from 33% for cases with clear margins to 80% in cases with positive margins. Similar results are reported in other studies.[9,86] Conversely, low recurrence rates have been reported in patients in whom histologically clear margins have been assured. Although several authors have reported higher local recurrence rates in cases treated by breast-conserving surgery compared to mastectomy,[8,73,96] other authors did not find a significant difference when conservative surgery is associated with clear margins.[3,11,92]

The role of tumor size is unclear. While most series have reported low local recurrence rates with tumors less than 2 cm in diameter, no correlation between tumor size and the risk of local recurrence has been demonstrated.[1,40,73] Most distant metastases develop from borderline or malignant tumors.[40]

Unlike in local recurrence, tumor size does appear to be an important factor in predicting metastatic spread.[8]

Many histological prognostic factors have been evaluated but no clear consensus exists for their role in the assessment of prognosis (see "Pathology" section above). Barth[88] performed a metaanalysis and demonstrated that strict adherence to histological criteria showed no distant metastases in lesions that were categorized as histologically benign or borderline. The use of a borderline category allows placement of tumors that usually do not act in a malignant fashion but may be more likely to recur locally.[78] Carter and Page have supported the use of three histological categories.[78] Some phyllodes tumors, although rare, are clinically malignant at presentation and have the ability to metastasize. These usually have a clear focus of easily recognizable sarcoma on histological exam. The vast majority of phyllodes tumors are benign and potentially curable by local excision when completely removed. A third subset of phyllodes tumors of indeterminate biology, some of which recur and a very few of which metastasize, also exists. It is this third group that probably makes up at least a slight majority of those tumors that were previously diagnosed as malignant but do not behave as such. In light of this knowledge, it seems unjustifiable to give a fully malignant diagnostic term to these lesions that only occasionally or rarely kill. By placing some phyllodes tumors in the borderline category, it will guide surgical colleagues to the need to achieve clearance and reduce the risk of recurrence in a particular patient.

Key points and authors' recommendations

• Phyllodes tumors are defined as fibroepithelial neoplasms of the breast, which show epithelial-lined clefted spaces with surrounding hypercellular stroma.
• Phyllodes tumors account for less than 1% of breast neoplasms in contrast to fibroadenomas which are common.
• They can be classified as benign, borderline, or malignant on the basis of histological features.
• There is no distinct boundary between fibroadenoma and phyllodes tumor at the benign end of the spectrum and both can be excised with breast conservation.
• Generally, phyllodes tumor presents as a rapidly growing and clinically benign breast lump in women within the fourth or fifth decade of life.
• No imaging techniques appear to be able to differentiate benign and malignant lesions.
• Core biopsy is the preferred nonoperative sampling technique.
• The majority of phyllodes tumors behave in a completely benign fashion in that they do not have metastatic potential, local recurrence being the only real concern.
• Local recurrence per se is not an indicator of malignancy because it has been described in benign, borderline, and malignant phyllodes tumors.
• The mainstay of treatment for phyllodes tumors remains excision with a safe surgical margin, taking advantage of breast-conserving surgery where amenable.
• Clear margin status is associated with a low local recurrence rate regardless of histological features of the lesion. We

recommend ensuring wide local excision even if this means mastectomy, especially in cases of borderline and malignant phyllodes tumor.

• Histological type is the most important predictor for metastatic spread; in particular, the presence of high-grade sarcoma, even in limited proportions, appears predictive of aggressive behavior.

• Axillary nodal dissection is not indicated in the management of phyllodes tumors.

• The prognosis of phyllodes tumors is favorable, with local recurrence occurring in approximately 15% of patients overall and distant recurrence in approximately 5–10% overall.

• Twenty percent of patients with malignant tumors develop distant metastases, the most common sites being the lung, bone, and abdominal viscera.

• Patients with locally recurrent disease should undergo wide excision of the recurrence with or without subsequent radiotherapy.

• The role of adjuvant radiotherapy and hormonal therapy remains to be defined.

• The role of adjuvant treatments is unproven and must be considered on a case-by-case basis. Following development of metastatic disease, palliation may be obtained with single-agent or combination chemotherapy (anthracycline-based regimens).

• Molecular analysis will potentially supplement classic histological examination in order to improve our management of these tumors.

References

1. Parker SJ, Harries SA. Phyllodes tumours. Postgrad Med J 2001; 77(909): 428–35.

2. Burga AM, Tavassoli FA. Periductal stromal tumor: a rare lesion with low-grade sarcomatous behavior. Am J Surg Pathol 2003; 27(3): 343–8.

3. Barth RJ Jr, Wells WA, Mitchell SE, Cole BF. A prospective, multi-institutional study of adjuvant radiotherapy after resection of malignant phyllodes tumors. Ann Surg Oncol 2009; 16(8): 2288–94.

4. Bernstein L, Deapen D, Ross RK. The descriptive epidemiology of malignant cystosarcoma phyllodes tumors of the breast. Cancer 1993; 71(10): 3020–4.

5. Macdonald OK, Lee CM, Tward JD, et al. Malignant phyllodes tumor of the female breast: association of primary therapy with cause-specific survival from the Surveillance, Epidemiology, and End Results (SEER) program. Cancer 2006; 107(9): 2127–33.

6. Moffat CJ, Pinder SE, Dixon AR, et al. Phyllodes tumours of the breast: a clinicopathological review of thirty-two cases. Histopathology 1995; 27(3): 205–18.

7. Tse GM, Niu Y, Shi HJ. Phyllodes tumor of the breast: an update. Breast Cancer 2010; 17(1): 29–34.

8. Pezner RD, Schultheiss TE, Paz IB. Malignant phyllodes tumor of the breast: local control rates with surgery alone. Int J Radiat Oncol Biol Phys 2008; 71(3): 710–13.

9. Pimiento JM, Gadgil PV, Santillan AA, et al. Phyllodes tumors: race-related differences. J Am Coll Surg 2011; 213(4): 537–42.

10. Rajan PB, Cranor ML, Rosen PP. Cystosarcoma phyllodes in adolescent girls and young women: a study of 45 patients. Am J Surg Pathol 1998; 22(1): 64–9.

11. Guillot E, Couturaud B, Reyal F, et al. Management of phyllodes breast tumors. Breast J 2011; 17(2): 129–37.

12. Campagnaro EL, Woodside KJ, Xiao SY, et al. Cystosarcoma phyllodes (phyllodes tumor) of the male breast. Surgery 2003; 133(6): 689–91.

13. Nielsen VT, Andreasen C. Phyllodes tumour of the male breast. Histopathology 1987; 11(7): 761–2.

14. Ansah-Boateng Y, Tavassoli FA. Fibroadenoma and cystosarcoma phyllodes of the male breast. Mod Pathol 1992; 5(2): 114–16.

15. Rosenfeld JC, DeLaurentis DA, Lerner H. Cystosarcoma phyllodes. Diagnosis and management. Cancer Clin Trials 1981; 4(2): 187–93.

16. Minkowitz S, Zeichner M, di Maio V, Nicastri AD. Cystosarcoma phyllodes: a unique case with multiple unilateral lesions and ipsilateral axillary metastasis. J Pathol Bacteriol 1968; 96(2): 514–17.

17. De Raeve H, Jeuris W, Wyndaele JJ, van Marck E. Cystosarcoma phyllodes of the prostate with rhabdomyoblastic differentiation. Pathol Res Pract 2001; 197(10): 657–62.

18. Chulia MT, Paya A, Niveiro M, et al. Phyllodes tumor in ectopic breast tissue of the vulva. Int J Surg Pathol 2001; 9(1): 81–3.

19. Oshida K, Miyauchi M, Yamamoto N, et al. Phyllodes tumor arising in ectopic breast tissue of the axilla. Breast Cancer 2003; 10(1): 82–4.

20. Lindquist KD, van Heerden JA, Weiland LH, Martin JK Jr. Recurrent and metastatic cystosarcoma phyllodes. Am J Surg 1982; 144(3): 341–3.

21. Mrad K, Driss M, Maalej M, Romdhane KB. Bilateral cystosarcoma phyllodes of the breast: a case report of malignant form with contralateral benign form. Ann Diagn Pathol 2000; 4(6): 370–2.

22. Treves N, Sunderland DA. Cystosarcoma phyllodes of the breast: a malignant and a benign tumor; a clinicopathological study of seventy-seven cases. Cancer 1951; 4(6): 1286–332.

23. Barrio AV, Clark BD, Goldberg JI, et al. Clinicopathologic features and long-term outcomes of 293 phyllodes tumors of the breast. Ann Surg Oncol 2007; 14(10): 2961–70.

24. Kuijper A, Buerger H, Simon R, et al. Analysis of the progression of fibroepithelial tumours of the breast by PCR-based clonality assay. J Pathol 2002; 197(5): 575–81.

25. Noguchi S, Aihara T, Koyama H, et al. Clonal analysis of benign and malignant human breast tumors by means of polymerase chain reaction. Cancer Lett 1995; 90(1): 57–63.

26. Kasami M, Vnencak-Jones CL, Manning S, et al. Monoclonality in fibroadenomas with complex histology and phyllodal features. Breast Cancer Res Treat 1998; 50(2): 185–91.

27. Noguchi S, Yokouchi H, Aihara T, et al. Progression of fibroadenoma to phyllodes tumor demonstrated by clonal analysis. Cancer 1995; 76(10): 1779–85.

28. Atherton AJ, Monaghan P, Warburton MJ, et al. Dipeptidyl peptidase IV expression identifies a functional subpopulation of breast fibroblasts. Int J Cancer 1992; 50(1): 15–19.

29. Kleer CG, Giordano TJ, Braun T, Oberman HA. Pathologic, immunohistochemical, and molecular features of benign and malignant phyllodes tumors of the breast. Mod Pathol 2001; 14(3): 185–90.

30. Sawhney N, Garrahan N, Douglas-Jones AG, Williams ED. Epithelial–stromal interactions in tumors. A morphologic study of fibroepithelial tumors of the breast. Cancer 1992; 70(8): 2115–20.

31. Karim RZ, Scolyer RA, Tse GM, et al. Pathogenic mechanisms in the initiation and progression of mammary phyllodes tumours. Pathology 2009; 41(2): 105–17.

32. Kracht J, Sapino A, Bussolati G. Malignant phyllodes tumor of breast with lung metastases mimicking the primary. Am J Surg Pathol 1998; 22(10): 1284–90.

33. West TL, Weiland LH, Clagett OT. Cystosarcoma phyllodes. Ann Surg 1971; 173(4): 520–8.

34. Belkacemi Y, Bousquet G, Marsiglia H, et al. Phyllodes tumor of the breast. Int J Radiat Oncol Biol Phys 2008; 70(2): 492–500.

35. Pietruszka M, Barnes L. Cystosarcoma phyllodes: a clinicopathologic analysis of 42 cases. Cancer 1978; 41(5): 1974–83.

36. Chen WH, Cheng SP, Tzen CY, et al. Surgical treatment of phyllodes tumors of the breast: retrospective review of 172 cases. J Surg Oncol 2005; 91(3): 185–94.

37. Hajdu SI, Espinosa MH, Robbins GF. Recurrent cystosarcoma phyllodes: a clinicopathologic study of 32 cases. Cancer 1976; 38(3): 1402–6.

38. Tan PH, Jayabaskar T, Chuah KL, et al. Phyllodes tumors of the breast: the role of pathologic parameters. Am J Clin Pathol 2005; 123(4): 529–40.

39. Taira N, Takabatake D, Aogi K, et al. Phyllodes tumor of the breast: stromal overgrowth and histological classification are useful prognosis-predictive factors for local recurrence in patients with a positive surgical margin. Jpn J Clin Oncol 2007; 37(10): 730–6.

40. Chaney AW, Pollack A, McNeese MD, et al. Primary treatment of cystosarcoma phyllodes of the breast. Cancer 2000; 89(7): 1502–11.

41. Sawyer EJ, Hanby AM, Ellis P, et al. Molecular analysis of phyllodes tumors reveals distinct changes in the epithelial and stromal components. Am J Pathol 2000; 156(3): 1093–8.

42. Kuijper A, Snijders AM, Berns EM, et al. Genomic profiling by array comparative genomic hybridization reveals novel DNA copy number changes in breast phyllodes tumours. Cell Oncol 2009; 31(1): 31–9.

43. Lu YJ, Birdsall S, Osin P, et al. Phyllodes tumors of the breast analyzed by comparative genomic hybridization and association of increased 1q copy number with stromal overgrowth and recurrence. Genes Chromosomes Cancer 1997; 20(3): 275–81.

44. Niezabitowski A, Lackowska B, Rys J, et al. Prognostic evaluation of proliferative activity and DNA content in the phyllodes tumor of the breast: immunohistochemical and flow cytometric study of 118 cases. Breast Cancer Res Treat 2001; 65(1): 77–85.

45. Singh Y, Hatano T, Uemura Y, et al. Immunohistochemical profile of phyllodes tumors of the breast. Oncol Rep 1996; 3(4): 677–81.

46. Lae M, Vincent-Salomon A, Savignoni A, et al. Phyllodes tumors of the breast segregate in two groups according to genetic criteria. Mod Pathol 2007; 20(4): 435–44.

47. Kim JH, Choi YD, Lee JS, et al. Borderline and malignant phyllodes tumors display similar promoter methylation profiles. Virchows Arch 2009; 455(6): 469–75.

48. Ang MK, Ooi AS, Thike AA, et al. Molecular classification of breast phyllodes tumors: validation of the histologic grading scheme and insights into malignant progression. Breast Cancer Res Treat 2010; 129(2): 319–29.

49. Birch JM, Alston RD, McNally RJ, et al. Relative frequency and morphology of cancers in carriers of germline TP53 mutations. Oncogene 2001; 20(34): 4621–8.

50. Tan PH, Jayabaskar T, Yip G, et al. p53 and c-kit (CD117) protein expression as prognostic indicators in breast phyllodes tumors: a tissue microarray study. Mod Pathol 2005; 18(12): 1527–34.

51. Tse GM, Putti TC, Kung FY, et al. Increased p53 protein expression in malignant mammary phyllodes tumors. Mod Pathol 2002; 15(7): 734–40.

52. Shpitz B, Bomstein Y, Sternberg A, et al. Immunoreactivity of p53, Ki-67, and c-erbB-2 in phyllodes tumors of the breast in correlation with clinical and morphologic features. J Surg Oncol 2002; 79(2): 86–92.

53. Yonemori K, Hasegawa T, Shimizu C, et al. Correlation of p53 and MIB-1 expression with both the systemic recurrence and survival in cases of phyllodes tumors of the breast. Pathol Res Pract 2006; 202(10): 705–12.

54. Ridgway PF, Jacklin RK, Ziprin P, et al. Perioperative diagnosis of cystosarcoma phyllodes of the breast may be enhanced by MIB-1 index. J Surg Res 2004; 122(1): 83–8.

55. Karim RZ, Gerega SK, Yang YH, et al. p16 and pRb immunohistochemical expression increases with increasing tumour grade in mammary phyllodes tumours. Histopathology 2010; 56(7): 868–75.

56. Sawyer EJ, Poulsom R, Hunt FT, et al. Malignant phyllodes tumours show stromal overexpression of c-myc and c-kit. J Pathol 2003; 200(1): 59–64.

57. Karim RZ, Gerega SK, Yang YH, et al. p16 and pRb immunohistochemical expression increases with increasing tumour grade in mammary phyllodes tumours. Histopathology; 56(7): 868–75.

58. Carvalho S, e Silva AO, Milanezi F, et al. c-KIT and PDGFRA in breast phyllodes tumours: overexpression without mutations? J Clin Pathol 2004; 57(10): 1075–9.

59. Wang X, Jones TD, Zhang S, et al. Amplifications of EGFR gene and protein expression of EGFR, Her-2/neu, c-kit, and androgen receptor in phyllodes tumor of the prostate. Mod Pathol 2007; 20(2): 175–82.

60. Tse GM, Tsang AK, Putti TC, et al. Stromal CD10 expression in mammary fibroadenomas and phyllodes tumours. J Clin Pathol 2005; 58(2): 185–9.

61. Tsai WC, Jin JS, Yu JC, Sheu LF. CD10, actin, and vimentin expression in breast phyllodes tumors correlates with tumor grades of the WHO grading system. Int J Surg Pathol 2006; 14(2): 127–31.

62. Noronha Y, Raza A, Hutchins B, et al. CD34, CD117, and Ki-67 expression in phyllodes tumor of the breast: an immunohistochemical study of 33 cases. Int J Surg Pathol 2011; 19(2): 152–8.

63. Moore T, Lee AH. Expression of CD34 and bcl-2 in phyllodes tumours, fibroadenomas and spindle cell lesions of the breast. Histopathology 2001; 38(1): 62–7.

64. Tse GM, Lee CS, Kung FY, et al. Hormonal receptors expression in epithelial cells of mammary phyllodes tumors correlates with pathologic grade of the tumor: a multicenter study of 143 cases. Am J Clin Pathol 2002; 118(4): 522–6.

65. Sapino A, Bosco M, Cassoni P, et al. Estrogen receptor-beta is expressed in stromal cells of fibroadenoma and phyllodes tumors of the breast. Mod Pathol 2006; 19(4): 599–606.

66. Tse GM, Lui PC, Vong JS, et al. Increased epidermal growth factor receptor (EGFR) expression in malignant mammary phyllodes tumors. Breast Cancer Res Treat 2009; 114(3): 441–8.

67. Kersting C, Kuijper A, Schmidt H, et al. Amplifications of the epidermal growth factor receptor gene (egfr) are common in phyllodes tumors of the breast and are associated with tumor progression. Lab Invest 2006; 86(1): 54–61.

68. Komenaka IK, El-Tamer M, Pile-Spellman E, Hibshoosh H. Core needle biopsy as a diagnostic tool to differentiate phyllodes tumor from fibroadenoma. Arch Surg 2003; 138(9): 987–90.

69. Parfitt JR, Armstrong C, O'Malley F, et al. In-situ and invasive carcinoma within a phyllodes tumor associated with lymph node metastases. World J Surg Oncol 2004; 2: 46.

70. Han AC, Soler AP, Knudsen KA, Salazar H. Distinct cadherin profiles in special variant carcinomas and other tumors of the breast. Hum Pathol 1999; 30(9): 1035–9.

71. Azzopardi JG. Problems in Breast Pathology, vol. 11. Philadelphia: WB Saunders, 1979.

72. Bellocq JP, Magro G. Pathology and genetics of tumors of the breast and female genital organs. In: Tavassoli FA, Devilee P (eds) World Health Organization Classification of Tumors. Lyon: IARC Press, 2003. pp. 100–103.

73. Cohn-Cedermark G, Rutqvist LE, Rosendahl I, Silfversward C. Prognostic factors in cystosarcoma phyllodes. A clinicopathologic study of 77 patients. Cancer 1991; 68(9): 2017–22.

74. Norris HJ, Taylor HB. Relationship of histologic features to behavior of cystosarcoma phyllodes. Analysis of ninety-four cases. Cancer 1967; 20(12): 2090–9.

75. Ward RM, Evans HL. Cystosarcoma phyllodes. A clinicopathologic study of 26 cases. Cancer 1986; 58(10): 2282–9.

76. Guerrero MA, Ballard BR, Grau AM. Malignant phyllodes tumor of the breast: review of the literature and case report of stromal overgrowth. Surg Oncol 2003; 12(1): 27–37.

77. Powell CM, Rosen PP. Adipose differentiation in cystosarcoma phyllodes. A study of 14 cases. Am J Surg Pathol 1994; 18(7): 720–7.

78. Carter BA, Page DL. Phyllodes tumor of the breast: local recurrence versus metastatic capacity. Hum Pathol 2004; 35(9): 1051–2.

79. Dunne B, Lee AH, Pinder SE, et al. An immunohistochemical study of metaplastic spindle cell carcinoma, phyllodes tumor and fibromatosis of the breast. Hum Pathol 2003; 34(10): 1009–15.

80. Wurdinger S, Herzog AB, Fischer DR, et al. Differentiation of phyllodes breast tumors from fibroadenomas on MRI. Am J Roentgenol 2005; 185(5): 1317–21.

81. Yabuuchi H, Soeda H, Matsuo Y, *et al.* Phyllodes tumor of the breast: correlation between MR findings and histologic grade. Radiology 2006; 241(3): 702–9.

82. Jara-Lazaro AR, Akhilesh M, Thike AA, *et al.* Predictors of phyllodes tumours on core biopsy specimens of fibroepithelial neoplasms. Histopathology 2010; 57(2): 220–32.

83. Lee AH, Hodi Z, Ellis IO, Elston CW. Histological features useful in the distinction of phyllodes tumour and fibroadenoma on needle core biopsy of the breast. Histopathology 2007; 51(3): 336–44.

84. Dillon MF, Quinn CM, McDermott EW, *et al.* Needle core biopsy in the diagnosis of phyllodes neoplasm. Surgery 2006; 140(5): 779–84.

85. Zurrida S, Bartoli C, Galimberti V, *et al.* Which therapy for unexpected phyllode tumour of the breast? Eur J Cancer 1992; 28(2–3): 654–7.

86. Mangi AA, Smith BL, Gadd MA, *et al.* Surgical management of phyllodes tumors. Arch Surg 1999; 134(5): 487–92; discussion 492–3.

87. Kapiris I, Nasiri N, A'Hern R, *et al.* Outcome and predictive factors of local recurrence and distant metastases following primary surgical treatment of high-grade malignant phyllodes tumours of the breast. Eur J Surg Oncol 2001; 27(8): 723–30.

88. Barth RJ Jr. Histologic features predict local recurrence after breast conserving therapy of phyllodes tumors. Breast Cancer Res Treat 1999; 57(3): 291–5.

89. Soumarova R, Seneklova Z, Horova H, *et al.* Retrospective analysis of 25 women with malignant cystosarcoma phyllodes – treatment results. Arch Gynecol Obstet 2004; 269(4): 278–81.

90. Chaney AW, Pollack A, McNeese MD, Zagars GK. Adjuvant radiotherapy for phyllodes tumor of breast. Radiat Oncol Invest 1998; 6(6): 264–7.

91. Telli ML, Horst KC, Guardino AE, *et al.* Phyllodes tumors of the breast: natural history, diagnosis, and treatment. J Natl Compr Canc Netw 2007; 5(3): 324–30.

92. McGowan TS, Cummings BJ, O'Sullivan B, *et al.* An analysis of 78 breast sarcoma patients without distant metastases at presentation. Int J Radiat Oncol Biol Phys 2000; 46(2): 383–90.

93. Eich PD, Diederich S, Eich HT, *et al.* Diagnostic radiation oncology: malignant cystosarcoma phylloides. Strahlenther Onkol 2000; 176(4): 192–5.

94. Hawkins RE, Schofield JB, Wiltshaw E, *et al.* Ifosfamide is an active drug for chemotherapy of metastatic cystosarcoma phyllodes. Cancer 1992; 69(9): 2271–5.

95. Morales-Vasquez F, Gonzalez-Angulo AM, Broglio K, *et al.* Adjuvant chemotherapy with doxorubicin and dacarbazine has no effect in recurrence-free survival of malignant phyllodes tumors of the breast. Breast J 2007; 13(6): 551–6.

96. Abdalla HM, Sakr MA. Predictive factors of local recurrence and survival following primary surgical treatment of phyllodes tumors of the breast. J Egypt Natl Canc Inst 2006; 18(2): 125–33.

97. Lester J, Stout AP. Cystosarcoma phyllodes. Cancer 1954; 7(2): 335–353.

98. Murad TM, Hines JR, Beal J, Bauer K. Histopathological and clinical correlations of cystosarcoma phyllodes. Arch Path Lab Med 1988; 112: 752–756.

99. Salvadori B, Cusumano F, del RBo, *et al.* Surgical treatment of phyllodes tumours of the breast. Cancer 1989; 63: 2532–2536.

100. Bartoli C, Zurrida S, Veronesi P, *et al.* Small sized phyllodes tumor of the breast. Eur J Surg Oncol 1990; 16(3): 215–219.

101. Grimes MM. Cystosarcoma phyllodes of the breast: histologic features, flow cytometry analysis and clinical correlations. Mod Pathol 1992; 5: 232–239.

102. Stebbing JF, Nash AG. Diagnosis and management of phyllodes tumour of the breast: experience of 33 cases at a specialist centre. Ann R Coll Surg Engl 1995; 77(3): 181–184.

103. Reinfuss M, Mitus J, Duda K, Stelmach A, Rys J, Smolak K. The treatment and prognosis of patients with phyllodes tumor of the breast: an analysis of 170 cases. Cancer 1996; 77(5): 910–916.

104. Yamada J, Iino Y, Yokoe T. Phyllodes tumors of the breast: a clinico-pathological study of 118 cases. Surg Today 1997; 27: 1137–1143.

105. Mokbel K, Price RK, Mostafa A, Wells CA, Carpenter R. Phyllodes tumour of the breast: a retrospective analysis of 30 cases. Breast 1999; 8(5): 278–281.

18 Carcinosarcoma of the Breast

Stacy L. Moulder,[1] Bryan T. Hennessy,[5] Michael Z. Gilcrease,[2] Gildy Babiera,[3] Wei Yang,[4] Vicente Valero,[1] and Gabriel N. Hortobagyi[1]

[1] Department of Breast Medical Oncology, [2] Department of Pathology, [3] Department of Surgical Oncology, [4] Department of Diagnostic Radiology, The University of Texas MD Anderson Cancer Center, Houston, TX, USA
[5] Department of Medical Oncology, Beaumont Hospital, Dublin, Ireland

Introduction

Carcinosarcoma of the breast is rare and accounts for less than 0.1% of all breast malignancies.[1,2] Though carcinosarcomas are considered a form of metaplastic breast cancer, these tumors warrant special discussion because of their aggressive and ominous prognosis. Carcinosarcomas consist of intraductal or infiltrating carcinoma contiguous or subtly merged with a highly cellular, often mitotically active malignant-appearing stroma (sarcomatous component).[3–6] The macroscopic appearance of these tumors is dependent on the variety of possible epithelial and mesenchymal components. By traditional definition, a "classic" carcinosarcoma has distinct demarcation between carcinomatous and sarcomatous components in all microscopic fields. If there is obvious microscopic transition between the epithelial and sarcomatoid components, then the term "biphasic sarcomatoid carcinoma" has often been employed to distinguish this tumor from a "classic" carcinosarcoma. Although the term "carcinosarcoma" has been used inconsistently in the literature, sometimes to describe only "classic" carcinosarcomas (Fig. 18.1) and in other instances to describe both "classic" carcinosarcomas and other metaplastic breast sarcomatoid carcinomas,[7,8] the less restrictive definition will be used in this chapter. Tumors that show both carcinomatous and sarcomatous features occur in various anatomical sites and, in spite of differences in terminology and exact microscopic composition, evidence suggests these are all similar tumors developing through a peculiar phenotypic transformation of carcinoma cells into sarcoma.[9–19] In the breast, the most popular theories regarding the histogenesis of the sarcomatous component of carcinosarcomas and sarcomatoid carcinomas propose the malignant transformation of myoepithelial cells or myofibroblastic metaplasia of malignant epithelial cells.[4,7,8,20–27]

Historical background

The issues of the histogenesis and clonality of carcinosarcomas of the breast have been debated for almost 100 years.[28] In fact, a search of the PubMed database reveals several articles dating back to the 1950s, presenting case reports, reviewing the literature, and discussing the origins of this rare tumor.[29–32] For years, a prevailing notion was that breast carcinosarcomas were derived from two distinct cells of origin which collided at some point during oncogenesis (collision hypothesis). However, modern-day molecular characterization has yielded rather compelling evidence to the contrary. Wargotz and Norris demonstrated in the 1980s that the sarcomatous component of carcinosarcoma is immunoreactive for cytokeratin in more than 50% of cases, regardless of the presence or absence of overt transitional areas between sarcomatous and epithelial areas.[4] In fact, they found that a majority of carcinosarcomas diagnosed using the traditional definition of a distinct demarcation between the carcinomatous and sarcomatous components contain, upon close inspection, foci of subtle transition between both components. These investigators were among the first to suspect a myoepithelial origin for these tumors, in part because of their demonstration of dual staining with epithelial and myoepithelial markers, including actin and S-100. A review of current ultrastructural, cytogenetic, and immunohistochemical data in fact supports a monoclonal origin for carcinosarcomas (see 'Molecular biology, genetics' section below).

Epidemiology

Carcinosarcoma of the breast is rare. Metaplastic breast cancers constituted 0.2% of all breast neoplasms seen at the University of Texas MD Anderson Cancer Center between

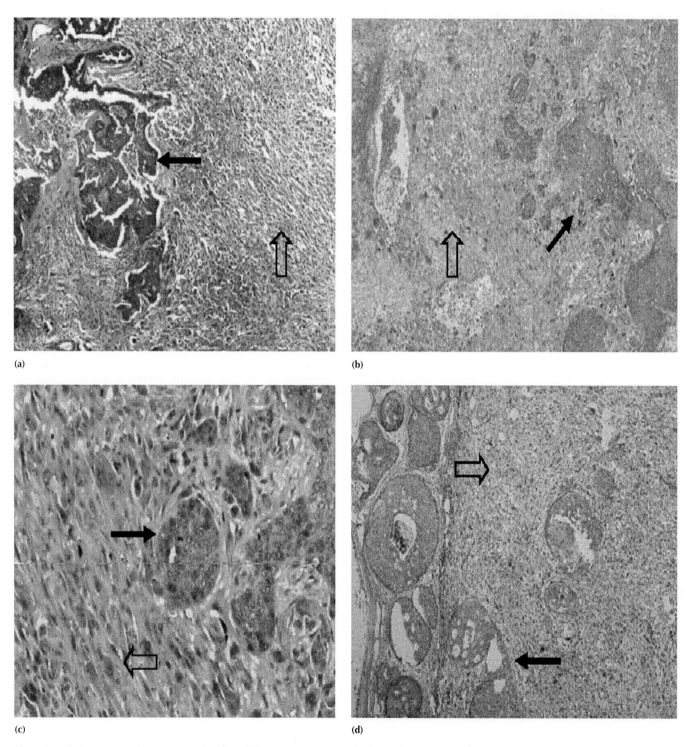

(a)

(b)

(c)

(d)

Figure 18.1 (a,b) Low-power photomicrographs of two different carcinosarcomas demonstrating invasive carcinoma (*solid arrows*) and distinct high-grade sarcomatous component (*open arrows*). (c) High-power photomicrograph of same tumor as in (b). (d) Carcinosarcoma with DCIS (*solid arrow*) and adjacent high-grade sarcomatous component (*open arrow*).

1948 and 1978. In the Surveillance, Epidemiology, and End Results (SEER) database, a population-based tumor registry sponsored by the US National Cancer Institute consisting of tumor registries that collect information on all newly diagnosed cancer cases that occur in persons residing in 11 SEER participating areas, of a total of 281,342 breast cancers registered between 1988 and 2001, there were 98 carcinosarcomas (0.03%; Table 18.1) and an additional 213 registered cases of metaplastic sarcomatoid carcinoma (0.08%). Of the 98 registered cases of breast carcinosarcoma, 83 occurred in Caucasians, 11 in African-Americans, and four in other races.

The etiology of breast carcinosarcomas is not known but chronic estrogenic stimulation may be involved, as with other breast cancers. In the uterus, tamoxifen has been implicated in the development of carcinosarcomas and adenocarcinomas.[33] A case of carcinosarcoma of the breast has also been reported in one patient who underwent breast augmentation by liquid silicone injection.[34]

Molecular biology, genetics

The monoclonality of carcinosarcomas is no longer in dispute.[8] More recent analysis of metaplastic carcinomas has clearly established the clonal relationship between morphologically distinct components of the same tumor, with some tumors showing no detectable differences in molecular characteristics while others harbored additional genetic aberrations, such as copy number changes, gene amplification and additional focal gene mutations or amplifications, leading some to suggest that further genetic changes may be responsible for "transdifferentiation" in selected tumors.[36]

Recently, the use of gene profiling has allowed the identification of a number of subtypes of breast cancer, each with differences in prognosis and therapy responsiveness.[37,38] Tumors characterized as basal or claudin-low subtypes usually, but not always, lack expression of estrogen, progesterone, and Her-2 receptors. The basal subtype of breast cancer is believed to arise from basal progenitor or myoepithelial cells in the ductal epithelium of the breast.[39,40] The claudin-low tumors are characterized by absent expression of luminal differentiation markers, enrichment of markers of epithelial-to-mesenchymal transition (EMT) and share similar features with cancer stem cells.[41] Metaplastic cancers, including carcinosarcomas, more closely resemble claudin-low tumors by molecular profiling and both claudin-low and metaplastic tumors demonstrate worse prognosis and increased resistance to therapy compared to basal-type tumors.[42–50]

Wargotz and Norris were among the first to suspect a myoepithelial origin for carcinosarcomas following their demonstration of dual staining of both tumor cell types with myoepithelial markers, including actin and S-100.[4] As further support for a myoepithelial origin, a second study found prominent p63 expression in sarcomatoid/metaplastic carcinomas of the breast.[51] ΔN isoforms of p63 are consistently expressed in the nuclei of normal breast myoepithelial and basal cells, as well as in basal cells of several multilayered epithelia, and may constitute a mechanism to overcome p53-driven cell cycle arrest and apoptosis.[51–54] Although myoepithelial cells and basal cells both express p63 isoforms, myoepithelial cells also express smooth muscle markers, whereas basal cells do not. These findings, along with staining of tumor cells for basal cell-type cytokeratins, provide support for some degree of myoepithelial differentiation in sarcomatoid carcinomas of the breast.[55] Other investigators have used genes significantly repressed in association with methylation (SRAM) to identify lineage-specific methylation signatures that segregate breast cancer cell lines into epithelial and mesenchymal lineages. In this study, both claudin-low and metaplastic tumors more closely resembled the mesenchymal expression signature, although the metaplastic tumors were also associated with expression of some epithelial markers.[56]

The loss of epithelial morphology and acquisition of mesenchymal characteristics (EMT) have been reported for some breast and other carcinoma cells in tumor progression.[21] Although originally thought to be restricted to mesenchymal cells and sarcomatoid epithelial neoplasms such as carcinosarcomas, in human infiltrating ductal breast carcinomas, correlated upregulation of the mesenchymal markers tenascin-C and vimentin is frequently observed and associated with increased malignancy and invasiveness.[57,58] Tenascin-C and vimentin expression also correlates with downregulation of estrogen receptors and increased tumor grade in breast cancer and epithelial tumor cells coexpressing vimentin and cytokeratins often have a spindle-shaped phenotype. Tenascin-C and vimentin may represent regulator genes involved in EMT during mammary carcinogenesis.[21] Thus, a sarcomatoid phenotype associated with breast cancer may reflect myofibroblastic metaplasia or transdifferentiation of adenocarcinoma cells during EMT. Several mechanisms have been implicated in EMT, including ras deregulation, by mutation or otherwise. Indeed, the transfection of transformed immortalized breast epithelial cells with a constitutively active form of ras can induce the acquisition of spindle morphology with loss of E-cadherin and other molecular changes.[59] E-cadherin, like N- and P-cadherin, is present in some areas of sarcomatoid breast cancers but is lost in the sarcomatous areas of carcinosarcomas.[5,60]

Molecular signatures obtained by large-scale transcriptional profiling of metaplastic tumors have also demonstrated upregulation of genes associated with extracellular matrix production and downregulation of genes associated with maintaining the epithelial phenotype, such as genes that encode for cell-cell adhesion molecules and tight junctions, particularly in tumors with predominant spindle cell morphology.[46] Hennessy et al. have published the largest molecular profiling series of metaplastic tumors which included predominantly squamous or sarcomatoid metaplasia.[47] In this series, significance analysis of microarray (SAM) was used to identify a molecular signature for metaplastic cancers compared to nonmetaplastic breast cancers and revealed upregulation of important regulators of EMT such as TWIST1 and SNAI2/SLUG in the metaplastic breast cancers.[61,62] Other investigators have demonstrated a close association of the metaplastic signature and claudin-low signature with an "EMT-core signature" derived by overexpressing EMT-inducing transcription factors in cell lines.[45] Metaplastic cancers also display high rates of Wnt pathway deregulation with aberrant expression of β-catenin within the nucleus or cytoplasm reported in 46–92% of metaplastic breast cancers.[63] Mutations in CTNNB1 (the gene encoding β-catenin) have been reported to occur in 26% of metaplastic cancers though this was not confirmed in two subsequent publications.[47,63,64]

Within the Hennessy series of metaplastic breast cancers, a high rate of mutations was noted in the phosphatidylinositol 3-kinase/Akt pathway: PIK3CA (47.4%) or PTEN (5%). Reverse-phase protein array demonstrated elevation in phosphorylation in PI3K/AKT pathway proteins in metaplastic breast cancers compared to other breast cancer subtypes, further suggesting the potential importance for this pathway in the

Table 18.1 Clinical studies of patients with carcinosarcoma of the breast and data extracted from the SEER population database. Only two studies and the SEER data included only breast carcinosarcoma using the traditional definition (*), while the others included all metaplastic high-grade sarcomatoid carcinomas of the breast. In the Gutman study, although the term carcinosarcoma was used, the tumors were defined as all epithelial carcinomas of the breast with "malignant sarcomatoid metaplasia".

Study	Cases	Symptom at diagnosis	Median age years (range)	Follow-up	Surgery (number cases)	Median T size mm (range)	ALN involvement at diagnosis	ER/PR	Adjuvant chemotherapy (cases)	Adjuvant radiotherapy (patients)	Cases with distant metastases at diagnosis (%)	Outcome	Site relapse (cases)
SEER*	98	No information	60 (33–91)	Patients registered from 1988 to 2001	Mastectomy/AD (50) Mastectomy (9) WLE/AD (23) WLE (10) None (6)	T1-16 T2-53 T3/4-20 TX-9	14 (14%) but unknown in 24 (24%)	4/68+ (6%)	No information	31	6 (6)	60% 5-year OS	No information
Wargotz[64]	70	Mass (70) Skin fixation (9) Chest wall fixation (2) Skin/nipple ulceration (7) Nipple retraction (3)	56 (29–95)	Mean 4.9 years	MRM (26) RM (28) SM (11) WLE (3) Excision (2)	50 (9–190)	26%	1/11+ (9%)	2 patients: CMF (1) ChlorMF (1)	11	0 (0)	49% 5-year OS Median RFS 10 months (range 1 month – 6.3 years)	Distant (24) Local (15)
Gutman[67]	50	No information	Mean 50 (25–76)	Median 27 months (4–240 months)	WLE (10) SM/MRM (31) RM (9); with AD (44)	Mean 46	9/44 (20.5%)	12.5% +	20 patients: all FAC	17	3 (6)	43% 5-year OS 32% 5-year DFS	Distant (19) Local (9)
Rayson[68]	27	Mass (24) MMG (5) Pain (1) Nipple discharge (1)	59 (39–90)	2.4-year median DFS time	RM (1) MRM (17) Lumpectomy (1) WLE/AD (6) SM (2)	34 (5–70)	13%	13% +	9 patients: AC (4) CMF (3) CAF (2)	5	1 (4)	40% 3-year DFS 70% 3-year OS	Lung (10) Local (4)
Kaufman[69]	26	Mass (26) Skin fixation (9) Chest wall fixation (6) Ulceration (1)	Mean 54 (27–80)	No information	RM/MRM (15) SM (8) Excision (3)	47 (12–130)	5/20 (25%)	?	4 patients	12	0 (0)	40% 5-year OS Mean OS 65 months	Distant (11) Local (4)

Oberman (2)[70] 15	No information	52 (32–88)	Median 3.3 years	MRM (5) RM (5) TM (4) Lumpectomy (1)	40 (15–190)	2/12 (17%)	1/5+ (20%)	None	1	0 (0)	7 relapses and 8 deaths	No information
Kurian[71] 12	No information	64 (46–82)	Minimum 12 years	Mastectomy (11) Axillary dissection (6)	52 (22–100)	1 (8%)	?	No information	No information	0 (0)	4 (33%) relapses	Lung (4) Bone (1)
Oberman (1)[70] 8	No information	64 (51–89)	Median 2.5 years	MRM (5) TM (2) RM (1)	50 (35–90)	1/6 (17%)	0	None	None	0 (0)	5 relapses and deaths	No information
Gersell[72] 6	Mass (6), 1 discovered by physician Nipple discharge (1)	68 (55–75)	2 months – 11 years	TM (3) Excision (2) RM (1)	50 (20–90)	0/4 (0%)	?	No information	No information	1 (17)	2 relapses and 4 dead	Lung (1) Local (1)
Ferrara[25] 4	Mass (3)	53 (39–81)	Median 1.75 years	RM (2) SM (1) MRM (1)	37 (30–60)	0 (0%)	?	1 patient	None	1 (25 bone)	2 relapses and 1 death	Lung (1) Local (1)
Gogas*[1] 2	Mass (2) MMG (1)	30, 67	–	MRM (2)	65, 50	Both patients	1/2 +	Both patients	None	0 (0)	Recurred at 3 months + 6 years	Lung, bone (1) Liver, brain (1)

Numbers may add up to greater than the number of patients in the study if more than one factor occurred in some patients.

The Oberman study examined 29 metaplastic breast cancer patients in total, of whom eight had "spindle cell carcinoma", 15 "carcinoma with pseudosarcomatous metaplasia", and six squamous metaplasia.

AC, doxorubicin and cyclophosphamide; ALN, axillary lymph node; CAF, AC and 5-fluorouracil; ChlorMF, chlorambucil and MF; CMF, cyclophosphamide, methotrexate, and 5-fluorouracil; DFS, disease-free survival; ER, estrogen receptor; MMG, mammogram; MRM, modified radical mastectomy; PR, progesterone receptor; OS, overall survival; RFS, relapse-free survival; RM, radical mastectomy; SM, simple mastectomy; TM, total mastectomy; WLE/AD, wide local excision and axillary dissection.

metaplastic subtype. The transcriptional signature generated for metaplastic cancer also showed high correlation with a "tumorigenic signature" heavily weighted for PI3K activity.[65]

Pathology

Azzopardi originally proposed the term "carcinosarcoma" of the breast for rare tumors containing discrete areas of carcinoma and sarcoma arising together within a fibroepithelial lesion, such as a phyllodes tumor.[66] Phyllodes tumors are true biphasic lesions.[3] The stromal component of malignant phyllodes tumors undergoes sarcomatous transformation, but only rarely does carcinoma arise from the ductal component. When it does, both the carcinomatous and sarcomatous components of the tumor represent distinct clonal proliferations arising from the separate components of the preexisting biphasic lesion. Azzopardi referred to these rare "collision" tumors as "carcinosarcomas."

Breast tumors containing areas of carcinoma admixed with sarcomatous-appearing elements are more frequently observed in the absence of a preexisting fibroepithelial lesion. Such tumors have been regarded most often as carcinomas with areas of sarcomatous metaplasia, or sarcomatoid carcinomas. On close examination, most are found to contain areas of transition between carcinomatous and sarcomatous components. The sarcomatoid cells often maintain expression of cytokeratin, an intermediate filament characteristic of epithelial cells but generally not expressed by stromal cells. Moreover, molecular analysis of some biphasic tumors has demonstrated monoclonality, supporting the concept that the keratin-positive sarcomatous-appearing elements are derived from the coexisting carcinomatous component.[20–27]

Azzopardi's strict definition of carcinosarcoma has not been maintained in the pathology literature. In their popular series of articles on the classification of metaplastic carcinomas, Wargotz and Norris referred to carcinosarcoma as a *subtype of metaplastic carcinoma*.[4] They considered tumors with a combination of overt carcinomatous elements and high-grade mesenchymal-appearing areas as carcinosarcomas, without regard to whether these elements arose within a preexisting fibroepithelial lesion. They believed the combined carcinomatous and sarcomatous behavior of these tumors supported their designation as carcinosarcomas, regardless of whether the sarcomatous-appearing elements appeared to be derived from the carcinomatous component. Although no consistent definition of carcinosarcoma has been used in the literature, most reports of carcinosarcomas appear to meet the definition provided by Wargotz and Norris, as such tumors clearly arising within preexisting fibroepithelial lesions are rare. It should be recognized that most carcinosarcomas and sarcomatoid carcinomas reported in the literature are essentially the same tumors.

The carcinomatous component of carcinosarcomas is generally similar in appearance to invasive ductal carcinomas (IDC), but it may be a poorly differentiated carcinoma or squamous carcinoma (see Fig. 18.1).[3–6] It may even be ductal carcinoma *in situ* (DCIS). The sarcomatous component is, by definition, intermediate to high grade and may have a variety of histological appearances. It is most often composed of a highly cellular arrangement of spindle cells. There may be varying amounts of myxoid matrix deposited among the tumor cells. Foci with osseous or cartilaginous differentiation or both are frequently observed, sometimes forming the bulk of the sarcomatous component and resembling osteosarcoma or chondrosarcoma. The gross appearance of these tumors is often deceptively well demarcated, but infiltrative growth is characteristic microscopically.

Differential diagnosis

It is important not to equate all types of metaplastic carcinomas with carcinosarcomas.[3,4] Metaplastic carcinoma is most often regarded as an aggressive form of breast cancer because most tumors contain at least focal intermediate- to high-grade mesenchymal-appearing areas, and such tumors are biologically aggressive. Other forms of metaplastic carcinoma have not been shown to be more aggressive than typical IDCs, and some appear to be more indolent. In particular, it is very important to distinguish low-grade fibromatosis-like metaplastic tumors from carcinosarcomas.[54] Fibromatosis-like metaplastic tumors resemble fibromatosis but express cytokeratin. They tend to recur locally, but most reported cases have not metastasized. Although not always explicitly stated, the term "spindle cell carcinoma" in the literature generally implies a low- to intermediate-grade tumor that should be distinguished from carcinosarcoma.

Carcinosarcomas should also be distinguished from malignant phyllodes tumors and other rare primary sarcomas of the breast.[3] Sarcomas have a high rate of hematogenous dissemination but, in contrast to carcinosarcomas, have a very low incidence of axillary lymph node involvement. Pure keratin-positive sarcomatoid tumors and those with only a minor (<5%) overt carcinomatous component should also be distinguished from carcinosarcomas, as pure or almost pure keratin-positive sarcomatoid tumors (excluding low-grade fibromatosis-like tumors) have a biological behavior similar to that of pure sarcomas.

Clinical aspects: presentation, diagnostic considerations, and techniques

Table 18.1 shows the clinical features associated with breast carcinosarcomas in a number of small published studies and in the SEER population database.[1,4,25,67–72] As stated, the definition of carcinosarcoma varies somewhat from study to study. In the largest study of 70 breast carcinosarcoma patients by Wargotz and Norris,[4] the definition used was "intraductal or infiltrating carcinoma contiguous or subtly merged with a highly cellular, mitotically active, pleomorphic spindle cell stroma", while the Gutman *et al.* study of 50 carcinosarcoma patients included cases with "coexistent infiltrating ductal carcinoma and sarcomatoid metaplasia."[67] Generally, the majority of patients present with a palpable breast lump or mass. Fine needle aspiration (FNA) is usually positive for malignancy in the case of metaplastic breast cancer, although ductal and metaplastic elements are both found in smear material in just over half of cases, allowing a definite diagnosis prior to definitive surgery.[73–75] The tumor is usually relatively large and well circumscribed at diagnosis.[4,7,22,23,25,67–72,76] As a result of large tumor size at presentation, skin or chest wall fixation, nipple retraction, and skin and nipple ulceration are relatively frequent. Occasionally, carcinosarcomas may manifest as inflammatory carcinomas.[77] Some studies have found tumor size to be the major predictor of patient outcome.[67,70]

In most series, the majority of breast carcinosarcomas and metaplastic sarcomatoid breast cancers have a high nuclear grade. Hormone receptors and Her-2/neu are usually negative. In most cases, the locoregional lymph nodes are not involved by tumor at presentation and the likelihood of regional lymph node involvement is related to the amount of overt carcinomatous component in the primary tumor.[49,78] Neither do most women have recognizable distant metastases at the time of diagnosis. Most reports suggest that hematogenous dissemination is more characteristic of breast carcinosarcoma than spread along lymphatic channels; this has traditionally been regarded as more in keeping with the sarcomatous rather than the carcinomatous phenotype. Consistent with this, certain investigators have noted that carcinosarcomas seem to behave biologically differently from conventional adenocarcinoma of the breast, with sarcomatoid characteristics dominating the clinical course.[67,78,79]

Generally, the prognosis is relatively poor, with most series suggesting that at least one-third of patients will die from the disease. This is in keeping with other carcinosarcomas such as uterine carcinosarcomas.[80] Locoregional recurrence of breast carcinosarcoma is relatively frequent (see Table 18.1).

Imaging of carcinosarcoma

Carcinosarcomas and other metaplastic breast carcinomas are frequently visible (up to 90% of patients) by mammography. A comparison of imaging features between invasive ductal and metaplastic carcinomas involving 86 patients reported that characteristic malignant imaging features of carcinomas, including irregular shape, spiculated margins, segmentally distributed pleomorphic calcifications, and posterior acoustic shadowing, are uncommon in metaplastic carcinomas.[81] Metaplastic carcinomas tend to show more benign imaging features, such as round or oval shape with circumscribed margins, when compared with ductal carcinomas (Fig. 18.2a).[82–86] Spiculated or partially spiculated margins can be present in up to 14% of the masses, and calcifications in up to 26%.

Other tumors that may present with similar mammographic features of round or oval-shaped masses with circumscribed margins include the triad of circumscribed carcinomas (medullary, papillary, and mucinous), phyllodes tumors, and high-grade IDCs in women with genetic mutations.[87–89]

Carcinosarcoma is most frequently seen on sonograms as a solid, hypoechoic, hypervascular, oval mass with indistinct margins and posterior acoustic enhancement (Fig. 18.2b). Mixed solid and cystic masses have been described in 19–50% of the patients.[83,85,86] On magnetic resonance (MR) imaging, T2-weighted images reveal fairly well-defined oval and lobular-shaped masses with internal high signal-intensity

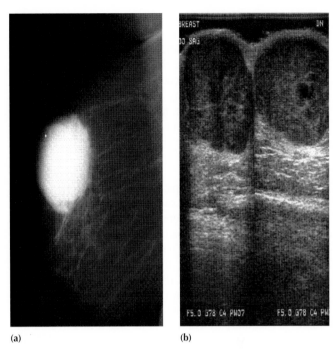

(a)   (b)

Figure 18.2 Radiographic appearance of a breast carcinosarcoma. (a) Right mediolateral oblique mammogram shows an oval high-density noncalcified mass with indistinct margins. (b) Right transverse ultrasound shows an oval heterogeneously hypoechoic solid mass with posterior acoustic enhancement.

necrotic or cystic components. On three-dimensional fast low-angle shot dynamic enhancement subtraction images, there is early enhancement and a delayed washout in a peripheral rim and nonenhancing internal components.[90,91] Despite these characteristic imaging features of carcinosarcoma and other metaplastic breast carcinomas on mammography, sonography, and MR imaging, there is overlap with other malignant and benign tumors. Therefore, biopsy is necessary. As with breast adenocarcinoma, the additional role of sonography is in the evaluation of regional lymph node status.

Treatment of breast carcinosarcomas

Carcinosarcomas seem to behave biologically differently from conventional adenocarcinoma of the breast, with sarcomatoid characteristics dominating the clinical course. These biological distinctions led one group to suggest that multimodality treatment including mastectomy and sarcoma-oriented adjuvant chemotherapy and radiotherapy should be considered in the treatment of this disease.[67] Mastectomy with adjuvant chemotherapy or radiotherapy or both was found to be superior to mastectomy alone and to wide local excision with or without adjuvant therapy, particularly for patients with stage II carcinosarcoma. Certain investigators also found complete surgical resection of recurrent disease to result in better outcomes than any other modality.[67,82] Conventional systemic chemotherapy appears to be less effective in these and other metaplastic breast cancers.[44,68] As a result of this and the inherent aggressiveness of the disease, the median survival of patients with metastatic disease is as low as 8 months.[71] As with breast carcinosarcomas, carcinosarcomas at other sites including the uterus are highly aggressive neoplasms that frequently recur after surgical treatment and adjuvant chemoradiotherapy, and also respond poorly to salvage chemotherapy and irradiation.[80] Some investigators therefore conclude that patients with metaplastic breast cancer including carcinosarcomas, particularly those with metastatic disease, are appropriate candidates for innovative therapeutic regimens.

Surgical management

Much of the literature groups breast carcinosarcomas with other subtypes of metaplastic carcinoma that may have different behaviors.[67,71,92,93] Therefore, defining surgical treatment for carcinosarcoma patients is often difficult. This is in contrast to surgical treatment for patients diagnosed with IDC, in whom multiple randomized trials have demonstrated that breast-conserving treatment (BCT) and mastectomy have equal efficacy.[94,95] Two studies in the literature specifically address surgical management of carcinosarcoma of the breast.[4,67] The study by Gutman et al. noted that overall and disease-free survival rates were not significantly different among patients treated by different surgical procedures (wide local excision 10 patients, simple mastectomy or modified radical mastectomy 31 patients, and radical mastectomy 9 patients). However, when mastectomy followed by adjuvant therapy (radiation therapy and/or chemotherapy) was compared with mastectomy alone and with wide local excision with or without adjuvant therapy, the local recurrence rate was much lower in patients undergoing surgery followed by adjuvant therapy (45 versus 89% ($p = 0.04$) and 78% ($p = 0.08$), respectively). Therefore, the authors recommended a multimodality approach that included mastectomy and sarcoma-oriented adjuvant chemotherapy and radiotherapy.

In the study by Wargotz and Norris, the majority of patients underwent mastectomy (65/70 patients), and only a minority had a partial mastectomy (wide local excision three patients, excisional biopsy two patients).[4] Only one patient underwent a partial mastectomy followed by adjuvant radiation therapy. Four of the five patients treated with partial mastectomy had a recurrence locally and were treated with subsequent mastectomy. One of the 65 patients who underwent some form of mastectomy experienced a local recurrence. Unfortunately, neither the tumor margin status nor the radiation therapy history of the specific patients who developed a local recurrence was clarified in the publication. In this study, those patients who developed a recurrence with distant metastases had an extremely poor prognosis compared with those patients experiencing only a local recurrence. Since the majority of patients underwent mastectomy, no conclusions could be drawn about the role of BCT. These authors also concluded by comparison with other subtypes of metaplastic carcinoma that carcinosarcoma seemed to be most aggressive.

Because these two studies are now relatively old and surgical treatments for breast cancer have improved considerably over the past 15 years, it is virtually impossible to interpret the data published by Gutman et al. and Wargotz and Norris in the current era so as to make surgical treatment recommendations.

In addition, the tumor margin status of those patients who underwent BCT (wide local excision, segmental mastectomy, partial mastectomy, or excisional biopsy, with or without radiation therapy) versus mastectomy was not assessed adequately. Both the tumor margin status and adjuvant treatment in patients undergoing BCT are extremely important to minimize local recurrence. Finally, the role of radiation therapy was not explored adequately in either study, specifically with regard to its use following wide local excision or segmental mastectomy. Presently, approximately 50–70% of patients diagnosed with primary breast cancer undergo BCT and it has been suggested that wide local excision may also be appropriate for patients with primary breast sarcoma.[96–98] Thus, on the basis of existing literature and considering current treatment strategies, it seems reasonable to suggest local excision of carcinosarcoma with "wide" margins (in the form of mastectomy, wide local excision, or partial mastectomy) followed by adjuvant chemoradiation. To actually determine an acceptable standard of care for patients with this rare tumor type, a multicenter prospective database needs to be established under the guidance of a multidisciplinary group of oncologists.

The role of surgery to the regional nodes is more apparent. Since the axillary lymph nodes will be involved in up to 20–25% of breast carcinosarcoma patients at presentation (see Table 18.1), and such involvement may be associated with a poorer prognosis, it is reasonable to suggest some form of axillary evaluation at the time of the primary breast surgery.[67] An exception to this applies to patients with pure or almost pure sarcomatous morphology (those with tumors having less than or equal to 5% carcinomatous component), in whom axillary lymph node involvement is exceedingly low and similar to patients with primary breast sarcoma.[78] There are no current data on the role of sentinel lymph node biopsy in the evaluation of regional lymph nodes in patients with breast carcinosarcoma.

Chemotherapy and radiotherapy

Conventional systemic chemotherapy appears to be less effective in carcinosarcomas and other metaplastic breast cancers.[44,68] In support of this, a retrospective analysis of patients treated with biphasic metaplastic sarcomatoid breast cancer ($n = 100$) at the University of Texas MD Anderson Cancer Center found the pathological complete response rate to neoadjuvant chemotherapy to be 10% and a clinical partial and complete response rate of 26% among the 21 patients treated with primary systemic chemotherapy, of which 15 had conventional anthracycline-containing breast cancer regimens, five anthracycline/taxane-based regimens, and one a "sarcoma-type" chemotherapy regimen – doxorubicin and ifosfamide (aromatase inhibitors – AI).[44] This is considerably lower than the response rates of breast adenocarcinoma to primary systemic chemotherapy, particularly when one considers that the majority of such metaplastic breast cancers are hormone receptor negative and of high nuclear grade. In the study by Rayson et al., of 10 chemotherapy regimens used in seven metaplastic breast cancer patients with metastatic disease, there was one partial response of 4 months' duration (to doxorubicin) and cases cases of stable disease (with doxorubicin and cyclophosphamide/5-fluorouracil/actinomycin-D).[68] Four patients with metastatic disease were treated with tamoxifen and two had stable disease (12 and 18 months), although there was no information provided on the hormone receptor status of these tumors. The median survival after disease recurrence in this study was just 8 months. Wargotz and Norris stated in their study that "chemotherapy for recurrence offered no significant advantage" but did not provide more detailed data to support this.[4] In the study by Gutman *et al.*, chemotherapy (mainly doxorubicin based) and hormonal therapy for metastatic breast carcinosarcoma also had minimal activity.[67]

Because of the small patient numbers in the studies presented in Table 18.1 and the lack of randomized controlled data, it is currently unknown if adjuvant chemotherapy or radiotherapy benefits patients with breast carcinosarcoma or other sarcomatoid breast cancers. In the Gutman *et al.* study, 14 patients with stage II disease given adjuvant chemotherapy, radiotherapy, or both had longer disease-free and overall survivals than six patients with stage II disease who did not receive adjuvant therapy.[67] However, the survival benefit for 17 patients with stage III disease treated with adjuvant therapy failed to reach statistical significance, probably because of small numbers and low power. Overall, of 17 patients given adjuvant radiotherapy and 29 patients not irradiated, there were two and nine local recurrences, respectively ($p=0.13$). Similarly, of 19 patients treated with adjuvant chemotherapy and 27 patients not so treated, there were five and 11 distant recurrences, respectively (p not significant). These statistical analyses are confounded by low patient numbers and also by lack of control for initial risk (one would expect patients chosen for adjuvant therapy to be at higher risk of recurrence). Most patients treated with adjuvant therapy in this study had 5-fluorouracil, doxorubicin, and cyclophosphamide (FAC) and/or "standard portal and standard dose radiotherapy." This group concluded that sarcoma-type chemotherapy combined with radiation therapy should be considered in the adjuvant treatment of patients with breast carcinosarcomas.

There is very little in the literature concerning the use of the currently popular sarcoma regimen AI (doxorubicin, ifosfamide) in patients with breast carcinosarcoma. In an MD Anderson analysis of 100 biphasic metaplastic sarcomatoid breast cancer patients, three patients given adjuvant AI chemotherapy were alive and recurrence free at a median follow-up of 55 months, in comparison to one of eight patients

treated with adjuvant cyclophosphamide, methotrexate, and 5-fluorouracil (CMF), 50% of 50 patients given adjuvant anthracycline-based therapy (predominantly FAC) and 54% of 13 patients given adjuvant anthracycline/taxane-based therapy.[44] Although limited statistical power again precludes definitive interpretation of these data, it is reasonable to consider at least an anthracycline-based regimen in the adjuvant treatment of breast carcinosarcoma patients.

Given the high rate of PI3K/PTEN mutations and activation of the PI3K pathway in metaplastic tumors, it is feasible that drugs which target the PI3K pathway may demonstrate activity against carcinosarcomas of the breast. In support of this, a small case series of five patients with metastatic metaplastic carcinoma treated in a phase 1 trial of liposomal doxorubicin (Doxil), bevacizumab (Avastin) and temsirolimus (Torisel) demonstrated a clinical benefit rate of 60%, including one durable complete response, one partial response and one patient with stable disease for 6 months.[99]

Prognosis

In the SEER database, the majority of breast carcinosarcoma patients (54; 55%) presented with American Joint Committee for Cancer (AJCC) stage II disease. As in other studies, and with breast adenocarcinoma, patient outcome deteriorates as the stage of disease at presentation becomes more advanced (Table 18.2).[67,69] Some studies suggest that tumor size at diagnosis is the most important determinant of patient outcome, with a tumor size greater than 5 cm having the most deleterious effect on prognosis.[4,67] Axillary nodal status appears to have less impact on outcome in some studies, but this is probably confounded by the relatively low frequency of nodal metastases seen in most studies. One study found that patients with macrometastases had a worse outcome than patients with negative lymph nodes or micrometastases.[98] In patients with stage I–II disease, Lester *et al.* reported that patients with tumors having a predominantly ($\geq$95%) sarcomatous morphology had worse disease-free survival.[49]

Prognostic factors described by Wargotz and Norris to be associated with a better prognosis in breast carcinosarcoma patients were complete microscopic circumscription of the tumor and the presence of an inflammatory infiltrate.[4] In the study by Rayson *et al.*, age greater than 60 years and no history of prior estrogen use were associated with a better outcome in a univariate analysis of 27 patients with metaplastic

Table 18.2 Five-year and median (in months) overall (OS) and disease-specific survival (DSS) rates for 98 breast carcinosarcoma patients registered in the SEER database between 1988 and 2001 by stage at diagnosis.

Stage	Patient number*	Median OS	5-year OS	5-year OS: 95% CI	Median DSS	5-year DSS	5-year DSS: 95% CI
I	20	NR	0.73	0.43–0.89	NR	0.87	0.57–0.97
II	54	96	0.59	0.44–0.71	NR	0.72	0.56–0.83
III	7	25	0.44	0.07–0.78	NR	0.53	0.07–0.86
IV	6	3	0.00	–	3	0.00	–

CI, confidence interval; NR, not reached.
* Outcome data were missing in 11 patients.

Stage	Patient number*	Median OS	5-year OS	5-year OS: 95% CI	Median DSS	5-year DSS	5-year DSS: 95% CI
I	45	NR	0.81	0.56–0.93	NR	0.93	0.74–0.98
II	122	97	0.59	0.46–0.69	NR	0.67	0.54–0.77
III	27	NR	0.67	0.40–0.84	NR	0.71	0.43–0.87
IV	14	5	0.18	0.03–0.43	5	0.20	0.03–0.46

Table 18.3 Five-year and median (in months) overall (OS) and disease-specific survival (DSS) rates for 213 metaplastic sarcomatoid breast cancer patients registered in the SEER database between 1988 and 2001 by stage at diagnosis.

CI, confidence interval; NR, not reached.
* Outcome data were missing in five patients.

breast cancer.[68] Conversely, Lester *et al.* found that patients greater than 50 years of age had a worse outcome.[49]

Table 18.1 indicates the generally poor prognosis associated with carcinosarcoma of the breast in the various reported studies. When the characteristics of breast carcinosarcomas and metaplastic sarcomatoid carcinomas in the SEER database are compared, it is apparent that clinical features and outcomes are very similar for both tumor types (Table 18.3). In the Wargotz and Norris study, the 5-year overall survival was 49%, and 43% in the Gutman *et al.* study.[4,67] The median survival after recurrence is as low as 8–15 months, and the prognosis is particularly ominous in those with distant metastases.[67,68] However, there is evidence that patients with only locoregional recurrence of disease may be cured, particularly with complete surgical resection.[4,67,100] In one study, the median survival after solitary recurrence was 22 months in those who underwent surgical resection, compared to 10 months in other patients after recurrence. Wargotz and Norris found a worse prognosis associated with carcinosarcoma compared to spindle cell carcinoma of the breast, with cumulative 5-year survival rates of 64% for 100 patients with the latter tumor type ($p = 0.056$), although the difference was less marked when survival was broken down by stage (Table 18.4). It may be that the larger size of the tumor at diagnosis in their carcinosarcoma series (mean 6.3 versus 4.4 cm) partly accounts for this difference, although, as stated earlier, the term spindle cell carcinoma also implies a less aggressive tumor to many pathologists, and this was reflected in their series where many of the spindle cell carcinomas were of a lower grade compared to the carcinosarcomas.

It is not entirely clear whether patients with carcinosarcoma have a worse clinical outcome compared to other patients with triple receptor-negative breast cancer. Although sarcomatoid carcinoma and carcinosarcoma of the breast are sometimes reported to have a clinical outcome similar to triple receptor-negative breast carcinoma,[93] a recent study with pathology review to exclude low-grade spindle cell carcinomas found that patients with sarcomatoid carcinomas of the breast had a significantly worse outcome compared to matched triple receptor-negative control patients.[49]

Conclusion and recommendations

Carcinosarcomas of the breast have traditionally been defined as biphasic tumors with a clear light microscopic demarcation

Table 18.4 Carcinosarcoma and spindle cell carcinoma of the breast.

	Stage	Patient number	5-year overall survival (%)
Carcinosarcoma	I	2	100
Spindle cell carcinoma		19	84
Carcinosarcoma	II	32	63
Spindle cell carcinoma		42	55
Carcinosarcoma	III	31	35
Spindle cell carcinoma		33	55

Reproduced from Wargotz and Norris[4] with permission from Wiley-Liss, Inc.

between epithelial and mesenchymal components but more recent studies have grouped them together with a more heterogeneous-appearing group of breast adenocarcinomas with varying degrees of high-grade sarcomatoid metaplasia. Although this would likely offend the traditional pathology purists, it may more accurately reflect the biology of many of these lesions. Evidence now suggests that these are similar tumors developing through a peculiar phenotypic transformation of carcinoma cells into sarcoma. These tumors are high-grade aggressive neoplasms that express mesenchymal, epithelial, and myoepithelial markers, and are usually negative for hormone receptors and Her-2/neu.

In truth, the most reasonable conclusion to draw from available studies is that there are currently not enough data available to justify treating breast carcinosarcomas differently from other high-grade breast adenocarcinomas. It seems reasonable to suggest local excision of carcinosarcoma with "wide" margins (in the form of mastectomy, wide local excision, or partial mastectomy) followed by adjuvant chemoradiation. The study of Gutman *et al.* certainly suggests that adjuvant radiation therapy may have some activity in terms of local tumor control.[67] Similarly, the data presented above suggest that although responsiveness to cytotoxic chemotherapy may be limited, adjuvant anthracycline-based chemotherapy is likely to be associated with some improvement in patient outcomes. It is not known whether this chemotherapy should be based on a sarcoma-type regimen such as AI or whether it should incorporate a taxane as with conventional breast adenocarcinomas. Clearly, the stage of the tumor is a major driver of prognosis and should be taken into account when making a therapy decision. If indeed carcinosarcoma sensitivity to cytotoxic chemotherapy is limited, this probably reflects molecular changes, most likely aberrations in the PI3K and EMT pathways. Participation in clinical trials incorporating targeted agents against PI3K and Wnt signaling should be strongly considered for the treatment of patients with carcinosarcoma.

References

1. Gogas J, Kouskos E, Markopoulos C, et al. Carcinosarcoma of the breast: report of two cases. Eur J Gynaecol Oncol 2003; 24: 93–5.
2. Aritas Y, Bedirli A, Karahan OI, Okten T, Sakrak O, Ince O. Carcinosarcoma of the breast: clinicopathologic and radiologic findings in an unusual case. Breast J 2003; 9: 323–4.
3. Tavassoli FA, ed. Pathology of the Breast, 2nd ed. Hong Kong, China: Appleton and Lang, 1999.
4. Wargotz ES, Norris HJ. Metaplastic carcinomas of the breast. III. Carcinosarcoma. Cancer 1989; 64: 1490–9.
5. Han AC, Soler AP, Knudsen KA, Salazar H. Distinct cadherin profiles in special variant carcinomas and other tumors of the breast. Hum Pathol 1999; 30: 1035–9.
6. Harris M, Persaud V. Carcinosarcoma of the breast. J Pathol 1974; 112: 99–105.
7. Foschini MP, Dina RE, Eusebi V. Sarcomatoid neoplasms of the breast: proposed definitions for biphasic and monophasic sarcomatoid mammary carcinomas. Semin Diagn Pathol 1993; 10: 128–36.
8. Wada H, Enomoto T, Tsujimoto M, Nomura T, Murata Y, Shroyer KR. Carcinosarcoma of the breast: molecular-biological study for analysis of histogenesis. Hum Pathol 1998; 29: 1324–8.
9. Nappi O, Wick MR. Sarcomatoid neoplasms of the respiratory tract. Semin Diagn Pathol 1993; 10: 137–47.
10. Colombi RP. Sarcomatoid carcinomas of the female genital tract (malignant mixed mullerian tumors). Semin Diagn Pathol 1993; 10: 169–75.
11. Iezzoni JC, Mills SE. Sarcomatoid carcinomas (carcinosarcomas) of the gastrointestinal tract: a review. Semin Diagn Pathol 1993; 10: 176–87.
12. Reuter VE. Sarcomatoid lesions of the urogenital tract. Semin Diagn Pathol 1993; 10: 188–201.
13. Siegal A, Freund U, Gal R. Carcinosarcoma of the stomach. Histopathology 1988; 13: 350–3.
14. Battifora H. Spindle cell carcinoma: ultrastructural evidence of squamous origin and collagen production by the tumor cells. Cancer 1976; 37: 2275–82.
15. Guarino M, Tricomi P, Giordano F, Cristofori E. Sarcomatoid carcinomas: pathological and histopathogenetic considerations. Pathology 1996; 28: 298–305.
16. George E, Manivel JC, Dehner LP, Wick MR. Malignant mixed mullerian tumors: an immunohistochemical study of 47 cases, with histogenetic considerations and clinical correlation. Hum Pathol 1991; 22: 215–23.
17. Fromowitz FB, Bard RH, Koss LG. The epithelial origin of a malignant mesodermal mixed tumor of the bladder: report of a case with long-term survival. J Urol 1984; 132: 978–81.
18. Guarino M. Epithelial-to-mesenchymal change of differentiation. From embryogenetic mechanism to pathological patterns. Histol Histopathol 1995; 10: 171–84.
19. Sonoda Y, Saigo PE, Federici MG, Boyd J. Carcinosarcoma of the ovary in a patient with a germline BRCA2 mutation: evidence for monoclonal origin. Gynecol Oncol 2000; 76: 226–9.
20. Teixeira MR, Qvist H, Bohler PJ, Pandis N, Heim S. Cytogenetic analysis shows that carcinosarcomas of the breast are of monoclonal origin. Genes Chromosomes Cancer 1998; 22: 145–51.
21. Dandachi N, Hauser-Kronberger C, More E, et al. Co-expression of tenascin-C and vimentin in human breast cancer cells indicates phenotypic transdifferentiation during tumour progression: correlation with histopathological parameters, hormone receptors, and oncoproteins. J Pathol 2001; 193: 181–9.
22. Wargotz ES, Deos PH, Norris HJ. Metaplastic carcinomas of the breast. II. Spindle cell carcinoma. Hum Pathol 1989; 20: 732–40.
23. Sapino A, Papotti M, Sanfilippo B, Gugliotta P, Bussolati G. Tumor types derived from epithelial and myoepithelial cell lines of R3230AC rat mammary carcinoma. Cancer Res 1992; 52: 1553–60.
24. Wargotz ES, Norris HJ. Metaplastic carcinomas of the breast. I. Matrix-producing carcinoma. Hum Pathol 1989; 20: 628–35.
25. Ferrara G. Sarcomatoid carcinoma of the breast: pathology of four cases. Breast Dis 1995; 8: 283–94.
26. Balercia G, Bhan AK, Dickersin GR. Sarcomatoid carcinoma: an ultrastructural study with light microscopic and immunohistochemical correlation of 10 cases from various anatomic sites. Ultrastruct Pathol 1995; 19: 249–63.
27. Yang GC, Yee HT, Waisman J. Metaplastic carcinoma of the breast with rhabdomyosarcomatous element: aspiration cytology with histological, immunohistochemical, and ultrastructural correlations. Diagn Cytopathol 2003; 28: 153–8.
28. Wick MR, Swanson PE. Carcinosarcomas: current perspectives and an historical review of nosological concepts. Semin Diagn Pathol 1993; 10: 118–27.
29. Tomasino RM, Verace V. [Rare tumors of the female breast (carcinosarcoma) and sarcomatous transformations of intracanalicular fibroadenoma]. Arch De Vecchi Anat Patol 1967; 49: 401–18.
30. Donegan WL. Sarcomas of the breast. Major Probl Clin Surg 1967; 5: 245–72.
31. Kruger J. [Carcinosarcoma of the breast]. Zentralbl Chir 1955; 80: 1238–41.
32. EIa S, Vadova AV, MIa PN, Ia C. [Carcinosarcoma of the breast developing in monkeys after hyperestrinization and the use of radioactive silver (Ag-110)]. Vopr Onkol 1960; 6(5): 35–42.
33. Kloos I, Delaloge S, Pautier P, et al. Tamoxifen-related uterine carcinosarcomas occur under/after prolonged treatment: report of five cases and review of the literature. Int J Gynecol Cancer 2002; 12: 496–500.
34. Cheung YC, Lee KF, Ng SH, Chan SC, Wong AM. Sonographic features with histologic correlation in two cases of palpable breast cancer after breast augmentation by liquid silicone injection. J Clin Ultrasound 2002; 30: 548–51.
35. Zhuang Z, Lininger RA, Man YG, Albuquerque A, Merino MJ, Tavassoli FA. Identical clonality of both components of mammary carcinosarcoma with differential loss of heterozygosity. Mod Pathol 1997; 10: 354–62.
36. Geyer FC, Weigelt B, Natrajan R, et al. Molecular analysis reveals a genetic basis for the phenotypic diversity of metaplastic breast carcinomas. J Pathol 2010; 220: 562–73.
37. Perou CM, Sorlie T, Eisen MB, et al. Molecular portraits of human breast tumours. Nature 2000; 406: 747–52.
38. Herschkowitz JI, Simin K, Weigman VJ, et al. Identification of conserved gene expression features between murine mammary carcinoma models and human breast tumors. Genome Biol 2007; 8: R76.
39. Chang CC, Sun W, Cruz A, Saitoh M, Tai MH, Trosko JE. A human breast epithelial cell type with stem cell characteristics as target cells for carcinogenesis. Radiat Res 2001; 155: 201–7.
40. Nielsen TO, Hsu FD, Jensen K, et al. Immunohistochemical and clinical characterization of the basal-like subtype of invasive breast carcinoma. Clin Cancer Res 2004; 10: 5367–74.
41. Prat A, Parker JS, Karginova O, et al. Phenotypic and molecular characterization of the claudin-low intrinsic subtype of breast cancer. Breast Cancer Res 2010; 12: R68.
42. Jung SY, Kim HY, Nam BH, et al. Worse prognosis of metaplastic breast cancer patients than other patients with triple-negative breast cancer. Breast Cancer Res Treat 2010; 120: 627–37.
43. Yamaguchi R, Horii R, Maeda I, et al. Clinicopathologic study of 53 metaplastic breast carcinomas: their elements and prognostic implications. Hum Pathol 2010; 41: 679–85.
44. Hennessy BT, Giordano S, Broglio K, et al. Biphasic metaplastic sarcomatoid carcinoma of the breast. Ann Oncol 2006; 17: 605–13.
45. Taube JH, Herschkowitz JI, Komurov K, et al. Core epithelial-to-mesenchymal transition interactome gene-expression signature is associated with claudin-low and metaplastic breast cancer subtypes. Proc Natl Acad Sci USA 2010; 107: 15449–54.

46. Lien HC, Hsiao YH, Lin YS, *et al*. Molecular signatures of metaplastic carcinoma of the breast by large-scale transcriptional profiling: identification of genes potentially related to epithelial-mesenchymal transition. Oncogene 2007; 26: 7859–71.

47. Hennessy BT, Gonzalez-Angulo AM, Stemke-Hale K, *et al*. Characterization of a naturally occurring breast cancer subset enriched in epithelial-to-mesenchymal transition and stem cell characteristics. Cancer Res 2009; 69: 4116–24.

48. Weigelt B, Kreike B, Reis-Filho JS. Metaplastic breast carcinomas are basal-like breast cancers: a genomic profiling analysis. Breast Cancer Res Treat 2009; 117: 273–80.

49. Lester TR, Hunt KK, Nayeemuddin KM, *et al*. Metaplastic sarcomatoid carcinoma of the breast appears more aggressive than other triple receptor-negative breast cancers. Breast Cancer Res Treat 2011 Jan;131(1): 41–8. Epub 2011 Feb 18.

50. Luini A, Aguilar M, Gatti G, *et al*. Metaplastic carcinoma of the breast, an unusual disease with worse prognosis: the experience of the European Institute of Oncology and review of the literature. Breast Cancer Res Treat 2007; 101: 349–53.

51. Reis-Filho JS, Schmitt FC. p63 expression in sarcomatoid/metaplastic carcinomas of the breast. Histopathology 2003; 42: 94–5.

52. Reis-Filho JS, Schmitt FC. Taking advantage of basic research: p63 is a reliable myoepithelial and stem cell marker. Adv Anat Pathol 2002; 9: 280–9.

53. Yang A, McKeon F. P63 and P73: P53 mimics, menaces and more. Nat Rev Mol Cell Biol 2000; 1: 199–207.

54. Barbareschi M, Pecciarini L, Cangi MG, *et al*. p63, a p53 homologue, is a selective nuclear marker of myoepithelial cells of the human breast. Am J Surg Pathol 2001; 25: 1054–60.

55. Leibl S, Gogg-Kammerer M, Sommersacher A, Denk H, Moinfar F. Metaplastic breast carcinomas: are they of myoepithelial differentiation?: immunohistochemical profile of the sarcomatoid subtype using novel myoepithelial markers. Am J Surg Pathol 2005; 29: 347–53.

56. Sproul D, Nestor C, Culley J, *et al*. Transcriptionally repressed genes become aberrantly methylated and distinguish tumors of different lineages in breast cancer. Proc Natl Acad Sci U S A 2011; 108: 4364–9.

57. Lightner VA, Marks JR, McCachren SS. Epithelial cells are an important source of tenascin in normal and malignant human breast tissue. Exp Cell Res 1994; 210: 177–84.

58. Ishihara A, Yoshida T, Tamaki H, Sakakura T. Tenascin expression in cancer cells and stroma of human breast cancer and its prognostic significance. Clin Cancer Res 1995; 1: 1035–41.

59. Rao K, Bryant E, O'Hara Larivee S, McDougall JK. Production of spindle cell carcinoma by transduction of H-Ras 61 L into immortalized human mammary epithelial cells. Cancer Lett 2003; 201: 79–88.

60. Peralta Soler A, Knudsen KA, Salazar H, Han AC, Keshgegian AA. P-cadherin expression in breast carcinoma indicates poor survival. Cancer 1999; 86: 1263–72.

61. Karreth F, Tuveson DA. Twist induces an epithelial-mesenchymal transition to facilitate tumor metastasis. Cancer Biol Ther 2004; 3: 1058–9.

62. Valsesia-Wittmann S, Magdeleine M, Dupasquier S, *et al*. Oncogenic cooperation between H-Twist and N-Myc overrides failsafe programs in cancer cells. Cancer Cell 2004; 6: 625–30.

63. Hayes MJ, Thomas D, Emmons A, Giordano TJ, Kleer CG. Genetic changes of Wnt pathway genes are common events in metaplastic carcinomas of the breast. Clin Cancer Res 2008; 14: 4038–44.

64. Lacroix-Triki M, Geyer FC, Lambros MB, *et al*. beta-catenin/Wnt signalling pathway in fibromatosis, metaplastic carcinomas and phyllodes tumours of the breast. Mod Pathol 2010; 23: 1438–48.

65. Creighton CJ, Li X, Landis M, *et al*. Residual breast cancers after conventional therapy display mesenchymal as well as tumor-initiating features. Proc Natl Acad Sci U S A 2009; 106: 13820–5.

66. Azzopardi JG, Ahmed A, Millis RR. Problems in breast pathology. Major Probl Pathol 1979; 11: i–xvi, 1–466.

67. Gutman H, Pollock RE, Janjan NA, Johnston DA. Biologic distinctions and therapeutic implications of sarcomatoid metaplasia of epithelial carcinoma of the breast. J Am Coll Surg 1995; 180: 193–9.

68. Rayson D, Adjei AA, Suman VJ, Wold LE, Ingle JN. Metaplastic breast cancer: prognosis and response to systemic therapy. Ann Oncol 1999; 10: 413–9.

69. Kaufman MW, Marti JR, Gallager HS, Hoehn JL. Carcinoma of the breast with pseudosarcomatous metaplasia. Cancer 1984; 53: 1908–17.

70. Oberman HA. Metaplastic carcinoma of the breast. A clinicopathologic study of 29 patients. Am J Surg Pathol 1987; 11: 918–29.

71. Kurian KM, Al-Nafussi A. Sarcomatoid/metaplastic carcinoma of the breast: a clinicopathological study of 12 cases. Histopathology 2002; 40: 58–64.

72. Gersell DJ, Katzenstein AL. Spindle cell carcinoma of the breast. A clinocopathologic and ultrastructural study. Hum Pathol 1981; 12: 550–61.

73. Stanley MW, Tani EM, Skoog L. Metaplastic carcinoma of the breast: fine-needle aspiration cytology of seven cases. Diagn Cytopathol 1989; 5: 22–8.

74. Gupta RK. Cytodiagnostic patterns of metaplastic breast carcinoma in aspiration samples: a study of 14 cases. Diagn Cytopathol 1999; 20: 10–2.

75. Nogueira M, Andre S, Mendonca E. Metaplastic carcinomas of the breast–fine needle aspiration (FNA) cytology findings. Cytopathology 1998; 9: 291–300.

76. Al-Nafussi A. Spindle cell tumours of the breast: practical approach to diagnosis. Histopathology 1999; 35: 1–13.

77. Kuo SH, Chen CL, Huang CS, Cheng AL. Metaplastic carcinoma of the breast: analysis of eight Asian patients with special emphasis on two unusual cases presenting with inflammatory-type breast cancer. Anticancer Res 2000; 20: 2219–22.

78. Davis WG, Hennessy B, Babiera G, *et al*. Metaplastic sarcomatoid carcinoma of the breast with absent or minimal overt invasive carcinomatous component: a misnomer. Am J Surg Pathol 2005; 29: 1456–63.

79. Gilcrease MZ. Sarcomatoid breast tumors have sarcomatoid behavior. Am J Surg Pathol 2007; 31: 326–7; author reply 7.

80. Raspollini MR, Susini T, Amunni G, *et al*. COX-2, c-KIT and HER-2/neu expression in uterine carcinosarcomas: prognostic factors or potential markers for targeted therapies? Gynecol Oncol 2005; 96: 159–67.

81. Yang WT, Hennessy B, Broglio K, *et al*. Imaging differences in metaplastic and invasive ductal carcinomas of the breast. AJR Am J Roentgenol 2007; 189: 1288–93.

82. Patterson SK, Tworek JA, Roubidoux MA, Helvie MA, Oberman HA. Metaplastic carcinoma of the breast: mammographic appearance with pathologic correlation. AJR Am J Roentgenol 1997; 169: 709–12.

83. Samuels TH, Miller NA, Manchul LA, DeFreitas G, Panzarella T. Squamous cell carcinoma of the breast. Can Assoc Radiol J 1996; 47: 177–82.

84. Brenner RJ, Turner RR, Schiller V, Arndt RD, Giuliano A. Metaplastic carcinoma of the breast: report of three cases. Cancer 1998; 82: 1082–7.

85. Park JM, Han BK, Moon WK, Choe YH, Ahn SH, Gong G. Metaplastic carcinoma of the breast: mammographic and sonographic findings. J Clin Ultrasound 2000; 28: 179–86.

86. Gunhan-Bilgen I, Memis A, Ustun EE, Zekioglu O, Ozdemir N. Metaplastic carcinoma of the breast: clinical, mammographic, and sonographic findings with histopathologic correlation. AJR Am J Roentgenol 2002; 178: 1421–5.

87. Sickles EA. Nonpalpable, circumscribed, noncalcified solid breast masses: likelihood of malignancy based on lesion size and age of patient. Radiology 1994; 192: 439–42.

88. Kaas R, Kroger R, Hendriks JH, *et al*. The significance of circumscribed malignant mammographic masses in the surveillance of BRCA 1/2 gene mutation carriers. Eur Radiol 2004; 14: 1647–53.

89. Liberman L, Bonaccio E, Hamele-Bena D, Abramson AF, Cohen MA, Dershaw DD. Benign and malignant phyllodes tumors: mammographic and sonographic findings. Radiology 1996; 198: 121–4.

90. Velasco M, Santamaria G, Ganau S, *et al*. MRI of metaplastic carcinoma of the breast. AJR Am J Roentgenol 2005; 184: 1274–8.

91. Chang YW, Lee MH, Kwon KH, *et al*. Magnetic resonance imaging of metaplastic carcinoma of the breast: sonographic and pathologic correlation. Acta Radiol 2004; 45: 18–22.

92. Chao TC, Wang CS, Chen SC, Chen MF. Metaplastic carcinomas of the breast. J Surg Oncol 1999; 71: 220–5.

93. Christensen L, Schiodt T, Blichert-Toft M. Sarcomatoid tumours of the breast in Denmark from 1977 to 1987. A clinicopathological and immuno-histochemical study of 100 cases. Eur J Cancer 1993; 29A: 1824–31.

94. Veronesi U, Cascinelli N, Mariani L, *et al*. Twenty-year follow-up of a randomized study comparing breast-conserving surgery with radical mas-tectomy for early breast cancer. N Engl J Med 2002; 347: 1227–32.

95. Jacobson JA, Danforth DN, Cowan KH, *et al*. Ten-year results of a com-parison of conservation with mastectomy in the treatment of stage I and II breast cancer. N Engl J Med 1995; 332: 907–11.

96. Morrow M, White J, Moughan J, *et al*. Factors predicting the use of breast-conserving therapy in stage I and II breast carcinoma. J Clin Oncol 2001; 19: 2254–62.

97. Staradub VL, Rademaker AW, Morrow M. Factors influencing outcomes for breast conservation therapy of mammographically detected malig-nancies. J Am Coll Surg 2003; 196: 518–24.

98. Zelek L, Llombart-Cussac A, Terrier P, *et al*. Prognostic factors in primary breast sarcomas: a series of patients with long-term follow-up. J Clin Oncol 2003; 21: 2583–8.

99. Moulder S, Moroney J, Helgason T, *et al*. Responses to liposomal Doxorubicin, bevacizumab, and temsirolimus in metaplastic carcinoma of the breast: biologic rationale and implications for stem-cell research in breast cancer. J Clin Oncol 2011; 29: e572–5.

100. Okushiba S, Minagawa H, Shimizu M, *et al*. A case of spindle cell carcinoma of the breast–long survival achieved by multiple surgical treatment. Breast Cancer 2001; 8: 238–42.

19 Tubular Carcinoma

Melinda E. Sanders,[1] Ingrid A. Mayer,[2] and A. Bapsi Chakravarthy[3]

[1] Department of Pathology, [2] Department of Medicine, [3] Department of Radiation Oncology, Vanderbilt University School of Medicine, Nashville, TN, USA

Introduction

Tubular carcinoma of the breast is a rare, well-differentiated invasive adenocarcinoma. It can be pure or mixed with other histological types of carcinoma. The term tubular carcinoma is used only to indicate the pure forms, where the tubular component represents more than 90% of the tumor. This particular subtype of invasive ductal carcinoma occurs with a prevalence of 1–10% of all mammary adenocarcinomas, with a reported mortality of 2%.[1]

Historical background

The morphological features of tubular carcinoma were first described over a century ago by Cornil and Ranvier but received little attention until the last 20 years because they are rarely symptomatic. Only recently with the advent of mammographic screening programs have these usually small, indolent, nonpalpable tumors regularly reached clinical attention.[2] The orderly histological pattern composed of small, angulated tubules resulted in the original diagnosis of "well-differentiated carcinoma." The term tubular carcinoma is now preferred as it describes the lesional architecture of this "special type" of breast cancer. There has been considerable debate regarding the precise histological criteria and proportion of tubular structures required to establish the diagnosis of a "pure" tubular carcinoma.[3] Several studies have now demonstrated that when >90% purity of pattern is observed an excellent prognosis can be expected, even in the presence of a positive lymph node.[4–6] Patients with pure tubular carcinoma can expect survival rates similar to the general population.[5]

Biology and epidemiology

Pure tubular carcinoma accounts for 1–2% of invasive cancers in premammographic era series.[3,7] The frequency of cases now reported by mammographic screening series is 9–19%,[2,8–13] with higher percentages noted in series of T1 lesions. It should also be noted that the definition of tubular carcinoma in some series was not as stringent as the 90% rule which we and others now standardly require. Tubular carcinomas have a reported mortality of 2%.[1]

The biological origin of tubular carcinoma is unknown; however, the resemblance of epithelial elements in some radial scars to cancer and the presence of cancer in some radial scars[14–16] has prompted several authors to propose that radial scars represent an early stage in the evolution of invasive mammary carcinoma,[17,18] which is usually of tubular histology. However, none of these authors has been able to provide definitive evidence to indicate that radial scars are in and of themselves premalignant. In addition, a large cohort of women who underwent benign breast biopsies and were diagnosed with radial scar were shown to have a modest risk elevation in subsequent breast cancer development. This risk, however, could be attributed to the category of coexistent proliferative disease.[19]

Molecular and genetic studies

Overall tubular carcinomas have a low frequency of genetic alterations. They are typically characterized by a high frequency of 16q loss and 1q gain, and lower frequency of 17p loss. They share these changes with most low-grade, luminal-type breast carcinomas.[20,21] Molecular studies have also reported these same chromosomal alterations to occur in atypical ductal hyperplasia, low-grade ductal carcinoma in situ (DCIS), atypical lobular hyperplasia, lobular carcinoma in situ and columnar cell lesions with atypia suggesting that they are related[22–24]; however, DCIS is the only established nonobligate precursor to invasive carcinoma.[25]

Pathology

Grossly, no specific features, except small size, distinguish tubular cancer from other "no special type," often referred to as "ductal" or mixed tumor types. Tubular carcinomas usually

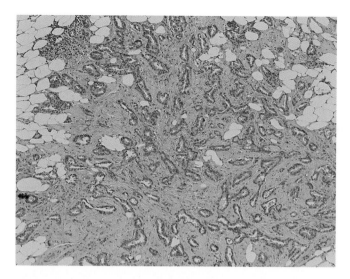

Figure 19.1 Low-power photomicrograph of tubular carcinoma showing the characteristic angulated tubules surrounded by desmoplastic and sclerotic stroma and invading adipose tissue at the periphery.

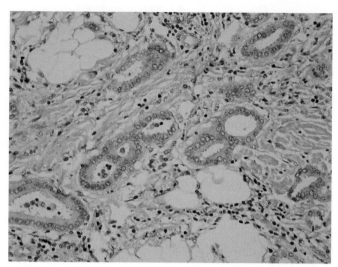

Figure 19.3 Higher power photomicrograph showing the small, round tumor cells lining the carcinomatous tubules to have minimal pleomorphism and essentially absent mitotic activity.

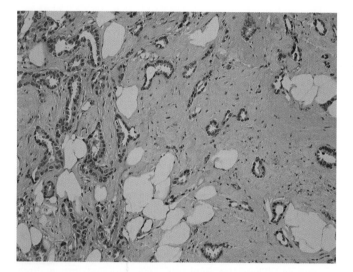

Figure 19.2 The characteristic round or bent teardrop shaped tubules of tubular carcinoma are lined by a single layer of epithelial cells. The intervening stroma shows areas of elastosis and sclerosis.

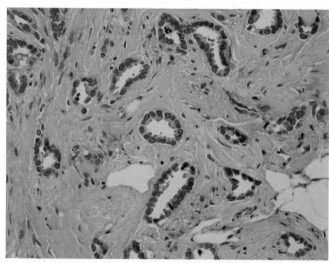

Figure 19.4 Higher power photomicrograph showing apical snouts which are present at the luminal aspect of the tumor cells in at least 30% of cases.

measure between 2.0 mm and 2.0 cm with the majority measuring less than 1.0 cm.[7,26,27] Occasional cases can reach 3.0 cm in size.

Histologically, tubular cancer is characterized by distinct tubular structures lined by a single layer of epithelial cells. The tubules may be round, oval, or "bent teardrop" shaped (Figs 19.1, 19.2). The epithelial cells lining the tubules are small and round with minimal pleomorphism and rare if any mitotic figures (Fig. 19.3). Many cases have a minority of the tumor with more than a single cell layer forming central lumina like those seen in invasive cribriform carcinoma. Apical snouts are seen in at least one-third of cases[28] but are not specific (Fig. 19.4). Fine calcifications may be present in the lumina in occasional cases.[26,29]

Historically, two morphological subtypes have been described which do not have any clinical significance. The "pure type" has a dominantly stellate configuration with radiating fibrous arms containing neoplastic tubules located peripherally, and stromal elastosis and hyalinized fibrosis present centrally. A consequence of this architecture is that the actual tumor volume of these lesions may be significantly less than that indicated by the overall tumor measurements mammographically and grossly. The "sclerosing type," which is more diffuse and ill defined, features a haphazard infiltration of tubules within a desmoplastic stroma without central hyalinization.[30,31] In approximately 90% of cases, varying combinations of low-grade cribriform or micropapillary DCIS, atypical ductal hyperplasia, and columnar cell lesions with and without atypia are found in association with tubular carcinoma.[22,24,32] They may be intimately associated with the carcinoma or present in the vicinity in the background breast. Tubular carcinoma is

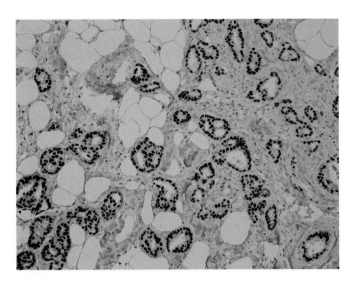

Figure 19.5 Immunohistochemical staining for estrogen receptor shows strong positivity in 100% of tubular carcinoma nuclei.

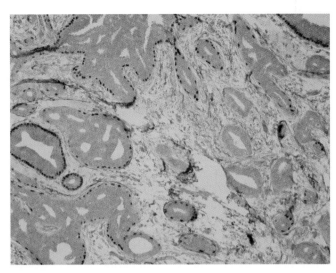

Figure 19.7 p63 Immunohistochemical stain for basal cells shows positive nuclear staining of myoepithelial cells in normal ducts and ductules as well as ducts with atypical ductal hyperplasia whereas the neoplastic tubules of tubular carcinoma show absence of staining.

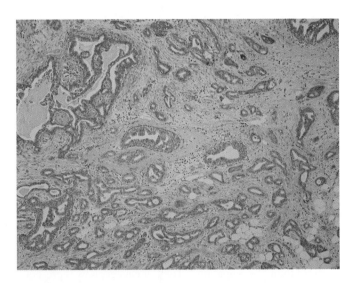

Figure 19.6 Low-power photomicrograph showing the neoplastic tubules of tubular carcinoma infiltrating among normal structures including usual type hyperplasia (*center*) and a papilloma (*upper left*) within a radial scar. Note the presence of a well-delineated myoepithelial layer surrounding the normal structures.

associated with atypical lobular hyperplasia or lobular carcinoma *in situ* in approximately 15% of cases.[22,27] Tubular carcinoma is essentially always estrogen (Fig. 19.5) and progesterone receptor positive, has a low growth phase fraction as demonstrated by Ki-67 staining and rare if any mitoses, and is Her 2/neu and EGFR negative.[5,33]

In some cases the tumor may be seen in association with a radial scar or complex sclerosing lesion. In such cases involvement is usually focal and recognized by the neoplastic tubules surrounding normal structures also associated with the radial scar/complex sclerosing lesion as well as extension of tubules into the adjacent adipose tissue (Fig. 19.6). Distinction of tubular carcinoma from adenosis or entrapped benign tubules in a sclerosing lesion may be facilitated by immunohistochemical

staining for myoepithelial cells. In our experience p63 (Fig. 19.7) and smooth muscle actin stains are the most useful. However, caution should be used during their interpretation as these stains are negative in tubular carcinoma but may also show loss of staining in benign glands entrapped in sclerosis.

Clinical aspects: presentation, diagnostic considerations, and techniques

Tubular carcinomas are increasingly encountered in recent years as a result of the widespread use of and advances in mammographic screening. Retrospective reviews of histologically proven tubular carcinomas suggest that this tumor usually presents as a small, nonpalpable lesion, with nonspecific imaging patterns.[34–36] Tubular carcinomas often are detected by their spiculated appearance and occasionally by the presence of microcalcifications but may have subtle mammographic findings.[26,29,34] They are usually incidental findings on screening mammography[35] and not associated with a palpable mass on physical exam. In comparison to "no special type" carcinomas, "pure" tubular carcinomas are more likely to occur in postmenopausal patients and be smaller in size. Axillary node metastases occur less frequently, in 0–13% of cases, and when observed usually involve a single node.[3,29,37,38] Multicentricity of tubular carcinoma in the ipsilateral breast has been reported[39] as well as an association with contralateral cancers occurring before and after the detection of the tubular cancer.[3,35,39] However, these contralateral cancers are not restricted to tubular carcinomas.[3,35] When several separate tubular carcinomas occur in a single breast, they are often in the same segment and are linked by a common, usually low-grade DCIS.

Because tubular areas are found focally in many breast cancers, strict criteria for the diagnosis of tubular carcinoma must be used so that the excellent prognosis applies. We reserve the diagnosis of "pure" tubular carcinoma for those tumors where the classic tubules represent 90% or greater of the tumor, and the remainder of the tumor shows the same well-differentiated morphology.[40] This is in agreement with the current WHO classification.[41] Tumors containing between 70% and 89% tubules we regard as tubular variants and tumors containing less than 70% of the classic tubules we designate as "no special type tumors" with tubular features. Note that this means that tubular carcinoma may be regarded as a special, more orderly, subset of tumors which would be assigned a grade of 1 for the tubular component of the Nottingham grade. Justification for these divisions comes from multiple studies indicating that tubular histology is of prognostic value, and that the greater the purity of the pattern, the more favorable the prognosis.

A series of 54 women reported by Cooper et al.[3] with tumors composed purely of the characteristic low-grade, angulated tubules were still alive after 15 years follow-up, regardless of tumor size. In contrast, almost half of the patients whose carcinomas were composed of a mixture of tubular and other areas of "no special type" carcinoma died within the 15-year follow-up period. This study showed the utility of recognizing tubular carcinoma by comparing outcome with that of other cases with similar but not precisely the same histological characteristics. This study was one of the first to demonstrate the importance of subset analysis in the prognostication of breast cancer.

A later study by Liebman et al. found no local or distant recurrences in 12 "pure" tubular carcinomas (defined as >90% tubules) after treatment by either lumpectomy or mastectomy to negative margins.[29] A study by Kader et al. of women in the Breast Cancer Outcomes Database (BCOD) maintained by the British Columbia Cancer Agency, Vancouver, British Columbia, compared outcomes in 171 "pure" tubular carcinomas, as defined using the current WHO criteria, to 386 low-grade ductal carcinomas. The investigators observed a lower rate of local recurrence in tubular carcinomas (0.8% versus 4.5%) and a trend toward a lower rate of systemic relapse (4.3% versus 9.7%) but no difference in disease-specific survival (95.7% versus 94.7%) over 6 years of follow-up.[42] The improved outcome was seen in the tubular group despite the fact that the low-grade ductal group was treated more aggressively. The women in the tubular group were almost twice as likely to have been treated by breast-conserving therapy alone. Also 38.6% of the low-grade ductal group received chemotherapy or chemotherapy plus tamoxifen versus 21.1% of the tubular group.

Several additional authors found the presence of a 75% tubular component to identify a more favorable prognosis than "no special type" carcinomas.[7,26,43] Although not as good a prognosis as those categorized as "pure,"[41] it justifies the recognition of the tubular variant category. Using these criteria, Elson found no patients with local or distant recurrence including four patients with positive lymph nodes at presentation.[26] In contrast, Cabral et al.[4] found no difference in presentation or outcome between pure tubular carcinomas and mixed tumors, using a definition of >95% tubularity for pure tubular carcinomas and 75–95% tubularity for mixed tumors. In this study of 22 pure and 22 mixed tumors, there were two local recurrences in the pure tubular group only, one managed by reexcision and another accompanied by systemic disease. These results are difficult to compare to other studies because their mixed group

contained cases placed in the pure category by other authors,[40,44] including cases with >90% tubules and mixed tubular and cribriform carcinomas as can be seen from the photomicrographs included in the paper.[4] Inclusion of cases regarded as pure by the current definition in their mixed group likely explains the lack of a difference in the outcome.

A recently published retrospective analysis of histologically well-characterized primary operable invasive breast carcinomas (2608 women age 70 years or less who presented with tumors <5 cm in diameter between 1989 and 2000; stage I and II) from the Nottingham Primary Breast Carcinoma Series[35] found, when compared with grade 1 ductal carcinoma ($n=212$), tubular carcinomas ($n=102$) were statistically significantly associated with longer 10-year disease-free survival (92% versus 63%) and 10-year breast cancer-specific survival (100% versus 36%). None of the patients with tubular carcinomas developed distant metastases or died from the disease without an intervening recurrence of an invasive carcinoma of a different histological type. Their findings reaffirm the excellent biological behavior of tubular carcinoma and its more favorable prognosis, emphasizing the importance of high-quality pathological assessment of tumor characteristics.

An additional diagnostic consideration is the coexistence of mixed tubular and invasive cribriform carcinomas.[40,44] Essentially, any combination of these two elements conveys the same excellent prognosis as a pure tubular carcinoma. This is an important consideration as many such cases may be assigned to the "no special type" group by an inexperienced pathologist or clinician and this potentially useful prognostic information is lost.

Treatment

The importance of tubular carcinoma lies with therapeutic decisions for individual patients. With the increasing use of mammographic screening, the number of tubular cancers has increased significantly and their average size is about half that of those found by palpation.[45] Tubular cancers now represent a significant proportion of incidental breast cancers.[11] The excellent prognostic implications of tubular carcinoma apply when strict criteria are used to make the diagnosis. Careful documentation of these histological features is critical to treatment decisions and avoids overtreatment. In fact, patients with pure tubular carcinoma can expect survival rates similar to the general population.[5]

Locoregional treatment: surgery and radiation

In most cases complete excision of the lesion to negative margins should be sufficient therapy for localized lesions.[35,46,47] The risk of local recurrence is so low that adjuvant radiation is unnecessary. This is further supported by the fact that any later events in these patients are regularly of low grade, also estrogen receptor positive, and more easily detected in the unirradiated breast. Rare local recurrences can usually be easily managed by reexcision. When lymph nodes are involved at presentation (8–17% of most series[3,37,38]), they tend to be confined to one or two nodes and these patients still have an excellent prognosis. Importantly, the presence of positive lymph nodes does not appear to affect disease-free survival and therefore a full lymph node dissection is not helpful in providing prognostic information in most cases of tubular carcinoma[5,6] and may introduce unnecessary morbidity.

A recent retrospective analysis from the Mayo Clinic of 105 cases of pure tubular carcinoma (from 1987 to 2009) confirmed that the incidence of nodal metastasis is very low (less than 7%), and none of the patients developed locoregional recurrence or metastases.[48] Similar trends have been confirmed by larger retrospective reviews, such as the one by Javid et al., which documented among 111 pure tubular carcinoma cases that less than 10% of these patients had nodal metastases, and when present, the primary tumor was always greater than 1 cm.[49] Akin to other series, no patients developed distant metastasis, and only one patient in the whole series developed a locoregional recurrence. These data suggest that nodal staging can indeed be omitted in smaller pure tubular carcinomas.

As a result of poor case definition, several studies have suggested that radiation and even chemotherapy may be necessary for some patients with tubular carcinoma given a small propensity for distant metastasis.[6,50–53] However, most of these studies did not have central pathology review,[8,52] did not list the percentage of tubular differentiation used to diagnose tubular carcinoma,[46] and several acknowledge inclusion of intermediate-grade[52,54] and ER-negative tumors.[51,53,54] In addition, the included cases were diagnosed over a 30–40-year period in these studies, a time during which criteria for diagnosis of tubular carcinoma have evolved considerably.[6,50,52] Despite the bias of poor classification, Livi et al.[52] showed no difference in locoregional failure between patients who had received adjuvant radiation therapy and those who had not.

Systemic treatment: endocrine therapy and chemotherapy

A series of 444 tubular cancers reported from the University of Texas Health Science Center in San Antonio, Texas, demonstrated 5-year disease-free survival (DFS) and 5-year overall survival (OS) rates of 95% and 91% for node-negative patients and rates of 94% and 92% for node-positive patients, respectively.[5] In addition, a subset analysis of patients who received adjuvant endocrine (29%) or chemotherapy (10%) demonstrated no significant difference in DFS or OS rates regardless of nodal status. The only study of patients with tubular carcinoma treated with breast-conserving therapy (lumpectomy followed by radiation) with central pathological review reports two of 28 patients as having a local recurrence and no distant failures at 10 years despite the fact that 17% of patients presented with positive lymph nodes.[55]

The recent analysis by Rakha et al.[35] comparing biological behavior and outcomes of tubular carcinomas versus low-grade ductal or mixed tubular carcinomas reaffirms the excellent prognosis of tubular carcinoma, as reflected by a significantly lower number of recurrences in the pure tubular carcinomas and no cancer-related deaths, despite the infrequent use of systemic therapy in their patient series. This difference was unrelated to tumor stage or early presentation. Interestingly,

five (5%) patients developed contralateral DCIS or invasive breast cancers, suggesting that adjuvant hormonal therapy may be a consideration for some patients; however, until the characteristic of such patients are better defined, the overall excellent prognosis of tubular carcinoma does not warrant endocrine therapy use in all tubular carcinoma cases. Patients should be informed that the risk of adverse effects may be much greater than the risk of death from breast cancer and that their life expectancy is close to normal after complete surgical excision.

Prognosis

When a strict definition is used, tubular carcinoma has an excellent long-term prognosis which in some series is similar to age-matched women without breast cancer.[5,35] Recurrence after mastectomy or breast-conserving therapy is rare. Thurman et al.[55] found no difference in site of first failure among cases of tubular, mucinous or medullary carcinomas treated by breast conservation therapy and followed for >10 years; however, rates of recurrence were lowest among tubular carcinomas, with only two of 28 patients with a local recurrence which was easily managed by reexcision and no examples of distant recurrence despite the fact that 17% of cases were associated with 1–3 positive lymph nodes. Thus, disease-specific survival was 100% for tubular carcinomas. Rakha et al.[35] confirm the same outcome.

We can find no examples of death from breast cancer after treatment for a clearly documented "pure" tubular carcinoma less than 1.0 cm in diameter. We would argue that the three studies in the literature reporting deaths from tubular carcinoma do not strictly define their criteria or include cases which are not "pure" by current definition. Cabral et al.[4] describe a woman with a 7.0 mm tubular carcinoma (defined as >95% tubules but with no mention of tumor grade) treated by modified radical mastectomy and 16 negative axillary nodes who developed a local recurrence and systemic disease, dying 87 months after her initial diagnosis.

Winchester et al.[54] also report a single death from a 6.0 mm pure tubular carcinoma. Although this study did include central pathology review, their criteria for tubular carcinoma required >80% tubularity and cases with intermediate-grade nuclei were included. Cases were then subdivided into pure tubular carcinoma and mixed pattern lesions, although neither definition was further defined. Three of the four cases which recurred were in the mixed pattern category and three of the four cases were intermediate combined histological grade, although it cannot be determined from the data the grades of individual tumors including the "pure" tubular carcinoma which resulted in death following metastasis to bone. In support of our contention, Peters et al. found distant metastases to occur only when the percentage of "no special type" carcinoma constituted over 25% of the lesion.[56]

Recommendations

For pure tubular carcinomas, the excellent prognosis indicates that conservative but complete surgical excision is adequate therapy for the overwhelming majority of cases. Since the addition of radiation or chemotherapy does not improve disease-free survival or overall survival, they should not be advocated. Similarly, involvement of axillary lymph nodes is an uncommon finding and does not adversely affect outcome. A full lymph node dissection is not helpful in providing prognostic information in most cases of tubular carcinoma[5,6] and may introduce unnecessary morbidity.

Because pure tubular carcinomas are estrogen receptor positive, endocrine therapy with tamoxifen or aromatase inhibitors (for postmenopausal women) is usually considered, although it should be recognized that such therapy likely benefits most women by reducing the incidence of subsequent contralateral tumors rather than affecting their survival. Adjuvant endocrine treatment may also be appropriate in patients with evidence of nodal metastases at presentation, but chemotherapy cannot be justified in patients without distant metastases.

References

1. Page DL. Special types of invasive breast cancer, with clinical implications. Am J Surg Pathol 2003; 27: 832–5.
2. Patchefsky AS, Shaber GS, Schwartz GF, Feig SA, Nerlinger RE. The pathology of breast cancer detected by mass population screening. Cancer 1977; 40: 1659–70.
3. Cooper HS, Patchefsky AS, Krall RA. Tubular carcinoma of the breast. Cancer 1978; 42: 2334–42.
4. Cabral AH, Recine M, Paramo JC, McPhee MM, Poppiti R, Mesko TW. Tubular carcinoma of the breast: an institutional experience and review of the literature. Breast J 2003; 9: 298–301.
5. Diab SG, Clark GM, Osborne CK, Libby A, Allred DC, Elledge RM. Tumor characteristics and clinical outcome of tubular and mucinous breast carcinomas. J Clin Oncol 1999; 17: 1442–8.
6. Kitchen PR, Smith TH, Henderson MA, et al. Tubular carcinoma of the breast: prognosis and response to adjuvant systemic therapy. ANZ J Surg 2001; 71: 27–31.
7. McDivitt RW, Boyce W, Gersell D. Tubular carcinoma of the breast. Clinical and pathological observations concerning 135 cases. Am J Surg Pathol 1982; 6: 401–11.
8. Anderson TJ, Alexander FE, Forrest PM. The natural history of breast carcinoma: what have we learned from screening? Cancer 2000; 88: 1758–9.
9. Anderson TJ, Lamb J, Alexander F, et al. Comparative pathology of prevalent and incident cancers detected by breast screening. Edinburgh Breast Screening Project. Lancet 1986; 1: 519–23.
10. Anderson TJ, Lamb J, Donnan P, et al. Comparative pathology of breast cancer in a randomised trial of screening. Br J Cancer 1991; 64: 108–13.
11. Anderson WF, Chu KC, Devesa SS. Distinct incidence patterns among in situ and invasive breast carcinomas,with possible etiologic implications. Breast Cancer Res Treat 2004; 88: 149–59.
12. Feig SA, Shaber GS, Patchefsky A, et al. Analysis of clinically occult and mammographically occult breast tumors. Am J Roentgenol 1977; 128: 403–8.
13. Rajakariar R, Walker RA. Pathological and biological features of mammographically detected invasive breast carcinomas. Br J Cancer 1995; 71: 150–4.
14. Douglas-Jones AG, Pace DP. Pathology of R4 spiculated lesions in the breast screening programme. Histopathology 1997; 30: 214–20.
15. Frouge C, Tristant H, Guinebretiere JM, et al. Mammographic lesions suggestive of radial scars: microscopic findings in 40 cases. Radiology 1995; 195: 623–5.
16. Sloane JP, Mayers MM. Carcinoma and atypical hyperplasia in radial scars and complex sclerosing lesions: importance of lesion size and patient age. Histopathology 1993; 23: 225–31.
17. Fisher ER, Palekar AS, Kotwal N, Lipana N. A nonencapsulated sclerosing lesion of the breast. Am J Clin Pathol 1979; 71: 240–6.
18. Linell F, Ljungberg O, Andersson I. Breast carcinoma. Aspects of early stages, progression and related problems. Acta Pathol Microbiol Scand Suppl 1980: 1–233.
19. Sanders M, Dupont W, Schuyler P, Simpson J, Page D. Interdependence of radial scar and proliferative disease with respect to invasive breast cancer risk in benign breast biopsies. Lab Invest 2002 82: 50A.
20. Roylance R, Gorman P, Harris W, et al. Comparative genomic hybridization of breast tumors stratified by histological grade reveals new insights into the biological progression of breast cancer. Cancer Res 1999; 59: 1433–6.
21. Waldman FM, Hwang ES, Etzell J, et al. Genomic alterations in tubular breast carcinomas. Hum Pathol 2001; 32: 222–6.
22. Abdel-Fatah TM, Powe DG, Hodi Z, Reis-Filho JS, Lee AH, Ellis IO. Morphologic and molecular evolutionary pathways of low nuclear grade invasive breast cancers and their putative precursor lesions: further evidence to support the concept of low nuclear grade breast neoplasia family. Am J Surg Pathol 2008; 32: 513–23.
23. Aulmann S, Elsawaf Z, Penzel R, Schirmacher P, Sinn HP. Invasive tubular carcinoma of the breast frequently is clonally related to flat epithelial atypia and low-grade ductal carcinoma in situ. Am J Surg Pathol 2009; 33: 1646–53.
24. Ellis IO. Intraductal proliferative lesions of the breast: morphology, associated risk and molecular biology. Mod Pathol 2010; 23(Suppl 2): S1–7.
25. Sanders ME, Schuyler PA, Dupont WD, Page DL. The natural history of low-grade ductal carcinoma in situ of the breast in women treated by biopsy only revealed over 30 years of long-term follow-up. Cancer 2005; 103: 2481–4.
26. Elson BC, Helvie MA, Frank TS, Wilson TE, Adler DD. Tubular carcinoma of the breast: mode of presentation, mammographic appearance, and frequency of nodal metastases. Am J Roentgenol 1993; 161: 1173–6.
27. Oberman HA, Fidler WJ Jr. Tubular carcinoma of the breast. Am J Surg Pathol 1979; 3: 387–95.
28. Tavassoli F. Infiltrating carcinomas, common and familiar special types. In: Tavassoli F (ed) Pathology of the Breast. Norwalk, CT: Appleton and Lange, 1992. pp.293–4.
29. Leibman AJ, Lewis M, Kruse B. Tubular carcinoma of the breast: mammographic appearance. Am J Roentgenol 1993; 160: 263–5.
30. Carstens PH, Huvos AG, Foote FW Jr, Ashikari R. Tubular carcinoma of the breast: a clinicopathologic study of 35 cases. Am J Clin Pathol 1972; 58: 231–8.
31. Parl FF, Richardson LD. The histologic and biologic spectrum of tubular carcinoma of the breast. Hum Pathol 1983; 14: 694–8.
32. Collins LC, Achacoso NA, Nekhlyudov L, et al. Clinical and pathologic features of ductal carcinoma in situ associated with the presence of flat epithelial atypia: an analysis of 543 patients. Mod Pathol 2007; 20: 1149–55.
33. Papadatos G, Rangan AM, Psarianos T, Ung O, Taylor R, Boyages J. Probability of axillary node involvement in patients with tubular carcinoma of the breast. Br J Surg 2001; 88: 860–4.
34. Gunhan-Bilgen I, Oktay A. Tubular carcinoma of the breast: mammographic, sonographic, clinical and pathologic findings. Eur J Radiol 2007; 61: 158–62.
35. Rakha EA, Lee AH, Evans AJ, et al. Tubular carcinoma of the breast: further evidence to support its excellent prognosis. J Clin Oncol 2010; 28: 99–104.
36. Zandrino F, Calabrese M, Faedda C, Musante F. Tubular carcinoma of the breast: pathological, clinical, and ultrasonographic findings. A review of the literature. Radiol Med 2006; 111: 773–82.
37. Berger AC, Miller SM, Harris MN, Roses DF. Axillary dissection for tubular carcinoma of the breast. Breast J 1996; 3: 204–8.
38. Deos PH, Norris HJ. Well-differentiated (tubular) carcinoma of the breast. A clinicopathologic study of 145 pure and mixed cases. Am J Clin Pathol 1982; 78: 1–7.

39. Lagios MD, Rose MR, Margolin FR. Tubular carcinoma of the breast: association with multicentricity, bilaterality, and family history of mammary carcinoma. Am J Clin Pathol 1980; 73: 25–30.

40. Page DL, Anderson TJ. Tubular Carcinoma. In: *Diagnostic Histopathology of the Breast*. Edinburgh: Churchill Livingstone, 1987. pp.193–235.

41. Tavassoli F, Devilee P (eds). *Tumors of the Breast and Female Genital Organs*. Lyon: IARC Press, 2003.

42. Kader HA, Jackson J, Mates D, Andersen S, Hayes M, Olivotto IA. Tubular carcinoma of the breast: a population-based study of nodal metastases at presentation and of patterns of relapse. Breast J 2001; 7: 8–13.

43. Carstens PH, Greenberg RA, Francis D, Lyon H. Tubular carcinoma of the breast. A long term follow-up. Histopathology 1985; 9: 271–80.

44. Elston CW, Ellis IO. *The Breast*, 3 rd edn. London: Churchill Livingstone, 1998.

45. Lagios MD. Multicentricity of breast carcinoma demonstrated by routine correlated serial subgross and radiographic examination. Cancer 1977; 40: 1726–34.

46. Leonard CE, Philpott P, Shapiro H, *et al*. Clinical observations of axillary involvement for tubular, lobular, and ductal carcinomas of the breast. J Surg Oncol 1999; 70: 13–20.

47. Baker RR. Unusual lesions and their management. Surg Clin North Am 1990; 70: 963–75.

48. Fedko MG, Scow JS, Shah SS, *et al*. Pure tubular carcinoma and axillary nodal metastases. Ann Surg Oncol 2010; 17(Suppl 3): 338–42.

49. Javid SH, Smith BL, Mayer E, *et al*. Tubular carcinoma of the breast: results of a large contemporary series. Am J Surg 2009; 197: 674–7.

50. Leonard CE, Howell K, Shapiro H, Ponce J, Kercher J. Excision only for tubular carcinoma of the breast. Breast J 2005; 11: 129–33.

51. Lim M, Bellon JR, Gelman R, *et al*. A prospective study of conservative surgery without radiation therapy in select patients with Stage I breast cancer. Int J Radiat Oncol Biol Phys 2006; 65: 1149–54.

52. Livi L, Paiar F, Meldolesi E, *et al*. Tubular carcinoma of the breast: outcome and loco-regional recurrence in 307 patients. Eur J Surg Oncol 2005; 31: 9–12.

53. Holland DW, Boucher LD, Mortimer JE. Tubular breast cancer experience at Washington University: a review of the literature. Clin Breast Cancer 2001; 2: 210–14.

54. Winchester DJ, Sahin AA, Tucker SL, Singletary SE. Predicting axillary nodal metastases and recurrence. Ann Surg 1996; 223: 342–7.

55. Thurman SA, Schnitt SJ, Connolly JL, *et al*. Outcome after breast-conserving therapy for patients with stage I or II mucinous, medullary, or tubular breast carcinoma. Int J Radiat Oncol Biol Phys 2004; 59: 152.

56. Peters GN, Wolff M, Haagensen CD. Clinical pathologic correlations based on 100 cases. Ann Surg 1981; 193: 138–49.

20 Thymoma and Thymic Carcinoma

Patrick J. Loehrer Sr.,[1] Mark R. Wick,[2] and Sunil Badve[3]

[1] Indiana University Melvin and Bren Simon Cancer Center, Indianapolis, IN, USA
[2] Department of Pathology, University of Virginia, Charlottesville, VA, USA
[3] Department of Pathology, Indiana University, Indianapolis, IN, USA

Historical background

The thymus is an enigmatic structure located in the anterior mediastinum whose function is to facilitate the differentiation and maturation of T lymphocytes. As such, the thymus requires a complex microenvironment and is composed of specialized epithelial cells. Thus, the thymus gland serves an integral role in the immune process and alteration of its controlled function has been associated with a protean array of disease manifestations. Thymic epithelial tumors are rare and the National Cancer Institute's Surveillance, Epidemiology, and End Results (SEER) tumor registry estimates the incidence of thymoma in the United States to be approximately 0.15 per 100,000 person-years.[1]

Thymomas, thymic carcinomas, thymic carcinoids, and thymolipomas contain epithelial components; however, only the first two are usually regarded as tumors exhibiting differentiation toward thymic epithelium. Accordingly, this chapter will solely concern itself with these lesions. Thymomas may be encapsulated tumors, which present as space-occupying lesions, or alternatively they can be locally invasive or systemically disseminated at presentation. Despite this, they still have a bland cytological appearance at all stages. In contrast, thymic carcinomas have overtly malignant cytological features. Thymic carcinomas can present in the same manner as thymomas, except that they usually present with invasive or metastatic disease and as such are associated with a much poorer prognosis.[2,3]

The traditional histological classification of thymomas was based on the proportion of nonneoplastic lymphoid cells to neoplastic epithelial cells. Using this system, there did not appear to be a correlation with prognosis. More recently, the World Health Organization (WHO) classification has been adopted by many pathologists. A discussion comparing and contrasting the WHO type, a clinicopathogical classification, and the more traditional descriptive terminology will be presented. Also in this chapter, thymomas and thymic carcinomas will be anatomically staged according to the system devised by Masaoka et al.[3] (Table 20.1). In this system, stage II and stage III tumors are further subdivided into those that are completely and incompletely resected. As a point of clarification, thymomas have been referred to as "encapsulated" and "benign" thymomas if there is no invasion, and "malignant" if there is infiltration into other intrathoracic structures or systemic dissemination. Furthermore, the term "type I malignant thymoma" has been used to label locally invasive or metastatic thymoma, whereas thymic carcinomas have been termed "type II malignant thymomas."[2] However, based on the observation that all histological subtypes of thymoma have the ability to locally invade and metastasize to distant sites, we prefer the more simple descriptors "thymoma" and "thymic carcinoma."

Anatomy

In the first trimester the thymus gland arises from the ventral portion of the third pharyngeal pouch as a paired epithelial structure, in close association with the parathyroid glands, which develop posteriorly.[4,5] The thymic epithelial cells are derived from the endoderm.[6] The rudimentary thymus enlarges and descends into the anterosuperior mediastinum by week 8. The thymus gland lies adjacent to the pericardium (inferiorly) and the great vessels (anteriorly), and its superior aspect is in the root of the neck. Precursor lymphocytes migrate to the thymus during week 8, at the time when the microscopic architecture becomes apparent. This features a cortex, a medulla, and perivascular spaces buttressed by fibrous septa. Moreover, the lymphoid cells are intimately admixed with the epithelial cells but are separated by the perivascular spaces. This partitioning forms the blood–thymus barrier. Ultrastructural evaluation of the epithelial cells in the thymus has shown that there is a close association between different types of epithelial cells and the

Table 20.1 Staging systems.

Stage	Description
Masaoka staging	
I	Macroscopically completely encapsulated and microscopically no capsular invasion
II	(1) Macroscopic invasion into surrounding fatty tissue, mediastinal pleura, or both
	(2) Microscopic invasion into capsule
III	Macroscopic invasion into neighboring organ, such as pericardium, great vessels, or lung
IVa	Pleural or pericardial dissemination
IVb	Lymphogenous or hematogenous metastasis
GETT classification	
Stage I	
IA	Encapsulated tumor, totally resected
IB	Macroscopically encapsulated tumor, totally resected, but the surgeon suspects mediastinal adhesions and potential capsular invasion
Stage II	Invasive tumor, totally resected
Stage III	
IIIA	Invasive tumor subtotally resected
IIIB	Invasive tumor, biopsy
Stage IV	
IVA	Supraclavicular metastasis or distant pleural implants
IVB	Distant metastasis
TNM	
T factor	
T1	Macroscopically completely encapsulated and microscopically no capsular invasion
T2	Macroscopic adhesion or invasion into surrounding fatty tissue or mediastinal pleura or microscopic invasion into the capsule
T3	Invasion into neighboring organs such as the pericardium, great vessels, or lung
T4	Pleural or pericardial dissemination
N factor	
N0	No lymph node metastasis
N1	Metastasis to anterior mediastinal lymph nodes
N2	Metastasis to intrathoracic lymph nodes except anterior mediastinal lymph nodes
N3	Metastasis to extrathoracic lymph nodes
M factor	
M0	No hematogenous metastasis
M1	Hematogenous metastasis

various steps in the maturation process of lymphocytes.[6,7] Six different types of thymic epithelium have been identified to date.[4] The outer cortex is the location for lymphoblastogenesis involving large immature lymphocytes, the inner cortex contains more mature thymocytes, and the medulla harbors the most mature T cells, which are similar to those in the peripheral blood.[6]

The thymus is the site of specialized lymphoid differentiation and "positive selection."[4,8] This gland generates large numbers of cortical thymocytes (lymphocytes) having both CD4 and CD8 molecules showing specificity for all major histocompatibility complex (MHC) molecules expressed in the human species. The thymus actively culls a small proportion of T cells, which recognize "self MHC" molecules. These immature elements, which coexpress CD4 and CD8, are thought to bind to epithelial (self) cells and receive a protective signal, which allows them to survive and be exported. Other CD4+ and CD8+ cells die and the surviving cells differentiate into either CD4 or CD8 cells. Physiologically, the latter classes of lymphocytes recognize peptides as foreign if they do not have the same "self MHC" repertoire and tolerate particles that possess the same determinants. Some of these T cells bind very avidly to the epithelial (self) cells, are thus recognized as "autoaggressive" and subsequently undergo apoptosis.[4,8] If not

eliminated, they can attack "self" and produce autoimmune disease.

In the neonate, the thymus has a maximal relative weight but it reaches a maximal absolute weight of roughly 35 g during puberty. The gland then undergoes gradual involution until it is only a small remnant structure in the adult, replaced mostly by adipocytes. Ectopic thymic tissue has been recognized in many locations in the mediastinum and neck, presumably due to aberrant or arrested migration.[5] The most common sites include retrocarinal and the aortopulmonary window.

Biology and epidemiology

Biology

The thymic microenvironment has been implicated in the genesis of thymomas and thymic carcinomas. Fibronectin and laminin are proteoglycans and are part of the ground substance of the extracellular matrix. They interact with T lymphocytes, thymic epithelial cells, various thymic hormones, and other factors. The absence of these ground substances may be associated with invasion more strongly than histological appearance alone, although they are more often lacking in "cortical" thymomas.[9]

The behavior of thymomas is determined by their epithelial components.[10] Although patients with lymphocyte-predominant tumors have a better survival compared with those who have epithelial-predominant tumors, lymphocyte content does not predict invasiveness.[11] Thymomas retain some functions of the normal thymus and may be able to induce the differentiation and homing of lymphocytes.[2] However, close observation reveals subtle differences.[12] Minor phenotypic abnormalities in Leu-2 and Leu-3 antigen expression were seen in three of 15 tumors in one series and six other cases showed aberrations of cortical and medullary differentiation. A lack of class II MHC antigens was associated with decreased lymphoid content and diminished Leu-1 expression in cortical thymocytes.[12] Moreover, a proliferation of the lymphocytes in thymomas has been documented with the Ki-67 antibody; it is 35–80% higher than age-matched controls. It is thought that this process may play a role in the pathogenesis of autoimmune diseases associated with thymoma.[13] Thymic carcinomas are less differentiated and functionally inert,[2] possibly explaining why they are rarely associated with autoimmune conditions.

Genetic abnormalities are poorly characterized. Several studies have shown loss of heterogeneity (LOH) in the long arm of chromosome 6 but at least two reports in the long arm of the chromosome 14A.[14–16] The presence of a translocation of 15 and 22 was observed in one case.[17] Cytogenetic abnormalities that have been observed include the presence of a translocation between chromosomes 15 and 19 in a cell line[18] and in three cases of thymic carcinoma[19–21] (WHO subtype – translocation associated carcinoma) in children and young adults which may represent a unique syndrome.[22].

Whether thymic carcinomas arise, at least sometimes, by clonal evolution from thymomas is under debate. A potential link is thymomas with modest cytological atypia, which some investigators classify as "well-differentiated thymic carcinmoma" (WDTC). This entity was initially described by Kirchner et al.[23]; WDTC otherwise retains most histological features of classic thymoma. This entity may represent the conceptual intermediary between thymoma and thymic carcinoma. Although the term "WDTC" has not been broadly accepted, proponents of this nomenclature argue that it is associated with invasive behavior in 83% of cases. On the other hand, critics point out that the frequency of paraneoplastic syndromes (predominantly myasthenia gravis – MG) that are associated with WDTC is incongruent with a diagnosis of carcinoma. Moreover, we consider it to be a variant of thymoma because it retains the general morphological features of this tumor.

One might posit a spectrum of genetic abnormality in thymic epithelial tumors, with marked karyotypic aberrancy conferring a greater degree of malignancy and a decreased likelihood of paraneoplasia. Anecdotal support for this notion comes from the observation that a small number of patients with biopsy-proven thymoma may later develop thymic carcinoma.[24–26] Although rare, thymic carcinoma may be associated with any histological type of thymoma, including the more benign histology of spindle cell thymoma. If necrosis is found in a thymoma, the pathologist should search for malignant changes such as specifically increased expression of epithelial membrane antigen (EMA), p53 protein, cytokeratin subtypes, or loss of CD99+ immature T lymphocytes.[25]

Epidemiology

The cause of thymoma is unknown.[182] Evidence implicating prior Epstein–Barr viral infection as a risk factor for thymic carcinoma includes the isolation of defective viral genomes in thymic carcinoma.[27–29] It is thought that defective virus can disrupt Epstein–Barr virus (EBV) latency, bring about EBV reactivation and an increase in EBV antibody levels, and result in malignant progression of infected cells, such as those in the thymus.[28] There may be geographical differences in this phenomenon, in analogy to EBV-associated nasopharyngeal cancer.[30] EBV is felt to be specifically associated with thymic lymphoepithelioma-like carcinomas in young individuals of Asian descent, but as will be discussed later, cellular EBV integration in thymic cancer is uncommon.[29,31,32] Support for this argument is built on the knowledge that nasopharyngeal carcinomas are also lymphoepithelial, can occur in younger patients and also arise from the primitive pharynx.[31] This raises the possibility that EBV causes thymic carcinoma only in people who are infected at an early age. However, the data are limited and cannot confirm whether there is increased incidence in Asian countries. Nonetheless, there is some evidence that the incidence is higher in Asians/Pacific islanders and African-Americans than in Caucasians.[1] These differences may arise from genetic polymorphisms. The distribution of alleles at the human leukocyte antigen (HLA) locus on chromosome 6 varies across racial groups.[33] Class I and class II HLA proteins are highly expressed on thymic epithelial cells and further studies need to be performed for a better understanding of a possible predisposition to thymoma.

Pathology

The nonneoplastic thymus

Microscopically, the thymus attains maturity during the first trimester of pregnancy. At that point, it has a multilobated appearance, with each lobule being composed of a cortex and a medulla (Fig. 20.1). The former of these two zones has a high lymphocyte-to-epithelial cell ratio, whereas the latter contains nearly an equal number of such elements. Clusters of epithelial cells in both subcompartments commonly undergo keratinization and microcystification, yielding the structures known as "Hassall's corpuscles." Mast cells are also found in abundance throughout both the cortex and medulla, and these become more notable with aging as the lymphocyte content of the gland decreases. Indeed, the postpubertal thymus contains relatively few thymocytes, and instead is represented by a large amount of mature adipose tissue in which residual epithelial cells are embedded (Fig. 20.2).[34,35]

Thymic epithelium demonstrates some degree of morphological variation, largely depending on whether it is located in one glandular subcompartment. Cortical epithelial cells have round-to-oval nuclear contours with vesicular chromatin and distinct small nucleoli, whereas those in the medulla more

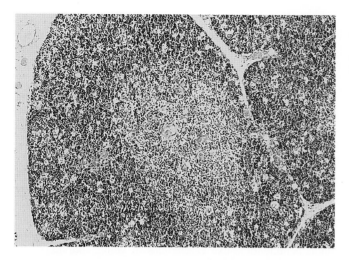

Figure 20.1 Normal thymic microarchitecture, showing peripheral, lymphocyte-rich cortical zone and a central medulla containing more numerous epithelial cells and Hassall's corpuscles.

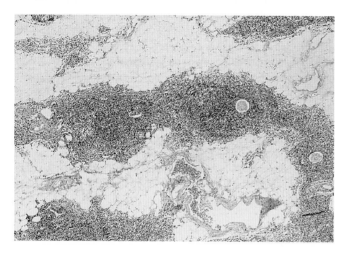

Figure 20.2 Photomicrograph of thymic atrophy in an adult, demonstrating replacement of a large portion of the glandular parenchyma by adipose tissue.

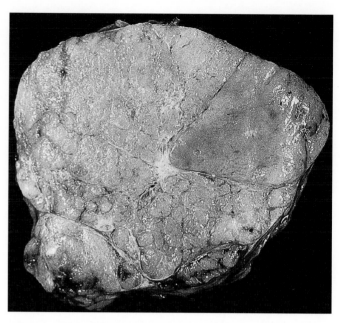

Figure 20.3 Gross photograph of a resected, bisected, encapsulated thymoma. The parenchyma demonstrates numerous fibrous septa that subdivide the tumor into angular lobules.

commonly assume a fusiform shape, contain dispersed chromatin, and manifest few, if any, nucleoli. In prepubescent individuals, thymocytes throughout the gland differ from the appearance of peripheral mature lymphocytes. The latter cells exhibit relatively enlarged nuclei with open chromatin patterns, discernible chromocenters, and folding of the nuclear membranes. Mitoses are commonly seen in thymocytes as well.[36]

The structural relationship between intrathymic lymphocytes and the thymic epithelium is an intimate one, wherein elongated and branched cytoplasmic processes of epithelial cells are closely apposed to the plasmalemma of resident thymocytes. Because of the overall constituency of the cortex, there are relatively more epithelial cell extensions than karyons, with the reverse pertaining to the thymic medulla.

Nonneoplastic morphological abnormalities in the thymus principally are represented by: (i) hyperplasia, which almost always involves proliferation of intrathymic lymphocytes but not epithelial cells, and (ii) dysplasia, where one observes only sparse thymocytes and abnormal aggregations of epithelium

into rosettes or arborizing cords. The first of these two conditions – which also features the formation of lymphoid germinal centers – is closely associated with MG or Graves disease, and the second is linked to congenital immunodeficiency states, although this feature can be seen adjacent to tumors.[37]

Thymoma

Thymomas generally take the form of well-localized, nodular, multilobated masses in the anterosuperior mediastinum, usually with at least partial fibrous encapsulation (Fig. 20.3). However, they have been reported to rarely occur as primary lesions in other sites as well, both inside and outside the thorax. Such locations include the middle and posterior mediastinal compartments, the intrapulmonary or extrapulmonary pleura, and the neck.[38–40] In fact, the term "SETTLE" (spindle cell epithelial tumors of thymic-like epithelium) has been named for intrathyroidal lesions with virtually all of the attributes of thymoma.[41,42] The cut surfaces of thymomas show subdivision of the lesions by fibrous bands, which generally intersect one another at acute angles. Spontaneous intralesional hemorrhage or necrosis is not usually apparent, but cystic changes may be prominent in selected examples. Indeed, such an alteration can be so striking in some instances – producing an image which simulates that of unilocular or multilocular thymic cysts – that the pathologist must undertake exhaustive tissue sampling to document the presence of a neoplastic cell population.[43]

Typically, all of the cytoarchitectural features described above, in reference to the nonneoplastic thymus, pertain to variants of thymoma as well. By definition, thymomas are primary tumors in which the neoplastic epithelial cells are cytologically bland or, at most, biologically indeterminate. With that fact in mind, it follows that other epithelial thymic

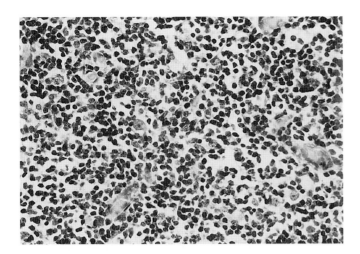

Figure 20.4 Photomicrograph of a "cortical" (lymphocyte-predominant) thymoma in which larger thymic epithelial tumor cells are widely separated. These show slightly vesicular chromatin and small nucleoli.

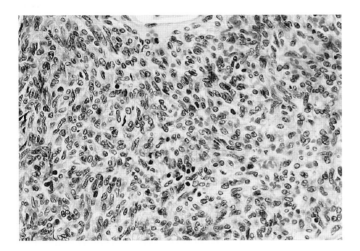

Figure 20.5 Histological image of a "medullary" (epithelial-predominant/spindle cell) thymoma. This lesion contains almost no lymphocytes, and the epithelial tumor cells have a fusiform appearance with dispersed nuclear chromatin and indistinct nucleoli.

tumors manifesting cytological malignancy must be classified differently (see below).

Some thymomas are composed of epithelium, which resembles that of the nonneoplastic thymic cortex, and accordingly have been termed "cortical" thymomas by some observers (Fig. 20.4).[44] On the other hand, others that are composed of spindle cells with fusiform nuclei and dispersed chromatin have the attributes of so-called "medullary" thymomas (Fig. 20.5). Still another subset exhibits a mixture of these two cytological morphotypes ("mixed" thymomas). However, it should be recognized that the microscopic variability of thymomas is considerable, perhaps second only to that of teratomas among all mediastinal neoplasms. Recognized secondary morphological findings in the former group of lesions include a vast predominance of intratumoral lymphocytes, microcystic change, pseudoglandular formations, perivascular pseudorosettes, assumption of an organoid, endocrine-like substructure, hemangiopericytoma-like growth with branched

stromal blood vessels, strikingly dense stromal vascularity with blood "lakes," zones of loose lymphocytic aggregation ("medullary" differentiation),[45] squamous metaplasia, storiform growth of spindle cells, rhabdomyoma-like differentiation, and focal nuclear atypia.[46] With regard to the last of these possibilities, it must be acknowledged that selected cases strain the morphological boundary between thymomas and thymic carcinomas (tumors with overt cytological malignancy), and it is likely that at least a theoretical continuum exists between those entities. Nevertheless, it is our opinion that the "well-differentiated thymic carcinoma" (WDTC) of Kirchner *et al.*[23] is more properly considered a form of thymoma with limited nuclear atypia.

Because of the many morphological differential diagnoses that are called to mind by the variations just cited, the pathologist may want to employ adjunctive diagnostic studies to solidify an interpretation of thymoma. These typically center on the use of electron microscopy and immunohistochemistry, the results of which serve to define the presence of an epithelial tumor, which lacks – in almost all cases – any evidence of neuroendocrine differentiation.[47]

Histological subclassification of thymomas

Histological classification of thymic tumors (Table 20.2), historically and currently, remains one of the most controversial areas in pathology. Historically, the histological subclassification of thymomas devised by Bernatz and colleagues[53] divided thymomas into four groups based on their microscopic features: lymphocyte predominant (>66% lymphocytes), epithelial predominant (>66% epithelial cells), mixed lymphoepithelial (34–66% epithelial cells), and spindle cell. The last of these categories pertains to epithelial-predominant thymoma featuring a virtually pure population of fusiform cells. It merits reemphasis that thymoma must first be defined as a cytologically bland epithelial neoplasm for this scheme to have histopathological utility. Its usefulness is in serving as a cue mechanism for well-defined histological differential diagnostic problems concerning thymomas. With the exception of spindle cell thymomas, which typically (but not universally) pursue a benign course, the Bernatz system does not present prognostic information.[54]

In 1985, a construct proposed by Marino and Muller-Hermelink (the MMH classification)[6] utilized the morphological resemblance of neoplastic epithelial cells to subtypes of normal epithelial cells in the thymus.[55] They presupposed that "medullary" thymomas carry a favorable prognosis, while "cortical" lesions have a relatively adverse evolution and "mixed cortical/medullary" thymomas have an intermediary behavior. As summarized by Shimosato and Mukai,[46] it appears that the MMH system actually represents a derivative array of information that would already be available if the Bernatz scheme were used, albeit with dissimilar terminology. Also, significant problems with interobserver reproducibility of the MMH system have been noted.[56] Because spindle cell ("medullary") thymomas have long been known to behave innocuously, regardless of what specific adjectives are attached to them, it would seem worthwhile to reevaluate the claims of MMH proponents,[57,58] after pure spindle cell neoplasms have

Table 20.2 Histology.

Study	Patients, n	Subgroups (%)	Clinical correlation
Thymoma Verley and Hollmann[110]	200	Type I: spindle and oval cell (30)	75*
		Type II: lymphocyte rich (30)	75*
		Type III: differentiated epithelial rich (33)	50*
		Type IV: undifferentiated epithelial rich (equivalent to thymic carcinoma) (7)	0*
Lewis et al.[64]	283	Predominantly lymphocytic (>66% lymphocytes) (25)	90†
		Mixed lymphoepithelial (33–66% lymphocytes) (43)	80†
		Predominantly epithelial (<33% lymphocytes) (25)	50†
		Spindle cell (predominantly epithelial cells with prominent fusiform cells) (6)	100†
Muller-Hermelink et al.[44]	58	Cortical (43)	67‡
		Mixed: predominantly cortical (8)	0‡
		Mixed: common (36)	0‡
		Medullary (5)	0‡
		Mixed: predominantly medullary (8)	0‡
Thymic carcinoma[30,31]			
High grade		Lymphoepithelial-like, small cell, large cell anaplastic, clear cell, sarcomatoid	11.3 months§
Low grade		Keratinizing squamous, basaloid squamous, mucoepidermoid	25.4 months§
WHO histological typing[48–52]		Predominant cells	
A	96	Epithelial cells (spindle)	37%¶
AB	237	Epithelial/lymphocyte	32%¶
B1	122	Lymphocyte	49%¶
B2	269	Polygonal neoplastic epithelial cells with immature lymphocytes	66%¶
B3	90	Neoplastic epithelial cells with minor portion of immature lymphocytes	86%¶
Carcinoma	92	Thymic carcinoma	91%¶

* 10-year survival (%).
† 15-year disease-specific survival.
‡ Subgroup with invasion (%).
§ Median survival.
¶ Percent invasive.

been excluded from formal statistical analyses. In our personal experience with a large number of thymoma cases, the MMH system has not attained independent significance as a prognostic factor under those conditions.

Although there is no means of pathologically classifying thymomas to correlate perfectly with biology (and hence prognosis), in 1999 the WHO agreed to a classification system based on the morphology of the epithelial cells, as well as the lymphocyte-to-epithelial cell ratio. The WHO classification separates the tumors into three types using letters A ("atrophic": the thymic cells of adult life), B ("bioreactive": the biologically active organ of the fetus and infant), and C (carcinoma). The more recent version of the WHO has dropped the term "C" in preference for "carcinoma".

Type A thymoma ("spindle cell: medullary")
Type A thymoma corresponds to the spindle cell thymoma and the medullary thymoma of prior classifications. Most type A thymomas are encapsulated.

Type AB thymoma (mixed)
Another subset exhibits a mixture of two cytological morphotypes: a lymphocyte-rich area (WHO type B-like component) and a lymphocyte-poor area (WHO type A, spindle cell component).

Type B thymoma
This tumor resembles the normal thymus. Type B thymomas are further subdivided (B1, B2, B3) based on the increasing epithelial:lymphocyte ratio and the emergence of atypia.

Type C thymoma (pathology of primary thymic carcinomas)
Thymic carcinomas have been well recognized only in relatively recent times.[24,59,60] Historically, it was often stated that the biological potential of thymic tumors could not be predicted by histology[60] but this opinion is only partially correct. It is true that conventional thymomas often demonstrate gross transcapsular invasion (invasive thymoma),[61–63] and a small proportion show extrathoracic (but idiosyncratic) spread ("metastasizing thymoma")[64] as well. Nevertheless, these biological events do not mandate a diagnosis of "carcinoma."

There is a distinctive subgroup of thymic epithelial neoplasms that exhibits obvious cellular anaplasia and aggressive behavior. This subgroup truly deserves the designation of "carcinomas." Thymic carcinomas commonly lack the encapsulation or fibrous septation of thymomas. Their parenchyma is firm-to-hard and has a white-gray appearance, with frequent necrosis and hemorrhage. Basaloid squamous thymic carcinoma may associate itself with multilocular thymic cysts[65]; another tumor variant, mucoepidermoid thymic carcinoma, has a gelatinous cut surface.[66]

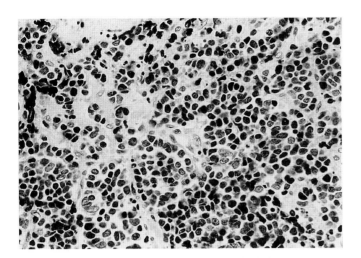

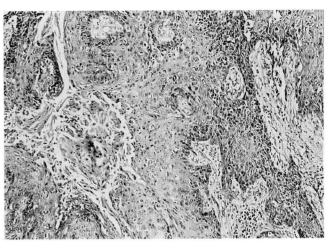

Figure 20.6 Microscopic photograph of primary small cell neuroendocrine carcinoma of the thymus. The neoplastic cells show dispersed nuclear chromatin, apoptosis, and "molding" of nuclear membranes on one another.

Figure 20.8 Histological image of keratinizing squamous cell carcinoma of the thymus. Interconnecting cords and nests of large tumor cells are present, with overtly atypical nuclei and foci of keratin deposition (*left center*).

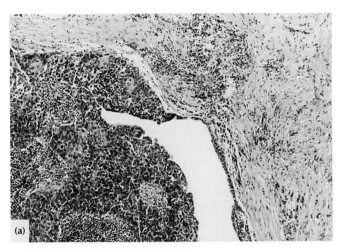

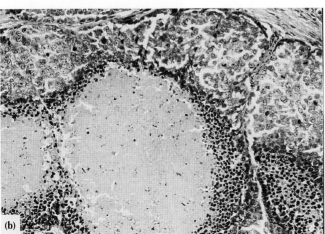

Figure 20.7 (a) Photomicrograph of basaloid thymic carcinoma, exhibiting an association with a preexisting multilocular thymic cyst (*right of figure*). (b) The tumor cells are arranged in lobules with prominent geographic necrosis.

The subtypes of thymic carcinoma recognized by the WHO include basaloid squamous cell carcinoma (BSCC), keratinizing squamous cell carcinoma, nonkeratinizing squamous cell carcinoma, lymphoepithelioma-like squamous carcinoma, mucoepidermoid carcinomas (MECs), clear cell carcinoma, undifferentiated carcinoma, papillary carcinoma, and sarcomatoid carcinoma.[67,68] These variants are discussed in some descriptive detail below, in light of their relative rarity and distinctive features.

Basaloid squamous cell carcinoma
BSCC has the potential to involve the thymus primarily or by metastasis. Potential origins for secondary lesions include the oropharynx, hypopharynx, larynx, esophagus, lungs, and anorectal region.[65] Thus, cautions should be exercised while concluding that BSCCs have originated in the mediastinum.

Histologically, BSCC is composed of polygonal cells with high nucleocytoplasmic ratios, hyperchromatic round nuclei, and brisk mitotic activity. Nuclear "molding" is absent (Fig. 20.6). Moreover, this lesion may include stromal mucin-containing pseudoglandular arrays resembling those of adenoid cystic carcinomas, as well as globular eosinophilic intercellular deposits of basement membrane material and areas of squamous differentiation with keratin "pearls."[60–65,69–72] The few cases reported as primary in the thymus had a tendency for association with multilocular thymic cysts (Fig. 20.7).[65]

Keratinizing squamous cell carcinoma
Keratinizing thymic squamous carcinoma (KTSC) is identical microscopically to its counterparts in other organs. It shows large polyhedral cells in nests and cords. Nuclei are vesicular or hyperchromatic, usually with obvious nucleoli (Fig. 20.8). Cytoplasm is eosinophilic, and incipient or well-formed keratin "pearls" are scattered throughout such lesions.[46,67,73,74]

A potential factor of consternation in cases of thymic KTSC concerns the concurrent presence of a histological pattern that is more consonant with that of conventional thymoma. The two

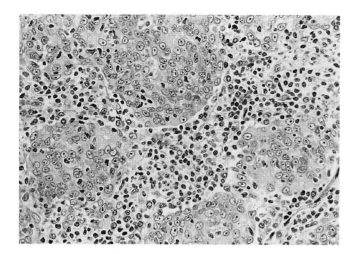

Figure 20.9 Photomicrograph of LETC, demonstrating syncytia of polygonal tumor cells with vesicular nuclear chromatin and prominent nucleoli. Lymphocytes are intimately interspersed throughout the lesion.

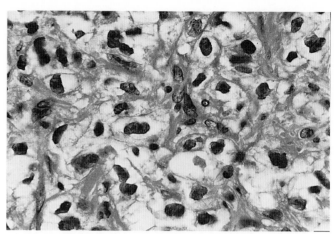

Figure 20.10 Microscopic photograph of clear cell carcinoma of the thymus, showing pleomorphic, hyperchromatic nuclei, and lucent cytoplasm.

components may be seen in widely separated tissue blocks, or in admixture. The authors have even seen rare cases in which a gradual transition between them was evident. These observations imply that some cases of KTSC may develop through the "clonal evolution" ("dedifferentiation") of thymomas.

Nonkeratinizing squamous cell carcinoma
The nonkeratinizing variant of squamous thymic carcinoma differs only in its lesser level of differentiation.[25,46,67] It is a tumor showing angular nests of polyhedral cells in a desmoplastic stroma. The distinct fibrous stromal septa of thymoma, however, are absent. The authors also include thymic neoplasms labeled by others as "large cell carcinomas"[46] in the category of nonkeratinizing squamous carcinoma.

Lymphoepithelioma-like squamous carcinoma
"Lymphoepitheliomas" of the nasopharynx and other anatomical sites are now known to represent distinctive forms of squamous cell carcinoma, some of which are associated with infection by the EBV.[75] Similar concepts apply to thymic neoplasia.[32] Lymphoepithelioma-like thymic carcinoma (LETC) has a peculiar histological appearance unlike that of KTSC or nonkeratinizing squamous carcinoma. LETCs contain syncytia of polygonal cells with ill-defined boundaries, vesicular nuclei, eosinophilic nucleoli, and an admixture of mature lymphocytes (Fig. 20.9).[46,32] Tumoral stroma is usually represented by narrow fibrovascular septa.

Mucoepidermoid carcinomas
Rare examples of primary thymic carcinoma have been reported that imitated MEC of the salivary glands[66] or adenosquamous carcinoma of the lung[46,65,76] in that they exhibited a partially squamous constituency. Obviously, concerns regarding the origin of such lesions within the thymus must be addressed once more. In MEC, foci that resemble well-differentiated KTSC are admixed with goblet cell-type epithelium that surrounds mucinous material. On the other hand, adenosquamous carcinoma is a high-grade tumor that resembles nonkeratinizing squamous

cancer histologically. The salient difference between those two lesions is the presence of glandular lumina in the adenosquamous carcinoma; these may contain material that is positive with the mucicarmine or periodic acid-Schiff (PAS)-diastase stains.

Clear cell carcinoma
Few examples of thymic clear cell carcinoma (TCCC) have been documented.[27,77] This lesion is uniformly composed of polyhedral cells with vesicular nuclei, distinct nucleoli, and clear cytoplasm (Fig. 20.10). In some cases, cellular lucency reflected the presence of abundant cytoplasmic glycogen; in others, hydropic change appeared to account for this finding. TCCC has a vaguely organoid growth pattern, inconspicuous vascularity, and an absence of "blood lakes" as expected in clear cell carcinomas in extrathymic sites such as the kidneys.[77]

Undifferentiated thymic carcinoma
Two "pure" adenocarcinomas of the thymus have been documented by Shimosato and Mukai.[46] One showed transition with an epithelial-predominant thymoma, as well as micropapillary growth and focal psammomatous calcification. The other lesion was also somewhat variable histologically, with foci of both micropapillary and solid growth.

Sarcomatoid carcinoma
Only rare examples of primary sarcomatoid thymic carcinoma (STC) have been reported.[58,74,78] At the risk of redundancy, it must again be said that metastases must be excluded rigorously before assigning a final diagnosis of primary STC.

Microscopically, this neoplasm manifests irregular fascicles of pleomorphic spindle cells. Nuclei are hyperchromatic, nucleoli are obvious, and mitoses are numerous. Occasional examples have contained cohesive epithelioid cell nests amongst the spindle cells,[59] and biphasic STCs with carcinoidal elements ("dedifferentiated" thymic carcinoids) have also been documented.[79,80]

Specialized pathological characteristics of thymic carcinomas
The major goals of ancillary pathological studies in cases of suspected thymic carcinoma are to provide information that

would exclude a nonepithelial lesion, and also to secure – if possible – data that would tend to support a primary intra-thymic nature for the mass in question. The cells of all thymic carcinomas are reactive for keratin and EMA; however, in sarcomatoid lesions these markers may be seen only focally.[81] This fact leaves open the possibility that a small biopsy speci-men might fail to demonstrate the true nature of the mass because of sampling artifact. The latter should be considered before accepting a final diagnosis of "mediastinal sarcoma."

Primary small cell neuroendocrine carcinoma of the thymus is distinguished from other forms of thymic carcinoma either by a distinctive pattern of intermediate filament expression, with perinuclear "globules" of keratin protein,[47] or by its poten-tial reactivity for one of several neuroendocrine markers. These include chromogranin A (a matrix protein of neurosecretory granules), synaptophysin, Leu-7 (CD57 antigen), and selected neuropeptides such as adrenocorticotropic hormone. There are, at present, no reliable markers that could be used to separate primary from secondary thymic small cell carcinomas.

In that context, it is notable that several studies have shown the expression of CD5 by epithelial cells of nonsmall cell thymic carcinomas,[82–84] but not thymomas. Other primary thymic malignancies, such as germ cell tumors and lympho-mas, are CD5 negative, as are metastatic mediastinal carcino-mas from other organs. This last fact obviously may be useful in excluding secondary tumors that might imitate thymic carci-nomas histologically.

At least some LETC cases show cellular EBV integration at a molecular level.[31,32] Using *in situ* hybridization and ribo-probes to Epstein–Barr virus early ribonucleic acid-1 (EBER-1), Wu and Kuo[29] observed positivity in only one of five LETCs and none of the other 15 thymic carcinomas for EBER-1 tran-scripts, markedly limiting the differential diagnostic utility of this technique. Evaluations for mutant p53 protein, as under-taken by Tateyama *et al.*, also show a broad range of expression by thymomas and PTC.[85] Nonetheless, common abnormalities in the *p53* gene in many other tumors preclude a meaningful role for that moiety in differential diagnosis.

One particular challenge for the pathologist is the distinction between primary mediastinal synovial sarcoma and STC; most specialized features of both those lesions are largely similar. The demonstration of t(X;18) chromosomal translocations in synovial sarcoma by fluorescence *in situ* hybridization has now made it recognizable with diagnostic certainty.[86]

Molecular markers in thymoma and thymic carcinoma

Flow cytometric analysis has been done of the nuclear DNA in epithelial cells of thymomas. In one study of 25 patients, diploidy was associated with lower stage and better 5-year survival although this was not true concerning the percentage of cells in S-phase.[87] Another evaluation showed that mean nuclear DNA exhibited a continuum of low values in noninva-sive thymomas but progressively higher DNA content was seen in invasive thymoma and thymic carcinomas.[88] This study was small in scope and showed an overlap between noninva-sive and invasive thymomas. However, a significant difference was found between the DNA content of thymic carcinomas and thymomas.

Several studies have assessed other factors such as the proliferative activity (proliferating cell nuclear antigen (PCNA), Ki-67, mitotic figures) and the activation of matrix metalloproteinase-2 (MMP-2).[89] Immunoreactivity for MMP-2 is low in WHO type AB thymoma, moderate in type B1, and high in types B2, BC, and C. These findings appear to correlate with the oncological behavior of each thymoma type.[90] Glycosylphosphatidyl inositol-anchored protein (GPI-80) gene expression is a secretory protein or cell surface protein that is also found in significantly higher concentrations in invasive thymoma (stage IV) versus earlier (stage I) thymoma.[91] Interestingly, GPI-80 was not elevated in thymic carcinomas. The exact mechanism for the overexpression of this protein during thymoma progression is not known.

The p53 protein has likewise been studied in thymic epithe-lial cells. There is some evidence that progression of thymic tumors may be associated with accumulation of mutant forms of this moiety.[85,92]

The protooncogene *bcl2* encodes a protein that inhibits apoptosis. It has been evaluated in 30 thymoma specimens.[93] Medullary thymocytes exhibited positivity for this marker, as shown in normal thymic medulla as well. Such findings cor-respond to a relative lack of apoptosis in the medullary com-partment and spindle cell thymomas, whereas cortical epithelial cells manifesting apoptosis did not stain. Similarly, "cortical" thymomas were bcl2 negative. These findings may support the concept that the neoplastic epithelial cells in thymomas are derived from different compartments and that the bcl2 protein may play a role in "medullary" (spindle cell) differentiation.

The MIC2 antibody 013 has also been investigated in this context.[94] This marker of immature T cells, which is almost always seen in cortical thymocytes and in only 5% of medullary lymphocytes, may assist in the diagnosis of thymoma in the mediastinum, or ectopic and metastatic sites. Thymic carcinoma is 013 negative but it should be recognized with caution that the lymphoid cells of both lymphocyte-predominant thymomas and lymphoblastic lymphomas are labeled with this marker.

Epidermal growth factor receptor (EGFR) is expressed in a high percentage of thymomas[95] and may be associated with invasive and/or advanced-stage disease.[96] There has been one case report of overexpression of mutated c-kit and a response to imatinib.[97] It appears that c-kit is present in thymic carcino-mas but not thymomas, and EGFR is present in thymomas but not thymic carcinomas.[98]

The expression of PAX8 has been recently studied in rela-tion to thymic tumors. Laury *et al.* analyzed the expression of PAX8 in a large number of human tumors.[99] They unexpect-edly found moderate diffuse expression in a large number of thymic tumors but importantly not in tumors of lung origin. Following this publication, Weissferdt and Moran analyzed a large series of thymic tumors and reported immunoreactivity for PAX8 in 77% of thymic carcinomas, 100% of WHO type A thymomas, and 93% of WHO type B thymomas.[100]

The 15,19 translocation reported in thymic carcinoma is associated with expression of the primitive protein NUT, which is normally expressed only in the testis.[22] French *et al.*[101] have generated an antibody against this protein and expression of this protein has been seen in some mediastinal tumors. The incidence of translocation-associated carcinoma might be significantly greater than has been reported to date.

Girard *et al.* have analyzed a series of thymomas and thymic carcinomas using array-based comparative genomic hybridization techniques.[102] They have identified the presence of mutations in c-kit, KRAS and HRAS that may be amenable to specific targeting using small molecular inhibitors. Our group and others have been using molecular analysis to better understand the genomic basis of thymomas and better ways of prognostication and to better understand the key differences between types of thymomas.[103]

Clinical presentation and diagnostic considerations

Clinical presentation

Thymoma is the most common tumor of the anterior mediastinum and most commonly affects people between the ages of 40 and 60 years (with a mean age of 50 years) but also may occur in the pediatric and geriatric populations and there is no sex predominance.[3,11,57,64,104–112] The same demographic features have been observed for thymic carcinoma.[24,67,74,113,114] The latter neoplasms account for about 5% of thymic epithelial tumors.[67] Manifestations associated with thymic epithelial tumors may be absent, they may be attributed to the tumor itself as a space-occupying lesion, or they may relate to systemic syndromes associated with such lesions.

Approximately 60% of patients with a thymoma or thymic carcinoma will have definite symptoms and signs of local disease or paraneoplastic syndromes. In contrast, about 30% of patients with thymoma[24,74] will be found to have a mediastinal mass on a chest x-ray, noted incidentally.[64,105,106] Local symptoms are manifested because of growth of tumors into the surrounding tissues. These include chest pain, dyspnea, hemoptysis, stridor, cough, dysphagia, fatigue, dysphonia, the superior vena cava syndrome, cardiac arrhythmias, and Horner syndrome. Rarely, thymic tumors may directly invade the spinal cord and cause neurological dysfunction.

Most thymomas (65% of cases) are locally invasive and rarely metastasize outside the thorax.[64,110] Noninvasive thymomas are characterized by an intact fibrous capsule, movability, and relatively easy resectability.

Invasive thymomas penetrate the capsule and may either grossly invade mediastinal structures and/or metastasize.[111] Metastases are most commonly seen on the pleural or pericardial surfaces and appear as "drop" lesions. Metastatic involvement of lymph nodes is uncommon in thymoma (3–7%).[115] Hematogenous spread is uncommon, but when it occurs, it may manifest with bony, hepatic, and pulmonary parenchymal lesions. These distant metastases occur in approximately 5% of patients with thymoma, but much more common in thymic carcinoma.[111]

The indolent and occasionally unpredictable nature of thymoma is exemplified in patients with fully resected disease who may have recurrent disease 5–10 years following resection even if the lesion was initially stage I.[64] Individuals with unresectable, locally advanced or metastatic disease may occasionally be alive with the disease for up to 20 years or more.[110]

In contrast, thymic carcinomas have a more aggressive clinical course. Thymic carcinomas also differ clinically from thymomas in that they are uncommonly associated with paraneoplastic syndromes such as MG or pure red cell aplasia (PRCA); however, some cases have been reported.[60,69,70] Patients with these malignant lesions usually present with complaints referring to structural displacement, or they are detected incidentally by chest radiography. Patients with thymic carcinomas characteristically are middle-aged or elderly adults; infrequent examples have affected children also. Because some lesions may resemble metastatic tumors from other organs, one must exclude an occult malignancy elsewhere before a final diagnosis is rendered.

In contrast to thymoma, thymic carcinoma presents with stage I or II disease in less than 50% of cases; stage III in roughly 30% and stage IV, usually with metastasis, in 20%.[24,74,113] Long-term survival in unresectable or advanced thymic carcinoma is rare.[114]

Metastatic lesions are grouped in the system of Masaoka *et al.*[3] into those with pericardial or pleural dissemination (stage IVa) or lymphogenous or hematogenous metastasis (IVb). As expected, high-stage disease is seen more frequently with thymic carcinomas.[115] Intrathoracic metastases are characterized by symptoms and signs of malignant effusions. These include chest pain, dyspnea, and, in the case of pericardial involvement, cardiac tamponade. Sites of lymphogenous spread may rarely include mediastinal, cervical, and axillary lymph nodes. Hematogenous metastases involve bones (especially the spine), liver, lung, brain (rarely), bone marrow, and kidney.[24,74]

Paraneoplastic syndromes

On account of the role of the thymus in the immunological and hematological systems, about 50–70% of thymomas are ultimately associated with one or more of a variety of systemic diseases (Box 20.1).[3,64,116,117] The most common and well recognized of these disorders is myasthenia gravis (MG) as observed in 30–50% of patients with thymomas. In contrast, only 10–12% of patients with MG have thymoma. The interplay between the two conditions is best illustrated by the fact that thymectomy can lessen MG manifestations in 50–60% of cases and can result in complete remissions (CRs) 8% of the time.[118] It has also been noted that the recurrence of MG can herald the progression, either locally or systemically, of a previously controlled tumor. It must be kept in mind that myasthenic crises are associated with significant medical stresses, such as myocardial infarction or sepsis, and may thus occur even though there may be no evidence of active thymomatous growth.

It is unclear if any paraneoplastic association may occur in patients with thymic carcinomas, but most series have reported no association. In one study, two patients were found to have had MG.[24] In both cases, however, there was a history of biopsy-proven thymoma. One other study has noted a 77% association of MG with "well-differentiated thymic carcinoma," a putative subtype of thymic carcinoma.[23] Nevertheless, as discussed below, we subscribe to the view that the latter

Box 20.1 Disorders associated with thymoma.

Neuromuscular syndromes

- Myasthenia gravis
- Myotonic dystrophy
- Limbic encephalopathy
- Eaton–Lambert syndrome
- Sensorimotor radiculopathy
- Stiff person syndrome

Immune deficiency syndromes

- Hypogammaglobulinemia
- T cell deficiency syndrome

Collagen diseases and autoimmune disorders

- Systemic lupus erythematosus
- Scleroderma
- Sarcoidosis
- Rheumatoid arthritis
- Polymyositis
- Cardiac disorders
- Myocarditis
- Acute pericarditis

Gastrointestinal disorders

- Ulcerative colitis

Malignancy

- Lymphoma, carcinoma, Kaposi sarcoma

Hematological syndromes

- Red cell aplasia/hypoplasia
- Pernicious anemia
- Agranulocytosis
- Erythrocytosis
- Multiple myeloma
- Hemolytic anemia
- Acute leukemia
- T cell lymphocytosis

Dermatological diseases

- Pemphigus
- Alopecia areata
- Chronic mucocutaneous candidiasis

Endocrine disorders

- Cushing syndrome
- Panhypopituitarism
- Addison disease
- Thyroiditis
- Hypertrophic osteoarthropathy

Renal disease

- Nephrotic syndrome
- Minimal change nephropathy

lesion is a thymoma variant, and in the WHO classification, this variant is now type B3 thymoma. More recently, our group analyzed the association of MG with thymic tumors and found that thymic carcinomas were as likely to have MG as thymomas.[119]

It is significant for the pathogenesis of paraneoplastic MG that there is no age nor gender predilection and almost no HLA association in paraneoplastic MG as opposed to the more frequent MG type that occurs in thymitis.[120] Theories attempting to explain the relationship between MG and thymoma include one or more of following: the autosensitization of T lymphocytes to acetylcholine receptors; thymic production of antibodies to acetylcholine receptors; T cell imbalances caused by thymic production of abnormal proportions of thymocytes; abnormal MHC II expression in the thymic stroma with abnormal thymocyte production; or thymic synthesis of hormones such as thymopoietin, which have been shown to bind to acetylcholine receptors and are found at their highest levels when thymoma or thymic hyperplasia is present.[4,121]

Myasthenia gravis

In earlier reviews, a decreased overall survival was observed in patients with MG and thymoma.[3,104] This was likely due to higher perioperative deaths and less effective medical management of these patients. Better control of MG and advances in perioperative management have made the prognosis of a patient with MG equivalent to other patients.[64,108,112,122] However, there are also data suggesting that MG portends a better prognosis. This may be due to earlier detection due to the symptoms of MG[123] yet there is evidence that stage for stage, patients with MG had higher rates of overall survival.[124]

The most common hematological condition associated with thymoma is PRCA. It is found in 5–10% of patients with such neoplasms. Conversely, 30–50% of patients with PRCA are found to have thymoma and approximately one-third will have improvement in their bone marrow function after thymectomy.[125,126] Examination of the bone marrow generally shows a decrease in all three hematopoietic cell lineages, with greatest involvement of the erythroid precursors. The cause of PRCA is thought to be autoimmune. A review of the literature detailed 10 instances of thymoma-associated agranulocytosis since 1967.[127] Three of these cases showed a complete absence of myelopoiesis and the remainder demonstrated promyelocyte arrest. Thymectomy was performed in five patients and was thought to be successful in two. Seven patients had associated hypogammaglobulinemia and two had MG. Four of six cases in which the serum was studied showed *in vitro* inhibition of myeloid colony growth. From this information, it can be speculated that thymoma-related agranulocytosis is also mediated by an autoimmune mechanism.

Another recognized disease association with thymoma is acquired hypogammaglobulinemia. It arises in 5–10% of patients with thymoma. In counterpoint, 10% of patients with hypogammaglobulinemia develop thymomas.[64,116]

Second malignancies

Thymomas appear to be associated with an increased risk of second neoplasms. One retrospective study using SEER data with 1334 patients demonstrated an incidence of second cancers in 11–65% of patients with prior radiation therapy and 12–35% of patients without prior radiotherapy ($p = 0.22$).[128]

Some authors have shown an association of thymoma and secondary tumors (usually malignancies) occurring in about 10–28% of cases.[116,129–131] However, in a more recent study of 2171 patients with thymoma from the SEER database, 306 (14%) had extrathymic malignancies (88 before the diagnosis of thymoma and 206 after the diagnosis). Extrathymic malignancies were significantly higher in patients with thymoma (8224 per 100,000 persons) than in the general population (459 per 100,000 persons; $p < 0.001$).[132] The single most important cancer association with thymoma was with non-Hodgkin lymphoma. The exact cause of this observation is not known but is thought to be due to abnormal regulation of B lymphocyte proliferation by dysfunctional T lymphocytes.

Diagnostic considerations

Imaging
After a general physical examination (with particular attention to the features listed above, including careful examination of the thyroid), plain posteroanterior and lateral chest radiographs should be obtained. These can identify a soft tissue density mass and the lateral chest film may clarify its location within the anterior mediastinum. Serum α-fetoprotein (AFP) and β-human chorionic gonadotropin (hCG) should be performed to rule out primary mediastinal germ cell tumor, particularly in young men presenting with large irregular mediastinal masses. Computed tomography (CT) using contrast should be performed to further define the nature of the lesion (cystic versus solid, the presence of calcium, its origin, and relationship to the surrounding anatomy).[133] Although magnetic resonance imaging (MRI) is more cumbersome and expensive, it is sometimes helpful preoperatively to evaluate neurovascular structures and the presence of invasion. MRI has been useful in distinguishing fibrosis from recurrent tumor and as an adjunct in resolving other confusing CT findings. It is also preferable to obtain an MRI if iodine contrast is contraindicated. Echocardiography (particularly the transesophageal technique) may detect possible cardiac involvement of the tumor.[134]

More recently, fluorodeoxyglucose positron emission tomography (FDG-PET) scans have been utilized and one study showed a high FDG uptake in thymic carcinomas (mean standardized uptake value (SUV) 7.2) with only a moderate uptake in noninvasive and invasive thymomas (mean SUV 3.0 and 3.8, respectively).[135] Routine PET is not recommended as uptake in small tumors and those tumors with low-grade malignancies such as most thymomas is not visualized. In patients with high-grade malignancies, such as thymic carcinoma, metastatic tumors may be ascertained via PET.[136,137]

Obtaining tissue for histological evaluation
Approximately two-thirds of patients with thymic epithelial neoplasms will present with a thymic mass, which on radiographic evaluation appears to be amenable to complete resection.[64,110] Some authors express concern that a biopsy will cause tumor seeding[112] and disruption of the capsule will result in a decreased chance of cure.[138] In circumstances where the tumor cannot be removed *en bloc* and the diagnosis is not readily apparent, a biopsy is required to direct therapeutic decisions. Owing to the many types of masses found in the mediastinum, adequate tissue must be obtained to enable the pathologist to make a proper assessment.

Cytological examination of CT-guided fine needle aspiration biopsies can identify obvious malignancies. Fine needle aspiration has a reported sensitivity and specificity of over 90% in the evaluation of mediastinal masses.[139] Core-cutting needle biopsies are required, however, to further refine the diagnosis of some malignancies, especially lymphoma and thymoma. Immunohistochemical, electron microscopic, and cytogenetic analysis can be employed with the latter procedure to determine the cell of origin. The major risks of these biopsy methods include pneumothorax, hemoptysis, and vascular injury. If the location of the lesion does not permit this approach or adequate tissue cannot be obtained, mediastinoscopy, anterior mediastinotomy, or video-assisted thoracoscopy can be employed.[138] Thoracotomy is occasionally required to procure suitable biopsy material. If thymoma is found, surgery will be required.

Staging
Several staging systems (see Table 20.1) have been described, but only three are in common use. Each has its own advantages and disadvantages. Such schemes were created primarily for thymomas but they are used for thymic carcinomas as well. The paradigm devised by Bergh *et al.*[140] is simple, but it fails to account for the tropism that thymomas have for the pleura and pericardium and their propensity for extrathoracic dissemination. The staging system of Masaoka and colleagues[3] does encompass these patterns of spread as seen with both thymoma and thymic carcinoma. For the most part, it serves as a rational template on which to base therapy. One pitfall is that all lymphatic metastases are grouped as IVb, regardless of whether they are intra- or extrathoracic. The intrathoracic lymph node metastases could generally be treated within a radiation port, but these are still grouped with extrathoracic lymph node metastases that cannot.

Yamakawa along with Masaoka and others proposed a tumor-node-metastasis (TNM) classification which takes these issues into consideration.[115] Involvement of intrathoracic lymph nodes constitutes N1 or N2 disease, but extrathoracic lymph node metastases are classified as N3. The authors contended that the metastatic sequence affected anterior mediastinal lymph nodes before other intrathoracic nodes and finally extrathoracic nodes. Their study of 207 patients was of insufficient size to determine whether the prognosis of patients with stage IVb, T1–2, N1, M0 disease is the same as that of others with stage IVb, Tx N3, and/or M1 lesions. The TNM system may be more applicable to thymic carcinomas because of their greater propensity for metastasis, especially to lymphatics.

Another area of uncertainty is the definition of "invasion." Masaoka *et al.* have described this phenomenon as infiltration of the tumor "into" its capsule.[3] Other investigators observed that recurrence was likely only if a thymoma breached its capsule and involved the mediastinal fat.[141] This distinction is clinically relevant with regard to staging and adjuvant therapy and highlights the fact that staging is based on pathology as well as the surgical assessment. Clarifications of some of the ambiguity of the Masaoka–Koga Staging System are published in a recent article by Detterbeck *et al*.[142]

Haniuda *et al*.[143] have suggested that further modification of the Masaoka system might be useful for stage II cases; these authors proposed appending a "p" designator to describe the precise status of the mediastinal pleura in the specified context. In such a construction, stage II-p0 tumors show no adhesion to the pleura; p1 tumors demonstrate fibrous adhesions between the tumor and pleura without true invasion of the latter structure; and p2 tumors manifest actual pleural infiltration. In their experience, an adverse breakpoint in behavior was seen at the stage II-p1 level (regardless of whether the lesions were stage IIA or IIB), and they therefore recommended adjuvant treatment with irradiation, or chemotherapy, or both at that point. These interventions appear to ameliorate the poorer prognosis that has attended thymomas which could not be completely resected surgically.

The greatest vindication of the Masaoka system is its correlation with therapy and outcome. Specifically, tumors with a low stage that are completely removed have a better prognosis than invasive lesions. As detailed above, histological grade pertains only to carcinomas. The incidence of recurrence that is associated with each stage is considered in many clinico-pathological reviews on thymoma. Caution must be exercised when interpreting such data, however, because the studies are heterogeneous with respect to whether staging was surgical or pathological in nature, and also regarding what adjuvant therapy was given.

The other staging system worth mentioning is the Groupe d'Etudes des Tumeurs Thymiques (GETT) classification (see Table 20.2).[144] It is based on the Masaoka system, as well as selected surgical findings and the extent of surgery that was performed. Some authors have also divided thymomas into "limited" and "extensive," based on whether all disease could be encompassed in a single radiotherapy portal. This may become more common parlance if combined modality therapy (radiation and chemotherapy) is proven to have a role.

Treatment

It must be kept in mind that thymoma and thymic carcinoma are rare disorders and there are no data from randomized controlled trials. Much of the data are conflicting and largely derived from retrospective reviews with different approaches regarding histological classification and treatments. Thymic carcinoma is even more rare with just over 300 cases reported in the literature.[145]

Thymoma

Noninvasive disease (stage I)
The important clinical questions best answered by the experienced pathologist are the following:
• Is invasion defined as "into" or "through" the capsule?
• Was the whole capsule evaluated for integrity?
• Was a portion of the capsule breached during handling?[146]

There is little doubt that surgery alone is the most effective way of curing a patient with a completely encapsulated tumor without evidence of microscopic invasion.

A median sternotomy incision is most commonly used and there are reports in the literature of video-assisted thorascopy being employed as a diagnostic and staging instrument and as a therapeutic tool if the disease is found to be well encapsulated.[147] The latter must be considered experimental at this stage until long-term results have been published. When the thymoma is laterally displaced, a thoracotomy may be required. It must also be emphasized that the whole thymus is removed at the time of surgery.

For stage I disease, radiation therapy has not been shown to increase survival as adjuvant therapy. One study of 132 stage I patients found a recurrence rate of 1.5%[122] and smaller studies concurred that radiotherapy following complete resection of a stage I thymoma is unlikely to add to overall survival.[123,146,148] Multiple outcome studies have shown that for stage I thymoma, nearly 90% of patients will be alive at 5 years and approximately 80% at 10 years after surgery. Nonetheless, there will occasionally be local recurrences.[122,123,149] Therefore lifelong surveillance is required, even for stage I disease. If the patient is deemed unfit for surgery, radiation therapy alone or observation (for slowly growing tumors) are alternative approaches.[150,151]

Locally invasive disease (stages II and III)
Complete resection
Surgery also plays a key role in locally invasive disease. It has been shown that if the whole tumor can be resected the survival is improved, even if invasion is found to be present.[123,124,144,150] Complete resection may require frozen section control to ensure that margins are clear and at times may require major resection and vascular reconstruction of mediastinal structures. These include lung, pleura, pericardium, and great vessels. For patients with locally advanced disease at the time of preoperative evaluation, the effectiveness of combination chemotherapy (see below) encourages the use of preoperative chemotherapy to downsize the tumor.

Incomplete resection
If residual disease remains after surgery, radiotherapy has been employed to maximize the chance of local control. In one report, CR with a mean dose of 50 Gy was obtained in approximately 80% of cases, and 80% of these patients have been shown to be disease free at about 9 years.[144] A crude analysis of several retrospective reviews comprising 225 patients with incomplete resection or unresectable tumors revealed a more pessimistic picture.[151] Thirty-five percent of cases developed local relapse.

There are two controversial issues in the scenario of incomplete resection. The first is, does the extent of surgery impact on survival? It has been established, as detailed above, that complete resection if at all possible does improve survival. However, retrospective series of patients with invasive disease report that radiotherapy after biopsy results in similar 5-year survival rates as debulking surgery (with residual disease) followed by radiation therapy.[152,153] Other studies have shown that partial resection and radiation portends a better prognosis than biopsy and radiation therapy.[122,123,144,150] For the reason that complete resection of tumor is important, for patients in whom doubt exists about the ability to conduct an R0 resection, preoperative chemotherapy should be strongly considered to downsize the tumor and potentially facilitate the resection.

Adjuvant radiotherapy for completely resected stage II tumors of the higher risk WHO subtypes B2, B3 and C is advocated by many authors.[149,154] In one review of eight series with a combined total of 115 completely resected stage II patients treated with postoperative radiation, the recurrence rate was decreased from 30% to 5%.[152] However, several more recent publications have disputed the role of adjuvant radiotherapy, especially those with a prior complete resection.[149]

Strobel et al. showed that thymomas of the WHO subtypes A, AB, and B1 in Masaoka stage I and II with R0 tumor resection do not require adjuvant therapy.[155] Kondo and Monden reported one of the largest retrospective series with 1320 patients and found that adjuvant radiation and/or chemotherapy was not helpful in patients with totally resected thymoma or thymic carcinoma.[156] A metaanalysis performed by Korst et al. also supported no benefit for adjuvant radiotherapy in those patients with stage II and III disease who had undergone complete resection though controversy remains in stage III and IV disease.[157,158]

Two additional papers evaluating the role of radiotherapy used data from the SEER database. In one paper by Fernandes et al., 1334 patients with thymoma evaluated from 1973 to 2005 showed no benefit to adjuvant radiotherapy for patients with stage I and IIA disease, with a benefit for overall survival for stage III and IV disease.[128] Forquer and colleagues reviewed 901 cases of thymoma and thymic carcinoma and separated patients into two groups: those with localized and regional disease.[159] The latter group likely included those patients with gross invasion into neighboring structures. The paper showed an adverse outcome with radiotherapy in patients with localized disease. Though a suggestion of some benefit was seen in patients with regional disease, no benefit was seen in those patients undergoing extirpative surgery.[159] In summary, current data suggest no role for adjuvant radiation in completely resected early-stage disease. For individuals undergoing an R0 resection for stage III disease, adjuvant radiotherapy has no proven benefit.

The second area of controversy concerns the optimal dose of radiation. Reported radiotherapy doses range from 30 to 60 Gy in 1.8 or 2.0 cGy fractions over 3–6 weeks. One retrospective study[160] of patients with invasive thymoma correlated doses of radiotherapy after surgery and outcome. Local recurrences at 2 years appeared similar regardless of dose range: 42% (5/12) for those given <48 Gy, 35% (6/17) between 49 and 59 Gy, and 0/3 locally relapsed if given more than 60 Gy. Notably, 21 patients (37.5%) recurred outside the radiation port. For macroscopic residual thymoma, it has been preferred that greater than 50 Gy be given, as less than this dose resulted in a recurrence rate of 34% in 90 patients with residual disease after surgery.[144] Although some investigators continue to do so, there are no data for or against treating a clinically negative supraclavicular fossa with radiation therapy.

The numbers from these series are small and no firm conclusion can be made. However, if one extrapolates data from subclinical breast carcinoma in which a dose–response curve (with 30–35 Gy controlling 60–70% of cases, 40 Gy 80–90%, and 50 Gy controlling greater than 90%[161]) appears to exist, then it is logical to consider higher-dose therapy for thymoma.

Dose fractions and treatment fields should be carefully planned to minimize complications such as fibrosis, pericarditis, and pneumonitis. It must be noted that the retrospective reviews have not demonstrated a consistent survival advantage for patients who received postoperative radiotherapy, despite improvements in local control.[149] This may be because of a selection bias and has not been studied in a prospective manner.

Furthermore, despite the obvious benefits of surgery and radiotherapy, the role of chemotherapy is yet to be answered. Data exist showing that even patients with completely resected stage II and III disease are at risk for relapse despite adjuvant radiotherapy.[162] A retrospective analysis reported that stage III–IV patients treated with local therapy (surgery, radiotherapy) plus cisplatin-based combination chemotherapy were associated with a longer disease-free survival than patients who did not receive chemotherapy.[150] Therefore, chemoradiotherapy after debulking surgery may have a role in this setting and a discussion regarding this is detailed below.

Local therapy for recurrent thymoma and/or metastatic thymoma

After primary local therapy, thymoma may recur with thoracic (pulmonary or pleural metastases) and/or extrathoracic disease. Given the indolent nature of the disease, with relatively long progression-free survival, surgical excision of recurrent disease is a reasonable approach in selected patients. Following surgery alone for recurrent disease, there are reports of patients free of disease up to 13 years.[149,163] There is some evidence that surgery provides a better survival than radiation in this setting.[149] If surgery is not possible and there has been no prior radiotherapy or the tissue tolerance allows, radiotherapy can be instituted for intrathoracic recurrences, with one study showing six of 10 patients alive at 7 years.[164]

In multifocal or extensive local recurrences, chemotherapy alone or followed by surgery or radiation therapy to residual disease is a reasonable therapeutic approach. This approach allows an in vivo evaluation of the sensitivity of the tumor to chemotherapy and may facilitate surgery. It should be noted that distant recurrences (intrathoracic pleural and extrathoracic) carry a worse prognosis than local recurrence, but that survival may be more dependent upon the intrinsic biology of the tumor as many patients with advanced disease may live decades with periodic systemic treatments.[149]

Chemotherapy for the treatment of thymoma and thymic carcinoma

Retrospective reviews show that 20–30% of patients may be candidates for systemic therapy at initial presentation. Relatively few prospective trials have been initiated to evaluate the role of chemotherapy in thymic malignancies. Any comments, however, must be prefaced by the knowledge that the optimal regimen and timing of chemotherapy has not yet been determined and enrollment in a clinical trial is still the favored approach. Availabe data can be divided into single-agent chemotherapy, combination chemotherapy, chemoradiotherapy, and corticosteroid and cytokine therapy.

Single-agent chemotherapy

The data from single-agent chemotherapy evaluations are limited to just a few small prospective trials, multiple case reports, and reviews. These limitations are compounded by the fact that most patients had differing regimens and/or had prior therapy. The most active agents appear to be cisplatin,[165] corticosteroids,[166,167] doxorubicin[168] and alkylating agents, but the activity of single agents remains limited.

The enthusiasm for cisplatin was based on case reports from 1973, in which objective remissions were observed and one response was maintained for more than 12 months.[165] This was followed up 20 years later with a study of cisplatin (50 mg/m^{-2}) given every 3 weeks in 20 patients with metastatic or recurrent thymoma.[165] Fifteen had received prior radiotherapy and three had received prior chemotherapy. Only two (10%) patients had a partial response, eight (44%) had stable disease and the remainder progressed.

Ifosfamide was evaluated in 15 patients with invasive thymoma by Highley et al.[169] Two different regimens of ifosfamide were given and 13 patients were assessable for response. Five patients had a complete response; one patient had a partial response. The median duration of complete response was 66+ months and the estimated survival rate at 5 years was 57%.

Pemetrexed was evaluated in 27 previously treated patients (16 thymoma and 11 thymic carcinoma). Two complete and two partial responses were observed among the patients with thymoma, and one partial response in a patient with thymic carcinoma was noted. The median overall survival was 29 months for all patients.[170]

Results of several agents from smaller series or case reports are worth mentioning. Suramin has been detailed in a case report to bring about a partial response for 8 months in a patient who had been treated with two previous courses of combination chemotherapy.[171] Doxorubicin as a single agent has been reported to result in two partial responses in three patients evaluated[166] and maytansine has resulted in five partial responses in seven patients.[168,172,173]

Other single agents that have been reported in series of two or more patients with no significant responses have included cyclophosphamide,[168,174] dacarbazine,[174] asparaginase,[175] azac-itidine,[175] chlorambucil,[168] chlormethine,[168] and vincristine.[176] Trials with targeted agents such as gefitinib, erlotinib plus bevacizumab, or imatinib have not shown major activity in multipatient trials.[177–181,183]

Because malignant thymic tumors were shown to express EGFR, gefitinib (an EGFR tyrosine kinase inhibitor) has been studied in patients with advanced thymic malignancies. This study included 26 previously treated patients and although the treatment was tolerable, only one patient had a partial response (response duration of 5 months) and 14 patients had stable disease. Five patient samples were analyzed for the EGFR

mutation and the mutation did not seem to be present in this small group of patients.[184] At least two investigators have found three partial responses with cetuximab in patients with recurrent thymoma.[185,186]

The histone deacetylase inhibitor belinostat was evaluated in 41 previously treated patients with thymoma ($n=25$) and thymic carcinoma ($n=16$). Two patients with thymoma achieved a partial response (8%), with 25 patients having stable disease. The median times for progression and survival were 5.8 and 19.1 months respectively.[187]

Isolated reports have demonstrated activity with a variety of targeted agents such as sorafenib, sunitinib, cixutumamab, cetuximab, and octreotide.[188] One case report[189] documented the ability of octreotide combined with prednisone to induce a CR in a patient with thymoma and PRCA who failed to respond to chemotherapy. This spurred a study of octreotide analogs with prednisone in advanced chemotherapy-refractory thymic tumors.[190] This study of 16 patients showed an overall response rate of 37%, with one patient with a complete response and five patients with partial responses. Median survival was 15 months. This combination had few side-effects and could be considered an effective palliative treatment in previously treated, refractory disease. The Eastern Cooperative Oncology Group conducted a phase 2 trial with octreotide with high-dose prednisone (0.6 mg/kg/day) for those not having a clear partial response after 2 months of octreotide therapy. Only four partial responses were seen in the first 2 months of octreotide alone, but ultimately two complete and 10 partial responses were seen in the group when prednisone was added (CR + PR = 32%).[189,191]

Combination chemotherapy

The optimal regimen has not been determined and the following is a review of the major studies. A summary of the other studies conducted can be found in Table 20.3.

Cisplatin (50 mg/m^{-2}), doxorubicin (50 mg/m^{-2}), and cyclophosphamide (500 mg/m^{-2}), or "PAC," was evaluated as a combination in 30 patients with metastatic disease, recurrent disease, or disease that could not be encompassed by one radiotherapy portal.[177] This group of patients received a mean of six cycles: three patients had complete responses, 12 had partial responses and 10 had stable disease. Median duration of response was 11.8 months and median survival was 37.7 months. Another Intergroup trial involved 23 patients with limited-stage unresectable thymoma (Masaoka stage III) who received 2–4 cycles of PAC followed by radiotherapy.[192] In this study, there were five CRs and 11 PRs to chemotherapy (70% response rate) with a median survival of 93 months. Five-year survival was 52.5%. Case reports have also described durable second remissions being obtained with this combination despite having been treated with these agents in the past.[193]

In a neoadjuvant setting, investigators treated patients with unresectable thymoma (Masaoka stage III or IVA) with three cycles of induction chemotherapy with PAC plus prednisone, followed by surgery and then radiotherapy.[194] These patients then went on to receive three more cycles of chemotherapy. There were 12 evaluable patients, and 11 patients underwent surgical resection. Among the 12 patients, response to inducion

Table 20.3 Results of chemotherapy in patients with thymoma.

Drug	Number of patients	Response*	Reference
Single agent			
Asparaginase	2	0	Chahinian et al.[175]
Azactidine	1	0	Chahinian et al.[175]
Belinostat	41	2	Giaccone et al.[187]
Chlorambucil	4	0	Boston[168]
Chlormethine	2	0	Boston[168]
Corticosteroids	13	3CR, 8PR	Hu and Levine[166]
Cisplatin	21	2PR	Bonomi et al.[165]
	5	3CR, 2PR	Harper and Addis [226]
	2	0	Donovan et al.[174]
Cyclophosphamide	3	0	Boston[168]
			Donovan et al.[174]
Dacarbazine	2	0	Donovan et al.[174]
Doxorubicin	2	0	Harper and Addis[226]
Docetaxel	1	1PR	Oguri et al.[211]
Erlotinib	1	1PR	Christodoulou et al.[212]
Ifosfamide	13	5CR, 1PR	Highley et al.[210]
Imatinib	33	2PR,	Strobel et al.[97]
			Buti et al.[213]
			Salter et al.[179]
			Giaccone et al.[178]
			Palmieri et al.[183]
Interleukin-2	1	1CR	Berthaud et al.[202]
	14	0	Gordon et al.[203]
Maytansine	7	5PR	Boston[168]
			Jaffrey[173]
			Chahinian et al.[175]
Pemetrexed	23	2CR, 2PR	Loehrer et al.[170]
Suramin	1	1PR	LaRocca et al.[171]
Vincristine	2	0	Stolinsky et al.[176]
Combination chemotherapy			
Noncisplatin-containing regimens			
Chlormethine, vincristine, procarbazine, vinblastine	2	1PR	Stolinsky et al.[176]
Cyclophosphamide, doxorubicin	1	1CR	Butler et al.[214]
Cyclophosphamide, doxorubicin, vincristine	2	2CR	Loehrer et al.[215]
	5	2CR, 3PR	Kosmidis et al.[216]
Cyclophosphamide, doxorubicin, vincristine, prednisone (CHOP)	13	5CR	Goldel et al.[217]
CHOP and cisplatin, etoposide	1	0	Hu and Levine[166]
Cyclophosphamide, vincristine, procarbazine, prednisone	5	0CR, 4PR	Evans et al.[218]
Lomustine, cyclophosphamide, vincristine, prednisone	9	4CR, 1PR	Daugaard et al.[219]
Cisplatin-containing regimens			
Cisplatin, doxorubicin	3	3CR	Klipstein et al.[220]
	9	1CR, 5PR	Mitrou et al.[221]
Cisplatin, doxorubicin, cyclophosphamide	30	3CR, 10PR	Loehrer et al.[177]
	1	1CR	Fornasiero et al.[222]
	23	5CR, 11PR	Loehrer et al.[192]
	1	1CR	Campbell et al.[223]
Cisplatin, doxorubicin, cyclophosphamide ± prednisone	22	3CR, 14PR	Kim et al.[194]
Cisplatin, etoposide, ifosfamide	28	0CR, 9PR	Loehrer et al.[197]
Cisplatin, doxorubicin, vincristine, cyclophosphamide	32	15CR, 14PR	Fornasiero et al.[195]
	16	7CR, 5PR	Rea et al.[200]
Cisplatin, doxorubicin, prednisone, bleomycin	9	1CR, 5PR	Chahinian et al.[224,225]
Cisplatin, etoposide	1	1PR	Harper and Addis[226]
	1	0	Hu and Levine[166]
	16	5CR, 1PR	Giaccone et al.[196]
Cisplatin, epirubicin, etoposide	7	4CR, 3PR	Macchiarini et al.[199]
Cisplatin, vinblastine, bleomycin	4	2CR, 1PR	Dy et al.[227]
Carboplatin, paclitaxel	44	3CR, 11PR	Lemma et al.[198]
	11	4PR	Igawa et al.[228]

*CR, complete remission; PR, partial remission.

chemotherapy revealed a 92% RR, with three CRs and eight partial responses. Two of the three CRs had 100% tumor necrosis at the time of resection, confirming the efficacy of chemotherapy.

Adriamycin (40 mg/m^{-2}), cisplatin (50 mg/m^{-2}), and cyclophosphamide (700 mg/m^{-2}) have been combined with vincristine (0.6 mg/m^{-2}) (ADOC) in a single-institution study of 37 patients with stage III or IV disease.[195] Responses were observed in 91.8% of patients with a 43% CR rate. The median durations of response and survival were 12 months and 15 months, respectively. The complete responses lasted for a median of 27 months and the partial responses lasted for 9.5 months. In this study etoposide, ifosfamide, and cisplatin used in combination as second-line therapy resulted in stable disease for 2 months and 6 months, in two out of three patients who relapsed.

The European Organization for Research and Treatment of Cancer (EORTC) evaluated the regimen of cisplatin (60 mg/m^{-2}) and etoposide (120 mg/m^{-2}).[196] Sixteen patients with metastatic or recurrent disease received a mean of six cycles and five CRs were noted with four partial responses (RR of 56%). A median response duration of 3.4 years was seen with a median survival of 4.3 years. Results of an Eastern Cooperative Group-coordinated intergroup trial evaluating etoposide, ifosfamide, and cisplatin (VIP) produced six partial responses out of 14 patients (43%). This study suggests that ifosfamide does not add to the combination of cisplatin and etoposide.[197] The Eastern Cooperative Oncology Group recently published a multicenter trial using carboplatin (AUC = 6) plus paclitaxel (225 mg/m^{-2}) in previously untreated patients with thymoma ($n = 21$) or thymic carcinoma ($n = 23$). Only three CRs and six partial responses were seen in the thymoma group (42.9%) and 5 partial responses in the thymic carcinoma cohort (21.7%).[198]

In summary, thymic malignancies respond to a broad range of systemic agents. Combination chemotherapy provides the highest response rates, but is not curative. Cumulative data strongly suggest that nonanthracycline-containing regimens produce inferior response rates compared to anthracycline-based regimens. In the salvage setting a number of different agents have activity (see Table 20.3).

Chemoradiotherapy

The concept of combined modality therapy is attractive for locally advanced thymoma and thymic carcinoma. Although several investigators have reported the feasibility and outcome of patients treated with chemoradiotherapy, there are no prospective randomized trials defining the optimal management of patients with locally advanced disease. Patients in whom a complete resection is accomplished appear to have a prolonged survival over patients with incomplete resection. Chemotherapy used in a neoadjuvant setting may enable a complete resection where it was not previously feasible or facilitate a surgery which is less morbid.[199]

The approach of preoperative radiotherapy was first reported by Macchiarini and colleagues. Three cycles of cisplatin, epirubicin, and etoposide were given in a neoadjuvant setting to seven patients with clinical stage III disease. All patients had a partial response following chemotherapy and underwent surgery, with four patients undergoing complete resection (two patients had microscopic disease and one had gross residual disease).[199] Similar results were then reported in another study of 16 patients with stage III and IVa, treated with cisplatin, doxorubicin, vincristine, and cyclophosphamide every 3 weeks for three or four cycles.[200] Postoperative radiation was given only if there was residual disease. If only fibrosis was present, the surgery was followed by three additional cycles of chemotherapy. Chemotherapy resulted in seven CRs and five partial responses. All patients received postoperative radiotherapy and the authors reported a projected 2-year survival of 80%.

A third study investigated three cycles of induction chemotherapy (PAC) combined with prednisone in 13 patients with stage III or IVa disease.[194] Twelve patients were evaluable for response: three had complete responses and eight had partial responses. Eleven patients had surgical resection, with complete resection in nine patients. Postoperative radiotherapy was given and followed by three cycles of consolidation chemotherapy. With a median follow-up of 43 months, all patients were alive, two with disease, and there was no excess morbidity despite the combination of three modes of therapy. These studies suggest that neoadjuvant chemotherapy with postoperative radiotherapy is a feasible approach.

A prospective intergroup trial of combined modality therapy in 23 patients with unresectable locally advanced disease was reported. Five complete and 11 partial responses were achieved with 2–4 cycles of PAC followed by 54 Gy of radiation therapy in 23 patients. The overall response rate was 69.6%.[164] The progression-free and overall survival rates at 5 years were 54.3% and 52.5% respectively. It should be noted that only four patients underwent major debulking prior to initiating chemotherapy. There are limitations, outlined in the paper, which prevent any definite conclusions. Specifically, the 95% confidence limits overlie the results of studies of radiotherapy as monotherapy; there may be as effective, if not more effective, regimens that are less toxic (i.e. radiation without an anthracycline).

Other agents

Responses to corticosteroid therapy have been reported in the literature. These are case reports or small retrospective reviews of patients with recurrent or metastatic disease.[166,201] This activity is thought to be due to a lympholytic effect against the lymphocyte component as the responses are usually brief in nature. There is no precedent to suggest that steroids would be active against the true malignant portion of thymomas, the epithelium. Unless the lymphocytes shown to be involved in the tumorigenesis or steroids are proven to be active against the epithelial malignancy, there is no primary role for corticosteroids at this time. However, in end-stage disease, corticosteroids may be used with palliative intent.

Interleukin-2 has been observed to bring about a CR in one patient who had been treated with prior chemotherapy.[202] A follow-up study of interleukin-2 in 14 relapsed or refractory patients did not reveal any response.[203] Further investigation with this drug is probably not warranted.

Thymic carcinoma

Most patients with thymic carcinoma present with locally advanced and/or metastatic disease. Sparse data exist regarding the optimal treatment of these patients. Most publications have employed the same approach used for the treatment of thymoma (surgery, radiation and chemotherapy). There is no reason to think that the principle of a multimodality approach should not apply to thymic carcinoma.[113,204–206]

Metastatic thymic carcinoma has been reported to respond to combination chemotherapy. In one series three out of five patients had responses to bleomycin, etoposide, and cisplatin with a median duration of remission of approximately 12 months.[207] Another small series found that two out of four patients responded to cyclophosphamide, doxorubicin, and vincristine.[67] A third series reported clinical response to cisplatin, doxorubicin, vincristine and cyclophosphamide (ADOC) with six partial remissions in eight treated patients with a median survival time of 19 months.[208] Three patients with thymic carcinoma were included in a prospective intergroup trial which evaluated cisplatin, doxorubicin, and cyclophosphamide (PAC) for thymoma.[192] One out of the three patients responded. The only retrospective review which investigated whether chemotherapy was beneficial found no survival advantage.[24]

One of the largest prospective trials in advanced thymic carcinoma was published by Lemma *et al.* who evaluated carboplatin plus paclitaxel.[198] In 23 patients, only five patients had a partial response (objective response rate 21.7%, 90% confidence interval (CI) 9–40.4%). However, the conclusions from this study are limited by the fact that the numbers were small and it was arbitrary as to which patients received chemotherapy.

Prognosis

The clinicopathological retrospective reviews are the best resource for determining the prognosis of various stages. It must be realized that some of the older data are flawed by the inclusion of patients with thymic carcinoma and that survival rates have been altered by improvements in perioperative care, especially of patients with MG.[11] Table 20.4 is from a series which covers a timespan of nearly four decades. The treatment for most cases has always been surgery, but refinements in radiation therapy and chemotherapy since the 1980s may have improved the outcome of patients with advanced disease that is not apparent from these data. Although there is some contention on whether to treat based on stage and histology type, the data from this are not strong and the one factor that has consistently been shown to be a prognostic factor useful for directing therapy is the stage of the tumor. Histology may have a limited role in prognosis. For example, stage I cortical thymoma is the only scenario for which one study has

Table 20.4 Survival for thymoma and thymic carcinoma.

Disease	3-year survival (%)	5-year survival (%)	10-year survival (%)
Thymoma	–	–	–
Stage I	–	94	75
Stage II	–	91	65
Stage III	–	70	50
Stage IV	–	38–56	10–30
Thymic carcinoma*	45	35	–

* Median survival 20 months.

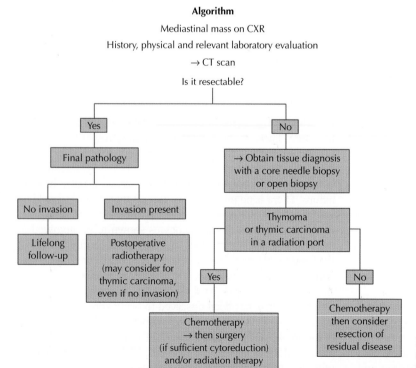

Algorithm

Mediastinal mass on CXR

History, physical and relevant laboratory evaluation

→ CT scan

Is it resectable?

Yes — Final pathology — No invasion — Lifelong follow-up / Invasion present — Postoperative radiotherapy (may consider for thymic carcinoma, even if no invasion)

No — → Obtain tissue diagnosis with a core needle biopsy or open biopsy — Thymoma or thymic carcinoma in a radiation port — Yes — Chemotherapy → then surgery (if sufficient cytoreduction) and/or radiation therapy / No — Chemotherapy then consider resection of residual disease

Figure 20.11 A suggested algorithm to guide the evaluation and management of a patient with a mediastinal mass who is found to have a thymoma or thymic carcinoma.

suggested the need for a change in therapy. It is argued that the prognosis is similar for patients with stage II and III mixed thymoma and thus patients may benefit from postoperative radiation therapy.[57]

Clinicopathological observations other than invasion which appear to be associated with a poor prognosis for patients with thymoma include the presence of tumor-related symptoms and signs at diagnosis, size greater than 15 cm, age under 30 years at diagnosis, and microscopic predominance of epithelial cells.[64,150,209]

Recommendations

Upon the diagnosis of an anterior mediastinal mass, it is our practice to obtain serum β-hCG, lactate dehydrogenase, and AFP to first rule out a germ cell tumor (Fig. 20.11). When suspicions of a thymic malignancy are high, an initial assessment of the surgical resectability should be made. For larger masses, a core biopsy should be performed, preferably without violation of the pleural space. If the mass is resectable, surgery is recommended. Histological evaluation by an experienced pathologist is necessary to obtain the correct diagnosis and to determine clear margins and the presence of local/capsular invasion.

If invasion through the capsule is noted, postoperative radiation therapy should be considered, especially for those patients with thymoma and positive surgical margins. The role of postoperative radiation therapy for patients with stage II and III thymoma and clear surgical margins is controversial. If clean surgical margins are seen, postoperative radiotherapy does not appear to improve prognosis. Postoperative radiation therapy should also be considered in all cases of thymic carcinoma, as most patients present with locally advanced disease.

Patients with unresectable thymic tumors should undergo core needle biopsy or open biopsy to confirm tissue diagnosis. For these tumors, neoadjuvant chemotherapy should be given, followed by consideration of surgical resection (or radiation for unresectable disease). For patients with advanced thymic malignancies, initial therapy should be anthracycline based (e.g. PAC, ADOC, CEE) which appears to provide the highest chance for objective response. In the salvage setting, strong consideration should be given to clinical trial or single-agent therapy. As many patients have an indolent course with or without chemotherapy, consideration for quality of life, with limitations of therapy, should be made. Because of the lack of data from adequately sized prospective studies, strong consideration should be given to referral to an academic center for enrollment on a clinical trial.

References

1. Engels EA, Pfeiffer RM. Malignant thymoma in the United States: demographic patterns in incidence and associations with subsequent malignancies. Int J Cancer 2003; 105: 546–51.
2. Levine GD, Rosai J. Thymic hyperplasia and neoplasia: a review of current concepts. Hum Pathol 1978; 9: 495–515.
3. Masaoka A, et al. Follow-up study of thymomas with special reference to their clinical stages. Cancer 1981; 48: 2485–92.
4. Muller-Hermelink HK, et al. Characterization of the human thymic microenvironment: lymphoepithelial interaction in normal thymus and thymoma. Arch Histol Cytol 1997; 60: 9–28.
5. Skandalakis JEGS, Todd NW. Embryology for Surgeons, 2nd edn. Baltimore, MD: Williams and Wilkins, 1994.
6. Marino M, Muller-Hermelink HK. Thymoma and thymic carcinoma. Relation of thymoma epithelial cells to the cortical and medullary differentiation of thymus. Virchows Arch A Pathol Anat Histopathol 1985; 407: 119–49.
7. Van de Wijngaert FP, et al. Heterogeneity of epithelial cells in the human thymus. An ultrastructural study. Cell Tissue Res 1984; 237: 227–37.
8. Sprent J, Kishimoto H. T cell tolerance and the thymus. Ann N Y Acad Sci 1998; 841: 236–45.
9. Mizuno T, Hashimoto T, Masaoka A. Distribution of fibronectin and laminin in human thymoma. Cancer 1990; 65: 1367–74.
10. Lauriola L, et al. Human thymoma: immunologic characteristics of the lymphocytic component. Cancer 1981; 48: 1992–5.
11. Bernatz PE, et al. Thymoma: factors influencing prognosis. Surg Clin North Am 1973; 53: 885–92.
12. Rouse RV, Weiss LM. Human thymomas: evidence of immunohistologically defined normal and abnormal microenvironmental differentiation. Cell Immunol 1988; 111: 94–106.
13. Chilosi M, et al. Immunohistochemical evidence of active thymocyte proliferation in thymoma. Its possible role in the pathogenesis of autoimmune diseases. Am J Pathol 1987; 128: 464–70.
14. Zettl A, et al. Recurrent genetic aberrations in thymoma and thymic carcinoma. Am J Pathol 2000; 157: 257–66.
15. Zhou R, et al. Thymic epithelial tumors can develop along two different pathogenetic pathways. Am J Pathol 2001; 159: 1853–60.
16. Inoue M, et al. Chromosome 6 suffers frequent and multiple aberrations in thymoma. Am J Pathol 2002; 161: 1507–13.
17. Cin PD, DeWolf-Peeters C, Deneffe G. Thymoma with a t(15;22) (p11;q11). Cancer Genetics Cytogen 1996; 89: 181–183.
18. Kuzume T, et al. Establishment and characterization of a thymic carcinoma cell line (Ty-82) carrying t(15;19)(q15;p13) chromosome abnormality. Int J Cancer 1992; 50: 259–64.
19. Lee AC, et al. Disseminated mediastinal carcinoma with chromosomal translocation (15;19). A distinctive clinicopathologic syndrome. Cancer 1993; 72: 2273–6.
20. Kees UR, Mulcahy MT, Willoughby ML. Intrathoracic carcinoma in an 11-year-old girl showing a translocation t(15;19). Am J Pediatr Hematol Oncology 1991; 13: 459–464.
21. Kubonishi I, et al. Novel t(15;19) (q15;p13) chromosome abnormality in a thymic carcinoma. Cancer Res 1991; 51: 3327–3328.
22. Toretsky JA, et al. Translocation (11;15;19): a highest specific chromosome rearrangement associated with poorly differentiated thymic carcinoma in young patients. Am J Clin Oncol 2003; 26(3): 300–306.
23. Kirchner T, et al. Well-differentiated thymic carcinoma. An organotypical low-grade carcinoma with relationship to cortical thymoma. Am J Surg Pathol 1992; 16: 1153–69.
24. Suster S, Rosai J. Thymic carcinoma. A clinicopathologic study of 60 cases. Cancer 1991; 67: 1025–32.
25. Kuo TT, Chan JK. Thymic carcinoma arising in thymoma is associated with alterations in immunohistochemical profile. Am J Surg Pathol 1998; 22: 1474–81.
26. Suster S, Moran CA. Primary thymic epithelial neoplasms: spectrum of differentiation and histological features. Semin Diagn Pathol 1999; 16: 2–17.
27. Hasserjian RP, Klimstra DS, Rosai J. Carcinoma of the thymus with clear-cell features. Report of eight cases and review of the literature. Am J Surg Pathol 1995; 19: 835–41.
28. Patton DF, et al. Thymic carcinoma with a defective Epstein–Barr virus encoding the BZLF1 trans-activator. J Infect Dis 1994; 170: 7–12.
29. Wu TC, Kuo TT. Study of Epstein–Barr virus early RNA 1 (EBER1) expression by in situ hybridization in thymic epithelial tumors of Chinese patients in Taiwan. Hum Pathol 1993; 24: 235–8.
30. Teoh R, et al. Increased incidence of thymoma in Chinese myasthenia gravis: possible relationship with Epstein–Barr virus. Acta Neurol Scand 1989; 80: 221–5.
31. Meyer M, et al. Lack of evidence for Epstein-Barr virus infection in myasthenia gravis thymus. Annal Neurol 2011; 70(3): 515–518.

32. Dimery IW, *et al*. Association of the Epstein–Barr virus with lymphoepithelioma of the thymus. Cancer 1988; 61: 2475–80.

33. Imanishi TGT. Diversity in human MHC genes among ethnic groups worldwide. In: Tajima KSS (ed) *Ethnoepidemiology of Cancer*. Tokyo, Japan: Scientific Societies Press, 1996. pp. 89–96.

34. Clark S. The intrathymic environment. In: Davies AJSCR (ed) *Contemporary Topics in Immunobiology*. New York: Plenum Press, 1973. pp. 77–9.

35. Shier KJ. The morphology of the epithelial thymus. Observations on lymphocyte-depleted and fetal thymus. Lab Invest 1963; 12: 316–26.

36. Shier KJ. The thymus according to Schambacher: medullary ducts and reticular epithelium of thymus and thymomas. Cancer 1981; 48: 1183–99.

37. Wick M. Mediastinum. In: Sternberg SS (ed) *Diagnostic Surgical Pathology*, 2nd edn. New York: Raven Press, 1994. pp. 1125–82.

38. Moran CA, *et al*. Thymomas presenting as pleural tumors. Report of eight cases. Am J Surg Pathol 1992; 16: 138–44.

39. Rosai J, Limas C, Husband EM. Ectopic hamartomatous thymoma. A distinctive benign lesion of lower neck. Am J Surg Pathol 1984; 8: 501–13.

40. Yeoh CB, *et al*. Intrapulmonary thymoma. J Thorac Cardiovasc Surg 1966; 51: 131–6.

41. Asa SL, *et al*. Primary thyroid thymoma: a distinct clinicopathologic entity. Hum Pathol 1988; 19: 1463–7.

42. Chan JK, Rosai J. Tumors of the neck showing thymic or related branchial pouch differentiation: a unifying concept. Hum Pathol 1991; 22: 349–67.

43. Suster S, Rosai J. Cystic thymomas. A clinicopathologic study of ten cases. Cancer 1992; 69: 92–7.

44. Muller-Hermelink HK, Marino M, Palestro G. Pathology of thymic epithelial tumors. Curr Top Pathol 1986; 75: 207–68.

45. Rosai J, Levine GD. Tumors of the thymus pathology. In: Hartmann WH (ed) *Atlas of Tumor Pathology*, Fascicle 13, Series 2. Washington, DC: Armed Forces Institute of Pathology, 1976. pp. 10–150.

46. Shimosato Y, Mukai K. Tumors of the thymus and mediastinum. In: Rosai J (ed) *Atlas of Tumor Pathology*. Washington, DC: Armed Forces Institute of Pathology, 1997. pp. 233–273.

47. Wick MRSR, Niehans GA, Scheithauer BW. Anterior mediastinal tumors: a clinicopathologic study of 100 cases, with emphasis on immunohistochemical analysis. Prog Surg Pathol 1990; 11: 79–119.

48. Chalabreysse L, *et al*. Correlation of the WHO schema for the classification of thymic epithelial neoplasms with prognosis: a retrospective study of 90 tumors. Am J Surg Pathol 2002; 26: 1605–11.

49. Chen G, *et al*. New WHO histologic classification predicts prognosis of thymic epithelial tumors: a clinicopathologic study of 200 thymoma cases from China. Cancer 2002; 95: 420–9.

50. Nakagawa K, *et al*. Thymoma: a clinicopathologic study based on the new World Health Organization classification. J Thorac Cardiovasc Surg 2003; 126: 1134–40.

51. Okumura M, *et al*. The World Health Organization histologic classification system reflects the oncologic behavior of thymoma: a clinical study of 273 patients. Cancer 2002; 94: 624–32.

52. Rieker RJHJ, *et al*. Histologic classification of thymic epithelial tumors: comparison of established classification schemes. Int J Cancer 2002; 98: 900–6.

53. Bernatz PE, Harrison EG, Clagett OT. Thymoma: a clinicopathologic study. J West Soc Periodontol Periodontal Abstr 1961; 42: 424–44.

54. Jain RK, *et al*. WHO types A and AB thymomas: not always benign. Mod Pathol 2010; 23(12): 1641–9.

55. Muller-Hermelink HK, Marx A. Pathological aspects of malignant and benign thymic disorders. Ann Med 1999; 2(Suppl 31): 5–14.

56. Dawson A, Ibrahim NB, Gibbs AR. Observer variation in the histopathological classification of thymoma: correlation with prognosis. J Clin Pathol 1994; 47: 519–23.

57. Quintanilla-Martinez L, *et al*. Thymoma. Histologic subclassification is an independent prognostic factor. Cancer 1994; 74: 606–17.

58. Ho FCFK, *et al*. Evaluation of a histogenetic classification for thymic epithelial tumors. Histopathology 1982; 25: 21–9.

59. Snover DC, Levine GD, Rosai J. Thymic carcinoma. Five distinctive histological variants. Am J Surg Pathol 1982; 6: 451–70.

60. Walker AN, Mills SE, Fechner RE. Thymomas and thymic carcinomas. Semin Diagn Pathol 1990; 7: 250–65.

61. McCart JA, *et al*. Predictors of survival following surgical resection of thymoma. J Surg Oncol 1993; 54: 233–8.

62. Morgenthaler TI, *et al*. Thymoma. Mayo Clin Proc 1993; 68: 1110–23.

63. Wick MR. Assessing the prognosis of thymomas. Ann Thorac Surg 1990; 50: 521–2.

64. Lewis JE, *et al*. Thymoma. A clinicopathologic review. Cancer 1987; 60: 2727–43.

65. Iezzoni JC, Nass LB. Thymic basaloid carcinoma: a case report and review of the literature. Mod Pathol 1996; 9: 21–5.

66. Moran CA, Suster S. Mucoepidermoid carcinomas of the thymus. A clinicopathologic study of six cases. Am J Surg Pathol 1995; 19: 826–34.

67. Shimizu J, *et al*. Primary thymic carcinoma: a clinicopathological and immunohistochemical study. J Surg Oncol 1994; 56: 159–64.

68. Dadmanesh F, Sekihara T, Rosai J. Histologic typing of thymoma according to the new World Health Organization classification. Chest Surg Clin North Am 2001; 11: 407–20.

69. Talwar J, Talwar V, Vaid AK. Thymic carcinoma presenting as myasthenia gravis. JIACM 2004; 5(4): 354–6.

70. Schmidt S, Padberg F. Late onset immunodeficiency in a patient with recurrent thymic carcinoma and myasthenia gravis. J Neurosci 1998; 157: 201–5.

71. Katzberg H, Miller RG, Katz J. Thymic carcinoma in myasthenia gravis developing years after thymectomy. Muscle Nerve 2009; 40: 137–8.

72. Morrison IM. Tumours and cysts of the mediastinum. Thorax 1958; 13: 294–307.

73. Kuo TT, *et al*. Thymic carcinomas: histopathological varieties and immunohistochemical study. Am J Surg Pathol 1990; 14: 24–34.

74. Wick MR, *et al*. Primary thymic carcinomas. Am J Surg Pathol 1982; 6: 613–30.

75. Weiss LM, Gaffey MJ, Shibata D. Lymphoepithelioma-like carcinoma and its relationship to Epstein–Barr virus. Am J Clin Pathol 1991; 96: 156–8.

76. Truong LD, *et al*. Thymic carcinoma. A clinicopathologic study of 13 cases. Am J Surg Pathol 1990; 14: 151–66.

77. Wick MR, *et al*. Clear cell neoplasms of the endocrine system and thymus. Semin Diagn Pathol 1997; 14: 183–202.

78. Nishimura M, *et al*. A case of sarcomatoid carcinoma of the thymus. Pathol Int 1997; 47: 260–3.

79. Kuo TT. Carcinoid tumor of the thymus with divergent sarcomatoid differentiation: report of a case with histogenetic consideration. Hum Pathol 1994; 25: 319–23.

80. Paties C, *et al*. Multidirectional carcinoma of the thymus with neuroendocrine and sarcomatoid components and carcinoid syndrome. Pathol Res Pract 1991; 187: 170–7.

81. Wick MR, Swanson PE. Carcinosarcomas: current perspectives and an historical review of nosological concepts. Semin Diagn Pathol 1993; 10: 118–27.

82. Berezowski K, *et al*. CD5 immunoreactivity of epithelial cells in thymic carcinoma and CASTLE using paraffin-embedded tissue. Am J Clin Pathol 1996; 106: 483–6.

83. Hishima T, *et al*. CD5 expression in thymic carcinoma. Am J Pathol 1994; 145: 268–75.

84. Kornstein MJ, Rosai J. CD5 labeling of thymic carcinomas and other non-lymphoid neoplasms. Am J Clin Pathol 1998; 109: 722–6.

85. Tateyama H, *et al*. p53 protein expression and p53 gene mutation in thymic epithelial tumors. An immunohistochemical and DNA sequencing study. Am J Clin Pathol 1995; 104: 375–81.

86. DeLeeuw BSR, *et al*. Distinct Xp11.2 breakpoint regions in synovial sarcoma revealed by metaphase and interphase FISH: relationship to histologic subtypes. Cancer Genet Cytogenet 1994; 73: 89–94.

87. Pollack A, *et al*. Thymoma. The prognostic significance of flow cytometric DNA analysis. Cancer 1992; 69: 1702–9.

88. Asamura H, *et al*. Degree of malignancy of thymic epithelial tumors in terms of nuclear DNA content and nuclear area. An analysis of 39 cases. Am J Pathol 1988; 133: 615–22.

89. Kondo K, *et al*. Activation of matrix metalloproteinase-2 is correlated with invasiveness in thymic epithelial tumors. J Surg Oncol 2001; 76: 169–75.

90. Sogawa K, *et al*. Increased expression of matrix metalloproteinase-2 and tissue inhibitor of metalloproteinase-2 is correlated with poor prognostic variables in patients with thymic epithelial tumors. Cancer 2003; 98: 1822–9.

91. Sasaki H, *et al*. Glycosylphosphatidyl inositol-anchored protein (GPI-80) gene expression is correlated with human thymoma stage. Cancer Sci 2003; 94: 809–13.

92. Puglisi F. p53 protein expression and p53 mutation in thymic epithelial tumors. Am J Clin Pathol 1996; 105: 657–8.

93. Brocheriou I, Carnot F, Briere J. Immunohistochemical detection of bcl-2 protein in thymoma. Histopathology 1995; 27: 251–5.

94. Chan JK, *et al*. The MIC2 antibody 013. Practical application for the study of thymic epithelial tumors. Am J Surg Pathol 1995; 19: 1115–23.

95. Henley JD, Koukoulis GK, Loehrer PJ Sr. Epidermal growth factor receptor expression in invasive thymoma. J Cancer Res Clin Oncol 2002; 128: 167–70.

96. Ionescu DN, *et al*. Protein expression and gene amplification of epidermal growth factor receptor in thymomas. Cancer 2005; 103: 630–6.

97. Strobel P, *et al*. Thymic carcinoma with overexpression of mutated KIT and the response to imatinib. N Engl J Med 2004; 350: 2625–6.

98. Henley JD, Cummings OW, Loehrer PJ Sr. Tyrosine kinase receptor expression in thymomas. J Cancer Res Clin Oncol 2004; 130: 222–4.

99. Laury A, *et al*. A comprehensive analysis of PAX8 expression in human epithelial tumors. Am J Surg Pathol 2011; 35(6): 816–26.

100. Weissferdt A, Moran CA. Pax8 expression in thymic epithelial neoplasms: an immunohistochemical analysis. Am J Surg Pathol 2011; 35(9): 1305–10.

101. French CA. NUT midline carcinoma. Cancer Genet Cytogenet 2010; 203(1): 16–20.

102. Girard N, *et al*. Comprehensive genomic analysis reveals clinically relevant molecular distinctions between thymic carcinomas and thymomas. Clin Cancer Res 2009; 15(22): 6790–9.

103. Strobel P, Hohenberger P, Marx A. Thymoma and thymic carcinoma: Molecular pathology and targeted therapy. J Thoracic Oncol 2010; 5(10): S286–S290.

104. Batata MA, *et al*. Thymomas: clinicopathologic features, therapy, and prognosis. Cancer 1974; 34: 389–96.

105. Legg MA, Brady WJ. Pathology and clinical behavior of thymomas. A survey of 51 cases. Cancer 1965; 18: 1131–44.

106. LeGolvan DP, Abell MR. Thymomas. Cancer 1977; 39: 2142–57.

107. Park HS, *et al*. Thymoma. A retrospective study of 87 cases. Cancer 1994; 73: 2491–8.

108. Pescarmona E, *et al*. Analysis of prognostic factors and clinicopathological staging of thymoma. Ann Thorac Surg 1990; 50: 534–8.

109. Salyer WR, Eggleston JC. Thymoma: a clinical and pathological study of 65 cases. Cancer 1976; 37: 229–49.

110. Verley JM, Hollmann KH. Thymoma. A comparative study of clinical stages, histologic features, and survival in 200 cases. Cancer 1985; 55: 1074–86.

111. Vladislav T, *et al*. Extrathoracic metastases of thymic origin: a review of 35 cases. Mod Pathol 2011; Nov 11 [Epub ahead of print].

112. Wilkins EW Jr, *et al*. J. Maxwell Chamberlain memorial paper. Role of staging in prognosis and management of thymoma. Ann Thorac Surg 1991; 51: 888–92.

113. Hsu CP, *et al*. Thymic carcinoma. Ten years' experience in twenty patients. J Thorac Cardiovasc Surg 1994; 107: 615–20.

114. Yano T, *et al*. Treatment and prognosis of primary thymic carcinoma. J Surg Oncol 1993; 52: 255–8.

115. Yamakawa Y, *et al*. A tentative tumor-node-metastasis classification of thymoma. Cancer 1991; 68: 1984–7.

116. Souadjian JV, *et al*. The spectrum of diseases associated with thymoma. Coincidence or syndrome? Arch Intern Med 1974; 134: 374–9.

117. Wilkins EW Jr. Thymoma. In: Pearson FG *et al*. (eds) *Thoracic Surgery*. New York: Churchill Livingstone, 1995. pp. 1419–27.

118. Blossom GB, *et al*. Thymectomy for myasthenia gravis. Arch Surg 1993; 128: 855–62.

119. Khawaja MR, Nelson RP, Miller N *et al*. Immune-mediated diseases and immunodeficiencies associated with thymic epithelial neoplasms. J Clin Immunol 2012; Jan 8 [Epub ahead of print].

120. Marx A, *et al*. Paraneoplastic autoimmunity in thymus tumors. Dev Immunol 1998; 6: 129–40.

121. Berrih-Aknin S, *et al*. The role of the thymus in myasthenia gravis: immunohistological and immunological studies in 115 cases. Ann N Y Acad Sci 1987; 505: 50–70.

122. Maggi G, *et al*. Thymoma: results of 241 operated cases. Ann Thorac Surg 1991; 51: 152–6.

123. Nakahara K, *et al*. Thymoma: results with complete resection and adjuvant postoperative irradiation in 141 consecutive patients. J Thorac Cardiovasc Surg 1988; 95: 1041–7.

124. Wilkins KB, *et al*. Clinical and pathologic predictors of survival in patients with thymoma. Ann Surg 1999; 230: 562–72; discussion 572–4.

125. Masaoka A, *et al*. Thymomas associated with pure red cell aplasia. Histologic and follow-up studies. Cancer 1989; 64: 1872–8.

126. Zeok JV, *et al*. The role of thymectomy in red cell aplasia. Ann Thorac Surg 1979; 28: 257–60.

127. Yip D, *et al*. Thymoma and agranulocytosis: two case reports and literature review. Br J Haematol 1996; 95: 52–6.

128. Fernandes, AT, *et al*. The role of radiation therapy in malignant thymoma: a surveillance, epidemiology, and end results data analysis. J Thor Oncol 2010; 5: 1454–60.

129. Welsh JS, *et al*. Association between thymoma and second neoplasms. JAMA 2000; 283: 1142–3.

130. Owe JF, Cvancarova M, Romi F, Gilhus NK. Extrathymic malignancies in thymoma patients with and without myasthenia gravis. J Neurosci 2010; 290: 66–9.

131. Gadalla SM, *et al*. A population-based assessment of mortality and morbidity among patients with thymoma. Int J Cancer 2011; 128: 2688–94.

132. Weksler B, *et al*. Thymomas and extrathymic cancers. Ann Thorac Surg 2011; Oct 1 [Epub ahead of print].

133. Batra P, *et al*. Mediastinal masses: magnetic resonance imaging in comparison with computed tomography. J Natl Med Assoc 1991; 83: 969–74.

134. Faletra F, *et al*. Transesophageal echocardiography in the evaluation of mediastinal masses. J Am Soc Echocardiogr 1992; 5: 178–86.

135. Sasaki M, *et al*. Differential diagnosis of thymic tumors using a combination of 11C-methionine PET and FDG PET. J Nucl Med 1999; 40: 1595–601.

136. Sung YM, *et al*. 18F-FDG PET/CT of thymic epithelial tumors: usefulness for distinguishing and staging tumor subgroups. J Nucl Med 2006; 47: 1628–34.

137. Marom EM. Imaging thymoma. J Thorac Oncol 2010; 5: S296–S303.

138. Ferguson MK, *et al*. Selective operative approach for diagnosis and treatment of anterior mediastinal masses. Ann Thorac Surg 1987; 44: 583–6.

139. Grief JSA, *et al*. Percutaneous core needle biopsy in the diagnosis of mediastinal tumors. Lung Cancer 1999; 25: 169–73.

140. Bergh NP, *et al*. Tumors of the thymus and thymic region: I. Clinicopathological studies on thymomas. Ann Thorac Surg 1978; 25: 91–8.

141. Kornstein MJ, *et al*. Cortical versus medullary thymomas: a useful morphologic distinction? Hum Pathol 1987; 19: 1335–9.

142. Detterback FC, Nicholson AG, Kondo K, van Schil P, Moran C. The Masaoka-Koga stage classification for thymic malignancies: clarification and definition of terms. J Thorac Oncol 2011; 6: S1710–S1716.

143. Haniuda M, *et al*. Adjuvant radiotherapy after complete resection of thymoma. Ann Thorac Surg 1992; 54: 311–15.

144. Mornex F, *et al*. Radiotherapy and chemotherapy for invasive thymomas: a multicentric retrospective review of 90 cases. The FNCLCC trialists. Federation Nationale des Centres de Lutte Contre le Cancer. Int J Radiat Oncol Biol Phys 1995; 32: 651–9.

145. Chung D. Thymic carcinoma. Analysis of nineteen clinicopathological studies. Thorac Cardiovasc Surg 2000; 48: 114–19.

146. Pollack A, *et al*. Thymoma: treatment and prognosis. Int J Radiat Oncol Biol Phys 1992; 23: 1037–43.

147. Roviaro GC, *et al*. Major thoracoscopic operations: pulmonary resection and mediastinal mass excision. Int Surg 1996; 81: 354–8.

148. Singhal S, *et al*. Comparison of stages I-II thymoma treated by complete resection with or without adjuvant radiation. Ann Thorac Surg 2003; 76: 1635–41; discussion 1641–2.

149. Ruffini E, *et al*. Recurrence of thymoma: analysis of clinicopathologic features, treatment, and outcome. J Thorac Cardiovasc Surg 1997; 113: 55–63.

150. Cowen D, *et al*. Thymoma: results of a multicentric retrospective series of 149 non-metastatic irradiated patients and review of the literature. FNCLCC trialists. Federation Nationale des Centres de Lutte Contre le Cancer. Radiother Oncol 1995; 34: 9–16.

151. Koh WJLP, Thomas C. Thymoma: radiation and chemotherapy. In: Wood DTC (ed) *Mediastinal Tumors: Update*. New York: Springer-Verlag, 1995. pp. 19–25.

152. Curran WJ Jr, *et al*. Invasive thymoma: the role of mediastinal irradiation following complete or incomplete surgical resection. J Clin Oncol 1988; 6: 1722–7.

153. Ciernik IF, Meier U, Lutolf UM. Prognostic factors and outcome of incompletely resected invasive thymoma following radiation therapy. J Clin Oncol 1994; 12: 1484–90.

154. Schmidt-Wolf IG, *et al*. Malignant thymoma: current status of classification and multimodality treatment. Ann Hematol 2003; 82: 69–76.

155. Strobel P, *et al*. Tumor recurrence and survival in patients treated for thymomas and thymic squamous cell carcinomas: a retrospective analysis. J Clin Oncol 2004; 22: 1501–9.

156. Kondo K, Monden Y. Therapy for thymic epithelial tumors: a clinical study of 1,320 patients from Japan. Ann Thorac Surg 2003; 76: 878–84; discussion 884–5.

157. Korst RJ, *et al*. Adjuvant radiotherapy for thymic epithelial tumors: a systemic review and meta-analysis. Ann Thor Surg 2009; 87: 1641–7.

158. Fuller CD, *et al*. Radiotherapy for thymic neoplasms. J Thorac Oncol 2010; 5: S327–S335.

159. Forquer JA, *et al*. Postoperative radiotherapy after surgical resection of thymoma and differing roles in localized and regional disease. Int J Radiat Oncol Biol Phys 2010; 76: 440–5.

160. Arriagada R, *et al*. Invasive carcinoma of the thymus. A multicenter retrospective review of 56 cases. Eur J Cancer Clin Oncol 1984; 20: 69–74.

161. Fletcher GH. Clinical dose response curves of human malignant epithelial tumours. Br J Radiol 1973; 46: 151.

162. Haniuda M, *et al*. Recurrence of thymoma: clinicopathological features, re-operation, and outcome. J Surg Oncol 2001; 78: 183–8.

163. Kirschner PA. Reoperation for thymoma: report of 23 cases. Ann Thorac Surg 1990; 49: 550–4; discussion 555.

164. Urgesi A, *et al*. Aggressive treatment of intrathoracic recurrences of thymoma. Radiother Oncol 1992; 24: 221–5.

165. Bonomi PD, *et al*. EST 2582 phase II trial of cisplatin in metastatic or recurrent thymoma. Am J Clin Oncol 1993; 16: 342–5.

166. Hu E, Levine J. Chemotherapy of malignant thymoma. Case report and review of the literature. Cancer 1986; 57: 1101–4.

167. Kirkove C, *et al*. Dramatic response of recurrent invasive thymoma to high doses of corticosteroids. Clin Oncol (R Coll Radiol) 1992; 4: 64–6.

168. Boston B. Chemotherapy of invasive thymoma. Cancer 1976; 38: 49–52.

169. Highley MS, *et al*. Treatment of invasive thymoma with single-agent ifosfamide. J Clin Oncol 1999; 17: 2737–44.

170. Loehrer PJ, *et al*. A phase II trial of pemetrexed in patients with recurrent thymoma or thymic carcinoma. ASCO Annual Meeting Proceedings. J Clin Oncol 2006; 24(Suppl): abstract 7079.

171. La Rocca RV, *et al*. Suramin therapy for malignant thymoma: a case report. Eur J Cancer 1994; 30A: 718–19.

172. Chahinian AP. Chemotherapy of thymomas and thymic carcinomas. Chest Surg Clin North Am 2001; 11: 447–56.

173. Jaffrey IS, Denefrio JM, Chahinian P. Response to maytansine in a patient with malignant thymoma. Cancer Treat Rep 1980; 64: 193–4.

174. Donovan PJ, Foley JF. Chemotherapy in invasive thymomas: five case reports. J Surg Oncol 1986; 33: 14–17.

175. Chahinian AP, *et al*. Phase I study of weekly maytansine given by iv bolus or 24-hour infusion. Cancer Treat Rep 1979; 63: 1953–60.

176. Stolinsky DC, *et al*. Clinical trial of weekly doses of vinblastine (NSC-49842) combined with vincristine (NSC-67574) in malignant lymphomas and other neoplasms. Cancer Chemother Rep 1973; 57: 477–80.

177. Loehrer PJ Sr, *et al*. The Eastern Cooperative Oncology Group, Southwest Oncology Group and Southeastern Cancer Study Group. Cisplatin plus doxorubicin plus cyclophosphamide in metastatic or recurrent thymoma: final results of an intergroup trial. J Clin Oncol 1994; 12: 1164–8.

178. Giaccone G, *et al*. Imatinib mesylate in patients with WHO B3 thymomas and thymic carcinomas. J Thor Oncol 2009; 4: 1270–3.

179. Salter JT, Lewis D, Yiannoutsos C, Loehrer PJ, Risley L, Chiorean EG. Imatinib for the treatment of thymic carcinoma. J Clin Oncol 2008; 26: abstract 8116.

180. Kurup A, Burns M, Dropcho S, Pao W, Loehrer PJ. Phase II study of gefitinib treatment in advanced thymic malignancies. J Clin Oncol 2005; 23: abstract 7068.

181. Bedano PM, *et al*. A phase II trial of erlotinib plus bevacizumab in patients with recurrent thymoma or thymic carcinoma. J Clin Oncol 2008; 26: abstract 19087.

182. Engel P, Pilsgaard B, Francis D. Thymomas and thymic carcinomas. A retrospective investigation with histological reclassification. Apmis 1995; 103: 671–8.

183. Palmieri G, *et al*. Imatinib mesylate in thymic epithelial malignancies. Cancer Chemother Pharmacol 2012; 69(2): 309–15.

184. Kurup ABM, *et al*. Phase II study of gefitinib treatment in advanced thymic malignancies. ASCO Annual Meeting Proceedings. J Clin Oncol 2005; 23 (16 Suppl): abstract 7068.

185. Palmieri G, *et al*. Cetuximab is an active treatment of metastatic and chemorefractory thymoma. Front Biosci 2007; 12:757–61.

186. Farina G, Garassino MC, Gambacorta M, La Verde N, Gherardi G, Scanni A. Response of thymoma to cetuximab. Lancet Oncol. 2007; 8: 449–50.

187. Giaccone G, *et al*. Phase II study of belinostat in patients with recurrent or refractory advanced thymic epithelial tumors. J Clin Oncol 2011; 29: 2052–9.

188. Rajan A, Giaccone G. Targeted therapy for advanced thymic tumors. J Thorac Oncol 2010; 5: 361–4.

189. Palmieri G, *et al*. Successful treatment of a patient with a thymoma and pure red-cell aplasia with octreotide and prednisone. N Engl J Med 1997; 336: 263–5.

190. Palmieri G, *et al*. Somatostatin analogs and prednisone in advanced refractory thymic tumors. Cancer 2002; 94: 1414–20.

191. Loehrer PJ, Wang W, Johnson DH, Ettinger DS. Octreotide alone or with prednisone in patients with advanced thymoma and thymic carcinoma: an Eastern Cooperative Oncology Group phase II trial. J Clin Oncol 2004; 22: 293–9.

192. Loehrer PJ Sr, *et al*. Cisplatin, doxorubicin, and cyclophosphamide plus thoracic radiation therapy for limited-stage unresectable thymoma: an intergroup trial. J Clin Oncol 1997; 15: 3093–9.

193. Lara PN Jr, Bonomi PD, Faber LP. Retreatment of recurrent invasive thymoma with platinum, doxorubicin, and cyclophosphamide. Chest 1996; 110: 1115–17.

194. Kim ES, *et al*. Phase II study of a multidisciplinary approach with induction chemotherapy, followed by surgical resection, radiation therapy, and consolidation chemotherapy for unresectable malignant thymomas: final report. Lung Cancer 2004; 44: 369–79.

195. Fornasiero A, *et al*. Chemotherapy for invasive thymoma. A 13-year experience. Cancer 1991; 68: 30–3.

196. Giaccone G, et al. Cisplatin and etoposide combination chemotherapy for locally advanced or metastatic thymoma. A phase II study of the European Organization for Research and Treatment of Cancer Lung Cancer Cooperative Group. J Clin Oncol 1996; 14: 814–20.

197. Loehrer PJ Sr, et al. Combined etoposide, ifosfamide, and cisplatin in the treatment of patients with advanced thymoma and thymic carcinoma: an intergroup trial. Cancer 2001; 91: 2010–15.

198. Lemma GL, Lee JW, Aisner SC et al. Phase II study of carboplatin and paclitaxel in advanced thymoma and thymic carcinoma. J Clin Oncol 2011; 29: 2060–5.

199. Macchiarini P, et al. Neoadjuvant chemotherapy, surgery, and postoperative radiation therapy for invasive thymoma. Cancer 1991; 68: 706–13.

200. Rea F, et al. Chemotherapy and operation for invasive thymoma. J Thorac Cardiovasc Surg 1993; 106: 543–9.

201. Tandan R, et al. Metastasizing thymoma and myasthenia gravis. Favorable response to glucocorticoids after failed chemotherapy and radiation therapy. Cancer 1990; 65: 1286–90.

202. Berthaud P, Le Chevalier T, Tursz T. Effectiveness of interleukin-2 in invasive lymphoepithelial thymoma. Lancet 1990; 335: 1590.

203. Gordon MS, et al. A phase II trial of subcutaneously administered recombinant human interleukin-2 in patients with relapsed/refractory thymoma. J Immunother Emphasis Tumor Immunol 1995; 18: 179–84.

204. Eng TY, et al. Thymic carcinoma: state of the art review. Int J Radiat Oncol Biol Phys 2004; 59: 654–64.

205. Lucchi M, et al. The multimodality treatment of thymic carcinoma. Eur J Cardiothorac Surg 2001; 19: 566–9.

206. Mayer R, et al. Radiotherapy for invasive thymoma and thymic carcinoma. Clinicopathological review. Strahlenther Onkol 1999; 175: 271–8.

207. Weide LG, et al. Thymic carcinoma. A distinct clinical entity responsive to chemotherapy. Cancer 1993; 71: 1219–23.

208. Koizumi T, et al. Chemotherapy for advanced thymic carcinoma: clinical response to cisplatin, doxorubicin, vincristine, and cyclophosphamide (ADOC chemotherapy). Am J Clin Oncol 2002; 25: 266–8.

209. Regnard JF, et al. Prognostic factors and long-term results after thymoma resection: a series of 307 patients. J Thorac Cardiovasc Surg 1996; 112: 376–84.

210. Highley MS, et al. Treatment of invasive thymoma with single-agent ifosfamide. J Clin Oncol 1999;17(9):2737–44.

211. Oguri T, et al. Efficacy of docetaxel as a second-line chemotherapy for thymic carcinoma. Chemotherapy 2004; 50(6): 279–82.

212. Christodoulou C, et al. Response of malignant thymoma to erlotinib. Ann Oncol 2008; 19(7): 1361–2.

213. Buti S, et al. Impressive response with imatinib in a heavily pretreated patient with metastatic c-KIT mutated thymic carcinoma. J Clin Oncol 2011; 29(33): e803–5.

214. Butler WM, et al. Metastatic thymoma with myasthenia gravis: complete remission with combination chemotherapy. Cancer 1982; 50: 419–22.

215. Loehrer PJ, et al. Remission of invasive thymoma due to chemotherapy. Two patients treated with cyclophosphamide, doxorubicin, and vincristine. Chest 1985; 87: 377–80.

216. Kosmidis PA, Iliopoulos E, Pentea S. Combination chemotherapy with cyclophosphamide, adriamycin, and vincristine in malignant thymoma and myasthenia gravis. Cancer 1988; 61: 1736–40.

217. Goldel N, et al. Chemotherapy of invasive thymoma. A retrospective study of 22 cases. Cancer 1989; 63: 1493–500.

218. Evans WKTD, et al. Combination chemotherapy in invasive thymoma: role of COPP. Cancer 1980; 46: 1523.

219. Daugaard G, Hansen HH, Rorth M. Combination chemotherapy for malignant thymoma. Ann Intern Med 1983; 99: 189–90.

220. Klippstein TH, et al. High-dose adriamycin (ADM) and cis-platinum (DDP) in advanced soft-tissue sarcomas and invasive thymomas. A pilot study. Cancer Chemother Pharmacol 1984; 13: 78–81.

221. Mitrou PS, Bergmann L, Tuengerthal S. Induction of complete remission with adriamycin and cis-platinum in invasive thymoma. Dtsch Med Wochenschr 1982; 107: 1667–70.

222. Fornasiero A, et al. Chemotherapy of invasive or metastatic thymoma: report of 11 cases. Cancer Treat Rep 1984; 68: 1205–10.

223. Campbell MG, Pollard R, Al-Sarraf M. A complete response in metastatic malignant thymoma to cis-platinum, doxorubicin and cyclophosphamide: a case report. Cancer 1981; 48: 1315–17.

224. Chahinian AP, et al. Treatment of invasive or metastatic thymoma: report of eleven cases. Cancer 1981; 47: 1752–61.

225. Chahinian AP, Holland JF, Bhardwaj S. Chemotherapy for malignant thymoma. Ann Intern Med 1983; 99: 736.

226. Harper P, Addis B. Unusual tumors of the mediastinum. In: William CJ, Krikorian JG, Green MR, Raghavan D (eds). *Textbook of Uncommon Cancer*. New York: John Wiley & Sons, 1988, p. 411.

227. Dy C, et al. Undifferentiated epithelial-rich invasive malignant thymoma: complete response to cisplatin, vinblastine, and bleomycin therapy. J Clin Oncol 1988; 6: 536–42.

228. Igawa S, et al. Efficacy of chemotherapy with carboplatin and paclitaxel for unresectable thymic carcinoma. Lung Cancer 2010; 67: 194–7.

Section 5: Thoracic Tumors

21 Primary Sarcomas of the Lung

Regan M. Duffy,[1] Amanda VanSandt,[2] and Alan B. Sandler[1]

[1] Division of Hematology and Medical Oncology, [2] Department of Pathology, Knight Cancer Institute, Oregon Health and Science University, Portland, OR, USA

Introduction

Soft tissue sarcomas are uncommon tumors, with an estimated incidence of approximately 10,520 cases and 3920 deaths in the United States in 2010.[1] Sarcomas are derived from mesenchymal tissues and three-fourths of all soft tissue sarcomas arise in the extremities. Sarcomas may also arise from the head and neck, retroperitoneum, or trunk but origin from a visceral structure is infrequent.[2] Although sarcomas may frequently metastasize to the lungs, primary pulmonary sarcomas (PPS) are very rare, accounting for less than 0.2% of all malignant pulmonary tumors.[2,3] The clinical course and treatment approaches for PPS differ from other primary pulmonary malignancies, thus the clinician needs to be aware to include PPS in the differential diagnosis during the evaluation of a pulmonary lesion.

This chapter reviews the available information on the different types of pulmonary sarcomas, focusing on differentiating pathological characteristics, clinical presentation, differential diagnosis, prognosis, and approaches to treatment.

Epidemiology and etiology

Primary pulmonary sarcomas occur at any age, being described in neonates and in the elderly. There is no evidence of a gender predilection and no racial predisposition, although the rarity of the tumors precludes the analysis of a large population database for reliable statistics. Most patients are middle aged at the time of diagnosis. In leiomyosarcoma, the most commonly diagnosed type of PPS, there are only 16 cases described in children under 16 years old in the literature.[4] Previously, the second most common type of PPS was fibrosarcoma. However, with better characterization by immunohistochemistry and a new classification of soft tissue sarcomas by the World Health Organization, tumors previously categorized as fibrosarcomas are now subdivided into specific types of fibrosarcoma or characterized as another type of soft tissue sarcoma.[5–8] Rhabdomyosarcoma has a bimodal age distribution, with the median age of diagnosis in children being 2 years old (usually embryonal and alveolar subtypes), and the median age of diagnosis in adults of 57 years (usually the pleomorphic subtype).[9] Primary pulmonary angiosarcoma is an extremely rare tumor and has not yet been described in children.[10]

Given the heterogeneity as well as the rarity of the subtypes of PPS, no large cohorts have been examined to suggest causative factors. Scattered associations with radiation exposure, thorotrast exposure, and chemical or insecticide exposures have been made, but no convincing evidence has been presented.

Pathology

Most histological subtypes of soft tissue sarcoma are represented in the literature on primary pulmonary sarcoma (Table 21.1). Pulmonary sarcomas, like soft tissue sarcomas, are generally categorized according to the normal mesenchymal tissues they mimic.[11] While some morphological features are distinctive, the different histological types of PPS have many similarities rendering definitive identification on the basis of microscopic examination alone unreliable. Immunohistochemistry and cytogenetics, however, often reveal features that aid in diagnosis. Despite histological characterization, tumor grade, size, and location correlate more strongly with outcome than individual histological subtypes.[12] At the time of diagnosis, PPS frequently demonstrates local invasion.[13] Similar to the more common soft tissue sarcomas, tumor invasion of the lymphatic system is unusual with the exception of a few subtypes such as synovial sarcoma. Metastatic spread occurs hematogenously, but is not usually found at the time of initial diagnosis.[13] Most PPS are grossly round to oval, well-circumscribed and pseudoencapsulated masses (Figs 21.1–21.3). Peripheral lesions may invade the adjacent pleura and thoracic wall.

Soft tissue sarcomas frequently have a distinctive spindle cell morphology separating them morphologically from most

Table 21.1 Histological subtypes of primary pulmonary sarcomas.

Primary	Subtype
Adipocytic sarcoma	Liposarcoma
Fibroblastic/ myofibroblastic tumors	Solitary fibrous Tumor/ hemangiopericytoma
	Adult fibrosarcoma
	Infantile fibrosarcoma
So-called fibrohistiocytic tumors	Undifferentiated pleomorphic sarcoma (pleomorphic "malignant fibrous histiocytoma")
	Undifferentiated pleomorphic sarcoma with giant cells (giant cell "malignant fibrous histiocytoma")
	Undifferentiated pleomorphic sarcoma with prominent inflammation (inflammatory "malignant fibrous histiocytoma")
Smooth muscle sarcoma	Leiomyosarcoma
Pericytic (perivascular) sarcoma	Glomus tumor
Skeletal muscle sarcoma	Rhabdomyosarcoma – embryonal, alveolar and pleomorphic
Vascular sarcoma	Kaposi sarcoma
	Epithelioid hemangioendothelioma
	Angiosarcoma
Chondroosseous sarcoma	Chrondrosarcoma
	Osteosarcoma
Sarcomas of uncertain differentiation	Synovial sarcoma
Intimal sarcoma	Pulmonary artery sarcoma
Sarcomas of peripheral nerves	Malignant peripheral nerve sheath tumor

carcinomas. Certain pulmonary carcinomas, such as spindle cell carcinomas and sarcomatoid mesotheliomas with spindle cell morphology, could be confused with PPS, requiring the use of immunohistochemical evaluation for diagnostic distinction.[14] PPS is typically vimentin positive and keratin and epithelial membrane antigen (EMA) negative, in addition to showing features of particular lineage differentiation (smooth muscle, vascular, etc.). Spindle cell carcinomas, carcinosarcomas, and sarcomatoid mesotheliomas are generally cytokeratin

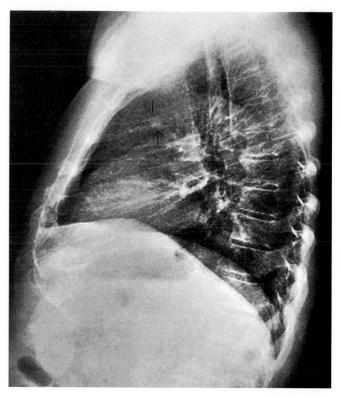

Figure 21.2 The lateral chest ratiograph of the same patient as in Figure 21.1 confirms the presence of a mass in the left upper lobe of the lung.

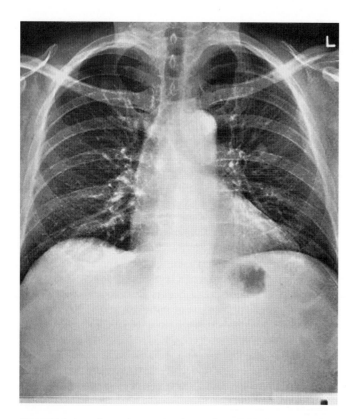

Figure 21.1 A routine posteroanterior chest radiograph in an asymptomatic patient detected this small mass in the left mid-lung field that was discovered to be a synovial sarcoma after biopsy.

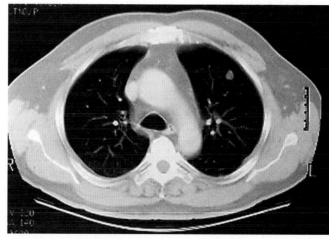

Figure 21.3 A CT scan of the chest of the same patient as in Figure 21.1 shows the peripheral location of the mass.

and EMA positive in addition to showing vimentin positivity. Given that sarcomas most commonly originate elsewhere in the body and subsequently metastasize to the lung, once a diagnosis of pulmonary sarcoma is made, careful exclusion of a primary lesion outside the lung is necessary before designating the sarcoma as PPS. Careful and routine follow-up with examination and imaging is necessary to evaluate for subsequent detection of a previously unapparent primary tumor.

In 2002 the World Health Organization's International Agency for Research on Cancer (IARC) issued a new classification scheme for soft tissue sarcomas.[8] In this new classification scheme, all soft tissue sarcomas, including PPS, were reorganized and arranged based on relevant and up-to-date pathology data including cytogenetic and molecular genetic data available for classification of soft tissue sarcomas. Earlier literature on soft tissue sarcomas, including PPS, grouped some tumors into vague and poorly defined categories. The new WHO classification clarifies many of the prior vague definitions and provides clear delineations for classification of soft tissue sarcomas.

Primary pulmonary sarcomas are represented by each of the new WHO classifications of soft tissue sarcomas. Prior iterations of this chapter on PPS have attempted to categorize PPS based on now outdated classification schemes. This current update attempts to summarize the new pathological classification from the WHO pertinent to PPS.

Smooth muscle tumors

Leiomyosarcoma

Leiomyosarcoma is one of the more common primary pulmonary sarcomas and may occur anywhere within the respiratory tract.[15] It tends to be peripheral and subpleural, but can be centrally located. The larger tumors are prone to extension into the chest wall, mediastinum, and diaphragm. Leiomyosarcomas are thought to arise from smooth muscle in either the blood vessels or the bronchi, and are commonly adherent to these structures. Leiomyosarcomas may also arise in large vessels such as the pulmonary veins and arteries; however, those arising from the arteries are rare and do not have typical features of leiomyosarcoma and fit better when classified as intimal sarcomas (see Pulmonary artery sarcoma, below).

Regardless of location, the morphology is the same. The spindle-shaped cells of leiomyosarcoma are arranged in prominent interlacing bundles and have long, blunt-ended darkly staining nuclei, with relatively abundant, often vacuolated cytoplasm and indistinct borders (Fig. 21.4). Rarely, epithelioid morphology is seen, with distinct cell borders and more abundant cytoplasm. Such tumors may be mistaken for carcinomas.[8,16–19]

Immunohistochemical studies are generally positive for smooth muscle actin (SMA), desmin and h-caldesmon (Table 21.2), although none is specific for leiomyosarcoma.[8] In one study of 18 primary pulmonary sarcomas, 75% stained with smooth muscle actin and only five (31%) stained with desmin.[20] Leu-7 (CD57) can be positive[21] but S-100 positivity is observed only rarely.[2,22]

Fibroblastic/myofibroblastic tumors

Extrapleural solitary fibrous tumor and hemangiopericytoma

Extrapleural solitary fibrous tumor (SFT) and hemangiopericytoma, once considered separate entities, are now thought to

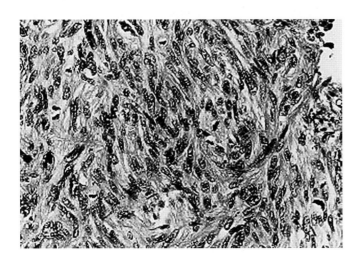

Figure 21.4 Cytological features of leiomyosarcoma.

Table 21.2 Immunohistochemical staining of PPS.

	VIM	Desmin	Actin	S-100	CD31	CD34	Myo	h-cald
LMS	+	+	+	+rare	–	–	–	+
SFT/HPC	+usually	+rare	+rare	+rare	–	+	–	–
IF	+	+rare	+focal	+rare	–	+rare	–	–
AF	+	–	+focal	-	–	+rare	–	–
Glomus	+	–	+	-	–	–	–	+
SS	+	–	–	+rare	–	–	–	–
RMS	+	+	+	+rare	–	–	+	–
AS	+	–	–	–	+	+	–	–
EH	+	–	–	–	+	+	–	–
KS	+	–	–	–	+	+	–	–

AF, adult fibrosarcoma; AS, angiosarcoma; EH, epithelioid hemangioendothelioma; h-cald, h-caldesmon; IF, infantile fibrosarcoma; KS, Kaposi sarcoma; LMS, leiomyosarcoma; Myo, myosin; RMS, rhabdomyosarcoma; SFT/HPC, solitary fibrous tumor/hemangiopericytoma; SS, synovial sarcoma; VIM, vimentin.

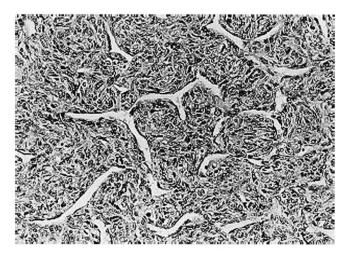

Figure 21.5 Histological section of hemangiopericytoma/solitary fibrous tumor.

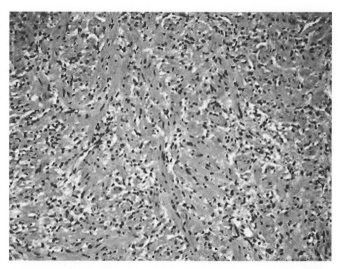

Figure 21.6 Histological section of solitary fibrous tumor, 200× magnification.

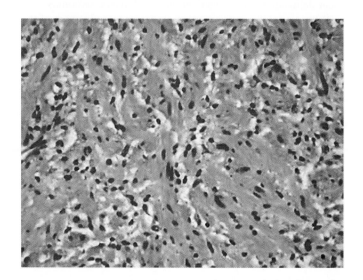

Figure 21.7 Histological section of solitary fibrous tumor, 400× magnification.

be overlapping diseases. SFT was first described as a pleural or subpleural tumor, but is now known to occur in any location.[22,23] The term hemangiopericytoma previously encompassed a variety of tumors with thin-walled branching vascular pattern. However, this vague definition makes a distinct entity of hemangiopericytoma elusive.[8] Most tumors included within the broad definition of hemangiopericytoma are now reclassified as another tumor based on improved immunohistochemistry and definitions of tumors. The remaining hemangiopericytoma tumors are notable as well-circumscribed masses with blunt, closely packed spindle cells resembling the cellular areas of SFT but with numerous thin-walled branching vessels often with staghorn configuration[8] (Fig. 21.5). The cytoplasm is scanty and pale or eosinophilic, with the oval nucleus filling the cell. Prior definitions of hemangiopericytoma have documented that the tumor cells often show features of an undifferentiated or fibroblastic cell type.[8,24] However, the updated WHO soft tissue sarcoma guidelines no longer use these terms to describe hemangiopericytoma.[8]

Solitary fibrous tumors are typically well circumscribed with patternless architecture on microscopic examination with alternating areas of hypo- and hypercellularity separated by hyalinized collagen and branching "hemangiopericytoma-like" vessels[8] (Figs 21.6, 21.7). SFT classically consists of atypical, round to spindle-shaped cells with little cytoplasm and frequently observed areas of fibrosis, interstitial mast cells, and myxoid change.[8] In addition to the previously described overlapping features with hemangiopericytoma, SFT was often also confused with fibrosarcoma, yet another previously vaguely defined tumor (see section below on updates to fibrosarcoma).

Both benign and malignant hemangiopericytomas have been described in the lung[8,25–27] and no convincing evidence for pericytic differentiation has been documented.[8] Immunohistochemistry of both SFT and hemangiopericytomas is generally positive for vimentin and CD34. Actin, desmin, and endothelial markers are negative[8,22] in hemangiopericytoma while a few SFT are positive for actin, desmin, and S-100.[8,28–30]

Criteria for malignancy of both SFT and hemangiopericytoma are proposed; mitotic count of >4/10 high-power fields (HPF)[8,31–33] is the most worrisome feature for malignancy. The presence of necrosis, tumor size >5 cm, and increased mitotic activity may also signify malignancy.[8] In a prior study of primary lung hemangiopericytomas, size >8 cm and mitotic count >3/10 HPF suggested a more aggressive clinical course.[34,35]

Fibrosarcoma

In the past many primary pulmonary sarcomas were defined as fibrosarcoma; however, with advances in pathological diagnosis and updates to WHO criteria for soft tissue sarcoma, fibrosarcoma alone is no longer acceptable terminology. Tumors composed of fibroblasts with variable collagen production are classically adult fibrosarcomas, which must be distinguished from infantile fibrosarcoma and other sarcomas composed of fibroblasts.[8] Classically, adult fibrosarcomas display a herringbone pattern of spindle-shaped cells arranged in sweeping fascicles.[8] Prior tumors diagnosed as fibrosarcomas have been retrospectively reclassified as synovial sarcoma or malignant fibrous histiocytoma (a subsequently outdated classification, see below).[20,25]

Both adult and infantile fibrosarcomas stain for vimentin, while adult fibrosarcoma stain focally for actin compared to the highly variable staining pattern for other markers. Notably, most infantile fibrosarcomas carry a chromosomal translocation, t(12;15), involving oncogenic activation of the NTRK3 receptor tyrosine kinase gene. There is no specific diagnostic gene rearrangement in adult fibrosarcoma; rather, these tumors can have multiple, complex chromosome rearrangements.[8]

Ultrastructurally, adult fibrosarcomas show fibroblastic differentiation with prominent nucleoli and dilated rough endoplasmic reticulum and absent myofilaments, external laminal or intercellular junctions. Intra- and extracellular collagen fibers are commonly seen. Infrequently, adult fibrosarcomas have peripheral filament bundles suggestive of myofibroblastic differentiation and are usually reclassified (based on histology) as either myofibrosarcomas or leiomyosarcoma.[8,36,37] Infantile fibrosarcomas display properties of fibroblasts and myofibroblasts, but the cells are similar in appearance to adult fibrosarcomas with large nuclei, dilated rough endoplasmic reticulum with dense material, and cytoplasmic filaments.[8]

There are other variants of fibrosarcoma, including low-grade fibromyxoid sarcoma and sclerosing epithelioid fibrosarcoma, under the WHO soft tissue sarcoma classification. These subtypes have not yet specifically been documented in PPS.

Undifferentiated pleomorphic sarcomas

In 2002, the WHO declassified malignant fibrous histiocytoma (MFH) as a formal diagnostic entity and the term MFH is now synonymous with undifferentiated pleomorphic sarcoma, a diagnosis of exclusion, representing less than 5% of adult sarcomas. First described in 1979, MFH was previously considered the most common soft tissue sarcoma.[38,39] However, advances in pathological diagnosis demonstrate that most (if not all) tumors that were once defined as MFH can now be further characterized and classified as another tumor.[8,40] While it remains unclear how to most accurately organize these tumors, the term malignant fibrous histiocytoma represents a diagnosis previously applied to thousands of patients and is still commonly used by both patients and physicians.

Pleomorphic malignant fibrous histiocytoma (synonymous with undifferentiated high-grade pleomorphic sarcoma) was previously thought of as the prototypical form of MFH and the most common soft tissue sarcoma in adults; however, the prior definition included pleomorphic spindle cell malignant neoplasm showing fibroblastic and facultative histiocytic differentiation which is a pattern shared by a wide variety of poorly differentiated malignant neoplasms. These tumors, in fact, do not show evidence of true histiocytic differentiation. Current use of the term undifferentiated high-grade pleomorphic sarcoma is reserved for a very small group of pleomorphic sarcomas showing no definable line of differentiation. Furthermore, previously described variants of MFH, giant cell malignant fibrous histiocytoma and inflammatory malignant fibrous histiocytoma, have

been reassessed and are now recognized as sharing morphology with other neoplasms; the terms undifferentiated pleomorphic sarcoma with giant cells and undifferentiated pleomorphic sarcoma with prominent inflammation are reserved for the rare tumors undifferentiated pleomorphic sarcomas with prominent osteoclastic giant cells and with prominent histiocytic and inflammatory cells, respectively.[8] Finally, some previously documented MFH tumors of the "myxoid" type carried an improved diagnosis over other MFH, and these tumors are now defined as myxofibrosarcoma, a distinct entity under WHO classification.[8,22]

Pericytic/perivascular tumors

Glomus tumors

Overall, glomus tumors (both typical and malignant) are exceedingly rare. They can be subcategorized as typical glomus tumors (further subdivided into solid glomus tumor, glomangioma, and glomangiomyoma), glomangiomatosis, simplistic glomus tumors, and malignant glomus tumors (including glomangiosarcomas and glomus tumors of uncertain malignant potential).[8] Glomus tumors may arise in the bronchus, mediastinum, or pulmonary parenchyma. They tend to be round, well-circumscribed tumors. Intratumoral hemorrhage is variably present. As opposed to the uniform epithelioid cells with distinct borders, scant clear to eosinophilic cytoplasm, and central, round nuclei seen in the glomus tumors, cases of glomangiosarcoma demonstrate focal cystic degeneration and prominent zones of necrosis, a high mitotic count, and diffuse cytological atypia.[8,41] Glomus tumors of all subtypes stain positively for SMA, vimentin, and h-caldesmon as well as collagen type IV (pericellular staining). Typically, glomus tumors stain negative for desmin, CD34, cytokeratin, and S-100.[8,41]

Skeletal muscle tumors

Rhabdomyosarcoma

Rhabdomyosarcoma occurring in the lung can be endobronchial or intraparenchymal and tends to fill an entire lobe of the lung and invade pulmonary veins and bronchi. It may be associated with a congenital adenomatoid malformation.[9] Rhabdomyosarcoma occurs in three subtypes: pleomorphic, embryonal, and alveolar. Embryonal rhabdomyosarcoma recapitulates the morphology of the embryonic myoblast. Alveolar rhabdomyosarcoma is a round cell neoplasm that cytologically resembles lymphoma and displays partial skeletal muscle differentiation. Pleomorphic rhabdomyosarcoma is a high-grade sarcoma made of bizarre polygonal, spindle and round cells with skeletal muscle differentiation without evidence of embryonal or alveolar components.[8,9]

The embryonal and alveolar rhabdomyosarcomas usually occur in the pediatric population (<15 years of age and 10–25 years of age, respectively)[22] while the pleomorphic subtype usually occurs in adults and resembles other pleomorphic sarcomas. In the lung, all three subtypes have been described. The majority of lung rhabdomyosarcomas are of the pleomorphic type.[9] Given the bimodal age distribution, it is possible that different etiologies exist for children compared with adults.[42] The histological features of rhabdomyosarcoma vary with the subtype. Embryonal rhabdomyosarcoma consists of primitive mesenchymal cells generally in different stages of myogenesis. At the primitive end of this spectrum, stellate cells with slight amphophilic cytoplasm and central, oval nuclei are present. As differentiation occurs, cells gain more cytoplasmic eosinophilia with elongated strap-like shape of cells. Cross-striations and multinucleation indicate terminal differentiation.[8]

Alveolar rhabdomyosarcoma has round cell cytological features with primitive myoblastic differentiation. Uniquely, alveolar rhabdomyosarcoma can exhibit three separate histological subtypes: typical alveolar rhabdomyosarcoma features, solid pattern, and mixed embryonal/alveolar features. Typical alveolar rhabdomyosarcomas have fibrovascular septa creating nests of cells compared to solid variant alveolar rhabdomyosarcoma, which do not have fibrovascular septa, therefore forming sheets of round cells. The mixed variant has both embryonal forms (spindle cell myoblasts with myxoid stroma) and additional alveolar areas (nests with fibrous stroma). Pleomorphic rhabdomyosarcoma, on the other hand, is a high-grade sarcoma composed of undifferentiated cells, round to spindle shaped, with additional mixture of polygonal cells with densely eosinophilic cytoplasm.[8,43–47]

Immunohistochemistry identifies the differentiation of embryonal rhabdomyosarcoma; vimentin is present in most primitive cells, desmin and actin are identifiable in developing rhabdomyoblasts, and fully differentiated cells stain positive for myoglobin and myosin (see Table 21.2).[8,9] Antibodies against myoD1 and myogenin are both specific and sensitive for rhabdomyosarcoma.[8] Ultrastructural features include myofilaments displaying the Z-disk of normal sarcomeres. In less differentiated cases, intermixtures of thin (actin) and thick (myosin) filaments may be identified, with varying representation of Z-bands.[2,8,43]

Vascular tumors

Kaposi sarcoma

Kaposi sarcoma (KS) is a tumor of vascular origin that usually affects the lung in patients with disseminated tumor beginning in the skin. However, AIDS patients can present with pulmonary KS in the absence of cutaneous or other visceral involvement. Diffuse interstitial infiltrates can be seen without a discrete mass. However, abnormalities may be extremely focal.[2,28,48–50]

The gross appearance of pulmonary KS demonstrates flat or slightly raised plaques of red, violaceous, or red-blue coloration. These plaques may coalesce to form nodules, and may additionally be seen in the bronchial airways on transbronchial examination.[51] Spindle tumor cells are found in concert with telangiectatic vessels, spreading along lymphatics and infiltrating vessel walls, airways, and pleural surfaces.[28] The spindle cells trap extravasated erythrocytes. Occasional spindle cells contain cytoplasmic vacuoles or eosinophilic, hyaline globules, a characteristic finding.[8] The lining cells of developed vascular structures generally stain positive for typical vascular markers (CD31, CD 34, and factor VIII), while the spindle cell component within the KS lesions are usually CD34 positive,

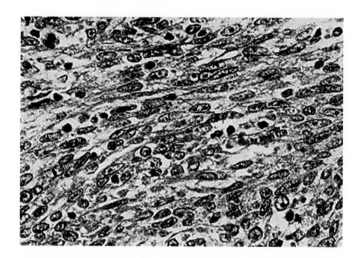

Figure 21.8 Histological section of epithelioid hemangioendothelioma.

often CD31 positive but FVIII negative (see Table 21.2). All tumors are human herpes virus-8 positive. KS also expresses FLi-1, similar to all vascular tumors.[8]

Epithelioid hemangioendothelioma

This tumor was initially termed intravascular "sclerosing" bronchioalveolar tumor or IVBAT as it was thought to demonstrate an aggressive variant of bronchioalveolar cell carcinoma.[28,52–55] It is a rare tumor and appears to be more frequent in young women. It is considered a low-intermediate grade vascular malignancy with clinical and radiological features overlapping those of angiosarcoma of the lung.[56] Patients often present with an indolent course and many are asymptomatic. Common symptoms include dyspnea, pleuritic chest pain, hemoptysis, and a nonproductive cough.[56] Up to 15% of patients may have liver involvement.[56] Imaging commonly shows multiple, peripheral multifocal nodules that occasionally appear calcified.

Histologically, the tumor is composed of round or oval-shaped nodules, and spreads into adjacent spaces in a micropolypoid manner. The cytoplasm of tumor cells is eosinophilic and may contain vacuoles, an attempt to form vascular channels. The tumor typically has a central sclerotic and hypocellular zone with a cellular peripheral zone. The central portion may ossify or calcify (Fig. 21.8). Immunohistochemical and ultrastructural analysis resembles that of angiosarcoma, including positive staining for vimentin, CD31, CD34, and factor VIII (von Willebrand factor), although recent studies have suggested that CD31, CD34 and FLi-1protein are more reliable than factor VIII.[52–56]

Angiosarcoma

Only a few reports of primary pulmonary angiosarcoma exist in the literature.[10] Angiosarcomas of the lung can assume a multifocal, bilateral, nodular appearance and hence are most likely to be confused with metastases. They can present as a fulminant hemorrhagic syndrome[57] and are characterized by extensive local invasion and hematogenous metastasis.[10] Some authorities consider primary pulmonary angiosarcoma to be metastatic from an unapparent primary lesion.[28] Two cases of angiosarcoma occurring along the pleural surface and mimicking mesothelioma have also been noted.[58]

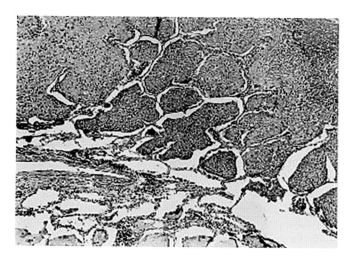

Figure 21.9 Microscopic appearance of angiosarcoma.

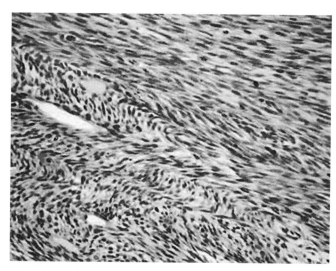

Figure 21.10 Histological section of synovial sarcoma magnification.

Histologically, angiosarcomas display anastomosing vascular channels lined by malignant endothelial cells and form sieve-like patterns (Fig. 21.9). Foci of necrosis, hemorrhage, and hemosiderin deposits are common. Peripheral spread along vascular channels may simulate the appearance of lymphangitic carcinomatosis.[28,42,59] The majority of angiosarcomas are high grade with increased mitotic activity.[8] The cells have scanty cytoplasm, and hobnail nucleoli often project into the vascular spaces.

Immunohistochemistry is important in angiosarcoma as some poorly differentiated tumors forming vascular channels can be difficult to categorize based on histology alone.[8] Angiosarcomas display typical vascular markers, such as CD34 and CD31 and von Willebrand factor. CD31 is more sensitive and specific, and although von Willebrand factor is most specific for angiosarcoma, it is the least sensitive marker (less than 50% of cases).[8,22] Vimentin is usually present in all angiosarcomas (see Table 21.2). More recently, FLi-1, a nuclear transcription factor, has shown positivity in almost all vascular tumors.[8,60] Ultrastructurally, angiosarcomas exhibit abundant intermediate filaments with sparse-to-moderate rough endoplasmic reticulum mitochondria and Golgi complexes; cells are connected by junctional attachments. Peculiar rod-like cytoplasmic inclusions (Weibel–Palade bodies) may be seen in a third of cases.[2,8,28,59]

Tumors of uncertain differentiation

Synovial sarcoma
Synovial sarcoma arising in the lung is not a classically recognized entity.[61–63] The morphology of this tumor (which does not actually arise from the synovium but from immature mesenchymal cells) is histologically identical to synovial sarcoma of the soft tissue and is divided into two general subtypes: biphasic and monophasic.[56,63] The monophasic subtype is the most commonly diagnosed primary pulmonary synovial sarcoma. The histology of the monophasic type is characterized by atypical spindle cell proliferation composed of densely cellular sheets of elongated cells with oval nuclei and indistinct cytoplasm (Figs 21.10, 21.11). There is often dense

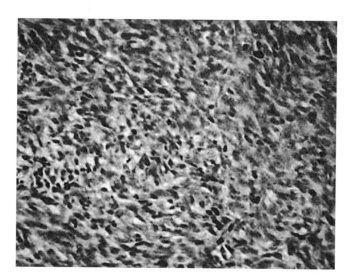

Figure 21.11 Histological section of synovial sarcoma, 600× magnification.

hyaline fibrosis and a prominent hemangiopericytomatous vascular pattern.[56] Mast cells are frequently seen in the surrounding stroma and calcification can be seen.[63,64] The biphasic subtype is characterized by both epithelial and spindle components; the cells are cuboid shaped and have eosinophilic cytoplasm and round nuclei. Mucoid secretions are common in the biphasic subtype.[56] Both subtypes of synovial sarcoma have varied mitotic activity and contain focal areas of necrosis.

Immunohistochemical staining is positive for vimentin as in all soft tissue sarcomas. However, unlike most other sarcomas, EMA and keratin reactivity are common in both subtypes of synovial sarcoma (see Table 21.2). Cytokeratins 7 and 19 can be very useful in this diagnosis because they are positive in synovial sarcoma but generally negative in other spindle cell neoplasms.[56] BCL-2 and CD99 are often positive and CD34 is generally negative.[25,56] In addition, up to 30% of synovial sarcomas are positive for S-100.[56] These features highlight the broad differential diagnosis of synovial sarcoma, including carcinoma, melanoma, and tumors with neural differentiation.

Cytogenetic analysis is specific for the diagnosis of synovial sarcoma. A unique chromosomal translocation, t(X;18)(p11;q11), results in the fusion of the *SYT* gene on chromosome 18 to either the *SSX1* or *SSX2* gene on chromosome X. This translocation is specific for synovial sarcoma and has been found in >90% of synovial sarcomas; it is used to confirm the diagnosis of primary pulmonary synovial sarcomas.[56,62,63,65,66] The diagnosis of the translocation can be made not only using conventional cytogenetic analysis, but now can be performed on paraffin-embedded tissue by either fluorescent *in situ* hybridization (FISH) or real-time polymerase chain reaction (PCR).[67–70] The *SYT-SSX* fusion gene is thought to function in transcription regulation, although the precise function has not yet been identified. Some data suggest that prognosis does not differ between monophasic or biphasic tumors; however, cases with the *SYT-SSX2* variant gene have shown better prognosis.[8] Identification of this chromosomal translocation and fusion gene products has led to increasing diagnoses of pulmonary synovial sarcoma in recent years.

Pulmonary artery sarcoma

Sarcomas of the pulmonary arteries are rare and distinct clinically and pathologically from parenchymal or endobronchial sarcomas. They clinically resemble congestive heart failure or pulmonary embolism and present with dyspnea. Imaging shows filling defects of the pulmonary artery tree with or without a hilar mass; solid expansion of the proximal pulmonary artery branches is very suggestive of sarcoma, increasingly if combined with cardiac enlargement, decreased vascularity, and pulmonary nodules.[56] They can extend outside the arterial lumen into the surrounding lung or mediastinum. Emboli are commonly present in the lung parenchyma owing to distal embolization of tumor along the arterial tree. Proximal extension can cause right heart failure.[2,13,28,71–73] Pulmonary arterial sarcomas tend to metastasize into the distal pulmonary vessels via tumor embolism, but rarely metastasize systemically.[74] Pulmonary arterial sarcomas have a very poor prognosis – mean overall survival <18 months.[56]

Thoracic vascular lesions are divided into intimal and mural sarcomas. Intimal sarcomas are most common in the large arteries (aorta, pulmonary artery), probably arising from pleuripotent mesenchymal cells in the intima.[75] Histologically, intimal sarcomas have a proliferation of spindle cells in a myxoid background with areas of hypocellular stroma interspersed.[56] There are some intimal sarcomas that have areas of differentiated sarcomas, including osteosarcoma, chondrosarcoma or rhabdomyosarcoma, but this is not common. Immunohistochemistry is consistent with myofibroblastic differentiation, staining positively for vimentin, with variable expression of desmin, factor VIII, CD31, and CD34.[56] Mural sarcomas occur most commonly in the pulmonary veins and inferior vena cava, and are usually leiomyosarcomas arising in the vascular smooth muscle wall. Immunohistochemistry and ultrastructural morphology resemble those for each of the histological subtypes.[28]

Other cases of primary pulmonary sarcoma

Rare cases of chondrosarcoma, including myxoid chondrosarcoma, mesenchymal chondrosarcoma, dedifferentiated chondrosarcoma, osteosarcoma, liposarcoma (including myxoid and pleomorphic types), malignant mesenchymoma, and "triton" tumor (neurogenic tumor with rhabdomyoblastic differentiation), have been described in the literature.[76–86] Histological, immunohistochemical, and ultrastructural features resemble those of primary osseous or soft tissue tumors.

Malignant peripheral nerve sheath tumor (MPNST) has also been described as a PPS. The term malignant peripheral nerve sheath tumor has replaced several previously used terms for neural malignancies, including neurogenic sarcoma and malignant schwannoma. MPNST arise from a peripheral nerve but when located in extraneural soft tissue, these tumors show nerve sheath differentiation. MPNST in the lungs is encountered usually in the setting of neurofibromatosis and arises in the posterior mediastinum.[28,87–89] MPNST is characterized by

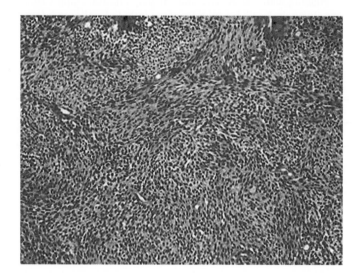

Figure 21.12 Histological section of malignant peripheral nerve sheath tumor, 200× magnification.

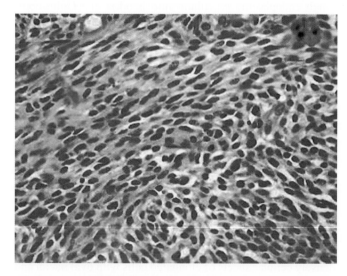

Figure 21.13 Malignant peripheral nerve sheath tumor, s98.

malignant spindle cells with elongated nuclei with tapered ends; cytoplasm displays a fascicular or whorled pattern, with alternating hypocellular and hypercellular areas ("marble-like" pattern) (Figs 21.12, 21.13). Immunohistochemistry for MPNST is only positive for S-100 in 50–70% of cases[90] (see Table 21.2). Triton tumors are MPNST with rhabdomyosarcomatous differentiation exhibiting mature rhabdomyoblasts scattered throughout sheets of schwannoma cells.[90,91]

Clinical presentation

Primary pulmonary sarcomas can affect any age group, although they are most commonly diagnosed in older adults. PPSs in children are usually found on workup for unrelenting pneumonia or dyspnea. Persistent symptoms prompt imaging evaluation that may reveal a large lung mass or fiberoptic bronchoscopy that may demonstrate an endobronchial lesion.

Most PPS are parenchymal, while a smaller proportion is endobronchial. Common presenting features in adults with PPS include dyspnea, cough, chest pain, or hemoptysis. Although hemoptysis may be a common presenting feature prompting initial diagnostic evaluation, PPSs do not have the exfoliative tendency that is present in primary pulmonary carcinomas. Patients may experience fever or weight loss from postobstructive pneumonia or, less frequently, from the primary malignancy. Clinical examination might demonstrate evidence of consolidation over the involved lungs due to postobstructive pneumonia or secondary to mass effect of the tumor. Sputum collection for cytology generally is of lower yield than even for primary pulmonary carcinomas, and a biopsy specimen is generally required for diagnosis.[2,92]

Symptomatic pulmonary thromboembolism can be evident, particularly with angiosarcomas and primary pulmonary artery sarcomas. Alternatively, patients may manifest with intrathoracic or pulmonary hemorrhage secondary to angiosarcoma or KS. More dramatic presentations with superior vena cava syndrome, massive hemoptysis, cyanosis, and acute respiratory failure have been documented. A case of hemangiopericytoma mimicking a Pancoast tumor has been published.[93]

Primary pulmonary artery sarcomas can produce symptomatic pulmonary hypertension or right heart failure as the initial presenting symptoms. Many patients are asymptomatic, with abnormalities detected on routine imaging for other reasons. Paraneoplastic syndromes are a rare phenomenon associated with hemangiopericytoma, manifest by hypoglycemia, hypertension, coagulopathy (both thrombotic and hemorrhagic diatheses), and pulmonary osteoarthropathy.[94] Hypoglycemia might also occur secondary to significant glucose utilization of the primary tumor.[95] Pulmonary osteoarthropathy has additionally been linked to cases of pulmonary angiosarcoma and pulmonary artery sarcoma.[2,13,28,71]

Sites of tumor metastasis may include the contralateral lung, liver, brain, bone, or soft tissues. Tumor detection outside the thorax should prompt an evaluation to determine whether the soft tissue tumor represents a previously indiscernible primary tumor with metastasis to the lung.

In patients with evidence of unilateral thromboembolism not responding to conventional therapy, the possibility of vascular involvement of malignancy must be considered. In angiosarcomas and primary pulmonary arterial sarcomas, the tumor origin may be intraluminal, mimicking thromboembolism on imaging studies.[96] Pulmonary KS can be mistaken on imaging for pulmonary infections, particularly opportunistic infections with unusual imaging findings, in immunocompromised patients. Indeed, the primary malignancy may be intermingled with opportunistic infections in these patients, and the partial response of a treated infection should cause suspicion for a concurrent malignancy.[51]

Differential diagnosis

See Boxes 21.1 and 21.2.

Lesions originating in the lung

Bronchogenic carcinoma
Bronchogenic carcinomas are a vastly more common pulmonary malignancy than sarcomas, with a great variety of histological

---

Box 21.1 Differential diagnosis of pulmonary tumor for the pathologist.

Spindle cell pathology

- Sarcomatoid carcinoma – including poorly differentiated squamous cell or adenocarcinoma
- Pulmonary blastoma
- Sarcomatoid mesothelioma
- Pleomorphic carcinoma
- Giant cell carcinoma
- Spindle cell carcinoma
- Carcinosarcoma
- Metastatic sarcoma
- Lymphangiomyomatosis
- Inflammatory pseudotumor
- Metastatic tumor with spindle pathology

Round cell

- Small cell carcinoma of the lung
- Lymphoma

Epithelioid

- Epithelioid mesothelioma
- Thymoma
- Chondroma

Other

- Squamous cell carcinoma of the lung
- Adenocarcinoma of the lung
- Large cell carcinoma of the lung
- Carcinoid tumor
- Hamartoma
- Melanoma

Box 21.2 Differential diagnosis of primary pulmonary sarcomas for the clinician.

Malignant lesions

- Bronchogenic carcinoma
- Sarcoma metastatic to lung
- Melanoma
- Lymphoma

Nonmalignant lesions

- Thromboembolism
- Opportunistic infection
- Interstitial lung disease

differences between different subtypes. Bronchogenic carcinomas of the spindle cell variant (sarcomatoid carcinoma) can resemble PPS. These are carcinomas composed entirely of spindled tumor cells. However, immunohistochemical staining of sarcomatoid carcinomas demonstrates cytokeratin and epithelial membrane antigen positivity, features not usually demonstrated in PPS. To exclude synovial sarcoma, electron microscopy or cytogenetics may be necessary. Ultrastructurally, characteristics of carcinomas rather than sarcomas are demonstrated.

Small cell carcinoma

Small cell carcinomas and atypical neuroendocrine tumors can also be confused with PPS on morphological examination. Small cell carcinoma is composed of small, malignant cells with high nuclear-to-cytoplasmic ratio. The differential diagnosis for small cell carcinoma includes PPSs such as Ewing sarcoma, primitive neuroectodermal tumor (PNET), synovial sarcoma, and nonsarcomatous malignancies such as lymphoma. Immunohistochemical staining, however, demonstrates at least focal cytokeratin, although less than most nonsmall cell carcinomas, with additional markers of neuroendocrine differentiation. These include neuron-specific enolase, chromogranin, synaptophysin, and neural cell adhesion molecule (N-CAM)/CD56. Small cell carcinoma of the lung is also positive for thyroid transcription factor (TTF-1) in up to 90% of cases.[56] Carcinomas are vimentin negative compared to the universally positive vimentin staining in sarcoma.[2,13,28,71]

Carcinosarcoma

Carcinosarcoma is composed of both epithelial and sarcomatous elements.[1,13,27,28,71,97–99] Pulmonary carcinosarcomas are considered a variant of sarcomatoid carcinomas.[100] Carcinosarcomas may contain elements of adenocarcinoma or squamous cell carcinoma in addition to leiomyosarcoma, rhabdomyosarcoma, chondrosarcoma, or osteosarcomas. Undifferentiated sarcomas may also be present.[100]

Carcinosarcomas more commonly occur in men (7.25–9:1 cases in men compared with women), versus the equal occurrence of PPS in women and men.[100] Lymph nodes are the most common site of metastasis in carcinosarcomas; PPSs do not usually metastasize to lymph nodes. Carcinosarcomas exhibit the very aggressive behavior of both tumor cell populations and tend to carry a poor prognosis, with 5-year survival reaching only 21.3%.[96–100]

Pulmonary blastoma

Pulmonary blastomas are rare tumors with bimodal distribution. In adults, pulmonary blastoma is a biphasic tumor that contains an epithelial component resembling fetal adenocarcinoma in addition to primitive mesenchymal elements, similar to a carcinosarcoma.[56,101–105] The fetal type of pulmonary blastoma, well-differentiated adenocarcinoma, is considered a monophasic, purely epithelial variant with a better prognosis than the biphasic form. Overall survival is only 25% at 1 year.[13,71]

Lymphoma and thymoma

Lymphoma may histologically resemble sarcoma, especially embryonal or alveolar cell rhabdomyosarcoma, Ewing sarcoma, and PNET. However, staining for leukocyte common antigen (LCA), T cell and B cell-associated antigens, and electron microscopy displaying absence of sarcomeric differentiation assist in differentiating a lymphoma from PPS.[2,13,28,71] Unusual cases of pulmonary thymomas resembling sarcoma have been reported.[106]

Benign lesions

Benign lesions may occasionally imitate PPS. Inflammatory pseudotumors can resemble sarcomas, although the presence of abundant inflammatory cells, lack of cellular atypia, and, more recently, lack of p53 immunostaining have been employed in making the distinction.[2,28,107]

Lymphangioleiomyomatosis is a disorder typified by the proliferation of bland-appearing smooth muscle in the bronchial, vascular, and lymphatic structures. Reticulonodular shadows are apparent radiologically and women of reproductive age are commonly affected.[28] Other benign lesions of the lung that can be confused with sarcomas include leiomyomas and chondromas.[2,28,108]

Metastatic disease originating in other sites

Metastatic sarcoma

Primary pulmonary sarcoma is a diagnosis of exclusion. The most common etiology of pulmonary sarcoma is secondary to metastatic disease from another primary. Therefore, in any patient with a diagnosed pulmonary sarcoma, a thorough clinical and radiographic evaluation to exclude another source of primary malignancy must be executed. This includes careful evaluation on follow-up exams, as the primary site may manifest later than the initial pulmonary lesion.

Melanoma

Malignant pulmonary melanoma is almost always a metastatic lesion, and histologically can mimic sarcoma.[2,13,28,71] Once again, immunohistochemistry (HMB-45 and S-100 positivity) and ultrastructural findings (premelanosomes) usually assist in distinguishing it from sarcoma. Of note, some poorly differentiated melanomas, particularly the spindled melanomas, can lose immunoreactivity for melanocytic markers, and ultrastructural features may become less well defined.[109] In those cases in which S-100 is the only positive marker, MPNST may be a diagnostic consideration.

See also Chapter 23.

Sarcomatoid renal cell carcinoma

When metastatic to the lung, the sarcomatoid variant of renal cell carcinoma can simulate PPS. However, a careful clinical evaluation and positive staining for epithelial antigens help to identify this entity.[28]

Diagnostic evaluation

Imaging studies may demonstrate evidence of pulmonary infarction from thromboembolism or secondary to tumor invasion of vascular structures. In one series of imaging studies, tumors arising from the pulmonary vascular system tended to be located more centrally compared with the more peripheral locations of pulmonary emboli, and more often caused complete occlusion of the vessel (as opposed to partial occlusion with pulmonary emboli).[110] In the same series, sarcomas arising from the vascular system were more often unilateral compared to the more frequently bilateral pulmonary emboli, and tended to cause an expansion of the involved pulmonary artery, while most emboli did not.[110] Any extension beyond the lumen of the vessel into the parenchymal space would indicate malignancy instead of benign emboli. Magnetic resonance imaging (MRI) or echocardiography may assist in the differentiation between a tumor of vascular origin and thromboembolism, but this requires suspicion of a vascular tumor at the time of imaging workup.[74]

Other radiographic findings may include nodules of varying sizes suspicious for carcinomas or, in the case of the tumors of vascular origin, patchy, diffuse infiltrates, with some resembling interstitial lung disease. Postobstructive pneumonia can be seen. Calcification of the lesion is not typical. As tumors are commonly very advanced at the time of diagnosis, invasion into the surrounding structures (e.g. mediastinum, chest wall) is frequent.

Utility of fine needle aspiration in primary pulmonary sarcomas

Adequate tumor biopsy frequently requires surgical intervention. However, in cases in which a fine needle aspiration (FNA) might be clinically preferred, a substantial amount of information can be gleaned from aspiration biopsies, in some cases yielding a definitive diagnosis.[6,15,111] In general, FNA of sarcomas yields cellular smears with atypia ranging from bland to obviously malignant. Certain cytological patterns can suggest a diagnosis. For example, tumors composed of atypical spindled cells include synovial sarcoma, leiomyosarcoma, and MPNST. Round cell morphology can be seen in synovial sarcoma, epithelioid leiomyosarcoma, Ewing sarcoma, PNET, embryonal or alveolar rhabdomyosarcoma, and round cell

liposarcoma. Pleomorphic spindle tumors are often undifferentiated high-grade pleomorphic sarcoma and pleomorphic rhabdomyosarcoma.[8,111,112] From these differential diagnoses, immunohistochemistry can be performed in a judicious manner on either the cytological smears or a cell block. Cases in which a definitive diagnosis is feasible usually consist of sufficient material to produce a cytological cell block preparation, upon which immunohistochemical stains and FISH can be performed, just as with larger histological samples. Tumors may contain areas of necrosis, requiring adequate or larger tissue samples containing viable tissue for morphological, immunohistochemical, and possibly cytogenetic evaluation.

Mediastinoscopy is generally not helpful in diagnosis or staging, as metastasis to the mediastinal lymph nodes is rare. In pulmonary KS, diagnosis is typically based upon the clinical appearance of lesions with airway inspection, as biopsy carries a high risk of hemorrhagic complications.[51]

Prognostic factors

The most important prognostic factor for any patient with PPS is whether the tumor is amenable to complete surgical resection. This includes evaluation for the presence of distant metastases. Among the majority of reported cases, surviving patients have undergone complete surgical resection of their tumors.

Histological grade is the next most important prognostic factor for PPS. Despite the lack of standardization for grading among institutions, attempts are made to classify tumors into categories of low-, intermediate- or high-grade malignancies. Moran and colleagues proposed a classification system for primary pulmonary leiomyosarcomas, with low-grade tumors demonstrating low mitotic rate (<3 mitoses per 10 HPF) and absence of pleomorphism, hyperchromism, hemorrhage, or necrosis. Intermediate-grade tumors demonstrate increased mitotic rate (3–8 mitoses per 10 HPF), increased cellularity, and mild-to-moderate nuclear pleomorphism. High-grade tumors were those with increased cellularity, high mitotic rate (>8 mitoses per 10 HPF), and marked nuclear atypia and pleomorphism.[18] Median survival time in this series of 18 patients differed based on grade, with the median survival time for eight patients with high-grade tumors of 5 months, while six patients with lower-grade tumors were alive and free of disease between 2 and 12 years after diagnosis.[18] The nonspecific determinations of the degree of tumor cellularity and nuclear atypia and polymorphism obviously leave a large amount of the assignment of tumor grade to the individual pathologist.

An endobronchial location of the primary lesion has been associated with better prognosis.[4,5,113] This is likely secondary to a relatively earlier stage at the time of symptomatic presentation, although an association with lower-grade tumors in this location has been suggested.[114]

Size of the primary tumor has been identified as a prognostic factor as well, with tumors greater than 5 cm demonstrating poorer prognosis when compared to smaller lesions.[95]

Different histological types of PPS and age at diagnosis may carry varying prognostic implications. In leiomyosarcomas, younger age at presentation portends a poorer prognosis, whereas for fibrosarcomas (defined prior to the WHO soft tissue sarcoma update in 2002), survival rates of 78% have been reported for childhood cases.[7,113] Adults with leiomyosarcomas tend to have a better outcome than adults with other types of PPS.[12] Pulmonary synovial sarcoma is thought to represent a more aggressive subtype, with overall 5-year survival of 50%.[115] Primary pulmonary angiosarcomas and pulmonary artery sarcomas are highly aggressive tumors, with patients dying within a few months of diagnosis.[10,116] In a series of nine patients with pulmonary arterial sarcomas seen at the Mayo Clinic, the longest survival time in seven evaluable patients was 3.5 years. The majority of patients died within 5 months of diagnosis.[74]

Epithelioid hemangioendotheliomas may exhibit a range of aggressiveness. Malignant triton tumors, in the few reported cases, seem to represent highly aggressive malignancies.

Molecular markers may play a role in the prognosis of PPS. Vascular endothelial growth factor (VEGF) has been identified as a potential prognostic factor in PPS. Retrospective review of PPS expressing strong VEGF (>50% positive cells) showed significantly reduced 5-year disease-free survival (13.2%) compared to PPS with absent or faint VEGF (83.3%, p <0.05) expression. This survival difference was confirmed on multivariate analysis. These data have not been replicated in other studies but this study provides promising data for potential new markers in PPS.[117]

Staging in primary pulmonary sarcoma

As PPSs do not typically involve regional lymphatic structures, the staging of PPS does not follow the common tumor-node-metastasis (TNM) staging system. One important factor in the prognosis of PPS is the presence or absence of metastases. Histological grade, including mitotic count, is the next most important prognostic factor. A standardized system of assessing grade for these rare and varied tumors does not exist, rendering evaluation of tumor grade highly variable among individual institutions. Gal and colleagues proposed that a high-grade pulmonary sarcoma is typified by a mitotic count greater than five per 50 HPF, the presence of giant cells, tumor necrosis, high cellularity, and poor tumor circumscription.[118]

Treatment

Definitive therapy for PPS involves complete surgical excision of tumor. Most commonly, this is accomplished with lobectomy or pneumonectomy, although reports of endobronchial resection for isolated endobronchial tumors exist (with varying degrees of success).[4,5] Frequently PPSs are very locally advanced at the time of presentation and diagnosis, with invasion of vital structures, precluding surgery. A report has been published of radical resection involving cardiopulmonary bypass and resection of the left atrium or pulmonary trunk, demonstrating that such approaches may be possible, but follow-up is short and overall outcome is not disclosed.[119]

Experience with neoadjuvant chemotherapy for PPS is limited to a few case reports in the literature. Neoadjuvant combination chemotherapy was attempted in a patient with advanced pulmonary fibrosarcoma (as described previously, this is an out-of-date diagnosis but further characterization is not available) as well as in a patient with advanced pulmonary hemangiopericytoma in order to render resection easier. However, no response to therapy was documented on imaging or at the time of surgical resections.[7,27] Combination chemoradiotherapy was administered preoperatively to a patient with primary pulmonary artery leiomyosarcoma with secondary superior vena cava syndrome. This patient demonstrated significant tumor response, with only microscopic residual disease demonstrated among tumor necrosis at pneumonectomy.[120]

Even for those patients who are able to undergo initial complete surgical resection, subsequent unresectable local relapse remains a significant problem. Chemotherapy and radiation therapy have been administered alone or in combination in the adjuvant setting; however, no definitive benefit has been shown given the short follow-up of all case reports. For patients with completely resected PPS, adjuvant therapy should be considered, in an approach similar to patients with completely resected extremity soft tissue sarcomas. No randomized trial exists to support the use of adjuvant chemotherapy or radiation for PPS, and given the rarity of the tumors, a randomized trial will not be possible.

Therefore, a benefit from adjuvant chemotherapy and radiation could be postulated to be similar to patients with resected nonpulmonary soft tissue sarcomas. Adjuvant chemotherapy should be considered for all stage II and III (<5 cm primary tumor with histological grade 2 or 3, or ≥5 cm primary tumor any grade) extremity soft tissue sarcomas after resection or as preoperative therapy, as well as consideration of postoperative radiation therapy in resected stage I soft tissue sarcomas with inadequate surgical margins (≤1 cm). Lastly, if the tumor is unresectable or metastatic, chemotherapy and radiation therapy are reasonable approaches to therapy, regardless of primary tumor size, and should be considered in a sequential manner rather than concurrent chemotherapy and radiation therapy (for which there is little evidence in soft tissue sarcoma).

Follow-up of surgically resected patients or patients treated with chemotherapy and/or radiation without surgery should include regular imaging in addition to history and physical examination. PPSs tend to recur locally rather than distantly, and early recognition of local recurrence may allow repeat resection for possible survival benefit. A proven standard of care for imaging follow-up does not exist, although the authors recommend chest radiograph with each clinic visit, as well as consideration of an annual chest CT.

Chemotherapy, either as single agent or in combination regimens, may have palliative benefit in the setting of unresectable disease. Experience with chemotherapy for PPS is predominantly gathered from patients with traditional soft tissue sarcomas and extrapolated to pulmonary sarcomas. The most commonly used agents include doxorubicin (20% response rate), ifosfamide, and dacarbazine.[121,122] A child with recurrent unresectable bronchopulmonary leiomyosarcoma treated with the combination of vincristine, dactinomycin, ifosfamide, and doxorubicin obtained complete response with three cycles of therapy, confirmed on subsequent surgical exploration.[123] The patient subsequently received a total of nine cycles of chemotherapy followed by involved-field radiation, with no evidence of relapse 16 months after disease recurrence.[123]

Immunotherapy with high-dose interleukin-2 was reported to induce tumor regression when used in combination with radiotherapy for a patient with unresectable pulmonary angiosarcoma.[10] It is unclear whether the combination, or one treatment modality over another, caused the tumor shrinkage. Interferon-α2B was administered to a patient with epithelioid hemangioendothelioma without response.[55]

In patients with AIDS and pulmonary KS, highly active antiretroviral therapy (HAART) has dramatically changed the outlook for this previously highly lethal disease (survival time less than 12 months). In a retrospective series of patients with pulmonary KS in the pre- and post-HAART eras, median survival was 8.9 weeks for patients before HAART and was not reached in the post-HAART era, findings that were highly statistically significant.[124] Patients previously receiving chemotherapy for pulmonary KS were able to obtain remission on HAART and discontinue chemotherapy.[124] This represents the first major breakthrough in the treatment of a type of pulmonary sarcoma, dramatically improving survival.

While many PPSs tend to be very aggressive if not completely surgically resected, reports of long-term survival even with recurrent or metastatic disease exist, including a patient surviving more than 7 years with local and metastatic disease who did not receive therapy beyond initial diagnostic surgery.[4] Partial spontaneous regression after long-term presence of disease has been described in a few patients with epithelioid hemangioendothelioma.[55]

Given the extreme rarity of all types of PPS, dedicated therapeutic trials for this group of diseases are not feasible. This is unfortunate as (with the exception of HAART for KS) no effective therapy has been demonstrated for advanced disease. If possible, enrollment in clinical trials with newer agents (phase 1 or phase 2 studies) should be recommended for patients with advanced unresectable disease.

Recommendations

Primary pulmonary sarcoma is a rare cause of pulmonary malignancy. It consists of a diverse collection of tumor subtypes with different tissue origins and wide-ranging clinical behavior. PPS tends to be very advanced at the time of diagnosis and the prognosis as a group is poor. Complete surgical resection remains the only potentially curative therapeutic modality. Surgical resection should be employed whenever possible, and radiation therapy should be employed for any positive surgical margins. Despite the lack of randomized clinical data in treating PPS, the addition of adjuvant chemotherapy should be considered for large primary tumors >5 cm, any size tumor with histological grade 2 or higher, and/or involved lymph nodes. For unresectable disease, sequential chemotherapy and radiation therapy should be considered as primary treatment modality for advanced and metastatic disease based on treatment data for soft tissue sarcomas of the extremities. Ideally, the dramatic increase in the understanding of

malignancies on a molecular level that has occurred in recent years and recent updates to the classification of soft tissue sarcomas by the WHO might lead to further progress in the treatment of PPS. Clinical trials, especially phase 1 and 2 studies, evaluating newer agents and treatment approaches should be considered for all patients with PPS.

Acknowledgments

The authors acknowledge the contributions of Adriana L. Gonzalez MD, Rachel E. Sanborn MD, and Thomas M. Ulbright MD to earlier editions of this chapter.

References

1. Jemal A, *et al*. Cancer statistics, 2010. CA: A Cancer Journal for Clinicians 2010; 60: 277–300.
2. Sonpavde G, Ulbright TM, Sandler A. Primary sarcomas of the lung. In: Raghavan D, Brecher ML, Johnson DH, *et al*. (eds) *Textbook of Uncommon Cancer*, 2nd edn. Chichester: Wiley, 1999. pp. 511–21.
3. Attanoos RL, Appelton MAC, Gibbs AR. Primary sarcomas of the lung: a clinicopathological and immunohistochemical study of 14 cases. Histopathology 1996; 29: 29–36.
4. Takeda F, *et al*. Leiomyosarcoma of the main bronchus in a girl: a long-time survivor with multiple lung metastases. Pediatr Pulmonol 2004; 37: 368–74.
5. Savas C, Candir O, Ozguner F. Acute respiratory distress due to fibrosarcoma of the carina in a child. Pediatr Pulmonol 2004; 38: 355–7.
6. Logrono R, *et al*. Diagnosis of primary fibrosarcoma of the lung by fine-needle aspiration and core biopsy: a case report and review of the literature. Arch Pathol Lab Med 1999; 123: 731–5.
7. Picard E, *et al*. Pulmonary fibrosarcoma in childhood: fiber-optic bronchoscopic diagnosis and review of the literature. Pediatr Pulmonol 1999; 27: 347–50.
8. World Health Organization. Pathology and genetics of tumours of soft tissue and bone. In: Fletcher CDM, Unni KK, Mertens F (eds) *World Health Organization Classification of Tumours*. Lyon: IARC Press, 2002.
9. Comin CE, *et al*. Primary pulmonary rhabdomyosarcoma: report of a case in an adult and review of the literature. Ultrastruct Pathol 2001; 25: 269–73.
10. Kojima K, *et al*. Successful treatment of primary pulmonary angiosarcoma. Chest 2003; 124: 2397–400.
11. Dail DH. Uncommon tumors. In: Dail DH, Hammar SP (eds) *Pulmonary Pathology*. New York: Springer, 1988. p. 847.
12. McCormack PM, Martini N. Primary sarcomas and lymphomas of the lung. In: Martini N, Vogt-Moykopf I (eds) *Thoracic Surgery: Frontiers and Uncommon Neoplasms*, vol 5. St Louis, MO: CV Mosby, 1989. p. 269.
13. Robinson PG, Shields TW. Uncommon Primary Malignant Tumors of the Lung. In: Shields TW, Locicero J III, Ronn RB, Rusch VW (eds). *General Thoracic Surgery*, 6th edn. Philadelphia; Lippincott, Williams & Wilkins, 2004. pp. 1801–1830.
14. Lucas DR, *et al*. Sarcomatoid mesothelioma and its histological mimics: a comparative immunohistochemical study. Histopathology 2003; 42: 270–9.
15. Ali SZ, *et al*. Solitary fibrous tumor. A cytologic-histologic study with clinical, radiologic, and immunohistochemical correlations. Cancer 1997; 81: 116–21.
16. Lillo-Gil R, Albrechtsson U, Jakobsson B. Pulmonary leiomyosarcoma appearing as a cyst: report of one case and review of the literature. Thoracic Cardiovasc Surg 1985; 33: 250–2.
17. Ramanathan T. Primary leiomyosarcoma of the lung. Thorax 1974; 29: 482–9.
18. Moran CA. Primary leiomyosarcoma of the lung: a clinicopathologic and immunohistochemical study of 18 cases. Mod Pathol 1997; 10: 121–8.
19. Shaw RR, *et al*. Primary pulmonary leiomyosarcomas. J Thoracic Cardiovasc Surg 1961; 41: 430.

20. Ono N, *et al*. Primary bronchopulmonary fibrosarcoma: report of a case. Surg Today 1998; 28: 1313–15.

21. Ockner DM, *et al*. Genital angiomyofibroblastoma. Comparison with aggressive angiomyxoma and other myxoid neoplasms of skin and soft tissue. Am J Clin Pathol 1997; 107: 36–44.

22. Weiss SW, Goldblum JR (eds). *Enzinger and Weiss's Soft Tissue Tumors*, 4th edn. St Louis, MO: Mosby, 2001.

23. Klemperer P, Rabin C. Primary neoplasm of the pleura: a report of five cases. Arch Pathol 1931; 11: 385.

24. Erlandson RA, Woodruff JM. Role of electron microscopy in the evaluation of soft tissue neoplasms, with emphasis on spindle cell and pleomorphic tumors. Hum Pathol 1998; 29: 1372–81.

25. Suster S, Moran CA. Primary synovial sarcomas of the mediastinum: a clinicopathologic, immunohistochemical, and ultrastructural study of 15 cases. Am J Surg Pathol 2005; 29: 569–78.

26. Brega Massone PP, *et al*. A particular case with long-term follow-up of rare malignant hemangiopericytoma of the lung with metachronous diaphragmatic metastasis. Thorac Cardiovasc Surg 2002; 50: 178–80.

27. Wu YC, *et al*. Primary pulmonary malignant hemangiopericytoma associated with coagulopathy. Ann Thorac Surg 1997; 64: 841–3.

28. Suster S. Primary sarcomas of the lung. Semin Diag Pathol 1995; 12: 140–57.

29. Yousem SA, Glynn SD. Intrapulmonary localized fibrous tumor. Am J Clin Pathol 1988; 89: 365–9.

30. Van de Rijn M, Lombard CM, Rouse RV. Expression of CD34 by solitary fibrous tumor of the pleura, mediastinum and lung. Am J Surg Pathol 1994; 18: 814–20.

31. England DM, Hochholzer L, McCarthy MJ. Localized benign and malignant fibrous tumors of the pleura. A clinicopathologic review of 223 cases. Am J Surg Pathol 1989; 13: 640–58.

32. Vallat-Decouvelaere AV, Dry SM, Fletcher CD. Atypical and malignant solitary fibrous tumors in extrathoracic locations: evidence of their comparability to intrathoracic tumors. Am J Surg Pathol 1998; 22: 1501–11.

33. Magdeleinat P, *et al*. Solitary fibrous tumors of the pleura: clinical characteristics, surgical treatment and outcome. Eur J Cardiothorac Surg 2002; 21: 1087–93.

34. Yousem SA, Hochholzer L. Primary pulmonary hemangiopericytoma. Cancer 1987; 59: 549–55.

35. Katz DS, *et al*. Primary malignant pulmonary hemangiopericytoma. Clin Imaging 1998; 22: 192–5.

36. Stembridge VA, Luibel FJ, Ashworth CT. Soft tissue sarcomas: electron microscopic approach to histogenic classification. South Med J 1964; 57: 772–9.

37. Van Haelst UJGM. General considerations on electron microscopy of soft tissues. In: Fenoglio CM, Wolff M (eds) *Progress in Surgical Pathology*, vol 2. New York: Masson, 1980. pp. 225–57.

38. Bedrossian CWM, *et al*. Pulmonary malignant fibrous histiocytoma. Chest 1979; 75: 186–9.

39. Kimizuka G, Okuzawa K, Yarita T. Primary giant cell malignant fibrous histiocytoma of the lung: a case report. Pathol Int 1999; 49: 342–6.

40. Fletcher CDM. The evolving classification of soft tissue tumors: an update based on the new WHO classification. Histopathology 2006;48: 3–12.

41. Gaertner EM, *et al*. Pulmonary and mediastinal glomus tumors: report of five cases including a pulmonary glomangiosarcoma: a clinicopathologic study with literature review. Am J Surg Pathol 2000; 24: 1105–14.

42. Spragg RG, *et al*. Angiosarcoma of the lung with fatal pulmonary hemorrhage. Am J Med 1983; 74: 1072–6.

43. Avignina A, *et al*. Pulmonary rhabdomyosarcoma with isolated small bowel metastases: a report of a case with immunohistological and ultrastructural studies. Cancer 1984; 53: 1948–51.

44. Lee SH, Reganchary SS, Paramesh J. Primary pulmonary rhabdomyosarcoma: a case report and review of the literature. Hum Pathol 1981; 12: 92–6.

45. Shariff S, *et al*. Primary pulmonary rhabdomyosarcoma in a child, with review of the literature. J Surg Oncol 1988; 38: 261–4.

46. Ueda K, *et al*. Rhabdomyosarcoma of lung arising in congenital cystic malformation. Cancer 1977; 40: 383–8.

47. Luck SR, Reynolds M, Raffensperger JG. Congenital bronchopulmonary malformations. Curr Probl Surg 1986; 23: 245–314.

48. Nash G, Fligel S. Kaposi's sarcoma presenting as pulmonary disease in the acquired immunodeficiency syndrome: diagnosis by lung biopsy. Hum Pathol 1984; 15: 999–1001.

49. Misra DP, Sunderrajan EV, Hurst DJ. Kaposi's sarcoma of the lung: radiography and pathology. Thorax 1982; 37: 155–6.

50. Epstein DM, Gefter WB, Conrad K. Lung disease in homosexual men. Radiology 1982; 143: 7–10.

51. Aboulafia DM. The epidemiologic, pathologic, and clinical features of AIDS-associated pulmonary Kaposi's sarcoma. Chest 2000; 117: 1128–45.

52. Weiss SW, Enzinger FM. Epithelioid hemangioendothelioma: a vascular tumor often mistaken for a carcinoma. Cancer 1982; 50: 970–81.

53. Weiss SW, *et al*. Epithelioid hemangioendothelioma and related lesions. Semin Diagn Pathol 1986; 3: 259–87.

54. Dail DH, *et al*. Intravascular, bronchiolar and alveolar tumor of the lung (IVBAT): an analysis of twenty cases of a peculiar sclerosing endothelial tumor. Cancer 1983; 51: 452–64.

55. Cronin P, Arenberg D. Pulmonary epithelioid hemangioendothelioma: an unusual case and a review of the literature. Chest 2004; 125: 789–92.

56. World Health Organization. Pathology and genetics of tumours of the lung, pleura, thymus and heart. In: Travis WD, Brambilla E, Muller-Hermelink HK, Harris CC (eds) *World Health Organization Classification of Tumours*. Lyon: IARC Press, 2004.

57. Colby TV, Koss MN, Travis WD. *Atlas of Tumor Pathology: Tumors of the Lower Respiratory Tract*, vol. fascicle 13. Washington DC: Armed Forces Institute of Pathology, 1995.

58. Falconieri G, *et al*. Pseudomesotheliomatous angiosarcoma: a pleuropulmonary lesion simulating malignant pleural mesothelioma. Histopathology 1997; 30: 419–24.

59. Ott RA, *et al*. Primary pulmonary angiosarcoma associated with multiple synchronous neoplasms. J Surg Oncol 1987; 35: 269–76.

60. Sebenik M, *et al*. Undifferentiated intimal sarcoma of large systemic blood vessels: report of 14 cases with immunohistochemical profile and review of the literature. Am J Surg Pathol 2005; 29: 1184–93.

61. Zeren H, *et al*. Primary pulmonary sarcomas with features of monophasic synovial sarcoma: a clinicopathological, immunohistochemical and ultrastructural study of 25 cases. Hum Pathol 1995; 26: 474–80.

62. Kaplan MA, *et al*. Primary pulmonary sarcoma with morphologic features of monophasic synovial sarcoma and chromosome translocation t(X;18). Am J Clin Pathol 1996; 105: 195–9.

63. Okamoto S, *et al*. Primary pulmonary synovial sarcoma: a clinicopathologic, immunohistochemical, and molecular study of 11 cases. Hum Pathol 2004; 35: 850–6.

64. Essary LR, Vargas SO, Fletcher CDM. Primary pleuropulmonary synovial sarcoma: reappraisal of a recently described anatomic subset. Cancer 2002; 94: 459–69.

65. De Leeuw B, Geurts VKA. Molecular cloning of the synovial sarcoma specific translocation breakpoint. Hum Mol Genet 1994; 3: 745–9.

66. Duran-Mendicuti A, Costello P, Vargas SO. Primary synovial sarcoma of the chest: radiographic and clinicopathologic correlation. J Thorac Imaging 2003; 18: 87–93.

67. Guillou L, *et al*. Detection of the synovial sarcoma translocation t(X;18) (SYT;SSX) in paraffin-embedded tissues using reverse transcriptase-polymerase chain reaction: a reliable and powerful diagnostic tool for pathologists. A molecular analysis of 221 mesenchymal tumors fixed in different fixatives. Hum Pathol 2001; 32: 105–12.

68. Coindre JM, *et al*. Should molecular testing be required for diagnosing synovial sarcoma? A prospective study of 204 cases. Cancer 2003; 98: 2700–7.

69. Hill DA, *et al*. Real-time polymerase chain reaction as an aid for the detection of SYT-SSX1 and SYT-SSX2 transcripts in fresh and archival pediatric synovial sarcoma specimens: report of 25 cases from St Jude Children's Research Hospital. Pediatr Dev Pathol 2003; 6: 24–34.

70. Hisaoka M, *et al*. Primary synovial sarcoma of the lung: report of two cases confirmed by molecular detection of SYT-SSX fusion gene transcripts. Histopathology 1999; 34: 205–10.

71. Miller DL, Allen MS. Rare pulmonary neoplasms. Mayo Clinic Proc 1993; 68: 492–8.

72. Nonomura A, et al. Primary pulmonary artery sarcoma: report of two autopsy cases studied by immunohistochemistry and electon microscopy and review of 110 cases reported in the literature. Acta Pathol Jpn 1988; 38: 883–96.

73. Gebauer C. The postoperative prognosis of primary pulmonary sarcomas: a review with a comparison between the histological forms and the other primary endothoracal sarcomas based on 474 cases. Scand J Thorac Cardiovasc Surg 1982; 16: 91–7.

74. Parish JM, et al. Pulmonary artery sarcoma: clinical features. Chest 1996; 110: 1480–8.

75. Yi ES. Tumors of the pulmonary vasculature. Cardiol Clin 2004; 22: 431–40, vi–vii.

76. Smith EAC, Cohen RV, Peale ARE. Primary chondrosarcoma of the lung. Ann Intern Med 1960; 53: 838.

77. Morgenroth A, et al. Primary chondrosarcoma of the left inferior lobar bronchus. Respiration 1989; 56: 241–4.

78. Morgan AD, Salama FD. Primary chondrosarcoma of the lung: case report and review of the literature. J Thorac Cardiovasc Surg 1972; 64: 460–6.

79. Loose JH, et al. Primary osteosarcoma of the lung: report of two cases and review of the literature. J Thorac Cardiovasc Surg 1990; 100: 867–73.

80. Sawamura K, et al. Primary lipsarcoma of the lung: report of a case. J Surg Oncol 1982; 19: 243–6.

81. Kalus M, et al. Malignant mesenchymoma of the lung. Arch Pathol 1973; 95: 199–202.

82. Moran CA, Suster S, Koss MN. Primary malignant "triton" tumor of the lung. Histopathology 1997; 30: 140–4.

83. Huang HY, et al. Primary mesenchymal chondrosarcoma of the lung. Ann Thorac Surg 2002; 73: 1960–2.

84. Ichimura H, et al. Primary chondrosarcoma of the lung recognized as a long-standing solitary nodule prior to resection. Jpn J Thorac Cardiovasc Surg 2005; 53: 106–8.

85. Tsunezuke Y, et al. Primary chondromatous osteosarcoma of the pulmonary aretery. Ann Thorac Surg 2004; 77: 331–4.

86. Kawano D, et al. Dedifferentiated chondrosarcoma of the lung: report of a case. Surg Today 2011; 41: 251–4.

87. Bartley TD, Arean VM. Intrapulmonary neurogenic tumors. J Thorac Cardiovasc Surg 1965; 50: 114–23.

88. McCluggage WG, Bharucha H. Primary pulmonary tumors of nerve sheath origin. Histopathology 1995; 26: 247–54.

89. Roviaro G, et al. Primary pulmonary tumors of neurogenic origin. Thorax 1983; 38: 842–5.

90. World Health Organization. Classification of tumors of the central nervous system. In: Louis DN, Ohgaki H, Wiestler OD, et al. (eds) World Health Organization Classification of Tumours. Lyon: IARC Press, 2007.

91. Bose AK, Deodhar AP, Duncan AJ. Malignant triton tumor of the right vagus. Ann Thorac Surg 2002; 74: 1227–8.

92. Martini N, Hadju DI, Beattie EJ. Primary sarcoma of the lung. J Thorac Cardiovasc Surg 1971; 61: 33–8.

93. Murad TM, von Haam E, Murthy MS. Ultrastructure of a hemangiopericytoma and a glomus tumor. Cancer 1968; 22: 1239–49.

94. Engelke C, et al. Pulmonary haemangiosarcoma with main pulmonary artery thrombosis imitating subacute pulmonary embolism with infarction. Br J Radiol 2004; 77: 623–5.

95. Nascimento AG, Unni KK, Bernatz PE. Sarcomas of the lung. Mayo Clinic Proc 1982; 57: 355–9.

96. Ishida T, et al. Carcinosarcoma and spindle cell carcinoma of the lung: clinicopathologic and immunohistochemical studies. J Thorac Cardiovasc Surg 1990; 100: 844–52.

97. Cabarcos A, Gomez DM, Lobo BJL. Pulmonary carcinosarcoma: a case study and review of the literature. Br J Dis Chest 1985; 79: 83–94.

98. Meade P, et al. Carcinosarcoma of the lung with hypertrophic pulmonary osteoarthropathy. Ann Thorac Surg 1991; 51: 488–90.

99. Davis MP, et al. Carcinosarcoma of the lung: Mayo Clinic experience and response to chemotherapy. Mayo Clinic Proc 1984; 59: 598–603.

100. Koss MN, Hochholzer L, Frommelt RA. Carcinosarcomas of the lung: a clinicopathologic study of 66 patients. Am J Surg Pathol 1999; 23: 1514–26.

101. Manivel JC, et al. Pleuropulmonary blastoma: the so-called blastoma of childhood. Cancer 1988; 62: 1516–26.

102. Francis D, Jacobsen M. Pulmonary blastoma. Curr Top Pathol 1983; 73: 265–94.

103. Kodama T, et al. Six cases of well differentiated adenocarcinoma simulating fetal lung tubules in pseudoglandular stage: comparison with pulmonary blastoma. Am J Surg Pathol 1984; 8: 735–44.

104. Koss MN, Hochholzer L, O'Leary T. Pulmonary blastomas. Cancer 1991; 67: 2368–81.

105. Spencer H. Pulmonary blastoma. J Pathol 1961; 82: 161.

106. Fukayama M, et al. Pulmonary and pleural thymoma: diagnostic application of lymphocytic markers to the thymoma of unusual site. Am J Clin Pathol 1988; 89: 617–21.

107. Ledet SC, Brown RW, Cagle PT. P53 immunostaining in the differentiation of inflammatory pseudotumor from sarcoma involving the lung. Mod Pathol 1995; 8: 282–6.

108. Aakhus T, Mylius EA. Leiomyoma of the lung. Acta Chirurg Scand 1962; 124: 372–6.

109. Winnepenninckx V, et al. New phenotypical and ultrastructural findings in spindle cell (desmoplastic/neurotropic) melanoma. Appl Immunohistochem Mol Morphol 2003; 11: 319–25.

110. Yi CA, et al. Computed tomography in pulmonary artery sarcoma: distinguishing features from pulmonary embolic disease. J Comput Assist Tomogr 2004; 28: 34–9.

111. McGee RS Jr, Ward WG, Kilpatrick SE. Malignant peripheral nerve sheath tumor: a fine-needle aspiration biopsy study. Diagn Cytopathol 1997; 17: 298–305.

112. DeMay RM. The Art and Science of Cytopathology. Vol. II. Aspiration Cytology. Chicago: ASCP Press, 1996.

113. Lai DS, et al. Primary bronchopulmonary leiomyosarcoma of the left main bronchus in a child presenting with wheezing and atelectasis of the left lung. Pediatr Pulmonol 2002; 33: 318–21.

114. Pettinato G, et al. Primary bronchopulmonary fibrosarcoma of childhood and adolescence: reassessment of a low-grade malignancy. Hum Pathol 1989; 20: 463–71.

115. Dennison S, Weppler E, Giacoppe G. Primary pulmonary synovial sarcoma: a case report and review of current diagnostic and therapeutic standards. Oncologist 204; 9: 339–42.

116. Choong CK, et al. Failure of medical therapy for pulmonary "thromboembolic" disease: beware the unsuspected primary sarcoma of the pulmonary artery. J Thorac Cardiovasc Surg 2004; 128: 763–5.

117. Iyoda A, et al. Expression of vascular endothelial growth factor in thoracic sarcomas. Ann Thorac Surg 2001; 71: 1635–9.

118. Gal AA, et al. Prognostic factors in pulmonary fibrohistiocytic lesions. Cancer 1994; 73: 1817–24.

119. Shimono T, et al. Pulmonary leiomyosarcoma extending into left atrium or pulmonary trunk: complete resection with cardiopulmonary bypass. J Thorac Cardiovasc Surg 1998; 115: 460–1.

120. Faul JL, et al. Superior vena cava syndrome caused by pulmonary artery sarcoma. J Thorac Cardiovasc Surg 1999; 118: 749–50.

121. Edmonson JH, et al. Randomized comparison of doxorubicin alone versus ifosfamide plus doxorubicin or mitomycin, doxorubicin and cisplatin against advanced soft tissue sarcomas. J Clin Oncol 1993; 11: 1269–75.

122. Santoro A, et al. Doxorubicin versus CYVADIC versus doxorubicin plus ifosfamide in first line treatment of advanced soft tissue sarcomas: a randomized study of the EORTC and Bone Sarcoma Group. J Clin Oncol 1995; 13: 1537–45.

123. Ferrari A, et al. Response to chemotherapy in a child with primary bronchopulmonary leiomyosarcoma. Med Pediatr Oncol 2002; 39: 55–7.

124. Holkova B, et al. Effect of highly active antiretroviral therapy on survival in patients with AIDS-associated pulmonary Kaposi's sarcoma treated with chemotherapy. J Clin Oncol 2001; 19: 3848–51.

22 Mesotheliomas

Giuseppe Giaccone, Anish Thomas, and Arun Rajan

Medical Oncology Branch, National Cancer Institute, Bethesda, MD, USA

Introduction

Malignant mesotheliomas (MM) are aggressive tumors originating from the serosa of the pleura, pericardium or peritoneum. The disease is strongly associated with exposure to certain forms of asbestos. However, a small proportion of patients do not have a history of asbestos exposure, leading to the search for other environmental and genetic factors that may play a role in the development of MM. The disease occurs more commonly in men (ratio of men to women, 3:1) with an even greater proportion of men being diagnosed with malignant pleural mesothelioma (MPM; ratio 5:1). The incidence of MM also increases steadily with age; MPM commonly develops between the fifth and seventh decades of life. This is probably a reflection of the long latent period between exposure to asbestos and the development of disease which can range from 20 to 60 years.

Histologically MM can present as epitheloid, biphasic or sarcomatoid tumors. New insights are being gained into the molecular changes that result in the development of MM and attempts are being made to develop serum biomarkers with prognostic and predictive value.

Malignant mesothelioma is an aggressive disease associated with poor survival with supportive care alone. Surgery in combination with multimodality therapies has the potential to provide long-term survival benefit. Various targeted therapies and immunological approaches are being evaluated in MM.

Biology and epidemiology

A number of studies have focused on the multiple genetic changes that take place in MM. A detailed and thorough review of molecular alterations in mesothelioma has been published recently.[1]

Alterations in the neurofibromatosis type II (*NF2*) gene and *ink4a* generate resistance to apoptosis. The *NF2* gene, which is located on chromosome 22, often lost in MM, was found to be mutated in 53% of 15 MM cell lines.[2] Inactivation of *NF2* in MM probably occurs via a two-hit mechanism.[3]

Frequent genetic losses involving specific regions of chromosome arms 1p, 3p, 6q, and 9p, and numerical losses of chromosome 22 have been described in MM. These chromosomal changes suggest the presence of multiple important genes involved in the molecular development of this disease.

Deletion of chromosome bands 9p13–p22 has been described cytogenetically in 50% of MMs;[4] in this region, two putative tumor suppressor genes, *p15* and *p16*, are located. Alterations of *p16* were found to be common in MM cell lines (homozygous deletions in 85% of 40 cell lines), but less in primary tumors (22% of 23 specimens).[5] Deletions of 9p21–p22 outside the *p16* locus may reflect the involvement of other putative tumor suppressor genes. Codeletion of *p15* and *p16* was observed in 72% of 50 cases by fluorescent in situ hybridization (FISH) analysis, including all the sarcomatoid cases (21 of 21).[6] This finding strongly suggests that *p15* and *p16* or other neighboring genes on chromosome 9p are the targets for the development of this tumor.

Frequent losses of 6q have been observed by cytogenetic analysis (about 40%). By using 32 microsatellite markers, loss of heterozygosity (LOH) was observed in 61% of 46 MMs. These deletions fall into four distinct locations, possibly loci of putative tumor suppressor genes.[7] Of the 28 cases with LOH of 6q, 23 (82%) also had LOH of 1p; therefore deletions of regions on both chromosomes occur frequently. LOH in 3p14 to 3p25 was also found in a total of 42% of MMs (cell lines and tumors).[8] The *Fhit* gene, located at 3p14.2, was found to be absent or reduced in 54% of 13 mesothelioma cases, which suggests a potential significance of *Fhit* inactivation in the pathogenesis of this tumor.[9]

Data obtained from comparative genomic hybridization identified a region on 15q which is deleted in 54% of mesotheliomas; this finding suggests that this region probably harbors a putative tumor suppressor gene that may contribute to the pathogenesis of MM.[10]

Textbook of Uncommon Cancer, Fourth Edition. Edited by Derek Raghavan, Charles D. Blanke, David H. Johnson, Paul L. Moots, Gregory H. Reaman, Peter G. Rose and Mikkael A. Sekeres.
© 2012 John Wiley & Sons, Inc. Published 2012 by John Wiley & Sons, Inc.

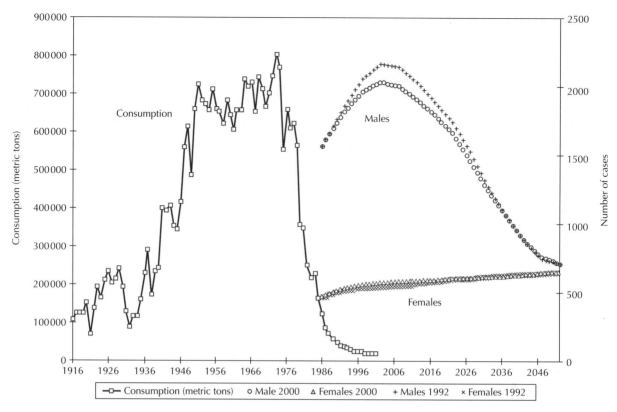

Figure 22.1 Asbestos use (consumption) in the United States and projected numbers of male and female mesothelioma cases based on a birth cohort and age model estimated from Surveillance, Epidemiology, and End Results (SEER) Program data for two periods, 1973–1992 and 1973–2000. Reproduced from Bianchi *et al.*[2] with permission from Oxford University Press.

Angiogenesis plays an important role in mesothelioma. Interleukin (IL)-8, a potent chemokine with angiogenesis function, has been shown to be an autocrine growth factor for mesothelioma cell lines.[11] A higher expression of vascular endothelial growth factor (VEGF) and higher microvessel density (MVD) were found in epithelial type mesothelioma,[12] supporting an important role in angiogenesis and lymphangiogenesis in mesothelioma.[12–14] Angiogenesis has also been shown to be a poor prognostic factor in this disease.[15]

Epigenetic alterations involving hypermethylation and histone regulation represent another important mechanism of tumorigenesis in malignant mesothelioma.[1] With the advent of new technologies, attempts have been made to discover novel candidate oncogenes and tumor suppressor genes using high-density oligonucleotide microarrays. These genes should be further validated in functional assays.[16] Differential patterns of gene expression may also aid in diagnosis, as different patterns have been observed between sarcomatoid and epithelial tumors.[17]

Asbestos is the major cause of MM localized to the pleura, peritoneum, and tunica vaginalis testis; a history of asbestos exposure can be obtained in about 75% patients. After the identification of asbestos as a major cause of pleural mesothelioma before 1960, an increased interest in MM led to better registration.[18] The incidence of MM in the United States and western Europe has shown a steep increase in the past decades and a modification of the ratio of incidence between the genders.[19,20] In western Europe, asbestos use remained high until

1980; men born in the period 1945–1950 suffered the highest risk, and of these 1 in 150 would die of mesothelioma.[20] In Europe, about 9000 deaths due to MM are expected by the year 2018, because of the very long latency period, followed by a decline in incidence.[20] In an update on the European epidemic by Pelucchi and colleagues, it appears that the incidence is indeed leveling off.[21] As shown in Figure 22.1, the incidence in the United States has leveled off after a peak at year ~2000 as a result of an earlier ban on asbestos.[22]

Over the past 40 years, the male:female ratio has changed from 1:1 to 3:1, as would be expected, considering the occupational relationship of exposure to asbestos.[19,20] According to Hillerdal, the incidence of MM in autopsy series varies from 0.02% to 0.7% and is closely related to the level of asbestos exposure.[23] However, there is no evidence of a threshold level below which there is no risk of developing mesothelioma.[23] The highest incidences are observed in areas with shipyards, and involve construction workers, asbestos miners, manufacturers of heating equipment, and insulation workers.[22] A major concern is the widespread use of asbestos in developing countries. Now that the western world has stringent regulations for the handling and manufacturing of asbestos products, companies have found their way to developing countries. Unrestricted and unprotected use of asbestos is unfortunately quite common, and people are not adequately informed about the risks of asbestos exposure.[24]

In the western industrialized countries a dramatic decrease in the incidence of MM is seen in the male population born

Table 22.1 Types of asbestos fibers and estimated risk of carcinogenicity.

Fiber type	Color	Exposure site	Specifications ratio length/diameter	Carcinogenicity
Crocidolite	Blue asbestos	Mining (South Africa, Australia)	High	High
		Factory workers	–	–
		Shipyards	–	–
Amosite	Brown asbestos	Mining and milling	High	High
		Insulators	–	–
		Factory workers	–	–
Erionite	–	As contaminant in chrysotile	High	High
Tremolite	–	Environmental (Greece)	–	Possibly high
Chrysotile	White asbestos	Mining and milling	Low	Low
		Insulators	–	–
		Factory workers	–	–
Anthophyllite	–	Miners (Finland)	Thick and coarse	Remote

after 1953 because of government restrictions on the use and handling of asbestos materials in the mid-1960s. In general, two-thirds of patients with MM are between 50 and 70 years of age. The partners of men employed in the asbestos industry also have an increased risk of developing MM. Cleaning of clothes contaminated with asbestos fibers is considered a major source of asbestos exposure in this setting.[25] MM occurs rarely in children and in those cases it is mostly localized to the peritoneal cavity. Finally, it must be emphasized that because of its occurrence at an older age and the difficulty of diagnosis, the real incidence of this disease is probably being underestimated.

The mechanism of induction of MM and the risk of developing this disease after exposure to different types of asbestos fibers have been the subject of a number of studies. Different asbestos fibers are known, with different physical properties and carcinogenicity. The length:diameter ratio is considered to be of importance in evading the neutralizing action of the immune system and leading to penetration of the fibers in the pleura. The needle-like configuration combined with the longevity and the presence of iron in the fiber leads to chronic irritation of phagocytic cells. Fibers with the highest ratio are considered to be the most carcinogenic. Active oxygen species and reactive metabolites of oxygen produced by phagocytic cells are probably also involved in the chronic irritation and cytotoxicity of the asbestos fibers.[26]

Serpentines, also known as *white asbestos* (*chrysotile*), and anthophyllite are curlier and can be broken down to some extent by the immune system and removed by the lymphatic system. The carcinogenicity is considered to be relatively low for the serpentines, of which chrysotile is the best-known fiber. The amphiboles have the highest malignant potential and have a high length:diameter ratio.[27] Crocidolite (blue asbestos), amosite (brown asbestos), and tremolite also contain more iron than the serpentines, and this probably increases their malignancy potential. In Table 22.1, a summary of the risk and some of the features of the fibers are presented.

Malignant peritoneal mesothelioma

Malignant peritoneal mesotheliomas (MPM) represent one-third to one-fifth of all MM.[28] Symptoms of MPM are usually the signs of advanced disease, and include abdominal pain, ascites, weight loss, and the presence of a palpable abdominal mass. In a large series of MM, of 180 patients, 37 (21%) had peritoneal localization.[29] MPM progresses almost exclusively within the abdominal cavity. Extraperitoneal spread into the diaphragm and pleural space occurs at very advanced stages of the disease. Noninvasive radiological findings are not very helpful; CT scan of the abdomen usually reveals only peritoneal thickenings and ascites. Distant metastases or intraabdominal metastases to abdominal organs are unusual. Definite diagnosis can only be performed by tissue examination and only very rarely by cytology. Also, in MPM, paraneoplastic syndromes, such as thrombocytosis, phlebitis, and disseminated intravascular coagulation, are common.

Until recently no formal staging system existed for MPM, largely due to the rarity of the tumor and limitations of quantifying diffuse peritoneal dissemination. A new TNM staging was proposed recently, based on outcomes of 294 patients who underwent cytoreductive surgery (CRS) and hyperthermic intraperitoneal chemotherapy (HIPEC).[29] For this staging, peritoneal tumor deposits were quantified intraoperatively, using the peritoneal cancer index (PCI),[30] which combined lesion size (0–3) with tumor distribution (abdominopelvic region 0–13) to quantify the extent of disease as a numerical score (PCI 0–39). The peritoneal cancer index was further categorized into T1 (PCI 1–10), T2 (PCI 11–20), T3 (PCI 21–30), and T4 (PCI 30–9).[31] Presence of positive lymph nodes and extraabdominal metastases were attributed N1 and M1 respectively. The 5-year survival associated with stages I (T1N0M0), II (T2,T3,N0M0), and III (T4,N1 and/or M1) were 87%, 53%, and 29% respectively. Prognostic factors independently associated with survival in the multivariate analysis were histological subtype, completeness of cytoreduction, and the proposed TNM staging.[29]

Because the tumor remains localized to the peritoneal cavity for most of the course of the disease, local therapy has been investigated. Although surgical resection may provide palliation, especially in the case of bowel obstruction, it can rarely be complete. In selected patients, CRS, which attempts to remove all gross disease, and HIPEC, which uses chemical cytoreduction to eradicate residual cancer cells and small implants, have achieved median overall survival of 34.2–92 months.[32–36]

Due to the rarity of disease, the number of patients is small and the results are mostly based on single-institution experiences. The only multi-institutional data registry published to date included 405 patients, of whom 46% underwent complete or near-complete cytoreduction and 92% HIPEC.[36] The procedure was associated with substantial morbidity: 127 patients (31%) had grades 3–4 complications, nine patients (2%) died perioperatively and mean length of hospital stay was 22 days. The overall median survival was 53 months, and 3- and 5-year survival rates were 60% and 47%, respectively. Four prognostic factors independently associated with improved survival in the multivariate analysis were epithelial subtype, absence of lymph node metastasis, completeness of cytoreduction, and HIPEC.[36]

More advanced cases have been treated with systemic chemotherapy. To date, few large studies of chemotherapy have been reported in MPM, and treatment of this disease has been largely extrapolated from the treatment of pleural mesothelioma. As part of an extended access program for pemetrexed in the United States, 73 assessable patients with peritoneal mesothelioma were treated with cisplatin-pemetrexed or pemetrexed alone.[37] The response rate was 19% to pemetrexed alone and 29% to the combination. A phase 2 study of combination of pemetrexed and gemcitabine in 20 patients with MPM observed a 20% partial response (PR) rate, but with a high rate of hematological toxicities.[38] The combination of cisplatin-irinotecan yielded a response rate of 24% in 17 patients treated.[39] Other chemotherapy agents that have been used alone or in combination for MPM include doxorubicin, mitomycin, and trimetrexate.[40,41] The predictive value of gene expression patterns is under active investigation in MPM.[42]

Malignant mesothelioma of the tunica vaginalis testis

There are fewer than 100 cases reported in the literature.[43] Patients present with a hydrocele or hernia, and sometimes diffuse involvement of abdominal lymph nodes is present at diagnosis. Initial aggressive surgery and adjuvant treatment appear to improve survival.

Malignant mesothelioma of the pericardium

There are fewer than 200 cases reported.[44] This tumor is usually not diagnosed prior to surgery or autopsy. Patients generally present with pericardial effusion, congestive heart failure, a mass, or tamponade, which often require urgent surgery.

Nonasbestos-related mesothelioma

Although in 70–87% of cases of MM direct or indirect exposure to asbestos can be found, only 10% of those with asbestos exposure develop mesothelioma, and therefore other etiologies have been suggested. Volcanic minerals like zeolite have been associated with an increased incidence of MM. Erionite, a respirable form of zeolite, was found in the soil and rocks of Anatolian villages and was identified as the causative agent, since asbestos fibers were absent, and because it has been shown to be carcinogenic in mice and rats.[45] Of special interest

are the man-made mineral fibers (MMMF), of which fiberglass (glass wool) is the best known. These fibers have been developed to replace asbestos fibers and are used for insulation and construction. Metaanalyses of epidemiological studies have not shown a clear association between exposure to MMMF and development of cancers of the lung and pleural mesothelioma.[46]

Familial aspects of MM have been the subject of some reports: in a study of 196 MM patients and 511 deceased controls, there was a twofold elevation in the risk of mesothelioma among men exposed to asbestos when reporting cancer in two or more first-degree relatives. However, no correlation among women and nonasbestos-exposed men was observed. This may suggest that a family history of cancer may enhance susceptibility to MM given asbestos exposure.[47] A recent study found germline mutations in the gene encoding for BRCA1-associated protein-1 (BAP1) in two families with a high incidence of mesothelioma. Aberrant expression of *BAP1* was also observed in cases of sporadic mesothelioma without germline mutations. Some carriers of the *BAP1* mutation developed uveal melanoma. The results of this study suggested the presence of a *BAP1*-related cancer syndrome in which mesothelioma predominates in the presence of asbestos exposure.[48]

The viral nature of MM has been the object of several controversial reports. SV40 induces mesotheliomas in hamsters and 60% of human mesotheliomas contain and express SV40 sequences, as published by Carbone *et al.*[49] Furthermore, SV40 large T antigen (Tag) retains its ability to bind and inactivate p53, which would then be an important way to inactivate p53 in the absence of mutations in MM.[50] SV40 Tag targets and inactivates growth suppressive proteins, such as those of the Rb family and p53. SV40 is able to initiate the transformation of mesothelial cells into malignant cells by blocking tumor suppressor proteins such as p53 and the products of the retinoblastoma-susceptibility gene. These transformations can occur easily in rodent cells, but the conversion of human cells is more complex. SV40 is not specific to the development of MM. It has been shown that different tumor types such as lymphoblastomas, sarcomas, ependymomas, and osteosarcomas can develop after infection with the SV40 virus. Some studies in humans have identified the presence of SV40 large T antigen in mesothelioma samples but others have observed a total absence. Contamination by plasmids during the sequencing or selection of patients might explain some of these differences. Given conflicting results from various studies, the role of SV40 in the pathogenesis of MM remains uncertain.[51–54]

Pathology

Histological material is obtained by thoracoscopic biopsies, pleurectomy, or pneumonectomy in the case of pleural mesothelioma, and by peritoneoscopy or preferably open directed biopsy in the case of peritoneal mesothelioma.[45] Diffuse MM is a biphasic tumor of the mesothelium, and three major variants can be distinguished by optic microscopy: epithelial (approximately 50% of cases), sarcomatoid (16%), and mixed (34%).[23] The frequency of diagnosis of the mixed type is dependent on the number of samples available, as biphasic features are often absent in a single sample.

The major difficulty in the diagnosis of MM is in differentiating it from pleural metastases of a tumor, usually an adenocarcinoma, originating elsewhere. There may also be difficulties in determining whether a pleural proliferation is benign or malignant. Several criteria have been developed to separate these entities,[55] and strong telomerase activity has been associated with MM and not benign mesothelial proliferations.[56] The presence of a biphasic aspect of predominant sarcomatoid features may make the diagnosis rather straightforward; however, immunohistochemistry is often necessary, and sometimes also electron microscopy, to differentiate epithelial mesothelioma from a metastasis of an adenocarcinoma. Hence a portion of the biopsy should be fixed in glutaraldehyde for electron microscopy in those cases where standard pathological assessment proves inconclusive. Periodic acid-Schiff (PAS) diastase-positive intracellular vacuoles are usually absent in mesotheliomas but present in adenocarcinomas; mucicarmine staining is also usually negative in mesotheliomas and positive in adenocarcinomas. Conversely, Alcian blue disappearance after digestion with hyaluronidase is characteristic of mesothelioma.

Immunohistochemistry may help in rendering evident the biphasic nature of diffuse mesothelioma, and can be used to differentiate it from adenocarcinoma and sarcomas. Carcinoembryonic antigen (CEA) expression is usually weak or absent in mesothelioma, but strongly expressed in several carcinomas. The calcium-binding protein calretinin was shown to be expressed in MM but not in metastatic adenocarcinomas.[57] However, this marker was exquisitely expressed in the epithelial type but was not expressed in the sarcomatoid type and the mixed type.[58] Immunostaining with surfactant protein B and thyroid transcription factor 1 (TTF-1) antibodies has been shown to be able to differentiate adenocarcinoma of the lung, which is often positive, from mesothelioma, which is always negative.[59] Other epithelial markers and cytokeratins can also distinguish adenocarcinomas from epithelial mesothelioma.[45,60,61] Of possible help in differentiating MM from nonsmall cell lung cancer is the expression of Wilms tumor 1 susceptibility (*WT1*) gene products; detection of WT1 expression (mRNA or protein) is frequent in MM but absent in nonsmall cell lung cancer.[61,62] N-cadherin staining has also been shown in most pleural MM.[63] Thus, a battery of immunohistochemical tests needs to be performed to make a diagnosis of MM.[64]

Electron microscopy can be considered as the reference method in doubtful cases.[65] Epithelial mesothelioma is characterized by numerous long, slender, branching surface microvilli, desmosomes, abundant tonofilaments, and intracellular lumen formation on polygonal cells; in the sarcomatous type, elongated nuclei and abundant rough endoplasmic reticulum are observed.

In recent years attempts have been made to identify serum biomarkers to screen individuals at risk for developing MM and to help monitor response to treatment in patients diagnosed with the disease.[66] Soluble mesothelin-related peptide (SMRP) is elevated in epithelioid mesothelioma and levels can decrease with a response to treatment whereas osteopontin can be elevated in both epithelioid and sarcomatoid mesothelioma but a change in levels may not correlate with response to treatment.[67]

Malignant pleural mesothelioma

Clinical presentation

Malignant pleural mesothelioma tends to remain confined to one hemithorax and is mainly characterized by locoregional growth and spread. However, at autopsy as many as 70% of cases have detectable tumor invasion in thoracic lymph nodes, and distant metastases are observed in liver, lungs, kidney, adrenals, and bones in approximately 50% of cases.[68]

It is generally believed that the initial growth rate of MM is slow and that therefore symptoms appear at a late stage. Sometimes, a pleuritic effusion is noted, which initially subsides but, after a few years, results in the development of mesothelioma. The tendency of mesothelioma to first grow along the pleural lining and finally invade adjacent structures like muscles, ribs, and diaphragm makes early diagnosis difficult. The most frequently reported complaints are pain, shortness of breath, and cough; unexplained fever is also encountered in a number of patients. In the majority of cases, there is a pleural effusion that can vary in volume, and a number of patients present with a large exudate, which causes compression of the lung and displacement of the mediastinum. The fluid is often a bloody exudate in which a provisional diagnosis of MM can be made.[45,69] A more typical feature of the tumor in advanced cases is the retraction of the chest wall on the involved side, which occurs after obliteration of the pleural space and encasement of the lung. Growth into the ribs and muscles leads to localized swelling and pain. Invasion of the mediastinum can result in dysphagia, superior vena cava syndrome, and pericardial effusion. When cardiac involvement is present, arrhythmias, nonspecific ST-T changes, conducting abnormalities, or atrial fibrillation can ensue.[70] Paraneoplastic symptoms are not frequently reported except for thrombocytosis, which has been observed in 40–90% of patients, depending on the stage of the disease.[71] Other paraneoplastic symptoms, such as diffuse intravascular coagulation, autoimmune hemolytic anemia, syndrome of inappropriate antidiuretic hormone (ADH) secretion, hypoglycemia, and hypercalcemia, have also been observed, albeit rarely.

Evaluation and staging

A wide variety of radiographic methods are used in MM to determine the extent of the disease. In some cases, the combination of the history and chest x-rays can lead to a presumptive diagnosis of MM. The diagnosis, however, can only be made with certainty on a histological specimen. The chest x-ray usually shows a unilateral effusion and pleural thickening that is often diffuse, circumferential in most cases, and presenting with nodules or masses. During the course of the disease, the tumor grows into the fissures of the lung and encases the lung, leading to the typical retracted hemithorax.[72,73] An additional clue to the diagnosis of MM is the finding of calcified pleural plaques, which are often seen in patients exposed to asbestos. It is, however, not believed that the tumor arises from these plaques.

Invasion of the mediastinum and diaphragm can be identified by computed tomography (CT) scan or magnetic resonance

Box 22.1 TNM staging system for malignant pleural mesothelioma developed by the International Mesothelioma Interest Group.[82]

T = Tumor

T1

T1a Tumor limited to the ipsilateral parietal including mediastinal and diaphragmatic pleura

No involvement of the visceral pleura

T1b Tumor involving the ipsilateral parietal including mediastinal and diaphragmatic pleura

Scattered foci of tumors also involving the visceral pleura

T2

Tumor involving each of the ipsilateral pleural surfaces (parietal, mediastinal, diaphragmatic, and visceral pleura) with at least one of the following features:

- Involvement of diaphragmatic muscle
- Confluent visceral pleural tumor (including the fissures), or extension of tumor from visceral pleura into the underlying pulmonary parenchyma

T3

Describes locally advanced but **potentially resectable** tumor. Tumor involving all the ipsilateral pleural surfaces (parietal, mediastinal, diaphragmatic, and visceral pleura) with at least one of the following features:

- Involvement of the endothoracic fascia
- Extension into the mediastinal fat
- Solitary, completely resectable focus of tumor extending into the soft tissue of the chest wall
- Nontransmural involvement of the pericardium

T4

Describes locally advanced **technically unresectable** tumor. Tumor involving all the ipsilateral pleural surfaces (parietal, mediastinal, diaphragmatic, and visceral pleura) with at least one of the following features:

- Diffuse extension or multifocal masses of tumor in the chest wall, with or without associated rib destruction
- Direct transdiaphragmatic extension of tumor to the peritoneum
- Direct extension of tumor to the contralateral pleura
- Direct extension of the tumor to one or more mediastinal organs
- Direct extension of tumor into the spine
- Tumor extending through the internal surface of the pericardium with or without a pericardial effusion; or tumor involving the myocardium

N = Lymph node

NX Regional lymph nodes cannot be assessed
N1 No regional lymph node metastases
N2 Metastases in the ipsilateral bronchopulmonary or hilar lymph nodes
N3 Metastases in the contralateral mediastinal, contralateral internal thoracic, ipsilateral, or contralateral supraclavicular lymph nodes

M = Metastases

MX Presence of distant metastases cannot be assessed
M0 No distant metastases
M1 Distant metastases present

Stage I	
Ia	T1a N0 M0
Ib	T1b N0 M0
Stage II	T2 N0 M0
Stage III	Any T3 N0
	Any N1 M0
	Any N2 M0
Stage IV	Any T4
	Any N3
	Any M1

imaging (MRI).[74–76] MRI has the advantage of generating sagittal images that are informative of the growth of the tumor in the sinuses. Also, invasion of the heart, pericardium, and diaphragm can be discriminated better by MRI than by CT scan. Additional imaging modalities can be helpful in staging as well. For example, the diaphragm can also be visualized by laparoscopic examination.[77] The use of ultrasound is of help in defining pleural effusions and possible involvement of the heart. Fluorodeoxyglucose (FDG) positron emission tomography (PET) scan can be used to differentiate between malignant and benign (fibrotic) tissue, and is a valuable addition to CT and MRI in detecting disease spreading outside the chest, especially in patients who are considered candidates for surgery.[78] PET scans can also yield prognostic information in patients with MM.[79] Newer molecular imaging techniques are currently in development with potential applications in mesothelioma such as single photon emission comuted tomography (SPECT) imaging utilizing ^{111}In-labeled antimesothelin antibodies.[80]

Staging of malignant pleural mesothelioma is challenging. The first staging system was developed by Butchart *et al.*[81] Since that initial effort six other staging systems have been proposed. The version developed by the International Mesothelioma Interest Group (IMIG) (Box 22.1),[82] based on a TNM modification, is considered the best framework for analyzing prospective clinical trials. Optimal staging is very important for selection of patients who have localized disease and could be candidates for surgery or combined modality treatments. Also, a more reliable comparison of data obtained from international studies can be made.

Treatment

Median survival of patients with MM treated with supportive care alone is approximately 7 months.[83] Attitudes toward the treatment of this disease vary greatly, and range from supportive treatment only to aggressive surgery and combined modality treatment.

Surgery

Local control in malignant pleural mesothelioma is important as the tumor tends to remain localized to the hemithorax for a large part of the course of the disease. In the presence of different staging systems, which did not provide very accurate estimates of prognosis, the role of surgery has been debated.

However, in general, patients with stage I disease according to the Butchart classification should be considered candidates for radical surgery.

There are two major types of operation that have been employed in patients with malignant pleural mesothelioma: pleurectomy and extrapleural pneumonectomy (EPP). Pleurectomy consists of stripping the pleura from the apex of the lung to the diaphragm, along with the pericardium, if necessary. This operation generally requires a thoracotomy. A summary of various surgical series is provided in Table 22.2. Operative mortality is only 1–2%, but complications include bronchopleural fistulas, hemorrhage, and subcutaneous emphysema. The value of pleural decortication as a palliative measure in the case of recurrent effusion has not been well established and might be taken into consideration in case pleurodesis fails repeatedly.

Extrapleural pneumonectomy is the *en bloc* removal of the parietal pleura, lung, pericardium, and hemidiaphragm. Diaphragmatic resection is followed by reconstruction to prevent herniation. In the hands of experienced thoracic surgeons, the operative mortality of this complex procedure is nowadays 5–9%, but serious complications are seen in 25% of patients or more, and include bronchopleural fistulas and empyema, vocal cord paralysis, chylothorax, arrhythmia, and respiratory insufficiency. EPP is a complex operation, which should be performed by skilled surgeons and in select centers with experience in the treatment of this disease. The results of the most representative series are summarized in Table 22.3.

Results of surgery are difficult to interpret because of differences in patient selection, the relatively small number of patients, the lack of randomized trials, and often the addition of another treatment modality to surgery. These factors and others are highlighted in a recently published review on the surgical management of malignant pleural mesothelioma.[101]

Radiotherapy

The role of radiotherapy in the management of malignant pleural mesothelioma is still unsettled.[102] Radiotherapy alone has only a limited role in disease control and survival. The most recent series do not indicate that irradiation improves survival in comparison to best supportive care. However, radiotherapy, given after EPP, has been used extensively as adjuvant treatment in several series in order to reduce the local recurrence rate.[100]

The treatment volume is a crucial aspect of radiation of malignant pleural mesothelioma, and treatment of the entire pleura is indicated. This is extremely difficult to achieve because tumoricidal doses cannot be delivered without causing serious side-effects in normal surrounding tissues, such as the lung, heart, and liver. Of course, these issues are less relevant post pneumonectomy, where higher doses can be given.[103] Several different irradiation techniques have been developed in order to spare normal tissue from the irradiated fields, including the use of intraoperative radiotherapy.[94,104] Radical irradiation delivers 40–50 Gy to the entire pleural space and the mediastinum, followed by boost irradiation up to 55–71 Gy to areas of gross disease; however, until now no specific technique has been developed that allows high-dose radiation without major risks for the adjacent normal tissues.

Radiotherapy is often used for palliation of pain, and it has often been added to surgery in an attempt to improve local control and reduce local failures. The results of the published literature are, however, difficult to interpret, because radiotherapy was used as part of a multimodality treatment in locally advanced cases of pleural mesothelioma, because of the small number of patients reported in single studies and because of the lack of randomized trials.

A randomized trial of radiotherapy proved that radiotherapy to the thoracoscopy entry tract significantly reduced the incidence of local relapse: in this study, of 20 patients who received 21 Gy delivered in three fractions 10–15 days after thoracoscopy, none had local recurrence, whereas local recurrence developed in eight of 20 (40%) patients who did not receive radiation.[105] However, two other randomized controlled trials showed that prophylactic radiotherapy to the entry tract did not reduce the incidence of local relapse.[102]

Table 22.2 Results of pleurectomy.

References	Patients	Two-year survival (%)	Median survival (months)
McCormack et al.[84]	95*	35	12.6
Law et al.[85]	28	32	20
Faber et al.[86]	35	12	10
DaValle et al.[87]	23	NA	11.2
Wanebo et al.[88]	17 epithelial	NA	21
	16 sarcomatous	NA	11
Achatzy et al.[89]	46	11	10
Ruffie et al.[90]	63	NA	9.8
Brancatisano et al.[91]	45	21	16
Rusch et al.[92]	51	40	18.3
Branscheid et al.[93]	82	25	315 days
Lee et al.[94]	32	32	18

NA, not available.
* With implant or external irradiation.

Table 22.3 Results of extrapleural pneumonectomy.

References	Patients	Two-year survival (%)	Median survival (months)	Operative mortality (%)
Worn et al.[95]	62	37	19	20–25
Bamler and Maassen[96]	17	35	NA	23
Butchart et al.[81]	29	10	4	31
DeLaria et al.[97]	11	NA	15	0
Branscheid et al.[93]	76	10	284 days	11.8
Faber[72]	33	27	13.5	9
Geroulanos et al.[98]	18	NA	20	7
Rush and Venkatraman[99]	50	20	9.9	6
Sugarbaker et al.[100]	183	38	19	3.8
Ruffie et al.[83]	23	17	9.3	14

NA, not available.

Chemotherapy and targeted therapy

A large number of chemotherapeutic agents have been investigated in MM. The level of activity of several of these agents is low and variable from study to study. Given the rarity of the disease, phase 2 studies have usually been performed in a small number of patients. Extensive reviews of chemotherapy and targeted therapy in MM have been published recently.[106–108] Since phase 2 trials often have assessment of response rate as a major objective, the measurability of disease becomes an important issue. In malignant pleural mesothelioma, even by CT scan it is sometimes difficult to assess the extent of disease extension accurately and therefore identify changes during treatment. Disease assessment by chest x-ray is unreliable, and this is the major reason for overestimation of treatment results in older studies.

The use of RECIST criteria in the assessment of response in solid tumors has raised some questions about the applicability of this system to mesothelioma, for which the maximum diameter is usually the pleural base of implant, which does not easily decrease even when a treatment is active.[109] Although modified RECIST criteria have been developed and are being used in MM, efforts are ongoing to develop and validate newer techniques to assess response to treatment in this disease.[110]

When used as single agents, the anthracyclines doxorubicin and epidoxorubicin, cisplatin, and high-dose methotrexate appear to have consistent albeit modest degrees of efficacy, with a major response rate in the order of 10–20% (Table 22.4). Although doxorubicin and cisplatin have been considered to be the most active agents against this disease in the past, there have been conflicting reports on their degree of activity. Most antimetabolites have also been reported to have some degree of activity. In a phase 2 study a response rate of 16% was observed with single-agent pemetrexed.[111] The drug is well tolerated when combined with folate and vitamin B_{12} supplementation, which significantly reduce side-effects without impairing antitumor activity. Gemcitabine has negligible activity as a single agent, but reproducible activity in combination with cisplatin.[112–119]

The use of novel targeted therapies has so far not been successful. Both gefitinib, a tyrosine kinase inhibitor (TKI) of epidermal growth factor receptor (EGFR), and imatinib, a TKI of c-kit, were ineffective in single-agent studies in chemotherapy-naive patients.[169,170] These disappointing results are likely due to the lack of patient selection. It is now known that mesotheliomas do not have EGFR mutations that confer sensitivity in nonsmall cell lung cancer,[173] and c-kit is poorly expressed in MM.[174,175] Interestingly, angiogenesis inhibitors may have some promise, as VEGF and VEGFR are frequently overexpressed in mesothelioma and VEGF appears to be a growth factor for this malignancy.[176,177] However clinical trials evaluating VEGF inhibitors have shown only modest results in mesothelioma so far. The combination of cisplatin, gemcitabine, and bevacizumab was comapared to cisplatin and gemcitabine alone in a randomized phase 2 trial. The primary endpoint of a statistically significant improvement in progression-free survival was not met (6.9 months versus 6 months, $p=0.88$).[178] Sorafenib and sunitinb have been evaluated as single agents in patients with MPM and shown modest activity (objective response rates of 6% with sorafenib and 10% with sunitinib).[171,172]

Table 22.4 Systemic single-agent therapy in series with ≥15 patients in the first-line setting.

Drug	Patients	Responses	Response rate (%)	References
Topoisomerase inhibitors				
Doxorubicin	66	7	11	120,121
Liposomal doxorubicin	55	2	4	122,123
Detorubicin	35	9	26	124
Pirarubicin	35	8	22	125
Epirubicin	59	8	14	126,127
Mitoxantrone	62	3	5	128,129
Menogaril	22	1	3	130
Etoposide	111	6	3	131,132
Amsacrine	19	1	5	133
Irinotecan	25	0	0	134
Alkylating agents				
Cyclophosphamide	16	0	0	121
Ifosfamide	133	9	7	135–138
Mitomycin	19	4	21	139
Cisplatin	59	8	14	140,141
Carboplatin	88	10	11	142–144
ZD0473*	43	0	0	145
Temozolomide	27	1	4	146
Antimetabolites				
High-dose methotrexate	60	22	37	147
Trimetrexate	51	6	12	148
Edatrexate	58	9	16	149
Di-deazofolic acid	18	1	6	150
5-Fluorouracil	20	1	5	151
Capecitabine	27	1	4	152
5-DHAC	56	7	13	153,154
Gemcitabine	44	2	5	119,134
Pemetrexed	64	9	14	111
Tubulin-interfering				
Vincristine	23	0	0	155
Vinblastine	20	0	0	156
Vindesine	38	1	3	157,158
Vinorelbine	29	7	24	159
Docetaxel	48	4	8	160,161
Paclitaxel	50	3	6	162,163
Others				
Aziridinylbenzoquinone	20	0	0	164
Acivicin	19	0	0	165
IL-2	29	2	8	166
Ranpirnase†	81	4	6	167
Thalidomide‡	40	0	0	168
Gefitinib	42	2	4	169
Imatinib	25	0	0	170
Sorafenib	50	3	6	171
Sunitinib*	51	5	10	172

DHAC, 5-Dihydroazacytidine.
* Second-line treatment.
† 37% had prior chemotherapy.
‡ 50% had prior chemotherapy.

Other targeted agents that are being evalutated in patients with mesothelioma include the proteosome inhibitor bortezomib, the histone deacetylase (HDAC) inhibitor vorinostat, and the mTOR inhibitor everolimus.

Table 22.5 Results of randomized trials in malignant pleural mesothelioma.

Regimen	Patients	Response rate (%)	Median survival (weeks)	One-year survival (%)	References
Doxorubicin + cyclophosphamide	36	11	30	NR	183
Doxorubicin + cyclophosphamide + dacarbazine (DTIC)	40	13	25	NR	
Doxorubicin	16	0	NR	NR	121
Cyclophosphamide	16	0	NR	NR	
Cisplatin	222	16.7	9.3 months	38	179
Cisplatin + pemetrexed	225	41.3 $p<0.001$	12.1 months $p=0.02$	50.3	
Cisplatin	124	14	8.8 months	39.6	180
Cisplatin + raltitrexed	126	24 $p=0.06$	11.4 months $p=0.048$	46.2	
Carboplatin continuous infusion	13	58	21.7	33	184
Cisplatin + etoposide	12	39	18.7 $p=0.0135$	0	

NR, not reported.

Combination chemotherapy

Combination chemotherapy has been extensively evaluated in the first-line setting. It results in a higher response rate and survival compared to single agents in nonrandomized comparisons.

Based on a large phase 3 study that compared a combination of pemetrexed and cisplatin to cisplatin alone in patients with MM, this combination has been established as the standard of care for front-line therapy of MM. In this study, 456 patients were randomized to receive either cisplatin alone (75 mg/m^2) or combination of pemetrexed (500 mg/m^2) and cisplatin (75 mg/m^2) every 3 weeks. The response rate, median time to progression and median overall survival with combination therapy were 41% versus 17% (p <0.0001), 5.7 months versus 3.9 months ($p=0.001$) and 12.1 months versus 9.3 months ($p=0.020$) respectively.[179] Another large phase 3 study compared the thymidine synthase inhibitor, raltitrexed in combination with cisplatin against cisplatin alone for first-line treatment of malignant pleural mesothelioma. Two hundred and fifty patients were randomized to receive either cisplatin alone at a dose of 80 mg/m^2 or a combination of raltitrexed at a dose of 3 mg/m^2 with cisplatin 80 mg/m^2 adminstered every 3 weeks. Two hundred and thirteen patients were evaluable for response. The response rate and median overall survival for the combination were 24% versus 14% ($p=0.06$) and 11.4 months versus 8.8 months (hazard ratio (HR) 0.76; 95% confidence interval (CI) 0.58–1.00; $p=0.048$) respectively. The most common grade 3 and 4 toxicities were neutropenia, nausea, emesis and fatigue which were observed twice as often in the combination arm.[180]

The results of these studies indicate that a clinically significant survival benefit can be achieved with combination therapy with better responses and improved quality of life (Table 22.5). These data led to a renewed interest in the chemotherapeutic treatment of patients with advanced mesothelioma and to the implementation of more effective chemotherapy in multimodality regimens and in the neoadjuvant setting. Furthermore, other studies were performed to investigate the role of systemic therapy in the second-line setting and beyond, either as single agent[145] or combination therapy.[181] The percentage of patients who received second-line chemotherapy varied between 37% and 47% in the cisplatin-pemetrexed randomized study.[182]

Combined modality treatment

Given the disappointing results of surgery alone, combined modality therapy has been attempted in order to reduce local recurrence and systemic spread. Several surgical procedures including pleurectomy and EPP in combination with various forms of radiation and chemotherapy have been used as part of combined modality treatment. In the absence of properly conducted controlled prospective and randomized trials, it is difficult to draw definitive conclusions regarding the superiority of one form of combined modality therapy over another.

The experience of the Memorial Sloan-Kettering Cancer Center with pleurectomy, intraoperative brachytherapy, and post-operative irradiation was reported in 1984, with a relatively short follow-up.[185] Rusch et al. reported a study of surgical resection with intrapleural and systemic chemotherapy.[186] The authors concluded that this cannot be considered routine treatment. Three other smaller studies with a similar design confirmed the limited indication for this approach and a high morbidity rate.[187–189] In an update of the Memorial experience,[190] it was reported that a total of 231 thoracotomies was performed between 1983 and 1998 for the treatment of pleural mesothelioma. In 115 cases, EPP was performed and only pleurectomy/decortication in 59 cases. A total of 142 patients received adjuvant therapy. By multivariate analysis stage, histology, gender, and adjuvant therapy had an impact on survival, but not the type of surgical resection.

The Dana Farber Cancer Institute has considerable experience with EPP combined with multiagent chemotherapy and postoperative radiation.[191] The operative mortality after 328 consecutive extrapleural pneumonectomies (performed from 1980 to 2003) was 3.4% with a morbidity rate (minor and major complications) of 60.4%.[191] The most common complications were atrial fibrillation (44.2%), prolonged intubation (7.9%), vocal cord paralysis (6.7%), deep vein thrombosis (6.4%), and technical complications (6.1%).[191] A total of 183 patients were treated between 1980 and 1997 by en bloc EPP, followed

4–6 weeks later by 4–6 cycles of doxorubicin-cyclophosphamide (with the addition of cisplatin after 1985), followed by ipsilateral hemithorax and mediastinum radiotherapy.[100] The median survival was 19 months with 2- and 5-year survival rates of 38 and 15%, respectively.[100] Epithelial cell type mesothelioma had better survival and nodal involvement was a negative prognostic factor. The conclusion of this group is that trimodality treatment is safe and effective for selected patients with malignant pleural mesothelioma without nodal involvement.

From the same group, Baldini *et al.* also analyzed the pattern of failure of 46 evaluable patients treated with trimodality therapy.[192] Twenty-five patients (54%) had recurrences; sites of recurrence were 35% local, abdominal in 26%, contralateral in 17%, and distant in 8%. Median time to first recurrence was 19 months. This and other studies clearly indicate that more effective strategies should be sought to increase local control. It is also well recognized that preoperative CT and MRI do not accurately stage patients preoperatively,[193] and better staging procedures need to be developed.

In a study performed at the National Cancer Institute (NCI), 36 patients received cisplatin at a dose of 25 mg/m^2 per week for 4 weeks, interferon-α 5 mU/m^2 subcutaneously three times weekly, and tamoxifen 20 mg orally twice a day for 35 days, for 1–5 cycles; 10 additional patients had debulking surgery followed by two cycles. The partial response rate was 19% and median survival was 8.7 months (14.7 months for responders and 8 months for for nonresponders).[194]

In another study 19 potentially resectable patients with pleural mesothelioma received three cycles of cisplatin 80 mg/m^2 on day 1 and gemcitabine 1000 mg/m^2 on days 1, 8, and 15, administered every 28 days as neoadjuvant treatment.[195] EPP was successfully performed in 16 patients, and 13 patients received postoperative radiotherapy. Median survival was 23 months.

Two recent multicenter phase 2 trials, one from the United States and another from Europe, suggest that trimodality treatment consisting of induction chemotherapy with cisplatin plus pemetrexed is feasible in selected patients with early-stage mesothelioma. In both trials, patients without disease progression after neoadjuvant chemotherapy (consisting of cisplatin 75 mg/m^2 plus pemetrexed 500 mg/m^2 once every 21 days, four cycles in the US study and three cycles in the European study) underwent EPP and hemithoracic radiation (54 Gy in 30 fractions). In the US trial (*n* = 77), forty patients who completed all three therapies had a median survival of 29.1 months compared to 16.8 months for the overall population and a 2-year survival rate of 61.2%. Three pathological complete responses (primary endpoint) were observed (5% of EPP) and radiological response to neoadjuvant chemotherapy was associated with improved survival.[196] In the European trial (*n* = 59), 37 patients completed trimodality therapy and had a median overall survival time of 33 months compared to 18.4 months for the overall population. Twenty-four (42%) patients met the primary endpoint of this trial which was labeled as "success of treatment" and defined as completion of all therapies within the defined time-frames with patient being alive 90 days after the end of treatment without progression or evidence of grade 3–4 toxicity.[197] The authors concluded that trimodality treatment

appeared feasible in selected patients with early-stage mesothelioma, but should be used in selected institutions with adequate experience, preferably in the setting of a prospective clinical trial.

The Mesothelioma and Radical Surgery (MARS) study was a randomized multicenter study performed to evaluate the benefit of performing EPP in the setting of trimodal therapy.[198] One hundred and twelve patients were registered, of whom 83 (74%) received three cycles of platinum-based chemotherapy (cisplatin plus gemcitabine was most commonly used; other combinations included cisplatin plus pemetrexed, and cisplatin plus mitomycin plus vinblastine). Subsequently 50 patients were randomized to EPP (*n* = 24) or to no EPP (*n* = 26). Sixteen out of 24 patients assigned to EPP completed surgery as planned. Eight out of 16 patients who completed EPP received radical radiotherapy. Median survival was 14.4 months in the EPP arm and 19.5 months in the non-EPP arm. One-year survival was 52% (95% CI 30.5–70.0) for patients in the EPP arm and 73% (95% CI 51.7–86.2) in the no EPP arm. The hazard ratio for overall survival between the EPP and no EPP groups was 1.9 (95% CI 0.92–3.93; *p* = 0.082). Median recurrence-free survival was 7.6 months (5.0–13.4 months) in the EPP group and median progression-free survival was estimated to be 9 months (7.2–14.7 months) in the no EPP group. Ten serious adverse events were reported in the EP group and two in the no EPP group. This trial showed that only a third of patients who were randomized to the EPP arm received trimodality therapy as planned and patients who underwent radical surgery as part of trimodal therapy did not do better, and possibly did worse than patients who did not undergo surgery.

Intracavitary therapy

Because mesothelioma of the pleural cavity tends to remain localized for a long time, local treatment with cytotoxic agents or other new approaches may be interesting. Different approaches have been tested, such as local instillation of interferon-γ,[199,200] IL-2,[201] tumor necrosis factor (TNF)-α,[202] and the use of radiocolloids, such as ^{198}Au or ^{32}P with limited success. In another study using IL-2 in 31 patients with pleural mesothelioma, the response rate was 22% and median survival 15 months, with only mild toxicity.[203]

Another approach to the problem of eliminating residual disease after surgery is the use of perioperative photodynamic therapy. The photosensitizer is administered a few days before the operation and is retained to some extent in the tumor tissue and vasculature. This treatment modality has been used in a few small studies.[204] A study of intraoperative photodynamic therapy after pleuropneumonectomy has been performed in 28 patients.[205] Considerable toxicity was encountered, including three perioperative deaths, associated with local control in 50% of cases. The same group of investigators attempted intraoperative hyperthermic intrathoracic chemotherapy with cisplatin and doxorubicin heated at 40–41°C after tumor debulking.[206] Although no postoperative deaths occurred, significant morbidity was observed in 65% of patients, and median survival was only 11 months. A small feasibility study in 10 patients demonstrated that pleural space perfusion with cisplatin was feasible and safe after operation.[207] A liposome-entrapped platinum compound was given to 33 patients with pleural mesothelioma and free-flowing pleural effusions.[208] After at least two cycles, a pathological complete response, ascertained by repeat biopsies, was obtained in 42% of cases, and median survival was 11 months. Although feasible, this approach demonstrated substantial morbidity and the instillation of the drug was unable to penetrate all tumor deposits.

Immunotherapy

Immunotherapies are still in the early stages of clinical investigation in mesothelioma. Immunotherapeutic agents being evaluated include dendritic cell vaccines, listeria-based, allogenic tumor cell and WT1 analog peptide vaccines and anti-mesothelin (SS1P and MORAb-009 or amatuximab) and anti-TGF monoclonal antibodies (GC1008).

Dendritic cells (DC) are potent antigen-presenting cells present in peripheral tissues, where they capture, process and transport antigens to naive T cells in secondary lymphoid organs. Tissue inflammation results in DC maturation, migration to draining lymph nodes and expression of peptide–MHC complexes as well as costimulatory molecules which allows priming of CD4+ T helper cells and CD8+ cytotoxic T lymphocytes, activation of B cells and initiation of an adaptive immune response.[209] In a phase 1 study of 10 mesothelioma patients with either PR or stable disease (SD) after prior combination chemotherapy, DC vaccination was safe and induced immune as well as radiographic responses (three PRs, one SD).[210] In this study, patients underwent leukapheresis 10 weeks after last dose of chemotherapy. Two weeks later and at subsequent 2-week intervals for a total of three doses, autologous tumor lysate-pulsed DC was administered intradermally (one-third of the dose) and intravenously (two-thirds of the dose).[210]

The Wilms tumor suppressor gene (WT1) is a transcription factor which is differentially overexpressed in leukemias and some solid tumors, including mesothelioma.[211] In a pilot trial in nine patients, six doses of a vaccine comprising four WT1 analog peptides were administered subcutaneously over 12 weeks followed by six additional monthly injections for responding patients. The vaccine was safe and induced an immune response: six out of nine patients tested demonstrated CD4 T cell proliferation to WT1 specific peptides, and five of the six HLA-A0201 patients tested mounted a CD8 T cell response.[212,213] Further evaluation of both WT1 analog peptide vaccine and DC vaccination in mesothelioma patients is ongoing.

Mesothelin is as an immunogenic glycoprotein which is highly expressed in malignant mesotheliomas with limited expression in normal mesothelial cells.[214] SS1(dsFv)PE38 (SS1P) is a chimeric recombinant immunotoxin comprising antimesothelin disulfide-stabilized murine antibody Fv fused to PE38, a 38 kD portion of *Pseudomonas* exotoxin A. In a trial of combination of SS1P with pemetrexed and cisplatin in frontline therapy for patients with advanced mesothelioma, escalating doses of SS1P were administered on days 1, 3, and

5 of cycles 1 and 2.[215] Of the 14 evaluable patients treated at all dose levels, seven PRs and three SDs were observed. Of the seven patients treated at maximum tolerated dose (MTD) (45 µg/kg), five had PR and one had SD.

MORAb-009 is a fully humanized high-affinity monoclonal chimeric IgG1/k antibody that targets mesothelin. MORAb-009 was well tolerated in a phase 1 study (*n* = 24) with low incidence of immunogenicity.[216] There were no objective responses but disease stabilization was observed in several heavily pretreated patients. An open-label multicenter phase 2 clinical trial of MORAb-009 plus pemetrexed and cisplatin for treatment of malignant pleural mesothelioma with progression-free survival as the primary endpoint has recently completed accrual.

Gene therapy

Gene therapy remains an experimental approach for treatment of mesothelioma at this time. Various strategies are being evaluated to enhance expression of immunostimulatory cytokines from tumor cells and introduce modified T cells via gene therapy in an effort to induce an *in vivo* antitumor immune response.[217,218]

Prognosis

A number of prognostic factors have been identified in large series of mainly advanced MM. Staging (in particular, nodal status) appears to be important in early onset of the disease.[99,100] In a database of 204 patients enrolled into sequential phase 2 studies of the European Organization for Research and Treatment of Cancer (EORTC), poor prognostic factors by multivariate analysis were a poor performance status, high white blood count, male gender, sarcomatous histology, and having a probable/possible histological diagnosis of MM.[219] Similarly, the Cancer and Leukemia Group B (CALGB) analyzed their database of 337 patients treated over a 10-year period. Multivariate analyses showed that poor prognostic factors included pleural involvement, lactate dehydrogenase (LDH) >500 IU/L, poor performance status, chest pain, platelet count >400,000/µL, nonepithelial histology, and age >75 years.[220] A subsequent retrospective analysis of an independent cohort of patients confirmed the prognostic value of both the EORTC and the CALGB scoring systems.[221,222] These identified risk groups might help in stratifying patients in future studies.

A number of biological factors have been investigated in MM. Among these, angiogenesis[15] has been shown to confer poor survival in retrospective series. High expression of p27 and low proliferation were associated with prolonged survival in a small study.[223] The advent of microarray technology has been used to investigate prognostic profiles and possibly identify targets for treatment.[16,17,224] cDNA expression profiling identified a 27-gene classifier that was highly predictive of survival in 21 patients who underwent cytoreductive surgery.[225] Another study was able to confirm the prognostic signature obtained in 39 cases, in another cohort of 52 tumors.[226] Of course, these studies will require larger sample sizes and prospective validation.

Benign forms of mesothelioma

Benign fibrous tumors of the pleura are also called *localized fibrous mesothelioma*; they are one-third as common as the diffuse pleural mesotheliomas.[227] Histological studies can provide the differential diagnosis with MM (see above). These tumors are usually pedunculated and can often be radically resected; however, local relapses have been described, even after many years.[228]

Well-differentiated papillary mesotheliomas or cystic mesotheliomas of the peritoneum have been described in young women and are associated with long survival and rare progression to a typical MM.[229]

Benign fibrous mesotheliomas of the genital tract and of the atrioventricular (AV) node have also been described; their histogenesis is not clearly related to the mesothelium.

Recommendations

Malignant mesothelioma is a rare but aggressive tumor that arises from the serosal lining of the pleura, pericardium, or peritoneum. Multimodality therapy that includes surgery, chemotherapy, and radiation therapy in carefully selected patients offers the best long-term outcome. Surgical options for malignant pleural mesothelioma include EPP and pleurectomy/decortication. Due to a lack of data from randomized control trials to ascertain the advantages of one procedure over another, the choice of surgical method remains contentious and is determined by a number of factors, including the stage of the disease, presence of other comorbidities, and the experience of the surgeon. Radiation therapy has a limited role when used alone but is frequently used as a component of multimodality therapy to improve local control. The combination of cisplatin and pemetrexed is the chemotherapeutic regimen of choice for first-line treatment. Biological agents that have been evaluated so far, including EGFR and VEGF inhibitors, have limited activity when used as single agents. Novel combinations of chemotherapy with targeted agents are currently under investigation and may have a role as part of multimodal therapy in the future. Immunotherapeutic approaches such as the use of anti-mesothelin antibodies are also being developed and may play a greater role in the treatment of MM in the future.

References

1. Zucali PA, *et al.* Advances in the biology of malignant pleural mesothelioma. Cancer Treat Rev 2011; 37(7): 543–58.
2. Bianchi AB, *et al.* High frequency of inactivating mutations in the neurofibromatosis type 2 gene (NF2) in primary malignant mesotheliomas. Proc Natl Acad Sci U S A 1995; 92: 10854–8.
3. Cheng JQ, *et al.* Frequent mutations of NF2 and allelic loss from chromosome band 22q12 in malignant mesothelioma: evidence for a two-hit mechanism of NF2 inactivation. Genes Chromosomes Cancer 1999; 24: 238–42.
4. Taguchi T, *et al.* Recurrent deletions of specific chromosomal sites in 1p, 3p, 6q, and 9p in human malignant mesothelioma. Cancer Res 1993; 53: 4349–55.
5. Cheng JQ, *et al.* Homozygous deletions within 9p21–p22 identify a small critical region of chromosomal loss in human malignant mesotheliomas. Cancer Res 1993; 53: 4761–3.
6. Xio S, *et al.* Codeletion of p15 and p16 in primary malignant mesothelioma. Oncogene 1995; 11: 511–5.
7. Bell DW, Jhanwar SC, Testa JR. Multiple regions of allelic loss from chromosome arm 6q in malignant mesothelioma. Cancer Res 1997; 57: 4057–62.
8. Zeiger MA, *et al.* Loss of heterozygosity on the short arm of chromosome 3 in mesothelioma cell lines and solid tumors. Genes Chromosomes Cancer 1994; 11: 15–20.
9. Pylkkanen L, *et al.* Reduced Fhit protein expression in human malignant mesothelioma. Virchows Arch 2004; 444: 43–8.
10. Balsara BR, *et al.* Comparative genomic hybridization and loss of heterozygosity analyses identify a common region of deletion at 15q11.1-15 in human malignant mesothelioma. Cancer Res 1999; 59: 450–4.
11. Galffy G, *et al.* Interleukin 8: an autocrine growth factor for malignant mesothelioma. Cancer Res 1999; 59: 367–71.
12. Konig JE, *et al.* Expression of vascular endothelial growth factor in diffuse malignant pleural mesothelioma. Virchows Arch 1999; 435: 8–12.
13. Ohta Y, *et al.* VEGF and VEGF type C play an important role in angiogenesis and lymphangiogenesis in human malignant mesothelioma tumours. Br J Cancer 1999; 81: 54–61.
14. Strizzi L, *et al.* Vascular endothelial growth factor is an autocrine growth factor in human malignant mesothelioma. J Pathol 2001; 193: 468–75.
15. Edwards JG, *et al.* Angiogenesis is an independent prognostic factor in malignant mesothelioma. Br J Cancer 2001; 85: 863–8.
16. Gordon GJ, *et al.* Identification of novel candidate oncogenes and tumor suppressors in malignant pleural mesothelioma using large-scale transcriptional profiling. Am J Pathol 2005; 166: 1827–40.
17. Sun X, *et al.* Molecular characterization of tumour heterogeneity and malignant mesothelioma cell differentiation by gene profiling. J Pathol 2005; 207: 91–101.
18. Working Group on Asbestos and Cancer. Report and recommendations of the working group convened under the auspices of the geographical pathology committee of the international union against cancer. Arch Environ Health 1965; 11: 221–9.
19. Price B, Ware A. Mesothelioma trends in the United States: an update based on surveillance, epidemiology, and end results program data for 1973 through 2003. Am J Epidemiol 2004; 159: 107–12.
20. Peto J, *et al.* The European mesothelioma epidemic. Br J Cancer 1999; 79: 666–72.
21. Pelucchi C, *et al.* The mesothelioma epidemic in Western Europe: an update. Br J Cancer 2004; 90: 1022–4.
22. Weill H, Hughes J, Churg A. Changing trends in US mesothelioma incidence. Occup Environ Med 2005; 62: 270.
23. Hillerdal G. Malignant mesothelioma 1982: review of 4710 published cases. Br J Dis Chest 1983; 77: 321–43.
24. LaDou J. The asbestos cancer epidemic. Environ Health Perspect 2004; 112: 285–90.
25. Smith AH, Wright CC. Chrysotile asbestos is the main cause of pleural mesothelioma. Am J Ind Med 1996; 30: 252–66.
26. Mossman BT, Kamp DW, Weitzman SA. Mechanisms of carcinogenesis and clinical features of asbestos-associated cancers. Cancer Invest 1996; 14: 466–80.
27. Roggli VL, *et al.* Malignant mesothelioma and occupational exposure to asbestos: a clinicopathological correlation of 1445 cases. Ultrastruct Pathol 2002; 26: 55–65.
28. Mohamed F, Sugarbaker PH. Peritoneal mesothelioma. Curr Treat Options Oncol 2002; 3: 375–86.
29. Antman K, *et al.* Malignant mesothelioma: prognostic variables in a registry of 180 patients, the Dana-Farber Cancer Institute and Brigham and Women's Hospital experience over two decades, 1965–1985. J Clin Oncol 1988; 6: 147–53.
30. Yan TD, *et al.* A novel tumor-node-metastasis (TNM) staging system of diffuse malignant peritoneal mesothelioma using outcome analysis of a multi-institutional database. Cancer 2011; 117: 1855–63.
31. Jacquet P, Sugarbaker PH. Clinical research methodologies in diagnosis and staging of patients with peritoneal carcinomatosis. Cancer Treatment Res 1996; 82: 359–74.

32. Feldman AL, *et al*. Analysis of factors associated with outcome in patients with malignant peritoneal mesothelioma undergoing surgical debulking and intraperitoneal chemotherapy. J Clin Oncol 2003; 21: 4560–7.

33. Loggie BW, *et al*. Prospective trial for the treatment of malignant peritoneal mesothelioma. Am Surg 2001;67: 999–1003.

34. Brigand C, *et al*. Peritoneal mesothelioma treated by cytoreductive surgery and intraperitoneal hyperthermic chemotherapy: results of a prospective study. Ann Surg Oncol 2006; 13: 405–12.

35. Sugarbaker PH, *et al*. Comprehensive management of diffuse malignant peritoneal mesothelioma. Eur J Surg Oncol 2006: 32: 686–91.

36. Yan TD, *et al*. Cytoreductive surgery and hyperthermic intraperitoneal chemotherapy for malignant peritoneal mesothelioma: multi-institutional experience. J Clin Oncol 2009; 27: 6237–42.

37. Jänne PA, *et al*. Open-label study of pemetrexed alone or in combination with cisplatin for the treatment of patients with peritoneal mesothelioma: outcomes of an expanded access program. Clin Lung Cancer 2005; 7: 40–6.

38. Simon GR, *et al*. Pemetrexed plus gemcitabine as first-line chemotherapy for patients with peritoneal mesothelioma: final report of a phase II trial. J Clin Oncol 2008; 26: 3567–72.

39. Le DT, *et al*. Cisplatin and irinotecan (CPT-11) for peritoneal mesothelioma. Cancer Invest 2003; 21: 682–9.

40. Chahinian AP, *et al*. Randomized phase II trial of cisplatin with mitomycin or doxorubicin for malignant mesothelioma by the Cancer and Leukemia Group B. J Clin Oncol 1993; 11: 1559–65.

41. Vogelzang NJ, *et al*. Trimetrexate in malignant mesothelioma: a Cancer and Leukemia Group B Phase II study. J Clin Oncol 1994; 12: 1436–42.

42. Varghese S, *et al*. Activation of the phosphoinositide-3-kinase and mammalian target of rapamycin signaling pathways are associated with shortened survival in patients with malignant peritoneal mesothelioma. Cancer 2011; 117: 361–71.

43. Gupta NP, *et al*. Malignant mesothelioma of the tunica vaginalis testis: a report of two cases and review of literature. J Surg Oncol 1999; 70: 251–4.

44. Vigneswaran WT, Stefanacci PR. Pericardial mesothelioma. Curr Treat Options Oncol 2000; 1: 299–302.

45. Pistolesi M, Rusthoven J. Malignant pleural mesothelioma: update, current management, and newer therapeutic strategies. Chest 2004; 126: 1318–29.

46. Lipworth L, *et al*. Occupational exposure to rock wool and glass wool and risk of cancers of the lung and the head and neck: a systematic review and meta-analysis. J Occup Environ Med 2009; 51: 1075–87.

47. Burdorf A, *et al*. Future increase of the incidence of mesothelioma due to occupational exposure to asbestos in the past. Ned Tijdschr Geneeskd 1997; 141: 1093–8.

48. Testa JR, *et al*. Germline BAP1 mutations predispose to malignant mesothelioma. Nat Genet 2011;43(10): 1022–5.

49. Carbone M, *et al*. Simian virus 40-like DNA sequences in human pleural mesothelioma. Oncogene 1994; 9: 1781–90.

50. Carbone M, *et al*. New developments about the association of SV40 with human mesothelioma. Oncogene 2003; 22: 5173–80.

51. Gee GV, *et al*. SV40 associated miRNAs are not detectable in mesotheliomas. Br J Cancer 2010; 103: 885–88.

52. Manfredi JJ, *et al*. Evidence against a role for SV40 in human mesothelioma. Cancer Res 2005; 65: 2602–9.

53. Lopez-Rios F, *et al*. Evidence against a role for SV40 infection in human mesotheliomas and high risk of false-positive PCR results owing to presence of SV40 sequences in common laboratory plasmids. Lancet 2004; 364: 1157–66.

54. Cristaudo A, *et al*. SV40 enhances the risk of malignant mesothelioma among people exposed to asbestos: a molecular epidemiologic case-control study. Cancer Res 2005; 65: 3049–52.

55. Churg A, *et al*. The separation of benign and malignant mesothelial proliferations. Am J Surg Pathol 2000; 24: 1183–200.

56. Kumaki F, *et al*. Expression of telomerase reverse transcriptase (TERT) in malignant mesotheliomas. Am J Surg Pathol 2002; 26: 365–70.

57. Doglioni C, *et al*. Calretinn a novel immunocytochemical marker for mesothelioma. Am J Surg Pathol 1996; 20: 1037–46.

58. Gotzos V, Vogt P, Celio MR. The calcium binding protein calretinin is a selective marker for malignant pleural mesotheliomas of the epithelial type. Pathol Res Pract 1996; 192: 137–47.

59. Bakir K, *et al*. TTF-1 and surfactant-B as co-adjuvants in the diagnosis of lung adenocarcinoma and pleural mesothelioma. Ann Diagn Pathol 2004; 8: 337–41.

60. Brockstedt U, *et al*. An optimized battery of eight antibodies that can distinguish most cases of epithelial mesothelioma from adenocarcinoma. Am J Clin Pathol 2000; 114: 203–9.

61. Ordonez NG. Value of thyroid transcription factor-1, E-cadherin, BG8, WT1, and CD44S immunostaining in distinguishing epithelial pleural mesothelioma from pulmonary and nonpulmonary adenocarcinoma. Am J Surg Pathol 2000; 24: 598–606.

62. Amin KM, *et al*. Wilms' tumor 1 susceptibility (WT1) gene products are selectively expressed in malignant mesothelioma. Am J Pathol 1995; 146: 344–56.

63. Thirkettle I, *et al*. Immunoreactivity for cadherins, HGF/SF, met, and erbB-2 in pleural malignant mesotheliomas. Histopathology 2000; 36: 522–8.

64. Hussain AN, *et al*. Guidelines for pathologic diagnosis of malignant mesothelioma: a consensus statement from the International Mesothelioma Interest Group. Arch Pathol Lab Med 2009; 133; 1317–31.

65. Oury TD, Hammar SP, Roggli VL. Ultrastructural features of diffuse malignant mesotheliomas. Hum Pathol 1998; 29: 1382–92.

66. Ray M, Kindler HL. Malignant pleural mesothelioma: an update on biomarkers and treatment. Chest 2009; 136: 888–96.

67. Wheatley-Price P, *et al*. Soluble mesothelin-related peptide and osteopontin as markers of response in malignant mesothelioma. J Clin Oncol 2010; 28: 3316–22.

68. Kannerstein M, *et al*. A critique of the criteria for the diagnosis of diffuse malignant mesothelioma. Mt Sinai J Med 1977; 44: 485–94.

69. Aisner J. Current approach to malignant mesothelioma of the pleura. Chest 1995; 107: 332S–344S.

70. Wadler S, *et al*. Cardiac abnormalities in patients with diffuse malignant pleural mesothelioma. Cancer 1986; 58: 2744–50.

71. De Pangher Manzini V, Brollo A, Bianchi C. Thrombocytosis in malignant pleural mesothelioma. Tumori 1990; 76: 576–8.

72. Faber LP. Surgical treatment of asbestos-related disease of the chest. Surg Clin North Am 1988; 68: 525–43.

73. DaValle MJ, *et al*. Extrapleural pneumonectomy for diffuse, malignant mesothelioma. Ann Thorac Surg 1986; 42: 612–18.

74. Gill RR. Imaging of mesothelioma. Recent Results Cancer Res 2011; 189: 27–43.

75. Patz EF Jr, *et al*. Malignant pleural mesothelioma: value of CT and MR imaging in predicting resectability. Am J Roentgenol 1992; 159: 961–6.

76. Lorigan JG, Libshitz HI. MR imaging of malignant pleural mesothelioma. J Comput Assist Tomogr 1989; 13: 617–20.

77. Conlon KC, Rusch VW, Gillern S. Laparoscopy: an important tool in the staging of malignant pleural mesothelioma. Ann Surg Oncol 1996; 3: 489–94.

78. Wang ZJ, *et al*. Malignant pleural mesothelioma: evaluation with CT, MR imaging, and PET. Radiographics 2004; 24: 105–19.

79. Sharif S, *et al*. Does positron emission tomography offer prognostic information in malignant pleural mesothelioma? Interact Cardiovasc Thorac Surg 2011; 12: 806–11.

80. Misri R, *et al*. Evaluation of (111)In labeled antibodies for SPECT imaging of mesothelin expressing tumors. Nucl Med Biol 2011; 38: 885–96.

81. Butchart EG, *et al*. Pleuropneumonectomy in the management of diffuse malignant mesothelioma of the pleura. Experience with 29 patients. Thorax 1976; 31: 15–24.

82. Rusch VW, for the International Mesothelioma Interest Group. A proposed new international TNM staging system for malignant pleural mesothelioma. Chest 1995; 108: 1122–8.

83. Ruffie P, *et al*. Diffuse malignant mesothelioma of the pleura in Ontario and Quebec: a retrospective study of 332 patients. J Clin Oncol 1989; 7: 1157–68.

84. McCormack PM, *et al*. Surgical treatment of pleural mesothelioma. J Thorac Cardiovasc Surg 1982; 84: 834–42.

85. Law MR, *et al.* Malignant mesothelioma of the pleura: a study of 52 treated and 64 untreated patients. Thorax 1984; 39: 255–9.

86. Faber LP. Surgical treatment of asbestos-related disease of the chest. Surg Clin North Am 1988; 68: 525–43.

87. DaValle MJ, *et al.* Extrapleural pneumonectomy for diffuse, malignant mesothelioma. Ann Thorac Surg 1986; 42: 612–18.

88. Wanebo HJ, *et al.* Pleural mesothelioma. Cancer 1976; 38: 2481–8.

89. Achatzy R, *et al.* The diagnosis, therapy and prognosis of diffuse malignant mesothelioma. Eur J Cardiothorac Surg 1989; 3: 445–7.

90. Ruffie P, *et al.* Diffuse malignant mesothelioma of the pleura in Ontario and Quebec: a retrospective study of 332 patients. J Clin Oncol 1989; 7: 1157–68.

91. Brancatisano RP, Joseph MG, McCaughan BC. Pleurectomy for mesothelioma. Med J Aust 1991; 154: 455–7, 460.

92. Rusch VW. Pleurectomy/decortication and adjuvant therapy for malignant mesothelioma. Chest 1993; 103: 382 S–4 S.74.

93. Branscheid D, *et al.* Diagnostic and therapeutic strategy in malignant pleural mesothelioma. Eur J Cardiothorac Surg 1991; 5: 466–72.

94. Lee TT, *et al.* Radical pleurectomy/decortication and intraoperative radiotherapy followed by conformal radiation with or without chemotherapy for malignant pleural mesothelioma. J Thorac Cardiovasc Surg 2002; 124: 1183–9.

95. Worn H. Chances and results of surgery of malignant mesothelioma of the pleura (author's transl). Thoraxchir Vask Chir 1974; 22: 391–3.

96. Bamler KJ, Maassen W. The percentage of benign and malign pleura-tumors among the patients of a clinic of lung surgery with special consideration of the malign pleuramesothelioma and its radical treatment, including results of a diaphragma substitution of preserved dura mater (author's transl). Thoraxchir Vask Chir 1974; 22: 386–91.

97. DeLaria GA, *et al.* Surgical management of malignant mesothelioma. Ann Thorac Surg 1978; 26: 375–82.

98. Geroulanos S, *et al.* Malignant pleural mesothelioma: diagnosis, therapy and prognosis. Schweiz Rundsch Med Prax 1990; 79: 361–7.

99. Rusch VW, Venkatraman E. The importance of surgical staging in the treatment of malignant pleural mesothelioma. J Thorac Cardiovasc Surg 1996; 111: 815–25.S.

100. Sugarbaker DJ, *et al.* Resection margins, extrapleural nodal status, and cell type determine postoperative long-term survival in trimodality therapy of malignant pleural mesothelioma: results in 183 patients. J Thorac Cardiovasc Surg 1999; 117: 54–63.

101. Kaufman AJ, Flores RM. Surgical treatment of malignant pleural mesothelioma. Curr Treat Options Oncol 2011; 12: 201–16.

102. Van Thiel ER, Surmont VF, van Meerbeeck JP. Malignant pleural mesothelioma: when is radiation therapy indicated? Expert Rev Anticancer Ther 2011; 11: 551–60.

103. Rusch VW, *et al.* A phase II trial of surgical resection and adjuvant high-dose hemithoracic radiation for malignant pleural mesothelioma. J Thorac Cardiovasc Surg 2001; 122: 788–95.

104. Rosenzweig KE, *et al.* A pilot trial of high-dose-rate intraoperative radiation therapy for malignant pleural mesothelioma. Brachytherapy 2005; 4: 30–3.

105. Boutin C, Rey F, Viallat JR. Prevention of malignant seeding after invasive diagnostic procedures in patients with pleural mesothelioma. A randomized trial of local radiotherapy. Chest 1995; 108: 754–8.

106. Bertino P, Carbone M, Pass H. Chemotherapy of malignant pleural mesothelioma. Expert Opin Pharmacother 2009; 10: 99–107.

107. Jakobsen JN, Sorensen JB. Review on clinical trials of targeted treatments in malignant mesothelioma. Cancer Chemother Pharmacol 2011; 68: 1–15.

108. Kelly RJ, Sharon E, Hassan R. Chemotherapy and targeted therapies for unresectable malignant mesothelioma. Lung Cancer 2011; 73: 256–63.

109. Van Klaveren RJ, *et al.* Inadequacy of the RECIST criteria for response evaluation in patients with malignant pleural mesothelioma. Lung Cancer 2004; 43: 63–9.

110. Ceresoli GL, *et al.* Assessment of tumor response in malignant pleural mesothelioma. Cancer Treat Rev 2007; 33: 533–41.

111. Scagliotti GV, *et al.* Phase II study of pemetrexed with and without folic acid and vitamin B12 as front-line therapy in malignant pleural mesothelioma. J Clin Oncol 2003; 21: 1556–61.

112. Kindler HL, *et al.* Gemcitabine for malignant mesothelioma: a phase II trial by the Cancer and Leukemia Group B. Lung Cancer 2001; 31: 311–17.

113. Aversa SM, Favaretto AG. Carboplatin and gemcitabine chemotherapy for malignant pleural mesothelioma: a phase II study of the GSTPV. Clin Lung Cancer 1999; 1: 73–5.

114. Favaretto AG, *et al.* Gemcitabine combined with carboplatin in patients with malignant pleural mesothelioma: a multicentric phase II study. Cancer 2003; 97: 2791–7.

115. Byrne MJ, *et al.* Cisplatin and gemcitabine treatment for malignant mesothelioma: a phase II study. J Clin Oncol 1999; 17: 25–30.

116. Nowak AK, *et al.* A multicentre phase II study of cisplatin and gemcitabine for malignant mesothelioma. Br J Cancer 2002; 87: 491–6.

117. Van Haarst JM, *et al.* Multicentre phase II study of gemcitabine and cisplatin in malignant pleural mesothelioma. Br J Cancer 2002; 86: 342–5.

118. Castagneto B, *et al.* Cisplatin and gemcitabine in malignant pleural mesothelioma: a phase II study. Am J Clin Oncol 2005; 28: 223–6.

119. Van Meerbeeck JP *et al.*, European Organization for Research and Treatment of Cancer Lung Cancer Cooperative Group. A Phase II study of gemcitabine in patients with malignant pleural mesothelioma. Cancer 1999; 85: 2577–82.

120. Lerner HJ, *et al.* Malignant mesothelioma. The Eastern Cooperative Oncology Group (ECOG) experience. Cancer 1983; 52: 1981–5.

121. Sorensen PG, *et al.* Randomized trial of doxorubicin versus cyclophosphamide in diffuse malignant pleural mesothelioma. Cancer Treat Rep 1985; 69: 1431–2.

122. Baas P, *et al.* Caelyx in malignant mesothelioma: a phase II EORTC study. Ann Oncol 2000; 11: 697–700.

123. Oh Y, *et al.* Phase II study of intravenous Doxil in malignant pleural mesothelioma. Invest New Drugs 2000; 18: 243–5.

124. Colbert N, *et al.* A prospective study of detorubicin in malignant mesothelioma. Cancer 1985; 56: 2170–4.

125. Kaukel E, *et al.* A phase II study of pirarubicin in malignant pleural mesothelioma. Cancer 1990; 66: 651–4.

126. Magri MD, *et al.* Epirubicin in the treatment of malignant mesothelioma: a phase II cooperative study. Tumori 1991; 77: 49–51.

127. Mattson K, *et al.* Epirubicin in malignant mesothelioma: a phase II study of the European Organization for Research and Treatment of Cancer Lung Cancer Cooperative Group. J Clin Oncol 1992; 10: 824–8.

128. Eisenhauer EA, *et al.* Phase II study of mitoxantrone in patients with mesothelioma: a National Cancer Institute of Canada Clinical Trials Group Study. Cancer Treat Rep 1986; 70: 1029–30.

129. Van Breukelen FJ, *et al.* Mitoxantrone in malignant pleural mesothelioma: a study by the EORTC Lung Cancer Cooperative Group. Eur J Cancer 1991; 27: 1627–9.

130. Hudis CA, Kelsen DP. Menogaril in the treatment of malignant mesothelioma: a phase II study. Invest New Drugs 1992; 10: 103–6.

131. Sahmoud T, *et al.* Etoposide in malignant pleural mesothelioma: two phase II trials of the EORTC Lung Cancer Cooperative Group. Eur J Cancer 1997; 33: 2211–15.

132. Tammilehto L, *et al.* Oral etoposide in the treatment of malignant mesothelioma. A phase II study. Ann Oncol 1994; 5: 949–50.

133. Falkson G, Vorobiof DA, Lerner HJ. A phase II study of m-AMSA in patients with malignant mesothelioma. Cancer Chemother Pharmacol 1983; 11: 94–7.

134. Kindler HL, *et al.* Irinotecan for malignant mesothelioma. A phase II trial by the Cancer and Leukemia Group B. Lung Cancer 2005; 48: 423–8.

135. Alberts AS, Falkson G, van Zyl L. Ifosfamide and mesna with doxorubicin have activity in malignant mesothelioma. Eur J Cancer 1990; 26: 1002.

136. Zidar BL *et al.*, A Southwest Oncology Group Study. A phase II evaluation of ifosfamide and mesna in unresectable diffuse malignant mesothelioma. Cancer 1992; 70: 2547–51.

137. Andersen MK, *et al.* Ifosfamide in malignant mesothelioma: a phase II study. Lung Cancer 1999; 24: 39–43.

138. Talbot SM, *et al.* High-dose ifosfamide with mesna and granuloctye-colony-stimulating factor (recombinant human G-CSF) in patients with unresectable malignant mesothelioma. Cancer 2003; 98: 331–6.

139. Bajorin D, Kelsen D, Mintzer DM. Phase II trial of mitomycin in malignant mesothelioma. Cancer Treat Rep 1987; 71: 857–8.

140. Mintzer DM, et al. Phase II trial of high-dose cisplatin in patients with malignant mesothelioma. Cancer Treat Rep 1985; 69: 711–12.

141. Zidar BL, et al. A phase II evaluation of cisplatin in unresectable diffuse malignant mesothelioma: a Southwest Oncology Group Study. Invest New Drugs 1988; 6: 223–6.

142. Mbidde EK, et al. Phase II trial of carboplatin (JM8) in treatment of patients with malignant mesothelioma. Cancer Chemother Pharmacol 1986; 18: 284–5.

143. Vogelzang NJ, et al. Carboplatin in malignant mesothelioma: a phase II study of the Cancer and Leukemia Group B. Cancer Chemother Pharmacol 1990; 27: 239–42.

144. Raghavan D, et al. Phase II trial of carboplatin in the management of malignant mesothelioma. J Clin Oncol 1990; 8: 151–4.

145. Giaccone G, et al. Phase II trial of ZD0473 as second-line therapy in mesothelioma. Eur J Cancer 2002; 38(Suppl 8): S19–24.

146. Van Meerbeeck JP, et al. A phase II EORTC study of temozolomide in patients with malignant pleural mesothelioma. Eur J Cancer 2002; 38: 779–83.

147. Solheim OP, et al. High-dose methotrexate in the treatment of malignant mesothelioma of the pleura. A phase II study. Br J Cancer 1992; 65: 956–60.

148. Vogelzang NJ, et al. Trimetrexate in malignant mesothelioma: a Cancer and Leukemia Group B Phase II study. J Clin Oncol 1994; 12: 1436–42.

149. Kindler HL, et al. Edatrexate (10-ethyl-deaza-aminopterin) (NSC #626715) with or without leucovorin rescue for malignant mesothelioma. Sequential phase II trials by the cancer and leukemia group B. Cancer 1999; 86: 1985–91.

150. Cantwell BM, Earnshaw M, Harris AL. Phase II study of a novel antifolate, N10-propargyl-5,8 dideazafolic acid (CB3717), in malignant mesothelioma. Cancer Treat Rep 1986; 70: 1335–6.

151. Harvey VJ, et al. Chemotherapy of diffuse malignant mesothelioma. Phase II trials of single-agent 5-fluorouracil and adriamycin. Cancer 1984; 54: 961–4.

152. Otterson GA, et al. Capecitabine in malignant mesothelioma: a phase II trial by the Cancer and Leukemia Group B (39807). Lung Cancer 2004; 44: 251–9.

153. Vogelzang NJ, et al. Cancer and Leukemia Group B. Dihydro-5-azacytidine in malignant mesothelioma. A phase II trial demonstrating activity accompanied by cardiac toxicity. Cancer 1997; 79: 2237–42.

154. Dhingra HM, et al. Phase II trial of 5,6-dihydro-5-azacytidine in pleural malignant mesothelioma. Invest New Drugs 1991; 9: 69–72.

155. Martensson G, Sorenson S. A phase II study of vincristine in malignant mesothelioma – a negative report. Cancer Chemother Pharmacol 1989; 24: 133–4.

156. Cowan JD, et al. Phase II trial of five day intravenous infusion vinblastine sulfate in patients with diffuse malignant mesothelioma: a Southwest Oncology Group study. Invest New Drugs 1988; 6: 247–8.

157. Kelsen D, et al. Vindesine in the treatment of malignant mesothelioma: a phase II study. Cancer Treat Rep 1983; 67: 821–2.

158. Boutin C, et al. Phase II trial of vindesine in malignant pleural mesothelioma. Cancer Treat Rep 1987; 71: 205–6.

159. Steele JP, et al. Phase II study of vinorelbine in patients with malignant pleural mesothelioma. J Clin Oncol 2000; 18: 3912–17.

160. Vorobiof DA, et al. Malignant pleural mesothelioma: a phase II trial with docetaxel. Ann Oncol 2002; 13: 412–15.

161. Belani CP, et al. Docetaxel for malignant mesothelioma: phase II study of the Eastern Cooperative Oncology Group. Clin Lung Cancer 2004; 6: 43–7.

162. Van Meerbeeck J, et al. Paclitaxel for malignant pleural mesothelioma: a phase II study of the EORTC Lung Cancer Cooperative Group. Br J Cancer 1996; 74: 961–3.

163. Vogelzang NJ, et al. High-dose paclitaxel plus G-CSF for malignant mesothelioma: CALGB phase II study 9234. Ann Oncol 1999; 10: 597–600.

164. Eagan RT, et al. Phase II trial of diaziquone in malignant mesothelioma. Cancer Treat Rep 1986; 70: 429.

165. Falkson G, et al. Phase II trial of acivicin in malignant mesothelioma. Cancer Treat Rep 1987; 71: 545–6.

166. Mulatero CW, et al. A phase II study of combined intravenous and subcutaneous interleukin-2 in malignant pleural mesothelioma. Lung Cancer 2001; 31: 67–72.

167. Mikulski SM, et al. Phase II trial of a single weekly intravenous dose of ranpirnase in patients with unresectable malignant mesothelioma. J Clin Oncol 2002; 20: 274–81.

168. Baas P, et al. Thalidomide in patients with malignant pleural mesothelioma. Lung Cancer 2005; 48: 291–6.

169. Govindan R, et al. Gefitinib in patients with malignant mesothelioma: a phase II study by the Cancer and Leukemia Group B. Clin Cancer Res 2005; 11: 2300–4.

170. Mathy A, et al. Limited efficacy of imatinib mesylate in malignant mesothelioma: a phase II trial. Lung Cancer 2005; 50(1): 83–6.

171. Dubey S, et al. A phase II study of sorafenib in malignant mesothelioma: results of Cancer and Leukemia Group B 30307. J Thoracic Oncol 2010; 5: 1655–61.

172. Nowak AK, et al. Final results of a phase II study of sunitinib as second-line therapy in malignant pleural mesothelioma. J Clin Oncol 2010; 28(Suppl): abstr 7036.

173. Cortese JF, et al. Common EGFR mutations conferring sensitivity to gefitinib in lung adenocarcinoma are not prevalent in human malignant mesothelioma. Int J Cancer 2006; 118: 521–2.

174. Butnor KJ, et al. The spectrum of Kit (CD117) immunoreactivity in lung and pleural tumors: a study of 96 cases using a single-source antibody with a review of the literature. Arch Pathol Lab Med 2004; 128: 538–43.

175. Horvai AE, et al. c-Kit is not expressed in malignant mesothelioma. Mod Pathol 2003; 16: 818–22.

176. Ohta Y, et al. VEGF and VEGF type C play an important role in angiogenesis and lymphangiogenesis in human malignant mesothelioma tumours. Br J Cancer 1999; 81: 54–61.

177. Strizzi L, et al. Vascular endothelial growth factor is an autocrine growth factor in human malignant mesothelioma. J Pathol 2001; 193: 468–75.

178. Karrison T, et al. Final analysis of a multi-center, double blind, placebo-controlled, randomized phase II trial of gemcitabine/cisplatin plus bevacizumab or placebo in patients with malignant mesothelioma. J Clin Oncol 2007; 25(Suppl): abstr 7526.

179. Vogelzang NJ, et al. Phase III study of pemetrexed in combination with cisplatin versus cisplatin alone in patients with malignant pleural mesothelioma. J Clin Oncol 2003; 21: 2636–44.

180. Van Meerbeeck JP, et al. A randomized phase III study of cisplatin with or without raltitrexed in patients with malignant pleural mesothelioma: an Intergroup Study of the European Organization for Research and Treatemnt of Cancer Lung Cancer Group and the National Cancer Institute of Canada. J Clin Oncol 2005; 23: 6881–9.

181. Porta C, et al. Raltitrexed-oxaliplatin combination chemotherapy is inactive as second-line treatment for malignant pleural mesothelioma patients. Lung Cancer 2005; 48: 429–34.

182. Manegold C, et al. Second-line (post-study) chemotherapy received by patients treated in the phase III trial of pemetrexed plus cisplatin versus cisplatin alone in malignant pleural mesothelioma. Ann Oncol 2005; 16: 923–7.

183. Samson MK, et al. Randomized comparison of cyclophosphamide, imidazole carboxamide, and adriamycin versus cyclophosphamide and adriamycin in patients with advanced stage malignant mesothelioma: a Sarcoma Intergroup Study. J Clin Oncol 1987; 5: 86–91.

184. White SC, et al. Randomised phase II study of cisplatin-etoposide versus infusional carboplatin in advanced non-small-cell lung cancer and mesothelioma. Ann Oncol 2000; 11: 201–6.

185. Hilaris BS, et al. Pleurectomy and intraoperative brachytherapy and postoperative radiation in the treatment of malignant pleural mesothelioma. Int J Radiat Oncol Biol Phys 1984; 10: 325–31.

186. Rusch V, et al. A phase II trial of pleurectomy/decortication followed by intrapleural and systemic chemotherapy for malignant pleural mesothelioma. J Clin Oncol 1994; 12: 1156–63.

187. Lee JD, *et al*. Intrapleural chemotherapy for patients with incompletely resected malignant mesothelioma: the UCLA experience. J Surg Oncol 1995; 60: 262–7.

188. Rice TW, *et al*. Aggressive multimodality therapy for malignant pleural mesothelioma. Ann Thorac Surg 1994; 58: 24–9.

189. Sauter ER, *et al*. Optimal management of malignant mesothelioma after subtotal pleurectomy: revisiting the role of intrapleural chemotherapy and postoperative radiation. J Surg Oncol 1995; 60: 100–5.

190. Rusch VW, Venkatraman ES. Important prognostic factors in patients with malignant pleural mesothelioma, managed surgically. Ann Thorac Surg 1999; 68: 1799–804.

191. Sugarbaker DJ, *et al*. Prevention, early detection, and management of complications after 328 consecutive extrapleural pneumonectomies. J Thorac Cardiovasc Surg 2004; 128: 138–46.

192. Baldini EH, *et al*. Patterns of failure after trimodality therapy for malignant pleural mesothelioma. Ann Thorac Surg 1997; 63: 334–8.

193. Maggi G, *et al*. Trimodality management of malignant pleural mesothelioma. Eur J Cardiothorac Surg 2001; 19: 346–50.

194. Pass HW, *et al*. A phase II trial investigating primary immunochemotherapy for malignant pleural mesothelioma and the feasibility of adjuvant immunochemotherapy after maximal cytoreduction. Ann Surg Oncol 1995; 2: 214–20.

195. Weder W, *et al*. Neoadjuvant chemotherapy followed by extrapleural pneumonectomy in malignant pleural mesothelioma. J Clin Oncol 2004; 22: 3451–7.

196. Krug LM, *et al*. Multicenter phase II trial of neoadjuvant pemetrexed plus cisplatin followed by extrapleural pneumonectomy and radiation for malignant pleural mesothelioma. J Clin Oncol 2009; 27: 3007–13.

197. Van Schil P, *et al*. Trimodality therapy for malignant pleural mesothelioma: results from an EORTC phase II multicentre trial. Eur Respir J 2010; 36: 1362–9.

198. Treasure T, *et al*. Extra-pleural pneumonectomy versus no extra-pleural pneumonectomy for patients with malignant pleural mesothelioma: clinical outcomes of the Mesothelioma and Radical Surgery (MARS) randomised feasibility study. Lancet Oncol 2011; 12:763–72.

199. Boutin C, *et al*. Intrapleural treatment with recombinant gamma-interferon in early stage malignant pleural mesothelioma. Cancer 1994; 74: 2460–7.

200. Monnet I, *et al*. Intrapleural infusion of activated macrophages and gamma-interferon in malignant pleural mesothelioma: a phase II study. Chest 2002; 121: 1921–7.

201. Goey SH, *et al*. Intrapleural administration of interleukin 2 in pleural mesothelioma: a phase I-II study. Br J Cancer 1995; 72: 1283–8.

202. Stam TC, *et al*. Intrapleural administration of tumour necrosis factor-alpha (TNFalpha) in patients with mesothelioma: cytokine patterns and acute-phase protein response. Eur J Clin Invest 2000; 30: 336–43.

203. Castagneto B, *et al*. Palliative and therapeutic activity of IL-2 immunotherapy in unresectable malignant pleural mesothelioma with pleural effusion: results of a phase II study on 31 consecutive patients. Lung Cancer 2001; 31: 303–10.

204. Ris HB. Photodynamic therapy as an adjunct to surgery for malignant pleural mesothelioma. Lung Cancer 2005; 49(Suppl 1): S65–8.

205. Schouwink H, *et al*. Intraoperative photodynamic therapy after pleuropneumonectomy in patients with malignant pleural mesothelioma: dose finding and toxicity results. Chest 2001; 120: 1167–74.

206. Van Ruth S, *et al*. Cytoreductive surgery combined with intraoperative hyperthermic intrathoracic chemotherapy for stage I malignant pleural mesothelioma. Ann Surg Oncol 2003; 10: 176–82.

207. Ratto GB, *et al*. Pleural space perfusion with cisplatin in the multimodality treatment of malignant mesothelioma: a feasibility and pharmacokinetic study. J Thorac Cardiovasc Surg 1999; 117: 759–65.

208. Lu C, *et al*. Phase II study of a liposome-entrapped cisplatin analog (L-NDDP) administered intrapleurally and pathologic response rates in patients with malignant pleural mesothelioma. J Clin Oncol 2005; 23: 3495–501.

209. Banchereau J, Palucka AK. Dendritic cells as therapeutic vaccines against cancer. Nat Rev Immunol 2005; 5: 296–306.

210. Hegmans JP, *et al*. Consolidative dendritic cell-based immunotherapy elicits cytotoxicity against malignant mesothelioma. Am J Respir Crit Care Med 2010; 181: 1383–90.

211. Keilholz U, *et al*. Wilms' tumour gene 1 (WT1) in human neoplasia. Leukemia 2005; 19: 1318–23.

212. Krug LM, *et al*. Randomized, double-blinded, phase II trial of a WT1 peptide vaccine as adjuvant therapy in patients with malignant pleural mesothelioma (MPM). J Clin Oncol 2011; 29(Suppl): abstr TPS139.

213. Krug LM, *et al*. WT1 peptide vaccinations induce CD4 and CD8 T cell immune responses in patients with mesothelioma and non-small cell lung cancer. Cancer Immunol Immunother 2010; 59: 1467–79.

214. Hassan R, *et al*. Mesothelin: a new target for immunotherapy. Clin Cancer Res 2004; 10: 3937–42.

215. Hassan R, *et al*. Antitumor activity of SS1P with pemetrexed and cisplatin for front-line treatment of pleural mesothelioma and utility of serum mesothelin as a marker of tumor response. J Clin Oncol 2011; 29(Suppl): abstr 7026.

216. Hassan R, *et al*. Phase I clinical trial of the chimeric anti-mesothelin monoclonal antibody MORAb-009 in patients with mesothelin-expressing cancers. Clin Cancer Res 2010; 16: 6132–8.

217. Sterman DH, *et al*. A phase I trial of repeated intra-pleural adenoviral-mediated interferon-beta gene transfer for mesothelioma and metastatic pleural effusions. Mol Ther 2010; 18: 852–60.

218. Vachani A, Moon E, Albelda SM. Gene therapy for mesothelioma. Curr Treat Options Oncol 2011; 12: 173–80.

219. Curran D, *et al*. Prognostic factors in patients with pleural mesothelioma: the European Organization for Research and Treatment of Cancer experience. J Clin Oncol 1998; 16: 145–52.

220. Herndon JE, *et al*. Factors predictive of survival among 337 patients with mesothelioma treated between 1984 and 1994 by the Cancer and Leukemia Group B. Chest 1998; 113: 723–31.

221. Edwards JG, *et al*. Prognostic factors for malignant mesothelioma in 142 patients: validation of CALGB and EORTC prognostic scoring systems. Thorax 2000; 55: 731–5.

222. Fennell DA, *et al*. Statistical validation of the EORTC prognostic model for malignant pleural mesothelioma based on three consecutive phase II trials. J Clin Oncol 2005; 23: 184–9.

223. Bongiovanni M, *et al*. p27(kip1) immunoreactivity correlates with long-term survival in pleural malignant mesothelioma. Cancer 2001; 92: 1245–50.

224. Roe OD, *et al*. Genome-wide profile of pleural mesothelioma versus parietal and visceral pleura: the emerging gene portrait of the mesothelioma phenotype. PLoS One 2009; 4: e6554.

225. Pass HI, *et al*. Gene expression profiles predict survival and progression of pleural mesothelioma. Clin Cancer Res 2004; 10: 849–59.

226. Gordon GJ, *et al*. Validation of genomics-based prognostic tests in malignant pleural mesothelioma. Clin Cancer Res 2005; 11: 4406–14.

227. Briselli M, Mark EJ, Dickersin GR. Solitary fibrous tumors of the pleura: eight new cases and review of 360 cases in the literature. Cancer 1981; 47: 2678–89.

228. Sung SH, *et al*. Solitary fibrous tumors of the pleura: surgical outcome and clinical course. Ann Thorac Surg 2005; 79: 303–7.

229. Sethna K, *et al*. Peritoneal cystic mesothelioma: a case series. Tumori 2003; 89: 31–5.

Section 5: Thoracic Tumors

23 Primary Melanoma of the Lung

Richard A. Scolyer,[1,2,3] **James F. Bishop,**[3,4] **and John F. Thompson,**[1,2,3]

[1] Melanoma Institute Australia, Sydney, NSW, Australia
[2] Tissue Pathology and Diagnostic Oncology, Royal Prince Alfred Hospital, Camperdown, NSW, Australia
[3] The University of Sydney, Sydney, NSW, Australia
[4] Victorian Comprehensive Cancer Centre and University of Melbourne, VIC, Australia

Introduction

Although most primary melanomas develop as cutaneous or ocular tumors and a few develop in recognized mucosal sites, the very occasional occurrence of primary melanomas in unusual noncutaneous sites, including the lung, is well documented.[1] Primary melanoma of the lung is undoubtedly a very rare tumor but its precise incidence is the subject of continuing debate. Some have even questioned whether the condition actually exists. The difficulty arises because an unrecognized primary cutaneous melanoma can occasionally undergo complete regression and disappear without trace, while a lung metastasis which has arisen from it continues to grow and may eventually present as an apparently isolated focus of melanoma.[2,3] Because melanocytes are not normally found in the tracheobronchial tree, it is also difficult to explain the histogenesis of a primary lung melanoma. In patients who do have a history of primary cutaneous melanoma and who subsequently present with metastatic disease, the lungs are the only clinically detectable site of metastasis in 7–9% of cases.[4] Melanoma has a predilection to metastasize to the lungs,[5,6] and approximately 70% of patients who die of melanoma are found to have pulmonary metastases at autopsy.[7,8]

The literature contains numerous reports of patients with melanomas that seem to be of primary lung origin. In many of these patients, their history and subsequent follow-up appear to exclude the possibility of metastasis to the lung from a primary site elsewhere.[7,9–51] Supporting evidence for a diagnosis of primary lung melanoma may be obtained from histopathological features of the tumor, from a pattern of subsequent involvement of regional lymph nodes which is consistent with that of other tumors of primary bronchial origin, and from failure to find a primary melanoma elsewhere in the body either during life or at the time of autopsy.

The occurrence of primary melanomas in other noncutaneous sites has long been recognized[1,12,52] and is much more comprehensively documented in the literature. Ocular and conjunctival melanomas are the most common, but noncutaneous melanomas are also well recognized to arise in the urethra, vulva, vagina, leptomeninges, adrenal gland, nasopharynx, oropharynx, esophagus, gall bladder, and occasionally in other parts of the gastrointestinal tract including the stomach, small bowel, large bowel, and anal canal.[53] An important difference, however, is that melanocytes have been identified in most of these sites in normal individuals, providing a plausible histogenetic basis for the origin of the melanomas.

Historical background

Although there have been numerous case reports claiming a diagnosis of primary lung melanoma, the patients described in many of the early publications did not fulfill the criteria subsequently accepted as being necessary to definitively establish the diagnosis. The first two recorded cases, reported by Todd in 1888,[9] were certainly based on insufficient evidence to warrant the diagnosis. Similarly, other early reports by Kunkel and Torrey in 1916[10] and by Carlucci and Schleussner in 1942[11] were deficient because full autopsies were not performed to exclude the possibility of a primary melanoma elsewhere. It was not until 1963 that a patient fulfilling subsequently accepted criteria for the diagnosis of primary lung melanoma was reported.[7] In a 1987 publication, Alghanem et al.[31] considered it appropriate to accept only seven previously reported cases as true primary lung melanomas, on the basis of stringent criteria for diagnosis. Reporting a series of eight new cases in 1997, Wilson and Moran suggested that there were fewer than 25 previous cases acceptable as primary pulmonary melanomas.[46] As far as could be determined from a comprehensive review of the literature by the present authors, the total number of reported cases for which the diagnosis had been established by appropriate criteria stood at 62 in 2011 (Table 23.1).

Textbook of Uncommon Cancer, Fourth Edition. Edited by Derek Raghavan, Charles D. Blanke, David H. Johnson, Paul L. Moots, Gregory H. Reaman, Peter G. Rose and Mikkael A. Sekeres.
© 2012 John Wiley & Sons, Inc. Published 2012 by John Wiley & Sons, Inc.

Table 23.1 Published reports of 62 patients with primary melanomas of the trachea, bronchi, lungs, and pleura fulfilling most or all of the currently accepted diagnostic criteria.

Reference	Sex/age	Site
Salm (1963)[6]	M/45	LL
Reed and Kent (1964)[13]	M/71	LL
Reid and Mehta (1966)[13]	F/60	Trachea
	M/35	LL
Jensen and Egedorf (1967)[15]	F/61	UL
Allen and Drash (1968)[16]	F/40	LL
Taboada et al. (1972)[17]	M/56	LL
	M/40	UL
Walter et al. (1972)[18]	M/33	LL
Mori et al. (1977)[19]	F/47	Trachea
Smith and Opipari (1978)[20]	M/49	Pleura
Adebonojo et al. (1979)[21]	F/55	UL
Robertson et al. (1980)[22]	F/70	Carina
Gephardt (1981)[24]	M/47	MSB
Verweij et al. (1982)[25]	M/46	Trachea, MSB
Angel and Prados (1984)[27]	F/41	ML
Cagle et al. (1984)[28]	M/80	ML
Carstens et al. (1984)[29]	F/29	UL
Alghanem et al. (1987)[30]	F/42	LL
Demeter et al. (1987)[31]	M/56	UL
Santos et al. (1987)[32]	M/58	LL
Bagwell et al. (1989)[33]	M/62	UL
Bertola et al. (1989)[35]	F/30	LL
Jennings et al. (1990)[37]	F/34	UK
Sanchez-Navarro et al. (1991)[38]	M/75	MSB
Miller and Allen (1993)[39]	M/56	LL
	M/67	ML
	F/77	LL
Barzó et al. (1994)[40]	F/43	UL
	F/81	LL
Pasquini et al. (1994)[41]	F/66	LL
Farrell et al. (1996)[42]	F/66	LL
Wilson and Moran (1997)[46]	M/71	LL
	M/45	UL
	M/UK	ML
	F/55	UL
	M/52	UL
	M/64	UL
	M/48	UL
	M/50	UL
Sekine et al. (1998)[45]	UK	UK
Ost et al. (1999)[47]	M/90	UL
Ozdemir et al. (2001)[48]	M/41	LL
Testini et al. (2002)[49]	M/44	LL
Dountsis et al. (2003)[50]	F/41	UL
Lie et al. (2005)[51]	F/44	LL
De Wilt et al. (2005)[44]	M/71	ML
	F/49	LL
	M/61	LL
	M/62	LL
	M/66	LL
	M/60	LL
	F/49	UL
Kundranda et al. (2006)[102]	M/60	UK
Reddy et al. (2007)[103]	M/74	LL
Kotoulas et al. (2007)[104]	M/67	UK
Saint-Blancard et al. (2009)[105]	M/82	UL
Shikuma et al. (2009)[106]	M/71	LL
Maeda et al. (2009)[107]	M/68	UL
Pan et al. (2010)[108]	M/81	LL
Neri et al. (2011)[109]	M/58	LL
Mochizuki et al. (2011)[110]	M/84	LL

LL, lower lobe; ML, middle lobe; MSB, main stem bronchus; UK, unknown; UL, upper lobe.

Biology and epidemiology

Biology

A histogenetic basis for the development of primary lung melanomas is not obvious, but several explanations have been proposed. Although melanocytes have not been demonstrated in the lower respiratory tract, some investigators hypothesize that there can be aberrant migration of these potential precursor cells to the lung, and suggest that this could explain the development of primary melanomas at this site.[16] This seems a plausible explanation because embryologically the respiratory tract develops from an outgrowth of the primitive foregut between the pharynx and esophagus, in the region of the larynx, and melanocytes have been identified in the mucosa of these sites.[54–56]

Because squamous metaplasia is occasionally observed in melanoma-affected epithelium, a proposed alternative explanation is that epithelial cells undergo metaplastic transformation into melanocytes.[14] However, it appears more likely that the squamous metaplasia is a consequence of bronchial involvement by melanoma. A condition described as "melanogenic metaplasia" of mucous glands in the oral cavity has also been reported[57] and it is possible that a similar process might occur in the mucous glands of the tracheobronchial tree. Another proposal, perhaps more plausible, is that neuroendocrine (Kulchitsky) precursor cells have the potential to undergo melanocytic differentiation; both cell types are histogenetically related, being of neural crest origin.[38] This theory is supported by the occasional occurrence of melanocytic differentiation in carcinoid tumors[58] and reports of malignant tumors displaying neuroendocrine and melanocytic differentiation.[59,60] A similar theory has been proposed to explain the origin of primary adrenal melanomas[30,61–63] since melanocytes have not been identified in this location either.

The occurrence of melanocytic differentiation within peripheral nerve sheath tumors, such as melanotic schwannomas, raises the possibility that primary pulmonary melanomas may also arise from native pulmonary neural elements.

Epidemiology

In a recent review from the Melanoma Institute Australia (formerly the Sydney Melanoma Unit) in Sydney, Australia, de Wilt and colleagues identified 27 patients who presented with pulmonary melanoma as their first sign of disease and in whom no foci of melanoma at other sites were found.[44] This was from a total of 19,000 patients with melanoma treated over a 50-year period. Following detailed analysis of clinical, pathological and follow-up data, the authors concluded that seven of these patients were likely to have had primary pulmonary melanomas. Reviewing 10,134 patients with primary lung tumors treated at the Mayo Clinic over a 10-year period, Miller and Allen[40] reported three patients with primary lung melanomas. In a report from Japan published in 1998, Sekine et al. identified one case of primary pulmonary melanoma from 3481 primary lung tumors resected over a 20-year period.[45] Each of these reports emphasizes the rarity of primary lung melanoma, but cannot be used to quantify its incidence since the patients seen at each of the institutions were referred for treatment and the data were therefore not population based.

Molecular biology and genetics

During the past decade, critical molecular alterations in melanomas have been identified that are important for development and progression.[64] Mutations in genes coding for proteins in the mitogen-activated protein (MAP) kinase signal transduction pathway have been found in about 70% of melanomas.[65] This pathway involves signalling through RAS-RAF-MEK-ERK and controls cellular proliferation, apoptosis, and migration. Mutant B-RAF, one of three types of RAF proteins, is present in approximately 50% of cutaneous melanomas[66] and mutant N-RAS occurs in approximately 20% of cases.[65] Mutant N-RAS also induces the phosphatidylinositol 3′ kinase (PI3K) cascade, which is another important pathway for control of cellular proliferation, apoptosis, and invasion. B-RAF mutant primary melanoma typically occurs in younger individuals at axial sites where there is a low degree of chronic sun damage.[67] In contrast, N-RAS mutant melanoma shows no age or anatomical site predilection.[68] Activating mutations or gene amplification of the tyrosine kinase receptor c-kit are present in 10–15% of acral and mucosal melanomas and occasionally in melanomas occurring at chronically sun-damaged anatomical sites.[69,70] Uveal melanomas typically show mutations in GNAQ or GNA11.[71] Many other less common mutation events implicated in the pathogenesis of melanoma have also been identified, including those affecting PIK3CA (PI3 kinase), FLT3, PDGFR, MET, and ERBB4.[72,73] However, the molecular pathogenesis of a significant proportion of cutaneous melanomas remains unknown and, to the best of our knowledge, the mutation profile of primary melanoma of the lung has not been reported to date. Because mutations in B-RAF and c-kit are now being successfully exploited by new targeted therapies, as discussed in more detail below, it would appear appropriate to perform relevant mutation testing of primary pulmonary melanoma in patients in whom systemic treatment is being considered.

Pathology

In 1968, Allen and Drash suggested that the surgical pathologist must always consider the possibility of melanoma when examining a lung tumor if the diagnosis is not to be missed.[17] More than 40 years later, this advice may still be appropriate. As melanoma remains "the great imitator" and unless the possibility is considered, primary lung melanoma may be misdiagnosed as a large cell carcinoma of the lung or as a sarcoma of the lung. Having considered the possibility of a melanoma, confirmation or exclusion of this possibility should then be achievable by careful examination for the classic features of melanoma, with support from immunohistochemistry.

A number of histological features (Fig. 23.1) have been suggested as being indicative of primary lung melanoma,[17,28,36] including:

- obvious melanoma cells, confirmed by immunohistochemical staining for S-100 and HMB-45 and possibly electron microscopy
- evidence of junctional change

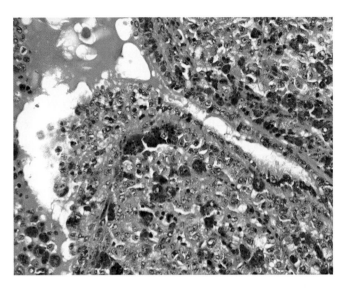

Figure 23.1 Primary pulmonary melanoma occurring in a male aged 61 years. Pleomorphic epithelioid melanoma cells are present, some of which are pigmented, beneath bronchial respiratory-type mucosa. There is focal mucosal surface erosion by the tumor. H & E stained section, original magnification ×100.

- "nesting" of cells beneath the bronchial epithelium
- invasion of the intact (i.e. nonulcerated) bronchial epithelium by melanoma cells.

However, these features were not demonstrated in many of the previously reported cases of primary pulmonary melanoma[46] and, furthermore, are probably not as specific as has been suggested. "*In situ* melanoma" changes, which the latter three criteria represent, may be absent in primary melanomas occurring at other sites, particularly ulcerated primary cutaneous melanomas. In addition, similar changes are sometimes observed in epidermotropic melanomas metastasizing to the skin[74] and an intraepithelial growth of melanoma metastatic to the lung has been documented previously.[75] Indeed, the results of one recent series of 15 patients suggests that distinguishing primary from metastatic melanoma is best performed on the basis of clinical behavior, particularly the pattern of metastatic spread, rather than on histopathological criteria.[44]

Clinical aspects

Presentation

The cases of lung melanoma reported in the literature are divided approximately equally into those which presented as a polypoid obstructing lesion within the tracheobronchial tree and those which presented as a mass within the lung parenchyma. The tumor is almost always unifocal, but multifocal primary lung melanomas have been described.[26,61] Primary pleural melanoma has also been reported.[21]

As expected, the presenting symptoms of a patient with a primary lung melanoma are determined by the site and size of the tumor. Initial recognition of an abnormality is sometimes made on a chest x-ray performed for an unrelated reason.[18,36] A definitive histological diagnosis of melanoma can usually be obtained for endobronchial lesions by bronchoscopy and biopsy, and for lesions in the peripheral lung parenchyma by fine needle aspiration biopsy. However, a diagnosis of primary (rather than metastatic) lung melanoma is unlikely to be made at this time, and may not be reached until after full staging investigations, pathological examination of the resected tumor, an appropriate period of follow-up and possibly at autopsy.

Patterns of metastasis

Primary melanoma of the lung metastasizes in a pattern consistent with that of other primary lung tumors – indeed, this is one of the points of evidence raised in support of the existence of lung melanoma as an entity. Thus involvement of regional lymph nodes in the lung hilum and mediastinum is likely to be observed. As with primary cutaneous melanomas, there is the additional possibility of systemic dissemination via the bloodstream to such sites as brain, liver, adrenal gland, and so on. Metastatic disease involving the pleura, pericardium and heart also occurs.[35,36]

Criteria for diagnosis

To define cases of primary lung melanomas with greater certainty, minimal criteria on which the diagnosis should be based have been proposed. The first such proposal was in 1967 by Jensen and Egedorf,[16] who suggested that a diagnosis of primary lung melanoma should be made in the following circumstances:
- no history suggestive of a previous melanoma (cutaneous or ocular)
- no demonstrable melanoma in any other organ at the time of operation
- a solitary tumor in the surgical specimen from the lung
- tumor morphology compatible with a primary tumor
- no evidence at autopsy of a primary melanoma elsewhere.

Other authors have since endorsed these criteria, with minor variations and additions.[17,26,31,43,76] However, detailed staging investigations and prolonged follow-up are also probably necessary before accepting a definitive diagnosis of primary pulmonary melanoma because, as recently reported by de Wilt et al.,[44] some patients presenting with apparently isolated pulmonary melanoma may subsequently develop cutaneous or nodal recurrences, suggesting that the tumor originated from a regressed primary cutaneous melanoma. Although the criteria proposed by Jensen and Egedorf are undoubtedly appropriate and desirable, it is nevertheless clear that there are instances in which they cannot all be satisfied yet in which the likelihood is high that a lung tumor is a primary melanoma.[38]

Treatment

Surgery

Based on experience with primary melanomas arising in other sites, the treatment of choice for primary lung melanoma is radical surgical excision. This will usually involve formal lobectomy or pneumonectomy. For primary cutaneous melanoma, elective regional lymph node dissection is no longer performed, having been superseded by sentinel lymph node biopsy. Now, in patients with clinical localized primary cutaneous melanoma, regional lymph node clearance is generally only performed in patients with a positive sentinel lymph node. Lymphatic mapping and sentinel lymphadenectomy have been performed in patients with primary and secondary lung tumors, including melanomas, and may provide more accurate pathological staging.[77] The major difficulty with this theoretically attractive approach is that the diagnosis of primary rather than secondary lung melanoma may not be established with reasonable certainty until after detailed pathological examination of the resected tumor. Furthermore, there is little possibility of performing satisfactory delayed regional lymph node clearance in the lung hilum and mediastinum following lobectomy and pneumonectomy. It therefore seems logical to clear these nodes at the time of the initial definitive lung surgery whenever possible.

In the absence of any evidence to indicate otherwise, the treatment of locally recurrent melanoma from a lung primary must be based on the standard treatment principles established for other forms of melanoma. If radical surgical excision is possible, it provides the best form of palliation and may even achieve cure. If whole-body imaging by computed tomography (CT) scanning or more reliably by positron emission tomography (PET) scanning with fluorine-18-fluorodeoxyglucose[62] does not reveal any evidence of metastatic disease elsewhere, radical surgery is certainly indicated. Because melanoma tissue almost always has a very high glucose uptake, whole-body PET/CT scans[62,63,78–83] have largely replaced CT and magnetic resonance imaging (MRI) scans as the staging investigation of choice in most major melanoma treatment centers. PET/CT is therefore likely to assist in determining whether a focus of melanoma in the lung is a primary or secondary tumor. If a diagnosis of primary lung melanoma is confirmed, PET/CT scanning should also demonstrate whether distant metastasis has occurred and, if it has, should prevent inappropriate surgery as treatment for primary lung melanoma from being performed.

Radiotherapy and systemic therapies (including targeted therapies and immunotherapy)

If surgical clearance of locally recurrent disease following resection of a primary lung melanoma is not feasible, systemic therapy may be considered, or radiotherapy if the tumor mass in the chest is causing troublesome symptoms. Foci of metastatic disease outside the chest must similarly be treated on their merits, according to general principles for the treatment of metastatic melanoma, since there are no data to indicate that any different form of treatment is likely to be more effective for metastases from primary lung melanomas. Recently, the identification of oncogenic mutations in melanoma and both the rapid development and application of active targeted therapies and immunotherapies are revolutionizing the treatment of patients with metastatic melanoma.[64–66] It is likely that these therapies will be as effective in metastatic pulmonary melanoma as they are in melanomas arising in other locations.

Highly potent inhibitors of oncogenic mutated B-RAF and c-kit proteins have shown remarkable clinical efficacy in the treatment of metastatic melanoma patients.[69,84,85] Clinical trials of the orally administered inhibitors of V600 mutant B-RAF, vemurafenib and GSK2118436, showed shrinkage of tumor in the majority of B-RAF mutant metastatic melanoma patients.[84–86] Furthermore, vemurafenib has demonstrated a clear survival benefit over standard chemotherapy with dacarbazine in advanced-stage metastatic melanoma patients.[85] However, drug resistance is a limiting factor and all but a few patients relapse, resulting in a progression-free survival of only 5–7 months. Nevertheless, it is likely that, in the near future, elucidation of the mechanisms of resistance to B-RAF inhibitor therapy will lead to new rational and effective multiagent/multimodality therapeutic approaches.[87] Most of the documented toxicities of BRAF inhibitors in humans appear mild and well tolerated. However, cutaneous squamous cell carcinomas and keratoacanthomas develop in a small percentage of patients. Inhibitors of MEK, another protein in the MAP kinase signaling pathway that is downstream of B-RAF, are also showing encouraging activity in clinical trials involving patients with mutant B-RAF metastatic melanoma, particularly when given in combination with a B-RAF inhibitor. Similarly, patients with c-kit mutant metastatic melanoma have been treated with c-kit inhibitors with some clinical responses.[88,89]

Systemic treatment may also be provided by immunotherapy. Ipilimumab is a potent targeted T cell antibody directed against the cytotoxic T lymphocyte antigen 4 (CTLA-4) and is administered intravenously. Activation of CTLA-4 normally suppresses immune responses and hence CTLA-4 blockage by ipilimumab enhances the tumoral immunoactivity. Ipilimumab was shown to extend survival in clinical trials in patients with advanced-stage melanoma, with 2-year survival of over 30%,[90,91] and the drug received approval from the FDA in March 2011. Serious immune-related systemic adverse reactions, some life threatening, occur in up to 15% of patients receiving ipilimumab and require specialized multidisciplinary care.[90,91]

Prognosis

The very limited information that can be gleaned from published reports of patients with primary lung melanomas indicates that the prognosis is generally very poor, with the principal determinant of outcome being the presence or absence of local (peribronchial and hilar) lymph node metastases. However, in one recent series of 15 patients who presented with isolated pulmonary melanoma with no known primary tumor, the overall actuarial survival was 42%.[44] This is remarkably high when compared with other studies reporting resection of pulmonary metastatic melanomas in which actuarial 5-year survival rates of about 20% were observed.[92–95] In addition, a number of long-term survivors after treatment of apparently primary pulmonary melanoma by radical surgery have been reported.[14,15,18,44] Long-term survival after treatment of primary lung melanoma by chemotherapy, immunotherapy or radiotherapy alone, however, has not been documented.

It is possible that some tumors diagnosed as primary lung melanomas may actually be metastases from totally regressed primary cutaneous melanomas. Thus, the results of treating foci of metastatic melanoma from an occult primary site

warrant review. Several recent large studies have suggested that the survival outcome for patients with metastatic disease from an occult primary tumor is somewhat more favorable compared with patients with known sites of primary disease.[96–101]

Recommendations

In patients presenting with apparently isolated pulmonary melanoma, if no other focus of primary or secondary melanoma in the body can be demonstrated by the best available imaging techniques, radical surgical treatment for a suspected primary lung melanoma is entirely logical and offers the patient the best chance of cure, even if it is subsequently shown to be a deposit of metastatic melanoma. The treatment will usually involve formal lobectomy or pneumonectomy and hilar and mediastinal lymphadenectomy. The treatment of locally recurrent and metastatic melanoma from a lung primary should be based on the standard treatment principles established for other forms of melanoma.

References

1. Dasgupta TK, Brasfield RD, Paglia MA. Primary melanomas in unusual sites. Surg Gynecol Obstet 1969; 128(4): 841–8.
2. Smith JL Jr, Stehlin JS Jr. Spontaneous regression of primary malignant melanomas with regional metastases. Cancer 1965; 18(11): 1399–415.
3. Milton GW, Lane Brown MM, Gilder M. Malignant melanoma with an occult primary lesion. Br J Surg 1967; 54(7): 651–8.
4. Gromet MA, Ominsky SH, Epstein WL, Blois MS. The thorax as the initial site for systemic relapse in malignant melanoma: a prospective survey of 324 patients. Cancer 1979; 44(2): 776–84.
5. Sutton FD Jr, Vestal RE, Creagh CE. Varied presentations of metastatic pulmonary melanoma. Chest 1974; 65(4): 415–19.
6. Webb WR, Gamsu G. Thoracic metastasis in malignant melanoma. A radiographic survey of 65 patients. Chest 1977; 71(2): 176–81.
7. Salm R. A primary malignant melanoma of the bronchus. J Pathol Bacteriol 1963; 85: 121–6.
8. Dasgupta T, Brasfield R. Metastatic melanoma. A clinicopathological study. Cancer 1964; 17: 1323–39.
9. Todd FW. Two cases of melanotic tumors in the lungs. JAMA 1888; 11: 53–4.
10. Kunkel OF, Torrey E. Report of a case of primary melanotic sarcoma of the lung presenting difficulties in differentiating from tuberculosis. N Y State J Med 1916; 16: 198–201.
11. Carlucci GA, Schleussner RC. Primary melanoma of the lung: case report. J Thorac Surg 1942; 11: 643–9.
12. Allen AC, Spitz S. Malignant melanoma; a clinicopathological analysis of the criteria for diagnosis and prognosis. Cancer 1953; 6(1): 1–45.
13. Hsu CW, Wu SC, Ch'En CS. Melanoma of lung. Chin Med J 1962; 81: 263–6.
14. Reed RJ, Kent EM. Solitary pulmonary melanomas: two case reports. J Thorac Cardiovasc Surg 1964; 48: 226–31.
15. Reid JD, Mehta VT. Melanoma of the lower respiratory tract. Cancer 1966; 19(5): 627–31.
16. Jensen OA, Egedorf J. Primary malignant melanoma of the lung. Scand J Respir Dis 1967; 48(2): 127–35.
17. Allen MS Jr, Drash EC. Primary melanoma of the lung. Cancer 1968; 21(1): 154–9.
18. Taboada CF, McMurray JD, Jordan RA, Seybold WD. Primary melanoma of the lung. Chest 1972; 62(5): 629–31.
19. Walter P, Fernandes C, Florange W. Melanome malin primitif pulmonaire. Ann Anat Pathol (Paris) 1972; 17(1): 91–9.

20. Mori K, Cho H, Som M. Primary "flat" melanoma of the trachea. J Pathol 1977; 121(2): 101–5.

21. Smith S, Opipari MI. Primary pleural melanoma. A first reported case and literature reivew. J Thorac Cardiovasc Surg 1978; 75(6): 827–31.

22. Adebonojo SA, Grillo IA, Durodola JI. Primary malignant melanoma of the bronchus. J Natl Med Assoc 1979; 71(6): 579–81.

23. Robertson AJ, Sinclair DJ, Sutton PP, Guthrie W. Primary melanocarcinoma of the lower respiratory tract. Thorax 1980; 35(2): 158–9.

24. Weshler Z, Sulkes A, Kopolovitch J, et al. Bronchial malignant melanoma. J Surg Oncol 1980; 15(3): 243–8.

25. Gephardt GN. Malignant melanoma of the bronchus. Hum Pathol 1981; 12(7): 671–3.

26. Verweij J, Breed WP, Jansveld CA. Primary tracheo-bronchial melanoma. Neth J Med 1982; 25(6): 163–6.

27. Roldan JG, Pla RV, Jac M. Nodulo puylmonar soitario en el curso de melanoma maligno. A proposito de cuatro observaciones. Arch Bronchoneumol 1983; 19: 128–31.

28. Angel R, Prados M. Primary bronchial melanoma. J La State Med Soc 1984; 136(6): 13–15.

29. Cagle P, Mace ML, Judge DM, et al. Pulmonary melanoma. Primary vs metastatic. Chest 1984; 85(1): 125–6.

30. Carstens PH, Kuhns JG, Ghazi C. Primary malignant melanomas of the lung and adrenal. Hum Pathol 1984; 15(10): 910–14.

31. Alghanem AA, Mehan J, Hassan AA. Primary malignant melanoma of the lung. J Surg Oncol 1987; 34(2): 109–12.

32. Demeter SL, Fuenning C, Miller JB. Primary malignant melanoma of the lower respiratory tract: endoscopic identification. Cleve Clin J Med 1987; 54(4): 305–8.

33. Santos F, Entrenas LM, Sebastian F, et al. Primary bronchopulmonary malignant melanoma. Case report. Scand J Thorac Cardiovasc Surg 1987; 21(2): 187–9.

34. Andre N, Leroyer C, Proust A, et al. [Malignant endobronchial melanoma, apparently primary. Apropos of a case]. Rev Pneumol Clin 1988; 44(3): 143–5.

35. Bagwell SP, Flynn SD, Cox PM, Davison JA. Primary malignant melanoma of the lung. Am Rev Respir Dis 1989; 139(6): 1543–7.

36. Bertola G, Pasquotti B, Morassut S, et al. Primary lung melanoma. Ital J Surg Sci 1989; 19(2): 187–9.

37. Cohen RE, Weaver MG, Montenegro HD, Abdul-Karim FW. Pulmonary blastoma with malignant melanoma component. Arch Pathol Lab Med 1990; 114(10): 1076–8.

38. Jennings TA, Axiotis CA, Kress Y, Carter D. Primary malignant melanoma of the lower respiratory tract. Report of a case and literature review. Am J Clin Pathol 1990; 94(5): 649–55.

39. Sanchez Navarro JJ, Galindo Jimeno M, et al. Melanoma maligno primitivo de pulmon. Rev Clin Esp 1991; 188: 68–9.

40. Miller DL, Allen MS. Rare pulmonary neoplasms. Mayo Clin Proc 1993; 68(5): 492–8.

41. Barzo P, Tuka P, Minik K, Kiss JI. [Primary malignant melanoma of the lung and lower respiratory tract]. Orv Hetil 1994; 135(5): 245–9.

42. Pasquini E, Rastelli E, Muretto P, et al. Primary bronchial malignant melanoma. A case report. Pathologica 1994; 86(5): 546–8.

43. Farrell DJ, Kashyap AP, Ashcroft T, Morritt GN. Primary malignant melanoma of the bronchus. Thorax 1996; 51(2): 223–4.

44. De Wilt JHW, Farmer SEJ, Scolyer RA, et al. Isolated melanoma in the lung when there is no known primary site: metastatic disease or primary lung tumour? Melanoma Res 2005; 15(6): 531–7.

45. Sekine I, Kodama T, Yokose T, et al. Rare pulmonary tumors – a review of 32 cases. Oncology 1998; 55(5): 431–4.

46. Wilson RW, Moran CA. Primary melanoma of the lung: a clinicopathologic and immunohistochemical study of eight cases. Am J Surg Pathol 1997; 21(10): 1196–202.

47. Ost D, Joseph C, Sogoloff H, Menezes G. Primary pulmonary melanoma: case report and literature review. Mayo Clin Proc 1999; 74(1): 62–6.

48. Ozdemir N, Cangir AK, Kutlay H, Yavuzer ST. Primary malignant melanoma of the lung in oculocutaneous albino patient. Eur J Cardiothorac Surg 2001; 20(4): 864–7.

49. Testini M, Trabucco S, di Venere B, Piscitelli D. Ileal intussusception due to intestinal metastases from primary malignant melanoma of the lung. Am Surg 2002; 68(4): 377–9.

50. Dountsis A, Zisis C, Karagianni E, Dahabreh J. Primary malignant melanoma of the lung: a case report. World J Surg Oncol 2003; 1(1): 26.

51. Lie CH, Chao TY, Chung YH, Lin MC. Primary pulmonary malignant melanoma presenting with haemoptysis. Melanoma Res 2005; 15(3): 219–21.

52. Scotto J, Fraumeni JF Jr, Lee JA. Melanomas of the eye and other noncutaneous sites: epidemiologic aspects. J Natl Cancer Inst 1976; 56(3): 489–91.

53. Ross MI, Henderson MA. Mucosal melanoma. In: Balch CM, Houghton AN, Sober AJ, et al. (eds) Cutaneous Melanoma. St Louis, MO: Quality Medical Publishing, 2009. pp. 337–50.

54. Fowler M, Sutherland HDA. Malignant melanoma of the oesophagus. J Pathol Bacteriol 1952; 64(3): 473–7.

55. Goldman JL, Lawson W, Zak FG, Roffman JD. The presence of melanocytes in the human larynx. Laryngoscope 1972; 82(5): 824–35.

56. Busuttil A. Dendritic pigmented cells within human laryngeal mucosa. Arch Otolaryngol 1976; 102(1): 43–4.

57. Batsakis JG, Regezi JA, Solomon AR, Rice DH. The pathology of head and neck tumors: mucosal melanomas, part 13. Head Neck Surg 1982; 4(5): 404–18.

58. Grazer R, Cohen SM, Jacobs JB, Lucas P. Melanin-containing peripheral carcinoid of the lung. Am J Surg Pathol 1982; 6(1): 73–8.

59. Rajaratnam R, Marsden JR, Marzouk J, Hero I. Pulmonary carcinoid associated with melanoma: two cases and a review of the literature. Br J Dermatol 2007; 156(4): 738–41.

60. Pilozzi E, Cacchi C, di Napoli A, et al. Primary malignant tumour of the lung with neuroendocrine and melanoma differentiation. Virchows Arch 2011; 459(2): 239–43.

61. Rosenberg LM, Polanco GB, Blank S. Multiple tracheobronchial melanomas with ten-year survival. JAMA 1965; 192: 717–19.

62. Damian DL, Fulham MJ, Thompson E, Thompson JF. Positron emission tomography in the detection and management of metastatic melanoma. Melanoma Res 1996; 6(4): 325–9.

63. Gritters LS, Francis IR, Zasadny KR, Wahl RL. Initial assessment of positron emission tomography using 2-fluorine-18-fluoro-2-deoxy-D-glucose in the imaging of malignant melanoma. J Nucl Med 1993; 34(9): 1420–7.

64. Scolyer RA, Long GV, Thompson JF. Evolving concepts in melanoma classification and their relevance to multidisciplinary melanoma patient care. Mol Oncol 2011; 5(2): 124–36.

65. Curtin JA, Fridlyand J, Kageshita T, et al. Distinct sets of genetic alterations in melanoma. N Engl J Med 2005; 353: 2135–47.

66. Long GV, Menzies AM, Nagrial AM, et al. Prognostic and clinicopathologic associations of oncogenic BRAF in metastatic melanoma. J Clin Oncol 2011; 29(10): 1239–46.

67. Bauer J, Büttner P, Murali R, et al. BRAF mutations in cutaneous melanoma are independently associated with age, anatomic site of the primary tumor, and the degree of solar elastosis at the primary tumor site. Pigment Cell Melanoma Res 2011; 24(2): 345–51.

68. Broekaert SM, Roy R, Okamoto I, et al. Genetic and morphologic features for melanoma classification. Pigment Cell Melanoma Res 2010; 23(6): 763–70.

69. Curtin JA, Busam K, Pinkel D, Bastian BC. Somatic activation of KIT in distinct subtypes of melanoma. J Clin Oncol 2006; 24(26): 4340–6.

70. Kong Y, Si L, Zhu Y, et al. Large-scale analysis of KIT aberrations in Chinese patients with melanoma. Clin Cancer Res. 2011; 17(7): 1684–91.

71. Van Raamsdonk CD, Griewank KG, Crosby MB, et al. Mutations in GNA11 in uveal melanoma. N Engl J Med. 2010; 363(23): 2191–9.

72. Carter CA, Pianova S, Synnott S, et al. BRAF mutation, NRAS mutation and absence of an immune-related expressed gene profile predict poor outcome in surgically resected stage III melanoma. In: P.C.M. Research (Ed.) Melanoma 2010 Congress, Vol. 23. Sydney, Australia: Blackwell Publishing Ltd, 2010, p. 6.

73. Schramm SJ, Campain AE, Scolyer RA, Yang YH, Mann GJ. Review and cross-validation of gene expression signatures and melanoma prognosis. J Invest Dermatol 2012; 132(2): 274–83.

74. Heenan PJ. Local recurrence of melanoma. Pathology 2004; 36(5): 491–5.

75. Littman CD. Metastatic melanoma mimicking primary bronchial melanoma. Histopathology 1991; 18(6): 561–3.

76. Carter D, Eggleston J. Tumors of the lower respiratory tract. In: *Atlas of Tumor Pathology,* series 2, fascicle 17. Washington, DC: Armed Forces Institute of Pathology, 1979. pp. 220.

77. Faries MB, Bleicher RJ, Ye X, *et al.* Lymphatic mapping and sentinel lymphadenectomy for primary and metastatic pulmonary malignant neoplasms. Arch Surg 2004; 139(8): 870–6; discussion 876–7.

78. Boni R, Boni RA, Steinert H, *et al.* Staging of metastatic melanoma by whole-body positron emission tomography using 2-fluorine-18-fluoro-2-deoxy-D-glucose. Br J Dermatol 1995; 132(4): 556–62.

79. Rigo P, Paulus P, Kaschten BJ, *et al.* Oncological applications of positron emission tomography with fluorine-18 fluorodeoxyglucose. Eur J Nucl Med 1996; 23(12): 1641–74.

80. Valk PE, Pounds TR, Tesar RD, *et al.* Cost-effectiveness of PET imaging in clinical oncology. Nucl Med Biol 1996; 23(6): 737–43.

81. Wagner JD, Schauwecker D, Hutchins G, Coleman JJ 3rd. Initial assessment of positron emission tomography for detection of nonpalpable regional lymphatic metastases in melanoma. J Surg Oncol 1997; 64(3): 181–9.

82. Gulec SA, Faries MB, Lee CC, *et al.* The role of fluorine-18 deoxyglucose positron emission tomography in the management of patients with metastatic melanoma: impact on surgical decision making. Clin Nucl Med 2003; 28(12): 961–5.

83. Dalrymple-Hay MJ, Rome PD, Kennedy C, *et al.* Pulmonary metastatic melanoma – the survival benefit associated with positron emission tomography scanning. Eur J Cardiothorac Surg 2002; 21(4): 611–14; discussion 614–15.

84. Flaherty KT, Puzanov I, Kim KB, *et al.* Inhibition of mutated, activated BRAF in metastatic melanoma. N Engl J Med 2010; 363: 809–19.

85. Chapman PB, Hauschild A, Robert C, *et al.* Improved Survival with Vemurafenib in Melanoma with BRAF V600E Mutation. N Engl J Med 2011; 364: 2507–16.

86. Kefford K, Arkenau H, Brown MP, *et al.* Phase I/II study of GSK2118436, a selective inhibitor of oncogenic mutant BRAF kinase, in patients with metastatic melanoma and other solid tumors. J Clin Oncol 2010; 28.

87. Bollag G, Hirth P, Tsai J, *et al.* Clinical efficacy of a RAF inhibitor needs broad target blockade in BRAF-mutant melanoma. Nature 2010; 467:596–9.

88. Carvajal RD, Antonescu CR, Wolchok JD, *et al.* KIT as a therapeutic target in metastatic melanoma. JAMA 2011; 305(22): 2327–34.

89. Handolias D, Hamilton AL, Salemi R, *et al.* Clinical responses observed with imatinib or sorafenib in melanoma patients expressing mutations in KIT. Br J Cancer 2010; 102: 1219–23.

90. Hodi FS, O'Day SJ, McDermott DF, *et al.* Improved Survival with Ipilimumab in Patients with Metastatic Melanoma. N Engl J Med 2010; 363: 711–23.

91. Robert C, Thomas L, Bondarenko I, *et al.* Ipilimumab plus Dacarbazine for Previously Untreated Metastatic Melanoma. N Engl J Med 2011; 364: 2517–26.

92. La Hei ER, Thompson JF, McCaughan BC, *et al.* Surgical resection of pulmonary metastatic melanoma: a review of 83 thoracotomies. Asia Pacific Heart 1996; 5: 111–14.

93. Harpole DH Jr, Johnson CM, Wolfe WG, *et al.* Analysis of 945 cases of pulmonary metastatic melanoma. J Thorac Cardiovasc Surg 1992; 103(4): 743–8; discussion 748–50.

94. Gorenstein LA, Putnam JB, Natarajan G, *et al.* Improved survival after resection of pulmonary metastases from malignant melanoma. Ann Thorac Surg 1991; 52(2): 204–10.

95. Chua TC, Scolyer RA, Kennedy CW, Yan TD, McCaughan BC, Thompson JF. Surgical Management of Melanoma Lung Metastasis: An Analysis of Survival Outcomes in 292 Consecutive Patients. Ann Surg Oncol 2012 Jan 31. [Epub ahead of print]

96. Norman J, Cruse CW, Wells KE, *et al.* Metastatic melanoma with an unknown primary. Ann Plast Surg 1992; 28(1): 81–4.

97. Cormier JN, Xing Y, Feng L, *et al.* Metastatic melanoma to lymph nodes in patients with unknown primary sites. Cancer 2006; 106(9): 2012–20.

98. Vijuk G, Coates AS. Survival of patients with visceral metastatic melanoma from an occult primary lesion: a retrospective matched cohort study. Ann Oncol 1998; 9(4): 419–22.

99. Lee CC, Faries MB, Wanek LA, Morton DL. Improved survival after lymphadenectomy for nodal metastasis from an unknown primary melanoma. J Clin Oncol 2008; 26(4): 535–41.

100. Prens SP, van der Ploeg AP, van Akkooi AC, *et al.* Outcome after therapeutic lymph node dissection in patients with unknown primary melanoma site. Ann Surg Oncol 2011; 18(13): 3586–92.

101. Rutkowski P, Nowecki ZI, Dziewirski W, *et al.* Melanoma without a detectable primary site with metastases to lymph nodes. Dermatol Surg 2010; 36(6): 868–76.

102. Kundranda MN, Clark CT, Chaudhry AA, *et al.* Primary malignant melanoma of the lung: a case report and review of the literature. Clin Lung Cancer 2006; 7(4): 279–81.

103. Reddy VS, Mykytenko J, Giltman LI, Mansour KA. Primary malignant melanoma of the lung: review of literature and report of a case. Am Surg 2007; 73(3): 287–9.

104. Kotoulas C, Skagias L, Konstantinou G, *et al.* Primary pulmonary melanoma diagnosis: the role of immunohistochemistry and immunocytochemistry. J BUON 2007; 12(4): 543–5.

105. Saint-Blancard P, Vaylet F, Jancovici R. [A rare pulmonary tumour, primary malignant melanoma]. Rev Mal Respir 2009; 26(1): 57–61.

106. Shikuma K, Omasa M, Yutaka Y, *et al.* Treatment of primary melanoma of the lung monitored by 5-S-cysteinyldopa levels. Ann Thorac Surg 2009; 87(4): 1264–6.

107. Maeda R, Isowa N, Onuma H, *et al.* Primary malignant melanoma of the lung with rapid progression. Gen Thorac Cardiovasc Surg 2009; 57(12): 671–4.

108. Pan XD, Zhang B, Guo LC, *et al.* Primary malignant melanoma of the lung in the elderly: case report and literature review. Chin Med J (Engl) 2010; 123(13): 1815–17.

109. Neri S, Komatsu T, Kitamura J, *et al.* Malignant melanoma of the lung: report of two cases. Ann Thorac Cardiovasc Surg 2011; 17(2): 170–3.

110. Mochizuki H, Chikui E, Tokumaru A, *et al.* [A case of pulmonary malignant melanoma mimicking lung abscess]. Nihon Kokyuki Gakkai Zasshi 2011; 49(6): 472–7.

Section 5: Thoracic Tumors

24 Large Cell Neuroendocrine Carcinoma

William D. Travis,[1] M. Catherine Pietanza,[2] and Inderpal (Netu) S. Sarkaria[3]

[1] Department of Pathology, [2] Department of Medicine, [3] Department of Thoracic Surgery, Memorial Sloan-Kettering Cancer Center, New York, NY, USA

Introduction and historical background

Large cell neuroendocrine carcinoma (LCNEC) of the lung was first described in 1991 as a form of high-grade nonsmall cell neuroendocrine carcinoma.[1] It is part of a family of pulmonary neuroendocrine tumors that includes the low-grade typical carcinoid (TC), intermediate-grade atypical carcinoid (AC) and the high-grade LCNEC and small cell lungcarcinoma (SCLC).[2,3]

In the 2004 WHO classification, LCNEC is classified as a variant of large cell carcinoma. Within large cell carcinoma there are four major categories of neuroendocrine differentiation that can occur (Table 24.1):
- LCNEC which has neuroendocrine features by light microscopy as well as immunohistochemistry and/or electron microscopy
- large cell carcinoma with neuroendocrine morphology (LCNEM) that has neuroendocrine morphology but lack neuroendocrine differentiation by electron microscopy or immunohistochemistry
- large cell carcinoma with neuroendocrine differentiation (LCC-NED) that has no neuroendocrine pattern by light microscopy but show neuroendocrine differentiation by immunohistochemistry or electron microscopy
- classic large cell carcinoma (LCC) that lacks both neuroendocrine morphology by light microscopy and neuroendocrine differentiation by immunohistochemistry or electron microscopy.[1,4]

In the past, LCNEC has been classified as a variety of other lung tumors including atypical carcinoid, the intermediate subtype of SCLC, large cell carcinoma, and large cell neuroendocrine tumor.[1,2] These tumors can also be confused with poorly differentiated adenocarcinomas, squamous cell carcinomas, and basaloid carcinomas.[2] These cases also frequently are confused with large cell carcinomas or nonsmall cell carcinomas with neuroendocrine differentiation that lack neuroendocrine morphology.[2]

The concept of LCNEC has been widely accepted, as reflected by the growing number of publications on this subject. Nevertheless, the literature has to be read critically because some authors have lumped the above subsets together or also included combined small cell carcinoma/large cell carcinoma into a single category of LCNEC.[5–8] This complicated our attempt to summarize some of the published data in Table 24.2. Until these distinct subsets of large cell carcinoma with neuroendocrine morphology/differentiation have been carefully characterized, it is premature to analyze them together.

Due to the rarity of LCNECs, little is known about their clinical behavior and how these tumors should be treated. No single institution has sufficient cases to address this issue. This chapter will review the existing literature on LCNEC and summarize the limited knowledge about therapy. Brief mention will be made about the scant data regarding large cell carcinoma with neuroendocrine morphology. Large cell carcinoma or NSCLC with neuroendocrine differentiation will not be specifically addressed in this chapter. The formation of an international registry of pulmonary neuroendocrine tumors intended to address the lack of knowledge about LCNEC is also presented.[9] We will summarize new data that have emerged in the past 5 years that give further insights into prognosis,[10,11] genetics,[12–15] and therapy[10,11,16–19] for this uncommon lung cancer.

Biology and epidemiology

Large cell neuroendocrine carcinomas are biologically very aggressive tumors that account for about 3% of surgically resected lung cancers (range 1–5%, see Table 24.2).[20] The vast majority of patients are cigarette smokers and most have over a 50 pack-year history of smoking.[1] Recent series of LCNEC report less of a male predominance probably due to the increased smoking in females (see Table 24.2).

Textbook of Uncommon Cancer, Fourth Edition. Edited by Derek Raghavan, Charles D. Blanke, David H. Johnson, Paul L. Moots, Gregory H. Reaman, Peter G. Rose and Mikkael A. Sekeres.
© 2012 John Wiley & Sons, Inc. Published 2012 by John Wiley & Sons, Inc.

Table 24.1 Neuroendocrine differentiation in large cell carcinoma.

Tumor name	Neuroendocrine morphology	Neuroendocrine special studies: immunohistochemistry or electron microscopy
Large cell carcinoma (LCC)	No	No
Large cell neuroendocrine carcinoma (LCNEC)	Yes	Yes
Large cell carcinoma with neuroendocrine morphology (LCNEM)	Yes	No
Large cell carcinoma with neuroendocrine differentiation (LCNED)	No	Yes

Molecular biology and genetics

In the spectrum of neuroendocrine lung tumors, LCNEC expresses many molecular abnormalities similar to SCLC but there are considerable differences with TC and AC. Identification of molecular alterations in tumors has become an attractive way to identify novel therapeutic approaches. As we do not have effective therapies for LCNEC, understanding of the molecular changes in the entire spectrum of pulmonary neuroendocrine tumors is important. Since these tumors are so uncommon, there are few molecular studies that have examined large numbers of LCNECs. The larger studies usually include the entire spectrum of pulmonary neuroendocrine tumors so cases of TC, AC, and SCLC are included with the LCNECs. Also since very few institutions have frozen tissue banks, most molecular studies of LCNECs have been retrospective studies performed on tissue samples that are formalin fixed and paraffin embedded, limiting the type of molecular studies that can be performed. As there are a large number of molecular pathways that have been studied in LCNEC, mostly using small numbers of cases, we will focus on a few major studies in this summary.

In LCNEC, Onuki et al. demonstrated a high percentage of P53 abnormalities by immunohistochemical overexpression (75%), loss of heterozygosity (67%), and mutation analysis (59%).[21] These findings were very similar to those seen in SCLC, but significantly higher than those seen in TC and AC.[21] Similar findings have been demonstrated by others with p53 expression ranging between 40% and 86% and P53 mutations from 27% to 59%.[22–27] Interestingly, Onuki et al. found that 58% of the point mutations found in high-grade neuroendocrine tumors were G:C to T:A or other transversions.[21] The G:C to T:A transversions are associated with carcinogens found in cigarette smoke, consistent with the high frequency of heavy cigarette smoking in LCNEC patients.[28]

Large cell neuroendocrine carcinomas have frequent abnormalities of the $P16^{INK4}$/cyclin D1/Rb pathway involved with regulation of G1 arrest in the cell cycle. Lack of Rb expression was found by Beasley et al. and Igarashi et al. in 49–68% of LCNEC, similar to SCLC (84–87%), but significantly more often than in TC (0%) and AC (0–21%).[29,30] Cyclin D1 overexpression and loss of p16 staining were found in 9.5–32% and 18–22% of LCNEC, respectively.[29,30] Igarashi also demonstrated overexpression of cyclin B1 in 84% of LCNEC and SCLC. Since an intact Rb pathway would demonstrate p16 positive, cyclin D1 positive and Rb positive, in 78–90% of LCNEC, the Rb pathway is disrupted.[29,30] The finding that virtually all cyclin D1-positive tumors are Rb positive indicates

that cyclin D1 overexpression characteristically occurs only in the presence of intact Rb. Loss of Rb is the most frequent mechanism of Rb cell cycle pathway deregulation in LCNEC and SCLC. The frequent expression of cyclin B1 in high-grade neuroendocrine carcinomas is consistent with the concept that regulation of cyclin B1 expression and G2/M arrest are consistently compromised in LCNEC and SCLC.[30]

Large cell neuroendocrine carcinomas have a high index (1.3–6.8%) of apoptosis compared to carcinoids that have a variable apoptotic index and SCLC that have almost no apoptosis.[22] LCNEC and SCLC have a high Bcl2:bax ratio in contrast to TC and AC that have predominant Bax expression.[22,31] These findings are consistent with the concept that the high rate of cell division in LCNEC could be worsened by abrogation of cell death which is favored by high Bcl2 and low Bax levels, leading to a short doubling time and tumor aggressiveness.[22]

C-kit protein expression by immunohistochemistry was demonstrated in 55–77% of LCNECs.[32–34] Differing criteria for interpretation of results have been used with at least 50% of tumor cells with 2 plus positive cytoplasmic and membrane staining of tumor cells used by Casali et al.[33] while Pelosi et al. separated the results of membranous versus cytoplasmic patterns of c-kit staining and found membrane immunoreactivity in 77% and cytoplasmic reactivity in 44% of LCNEC, using a cutoff of 5% or more immunoreactivity for a positive result.[35] Casali et al. found a significantly worse prognosis ($p = 0.046$) as well as a higher rate of recurrence (0.037) for patients with c-kit-positive tumors.[33] However, neither Pelosi et al. nor Araki et al. found any prognostic significance to c-kit expression in LCNEC or SCLC.[32,35]

In contrast to lung carcinoids, multiple endocrine neoplasia (MEN) 1 gene mutations are very rare in LCNEC. Debelenko et al. found a somatic frameshift in the MEN 1 gene (1226delC) in one of 13 tumors. This represented the first mutation observed outside the spectrum of neoplasms associated with MEN 1. On the other allele, neither a deletion or mutation was detected and wild-type mRNA sequence was expressed, suggesting that the typical two-hit mechanism of MEN 1 gene inactivation did not occur.[36]

Several recent studies have shown a variety of molecular differences between LCNEC and SCLC. Rekhtman et al. analyzed 81 SCLC and 51 LCNEC cases for hot-spot point mutations EGFR, KRAS, AKT1, BRAF, HER2, MEK1, and PIK3CA by Sequenom mass spectrometry genotyping and EGFR Exon 19 deletions by standard methods. Of 82 SCLC, two (2.4%) harbored EGFR, one (1.2%) KRAS, and one (1.2%) PIK3CA mutations yet these cases were restricted to SCLC associated with either prior or combined adenocarcinoma, whereas none

Table 24.2 Large cell neuroendocrine carcinoma: demographics and survival.

Author	Year	N	% cases	Median Age	Male (%)	Smoking history %	5-year survival (%)				
							Overall	Stage I	Stage II	Stage III	Stage IV
Jiang[42]	1998	22	2.9	63 (51–77)	83	NA	44.8	NA	NA	NA	NA
Travis[3]	1998	37	NA	58 (21–75)	67	100	27	35	0	0	0
Garcia-Yuste[74]	2000	22	NA	67 (47–70)	77	NA	21	NA	NA	NA	NA
Iyoda[40]	2001	50	2.4	64 (38–82)	84	NA/906.8*	35.3	NA	NA	NA	NA
Mazieres[80]	2002	18	1.6	63 (49–78)	100	94	NA	NA	NA	NA	NA
Takei[43]	2002	87	3.1	68 (37–82)	89	98	57	67	75	4	0
Kakinuma[52]	2003	38	4.1	63 (51–74)	85	NA	NA	NA	NA	NA	NA
Zacharias[8]	2003	15	NA	64 (45–79)	60	NA	52	88†	28†	NA	NA
Ab'Saber[79]	2004	24	5	58 (44–84)	58	NA	13 m‡	NA	NA	NA	NA
Casali[33]	2004	33	NA	65 (42–80)	94	97	51	NA	NA	NA	NA
Daddi[37]	2004	18	1	69 (58–77)	72	94.4	37.5	NA	NA	NA	NA
Doddoli[81]	2004	20	NA	62 (43–80)	90	100	36	54	NA	25	NA
Oshiro[38]	2004	38	NA	66 (45–82)	95	100	NA	NA	NA	NA	NA
Paci[47]	2004	48	3.5	64 (39–81)	87	87	21	IA:66% IB:10	IIB:18%	0	NA
Battafarano[5]	2005	45	2.1	NA§	NA§	NA§	30.2§	32§	NA	NA	NA
Filosso[89]	2005	18	1.2	63 (48–71)	61	78	35	NA	NA	NA	NA
Rossi[88]	2005	83	1.7	67 (41–89)	88	96	28	33	23	8	NA
Yamazaki[90]	2005	20	3	58 (37–74)	90	95	NA; 1 yr survival 35%; 2 yr survival:15%				
Asamura[91]	2006	141	44	66 (38–88)	90	99	40	58	32	NA	NA
Iyoda[87]	2006	15	NA	64 (52–73)	100	NA/985*	89	NA	NA	NA	NA
Adjuv Control	2006	23	NA	67 (53–79)	96	NA/1148*	47	NA	NA	NA	NA
Veronesi[85]	2006	144	NA	64 (35–80)	81	94	43	52	59	20	NA
Fujiwara[19]	2007	22	NA	65 (47–78)	95	95	NA; Median Survival: 10mo; 1 yr survival: 43%				NA
Skov[92]	2008	27	NA	65 (31–79)	59	NA	30	NA	NA	NA	NA
Sarkaria[10]	2011	100	NA	64 (41–86)	54	98	30	53 IA:72 IB:26	65	24	NA
Varlotto[11]	2011	1211	1	67 (23–85)	57	NA	41¶	NA	NA	NA	NA

* Smoking index.
† Three-year survival.
‡ Median survival.
§ Lumped large cell neuroendocrine carcinoma, large cell carcinoma with neuroendocrine morphology and large cell carcinoma with neuroendocrine differentiation together (personal communication).
¶ Four-year overall survival (not five year).
Adjuv, adjuvant chemotherapy; m, months; NA, not applicable.

occurred in pure SCLC. In contrast to SCLC, pure LCNEC harbored *KRAS* mutations in seven of 51 (14%; 95% confidence interval (CI) 4–23%) cases (*p* = 0.0017). Similar to adenocarcinoma in smokers, *KRAS* mutations in LCNEC were predominantly smoking-related G-T or G-C transversions (5/7; 71%), suggesting a histogenetic link between a subset of LCNEC and adenocarcinoma.[13] Nomura *et al.* used liquid chromatography tandem mass spectrometry for global proteomic analysis of formalin-fixed paraffin-embedded tissues of lung neuroendocrine tumors to identify four cancer stem cell protein markers including aldehyde dehydrogenase 1 family member A1 (AL1A1), aldo-keto reductase family 1 members C1 (AK1C1) and C3 (AK1C3) as well as CD44, that were present in LCNEC rather than SCLC.[12] Sun *et al.* showed that CK7, CK18, P-cadherin, E-cadherin, β-catenin, villin, c-Met, and α-enolase were significantly more commonly expressed in LCNEC compared to SCLC.[15] Skov *et al.* also showed more frequent expression of *ERCC1* in LCNEC (19%) compared to SCLC (10%, *p* <0.009).[14] All of these show genetic differences between LCNEC and SCLC.

Pathology

Gross features

Most LCNEC are peripheral (66–100%) with the remainder being centrally located.[37–39] The average size is 3–4.0 cm with a range from 0.9 up to 12 cm.[3,37–40] They are usually circumscribed, nodular masses with a necrotic, tan, red cut surface. In larger tumors the necrosis tends to be confluent and more extensive.[38]

Histological features

The diagnostic criteria for LCNEC are:
• neuroendocrine morphology with organoid nesting, palisading or rosette-like structures (Fig. 24.1)

• high mitotic rate greater than 10 mitoses per 2 mm^2 (average 60–80 mitoses per 2 mm^2)
• nonsmall cell cytological features including large cell size, low nuclear:cytoplasmic ratio, nucleoli, or vesicular chromatin (Fig. 24.2)
• neuroendocrine differentiation by immunohistochemistry (chromogranin, CD56 or synaptophysin) or electron microscopy (Fig. 24.3).[2,3]

Combined LCNEC consists of a LCNEC with components of adenocarcinoma, squamous cell carcinoma, giant cell carcinoma, and/or spindle cell carcinoma.[2,3] Most often, this represents a component of adenocarcinoma, but squamous cell, giant cell or spindle cell carcinoma can be present. If there is a

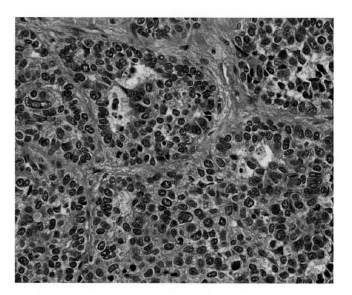

Figure 24.2 The tumor cells demonstrate rosette-like structures, abundant cytoplasm, nuclei with vesicular chromatin and scattered nucleoli. Several mitotic figures are present in this high-power field.

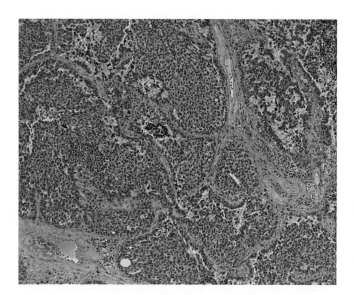

Figure 24.1 Large cell neuroendocrine carcinoma shows organoid nesting pattern with prominent palisading at the periphery of the tumor cell nests. A few rosette-like structures are present. Focal necrosis is seen.

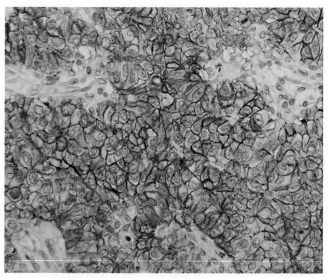

Figure 24.3 The tumor cells strongly express CD56 with a membranous pattern of staining, indicating neuroendocrine differentiation.

component of SCLC the tumor becomes a combined SCLC and LCNEC.

It is very difficult to make the diagnosis of LCNEC based on small biopsies or cytology (see "Cytology" section below). This is because of the problems in recognizing the neuroendocrine morphological pattern and demonstrating neuroendocrine differentiation by immunohistochemistry in small pieces of tissue. Therefore in the vast majority of cases, a definite diagnosis of SCLC will require a surgical lung biopsy.

Large cell carcinoma with neuroendocrine morphology

Except for the lack of neuroendocrine differentiation by immunohistochemistry, few data exist to suggest that the pathological characteristics of LCNEM are much different from LCNEC. The only major difference was reported by Iyoda et al. who found the mitotic rate of LCC-NEM was significantly higher than that of LCNEC.[40]

Immunohistochemistry/electron microscopy

The presence of neuroendocrine differentiation by immunohistochemistry or electron microscopy is required for the diagnosis of LCNEC.[2,3] By immunohistochemistry LCNEC stain positively with cytokeratin antibodies such as AE1/AE3 and CAM5.2.[39,41] LCNEC stain immunohistochemically with chromogranin (55–82%), cd56/NCAM (73–100%), synaptophysin (40–91%), and pancytokeratin (100%).[1,42–44] A panel of neuroendocrine markers is useful rather than stain with a single antibody. Currently the most useful antibodies include chromogranin, CD56, and synaptophysin. TTF-1 is positive in 41–75% of LCNECs.[41,45,46] The adenocarcinoma component of combined LCNEC and adenocarcinomas is likely to express TTF-1.[41]

A variety of different criteria have been applied regarding the minimum positive staining for neuroendocrine markers. Most studies have required only one neuroendocrine marker (excluding neuron-specific enolase – NSE) to be positive[43,47] but others have required two positive stains.[42] Some have required as much as 10%[47] or as little as a single definite positive cell.[43] In general, the distribution and intensity of immunohistochemical staining for neuroendocrine markers are less for LCNEC than for typical and atypical carcinoid tumors. However, neuroendocrine markers may be diffusely and strongly positive. Staining for neuroendocrine markers is often focal since these are poorly differentiated tumors. Takei et al. found that less than half of their cases stained diffusely.[43] They found all three neuroendocrine markers, synaptophysin, NCAM (CD56), and chromogranin, to be positive in 68% of cases, two markers in 85%, and at least one marker in 100% of cases.[43] NSE is not regarded to be a reliable marker for neuroendocrine differentiation since it will stain up to 60% of nonsmall cell carcinomas.[48] Hormonal markers such as adrenocorticotropic hormone (ACTH) and calcitonin are positive in only a minority of cases. A higher percentage of LCNECs stain for keratin and CEA, in contrast to typical carcinoid and atypical carcinoid.[1]

By electron microscopy, LCNECs show dense core granules and may have cytoplasmic lumina and/or desmosomes.[1]

The proliferation index by Ki-67 is very high in LCNEC (usually 70–100%), similar to that for SCLC. However, it is usually much lower for typical carcinoid (<5%) and atypical carcinoid (<5–15%). Tsuta et al. proposed using the mitotic-specific antibody to phosphohistone H3 (PHH3) as a surrogate to identify mitotic figures, although this approach needs more validation before it can be accepted as a replacement for counting mitoses.[49]

Cytology

It is very difficult to diagnose LCNEC based on cytology specimens, but several groups have addressed this subject.[50–55] The difficulty in making this diagnosis is reflected by the study of Kakinuma et al. in which the diagnosis of LCNEC was not made in any of the 20 cases that they reported.[52] Instead, the most common diagnosis rendered was carcinoma, histological type undetermined, or, less often, squamous cell carcinoma, atypical carcinoid, small cell carcinoma, and large cell carcinoma.[52] Similarly, in a retrospective review of 100 resected LCNECs from the Memorial Sloan-Kettering Cancer Center, the correct preoperative diagnosis was not discerned in cytological specimens obtained in any of the 57 patients undergoing fine needle aspiration or bronchoscopy.[10]

Wiatrowska et al. found the most characteristic features were (i) a bloody, inflammatory and necrotic background, (ii) flattened three-dimensional clusters of large cells with peripheral palisading, and many single cells, (iii) cytological characteristics including a moderate to high nuclear to cytoplasmic ratio, and nuclei that are large, oval/round to polygonal and show nucleoli in most cases.[54] Mitoses were seen in only one-third of cases.[54] Immunohistochemistry for neuroendocrine markers was positive in 87% of cases using a panel of chromogranin (5/16 positive, 31%) and synaptophysin (12/16 positive, 75%).

Kakinuma et al. reported bronchial brush cytology in 20 LCNECs and compared the findings with poorly differentiated adenocarcinomas, squamous cell carcinomas, and small cell carcinomas.[52] Characteristic features included abundant necrotic debris (90%), large tumor cell size (90%), naked nuclei (90%), and nuclear streaking (90%). Nuclear features consisted of thin nuclear membranes, finely granular nuclear chromatin and one or a few nucleoli. Less than one-half of the cases showed Indian filing and rosette-like structures. These features were less frequent in poorly differentiated adenocarcinomas and squamous cell carcinomas that more often showed thick nuclear membranes.[52] Immunohistochemistry for neuroendocrine markers was less sensitive in cytology specimens compared to biopsy specimens. In cytological specimens obtained by transbronchial aspiration and/or imprint from resected specimens, Hoshi et al. formulated a logistic discriminant model based on scatter plots identifying large clusters of cells (consisting of >60 tumor cells) with tight cohesion versus small tumor cells without prominent nucleoli (showing <120 μm) as parameters distinguishing LCNEC from SCLC. In addition, palisading was more characteristic of LCNEC than SCLC. Using this model, the authors reported a high degree of sensitivity, specificity, and accuracy (100% for all) in differentiating these histological types in 29 LCNEC and SCLC specimens.[56]

Hiroshima *et al.* reported cytology of 14 touch imprint and 11 curettage specimens from 25 histologically confirmed LCNECs.[50] Their specimens were characterized by medium to large-sized, round or polygonal tumor cells with nuclear pleomorphism. Naked nuclei were frequent. The nuclear chromatin was finely or coarsely granular. Most cases had one or two nucleoli, but they were inconspicuous in some cases. Tumor cells were in clusters with some rosette-like structures or single cells. A necrotic background and nuclear streaking were common. The diagnosis of LCNEC could be suspected in cases where the neuroendocrine morphological pattern was identifiable.

Maleki compared LCNEC with SCLC and basaloid carcinoma.[57] LCNEC showed flattened three-dimensional clusters of tumor cells with a high nuclear:cytoplasmic ratio and medium to large cells with peripheral palisading, rosette-like structures with a background that was bloody, inflammatory, and necrotic. They also found that tumor cells in LCNEC are larger than those in classic SCLC with some nucleoli although the tumor cells had scant cytoplasm and finely granular nuclear chromatin. Prominent nucleoli were characteristic of LCNEC and against SCLC or basaloid carcinoma. Tumor cells showed marked nuclear pleomorphism, moderate to abundant cytoplasm, large oval or round nuclei, finely or coarsely granular chromatin, and some with one or two nucleoli.[57] Rosette-like structures were more common in LCNEC than SCLC or basaloid carcinoma.

Differential diagnosis

Large cell neuroendocrine carcinomas must be distinguished from AC, SCLC, large cell carcinoma, large cell carcinoma with neuroendocrine differentiation (LCC-ND), large cell carcinoma with neuroendocrine morphology (LCC-NEM), and classic large cell carcinoma (LCC) with no neuroendocrine features (see Table 24.1). Mitotic counts are one of the most useful criteria for distinguishing AC from LCNEC.[1] According to the new WHO criteria for AC, the upper limit of mitoses should be 10 mitoses per $2\,mm^2$.[2] This contrasts with LCNEC, which should have a mitotic count greater than 11 per $2\,mm^2$ but typically ranges between 50 and 100 mitoses per 10 high-power field (HPF).[2] Necrosis in LCNEC is generally more extensive than in AC where it usually consists of punctate foci within organoid nests of tumor cells. Nuclei of AC usually show a finely granular chromatin while most LCNEC have a vesicular or coarse chromatin.

Separation of LCNEC from SCLC requires consideration of multiple histological features such as cell size, nucleoli, chromatin pattern, and nuclear:cytoplasmic ratio, rather than a single criterion. Artifacts, such as those introduced by frozen sections, can distort cellular morphology, resulting in confusion with SCLC. The difficulty in making this distinction is reflected in the retrospective review of a group of previously diagnosed SCLC where up to 44% of cases were reclassified as LCNEC.[43,58]

If a large cell carcinoma has no neuroendocrine pattern by light microscopy but immunohistochemistry or electron microscopy demonstrates neuroendocrine features, the tumor is classified as large cell carcinoma with neuroendocrine differentiation (LCC-NED). These cases are similar to the 10–15% of nonsmall cell lung carcinomas (NSCLC) in which neuroendocrine differentiation (NSCLC-NED) can be found by electron microscopy and/or immunohistochemistry despite the absence of neuroendocrine morphology by light microscopy.[20,59–73] All the published studies are retrospective and there is no consensus on whether these patients have a better or worse prognosis or if their tumors are more or less responsive to chemotherapy compared to NSCLC without neuroendocrine differentiation.

Separation of LCNEC from LCC is based on whether or not a light microscopic neuroendocrine pattern is present. In most cases this is not difficult because the neuroendocrine morphological features are so distinctive. However, in some tumors the morphological neuroendocrine features may be more subtle and separation from LCC or LCC-NE may be more difficult.

Further data regarding the spectrum of clinical and pathological features of LCNEC are awaiting larger series of cases. Hopefully this will further define the differences in survival and response to therapy for LCNEC compared to AC, LCNEM, LCC-NE, LCC, and SCLC.

Clinical aspects: presentation and diagnostic considerations and techniques

In previously reported series (see Table 24.2), LCNEC patients have a median age of 62 years (range 33–87 years).[1] The vast majority of patients are male smokers (see Table 24.2).

The most common presenting symptom is chest pain, followed by hemoptysis, dyspnea, cough, fever, and weight loss. Up to 24% may be asymptomatic.[8] Paraneoplastic syndromes are typically absent,[43,74] a significant clinical difference with SCLC. Because surgical resection is usually required to establish the diagnosis, the stage distribution in most series is weighted towards early-stage resectable tumors rather than advanced disease.

Several studies have reported computed tomography (CT) findings of LCNEC.[38,75,76] Sarkaria *et al.* reported on 100 cases in which most tumors were on the right side (63%), in the lung periphery (79%), and in the upper lobes (75%).[10] Oshiro *et al.*, in a detailed radiological review of 28 patients, identified endobronchial growth in 5% of cases, obstructive pneumonia in 8%, and pleural effusion in 24%.[38] With high-resolution CT, the tumor–lung interface was well defined in 74% of cases and lobulation was present in 79%. Spiculation is reported in 32–73% of cases.[38,75] Cavitation was rare (3%).[38] The enhancement pattern on contrast-enhanced CT is more inhomogeneous in larger tumors.[38] LCNEC typically have homogeneously high fluorodeoxyglucose (FDG) uptake on positron emission tomography (PET) scans, which are helpful in locating extrathoracic metastases.[13,77] These tumors also contain somatostatin receptors and can be OctreoScan™ positive, yet this imaging modality is not used frequently for the evaluation of this malignancy.

Serum tumor markers have been reported in a few series. Kozuki *et al.* found elevated serum levels of serum soluble fragments of cytokeratin 19 (CYFRA) in 67% of patients, NSE in 63%, lactate dehydrogenase (LDH) in 55%, sialyl Lewis X-I (SLX) in 50%, carcinoembryonic antigen (CEA) in 42%, and pro gastrin-related polypeptide (ProGRP) in 33%, while no patients had elevations in carbohydrate antigen 19-9 (CA19-9) or squamous cell carcinoma-related antigen (SCC). All patients with elevated CYFRA, NSE and ProGRP) had stage IV disease.[78] Takei et al. found elevated serum CEA in 49% of patients while NSE and pro-gastrin-releasing peptide were elevated in 19% and 11% of patients, respectively.[43]

Large cell carcinoma with neuroendocrine morphology

There is little information available regarding the clinical characteristics of patients with large cell carcinoma with neuroendocrine morphology.[8,40,79] However, the data suggest that the clinical features such as age, gender predilection, smoking history, stage distribution, and survival are very similar.[8,40,79] Iyoda et al. demonstrated that LCC-NEM had similar clinical properties to LCNEC with the exception that LCC-NEM had a more significantly elevated serum tissue polypeptide antigen (TPA) compared to LCNEC and a higher LDH than classic large cell carcinomas.

Treatment

Surgery

The vast majority of patients with LCNEC have had surgical resections usually consisting of lobectomy or pneumonectomy, with some cases requiring intrapericardial resections, chest wall resection and reconstruction, phrenic nerve resection, and rare major vascular reconstruction.[10] Smaller numbers of patients have only had wedge or segmental resections, sleeve resections or excisional biopsies of metastatic lesions. Even fewer cases are diagnosed by small biopsies such as bronchoscopic or needle biopsies. Part of the reason for this is that the diagnosis of LCNEC is very difficult to establish in small specimens due to the requirement of identifying the neuroendocrine morphological pattern as well as the need for immunohistochemistry to confirm neuroendocrine differentiation.

For patients with early-stage LCNEC, resection is recommended. The modalities of choice are either lobectomy or pneumonectomy, with systematic nodal dissection.[8] Zacharias et al. and Sarkaria et al. reported independent series of patients with LCNEC where they performed a meticulous systematic nodal dissection in the majority of their patients. This careful approach to staging has been suggested as a possible cause for the relatively favorable survival found in their stage I patients compared to other studies.[8,10]

Surgical complications do not appear to be increased or significantly different than those for operations performed for other nonsmall cell carcinomas. Mazieres et al. reported a 5% perioperative mortality.[80] Most studies do not report major operative complications, but acute respiratory failure and hemothorax have been reported.[80,81]

Radiotherapy

Radiation has been administered to a subset of patients in some studies,[5,40,43,47,81] but there is insufficient information to establish whether this modality is effective or not. In some cases it has been given only in a palliative setting.[43] No studies have attempted to specifically determine the optimal approach to radiation and to document tumor responsiveness.

Chemotherapy

Adjuvant chemotherapy

In nonsmall cell lung cancer, multiple large randomized trials have now confirmed that adjuvant chemotherapy after surgery confers a survival advantage.[82,83] Given the aggressive nature of LCNEC, surgery alone is not sufficient for its treatment. Several studies have attempted to discern the role of adjuvant chemotherapy in LCNEC yet the majority of these are retrospective and include small numbers of patients. Thus, the benefit of chemotherapy after surgical resection has not been established specifically for LCNEC. Further, the most appropriate regimens have not been clearly delineated and there is controversy on whether to treat LCNEC, based on the neuroendocrine features, in the same manner as small cell lung cancer or nonsmall cell lung cancer. Certainly the aggressive natural history and propensity to metastasize are similar to small cell lung cancer, yet LCNEC clearly does not demonstrate the same chemosensitivity.

A Japanese group compiled data on 16 patients who received postoperative chemotherapy and 57 who did not.[84] For most patients, the chemotherapy regimens administered included combinations typically used for SCLC, such as cisplatin or carboplatin with etoposide, or cyclophosphamide, doxorubicin, and vincristine. For all patients, the 5-year survival was 62% for stage I, 18% for stage II, and 17% for stage III. The authors note that the 5-year survival for the five patients with stage I disease who received adjuvant chemotherapy was 100% while it was 51% for the 23 patients who did not. Postoperative chemotherapy did not affect survival for other stages.[84] In a retrospective analysis of 144 surgical cases, Veronesi et al. showed a trend toward improved survival in stage I patients who received neoadjuvant or adjuvant chemotherapy. Preoperative and postoperative chemotherapy was given to 21 and 24 patients, respectively, with half receiving standard SCLC regimens and the other half receiving regimens recommended for NSCLC.[85] A statistically significant survival benefit was found for patients with LCNEC who received perioperative chemotherapy compared to surgery alone across all stages ($p = 0.04$).[85] In a retrospective review of 45 surgically resected patients with LCNEC, 23 received perioperative chemotherapy, 91% of which was cisplatin based.[86] Further, surgery with or without chemotherapy demonstrated an independent prognostic influence on survival in multivariate analysis; patients who did not receive chemotherapy after surgery were more likely to die than patients who underwent surgery plus chemotherapy (hazard ratio (HR) 9.472; 95% CI 1.050–85.478; $p = 0.0457$).[86]

Importantly, several studies support the use of SCLC-based regimens in the adjuvant treatment of LCNEC. Iyoda et al.

performed a prospective analysis on 15 LCNEC patients who received adjuvant chemotherapy with cisplatin and etoposide and compared outcomes to a historical cohort of LCNEC patients treated without platinum-based adjuvant therapy. Prolonged survival was noted for the patients who received at least two cycles of SCLC-based regimens; the 5-year overall survival rates were 88.9% and 47.4% in the adjuvant chemotherapy group and the control group, respectively.[87] Further, those receiving platinum-based adjuvant chemotherapy were noted to have a significantly lower rate of tumor recurrence when compared to patients receiving nonplatinum-based or no adjuvant chemotherapy.[18] In an Italian retrospective series of 83 LCNEC cases, the 13 patients who received SCLC-based regimens had significantly better survival than the 15 patients who received drug combinations used in NSCLC (median survival, 42 versus 11 months, respectively; p <0.0001). The best prognosis was noted in stage I LCNEC patients who received SCLC-based adjuvant chemotherapy. In univariate and multivariate analysis, the administration of adjuvant chemotherapy with cisplatin or carboplatin plus etoposide was the most important variable correlating with survival.[88]

In a report of 100 surgically resected patients with LCNEC at the Memorial Sloan-Kettering Cancer Center, Sarkaria et al. could not identify a significant impact on overall survival, disease-free survival, or recurrence rates in patients receiving neoadjuvant or adjuvant chemotherapy in the study group as a whole.[10] This disparity with other studies may have been due to the relatively large numbers of stage I patients who did not receive chemotherapy and who did not reach median survival. In a subset analysis of stage IB to IIIA surgical patients who would typically be considered for pre- or postresection adjuvant chemotherapy, a trend towards improved survival was seen in those patients receiving a complete resection and platinum-based combination therapy. In the multivariate analysis, only male sex, comorbid pulmonary disease, and advanced tumor stage were significantly associated with worse survival. The presence or absence of etoposide as a second agent in combination with platinum regimens did not affect survival rates in this study.

Interpretation of these reports is limited by their retrospective nature and the small sample size. However, these data, along with the known poor natural history and the routine use of adjuvant chemotherapy for SCLC and NSCLC, suggest that postoperative treatment with etoposide and cisplatin is appropriate in patients with completely resected LCNEC, including patients with stage I disease.

Adjuvant treatment with octreotide for patients with LCNEC was evaluated by Filosso and colleagues.[89] Retrospectively, 18 patients were identified who had surgery for LCNEC. Ten patients had positive octreotide scans preoperatively and were given octreotide as adjuvant therapy. No patient received adjuvant chemotherapy, but patients with greater than stage IB disease received radiation. At the time of their report, 90% of patients were alive and free of disease.[89]

Stage IV

The optimal chemotherapeutic regimen in relapsed or stage IV disease is not defined. Again, the controversy centers on whether to treat LCNEC in the same manner as small cell lung cancer or nonsmall cell lung cancer.

In the study by Mazieres et al., 13 patients with relapsed disease received chemotherapy with etoposide plus cisplatin or carboplatin.[80] Partial responses were noted only in two of the 10 evaluable patients. Kozuki and colleagues described five patients with stage IV disease treated with chemotherapy.[78] Three of these patients received platinum-based regimens, without any objective response. Subsequent regimens including paclitaxel, docetaxel, irinotecan, gemcitabine, vinorelbine, or amrubicin were equally ineffective. Five patients were treated with gefitinib, an epidermal growth factor tyrosine kinase inhibitor, and one (a male with a 114 pack-year smoking history) achieved a partial response. In 22 patients receiving platinum-based doublet chemotherapy with standard second agents, Sarkaria et al. reported a 68% partial response rate, with the remaining patients having stable disease. Two additional patients receiving nonplatinum monotherapy progressed or had stable disease.[10]

In contrast, several studies have shown that the response rate of LCNEC to cisplatin-based chemotherapy is comparable to SCLC. A retrospective series of 20 patients with advanced LCNEC (stage IIIA, 3; stage IIIB, 6; stage IV, 6; postoperative recurrence, 5) treated with platinum-based therapy showed a response rate of 50% (complete response, 1; partial response, 9).[90] Interestingly, the response rate for chemotherapy-naïve patients (64%) was better than for those patients who were previously treated (17%).[90] Rossi et al. showed that in metastatic disease, the 12 patients who received SCLC-based chemotherapy (three also received radiation therapy) had a significantly better survival than the 15 patients who received common NSCLC regimens (gemcitabine and carboplatin, 10; carboplatin and paclitaxel, 3; gemcitabine, 2; six also received radiation therapy); median survival, 51 versus 21 months, respectively (p <0.001).[88] Only the patients who received SCLC-based chemotherapy had a complete ($n = 2$) or partial ($n = 4$) response.[88]

In a recent Japanese study of advanced previously treated LCNEC, Yoshida et al. showed a 28% objective response rate using amrubicin.[16]

As can be seen from the above, information regarding the treatment of LCNEC has been derived from small retrospective studies for the most part. Larger, randomized prospective studies are needed to determine the optimal treatment regimen for this disease. Only recently has a prospective trial, selectively enrolling patients with LCNEC (a Japanese phase 2 trial of irinotecan and cisplatin), just begun. Further, as more information regarding the molecular biology of this disease is elucidated, it can help guide our treatment recommendations.

Prognosis

The survival for patients with LCNEC is poor. Overall 5-year survival ranges from 15% to 57% (see Table 24.2). The variation in survival is probably due to several factors including the distribution of lower versus higher stage or the thoroughness of the staging methods in the study. Given the lack of clear responses to chemotherapy or radiation, it is unlikely that differences in survival has been due to variation in approach to treatment with these modalities. It is likely that the favorable survival data stage for stage in some series can be attributed to the careful approach to surgical staging such as systematic nodal dissection.[8] However, even the studies with more favorable outcomes for LCNEC have not been able to demonstrate a significant difference in survival for SCLC treated in the same fashion.

Several studies have demonstrated that survival for LCNEC is significantly worse than that for nonneuroendocrine nonsmall cell carcinomas. With such poorly differentiated and aggressive tumors, these survival differences are best observed in comparing survival of patients with lower stage tumors, because the higher stage patients die so rapidly that there is little chance to see survival differences in small series of patients. Jiang et al. found 58.8% and 44.8% 1- and 5-year survival rates in 22 patients with a significantly worse prognosis than patients with other nonsmall cell carcinomas ($p = 0.046$).[42] Iyoda also found that the survival for LCNEC was significantly worse than that for classic large cell carcinoma.[40] Takei et al. found that in patients with only stage I tumors, survival rates for LCNEC, poorly differentiated NSCLC, and LCC were 67%, 88%, and 92% with significant differences between LCNEC and NSCLC ($p = 0.003$), LCNEC, and LCC ($p = 0.03$) but not between LCNEC and SCLC.[43] However, they found LCNEC to have no significant difference in survival compared with all stages of patients with poorly differentiated NSCLC, LCC or SCLC.

Within LCNEC itself, Sarkaria et al., in a subset analysis of stage I patients, found that stage IB patients fared far worse (5-year overall survival 26%) than stage IA patients (5-year overall survival 72%), which may partially explain disparities in early-stage survival rates seen between studies where stage I patients were lumped together.[10] Sarkaria et al. reported recurrence in 38% of patients, with 60% of those recurring at distant sites, 27% at local or regional sites, and 13% simultaneously at both.[10] Similarly, of the 40% of patients who developed recurrence in the study by Takei et al., distant metastases occurred in 56% in the brain, liver, bone, and lung and locoregional recurrence occurred in 35% either in mediastinal or supraclavicular lymph nodes or in the bronchial stump.[43] In 9% of cases both distant and locoregional recurrences occurred simultaneously.[43] Recurrence occurred within the first 6 months in 50% of patients, at 7–12 months in 32%, at 13–24 months in 9%, and after 24 months in 9%.[43]

Using the National Cancer Institute (NCI) Surveillance, Epidemiology, and End Results (SEER) data, Varlotto et al. analyzed 1211 LCNEC patients and showed that the overall and lung cancer-specific survival for LCNEC was signifcantly better than that for SCLC and similar to that of other large cell carcinomas in patients who received definitive surgery without radiation.[11] These data support continuing to classify LCNEC as a subtype of large cell carcinoma, rather than being classified with SCLC.

Recommendations

Large cell neuroendocrine carcinoma is an aggressive disease with distinct pathological and biological features shared by both SCLC and NSCLC. Since a surgical specimen is required to establish a definitive pathological diagnosis in virtually all cases, most patients will undergo a surgical resection. Because of the aggressive behavior of this tumor adjunctive chemotherapy or radiation will be given in many cases.

Treatment with chemotherapy has marginal benefit. The optimal chemotherapy regimen for LCNEC remains unknown, but regimens used for small cell lung cancer, such as etoposide and cisplatin, seem to have the most data supporting their use. In line with standard therapy for both small cell and nonsmall cell lung cancer, patients with resected LCNEC should be offered adjuvant chemotherapy. Clinical trials designed specifically for patients with LCNEC are sorely needed to better define the role of chemotherapy and other treatment modalities.

References

1. Travis WD, Linnoila RI, Tsokos MG, et al. Neuroendocrine tumors of the lung with proposed criteria for large-cell neuroendocrine carcinoma. An ultrastructural, immunohistochemical, and flow cytometric study of 35 cases. Am J Surg Pathol 1991; 15: 529–53.
2. Travis WD, Brambilla E, Müller-Hermelink HK, Harris CC. Pathology and Genetics: Tumours of the Lung, Pleura, Thymus and Heart. Lyon: IARC, 2004.
3. Travis WD, Rush W, Flieder DB, et al. Survival analysis of 200 pulmonary neuroendocrine tumors with clarification of criteria for atypical carcinoid and its separation from typical carcinoid. Am J Surg Pathol 1998; 22(8): 934–44.
4. Travis WD, Colby TV, Corrin B, et al. Histological Typing of Lung and Pleural Tumors, 3 rd edn. Berlin: Springer, 1999.
5. Battafarano RJ, Fernandez FG, Ritter J, et al. Large cell neuroendocrine carcinoma: an aggressive form of non-small cell lung cancer. J Thorac Cardiovasc Surg 2005; 130(1): 166–72.
6. Dresler CM, Ritter JH, Patterson GA, Ross E, Bailey MS, Wick MR. Clinical-pathologic analysis of 40 patients with large cell neuroendocrine carcinoma of the lung. Ann Thorac Surg 1997; 63(1): 180–5.
7. Rusch VW, Klimstra DS, Venkatraman ES. Molecular markers help characterize neuroendocrine lung tumors. Ann Thorac Surg 1996; 62(3): 798–809.
8. Zacharias J, Nicholson AG, Ladas GP, Goldstraw P. Large cell neuroendocrine carcinoma and large cell carcinomas with neuroendocrine morphology of the lung: prognosis after complete resection and systematic nodal dissection. Ann Thorac Surg 2003; 75(2): 348–52.
9. Lim E, Goldstraw P, Nicholson AG, et al. Proceedings of the IASLC International Workshop on Advances in Pulmonary Neuroendocrine Tumors 2007. J Thorac Oncol 2008; 3(10): 1194–201.
10. Sarkaria IS, Iyoda A, Roh MS, et al. Neoadjuvant and adjuvant chemotherapy in resected pulmonary large cell neuroendocrine carcinomas: a single institution experience. Ann Thorac Surg 2011; 92(4): 1180–7.
11. Varlotto JM, Medford-Davis LN, Recht A, et al. Should large cell neuroendocrine lung carcinoma be classified and treated as a small cell lung cancer or with other large cell carcinomas? J Thorac Oncol 2011; 6(6): 1050–8.
12. Nomura M, Fukuda T, Fujii K, et al. Preferential expression of potential markers for cancer stem cells in large cell neuroendocrine carcinoma of the lung. An FFPE proteomic study. J Clin Bioinform 2011; 1(1): 23.
13. Rekhtman N, Marchetti A, Lau C, et al. Analysis of EGFR and KRAS mutations in small cell carcinoma and large cell neuroendocrine carcinoma of lung. J Thoracic Oncol 2011; 6: S346.
14. Skov BG, Holm B, Erreboe A, Skov T, Mellemgaard A. ERCC1 and Ki67 in small cell lung carcinoma and other neuroendocrine tumors of the lung: distribution and impact on survival. J Thorac Oncol 2010; 5(4): 453–9.

15. Sun L, Sakurai S, Sano T, Hironaka M, Kawashima O, Nakajima T. High-grade neuroendocrine carcinoma of the lung: comparative clinicopathological study of large cell neuroendocrine carcinoma and small cell lung carcinoma. Pathol Int 2009; 59(8): 522–9.

16. Yoshida H, Sekine I, Tsuta K, et al. Amrubicin monotherapy for patients with previously treated advanced large-cell neuroendocrine carcinoma of the lung. Jpn J Clin Oncol 2011; 41(7): 897–901.

17. Igawa S, Watanabe R, Ito I, et al. Comparison of chemotherapy for unresectable pulmonary high-grade non-small cell neuroendocrine carcinoma and small-cell lung cancer. Lung Cancer 2010; 68(3): 438–45.

18. Iyoda A, Hiroshima K, Moriya Y, et al. Postoperative recurrence and the role of adjuvant chemotherapy in patients with pulmonary large-cell neuroendocrine carcinoma. J Thorac Cardiovasc Surg 2009; 138(2): 446–53.

19. Fujiwara Y, Sekine I, Tsuta K, et al. Effect of platinum combined with irinotecan or paclitaxel against large cell neuroendocrine carcinoma of the lung. Jpn J Clin Oncol 2007; 37(7): 482–6.

20. Iyoda A, Hiroshima K, Baba M, Saitoh Y, Ohwada H, Fujisawa T. Pulmonary large cell carcinomas with neuroendocrine features are high-grade neuroendocrine tumors. Ann Thorac Surg 2002; 73(4): 1049–54.

21. Onuki N, Wistuba II, Travis WD, et al. Genetic changes in the spectrum of neuroendocrine lung tumors. Cancer 1999; 85(3): 600–7.

22. Brambilla E, Negoescu A, Gazzeri S, et al. Apoptosis-related factors p53, Bcl2, and Bax in neuroendocrine lung tumors. Am J Pathol 1996; 149(6): 1941–52.

23. Hiroshima K, Iyoda A, Shibuya K, et al. Genetic alterations in early-stage pulmonary large cell neuroendocrine carcinoma. Cancer 2004; 100(6): 1190–8.

24. Iyoda A, Hiroshima K, Moriya Y, et al. Pulmonary large cell neuroendocrine carcinoma demonstrates high proliferative activity. Ann Thorac Surg 2004; 77(6): 1891–5.

25. Jiang SX, Kameya T, Shinada J, Yoshimura H. The significance of frequent and independent p53 and bcl-2 expression in large-cell neuroendocrine carcinomas of the lung. Mod Pathol 1999; 12(4): 362–9.

26. Przygodzki RM, Finkelstein SD, Langer JC, et al. Analysis of p53, K-ras-2, and C-raf-1 in pulmonary neuroendocrine tumors. Correlation with histological subtype and clinical outcome. Am J Pathol 1996; 148: 1531–41.

27. Sampietro G, Tomasic G, Collini P, et al. Gene product immunophenotyping of neuroendocrine lung tumors. No linking evidence between carcinoids and small-cell lung carcinomas suggested by multivariate statistical analysis. Appl Immunohistochem Mol Morphol 2000; 8(1): 49–56.

28. Hollstein M, Sidransky D, Vogelstein B, Harris CC. p53 mutations in human cancers. Science 1991; 253: 49–53.

29. Beasley MB, Lantuejoul S, Abbondanzo S, et al. The P16/cyclin D1/Rb pathway in neuroendocrine tumors of the lung. Hum Pathol 2003; 34(2): 136–42.

30. Igarashi T, Jiang SX, Kameya T, et al. Divergent cyclin B1 expression and Rb/p16/cyclin D1 pathway aberrations among pulmonary neuroendocrine tumors. Mod Pathol 2004; 17(10): 1259–67.

31. Kobayashi Y, Tokuchi Y, Hashimoto T, et al. Molecular markers for reinforcement of histological subclassification of neuroendocrine lung tumors. Cancer Sci 2004; 95(4): 334–41.

32. Araki K, Ishii G, Yokose T, et al. Frequent overexpression of the c-kit protein in large cell neuroendocrine carcinoma of the lung. Lung Cancer 2003; 40(2): 173–80.

33. Casali C, Stefani A, Rossi G, et al. The prognostic role of c-kit protein expression in resected large cell neuroendocrine carcinoma of the lung. Ann Thorac Surg 2004; 77(1): 247–52.

34. Iyoda A, Travis WD, Sarkaria IS, et al. Expression profiling and identification of potential molecular targets for therapy in pulmonary large cell neuroendocrine carcinoma. Exp Therapeut Med 2011; [Epub ahead of print].

35. Pelosi G, Masullo M, Leon ME, et al. CD117 immunoreactivity in high-grade neuroendocrine tumors of the lung: a comparative study of 39 large-cell neuroendocrine carcinomas and 27 surgically resected small-cell carcinomas. Virchows Arch 2004; 445(5): 449–55.

36. Debelenko LV, Swalwell JI, Kelley MJ, et al. MEN1 gene mutation analysis of high-grade neuroendocrine lung carcinoma. Genes Chromosomes Cancer 2000; 28(1): 58–65.

37. Daddi N, Ferolla P, Urbani M, et al. Surgical treatment of neuroendocrine tumors of the lung. Eur J Cardiothorac Surg 2004; 26(4): 813–17.

38. Oshiro Y, Kusumoto M, Matsuno Y, et al. CT findings of surgically resected large cell neuroendocrine carcinoma of the lung in 38 patients. Am J Roentgenol 2004; 182(1): 87–91.

39. Rossi G, Marchioni A, Milani M, et al. TTF-1, cytokeratin 7, 34betaE12, and CD56/NCAM immunostaining in the subclassification of large cell carcinomas of the lung. Am J Clin Pathol 2004; 122(6): 884–93.

40. Iyoda A, Hiroshima K, Toyozaki T, Haga Y, Fujisawa T, Ohwada H. Clinical characterization of pulmonary large cell neuroendocrine carcinoma and large cell carcinoma with neuroendocrine morphology. Cancer 2001; 91(11): 1992–2000.

41. Sturm N, Lantuejoul S, Laverriere MH, et al. Thyroid transcription factor 1 and cytokeratins 1, 5, 10, 14 (34betaE12) expression in basaloid and large-cell neuroendocrine carcinomas of the lung. Hum Pathol 2001; 32(9): 918–25.

42. Jiang SX, Kameya T, Shoji M, Dobashi Y, Shinada J, Yoshimura H. Large cell neuroendocrine carcinoma of the lung: a histologic and immunohistochemical study of 22 cases. Am J Surg Pathol 1998; 22(5): 526–37.

43. Takei H, Asamura H, Maeshima A, et al. Large cell neuroendocrine carcinoma of the lung: a clinicopathologic study of eighty-seven cases. J Thorac Cardiovasc Surg 2002; 124(2): 285–92.

44. Lantuejoul S, Moro D, Michalides RJ, Brambilla C, Brambilla E. Neural cell adhesion molecules (NCAM) and NCAM-PSA expression in neuroendocrine lung tumors. Am J Surg Pathol 1998; 22(10): 1267–76.

45. Folpe AL, Gown AM, Lamps LW, et al. Thyroid transcription factor-1: immunohistochemical evaluation in pulmonary neuroendocrine tumors. Mod Pathol 1999; 12(1): 5–8.

46. Sturm N, Rossi G, Lantuejoul S, et al. Expression of thyroid transcription factor-1 in the spectrum of neuroendocrine cell lung proliferations with special interest in carcinoids. Hum Pathol 2002; 33(2): 175–82.

47. Paci M, Cavazza A, Annessi V, et al. Large cell neuroendocrine carcinoma of the lung: a 10-year clinicopathologic retrospective study. Ann Thorac Surg 2004; 77(4): 1163–7.

48. Said JW, Vimadalal S, Nash G, et al. Immunoreactive neuron-specific enolase, bombesin, and chromogranin as markers for neuroendocrine lung tumors. Hum Pathol 1985; 16: 236–40.

49. Tsuta K, Liu DC, Kalhor N, Wistuba II, Moran CA. Using the mitosis-specific marker anti-phosphohistone h3 to assess mitosis in pulmonary neuroendocrine carcinomas. Am J Clin Pathol 2011; 136(2): 252–9.

50. Hiroshima K, Abe S, Ebihara Y, et al. Cytological characteristics of pulmonary large cell neuroendocrine carcinoma. Lung Cancer 2005; 48(3): 331–7.

51. Iyoda A, Baba M, Hiroshima K, et al. Imprint cytologic features of pulmonary large cell neuroendocrine carcinoma: comparison with classic large cell carcinoma. Oncol Rep 2004; 11(2): 285–8.

52. Kakinuma H, Mikami T, Iwabuchi K, et al. Diagnostic findings of bronchial brush cytology for pulmonary large cell neuroendocrine carcinomas: comparison with poorly differentiated adenocarcinomas, squamous cell carcinomas, and small cell carcinomas. Cancer 2003; 99(4): 247–54.

53. Nicholson SA, Ryan MR. A review of cytologic findings in neuroendocrine carcinomas including carcinoid tumors with histologic correlation. Cancer 2000; 90(3): 148–61.

54. Wiatrowska BA, Krol J, Zakowski MF. Large-cell neuroendocrine carcinoma of the lung: proposed criteria for cytologic diagnosis. Diagn Cytopathol 2001; 24(1): 58–64.

55. Yang YJ, Steele CT, Ou XL, Snyder KP, Kohman LJ. Diagnosis of high-grade pulmonary neuroendocrine carcinoma by fine-needle aspiration biopsy: nonsmall-cell or small-cell type? Diagn Cytopathol 2001; 25(5): 292–300.

56. Hoshi R, Furuta N, Horai T, Ishikawa Y, Miyata S, Satoh Y. Discriminant model for cytologic distinction of large cell neuroendocrine carcinoma from small cell carcinoma of the lung. J Thorac Oncol 2010; 5(4): 472–8.

57. Maleki Z. Diagnostic issues with cytopathologic interpretation of lung neoplasms displaying high-grade basaloid or neuroendocrine morphology. Diagn Cytopathol 2011; 39(3): 159–67.

58. Travis WD, Gal AA, Colby TV, Klimstra DS, Falk R, Koss MN. Reproducibility of neuroendocrine lung tumor classification. Hum Pathol 1998; 29(3): 272–9.

59. Howe MC, Chapman A, Kerr K, Dougal M, Anderson H, Hasleton PS. Neuroendocrine differentiation in non-small cell lung cancer and its relation to prognosis and therapy. Histopathology 2005; 46(2): 195–201.

60. Hiroshima K, Iyoda A, Shibuya K, et al. Prognostic significance of neuroendocrine differentiation in adenocarcinoma of the lung. Ann Thorac Surg 2002; 73(6): 1732–5.

61. Carnaghi C, Rimassa L, Garassino I, Santoro A. Clinical significance of neuroendocrine phenotype in non-small-cell lung cancer. Ann Oncol 2001; 12(Suppl 2): S119–23.

62. Baldi A, Groger AM, Esposito V, di Marino MP, Ferrara N, Baldi F. Neuroendocrine differentiation in non-small cell lung carcinomas. In Vivo 2000; 14(1): 109–14.

63. Abbona G, Papotti M, Viberti L, Macri L, Stella A, Bussolati G. Chromogranin A gene expression in non-small cell lung carcinomas. J Pathol 1998; 186(2): 151–6.

64. Hage R, Elbers HR, Brutel R, van den Bosch JM. Neural cell adhesion molecule expression: prognosis in 889 patients with resected non-small cell lung cancer. Chest 1998; 114(5): 1316–20.

65. Kwa HB, Michalides RJ, Dijkman JH, Mooi WJ. The prognostic value of NCAM, p53 and cyclin D1 in resected non-small cell lung cancer. Lung Cancer 1996; 14(2–3): 207–17.

66. Schleusener JT, Tazelaar HD, Jung SH, et al. Neuroendocrine differentiation is an independent prognostic factor in chemotherapy-treated nonsmall cell lung carcinoma. Cancer 1996; 77: 1284–91.

67. Senderovitz T, Skov BG, Hirsch FR. Neuroendocrine characteristics in malignant lung tumors: implications for diagnosis, treatment, and prognosis. Cancer Treat Res 1995; 72: 143–54.

68. Linnoila RI, Piantadosi S, Ruckdeschel JC. Impact of neuroendocrine differentiation in non-small cell lung cancer. The LCSG experience. Chest 1994; 106: 367S–371S.

69. Carles J, Rosell R, Ariza A, et al. Neuroendocrine differentiation as a prognostic factor in non-small cell lung cancer. Lung Cancer 1993; 10: 209–19.

70. Pujol JL, Simony J, Demoly P, et al. Neural cell adhesion molecule and prognosis of surgically resected lung cancer. Am Rev Respir Dis 1993; 148: 1071–5.

71. Skov BG, Sorensen JB, Hirsch FR, Larsson LI, Hansen HH. Prognostic impact of histologic demonstration of chromogranin A and neuron specific enolase in pulmonary adenocarcinoma. Ann Oncol 1991; 2: 355–60.

72. Sundaresan V, Reeve JG, Stenning S, Stewart S, Bleehen NM. Neuroendocrine differentiation and clinical behaviour in non-small cell lung tumours. Br J Cancer 1991; 64: 333–8.

73. Berendsen HH, de Leij L, Poppema S, et al. Clinical characterization of non-small-cell lung cancer tumors showing neuroendocrine differentiation features. J Clin Oncol 1989; 7: 1614–20.

74. Garcia-Yuste M, Matilla JM, Alvarez-Gago T, et al. Prognostic factors in neuroendocrine lung tumors: a Spanish Multicenter Study. Spanish Multicenter Study of Neuroendocrine Tumors of the Lung of the Spanish Society of Pneumonology and Thoracic Surgery (EMETNE–SEPAR). Ann Thorac Surg 2000; 70(1): 258–63.

75. Jung KJ, Lee KS, Han J, et al. Large cell neuroendocrine carcinoma of the lung: clinical, CT, and pathologic findings in 11 patients. J Thorac Imaging 2001; 16(3): 156–62.

76. Shin AR, Shin BK, Choi JA, Oh YW, Kim HK, Kang EY. Large cell neuroendocrine carcinoma of the lung: radiologic and pathologic findings. J Comput Assist Tomogr 2000; 24(4): 567–73.

77. Chong S, Lee KS, Kim BT, et al. Integrated PET/CT of pulmonary neuroendocrine tumors: diagnostic and prognostic implications. Am J Roentgenol 2007; 188(5): 1223–31.

78. Kozuki T, Fujimoto N, Ueoka H, et al. Complexity in the treatment of pulmonary large cell neuroendocrine carcinoma. J Cancer Res Clin Oncol 2005; 131(3): 147–51.

79. ab' Saber AM, Massoni Neto LM, Bianchi CP, et al. Neuroendocrine and biologic features of primary tumors and tissue in pulmonary large cell carcinomas. Ann Thorac Surg 2004; 77(6): 1883–90.

80. Mazieres J, Daste G, Molinier L, et al. Large cell neuroendocrine carcinoma of the lung: pathological study and clinical outcome of 18 resected cases. Lung Cancer 2002; 37(3): 287–92.

81. Doddoli C, Barlesi F, Chetaille B, et al. Large cell neuroendocrine carcinoma of the lung: an aggressive disease potentially treatable with surgery. Ann Thorac Surg 2004; 77(4): 1168–72.

82. Arriagada R, Bergman B, Dunant A, Le CT, Pignon JP, Vansteenkiste J. Cisplatin-based adjuvant chemotherapy in patients with completely resected non-small-cell lung cancer. N Engl J Med 2004; 350(4): 351–60.

83. Winton T, Livingston R, Johnson D, et al. Vinorelbine plus cisplatin vs. observation in resected non-small-cell lung cancer. N Engl J Med 2005; 352(25): 2589–97.

84. Iyoda A, Hiroshima K, Toyozaki T, et al. Adjuvant chemotherapy for large cell carcinoma with neuroendocrine features. Cancer 2001; 92(5): 1108–12.

85. Veronesi G, Morandi U, Alloisio M, et al. Large cell neuroendocrine carcinoma of the lung: a retrospective analysis of 144 surgical cases. Lung Cancer 2006; 53(1): 111–15.

86. Saji H, Tsuboi M, Matsubayashi J, et al. Clinical response of large cell neuroendocrine carcinoma of the lung to perioperative adjuvant chemotherapy. Anticancer Drugs 2010; 21(1): 89–93.

87. Iyoda A, Hiroshima K, Moriya Y, et al. Prospective study of adjuvant chemotherapy for pulmonary large cell neuroendocrine carcinoma. Ann Thorac Surg 2006; 82(5): 1802–7.

88. Rossi G, Cavazza A, Marchioni A, et al. Role of chemotherapy and the receptor tyrosine kinases KIT, PDGFRalpha, PDGFRbeta, and met in large-cell neuroendocrine carcinoma of the lung. J Clin Oncol 2005; 23(34): 8774–85.

89. Filosso PL, Ruffini E, Oliaro A, et al. Large-cell neuroendocrine carcinoma of the lung: a clinicopathologic study of eighteen cases and the efficacy of adjuvant treatment with octreotide. J Thorac Cardiovasc Surg 2005; 129(4): 819–24.

90. Yamazaki S, Sekine I, Matsuno Y, et al. Clinical responses of large cell neuroendocrine carcinoma of the lung to cisplatin-based chemotherapy. Lung Cancer 2005; 49(2): 217–23.

91. Asamura H, Kameya T, Matsuno Y, et al. Neuroendocrine neoplasms of the lung: a prognostic spectrum. J Clin Oncol 2006; 24(1): 70–6.

92. Skov BG, Krasnik M, Lantuejoul S, Skov T, Brambilla E. Reclassification of neuroendocrine tumors improves the separation of carcinoids and the prediction of survival. J Thorac Oncol 2008; 3(12): 1410–15.

93. Rusch VW, Appleman HD, Blackstone E, et al. Lung. In: Edge SB, Byrd DR, Compton C, et al. (eds) AJCC Cancer Staging Manual, 7th edn. Chicago: American Joint Commission on Cancer/Springer, 2009. pp.253–70.

Section 5: Thoracic Tumors

25 Bronchioloalveolar Carcinoma of the Lung

Gregory J. Riely and Vincent A. Miller

Thoracic Oncology Service, Division of Solid Tumor Oncology, Department of Medicine, Memorial Sloan-Kettering Cancer Center, New York, NY, USA

Introduction

Bronchioloalveolar carcinoma (BAC) is a widely used descriptive term that encompasses a subset of adenocarcinomas of the lung commonly characterized by particular clinical presentation, natural history, radiographic appearances, response to treatment, and molecular biology. Interest in BAC has increased due to recognition of a subset of patients with a protracted clinical course as well as results from clinical trials which showed that epidermal growth factor (EGF) receptor tyrosine kinase inhibitors (such as erlotinib and gefitinib) showed preferential efficacy in these patients. This clinical observation preceded and, in some cases, aided the identification of somatic mutations in the EGF gene which are known to identify patients who will benefit from erlotinib and gefitinib. In this chapter, we review the current understanding of the biology, pathology, radiology, and treatment of BAC.

Historical background

The entity now described as bronchioloalveolar carcinoma (synonyms include bronchiolar carcinoma, alveolar carcinoma, pulmonary adenomatosis, and bronchoalveolar carcinoma; henceforth referred to as BAC) was first described in the late 19th and early 20th centuries (reviewed in Liebow[1]). Malassez is credited with the first report of what has become multifocal BAC in 1876. In 1903, Musser was the first to characterize pneumonic BAC. The first application of the term bronchioloalveolar carcinoma came in 1960 by Dr Averill A. Liebow.[1] In this report, he described the pathology of patients with "peripheral pulmonary neoplasms which pursue a rather characteristic course when permitted to progress untreated." Acknowledging some controversy in describing BAC, Liebow defined it as "well-differentiated adenocarcinomas primary in the periphery of the lung … with a tendency to spread chiefly within the confines of the lung by aerogenous and lymphatic routes, the walls of the distal air spaces often acting as supporting stroma for the neoplastic cells." Since there were such widely varied definitions of BAC, he noted that the one finding that grouped these patients together was that patients with BAC were more likely to have spread within the lung, with many patients dying from respiratory failure without metastatic disease.

For the first century of study, BAC was diagnosed using a variety of criteria. Some standardization was achieved with the 1981 World Health Organization (WHO) lung tumor classification which designated BAC as an "adenocarcinoma in which cylindrical tumor cells grow upon the pre-existing alveoli."[2] The more recent and specific definition of BAC comes from the 1999 WHO criteria (repeated again in 2004).[2] These criteria define BAC as "an adenocarcinoma with a pure bronchioloalveolar growth pattern and no evidence of stromal, vascular, or pleural invasion." Specific note is made in this classification system that the diagnosis of BAC cannot be made with cytological material alone.

The most dramatic changes in the history of BAC came with the adoption of the International Association for the Study of Lung Cancer/American Thoracic Society/European Respiratory Society International Multidisciplinary Classification of Lung Adenocarcinoma which was published in 2011.[3] This classification system (described further under Pathology, below) recommended complete abolition of the use of the term BAC. This recommendation was based upon the observation that BAC had come to be used to describe several different clinical entities, many of which would not fit into the WHO classification system for BAC. This classification recommends that those tumors which were formerly classified as BAC be moved into a variety of different categories based upon their unique clinical behaviors. Tumors which were pure BAC tumors without invasion are classified as adenocarcinoma *in situ* (AIS) while tumors previously described as adenocarcinoma with BAC features are now described as lepidic predominant adenocarcinoma (LPA).

Textbook of Uncommon Cancer, Fourth Edition. Edited by Derek Raghavan, Charles D. Blanke, David H. Johnson, Paul L. Moots, Gregory H. Reaman, Peter G. Rose and Mikkael A. Sekeres.
© 2012 John Wiley & Sons, Inc. Published 2012 by John Wiley & Sons, Inc.

Biology and epidemiology

Epidemiology

Estimates of the proportion of patients with non-small cell lung carcinoma (NSCLC) who have BAC (also known as AIS) range widely and depend heavily on the time period during which the epidemiological study was performed, the pathological definition used, and the means of detection of NSCLC (i.e. screen detected or symptom related). While evaluations of the Surveillance, Epidemiology, and End Results (SEER) population-based cancer registry have supported a relatively stable incidence of BAC, both in absolute number and as a proportion of patients with NSCLC, the uncertainty of what can be called BAC makes interpretation of these findings difficult.[4] More recent studies, with pathological reevaluation of lung adenocarcinomas compared with contemporary lung adenocarcinomas, suggest that the number of patients with BAC and the proportion of patients with lung adenocarcinomas who have BAC are rising.[5–7]

The only clearly identified risk factor for BAC is a history of cigarette smoking. While the odds ratio for BAC in patients with a smoking history is not as high as that found for either non-BAC adenocarcinomas or squamous cell carcinoma, smoking remains the only clear risk factor.[8] An estimated 60–70% of patients with BAC are either former or current smokers.[8] Since nearly 40% of patients with BAC are never smokers and have not had long-term exposure to mutagenic carcinogens, this population provides an ideal venue to study the molecular biology of lung cancer.

Biology

In order to understand the biology of BAC, a number of animal models have been explored. Ovine pulmonary adenomatosis (OPA, also known as jaagsiekte, sheep pulmonary adenomatosis, or ovine pulmonary carcinoma) is a widely studied model of BAC that was discussed in Liebow's initial description of BAC[9,10] and probably most closely resembles the entity of mucinous BAC. Similarities in sheep and human disease include presence of peripheral, multifocal lesions, the production of large amounts of mucus, and tumors that originate from type II pneumocytes and Clara cells. By WHO criteria, OPA would be classified as mixed adenocarcinoma showing acinar, papillary, and bronchioloalveolar growth patterns. OPA is caused by a retrovirus (the Jaagsiekte sheep retrovirus, JSRV) and its transforming element was recently identified as the Env protein.[11] Despite its histological similarities, no virus has been isolated from human BAC. The human disease does not appear to be transmissible.

Explorations of tumorigenesis mechanisms of BAC (AIS) have focused on atypical adenomatous hyperplasia (AAH) as a possible precursor lesion. AAH is "a localized proliferation of mild to moderately atypical cells lining involved alveoli …"[2] While etiological and molecular evidence that AAH is a precursor of BAC and invasive adenocarcinoma is lacking, there is evidence that genetic changes become more prevalent with greater invasiveness of tumors. The best example of this is the identification of allelic loss corresponding to the Noguchi classification.[12] As described below, the Noguchi classification of tumors classifies adenocarcinomas with BAC components into subgroups: type A (localized BAC, LBAC), type B (LBAC with focal alveolar collapse), and type C (invasive adenocarcinoma with BAC). Aoyagi et al. determined the allelic loss of 66 tumors which had been classified as type A, B, or C.[13] They found that allelic loss increased from 17% in type A tumors to 39% in type B tumors, and 96% in type C tumors. More recently, Yoshida et al. noted that only 3% (1/35) patients with AAH had activating mutations in epidermal growth factor receptor (EGFR), while 11% (4/37) patients with BAC had such mutations.[14] EGFR mutations were seen in 42% (13/31) of invasive adenocarcinomas. In contrast, 27% (8/30) of AAH had KRAS mutations whereas 16% (5/30) of BAC tumors and 10% (3/30) of invasive adenocarcinomas had KRAS mutations. These data support a possible role for BAC as an intervening stage of tumorigenesis between AAH and invasive adenocarcinoma. In such a model, EGFR mutations arise later in tumorigenesis while KRAS mutations occur relatively early. Another oncogene, squamous cell carcinoma-related oncogene (SCCRO), also occurs as a relatively late lesion, with SCCRO expression (detected by immunohistochemistry) uncommon in pure BAC but found in 29% of adenocarcinomas.[15]

Molecular biology

Similar to our understanding of the molecular genetics of NSCLC in general, the molecular genetics of BAC tumors appears to be heterogeneous, with no identified single-gene mutation leading to this clinical entity. The most commonly identified somatic mutations described in lung cancer are those in KRAS, with approximately 25% of patients with NSCLC having KRAS mutations. Looking specifically at BAC patients, Rusch et al. found KRAS mutations in 10% (2/20) of BAC tumors (both occurred in smokers with codon 12 mutations).[16] Separately, Marchetti et al. looked at 58 BAC tumors (10 mucinous BAC, 40 nonmucinous, and eight with "sclerosing" BAC).[17] They found that 36% of BAC tumors had KRAS mutations. In contrast, just 26% of adenocarcinomas had evidence of KRAS mutations. Of the 10 mucinous BACs evaluated, all had mutations in KRAS whereas only 23% (9/40) of nonmucinous BAC had KRAS mutations.

Frequency of EGFR and KRAS mutations is significantly different when comparing nonmucinous BAC (AIS or LPA nonmucinous) to mucinous BAC (invasive mucinous adenocarcinoma).[18] For example, Finberg et al. evaluated EGFR and KRAS mutation status in tumors that were BAC or adenocarcinoma with BAC features (AWBF) from 43 patients. In their analysis, 47% of nonmucinous BAC tumors had EGFR mutations while none of 13 mucinous tumors had an EGFR mutation ($p = 0.003$) Of mucinous tumors, 6/7 tumors had a KRAS mutation, suggesting that one could reliably predict that tumors with mucinous BAC would be very unlikely to have an EGFR mutation and may not even be worth testing.

Table 25.1 Systems of classification of bronchioloalveolar carcinoma and adenocarcinomas.

Noguchi[12]	Ebright[60]	Terasaki[30]	Higashiyama[29]	WHO[2]	IASLC/ATS/ERS[3]
Type A – localized BAC (LBAC)	BAC	BAC	100% BAC	BAC	AIS
Type B – LBAC with foci of alveolar collapse	BAC with focal invasion	Adenocarcinoma with BAC	>50% BAC	Adenocarcinoma mixed subtype	Minimally invasive BAC
Type C – LBAC with foci of fibroblast proliferation	Adenocarcinoma with BAC features	Adenocarcinoma without BAC	<50% BAC	Adenocarcinoma	
Type D – poorly differentiated adenocarcinoma	Adenocarcinoma		0% BAC		Lepidic predominant adenocarcinoma
Type E – tubular adenocarcinoma					
Type F – papillary adenocarcinoma					

AIS, adenocarcinoma in situ; ATS, American Thoracic Society; BAC, bronchioloalveolar carcinoma; ERS, European Respiratory Society; IASLC, International Association for the Study of Lung Cancer; WHO, World Health Organization.

Pathology

The pathology of BAC has been controversial from the time of the original description of this disease. The greatest disagreements arise over what histological patterns should correctly be called BAC, whether evidence of an invasive adenocarcinoma component precludes the diagnosis of BAC, and the material required to make the diagnosis (i.e. cytology versus histological section).

The strictest criteria for diagnosis of BAC have emanated from the WHO lung tumor classification system. In 1999 (and repeated in 2004), these guidelines defined BAC as "growth of neoplastic cells along pre-existing alveolar structures (lepidic growth) without evidence of stromal, vascular, or pleural invasion."[2] These guidelines specifically preclude diagnosis of BAC based upon cytological specimens, stating that "the diagnosis of BAC requires thorough histologic evaluation to exclude the presence of invasive growth." The clinical utility of the WHO guidelines is limited by the fact that the majority of advanced lung cancers are diagnosed based solely upon cytology. While some pathologists have great confidence in a diagnosis of BAC based upon cytology, systematic studies have failed to agree upon specific cytological features which can make the diagnosis.[19–28] Some features that have been suggested to support a cytological diagnosis of BAC include absence of three-dimensional clusters, neoplastic cells in flat sheets, orderly arrangement of cells with round uniform nuclei, predominance of mucinous cells, absence of nuclear overlap, absence of irregular nuclear membranes, fine granular chromatin, and presence of nuclear grooves.[20]

Since the criteria proposed by the WHO had not been correlated with clinical outcomes, some investigators have developed more descriptive categories of BAC. Noguchi et al. studied 236 small peripheral adenocarcinomas and subdivided them into six categories (Table 25.1).[12] Of the BAC subtypes (types A–C), patients with type A and type B tumors had 100% 5-year survival. Patients with type A, B, and C tumors had an improved survival when compared with patients with types D, E, or F. Higashiyama subclassified BAC by examining 206 peripheral lung adenocarcinomas and classifying them based on the proportion of BAC (see Table 25.1).[29] Similar to Noguchi's series, among 17 patients with 100% BAC (type IV), none had nodal involvement and 5-year overall survival (OS) was 100%. Ebright et al. evaluated 100 resected tumors with some component of BAC and classified them based on the degree of invasive adenocarcinoma.[29] They classified tumors into four groups: pure BAC, BAC with focal invasion (BWFI), adenocarcinoma with bronchioloalveolar features (AWBF), and adenocarcinoma without evidence of BAC features. Overall survival was improved for patients with any component of BAC, emphasizing the importance of examining and subclassifying all NSCLC containing any element of BAC.

The largest pathological review yet performed examined 484 adenocarcinomas and divided them into BAC, adenocarcinoma with BAC, and adenocarcinoma without BAC.[30] Patients with pure BAC had no vascular, lymphatic, or pleural invasion. While there was more invasive disease in the adenocarcinoma with BAC features group (5.5% vascular invasion, 14.8% lymphatic invasion and 1.9% pleural invasion), the adenocarcinoma group without BAC showed the most invasion, with 84.9%, 61.4%, and 60.8% of tumors with vascular, lymphatic, and pleural invasion respectively. Unfortunately, no data were provided about clinical outcomes.

In 2011, a committee sponsored by the International Association for the Study of Lung Cancer, American Thoracic Society, and European Respiratory Society proposed a new classification system for lung adenocarcinomas.[3] The classification system proposes a variety of clinically useful standards for evaluation and management of lung adenocarcinomas but probably its most striking recommendation is to discontinue use of the term BAC. To support this recommendation, the committee notes that in common usage the term BAC refers to many disparate entities, including small noninvasive tumors with 100% 5-year overall survival, small invasive adenocarcinomas, mixed subtype invasive adenocarcinomas, invasive mucinous adenocarcinoma, as well as metastatic disease, all of which have different clinical presentations and courses. As a substitute, this committee recommends a new system of classification (Box 25.1). The organizing characteristics are the

Box 25.1 International Association for the Study of Lung Cancer/
American Thoracic Society/European Respiratory Society
classification of lung adenocarcinoma in resection specimens.

Preinvasive lesions

- Atypical adenomatous hyperplasia
- Adenocarcinoma in situ (≤3 cm formerly BAC)
  - Nonmucinous
  - Mucinous
  - Mixed mucinous/nonmucinous

Minimally invasive adenocarcinoma (≤3 cm lepidic predominant tumor with≤5 mm invasion)

- Nonmucinous
- Mucinous
- Mixed mucinous/nonmucinous

Invasive adenocarcinoma

- Lepidic predominant (formerly nonmucinous BAC pattern, with >5 mm invasion)
- Acinar predominant
- Papillary predominant
- Micropapillary predominant
- Solid predominant with mucin production

Reproduced with permission from Travis et al.[3]

Table 25.2 Presenting symptoms in bronchioloalveolar carcinoma.

Symptom	Frequency[31–35]
Asymptomatic	32–71%
Cough	20–42%
Dyspnea	4–27%
Hemoptysis	9–17%
Chest pain	6–26%
Pneumonia	2–19%
Bronchorrhea	3–11%

invasiveness of the tumors. Whether this new classification is widely adopted will depend upon its validation in several samples to confirm interobserver variability as well as clinical significance. Ultimately, if this classification system is found to be useful, it may be incorporated into the next iterations of the WHO classification system.

Clinical aspects: presentation, diagnostic considerations, and techniques

The clinical presentation of patients with BAC is similar to patients with other NSCLC tumors. The most common symptoms (Table 25.2) at the time of presentation are cough, hemoptysis, chest pain, dyspnea, weight loss, and bronchorrhea.[31–35] A symptom which is relatively unique to BAC is bronchorrhea, the production of large amounts of sputum which is often quite bothersome to the patient. The majority of retrospective reviews have suggested that patients with BAC are more likely than patients with other forms of adenocarcinoma to be women and to have never smoked cigarettes.[31–41]

The most comprehensive retrospective report to date described the experience of the Lung Cancer Study Group (LCSG) from 1977 to 1988. They identified 235 patients with BAC histology and compared their clinical characteristics with those of 710 patients with other adenocarcinomas and 608 patients with squamous cell tumors.[37] While patients with BAC were more likely than patients with squamous cell tumors to be women (42% versus 14%, p <0.001), the difference when compared to other

adenocarcinomas was less striking (42% versus 37%). Patients with BAC were more likely to present at an earlier stage (with smaller tumors and less frequent nodal involvement), with no history of smoking, and with no weight loss or weight loss <10%. The median age at diagnosis is not significantly different from patients with other forms of adenocarcinoma.

Just as patients with BAC have diverse clinical characteristics, the pattern of disease which is observed in such patients can vary widely and can be described as multifocal, pneumonic, or nodular. Multifocal disease refers to multiple sites of BAC within the lung. Pneumonic BAC has a consolidative radiographic appearance and is often bilateral. Nodular BAC is a multifocal process which has the radiographic appearance of multiple nodules.

Given the potential importance of distinguishing and classifying BAC from other adenocarcinomas, a number of investigators have attempted to correlate radiographic features with pathological findings at the time of surgery. Most work has focused on small peripheral tumors where the goal is to differentiate pure BAC from invasive adenocarcinoma. With more frequent high-resolution computed tomography (CT) screening, it became apparent that patients with BAC had unique radiographic findings, most commonly ground glass opacities (GGO).[42] In multifocal BAC, high-resolution CT can reveal a variety of patterns, including GGO, areas of consolidation, centrilobular and peripheral nodules, and air bronchograms.[43] Kim et al. studied 224 resected small peripheral adenocarcinomas. In correlating CT scan findings with the pathology of the tumors by Noguchi classification, they noted a correlation between the Noguchi classification and the mean proportion of GGO. Noguchi type A tumors had a mean proportion of GGO of 49% while Noguchi type C tumors had a mean of 23% GGO and Noguchi E tumors had a mean of 8% GGO.[44] Similarly, others have demonstrated that the higher the proportion of GGO on CT images of the tumor, the more likely it is to represent pure BAC.[45]

Quantification of the proportion of GGO is difficult to reproduce and would benefit from development of standardized criteria and methodology. Nakata et al. used NIH image software to reproducibly determine the percentage of GGO on high-resolution CT scans of tumors <3 cm.[46] By doing this, they found that among lesions with more than 90% GGO component, 87% had pure BAC as defined by the WHO, while in lesions with less than 50% GGO in the tumor, only 5% were pure BAC. In the intermediate range of 50–89%, 44% (20/45) tumors were pure BAC. Nomori et al. compared the Hounsfield units histograms of CT images of 10 patients with nonmucinous BAC and nine patients with AAH, arguing that AAH could be discerned from BAC based upon this relatively simple measurement.[47]

Fluorodeoxyglucose positron emission tomography (FDG-PET) imaging of BAC has only recently been explored. Initial reports all described a relatively low FDG avidity of BAC, with many lesions showing no uptake.[48–50] Further subclassification of patients with BAC revealed that the greater the percentage of BAC within a tumor, the more likely that the nodule will not show FDG avidity.[51] In a recent series of 22 peripheral tumors found as part of a screening project, of seven tumors that were not FDG avid, four were BAC.[85] Similarly, in a study of 192 early-stage lung tumors, nine tumors were found to be PET negative, and four of these tumors were BAC.[52] PET scanning of patients with known pure BAC have found that 42–63% of tumors are FDG avid compared with 97% of patients with NSCLC.[50,53–55] Some investigators are exploring other tracers that might be more reliably imaged in BAC.

Treatment

Surgery

Patients with early-stage disease are generally offered surgical resection of the tumor. Some controversy exists over the procedure of choice for patients with a unifocal presentation of BAC. Most early-stage NSCLC has been treated with lobectomy based upon the LCSG trial which showed a higher rate of recurrence for NSCLC patients treated with wedge resection compared with those who had a lobectomy.[56] Given the propensity for some BAC tumors to present at a relatively early stage and the decreased likelihood of lymph node involvement, wedge resections may be appropriate for some BAC patients. In a retrospective review of 33 patients with stage I BAC, no significant difference in survival was noted for patients treated with wedge or lobectomy.[36] Prospective evaluation of the use of limited resection for patients with small, peripheral adenocarcinomas with features of BAC (including GGO) was carried out by Koike et al. who performed limited resections on 46 patients (44 wedge resections and two segmentectomies) who were diagnosed with noninvasive BAC (AIS).[57] For these patients, the 5-year cancer-specific survival rate was 100%.

A second controversy in the management of BAC surrounds patients with multifocal BAC. BAC patients frequently present with multiple nodules without lymph node involvement or develop metachronous lesions in short periods of time. While these patients might be classified as having stage IV disease and therefore are not approached surgically, these nodules could also represent multiple primary tumors.[58] Thus, some groups have explored surgical resection in this setting. While Daly et al. reported a dismal 5-year survival for patients with bilateral multifocal BAC who underwent resection, a later series, which included both BAC and adenocarcinoma with BAC features, found that there was no significant difference in survival between patients with multifocal and unifocal disease.[59,60] These data suggest that if, after rigorous staging

evaluation, a multifocal BAC appears to represent individual primary tumors, surgical resection is a reasonable approach.

A more radical approach to management of multifocal BAC is lung transplantation.[61,62] De Perrot and colleagues did a worldwide survey of lung transplantations and identified a total of 26 patients who had lung transplantation for the diagnosis of multifocal BAC.[61] They found that, of 22 patients who survived the postoperative period, 13 had disease recurrence at a median of 12 months, with nine patients dying a median of 22 months after transplantation. Similarly, Zorn et al. reported a prospective study of lung transplantation in patients with multifocal BAC. Among eight patients who underwent transplant, six had disease recurrence and four died of BAC.[62] Disease recurrence in patients with BAC who have undergone transplantation is thought to be due to recurrence of host tumor and not related to new BAC forming from donor lung tissue.[63] Lung transplantation remains an investigative approach for the treatment of BAC.

Systemic therapy

Historical knowledge about systemic therapy for BAC has largely relied upon single-institution retrospective reviews and subset analyses of larger trials. Feldman et al. performed a retrospective examination of response to chemotherapy in patients with BAC treated at the Mayo Clinic from 1975 to 1985.[64] They identified 25 patients with BAC and compared those with 223 patients with other adenocarcinoma subtypes. There was no difference in response rate to chemotherapy, time to progression, or overall survival. Similarly, Breathnach et al. collected information on 28 patients with BAC and compared their course with 124 patients with other forms of NSCLC.[65] BAC patients treated with systemic chemotherapy (most with cisplatin-based combination chemotherapy regimens) had a median survival of 12 months compared to 8 months for patients other forms of NSCLC or 10 months for patients with other adenocarcinomas. The 1-year survival for patients with BAC was 48%. A Japanese retrospective identified 16 patients with BAC and 70 control patients with other variants of NSCLC.[66] The authors noted a 50% response rate to chemotherapy for BAC patients compared to a 27% response rate in controls ($p = 0.076$). The median survival for patients with BAC was 10 months compared to 8 months for controls ($p = 0.025$).

Subset analysis of ECOG 1594, a randomized trial of a four platinum-based doublet regimens, identified just 17 patients with BAC, though no specific pathological criteria were reported.[67] Of the 17 patients, the response rate was 6% compared to the overall response rate of 20%. The median survival for this group was 12 months.

The first prospective trial exclusively for patients with BAC was SWOG 9714.[68] This trial enrolled 58 patients from 1997 to 2000 and treated patients with a 96-h infusion of paclitaxel every 21 days. The definition of BAC was that chosen by local pathologists but subsequent central pathology review was performed. Three patients enrolled and treated were found to have adenocarcinoma without any BAC features. Further correlation between hospital pathology and central pathology review was not reported. The response rate for this treatment was 9%, with 40% of patients having stable disease. The median progression-free survival (PFS) was 5 months and the median overall survival was 12 months. Survival at 3 years was 13%. Two-thirds of patients had one grade 3 toxicity, with 43% having grade 3 or 4 neutropenia. Patients with mucinous BAC ($n=16$) had a median survival of 17 months compared to 9 months for nonmucinous BAC and 18 months for adenocarcinoma with BAC features ($n=17$).

A second trial of paclitaxel in BAC was undertaken by the European Organization for Research and Treatment of Cancer (EORTC).[69] Enrollment in this trial of BAC was limited to patients who fulfilled the following criteria: they did not have a primary adenocarcinoma elsewhere, had a peripheral tumor within the lung parenchyma, histological appearance with cells lining the alveolar septa with preservation of basic pulmonary architecture. Due to a poor response to treatment, EORTC 08956 was discontinued after 19 patients had been treated for a median of three cycles. After central review of all radiology, partial responses were seen in just 2/17 (11%) patients. The median progression-free survival was 2 months.

Recent data have examined the role of the EGFR tyrosine kinase inhibitors erlotinib and gefitinib in the treatment of BAC. In the trials examining the treatment of NSCLC with erlotinib or gefitinib, a subset of patients had dramatic radiographic responses.[70,71] A retrospective review of patients treated with gefitinib identified improved response rates for patients with adenocarcinoma with BAC features (38% versus 14% for other adenocarcinomas), never smokers (36% versus 8% for former or current smokers), and patients with Karnofsky performance status $\geq 80\%$ (22% versus 8% for patients with $\leq 70\%$).[72]

Gefitinib was the first EGFR tyrosine kinase inhibitor to be prospectively studied in patients with BAC. The South West Oncology Group (SWOG) conducted a phase 2 trial of gefitinib (500 mg daily) in 136 patients with metastatic, recurrent, or inoperable BAC.[73] Patients who had no prior treatment had a 17% response rate, compared to 9% for previously treated patients. Median overall survival was 13 months for both previously treated and untreated patients. The authors concluded that further evaluation of EGFR tyrosine kinase inhibitors was worthwhile for this patient population, potentially in combination with other drugs. Similarly, Cadranel *et al.* reported the Intergroupe Francophone de Cancérologie Thoracique (IFCT) experience with gefitinib in BAC in European patients.[74] In 88 previously untreated patients who had adenocarcinoma with BAC subtype, there was a disease control rate of 29%, with 13% of patients having a partial response. The median OS was 13 months and they noted a dramatically worse median PFS for mucinous (2.6 months) versus nonmucinous BAC (11 months).

Simultaneously, investigators at the Memorial Sloan-Kettering Cancer Center and Vanderbilt-Ingram Cancer Center commenced a multiinstitutional phase 2 trial of erlotinib in patients with BAC.[75] To be eligible, all patients needed pathological evidence of adenocarcinoma with some bronchioloalveolar features or pure BAC. Patients had measurable disease and were either chemotherapy naïve or had refractory disease after one therapeutic regimen. In this trial, partial responses were seen in 22% of patients and median survival exceeded 1 year. In patients with "pure BAC" (AIS), there was a 20% response rate and median OS of just 4 months compared with a response rate of 23% and median OS of 19 months in those with adenocarcinomas. Patients with *EGFR* mutations in this study had a response rate of 83% with a median OS of 23 months. There were no responses among patients with *KRAS* mutations.

An alternative strategy to blocking EGFR signaling by small molecule tyrosine kinases is to use antibodies such as cetuximab directed at the extracellular domain.[76] The use of cetuximab was evaluated in 68 patients with advanced-stage pure BAC or adenocarcinoma with BAC features who had received fewer than two prior chemotherapy regimens. The confirmed response rate was 7% and stable disease was observed in 35%. One of seven patients with a *KRAS* mutation had a response to therapy.

Building on the observation that there is a high frequency of somatic mutations in *p53* in BAC, the Eastern Cooperative Oncology Group (ECOG) (E6597) investigated adenovirus p53 administered by bronchoalveolar lavage every 2 weeks.[77] Twenty-five patients were treated, with 10 of them treated at the recommended phase 2 dose. Twenty-three patients were assessable, 16 of whom had stable disease.

A variety of treatments whose aim is to treat bronchorrhea, an often debilitating symptom of BAC, have also been reported. Treatment of the underlying malignancy is the most effective treatment of this symptom but symptomatic relief can be obtained with some agents. Limited reports support the efficacy of macrolide antibiotics, epidermal growth factor tyrosine kinase inhibitors, and inhaled indomethacin for the reduction of bronchorrhea.[78–82] No prospective studies have been reported for the treatment of this troublesome symptom.

Prognosis

With the continually changing pathological definition of BAC, evaluating consistent groups of patients to give a sense of prognosis is difficult. While the data are modest, there is an overall sense that patients with a clinical diagnosis of BAC have a more protracted clinical course than patients with other subtypes of adenocarcinoma. The prognostic significance of a diagnosis of BAC (AIS or LPA) can differ dramatically based on a variety of pathological features. Patients with adenocarcinoma with BAC features (LPA) have a prognosis which is dependent upon stage but closer to the prognosis associated with other subtypes of lung adenocarcinoma.[83] In contrast, patients with peripheral lung lesion without invasion, the prototype of the pure BAC (AIS), can have 5-year disease-free survivals of 100% after surgical reseaction.[12]

Recommendations

In the management of patients with entities previously known as BAC, we begin with a complete description of the pathology for each patient through close consultation with the pathologist. At a minimum, the pathology report for all patients should include the type of NSCLC (e.g. squamous, adenocarcinoma, large cell, etc.) and if any subtypes (e.g. lepidic) are present, an estimation of the relative proportions should be clearly stated. If multiple foci of disease are present, the pathology from each site of disease should be rigorously compared to exclude multiple primary lung cancers. If adequate tissue is available, molecular analysis for *EGFR* mutations can also be helpful in the pathological analysis. Initial treatment decisions focus on whether the patient can be rendered disease free by surgery. Complete staging evaluation including CT chest and upper abdomen, PET scan, magnetic resonance imaging of the brain and, when necessary, mediastinoscopy is performed to identify whether patients with single lesions have distant metastases and determine whether those patients with multifocal disease can or should have surgical treatment as their primary treatment. If surgical treatment is not feasible, discussion of systemic therapies focuses on the goal of prolonging life and controlling symptoms.

Choice of therapy can be aided by understanding the patient's *EGFR* and *KRAS* mutation status, when available. In patients with minimal or no smoking history or those with known *EGFR* mutations, we begin treatment with erlotinib alone or erlotinib with cytotoxic chemotherapy.[84] Additional systemic therapy options are guided by good clinical practices in the treatment of patients with lung adenocarcinoma. In patients suitable for disease-specific clinical trials, adequate tissue should be obtained to allow detailed pathological description, *EGFR* and *KRAS* determination, and assessment of other molecular markers of interest.

References

1. Liebow AA. Bronchiolo-alveolar carcinoma. Adv Intern Med 1960; 10: 329–58.

2. Travis WD, Brambilla E, Muller KM, Harris CC. *Pathology and Genetics of Tumours of the Lung, Pleura, Thymus and Heart*. Lyon, France: IARC Press, 2004.

3. Travis WD, Brambilla E, Noguchi M, *et al*. International Association for the Study of Lung Cancer/American Thoracic Society/European Respiratory Society international multidisciplinary classification of lung adenocarcinoma. J Thorac Oncol 2011; 6: 244–85.

4. Read WL, Page NC, Tierney RM, Piccirillo JF, Govindan R. The epidemiology of bronchioloalveolar carcinoma over the past two decades: analysis of the SEER database. Lung Cancer 2004; 45: 137–42.

5. Auerbach O, Garfinkel L. The changing pattern of lung carcinoma. Cancer 1991; 68: 1973–7.

6. Barsky SH, Cameron R, Osann KE, Tomita D, Holmes EC. Rising incidence of bronchioloalveolar lung carcinoma and its unique clinicopathologic features. Cancer 1994; 73: 1163–70.

7. Falk RT, Pickle LW, Fontham ET, *et al*. Epidemiology of bronchioloalveolar carcinoma. Cancer Epidemiol Biomarkers Prev 1992; 1: 339–44.

8. Rolen KA, Fulton JP, Tamura DJ, Strauss GM. *Bronchoalveolar carcinoma (BAC) of the lung is related to cigarette smoking: a case control study from Rhode Island*. Presented at the ASCO Meeting, New Orleans, 2003. p.2711.

9. Palmarini M, Fan H. Molecular biology of jaagsiekte sheep retrovirus. Curr Top Microbiol Immunol 2003; 275: 81–115.

10. Palmarini M, Fan H, Sharp JM. Sheep pulmonary adenomatosis: a unique model of retrovirus-associated lung cancer. Trends Microbiol 1997; 5: 478–83.

11. Wootton SK, Halbert CL, Miller AD. Sheep retrovirus structural protein induces lung tumours. Nature 2005; 434: 904–7.

12. Noguchi M, Morikawa A, Kawasaki M, *et al*. Small adenocarcinoma of the lung. Histologic characteristics and prognosis. Cancer 1995; 75: 2844–52.

13. Aoyagi Y, Yokose T, Minami Y, *et al*. Accumulation of losses of heterozygosity and multistep carcinogenesis in pulmonary adenocarcinoma. Cancer Res 2001; 61: 7950–4.

14. Yoshida Y, Shibata T, Kokubu A, *et al*. Mutations of the epidermal growth factor receptor gene in atypical adenomatous hyperplasia and bronchioloalveolar carcinoma of the lung. Lung Cancer 2005; 50(1): 1–8.

15. Sarkaria IS, Pham D, Ghossein RA, *et al*. SCCRO expression correlates with invasive progression in bronchioloalveolar carcinoma. Ann Thorac Surg 2004; 78: 1734–41.

16. Rusch VW, Reuter VE, Kris MG, *et al*. Ras oncogene point mutation: an infrequent event in bronchioloalveolar cancer. J Thorac Cardiovasc Surg 1992; 104: 1465–9.

17. Marchetti A, Buttitta F, Pellegrini S, *et al*. Bronchioloalveolar lung carcinomas: K-ras mutations are constant events in the mucinous subtype. J Pathol 1996; 179: 254–9.

18. Garfield DH, Cadranel J, West HL. Bronchioloalveolar carcinoma: the case for two diseases. Clin Lung Cancer 2008; 9: 24–9.

19. Atkins KA. The diagnosis of bronchioloalveolar carcinoma by cytologic means. Am J Clin Pathol 2004; 122: 14–16.

20. Ohori NP, Santa Maria EL. Cytopathologic diagnosis of bronchioloalveolar carcinoma: does it correlate with the 1999 World Health Organization definition? Am J Clin Pathol 2004; 122: 44–50.

21. Auger M, Katz RL, Johnston DA. Differentiating cytological features of bronchioloalveolar carcinoma from adenocarcinoma of the lung in fine-needle aspirations: a statistical analysis of 27 cases. Diagn Cytopathol 1997; 16: 253–7.

22. Lozowski W, Hajdu SI. Cytology and immunocytochemistry of bronchioloalveolar carcinoma. Acta Cytol 1987; 31: 717–25.

23. MacDonald LL, Yazdi HM. Fine-needle aspiration biopsy of bronchioloalveolar carcinoma. Cancer 2001; 93: 29–34.

24. Morishita Y, Fukasawa M, Takeuchi M, Inadome Y, Matsuno Y, Noguchi M. Small-sized adenocarcinoma of the lung. Cytologic characteristics and clinical behavior. Cancer 2001; 93: 124–31.

25. Silverman JF, Finley JL, Park HK, Strausbauch P, Unverferth M, Carney M. Fine needle aspiration cytology of bronchioloalveolar cell carcinoma of the lung. Acta Cytol 1985; 29: 887–94.

26. Tao LC, Delarue NC, Sanders D, Weisbrod G. Bronchiolo-alveolar carcinoma: a correlative clinical and cytologic study. Cancer 1978; 42: 2759–67.

27. Tao LC, Weisbrod GL, Pearson FG, Sanders DE, Donat EE, Filipetto L. Cytologic diagnosis of bronchioloalveolar carcinoma by fine-needle aspiration biopsy. Cancer 1986; 57: 1565–70.

28. Zaman SS, van Hoeven KH, Slott S, Gupta PK. Distinction between bronchioloalveolar carcinoma and hyperplastic pulmonary proliferations: a cytologic and morphometric analysis. Diagn Cytopathol 1997; 16: 396–401.

29. Higashiyama M, Kodama K, Yokouchi H, *et al*. Prognostic value of bronchiolo-alveolar carcinoma component of small lung adenocarcinoma. Ann Thorac Surg 1999; 68: 2069–73.

30. Terasaki H, Niki T, Matsuno Y, *et al*. Lung adenocarcinoma with mixed bronchioloalveolar and invasive components: clinicopathological features, subclassification by extent of invasive foci, and immunohistochemical characterization. Am J Surg Pathol 2003; 27: 937–51.

31. Carretta A, Canneto B, Calori G, *et al*. Evaluation of radiological and pathological prognostic factors in surgically-treated patients with bronchoalveolar carcinoma. Eur J Cardiothorac Surg 2001; 20: 367–71.

32. Martini N, Khafagy MM, Melamed MR, Golbey RB, Beattie EJ. Bronchiolar carcinoma: a review of 152 patients. Clin Bull 1973; 3: 98–101.

33. Okubo K, Mark EJ, Flieder D, *et al*. Bronchoalveolar carcinoma: clinical, radiologic, and pathologic factors and survival. J Thorac Cardiovasc Surg 1999; 118: 702–9.

34. Regnard JF, Santelmo N, Romdhani N, *et al*. Bronchioloalveolar lung carcinoma: results of surgical treatment and prognostic factors. Chest 1998; 114: 45–50.

35. Volpino P, Cavallaro A, Cangemi R, et al. Comparative analysis of clinical features and prognostic factors in resected bronchioloalveolar carcinoma and adenocarcinoma of the lung. Anticancer Res 2003; 23: 4959–65.

36. Breathnach OS, Kwiatkowski DJ, Finkelstein DM, et al. Bronchioloalveolar carcinoma of the lung: recurrences and survival in patients with stage I disease. J Thorac Cardiovasc Surg 2001; 121: 42–7.

37. Grover FL, Piantadosi S. Recurrence and survival following resection of bronchioloalveolar carcinoma of the lung. The Lung Cancer Study Group experience. Ann Surg 1989; 209: 779–90.

38. Liu YY, Chen YM, Huang MH, Perng RP. Prognosis and recurrent patterns in bronchioloalveolar carcinoma. Chest 2000; 118: 940–7.

39. Rena O, Papalia E, Ruffini E, et al. Stage I pure bronchioloalveolar carcinoma: recurrences, survival and comparison with adenocarcinoma of the lung. Eur J Cardiothorac Surg 2003; 23: 409–14.

40. Sakurai H, Dobashi Y, Mizutani E, et al. Bronchioloalveolar carcinoma of the lung 3 centimeters or less in diameter: a prognostic assessment. Ann Thorac Surg 2004; 78: 1728–33.

41. Volpino P, d'Andrea N, Cangemi R, Mingazzini P, Cangemi B, Cangemi V. Bronchioloalveolar carcinoma: clinical, radiographic, and pathological findings. Surgical results. J Cardiovasc Surg (Torino) 2001; 42: 261–7.

42. Jang HJ, Lee KS, Kwon OJ, Rhee CH, Shim YM, Han J. Bronchioloalveolar carcinoma: focal area of ground-glass attenuation at thin-section CT as an early sign. Radiology 1996; 199: 485–8.

43. Akira M, Atagi S, Kawahara M, Iuchi K, Johkoh T. High-resolution CT findings of diffuse bronchioloalveolar carcinoma in 38 patients. Am J Roentgenol 1999; 173: 1623–9.

44. Kim EA, Johkoh T, Lee KS, et al. Quantification of ground-glass opacity on high-resolution CT of small peripheral adenocarcinoma of the lung: pathologic and prognostic implications. Am J Roentgenol 2001; 177: 1417–22.

45. Matsuguma H, Nakahara R, Anraku M, et al. Objective definition and measurement method of ground-glass opacity for planning limited resection in patients with clinical stage IA adenocarcinoma of the lung. Eur J Cardiothorac Surg 2004; 25: 1102–6.

46. Nagata M, Shijubo N, Walls AF, Ichimiya S, Abe S, Sato N. Chymase-positive mast cells in small sized adenocarcinoma of the lung. Virchows Arch 2003; 443: 565–73.

47. Nomori H, Ohtsuka T, Naruke T, Suemasu K. Differentiating between atypical adenomatous hyperplasia and bronchioloalveolar carcinoma using the computed tomography number histogram. Ann Thorac Surg 2003; 76: 867–71.

48. Hidaka N, Nagao T, Asoh A, Kondo Y, Nagao K. Expression of E-cadherin, alpha-catenin, beta-catenin, and gamma-catenin in bronchioloalveolar carcinoma and conventional pulmonary adenocarcinoma: an immunohistochemical study. Mod Pathol 1998; 11: 1039–45.

49. Kim BT, Kim Y, Lee KS, et al. Localized form of bronchioloalveolar carcinoma: FDG PET findings. Am J Roentgenol 1998; 170: 935–9.

50. Smith GT, Hubner KF, Peterson A, Hunter K, Neff J. FDG PET for evaluation of bronchioloalveolar cell carcinoma (BAC) of the lung. Clin Positron Imaging 1998; 1: 260.

51. Yap CS, Schiepers C, Fishbein MC, Phelps ME, Czernin J. FDG-PET imaging in lung cancer: how sensitive is it for bronchioloalveolar carcinoma? Eur J Nucl Med Mol Imaging 2002; 29: 1166–73.

52. Marom EM, Sarvis S, Herndon JE 2nd, Patz EF Jr. T1 lung cancers: sensitivity of diagnosis with fluorodeoxyglucose PET. Radiology 2002; 223: 453–9.

53. Heyneman LE, Patz EF. PET imaging in patients with bronchioloalveolar cell carcinoma. Lung Cancer 2002; 38: 261–6.

54. Higashi K, Nishikawa T, Seki H, et al. Comparison of fluorine-18-FDG PET and thallium-201 SPECT in evaluation of lung cancer. J Nucl Med 1998; 39: 9–15.

55. Gould MK, Maclean CC, Kuschner WG, Rydzak CE, Owens DK. Accuracy of positron emission tomography for diagnosis of pulmonary nodules and mass lesions: a meta-analysis. JAMA 2001; 285: 914–24.

56. Ginsberg RJ, Rubinstein LV. Randomized trial of lobectomy versus limited resection for T1 N0 non-small cell lung cancer. Lung Cancer Study Group. Ann Thorac Surg 1995; 60: 615–22; discussion 22–3.

57. Koike T, Togashi K, Shirato T, et al. Limited resection for noninvasive bronchioloalveolar carcinoma diagnosed by intraoperative pathologic examination. Ann Thorac Surg 2009; 88: 1106–11.

58. Martini N, Melamed MR. Multiple primary lung cancers. J Thorac Cardiovasc Surg 1975; 70: 606–12.

59. Daly RC, Trastek VF, Pairolero PC, et al. Bronchoalveolar carcinoma: factors affecting survival. Ann Thorac Surg 1991; 51: 368–76; discussion 76–7.

60. Ebright MI, Zakowski MF, Martin J, et al. Clinical pattern and pathologic stage but not histologic features predict outcome for bronchioloalveolar carcinoma. Ann Thorac Surg 2002; 74: 1640–6; discussion 1646–7.

61. De Perrot M, Chernenko S, Waddell TK, et al. Role of lung transplantation in the treatment of bronchogenic carcinomas for patients with end-stage pulmonary disease. J Clin Oncol 2004; 22: 4351–6.

62. Zorn GL Jr, McGiffin DC, Young KR Jr, Alexander CB, Weill D, Kirklin JK. Pulmonary transplantation for advanced bronchioloalveolar carcinoma. J Thorac Cardiovasc Surg 2003; 125: 45–8.

63. Garver RI Jr, Zorn GL, Wu X, McGiffin DC, Young KR Jr, Pinkard NB. Recurrence of bronchioloalveolar carcinoma in transplanted lungs. N Engl J Med 1999; 340: 1071–4.

64. Feldman ER, Eagan RT, Schaid DJ. Metastatic bronchioloalveolar carcinoma and metastatic adenocarcinoma of the lung: comparison of clinical manifestations, chemotherapeutic responses, and prognosis. Mayo Clin Proc 1992; 67: 27–32.

65. Breathnach OS, Ishibe N, Williams J, Linnoila RI, Caporaso N, Johnson BE. Clinical features of patients with stage IIIB and IV bronchioloalveolar carcinoma of the lung. Cancer 1999; 86: 1165–73.

66. Fujimoto N, Segawa Y, Takigawa N, et al. Clinical investigation of bronchioloalveolar carcinoma: a retrospective analysis of 53 patients in a single institution. Anticancer Res 1999; 19: 1369–73.

67. Schiller JH, Harrington D, Belani CP, et al. Comparison of four chemotherapy regimens for advanced non-small-cell lung cancer. N Engl J Med 2002; 346: 92–8.

68. West HL, Crowley JJ, Vance RB, et al. Advanced bronchioloalveolar carcinoma: a phase II trial of paclitaxel by 96-hour infusion (SWOG 9714): a Southwest Oncology Group study. Ann Oncol 2005; 16: 1076–80.

69. Scagliotti GV, Smit E, Bosquee L, et al. A phase II study of paclitaxel in advanced bronchioloalveolar carcinoma (EORTC trial 08956). Lung Cancer 2005; 50: 91–6.

70. Fukuoka M, Yano S, Giaccone G, et al. Multi-institutional randomized phase II trial of gefitinib for previously treated patients with advanced non-small-cell lung cancer (the IDEAL 1 Trial). J Clin Oncol 2003; 21: 2237–46.

71. Kris MG, Natale RB, Herbst RS, et al. Efficacy of gefitinib, an inhibitor of the epidermal growth factor receptor tyrosine kinase, in symptomatic patients with non-small cell lung cancer: a randomized trial. JAMA 2003; 290: 2149–58.

72. Miller VA, Kris MG, Shah N, et al. Bronchioloalveolar pathologic subtype and smoking history predict sensitivity to gefitinib in advanced non-small-cell lung cancer. J Clin Oncol 2004; 22: 1103–9.

73. West HL, Franklin WA, McCoy J, et al. Gefitinib therapy in advanced bronchioloalveolar carcinoma: Southwest Oncology Group Study S0126. J Clin Oncol 2006; 24: 1807–13.

74. Cadranel J, Quoix E, Baudrin L, et al. IFCT–0401 Trial: a phase II study of gefitinib administered as first-line treatment in advanced adenocarcinoma with bronchioloalveolar carcinoma subtype. J Thorac Oncol 2009; 4: 1126–35.

75. Miller VA, Riely GJ, Zakowski MF, et al. Molecular characteristics of bronchioloalveolar carcinoma and adenocarcinoma, bronchioloalveolar carcinoma subtype, predict response to erlotinib. J Clin Oncol 2008; 26: 1472–8.

76. Ramalingam SS, Lee JW, Belani CP, *et al.* Cetuximab for the treatment of advanced bronchioloalveolar carcinoma (BAC): an Eastern Cooperative Oncology Group phase II study (ECOG 1504). J Clin Oncol 2011; 29: 1709–14.

77. Keedy V, Wang W, Schiller J, *et al.* Phase I study of adenovirus p53 administered by bronchoalveolar lavage in patients with bronchioloalveolar cell lung carcinoma: ECOG 6597. J Clin Oncol 2008; 26: 4166–71.

78. Milton DT, Kris MG, Gomez JE, Feinstein MB. Prompt control of bronchorrhea in patients with bronchioloalveolar carcinoma treated with gefitinib (Iressa). Support Care Cancer 2005; 13: 70–2.

79. Suga T, Sugiyama Y, Fujii T, Kitamura S. Bronchioloalveolar carcinoma with bronchorrhoea treated with erythromycin. Eur Respir J 1994; 7: 2249–51.

80. Takao M, Inoue K, Watanabe F, *et al.* Successful treatment of persistent bronchorrhea by gefitinib in a case with recurrent bronchioloalveolar carcinoma: a case report. World J Surg Oncol 2003; 1: 8.

81. Tamaoki J, Kohri K, Isono K, Nagai A. Inhaled indomethacin in bronchorrhea in bronchioloalveolar carcinoma: role of cyclooxygenase. Chest 2000; 117: 1213–14.

82. Homma S, Kawabata M, Kishi K, *et al.* Successful treatment of refractory bronchorrhea by inhaled indomethacin in two patients with bronchioloalveolar carcinoma. Chest 1999; 115: 1465–8.

83. Ebbert JO, Chhatwani L, Aubry MC, *et al.* Clinical features of bronchioloalveolar carcinoma with new histologic and staging definitions. J Thorac Oncol 2010; 5: 1213–20.

84. Herbst RS, Prager D, Hermann R, *et al.* TRIBUTE: a phase III trial of erlotinib hydrochloride (OSI-774) combined with carboplatin and paclitaxel chemotherapy in advanced non-small-cell lung cancer. J Clin Oncol 2005; 23: 5892–9.

85. Lindell RM, *et al.* Lung cancer screening experience: a retrospective review of PET in 22 non-small cell lung carcinomas detected on screening chest CT in a high-risk population. Am J Roentgenol 2005; 185(1): 126–131.

26 Primary Adenoid Cystic Carcinoma of the Lung

John G. Devlin[1] and Corey J. Langer[2]

[1] Hematology/Oncology Section, Bryn Mawr Medical Specialists Associates, Bryn Mawr, PA, USA
[2] Abramson Cancer Center, University of Pennsylvania, Philadelphia, PA, USA

Introduction

Primary bronchogenic adenoid cystic carcinoma (ACC) is a rare cancer, estimated to represent only 0.2% of all primary pulmonary malignancies. Compared to the more common small cell or nonsmall cell lung cancers, this rare tumor typically displays a more indolent clinical behavior; as such, recognition of this uncommon tumor has important clinical implications. Despite the successful development of targeted therapies for many other cancers, the mainstay of treatment remains surgical resection, though recurrences frequently occur despite this intervention. Interventional bronchoscopy, radiation therapy, systemic chemotherapy, and newer targeted therapies may ultimately provide additional benefit, although adequately powered prospective studies are unfortunately lacking. The identification of genetic and environmental risk factors, and the development of optimal treatment strategies, will likely remain active areas of ongoing research to the extent made possible by such a rare clinical entity.

Background

Adenoid cystic carcinoma is an uncommon epithelial tumor, first reported by Billroth in the mid-19th century. It typically arises in the minor salivary glands, though it has also been reported rarely to arise in the breast, cervix, skin, prostate, upper aerodigestive tract, and lung.[1–5] Published literature is unfortunately riddled with misclassification and misnomers for this rare tumor, which in past years has been called basaloid squamous carcinoma, cylindroma, pseudoadenomatous basal cell carcinoma, adenomyoepithelioma, and even adenoma (among other less common terms), making interpretation of the literature confusing and difficult. Although very low in incidence, recognition of this uncommon bronchial tumor has important clinical implications, given the very different natural history and treatment of this tumor compared to more common primary lung cancers.[6] This chapter takes into account hundreds of reported cases of this rare bronchogenic tumor in roughly 70 years of world literature.

Pathology

Bronchial adenoid cystic carcinomas are typically discovered in a submucosal location, where they are often associated with mucous glands,[7] a likely site of origin, though a dual origin of ductal and myoepithelial cells has also been suggested, similar to their salivary gland counterparts.[8] Grossly, typical adenoid cystic carcinomas are small, infiltrative lesions with a poorly defined capsule, usually tan, pink, or gray in color.[9] Histologically, perineural invasion is a common and prominent feature; angiolymphatic invasion is rarer.[6,8,9] Tumor cells are usually small and uniform, possessing densely compact nuclei and very little basophilic cytoplasm; mitoses or necrosis are rarely seen.[9] Cells may grow in solid sheets, in tubular clusters, or in the classic cribriform structure, giving rise to the previously used "cylindroma" descriptor.[9] Clinical tumor behavior and prognosis may correlate with the pattern of tumor clustering (see below),[10,11] though this has not been consistently observed.[8] Intracellular periodic acid-Schiff (PAS)-positive mucin is often found but is even more prominent in the extracellular lumen.[8,9,12] The surrounding stroma is characteristically myxoid or extensively hyalinized, and may be composed of excess basement membrane.[9] Light microscopy typically reveals bronchial submucosal spread as reported by Payne et al.,[13] Conlan et al.,[14] Reid et al.,[15] and later by Moran et al.,[8] who additionally described a predominantly cribriform pattern in resected metastases, which resembled the primary tumor in nearly every case.

Immunohistochemical studies reported by Nomori and colleagues[10] have shown that the tubular and cribriform subtypes stain with antibodies to keratin (similar to normal tracheal duct epithelium and myoepithelial cells), Schwann (S-100) protein, human secretory component (SC), and lactoferrin (similar to

Table 26.1 Growth pattern and prognosis of 12 patients based on histological grade for adenoid cystic carcinoma of the tracheobronchial tree.

Tumor grade	Grade I (tubular or cribriform with no solid component)	Grade II (tubular or cribriform with solid <20%)	Grade III (>20% solid component)
Growth pattern	50% entirely intraluminal, 50% partially infiltrating	100% partially infiltrating	33% partially infiltrating, 66% extensively infiltrating
Prognosis	All 4 patients alive (4–86 months postoperatively)	Four patients alive (36–87 months postoperatively); 1 patient deceased (63 months postoperatively)	One patient alive (49 months postoperatively); 2 patients deceased (41–78 months postoperatively)

Source: Nomori et al.[10]

normal tracheobronchial serous acinar cells). The solid subtype typically does not stain with these markers, perhaps implying a more poorly differentiated subtype.[10] In addition, necrosis, mitoses, angiolymphatic invasion, and a higher synthetic-phase fraction are more likely to be observed.[16] In the same study,[10] a strong correlation was observed between the histological tumor grade (defined as grade I being tubular or cribriform with no solid component, grade II identical but with solid component <20%, grade III identical but with solid component >20%) and the gross tumor growth pattern, with the grade I tumors more likely to show an intraluminal growth pattern, and the solid component/grade III tumors far more likely to invade the tracheobronchial architecture (Table 26.1). Moran et al.[8] reported tumor staining with actin, keratin, and vimentin, which should differentiate adenoid cystic carcinomas from a histologically similar adenocarcinoma, which does not typically stain for such myoepithelial markers.

Potential molecular therapeutic targets have been investigated. In contrast to the more common nonsmall cell lung cancers, expression of p53, cyclooxygenase-2 (COX-2), and Her-2-neu (erb2) has generally not been observed in adenoid cystic bronchial carcinoma,[16] although some authors have proposed that "de-differentiated" variants may exist that overexpress Her-2-neu, and, as in the case of "transformed" adenoid cystic carcinomas of nonpulmonary sites, probably behave more aggressively.[17,18] Expression of CD117, marking the presence and function of the protooncogene c-kit, has been reported in all 13 patients evaluated by Albers et al.,[7] which is consistent with that of adenoid cystic carcinomas in the upper aerodigestive tract. In the same study, CD117 expression did not correlate with Ki-67 expression or with tumor grade.[7] Recent data indicate absence of activating c-kit mutations despite c-kit expression, perhaps explaining this observation, as well as the typically poor response of these tumors to c-kit inhibition.[19] Similarly, expression of epidermal growth factor receptor (EGFR) has been noted, though without EGFR gene amplification or activating mutations in exons 18–21 in at least one study.[20] Mutations in the Wnt signaling pathway have also been described.[21]

The poorly differentiated, solid subtype of adenoid cystic carcinoma is often confused with the more common basaloid squamous carcinoma, probably as a result of similar histopathological and immunohistochemical features (though the latter are somewhat variable). Emanuel et al.[22] reported that immunohistochemistry for p63 may help distinguish between the two, however. Ultrastructural studies[23–25] have also shown subtle differences between the two tumors. Hewan-Lowe and Dardick[23] found in a review of six cases (only one of which was bronchial) that adenoid cystic carcinoma is more likely to display oligocilia, a combination of large and small compressed lumina, and cytoplasmic filaments that displace organelles, whereas the basaloid squamous carcinoma is more likely to show focal squamous differentiation, including keratin "pearl" formation. Additionally, basaloid squamous carcinomas (particularly esophageal variants) are often associated with dysplasia in overlying or adjacent mucosa,[26] and direct contiguity is sometimes discovered between the tumor and overlying squamous carcinoma in situ.[27] Ultrastructural studies of exclusively bronchial adenoid cystic carcinomas are lacking, however.

Clinical aspects

Adenoid cystic carcinoma is estimated to comprise 0.2% of all primary pulmonary tumors.[28,29] In a study of 50 patients by Xu et al.,[30] adenoid cystic carcinomas occurred in the trachea with the same frequency as squamous cell carcinomas (together the two most common primary tracheal tumors), and were the most common primary bronchial tumor, along with carcinoid tumors.

The natural history of adenoid cystic carcinomas of any primary body tissue is generally very different from that of more common tumors of different histology arising in the same anatomical location. Classically, adenoid cystic cancers behave in indolent fashion, typically growing over years to decades.[6] Indeed, 5-year survival rates are probably an inadequate way to describe prognosis, and recurrence may ultimately occur beyond 5 years.[6] Regional nodal involvement upon diagnosis is uncommon. In one representative older study it was estimated to be 2%, though the rate of distant metastasis was still 26%,[31] implying a higher chance of hematogenous spread. In other series,[32] the metastatic rates have been higher. Metastatic involvement in the lungs is generally observed whether the primary site originates in the lung or the far more common primary salivary gland. The lungs are preferentially involved at some point in the natural history of nonpulmonary adenoid cystic tumors in about 40% of patients, though long-term survival of years or even decades despite lung metastases has been reported.[6] Involvement of visceral organs or bone portends a prognosis that is far worse.[6,8]

Median age of onset for primary bronchial adenoid cystic carcinoma is in the fifth decade of life, with a range from 29 to 76 years old, though most published cases describe patients between ages 35 and 50. There may be a slight predilection for females,[6,7] though most studies of bronchial variants report a relatively even gender distribution. Further demographic study has not been performed, though Asians and Caucasians are the best represented racial groups in studies that have reported ethnicity.

Risk factors for this uncommon bronchial tumor have not clearly been identified. Occasional reports[12,28] have described patients with a prior history of pulmonary tuberculosis and suspicious multinodular lungs, which on final surgical pathology specimens contained both tuberculomas and tumor. No formal causal or correlative relationship, however, has been established between these two diseases. Importantly, tobacco smoking is not felt to be a risk factor for this disease, unlike the more common bronchogenic carcinomas.[6] This observation is consistent with reported data on risk factors for adenoid cystic carcinomas of other primary sites,[2–5] including the upper aerodigestive tract. There are no data regarding environmental exposures or known genetic abnormalities that may predispose to these bronchial lesions.

Patients often present with symptoms of bronchial irritation, including hemoptysis, wheezing, or cough, typically of subacute or even chronic duration. Kanematsu et al.[33] found that 80% of 16 patients were symptomatic. The 50-year, 20-patient, seminal Mayo Clinic series reported by Conlan et al.[14] found an average duration of such symptoms before diagnosis to be 4.5 years, underscoring the symptomatic chronicity and indolent but locally disruptive behavior of this entity. On occasion, a history of recurrent pulmonary infections can be elicited, particularly during very early childhood,[34,35] probably from partial airway obstruction with recurrent subtle postobstructive infection.

Given the more common diseases responsible for these generic pulmonary symptoms, delay of diagnosis and even frank misdiagnosis occur frequently. For example, Wright et al.[36] reported the case of a 23-year-old woman found to have an adenoid cystic carcinoma occluding the left main bronchus, after presenting with subacute exertional dyspnea and chest tightness and a 10-year history of recurrent pulmonary infections. The woman carried a diagnosis of MacLeod (or Swyer-James) syndrome based on an abnormally hyperlucent left lung found on chest roentgogram at the age of 15. Swyer-James syndrome is a manifestation of postinfectious obliterative bronchiolitis. Stalpaert et al.[37] described a 23-year-old woman who suffered from recurrent bronchitis, dyspnea, and intermittent stridor for at least 3 years before diagnosis. Toole et al.[38] reported the case of a 31-year-old woman with recurrent pneumonitis for 8 years, which for unclear reasons seemed to flare during three of her four pregnancies. She was later found to have adenoid cystic carcinoma in her lower trachea and right mainstem bronchus. Older patients are often erroneously treated empirically for presumed chronic obstructive pulmonary disease or asthma but their symptoms persist despite bronchodilator and antiinflammatory therapy.[39]

Other presentations have been described. Cases of acute pneumonitis and even life-threatening stridor have been reported as a result of frank airway obstruction, occasionally necessitating emergency intervention.[40] A single report exists of a patient presenting with right scapular pain radiating down the right arm, Horner syndrome, and classic physical examination findings for a Pancoast tumor, who was later found to have an adenoid cystic carcinoma of the right lung apex.[41]

Xu et al. reviewed the typical symptoms of 50 patients with various tracheobronchial tumors, 31 of which were malignant.[30] Of the 24 patients with primary tumors arising in the trachea, 18 were malignant, and 10 patients had adenoid cystic carcinoma. Signs and symptoms from primary tracheal tumors (benign or malignant) included stridor, respiratory distress, and cyanosis. Patients were typically misdiagnosed with asthma, as often seen in other studies.[30,40] In the same study, patients with primary bronchus tumors were most likely to present with atelectasis (with complete obstruction) or recurrent suppurative pulmonary infections (with incomplete obstruction).[30] In a review of 14 patients with predominantly tracheal adenoid cystic carcinomas reported by Albers et al.,[7] dyspnea was the presenting symptom in 10 patients, cough was present in eight patients, and seven patients were found to have stridor or wheezing. Although patients with adenocystic carcinoma are usually symptomatic, some tumors may be found incidentally on chest imaging for other purposes such as those undergoing surveillance post resection of prior sarcoma or as follow-up to previous infections.[42–44]

Radiographic appearance and diagnosis

Diagnosis is usually made via bronchoscopy; the gross appearance is often similar to that of conventional bronchogenic carcinoma. Conlan et al.[14] described the usual appearance of this tumor as a polypoid mass with a broad base and superficial necrosis, partially or even totally obstructing the airway lumen. Bronchoscopic debulking may be required to restore the airway function. Albers et al.[7] have described multiple lobulated whitish-yellow masses with increased vascularity, covered by intact bronchial mucosa. In earlier stage disease, the overlying mucosa is often uninvolved, though fine needle aspiration of suspiciously prominent submucosa has been reported to concur with definitive surgical pathological examination in one study.[45]

Pulmonary ACC classically arises in the proximal tracheobronchial tree, where the usual extensive submucosal spreading is often observed.[13,15,32,46] Promegger et al.[46] reported a review of 16 patients with primary adenoid cystic carcinomas of the trachea and bronchus; nine occurred in the tracheal bifurcation, five in the trachea itself, one in the middle-lobe bronchus, and only one was truly parenchymal. ACC in the lung periphery has been reported; however, the incidence of peripheral tumors is felt to be only 10%.[28,43,47] Peripheral lesions form an intraluminal polypoid mass more readily, and perhaps at an earlier stage, though at least one case of submucosal extension to the proximal bronchus has been reported.[28] Additionally, ACC may rarely assume the form of multiple peripheral pulmonary nodules.[14]

On chest radiographs, endobronchial tumors are typically suspected when opacification and/or atelectasis of a section of lung is found.[14] However, small tracheal tumors may be missed on chest films.[30] Computed tomography (CT) scanning typically confirms a central mass and postobstructive pneumonitis, and may or may not show localized mediastinal invasion in advanced cases. Pleural effusion, pneumothorax, solitary lung masses, multifocal metastatic disease, and other patterns are far rarer. Primary adenoid cystic carcinoma of the lung is fluorodeoxyglucose (FDG) avid on positron emission tomography (PET) scanning.[48] Pulmonary function tests (PFTs) may provide evidence of an obstructive defect that does not improve with bronchodilators.

Laboratory evaluation is not helpful. No tumor markers have been reported to be sufficiently reliable to aid in the diagnosis, assessment of treatment response, or surveillance after a potentially curative treatment. There is a single case report of a tumor producing CA19-9,[49] describing a trend in serum levels of CA19-9 that seemed to correlate with clinical events. Serum CA125 and SLX, however, were not helpful.[49,50]

Treatment

Surgical resection

Surgical resection remains the current standard of care for tracheobronchial adenoid cystic carcinoma. The goals of surgery are complete resection of the tumor (if feasible), relief of obstruction, and restoration of ventilation.[30] Surgery can provide a cure or at least a long interval until recurrence, though often the goals of surgery are ultimately palliative in nature. Early authors advocated exploratory surgery to evaluate candidacy for total resection,[51] even when palliative excision was all that could be accomplished. Near-unanimous agreement exists in the literature, however, that carinal involvement with simultaneous bilateral mainstem bronchus invasion precludes an attempt at optimal curative resection.[52]

Complete surgical excision is mandatory to prevent recurrence.[14,53] Most authors recommend intraoperative frozen section of margins to assure the highest chance of complete surgical resection.[14] Unfortunately, complete resection is often not possible, due to the submucosal location, pattern of local spread, central nature of this tumor, and the advanced stage at diagnosis.[13,14] More recently, presentation at an earlier stage of disease has become more common, perhaps as a result of improved preoperative radiographic staging, which probably allows for better assessment of surgical candidacy.[14] Additionally, the usual absence of tobacco-associated comorbidity may allow more patients to be medically operable.

Surgical approaches have been evaluated and described extensively,[54–57] particularly in the case of tracheal tumors by Grillo et al.[54–56] Transverse cervical incision is the preferred approach for upper tracheal tumors, and a right posterolateral thoracotomy provides access to the lower half. Median sternotomy and a cervical incision allow for visualization and manipulation of the entire trachea. Ideally, the extent of tracheal resection is determined preoperatively, and the tracheal anastomosis, done with absorbable suture, is kept under little tension postoperatively to avoid complications.[52]

Given the central location of most proximal bronchial tumors, unilateral sleeve pneumonectomy is the most common procedure reported, although certainly small peripheral tumors have been successfully excised by less extensive resection, such as lobectomy.[8] Mixed results have been reported with combined tracheal and carinal resections, with poorer outcomes occurring more frequently when greater than 6.6 cm of trachea was resected.[30,37,52,54–56] Some authors recommend a two-stage procedure when bilateral thoracotomy is needed, to minimize perioperative morbidity.[52]

Even with adequate resection, adenoid cystic carcinomas often recur, either locally or distantly. Moran et al.,[8] Houston et al.,[58] and Wilkins et al.[59] have each separately reported recurrence of primary tracheobronchial adenoid cystic carcinomas decades after initial resection. Promegger et al.[46] reported the rates of recurrence in 16 patients with surgically resected adenoid cystic carcinomas of the trachea and bronchus, most of which were central lesions requiring pneumonectomy and/or carinotracheal resection. Of the 11 patients available in follow-up, three had suffered a local recurrence at a median time of over 14 years after surgery (range 10–16 years), and six patients had experienced a distant recurrence at a median time of 8 years (range 2–16.5 years) postoperatively.[46] However, second long-term remissions can potentially be achieved with resection of the recurrence. For example, of 10 patients followed on average for 5.5 years by Xu and colleagues (range 1–10 years), one patient experienced a local recurrence 2 years after a lateral tracheal wall resection, which was again successfully resected (no information was available on initial margins).[30]

Long-term survival has occasionally been reported, even after suboptimal resection, perhaps due to the tumor's indolent growth rate.[10,12,30,58,59] An illustrative case was reported by Schoenfeld et al.[12] A 42-year-old patient presented with a tubular variant adenoid cystic carcinoma involving the left mainstem bronchus and near-total atelectasis of the left lung (T4N0M0). Pneumonectomy failed to remove all gross tumor; the aortic wall and bronchial margin were noted to contain residual carcinoma. Twenty-two years later, the patient was readmitted with a 2-week history of moderately severe dyspnea at rest, ultimately attributed to occlusion of the bronchus intermedius and right mainstem bronchus caused by recurrent tumor, which on biopsy resembled the original adenoid cystic carcinoma. Endobronchial laser and radiation treatments were administered, with some success, though a new right lower lobe metastasis appeared soon after. Interestingly, this patient eventually succumbed to unrelated ileus and pancreatitis, and not from respiratory difficulties or tumor, though no autopsy was permitted.

Though debate exists regarding the actual chance of cure, surgery, when done successfully, usually affords most patients a long disease-free interval, which is often of the order of years to decades as noted in case reports and small series. For example, a patient reported by Xu et al.[30] died 8 years after an initial carinal resection, and 3 years after he was found to have bilateral pulmonary metastases, though "unrelated causes" were reportedly the cause of death. Promegger et al.[46] reported survival rates of 79% at 5 years and 57% at 10 years, with surgical treatment. Gaissert et al.[60] reported a retrospective experience with 270 patients (135 of whom had tracheal adenoid cystic carcinoma) treated surgically; most also received additional radiation. A statistically significant association with long-term survival was observed for completeness of resection, negative surgical margins, or adenoid cystic histology.[60] Interestingly, nodal status, tumor length, and type of resection were not significantly associated with survival.[60] In the rare studies that have reported survival rates,[32,61] 5-year and 10-year survival rates with surgical resection appear to be in the range of 50–80% and 30–60%, respectively.

Interventional bronchoscopy

For patients with symptomatic partial or near-total airway obstruction who are not surgical candidates, palliative endobronchial laser resection has become a standard measure. Albers et al.[7] reported on 14 patients (nine women and five men), 12 of whom were primarily treated with palliative laser resection and radiation therapy; the other two patients were treated with radiation alone and with tracheal resection followed by radiation, respectively. Recurrence was documented in 11 of the 14, with an average time to recurrence or metastasis of 4.6 years. Half of all recurrences were localized to the trachea or bronchi; five patients had multiple recurrences in different sites. Metastases occurred in four patients, primarily to the lungs, and five patients died of the disease. Three of the 12 patients initially treated with laser resection later required tracheal resection with anastomosis. Single case reports note similar results using laser therapy.[62,63]

Radiation therapy

The lack of adequately powered clinical trials precludes an accurate assessment of radiation therapy's survival impact in ACC. In one 10-year review of salivary gland ACC,[64] surgical resection followed by radiation therapy provided excellent local control but was not found to affect survival. Kanematsu et al.[33] reported a retrospective experience of 16 patients with tracheobronchial adenoid cystic carcinomas from 1972 to 1998, 11 of whom underwent resection. Microscopic residual disease remained in six of the 11 resected patients, who were then treated with palliative radiotherapy. Five additional patients were medically inoperable, had unresectable tumors, and/or had refused surgery, and were treated with radiation therapy alone. Five-year survival (91% versus 40%) and ten-year survival (76% versus 0%) was superior for the patients who underwent surgery followed by radiation versus radiation alone, though patients who had only received radiation may still have derived some benefit.

Refaely et al.[52] reported results of 13 patients with resected adenoid cystic carcinomas of the tracheobronchial tree, 10 of whom received adjuvant radiation therapy; of the remaining three, one died intraoperatively and two did not receive radiation. One patient who had received radiation died of myocardial infarction 3 years postoperatively (with no sign of recurrence), and the other nine patients were still alive without recurrence as of publication date (range 4 years to 12 years 2 months postoperative). The two patients who did not receive radiation both suffered fatal "metastatic spread" at 5 years 2 months and 7 years after the operation, respectively, though sites of recurrence were not further anatomically defined. Andou et al.[65] reported a 5-year survival rate of 68.6% in seven patients treated surgically; six had also received either adjuvant or neoadjuvant radiation. In the study by Gaissert et al.,[60] most patients had received radiation (as reviewed above), and fared quite well.

Based on extant literature and personal experience, we recommend local postoperative radiotherapy for those patients with positive surgical margins and/or residual disease. Radiotherapy likely reduces local recurrence and may provide a survival benefit.

Chemotherapy

There have been no trials evaluating chemotherapy alone in bronchial adenoid cystic carcinomas. Extrapolating from upper aerodigestive tract variants, however, would suggest that chemotherapy is generally reserved for locoregionally recurrent disease without further surgical or radiation options, or for frank metastatic disease.[66] Dreyfuss et al.[67] reported a response rate of 40–50% and an average response duration of 3–7 months with the CAP regimen (cyclophosphamide, doxorubicin, cisplatin), one of the most commonly reported regimens. Adding 5-fluorouracil to this regimen increased the duration of response to 8 months, albeit with increased toxicity.[68] A review by Laurie et al., however, has cited a somewhat lower response rate of 30%.[69] Vinorelbine, mitoxantrone, and 5-fluorouracil each have yielded roughly a 10% response rate.[69] Taxanes have rarely been reported to provide benefit.[70] Overall combination chemotherapy has not clearly improved survival, although responses may provide benefits in symptom palliation.[69] Data are scarce for more "modern" chemotherapeutic agents, such as pemetrexed or nab-paclitaxel, in the management of this cancer.

Though often responsive initially, these tumors tend not to be controlled by chemotherapy. Moreover, since ACC patients may live for years despite recurrence and/or metastases, it is difficult to define the optimal time to initiate such therapy, and reliance on clinical judgment is essential (i.e. patients with symptoms requiring palliation or with evidence of rapid progression may benefit the most). We recommend a conservative approach and choose to employ chemotherapy only in the face of tumor-related symptoms and in the absence of alternative therapies. The mere presence of asymptomatic metastases does not in itself require initiation of chemotherapy particularly if slow growth is observed.

Targeted therapy

Unfortunately, there are no targeted therapy trials exclusive to bronchial variants. One of the most commonly tested targeted approaches in adenoid cystic carcinoma of salivary glands has been the inhibition of c-kit.[71,72] Imatinib mesylate

Table 26.2 Prognosis based on clinical stage at diagnosis for 16 patients with adenoid cystic carcinoma (ACC) of the lung and tracheobronchial tree.

Clinical stage (by TNM[3])	I (T1–2N0M0)	II (T1–2N1M0 or T3N0M0)	III (T1–2 N2–3 M0, T3N1–3 M0, or T4N1–3 M0)	IV (anyT,anyN, M1)	Unknown
Prognosis	five of 8 patients alive 5–12 years postoperatively; 3 patients deceased 3–9 years postoperatively	NA	Only a single patient, alive with "massive" local recurrence 2 years postoperatively	Two of 2 patients deceased, 2–12 months after diagnosis	Of 4 patients, 1 alive (3 lost to follow-up)
Follow-up information	One alive patient has metastasis to contralateral lung; 3 deceased patients died from other causes	NA	Patient had regional lymph node metastasis at diagnosis	One patient with liver metastasis died 2 months later of ACC; 1 patient with rib and lymph node metastasis died 12 months later of ACC	The single patient with follow-up is alive but experienced a stump recurrence

Source: Moran *et al.*[8]

(Gleevec©) inhibits platelet-derived growth factor receptor β (PDGFR-β), the Philadelphia chromosome protein bcr-abl, and the c-kit protein (CD117), which is often overexpressed in adenoid cystic tumors[71,72] (including bronchial variants as reported by Albers *et al.*[7]). One study reported objective responses to imatinib mesylate in two patients with salivary gland adenoid cystic carcinomas, allowing one to have potentially curative resection.[71] However, a subsequent phase 2 study of 16 patients with unresectable or metastatic adenoid cystic carcinomas of the salivary glands found no objective responses to imatinib mesylate in any of the 15 evaluable patients, leading to early termination of the study.[72] Dual inhibition of Her-1/EGFR and Her-2 with lapatinib produced no meaningful responses in one study.[73] In another study, Akt signaling inhibition with the anti-HIV drug nelfinavir resulted in growth inhibition of adenoid cystic tumor cells, though to date only preclinical data exist in that regard.[74] Further investigation of targeted therapies will no doubt continue, though reports are only sporadic.

In light of these findings, we do not recommend using imatinib or lapatinib in patients with pulmonary ACC. It is unlikely that other Her-2-targeted agents will provide benefit.

Prognosis

There have been efforts to assign value to various prognostic factors. Some authors have advocated that overall survival may be influenced by pathological factors, such as tumor grade or level of differentiation.[10] Data from upper aerodigestive tract adenoid cystic carcinoma[11,75–78] had already suggested this correlation, most notably from Spiro *et al.*[75] Although patients can survive for years to decades despite recurrence and metastases, long-term survival was rare in patients with grade III tumors. Additionally, patients with tubular tumors tended to have a better prognosis, which was also observed by Ishida *et al.*[76] in primary adenoid cystic carcinomas of the lung.[11,75–78] Nomori *et al.*[10] described 12 patients with adenoid cystic carcinomas of the tracheobronchial tree, all of whom were treated surgically, eight of whom also received radiation. In addition

to observing that grade I/tubular tumors tended to grow intraluminally, and that grade III/solid tumors tended to invade extraluminally, the authors also observed that the two patients who died of distant metastasis had grade III tumors (see Table 26.1). A preliminary correlation between prognosis and tumor grade was thus hypothesized.

Other studies, though obviously handicapped by the small number of cases, have suggested similar associations between histology and prognosis. Interestingly, the single patient overexpressing Her-2-neu (erb2) reported in the study by Lin *et al.*[16] was the single patient to develop distant metastases, roughly 4 years after surgery. Albers *et al.*[7] reported that perineural invasion could not be correlated with impaired survival in the three patients in whom it was observed.

Some authors have disputed these assumptions.[7,8] Most notably, Moran *et al.*[8] assigned clinical stage at diagnosis as the most important prognostic factor in their study of 16 patients with predominantly (*n* = 14) tracheal adenoid cystic carcinomas (Table 26.2). Two patients who presented with liver and/or bone metastasis died in 2 and 12 months, respectively. In contrast, three patients who had well-circumscribed endobronchial lesions were alive at 5, 10, and 12 years after surgery, respectively. Thus, earlier stage disease portended a better prognosis, despite tumor grade.

Recommendations

Primary adenoid cystic carcinoma of the tracheobronchial tree is a very rare cancer. Recognition of ACC as an entity distinct from the more common lung cancers is essential, given its dramatically different natural history. Its indolent growth rate explains both its insidious symptoms and its prolonged natural history; higher-grade tumors probably behave more aggressively but are relatively rare. Long-term survival has been reported, most often with surgical resection, which remains the current standard of care. Radiotherapy may provide a reduction in the rates of local recurrence, although trials have not demonstrated a clear survival benefit to date. Systemic chemotherapy and targeted therapy have yielded mixed results.

Future studies to develop better treatment recommendations will be hampered by the small numbers of available patients. Eventual recurrence and/or metastasis are the rule rather than the exception. In spite of the high likelihood of disease recurrence, patients may live for years to decades and should be managed accordingly. Future areas for research include the identification of risk factors and the development of potential molecular targets of systemic therapy as well as optimal treatment strategies.

References

1. Billroth T. Die cylindergeschwalst. In: *Untersuchungen ueber die Entwicklung der Blutgefasse*. Berlin: G Reimer, 1856. pp.55–69.

2. Cavanzo FJ, Taylor HB. Adenoid cystic carcinoma of the breast: an analysis of 21 cases. Cancer 1969; 24: 740–746.

3. Fowler WC, Miles PA, Surwit EA, et al. Adenoid cystic carcinoma of the cervix: report of 9 cases and a reappraisal. Obstet Gynecol 1978; 52: 337–9.

4. Olaffsson J, VanNostrand A. Adenoid cystic carcinoma of the larynx: a report of four cases and a review of the literature. Cancer 1977; 40: 1307–12.

5. Lawrens JB, Mazur MT. Adenoid cystic carcinoma: a comparative pathologic study of tumors in the salivary glands, breast, lung, and cervix. Hum Pathol 1982; 13: 916–24.

6. Sessions RB, Harrison LB, Forastiere AA. Tumors of the salivary glands and paragangliomas. In: DeVita VT, Hellman S, Rosenberg SA (eds) *Cancer. Principles and Practice of Oncology*, 6th edn. Philadelphia: Lippincott, 2001. pp.886–900.

7. Albers E, Lawrie T, Harrell JH, et al. Tracheobronchial adenoid cystic carcinoma: a clinicopathologic study of 14 cases. Chest 2004; 125: 1160–5.

8. Moran CA, Suster S, Koss MN. Primary adenoid cystic carcinoma of the lung: a clinical and immunohistochemical study of 16 cases. Cancer 1994; 73: 1390–7.

9. Cotran RS, Kumar V, Robbins SL, et al. Head and neck. In: Schoen FJ (ed) *Robbins Pathologic Basis of Disease*, 5th edn. Philadelphia: WB Saunders, 1994. pp.752–3.

10. Nomori H, Kaseda S, Kobayashi K, et al. Adenoid cystic carcinoma of the trachea and mainstem bronchus: a clinical, histopathologic, and immunohistochemical study. J Thorac Cardiovasc Surg 1988; 96: 271–7.

11. Szanto PA, Luna MA, Tortoledo ME, et al. Histologic grading of adenoid cystic carcinoma of the salivary glands. Cancer 1984; 54: 1062–9.

12. Schoenfeld N, Rahn W, Loddenkemper R. Twenty-two year survival after incomplete resection of advanced adenoid cystic bronchogenic carcinoma. Eur Respir J 1996; 9: 1560–1.

13. Payne WS, Ellis FH Jr, Woolner LB, et al. The surgical treatment of cylindroma (adenoid cystic carcinoma) and muco-epidermoid tumors of the bronchus. J Thorac Cardiovasc Surg 1959; 38: 709–26.

14. Conlan AA, Payne WS, Woolner LB, et al. Adenoid cystic carcinoma (cylindroma) and mucoepidermoid carcinoma of the bronchus: factors affecting survival. J Thorac Cardiovasc Surg 1978; 76: 369–77.

15. Reid JD. Adenoid cystic carcinoma (cylindroma) of the bronchial tree. Cancer 1952; 5: 685–94.

16. Lin CM, Li AF, Wu LH, et al. Adenoid cystic carcinoma of the trachea and bronchus – a clinicopathologic study with DNA flow cytometric analysis and oncogene expression. Eur J Cardiothorac Surg 2002; 22: 621–5.

17. Nagao T, Gaffey TA, Serizawa H, et al. Dedifferentiated adenoid cystic carcinoma: a clinicopathologic study of 6 cases. Mod Pathol 2003; 16: 1265–72.

18. Seethala RR, Hunt JL, Baloch ZW, et al. Adenoid cystic carcinoma with high-grade transformation: a report of 11 cases and a review of the literature. Am J Surg Pathol 2007; 31(11): 1683–94.

19. Aubry MC, Heinrich MC, Molina J, et al. Primary Adenoid cystic carcinoma of the lung: absence of KIT mutations. Cancer 2007; 110(11): 2507–10.

20. Macarenco RS, Uphoff TS, Gilmer HF, et al. Salivary gland-type lung carcinomas: an EGFR immunohistochemical, molecular genetic, and mutational analysis study. Mod Pathol 2008; 21(9): 1168–75.

21. Daa T, Kashima K, Kaku N, et al. Mutations in components of the Wnt signaling pathway in adenoid cystic carcinoma. Mod Pathol 2004; 17: 1475–82.

22. Emanuel P, Wang B, Wu M, et al. p63 Immunohistochemistry in the distinction of adenoid cystic carcinoma from basaloid squamous carcinoma. Mod Pathol 2005; 18: 645–50.

23. Hewan-Lowe K, Dardick I. Ultrastructural distinction of basaloid squamous carcinoma and adenoid cystic carcinoma. Ultrastruct Pathol 1995; 19: 371–81.

24. Wain SL, Kier R, Vollmer RT, et al. Basaloid-squamous carcinoma of the tongue, hypopharynx and larynx: report of 10 cases. Hum Pathol 1986; 17: 1158–66.

25. Tandler B. Ultrastructure of adenoid cystic carcinoma of salivary gland origin. Lab Invest 1971; 24: 504–12.

26. Epstein JI, Sears DL, Tucker RS, et al. Carcinoma of the esophagus with adenoid cystic differentiation. Cancer 1984; 53: 1131–6.

27. Azzopardi JG, Menzies T. Primary oesophageal adenocarcinoma. Br J Surg 1962; 49: 497–506.

28. Inoue H, Iwashita A, Kanegae H, et al. Peripheral pulmonary adenoid cystic carcinoma with substantial submucosal extension to the proximal bronchus. Thorax 1991; 46: 147–8.

29. DeLima R. Bronchial adenoma: clinicopathologic study and results of treatment. Chest 1980; 77: 81–4.

30. Xu LT, Sun ZF, Li ZJ. Clinical and pathologic characteristics in patients with tracheobronchial tumor: report of 50 patients. Ann Thorac Surg 1987; 43: 276–8.

31. Goldstraw P, Lamb D, McCormack RJM, et al. The malignancy of bronchial adenomas. J Thorac Cardiovasc Surg 1976; 72: 309–14.

32. Molina JR, Aubry MC, Lewis JE, et al. Primary salivary gland-type lung cancer: spectrum of clinical presentation, histopathologic, and prognostic factors. Cancer 2007; 110(10): 2253–9.

33. Kanematsu T, Yohena T, Uehara T, et al. Treatment outcome of resected and nonresected primary adenoid cystic carcinoma of the lung. Ann Thorac Cardiovasc Surg 2002; 8: 74–7.

34. Scott BF. Cylindromatous adenoma of the bronchus in a 4-year old child. Dis Chest 1963; 44: 547.

35. Ahel V, Zubovic I, Rozmanic V. Bronchial adenoid cystic carcinoma with saccular bronchiectasis as a cause of recurrent pneumonia in children. Pediatr Pulmonol 1992; 12: 260–2.

36. Wright CL, Gandhi M, Mitchell CA. Adenoid cystic carcinoma of the left main bronchus mimicking MacLeod's syndrome. Thorax 1996; 51: 451–2.

37. Stalpaert G, Deneffe G, van Maele R. Surgical treatment of adenoid cystic carcinoma of the left main bronchus and trachea by left pneumonectomy, resection of 7.5 cm of trachea, and direct reanastomosis of right lung. Thorax 1979; 34: 554–6.

38. Toole AL, Stern H. Carcinoid and adenoid cystic carcinoma of the bronchus. Ann Thorac Surg 1972; 13: 63–81.

39. Nakayama M, Hosomura M, Yamahata T, et al. A case of adenoid cystic carcinoma of the left main bronchus, which was performed carinal resection and reconstruction while the aortic arch is pulled down. [Article in Japanese] Kyobu Geka 2001; 54: 31–5.

40. Takenaka H, Choh S, Ikoma Y, et al. A case of adenoid cystic carcinoma presenting with stridor and which was treated by reversed gamma type stent placement. [Article in Japanese] Nihon Kokyuki Gakkai Zasshi 1998; 36: 106–10.

41. Hatton MQ, Allen MB, Cooke NJ. Pancoast syndrome: an unusual presentation of adenoid cystic carcinoma. Eur Respir J 1993; 6: 271–2.

42. Azukari K, Yoshioka K, Seto S, et al. Adenoid cystic carcinoma arising in the intrapulmonary bronchus. Intern Med 1996; 35: 407–9.

43. Okura T, Shiode M, Tanaka R, et al. A case of peripheral adenoid cystic carcinoma. [Article in Japanese] Nihon Kyobu Shikkan Gakkai Zasshi 1990; 28: 773–6.

44. Dohba S, Fujita H, Kawamura T, *et al*. Adenoid cystic carcinoma of the lower lobe of right lung: report of a case. [Article in Japanese] Kyobu Geka 2003; 56: 977–80.

45. Qiu S, Nampoothiri MM, Zaharopoulos P, *et al*. Primary pulmonary adenoid cystic carcinoma: report of a case diagnosed by fine-needle aspiration cytology. Diagn Cytopathol 2004; 30: 51–6.

46. Prommegger R, Salzer GM. Long-term results of surgery for adenoid cystic carcinoma of the trachea and bronchi. Eur J Surg Oncol 1998; 24: 440–4.

47. Tolis GA, Fry WA, Head L, *et al*. Bronchial adenomas. Surg Gynec Obstet 1972; 134: 605–10.

48. Campistron M, Rougette I, Courbon F, *et al*. Adenoid cystic carcinoma of the lung: interest of 18FDG PET/CT in the management of an atypical presentation. Lung Cancer 2008; 59(1): 133–6.

49. Tamura S, Nakano T, Yamaguchi K, *et al*. A case of adenoid cystic carcinoma of the bronchus producing cancer-associated antigen, CA19-9. Intern Med 1992; 31: 363–7.

50. Tamura S, Yamaguchi K, Terada M, *et al*. Immunohistochemical analysis of CA19-9, SLX, and CA125 in adenoid cystic carcinoma of the trachea and bronchus. [Article in Japanese] Nihon Kyobu Shikkan Gakkai Zasshi 1992; 30: 407–11.

51. Thompson DT, Doyle JA, Roncoroni AJ. Carinal resection, left pneumonectomy, and right lung anastomosis for adenocystic basal cell carcinoma (cylindroma). Thorax 1969; 24: 752–5.

52. Refaely Y, Weissberg D. Surgical management of tracheal tumors. Ann Thorac Surg 1997; 64: 1429–32.

53. Yang, PY, Liu MS, Chen CH, *et al*. Adenoid cystic carcinoma of the trachea: a report of seven cases and literature review. Chang Gung Med J 2005; 28(5): 357–62.

54. Grillo HC. Reconstruction of the trachea. Thorax 1973; 28: 667–79.

55. Grillo, HC. Circumferential resection and reconstruction of the mediastinal and cervical trachea. Ann Surg 1965; 162: 374–88.

56. Grillo HC, Dignan EF, Miura T, *et al*. Extensive resection and reconstruction of mediastinal trachea without prosthesis or graft: an anatomical study in man. J Thorac Cardiovasc Surg 1964; 48: 741–9.

57. Pearson FG, Todd TRJ, Cooper JD. Experience with primary neoplasms of the trachea and carina. J Thorac Cardiovasc Surg 1984; 88: 511–18.

58. Houston HE, Payne WS, Harrison EG, *et al*. Primary cancers of the trachea. Arch Surg 1969; 99: 132–40.

59. Wilkins EW, Darling RC, Soutter L, *et al*. A continuing clinical survey of adenomas of the trachea and bronchus in a general hospital. J Thorac Cardiovasc Surg 1963; 46: 279–91.

60. Gaissert HA, Grillo HC, Shadmehr MB, *et al*. Long-term survival after resection of primary adenoid cystic and squamous cell carcinoma of the trachea and carina. Ann Thorac Surg 2004; 78: 1889–96.

61. Kang DY, Yoon YS, Kim HK, *et al*. Primary salivary gland-type lung cancer: surgical outcomes. Lung Cancer 2011; 72(2): 250–4.

62. Diaz-Jimenez JP, Canela-Cordona M, Maestre-Alcacer J. Nd:YAG laser photoresection of low-grade malignant tumors of the tracheobronchial tree. Chest 1990; 97: 20–2.

63. Rau BK, Harikrishnan KM, Krishna S. Neodymium:YAG laser therapy for obstructing tracheobronchial tumors. Ann Acad Med Singapore 1994; 23: 29–31.

64. Sur RK, Donde B, Levin V, *et al*. Adenoid cystic carcinoma of the salivary glands: a review of 10 years. Laryngoscope 1997; 107: 1276–80.

65. Andou A, Shimizu N, Okabe K, *et al*. A clinical study of resected adenoid cystic carcinoma of the tracheobronchial tree. [Article in Japanese] Kyobu Geka 1993; 46: 134–9.

66. Laurie SA, Ho AL, Fury MG, *et al*. Systemic therapy in the management of metastatic or locally recurrent adenoid cystic carcinoma of the salivary glands: a systematic review. Lancet Oncol 2011; 12(8): 815–24.

67. Dreyfuss AI, Clark JR, Fallon BG, *et al*. Cyclophosphamide, doxorubicin and cisplatin combination chemotherapy for advanced carcinomas of salivary gland origin.Cancer 1987: 60: 2869–72.

68. Dimery IW, Legha SS, Shirinian M, *et al*. Fluorouracil, doxorubicin, cyclophosphamide and cisplatin combination chemotherapy for advanced or recurrent salivary gland carcinoma. J Clin Oncol 1990: 8: 1056–62.

69. Laurie SJ, Su YB, Pfister DG. Chemotherapy in the management of metastatic adenoid cystic carcinoma: a systematic review. ASCO Annual Meeting Proceedings. J Clin Oncol 2005; 23(16 S): 5581.

70. Perrot E, Davy N, Poubeau P, *et al*. Chemotherapy with paclitaxel for lung metastases of cystic adenoid carcinoma. A case report and review of the literature. Rev Pneumol Clin 2003; 59: 371–4.

71. Alcedo JC, Fabrega JM, Arosemena JR, *et al*. Imatinib mesylate as treatment for adenoid cystic carcinoma of the salivary glands: report of two successfully treated cases. Head Neck 2004; 26: 829–31.

72. Hotte SJ, Winquist EW, Lamont E, *et al*. Imatinib mesylate in patients with adenoid cystic cancers of the salivary glands expressing c-kit: a Princess Margaret Hospital Phase II Consortium Study. J Clin Oncol 2005; 23: 585–90.

73. Aqulnik M, Cohen EW, Cohen RB, *et al*. Phase II study of lapatinib in recurrent or metastatic epidermal growth factor receptor and/or erbB2 expressing adenoid cystic carcinoma and non adenoid cystic carcinoma malignant tumors of the salivary glands. J Clin Oncol 2007; 25(25): 3978–84.

74. Aqulnik M, Cohen EW, Cohen RB, *et al*. Phase II study of lapatinib in recurrent or metastatic epidermal growth factor receptor and/or erbB2 expressing adenoid cystic carcinoma and non adenoid cystic carcinoma malignant tumors of the salivary glands. J Clin Oncol 2007; 25(25): 3978–84.

75. Spiro RH, Huvos AG, Strong EW. Adenoid cystic carcinoma: factors influencing survival. Am J Surg 1979; 138: 579–83.

76. Ishida T, Yano T, Sugimachi K, *et al*. Clinical applications of the pathologic properties of small cell carcinoma, large cell carcinoma, and adenoid cystic carcinoma of the lung. Semin Surg Oncol 1990; 6: 53–63.

77. Fordice J, Kershaw C, El-Neggar A, *et al*. Adenoid cystic carcinoma of the head and neck: predictors of morbidity and mortality. Arch Otolaryngol Head Neck Surg 1999; 125: 149–52.

78. Perzin KH, Gullane P, Clairmont AC. Adenoid cystic carcinoma arising in salivary glands: a correlation of histological features and clinical outcome. Cancer 1978; 42: 265–82.

Section 6: Gastrointestinal Tumors

27 Uncommon Tumors of the Esophagus

Lawrence Leichman[1] and Robert Rosser[2]

[1] Aptium GI Cancer Consortium, Palm Springs, CA, USA
[2] Anatomic Pathology, Desert Regional Medical Center, Palm Springs, CA, USA

Introduction

Esophageal cancers continue to rank among the eight most common malignancies in the world. However, the incidence of esophageal tumors tends to be far lower in western than in Middle Eastern and Far Eastern countries.[1] While the overall worldwide incidence of esophageal cancer may not have changed, in developed western countries, a marked shift in histology has taken place: the incidence of adenocarcinoma of the esophagus, with etiological roots in Barrett esophagus, is now greater than squamous cell cancer.[2] Still, in parts of the United States, Europe, Africa, Middle Eastern and Far Eastern countries, squamous cell tumors of the esophagus continue to predominate.[3] Although the incidence of esophageal cancer is lower in women than men, the death rates for men and women are equal. Furthermore, it has yet to be proven that treatment options ought to differ for those afflicted with esophageal squamous versus those with adenocarcinomas. Indeed, despite differing populations and separate molecular etiologies, the prognosis for typical squamous cell cancers and adenocarcinomas of esophagus, which represent greater than 92% of all esophageal cancers, is quite similar.[4]

This chapter will review the data for etiology and treatment options for the remaining 7–8% of esophageal tumors. These include unusual variants of esophageal squamous cell and adenocarcinomas, mesenchymal tumors of the esophagus, neural crest tumors originating in the esophagus, lymphoid tumors of the esophagus, choriocarcinomas, melanomas, and tumors that have a propensity to metastasize to the esophagus. At the conclusion of each section, we give advice on what we consider to be the best therapy. However, it should be noted that the evidence for "best treatment" or "standard treatment" for these uncommon tumors of the esophagus will be based, at best, on limited data.

Esophageal embryology

The esophagus comes directly from the cranial portion of the foregut. By the third week of fetal development, the embryo becomes a trilaminate structure that will allow the formation of ectoderm, mesoderm, and endoderm. The pleuripotent endodermal layer is responsible for the development of the epithelial lining of the esophagus. The mesoderm plays an important role in the formation of the gut, as it brings together connective tissue, angioblasts, smooth muscles, the interstitial tissues of Cajal, and the serosal layers of the gut. Although the esophagus does not have a serosal layer, the mesodermal portion of the gut is the derivation for most of the nonepithelial tumors of the esophagus. The neural tissue innervating the esophagus comes from the ectodermal layer of the trilaminate embryo.[5]

Unusual tumors related to squamous cell cancers of the esophagus

Early or superficial esophageal tumors

These tumors have been defined by Japanese and Chinese investigators as squamous cell malignancies that have no propensity to metastasize beyond lymph nodes. Indeed, the Japanese have defined early esophageal cancers as those which invade the lamina propria but not the muscularis mucosa (Fig. 27.1). Patients with early or superficial esophageal cancers have a 95% 5-year survivorship.[6] Although open surgical esophagectomy remains the gold standard for the treatment for early squamous cell tumors, current reports demonstrate excellent results for submucosal endoscopic resections.[7] In the authors' opinion, submucosal esophagectomy is ideal *only* in the hands of experienced endoscopists. Otherwise the best therapy is a thoracoscopic esophagectomy.

Carcinosarcomas

Carcinosarcomas of the esophagus, first described by Virchow in 1865, are epithelial tumors that can be difficult to distinguish from true sarcomatoid lesions originating in the esophagus. Among cancers of the esophagus, the incidence of carcinosarcomas varies between 0.5% and 2.5%.[8,9] Carcinosarcomas

Textbook of Uncommon Cancer, Fourth Edition. Edited by Derek Raghavan, Charles D. Blanke, David H. Johnson, Paul L. Moots, Gregory H. Reaman, Peter G. Rose and Mikkael A. Sekeres.
© 2012 John Wiley & Sons, Inc. Published 2012 by John Wiley & Sons, Inc.

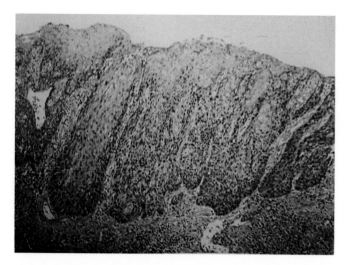

Figure 27.1 Squamous cell carcinoma with possible incipient invasion at the base. The long prongs of dysplastic epithelium extend deeply into the lamina propria, but only at the base of the epithelium. In the center there is invasion with irregularity of the basal epithelium and separation of small clusters of cells from the main prongs. Serial sections might be necessary to ensure that these nests are truly separated from the basal epithelium.

generally present in men as bulky tumors (causing dysphagia), but without complete esophageal obstruction. Over 90% of carcinosarcomas are found in the mid or distal esophagus.

Over the years, the various terminologies used for carcinosarcomas (sarcomatoid carcinoma, pseudosarcoma, psuedosarcomatous squamous cell carcinoma, spindle cell carcinoma and polypoid carcinoma) have reflected the uncertain histogenesis of the tumor. Whether histogenesis comes from two distinct entities or from a metaplastic change of squamous cell elements remains an active discussion among pathologists. However, the common p53 point mutations that have been found in both the squamous and sarcomatoid portions of the same tumor suggest a common etiologic stem cell rather than a collision of two separate tumors.[10] Although the squamous component of the tumor may be well differentiated, the spindle component of the malignancy is generally poorly differentiated with many mitoses visible per high-power field. Unless a clear area of transition from squamous cell to spindle cell histology is found on biopsy, other means may be necessary to define an esophageal carcinosarcoma.[11]

Positive immunohistochemical (IHC) staining for cytokeratin will generally distinguish carcinosarcomas from the true primary sarcomas of the esophagus. As expected, the cytokeratin stain is positive in the squamous portion of the tumor. However, the spindle cell portion may also stain positively for cytokeratin and vimentin. If IHC cannot adequately demonstrate a carcinosarcoma, electron microscopy may be useful to demonstrate epithelial components, such as bridging at the transitional point between the squamous cell malignancy and the sarcomatoid portion of the tumor.[12] See Figure 27.2.

While the literature suggests that carcinosarcomas have a poor prognosis, with reported 5-year survivals between 10% and 15%, it is unclear whether this is actually worse than squamous cell tumors found at the same stage. In a recent review of

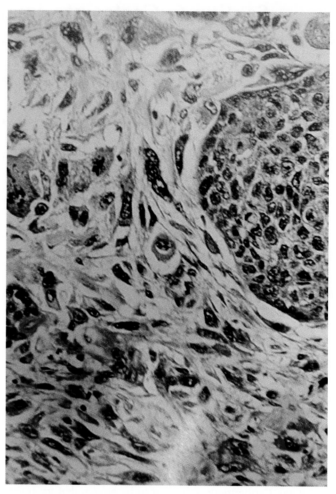

Figure 27.2 Pseudosarcomatous squamous cell carcinoma. In this high-power field, there is a nest of poorly differentiated squamous cancer at the right, while the entire left has the bizarre stroma.

20 Japanese patients diagnosed with carcinosarcoma compared with 142 patients with pure squamous cell tumor, the authors noted that the carcinosarcoma patients with T1 lesions had a significantly worse prognosis than patients with pure squamous cell malignancies ($p=0.008$). However, when all patients were included in their analysis, there was no difference in 5-year survival.[13]

Although carcinosarcomas tend to present as bulky tumors, their predilection for having a pedunculated stalk has led to successful resection by endoscopic means. For those carcinosarcoma patients with ultrasonographic evidence of T1N0 staging, endoscopic resection may be an acceptable alternative to esophagectomy.[14] Some have suggested that neoadjuvant chemotherapy and radiation would be an acceptable approach to invasive esophageal carcinosarcomas. Nevertheless, a series of patients with esophageal carcinosarcoma treated this way has not been published. Thus, while the standard of care remains surgical resection for those patients whose tumors are T1N0, neoadjuvant therapy prior to surgery with a combination of chemotherapy and external beam radiation for locally advanced tumors is acceptable and may be preferred over esophagectomy alone.

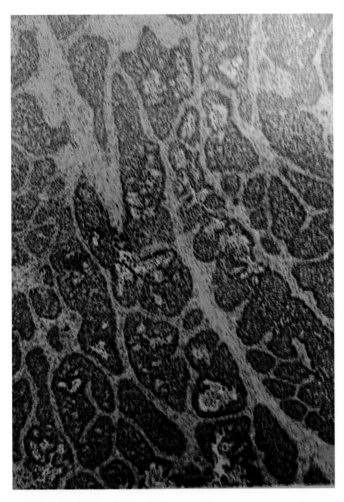

Figure 27.3 Basaloid squamous cell carcinoma. The small dark carcinoma cells form strands, trabeculae, and nests, some with central holes. The stromal spaces separating the cell groups are often uniform, as in typical adenoid cystic carcinomas.

Basaloid carcinomas

Histologically, basaloid carcinomas appear in cellular nests or trabeculae with marked peripheral palisading and hyperchromasia that may resemble neuroendocrine tumors or adenoid cystic tumors of the esophagus (Fig. 27.3). Pathologists describe these cells as "basaloid" with moderate to scant basophilic cytoplasm. Estimates of the incidence of basaloid tumor variant of squamous cell malignancies vary from 1% to 11%.[15,16] Because basaloid tumors frequently show histological features similar to neuroendocrine tumors, adenocarcinomas, small cell carcinomas and adenocystic carcinomas, they are believed to come from pleuripotent stem cells.[17]

Basaloid carcinomas of the esophagus (Fig. 27.4) show a relatively weak predilection for positive IHC staining with cytokeratin. Furthermore, they do not stain with typical neuroendocrine markers such as neuron-specific enolase (NSE) and S-100. However, the mucoid matrix stain with periodic acid-Schiff and alcian blue may be present in the cribiform spaces of the tumor cell nests. The basal cell component of these tumors generally stains quite strongly for CK14 and CK19.[18] Those staining characteristics are important in

distinguishing basaloid tumors from less biologically aggressive adenoid cystic tumors, which will stain positively for S-100 and actin.[19] On a molecular level, basaloid tumors are quite similar to squamous cell malignancies as both show the same frequency of mutations for p53 and the retinoblastoma (RB) tumor suppressor genes.[20]

In a study of head and neck tumors, it was found that basaloid tumors appeared to be more aggressive than purely squamous cell malignancies.[21] However, further studies for patients with esophageal cancer have suggested the basaloid and squamous tumors have a similar biological behavior.[22] Basaloid tumors share a similar demographic with squamous cell malignancies as they mainly affect men over the age of 60; they also share a predilection for the middistal esophagus with symptoms of dysphagia and odynophagia.

Most reports of therapy for basaloid esophageal tumors have emanated from the Far East where squamous cell tumors predominate. Even then, single institutions are likely to see only a few of these rare tumors. However, there was enough interest in the molecular differences between basaloid and squamous cell esophageal malignancies for a Japanese group to note that thymidylate synthase (TS) activity in basaloid tumors is higher than those found in pure squamous malignancies. Since TS is not only necessary for DNA replication but is also the target for the commonly used chemotherapy 5-fluorouracil (5-FU), the group postulated that basaloid tumors are more aggressive than most squamous cell malignancies and would be likely to demonstrate resistance to 5-FU.[23] That noted, other investigators have reported brief success using 5-FU in combination with cisplatin for patients with metastatic basaloid tumors.[24] Still others have reported success in treating basaloid esophageal tumors with cisplatin and 5-FU prior to surgery with the hope of enhancing the surgical cure rate.[25] Nevertheless, if preoperative neoadjuvant therapy is to be considered, the authors recommend treatment with low-dose carboplatin (AUC 2) + weekly paclitaxel 80 mg/m^2 in combination with external beam radiation.

Verrucous carcinomas

Verrucous carcinomas, first described in the oral cavity in 1948, may be found in the esophagus as well.[26,27] The few esophageal cases that have been reported are usually found in men and have been associated with chronic caustic injury such as lye, achalasia, diverticular disease or reflux.[28] Indeed, Spanish pathologists have suggested that verrucous tumors can mimic tuberculosis of the esophagus.[29] In one report, the authors noted an association between verrucous esophageal cancers and the human papillomavirus 51.[30]

Verrucous tumors are generally slow growing, warty, and exophytic in appearance (Fig. 27.5). Under the microscope, these tumors are well differentiated with abundant keratin and "pushing" margins that may make depth of invasion difficult to interpret. The key differential diagnosis is benign squamous papilloma. The endoscopist's visual description will help, as benign papillomas are seen as discrete lesions that are generally less than 3 cm. Verrucous carcinomas are more extensive and generally circumferential.[31] Although esophageal verrucous

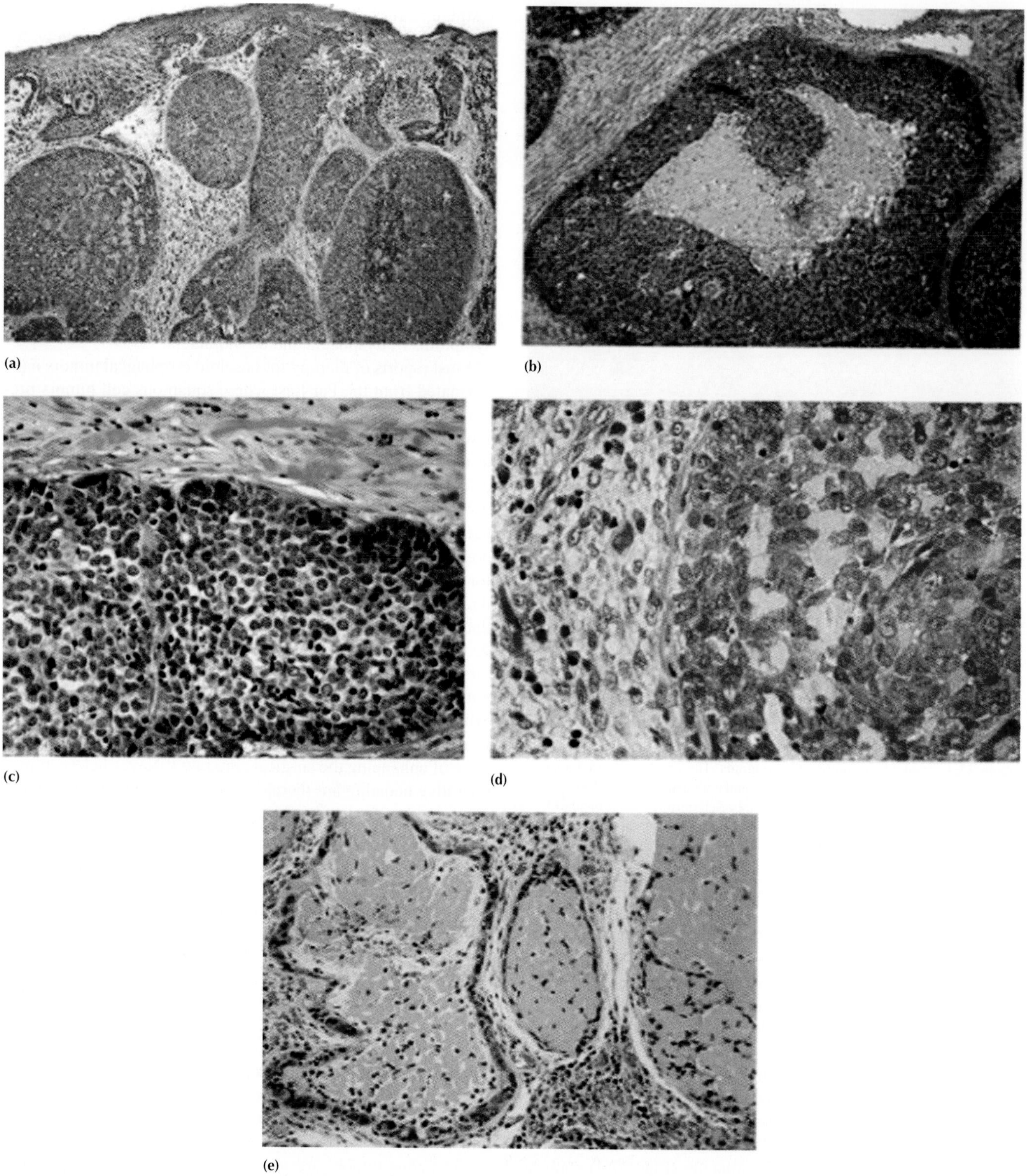

(a)

(b)

(c)

(d)

(e)

Figure 27.4 Basaloid carcinoma of the esophagus. (a) Low-power image shows a proliferation of well-circumscribed nodules of basaloid cells extending beneath mildly dysplastic squamous epithelium. (b) Nest of tumor cells with central necrosis. (c) Basaloid carcinomas are characterized by cells with oval to round nuclei, an open chromatin pattern, small nucleoli, and scant cytoplasm. (d) A mucoid hyaline-like substance is noted in some intercellular spaces. (e) In some cases, basaloid carcinomas show marked intratumoral necrosis, which gives the false appearance of gland formation and an adenocystic carcinoma-like quality to the tumor nodules.

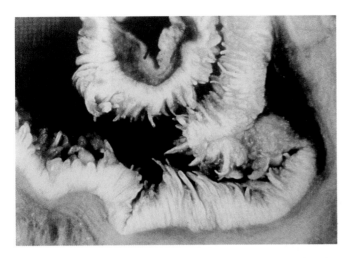

Figure 27.5 Verrucous squamous cell carcinoma. In this gross view, there is a very long plaque of carcinoma with its base in the lamina propria. Its luminal aspect has many spike-like projections: these are the epithelial spikes covered by thick keratin. Courtesy of Dr Karel Geboes, Leuven, Belgium.

tumors are not known to metastasize to distant organs, they may be locally aggressive, forming fistulous tracts into the trachea.[32] Almost 45 years after the first description of verrucous esophageal cancers, there are fewer than 30 reported in the world's literature. Because these lesions tend to grow rather large before diagnosis, optimal treatment requires surgery. As distant disease is not an issue for patients with these tumors, there is no role for systemic chemotherapy.

Intraepithelial neoplasia or squamous cell dysplasia

To resolve the differences in diagnostic criteria of "reactive changes," "low-grade dysplasia" and "high-grade dysplasia," the 1998 meeting of the World Congress of Gastroenterology in Vienna devised a new classification for epithelial neoplasia. They collapsed the diagnoses of "high-grade adenoma/dysplasia" and "noninvasive carcinoma (carcinoma *in situ*)" into "noninvasive high-grade dysplasia." In turn, "dysplasia" was then modified by the World Health Organization into "intraepithelial neoplasia."[33]

Squamous dysplasia of the esophagus has been linked to malignancy. The issue of concern for the clinician and patient is the time that it will take for cancer to appear: for each patient, this is an unknown. Low-grade dysplasia is limited to less than half of the epithelial basal layer while high-grade dysplasia shows a lack of maturation and cytological atypia generally extending to more than half the epithelial thickness (Fig. 27.6).[34] As the degree of dysplasia increases from mild to moderate to severe or high grade, the statistical risk of squamous cell malignancies of the esophagus increases.[35] Only high-grade dysplasia harbors a close temporal association with cancer.

Although screening for esophageal squamous cell cancers is not performed in the west, in high-risk Far Eastern and Middle Eastern countries efforts have been made to conduct screening to detect early, potentially curable tumors. Squamous dysplasia is generally visible by endoscopy, especially if the esophagus is sprayed with iodine. In a study conducted in Linxian, China,

59 of 682 (8.6%) screened subjects developed invasive squamous cell tumors within 3 years of screening if dysplasia was identified. In Japan, where 90% of invasive esophageal are squamous cell malignancies, intraepithelial carcinomas account for almost 20% of cases.[36]

Japanese endoscopists are now expected to find intraepithelial malignancies less than 1 mm in size.[37] These lesions are being found by new types of endoscopic procedures including magnifying endoscopy, narrow-band (NB) imaging, and endocytoscopy. Where the endoscopists have appropriate training, these very early low-grade lesions are easily removed by endoscopic procedures. However, in many centers where these lesions are frequently encountered, surgical extirpation is still the treatment of choice for high-grade intraepithelial lesions.[38] Once again, it is the authors' opinion that if endoscopic extirpation is considered, it should be done by experienced operators.

Heterotopic tumors of the esophagus

It is well accepted that the intestinal metaplasia found in the lining of the distal esophagus, known as Barrett esophagus, is a premalignant condition associated with esophageal reflux, obesity, tobacco use, and male gender.[39] However, adenocarcinomas arising independently of Barrett esophagus may result from misplacement of embryonic tissue lodged in the esophagus, eventually maturing within the esophagus. These heterotopic or ectopic tissues are generally found incidentally within the esophageal submucosa as benign lesions in the upper and middle esophagus.[40]

Patients with true gastric mucosa in the esophagus or gastric heterotopia may have symptoms from acid produced by parietal cells. A few patients are known to have coughing and mild dysphagia.[41] There are reports of rare malignant esophageal cancers occurring in these so-called "inlet patches." These cancers may be treated as if they were typical esophageal cancers. Indeed, one report of chemotherapy and radiation to a cervical adenocarcinoma occurring from an area of gastric heterotopia was so successful that no cancer was found upon resection.[42] Pancreatic heterotopia of the esophagus appears to occur most often in the distal esophagus. It has been associated with esophageal atresia in infants, with inflammation in the distal esophagus and hiatal hernias.[43,44] A tumor formed by pancreatic heterotopia in the esophagus is present in the submucosa (Fig. 27.7). As such, these tumors must be differentiated from gastrointestinal stromal tumors (GISTs) and other submucosal lesions that may occur in the esophagus.[45]

Salivary gland tumors arising from the esophagus represent less than 1% of all adenocarcinomas of the esophagus. These tumors appear to arise from submucosal glands located in the esophagus or from the epithelium of tracheobronchial rests.[46] They are classified as adenoid cystic carcinoma and mucoepidermoid carcinoma. Adenoid cystic tumors of the esophagus may present in any portion of the esophagus. These tumors, which are more common in women, exhibit two cell lineages. The majority of cells demonstrate a basaloid or myoepithelial differentiation; the second type of cells are ductal in nature, represented by scattered foci of ductal epithelial cells which surround tiny lumens.[47]

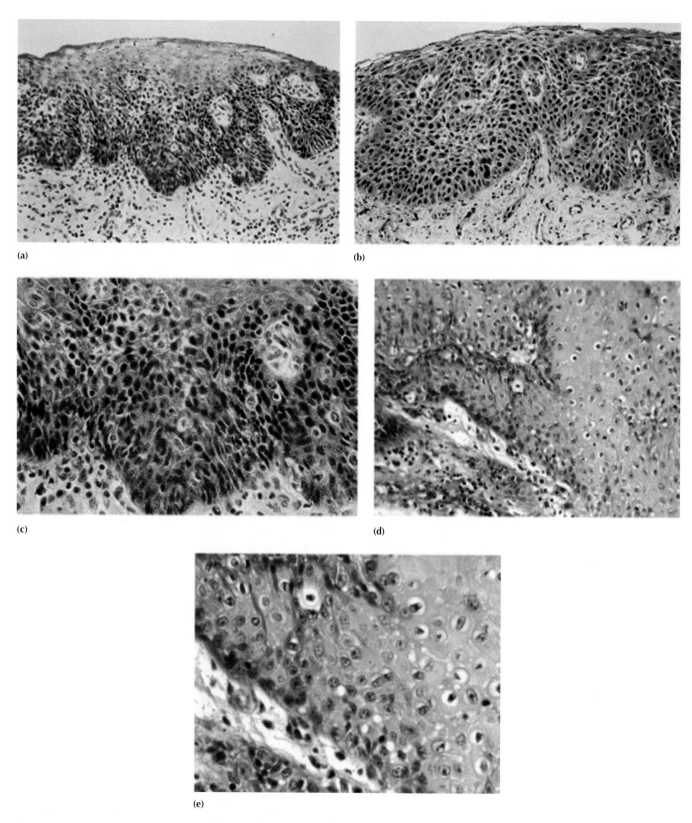

Figure 27.6 Squamous dysplasia of the esophagus. (a) Low-grade squamous dysplasia characterized by a proliferation of neoplastic cells involving about one-third to one-half of the thickness of the epithelium. (b) In contrast to (a), dysplastic cells extend to the surface of the epithelium and are associated with a significant loss of surface maturation (high-grade dysplasia). (c) In this high-power image, dysplastic cells are noted to have an increased nucleus-to-cytoplasm ratio, marked hyperchromatic nuclei, significant loss of polarity, and overlapping of the cells and their nuclei. (d) An unusual morphological appearance of squamous dysplasia, characterized by disorganized large cells with open nuclei. (e) High-power photomicrograph of the dysplastic cells seen in (d).

Immunohistochemically, adenoid cystic carcinomas demonstrate intense keratin and carcinoembryonic antigen staining in the ductal cells with S-100, actin and vimentin positivity in the basaloid or myoepithelial cells.[48,49] Because these tumors are very rare, it is difficult to generalize about the biology of adenoid cystic tumors. One group of investigators has suggested that they have an aggressive biology with distant metastatic lesions commonly found. Others have reported a less aggressive biology.[50,51] For locally advanced tumors, the treatment of choice remains surgical excision.

Mucoepidermoid carcinoma

Mucoepidermoid tumors of the esophagus have their origin in heterotopic salivary glands. These tumors can easily be confused with adenosquamous carcinomas. Mucoepidermoid

tumors are graded on the basis of morphology as low, intermediate, and high grade. They are staged just as other epithelial esophageal tumors. Although pathologists consider mucoepidermoid histology to be less aggressive than adenosquamous carcinoma, they are generally detected quite late because they originate beneath the esophageal mucosa.[52] Histologically, mucoepidermoid tumors demonstrate mucus-secreting cells within islands of squamous carcinoma (Fig. 27.8). In contradistinction, adenosquamous carcinomas have distinct areas of squamous cancer and glandular cancer.[53] Thus, the therapy of choice for patients with locally advanced tumors should be combined-modality chemotherapy plus external beam radiation followed by surgery.

Tumors of mixed cellularity: adenosquamous cell carcinomas

Epithelial esophageal cancers have a strong tendency to exhibit distinct and different histologies within the same tumor.[54] Most pathologists have suggested that disparate histologies within the same tumor are a result of neoplastic transformation of a totipotent stem cell in the basal region of the esophageal squamous mucosa. Clonality studies of these tumors have supported this theory.[55] In an ultrastructural study of 43 esophageal cancers, one-quarter showed "multidirectional" differentiation. These included tumors initially thought to be purely squamous cancers, adenocarcinomas or small cell tumors.[56] To find these truly mixed tumors, readily available markers for squamous differentiation have been sought. Immunohistochemical staining for CD44 has been shown to be an excellent marker for squamous differentiation in well-differentiated adenosquamous carcinomas. However, when the squamous component is poorly differentiated and more difficult to identify under light microscopy, the immunohistochemical stain is not as useful.[57] Recently, studies on tumors that clearly originate in a Barrett esophagus mucosa have been shown to have heterogeneity.[58] Most likely, the biological behavior of these mixed cellularity

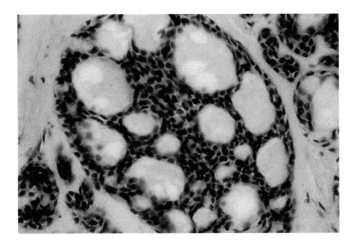

Figure 27.7 True adenoid cystic carcinoma of the esophagus. In contrast to basaloid carcinomas, adenoid cystic carcinomas show a proliferation of small hyperchromatic cells with less variation of nuclear size, infrequent mitoses, and no necrosis. The glandular lumina contain basement membrane-like extracellular material.

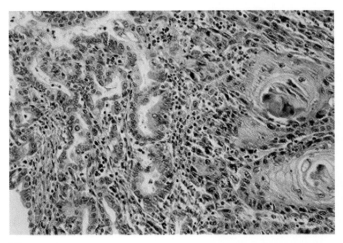

(a)

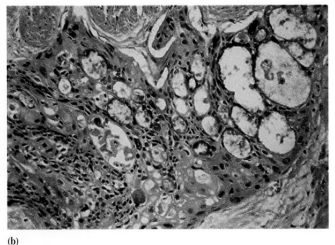

(b)

Figure 27.8 (a) Adenosquamous carcinoma of the esophagus characterized by a proliferation of malignant glands *(left side)* adjacent to malignant squamous epithelium *(right side)*. (b) Mucoepidermoid carcinoma characterized by large aggregates of cells, which have features of malignant squamous cells toward the periphery of the cellular units intimately mixed with centrally located cells that contain mucin.

tumors is similar to "pure" squamous cell cancers or "pure" adenocarcinomas, i.e. it is stage dependent.[59]

As noted above, in adenosquamous tumors, the squamous and glandular elements usually appear side by side but are not admixed (see Fig. 27.8). Adenoacanthomas represent a variation of adenosquamous tumors: these are tumors in which mature but nonmalignant squamous elements are found within an adenocarcinoma.[60]

Japanese investigators have enriched the literature on the treatment of adenosquamous cell tumors of the esophagus. In general, these tumors are responsive to the same type of chemotherapeutic agents as squamous cell carcinomas or adenocarcinomas arising from Barrett esophagus.[61] In one retrospective review, the investigators noted that over a 30-year period, the incidence of these tumors was 1% of their esophageal cancer cases. The tumors were successfully treated with radiation and/or surgery and appeared to have a better prognosis because they were found at a lower stage than the usual squamous cell tumors treated at their institution.[62] However, for tumors that are more locally invasive, i.e. T2–4 NanyM0, optimal therapy would include preoperative chemotherapy and external beam radiation prior to surgery.

Choriocarcinomas of the esophagus

Choriocarcinoma is a malignant tumor that generates trophoblastic tissue. Although commonly found in the genital tract, there are rare cases of these tumors appearing in the gastrointestinal (GI) tract, including the esophagus. This chapter places choriocarcinoma in the section of heterotopic tumors; choriocarcinoma of the esophagus does not appear to come from misplaced trophoblastic tissue but from "dedifferentiation" of glandular tissue, as several have been found to be admixed with adenocarcinomas.[63] Indeed, recent reports have shown choriocarcinomas to be associated with squamous cell malignancies of the esophagus.[64]

In general, patients tend to be younger than those with epithelial esophageal carcinomas. Moreover, while acute bleeding is not usually a presenting finding for typical squamous or adenocarcinomas, esophageal choriocarcinomas tend to present with massive bleeding.[65] As germ cell malignancies are quite sensitive to cisplatin, a combination of cisplatin and etoposide should produce an excellent response. Indeed, at least one report of disseminated choriocarcinoma of the esophagus suggested an excellent, if short-lived response to this combination.[66]

Malignant mesenchymal tumors of the esophagus

Leiomyoma of the esophagus

Leiomyomas are the most common mesenchymal tumors found in the esophagus. Almost all leiomyomas of the esophagus are benign; they are usually incidental discoveries by the endoscopist. Leiomyomas have a male-to-female predilection of 2:1 and they affect younger patients (average age for men, 33 years and women 44 years).[67] In a review of a 40-year experience at Massachusetts General Hospitals, 53 patients with esophageal leiomyoma were found. Although most patients are asymptomatic, as the average size of esophageal leiomyomas is 5.3 cm, the most common symptom is dysphagia.[68]

Histologically, leiomyomas exhibit low to moderate cellularity with bundles of interlacing spindle-shaped smooth muscle cells with cigar-shaped nuclei (Fig. 27.9). Mitoses are infrequent. Leiomyomas do not stain positively for for CD34

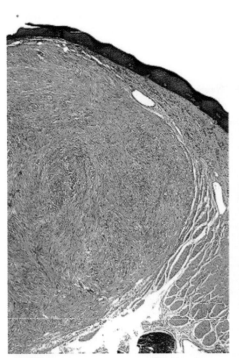
(a)

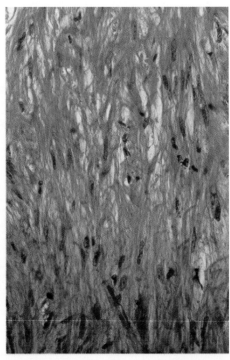
(b)

Figure 27.9 Leiomyoma. (a) This leiomyoma arose from the muscularis mucosae and presented as an intraluminal nodule. (b) Histologically, this leiomyoma is paucicellular. The tumor cells are bland and have abundant, fibrillar, brightly eosinophilic cytoplasm without nuclear atypia.

and CD117, GIST markers or S-100, a neural marker.[69] Therapy depends on the clinical picture that is presented. Regardless of its benign nature, patients with symptoms secondary to a leiomyoma will need resection. As these tumors average over 5 cm in size, transthoracic open surgical procedures are most commonly employed. For smaller tumors that do not cause symptoms, endoscopic resection is the treatment of choice.[70] In the authors' opinion, there is no role for neoadjuvant chemotherapy or radiation.

Gastrointestinal stromal tumor

Gastrointestinal stromal tumors, accounting for between 1% and 3% of all gastrointestinal malignancies, are the most common mesenchymal tumor found in the GI tract. The term GIST was first descriptively coined in 1983 by Clark and Mazur who noted (as did others) that these tumors had features that distinguished them from smooth muscle and/or nerve tumors.[71]

The modern definition of GIST came from a Japanese group of investigators who were interested in the role of interstitial cells of Cajal (ICC), neurological pacemaker cells found in the myenteric plexus of the GI tract. ICC cells and GIST cells both expressed the KIT tyrosine kinase receptor. The investigators noted that GIST cells exhibited mutations in the GIST protooncogene that seemed to allow for unregulated growth of GISTs. Indeed, the Japanese team discovered that five of six cases they studied had *KIT* gene mutations. These mutations led to uncontrolled, ligand-independent phosphorylation by KIT kinase.[72] The increased protein produced by the mutation can be found by immunohistochemistry using a stain for the CD117 antigen. Approximately 95% of all GISTs stain positively with CD117. The 5% that do not contain mutation of the platelet-derived growth factor receptor-α (PDGFRA).[73]

Rational, scientifically based therapy for GIST came about because of investigations of the signal transduction inhibitor-571 (STI-571). This agent was of interest because it had the property of inhibiting platelets from clogging coronary arterial graft stents. While these investigations were ongoing, the agent was also found to have profoundly effective activity in chronic myelocytic leukemia (CML) as it acted against dysregulated BCR-ABL.[74] In turn, the investigators noted that the agent STI-571 (subsequently named imatinib mesylate) had activity against wild-type and mutant KIT protein.[75] Imatinib (Glivec[R]) was developed by Novartis Pharmaceuticals (Basel, Switzerland) as a targeted therapy against CML and GISTs. This was a major advance in the development of specific molecular therapy targeted against a mutation driving a malignant disease.[76]

Only 1% of all GISTs are found in the esophagus. Localized GISTs are categorized as having low, intermediate or high risk depending on their size and mitotic index. GISTs 5 cm or greater and those with two or more mitoses/high-power field (HPF) are most likely to metastasize. In a series of 17 esophageal GISTs, 12 (70.5%) were in the high-risk category.[77] Although unusual, GISTs have been reported to metastasize to lymph nodes draining the esophagus.[78] However, the liver is the organ most likely to harbor metastatic GIST. Despite their rarity as an esophageal tumor, patients with a GIST generally present with the protean symptoms of dysphagia, odynophagia, and weight loss. Because of the submucosal nature of the tumor, most patients are operated upon without a histological diagnosis before the surgery.[79] For those patients at high risk for recurrence following resection of a GIST, postoperative therapy with imatinib is now recommended. The authors concur with this approach. However, current trials will have to determine the optimal duration of treatment.[80]

Sarcomas of the esophagus

Leiomyosarcomas account for approximately 90% of esophageal sarcomas. However, esophageal leiomyosarcomas are very rare tumors, accounting for 0.3% of a Mayo Clinic series of 6359 patients with esophageal malignancies over a 76-year history.[81] Leiomyosarcomas are found in the cervical, thoracic, and distal esophagus. Their cellular characteristics are generally pleomorphic and they are almost always high grade. Most often, they stain positively for desmin and smooth muscle antigen (SMA). Most common metastatic sites are liver and lung. Most esophageal leiomyosarcomas are not readily available for biopsy. However, it is thought that the few exophytic lesions that are discovered have a better prognosis than the large lesions that grow under the esophageal mucosa.[82]

Rhabdomyosarcomas, synovial cell sarcoma, malignant schwanommas, fibrosarcoma, Ewing sarcoma, and liposarcomas of the esophagus have been documented in the literature.[83] Clinically, these tumors generally grow to large size and then present with typical symptoms of odynophagia, dysphagia, and weight loss. For these tumors, presenting as locally advanced, surgical excision followed by combination chemotherapy is recommended. Although doxorubicin has been a mainstay of sarcoma therapy, the authors recommend therapy with gemcitabine and docetaxel for patients with leiomyosarcoma.[84] See Figure 27.10.

Schwannoma of the esophagus

Schwannomas are rare GI tract malignancies, of which esophageal schwannomas represent a tiny fraction. Those reported in the GI tract may grow to rather large size, causing dysphagia and weight loss. Nevertheless, even large schwannomas are generally benign. The majority of schwannomas occur in women.[85] They are highly vascular tumors composed of homogeneous biphasic fusiform-shaped cells with a palisading appearance. Immunohistochemical examination of schwannomas is positive for S-100 and negative for CD117, CD34 and SMA.[86] As expected, large schwannomas will present with symptoms of dysphagia. However, because of their vascular nature, these tumors may also present with an acute upper GI bleeding episode.[87] Regardless of their size, if these tumors remain localized, the optimal therapy is surgery alone.

Neuroendocrine neoplasms of the esophagus

Because of an increasing incidence of these tumors in the GI tract, neuroendocrine neoplasms (NEN) have received

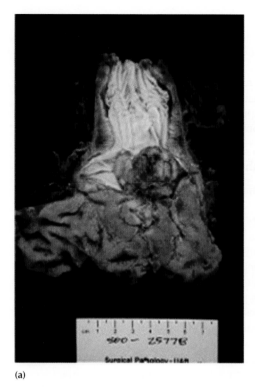

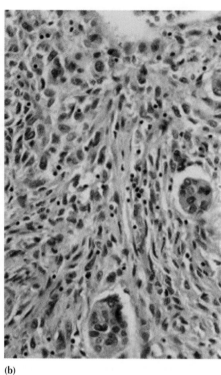

(a)   (b)

Figure 27.10 Spindle cell carcinoma. (a) This spindle cell carcinoma formed a polypoid intraluminal mass located above the gastroesophageal junction. (b) These tumors reveal biphasic histology, typically with a predominance of malignant spindle cells, and with only focal areas of carcinoma.

significant recent attention, which has helped to clarify classification and improve understanding of prognosis and therapeutic options. In part, the increased incidence of these tumors is due to the increased use of endoscopy (both upper and lower) and the improvement in imaging studies of the GI tracts.[88,89] However, when these tumors appear in the esophagus, their biological behavior is no different from that of tumors discovered and treated in other areas of the GI tract.

The varied, almost idiosyncratic nomenclature attached to the different types of neuroendocrine tumors has created confusion for the average pathologist and clinician. Whether these efforts to consolidate the classification of NENs have succeeded in creating more clarity or more confusion remains to be determined.

Low-grade NEN cancers are generally referred to as carcinoid tumors. Esophageal carcinoids are very rarely reported. High-grade neuroendocrine carcinomas (HGNECs) of the esophagus represent approximately 1–2.8% of all esophageal carcinomas.[90] HGNECs are more heterogeneous in appearance and biology than carcinoids. In 2010, the WHO classified NENs into three categories by grade: well-differentiated neuroendocrine tumors (NETs) which are essentially carcinoids (Fig. 27.11). The well-differentiated NETs or carcinoids are themselves subclassified into grades I or II. Grade III neuroendocrine carcinomas (NECs) are poorly differentiated.

Neuroendocrine carcinomas are divided into two categories: small cell and large cell neoplasms. Within these categories, there are two more strata: tumors that are "pure" NECs and those tumors in which 30% or more of the tumor has features of adenocarcinomas, referred to as "mixed adenoneuroendocrine carcinomas" (MANECs).[91] Although carcinoids and

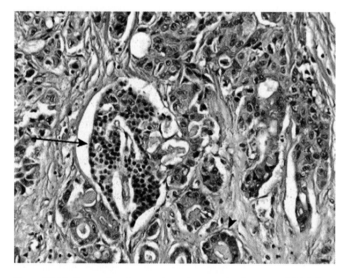

Figure 27.11 Composite adenocarcinoma/neuroendocrine tumor (NET). In the center of moderately differentiated adenocarcinoma glands is a nest of monomorphous polygonal NET cells *(arrow)* that blend imperceptibly with the adjacent adenocarcinoma. *Arrowhead* denotes gland with central mucin.

HGNECs express neuroendocrine markers such as chromogranin and synaptophysin, most investigators have stated that these tumors come from different cell lineages: carcinoids arise from the diffuse neuroendocrine cell system of the GI tract and HGNECs come from the surface epithelium of the GI tract.[92]

There are not enough cases of large cell HGNECs of the esophagus to draw definitive conclusions regarding therapy. Recent reports have shown these tumors in other GI sites to be susceptible to alkylating agents such as temozolomide and the

Figure 27.12 Granular cell tumor.
(a) Endoscopically, granular cell tumors appear as small white to yellow subepithelial nodules. (b) Histologically, these lesions are composed of large cells with abundant eosinophilic granular cytoplasm and pyknotic nuclei. (c) If the diagnosis is in question, a positive immunoperoxidase stain for S-100 can help confirm the diagnosis. Courtesy of Dr Christopher Truss.

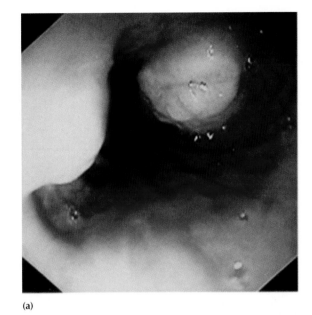

(a)

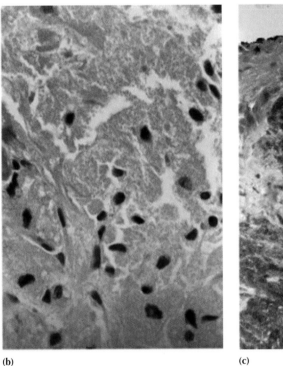

(b)

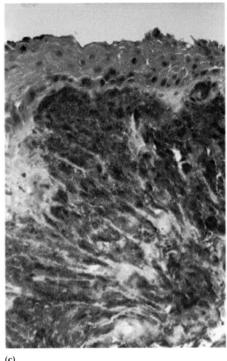

(c)

combination of streptozotocin and 5-fluorouracil, as well as targeted agents such as sunitinib and everolimus.[93] Unfortunately, the small cell variant of HGNEC is diagnosed most often. These tumors strongly resemble small cell cancers of the lung. They form diffusely infiltrating masses in solid sheets, ribbons or nests. Silver stains demonstrate occasional argyrophilic cells. However, the cells of small cell carcinomas are not argentaffinic.[94] Locally advanced small cell HGNEC esophageal tumors are treated with combined chemotherapy (cisplatin and etoposide) and radiation. Disseminated small cell esophageal cancers are uniformly fatal but generally respond for a short period to the combination of cisplatin and etoposide.[95]

Granular cell tumors

Since the first report identifying granular cell tumors of the esophagus came out in 1928, the tumor has been found to be the second most common esophageal stromal tumor after leiomyoma.[96] These submucosal tumors, thought to arise from neural tissue, are almost always benign. In some series, the esophagus is the most common site of GI tract granular tumors.[97] Unlike malignant epithelial tumors of the esophagus, the incidence of granular tumors in women is twice that of men.[98]

Approximately 75% of granular tumors are found to be 2 cm in size or less (Fig. 27.12). As patients with granular tumors

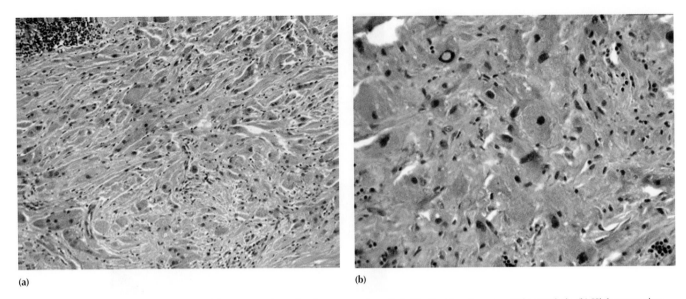

(a)   (b)

Figure 27.13 Malignant granular cell tumor. (a) Low-power view of malignant granular cells infiltrating the submucosa and muscularis. (b) High-power view showing granular cells with enlarged, irregular, and hyperchromatic nuclei. Mitoses were present in other areas of the tumor.

are rarely symptomatic, these tumors are generally found incidentally when endoscopy is performed for another reason.[99] Some patients with these tumors have been followed for years after biopsy with little change in size.[100] Nevertheless, there have been a few reports of malignant granular cell tumors (Fig. 27.13). The diagnosis of malignancy is made on the basis of infiltrative growth into adjacent structures without evidence of widespread metastatic cancer.[101]

Management of granular tumors depends on their size. The treatment of choice is endoscopic resection (in the hands of experienced operators). Those tumors causing no symptoms may be followed without resection. However, large granular tumors causing symptoms of dysphagia should be treated with surgery alone. Postoperative or neoadjuvant therapy has no role in the treatment of granular esophageal tumors.

Lymphoepithelial-like carcinoma and extramedullary plasmacytoma of the esophagus

Lymphoepithelial tumors of the esophagus have a similar histology and possibly a less aggressive biology than lymphoepithelial tumors of the nasopharynx or epithelial tumors of the esophagus.[102,103] Lymphoepithelial tumors exhibit a lymphoid stroma. These tumors may also appear in the breast, uterine cervix, stomach, salivary gland, skin, lung, and urinary bladder.[104–110] Most cases of lymphoepithelial tumors in which the esophagus is the primary organ have been reported from Japan. As suggested by the name, these tumors are undifferentiated, composed chiefly of lymphoid infiltrate with many surrounding plasma cells. Depending on the organ, the association with the Epstein–Barr virus varies from 44% to 92%. Less than 50% of esophageal lymphoepithelial tumors show an affiliation with the Epstein–Barr virus.[111] As reported in Japan, treatment almost always involves surgery as the primary curative modality. Chemotherapy and radiation prior to surgery have been used in Japan as well.[112] The

authors recommend surgery alone for tumors that appear to be T1N0M0 and preoperative neoadjuvant therapy with chemotherapy (a platinum compound and a fluoropyrimidine) plus external beam radiation for large tumors that appear to be locally advanced.

Malignant lymphomas of the esophagus

Although lymphomas of the GI tract are not considered rare, less than 1% of all GI lymphomas originate in the esophagus.[113] Indeed, in a series examining over 1400 cases of extranodal lymphomas, only three were reported from the esophagus.[114] The majority of lymphomas diagnosed with an esophageal biopsy are infiltrating from an organ or lymph nodes outside the esophagus (Fig. 27.14). As with other lymphomas, esophageal lymphomas are classified by their cell of origin as defined by light microscopy, flow cytometry, and/or immunohistochemistry. Non-Hodgkin B cell lymphomas are those most commonly reported in the esophagus. Hodgkin lymphoma represents 11% of all reported esophageal lymphomas.[115] The criteria for diagnosis of a primary esophageal lymphoma include no superficial or palpable lymphadenopathy, normal white blood cell count, no mediastinal lymphadenopathy, and a primary lesion found in the esophagus with only local or continuous lymph nodes involved.[116]

Esophageal lymphomas are commonly associated with conditions in which the patient exhibits chronic immunosuppression such as infection with human immunodeficiency virus (HIV) and hepatitis C.[117,118] Also, there have been reports of T cell lymphomas originating in the esophagus.[119] Clinical presentation of esophageal lymphomas is similar to epithelial tumors. Most patients complain of dysphagia and odynophagia with weight loss. Tracheoesophageal fistulas have also been reported.[120] As noted above, if lymph nodes are palpable in the axillary or supraclavicular regions, the diagnosis of a primary esophageal lymphoma is most unlikely. While endoscopic

Figure 27.14 Large cell lymphoma of the esophagus. (a) Low-power magnification of a lymphomatous infiltrate extending to the squamous epithelium. (b) High-power magnification of the atypical large lymphocytes admixed with numerous smaller lymphocytes, many of which appear normal.

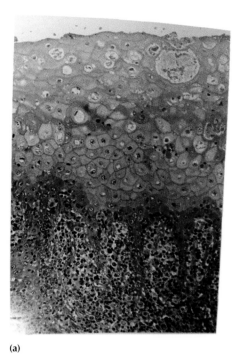

(a)

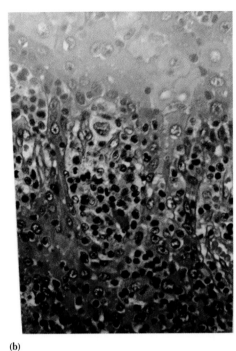

(b)

biopsy is the most common method of obtaining tissue for diagnosis, the false-negative rate of endoscopic biopsies for patients with primary esophageal lymphomas is approximately 30%.[121]

There is no agreed standard therapy for esophageal lymphomas. Surgery alone or surgery followed by radiation has been used, external beam radiation has been used successfully, and radiation and chemotherapy with the standard combination of cyclophosphamide, doxorubicin, vincristine and prednisone (CHOP) have been employed as well.[122] Primary esophageal Hodgkin lymphoma treated with either mechlorethamine, procarbazine, vincristine and prednisone (MOPP) or doxorubicin (adriamycin), bleomycin, vincristine and dacarbazine (ABVD) has a relatively good prognosis or at least a prognosis similar to this disease when found in other extranodal sites.[123] Essentially, our recommendation for therapy of an esophageal lymphoma depends on the clinical stage at presentation. Thus, for advanced, bulky lymphomas that have been resected, a postoperative course of standard systemic therapy plus radiation would be appropriate. For smaller but aggressive lymphomas, chemotherapy without radiation after surgery is recommended. For tumors that are beyond surgical resection, definitive combination chemotherapy followed by radiation is most appropriate.

Malignant melanoma

The thin basal layer of the esophageal mucosa contains melanocytes.[124] Malignant melanoma of the esophagus is generally considered a disease of older individuals. Patients present with a visible tumor in the mid or distal esophagus, causing dysphagia.[125] As making the correct diagnosis via endoscopic biopsy can be challenging, at least 25% of esophageal melanomas require esophagectomy for diagnosis.[126] Melanomas of the esophagus are almost always positive for typical melanocyte markers such as S-100 and HMB-45.[127] As with any melanoma, curative surgery is the treatment of choice. It cannot be said that esophageal melanomas are more aggressive than those found in the skin or other organs. Nevertheless, average survival following esophagectomy is less than 1 year. Less than 2% of patients with esophageal melanoma are alive 5 years after diagnosis.[128]

At this time, it is difficult for us to recommend a preferred postoperative therapy. However, for stage III patients with esophageal melanoma that has been successfully resected, postoperative systemic therapy with interferon-α2b would be appropriate.

Metastatic cancer to the esophagus

While the diagnosis of metastatic cancer to the esophagus is rarely made, autopsy series have demonstrated that esophageal metastases can be found in 6% of patients dying of cancer. Most metastatic lesions find their way to the esophagus either by direct extension (45%) or lymphatic spread (36%). Nineteen percent spread by a hematogenous route. In the west, breast cancer is the most common tumor to metastasize to the esophagus. In Japan, lung cancer metastases to the esophagus are found in 11% of autopsy cases.[129–131] In general, lung and breast cancer spread via the extensive esophageal submucosal lymphatics. However, some lung cancers may spread directly. The tumors that most commonly spread through the blood are breast, renal cell, malignant melanoma, endometrial, ovarian, colorectal, and prostate cancers.[132–134]

Metastatic lesions to the esophagus generally appear as smooth strictures by endoscopic examination.[135] These lesions are best diagnosed by endoscopic ultrasonography.[136] Therapy of tumors that metastasize to the esophagus is tailored to the primary. Although there are reports of surgical therapy, esophagectomy is rarely employed for these metastatic lesions.[137] Systemic therapy directed to the primary tumor is appropriate.

Conclusion

The so-called rare tumors of the esophagus that have been briefly discussed in this chapter are found in less than 8% of patients with esophageal malignancies. As such, they present diagnostic challenges for the endoscopist, the pathologist, and the treating clinician. However, as endoscopic procedures are becoming more widespread, with increased utilization of immunohistochemistry and molecular probes, recognition of the rare tumors will likely increase as well.

References

1. Ferlay J, *et al. Globocan 2002. Cancer Incidence, Mortality and Prevalence*. IARC Cancer Base No. 5 [version 2.0]. Lyon: IARC Press, 2004.

2. Devesa S, *et al.* Changing patterns in the incidence of esophageal and gastric carcinoma in the United States. Cancer 1998; 83: 2049–53.

3. Jemal A, *et al.* Cancer statistics 2008. CA Cancer J Clin 2008; 58–71.

4. Edwards BK, *et al.* Annual report to the nation on the status of cancer, 1975–2002, featuring population trends in cancer treatment. J Natl Cancer Inst 2005; 97: 1407–27.

5. Gaman A, *et al.* Esophageal embryology and congenital disorders. In: Jobe BA, Thomas CR Jr, Hunter JG (eds) *Esophageal Cancer: Principles and Practice*. New York: Demos Medical Publishing, 2009.

6. Takubo K, *et al.* Early squamous cell carcinoma of the esophagus: the Japanese view point. Histopathology 2007; 51: 733–42.

7. Low DE. Open versus minimally invasive esophagectomy: what is the best approach? Frame the issue. J Gastrointest Surg 2011; 15(9): 1497–9.

8. Xu LT, *et al.* Clinical and pathological characteristics of carcinosarcomas of the esophagus: report of four cases. Ann Thorac Surg 1984; 37: 197–203.

9. Lyomasa S, *et al.* Carcinosarcoma of the esophagus: a twenty-case study. Jpn J Clin Oncol 1990; 20: 99–106.

10. Mills *et al.* Variants of squamous cell carcinoma. In: Mills SE, Carter D, Greenson JK, Reuter VE, Stoler MH (eds) *Steinberg's Diagnostic Surgical Pathology*, 5th edn. Philadelphia: Lippincott Williams and Wilkins, 2009. pp.1268–9.

11. Gatter KM, *et al.* Malignant: squamous cell carcinoma and variants. In: Jobe BA, Thomas CR Jr, Hunter JG (eds) *Esophageal Cancer: Principles and Practice*. New York: Demos Medical Publishing, 2009.

12. Balercia G, *et al.* Sarcomatoid carcinoma: an ultrastructural study with light microscopic and immunohistochemical correlation of 10 cases from various anatomic sites. Ultrastruct Pathol 1995; 19: 249–63.

13. Sakurai SA, *et al.* Clinicopathological and immunohistochemical characteristics of esophageal carcinosarcoma. Anticancer Res 2009; 29(8): 3375–80.

14. Feng J *et al.* Endoscopic polypectomy: a promising therapeutic choice for esophageal carcinosarcoma. World J Gastroenterol 2009; 15(27): 3448–50.

15. Sarbia M, *et al.* Basaloid squamous cell carcinoma of the esophagus: diagnosis and prognosis. Cancer 1997; 79: 1871–8.

16. Cho KJ, *et al.* Basaloid squamous carcinoma of the oesophagus: a distinct neoplasm with multipotential differentiation. Histopathology 2000; 36: 331–40.

17. Abe K, *et al.* Basaloid-squamous carcinoma of the esophagus: a clinicopathologic, DNA ploidy, and immunohistochemical study of seven cases. Am J Surg Pathol 1996; 20: 453–61.

18. Tsubochi H, *et al.* Immunohistochemical study of basaloid squamous cell carcinoma, adenoid cystic and mucoepidermoid carcinoma in the upper aerodigestive tract. Anticancer Res 2000; 20: 1205–11.

19. Li TJ, *et al.* Basaloid squamous cell carcinoma of the esophagus with or without adenoid cystic features. Arch Pathol Lab Med 2004; 128: 1124–30.

20. Owonikoko T, *et al.* Comparative analysis of basaloid and typical squamous cell carcinoma of the oesophagus: a molecular biological and immunohistochemical study. J Pathol 2001; 193(2): 155–61.

21. De Sampaio, G, *et al.* Prognoses of oral basaloid squamous cell carcinoma and squamous cell carcinoma: a comparison. Arch Otolaryngol Head Neck Surg 2004; 130(1): 83–6.

22. Sarbia M, *et al.* Basaloid squamous cell carcinoma of the esophagus: diagnosis and prognosis. Cancer 1997; 79: 1871–8.

23. Takemura M, *et al.* Four resected cases with basaloid carcinoma of the esophagus – comparison of 5-FU-related enzymes (thymidylate synthase (TS), dihydropyrimidine dehydrogenase (DPD), orotate phosphoribosyl transferase ((OPRT) between basaloid carcinoma and squamous cell carcinoma. Gan To Kagaku Ryoho 2010; 37(11): 2143–6.

24. Shibata Y, *et al.* Metastatic basaloid-squamous cell carcinoma of the esophagus treated by 5–fluorouracil and cisplatin. World J Gastroenterol 2007; 13(26): 3634–7.

25. Koide N, *et al.* Basaloid-squamous carcinoma of the esophagus treated by preoperative chemotherapy: report of two cases. Surg Today 2003; 33(6): 444–7.

26. Ackerman LV. Verrucous carcinoma of the oral cavity. Surgery 1948; 23: 670–8.

27. Minelli JA, *et al.* Verrucous squamous cell carcinoma of the esophagus. Cancer 1967; 20: 2078–87.

28. Kavin H, *et al.* Chronic esophagitis evolving to verrucous squamous cell carcinoma: possible role of exogenous chemical carcinogens. Gastroenterology 1996; 110: 904–14.

29. Fernandez-Ananin S, *et al.* Carcinoma verrucoso esofagicio: un diagnostico problematico. Cir Esp 2009; 85(3): 181–2.

30. Tonna J, *et al.* Esophageal verrucous carcinoma arising from hyperkeratotic plaques associated with human papilloma virus type 51. Dis Esophagus 2010; 23(5): e17–20.

31. Tajiri H *et al.* Verrucous carcinoma of the esophagus completely resected by endoscopy. Am J Gastroenterol 2000; 95: 1076–7.

32. Biemond P, *et al.* Esophageal verrucous carcinoma: histologically a low-grade malignancy but clinically a fatal disease. J Clin Gastroenterol 1991; 13: 102–7.

33. Stolte M. The new Vienna classification of epithelial neoplasia of the gastrointestinal tract: advantages and disadvantages. Virchows Arch 2003; 442(2): 99–106.

34. Gabbert HE, *et al.* WHO classification of tumours: pathology and genetics tumours of the digestive system squamous cell carcinoma of the oesophagus. Lyon: IARC Press, 2000.

35. Dawsey SM, *et al.* Squamous esophageal histology and subsequent risk of squamous cell carcinoma of the esophagus. A prospective follow-up study from Linxian, China. Cancer 1994; 76(15): 1686–92.

36. Dry SM, *et al.* Esophageal squamous dysplasia. Semin Diagn Pathol 2002; 1: 2–11.

37. Takubo K, *et al.* Early squamous cell carcinoma of the oesophagus: the Japanese viewpoint. Histopathology 2007; 51(6): 733–42.

38. Shimizu M, *et al.* Squamous intraepithelial neoplasia of the esophagus: past, present and future. J Gastroenterol 2009; 44(2): 103–12.

39. Sampliner R. *Barrett's Esophgagus: Screening and Surveillance in Esophageal Cancer: Principles and Practice*. New York: Demos Medical, 2009. pp.69–72.

40. Von Rahden BH, *et al.* Heterotropic gastric mucosa of the esophagus: literature review and proposal of clinicopathologic classification. Am J Gastroenterol 2004; 99: 543–51.

41. Tang P, *et al.* Inlet patch: prevalence, histologic type, and association with esophagitis, Barrett's esophagus and antritis. Arch Pathol Lab Med 2004; 128: 444–7.

42. Von Rahden BH *et al.* Esophageal adenocarcinomas in heterotopic gastric mucosa: review and report of a case with complete response to neoadjuvant radiochemotherapy. Dig Surg 2005; 22(1–2): 107–12.

43. Park J. Heterotopic pancreas of the esophagus and stomach associated with pure esophageal atresia. J Pediatr Surg 2010; 45(3): E25–7.

44. Guillou L, et al. Ductal adenocarcinoma arising in a heterotopic pancreas situated in a hiatal hernia. Arch Pathol Lab Med 1994; 118(5): 568–71.

45. Noffingsinger AE, et al. Esophageal heterotopic pancreas presenting as an inflammatory mass. Dig Dis Sci 1995; 40(11): 2373–9.

46. Bergmann M, et al. Tracheobronchial rests in the esophagus; their relation to some benign strictures and certain types of cancer of the esophagus. J Thorac Surg 1958; 35: 97–104.

47. Cerar A, et al. Adenoid cystic carcinoma of the esophagus: a clinicopathologic study of three cases. Cancer 1991; 67: 2159–64.

48. Tsubochi H, et al. Immunohistochemical study of basaloid squamous cell carcinoma, adenoid cystic and mucoepidermoid carcinoma in the upper aerodigestive tract. Anticancer Res 2000; 20: 1205–11.

49. Owonikoko T, et al. Comparative analysis of basaloid and typical squamous cell carcinoma of the oesophagus: a molecular biological and immunohistochemical study. J Pathol 2001; 193: 155–61.

50. Morisaki Y, et al. Adenoid cystic carcinoma of the esophagus: report of a case and a review of the Japanese literature. Surg Today 1996; 26: 1006–9.

51. Kabuto T, et al. Primary adenoid cystic carcinoma of the esophagus: report of a case. Cancer 1979; 43: 2152–6

52. Hagiwara N, et al. Biologic behavior of mucoepidermoid carcinoma of the esophagus. J Nippon Med Sch 2003; 70: 401–7.

53. Lewin, et al. Barrett's esophagus, columnar dysplasia and adenocarcinoma of the esophagus. In: Atlas of Tumor Pathology: Tumors of the Esophagus and Stomach. Washington, DC: Armed Forces Institute of Pathology, 1996. pp.99–144.

54. Kanamoto A, et al. A case of small polypoid esophageal carcinoma with multidirectional differentiation, including neuroendocrine, squamous, ciliated glandular, and sarcomatous components. Arch Pathol Lab Med 2000; 124: 1685–7.

55. Van Rees BP, et al. Molecular evidence for the same clonal origin of both components of an adenosquamous Barrett carcinoma. Gastroenterology 2002; 122: 784–8.

56. Newman J, et al. The ultrastructure of oesophageal carcinomas: multidirectional differentiation – a transmission electron microscopic study of 43 cases. J Pathol 1992; 167: 193–8.

57. Ylagan LR, et al. Cd44: a marker of squamous differentiation in adenosquamous neoplasms. Arch Pathol Lab Med 2000; 124(2): 212–15.

58. Wilson CI, et al. Esophageal collision tumor (large cell neuroendocrine carcinoma and papillary carcinoma) arising in a Barrett esophagus. Arch Pathol Lab Med 2000; 124: 411–15.

59. Lam KY, et al. Squamous cell carcinoma of the oesophagus with mucin-secreting component (mucoepidermoid carcinoma and adenosquamous carcinoma): a clinicopathologic study and a review of literature. Eur J Surg Oncol 1994; 20: 25–31.

60. Montero GM, et al. Adenoacanthoma of the esophagus. Report of case. Rev Esp Enferm Apar Dig 1978; 54(7): 737–42.

61. Ohchi T, et al. A 6-year survival case of esophageal adenosquamous cancer with liver metastases cured by multidisciplinary therapy. Gan To Kagaku Ryoho 2006; 33(2): 231–4.

62. Yachida S, et al. Adenosquamous carcinoma of the esophagus. Clinicopathologic study of 18 cases. Oncology 2004; 66(3): 218–25.

63. McKechnie JC, et al. Choriocarcinoma and adenocarcinoma of the esophagus with gonadotropin secretion. Cancer 1971; 27: 694–702.

64. Ramakrishna PS et al. Choriocarcinoma – a rare association with squamous cell carcinoma of the esophagus. Indian J Gastroenterol 2006; 25(1): 42–3.

65. Trillo AA, et al. Choriocarcinoma of the esophagus: histologic and cytologic findings. A case report. Acta Cytol 1979; 23: 69–74.

66. Merimsky O, et al. Choriocarcinoma arising in a squamous cell carcinoma of esophagus. Am J Clin Oncol 2000; 23(2): 203–6.

67. Punpal A, et al. Leiomyomas of the esophagus. Ann Thorac Cardiovasc Surg 2007; 13: 78–87.

68. Mutrie CJ, et al. Esophageal leiomyoma: a 40 year experience. Ann Thorac Surg 2005; 70(4): 1122–5.

69. Klaase JM, et al. Surgery for unusual histopathologic variants of esophageal neoplasms: a report of 23 cases with emphasis on histologic characteristics. Ann Surg Oncol 2003; 10: 261–7.

70. Benedetti G, et al. Fiberoptic endoscopic resection of symptomatic leiomyoma of the upper esophagus. Acta Chirurg Scand 1990; 156: 807–8.

71. Mazur MT, et al. Gastric stromal tumors. Reappraisal of histogenesis. Am J Surg Pathol 1983; 7: 507–20.

72. Hirota S, et al. Gain of function mutations of c-kit in human gastrointestinal stromal tumors. Science 1998; 279: 577–80.

73. Heinrich M, et al. PDGFRA activating mutation in gastrointestinal stromal tumors. Science 2003; 229: 708–10.

74. Druker BJ, et al. Effects of a selective inhibitor of the Abl-tyrosine kinase on the growth of Bcr-Abl positive cells. Nat Med 1996; 2: 561–6.

75. Heinrich MC, et al. Inhibition of cKit tyrosine kinase activity by STI-571, a selective tyrosine kinase inhibitor. Blood 2000; 96: 925–32.

76. Joensuu H, et al. Effect of tyrosine kinase inhibitor STI571 in a patient with metastatic gastrointestinal stromal tumor. N Engl J Med 2001; 344: 1052–6.

77. Miettinen M, et al. Esophageal stromal tumors: a clinicopathologic, immunohistochemical and molecular genetic study of 17 cases and comparison with esophageal leiomyomas and leiomyosarcomas. Am J Surg Pathol 2000; 24: 211–22.

78. Masuda T, et al. Overt lymph node metastases from a gastrointestinal stromal tumor of the esophagus. J Thorac Cardiovasc Surg 2007; 134: 1810–11.

79. Efron DT, et al. The current management of gastrointestinal stromal tumors. Adv Surg 2005; 39: 193–221.

80. Eisenberg BL, et al. Adjuvant and neoadjuvant therapy for primary GIST. Cancer Chemother Pharmacol 2011; 67(Suppl 1): S3–S8.

81. Rocco G, et al. Leiomyosarcoma of the esophagus: results of surgical treatment. Ann Thorac Surg 1998; 66: 894–6.

82. Kimura H. Smooth muscle tumors of the esophagus: clinicopathologic findings in six patients. Dis Esoph 1999; 12: 77–81.

83. Ginsberg GG. Esophageal imaging: anatomic. In: Jobe BA, Thomas CR Jr, Hunter JG (eds) Esophageal Cancer: Principles and Practice. New York: Demos Medical Publishing, 2009. pp. 153–65.

84. Hesley ML. Role of chemotherapy and biomolecular therapy in the treatment of uterine sarcomas. Best Pract Res Clin Obstet Gynaecol 2011; 25(6): 773–82.

85. Saito R, et al. Esophageal schwannoma. Ann Thorac Surg 2000; 69: 1947–9.

86. Daimaru Y, et al. Benign schwannoma of the gastrointestinal tract: a clinicopathologic and immunohistochemical study. Hum Pathol 1988; 19: 257–64.

87. Dutta R, et al. Concurrent benign schwannoma of oesophagus and posterior mediastinum. Interact Cardiovasc Thorac Surg 2009; 9: 1032–4.

88. Yao JC, et al. One hundred years after "carcinoid" epidemiology of and prognostic factors for neuroendocrine tumors in 35,825 cases in the United States. J Clin Oncol 2008; 26: 3063–72.

89. Kloppel G, et al. ENETS consensus guidelines for the standards of care in neuroendocrine tumors towards a standardized approach to the diagnosis of gastroenteropancreatic neuroendocrine tumors and their prognostic significance. Neuroendocrinology 2009; 90: 162–6.

90. Brenner B, et al. Small cell carcinomas of the gastrointestinal tract: clinicopathological features and treatment approach. Semin Oncol 2007; 34: 43–50.

91. Scherubi H, et al. Management of early gastrointestinal neuroendocrine neoplasms. World J Gastrointest Endosc 2011; 3(7): 133–9.

92. Shia J, et al. Is non-small cell type high grade neuroendocrine carcinoma of the tubular gastrointestinal tract a distinct disease entity? Am J Surg Pathol 2008; 32(5): 719–31.

93. Kulke M, et al. Future directions in the treatment of neuroendocrine tumors: consensus report of the National Cancer Institute neuroendocrine tumor clinical trials planning meeting. J Clin Oncol 2011; 39: 934–43.

94. Reid HA, et al. Oat cell carcinoma of the esophagus. Cancer 1980; 45: 2342–7.

95. Medgyesy DC *et al.* Small cell carcinoma of the esophagus: the University of Texas M.D. Anderson Cancer Center experience and literature review. Cancer 2000; 88(2); 262–7.

96. Abrikossoff A. Ueber Myome, augsehend von der quergestreiften willkurlichen muskulatur. Virchows Arch Pathol Anat 1926; 260: 215–33.

97. Orlowska J, *et al.* A conservative approach to granular cell tumors of the esophagus: four case reports and literature review. Am J Gastroenterol 1993; 88: 311–15.

98. Johnston J, *et al.* Granular cell tumor of the gastrointestinal tract and the perianal region. A study of 74 cases. Dig Dis Sci 1981; 26: 807–16.

99. Countinho DS, *et al.* Granular cell tumors of the esophagus: report of two cases and review of the literature. Am J Gastroenterol 1985; 80: 758–62.

100. Brady PG, *et al.* Granular cell tumor of the esophagus: natural history, diagnosis and therapy. Dig Dis Sci 1988; 33: 1329–33.

101. Ohmori T, *et al.* Malignant granular cell tumor of the esophagus. A case report with light and electron microscopic, histochemical and immunohistochemical study. Acta Pathol Jpn 1987; 37: 775–83.

102. Sashiyama H, *et al.* Case report: a case of lymphoepithelioma-like carcinoma of the esophagus and review of the literature. J. Gastroenterol Hepatol 1999; 14(6): 534–9.

103. Mori M, *et al.* Ten-year survivors after surgical treatment and peri-operative irradiation for esophageal carcinoma. J Surg Oncol 1991; 47: 71–4.

104. Moore OS, *et al.* The relatively favorable prognosis of medullary carcinoma of the breast. Cancer 1949; 2: 635–42.

105. Bramdev CR, *et al.* Primary extramedullary plasmacytoma of the esophagus. Ann Diagn Pathol 2003; 7(3): 174–9.

106. Watanabe H, *et al.* Gastric carcinoma with lymphoid stroma. Cancer 1976; 38: 232–43.

107. Hasumi K, *et al.* Circumscribed carcinoma of the uterine cervix, with marked lymphocytic infiltration. Cancer 1977; 39: 2503–27.

108. Saemundsen AK, *et al.* Epstein Barr Virus in nasopharyngeal and salivary gland carcinomas of Greenland Eskimos. Br J Cancer 1982; 46: 721–8.

109. Leyvraz S, *et al.* Association of Epstein–Barr virus with thymic carcinoma. N Engl J Med 1985; 312: 1296–9.

110. Swanson SA, *et al.* Lymphoepithelioma-like carcinoma of the skin. Mod Pathol 1988; 1: 359–65.

111. Iezzoni JC, *et al.* The role of Epstein–Barr virus in lymphoepithelioma-like carcinomas. Am J Clin Pathol 1995; 103: 308–14.

112. Kamiyoshi K, *et al.* A case of esophageal non-small cellular undifferentiated carcinoma with lymphoid stroma. Jpn J Gastroenterol Surg 1994; 27: 446–8.

113. Herrmann R, *et al.* Gastrointestinal involvement in non-Hodgkin's lymphoma. Cancer 1980; 46: 215–22.

114. Freeman C, *et al.* Occurrence and prognosis of extranodal lymphomas. Cancer 1972; 29: 252–60.

115. Orvidas LJ, *et al.* Lymphoma involving the esophagus. Ann Otol Rhinol Laryngol 1994; 103: 843–8.

116. Dawson JM, *et al.* Primary malignant lymphoid tumors tumors of the intestinal tract. Report of 37 cases with a study of factors influencing prognosis. Br J Surg 1961; 49: 80–9.

117. Weeratunge CN, *et al.* Primary esophageal lymphoma: a diagnostic challenge in acquired immunodeficiency syndrome – two case reports and review. South Med J 2004; 97: 383–7.

118. Golioto M, *et al.* Primary lymphoma of the esophagus in a chronically immunosuppressed patient with hepatitis C: case report and review of the literature. Am J Med Sci 2001; 321: 203–5.

119. George MK, *et al.* Primary esophageal T-cell lymphoma. Indian J Gastroenterol 1005; 24: 119–24.

120. Perry RR, *et al.* Tracheoesophageal fistula in the patient with lymphoma: case report and review of the literature. Surgery 1989; 105(6): 770–7.

121. Doki T, *et al.* Primary malignant lymphoma of the esophagus. A case report. Endoscopy 1984; 16: 189–92.

122. Chadha KS, *et al.* Primary esophageal lymphoma: case series and review of the literature. Dig Dis Sci 2006; 51: 77–83.

123. Taal BG, *et al.* Isolated primary oesophageal involvement by lymphoma: a rare cause of dysphagia and a review of other published data. Gut 1993; 34: 994–8.

124. DiCostnazo DP, *et al.* Primary malignant melanoma of the esophagus. Am J Surg Pathol 1897; 11: 46–7.

125. Sharma SS, *et al.* Melanosis of the esophagus. An endoscopic, histochemical and ultrastructural study. Gastroenterology 1991; 100(1): 13–16.

126. Mills SE, *et al.* Malignant melanoma of the digestive system. Pathol Annu 1983; 18: 1–26.

127. Symmans WF, *et al.* Malignant melanoma of the esophagus: histologic variants and immunohistochemical findings in four cases. Surg Pathol 1991; 4: 222–34.

128. Sabanathan S, *et al.* Primary melanoma of the esophagus. Am J Gastroenterol 1989; 84: 1475–81.

129. Agha FP. Secondary neoplasms of the esophagus. Gastrointest Radiol 1987; 12: 187–93.

130. Mizobuchi S *et al.* Metastatic esophageal tumors from distant primary lesions: report of three esophagectomies and study of 1835 cases. Jap J Clin Oncol 1997; 27: 410–14.

131. Holyoke ED *et al.* Esophageal metastases and dysphagia in patients with carcinoma of the breast. J Surg Oncol 1969; 1: 97–107.

132. Trentino P, *et al.* Esophageal metastasis from clear cell carcinoma of the kidney. Am J Gastroenterol 1997; 1381–2.

133. Eng J, *et al.* Malignant melanoma metastatic to the esophagus. Ann Thorac Surg 1989; 48: 287–8.

134. Zarian LP, *et al.* Metastatic endometrial carcinoma to the esophagus. Am J Gastroenterol 1983; 78: 9–11.

135. Rampado S, *et al.* Mediastinal carcinosis involving the esophagus in breast cancer: the "breast-esophagus" syndrome. Report on 25 cases and guidelines for diagnosis and treatment. Ann Surg 2007; 246: 316–22.

136. Sobel JM, *et al.* The utility of EUS-guided FNA in the diagnosis of metastatic breast cancer to the esophagus and mediastinum. Gastrointest Endosc 2005; 61: 416–20.

137. Haney JC, *et al.* Transhiatal esophagogastrectomy for an isolated ovarian cancer metastasis to the esophagus. J Thorac Cardiovasc Surg 2004; 127(6): 1835–6.

28 Uncommon Cancers of the Stomach

Elizabeta Popa,[1] Felice Schnoll-Sussman,[2] Arun Jesudian,[2] Govind Nandakumar,[3] and Manish A. Shah[1]

[1] Division of Hematology and Medical Oncology, Gastrointestinal Oncology, Department of Medicine, [2] Division of Gastroenterology and Hepatology, Department of Medicine, [3] Department of Surgery, Colorectal Surgery, Center for Advanced Digestive Care, New York-Presbyterian Hospital, Weill Cornell Medical College of Cornell University, New York, NY, USA

Introduction

Gastric cancer is the second leading cause of cancer-related mortality worldwide.[1] The Surveillance, Epidemiology and End Results (SEER) database reports an incidence of gastric cancer at 10.8 per 100,000 among men and 5.4 per 100,000 among women in the US.[2] Over the past several decades, there has been a slight decline in both the incidence and mortality of gastric cancer, attributable to increased treatment and recognition of chronic inflammation secondary to acid reflux and *Helicobacter pylori* as well as improvements in food processing and storage systems.[3] In the US, patients with gastric cancer present in equal distribution of stages with roughly one-third of patients diagnosed with localized, regional or metastatic disease and associated with 5-year overall survival rates of 61%, 28%, and 4%, respectively.[2]

Several different histological types of malignancy can be found in the stomach. These different tumor types have widely differing biological behaviors and prognoses. Adenocarcinomas constitute the overwhelming majority of gastric cancers, accounting for more than 90%. Gastric adenocarcinomas have been traditionally classified into two histological subtypes by the Lauren classification, intestinal and diffuse, which portend different biological behavior. More recently, three distinct gastric cancer subtypes have been promoted – proximal/gastric cardia nondiffuse gastric cancer, diffuse gastric cancer, and distal/body nondiffuse gastric cancer – each with different risk factors and epidemiology.[4] These gastric cancer subtypes have distinct molecular profiles, suggesting unique biology.[5]

Proximal gastric cancer is commonly grouped together with gastroesophageal junction (GEJ) and distal esophageal adenocarcinoma. There is a notable differential effect of *H. pylori* infection on the development of proximal versus distal intestinal gastric cancers. Specifically, *H. pylori* infection is associated with increased risk of developing noncardia gastric adenocarcinoma, whereas infection with *H. pylori* appears to be protective for the development of more proximal tumors in some case–control cohort studies.[6,7] The stepwise development

of proximal gastric cancer has not been specifically described, although it may be related to chronic inflammation as in reflux disease and Barrett esophagus. The pathogenesis of noncardia intestinal gastric cancer, however, has been well described. Distal/body intestinal gastric cancer follows a multistep progression that is likely initiated by chronic inflammation (e.g. as a result of *H. pylori* infection,[8,9] chronic gastritis, or autoimmune gastritis). The disease progresses through chronic gastritis, intestinal metaplasia, and dysplasia.[10] Environmental factors that increase the risk of developing noncardia gastric cancer include tobacco, high salt intake (reviewed by Wang[11]), and alcohol consumption.

Diffuse gastric cancer, in contrast, has no known precursor lesion, although mutation or epigenetic silencing of the *E-cadherin* gene appears to be a key carcinogenic event. *E-cadherin* loss is observed by immunohistochemistry in approximately 50% of patients with sporadic diffuse gastric cancer and confirmed by genome sequencing,[12] suggesting that this pathway may present a common precursor event in the development of diffuse gastric cancer, distinct from chronic inflammation and gastric atrophy that characterizes intestinal noncardia gastric cancer.

Hereditary diffuse gastric cancer (HDGC) is a genetic predisposition syndrome that was defined in 1999 by the International Gastric Cancer Linkage Consortium (IGCLC). Clinical criteria for genetic testing have recently been updated, and include the diagnosis of diffuse gastric cancer before the age of 40, or having one or more first-degree relatives or two or more second-degree relatives with diffuse gastric cancer.[13] HDGC is caused by loss of function mutations in the E-cadherin (*CDH1*) gene. The current recommendations for patients harboring a *CDH1* mutation is prophylactic gastrectomy, which is felt to dramatically reduce the risk of developing gastric cancer.[13] Notably, HDGC represents approximately 30% of all familial gastric cancers.

About 10% of gastric cancers are not the adenocarcinomas as described above. These unusual tumors of the stomach come

Textbook of Uncommon Cancer, Fourth Edition. Edited by Derek Raghavan, Charles D. Blanke, David H. Johnson, Paul L. Moots, Gregory H. Reaman, Peter G. Rose and Mikkael A. Sekeres.
© 2012 John Wiley & Sons, Inc. Published 2012 by John Wiley & Sons, Inc.

in a wide variety and are of clinical significance despite their relative rarity. These include neuroendocrine cancers of the stomach, gastric gastrointestinal stromal tumors (GISTs), gastric tumors related to pathogenic infection (i.e. mucosa-associated lymphoid tissue (MALT) lymphomas and Epstein–Barr virus (EBV)-associated gastric cancer), as well as other even more rare gastric cancer subtypes. Their biology and treatments are outlined below.

Neuroendocrine tumors of the stomach

Neuroendocrine tumor (NET) is a broad term that encompasses a spectrum of epithelial malignancies possesing predominantly neuroendocrine characteristics. These tumors tend to be relatively indolent malignancies and are characterized by secretion of proteins leading to specific clinical syndromes. However, more aggressive forms of NETs exist with a much more aggressive course and associated with a high mortality. The term neuroendocrine tumor has been historically interchangeably used with the term carcinoid. However, given an increasing understanding of histological subtypes and their associated clinical behavior, the use of that term has fallen out of favor.

The annual incidence of digestive NETs, also known as gastroenteropancreatic NETs (GEP-NETs), is 3.65 per 100,000 population. The reported incidence of gastric NETs varies according to geographic area and analysis type. In a recent SEER registry analysis, gastric NETs accounted for 4–6% of all neuroendocrine tumors in the US, with an annual incidence of 0.3 per 100,000 people.[14] In addition, the incidence of GEP-NETs is increasing, with a recent analysis reporting a 10-fold rise.[15] Gastric NETs are typically classified as foregut tumors, which are composed of neuroendocrine tumors of the stomach and proximal duodenum. Recent reports suggest significant geographic differences, including that the stomach may be the most common site of disease in European populations.[16] Gastric NETs are generally diagnosed at an early stage as localized disease, though somewhat later by comparison than GEP-NETs of the rectum and duodenum.

Classification

The 2010 WHO classification of NETs established a new staging schema for GEP-NETs. The European Neuroendocrine Tumor Society (ENETS) guidelines recommends incorporation of this staging schema into the most recent 2009 American Joint Commission on Cancer (AJCC)/International Union against Cancer (UICC) staging system.[17,18] The WHO schema separates tumors into well-differentiated, intermediate-grade and poorly differentiated tumors (G1–G3 respectively), based on mitotic count and Ki-67 staining (Table 28.1). There is further stratification of GEP-NETs into pure and mixed histology if more or less than 30% of all tumor cells have nonendocrine components. The AJCC staging system has a separate schema for pancreatic NETs (P-NETs) due to a somewhat better prognosis conferred by that location.[19] This can be seen in the fact that lymph node-positive disease for P-NETs is considered stage IIb rather than IIIb. Gastric NETs (G-NETs), however, continue to be segregated with the other GEP-NETs with no individual staging schema. In addition, the WHO further stratifies GEP-NETs into pure and mixed histology, if more or less than 30% of all tumor cells have nonendocrine components.

A secondary, older embryological classification remains useful, as it takes into account the foregut origin of the stomach as well as associated clinical characteristics. According to this schema, G-NETs were initially classified into three groups named types I–III tumors respectively with a fourth type recently added to incorporate small cell histology[20] (see Table 28.1).

Type I and II tumors are often multifocal and account for approximately 80% of all G-NETs. These two subtypes are thought to arise from enterochromaffin-like (ECL) cells that are hyperstimulated by chronically elevated gastrin levels.[21] These tumors often arise in the setting of atrophic gastritis with associated hypergastrinemia. More recently, ghrelin-containing cells have also been found to be involved.[22] Type I and II tumors have a generally indolent behavior. Type I G-NETs are the most common subtype (>70% of all G-NETs) and are associated with chronic atrophic gastritis while type II tumors

Table 28.1 TNM staging neuroendocrine.

Stage	T (tumor size/invasion)	N (nodal status)	M (metastasis)
AJCC 2010			
0	Tis	N0	M0
I	T1	N0	M0
IIA	T2	N0	M0
IIB	T3	N0	M0
IIIA	T4	N0	M0
IIIB	T1–T4	N1	M0
IV	T1–T4	N0–N1	M1
WHO 2010			
	Grade	Mitoses per 10 HPF	Ki-67/MIB-1 index
Neuroendocrine tumor	G1	<2	<2%
Neuroendocrine tumor	G2	2–20	3–20%
Neuroendocrine carcinoma (large or small cell)	G3	>20	>20%

HPF, high-power field.

occur in the setting of Zollinger–Ellison syndrome (ZES) and multiple endocrine neoplasia type I (MEN 1).[23] Patients with type I G-NETs are usually found to have multiple small nodules in the body of the stomach and limited to the mucosa and submucosa. Type 1 G-NETs tend to be very indolent, and may regress following antrectomy.

Lymph node metastases are rare (occurring only when tumors are >2 cm, and when infiltrating through the muscularis propria). Type II G-NETs are more rare, commonly presenting as multifocal, small tumors (generally <1.5 cm), developing in the body of the stomach and confined to the mucosa or submucosa.[24] In contrast to type I G-NET, type II G-NETs have a modest risk of developing metastases (30%), with increased risk in tumors >2 cm, invading the muscularis propria, and exhibiting vascular invasion.

Type III Ga-NETs are the second most common and are also known as sporadic G-NETs. These NETs have no association with gastrin overproduction, are composed of a more heterogeneous population of cells and thus can be rarely associated with an atypical secretory syndrome characterized by cutaneous flushing without diarrhea due to release of histamine and 5-hydroxytryptophan.[23] Type III tumors are more aggressive, have >30% incidence of lymph node metastases and are often diagnosed with hepatic metastases. These tumors may occur throughout the stomach.

Type IV tumors are poorly differentiated (high-grade) tumors with no secretory component, extensive metastatic disease at presentation and usually with small or large cell histology akin to that found in lung tumors and they represent a rare group of G-NETs with only a few hundred cases reported in the literature.[25]

Clinical features and usual presentation

Patients diagnosed with a G-NET (type I) often present with vague abdominal symptoms, undergo upper endoscopy, and are found to have multifocal, subcentimeter, well-differentiated gastric corpus lesions with no secretory syndrome. Indeed, endoscopy is done for symptoms unrelated to the presence of G-NETs in the majority of cases. Another common presentation (type III) would be that of a middle-aged male with a larger lesion, T2 or greater stage, low to intermediate grade and significant rate of metastatic disease (>50% in one series). Type IV G-NETs, which are very rarely encountered, have been traditionally classified into two subcategories, pure and composite type, depending on the absence or presence of a mixture of adenocarcinoma and/or squamous cell carcinoma along with small cell carcinoma. Only case reports or small case series exist of type IV G-NETs but all agree on the dismal prognosis with rapid and early progressive metastatic disease.

The flushing in G-NETs is not associated with diaphoresis and has an intense purplish or violet hue in contrast to the common red/pink hue seen in other NET-related carcinoid syndromes. Telangiectasias and thickening of the skin of the face and upper neck can occur with lasting change in appearance after repeated episodes.[26] The syndrome is due to release of histamine and to absence of dopa-decarboxylase in the tumor cells, leading to secretion of 5-hydroxytryptophan rather than serotonin.

Pathology

Pathological diagnosis of GEP-NETs requires a description of tumor morphology as well as immunohistochemical characteristics and grade of the tumor. Sequential progression from hyperplastic to neoplastic lesions has been described only for type I and II tumors derived from ECL cells. Most G-NETs are type I, well-differentiated, low-grade tumors (Fig. 28.1).

Immunohistochemical characteristics recommended by the WHO classification for histological diagnosis include positive staining for chromogranin-A (CGA) and synaptophysin (SP). CGA is a functional component of the membrane of intracellular neurosecretory vesicles and as such is more often expressed on well-differentiated tumors that contain them. SP, on the other hand, is a component of small synaptic vesicles that are found in all neuroendocrine tumors. Neuron-specific enolase (NSE), CD56 antigen or CDX-2 can have variable expression in G-NETs and are sometimes used to aid in diagnosis of very poorly differentiated tumors. More recently, vesicular monoamine transporter 2 (VMAT2) and somatostatin receptor 2A (SSTR-2A) have been discovered as GEP-NET specific markers with possible clinical utility[27,28] (Table 28.2).

Histamine is formed by ECL cells and is concentrated in the neurosecretory vesicles by VMAT2.[29] SSTR-2A has the greatest binding affinity to somatostatin analogs and can be found in a majority of G-NETs. VMAT2 can also be used as a marker of G-NETs when trying to identify the origin of a metastatic tumor. SSTR-2A expression has implications for the utility of somatostatin analogs (SSAs) both for diagnostic testing (In[111]-DTPA octreotide imaging) and therapeutic purposes.[30]

Proliferation-based grading is an essential part of the characterization and staging of all GEP-NETs. The Ki-67/MIB index groupings adopted by the WHO are composed of low-grade (G1) with an index of <2%, intermediate grade (G2) 2–20% and high grade (G3) >20% neoplasms.[31] Histological

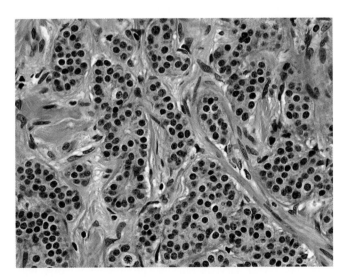

Figure 28.1 Type I neuroendocrine tumor of the stomach.

	Type I	Type II	Type III	Type IV
Disease frequency	70–80%	~5%	~15%	<5%
Lymph node metastases	Rare	Rare	Common	Common
Distribution	Multifocal, ≤1 cm	Multifocal, ≤1 cm	Solitary, ≥2 cm	Solitary, ulcerated
Location	Corpus	Corpus	Nonspecific	Nonspecific
Serum gastrin	High	High	Normal	Normal
Gastric pH	High	Low	Normal	Normal
Tumor grade	G1	G1	G1/2	G3
IHC markers				
CGA	Yes	Yes	Yes	Variable
SP	Yes	Yes	Yes	Yes
NSE	Variable	Variable	Variable	Yes
VMAT2	Yes	Yes	Variable	No
Ki-67	<2%	<2%	2–20%	>20%
SSTR	Positive	Positive	Variable	Variable

Table 28.2 Clinicopathological characteristics of gastric neuroendocrine tumors.

CGA, chromogranin-A; IHC, immunohistochemistry; NSE, neuron-specific enolase; SP, synaptophysin; SSTR, somatostatin receptor; VMAT, vesicular monoamine transporter.

grading can provide information regarding the utility of diagnostic tests such as fluorodeoxyglucose positron emission tomography (FDG-PET) as it has been established that Ki-67 index is closely correlated with FDG uptake.

Of note, exocrine-endocrine (amphicrine) differentiated carcinomas of the stomach have been described that contain both neuroendocrine and exocrine tumor components due to either dual histological characteristics or anatomical collision.[32] In general, these tumors are to be managed as gastric adenocarcinomas.

Genetic associations

Gastric NETs, most often type II, develop in up to 30% of patients with MEN 1/ZES. In this setting, G-NETs usually develop after decades of disease. Though thymic and bronchial NETs are more common in MEN 1, there is an increased incidence of G-NETs as well in this setting.[33] A case series of 57 patients with MEN 1/ZES was prospectively evaluated for the development of G-NETs and associated risk factors.[34] There was an almost 25% incidence of G-NETs reported, with high fasting serum gastrin levels and long disease duration associated with a higher risk. The authors suggest regular surveillance of these patients for G-NETs. Interestingly, loss of heterozygosity at the MEN 1 gene locus 11q13 is found commonly in type I G-NETs as well as predictably in 100% of type II tumors.[35]

Prognostic implications

As mentioned above, the new classifications systems were updated to better define prognostic groups. Five-year survival rates for G-NETs range from 21% to 74% depending on AJCC/UICC stage. Long-term survival data by tumor type utilizing the more modern classification system have been reported largely in retrospective series. Five-year survival for type I G-NETs approximates that of the general population. As expected, 5-year survival rates are progressively worse with higher grade and tumor type number, ranging from 70% for

type II to less than 50% for type III. Type IV G-NETs have a median overall survival (OS) of approximately 12 months.[14]

Diagnostic considerations

As noted above, most G-NETs are found incidentally.[16] For complete evaluation and for accurate staging and treatment planning, one must obtain serum gastrin levels. There is dissociation of gastric pH and gastrin levels between types I and II tumors, with the former being associated with achlorhydria while the latter is associated with a very low gastric pH.[36] If a gastric pH <2 and elevated gastrin levels are found, a secretin stimulation test should be performed to confirm the diagnosis of ZES, if not previously made. Plasma CGA levels are frequently elevated in types I–III G-NETs and are useful for surveillance. In patients with metastatic disease, high CGA levels may have prognostic value. CGA levels are known to decline in patients on SSA therapy and may reflect decrease in hormonal synthesis rather than decline in tumor mass. Conversely, a rise in CGA level while on SSA therapy may indicate autonomous hypersecretion versus progression of tumor. More recently, CGA level change has been shown to be a poor surrogate measure for changes in tumor burden.[37]

G-NETs are usually detected during endoscopy (Fig. 28.2). Surgical management depends on the identification of T and N stage and endoscopic ultrasound (EUS). EUS is useful in determining T stage and depth of invasion. Recent prospective case series suggest usefulness in selecting tumors for endoscopic and/or limited surgical resections based on results of EUS staging.[38]

Gastric NET liver metastases are hypervascular and dual-phase computed tomography (CT) imaging to assess for metastases is recommended in patients with type I or II G-NETs >2 cm as well as for most patients with types III and IV tumors.[39] Lastly, somatostatin receptor scintigraphy (SRS) has been recommended as an adjunct to staging high-risk disease. For G-NETs, sensitivities range around 75% but there is high >90% sensitivity. Reduced sensitivity of SRS is noted for sub-centimeter lesions.[40] ^{111}In-diethylene triamine pentaacetic acid

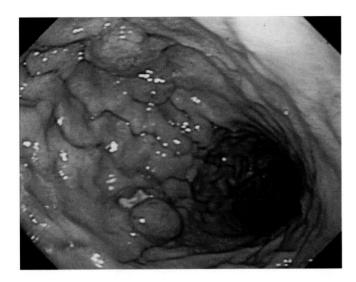

Figure 28.2 Endoscopic appearance of type I G-NET.

(DTPA) octreotide is the only registered radiopharmaceutical for SRS of GEP-NETs. As described above, the expression of multiple subtypes of SSTRs by tumor cells allows for visualization and the amount of radionuclide uptake can help predict therapeutic effect of SSAs. SSA therapy can affect accuracy of SRS and official guidelines recommend withdrawal of long-acting SSAs before imaging is carried out.[41]

New SRS techniques are under advanced clinical testing but none has yet been approved by the European Medicines Agency (EMA)/Food and Drug Administration (FDA).[40] Radiolabeled somatostatin analogs that are used for both diagnostic and therapeutic purposes consist of three parts: a cyclic octapeptide, a chelator, and a radionuclide. Modifications to ^{111}In-DTPA have included changing the chelator to dodecanetetraacetic acid[42] instead of DTPA, allowing for stable conjugation with the newer β-emitting radionuclides such as yttrium-90 (^{90}Y) and lutetium-177 (^{177}Lu), which are used in peptide receptor radionuclide therapy (PRRT) (see below). PET using 18 F-FDG is only useful in tumors with high proliferative activity and low differentiation grade.[43] FDG-PET is only indicated in staging small cell and large cell G-NETs as well as in the rare cases of nontype IV G-NETs that are negative on ^{111}In-DTPA imaging.

Treatment of localized disease

Type I G-NETs have a very low frequency of direct invasion into the muscularis or of distant metastasis. Conservative strategies are warranted, including observation only for the elderly with small tumors, limited surgeries with endoscopic mucosal resection (EMR) or antrectomy.[44] If EMR is performed, surveillance by endoscopy is necessary every 1–2 years. In addition, lymphovascular invasion needs to be assessed as completion surgery may be warranted. Antrectomy has been reported to abolish hypergastrinemia and cause regression of unresected tumors, likely due to withdrawal of the paracrine stimulation.[45] In general, antrectomy is reserved for tumors >2 cm or multifocal disease. Endoscopic techniques are being explored, including endoscopic mucosal dissection (EMD)

that allows for *en bloc* R0 resection of multifocal disease. In general, surgical resection is not considered for G-NETs smaller than 2 cm unless they show grade 2 characteristics, higher T stage or lymphovascular invasion. Long-term treatment with somatostatin analogs has been reported to cause regression of subcentimeter G-NETs and may be a consideration for elderly patients. This latter approach has no prospective studies regarding survival outcomes while retrospective data suggest equivalent outcomes. None of the above approaches has been studied in a randomized or controlled manner.[16,20]

Treatment options for type II G-NETs are even more controversial given the coexistence of a gastrinoma. An antrectomy does not improve hypergastrinemia and total gastrectomy is more likely to be recommended given the increased risk for recurrence and metastasis.[46] Another indication for total gastrectomy includes G-NETs of any type or grade with evidence of recurrence on surveillance endoscopy. Type III G-NETs are usually surgically resected given that they are present as solitary tumors. Localized type IV small or large cell NETs have minimal data regarding optimal therapies as they are often diagnosed with metastatic disease. Therapeutic strategies have been extrapolated from those of the more common pulmonary tumors, including systemic therapies, with a recent report supporting this strategy.[47] In contrast to chemoradiation which is recommended for limited-stage small cell lung cancer, localized poorly differentiated neuroendocrine tumors of the stomach are surgically resected.

Treatment of metastatic disease

Most nonsurgical treatment strategies for G-NETs, including SSA therapy, are extrapolated from results of large studies including all GEP-NETs. Resection of metastatic disease to the liver is recommended when possible. Overall, a 10% of all GEP-NETs with liver metastases can achieve a long-term remission with resection if there is unifocal metastatic disease.[48,49]

Despite being more aggressive phenotypically, hepatic metastasectomy can be recommended for type III G-NETs as well as for types I and II, given their relatively indolent course. Criteria defining what metastatic tumor burden is appropriate for surgical resection have not been defined. Locoregional ablative therapies are used for multifocal or unresectable hepatic metastases. Current radiofrequency ablation (RFA) technology can be used for hepatic metastases up to 4–5 cm in diameter. In 2008, a classification was proposed to stratify patients most appropriate for RFA. It was determined that oligometastatic disease is appropriate for RFA, which is to be used as an adjunct to resection or to SSA therapy.[50,51]

Lastly, transhepatic artery embolization (TAE) techniques with particle embolization, chemoembolization (anthracycline or platinum chemotherapy), and selective internal radiation microsphere therapies (^{90}Y) are used mostly to palliate symptoms of carcinoid syndrome.[50] Several case series have been published showing 5-year postembolization survival rates of 28–44% for GEP-NET liver metastases.[52]

The mainstay of treatment, however, for metastatic GEP-NETs that are unresectable is SSA therapy in all but type IV tumors.[53] There are minimal data, however, to support the use of SSAs in nonfunctioning tumors, which represent the majority of G-NETs. SSAs bind mostly to SSTR subtypes 2 and 5. They are of most use in controlling hormonal symptoms of secretory GEP-NETs. Nevertheless, SSAs for G-NETs are routinely given for growth factor antagonism effects. At very high dosage SSAs have been shown to induce apoptosis.[54]

The PROMID study (Placebo-controlled, double-blind, prospective, Randomized study on the effect of Octreotide LAR in the control of tumour growth in patients with metastatic neuroendocrine MIDgut tumors) revealed a significant improvement in progression-free survival (PFS), from 6 months in the placebo group to 14.3 months in patients with metastatic GEP-NETs of midgut origin receiving octreotide long-acting release (LAR).[55] Octreotide and lanreotide are the two commercially available SSAs. Both short- and long-acting formulations exist. SSAs are well tolerated with mild symptoms attributable to absorptive dysfunction (flatulence, cramps, diarrhea or steatorrhea) but may predispose to gallstones, prompting removal of the gallbladder at the time of metastasectomy, when feasible. Rarely can bradycardia or alopecia can occur.[44] There is ongoing interest in the development of new SSAs, such as pasireotide, with different SSTR subtype affinities.[56]

Although G-NETs are rarely associated with carcinoid syndrome, SSAs should be available perioperatively as well as before locoregional therapies such as RFA or TAE procedures as these therapies may trigger massive release of hormones from necrotic tumor which rarely can provoke a carcinoid crisis, depending on the size of targeted tumor volume.

Treatment with PRRT is an emerging option for metastatic GEP-NETs. Agents used include [90]Y- and ^{177}Lu-labeled peptide analogs with varying affinities for the SSTR subtypes.[57] Selection of therapeutic agent can be done based on pretreatment imaging (see above). Most trials to date are single-arm phase 2 studies. They have revealed variable response rates ranging from 0–29% with stable disease (SD) in 35–81%. Toxicities could be severe, including significant myelosuppression and renal toxicity as well as a few cases of myelodysplastic syndrome (MDS) and overt leukemic transformation. Various modalities are described to mitigate the hematological and renal toxicities of PRRT therapies, including the coadministration of amino acids such as D-lysine to reduce renal tubular peptide binding but currently no standardized approach is in use.[58,59]

Systemic therapies with cytotoxic chemotherapy or interferon have been traditionally used with minimal impact on survival after failure of SSA therapy. In a prospective study for assessment of the antiproliferative activity of SSA and interferon (IFN), no superiority of a combination therapy of lanreotide and IFN to either drug alone could be demonstrated.[60] Lanreotide alone is currently under further evaluation in an ongoing placebo-controlled trial (the CLARINET study[61]) in nonfunctioning well-differentiated GEP-NETs.[62]

Streptozotocin-based chemotherapeutic regimens have been the mainstay of therapy for SSA-refractory types I–III GEP-NETs since the 1970s. Two retrospective analyses and one more recent prospective study demonstrated response rates of 39% and 36% respectively, at the cost of significant toxicity, with no randomized studies ever done to document survival benefit.[63,64] Systemic therapies are only starting to show efficacy in GEP-NETs with the advent of new targeted agents such as the tyrosine kinase inhibitor sunitinib malate and the mTOR inhibitor everolimus.[65,66] Both these agents have recently been FDA approved only for the treatment of P-NETs. Even in older studies, increased responsiveness of P-NETs to systemic therapies has been noted. In 2006, a trial with one of the earliest antiangiogenic agents, thalidomide, combined with temozolomide, reported a relative risk (RR) of 45% among P-NETs as opposed to 7% for other GEP-NETs.[67]

Extrapolating results of these trials to formulate a management strategy for G-NETs is not advised. P-NETs derive from precursors in the ductal epithelium, and commonly are diagnosed with metastatic disease (64% versus 15% for G-NETs).[14] Phase 2 studies have not enrolled a significant number of G-NETs, suggesting that further studies are warranted. Other agents under current scrutiny include bevacizumab, sorafenib, and pazopanib. All these agents are multitargeted and attempt to exploit an antiangiogenic mechanism of action. Notably, bevacizumab combined with octreotide LAR was compared to IFN-α2b in a random assignment study.[68] Investigators observed a response rate of 18% with bevacizumab + octreotide LAR versus 0% for the IFN arm, as well as a clinically significant improvement in PFS, leading to a presently ongoing phase 3 trial (SWOG S0518[69]). Smaller studies using the classic colorectal cancer regimen of FOLFOX or XELOX (5-fluorouracil or capecitabine and oxaliplatin) and bevacizumab have demonstrated RR of up to 33% with arguably better tolerability than streptozotocin-based therapies.[70] At present, drugs targeting epidermal growth factor receptor (EGFR) or insulin-like growth factor (IGF)-1/insulin-like growth factor receptor (IGFR) pathways are also being evaluated as there are in vitro correlates between EGFR expression and prognosis as well as a suggestion that IGF-mediated pathways are involved in GEP-NET proliferation via an autocrine loop mechanism.[71]

Most of the above therapeutic options apply to types I–III G-NETs. Type IV G-NETs present different sensitivity to therapies with no role for SSAs and a minimal role for locoregional ablative therapies. Small or large cell histology is associated, as noted before, with rapid systemic proliferation and sensitivity to platinum-doublets used as first-line therapy for small cell carcinomas of the lung.

Summary and recommendations

The classic and most common G-NETs subtype I can be managed conservatively or with surgery only when identified as localized disease. More aggressive surgical resection needs to be pursued for type III G-NETs. The much rarer types II and IV disease require multidisciplinary team management to determine the sequence of therapies to be used, including surgical and systemic therapies when found at an early stage.

Metastatic G-NETs of all types excluding type IV may be managed with antihormonal therapies for years with minimal toxicity. Novel radiolabeled or targeted systemic therapies need to be approached with caution given the lack of mature data in most cases and significant toxicities. The risks of therapy need to be carefully balanced against the generally indolent course of disease. Newer combinations of targeted therapies such as FOLFOX-A can be considered when disease response is paramount due to symptoms caused by disease bulk.

Gastrointestinal stromal tumors

Most subepithelial tumors of the gastrointestinal (GI) tract are stromal or mesenchymal neoplasms which are traditionally divided into two broad categories: the more common gastrointestinal stromal tumors (GISTs) and the rarer soft tissue and neural origin tumors including leiomyomas, leiomyosarcomas, schwannomas, and nerve sheath tumors.[72] The term GIST was introduced in 1983 to describe those mesenchymal tumors of the GI tract of neither neurogenic nor smooth muscle origin. Gastrointestinal stromal tumors most commonly arise in the stomach (60–70%), followed by the small intestine (20–30%), and rarely elsewhere in the GI tract or at extraintestinal sites such as the omentum, mesentery, or retroperitoneum.[73]

Estimating the true frequency of GISTs has been difficult as much of the available epidemiological data was collected prior to the use of molecular diagnostics and therefore based on incorrect definitions. Informal estimates based on recruiting into therapeutic trials yield an approximate annual incidence of 5000–6000 new cases of GISTs per year in the United States.[74] Although reported in patients of all ages, GISTs occur primarily in adults with a median age of around 60 years, with a slight male predominance.[75] GIST tumors are characterized by overexpression of the c-kit receptor. Although some families with heritable GISTs have been identified, the vast majority of GIST tumors arise sporadically.[76]

Classification

The National Institutes of Health (NIH) consensus statement from 2002 stratifies patients into very low, low, intermediate, and high risk based on tumor size and mitotic index.[77] In 2011, a modified NIH classification incorporated tumor rupture into the stratification system as a high-risk tumor irrespective of other features as well as some refinements in classification of nongastric tumors into various risk groups.[78] In 2010, the AJCC/UICC TNM schema was created by incorporating findings both from the NIH as well as from two large retrospective clinicopathological case series carried out by the Armed Forces Institute of Pathology (AFIP), in which almost 3000 cases were reviewed.[73]

All GISTs have potential for aggressive behavior. Gastric GISTs have a better outcome than intestinal GISTs and as such have a separate AJCC/UICC stage grouping. Mutational status of the gene encoding the KIT receptor is not yet incorporated into risk stratification but patients with certain mutations are more likely to respond to antireceptor tyrosine kinase (RTK) therapy with imatinib, which has a significant impact upon overall survival in the unresectable disease setting.[79]

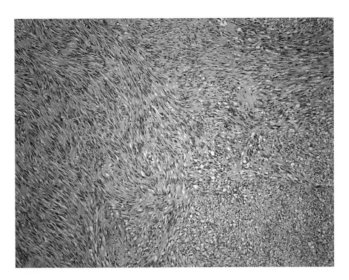

Figure 28.3 Low-power H&E microscopic appearance of GIST.

Clinical pathology

Gastrointestinal stromal tumors likely originate from the interstitial cells of Cajal (ICCs), distributed in specific locations within the tunica muscularis of the gastrointestinal tract, which act as electrical pacemakers and mediators of enteric neurotransmission.[80] Prior to the discovery of the CD117 antigen, GISTs were defined histologically as a heterogeneous group of spindle cell neoplasms with morphological variations including epithelioid and mixed subtypes of unclear prognostic significance with bland morphological features not predictive of benign clinical behavior (Fig. 28.3).

CD117, otherwise known as KIT, is pathognomonic for a GIST tumor.[81] It is one of a family of membrane RTKs that includes platelet-derived growth factor receptors (PDGFRA, PDGFRB), macrophage colony-stimulating factor receptor (CSF1R), and Fl cytokine receptor (FLT3). Mutations in the KIT receptor constitute primary oncogenic events that result in ligand-independent receptor dimerization and constitutive kinase activation. GISTs may be further classified by mutational type that is relevant to therapeutic efficacy.[82] Over 60% of mutations occur in exon 11 of the *KIT* gene on chromosome 4 that encodes the juxtamembrane region. Tumors are usually heterozygous for the mutation though in a minority there is loss of the wild-type allele.[83] A less common mutation at exon 9 of the gene that encodes part of the extracellular domain of the receptor occurs in approximately 10% of GISTs but is rare in gastric GISTs. This second type of mutation identified in GIST tumors causes a conformational change similar to that provoked by the natural ligand, stem cell factor, retaining a relatively normal kinase domain.[84] Between 5% and 10% of GISTs have mutations in the related *PDGFRA* gene in exons 12, 14 or 18. By similar mechanisms, these mutations cause constitutive activation of PDGFRA, are mutually exclusive with *KIT* mutations and are associated with a less aggressive malignancy.[85] *PDGFRA* mutations are commonly found in gastric GISTs and may explain the relatively better prognosis of resectable GISTs of the stomach as compared to other sites of disease. However, the most common *PDGFRA* mutation in

GISTs, *D842V*, confers resistance to imatinib, inducing the active conformation of the intracellular kinase segment and thereby bypassing the effects of imatinib binding. Another 15% of GISTs do not have these RTK mutations even though they express KIT with high levels of phosphorylation.[80]

Mutations in downstream signaling pathway components, BRAF and RAS, have been identified in some of these tumors, explaining KIT-independent growth and resistance to receptor tyrosine kinase inhibitor (RTKI) therapy.[86] *BRAFV600E* mutation can occur in 10% of these non-*KIT* mutant tumors. Other oncogenic changes currently under investigation include mutations in Krebs cycle complex II proteins, the succinate dehydrogenases (SDHs), as well as overexpression of IGF-1R, the latter noted primarily in non-*KIT* mutated GISTs.[87,88] Presence or absence of these mutations has therapeutic implications in the use of targeted therapies such as imatinib. Patients with exon 11 mutations are most likely to respond to RTKI therapy with imatinib in general, while those tumors that harbor exon 9 mutations seem to have better disease-free survival when treated with higher imatinib doses (800 versus 400 mg). Moreover, dedifferentiation can occur with loss of KIT expression in time without correlation to previous imatinib exposure or mutational type.[89]

Genetic associations

Germline mutations in *KIT* and *PDGFRA* have been described. Familial GIST syndromes are usually inherited in an autosomal dominant manner with mutations identical to those found in sporadic tumors. Only a few small kindreds have been evaluated and clinical behavior of GISTs is hard to assess. There are various associated abnormalities including cutaneous findings and increased numbers of mast cells. Two specific syndromes have been defined, known as the Carney triad and the Carney–Stratakis (CS) syndrome.[90,91] The former is not associated with known mutations and clinically manifests as multiple GISTs, especially gastric, paragangliomas and pulmonary chrondromatae in young women. The CS syndrome is related to mutations in the SDH proteins described above, again presenting clinically with GISTs preferentially localized in the stomach and paragangliomas. Lastly, GISTs can arise in the setting of neurofibromatosis (NF) type I, occurring in approximately 7% of patients.[92] NF1-related GISTs are notable for lack of known mutations and multifocal disease with early but overexpression of KIT. Notwithstanding these characteristics, NF1 GISTs appear to be clinically indolent.

Prognostic implications

In the pre-imatinib era, between 1992 and 2000, the 5-year survival rate for localized GIST was estimated to be about 45%, ranging from 64% for early disease to 30% for locally invasive disease. Metastatic GIST had a 5-year survival of 13%. The 2005 AFIP retrospective analysis of over 1700 patients with gastric GIST recommended five prognostic groups according to size and mitotic activity.[73] These findings form the basis of the current updated NIH classification schema.[93] Findings of the AFIP study included a median survival over 14 years with an approximately 20-year median

follow-up. Tumor-related mortality (TRM) for all tumors with mitotic activity not greater than 5/50 high-power field (HPF) was 3% (range 0–11%). There was no mortality for patients with tumors ≤2 cm. TRM for tumors ≥5/50 HPF ($p < 0.0001$) was significantly higher at 46% (range, 0–86%), while it was up to 86% for tumors ≥10 cm. A "saturation point" with equally low survivals with any mitotic cell counts of over 10/50 HPF for tumors ≥10 cm was noted. More aggressive lesions were located in the gastric fundus and gastroesophageal junction–cardia region as compared with GISTs of the antrum that have been shown to correlate with epithelioid histology.

A recent evaluation of survival and costs of localized GISTs, which used pre-imatinib SEER data, revealed a median survival for patients with tumors ≤6 cm of 87.6 months, 6–10 cm 74 months, ≥10 cm 50 months.[94] A more recent analysis of pooled population-based cohorts published in December 2011, using more recent data from 2000–2010, concluded that approximately half of all operable GIST patients were cured by surgery alone with similar accuracy of risk stratification when using any of the schemas discussed above.[95] Postoperative risk assessment now uses the NIH consensus criteria in view of recommendations for surveillance and adjuvant therapy.

Diagnostic considerations

The clinical presentation of gastric GISTs is variable, with some patients diagnosed incidentally during endoscopic or radiographic studies. Small tumors, in particular, are usually asymptomatic.[96] As the GIST grows to >5 cm and compresses neighboring structures, nonspecific symptoms develop, including abdominal pain, bloating, fullness or mass and early satiety. Many patients will have occult GI bleeding from the GIST and a minority present with overt GI bleeding or obstructive symptoms.[97] If metastatic disease is present at the time of diagnosis, it is usually intraabdominal, affecting the liver or peritoneum and far less commonly distant sites such as the lung. Lymphatic spread is exceedingly rare.[98]

Patients with gastric GISTs typically undergo upper endoscopy, either at the time of discovery or as further evaluation of a mass identified by barium study, CT or magnetic resonance imaging (MRI). Endoscopically, GISTs appear as a submucosal smooth-contoured mass with normal overlying mucosa protruding into the gastric lumen (Fig. 28.4). Routine endoscopic biopsies are commonly unrevealing, demonstrating only intact mucosa.[99,100]

Endoscopic ultrasonography has become the preferred method of evaluating suspected gastric GISTs given the submucosal location and the ability to perform guided fine needle aspiration (FNA) or core needle biopsies at the time of evaluation.[101] The typical appearance of a GIST on EUS is a round, hypoechoic mass contiguous with the fourth (muscularis propria) or less commonly second (muscularis mucosae) or third (submucosa) layers[102] (Fig. 28.5). While all GISTs have malignant potential, 20–25% of gastric GISTs are malignant. Certain EUS characteristics have been shown to be more predictive of malignancy such as diameter greater than 4 cm, irregular borders, echogenic foci larger than 3 mm, or cystic spaces larger than 4 mm.[103] Findings suggestive of benign

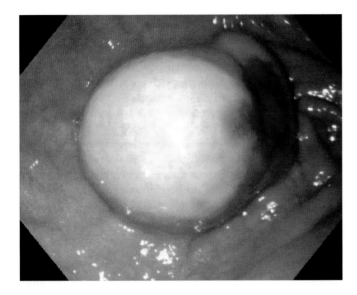

Figure 28.4 Endoscopic appearance of GIST.

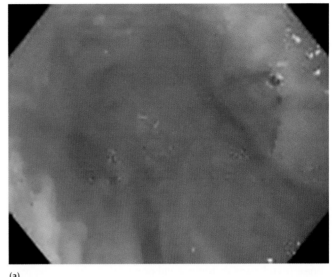

(a)

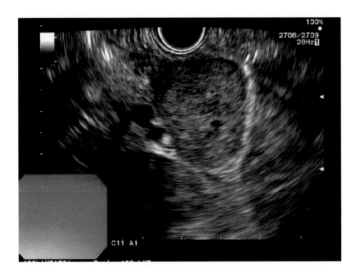

Figure 28.5 EUS appearance of GIST.

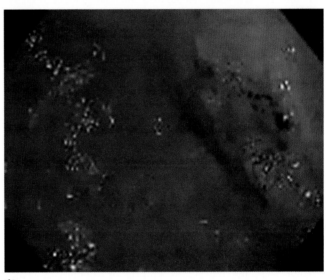

(b)

Figure 28.6 Endoscopic appearance of MALT. (a) Patch of erythema (fundus). (b) Narrow band imaging (fundus).

pathology include regular margins, tumor size ≤3 cm, and a homogeneous echo pattern (Fig. 28.6). Definitive determination of malignant potential, however, requires tissue sampling.

Preoperative biopsy is generally not required in a surgically resectable highly suspected GIST based on endoscopic and radiographic appearance. When the diagnosis is uncertain or there is concern for metastatic disease, EUS-FNA is the preferred method for tissue collection as percutaneous biopsy carries with it the theoretical risk of tumor capsule rupture and peritoneal dissemination. Based on numerous studies, the diagnostic yield of EUS-FNA in GISTs is estimated to be 78–84%. Utilizing EUS-guided core needle sampling can obtain larger biopsy specimens in selected cases where specialized histopathological studies such as mitotic index are required, although in general the yield is not superior to EUS-FNA and smaller lesions or those in difficult anatomical locations are

harder to access via this method. Staging of GISTs is best carried out with combined FDG-PET/CT imaging. If both studies are not available either separately or as a combined imaging technique, CT scanning should be used. CT scans have the highest sensitivity of around 90% for detecting GISTs. Better preoperative evaluation is needed, however, due to the small but real risk of malignant behavior even for low-grade tumors.

An attempt at more refined criteria than RECIST for measuring response to therapy was developed by Choi *et al.* and known as the Choi criteria.[104] These criteria measured change in both tumor size and tumor density on CT scan and were shown to correlate well with positive responses by PET. PET scanning is known to be A sensitive imaging technique for metabolically active lesions, which usually correlate with high proliferative index tumors. PET has been accepted for monitoring for response to imatinib therapy. An FDG-PET response, which is characterized by a marked decrease in the glycolytic metabolism of GISTs, can be seen as early as 24 h after treatment is initiated. Several series have confirmed correlation between standardized uptake value (SUV) levels and Ki-67 index in GIST tumors. Defining mean standard uptake (MSU) values to accurately predict risk categories preoperatively as defined by the NIH has proven more challenging. It should be noted that overall, less than 10% of patients will show a complete response on imaging. In imatinib therapy for GIST, response rate does not correlate with clinical benefit in patients with advanced disease, with nonresponders deriving similar disease-free survival (DFS) benefits as responders.

Treatment of localized disease

Localized GISTs >2–3 cm should be resected in patients who are acceptable surgical candidates with care taken to avoid tumor pseudocapsule rupture and potential seeding of the peritoneum. There is some debate over the management of GISTs 2–3 cm in size, with the National Comprehensive Cancer Network advising resection of all GISTs >2 cm and the American Gastroenterological Association advocating resection for GISTs >3 cm or <3 cm with concerning endosonographic features.[105] Tumors <2 cm without concerning endosonographic features can be followed with EUS surveillance at 6–12-month intervals given their lower malignant potential. Segmental surgical resection with clear macroscopic (but not wide) margins is adequate for localized gastric GIST, without the need for lymph node dissection.[57]

Laparoscopic resection is being increasingly utilized in the surgical management of gastric GISTs and can yield equivalent results to laparotomy in the hands of experienced surgeons, especially for those tumors <5 cm or larger with favorable shape or location. In addition, advances in endoscopic technology have enabled gastroenterologists to begin developing expertise in *en bloc* endoscopic resection of smaller GISTs arising from the muscularis propria or submucosa layers. Endoscopic techniques for gastric GIST resection include band ligation of tumors, submucosal dissection, and electrosurgery.[27] Based on risk stratification systems discussed above, much effort has been made to define groups of patients who would benefit from adjuvant anti-TKR therapy.[106] The first tyrosine kinase inhibitor (TKI) imatinib was developed in the early 1990s as a therapy for chronic myelogenous leukemia (CML), owing to its ability to inhibit the fusion oncoprotein BCR-ABL which is structurally similar to KIT. Imatinib inhibits KIT by direct competitive inhibition of the ATP-binding site, stabilizing the kinase in the inactive conformation.

Two large randomized trials of adjuvant imatinib have been completed. ACOSOG Z9001 compared imatinib to surgery alone in a randomized fashion.[107] In the initial results, recurrence-free survival (RFS) was significantly longer for all risk groups in the imatinib group, prompting early stopping of the trial to allow patients to cross over from the placebo arm to the treatment arm. In a 2010 follow-up analysis, clinically significant 2-year RFS improvement was shown mostly for high-risk patients (77% versus 41%, $p < 0.0001$). Based on the results of this trial, the FDA approved imatinib in 2008 for

adjuvant use at 400 mg/day. The SSG XVIII trial attempted to determine the appropriate length of adjuvant therapy with imatinib, comparing 12 to 36 months of therapy in high-risk patients only.[33] There was a significant improvement in RFS and OS at the first interim report presented at ASCO 2011. After discontinuation of drug, recurrence rates were noted to rise in both treatment groups, suggesting that imatinib therapy simply delays recurrence rather than inducing a cure.

Results of EORTC 62024, which is evaluating imatinib versus surgery alone for 2 years, are pending and are likely to take some time because the primary endpoint of that trial is OS rather than RFS. In the pre-imatinib era, most recurrences were noted to occur with 2 years of resection.[95] Imatinib is also being studied in the neoadjuvant setting, mostly for borderline or unresectable tumors. Major guidelines agree on the neoadjuvant use of imatinib for cytoreduction to reduce surgical morbidity, facilitate R0 resection and reduce associated complications. The RTOG 0132/ACRIN 6665 trial of neoadjuvant imatinib for primary and recurrent operable GIST tumors reported modest response rates by RECIST criteria – between 4–7% partial responses.[108] A 2011 update of this trial revealed estimated 5-year PFS and OS rates for patients with primary disease of 57% and 77% respectively; PFS and DFS rates of 30% and 68% were reported for resected metastatic/recurrent disease.[109] A metaanalysis of adjuvant trials supports an improvement in RFS but no OS benefit.[110] Of note is that most studies of imatinib in metastatic disease require several months of therapy to obtain maximal radiographic response, while the course of neoadjuvant therapy in this trial was only 2–3 months, suggesting that longer preoperative therapy may be more beneficial. Conversely, another report suggests that a 1-week course of imatinib could be enough to determine sensitivity of the tumor to the drug when followed by assessment with a panel of techniques including FDG-PET, dynamic (d)CT, and terminal deoxynucleotidyl transferase mediated dUTP nick end labeling (TUNEL) assay.[111] How this translates into improved outcomes or stratification for surgery versus neoadjuvant chemotherapy is unknown.

Treatment of metastatic disease

Imatinib was first approved for use in the metastatic setting in 2001 by the FDA, based on the results of two phase 2 trials (B2222 US-Finland study and the EORTC Soft Tissue and Bone Sarcoma Group trials).[112–114] A pooled response rate of 38% observed in the study (33% for the 400 mg dose group and 43% for the 600 mg dose group) served as the basis for accelerated approval. Several subsequent studies have attempted to determine the optimal dose of imatinib. Two phase 3 trials, the EU-AUS and the US-CDN studies, compared response rates and PFS rates for either daily doses of 400 mg versus 800 mg or 400 mg versus 600 mg respectively.[113,115] Notable results included lack of PFS benefit from doses higher than 400 mg, and improved response rates with higher doses in the exon 9 mutation subset of patients when they progressed on 400 mg daily and were allowed to cross over to the higher dose. An additional 30% of patients thus had either a partial response or SD at the higher dose, suggesting some dose–response relationship for this subset. This has prompted formal recommendation that patients with exon 9 mutation be treated with 800 mg daily. The Meta-GIST Study Group confirmed this recommendation in 2010 but noted that no overall survival benefit to this strategy was conferred even in these patients.[116]

Though almost 80% of GIST patients with advanced disease receive some benefit from imatinib therapy, a significant proportion eventually become resistant, with a median time to progression of 2 years.[117] The probability of primary resistance to imatinib for *KIT exon 11, KIT exon 9*, and non-*KIT* mutated GISTs is 5%, 16%, and 23%, respectively. Secondary resistance is thought to occur due to new KIT mutations in more than half of cases. However, progress has been observed. A 2008 analysis of SEER data reported a significant increase in median survival from 12 to 33 months, respectively ($p < 0.001$) and a 3-year OS increased from 24% to 48%, respectively ($p < 0.001$) between 1995–2001 and 2001–2004 time groups, suggesting the effect of imatinib on outcomes.[118]

In 2006, the FDA approved sunitinib, another multitargeting RTKI, as second-line therapy for unresectable GIST. Sunitinib targets both vascular endothelial growth factor receptor (VEGFR)1 and VEGFR2 in addition to PDGFRA and KIT. Given the accumulation of various mutations in the KIT gene that cause changes in the ATP-binding region as well as other domains, mixed responses to therapy are often observed with second-line therapy. The phase 3 trial of sunitinib versus placebo that led to the new indication also revealed that the time to progression (TTP), which was the primary endpoint, was significantly longer with sunitinib compared with placebo (6.8 versus 1.6 months, hazard ratio (HR) 0.33, $p \leq 0.0001$).[119] Treatment with either imatinib or sunitinib is overall well tolerated though far from innocuous. Toxicities reported in both perioperative and metastatic settings include gastrointestinal and hematological problems, with 3% or less reporting grade 3 or higher severity. The most common symptoms of both include diarrhea, nausea, neutropenia, hand foot syndrome, and fatigue. Myelosuppression and hypertension are both more common with sunitinib.[120]

Current drugs under evaluation that attempt to exploit multitarget inhibition include second-generation PDGFR/KIT inhibitors such as nilotinib, masitinib, and dasatinib. Sorafenib, a small molecule with a broad spectrum of targets including the serine/threonine Raf kinases, KIT, PDGFRb, VEGFR(2,3), Flt3, and Ret, has shown activity in the third-line setting after failure of imatinib and sunitinib. At ASCO GI 2011, a small phase 2 study was reported in which 13% of patients achieved a partial response and 55% had stable disease.[50] Median PFS was 5.2 months and OS was 11.6 months. Perifosine, an oral inhibitor of Akt phosphorylation, was noted to induce stable disease in non-KIT mutated patients, consistent with the mechanism described in which IGF-1R signals through the PI3K/AKT pathway which is overexpressed in this GIST subtype.[121]

Summary and recommendations

Localized gastric GISTs are best treated by minimally invasive endoscopic resection techniques or by classic surgical resection. Prognosis is generally excellent despite non-negligible local and metastatic recurrence rates. Adjuvant targeted therapy with imatinib is to be considered on a case-by-case basis after risk assessment and a thorough review of risks to the patient given the drug's known side-effect profile. If neoadjuvant imatinib is pursued, it should be continued postoperatively for a total treatment time of 3 years especially if response was seen on preoperative imaging or on pathological review of the resected specimen. Less than R1 resections should prompt either a repeat attempt at resection, given overall excellent results with complete surgical resection, or a trial of imatinib if resection is not feasible. Several lines of therapy are becoming available for metastatic disease, the existence of which is translating into significantly improved survival.

Mucosa-associated lymphoid tissue

The stomach is the most common site for extranodal lymphoma. Gastric lymphomas account for over 70% of all gastrointestinal lymphomas.[51] They constitute approximately 5% of all malignant gastric tumors and 8% of all non-Hodgkin lymphomas (NHLs).[49] The majority of gastric lymphomas are of B cell origin, of which the most common are diffuse large B cell lymphomas (DLBCL) and extranodal marginal zone lymphomas of the mucosa-associated lymphoid tissue (MALT) type.[58] Extranodal MALT lymphomas account for 50% of gastric lymphomas.[122] They comprise a group of neoplasms that result from lymphoid proliferation in mucosal sites, most commonly the gastrointestinal tract but rarely in other extranodal sites. In the vast majority of cases, the development of gastric MALT lymphoma (G-MALTL) is preceded by *Helicobacter pylori*-associated chronic gastritis.[123]

Gastric MALTs are primarily seen in adult patients with a very slight male predominance. Increased identification and treatment of *H. pylori* led to decreased incidence of G-MALT in the 1990s, but this incidence has subsequently stabilized.[61]

Classification

Primary gastric lymphomas are typically NHLs. G-MALTs are mature B cell lymphomas with a unique association to an infectious agent as noted above.[124] The latest WHO classification of hematopoietic neoplasms includes three categories of marginal zone lymphomas: nodal, splenic, and MALT. The latter is the most prevalent.[125] The first staging system for G-MALT lymphomas consisted of the Ann Arbor system for NHLs that subsequently became the Blackledge or "Lugano" staging system. Staging evolved as importance of lymph node region (regional versus distant) and depth of tumor invasion (submucosa to serosa) was identified. The most recent AJCC/UICC TNM staging system, the so-called "Paris" staging system, combines the stratification for gastric cancer with depth of invasion as measured by EUS.[126] *H. pylori* infection is associated with 50–100% of cases in various series. Though most G-MALTs are "low grade," in part by definition, there is a 20–30% reported incidence of "high-grade" cases. Currently discussing grade of MALT lymphomas is probably inaccurate, as the old Kiel and IWF classification systems that used grading definitions have largely been abandoned. They have been replaced by the WHO system that classifies neoplasms by cell of origin as noted above, but the terminology lingers and "high-grade" lesions are still referred to in the literature, describing gastric lymphomas that harbor large cell features and a higher frequency of genetic translocations.[127] These tumors can be considered for all intents and purposes DLBCL with MALT features. *H. pylori* infection is generally associated with classic MALT lymphoma, i.e. low-grade lesions, and prevalence of infection is much lower in neoplasms extending beyond the lamina propria (higher T stage).[125] An interesting observation has been that as lesions progress and undergo large cell or blastic transformation, there is associated loss of *H. pylori* infection. This observation explains the lack of association between "pure" DLBCL and *H. pylori*. The subset of MALT lymphomas with clearly no *H. pylori* association may represent an entity that bridges the spectrum of gastric lymphomas from classic MALT to DLBCL.

Clinical pathology

Gastric MALT is derived from marginal zone B cells and resembles native MALT as found in the tonsils and in Peyer's patches in the terminal ileum. Lymphatic tissue is otherwise absent from the gastrointestinal tract in the absence of inflammation. Follicular architecture is maintained as disease progresses, but there is a characteristic infiltrate into the gastric epithelium manifesting as lymphoepithelial lesions. These are destructive lesions involving the gastric glands, which are virtually pathognomonic for neoplasia.[128] There is a variable admixture of large and small cells and an often conspicuous plasma cell infiltrate. Features that distinguish a G-MALTL from reactive infiltrates or DLBCL include a preponderance of small monotonous cells clustering in follicles with poorly demarcated edges.[123,129] CD43 staining is useful as it is absent in reactive lesions. A characteristic flow cytometry profile would show CD20+, CD5-, CD23-, cyclin D1-cells. There is rare overlap in profile with chronic lymphocytic leukemia (CLL) cells (CD5+, CD23+) or mantle cell lymphoma (CD5+, CD23+). Bcl-2 staining is also usually positive. The tumor cells usually express IgM.

Endoscopic biopsy with adequate tissue to determine tissue architecture, presence of *H. pylori* and flow cytometry is essential and recommended by the latest EGILS consensus report from 2011. This may require a minimum of 10 samples from involved and uninvolved mucosa to establish diagnosis. Evaluation of extrafollicular tissue is important to detect any possible DLBCL component. PCR to demonstrate monoclonality is not essential to diagnosis as it may fail to detect this feature in up to 15% of MALT lymphomas due to high frequency of immunoglobulin heavy chain variable (IGHV) mutations. This latter finding correlates with antigen-driven selection of the tumor clone in response to the infective agent. Note that MALT lymphomas can occur secondary to noninfectious, autoimmune processes such as Hashimoto thyroiditis or Sjögren syndrome in the thyroid or salivary glands respectively.

Mucosa-associated lymphoid tissue lymphomas may be multicentric and each extranodal subsite can be managed separately. Disseminated nodal involvement portends a poorer prognosis with behavior resembling that of classic follicular or nodal marginal zone lymphomas. Lastly, several case reports document simultaneous occurrence of gastric adenocarcinoma and MALT lymphoma. Common features of these cases include early stage of adenocarcinoma on diagnosis and evidence that the MALT lymphoma preceded development of the adenocarcinoma. A 2008 epidemiological study documented a six-fold increased risk of gastric adenocarcinoma in patients with MALT lymphoma as compared to the general population but other studies have not noted statistical significance.[122] Endoscopic surveillance recommendations after successful therapy for MALT lymphoma should be done with the additional care for a possibly increased risk of gastric adenocarcinoma. Though used for other hematological neoplasms, demonstration of complete molecular response or surveillance by means of polymerase chain reaction (PCR) for clonality is not recommended. Several investigators have noted that there is persistence of translocation-positive lymphocytes or of monoclonal IGHV gene rearrangements after eradication of *H. pylori* and tumoral regression. There have been conflicting reports regarding risk of relapse in patients found to have this minimal residual disease, therefore the significance of this finding is unknown and it cannot be used to start systemic therapy nor to decrease the frequency of surveillance endoscopies.

Genetic associations

The pathogenic role of *H. pylori* (or very rarely other *Helicobacter* species) in the development of gastric MALT lymphoma has been well described, including many of the molecular changes involved in the progression from *H. pylori*-associated gastritis to MALT lymphoma. A predilection for *Helicobacter* of this particular species and not others to stimulate proliferation of IL-2 receptor positive B cells suggests a role for T cell-mediated proliferation. Chronic immune stimulation from bacterial antigens is postulated to cause clonal B cell proliferation that can extend beyond the gastric mucosa in the setting of certain genetic mutations.[130,131] Four recurrent chromosomal translocations have been identified: *t(11;18) (q21;q21)*, *t(14;18)(q32;q21)*, *t(1;14)(p22;q32)*, and *t(3;14) (p13;q32)*. These translocations cause eventual activation of NF-κB, a transcription factor with a central role in immunity including B cell survival.[132] The most common translocation, *t(11;18)*, causes reciprocal fusion of the apoptosis inhibitor-2 gene on chromosome 11 with the *MALT1* gene on chromosome 18 and is associated with *H. pylori*-negative MALT lymphomas and with more advanced disease.[133,134] The *t(14;18)(q32;q21)* translocation causes fusion of MALT1 with the promoter region of the immunoglobulin heavy chain (IgH) genes whereas the much rarer *t(1;14)(p22;q32)* translocation causes overexpression of the BCL-10 gene.[135] Finally, the *t(3;14)(p13;q32)* translocation fuses the *FOXP1* gene on chromosome 3 to the IgH gene, increasing the amount of *FOXP1* transcription factor.[136] This translocation causes transformation to DLBCL much more frequently than the others.

Prognostic implications

Several of the genetic changes noted above have significant prognostic value. Most series note a 5-year OS over 85%. Gastric MALTs can disseminate to the small intestine or spleen. Bone marrow involvement occurs in approximately 20% of cases. Though presenting earlier with more localized disease than non-GI MALT lymphomas, gastric MALTs have the same OS.[137] Histological transformation to DLBCL occurs in 10% of cases and does not correlate with stage at the time of transformation. A 2010 series notes that lower stage at diagnosis, submucosal involvement only and distal stomach location as well as lack of API2-MALT1 translocation all portend a higher remission rate after primary *H. pylori* therapy.[137] Cure of gastric MALT is achieved in fewer patients with local lymph node involvement (i.e. stages T1–T4N0 versus T1–T4N1), remission rates being 78.4% versus 55.6% respectively.[129] Recurrence of MALT can occur years later and *H. pylori* reinfection is not a necessary prerequisite for this occurrence. Reinfection has been documented in relapsed cases in 25–50% of cases only. Interpretation of recurrence risk is further complicated by a relatively high incidence of spontaneous regression of disease in approximately 25% of relapsed cases. Overall, 5-year OS, recurrent-free survival, and disease-free survival rates for stage I and II MALT lymphoma patients who received radiation therapy and systemic therapy have been reported to be 95%, 82%, and 79%, respectively.[138]

Diagnostic considerations

The most common presenting symptoms of gastric MALT lymphoma are epigastric pain and dyspepsia, followed by nausea, vomiting, anorexia, and weight loss. Occult or overt gastrointestinal bleeding can occur in up to 30% of patients. Systemic B-symptoms (fevers, night sweats, weight loss) or gastric obstruction and perforation are rare.[139,140] Few patients present with elevated lactate dehydrogenase (LDH) or β2-microglobulin levels.

The diagnosis of gastric MALT lymphoma is made by accurate histopathological analysis of endoscopic gastric biopsy. Endoscopic appearance of MALT lymphoma is variable and often subtle. Findings include but are not limited to thickened gastric folds, gastric erythema, ulceration, polypoid, and other mass lesions. Anatomically, gastric MALT lymphomas occur most commonly at the antrum, body, and gastric cardia, although they are often multifocal. Two methods of detection for *H. pylori* should be used as many false-negative results can occur with reliance on histological assessment alone.[129] This is mostly due to patchy involvement of the mucosa by *H. pylori*, thereby allowing for sampling error. Noninvasive testing such as serology or 13 C-urea breath testing can be done if MALT lymphoma is diagnosed with negative testing for *H. pylori*.

Once the diagnosis of gastric MALT lymphoma is made, local staging via repeat upper endoscopy should be performed with multiple biopsies taken of the duodenum, all segments of the stomach, the gastroesophageal junction, and any endoscopically abnormal area. EUS is being increasingly employed for accurate evaluation of regional lymph nodes and depth of gas-

tric invasion in the staging of MALT lymphoma (see Figs 28.5, 28.6). There is also burgeoning evidence for the use of EUS to evaluate treatment response.[141] Controversy exists, however, over the accuracy of EUS for surveillance of treated disease and at present EUS does not supplant endoscopy with mapping biopsies.[142] Obtaining CT of the chest and abdomen should complete staging. FDG-PET scans are routinely used for staging and assessment of response to therapy in high-grade lymphomas. Sensitivity of PET imaging ranges from 38% to 70% for MALT lymphoma and varies widely as can be expected from the biological behavior. Background uptake in the inflamed gastric mucosa makes detection difficult. More recent reports suggest the ability of PET to upstage disease in 20% of cases.[143] It is currently not recommended for routine staging or surveillance.

As per EGILS criteria, bone marrow biopsy should be reserved for staging of occult disseminated disease if there is no regression of G-MALTL in response to *H. pylori* eradication.[129]

Treatment of localized disease

Gastric MALT lymphomas remain localized in 70–80% of cases. The treatment of localized gastric MALT lymphoma in patients who are *H. pylori* positive consists of eradication of *H. pylori* through a combination of antibiotics and proton pump inhibitors (PPIs) and can lead to remission in 60–100% of patients.[144] The most commonly utilized regimens are triple therapy with a PPI twice daily + amoxicillin 1 g twice daily + clarithromycin 500 mg twice daily for 14 days or quadruple therapy with PPI twice daily + bismuth 525 mg four times daily + metronidazole 250 mg four times daily + tetracycline 500 mg four times daily for 10–14 days in patients who fail to respond to triple therapy or who live in a geographic area with a high prevalence of resistance to clarithromycin.

A histological system for assessing response to *H. pylori* treatment in gastric MALT lymphoma was developed by the Groupe d'Etude des Lymphomes de l'Adult (GELA).[145,146] Treatment response is divided into complete histological remission (CR), probable minimal residual (pMRD), residual disease in regression (rRD), or no change (NC) based on histological characteristics. Demonstration of the *API2/MALT1* translocation, found in 20–30% of G-MALTLs, requires close follow-up given a high incidence of lack of response to *H. pylori* therapy with this translocation, even in *H. pylori* + cases. There is an 80% overall response rate to *H. pylori* therapy in low-grade MALT lymphomas. Histological response to therapy takes several months, with complete response taking up to 12 months. Relapses occur in 3–10% of cases. A second course of *H. pylori* therapy is recommended as above, even if no further lymphoma is identified, while if *H. pylori* has been cleared but residual disease is noted, as occurs in *API2/MALT1*+ tumors, further therapy with radiation or systemic therapy is indicated.

Consensus guidelines recommend that *H. pylori* eradication should be checked by urea breath test at least 6 weeks after eradication therapy and at least 2 weeks after withdrawal of PPI medication. Follow-up endoscopy to assess for histological response should be done after 3 months at the earliest. In addition, some patients have evidence of residual lymphoid aggregates in the mucosa on surveillance endoscopy, despite *H. pylori* eradication. A third of these cases eventually clear in the year following therapy while the majority simply remain stable.[147,148] Recommendations are to observe these patients rather than to consider them refractory to therapy.

About 10% of MALT lymphomas are *H. pylori* negative. These should be treated with either radiation therapy (RT) or systemic therapy. There is controversy regarding *H. pylori*-negative low-grade MALT as several series have published a median rate of 20% to anti-*H. pylori* therapy.[149] Speculation regarding these findings includes that these are falsely negative *H. pylori* cases or that other infectious agents are involved. Conversely, high-grade gastric MALT or DLBCL has been shown to retain antigen-driven proliferative capacity. Complete remission has been achieved in up to 60% of cases of *H. pylori*+high-grade gastric lymphoma with antiinfective therapy.

Radiation therapy is preferred for the treatment of localized disease though there are no randomized trials comparing it to modern agents such as rituximab. It has supplanted surgical resection out of consideration for long-term morbidities though surgery traditionally achieved up to 90% long-term survival. MALT lymphomas are radiosensitive tumors. Radiation therapy doses ranging from 30 Gy to 45 Gy achieve 5-year event-free survival rates of 80–90%. Gastric MALT lymphomas in particular are the most amenable to RT of all gastrointestinal MALT lymphoma subsites due to the very low incidence of nonregional lymph node involvement (<5%).[150] Controversy exists regarding the management of rare cases where RT is contraindicated for localized disease.[147] In this setting, the NCCN guidelines recommend monotherapy with rituximab, an anti-CD20 monoclonal antibody, largely based on the selection of the least toxic systemic agent that has some evidence of efficacy but not any randomized data.

Metastatic disease

Systemic therapy is usually reserved for patients with disseminated disease including distant lymph node metastases.[137] Monotherapy with alkylating agents such as chlorambucil or the purine analog cladribine has been reported to achieve significant remission rates depending on *ALP2-MALT1* status.[151] Given the fact that gastric MALT lymphomas are indolent lymphomas, aggressive therapy with regimens such as R-CHOP is not recommended in the absence of symptoms or transformation with rapid progression. Rituximab has shown an overall RR of 71% in a small phase 2 study, with a 50% CR rate. However, rituximab has been shown in two small studies to add significant efficacy against *ALP2-MALT1*-positive tumors when combined with chlorambucil or the other purine analog, fludarabine.[152]

IELSG-19, the largest prospective randomized trial ever conducted in MALT lymphoma, is a three-arm study with interim results presented at ASH 2010. It compared chlorambucil versus rituximab versus the combination.[153] Out of 424 patients, 40% had gastric MALT lymphomas either refractory to therapy or unsuitable for RT. Five-year OS was no different between chlorambucil alone or with rituximab. Results are pending regarding the rituximab monotherapy arm. Of note, there were no differences in outcome between patients with gastric or nongastric MALT lymphomas.

Summary and recommendations

Gastric MALT lymphomas represent a subset of indolent B cell lymphomas with an overall good prognosis. Cure may be achieved by nonneoplastic therapy as above. Second-line treatment options exist but care must be taken not to diagnose residual disease due to inadequate short follow-up times. Characterization of cytogenetics appears important for prognostic purposes though no differences in endoscopic surveillance or management recommendations exist for those patients with higher risk, translocation-bearing disease. PET imaging is not routinely recommended and at this time does not supplant CT imaging though data are scarce regarding sensitivity of either technique for gastric MALT. The recommendation is based on sensitivities for staging of gastric adenocarcinoma. *H. pylori* therapy should be strongly considered for all patients with localized disease irrespective of cytogenetics and may even be considered for selected patients who are poor candidates for RT and who are negative for *H. pylori*.

Epstein–Barr virus-associated gastric carcinoma

In the past decade, increasing knowledge has accumulated regarding an uncommon subtype of gastric adenocarcinoma characterized by lymphoepitheliomatoid (LE) histology.[154] While classic gastric adenocarcinoma with either diffuse or intestinal histology has been associated with *H. pylori* infection, gastric carcinoma associated with lymphoid stroma (GCLS) is highly associated with Epstein–Barr virus (EBV) infection. These tumors are moderate to poorly differentiated neoplasms that account for less than 5% of all gastric carcinomas and have relatively better prognoses than the more commonly occurring gastric adenocarcinomas, with a lower incidence of lymph node involvement and earlier stage at presentation.[155] EBV-associated gastric carcinoma is the most common EBV-associated cancer worldwide. These tumors tend to occur in males more often and there has been a suggestion of a slightly younger age predilection as compared to non-EBV-associated gastric cancers. There is equal geographic distribution of cases with a predilection for proximal stomach localization, a tendency toward multifocal submucosal disease, and association with atrophic gastritis. A 2009 metaanalysis of EBV-associated gastric carcinomas revealed in addition that up to 20% of gastric adenocarcinomas may be associated with EBV as described below, but without the marked lymphocytic infiltrate that defines classic GCALS or LE histology.[156] Coinfection with *H. pylori* is common. A recent case series noted peptic ulcer disease as a risk factor for development of EBV+gastric carcinoma among 247 studied.[29] Alcohol and tobacco use were not related to the development of this subtype of gastric cancer. It is, however, the expression of latent viral proteins that makes this subtype distinct.

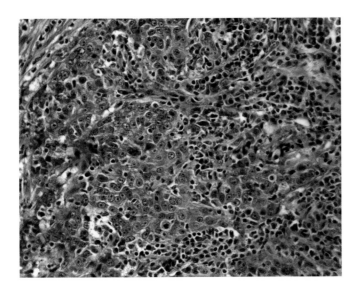

Figure 28.7 H&E microscopy of gastric carcinoma with lymphoid stroma.

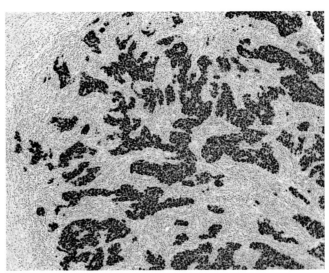

Figure 28.8 EBER staining of EBV-associated gastric carcinoma.

Classification

The staging for this histological subtype is the same as for conventional gastric adenocarcinomas. So far no histological or molecular stratification has provided prognostic information strong enough to change management algorithms. Subtypes of EBV-associated gastric carcinomas are still being classified by descriptive histology and include gastric carcinoma with lymphoid stroma (GCLS) and lymphocyte-rich gastric cancer which has varying degrees of lymphocyte involvement.[157] Of note, EBV positivity of intestinal adenocarcinomas has been associated with poorer outcomes, the converse being true of EBV + diffuse-type cancers. Lastly, there is an unusually high incidence of EBV involvement in gastric remnant cancers. Diagnostically these tumors are identifiable by the same means as the more common histological subtypes with occasionally hypoechoic submucosal masses visible on endoscopic ultrasound due to the lymphocytic component of the lesions.

Pathology

This variant of gastric adenocarcinoma has only recently been more thoroughly defined and still remains largely of interest due to the unique mechanisms of disease involved.

Lymphoepithelioma-like carcinoma is notable for a markedly high lymphocyte to carcinoma cell ratio and well-defined tumor margins (Fig. 28.7).[158] It is defined by the presence of EBV-encoded RNA (EBER) in the malignant gastric mucosal cells (Fig. 28.8).[159] The EBV latent viral protein expression pattern of EBV-associated gastric carcinomas is similar to that in Burkitt lymphoma. Infiltrating lymphocytes consist of CD8- or CD4-positive T lymphocytes[160] and CD68-positive macrophages, in a ratio of 2:1:1. Among the infiltrating lymphocytes, EBV infects very few cells. The latent viral protein LMP1 has been shown to be essential for clonal expansion of cells in both epithelial and lymphoid malignancies associated with EBV, inhibiting apoptosis by induction of Bcl-2.[161–163] Recent studies suggest that chronic inflammation may be expanding groups of

cells which are epigenetically altered by LMP2A, one of the EBV latent viral proteins.[24,164] Deregulation of cell cycle-regulating pathways such as PI3K/Akt occurs due to changes in CpG methylation and may play a role in immortalizing progenitor cells.[165]

Summary and recommendations

Despite a trend towards improved overall survival in univariate analyses, for now treatment recommendations remain the same irrespective of gastric adenocarcinoma subtype for both localized and metastatic disease. The fascinating link to viral pathogenesis in EBV-associated tumors offers the potential for novel EBV-targeted therapies. Several drugs can induce the lytic cycle in EBV-infected cells, including gemcitabine and doxorubicin, and synergistic *in vitro* effects of antiviral therapy with ganciclovir following therapy with cisplatin or 5-FU have been demonstrated.[166] Current investigative efforts concern further elucidation of interaction between viral and host cellular processes. In addition, interactions between viral protein products and chemotherapeutic agents are being studied in an attempt to identify a weakness uniquely associated with EBV-associated neoplasms.

Gastric tumors with hepatic and germ cell differentiation

a-Fetoprotein (AFP)-producing gastric carcinoma (AFPGC) is a rare type of gastric adenocarcinoma first described in the 1970s. AFP is fetal serum protein produced by fetal liver and yolk sac cells, and by some fetal gastrointestinal cells. Serum AFP is a marker routinely used for surveillance of patients with certain germ cell and hepatocellular tumors. The incidence of AFPCG has been reported to be 1.3–15% of all gastric tumors.[167] Its etiology is still obscure and there is overlap with another entity termed hepatoid adenocarcinoma though other histological types of gastric cancer have been associated with a high serum AFP level. Conversely, hepatoid adenocarcinoma of the stomach is associated with elevated serum AFP levels in approximately half of cases.[168] Further complicating matters, several gastric carcinoma cases have been reported to be AFP positive on immunohistochemistry in the absence of elevated serum levels. A recent case series of 23 patients with AFPGCs revealed yolk sac differentiation, enteroblastic growth patterns as well as conventional adenocarcinoma morphology. There was evidence that premalignant lesions had a predominantly conventional phenotype while hepatoid differentiation was seen only in advanced, invasive lesions.[169] AFPGCs as defined by elevated serum levels are associated with advanced stage at diagnosis, frequent liver metastasis, richer neovascularization, and a worse prognosis.[170] Hepatoid adenocarcinomas defined on the basis of histology rather than AFP positivity have the same clinical characteristics. This observation suggests a spectrum of aberrant expression of hepatocyte features by a minority of gastric adenocarcinomas which universally confers poor prognosis.

Given the paucity of data for these tumors, only the same management recommendations as for conventional gastric adenocarcinoma can be made, even given the occasional observation of metastatic disease associated with T1 lesions. Also worthy of mention in this context are germ cell tumors of the stomach, most commonly nonseminomas, choriocarcinomas or yolk sac tumors.[171] These entities are even more rare than the variants above, with most cases reported in the literature describing neoplasms with mixed histology, including features of adenocarcinoma. A handful of pure yolk sac tumors have been described and their origin is under debate.[172,173] They are associated with elevated serum AFP. Prognosis of these tumors is very poor because of usual metastatic disease at presentation but they seem to be treated as far as possible as testicular germ cell tumors, with resection when possible. The same recommendation exists for choriocarcinomas, which have similar clinical and prognostic features, with the exception of elevated serum hCG levels as opposed to AFP.

Metastases to the stomach

Gastric metastases from other sites are extremely rare findings. The most common sites of origin reported in the literature are the breast, lungs, and skin (melanoma).[174] Most reports are either from endoscopies or from autopsy case series with an incidence of less than 1% to over 20% with a higher incidence in patients evaluated with known malignancy.[175–178] Metastatic foci were usually isolated and both submucosal as well as transmural in location. Autopsy series tend to show a much higher incidence of occult gastric metastasis but as endoscopic techniques and survival improve, there is likely to be an increased incidence of clinically relevant, symptomatic metastases to the stomach. In two large autopsy series, gastric metastases were found in about 20% of cases. There is also evidence for a propensity for single metastases to occur in the upper two-thirds of the stomach.

Metastatic melanoma to the stomach merits separate mention. Primary GI melanoma can arise in most other sites of the gastrointestinal tract in the absence of prior cutaneous melanoma due to the known presence of melanocytes.[179,180] The stomach is a notable exception to this observation. Most gastric melanomas are likely to be metastatic in nature. The gastrointestinal tract, in fact, represents the second most common site of metastasis for melanoma after the lung. In a large autopsy series from Johns Hopkins, there was an over 40% incidence of GI metastases, with almost 23% involvement of the stomach.

More recent series include reports of renal cell carcinoma metastasizing to the GI tract. In an Austrian report from a single institution, out of over 2000 patients with renal cell carcinoma, 22 cases of gastric metastases were noted.[181] All had clear cell histology and there were synchronous metastases to other organs. There was no distinct correlation to worse overall survival when compared to the average OS of patients with metastatic renal cell carcinoma to other sites.

A case series from Taiwan found only 18 cases of secondary gastric cancers out of a total of over 48,000 patients over a 10-year period, with a majority being hepatocellular carcinoma. This likely reflects the geographic bias.[182]

Presenting symptoms of metastatic disease to the stomach are similar irrespective of etiology, including melena and epigastric pain. If detected clinically, due to symptoms, gastric metastases have a universally poor prognosis as a consequence of widespread disease.

Conclusion

Rare tumors of the stomach, including neuroendocrine cancers, GIST tumors, MALT, and EBV-associated gastric tumors as well as several others, collectively may be seen with some frequency. Recognizing these entities and having a working knowledge of these diseases is important because their management may be very different from the usual adenocarcinoma of the stomach.

References

1. Parkin DM, *et al*. Global cancer statistics, 2002. CA Cancer J Clin 2005; 55(2): 74–108.
2. Howlader N, *et al* (eds). SEER Cancer Statistics Review, 1975–2008, National Cancer Institute. Bethesda, MD, http://seer.cancer.gov/csr/1975_2008/.
3. Crew KD, Neugut AI. Epidemiology of gastric cancer. World J Gastroenterol 2006; 12(3): 354–62.
4. Shah MA, Kelsen DP. Gastric cancer: A primer on the epidemiology and biology of the disease and an overview of the medical management of advanced disease. J Natl Compr Canc Netw 2010; 8(4): 437–47.
5. Shah MA, *et al*. Molecular classsification of gastric cancer: a new paradigm. Clin Cancer Res 2011; 17(9): 2693–701.
6. Kamangar F, Dores GM, Anderson WF. Patterns of cancer incidence, mortality, and prevalence across five continents: defining priorities to reduce cancer disparities in different geographic regions of the world. J Clin Oncol 2006; 24(14): 2137–50.
7. Ye W, *et al*. Helicobacter pylori infection and gastric atrophy: risk of adenocarcinoma and squamous-cell carcinoma of the esophagus and adenocarcinoma of the gastric cardia. J Natl Cancer Inst 2004; 96: 388–96.
8. Peek RM, Blaser MJ. Helicobacter pylori and gastrointestinal tract adenocarcinomas. Nature Rev Cancer 2002; 2: 28–37.
9. Uemura N, *et al*. Helicobacter pylori infection and the development of gastric cancer. N Engl J Med 2001; 345(11): 784–9.

10. Correa P, Shiao YH. Phenotypic and genotypic events in gastric carcinogenesis. Cancer Res 1994; 54 (7 Suppl): 1941s–3s.

11. Wang XQ, Terry PD, Yan H. Review of salt consumption and stomach cancer risk: epidemiological and biological evidence. World J Gastroenterol 2009; 15(18): 2204–13.

12. Hennies HC, Hagedorn M, Reis A. Palmoplantar keratoderma in association with carcinoma of the esophagus maps to chromosome 17q distal to the keratin gene cluster. Genomics 1995; 29(2): 537–40.

13. Fitzgerald RC, et al. Hereditary diffuse gastric cancer: updated consensus guidelines for clinical management and directions for future research. J Med Genet 2010; 47(7): 436–44.

14. Yao JC, et al. One hundred years after "carcinoid": epidemiology of and prognostic factors for neuroendocrine tumors in 35,825 cases in the United States. J Clin Oncol 2008; 26(18): 3063–72.

15. Scherubl H, et al. Neuroendocrine tumors of the stomach (gastric carcinoids) are on the rise: small tumors, small problems? Endoscopy 2010; 42(8): 664–71.

16. Vinik AI, et al. NANETS consensus guidelines for the diagnosis of neuroendocrine tumor. Pancreas 2010; 39(6): 713–34.

17. Niederle MB, et al. Gastroenteropancreatic neuroendocrine tumours: the current incidence and staging based on the WHO and European Neuroendocrine Tumour Society classification: an analysis based on prospectively collected parameters. Endocr Relat Cancer 2010; 17(4): 909–18.

18. Pape UF, et al. Prognostic relevance of a novel TNM classification system for upper gastroenteropancreatic neuroendocrine tumors. Cancer 2008; 113(2): 256–65.

19. Klöppel G, et al. The ENETS and AJCC/UICC TNM classifications of the neuroendocrine tumors of the gastrointestinal tract and the pancreas: a statement. Virchows Arch 2010; 456(6): 595–7.

20. Ramage JK, et al. Guidelines for the management of gastroenteropancreatic neuroendocrine (including carcinoid) tumours (NETs). Gut 2012; 61(1): 6–32.

21. Solcia E, et al. Enterochromaffin-like (ECL) cells and their growths: relationships to gastrin, reduced acid secretion and gastritis. Baillieres Clin Gastroenterol 1993; 7(1): 149–65.

22. Tsolakis AV, et al. Ghrelin immunoreactive cells in gastric endocrine tumors and their relation to plasma ghrelin concentration. J Clin Gastroenterol 2008; 42(4): 381–8.

23. Rindi G, Inzani F, Solcia E. Pathology of gastrointestinal disorders. Endocrinol Metab Clin North Am 2010; 39(4): 713–27.

24. Sullivan TC. Anorectal carcinoid tumors: is aggressive surgery warranted? Ann Surg 1990; 212(5): 650–1.

25. Richards D, et al. Unusual case of small cell gastric carcinoma: case report and literature review. Dig Dis Sci 2011; 56(4): 951–7.

26. Cho MY, et al. Relationship between Epstein–Barr virus-encoded RNA expression, apoptosis and lymphocytic infiltration in gastric carcinoma with lymphoid-rich stroma. Med Princ Pract 2004; 13(6): 353–60.

27. Grozinsky-Glasberg S, et al. Somatostatin analogues in the control of neuroendocrine tumours: efficacy and mechanisms. Endocr Relat Cancer 2008; 15(3): 701–20.

28. Rindi G, et al. Gastroenteropancreatic (neuro)endocrine neoplasms: the histology report. Dig Liver Disase 2011; 43(Suppl 4): S356–60.

29. Uccella S, et al. Histidine decarboxylase, DOPA decarboxylase, and vesicular monoamine transporter 2 expression in neuroendocrine tumors: immunohistochemical study and gene expression analysis. J Histochem Cytochem 2006; 54(8): 863–75.

30. Krenning EP, et al. Somatostatin receptor scintigraphy with [111In-DTPA-D-Phe1]- and [123I-Tyr3]-octreotide: the Rotterdam experience with more than 1000 patients. Eur J Nucl Med 1993; 20(8): 716–31.

31. Anlauf M. Neuroendocrine neoplasms of the gastroenteropancreatic system: pathology and classification. Horm Metab Res 2011; 43(12): 825–31.

32. Faverly DR, et al. Adeno-carcinoid or amphicrine tumors of the middle ear a new entity? Pathol Res Pract 1992; 188(1-2): 162–71.

33. Thakker RV. Multiple endocrine neoplasia type 1 (MEN1). Best Pract Res Clin Endocrinol Metab 2010; 24(3): 355–70.

34. Berna MJ, et al. A prospective study of gastric carcinoids and enterochromaffin-like cell changes in multiple endocrine neoplasia type 1 and Zollinger–Ellison syndrome: identification of risk factors. J Clin Endocrinol Metab 2008; 93(5): 1582–91.

35. D'Adda T, et al. Loss of heterozygosity in 11q13-14 regions in gastric neuroendocrine tumors not associated with multiple endocrine neoplasia type 1 syndrome. Lab Invest 1999; 79(6): 671–7.

36. Hung OY, et al. Hypergastrinemia, type 1 gastric carcinoid tumors: diagnosis and management. J Clin Oncol 2011; 29(25): e713–15.

37. Walter T, et al. Is the combination of chromogranin A and pancreatic polypeptide serum determinations of interest in the diagnosis and follow-up of gastro-entero-pancreatic neuroendocrine tumours? Eur J Cancer 2011; Nov 29 [Epub ahead of print].

38. Varas MJ, et al. Usefulness of endoscopic ultrasonography (EUS) for selecting carcinoid tumors as candidates to endoscopic resection. Rev Esp Enferm Dig 2010; 102(10): 577–82.

39. Rockall AG, Reznek RH. Imaging of neuroendocrine tumours (CT/MR/US). Best Pract Res Clin Endocrinol Metab 2007; 21(1): 43–68.

40. Gibril F, et al. Ability of somatostatin receptor scintigraphy to identify patients with gastric carcinoids: a prospective study. J Nucl Med 2000; 41(10): 1646–56.

41. Teunissen JJ, et al. Nuclear medicine techniques for the imaging and treatment of neuroendocrine tumours. Endocr Relat Cancer 2011; 18(Suppl 1): S27–51.

42. Nisa L, Savelli G, Giubbini R. Yttrium-90 DOTATOC therapy in GEP-NET and other SST2 expressing tumors: a selected review. Ann Nucl Med 2011; 25(2): 75–85.

43. Binderup T, et al. 18F-fluorodeoxyglucose positron emission tomography predicts survival of patients with neuroendocrine tumors. Clin Cancer Res 2010; 16(3): 978–85.

44. Kulke MH, et al. NANETS treatment guidelines: well-differentiated neuroendocrine tumors of the stomach and pancreas. Pancreas 2010; 39(6): 735–52.

45. Kubota T, et al. Endocrine carcinoma of the stomach: clinicopathological analysis of 27 surgically treated cases in a single institute. Gastric Cancer 2012; Jan 18 [Epub ahead of print].

46. Norton JA, et al. Gastric carcinoid tumors in multiple endocrine neoplasia-1 patients with Zollinger–Ellison syndrome can be symptomatic, demonstrate aggressive growth, and require surgical treatment. Surgery 2004; 136(6): 1267–74.

47. Okita NT, et al. Neuroendocrine tumors of the stomach: chemotherapy with cisplatin plus irinotecan is effective for gastric poorly-differentiated neuroendocrine carcinoma. Gastric Cancer 2011; 14(2): 161–5.

48. Kim SJ, et al. Biological characteristics and treatment outcomes of metastatic or recurrent neuroendocrine tumors: tumor grade and metastatic site are important for treatment strategy. BMC Cancer 2010; 10: 448.

49. Saxena A, et al. Progression and survival results after radical hepatic metastasectomy of indolent advanced neuroendocrine neoplasms (NENs) supports an aggressive surgical approach. Surgery 2011; 149(2): 209–20.

50. Shaheen M, et al. Predictors of response to radio-embolization (TheraSphere(R)) treatment of neuroendocrine liver metastasis. HPB (Oxford) 2012; 14(1): 60–6.

51. Gamblin TC, Christians K, Pappas SG. Radiofrequency ablation of neuroendocrine hepatic metastasis. Surg Oncol Clin North Am 2011; 20(2): 273–9, vii–viii.

52. Harring TR, et al. Treatment of liver metastases in patients with neuroendocrine tumors: a comprehensive review. Int J Hepatol 2011; 154541 [Epub ahead of print].

53. Modlin IM, et al. Review article: somatostatin analogues in the treatment of gastroenteropancreatic neuroendocrine (carcinoid) tumours. Aliment Pharmacol Ther 2010; 31(2): 169–88.

54. Chadha MK, et al. High-dose octreotide acetate for management of gastroenteropancreatic neuroendocrine tumors. Anticancer Res 2009; 29(10): 4127–30.

55. Rinke A, et al. Placebo-controlled, double-blind, prospective, randomized study on the effect of octreotide LAR in the control of tumor growth in patients with metastatic neuroendocrine midgut tumors: a report from the PROMID Study Group. J Clin Oncol 2009; 27(28): 4656–63.

56. Walter T, *et al*. New treatment strategies in advanced neuroendocrine tumours. Dig Liver Dis 2012; 44(2): 95–105.

57. Van Vliet EI, *et al*. Treatment of gastroenteropancreatic neuroendocrine tumors with peptide receptor radionuclide therapy. Neuroendocrinology 2012; Jan 10 [Epub ahead of print].

58. Bodei L, *et al*. Peptide receptor radionuclide therapy with (1) Lu-DOTATATE: the IEO phase I-II study. Eur J Nucl Med Mol Imaging 2011; 38(12): 2125–35.

59. Vegt E, *et al*. Renal toxicity of radiolabeled peptides and antibody fragments: mechanisms, impact on radionuclide therapy, and strategies for prevention. J Nucl Med 2010; 51(7): 1049–58.

60. Faiss S, *et al*. Prospective, randomized, multicenter trial on the antiproliferative effect of lanreotide, interferon alfa, and their combination for therapy of metastatic neuroendocrine gastroenteropancreatic tumors – the International Lanreotide and Interferon Alfa Study Group. J Clin Oncol 2003; 21(14): 2689–96.

61. http://clinicaltrials.gov/ct2/show/NCT00353496.

62. Strosberg J, Kvols L. Antiproliferative effect of somatostatin analogs in gastroenteropancreatic neuroendocrine tumors. World J Gastroenterol 2010; 16(24): 2963–70.

63. Turner NC, *et al*. Chemotherapy with 5-fluorouracil, cisplatin and streptozocin for neuroendocrine tumours. Br J Cancer 2010; 102(7): 1106–12.

64. Kouvaraki MA, *et al*. Fluorouracil, doxorubicin, and streptozocin in the treatment of patients with locally advanced and metastatic pancreatic endocrine carcinomas. J Clin Oncol 2004; 22(23): 4762–71.

65. Yao JC, *et al*. Daily oral everolimus activity in patients with metastatic pancreatic neuroendocrine tumors after failure of cytotoxic chemotherapy: a phase II trial. J Clin Oncol 2010; 28(1): 69–76.

66. Raymond E, *et al*. Sunitinib malate for the treatment of pancreatic neuroendocrine tumors. N Engl J Med 2011; 364(6): 501–13.

67. Kulke MH, *et al*. Phase II study of temozolomide and thalidomide in patients with metastatic neuroendocrine tumors. J Clin Oncol 2006; 24(3): 401–6.

68. Yao JC, *et al*. Targeting vascular endothelial growth factor in advanced carcinoid tumor: a random assignment phase II study of depot octreotide with bevacizumab and pegylated interferon alpha-2b. J Clin Oncol 2008; 26(8): 1316–23.

69. www.swog.org/Visitors/ViewProtocolDetails.asp?ProtocolID=2076.

70. Venook AP, *et al*. Phase II trial of FOLFOX plus bevacizumab in advanced, progressive neuroendocrine tumors. J Clin Oncol 2008; 26(Suppl): abstr 15545.

71. Raymond E, *et al*. Therapy innovations: tyrosine kinase inhibitors for the treatment of pancreatic neuroendocrine tumors. Cancer Metastasis Rev 2011; 30(Suppl 1): 19–26.

72. Mazur MT, Clark HB. Gastric stromal tumors: reappraisal of histogenesis. Am J Surg Pathol 1983; 7(6): 507–19.

73. Miettinen M, Sobin LH, Lasota J. Gastrointestinal stromal tumors of the stomach: a clinicopathologic, immunohistochemical, and molecular genetic study of 1765 cases with long-term follow-up. Am J Surg Pathol 2005; 29(1): 52–68.

74. Tran T, Davila JA, El-Serag HB. The epidemiology of malignant gastrointestinal stromal tumors: an analysis of 1,458 cases from 1992 to 2000. Am J Gastroenterol 2005; 100: 162–8.

75. Tryggvason G, *et al*. Gastrointestinal stromal tumors in Iceland, 1990–2003: the Icelandic GIST study, a population-based incidence and pathologic risk stratification study. Int J Cancer 2005; 117(2): 289–93.

76. Maeyama H, *et al*. Familial gastrointestinal stromal tumor with hyperpigmentation: association with a germline mutation of the c-kit gene. Gastroenterology 2001; 120: 210–15.

77. Fletcher CD, *et al*. Diagnosis of gastrointestinal stromal tumors: a consensus approach. Hum Pathol 2002; 33(5): 459–65.

78. Rutkowski P, *et al*. Clinical utility of the new American Joint Committee on Cancer staging system for gastrointestinal stromal tumors: current overall survival after primary tumor resection. Cancer 2011; 117(21): 4916–24.

79. Patil DT, Rubin BP. Gastrointestinal stromal tumor: advances in diagnosis and management. Arch Pathol Lab Med 2011; 135(10): 1298–310.

80. Corless CL, Barnett CM, Heinrich MC. Gastrointestinal stromal tumours: origin and molecular oncology. Nat Rev Cancer 2011; 11(12): 865–78.

81. Hirota S, *et al*. Gain-of-function mutations of c-kit in human gastrointestinal stromal tumors. Science 1998; 279(5350): 577–80.

82. Gajiwala KS, *et al*. KIT kinase mutants show unique mechanisms of drug resistance to imatinib and sunitinib in gastrointestinal stromal tumor patients. Proc Natl Acad Sci USA 2009; 106(5): 1542–7.

83. Zheng S, *et al*. Secondary C-kit mutation is a cause of acquired resistance to imatinib in gastrointestinal stromal tumor. Scand J Gastroenterol 2009; 44(6): 760–3.

84. Hirota S, *et al*. Gain-of-function mutations of platelet-derived growth factor receptor alpha gene in gastrointestinal stromal tumors. Gastroenterology 2003; 125(3): 660–7.

85. Pauls K, *et al*. PDGFRalpha- and c-kit-mutated gastrointestinal stromal tumours (GISTs) are characterized by distinctive histological and immunohistochemical features. Histopathology 2005; 46(2): 166–75.

86. Hostein I, *et al*. BRAF mutation status in gastrointestinal stromal tumors. Am J Clin Pathol 2010; 133(1): 141–8.

87. Janeway KA, *et al*. Defects in succinate dehydrogenase in gastrointestinal stromal tumors lacking KIT and PDGFRA mutations. Proc Natl Acad Sci USA 2011; 108(1): 314–18.

88. Pantaleo MA, *et al*. The emerging role of insulin-like growth factor 1 receptor (IGF1r) in gastrointestinal stromal tumors (GISTs). J Transl Med 2010; 8: 117.

89. Agaram NP, *et al*. Novel V600E BRAF mutations in imatinib-naive and imatinib-resistant gastrointestinal stromal tumors. Genes Chromosomes Cancer 2008; 47(10): 853–9.

90. Carney JA. Gastric stromal sarcoma, pulmonary chondroma, and extraadrenal paraganglioma (Carney triad): natural history, adrenocortical component, and possible familial occurrence. Mayo Clinic proceedings. Mayo Clin Proc 1999; 74(6): 543–52.

91. Stratakis CA, Carney JA. The triad of paragangliomas, gastric stromal tumours and pulmonary chondromas (Carney triad), and the dyad of paragangliomas and gastric stromal sarcomas (Carney–Stratakis syndrome): molecular genetics and clinical implications. J Intern Med 2009; 266(1): 43–52.

92. Andersson J, *et al*. NF1-associated gastrointestinal stromal tumors have unique clinical, phenotypic, and genotypic characteristics. Am J Surg Pathol 2005; 29(9): 1170–6.

93. Rutkowski P, *et al*. Validation of the Joensuu risk criteria for primary resectable gastrointestinal stromal tumour – the impact of tumour rupture on patient outcomes. Eur J Surg Oncol 2011; 37(10): 890–6.

94. Rubin JL, *et al*. Epidemiology, survival, and costs of localized gastrointestinal stromal tumors. Int J Gen Med 2011; 4: 121–30.

95. Joensuu H, *et al*. Risk of recurrence of gastrointestinal stromal tumour after surgery: an analysis of pooled population-based cohorts. Lancet Oncol 2011; Dec 6 [Epub ahead of print].

96. Ven der Zwan SM, de Matteo RP. Gastrointestinal stromal tumour: 5 years later. Cancer 2005; 104: 1781–8.

97. DeMatteo RP, *et al*. Two hundred gastrointestinal stromal tumors: recurrence patterns and prognostic factors for survival. Ann Surg 2000; 231(1): 51–8.

98. Nowain A, *et al*. Gastrointestinal stromal tumors: clinical profile, pathogenesis, treatment strategies and prognosis. J Gastroenterol Hepatol 2005; 20(6): 818–24.

99. Ha CY, *et al*. Diagnosis and management of GI stromal tumors by EUS-FNA: a survey of opinions and practices of endosonographers. Gastrointest Endosc 2009; 69(6): 1039–44 e1.

100. Yasuda K, *et al*. The diagnosis of submucosal tumors of the stomach by endoscopic ultrasonography. Gastrointest Endosc 1989; 35(1): 10–15.

101. Palazzo L, *et al*. Endosonographic features predictive of benign and malignant gastrointestinal stromal cell tumours. Gut 2000; 46(1): 88–92.

102. Sepe PS, *et al*. EUS-guided FNA for the diagnosis of GI stromal cell tumors: sensitivity and cytologic yield. Gastrointest Endosc 2009; 70(2): 254–61.

103. Tsai TL, *et al*. Differentiation of benign and malignant gastric stromal tumors using endoscopic ultrasonography. Chang Gung Med J 2001; 24(3): 167–73.

104. Dudeck O, *et al.* Comparison of RECIST and Choi criteria for computed tomographic response evaluation in patients with advanced gastrointestinal stromal tumor treated with sunitinib. Ann Oncol 2011; 22(8): 1828–33.

105. Demetri GD, *et al.* NCCN Task Force report: update on the management of patients with gastrointestinal stromal tumors. J Natl Compr Canc Netw 2010; 8(Suppl 2): S1–41; quiz S42–4.

106. DeMatteo RP, *et al.* Two hundred gastrointestinal stromal tumors: recurrence patterns and prognostic factors for survival. Ann Surg 2000; 231(1): 51–8.

107. DeMatteo RP, *et al.* Adjuvant imatinib mesylate after resection of localised, primary gastrointestinal stromal tumour: a randomised, double-blind, placebo-controlled trial. Lancet 2009; 373(9669): 1097–104.

108. Eisenberg BL, *et al.* Phase II trial of neoadjuvant/adjuvant imatinib mesylate (IM) for advanced primary and metastatic/recurrent operable gastrointestinal stromal tumor (GIST): early results of RTOG 0132/ACRIN 6665. J Surg Oncol 2009; 99(1): 42–7.

109. Wang D, *et al.* Phase II trial of neoadjuvant/adjuvant imatinib mesylate for advanced primary and metastatic/recurrent operable gastrointestinal stromal tumors: long-term follow-up results of Radiation Therapy Oncology Group 0132. Ann Surg Oncol 2011; Dec 28 [Epub ahead of print].

110. Essat M, Cooper K. Imatinib as adjuvant therapy for gastrointestinal stromal tumors: a systematic review. International journal of cancer. Int J Cancer 2011; 128(9): 2202–14.

111. McAuliffe JC, *et al.* A randomized, phase II study of preoperative plus postoperative imatinib in GIST: evidence of rapid radiographic response and temporal induction of tumor cell apoptosis. Ann Surg Oncol 2009; 16(4): 910–19.

112. Blanke CD, *et al.* Long-term results from a randomized phase II trial of standard- versus higher-dose imatinib mesylate for patients with unresectable or metastatic gastrointestinal stromal tumors expressing KIT. J Clin Oncol 2008; 26(4): 620–5.

113. Verweij J, *et al.* Progression-free survival in gastrointestinal stromal tumours with high-dose imatinib: randomised trial. Lancet 2004; 364(9440): 1127–34.

114. Demetri GD, *et al.* Efficacy and safety of imatinib mesylate in advanced gastrointestinal stromal tumors. N Engl J Med 2002; 347(7): 472–80.

115. Blanke CD, *et al.* Phase III randomized, intergroup trial assessing imatinib mesylate at two dose levels in patients with unresectable or metastatic gastrointestinal stromal tumors expressing the kit receptor tyrosine kinase: S0033. J Clin Oncol 2008; 26(4): 626–32.

116. Gastrointestinal Stromal Tumor Meta-Analysis Group. Comparison of two doses of imatinib for the treatment of unresectable or metastatic gastrointestinal stromal tumors: a meta-analysis of 1,640 patients. J Clin Oncol 2010; 28(7): 1247–53.

117. Kim EJ, Zalupski MM. Systemic therapy for advanced gastrointestinal stromal tumors: beyond imatinib. J Surg Oncol 2011; 104(8): 901–6.

118. Artinyan A, *et al.* Metastatic gastrointestinal stromal tumors in the era of imatinib: improved survival and elimination of socioeconomic survival disparities. Cancer Epidemiol Biomarkers Prev 2008; 17(8): 2194–201.

119. Demetri GD, *et al.* Efficacy and safety of sunitinib in patients with advanced gastrointestinal stromal tumour after failure of imatinib: a randomised controlled trial. Lancet 2006; 368(9544): 1329–38.

120. George S, *et al.* Clinical evaluation of continuous daily dosing of sunitinib malate in patients with advanced gastrointestinal stromal tumour after imatinib failure. Eur J Cancer 2009; 45(11): 1959–68.

121. Conley AP, *et al.* A randomized phase II study of perifosine (P) plus imatinib for patients with imatinib-resistant gastrointestinal stromal tumor (GIST). J Clin Oncol 2009; 27 (15 s suppl; abstr 10563).

122. Capelle LG, *et al.* Gastric MALT lymphoma: epidemiology and high adenocarcinoma risk in a nationwide study. Eur J Cancer 2008; 44(16): 2470–6.

123. Zullo A, *et al.* Gastric low-grade mucosal-associated lymphoid tissue-lymphoma: Helicobacter pylori and beyond. World J Gastrointest Oncol 2010; 2(4): 181–6.

124. Thieblemont C. Clinical presentation and management of marginal zone lymphomas. Hematology Am Soc Hematol Educ Program 2005; 307–13.

125. Boot H. Diagnosis and staging in gastrointestinal lymphoma. Best Pract Res Clin Gastroenterol 2010; 24(1): 3–12.

126. Ruskoné-Fourmestraux A, *et al.* Paris staging system for primary gastrointestinal lymphomas. Gut 2003; 52(6): 912–13.

127. Zullo A, *et al.* Primary low-grade and high-grade gastric MALT-lymphoma presentation. J Clin Gastroenterol 2010; 44(5): 340–4.

128. Doglioni C, *et al.* Gastric lymphoma: the histology report. Dig Liver Dis 2011; 43(Suppl 4): S310–18.

129. Ruskoné-Fourmestraux A, *et al.* EGILS consensus report. Gastric extranodal marginal zone B-cell lymphoma of MALT. Gut 2011; 60(6): 747–58.

130. Bertoni F, *et al.* Genetic alterations underlying the pathogenesis of MALT lymphoma. Hematol J 2002; 3(1): 10–13.

131. Ruefli-Brasse AA, French DM, Dixit VM. Regulation of NF-kappaB-dependent lymphocyte activation and development by paracaspase. Science 2003; 302(5650): 1581–4.

132. Farinha P, Gascoyne RD. Molecular pathogenesis of mucosa-associated lymphoid tissue lymphoma. J Clin Oncol 2005; 23: 6370–8.

133. Dierlamm J, *et al.* The apoptosis inhibitor gene API2 and a novel 18q gene, MLT, are recurrently rearranged in the t(11;18)(q21;q21) associated mucosa-associated lymphoid tissue lymphomas. Blood 1999; 93: 3601–9.

134. Liu H, Ye H, Ruskoné-Fourmestraux A. T(11;18) is a marker for all stage gastric MALT lymphomas that will not respond to H. pylori eradication. Gastroenterology 2002; 122: 1286–94.

135. Streubel B, Lamprecht A, Dierlamm J. T(14;18)(q32;q21) involving IGH and MALT1 is a frequent chromosomal aberration in MALT lymphoma. Blood 2003; 101(6): 2335–9.

136. Wlodarska I, *et al.* FOXP1, a gene highly expressed in a subset of diffuse large B-cell lymphoma, is recurrently targeted by genomic abberations. Leukemia 2005; 19: 1299–305.

137. Bertoni F, *et al.* MALT lymphomas: pathogenesis can drive treatment. Oncology 2011; 25(12): 1134–42, 1147.

138. Nakamura T, *et al.* Clinical features and prognosis of gastric MALT lymphoma with special reference to responsiveness to H. pylori eradication and API2-MALT1 status. Am J Gastroenterol 2008; 103(1): 62–70.

139. Koch P, *et al.* Primary gastrointestinal non-Hodgkin's lymphoma: II. Combined surgical and conservative or conservative management only in localized gastric lymphoma – results of the prospective German Multicenter Study GIT NHL 01/92. J Clin Oncol 2001; 19(18): 3874–83.

140. Radaszkiewicz T, Dragosics B, Bauer P. Gastrointestinal malignant lymphomas of the mucosa-associated lymphoid tissue: factors relevant to prognosis. Gastroenterology 1992; 102: 1628–38.

141. Ozao-Choy J, *et al.* Laparoscopic antrectomy for the treatment of type I gastric carcinoid tumors. J Surg Res 2010; 162(1): 22–5.

142. Pavic T, Hrabar D, Duvnjak M. The role of endoscopic ultrasound in evaluation of gastric subepithelial lesions. Coll Antropol 2010; 34(2): 757–62.

143. Hirose Y, *et al.* Comparison between endoscopic macroscopic classification and F-18 FDG PET findings in gastric mucosa-associated lymphoid tissue lymphoma patients. Clin Nucl Med 2012; 37(2): 152–7.

144. Zullo A, *et al.* Effects of Helicobacter pylori eradication on early stage gastric mucosa-associated lymphoid tissue lymphoma. Clin Gastroenterol Hepatol 2010; 8(2): 105–10.

145. Copie-Bergman C, Wotherspoon A. MALT lymphoma pathology, initial diagnosis, and posttreatment evaluation. In: Cavalli F, Stein H, Zucca E (eds) *Extranodal Lymphomas: Pathology and Management.* London: Informa Health Care, 2008. pp.114–23.

146. Copie-Bergman C, *et al.* Proposal for a new histological grading system for post-treatment evaluation of gastric MALT lymphoma. Gut 2003; 52: 1656.

147. Gisbert JP, Calvet X. Review article: common misconceptions in the management of Helicobacter pylori-associated gastric MALT-lymphoma. Aliment Pharmacol Ther 2011; 34(9): 1047–62.

148. Stathis A, *et al.* Long-term outcome following Helicobacter pylori eradication in a retrospective study of 105 patients with localized gastric marginal zone B-cell lymphoma of MALT type. Ann Oncol 2009; 20(6): 1086–93.

149. Nakamura S, *et al.* Long-term clinical outcome of gastric MALT lymphoma after eradication of Helicobacter pylori: a multicentre cohort follow-up study of 420 patients in Japan. Gut 2011; Sept 2 [Epub ahead of print].

150. Yahalom J. MALT lymphomas: a radiation oncology viewpoint. Ann Hematol 2001; 80(Suppl 3): B100–5.

151. Levy M, *et al.* Treatment of t(11;18)-positive gastric mucosa-associated lymphoid tissue lymphoma with rituximab and chlorambucil: clinical, histological, and molecular follow-up. Leuk Lymphoma 2010; 51(2): 284–90.

152. Salar A, *et al.* Combination therapy with rituximab and intravenous or oral fludarabine in the first-line, systemic treatment of patients with extranodal marginal zone B-cell lymphoma of the mucosa-associated lymphoid tissue type. Cancer 2009; 115(22): 5210–17.

153. www.ielsg.org/documents/ielsg19ash00.pdf.

154. Fukayama M, Ushiku T. Epstein–Barr virus-associated gastric carcinoma. Pathol Res Pract 2011; 207(9): 529–37.

155. Song HJ, Kim KM. Pathology of Epstein–Barr virus-associated gastric carcinoma and its relationship to prognosis. Gut Liver 2011; 5(2): 143–8.

156. Murphy G, *et al.* Meta-analysis shows that prevalence of Epstein–Barr virus-positive gastric cancer differs based on sex and anatomic location. Gastroenterology 2009; 137(3): 824–3.

157. Li S, *et al.* Meta-analysis of the relationship between Epstein–Barr virus infection and clinicopathological features of patients with gastric carcinoma. Sci China Life Sci 2010; 53(4): 524–30.

158. Chang MS, *et al.* Epstein–Barr virus in gastric carcinomas with lymphoid stroma. Histopathology 2000; 37(4): 309–15.

159. Oda K, *et al.* Association of Epstein–Barr virus with gastric carcinoma with lymphoid stroma. Am J Pathol 1993; 143(4): 1063–71.

160. Lee JM, *et al.* Expression of Epstein–Barr virus gene and clonality of infiltrated T lymphocytes in Epstein–Barr virus-associated gastric carcinoma. Immune Netw 2011; 11(1): 50–8.

161. Hino R, *et al.* Survival advantage of EBV-associated gastric carcinoma: survivin up-regulation by viral latent membrane protein 2A. Cancer Res 2008; 68(5): 1427–35.

162. Hino R, *et al.* Activation of DNA methyltransferase 1 by EBV latent membrane protein 2A leads to promoter hypermethylation of PTEN gene in gastric carcinoma. Cancer Res 2009; 69(7): 2766–74.

163. Kume T, *et al.* Low rate of apoptosis and overexpression of bcl-2 in Epstein–Barr virus-associated gastric carcinoma. Histopathology 1999; 34(6): 502–9.

164. Ito H, *et al.* Gastric carcinoma with lymphoid stroma: pathological and immunohistochemical analysis. Hiroshima J Med Sci 1990; 39(2): 29–37.

165. Chang MS, *et al.* CpG island methylation status in gastric carcinoma with and without infection of Epstein–Barr virus. Clin Cancer Res 2006; 12(10): 2995–3002.

166. Ji Jung E, *et al.* Ganciclovir augments the lytic induction and apoptosis induced by chemotherapeutic agents in an Epstein–Barr virus-infected gastric carcinoma cell line. Anticancer Drugs 2007; 18(1): 79–85.

167. Chun H, Kwon SJ. Clinicopathological characteristics of alpha-fetoprotein-producing gastric cancer. J Gastric Cancer 2011; 11(1): 23–30.

168. Zhang JF, *et al.* Clinicopathological and prognostic features of hepatoid adenocarcinoma of the stomach. Chin Med J (Engl) 2011; 124(10): 1470–6.

169. Inoue M, *et al.* Long-term results of gastrectomy for alpha-fetoprotein-producing gastric cancer. Br J Surg 2010; 97(7): 1056–61.

170. Liu X, *et al.* Clinicopathologic features and prognostic factors in alpha-fetoprotein-producing gastric cancers: analysis of 104 cases. J Surg Oncol 2010; 102(3): 249–55.

171. Liu Z, Mira JL, Cruz-Caudillo JC. Primary gastric choriocarcinoma: a case report and review of the literature. Arch Pathol Lab Med 2001; 125(12): 1601–4.

172. Kim YS, *et al.* Gastric yolk sac tumor: a case report and review of the literature. Korean J Intern Med 2009; 24(2): 143–6.

173. Kanai M, *et al.* Pure gastric yolk sac tumor that was diagnosed after curative resection: case report and review of literature. Int J Gastrointest Cancer 2005; 35(1): 77–81.

174. De Palma GD, *et al.* Metastatic tumors to the stomach: clinical and endoscopic features. World J Gastroenterol 2006; 12(45): 7326–8.

175. Oda I, *et al.* Metastatic tumors to the stomach: analysis of 54 patients diagnosed at endoscopy and 347 autopsy cases. Endoscopy 2001; 33(6): 507–10.

176. Trouillet N, *et al.* Gastric metastases. An endoscopic series of ten cases. Gastroenterol Clin Biol 2010; 34(4–5): 305–9.

177. Kobayashi O, *et al.* Clinical diagnosis of metastatic gastric tumors: clinicopathologic findings and prognosis of nine patients in a single cancer center. World J Surg 2004; 28(6): 548–51.

178. Green LK. Hematogenous metastases to the stomach. A review of 67 cases. Cancer 1990; 65(7): 1596–600.

179. Ravi A. Primary gastric melanoma: a rare cause of upper gastrointestinal bleeding. Gastroenterol Hepatol 2008; 4(11): 795–7.

180. Dasgupta TK, Brasfield RD. Metastatic melanoma of the gastrointestinal tract. Arch Surg 1964; 88: 969–73.

181. Pollheimer MJ, *et al.* Renal cell carcinoma metastatic to the stomach: single-centre experience and literature review. BJU Int 2008; 102(3): 315–19.

182. Wu MH, Lin MT, Lee PH. Clinicopathological study of gastric metastases. World J Surg 2007; 31(1): 132–6.

Section 6: Gastrointestinal Tumors

29 Unusual Cancers of the Pancreas

Chanjuan Shi,[1] John S. Macdonald,[2] and Jordan D. Berlin[1]

[1] Vanderbilt University Medical Center, Nashville, TN, USA
[2] Aptium Oncology, Los Angeles, CA, USA

Introduction

Tumors of the pancreas collectively are the fourth leading cause of neoplastic death despite being only the 10th most common site of cancer in the United States.[1] In 2011, it is expected that over 44,000 Americans will be diagnosed with pancreatic cancer and 37,660 will die from this disease. Approximately 95% of pancreatic cancers arise from the ductal epithelium, and another 3–4% arise from the islet cells. This chapter will review the unusual, remaining 1–2% (Box 29.1), particularly epithelial malignancies of nonneuroendocrine origin. The nonepithelial pancreatic malignancies, including lymphomas, sarcomas, primitive neuroectodermal tumor, and desmoplastic small round cell tumor, are treated similarly to those arising from other sites and will not be addressed in this chapter.

Uncommon exocrine tumors of the pancreas

Cystic neoplasms

Both malignant and benign cystic neoplasms may arise in the pancreas. Each has unique features but the evaluation and diagnostic workup are common for these lesions. It is important to try to distinguish these lesions, because of the impact on management.

Cystic neoplasms are classified as serous (benign or malignant), mucinous (benign or malignant), and intraductal papillary mucinous neoplasm (IPMN), a premalignant lesion that appears to lead to adenocarcinomas. Two recent reviews of all cystic neoplasms have been published.[2]

The most common clinical presentation for cystic neoplasms is an incidental finding on radiographic studies performed for other reasons.[2,3] Symptoms, when they occur, are nonspecific and include bloating, abdominal discomforts and other symptoms of mass effect from the lesions. Most commonly, the patients have had either a computed tomography (CT) scan or magnetic resonance imaging (MRI). These tests can differentiate cystic neoplasms from nonneoplastic lesions such as pancreatic pseudocyst. Pseudocyst generally presents with history of pancreatitis and on CT or MRI inflammation of the pancreas is usually seen.[4] Magnetic resonance cholangiopancreatography can help determine the etiology of the cystic lesion as well, showing biliary and pancreatic ductal structure. Endoscopic retrograde cholangiopancreatography (ERCP) may also be useful. One finding, that of a swollen papilla with mucin oozing from the papilla, is considered pathogenomic of IPMN but is not a common finding.[4]

Surgery is the diagnostic test of choice for cystic neoplasms but among less invasive testing, endoscopic ultrasound (EUS) should be considered. This procedure allows evaluation of the cyst, biopsy and aspiration of the cystic fluid for diagnostic testing. Cyst fluid analysis had been utilized prior to EUS but EUS provided a new modality for evaluating size, structure, and cyst fluid. In the Cooperative Pancreatic Cyst Study, 341 patients underwent EUS and cyst fluid aspiration, 112 of whom had subsequent surgical resection. The study demonstrated that cyst fluid carcinoembryonic antigen (CEA) was more accurate (79% accuracy) than cyst morphology (51% accuracy) or cytology (59% accuracy) in distinguishing mucinous from nonmucinous cysts.[5] In this study, a cut-off of 192 ng/mL was used for CEA levels but the sensitivity and specificity of this test can be changed by using a different CEA level. It is clear that a CEA level of <3.1 ng/mL is almost diagnostic of a serous cyst while levels above 480 ng/mL are diagnostic of a mucinous neoplasm.[6] However, it is more complex to determine malignant versus nonmalignant cystic neoplasms. Very high levels of CEA of ≥6000 ng/mL are suggestive of malignancy.[7]

Textbook of Uncommon Cancer, Fourth Edition. Edited by Derek Raghavan, Charles D. Blanke, David H. Johnson, Paul L. Moots, Gregory H. Reaman, Peter G. Rose and Mikkael A. Sekeres.
© 2012 John Wiley & Sons, Inc. Published 2012 by John Wiley & Sons, Inc.

Box 29.1 Classification of pancreatic neoplasms.

Epithelial malignancies

Exocrine neoplasms

1. Serous cystadenocarcinoma
2. Invasive carcinoma associated with mucinous cystic neoplasm (mucinous cystadenocarcinoma)
3. Invasive carcinoma associated with intraductal papillary mucinous neoplasm
4. Adenocarcinoma variants:
   - Adenosquamous carcinoma
   - Colloid carcinoma (mucinous noncystic adenocarcinoma)
   - Medullary carcinoma
   - Hepatoid carcinoma
   - Undifferentiated carcinoma
   - Undifferentiated carcinoma with osteoclast-like giant cells
5. Acinar cell carcinoma
6. Acinar cell cystadenocarcinoma

Endocrine malignancies

1. Well-differentiated pancreatic neuroendocrine tumor:
   - Oncocytic carcinoma
2. Poorly differentiated neuroendocrine carcinoma:
   - Small cell carcinoma
   - Large cell endocrine carcinoma

Epithelial malignancies with multiple directions of differentiation

1. Mixed acinar-neuroendocrine carcinoma
2. Pancreatoblastoma

Epithelial neoplasms of uncertain direction of differentiation

1. Solid-pseudopapillary neoplasm

Nonepithelial malignancies

1. Leiomyosarcoma and other sarcomas
2. Primitive neuroectodermal tumor
3. Desmoplastic small round cell tumor
4. Non-Hodgkin lymphoma

Cystadenocarcinoma

Serous cystic neoplasms

Most serous cystic neoplasms (SCNs) are benign, and malignant transformation is thought to be very rare.[8,9] Serous cystic neoplasms make up approximately 1.1% of exocrine pancreas tumors.[8] However, in a single-institution experience of 158 resected SCNs, only one was initially diagnosed as malignant although a second later presented with metastatic disease, demonstrating that cystadenocarcinoma represent fewer than 1% of serous cystic neoplasms.[9]

Serous cystic neoplasms can present at almost any age, although the median age at presentation is 61–2.[9,10] The majority of patients are female (75–80%) and one study suggested that female patients tend to present at a lower median age.[10]

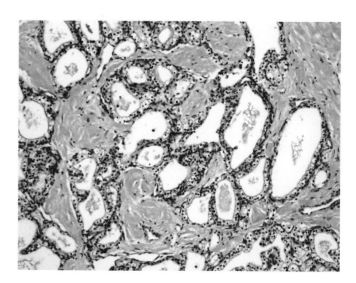

Figure 29.1 Serous cystadenocarcinoma is composed of uniform cuboidal cells with clear cytoplasm forming microcysts.

In single-institution studies, 36–47% of patients were asymptomatic with the finding arising from diagnostic workup for a separate problem.[9,10] SCNs are more likely to be found in asymptomatic patients as the use of CT and MRI imaging has increased in recent years. Both studies found the most common symptom was abdominal pain with other symptoms being weight loss, fatigue, abdominal fullness, jaundice, and gastrointestinal bleed. The majority of patients were Caucasian. In a Mayo Clinic review of 21 cases collected over 48 years, median age for cystadenocarcinoma was also 61 but a higher percentage of patients were males.[11] A higher percentage of patients presented with symptoms, with 81% having abdominal pain and nearly half presenting with weight loss. Jaundice, belching, nausea/vomiting, diarrhea, and fatigue were also reported.

As previously noted, cystadenocarcinoma is rare among the SCNs. By definition, serous cystadenocarcinoma is a serious cystic neoplasm of the pancreas with unequivocal metastases to extrapancreatic organs or tissues.[12] Grossly, they usually present with a large mass with multiple compartments filled with numerous microcysts. They frequently invade adjacent organs. Histologically, serous cystadenocarcinomas are identical to serous cystadenoma, being composed of uniform cuboidal, glycogen-rich cells that form numerous cysts containing serous fluid (Fig. 29.1). The presence of local invasion, involvement of regional nodes, cyst wall invasion, and/or histological dedifferentiation separate malignant from benign SCNs.

Diagnosis of cystic neoplasms is discussed above. For SCNs, CT and MRI of are variable accuracy.[13] Endoscopic ultrasound may also be helpful, particularly because fluid can be obtained for evaluation. The diagnostic accuracy of EUS is as low as 40%, and it cannot evaluate benign versus malignant lesions. As mentioned above, cyst fluid analysis adds to the diagnostic accuracy of EUS, and low CEA (<5 ng/mL) and low viscosity are among the most consistent tests for differentiating SCNs from mucinous cysts.[7,13]

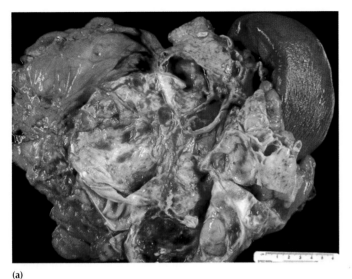
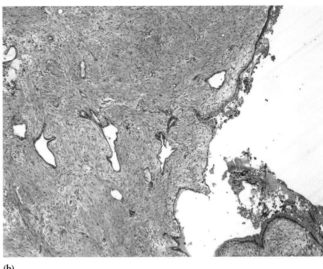

(a)

(b)

Figure 29.2 (a) Grossly, mucinous cystadenocarcinoma is a well-circumscribed, multilocular cystic mass with solid areas. (b) Microscopically, an invasive carcinoma (*left*) with ductal differentiation arises from cysts (*right*) lined by atypical epithelium associated with an underlying subepithelial ovarian-like stroma.

Therapy of SCNs is surgical. Tumors smaller than 4 cm can be observed, although the frequency of follow-up scans ranges from 6 months to 2 years.[13,14] If lesions show evidence of symptoms or rapid growth, or a definitive diagnosis cannot be obtained, surgery should also be considered. However, comorbidities and other risks for the surgery should be considered, due to the normally slow-growing, benign behavior of SCNs. For serous cystadenocarcinoma, with only one report of over 20 patients, there are few data as to the proper therapy.[11] Surgery is still the treatment of choice. For patients with fully resected lesions (*n* = 13), 5-year survival was much better than for those with partial excisions (*n* = 7) (68% versus 14%, respectively). As the 5-year survival for resected cystadenocarcinoma appears to be much better than that for typical adenocarcinoma, it is difficult to recommend adjuvant therapy. However, typical regimens for pancreatic adenocarcinoma could be used if the clinician opts for therapy. Of note, the survival curve for partially excised tumors indicates that five of the seven patients died within the first year after surgery, which does not match the table that suggests that four patients survived for more than 1 year.[11] The most common site of metastasis (5/7 patients) was the liver. For those with metastatic disease, there is no reason to believe that chemotherapy regimens used for pancreatic adenocarcinoma would be any more or less effective in cystadenocarcinoma, and treatment using standard regimens for pancreatic adenocarcinoma is recommended, based on performance status and comorbidities.

Mucinous cystadenocarcinoma

Mucinous cystic neoplasms represent 10–45% of cystic neoplasms.[5] In contrast to serous cystic neoplasms, mucinous cystic neoplasms are more prone to malignant transformation. Mucinous cystadenocarcinomas may represent 8–39% of mucinous cystic neoplasms.[15–17] Overall, they are felt to represent ~1% of pancreatic cancers.[18] This variabil-

ity may be due to methods for collecting patient data as well as the size of the series.

Mucinous cystadenocarcinoma of the pancreas is an invasive adenocarcinoma arising in mucinous cystadenoma. Grossly, it is a well-circumscribed, multilocular cystic lesion that does not communicate with the pancreatic duct (Fig. 29.2a). The majority of mucinous cystic neoplasms are located in the body or tail of the pancreas.[15,19] Benign mucinous cystadenomas have smooth cystic walls. Intracystic papillary excrescence and solid mural nodules are seen in mucinous cystadenocarcinomas. Microscopically, the cysts are lined with columnar epithelium with/without mucin, showing variable degrees of architectural and cytological atypia (Fig. 29.2b). The cystic walls contain ovarian stroma. Most mucinous cystadenocarcinomas are either undifferentiated carcinoma or adenocarcinoma similar to conventional ductal adenocarcinoma (see Fig. 29.2b).[20]

There is a female predominance for both mucinous cystadenoma (86–100% female) and mucinous cystadenocarcinoma (71–100% female). Cystadenomas tend to present at an earlier age than cystadenocarcinomas. In the largest series, mucinous cystadenoma presented at a median age of 52 while cystadenocarcinomas presented at a median age of 63.6 years.[15] In case series, the majority of patients with mucinous cystadenocarcinoma present with symptoms, the most common being abdominal pain in 41–64%, while only 11–25% presented as an incidental finding in patients without symptoms from the tumor.[15,16,21] Mucinous cystadenoma presented without symptoms more often (26%) than mucinous cystadenocarcinomas (14%) in one series.[15] Other series did not show a difference, with 25% of malignant and 28% of benign mucinous cystic neoplasms presenting as asymptomatic.[21] However, most of these series do not account for the greater availability of CT scans and other tests that will likely increase the percentage of asymptomatic patients over time. Other presenting symptoms or findings include mass, fatigue, weight loss, and pancreatitis. Few data exist on CA 19-9 elevations but in one series, there were elevations in 21% of mucinous cystadenoma cases while mucinous cystadenocarcinoma patients presented with CA 19-9 elevations 70% of the time.[15] However, other series have not shown a difference in CA 19-9 levels between benign and malignant lesions.[21]

Consistently, malignant lesions present on average at larger sizes. In one study, the differences were 82.5 mm versus 45 mm (p <0.001) for malignant versus benign.[21] In a pooled analysis of multiple studies, mean size of malignant tumors was 10.2 cm with only one malignant tumor under 4.5 cm.[22] Mucinous cystadenoma and cystadenocarcinomas predominantly develop in the body and tail of the pancreas with some studies reporting no head lesions.[21,22]

Treatment of mucinous cystic neoplasms is surgical. Mucinous cystadenomas appear to all be cured with surgical resection, with 99–100% surviving the disease.[21,22] The prognoses for resected mucinous cystadenocarcinoma patients are fairly good but only 57–62% are disease free at 5 years. One series reported 23% of patients alive at 10 years.[23] An analysis of pathological features predicting recurrence suggested that patients with peritumoral invasion were more likely to experience recurrence than those with only tumor wall invasion.[16] Those with no evidence of invasion had no recurrences. Recurrences tend to be in the peritoneum and liver when they occur. Once disease recurs, mean survival is as short as 6.5 months.[21] In addition, patients undergoing resection can subsequently develop exocrine or endocrine insufficiency, with both being more likely in patients with cystadenocarcinoma than those with cystadenoma.[21] Subsequent exocrine insufficiency occurred in 21.5% versus 4.5% malignant versus benign lesions ($p=0.007$) and subsequent endocrine insufficiency developed in 43% versus 18.5% malignant versus benign lesions ($p=0.005$).

Little is known about patients with unresectable disease or the effects of systemic therapy. One small series suggested that patients with subtotal resections may also have a long survival, 30 months from diagnosis to death.[24] However, patients unable to undergo any resection tend to have poor prognoses, with a 1-year survival rate of only 10% in one study.[15] Little is known about the effects of radiotherapy and chemotherapy in this entity. In the absence of any data, it is likely best to treat these patients with chemotherapy and/or chemoradiotherapy regimens used for adenocarcinoma of the pancreas.

Intraductal papillary mucinous neoplasm

Intraductal papillary mucinous neoplasm (IPMN) is not a malignant neoplasm of the pancreas but it remains in the differential diagnosis with other cystic neoplasms of the pancreas. This entity has been known for almost 30 years but was not well defined until 1996.[13] The incidence of IPMN is increasing but this most likely reflects increased awareness and improved technology as well as increased access to technology.[25] IPMNs represent 20–50% of pancreatic cystic neoplasms. They are of significant importance because they appear to be precursor lesions to the common form of pancre-

atic cancer. Most recently, three families were described with what appears to be a familial pattern of IPMN.[26] None of the mutations already known for familial pancreatic cancer (BRCA2, P16, and CDKN2A) were found in these families. An additional report suggested that this entity may occur with greater frequency in patients with Carney complex, a disorder most commonly associated with a germline PRKAR1A mutation.[27]

As expected for a precursor lesion of pancreatic cancer, IPMN most often occurs in older age and is more common in the head of the pancreas than in the body or tail.[13] There is also a male predominance. IPMNs are divided into those of branch duct origin and those of main duct origin. Main duct IPMNs appear more likely to undergo malignant transformation. In a study of 349 Japanese patients with branch duct IPMNs followed closely, the median age for these lesions was 66 years with only a slight male predominance of 51%.[28] Of note, only 1.7% of patients were symptomatic. Median cyst size was 19 mm. While 55% of the lesions were found in the head of the pancreas, 66% of those that progressed during the observation period arose in the head. Patients were observed for a median of 3.7 years and during that time, 17% exhibited progression. Surgery was performed on 29 patients on the study. During the observation period, a total of seven (2%) patients developed pancreatic ductal adenocarcinoma. A separate report of 46 patients with main duct IPMNs showed very different results.[29] Median age was 74.6 years with male predominance (59%). Half the lesions were located in the pancreatic head and 30% presented with symptoms. Twenty patients (43%) underwent resection of their IPMNs. Those patients who underwent resection were more likely to have symptoms, be of younger age and have lesions in the head of the pancreas. Malignancy was found in 35% of patients with main duct IPMNs. Data suggesting that main duct IPMNs have greater potential for malignancy than branch-type IPMNs have been shown elsewhere, with 23–57% of main duct IPMNs and only 0–31% of branch duct IPMNs demonstrating invasive carcinoma (adenocarcinoma and IPMN with invasion).[30]

Pathologically, IPMNs are characterized by proliferation of mucinous cells within the ducts[13] and the formation of papillae. There are four histological subtypes of IPMNs: intestinal, pancreatobiliary, oncocytic, and gastric.[25] These four subtypes have different expressions of MUC 1, MUC 2, MUC5AC, and MUC6 gastric.[25,31] The intestinal type is most common in main duct IPMN gastric.[25] It most frequently is associated with a colloid carcinoma that has a fairly favorable prognosis (57% 5-year survival rate). The pancreatobiliary variant occurs more often in main duct IPMN but overall is less common than the intestinal type. The oncocytic variant was once called intraductal oncocytic papillary neoplasm and is the rarest form. It usually has high-grade dysplasia.[31] In contrast, the gastric type of IPMN is the most common form and is largely associated with branch-type IPMN.[25] Gastric and pancreatobiliary subtypes are associated with ductal adenocarcinoma and oncocytic forms are associated with oncocytic adenocarcinoma (discussed below). A consensus conference determined that IPMNs are characterized by a lack of ovarian stroma as is seen in mucinous cystic neoplasms of the pancreas.[32] IPMNs can have mutations of kRas, BRAF, and PIK3CA as well as loss of SMAD4 expression and overexpression of p53, similar to pancreatic ductal adenocarcinoma but not necessarily with the same incidence.[25,31] These findings have now been detected in all subtypes of IPMN although the results thus far are highly variable. They can present with dilation of the pancreatic duct as well as accumulation of mucus.

Management of IPMNs is observation or surgery. Indications that have been used for resection include invasive component on biopsy, symptoms, and progression on radiographic imaging. In addition, presence of mural nodules in pancreatic cysts is more likely to predict dysplasia or invasive carcinoma than lack of mural nodules (23% versus 3%, respectively, $p = 0.02$).[33] Observation is much more likely to be used in branch-type than in main duct IPMNs.[13] It appears that the survival for resected IPMNs with invasion is much better than that for resected pancreatic ductal adenocarcinoma.[13,34] Although 5-year survival for resected IPMN without invasive component is at least 70%, historically 5-year survival with invasive component is only 30–50%.[13] However, a more recent report of 59 patients had 5-year survival for IPMN with an invasive carcinoma at 68%.[34] In that study, multivariate analysis showed that nodal involvement and tubular carcinoma subtype predicted poorer prognosis. Other authors have found that when controlled for T and N staging, carcinoma arising from IPMN has no better prognosis than pancreatic ductal adenocarcinoma.[35,36]

There are no guidelines on the frequency of follow-up for patients for whom observation is chosen rather than surgical resection. There is also no consensus on follow-up of patients with resected IPMNs but it is common to perform at least annual imaging (either CT or MRI).[13] Tumor markers appear of limited utility. There are no data on adjuvant therapy with either chemotherapy or chemoradiation. It is not currently recommended that these patients receive adjuvant therapy.

Adenocarcinoma variants

Adenosquamous carcinoma

Adenosquamous carcinoma is one of the more frequently occurring of the adenocarcinoma variants, ranging in autopsy and case series from <1% to as much as 11% of all pancreatic tumors.[8,14,37–40] The largest series place the incidence at less than 1%.[14,37,38] In the larger case series, adenosquamous carcinomas have a male predominance (~60% or more male).[14,39] Seventy-five to 88% were Caucasian and median age was 65–68.[14,39,41] There appears to be predominance for head of pancreas primaries. Patients most often present with metastatic disease (53%) and less often with regional (38%) or localized (9%) disease. Using the California Cancer Registry database, researchers compared 95 adenosquamous carcinoma patients to pancreatic adenocarcinoma patients and found that the two populations were very similar in presentation, demographics, and outcomes.[14]

Adenosquamous carcinoma is a rare variant of pancreatic adenocarcinoma with both glandular and squamous differentiation. The gross appearance is similar to that of conventional ductal adenocarcinoma and it usually presents as a large, firm, ill-defined mass. Microscopically, there are adenocarcinoma and squamous cell carcinoma components, which can be intimately admixed (Fig. 29.3a) or topographically separate within the neoplasm (Fig. 29.3b). When they are separated, the adenocarcinoma portion is indistinct from conventional ductal adenocarcinoma (see Fig. 29.3b). The squamous component can be either keratinizing or nonkeratinizing. In adenosquamous carcinoma, at least 30% of the neoplasm should be squamous cell carcinoma.[12] In a single analysis of immunohistochemical staining of 19 primary cases of adenosquamous carcinoma, 100% stained with cytokeratin (AE1/AE3 and CK1), 84% stained for CA 19-9, and 74% for CEA.[41] In addition, 68% stained for CK7 and 26% for CK20. Only six

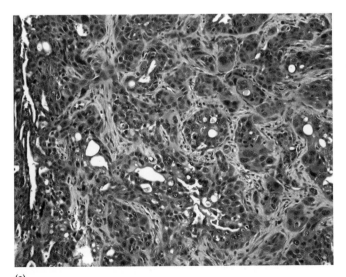

(a)

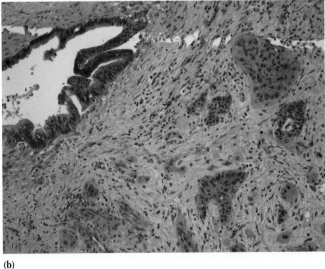

(b)

Figure 29.3 Adenosquamous carcinoma has two growth patterns: squamous cell carcinoma component intimately intermixed with adenocarcinoma with luminal formation (a), and nests of squamous cell carcinoma (*right lower half*) separated from adenocarcinoma (*left upper corner*) (b).

metastases were evaluated but staining patterns were similar to the primary tumors. Mutations in KRas have been identified in 50–100% of adenosquamous carcinoma.[39,42] A detailed analysis found similar mutations to pancreatic adenocarcinoma, including frequent loss of DPC4, and p16 proteins as well as strong nuclear positivity for p53.[42] However, the squamous component stained for p63, which does not happen in adenocarcinoma of the pancreas.

Several series have suggested a worse outcome for patients with adenosquamous carcinomas versus those with adenocarcinomas.[39,41] However, in the largest series the outcomes for adenosquamous carcinoma were similar provided that similar treatments were used.[14]

Treatment for localized disease is surgery. When surgery is performed, nodal involvement is common, occurring in 57–76% of cases.[14,41] In one study, margin involvement was found in 37% of cases.[41] Patients with locoregional disease treated with surgical resection have a median survival of 10.9–12 months. This may be better than in older, smaller series as a review of case reports and series from 1980 to 2007 revealed a median survival after surgery of only 6.7 months.[43] Adjuvant chemoradiation was associated with an improved overall survival compared to those patients who underwent surgical resection alone. Patients with locoregional disease who did not have resection had much shorter survival, in the range of 5 months.[14] Survival for metastatic disease patients is particularly poor, with a median of 4.5 months for those receiving chemotherapy and only 2 months for those who do not.

Stage for stage, the treatment of adenosquamous carcinoma should be the same as for patients with adenocarcinoma of the pancreas. Of note, the data for adjuvant therapy, though limited, exist only for chemoradiation and not for either therapy alone. No data exist for the use of FOLFIRINOX in patients with unresectable adenosquamous carcinoma but data suggest that patients benefit from chemotherapy.[14] Considering the squamous component of the disease, there may be a good

rationale for using a platinum-containing regimen in this setting to improve outcomes.

Colloid carcinoma (mucinous noncystic carcinoma)

Colloid carcinoma, a variant of pancreatic adenocarcinoma with abundant mucin pools, arises in association with IPMN. With recognition of the IPMN as the precursor lesion for this adenocarcinoma variant, less literature is available separating this entity from its apparent precursor, already discussed. The frequency of this lesion is not certain, as it is a variant of adenocarcinoma and includes both IPMN with minimally invasive disease and true invasive carcinoma, although IPMN can progress to pancreatic ductal adenocarcinoma, whereas colloid carcinoma appears to arise from the intestinal form of IPMN.[30,44]

Radiographic imaging of colloid carcinoma can include EUS, CT, and/or MRI. On CT, one small study described "peripheral and internal mesh-like progressive delayed enhancement," with contrast administration as well as multiple small cystic areas.[45] Similarly, a study of eight patients with colloid carcinoma who underwent MRI found a mesh-like appearance to the tumors as well as high intensity on T2-weighted images and nondistinct borders.[46]

Colloid carcinoma is usually larger than conventional ductal adenocarcinoma, with a mean size of 5.3 cm in one series.[47] On cross-section, they are well circumscribed with a soft gelatinous appearance (Fig. 29.4a). Microscopically, colloid carcinoma is predominantly composed of pools of extracellular mucin with few strips of neoplastic epithelium (Fig. 29.4b). Pools of mucin infiltrate and dissect through the stroma. Mucin-producing neoplastic epithelial cells are usually well differentiated. Strips of the cells may float freely in or partially line the pools. Signet ring cells are frequently present in the mucin pool. Careful examination of the specimens always reveals associated IPMN. A minor component of conventional duct adenocarcinoma may be

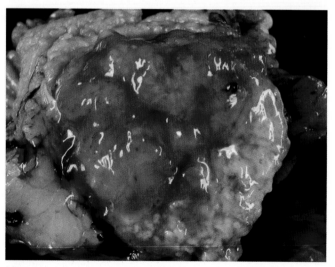

(a)

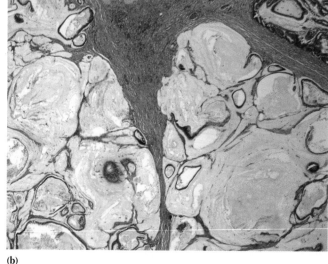

(b)

Figure 29.4 (a) Grossly, colloid carcinoma presents as a well-circumscribed mass with a soft gelatinous appearance. (b) Microscopically, there are pools of mucin associated with strips of neoplastic epithelium dissecting the stroma.

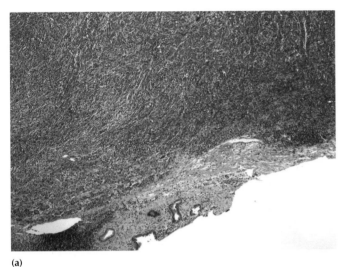

(a)

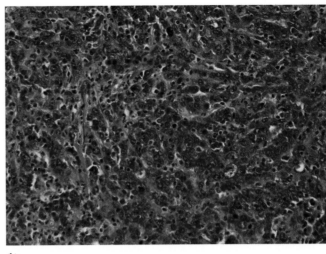

(b)

Figure 29.5 Medullary carcinoma is a poorly differentiated carcinoma with a pushing border (a) and prominent intratumoral lymphocytes (b).

present. However, at least 80% of the neoplasm should be colloid component.[47] Unlike conventional ductal adenocarcinoma which expresses MUC1 and is negative for CDX2, colloid carcinoma strongly expresses MUC2 and CDX2, indicating intestinal differentiation.[44]

As mentioned earlier, the historical 5-year survival rate for IPMN with an invasive component is 30–50% with more recent articles suggesting a rate as high as 68%. The latter may reflect increased recognition of IPMNs and/or more aggressive surgical management.[13,34] However, these figures likely include minimally invasive IPMN, colloid carcinoma and early forms of pancreatic ductal adenocarcinoma. A study that focused on only colloid carcinoma suggested a 5-year survival rate of 57%.[47]

Treatment data for colloid carcinoma are lacking. The majority of cases appear to remain localized with only ~30% presenting with metastases to lymph nodes and beyond.[35] For localized disease, the treatment of choice is surgery. In the face of limited efficacy data, standard chemotherapy regimens for pancreatic ductal adenocarcinoma are appropriate alternatives for unresectable disease; radiation may be considered as part of the therapy of localized, unresectable colloid carcinoma.

Medullary carcinoma

Medullary carcinoma is a more recently described variant of pancreatic carcinoma. In one analysis of 18 patients, 67% were male and all but one were Caucasian.[48] Age ranged from 33 to 85 years with a median of 69. A significant number of cancers were identified in other family members of patients with medullary pancreatic cancers. In fact, only one of the 18 patients had no family history of cancers while four others had unknown histories. Five-year survival for this cohort was 13%.

Medullary carcinoma of the pancreas is morphologically and genetically very similar to its counterpart in the colon. Grossly, medullary carcinomas are well circumscribed with a soft consistency. Microscopically, they have pushing rather than infiltrating borders. Dense lymphocytic infiltrates and/or

lymphoid aggregates may be observed in the peripheral area (Fig. 29.5a). Prominent intratumoral lymphocytes may also be seen in some cases. Medullary carcinomas are frequently poorly differentiated with a syncytial growth pattern (Fig. 29.5b). Immunohistochemical studies may show loss of expression of mismatch repair genes.[49] An evaluation of 18 patients with medullary carcinoma demonstrated that the majority (67%) had wild-type Ras tumors and a significant portion (22%) had microsatellite instability, including a case with hereditary nonpolyposis colorectal cancer.[48] Subsequently, a case report identified another medullary pancreatic carcinoma in a patient with hereditary nonpolyposis colorectal cancer (HNPCC) and MSH2 mutation.[50]

As with other rare tumors, there are no data on treatment. Surgical resection is recommended when able to be performed. Single-agent fluoropyrimidines may be considered, if these tumors behave like HNPCC-associated colorectal cancers.

Hepatoid carcinoma

Hepatoid carcinoma is extremely rare. It occurs in a variety of locations and is characterized by varying degrees of hepatic differentiation. There are only about 12 case reports of pancreatic hepatoid carcinoma but when reviewed, the majority of these stained for α-fetoprotein (AFP) and many had elevated serum levels of AFP.[51] However, little else is really known. In one case report, sorafenib was attempted as therapy for this disease; it would be as reasonable to treat this similarly to hepatocellular carcinoma as it is to try proven therapies for standard pancreatic cancer.

Undifferentiated carcinoma

Undifferentiated carcinoma of the pancreas is an aggressive variant of pancreatic carcinoma with no definable direction of differentiation. Grossly, it is similar to classic ductal adenocarcinoma with infiltrating borders. Microscopically, the neoplastic cells can have anything from an epithelioid appearance to a spindle cell appearance, and frequently infiltrate as individual

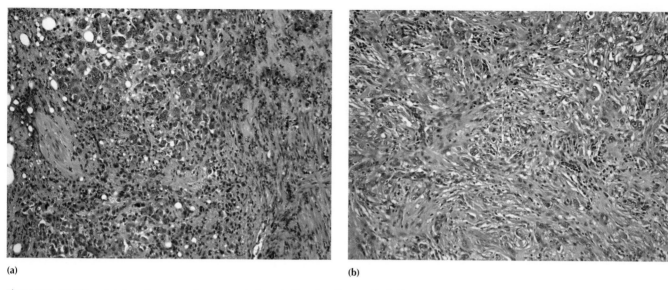

(a)   **(b)**

Figure 29.6 Undifferentiated carcinoma may be composed of neoplastic cells with an epithelioid appearance(a) or a spindle cell appearance (b).

cells (Fig. 29.6). Mitosis and necrosis are the prominent features of undifferentiated carcinoma. A minor component of conventional ductal adenocarcinoma may be present.

Undifferentiated carcinoma with osteoclast-like giant cells

Undifferentiated carcinomas with osteoclast-like giant cells are a variant of undifferentiated carcinoma with reactive osteoclast-like giant cells. Grossly, they tend to be soft and hemorrhagic. Microscopically, they are mainly composed of two groups of cells: large, reactive multinucleated osteoclast-like giant cells with multiple uniform small nuclei and atypical mononuclear cells with single large pleomorphic nuclei. Classic ductal adenocarcinoma or mucinous cystic neoplasm can be focally present. The presence of *KRAS2* mutations in the neoplastic cells establishes the ductal origin of this neoplasm.

Acinar cell carcinoma

Acinar cell carcinoma represents 1–2% of pancreatic cancers.[8,52,53] These lesions tend to be large (up to 15 cm) upon presentation. In a review of the Surveillance, Epidemiology, and End Results (SEER) database, of 672 patients with acinar cell carcinoma over 53% were male, while the majority with adenocarcinoma were female.[53] The average age at presentation is much younger than for pancreatic adenocarcinoma (70.2 versus 56.7 years, *p* <0.0001). These patients were more likely to present either unstaged or with localized disease and were far more likely to have resection (38.7% versus 11.0%, *p* <0.0001) than patients with adenocarcinoma. Location of the primary also differed, with head and body/tail occurring in 28% and 42% of cases of acinar cell respectively but 77% and 12% of cases of adenocarcinoma.

Common clinical presentations (generally listed as occurring >20% of the time) include pain (usually listed in >60% of patients), weight loss, anorexia, jaundice, and nausea/vomiting.[54–58] However, acinar cell carcinoma has been associated with two unique situations: a syndrome of panniculitis,

polyarthritis and pancreatic disease, and presentation without a primary lesion. Several decades ago, a syndrome including malaise, eosinophilia, nodular skin lesions, and polyarthritis was described in association with pancreatic disease including neoplasm.[59–62] The panniculitis comes with fat necrosis and has been observed to regress with treatment of the underlying pancreatic disease.[62] The skin lesions can be mistaken for erythema nodosum, initially presenting on the lower extremities but then they tend to become more widespread which is not typical for erythema nodosum.[59–61] The arthritis or synovitis has been described in both small and large joints without significant swelling, erythema or warmth in affected joints. Eosinophilia of up to 21% has been reported in this syndrome.[60] Elevated lipase was associated with this syndrome in at least one patient.[61] The other syndrome is one of presenting without an obvious pancreatic primary. In one small series of three patients, all had nodal disease, while liver and colon were also involved.[63] A paraneoplastic syndrome with thrombotic non-bacterial endocarditis has also been reported in association with acinar cell carcinoma.[54]

Diagnostic evaluation can include CA 19-9 and CEA, both of which have been reported to be elevated in some cases.[54,64] Imaging has been described in a few series. CT demonstrates a large, exophytic lesion with a cystic or necrotic component in 53% of cases and an enhancing capsule in 53% of cases.[64] In one study, ultrasound showed a heterogeneous, hyperechoic mass and MRI showed hypervascular lesions in the majority of cases.[58]

Acinar cell carcinoma is characterized by exocrine enzyme production by the neoplastic cells. Acinar cell carcinomas tend to present as a large, well-circumscribed mass. The cut surface is typically soft, fleshy, and focally necrotic and hemorrhagic. Unlike ductal adenocarcinoma, acinar cell carcinomas feature high neoplastic cellularity and a paucity of fibrous stroma. The neoplastic cells have abundant eosinophilic and granular cytoplasm, and are generally arranged in acinar or solid patterns (Fig. 29.7). The nuclei in acinar cell carcinomas are relatively uniform with prominent nucleoli. Mitosis is frequent. Immunohistochemical studies demonstrate that the neoplastic cells produce exocrine enzymes including trypsin, chymotrypsin,

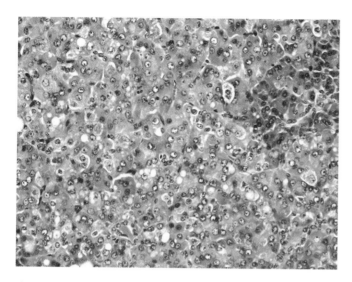

Figure 29.7 Neoplastic cells in acinar cell carcinoma have abundant eosinophilic cytoplasm and prominent nucleoli. Note: cells with dark eosinophilic cytoplasm (*upper right*) are benign acinar cells.

and lipase. On electron microscopy, the cytoplasm contains abundant rough endoplasmic reticulum, numerous mitochondria and, usually, electron-dense zymogen granules.[54] Although ductal components are seen in acinar cell carcinoma, there is also an entity of mixed acinar and neuroendocrine tumor.[56]

Mixed acinar-neuroendocrine carcinoma exhibits both acinar cell and neuroendocrine differentiation. However, the acinar cell component is always predominant. Most mixed acinar-neuroendocrine carcinomas are grossly solid, well circumscribed with a fleshy consistency. Microscopically, two cell types may be recognizable: cells with neuroendocrine differentiation with salt and pepper chromatin and cells with acinar cell differentiation with granular eosinophilic cytoplasm and prominent nucleoli (Fig. 29.8). Immunohistochemical labeling shows regions with acinar cell differentiation (trypsin, chymotrypsin, and lipase) and neuroendocrine differentiation (chromogranin and synaptophysin). Occasionally, the neoplastic cells demonstrate both acinar cell and neuroendocrine differentiation.

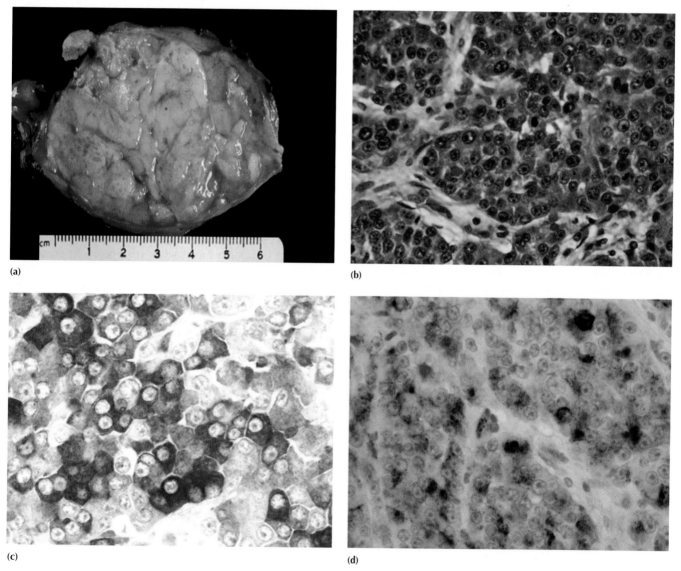

(a)   (b)   (c)   (d)

Figure 29.8 (a) Grossly, mixed acinar-neuroendocrine carcinomas present as a large, well-circumscribed mass with a fleshy consistency. (b) Microscopically, there are neoplastic cells with D-PAS positive granules in cytoplasm and prominent nucleoli and (c) labeled with chymotrypsin, and (d) neoplastic cells labeled with chromogranin.

Table 29.1 Comparison of survivals for acinar cell and adenocarcinoma of the pancreas from SEER data.

	Acinar cell*			Adenocarcinoma		
	Overall	Resected	Unresected	Overall	Resected	Unresected
Median survival	47 months	123 months	25 months	4 months	15 months	3 months
1 year survival	78.5%	92.3%	69%	19.8%	57.3%	16%
2 year survival	67.0%	88.2%	52%	8.2%	33.6%	6%
5 year survival	42.8%	71.6%	22%	3.8%	16.3%	2%

*p <0.0001 for differences in survival in every category.

Acinar cell carcinoma cytogenetics has been evaluated. Mutations in *KRAS* have not really been seen.[65,66] Additionally, *p53* mutations, loss of *DPC4* and mutations in *LKB1* are rare.[66,67] However, in one study of five patients, amplifications of chromosomes 20q and 19p occurred in 100% and 80% of cases respectively, and 80% had hypermethylation of at least one tumor suppressor gene.[66] An analysis of acinar cell carcinoma patients looking for changes in the APC/β-catenin pathway found alterations in 23.5% of cases.[67] The most common alteration found was allelic loss of 11p in 50% of analyzable cases. One patient with microsatellite instability-high phenotype had medullary features.

Acinar cell carcinoma is more indolent than adenocarcinoma. In the SEER database, overall median survival was much better for both resectable and unresectable acinar cell carcinoma (Table 29.1).[53] Surgery remains the treatment of choice when possible. Aggressive approaches including resecting patients with regional lymph nodes and limited metastatic disease have been undertaken and results were promising, although some of this may be due to the indolent nature of this disease.[55] A multimodality approach has been recommended for advanced disease.[55,58] The treatment of metastatic disease usually parallels that for metastatic adenocarcinoma of the pancreas, though reports have noted little effect from radiation or chemotherapy.[57] However, with mixed acinar and endocrine carcinoma, treatment of the endocrine component should be considered, especially in cases where the endocrine component is high grade, requiring a platinum-based regimen similar to small cell carcinoma.

Pancreatoblastoma

Pancreatoblastoma is a very uncommon pancreatic malignancy, representing less than 1% of pancreatic cancers.[51] It presents in a very young population, with an age range of 15 months to 13 years in one series.[68,69] Common presentations include abdominal mass and discomfort. Vomiting, jaundice, and weight loss have also been reported in more recent series.[69] The primary lesions are distributed throughout the pancreas without a predominant location. The majority of tumors were large (>5 cm) in 85% of cases and metastatic in 45% of patients. AFP was significantly elevated in 70% of patients. Imaging, including CT and MRI, shows large, heterogeneous masses with calcifications.[70]

Pancreatoblastomas are mostly solid, well-circumscribed, lobulated masses present in the head or tail of the pancreas. They tend to be large with an average size of 10.6 cm. They can be soft and fleshy or firm and fibrotic, depending on the proportion of stromal component. Microscopically, they are mainly composed of three cell types: cells with acinar differentiation, squamoid nests, and cells with neuroendocrine differentiation. A distinct ductal component may be seen in some cases. The neoplastic cells grow in a nested or organoid pattern separated by a relatively acellular stroma. Occasionally, focal osseous and cartilaginous differentiation may be seen in the stroma.

Immunohistochemically, acinar component labels with trypsin, chymotrypsin, and lipase, the neuroendocrine component with chromogranin and synpatophysin. The squamoid component usually does not express these markers.

Pancreatoblastoma is occasionally associated with Beckwith–Wiedemann syndrome and has been reported at least once in a patient with familial adenomatous polyposis.[67,69] In an assessment of nine cases of pancreatoblastoma, allelic chromosome loss of 11p was the most common finding.[67] Alterations of p53 and kRas were not observed and DPC4 loss occurred in two of seven cases. In contrast, five of nine patients had activating mutations in the β-catenin oncogene and seven showed accumulation of the β-catenin protein.

Standard therapy is multimodal, including chemotherapy, radiation therapy, and surgery. Neoadjuvant therapy is commonly used for stages II–IV. Surgery is the definitive therapy for this disease. Chemotherapy regimens used have multiple cytotoxic agents including dacarbazine, vincristine, cisplatin, gemcitabine, ifosfamide, cyclophosphamide, and/or doxorubicin, although there is no single standard regimen. In one series, this type of aggressive approach to therapy resulted in 5-year event-free survival of 58.8% and 5-year overall survival of 79.4%.[69]

Solid-pseudopapillary neoplasm

Solid-pseudopapillary neoplasm is a low-grade malignant epithelial neoplasm of the pancreas with unknown direction of differentiation. Grossly, solid-pseudopapillary neoplasms are well demarcated, solid and cystic masses with a soft consistency (Fig. 29.9). Recent or remote hemorrhage is common. Microscopically, the tumor is composed of sheets of relatively uniform polygonal cells admixed with delicate capillary-sized vessels. The neoplastic cells away from the vessels become loosely cohesive, thereby forming pseudopapillary structures (see Fig. 29.9). The nuclei of the neoplastic cells are round to oval with frequent longitudinal nuclear grooves. Prominent extracellular eosinophilic hyaline globules are often present. Immunohistochemically, solid-pseudopaillary neoplasms express α1-antitrypsin, CD10, progesterone receptors, and

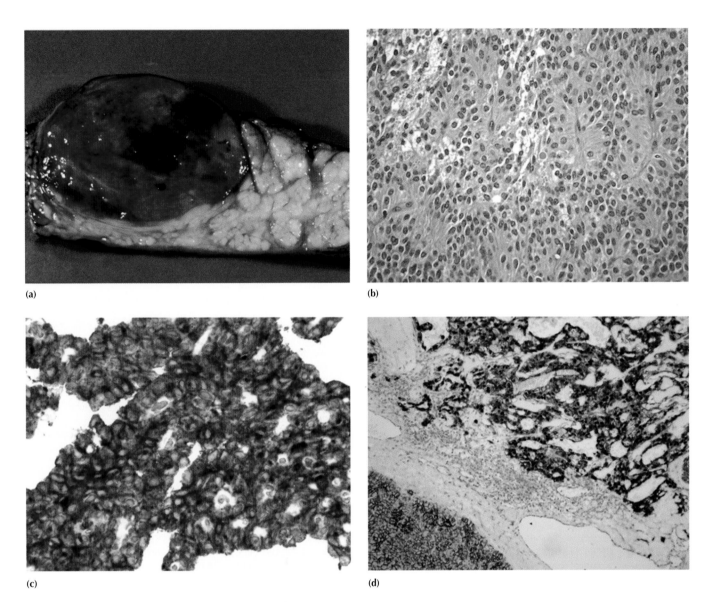

(a)

(b)

(c)

(d)

Figure 29.9 (a) Grossly, solid-pseudopapillary tumor is well circumscribed, with cystic and hemorrhagic areas on the cut surface. (b) Microscopically, it is composed of sheets of relatively uniform polygonal cells admixed with delicate capillary-sized vessels. Extracellular hyaline globes are common.

(c) Immunohistochemistry shows membranous labeling for CD10 and (d) nuclear labeling for β-catenin in the neoplastic cells. Note: predominantly membranous labeling for β-catenin in the bengin acinar cells (*left lower corner*).

synaptophysin. In contrast to pancreatic neuroectodermal tumors, solid-pseudopapillary neoplasms do not express chromogranin. In addition, almost all solid-pseudopapillary neoplasms have somatic mutations in β-catenin genes. Immunohistochemical labeling shows nuclear accumulation of β-catenin in the neoplastic cells.

Conclusion

Rare, nonendocrine tumors of the pancreas are heterogeneous in origin, presentation, and prognosis. Many of these rare tumors can be difficult to diagnose on histology alone and special immunohistochemistry or consultation with specialty centers may be crucial in confirming these rare disorders. These tumors are largely treated similarly to adenocarcinoma of the pancreas, though many have unqiue features that may

suggest other therapies, such as treating hepatoid carcinoma like hepatocellular cancer.

References

1. Siegel R, Ward E, Brawley O, Jemal A. Cancer statistics, 2011: the impact of eliminating socioeconomic and racial disparities on premature cancer deaths. CA Cancer J Clin 2011; 61(4): 212–36.
2. Tran Cao HS, Kellogg B, Lowy AM, Bouvet M. Cystic neoplasms of the pancreas. Surg Oncol Clin North Am 2010; 19(2): 267–95.
3. Sakorafas GH, Sarr MG. Cystic neoplasms of the pancreas; what a clinician should know. Cancer Treat Rev 2005; 31(7): 507–35.
4. Lai EC, Lau WY. Diagnosis and management strategy for cystic neoplasm of the pancreas. Int J Surg 2009; 7(1): 7–11.
5. Brugge WR, Lewandrowski K, Lee-Lewandrowski E, *et al*. Diagnosis of pancreatic cystic neoplasms: a report of the Cooperative Pancreatic Cyst Study. Gastroenterology 2004; 126(5): 1330–6.

6. Brugge WR. The use of EUS to diagnose cystic neoplasms of the pancreas. Gastrointest Endosc 2009; 69(2 Suppl): S203–9.

7. Linder JD, Geenen JE, Catalano MF. Cyst fluid analysis obtained by EUS-guided FNA in the evaluation of discrete cystic neoplasms of the pancreas: a prospective single-center experience. Gastrointest Endosc 2006; 64(5): 697–702.

8. Morohoshi T, Held G, Kloppel G. Exocrine pancreatic tumours and their histological classification. A study based on 167 autopsy and 97 surgical cases. Histopathology. 1983; 7(5): 645–61.

9. Galanis C, Zamani A, Cameron JL, et al. Resected serous cystic neoplasms of the pancreas: a review of 158 patients with recommendations for treatment. J Gastrointest Surg 2007; 11(7): 820–6.

10. Tseng JF, Warshaw AL, Sahani DV, Lauwers GY, Rattner DW, Fernandez-del Castillo C. Serous cystadenoma of the pancreas: tumor growth rates and recommendations for treatment. Ann Surg 2005; 242(3): 413–19; discussion 19–21.

11. Hodgkinson DJ, ReMine WH, Weiland LH. A clinicopathologic study of 21 cases of pancreatic cystadenocarcinoma. Ann Surg 1978; 188(5): 679–84.

12. Hruban RH, Pitman MB, Klimstra DS (eds). *AFIP Atlas of Tumor Pathology*. Washington, DC: Armed Forces Institute of Pathology, 2007.

13. Sakorafas GH, Smyrniotis V, Reid-Lombardo KM, Sarr MG. Primary pancreatic cystic neoplasms of the pancreas revisited. Part IV: Rare cystic neoplasms. Surg Oncol 2011: Aug 2 [Epub ahead of print].

14. Katz MH, Mortenson MM, Wang H, et al. Diagnosis and management of cystic neoplasms of the pancreas: an evidence-based approach. J Am Coll Surg 2008; 207(1): 106–20.

15. Le Borgne J, de Calan L, Partensky C. Cystadenomas and cystadenocarcinomas of the pancreas: a multiinstitutional retrospective study of 398 cases. French Surgical Association. Ann Surg 1999; 230(2): 152–61.

16. Zamboni G, Scarpa A, Bogina G. Mucinous cystic tumors of the pancreas: clinopathological features, prognosis, and relationship to other mucinous cystic tumors. Am J Surg Pathol 1999; 23: 410–22.

17. Sarr MG, Carpenter HA, Prabhakar LP, et al. Clinical and pathologic correlation of 84 mucinous cystic neoplasms of the pancreas: can one reliably differentiate benign from malignant (or premalignant) neoplasms? Ann Surg 2000; 231(2): 205–12.

18. Jeurnink SM, Vleggar FP, Siersema PD. Overview of the clinical problem: facts and current issues of mucinous cystic neoplasms of the pancreas. Digest Liver Dis 2008; 40: 837–46.

19. Wilentz RE, Albores-Saavedra J, Zahurak M, et al. Pathologic examination accurately predicts prognosis in mucinous cystic neoplasms of the pancreas. Am J Surg Pathol 1999; 23(11): 1320–7.

20. Wilentz RE, Albores-Saavedra J, Hruban RH. Mucinous cystic neoplasms of the pancreas. Semin Diagnost Pathol 2000; 17(1): 31–42.

21. Crippa S, Salvia R, Warshaw AL. Mucinous cystic neoplasms of the pancreas is not an aggressive entity: lessons from 163 resected patients. Ann Surg 2008; 247: 571–9.

22. Goh B, Tan YM, Chung YF, et al. A review of mucinous cystic neoplasms of the pancreas defined by ovarian-type stoma: clinicopathological features of 344 patients. World J Surg 2006; 30: 2236–45.

23. Warren KW, Hardy KJ. Cystadenocarcinoma of the pancreas. Surg Gynecol Obstet 1968; 127(4): 734–6.

24. Hodgkinson DJ, ReMine WH, Weiland LH. A clinicopathologic study of 21 cases of pancreatic cystadenocarcinoma. Ann Surg 1978; 188: 679–84.

25. Grutzmann R, Niedergethmann M, Pilarsky C. Intraductal papillary mucinonous tumors of the pancreas: biology, diagnosis, and treatment. Oncologist 2010; 15: 1294–309.

26. Rebours V, Couvelard A, Peyroux JL, et al. Familial intraductal papillary mucinous neoplasms of the pancreas. Dig Liver Dis 2011; Aug 6 [Epub ahead of print].

27. Gaujoux S, Tissier F, Ragazzon B, et al. Pancreatic ductal and acinar cell neoplasms in Carney complex: a possible new association. J Clin Endocrinol Metab 2011; 96(11): E1888–95.

28. Maguchi H, Tanno S, Mizuno N, et al. Natural history of branch duct intrapapillary mucinous neoplasms of the pancreas. Pancreas 2011; 40: 364–70.

29. Takuma K, Kamisawa T, Anjiki H, et al. Predictors of malignancy and natural histoy of main-duct intrapapillary mucinos neoplasms of the pancreas. Pancreas 2011; 40: 371–5.

30. Nakajima Y, Yamada T, Sho M. Malignant potential of intraductal papillary mucionous neoplasms of the pancreas. Surg Today 2010; 40: 816–24.

31. Xiao HD, Yamaguchi H, Dias-Santagata D, et al. Molecular characteristics and biological behaviours of the oncocytic and pancreatiobiliary subtypes of intraductal papillary mucinous neoplasms. J Pathol 2011; 222: 508–16.

32. Tanaka M, Chari S, Adsay V, et al. International consensus guidelines for management of intraductal papillary mucinous neoplasms and mucinous cystic neoplasms of the pancreas. Pancreatology 2006; 6(1–2): 17–32.

33. Zhong N, Zhang L, Takahashi N, et al. Histologic and imaging features of mural nodules in mucinous pancreatic cysts. Clin Gastroenterol Hepatol 2012; 10(2): 192–8.

34. Yopp AC, Katabi N, Janakos M, et al. Invasive carcinoma arising in intraductal papillary mucinous neoplasms of the pancreas: a matched control study with conventional pancreatic ductal adenocarcinoma. Ann Surg 2011; 253(5): 968–74.

35. Poultsides GA, Reddy S, Cameron JL, et al. Histopathologic basis for the favorable survival after resection of intraductal papillary mucinous neoplasm-associated invasive adenocarcinoma of the pancreas. Ann Surg 2010; 251(3): 470–6.

36. Woo SM, Ryu JK, Lee SH, et al. Survival and prognosis of invasive intraductal papillary mucinous neoplasms of the pancreas: comparison with pancreatic ductal adenocarcinoma. Pancreas 2008; 36(1): 50–5.

37. Fitzgerald TL, Hickner ZJ, Schmitz M, Kort EJ. Changing incidence of pancreatic neoplasms: a 16-year review of statewide tumor registry. Pancreas 2008; 37(2): 134–8.

38. Baylor SM, Berg JW. Cross-classification and survival characteristics of 5,000 cases of cancer of the pancreas. J Surg Oncol 1973; 5(4): 335–58.

39. Kardon DE, Thompson LD, Przygodzki RM, Heffess CS. Adenosquamous carcinoma of the pancreas: a clinicopathologic series of 25 cases. Mod Pathol 2001; 14(5): 443–51.

40. Ishikawa O, Matsui Y, Aoki I, Iwanaga T, Terasawa T, Wada A. Adenosquamous carcinoma of the pancreas: a clinicopathologic study and report of three cases. Cancer 1980; 46(5): 1192–6.

41. Voong KR, Davison J, Pawlik TM, et al. Resected pancreatic adenosquamous carcinoma: clinicopathologic review and evaluation of adjuvant chemotherapy and radiation in 38 patients. Human Pathol 2010; 41: 113–22.

42. Brody JR, Costantino CL, Potoczek M, et al. Adenosquamous carcinoma of the pancreas harbors KRAS2, DPC4 and TP53 molecular alterations similar to pancreatic ductal adenocarcinoma. Mod Pathol 2009; 22(5): 651–9.

43. Okabayashi T, Hanazaki K. Surgical outcome of adenosquamous carcinoma of the pancreas. World J Gastroenterol 2008; 14(44): 6765–70.

44. Adsay NV, Merati K, Basturk O, et al. Pathologically and biologically distinct types of epithelium in intraductal papillary mucinous neoplasms: delineation of an "intestinal" pathway of carcinogenesis in the pancreas. Am J Surg Pathol 2004; 28(7): 839–48.

45. Ren FY, Shao CW, Zuo CJ, Lu JP. CT features of colloid carcinomas of the pancreas. Chinese Med J 2010; 123(10): 1329–32.

46. Yoon MA, Lee JM, Kim SH, et al. MRI features of pancreatic colloid carcinoma. Am J Roentgenol 2009; 193(4): W308–13.

47. Adsay NV, Pierson C, Sarkar F, et al. Colloid (mucinous noncystic) carcinoma of the pancreas. Am J Surg Pathol 2001; 25(1): 26–42.

48. Wilentz RE, Goggins M, Redston M. Genetic, immunohisto-chemical and clinical features of medullary carcinoma of the pancreas. Am J Pathol 2000; 156: 1641–51.

49. Shi C, Hruban RH, Klein AP. Familial pancreatic cancer. Arch Pathol Lab Med 2009; 133(3): 365–74.

50. Banville N, Geraghty R, Fox E, et al. Medullary carcinoma of the pancreas in a man with herditary nonpolyposis colorectal cancer due to mutation of the MSH2 mismatch repair gene. Human Pathol 2006; 37: 1498–502.

51. Petrelli F, Ghilardi M, Colombo S, *et al*. A rare case of metastatic pancreatic hepatoid carcinoma treated with sorafenib. J Gastrointest Cancer 2012; 43(1): 97–102.

52. Cubilla AL, Fitzgerald PJ. Cancer of the pancreas (neuroendocrine): a suggested morphologic classification. Semin Oncol 1979; 6: 285–97.

53. Wisnoski NC, Townsend CM Jr, Nealon WH, Freeman JL, Riall TS. 672 patients with acinar cell carcinoma of the pancreas: a population-based comparison to pancreatic adenocarcinoma. Surgery 2008; 144(2): 141–8.

54. Webb JN. Acinar cell neoplasms of the exocrine pancreas. J Clin Pathol 1977; 30(2): 103–12.

55. Hartwig W, Danneberg M, Bergmann F, *et al*. Acinar cell carcinoma of the pancreas: is resection justified even in limited metastatic disease? Am J Surg 2011; 202: 23–7.

56. Stelow EB, Shaco-Levy R, Bao F, Garcia J, Klimstra DS. Pancreatic acinar cell carcinomas with prominent ductal differentiation: mixed acinar ductal carcinoma and mixed acinar endocrine ductal carcinoma. Am J Surg Pathol. 2010; 34(4): 510–18.

57. Mansfield A, Tafur A, Smithedajkul P, Corsini M, Quevedo F, Miller R. Mayo Clinic experience with very rare exocrine pancreatic neoplasms. Pancreas 2010; 39(7): 972–5.

58. Butturini G, Pisano M, Scarpa A, d'Onofrio M, Auriemma A, Bassi C. Aggressive approach to acinar cell carcinoma of the pancreas: a single-institution experience and a literature review. Langenbeck Arch Surg/ Deutsche Gesellsch Chirurg 2011; 396(3): 363–9.

59. MacMahon HE, Brown PA, Shen EM. Acinar cell carcinoma of the pancreas with subcutaneous fat necrosis. Gastroenterology 1965; 49(5): 555–9.

60. Mullin GT, Erskine MC, Crespin SR, Williams RC. Arthritis and skin lesion resembling erythema nodosum in pancreatic disease. Ann Intern Med 1968; 68: 76–87.

61. Burns WA, Matthews MJ, Hamosh M, Weide GV, Blum R, Johnson FB. Lipase-secreting acinar cell carcinoma of the pancreas with polyarthropathy. A light and electron microscopic, histochemical, and biochemical study. Cancer 1974; 33(4): 1002–9.

62. Moro M, Moletta L, Blandamura S, Sperti C. Acinar cell carcinoma of the pancreas associated with subcutaneous panniculitis. JOP 2011; 12(3): 292–6.

63. Terris B, Genevay M, Rouquette A, *et al*. Acinar cell carcinoma: a possible diagnosis in patients without intrapancreatic tumour. Dig Liver Dis 2011; 43(12): 971–4.

64. Raman SP, Hruban RH, Cameron JL, Wolfgang CL, Kawamoto S, Fishman EK. Acinar cell carcinoma of the pancreas: computed tomography features – a study of 15 patients. Abdom Imaging 2012; Feb 18 [Epub ahead of print].

65. Ohori NP, Khalid A, Etemad B, Finkelstein SD. Multiple loss of heterozygosity without K-ras mutation identified by molecular analysis on fine-needle aspiration cytology specimen of acinar cell carcinoma of pancreas. Diagnost Cytopathol 2002; 27(1): 42–6.

66. De Wilde RF, Ottenhoff NA, Jansen M, *et al*. Analysis of LKB1 mutations and other molecular alterations in pancreatic acinar cell carcinmona. Mod Pathol 2011; 24: 1229–36.

67. Abraham SC, Wu TT, Hruban RH, *et al*. Genetic and immunohistochemical analysis of pancreatic acinar cell carcinoma: frequent allelic loss on chromosome 11p and alterations in the APC/beta-catenin pathway. Am J Pathol 2002; 160(3): 953–62.

68. Buchino JJ, Castello FM, Nagaraj HS. Pancreatoblastoma. A histochemical and ultrastructural analysis. Cancer 1984; 53(4): 963–9.

69. Bien E, Godzinski J, Dall'igna P, *et al*. Pancreatoblastoma: a report from the European Cooperative Study Group for Paediatric Rare Tumours (EXPeRT). Eur J Cancer 2011; 47(15): 2347–52.

70. Yang X, Wang X. Imaging findings of pancreatoblastoma in 4 children including a case of ectopic pancreatoblastoma. Pediatr Radiol 2010; 40(10): 1609–14.

Section 6: Gastrointestinal Tumors

30 Uncommon Hepatobiliary Tumors

Abby B. Siegel,[1] Vladimir Sheynzon,[2] and Benjamin Samstein[3]

[1] Department of Medicine, [2] Clinical Radiology, [3] Department of Surgery, Columbia University Medical Center, New York, NY, USA

Introduction

This chapter reviews uncommon gallbladder, bile duct, and liver malignant tumors. A diagram showing anatomy of the liver, gallbladder, and biliary system is shown in Figure 30.1. In general, these tumors may be curable if recognized early. Advanced disease remains challenging, although progress has been made with novel, often multidisciplinary, treatment regimens. This chapter includes a final section on supportive care, which is applicable to most of the tumors described below.

Gallbladder tumors

Epidemiology and risk factors

There are about 6000 new cases of gallbladder cancers per year in the United States.[1,2] Incidence rates are highest worldwide (approximately 10–20/100,000) in northern India, where salmonella and chronic typhoid lead to bacterial infection of the bile.[3,4] Rates are also high in areas with high numbers of indigenous Indian populations, like Chile, Ecuador, and New Mexico. In these regions, gallbladder cancer risk is thought to be primarily due to gallstones.[5] Women are about three times as likely to develop gallbladder cancer as men.[6–8] Other risk factors include obesity, choledochal cysts, and anomalous pancreaticobiliary junctions. The latter seem to be more prevalent in Japanese patients who may have increased pancreatic secretions refluxing into the biliary tract, causing epithelial hyperplasia and then dysplasia.[9–11]

Pathology

Over 90% of gallbladder cancers are adenocarcinomas. Less common epithelial subtypes include squamous and adenosquamous variants, papillary, mucinous, signet ring, clear cell, and carcinosarcoma subtypes.[12] In addition, many nonepithelial subtypes have been reported, including melanomas, neuroendocrine tumors, mesenchymal tumors, and lymphomas.

Pathogenesis

In contrast to many other malignancies, transformation from adenoma to carcinoma is thought to be rare in epithelial gallbladder cancers.[13] A sequence of carcinogenesis has been identified for some patients with cholelithiasis, with flat epithelial changes leading to dysplasia, then carcinoma *in situ*, and finally frank malignancy (Fig. 30.2). In a study from Chile where specimens with dysplasia, less advanced, and more advanced carcinomas were examined, the time course from the development of dysplasia to advanced cancer was estimated to be about 15 years.[14]

Oncogenic p53 mutations are a common early change in patients with underlying gallstone-related inflammation, followed by mutations in *CDKN2A*. *KRAS* mutations are relatively rare, and when they occur, tend to appear later in

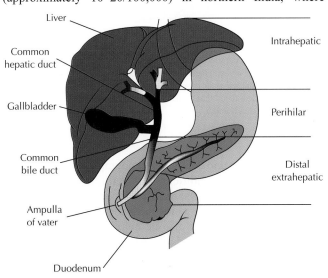

Figure 30.1 Biliary anatomy. Adapted from De Groen *et al.*, NEJM 1999 Oct 28; 341(18): 1368–78.

Liver
Common hepatic duct
Gallbladder
Common bile duct
Ampulla of vater
Duodenum
Intrahepatic
Perihilar
Distal extrahepatic

Textbook of Uncommon Cancer, Fourth Edition. Edited by Derek Raghavan, Charles D. Blanke, David H. Johnson, Paul L. Moots, Gregory H. Reaman, Peter G. Rose and Mikkael A. Sekeres.
© 2012 John Wiley & Sons, Inc. Published 2012 by John Wiley & Sons, Inc.

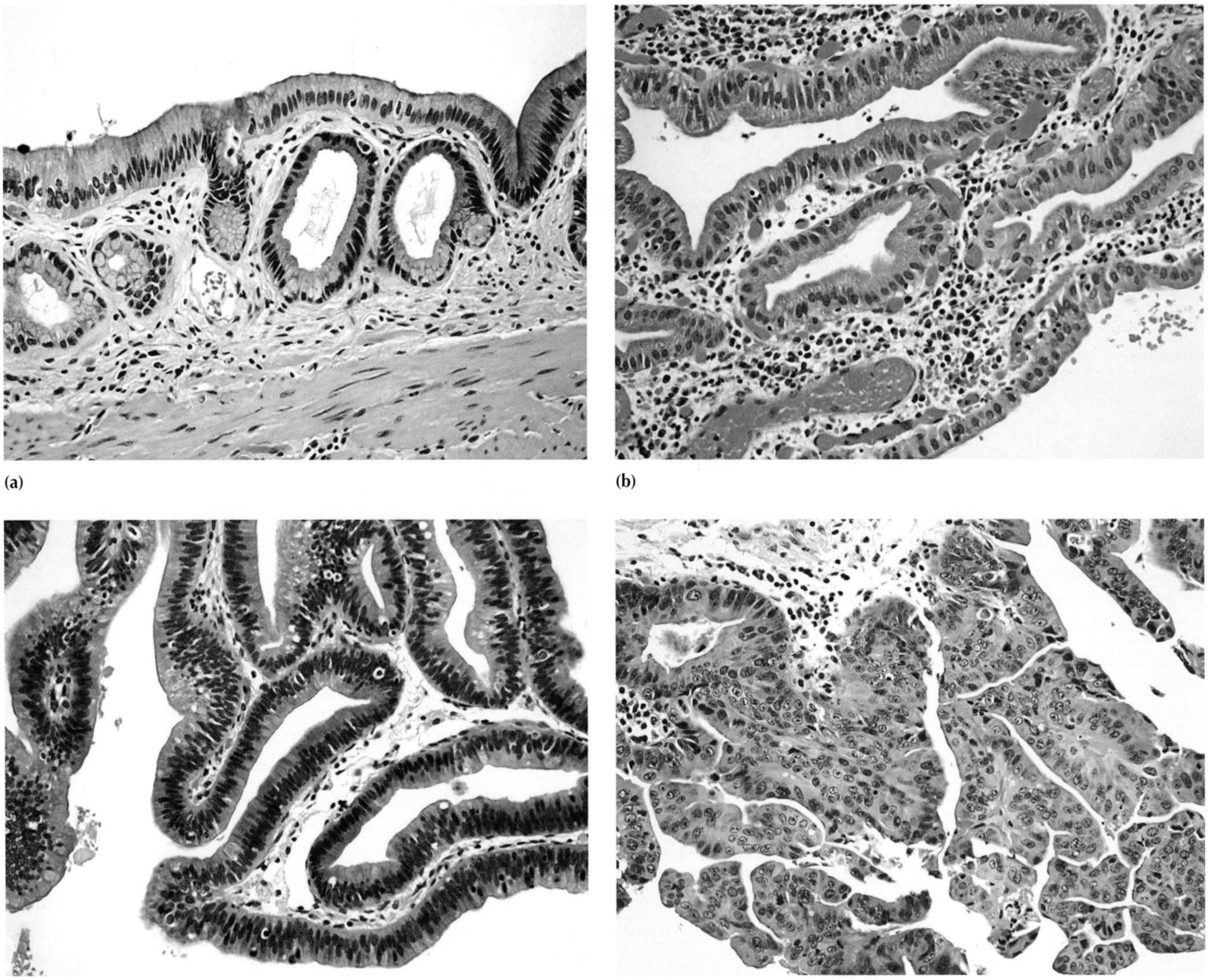

(a)

(b)

(c)

(d)

Figure 30.2 Spectrum of histological changes in the gallbladder epithelium in normal, reactive, and low- and high-grade dysplasia. (a) Normal gallbladder mucosa (×100). (b) Reactive gallbladder mucosa in chronic cholecystitis. (c) Gallbladder mucosa with low-grade dysplasia showing increased nuclear size, hyperchromasia, and nuclear stratification with general retained basal orientation of nuclei. (d) Gallbladder mucosa with high-grade dysplasia showing increased architectural complexity with haphazardly oriented nuclei that no longer show basal orientation. In high-grade dysplasia, cytological atypia is more marked, often with irregular nuclear membranes, enlarged vesicular nuclei, and distinct nucleoli. Courtesy of Dr Helen Remotti.

pathogenesis.[2] In contrast, *KRAS* mutations in codon 12 are more commonly seen as an early mutation in Japanese patients with anomalous pancreaticobiliary ducts.[15–17] Activating mutations cause resistance to drugs which target this pathway, so testing for these mutations will be a crucial component of ongoing trials in biliary malignancies using epidermal growth factor receptor (EGFR).

Clinical presentation and workup

Incidental findings at surgery account for most early-stage gallbladder cancers.[18] Computed tomography (CT) and magnetic resonance imaging (MRI) are superior to ultrasound for the detection of local liver extension and metastases.[19–21]

Positron emission and computed tomography (PET-CT) may add information to traditional CT with respect to nodal involvement and distant spread.[22] Endoscopic ultrasound is used at many centers to confirm depth of tumor invasion, and serum CA-19-9 may also be helpful in confirming the diagnosis. In one study of high-risk patients in Mexico and Bolivia, a CA-19-9 cutoff of 20 units/mL yielded a sensitivity and specificity of about 80% in diagnosing gallbladder cancer.[23] For patients with distant metastases, biopsy of the metastatic lesion (rather than the primary) is preferred to confirm the diagnosis and stage. Surgical consultation should be obtained if there is any question about resectability, since it is the only modality associated with long-term survival.

Epithelial tumors

Local disease

Approximately 1–2% of cholecystectomies for presumed benign gallbladder disease will yield malignancy. Treatment is guided by TNM staging, shown in Box 30.1.[24]

For T1a lesions, no additional surgery is recommended. Based on retrospective studies,[25,26] the current National Comprehensive Cancer Network (NCCN) guidelines recommend radical cholecystectomy for patients with stages Ib to IIIb gallbladder cancer.[27,28] Radical operation includes hepatic resection of liver segments IVb and V, and lymph node dissection of the hepatoduodenal ligament (Fig. 30.3). The cystic duct margin should be assessed, and if positive, a common bile duct resection with reconstructive hepaticojejunostomy should be performed. If patients need to return to the operating room for definitive surgery, it is helpful to know whether the gallbladder wall was perforated, and if the specimen was placed in a protective bag before removal to prevent tumor seeding.[29]

Adjuvant therapy

There are no definitive data to guide adjuvant treatment after resection of epithelial gallbladder cancer. The NCCN guidelines support either fluoropyrimidine-based chemoradiation or adjuvant chemotherapy alone with a fluoropyrimidine or gemcitabine.[28] In contrast to cholangiocarcinomas, gallbladder carcinomas are more likely to recur at distant sites (85% versus 41%),[30] suggesting that systemic therapy may be more effective than local therapy for gallbladder cancer. A small retrospective analysis from Korea showed improvements in disease-free survival (DFS) in 41 patients treated with chemotherapy, chemoradiotherapy, or radiotherapy alone. There was a suggestion that for patients with stage II disease, the chemotherapy alone group had better survivals.[31] Adjuvant chemoradiation (50.4 Gy with concurrent 5-fluorouracil) compared with no treatment was shown to be an independent prognostic factor in overall survival, and nomograms have been developed to predict who might benefit from such an approach.[32,33] Radiation alone as adjuvant therapy has also been studied, but with conflicting results.[34–36]

Advanced disease

Chemotherapy, local therapies, and palliative interventions are all possible components of management of patients with advanced gallbladder cancers. Chemotherapy will be discussed here, and local and palliative therapies in the cholangiocarcinoma section. Because most studies combine bile duct and gallbladder cancers, these sections are applicable to both types of tumors.

A new standard of care for advanced epithelial biliary cancers was established with the publication of randomized trial of 410 patients with gallbladder (37%), cholangiocarcinoma (58%), and ampullary cancers (5%). This study compared gemcitabine to gemcitabine and cisplatin.[37] The median overall survival in the combination group was 11.7 months, while in the gemcitabine alone arm it was 8.1 months ($p < 0.001$). Response rates for the combination were 26%, versus 16% in the gemcitabine alone arm ($p = 0.26$). Significantly higher rates of many expected cisplatin toxicities like alopecia or renal dysfunction were not seen and the number of neutropenic infections was similar.

Box 30.1 TNM staging of gallbladder cancer.

Primary tumor (T)

TX	Primary tumor cannot be assessed
T0	No evidence of primary tumor
Tis	Carcinoma *in situ*
T1	Tumor invades lamina propria or muscular layer
T1a	Tumor invades lamina propria
T1b	Tumor invades muscular layer
T2	Tumor invades perimuscular connective tissue; no extension beyond serosa or into liver
T3	Tumor perforates the serosa (visceral peritoneum) and/or directly invades the liver and/or one other adjacent organ or structure, such as the stomach, duodenum, colon, pancreas, omentum, or extrahepatic bile ducts
T4	Tumor invades main portal vein or hepatic artery or invades two or more extrahepatic organs or structures

Regional lymph nodes (N)

NX	Regional lymph nodes cannot be assessed
N0	No regional lymph node metastasis
N1	Metastases to nodes along the cystic duct, common bile duct, hepatic artery, and/or portal vein
N2	Metastases to periaortic, pericaval, superior mesenteric artery, and/or celiac artery lymph nodes

Distant metastasis (M)

M0	No distant metastasis
M1	Distant metastasis

Anatomical stage/prognostic groups			
Stage 0	Tis	N0	M0
Stage I	T1	N0	M0
Stage II	T2	N0	M0
Stage IIIA	T3	N0	M0
Stage IIIB	T1-3	N1	M0
Stage IVA	T4	N0-1	M0
Stage IVB	Any T	N2	M0
Any T	Any N	M1	

Note: cTNM is the clinical classification, pTNM is the pathological classification.

Reproduced from Edge *et al.*[24] Used with the permission of the American Joint Committee on Cancer (AJCC), Chicago, Illinois. The original source for this material is the AJCC Cancer Staging Manual, Seventh Edition (2010) published by Springer Science and Business Media LLC, www.springer.com.

Supporting the combination of a platin and gemcitabine is one of the few randomized studies specifically including patients with only gallbladder cancer.[38] Eighty-one patients were randomized to one of three arms from a single center in India: best supportive care (BSC), fluorouracil and folinic acid, or gemcitabine and oxaliplatin (G 900/m^2 and O 80 mg/m^2 IV day 1 and 8 q 3 weeks). Overall, complete or partial response rates in the three groups were 0%, 14.3%, and 30.7% respectively ($p = 0.03$), and overall survivals were 4.5 months, 4.6 months,

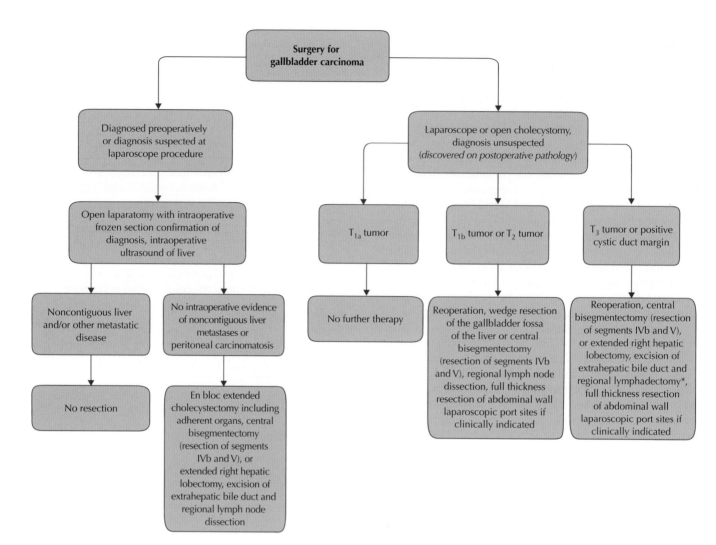

Figure 30.3 Algorithm for resectable gallbladder cancer. Reproduced with permission from Abbruzzese J, *et al.* (eds) *Gastrointestinal Oncology.* New York: Oxford University Press, 2004, p. 449.

and 9.5 months. The combination of capecitabine and gemcitabine yields response rates of 13–32%, and overall survivals of 7–14 months.[40-44] Other active chemotherapies include taxotere and irinotecan.[45-48] Few studies have been completed in the second-line setting but the oral fluoropyrimidene S-1 was studied in 22 Japanese patients refractory to gemcitabine, and a 22% response rate was seen.[49] Unfortunately, this agent is not yet available in the United States.

Targeted therapies are also undergoing broad evaluation in biliary cancers. Provocative results were seen in a phase 2 trial of cetuximab (500 mg/m² biweekly) with GEMOX. Objective responses were seen in 63% of patients, of whom 10% obtained a complete response, and 30% underwent resection after treatment; 90% of patients were wild-type for *KRAS*. Of the three with *KRAS* mutations, two had a partial response, and one had stable disease. A higher grade of skin rash was associated with a positive response to cetuximab therapy.[39] One intriguing report from France suggested that cetuximab could resensitize patients who had become resistant to GEMOX, similar to the resensitization seen in patients with colon cancer treated with cetuximab and irinotecan.[50,51]

In gastric and breast cancer, targeting the *HER-2/neu* pathway has led to significant improvements in survival.[52,53] Overexpression of *HER-2/neu* has been found in up to 20% of biliary cancers.[54] Studies are ongoing to evaluate this target by giving trastuzumab, a monoclonal antibody targeted against *HER-2*, to patients with advanced biliary cancers. Interestingly, a trial of lapatinib (a dual *HER-2* and EGFR tyrosine kinase inhibitor) showed no responses in patients with biliary cancers.[55] A MEK inhibitor, selumetinib, showed a promising 12% response rate in patients with biliary cancers.[56]

Angiogenic pathways also play a role in the pathogenesis of biliary cancers. Higher levels of expression of vascular endothelial growth factor (VEGF) in tissue of patients with extrahepatic biliary cancers predict a worse prognosis.[57] This has led to several trials examining both antibodies to VEGF ligand (bevacizumab) and small molecule tyrosine kinase inhibitors of VEGF receptor (VEGFR). A phase 2 trial of gemcitabine, oxaliplatin, and bevacizumab yielded a response rate of 40%, and overall survival of 12.7 months; 14.2 months for those with intrahepatic cholangiocarcinomas, and 8.5 months in patients with gallbladder cancer.[58]

Uncommon histologies: epithelial subtypes

Squamous and adenosquamous

Squamous cell (SCC) or adenosquamous (AC) cell features are seen in 5–10% of gallbladder malignancies.[12,59,60] Adenosquamous pathology typically is defined as having greater than 25% squamous differentiation.[60] Those without glandular features are labeled squamous and are characterized by keratinization and peritumoral eosinophils.[60] Those with squamous differentiation may be more likely to have nodal involvement, liver infiltration, and advanced-stage disease.[60–62] Nishihara and colleagues showed higher rates of staining for proliferating nuclear cell antigen in SCC components of mixed tumors compared with AC components, suggesting that SCC may have greater proliferative capacity.[63] Stage for stage, survival is usually worse for SCC than for adenocarcinomas, with median survivals in the 4–5-month range.[59,60,63] Treatments are similar for patients with other epithelial gallbladder cancers; surgery should be performed for localized disease.[62,64] These histologies were included in the large randomized trial of gemcitabine versus gemcitabine plus cisplatin for biliary cancers, so this chemotherapy combination is reasonable for patients with advanced disease.

Papillary

Papillary carcinomas account for 4–5% of gallbladder cancers, and tend to have a better prognosis than other histologies. Because they are often exophytic, they may cause obstructive symptoms earlier in the course of disease, leading to earlier diagnosis.[12,36,65,66] They are also often associated epidemiologically with an anomalous pancreaticobiliary junction.[67,68] They may be grouped into invasive (versus noninvasive) subtypes based on tumor size >1 cm, percentage of papillary architecture <80%, and infiltration into the gallbladder wall.[66] The expression of MK-1 antigen is more common in papillary gallbladder cancers, and predicts for a better prognosis.[66,69] For papillary carcinomas involving the biliary wall, patients had significantly better 10-year survival rates than those with other histologies (52%, versus 30%). For those with lymph node involvement, however, even those with papillary carcinoma had 10-year survival rates of only about 10%.[65,66] Factors prognostic for poorer outcomes include invasion of the duct wall and dedifferentiated pathology.[65] In general, papillary cancers should be treated like other gallbladder and biliary cancers.

Clear cell, mucinous, and signet ring carcinomas

Clear cell carcinomas are rare, and have epidemiology, workup, and treatment similar to adenocarcinomas.[70–73] Most are seen in women with underlying gallstones. The clear cells typically contain periodic acid-Schiff (PAS)-positive cytoplasmic granules, and patients may make α-fetoprotein (AFP) peripherally. They often are locally advanced on presentation, leading to a poor prognosis.[70,74] Primary tumors may be differentiated from metastatic renal cell cancers because primaries usually have pathological foci of adenocarcinoma or squamous cell carcinoma. Mucinous carcinomas are another rare variant, with just a few case reports in the literature without consistent epidemiological risk factors. Radiologically, mucinous gallbladder cancers often present with localized thickening along the wall of the gallbladder, with near water density on CT scan, and calcifications.[75] One report suggested an association with primary sclerosing cholangitis and ulcerative colitis in a 74-year-old woman.[71] Another report described an aggressive tumor with perineural and lymphovascular invasion in a 22-year-old African-American male with underlying hepatitis B and no gallstones.[76] Rokitansky–Aschoff sinuses, which are benign epithelial invaginations which extend down the gallbladder wall, can also contain extracellular mucin and may mimic mucinous carcinoma, sometimes leading to unnecessary surgery.[73] These subtypes should be worked up and treated like other epithelial gallbladder carcinomas. Signet ring carcinomas have only been reported in a few cases, and are notable for containing characteristic signet ring cells, often with intracellular mucin, which also stain positive with PAS stain.[72] They are always characterized pathologically as grade 3 tumors,[77] and have an aggressive phenotype.[72,78]

Carcinosarcomas

These tumors are characterized by both epithelial and mesenchymal components which are intermingled. The epithelial areas are typically made up of either adenocarcinoma or squamous cells. If the components do not intermingle, then the tumor is considered to be synchronous carcinoma and sarcoma, not a carcinosarcoma.[79] As with other gallbladder cancers, they most commonly present with right upper quadrant pain, and are worked up and treated like other epithelial variants.[80] Prognosis is thought to be worse than with other epithelial variants because of a high frequency of locally advanced disease, with mean survivals of typically a few months.[81–82]

Uncommon histologies: nonepithelial

Melanoma

Primary melanoma of the gallbladder has been reported, but is rare.[83] Melanoma is the most common malignancy to metastasize to the gallbladder, and about 15% of autopsy cases of melanoma involve the gallbladder. Because of this, evaluation of skin, eyes, and viscera is necessary to exclude a primary.[84] Differentiating primary from metastatic melanoma is difficult. Some have suggested that primary tumors display junctional activity, defined as the presence of pigmented dendritic cells at the junction of the epithelium and lamina propria, together with absence of other lesions.[85]

Melanoma of the gallbladder is thought to arise because of migration of melanin-producing cells from the neural crest to endodermal derivatives like the gallbladder.[86] The immunoperoxidase stain for S-100 is typically positive, as with most melanomas. The majority of patients with gallbladder melanoma present with cholecystitis, but fewer than 25% have associated gallstones.[83,86–87] Surgical evaluation is important for those with symptoms.[86,87] Marone and colleagues note that open surgery allows examination of the abdominal cavity, which often leads to the diagnosis of other metastatic lesions.[88] Prognosis is poor even after surgical resection of primary tumors.[86] It is not clear whether any adjuvant therapy improves prognosis. For those found to have metastatic disease, treatment should be similar to that for other metastatic melanomas, and testing undertaken for a V600 *BRAF* mutation. If this is present, patients may be offered vemurafenib[89]; ipilimumab and IL-2 may also be considered.[90]

Neuroendocrine tumors

Neuroendocrine tumors (NET) of the gallbladder account for about 2–3% of all gallbladder cancers, and fewer than 1% of neuroendocrine tumors.[18,91] These range in histology from very well-differentiated (WHO 1) to poorly differentiated tumors which act like small cell carcinomas (WHO 3). Biliary NETs tend to have a higher proportion of high-grade features compared with other sites in the gastrointestinal tract, leading to a generally poorer prognosis.[92] Most gallbladder neuroendocrine tumors are found in women, and occasionally are associated with genetic syndromes like von Hippel–Lindau and Zollinger–Ellison.[93,94]

Gallbladder and biliary neuroendocrine tumors usually are not functional,[92,95] and are typically identified after surgical resection. Tumors usually stain positive for neuroendocrine markers, including chromogranin and synaptophysin. For low- and intermediate-grade neuroendocrine tumors, staging should include octreotide scan, assessing serum chromogranin and urine 5-hydroxyindoleacetic acid (5-HIAA), and an echocardiogram to rule out right-sided valvular disease. Low-grade tumors are usually more indolent than adenocarcinomas, and there are no data to support adjuvant therapy for these tumors after resection. They typically have 5-year survivals in the range of 50%.[92,96] No guidelines exist for surveillance after surgery, so it is reasonable to follow the National Comprehensive Cancer Center (NCCC) recommendations established for pancreatic neuroendocrine tumors, including exam, serum markers, and scans at 3 months post surgery, then markers every 6 months for 3 years, then yearly.[28] Metastatic disease is discussed in more detail below in the section on primary hepatic neuroendocrine tumors. For poorly differentiated tumors, workup and treatment should mirror those for small cell cancers, including PET scan rather than octreotide scan, and imaging of the brain. Combinations of surgery together with chemotherapy used for pulmonary small cell cancers typically yield 5-year survivals of less than 10%.[92,97]

Mesenchymal tumors

About 2% of gallbladder cancers are mesenchymal.[18] They include leiomyosarcomas, rhabdomyosarcomas, angiosarcomas, Kaposi sarcoma, malignant fibrous histiocytomas (also known as high-grade pleomorphic sarcomas), and gastrointestinal stromal tumors (GISTs).[98–100] The median age is approximately 70, with more women affected than men; most present with symptoms of cholecystitis.[98] Leiomyosarcomas and malignant fibrous histiocytoma variants are the most common subtypes in adults, with most patients dying within 2 years.[99] Pathogenesis is unclear, but the different varieties can usually be differentiated by immunohistochemistry.[99]

Leiomyosarcomas account for about 7% of reported gallbladder sarcomas. Cells are usually fusiform, with atypical cytoplasm, and desmin and smooth muscle actin positivity.[99,101] Surgical resection, if possible, is appropriate. There are no

large randomized studies to support either adjuvant radiation or chemotherapy. However, one prospective trial of four cycles of adjuvant gemcitabine and docetaxel for patients with uterine leiomyosarcoma yielded promising 2-year disease-free survival rates and may be considered.[102] For advanced disease, it is reasonable to extrapolate from uterine leimyosarcoma regimens which often include docetaxel and gemcitabine.[103]

Malignant fibrous histiocytomas, or high-grade pleomorphic sarcomas, are often a diagnosis of exclusion: they lack markers which suggest other diagnoses, including desmin, *c-kit* (*CD117*), and *CD31*. They have a poor prognosis, with usual survivals of less than a year.[98,104] Agents which have shown some responses include doxorubicin, ifosfamide, and epirubicin. A recent paper showed a response in a patient with this subtype to the *mTOR* inhibitor ridaforolimus.[105]

Angiosarcomas of the gallbladder often present in patients in their 70s, and are equally divided among men and women.[106] Pathology reveals endothelial cells with nuclear atypia, mitoses, and immunostaining for *CD31*.[106] Surgery is performed for localized disease, and pathology is usually not recognized preoperatively. For metastatic disease, taxanes, anthracyclines, and antiangiogenics have all shown responses.[107,108]

Children diagnosed with rhabdomyosarcomas have a good prognosis, and should be referred to centers with expertise in multimodality therapy for these tumors.[98] Those that arise in the biliary tract have a particularly good prognosis, and some data suggest that extensive resection may not be necessary given their exquisite sensitivity to chemotherapy and radiation when localized.[109,110]

Gallbladder GISTs are extremely rare. They usually express *CD177* (*c-kit*), or platelet-derived growth factor receptor (PDGFR) by immunohistochemistry.[111] GISTs are negative for cytokeratin which helps to distinguish them from carcinomas.[112] One case report described a 34-year-old woman with gallstones who was found to have a 1.5 cm lesion composed of spindled to oval epithelioid cells which were positive for *CD117* (*c-kit*) and vimentin, but negative for cytokeratin, with 28 mitotic figures per 10 high-power fields (HPF).[100] Those with larger tumors (>3 cm), higher mitotic rates (>5/HPF), and tumor rupture could be considered for adjuvant therapy with imatinib for at least 3 years after resection.[113,114] In the metastatic setting, imatinib or similar drugs should be tried.[113]

Lymphomas

About 40% of lymphomas present in extranodal locations, with the gastrointestinal tract being the most common site.[115] However, lymphomas of the gallbladder are rare. The majority of patients present with cholecystitis; they are also immunosuppressed in some cases. The most common histologies include diffuse large B cell, extramarginal zone, and follicular histologies.[116] The gallbladder usually has minimal lymphoid tissue, so some have speculated that mucosa-associated lymphoid tissue (MALT) may arise from chronic inflammation in the setting of cholecystitis. Others have suggested that a malignant clone may develop outside the gallbladder and "home" to the gallbladder via adhesion molecules.[117] Staging should follow patterns established for other lymphomas, typically including a PET scan, bone marrow biopsy, and serum lactate dehydrogenase (LDH) level. Treatment should also follow standard guidelines for the underlying lymphoma type.

Bile duct tumors

Epidemiology and risk factors

There are about 5000 new cases of bile duct tumors yearly in the United States.[118,119] About two-thirds are extrahepatic and one-third are intrahepatic.[118] Primary sclerosing cholangitis (PSC) is the most closely linked risk factor in the United States, leading to a 6–30% lifetime risk of developing cholangiocarcinoma. Inflammatory bowel disease is often seen with PSC, and may also be an independent risk factor for cholangiocarcinoma.[120–124] Careful surveillance should be undertaken in patients with PSC for liver tumors and for bowel malignancies. In Asia, and particularly in northern Thailand, the liver flukes *Opisthorchis viverrini* and *Clonorchis sinensis* are strongly associated with biliary cancers. They are usually transmitted to humans from consumption of undercooked freshwater fish.[125,126] Elevated antibody titers to these flukes lead to odds ratios of 3–30 of developing cholangiocarcinoma in several case–control studies.[127–129]

Other risk factors for biliary cancers include choledochal cysts, which are often associated with anomalous pancreatico-biliary junctions and are thought to be more common in Asians. These cysts may lead to the development of biliary cancers at relatively early ages, with lifetime incidences ranging up to 30%.[130,131] Hepatolithiasis is another risk factor, also seen primarily in Asia. More recently, hepatitis C and the metabolic syndrome have also been linked to bile duct cancers.[132,133] A careful family history for patients with biliary cancer should be taken to identify genetic syndromes such as hereditary nonpolyposis colon cancer (HNPCC)[134] or biliary papillomatosis.[135] Ampullary cancers are associated with both traditional and attenuated familial adenomatous polyposis syndromes (FAP).[136]

Pathology

Bile duct tumors consist of perihilar (Klatskin) tumors, intrahepatic, and distal tumors. Intrahepatic bile duct tumors extend to the second-order bile ducts, while extrahepatic tumors include hilar tumors and tumors from the common hepatic ducts (see Fig. 30.1). Epithelial and nonepithelial variants of adenocarcinoma were described for gallbladder cancers and are approached similarly for cholangiocarcinomas.

Pathogenesis

Epithelial cholangiocarcinomas likely develop from the malignant transformation of cholangiocytes in the setting of inflammation and cholestasis.[137,138] Pathogenesis involves inflammatory cascades which lead to resistance to apoptotic pathways. Ironically, the death ligand TRAIL (tumor necrosis factor apoptosis inducing ligand) causes increased invasiveness of cholangiocarcinomas via activation of nuclear factor κ light chain enhancer of activated B cells (NFκB).[139] Another related mechanism of carcinogenesis may be resistance to Fas-mediated cell killing.[140] The inflammatory cytokine IL-6 is also thought to modulate downstream signaling pathways in cholangiocarcinomas, including upregulation of the antiapoptotic protein bcl-2, and mitogen-activated protein kinases which lead to cell proliferation.[141,142]

KRAS mutations have been described in 20–54% of bile duct tumors.[143–145] Tumor suppressor genes like *RASSF1A*, *P16*, and *APC* also are commonly inactivated in cholangiocarcinomas, often by promoter hypermethylation.[137] About 15% of biliary cancers have mutations in the tyrosine kinase domain of EGFR, suggesting a subgroup of patients who may respond particularly well to anti-EGFR therapy.[146,147] *HER-2* expression also varies widely, but is in the 5–20% range.[148] The C-MET receptor is also frequently overexpressed in biliary cancers.[149,150]

Clinical presentation and workup

Patients with extrahepatic cholangiocarcinoma often present with obstructive jaundice while intrahepatic lesions frequently present with constitutional symptoms, loss of appetite, and malaise, or a mass found on routine imaging.[118]

Workup includes an abdominal ultrasound, CT scan, and, increasingly, magnetic resonance cholangiopancreatography (MRCP). MRCP allows detailed imaging of the biliary ducts without the invasiveness of endoscopic retrograde cholangio-pancreatography (ERCP).[151,152] Imaging studies often reveal a discrete mass for intrahepatic cholangiocarcinomas, but often only ductal dilation for extrahepatic lesions. CA-19-9 is elevated in most patients with cholangiocarcinoma, but is not a sensitive marker, particularly in patients with underlying PSC.[153]

For epithelial variants in particular, surrounding desmoplasia is common and often makes the diagnosis of bile duct cancers difficult. Cytology yield with ERCP is typically less than 50%.[154] Other methods of diagnosis are being examined to try to improve diagnostic accuracy. For instance, fluorescence *in situ* hybridization (FISH) uses labeled DNA probes to evaluate cells for chromosomal abnormalities. Digital image analysis (DIA) evaluates for aneuploidy by assessing the DNA content of cells. Both of these techniques have been shown to improve sensitivity and specificity of carcinoma diagnosis compared with cytology alone.[155] Because of the difficulties in obtaining a tissue diagnosis, surgical exploration is often performed without definitive pathology. For those with cholangiocarcinomas being considered for transplant, tissue should be obtained via ERCP (not via a transperitoneal approach) to decrease the risk of tumor seeding.[156]

For a solitary intrahepatic adenocarcinoma, a physical exam, CT scan of chest, abdomen, and pelvis, mammography (women), and upper and lower endoscopy are reasonable to rule out another primary. In the absence of distant disease, a solitary liver lesion with pathology consistent with a cholangiocarcinoma should be treated with curative surgery. Immunostains can help to define the tissue of origin, with cholangiocarcinomas typically staining positive for CK7 and often for CK20, but negative for markers of hepatocellular carcinoma, lung, breast, and prostate cancer.[157]

Treatment considerations

Resectable disease

Patients with negative margins (R0 resections) have a significant rate of disease-free survival.[158,159] However, aggressive surgical management of these cases can also lead to higher rates of complications, including bleeding, liver failure, and infections.[160] When the remnant liver after the resection is expected to be less than 20% of standard liver volume, some centers use portal vein embolization (PVE) to induce growth in the remnant to enable more patients to undergo potentially curative resection.[160–165] Contraindications to surgical resection of cholangiocarcinomas include distant disease, bilobar liver involvement, and usually, hepatic artery or portal vein invasion. For resected patients, 5-year survival ranges broadly from 25% to 60%.[53,166] Adverse prognostic features include vascular invasion, nodal involvement, multiple tumors, and a positive margin.[54,167]

As with gallbladder cancers, it is unknown whether adjuvant (or neoadjuvant) therapy is helpful. Adjuvant chemoradiation is commonly offered if there is a positive margin after resection with either a fluoropyrimidine or gemcitabine, and 6 months of adjuvant gemcitabine or a fluoropyrimidine without radiation after resection if margins are clear. Neoadjuvant therapy with gemcitabine and a platin or a fluoropyrimidine may be considered, to try to downstage patients prior to resection. In very selected cases, particularly in patients with an initially positive margin, some experts advocate a few months of adjuvant chemotherapy, then repeat surgery, with the hope of subsequently obtaining clear margins. If this is thought to be a possibility, radiation is not given as part of initial adjuvant therapy.

Liver transplantation has been used in selected centers after the Mayo Clinic published favorable results in patients with unresectable hilar cholangiocarcinomas using a neoadjuvant protocol including chemotherapy, brachytherapy, and external beam radiation.[168] Contraindications include extrahepatic disease, prior attempted resection of the tumor, prior chemotherapy or radiation, and regional lymph node involvement.[169] Some reports indicate that transplantation may be applicable to patients with intrahepatic cholangiocarcinomas as well.[170,171]

Advanced disease

Systemic chemotherapy is similar to that described in the gallbladder section, with gemcitabine and a platin as reasonable first-line chemotherapy options for epithelial cholangiocarcinomas. For unresectable disease, locoregional therapies also are increasingly used after progression on chemotherapy. Modalities include embolization, ablation, and yttrium 90 (^{90}Y) particles. External beam radiation is another emerging area but will not be discussed here.

Transcather arterial embolization (TAE) selectively blocks the hepatic arterial supply to the tumor with various types of obstructing particles. When given with chemotherapy (TACE), this delivers high doses of chemotherapy to the tumor bed while sparing the surrounding hepatic parenchyma.[172] Bland embolization has never been definitively shown to be inferior to TACE[173] and both have been used as palliative treatment of unresectable biliary cancers, neuroendocrine tumors, and liver metastases.[174–176] Early data suggest that TACE treatment of mass-forming cholangiocarcinomas may lead to median survivals of almost 2 years, as compared to historical controls of 6–8 months.[174] Drug-eluting beads (DEBs) are a novel type of TACE. DEBs are loaded with chemotherapeutic agent such as doxorubicin or irinotecan by immersing them in a drug solution. Locoregional delivery of the DEBs using transcatheter techniques causes targeted tissue damage with minimal systemic impact. It is not clear whether beads yield better outcomes than other embolic techniques in biliary cancers.[177,178]

Contraindications to embolization include systemic infection in the settings of poor synthetic function (Child–Pugh class C), and severe portal vein occlusion. Following the procedure, fever, pain, malaise, nausea, and elevated liver enzymes are common. This constellation of symptoms is commonly referred as postembolization syndrome and usually requires only supportive care. Postprocedure evaluation includes triple-phase abdominal CT or gadolinium-enhanced MRI to evaluate deposition of embolization material, and then typically scans 6–8 weeks later to assess response.

Ablation

Radiofrequency ablation (RFA) causes cell death via heat surrounding the RF electrode (Fig. 30.4). Irreversible cellular injury occurs when cells are heated to 46°C for 60 min, and occurs more rapidly as the temperature increases.[179] A probe is usually inserted into the liver lesion under either ultrasound or CT guidance. Probe selection should be such that the probe covers the lesion with an additional margin of up to 1 cm to decrease local tumor recurrence. A Korean group reported overall survivals of unresectable cholangiocarcinomas of 38 months using RFA.[180,181] RFA is well tolerated and is associated with low mortality ranging from 0.1% to 0.5%.[182] Usually we use RFA for tumors which are small, typically less than 2–3 cm, in order to allow complete necrosis. For those which are larger, we usually use chemoembolization or ^{90}Y.

Yttrium 90

Yttrium 90 microspheres are 20–40 micron particles that emit β radiation, which are delivered via the hepatic artery. Two radioembolization devices are commercially available, both of which contain ^{90}Y. Theraspheres are glass particles, while Sir-Spheres are resin. Patients considered for radioembolization therapy include those with unresectable hepatic primary or metastatic cancer, liver-dominant tumor burden, and a life expectancy of at least 3 months. Yttrium 90 may be considered for patients who have portal vein involvement where TACE cannot be used,[183] although patients with irreversible elevations in serum bilirubin (>2 mg/dL) should be excluded. Pretreatment hepatic artery ^{99m}Tc macroaggregated albumin (MAA) scan is performed to evaluate hepatopulmonary shunting.[184]

Once a patient is deemed to be a candidate for radioembolization, an initial angiographic evaluation is performed, with prophylactic embolization of all extrahepatic vessels to avoid extrahepatic deposition of microspheres.[184] Side-effects include

Figure 30.4 RFA treatment for biliary cancer. Courtesy of Dr Vladimir Sheynzon.

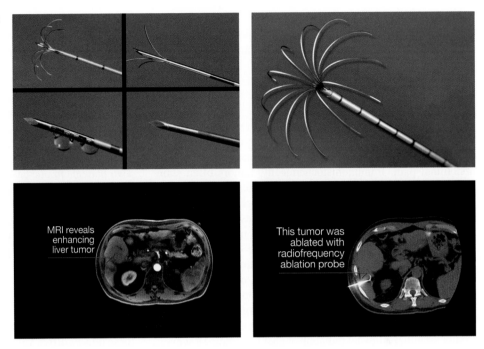

nontarget embolization/radiation, radiation pneumonitis, and radiation hepatitis.[185] One study showed a response rate of 36%, with survival of 22 months post treatment for patients with intrahepatic cholangiocarcinomas.[186]

Uncommon histologies: epithelial subtypes

Papillary

Papillary carcinomas comprise about 5–24% of bile duct epithelial tumors.[65] In one series of 13 extrahepatic papillary bile duct carcinomas, there was an equal male-to-female ratio, and most tumors were located in the proximal portion of the common bile duct. Patients presented with obstructive jaundice and abdominal pain[65] and, as with gallbladder cancers, tended to have a more indolent course than those with adenocarcinomas.[187] Jarnagin and colleagues reported on a series of 215 operations for hilar cholangiomas; 24% of tumors had a papillary component, and these were found to be better differentiated and found at an earlier stage.[188] Survival after resection was 56 months, almost twice as long as for other subtypes. These are treated in similar fashion as other epithelial subtypes.

Squamous

Squamous cell carcinomas of the biliary tract often involve the intrahepatic biliary tree.[189] Many are associated with liver fluke infestation, intrahepatic lithiasis, and PSC. Mixed adenosquamous carcinomas comprise approximately 5% of extrahepatic bile duct tumors. One series from Korea described six patients with adenosquamous histology. Five were men and the mean age was 64. All presented with obstructive jaundice and none had underlying gallstones or a biliary tract anomaly.[190] Five of

the six underwent radical surgery, and four had adjuvant chemoradiation, yielding a 5-year survival rate of 40%. Other studies have suggested 5-year survivals of about 15%, with pancreatic invasion and extensive lymph node metastases being negative prognostic features.[191] Squamous cancers are treated similarly to other epithelial subtypes.

Sarcomatous

About 5% of the time, intrahepatic cholangiocarcinomas may present with sarcomatous changes.[192] In a review of 17 cases, the mean age of patients was 65, with about equal numbers of men and women. Patients presented most commonly with fever and abdominal pain.[193] These combined tumors tend to have vascular invasion and a high propensity to metastasize.[193–195] Surgery should be performed when possible, and responses to gemcitabine and cisplatin have been reported in the advanced setting, as with other epithelial biliary histologies.[193] It is not clear whether adjuvant therapy after resection is helpful, but it can be considered as with other epithelial subtypes.

Uncommon histologies: nonepithelial

Melanomas

Bile duct melanomas are rare. Of reported cases, most were male, and patients usually presented with obstructive jaundice. Cells are typically positive for S-100 and HMB-45, and as with gallbladder melanomas, often have a junctional component.[196,197] As with gallbladder melanomas, it is important to search for a primary. These tumors are usually resected when possible when they are considered primary, and there are some data to support resecting an isolated site of metastasis for selected patients.[198] For metastatic disease, as for all metastatic melanomas, with the advent of new drugs, evaluation for a V600 mutation in *BRAF* is important for possible treatment with vemurafenib.[89] For those without a mutation, other agents such as ipilimumab may be tried.[199]

Mesenchymal tumors

Rhabdomyosarcoma (RMS) is important to recognize because with multidisciplinary treatment, it is often curable. Patients (usually children) may present with a hilar mass, jaundice, and abdominal pain. Immunohistochemically, tumors often stain positive with the transcription factors myogenin and MyoD1. In one series of 25 cases of RMS, the average age was 3, with the oldest patient being 10.[200] For patients with localized tumors, almost all survive after combined modality therapy with chemotherapy and radiation. Because of this, patients with biliary tract RMS may not need aggressive surgery.[110]

As in the gallbladder, leiomyosarcomas of the bile ducts have been reported.[201] Cells are usually fusiform, with desmin and smooth muscle actin positivity.[99,101] Surgical resection, if possible, is appropriate. There are no large randomized studies to support either adjuvant radiation or chemotherapy. However, one prospective trial of four cycles of adjuvant gemcitabine and docetaxel for patients with uterine leiomyosarcoma yielded promising 2-year disease-free survival rates and may be considered.[102] For advanced disease, it is reasonable to extrapolate from uterine leimyosarcoma regimens which also often include docetaxel and gemcitabine.[103]

Neuroendocrine tumors

Biliary neuroendocrine tumors have been reported, usually found incidentally on pathology, often presenting with painless jaundice.[95,202] In one series, 75% of patients were male.[203] Well-differentiated tumors (determined by low or intermediate grade, mitotic rate <20/10 HPF, and Ki-67 index <20%) usually stain positive for neuroendocrine markers, including chromogranin and synaptophysin. Serum chromogranin and urine 5-HIAA should be assessed. Staging includes CT or MRI scanning, octreotide scan, upper and lower endoscopy, and evaluation of the small bowel. An echocardiogram should be obtained to rule out right-sided valvular disease.

Prognosis is typically good for patients undergoing complete resection of low- and intermediate- grade tumors, and there are no data to support adjuvant therapy for these tumors.[92,95] Surveillance after surgery can be extrapolated from that for pancreatic neuroendocrine tumors, including exam, serum markers, and scans at 3 months post surgery, then markers every 6 months for 3 years, then yearly.[28] For those with unresectable disease, there is a progression-free survival benefit for everolimus and octreotide compared with octreotide alone for patients with advanced neuroendocrine tumors and carcinoid syndrome.[204] Octreotide has been shown to provide a benefit in progression-free survival for those with midgut neuroendocrine tumors.[205]

As with gallbladder cancers, high-grade biliary neuroendocrine tumors should be worked up and treated like small cell lung cancers, including PET scan rather than octreotide scan,

and MRI of the brain. Survival is dismal, with one series reporting 0% alive at 2 years.[95] Treatment for metastatic disease follows general guidelines for small cell tumors at other sites, as discussed above.

Lymphomas

Most patients with bile duct lymphomas present with obstructive jaundice, and are typically in their 40s; about 60% are women. The majority of tumors are diffuse large B cell lymphomas (DLBCL) and about 25% are follicular lymphomas. Two patients in one case series had EBV-associated posttransplant lymphoproliferative disorder in the context of solid organ transplantation.[116] Usually the diagnosis is made postoperatively and, as with gallbladder lymphomas, it is crucial to work patients up systemically and give chemotherapy if it is a lymphoma type which would typically require systemic chemotherapy.[206,207]

Hepatic tumors

The epidemiology, risk factors, workup, and treatment for these tumors differ. Uncommon primary hepatic tumors including fibrolamellar carcinoma (FC), combined hepatocellular cholangiocarcinoma, mesenchymal tumors, neuroendocrine tumors, hepatoblastomas, and lymphomas will be considered below. Treatment of hepatocellular carcinomas (HCC) is complex and multidisciplinary, often incorporating locoregional therapies together with surgery and, increasingly, systemic therapies.[208,209]

Fibrolamellar carcinoma

Fibrolamellar carcinoma accounts for less than 5% of hepatocellular carcinoma and usually is seen in younger patients in their second to third decades. It is equally distributed among men and women, and often arises in an otherwise normal liver, in contrast to most patients with HCC.[210,211] Pathologically, FC has large cells with eosinophilic cytoplasm, macronucleoli, and fibrous stroma with lamellae surrounding the tumor cells. They usually stain positive for HepPar1, CK7, and CD99.[211,212] CK7 is a marker commonly seen in cholangiocarcinomas and has led to speculation that FC may derive from a more primitive stem cell precursor. Recently, investigators have found that FC does express stem cell markers like CD133 more than traditional HCC.[213] In addition, FC has fewer overall chromosomal alterations than traditional HCC,[214] and epigenetic studies suggest that FCs lack global hypomethylation which is often seen in traditional HCCs.[215]

Most patients present with local symptoms, such as right upper quadrant pain. Imaging may reveal a large, lobulated, heterogeneous mass often with a central scar.[216] AFP levels are usually normal. Five-year survival based on registry data from SEER is about 32%, compared with about 7% for traditional HCC.[210] No prospective data compare resection versus transplant for FC. In one small series, patients undergoing resection had 3-year survivals of 100% (n=11), compared with 76% with liver transplantation (n=9). Overall survival was 50% at 5 years. Prognostic features, as expected, included stage, positive lymph nodes, and vascular invasion.[217] However, FC can metastasize and may be more likely to spread to lymph nodes and peritoneum than traditional HCC.[218] For those who are unresectable at presentation, median survival is only about 12 months.[219]

Despite resection or transplantation, many patients will have a recurrence. There are no clear data to guide systemic therapy. For HCC, sorafenib is now the initial treatment of choice based on two large randomized trials.[220,221] It is not clear if sorafenib is effective in patients with FC. Since most patients with FC do not have underlying liver disease, systemic chemotherapy may also be tried, and there are reports of benefit using platinum-based treatments.[222] In addition, about 30% of patients with FC overexpress *mTOR*, suggesting the possible efficacy of *mTOR* inhibitors.[223] For locally advanced, unresectable FC, locoregional therapy can also be considered, as discussed below.

Hepatocellular cholangiocarcinoma

These tumors are defined by expression of both hepatocellular and bile duct immunohistochemical stains on pathology, and account for 1–5% of primary liver tumors. A study from the United States suggested that these tumors have an epidemiology similar to cholangiocarcinomas,[224] while studies from Asia suggest that they are more similar epidemiologically to HCC, with a high male-to-female ratio and high prevalence of underlying hepatitis B virus (HBV).[225,226] Many express *c-kit*, a stem cell marker, again suggesting possible derivation from a common progenitor cell.[227,228] These tumors can be categorized into a "separate" type, where the HCC trabecular appearance and cholangiocarcinoma tubular components are discrete, a "transitional" type, where the two pathological types are contiguous, and an intermediate type, where the pathological characteristics are blended, with characteristic oval-shaped cells, hyperchromatic nuclei, and desmoplastic stroma.[226]

There are no radiographic features which distinguish hepatocellular cholangiocarcinoma (HCC-CC) from either HCC or cholangiocarcinomas.[229] This diagnosis should be considered in patients with adenocarcinoma in a liver biopsy with an elevated AFP. Resection should be undertaken if possible, but often these are discovered at explant after transplantation. One review demonstrated a median survival of 1.8 years, with 5- and 10-year survivals of 23% and 11% respectively.[230] An American cohort of 12 patients who had undergone liver transplant demonstrated 5-year survivals of about 15%; this is significantly worse than expected for patients with hepatocellular carcinoma falling within the Milan criteria.[229] For this reason, we sometimes offer adjuvant gemcitabine after transplantation, and often switch the immunosuppressive regimen to sirolimus if feasible, with early data suggesting a possible decrease in HCC recurrence after transplant and the *mTOR*-inhibiting properties of the drug.[231]

For locally unresectable disease, chemoembolization is reasonable.[173] For multifocal or metastatic disease, consideration of platinum-based chemotherapy or sorafenib are both reasonable options. Given the positivity for *c-kit* in some patients, it is reasonable to test for this marker and try imatinib if positive.[228]

Mesenchymal tumors

Primary liver angiosarcomas account for 2% of primary liver tumors. Many are associated with chemical exposures, including vinyl chloride, Thorotrast, and arsenic.[232] Patients often present with abdominal pain, weakness, and fatigue. Responses may be seen with ifosfamide- and doxorubicin-containing regimens, and paclitaxel.[233] Because these lesions tend to be vascular, antiangiogenic agents have been tried with chemotherapy and as single agents with some success.[107,234–236] Prognosis is usually poor because of limited resectability. Patients often die of liver failure or tumor rupture with hemorrhage.

Hepatic epithelioid hemangioendotheliomas are vascular tumors of endothelial origin. More than 200 cases have been reported, with a possible link to oral contraceptives.[237] There is a female predominance, and patients often present with nonspecific symptoms such as right upper quadrant pain and weight loss. In over 40% of patients, the tumor is found incidentally. Tumors usually contain dendritic and epithelioid cells with immunohistochemistry positive for at least one endothelial cell marker (FVIII-RAg, CD34, and/or CD31).[238] Clinical course is variable; resection or liver transplantation can be curative, with about half of patients alive at 5 years.[239] In a large series, 27% of patients developed metastases, and nearly half of all deaths occurred within 16 months of diagnosis.[238] Antiangiogenic agents like thalidomide and bevacizumab have also been tried in patients with advanced disease, with some benefit.[240,241]

Approximately 50 primary liver leiomyosarcomas have been documented. Patients typically present in their 50s. There is sometimes an associated immunosuppression, either due to HIV or solid organ transplantation.[242,243] Presenting symptoms relate to a hepatic mass (usually right lobe) and ascites. CT scans demonstrate heterogeneous enhancement, in contrast to metastatic liver leiomyosarcomas.[244] Metastatic disease is present in about 40% of patients at diagnosis. Supportive care typically yields median survivals of less than 1 year, while patients undergoing resection usually have survival of more than 3 years, supporting resection when possible. For advanced disease, it is reasonable to extrapolate from uterine leiomyosarcoma regimens which often include docetaxel and gemcitabine.[103] For those who have tumors in the setting of solid organ transplant, modulation of immunosuppression has sometimes led to responses.[245]

Malignant fibrous histiocytomas are also known as high-grade pleomorphic sarcomas. These are usually large, have storiform histology, and often invade adjacent organs. Surgical resection is recommended, although only one-fourth of patients are disease free long term.[246,247] Ezrin expression by immunohistochemistry predicts worsened prognosis.[248] The impact of chemotherapy is not clearly defined, but standard regimens for soft tissue sarcomas are reasonable for those with unresectable disease and preserved liver function.

Rhabdomyosarcomas (RMS) of liver typically appear in children and present with early jaundice due to biliary obstruction. Cure is possible with resection and multimodality therapy, so it is important to refer these patients to centers with experience in treating these tumors.[200]

Primary gastrointestinal stromal tumors (GISTs) of the liver are extremely rare, with only three reported cases in the literature.[112,249] They usually express *CD177* (*c-kit*) or PDGFR by immunohistochemisty, allowing treatment with imatinib, a tyrosine kinase inhibitor which targets these pathways.[111] GISTs are negative for cytokeratin which helps to distinguish them from carcinomas.[112] Downstaging with imatinib could be considered prior to resection. Those with larger tumors, higher mitotic rates, and tumor rupture may be considered for adjuvant therapy with imatinib for at least 3 years after resection.[113,114]

Neuroendocrine tumors

Primary liver neuroendocrine tumors account for about 4% of NETs in a SEER analysis, and are relatively equally distributed in terms of gender.[250] Well-differentiated tumors (determined by low or intermediate grade, mitotic rate <20/10 HPF, and Ki-67 index <20%) usually stain positive for neuroendocrine markers, including chromogranin and synaptophysin. Serum chromogranin and urine 5-HIAA should be assessed. Evaluating for a primary site is crucial, including CT or MRI scanning, octreotide scan, upper and lower endoscopy, and evaluation of the small bowel. One group noted that surgical exploration with attention to the small bowel is often necessary to identify and resect the primary.[251] An echocardiogram should be obtained to rule out right-sided valvular disease, although usually primary liver NETs are nonfunctional.

Liver transplantation is being examined for patients with low- and intermediate-grade neuroendocrine tumors, together with resection and locoregional therapies. No consensus has yet been reached with respect to optimal treatment of these tumors. Local therapies are commonly used because neuroendocrine tumors typically derive much of their blood supply from the hepatic artery, and receive a larger proportion of drug and embolic material than the surrounding liver parenchyma.[252,253] When treating NETs with surgery or local therapy, the operator should be aware of the risk of provoking carcinoid crisis due to the release of vasoactive substances.[254] Typically surgery leads to longest survival, but this may relate to selection bias. Some suggest that locoregional therapy is preferable for those who are asymptomatic and have a relatively large (>25% involvement) burden of disease.[252,255]

For patients with metastatic low- and intermediate-grade NET, an immunohistochemical stain, PAX-8, may help to differentiate pancreatic from other sites of neuroendocrine differentiation, particularly in the liver.[256] Pancreatic primary neuroendocrine tumors may be more responsive to *mTOR* inhibitors and the antiangiogenic agent sunitinib than other primaries, so this information may help to guide therapy, particularly for patients with advanced disease.[257,258] Recent data suggest a progression-free survival benefit for everolimus and octreotide compared with octreotide alone for patients with advanced neuroendocrine tumors and carcinoid syndrome.[204] This trial did include patients with primary liver tumors. Octreotide can also be tried and has been also shown to provide a benefit in progression-free survival for those with midgut neuroendocrine tumors.[205]

Patients with primary high-grade neuroendocrine tumors should be staged with PET/CT scans and brain MRI rather than octreotide scanning. For localized disease, resection followed by chemotherapy has occasionally led to long-term survivors, although this is unusual.[259] For those with unresectable disease, combinations of platinum-containing chemotherapy similar to those given for small cell lung cancer are reasonable.[260] These tumors need to be differentiated from less aggressive neuroendocrine tumors, based on mitotic rate, grade, and Ki-67 index.

Hepatoblastomas

Hepatoblastomas are usually found in children between 6 months and 3 years of age, and have a male predominance. They are thought to develop from pluripotent hepatic stem cells[261] and are found more commonly in families with familial adenomatous polyposis.[262] Patients typically present with an asymptomatic abdominal mass, with weight loss, anorexia, and abdominal pain.

Curative therapy involves surgery but given the chemosensitivity of this tumor, preoperative chemotherapy has become a standard. In one study, preoperative cisplatin and doxorubicin resulted in a less extensive liver resection in approximately one-fourth of patients. Five-year survival for all patients is over 70%.[263]

For patients in whom complete resection is not possible, or for those with intrahepatic recurrence, liver transplantation can result in long-term survival. In one large analysis, 6-year survival was 82% in 106 patients undergoing initial liver transplantation, and 30% for 41 patients undergoing salvage transplant.[264] For patients with metastatic disease, chemotherapy agents with activity include cisplatin, doxorubicin, cyclophosphamide, vincristine, and 5-FU.[261,265] The use of platins and anthracyclines in childhood can result in hearing and cardiac problems. This has led to new chemotherapy regimens and schedules to try to limit these toxicities.[266,267]

Lymphomas

Primary hepatic non-Hodgkin lymphoma (NHL) constitutes 0.02% of all NHL, and may be associated with hepatitis C.[268] Typical symptoms include abdominal pain, fevers, and sweats in middle-aged patients, with a male predominance. Imaging often reveals a solitary liver mass and the most common histology is diffuse large B cell. Typical chemotherapy for NHL, including CHOP plus rituximab, is often used.[268] A separate entity which has been reported is hepatosplenic T cell lymphoma. In one series of 21 patients from France, patients were often referred for cytopenias and splenomegaly, but no other involved nodes on imaging. All had bone marrow involvement. Five patients were immunosuppressed, because of either prior organ transplant or rheumatological disease. The patients all expressed γδTCR in tissue specimens, as well as CD2 and CD3 (T cell markers). Median survival, despite chemotherapy and transplantation in some patients, was only 16 months.[269]

References

1. Jemal A, Siegel R, Xu J, *et al.* Cancer statistics, 2010. CA Cancer J Clin 2010; 60: 277–300.

2. Wistuba, II, Gazdar AF. Gallbladder cancer: lessons from a rare tumour. Nat Rev Cancer 2004; 4: 695–706.

3. Nath G, Singh H, Shukla VK. Chronic typhoid carriage and carcinoma of the gallbladder. Eur J Cancer Prev 1997; 6: 557–9.

4. Dutta U, Garg PK, Kumar R, *et al.* Typhoid carriers among patients with gallstones are at increased risk for carcinoma of the gallbladder. Am J Gastroenterol 2000; 95: 784–7.

5. Zatonski WA, Lowenfels AB, Boyle P, *et al.* Epidemiologic aspects of gallbladder cancer: a case-control study of the SEARCH Program of the International Agency for Research on Cancer. J Natl Cancer Inst 1997; 89: 1132–8.

6. Randi G, Franceschi S, La Vecchia C. Gallbladder cancer worldwide: geographical distribution and risk factors. Int J Cancer 2006; 118: 1591–602.

7. Lazcano-Ponce EC, Miquel JF, Munoz N, *et al.* Epidemiology and molecular pathology of gallbladder cancer. CA Cancer J Clin 2001; 51: 349–64.

8. Black WC, Key CR, Carmany TB, *et al.* Carcinoma of the gallbladder in a population of Southwestern American Indians. Cancer 1977; 39: 1267–79.

9. Hasumi A, Matsui H, Sugioka A, *et al.* Precancerous conditions of biliary tract cancer in patients with pancreaticobiliary maljunction: reappraisal of nationwide survey in Japan. J Hepatobiliary Pancreat Surg 2000; 7: 551–5.

10. Kumar S. Infection as a risk factor for gallbladder cancer. J Surg Oncol 2006; 93: 633–9.

11. Chao TC, Wang CS, Jan YY, *et al.* Carcinogenesis in the biliary system associated with APDJ. J Hepatobiliary Pancreat Surg 1999; 6: 218–22.

12. Henson DE, Albores-Saavedra J, Corle D. Carcinoma of the gallbladder. Histologic types, stage of disease, grade, and survival rates. Cancer 1992; 70: 1493–7.

13. Kozuka S, Tsubone N, Yasui A, *et al.* Relation of adenoma to carcinoma in the gallbladder. Cancer 1982; 50: 2226–34.

14. Roa I, Araya JC, Villaseca M, *et al.* Preneoplastic lesions and gallbladder cancer: an estimate of the period required for progression. Gastroenterology 1996; 111: 232–6.

15. Hanada K, Tsuchida A, Iwao T, *et al.* Gene mutations of K-ras in gallbladder mucosae and gallbladder carcinoma with an anomalous junction of the pancreaticobiliary duct. Am J Gastroenterol 1999; 94: 1638–42.

16. Kim YT, Kim J, Jang YH, *et al.* Genetic alterations in gallbladder adenoma, dysplasia and carcinoma. Cancer Lett 2001; 169: 59–68.

17. Rashid A, Ueki T, Gao YT, *et al.* K-ras mutation, p53 overexpression, and microsatellite instability in biliary tract cancers: a population-based study in China. Clin Cancer Res 2002; 8: 3156–63.

18. Duffy A, Capanu M, Abou-Alfa GK, *et al.* Gallbladder cancer (GBC): 10-year experience at Memorial Sloan–Kettering Cancer Centre (MSKCC). J Surg Oncol 2008; 98: 485–9.

19. Schwartz LH, Black J, Fong Y, *et al.* Gallbladder carcinoma: findings at MR imaging with MR cholangiopancreatography. J Comput Assist Tomogr 2002; 26: 405–10.

20. Gore RM, Thakrar KH, Newmark GM, *et al.* Gallbladder imaging. Gastroenterol Clin North Am 2010; 39: 265–87, ix.

21. Rodriguez-Fernandez A, Gomez-Rio M, Medina-Benitez A, *et al.* Application of modern imaging methods in diagnosis of gallbladder cancer. J Surg Oncol 2006; 93: 650–64.

22. Lee SW, Kim HJ, Park JH, *et al.* Clinical usefulness of 18F-FDG PET-CT for patients with gallbladder cancer and cholangiocarcinoma. J Gastroenterol 2010; 45: 560–6.

23. Strom BL, Maislin G, West SL, *et al.* Serum CEA and CA 19-9: potential future diagnostic or screening tests for gallbladder cancer? Int J Cancer 1990; 45: 821–4.

24. Edge S, Byrd, DR, Compton, CC, *et al.* (eds). *AJCC (American Joint Committee on Cancer) Cancer Staging Manual.* New York: Springer, 2010. p. 211.

25. Dixon E. An aggressive surgical approach leads to improved survival in patients with gallbladder cancer: a 12-year study at a North American Center. Ann Surg 2005; 241: 385–94.

26. Glauser PM. Incidence, management, and outcome of incidental gallbladder carcinoma: analysis of the database of the Swiss association of laparoscopic and thoracoscopic surgery. Surg Endosc 2010; 24: 2281–6.

27. Mayo SC, Shore AD, Nathan H, *et al.* National trends in the management and survival of surgically managed gallbladder adenocarcinoma over 15 years: a population-based analysis. J Gastrointest Surg 2010; 14: 1578–91.

28. Morgan RJ Jr, Alvarez RD, Armstrong DK, *et al.* NCCN Clinical Practice Guidelines in Oncology: epithelial ovarian cancer. J Natl Compr Canc Netw 2011; 9: 82–113.

29. Yokomizo H, Yamane T, Hirata T, *et al.* Surgical treatment of pT2 gallbladder carcinoma: a reevaluation of the therapeutic effect of hepatectomy and extrahepatic bile duct resection based on the long-term outcome. Ann Surg Oncol 2007; 14: 1366–73.

30. Jarnagin WR, Ruo L, Little SA, *et al.* Patterns of initial disease recurrence after resection of gallbladder carcinoma and hilar cholangiocarcinoma: implications for adjuvant therapeutic strategies. Cancer 2003; 98: 1689–700.

31. Park HS, Lim JY, Yoon DS, *et al.* Outcome of adjuvant therapy for gallbladder cancer. Oncology 2010; 79: 168–73.

32. Gold DG, Miller RC, Haddock MG, *et al.* Adjuvant therapy for gallbladder carcinoma: the Mayo Clinic Experience. Int J Radiat Oncol Biol Phys 2009; 75: 150–5.

33. Wang SJ, Lemieux A, Kalpathy-Cramer J, *et al.* Nomogram for predicting the benefit of adjuvant chemoradiotherapy for resected gallbladder cancer. J Clin Oncol 2011; 29: 4627–32.

34. Lindell G, Holmin T, Ewers SB, *et al.* Extended operation with or without intraoperative (IORT) and external (EBRT) radiotherapy for gallbladder carcinoma. Hepatogastroenterology 2003; 50: 310–14.

35. Itoh H, Nishijima K, Kurosaka Y, *et al.* Magnitude of combination therapy of radical resection and external beam radiotherapy for patients with carcinomas of the extrahepatic bile duct and gallbladder. Dig Dis Sci 2005; 50: 2231–42.

36. Wang SJ, Fuller CD, Kim JS, *et al.* Prediction model for estimating the survival benefit of adjuvant radiotherapy for gallbladder cancer. J Clin Oncol 2008; 26: 2112–17.

37. Valle J, Wasan H, Palmer DH, *et al.* Cisplatin plus gemcitabine versus gemcitabine for biliary tract cancer. N Engl J Med 2010; 362: 1273–81.

38. Sharma A, Dwary AD, Mohanti BK, *et al.* Best supportive care compared with chemotherapy for unresectable gall bladder cancer: a randomized controlled study. J Clin Oncol 2010; 28: 4581–6.

39. Gruenberger B, Schueller J, Heubrandtner U, *et al.* Cetuximab, gemcitabine, and oxaliplatin in patients with unresectable advanced or metastatic biliary tract cancer: a phase 2 study. Lancet Oncol 2010; 11: 1142–8.

40. Iqbal S, Rankin C, Lenz HJ, *et al.* A phase II trial of gemcitabine and capecitabine in patients with unresectable or metastatic gallbladder cancer or cholangiocarcinoma: Southwest Oncology Group study S0202. Cancer Chemother Pharmacol 2011; 68: 1595–602.

41. Knox JJ, Hedley D, Oza A, *et al.* Combining gemcitabine and capecitabine in patients with advanced biliary cancer: a phase II trial. J Clin Oncol 2005; 23: 2332–8.

42. Cho JY, Paik YH, Chang YS, *et al.* Capecitabine combined with gemcitabine (CapGem) as first-line treatment in patients with advanced/metastatic biliary tract carcinoma. Cancer 2005; 104: 2753–8.

43. Riechelmann RP, Townsley CA, Chin SN, *et al.* Expanded phase II trial of gemcitabine and capecitabine for advanced biliary cancer. Cancer 2007; 110: 1307–12.

44. Iyer RV, Gibbs J, Kuvshinoff B, *et al.* A phase II study of gemcitabine and capecitabine in advanced cholangiocarcinoma and carcinoma of the gallbladder: a single-institution prospective study. Ann Surg Oncol 2007; 14: 3202–9.

45. Papakostas P, Kouroussis C, Androulakis N, *et al.* First-line chemotherapy with docetaxel for unresectable or metastatic carcinoma of the biliary tract. A multicentre phase II study. Eur J Cancer 2001; 37: 1833–8.

46. Kuhn R, Hribaschek A, Eichelmann K, *et al.* Outpatient therapy with gemcitabine and docetaxel for gallbladder, biliary, and cholangio-carcinomas. Invest New Drugs 2002; 20: 351–6.

47. Chung MJ, Kim YJ, Park JY, *et al.* Prospective phase II Trial of gemcitabine in combination with irinotecan as first-line chemotherapy in patients with advanced biliary tract cancer. Chemotherapy 2011; 57: 236–43.

48. Feisthammel J, Schoppmeyer K, Mossner J, *et al.* Irinotecan with 5-FU/FA in advanced biliary tract adenocarcinomas: a multicenter phase II trial. Am J Clin Oncol 2007; 30: 319–24.

49. Sasaki T, Isayama H, Nakai Y, *et al.* Multicenter phase II study of S-1 monotherapy as second-line chemotherapy for advanced biliary tract cancer refractory to gemcitabine. Invest New Drugs 2012; 30: 708–13.

50. Cunningham D, Humblet Y, Siena S, *et al.* Cetuximab monotherapy and cetuximab plus irinotecan in irinotecan-refractory metastatic colorectal cancer. N Engl J Med 2004; 351: 337–45.

51. Paule B, Herelle MO, Rage E, *et al.* Cetuximab plus gemcitabine-oxaliplatin (GEMOX) in patients with refractory advanced intrahepatic cholangiocarcinomas. Oncology 2007; 72: 105–10.

52. Slamon DJ, Leyland-Jones B, Shak S, *et al.* Use of chemotherapy plus a monoclonal antibody against HER2 for metastatic breast cancer that overexpresses HER2. N Engl J Med 2001; 344: 783–92.

53. Bang YJ, Van Cutsem E, Feyereislova A, *et al.* Trastuzumab in combination with chemotherapy versus chemotherapy alone for treatment of HER2-positive advanced gastric or gastro-oesophageal junction cancer (ToGA): a phase 3, open-label, randomised controlled trial. Lancet 2010; 376: 687–97.

54. Nakazawa K, Dobashi Y, Suzuki S, *et al.* Amplification and overexpression of c-erbB-2, epidermal growth factor receptor, and c-met in biliary tract cancers. J Pathol 2005; 206: 356–65.

55. Ramanathan RK, Belani CP, Singh DA, *et al.* A phase II study of lapatinib in patients with advanced biliary tree and hepatocellular cancer. Cancer Chemother Pharmacol 2009; 64: 777–83.

56. Bekaii-Saab T, Phelps MA, Li X, *et al.* Multi-institutional phase II study of selumetinib in patients with metastatic biliary cancers. J Clin Oncol 29: 2357–63.

57. Hida Y, Morita T, Fujita M, *et al.* Vascular endothelial growth factor expression is an independent negative predictor in extrahepatic biliary tract carcinomas. Anticancer Res 1999; 19: 2257–60.

58. Zhu AX, Meyerhardt JA, Blaszkowsky LS, *et al.* Efficacy and safety of gemcitabine, oxaliplatin, and bevacizumab in advanced biliary-tract cancers and correlation of changes in 18-fluorodeoxyglucose PET with clinical outcome: a phase 2 study. Lancet Oncol 2010; 11: 48–54.

59. Roa JC, Tapia O, Cakir A, *et al.* Squamous cell and adenosquamous carcinomas of the gallbladder: clinicopathological analysis of 34 cases identified in 606 carcinomas. Mod Pathol 2011; 24: 1069–78.

60. Roa JC, Tapia O, Cakir A, *et al.* Squamous cell and adenosquamous carcinomas of the gallbladder: clinicopathological analysis of 34 cases identified in 606 carcinomas. Mod Pathol 2011; 24: 1069–78.

61. Kim WS, Jang KT, Choi DW, *et al.* Clinicopathologic analysis of adenosquamous/squamous cell carcinoma of the gallbladder. J Surg Oncol 2011; 103: 239–42.

62. Chan KM, Yu MC, Lee WC, *et al.* Adenosquamous/squamous cell carcinoma of the gallbladder. J Surg Oncol 2007; 95: 129–34.

63. Nishihara K, Nagai E, Izumi Y, *et al.* Adenosquamous carcinoma of the gallbladder: a clinicopathological, immunohistochemical and flow-cytometric study of twenty cases. Jpn J Cancer Res 1994; 85: 389–99.

64. Oohashi Y, Shirai Y, Wakai T, *et al.* Adenosquamous carcinoma of the gallbladder warrants resection only if curative resection is feasible. Cancer 2002; 94: 3000–5.

65. Hoang MP, Murakata LA, Katabi N, *et al.* Invasive papillary carcinomas of the extrahepatic bile ducts: a clinicopathologic and immunohistochemical study of 13 cases. Mod Pathol 2002; 15: 1251–8.

66. Albores-Saavedra J, Tuck M, McLaren BK, *et al.* Papillary carcinomas of the gallbladder: analysis of noninvasive and invasive types. Arch Pathol Lab Med 2005; 129: 905–9.

67. Nuzzo G, Clemente G, Cadeddu F, *et al.* Papillary carcinoma of the gallbladder and anomalous pancreatico-biliary junction. Report of three

68. Yoshida T, Shibata K, Matsumoto T, *et al.* Carcinoma of the gallbladder associated with anomalous junction of the pancreaticobiliary duct in adults. J Am Coll Surg 1999; 189: 57–62.

69. Ikeda T, Nakayama Y, Hamada Y, *et al.* FU-MK-1 expression in human gallbladder carcinoma: an antigenic prediction marker for a better postsurgical prognosis. Am J Clin Pathol 2009; 132: 111–17.

70. Vardaman C, Albores-Saavedra J. Clear cell carcinomas of the gallbladder and extrahepatic bile ducts. Am J Surg Pathol 1995; 19: 91–9.

71. Noda H, Chiba F, Toyama N, *et al.* Mucin-producing carcinoma of the gallbladder associated with primary sclerosing cholangitis and ulcerative colitis. J Hepatobiliary Pancreat Surg 2009; 16: 83–5.

72. Mondal SK. Signet ring cell carcinoma of gallbladder with celiac lymph node metastasis in a young man. J Cancer Res Ther 2010; 6: 379–81.

73. Albores-Saavedra J, Galliani C, Chable-Montero F, *et al.* Mucin-containing Rokitansky–Aschoff sinuses with extracellular mucin deposits simulating mucinous carcinoma of the gallbladder. Am J Surg Pathol 2009; 33: 1633–8.

74. Watanabe M, Hori Y, Nojima T, *et al.* Alpha-fetoprotein-producing carcinoma of the gallbladder. Dig Dis Sci 1993; 38: 561–4.

75. Tian H, Matsumoto S, Takaki H, *et al.* Mucin-producing carcinoma of the gallbladder: imaging demonstration in four cases. J Comput Assist Tomogr 2003; 27: 150–4.

76. Czyszczon IA, Alatassi H. Signet ring cell carcinoma of the gallbladder in a 22-year-old man: a case report and review of the literature. Int J Surg Pathol 2010; 18: 358–62.

77. Henson DE, Albores-Saavedra J, Compton CC. Protocol for the examination of specimens from patients with carcinomas of the gallbladder, including those showing focal endocrine differentiation: a basis for checklists. Cancer Committee of the College of American Pathologists. Arch Pathol Lab Med 2000; 124: 37–40.

78. Karabulut Z, Yildirim Y, Abaci I, *et al.* Signet-ring cell carcinoma of the gallbladder: a case report. Adv Ther 2008; 25: 520–3.

79. Huguet KL, Hughes CB, Hewitt WR. Gallbladder carcinosarcoma: a case report and literature review. J Gastrointest Surg 2005; 9: 818–21.

80. Uzun MA, Koksal N, Gunerhan Y, *et al.* Carcinosarcoma of the gallbladder: report of a case. Surg Today 2009; 39: 168–71.

81. Takahashi Y, Fukushima J, Fukusato T, *et al.* Sarcomatoid carcinoma with components of small cell carcinoma and undifferentiated carcinoma of the gallbladder. Pathol Int 2004; 54: 866–71.

82. Okabayashi T, Sun ZL, Montgomery RA, *et al.* Surgical outcome of carcinosarcoma of the gall bladder: a review. World J Gastroenterol 2009; 15: 4877–82.

83. Verbanck JJ, Rutgeerts LJ, van Aelst FJ, *et al.* Primary malignant melanoma of the gallbladder, metastatic to the common bile duct. Gastroenterology 1986; 91: 214–18.

84. Dasgupta T, Brasfield R. Metastatic melanoma. A clinicopathological study. Cancer 1964; 17: 1323–39.

85. Heath DI, Womack C. Primary malignant melanoma of the gall bladder. J Clin Pathol 1988; 41: 1073–7.

86. Dong XD, DeMatos P, Prieto VG, *et al.* Melanoma of the gallbladder: a review of cases seen at Duke University Medical Center. Cancer 1999; 85: 32–9.

87. Katz SC, Bowne WB, Wolchok JD, *et al.* Surgical management of melanoma of the gallbladder: a report of 13 cases and review of the literature. Am J Surg 2007; 193: 493–7.

88. Marone U, Caraco C, Losito S, *et al.* Laparoscopic cholecystectomy for melanoma metastatic to the gallbladder: is it an adequate surgical procedure? Report of a case and review of the literature. World J Surg Oncol 2007; 5: 141.

89. Flaherty KT, Puzanov I, Kim KB, *et al.* Inhibition of mutated, activated BRAF in metastatic melanoma. N Engl J Med 2010; 363: 809–19.

90. Robert C, Thomas L, Bondarenko I, *et al.* Ipilimumab plus dacarbazine for previously untreated metastatic melanoma. N Engl J Med 2011; 364: 2517–26.

91. Eltawil KM, Gustafsson BI, Kidd M, *et al.* Neuroendocrine tumors of the gallbladder: an evaluation and reassessment of management strategy. J Clin Gastroenterol 2010; 44: 687–95.

92. Albores-Saavedra J, Batich K, Hossain S, *et al.* Carcinoid tumors and small-cell carcinomas of the gallbladder and extrahepatic bile ducts: a comparative study based on 221 cases from the Surveillance, Epidemiology, and End Results Program. Ann Diagn Pathol 2009; 13: 378–83.

93. Sinkre PA, Murakata L, Rabin L, *et al.* Clear cell carcinoid tumor of the gallbladder: another distinctive manifestation of von Hippel–Lindau disease. Am J Surg Pathol 2001; 25: 1334–9.

94. Barone GW, Schaefer RF, Counce JS, *et al.* Gallbladder and gastric argyrophil carcinoid associated with a case of Zollinger–Ellison syndrome. Am J Gastroenterol 1992; 87: 392–4.

95. Kim J, Lee WJ, Lee SH, *et al.* Clinical features of 20 patients with curatively resected biliary neuroendocrine tumours. Dig Liver Dis 2011; 43: 965–70.

96. Modlin IM, Shapiro MD, Kidd M. An analysis of rare carcinoid tumors: clarifying these clinical conundrums. World J Surg 2005; 29: 92–101.

97. Moskal TL, Zhang PJ, Nava HR. Small cell carcinoma of the gallbladder. J Surg Oncol 1999; 70: 54–9.

98. Al-Daraji WI, Makhlouf HR, Miettinen M, *et al.* Primary gallbladder sarcoma: a clinicopathologic study of 15 cases, heterogeneous sarcomas with poor outcome, except pediatric botryoid rhabdomyosarcoma. Am J Surg Pathol 2009; 33: 826–34.

99. Husain EA, Prescott RJ, Haider SA, *et al.* Gallbladder sarcoma: a clinicopathological study of seven cases from the UK and Austria with emphasis on morphological subtypes. Dig Dis Sci 2009; 54: 395–400.

100. Mendoza-Marin M, Hoang MP, Albores-Saavedra J. Malignant stromal tumor of the gallbladder with interstitial cells of Cajal phenotype. Arch Pathol Lab Med 2002; 126: 481–3.

101. Fotiadis C, Gugulakis A, Nakopoulou L, *et al.* Primary leiomyosarcoma of the gallbladder. Case report and review of the literature. HPB Surg 1990; 2: 211–14.

102. Hensley ML, Ishill N, Soslow R, *et al.* Adjuvant gemcitabine plus docetaxel for completely resected stages I-IV high grade uterine leiomyosarcoma: Results of a prospective study. Gynecol Oncol 2009; 112: 563–7.

103. Hensley ML, Blessing JA, Mannel R, *et al.* Fixed-dose rate gemcitabine plus docetaxel as first-line therapy for metastatic uterine leiomyosarcoma: a Gynecologic Oncology Group phase II trial. Gynecol Oncol 2008; 109: 329–34.

104. Gruttadauria S, Doria C, Minervini MI, *et al.* Malignant fibrous histiocytoma of the gallbladder: case report and review of the literature. Am Surg 2001; 67: 714–7.

105. Chawla SP, Staddon AP, Baker LH, *et al.* Phase II Study of the mammalian target of rapamycin inhibitor ridaforolimus in patients with advanced bone and soft tissue sarcomas. J Clin Oncol 2012; 30: 78–84.

106. Odashiro AN, Pereira PR, Odashiro Miiji LN, *et al.* Angiosarcoma of the gallbladder: case report and review of the literature. Can J Gastroenterol 2005; 19: 257–9.

107. Rosen A, Thimon S, Ternant D, *et al.* Partial response to bevacizumab of an extensive cutaneous angiosarcoma of the face. Br J Dermatol 2010; 163: 225–7.

108. Skubitz KM, Haddad PA. Paclitaxel and pegylated-liposomal doxorubicin are both active in angiosarcoma. Cancer 2005; 104: 361–6.

109. Meza JL, Anderson J, Pappo AS, *et al.* Analysis of prognostic factors in patients with nonmetastatic rhabdomyosarcoma treated on intergroup rhabdomyosarcoma studies III and IV: the Children's Oncology Group. J Clin Oncol 2006; 24: 3844–51.

110. Spunt SL, Lobe TE, Pappo AS, *et al.* Aggressive surgery is unwarranted for biliary tract rhabdomyosarcoma. J Pediatr Surg 2000; 35: 309–16.

111. De Chiara A, De Rosa V, Lastoria S, *et al.* Primary gastrointestinal stromal tumor of the liver with lung metastases successfully treated with STI-571 (imatinib mesylate). Front Biosci 2006; 11: 498–501.

112. Yamamoto H, Miyamoto Y, Nishihara Y, *et al.* Primary gastrointestinal stromal tumor of the liver with PDGFRA gene mutation. Hum Pathol 2010; 41: 605–9.

113. Dematteo RP, Ballman KV, Antonescu CR, *et al.* Adjuvant imatinib mesylate after resection of localised, primary gastrointestinal stromal tumour: a randomised, double-blind, placebo-controlled trial. Lancet 2009; 373: 1097–104.

114. Joensuu H, DeMatteo RP. The management of gastrointestinal stromal tumors: a model for targeted and multidisciplinary therapy of malignancy. Annu Rev Med 2012; 63: 247–58.

115. Harris NL, Jaffe ES, Stein H, *et al.* A revised European–American classification of lymphoid neoplasms: a proposal from the International Lymphoma Study Group. Blood 1994; 84: 1361–92.

116. Mani H, Climent F, Colomo L, *et al.* Gall bladder and extrahepatic bile duct lymphomas: clinicopathological observations and biological implications. Am J Surg Pathol 2010; 34: 1277–86.

117. Angelopoulou MK, Kontopidou FN, Pangalis GA. Adhesion molecules in B-chronic lymphoproliferative disorders. Semin Hematol 1999; 36:178–97.

118. Lazaridis KN, Gores GJ. Cholangiocarcinoma. Gastroenterology 2005; 128: 1655–67.

119. Shaib YH, Davila JA, McGlynn K, *et al.* Rising incidence of intrahepatic cholangiocarcinoma in the United States: a true increase? J Hepatol 2004; 40: 472–7.

120. Claessen MM, Vleggaar FP, Tytgat KM, *et al.* High lifetime risk of cancer in primary sclerosing cholangitis. J Hepatol 2009; 50: 158–64.

121. Burak K, Angulo P, Pasha TM, *et al.* Incidence and risk factors for cholangiocarcinoma in primary sclerosing cholangitis. Am J Gastroenterol 2004; 99: 523–6.

122. Kornfeld D, Ekbom A, Ihre T. Survival and risk of cholangiocarcinoma in patients with primary sclerosing cholangitis. A population-based study. Scand J Gastroenterol 1997; 32: 1042–5.

123. LaRusso NF, Shneider BL, Black D, *et al.* Primary sclerosing cholangitis: summary of a workshop. Hepatology 2006; 44: 746–64.

124. Welzel TM, Mellemkjaer L, Gloria G, *et al.* Risk factors for intrahepatic cholangiocarcinoma in a low–risk population: a nationwide case-control study. Int J Cancer 2007; 120: 638–41.

125. Kaewpitoon N, Kaewpitoon SJ, Pengsaa P, *et al.* Opisthorchis viverrini: the carcinogenic human liver fluke. World J Gastroenterol 2008; 14: 666–74.

126. Upatham ES, Viyanant V. Opisthorchis viverrini and opisthorchiasis: a historical review and future perspective. Acta Trop 2003; 88: 171–6.

127. Honjo S, Srivatanakul P, Sriplung H, *et al.* Genetic and environmental determinants of risk for cholangiocarcinoma via Opisthorchis viverrini in a densely infested area in Nakhon Phanom, northeast Thailand. Int J Cancer 2005; 117: 854–60.

128. Shin HR, Lee CU, Park HJ, *et al.* Hepatitis B and C virus, Clonorchis sinensis for the risk of liver cancer: a case-control study in Pusan, Korea. Int J Epidemiol 1996; 25: 933–40.

129. Parkin DM, Srivatanakul P, Khlat M, *et al.* Liver cancer in Thailand. I. A case-control study of cholangiocarcinoma. Int J Cancer 1991; 48: 323–8.

130. Soreide K, Korner H, Havnen J, *et al.* Bile duct cysts in adults. Br J Surg 2004; 91: 1538–48.

131. Blechacz BR, Gores GJ. Cholangiocarcinoma. Clin Liver Dis 2008; 12: 131–50, ix.

132. Welzel TM, Graubard BI, Zeuzem S, *et al.* Metabolic syndrome increases the risk of primary liver cancer in the United States: A population-based case-control study. Hepatology 2011; 54: 463–71.

133. Welzel TM, Graubard BI, El-Serag HB, *et al.* Risk factors for intrahepatic and extrahepatic cholangiocarcinoma in the United States: a population-based case-control study. Clin Gastroenterol Hepatol 2007; 5: 1221–8.

134. Koornstra JJ, Mourits MJ, Sijmons RH, *et al.* Management of extracolonic tumours in patients with Lynch syndrome. Lancet Oncol 2009; 10: 400–8.

135. Lee SS, Kim MH, Lee SK, *et al.* Clinicopathologic review of 58 patients with biliary papillomatosis. Cancer 2004; 100: 783–93.

136. Trimbath JD, Griffin C, Romans K, *et al.* Attenuated familial adenomatous polyposis presenting as ampullary adenocarcinoma. Gut 2003; 52: 903–4.

137. Boberg KM, Schrumpf E, Bergquist A, *et al.* Cholangiocarcinoma in primary sclerosing cholangitis: K-ras mutations and Tp53 dysfunction are implicated in the neoplastic development. J Hepatol 2000; 32: 374–80.

138. Jaiswal M, LaRusso NF, Burgart LJ, *et al.* Inflammatory cytokines induce DNA damage and inhibit DNA repair in cholangiocarcinoma cells by a nitric oxide-dependent mechanism. Cancer Res 2000; 60: 184–90.

139. Ishimura N, Isomoto H, Bronk SF, *et al.* Trail induces cell migration and invasion in apoptosis-resistant cholangiocarcinoma cells. Am J Physiol Gastrointest Liver Physiol 2006; 290: G129–36.

140. Humphreys EH, Williams KT, Adams DH, *et al.* Primary and malignant cholangiocytes undergo CD40 mediated Fas dependent apoptosis, but are insensitive to direct activation with exogenous Fas ligand. PLoS One 2010; 5: e14037.

141. Kobayashi S, Werneburg NW, Bronk SF, *et al.* Interleukin-6 contributes to Mcl-1 up-regulation and TRAIL resistance via an Akt-signaling pathway in cholangiocarcinoma cells. Gastroenterology 2005; 128: 2054–65.

142. Yokomuro S, Lunz JG 3rd, Sakamoto T, *et al.* The effect of interleukin-6 (IL-6)/gp130 signalling on biliary epithelial cell growth, in vitro. Cytokine 2000; 12: 727–30.

143. Isa T, Tomita S, Nakachi A, *et al.* Analysis of microsatellite instability, K-ras gene mutation and p53 protein overexpression in intrahepatic cholangiocarcinoma. Hepatogastroenterology 2002; 49: 604–8.

144. Tannapfel A, Benicke M, Katalinic A, *et al.* Frequency of p16(INK4A) alterations and K–ras mutations in intrahepatic cholangiocarcinoma of the liver. Gut 2000; 47: 721–7.

145. Furubo S, Harada K, Shimonishi T, *et al.* Protein expression and genetic alterations of p53 and ras in intrahepatic cholangiocarcinoma. Histopathology 1999; 35: 230–40.

146. Leone F, Cavalloni G, Pignochino Y, *et al.* Somatic mutations of epidermal growth factor receptor in bile duct and gallbladder carcinoma. Clin Cancer Res 2006; 12: 1680–5.

147. Lubner SJ, Mahoney MR, Kolesar JL, *et al.* Report of a multicenter phase II trial testing a combination of biweekly bevacizumab and daily erlotinib in patients with unresectable biliary cancer: a phase II Consortium study. J Clin Oncol 2010; 28: 3491–7.

148. Kim HJ, Yoo TW, Park DI, *et al.* Gene amplification and protein overexpression of HER-2/neu in human extrahepatic cholangiocarcinoma as detected by chromogenic in situ hybridization and immunohistochemistry: its prognostic implication in node-positive patients. Ann Oncol 2007; 18: 892–7.

149. Aishima SI, Taguchi KI, Sugimachi K, *et al.* c-erbB-2 and c-Met expression relates to cholangiocarcinogenesis and progression of intrahepatic cholangiocarcinoma. Histopathology 2002; 40: 269–78.

150. Terada T, Nakanuma Y, Sirica AE. Immunohistochemical demonstration of MET overexpression in human intrahepatic cholangiocarcinoma and in hepatolithiasis. Hum Pathol 1998; 29: 175–80.

151. Zidi SH, Prat F, Le Guen O, *et al.* Performance characteristics of magnetic resonance cholangiography in the staging of malignant hilar strictures. Gut 2000; 46: 103–6.

152. Maccioni F, Martinelli M, Al Ansari N, *et al.* Magnetic resonance cholangiography: past, present and future: a review. Eur Rev Med Pharmacol Sci 2010; 14: 721–5.

153. Levy C, Lymp J, Angulo P, *et al.* The value of serum CA 19-9 in predicting cholangiocarcinomas in patients with primary sclerosing cholangitis. Dig Dis Sci 2005; 50: 1734–40.

154. Kipp BR, Stadheim LM, Halling SA, *et al.* A comparison of routine cytology and fluorescence in situ hybridization for the detection of malignant bile duct strictures. Am J Gastroenterol 2004; 99: 1675–81.

155. Fritcher EG, Kipp BR, Halling KC, *et al.* A multivariable model using advanced cytologic methods for the evaluation of indeterminate pancreatobiliary strictures. Gastroenterology 2009; 136: 2180–6.

156. Heimbach JK, Sanchez W, Rosen CB, *et al.* Trans-peritoneal fine needle aspiration biopsy of hilar cholangiocarcinoma is associated with disease dissemination. HPB (Oxford) 2011; 13: 356–60.

157. Sempoux C, Jibara G, Ward SC, *et al.* Intrahepatic cholangiocarcinoma: new insights in pathology. Semin Liver Dis 2011; 31: 49–60.

158. Jarnagin WR, Fong Y, DeMatteo RP, *et al.* Staging, resectability, and outcome in 225 patients with hilar cholangiocarcinoma. Ann Surg 2001; 234: 507–17.

159. Dinant S, Gerhards MF, Rauws EA, *et al.* Improved outcome of resection of hilar cholangiocarcinoma (Klatskin tumor). Ann Surg Oncol 2006; 13: 872–80.

160. Ito F, Cho CS, Rikkers LF *et al.* Hilar cholangiocarcinoma: current management. Ann Surg 2009; 250: 210–18.

161. Azoulay D, Castaing D, Krissat J, *et al.* Percutaneous portal vein embolization increases the feasibility and safety of major liver resection for hepatocellular carcinoma in injured liver. Ann Surg 2000; 232: 665–72.

162. Farges O, Belghiti J, Kianmanesh R, *et al.* Portal vein embolization before right hepatectomy: prospective clinical trial. Ann Surg 2003; 237: 208–17.

163. Vauthey JN, Chaoui A, Do KA, *et al.* Standardized measurement of the future liver remnant prior to extended liver resection: methodology and clinical associations. Surgery 2000; 127: 512–19.

164. Ijichi M, Makuuchi M, Imamura H, *et al.* Portal embolization relieves persistent jaundice after complete biliary drainage. Surgery 2001; 130: 116–18.

165. Madoff DC, Hicks ME, Vauthey JN, *et al.* Transhepatic portal vein embolization: anatomy, indications, and technical considerations. Radiographics 2002; 22: 1063–76.

166. Neuhaus P, Jonas S, Bechstein WO, *et al.* Extended resections for hilar cholangiocarcinoma. Ann Surg 1999; 230: 808–18; discussion 819.

167. De Jong MC, Nathan H, Sotiropoulos GC, *et al.* Intrahepatic cholangiocarcinoma: an international multi-institutional analysis of prognostic factors and lymph node assessment. J Clin Oncol 2011; 29: 3140–5.

168. Rea DJ, Heimbach JK, Rosen CB. Liver transplantation with neoadjuvant chemoradiation is more effective than resection for hilar cholangiocarcinoma. Ann Surg 2005; 242: 451.

169. Rosen CB. Liver transplantation for cholangiocarcinoma. Transplant Int 2010; 23: 692–7.

170. Hong JC, Petrowsky H, Kaldas FM, *et al.* Predictive index for tumor recurrence after liver transplantation for locally advanced intrahepatic and hilar cholangiocarcinoma. J Am Coll Surg 2011; 212: 514–20.

171. Hong JC, Jones CM, Duffy JP, *et al.* Comparative analysis of resection and liver transplantation for intrahepatic and hilar cholangiocarcinoma: a 24-year experience in a single center. Arch Surg 2011; 146: 683–9.

172. Yamada R, Nakatsuka H, Nakamura K, *et al.* Hepatic artery embolization in 32 patients with unresectable hepatoma. Osaka City Med J 1980; 26: 81–96.

173. Llovet JM, Real MI, Montana X, *et al.* Arterial embolisation or chemoembolisation versus symptomatic treatment in patients with unresectable hepatocellular carcinoma: a randomised controlled trial. Lancet 2002; 359: 1734–9.

174. Burger I, Hong K, Schulick R, *et al.* Transcatheter arterial chemoembolization in unresectable cholangiocarcinoma: initial experience in a single institution. J Vasc Interv Radiol 2005; 16: 353–61.

175. Park SY, Kim JH, Yoon HJ, *et al.* Transarterial chemoembolization versus supportive therapy in the palliative treatment of unresectable intrahepatic cholangiocarcinoma. Clin Radiol 2011; 66: 322–8.

176. Liapi E, Geschwind JF, Vossen JA, *et al.* Functional MRI evaluation of tumor response in patients with neuroendocrine hepatic metastasis treated with transcatheter arterial chemoembolization. Am J Roentgenol 2008; 190: 67–73.

177. Martin RC, Howard J, Tomalty D, *et al.* Toxicity of irinotecan-eluting beads in the treatment of hepatic malignancies: results of a multi-institutional registry. Cardiovasc Intervent Radiol 2010; 33: 960–6.

178. Aliberti C, Tilli M, Benea G, *et al.* Trans-arterial chemoembolization (TACE) of liver metastases from colorectal cancer using irinotecan-eluting beads: preliminary results. Anticancer Res 2006; 26: 3793–5.

179. Goldberg SN, Charboneau JW, Dodd GD 3rd, *et al.* Image-guided tumor ablation: proposal for standardization of terms and reporting criteria. Radiology 2003; 228: 335–45.

180. Kim JH, Won HJ, Shin YM, *et al*. Radiofrequency ablation for the treatment of primary intrahepatic cholangiocarcinoma. Am J Roentgenol 2011; 196: W205–9.

181. Sironi S, Livraghi T, Meloni F, *et al*. Small hepatocellular carcinoma treated with percutaneous RF ablation: MR imaging follow-up. Am J Roentgenol 1999; 173: 1225–9.

182. Rhim H. Complications of radiofrequency ablation in hepatocellular carcinoma. Abdom Imaging 2005; 30: 409–18.

183. Salem R, Hunter RD. Yttrium-90 microspheres for the treatment of hepatocellular carcinoma: a review. Int J Radiat Oncol Biol Phys 2006; 66: S83–8.

184. Salem R, Thurston KG. Radioembolization with 90Yttrium microspheres: a state-of-the-art brachytherapy treatment for primary and secondary liver malignancies. Part 1: Technical and methodologic considerations. J Vasc Interv Radiol 2006; 17: 1251–78.

185. Salem R, Parikh P, Atassi B, *et al*. Incidence of radiation pneumonitis after hepatic intra-arterial radiotherapy with yttrium-90 microspheres assuming uniform lung distribution. Am J Clin Oncol 2008; 31: 431–8.

186. Hoffmann RT, Paprottka PM, Schön A, *et al*. Transarterial hepatic yttrium-90 radioembolization in patients with unresectable intrahepatic cholangiocarcinoma: factors associated with prolonged survival. Cardiovasc Intervent Radiol 2012; 35: 105–16.

187. Albores Saavedra J, Murakata L, Krueger JE, *et al*. Noninvasive and minimally invasive papillary carcinomas of the extrahepatic bile ducts. Cancer 2000; 89: 508–15.

188. Jarnagin WR, Bowne W, Klimstra DS, *et al*. Papillary phenotype confers improved survival after resection of hilar cholangiocarcinoma. Ann Surg 2005; 241: 703–12; discussion 712–14.

189. Sewkani A, Kapoor S, Sharma S, *et al*. Squamous cell carcinoma of the distal common bile duct. JOP 2005; 6: 162–5.

190. Kim KW, Kim SH, Kim MA, *et al*. Adenosquamous carcinoma of the extrahepatic bile duct: clinicopathologic and radiologic features. Abdom Imaging 2009; 34: 217–24.

191. Okabayashi T, Kobayashi M, Nishimori I, *et al*. Adenosquamous carcinoma of the extrahepatic biliary tract: clinicopathological analysis of Japanese cases of this uncommon disease. J Gastroenterol 2005; 40: 192–9.

192. Nakajima T, Tajima Y, Sugano I, *et al*. Intrahepatic cholangiocarcinoma with sarcomatous change. Clinicopathologic and immunohistochemical evaluation of seven cases. Cancer 1993; 72: 1872–7.

193. Malhotra S, Wood J, Mansy T, *et al*. Intrahepatic sarcomatoid cholangiocarcinoma. J Oncol 2010; 2010: 701476.

194. Aishima S, Kuroda Y, Asayama Y, *et al*. Prognostic impact of cholangiocellular and sarcomatous components in combined hepatocellular and cholangiocarcinoma. Hum Pathol 2006; 37: 283–91.

195. Kaibori M, Kawaguchi Y, Yokoigawa N, *et al*. Intrahepatic sarcomatoid cholangiocarcinoma. J Gastroenterol 2003; 38: 1097–101.

196. Wagner MS, Shoup M, Pickleman J, *et al*. Primary malignant melanoma of the common bile duct: a case report and review of the literature. Arch Pathol Lab Med 2000; 124: 419–22.

197. Gates J, Kane RA, Hartnell GG. Primary biliary tract malignant melanoma. Abdom Imaging 1996; 21: 453–5.

198. Wong JH, Skinner KA, Kim KA, *et al*. The role of surgery in the treatment of nonregionally recurrent melanoma. Surgery 1993; 113: 389–94.

199. Hodi FS, O'Day SJ, McDermott DF, *et al*. Improved survival with ipilimumab in patients with metastatic melanoma. N Engl J Med 2010; 363: 711–23.

200. Nicol K, Savell V, Moore J, *et al*. Distinguishing undifferentiated embryonal sarcoma of the liver from biliary tract rhabdomyosarcoma: a Children's Oncology Group study. Pediatr Dev Pathol 2007; 10: 89–97.

201. Jin J, Wei QY, Zhuang ZG, *et al*. Leiomyosarcoma of the common bile duct. Chin Med J (Engl) 1990; 103: 778–80.

202. Chamberlain RS, Blumgart LH. Carcinoid tumors of the extrahepatic bile duct. A rare cause of malignant biliary obstruction. Cancer 1999; 86: 1959–65.

203. Kim J, Lee WJ, Lee SH, *et al*. Clinical features of 20 patients with curatively resected biliary neuroendocrine tumours. Dig Liver Dis 2011; 43: 965–70.

204. Pavel ME, Hainsworth JD, Baudin E, *et al*. Everolimus plus octreotide long-acting repeatable for the treatment of advanced neuroendocrine tumours associated with carcinoid syndrome (RADIANT-2): a randomised, placebo-controlled, phase 3 study. Lancet 2011; 378: 2005–12.

205. Rinke A, Muller HH, Schade-Brittinger C, *et al*. Placebo-controlled, double-blind, prospective, randomized study on the effect of octreotide LAR in the control of tumor growth in patients with metastatic neuroendocrine midgut tumors: a report from the PROMID Study Group. J Clin Oncol 2009; 27: 4656–63.

206. Luigiano C, Ferrara F, Fabbri C, *et al*. Primary lymphoma of the common bile duct presenting with acute pancreatitis and cholangitis. Endoscopy 2010; 42 Suppl 2: E265–6.

207. Hwang DW, Lim CS, Jang JY, *et al*. Primary hematolymphoid malignancies involving the extrahepatic bile duct or gallbladder. Leuk Lymphoma 2010; 51: 1278–87.

208. El-Serag HB. Hepatocellular carcinoma. N Engl J Med 2011; 365: 1118–27.

209. Siegel AB, Olsen SK, Magun A, *et al*. Sorafenib: where do we go from here? Hepatology 2010; 52: 360–9.

210. El-Serag HB, Davila JA. Is fibrolamellar carcinoma different from hepatocellular carcinoma? A US population-based study. Hepatology 2004; 39: 798–803.

211. Liu S, Chan KW, Wang B, *et al*. Fibrolamellar hepatocellular carcinoma. Am J Gastroenterol 2009; 104: 2617–24; quiz 2625.

212. Klein WM, Molmenti EP, Colombani PM, *et al*. Primary liver carcinoma arising in people younger than 30 years. Am J Clin Pathol 2005; 124: 512–18.

213. Zenali MJ, Tan D, Li W, *et al*. Stemness characteristics of fibrolamellar hepatocellular carcinoma: immunohistochemical analysis with comparisons to conventional hepatocellular carcinoma. Ann Clin Lab Sci 2010; 40: 126–34.

214. Kakar S, Chen X, Ho C, *et al*. Chromosomal changes in fibrolamellar hepatocellular carcinoma detected by array comparative genomic hybridization. Mod Pathol 2009; 22: 134–41.

215. Trankenschuh W, Puls F, Christgen M, *et al*. Frequent and distinct aberrations of DNA methylation patterns in fibrolamellar carcinoma of the liver. PLoS One 2010; 5: e13688.

216. Tanaka J, Baba N, Arii S, *et al*. Typical fibrolamellar hepatocellular carcinoma in Japanese patients: report of two cases. Surg Today 1994; 24: 459–63.

217. El-Gazzaz G, Wong W, El-Hadary MK, *et al*. Outcome of liver resection and transplantation for fibrolamellar hepatocellular carcinoma. Transpl Int 2000; 13(Suppl 1): S406–9.

218. Craig JR, Peters RL, Edmondson HA, *et al*. Fibrolamellar carcinoma of the liver: a tumor of adolescents and young adults with distinctive clinico-pathologic features. Cancer 1980; 46: 372–9.

219. Stipa F, Yoon SS, Liau KH, *et al*. Outcome of patients with fibrolamellar hepatocellular carcinoma. Cancer 2006; 106: 1331–8.

220. Llovet JM, Ricci S, Mazzaferro V, *et al*. Sorafenib in advanced hepatocellular carcinoma. N Engl J Med 2008; 359: 378–90.

221. Cheng AL, Kang YK, Chen Z, *et al*. Efficacy and safety of sorafenib in patients in the Asia-Pacific region with advanced hepatocellular carcinoma: a phase III randomised, double-blind, placebo-controlled trial. Lancet Oncol 2009; 10: 25–34.

222. Maniaci V, Davidson BR, Rolles K, *et al*. Fibrolamellar hepatocellular carcinoma: prolonged survival with multimodality therapy. Eur J Surg Oncol 2009; 35: 617–21.

223. Sahin F, Kannangai R, Adegbola O, *et al*. mTOR and P70 S6 kinase expression in primary liver neoplasms. Clin Cancer Res 2004; 10: 8421–5.

224. Jarnagin WR, Weber S, Tickoo SK, *et al*. Combined hepatocellular and cholangiocarcinoma: demographic, clinical, and prognostic factors. Cancer 2002; 94: 2040–6.

225. Ng IO, Shek TW, Nicholls J, *et al*. Combined hepatocellular-cholangiocarcinoma: a clinicopathological study. J Gastroenterol Hepatol 1998; 13: 34–40.

226. Park HS, Bae JS, Jang KY, *et al*. Clinicopathologic study on combined hepatocellular carcinoma and cholangiocarcinoma: with emphasis on the intermediate cell morphology. J Korean Med Sci 2011; 26: 1023–30.

227. Bhagat V, Javle M, Yu J, *et al*. Combined hepatocholangiocarcinoma: case-series and review of literature. Int J Gastrointest Cancer 2006; 37: 27–34.

228. Kim H, Park C, Han KH, *et al*. Primary liver carcinoma of intermediate (hepatocyte-cholangiocyte) phenotype. J Hepatol 2004; 40: 298–304.

229. Panjala C, Senecal DL, Bridges MD, *et al*. The diagnostic conundrum and liver transplantation outcome for combined hepatocellular-cholangiocarcinoma. Am J Transplant 2010; 10: 1263–7.

230. Yano Y, Yamamoto J, Kosuge T, *et al*. Combined hepatocellular and cholangiocarcinoma: a clinicopathologic study of 26 resected cases. Jpn J Clin Oncol 2003; 33: 283–7.

231. Chinnakotla S, Davis GL, Vasani S, *et al*. Impact of sirolimus on the recurrence of hepatocellular carcinoma after liver transplantation. Liver Transpl 2009; 15: 1834–42.

232. Mani H, van Thiel DH. Mesenchymal tumors of the liver. Clin Liver Dis 2001; 5: 219–57, viii.

233. Kim HR, Rha SY, Cheon SH, *et al*. Clinical features and treatment outcomes of advanced stage primary hepatic angiosarcoma. Ann Oncol 2009; 20: 780–7.

234. Donghi D, Dummer R, Cozzio A. Complete remission in a patient with multifocal metastatic cutaneous angiosarcoma with a combination of paclitaxel and sorafenib. Br J Dermatol 2010; 162: 697–9.

235. Fuller CK, Charlson JA, Dankle SK, *et al*. Dramatic improvement of inoperable angiosarcoma with combination paclitaxel and bevacizumab chemotherapy. J Am Acad Dermatol 2010; 63: e83–4.

236. Yoo C, Kim JE, Yoon SK, *et al*. Angiosarcoma of the retroperitoneum: report on a patient treated with sunitinib. Sarcoma 2009; 2009: 360875.

237. Dean PJ, Haggitt RC, O'Hara CJ. Malignant epithelioid hemangioendothelioma of the liver in young women. Relationship to oral contraceptive use. Am J Surg Pathol 1985; 9: 695–704.

238. Makhlouf HR, Ishak KG, Goodman ZD. Epithelioid hemangioendothelioma of the liver: a clinicopathologic study of 137 cases. Cancer 1999; 85: 562–82.

239. Grossman EJ, Millis JM. Liver transplantation for non-hepatocellular carcinoma malignancy: Indications, limitations, and analysis of the current literature. Liver Transpl 2010; 16: 930–42.

240. Salech F, Valderrama S, Nervi B, *et al*. Thalidomide for the treatment of metastatic hepatic epithelioid hemangioendothelioma: a case report with a long term follow-up. Ann Hepatol 2011; 10: 99–102.

241. Trautmann K, Bethke A, Ehninger G, *et al*. Bevacizumab for recurrent hemangioendothelioma. Acta Oncol 2011; 50: 153–4.

242. Ross JS, del Rosario A, Bui HX, *et al*. Primary hepatic leiomyosarcoma in a child with the acquired immunodeficiency syndrome. Hum Pathol 1992; 23: 69–72.

243. Brichard B, Smets F, Sokal E, *et al*. Unusual evolution of an Epstein–Barr virus-associated leiomyosarcoma occurring after liver transplantation. Pediatr Transplant 2001; 5: 365–9.

244. Soyer P, Bluemke DA, Riopel M, *et al*. Hepatic leiomyosarcomas: CT features with pathologic correlation. Eur J Radiol 1995; 19: 177–82.

245. Shamseddine A, Faraj W, Mukherji D, *et al*. Unusually young age distribution of primary hepatic leiomyosarcoma: case series and review of the adult literature. World J Surg Oncol 2010; 8: 56.

246. Anagnostopoulos G, Sakorafas GH, Grigoriadis K, *et al*. Malignant fibrous histiocytoma of the liver: a case report and review of the literature. Mt Sinai J Med 2005; 72: 50–2.

247. Ye MF, Zheng S, Xu JH, *et al*. Primary hepatic malignant fibrous histiocytoma: a case report and review of the literature. Histol Histopathol 2007; 22: 1337–42.

248. Li YR, Akbari E, Tretiakova MS, *et al*. Primary hepatic malignant fibrous histiocytoma: clinicopathologic characteristics and prognostic value of ezrin expression. Am J Surg Pathol 2008; 32: 1144–58.

249. Hu X, Forster J, Damjanov I. Primary malignant gastrointestinal stromal tumor of the liver. Arch Pathol Lab Med 2003; 127: 1606–8.

250. Yao JC, Hassan M, Phan A, *et al*. One hundred years after "carcinoid": epidemiology of and prognostic factors for neuroendocrine tumors in 35,825 cases in the United States. J Clin Oncol 2008; 26: 3063–72.

251. Wang SC, Parekh JR, Zuraek MB, *et al*. Identification of unknown primary tumors in patients with neuroendocrine liver metastases. Arch Surg 2010; 145: 276–80.

252. Ramage JK, Davies AH, Ardill J, *et al*. Guidelines for the management of gastroenteropancreatic neuroendocrine (including carcinoid) tumours. Gut 2005; 54(Suppl 4): iv, 1–16.

253. Ruutiainen AT, Soulen MC, Tuite CM, *et al*. Chemoembolization and bland embolization of neuroendocrine tumor metastases to the liver. J Vasc Interv Radiol 2007; 18: 847–55.

254. Warner RR, Mani S, Profeta J, *et al*. Octreotide treatment of carcinoid hypertensive crisis. Mt Sinai J Med 1994; 61: 349–55.

255. Mayo SC, de Jong MC, Bloomston M, *et al*. Surgery versus intra-arterial therapy for neuroendocrine liver metastasis: a multicenter international analysis. Ann Surg Oncol 2011; 18: 3657–65.

256. Sangoi AR, Ohgami RS, Pai RK, *et al*. PAX8 expression reliably distinguishes pancreatic well-differentiated neuroendocrine tumors from ileal and pulmonary well-differentiated neuroendocrine tumors and pancreatic acinar cell carcinoma. Mod Pathol 2011; 24: 412–24.

257. Yao JC, Shah MH, Ito T, *et al*. Everolimus for advanced pancreatic neuroendocrine tumors. N Engl J Med 2011; 364: 514–23.

258. Raymond E, Dahan L, Raoul JL, *et al*. Sunitinib malate for the treatment of pancreatic neuroendocrine tumors. N Engl J Med 2011; 364: 501–13.

259. Choi SJ, Kim JM, Han JY, *et al*. Extrapulmonary small cell carcinoma of the liver: clinicopathological and immunohistochemical findings. Yonsei Med J 2007; 48: 1066–71.

260. Morikawa H, Nakayama Y, Maeda T, *et al*. A case of primary small cell carcinoma of the liver that was treated with chemotherapy. Hepatol Int 2008; 2: 500–4.

261. Schnater JM, Kohler SE, Lamers WH, *et al*. Where do we stand with hepatoblastoma? A review. Cancer 2003; 98: 668–78.

262. Groen EJ, Roos A, Muntinghe FL, *et al*. Extra-intestinal manifestations of familial adenomatous polyposis. Ann Surg Oncol 2008; 15: 2439–50.

263. Roebuck DJ, Perilongo G. Hepatoblastoma: an oncological review. Pediatr Radiol 2006; 36: 183–6.

264. Otte JB, Pritchard J, Aronson DC, *et al*. Liver transplantation for hepatoblastoma: results from the International Society of Pediatric Oncology (SIOP) study SIOPEL-1 and review of the world experience. Pediatr Blood Cancer 2004; 42: 74–83.

265. Lederman SM, Martin EC, Laffey KT, *et al*. Hepatic neurofibromatosis, malignant schwannoma, and angiosarcoma in von Recklinghausen's disease. Gastroenterology 1987; 92: 234–9.

266. Grewal S, Merchant T, Reymond R, *et al*. Auditory late effects of childhood cancer therapy: a report from the Children's Oncology Group. Pediatrics 2010; 125: e938–50.

267. Sivaprakasam P, Gupta AA, Greenberg ML, *et al*. Survival and long-term outcomes in children with hepatoblastoma treated with continuous infusion of cisplatin and doxorubicin. J Pediatr Hematol Oncol 2011; 33: e226–30.

268. Noronha V, Shafi NQ, Obando JA, *et al*. Primary non-Hodgkin's lymphoma of the liver. Crit Rev Oncol Hematol 2005; 53: 199–207.

269. Belhadj K, Reyes F, Farcet JP, *et al*. Hepatosplenic gammadelta T-cell lymphoma is a rare clinicopathologic entity with poor outcome: report on a series of 21 patients. Blood 2003; 102: 4261–9.

31 Cancers of the Small Bowel

Kanwal Raghav,[1] **Matthew H. G. Katz,**[2] **and Michael J. Overman**[3]

[1] Division of Cancer Medicine, [2] Department of Surgical Oncology, [3] Department of Gastrointestinal Medical Oncology, The University of Texas MD Anderson Cancer Center, Houston, TX, USA

Introduction

Small bowel tumors are exceedingly rare.[1,2] They account for about 0.4% of all cancers in the United States and nearly 2% of all gastrointestinal malignancies.[3] Approximately 6960 new cases of small bowel cancers and 1100 patient deaths were expected to occur in the United States in 2010.[2] Both benign and malignant tumors may arise throughout the small intestine; in addition, metastatic lesions from various primary tumors can also be seen. Small bowel cancer is a compendium of exceptionally diverse tumors with regard to histology, presentation, prognosis, and management.[4]

The vast disparity in the incidence between cancers of the large bowel (~50/100,000 population) and small bowel (~3/100,000 population) is remarkable.[2] Several theories have been proposed to explain this difference, based chiefly on the premise that the unique microenvironment of the small bowel protects against carcinogenic stimuli. The relative alkaline dilution of the food and secretions coupled with a rapid transit and low bacterial load minimizes exposure to potential carcinogens.[5] In addition, it is hypothesized that the abundant lymphoid tissue and IgA levels in the small bowel provide an enhanced tumor immunity.[6] Recently, the differing rate of mutations in the adenomatous polyposis coli gene have been suggested to explain this discrepancy in incidence for adenocarcinomas of the small (rare mutations) and large (near universal mutations) intestine.[7-10]

The small intestine is 6–7 meters long, representing approximately 75% of the length and over 90% of the surface area of the alimentary tract. It extends from the pylorus to the ileocolic valve. The small intestine is divided into three portions: the duodenum, the jejunum, and the ileum.[11] The duodenum represent the first 25 cm of the small intestine and is further divided into four portions: the superior portion (first portion), the descending portion (second portion), the horizontal portion (third portion), and the ascending portion (fourth portion). Aside from the proximal aspect of the first portion of the duodenum, the duodenum is a retroperitoneal structure with no mesentery. The duodenum ends at the duodenojejunal flexure which is surrounded by a fold of peritoneum called the ligament of Treitz. The remaining part of the small bowel is divided into jejunum (proximal two-fifths) and ileum (distal three-fifths) based on histological and structural differences. The jejunum is wider, has larger mucosal circular folds (plicae circulares), longer terminal arteries (vasa recta), and more villi compared to the ileum. The ileum has larger lymphoid aggregates (Peyer's patches), more mesenteric fat, and more prominent arterial arcades.[11] Overall, small bowel cancers tend to occur most commonly in the ileum (33%) followed by duodenum (25%) and jejunum (16%).[12] However, histological subtypes vary in their distribution (Fig. 31.1).[3]

In this chapter we will discuss the unusual malignant neoplasms of the small bowel. Since carcinoid tumors (44%) have surpassed adenocarcinomas (33%) as the most common small bowel tumors, these will be discussed only as background.[4] To provide an overall assessment of the various histological subtypes of small bowel cancer, the distribution of 1360 small bowel cancer cases seen at the University of Texas, MD Anderson Cancer Center from 2000 to 2010 is presented in Table 31.1.

Epidemiology

The incidence of small bowel cancers has been increasing over the past two decades, rising from 10.5 cases in 1980–1986 to 14.9 cases in 1994–2000 per 100,000 individuals.[3] This clearly has resulted from an increase in incidence of carcinoid tumors, as there has been no evident change in rates of adenocarcinomas and other cancers.[4] The incidence of small bowel cancers increases with age with minor variations depending on the histology.[12,13] The median age of presentation for small bowel adenocarcinomas is 65 years, with nearly 90% of cases occurring over the age of 40 years.[3,12,14]

Textbook of Uncommon Cancer, Fourth Edition. Edited by Derek Raghavan, Charles D. Blanke, David H. Johnson, Paul L. Moots, Gregory H. Reaman, Peter G. Rose and Mikkael A. Sekeres.

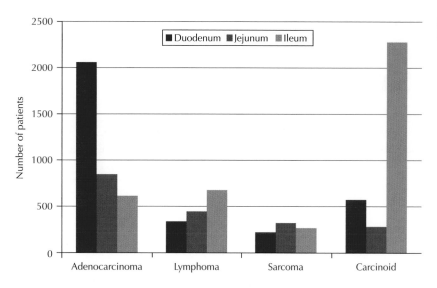

Figure 31.1 Small bowel cancer by site and histology. Data derived from Shottenfeld *et al.*[93]

Table 31.1 Malignant tumors of the small bowel, MD Anderson Cancer Center 2000–2010 (*n* = 1360).

Histological subtype	Number	Percentage
Adenocarcinoma	332	24%
Not otherwise specified	251	
Signet ring	24	
Mucinous	52	
Squamous variant	3	
Sarcomatoid variant	2	
Lymphoma	66	5%
Diffuse large B cell	29	
Follicular	25	
Mucosa-associated lymphoid tissue	4	
Peripheral T cell lymphoma	4	
Other	4	
Neuroendocrine	613	45%
Well differentiated, carcinoid	547	
Moderately differentiated	61	
Poorly differentiated, small cell	4	
Islet cell	1	
Sarcoma	345	25%
Gastrointestinal stromal tumor	261	
Leiomyosarcoma	42	
Desmoid	9	
Unclassified	20	
Other	13	
Melanoma	4	<1%

Lymphomas and sarcomas tend to occur at a slightly younger age (60 years and 62 years, respectively) as compared to adenocarcinomas, but then show a more gradual increase with age.[12,13] Small bowel cancers have a slight male predominance with a male-to-female ratio of 1.5:1.[12] Males have a higher incidence of all histological subtypes, especially lymphomas, which are diagnosed twice as frequently in men as in women.[13] While African-Americans have a 40% higher risk than whites for small bowel adenocarcinoma, their risk for small bowel lymphoma is approximately one-half that for Caucasians.[1]

Though a number of studies have investigated the role of various environmental and dietary factors in the causation of small bowel cancer, no consistent relationships have been identified.[15–19] The strongest predisposition to small bowel cancer relates to the presence of either a familial cancer syndrome, such as hereditary nonpolyposis colorectal cancer (HNPCC), familial adenomatous polyposis (FAP) and Peutz–Jeghers syndrome, or the presence of chronic small bowel inflammation, such as seen with celiac disease and inflammatory bowel disease (IBD).

Clinical presentation

Small bowel tumors are difficult to diagnose, due to their relative rarity and nonspecific and variable symptomatology. Delays from symptom initiation to diagnosis of 4–7 months are common and frequently result in patients presenting with advanced stages of disease.[4,20–22] The most commonly reported symptoms are abdominal pain (44–63%), nausea and vomiting (17–48%), weight loss (12–44%), and gastrointestinal bleeding (14–37%).[21,23,24] In general, malignant tumors of the small bowel are more likely to be symptomatic than are benign tumors. This is reflected in autopsy series, in which benign tumors represent a much higher percentage of small intestinal tumors. About one-quarter of patients with malignant small bowel tumors present with obstruction and less than 10% present with perforation.%).[24–27] Patients may also present with nonspecific symptoms such as early satiety, fatigue, lethargy, constipation, and anorexia. Patients with metastatic carcinoids, and in particular patients with extensive liver metastases, may demonstrate symptoms of the carcinoid syndrome, which is characterized by flushing, diarrhea, wheezing, abdominal cramping, and right-sided cardiac valvular dysfunction.

Diagnosis

Early diagnosis entails a high index of suspicion. Because imaging of the small intestine is difficult, multiple tests may be

Figure 31.2 (a) Small bowel follow-through (SBFT) showing intussuseption (*arrows*) from a diffuse large B cell lymphoma in the small bowel. (b) SBFT showing an "apple core" stricture (*arrow*) from a jejunal adenocarcinoma. (c) CT showing a mesenteric mass (*arrows*) with tethering of small bowel loops due to desmoplastic reaction representing mesenteric nodal metastasis from a small bowel carcinoid. (d) CT showing multiple heterogeneously enhancing liver metastases from a small bowel GIST metastatic to liver.

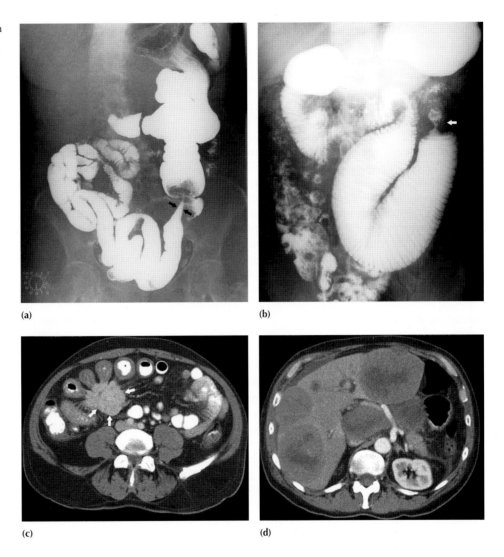

(a)

(b)

(c)

(d)

needed. Excluding patients presenting with the carcinoid syndrome, the nonspecific nature of small bowel cancer symptoms rarely suggests a specific histological subtype. Hence the preoperative diagnosis of small bowel cancers relies heavily upon radiographic and endoscopic evaluations.

Plain abdominal radiography is of limited utility but may demonstrate small bowel obstruction. The upper gastrointestinal (GI) series with small bowel follow-through has historically represented the gold standard for small bowel evaluation. In patients with advanced-stage disease, this technique has a sensitivity of approximately 60% for diagnosing small bowel tumors (Fig. 31.2a,b).[28,29] However, cross-sectional imaging and capsule endoscopy have now supplanted this modality in the diagnosis of small bowel tumors. Enteroclysis, in which contrast material is infused directly into the small intestine through a nasogastric tube, provides a slightly higher sensitivity than small bowel follow-through (sensitivity 61–95%).[28] Newer computed tomography (CT) or magnetic resonance imaging (MRI)-based enterography, utilizing negative oral contrast agents such as water or mannitol substituted for positive contrast media such as barium or gastrografin, are able to achieve adequate small bowel distension and evaluate both the

luminal as well as extraluminal extent of disease.[30,31] In a series of 219 patients, CT enterography showed sensitivity, specificity, negative predictive, and positive predictive values of 85%, 97%, 95%, and 91% respectively.[32] Three-dimensional imaging with either CT or MRI is critical to identifying locoregional lymph node involvement and the presence of distant metastatic disease (Fig. 31.2c,d).[25,33] For neuroendocrine tumors, an OctreoScan, which utilizes indium 111-labeled octreotide, is able to image somatostatin receptor-positive tumors and can detect additional metastatic disease beyond standard cross-sectional imaging in approximately 5–10% of patients.[34]

Endoscopic evaluation of the small bowel has been limited by the length of the small intestine which can measure up to 7 meters. Push enteroscopy, which involves the examination of the small bowel with a long enteroscope, is generally only able to visualize into the proximal jejunum. Double-balloon enteroscopy is able to visualize the entire small bowel, though it is technically challenging and only available at specialized centers.[35–37] The recent incorporation of wireless capsule endoscopy has dramatically improved the ability to visualize the entire small bowel lumen. In a metaanalysis evaluating 32 studies in which capsule endoscopy was prospectively compared to a comparator technique (push enteroscopy, small bowel series, or colonoscopy with ileoscopy), a total of 106 neoplasms was identified.[36] Capsule endoscopy identified 81% of these lesions while the comparator technique identified only 37%. Tissue acquisition is not possible with capsule endoscopy and the presence of small bowel obstruction is a contraindication to its use.

Laboratory testing can reveal iron deficiency anemia resulting from either overt or occult gastrointestinal tract bleeding. Approximately 30% of cases will test positive for fecal occult blood.[21] Both carcinoembryonic antigen (CEA) and carbohydrate antigen 19-9 (CA-19-9) are elevated in about 30% and 40% of patients with advanced small bowel adenocarcinomas, but these are neither specific nor sensitive enough for diagnosis.[38] Because neuroendocrine carcinomas have the ability to secrete bioactive amines and peptides, laboratory tests for elevated levels of chromogranin A in the blood and 5-hydroxyindoleacetic acid (5-HIAA) in a 24-h urine collection are useful. Elevated levels of 5-HIAA are frequently seen in patients with the carcinoid syndrome.[39]

Staging

The staging of small bowel cancer is dependent upon the tumor type. Small bowel adenocarcinomas and gastrointestinal stromal tumors are staged according to specific American Joint Committee on Cancer (AJCC) 7th edition TNM staging systems.[40] Lymphomas are staged according to the standard Ann Arbor staging system or the Lugano staging system for gastrointestinal lymphomas.[41] Carcinoids are generally staged according to the disease categories of localized, regional, or metastatic, although a specific AJCC TNM 7th edition staging system does exist. Non-GIST sarcomas are staged according to the AJCC 7th edition TNM staging for soft tissue sarcomas.

Adenocarcinoma

Biology

Carcinogenesis for small bowel adenocarcinoma appears to occur via a similar phenotypic adenoma to carcinoma transformation as occurs in colorectal cancers.[42,43] From a molecular perspective, a number of alterations, such as 18q loss,[44] p53 loss,[45,46] and activating mutations in kras[7,47] occur at similar rates in both small and large bowel adenocarcinoma. Surprisingly, mutations in the adenomatous polyposis coli (APC) gene differ markedly between small bowel adenocarcinoma (7–13%)[7,8] and large bowel adenocarcinoma (60–68%).[9,10] In addition, this molecular difference correlates with the lower rate of adenomas within the small intestine and suggests that adenoma initiation may be partially responsible for the differing incidence between these two intestinal adenocaricnomas.[48] Despite the lack of APC mutations, abnormalities in the WNT pathway are seen with frequent loss of E-cadherin expression and nuclear localization of β-catenin.[49,50] In addition, as is seen in colorectal cancer, a subset of small bowel adenocarcinomas are characterized by defects in mismatch repair or microsatellite instability-high phenotype

(MSI-H). This rate appears slightly higher than that seen in colorectal cancer at 18–35%,[50,51] which may reflect the high rate of MSI-H in small bowel adenocarcinoma patients with coexisting celiac disease, 67–73%.[52,53] In all celiac-associated MSI-H small bowel adenocarcinomas, hypermethylation of the hMLH1 promoter was responsible.[52]

The majority of small bowel adenocarcinomas are sporadic and localized to either the duodenum, potentially reflecting the possible carcinogenic effects of pancreaticobiliary secretions, or sites of small bowel inflammation. In particular, both celiac disease and IBD are characterized by an increased risk of small bowel adenocarcinoma.[54,55] For patients with IBD, the increase in risk varies depending on both the extent and duration of small bowel involvement. In one study, the cumulative risk of small bowel adenocarcinoma in patients with Crohn's disease was 0.2% at 10 years and 2.2% at 25 years.[56] Because Crohn's disease frequently involves the ileum, 70% of the small bowel cancers in patients with Crohn's disease will occur in the ileum. Gluten-sensitive enteropathy or celiac disease is an autoimmune disorder of the small bowel triggered by the environmental agent, gluten. Chronic small bowel inflammation leads to villous atrophy and an increased risk for the development of both adenocarcinoma (hazard ratio 1.9) and lymphoma (hazard ratio 4.8).[57]

A number of familial cancer syndromes, including HNPCC, FAP, and Peutz–Jeghers, have been associated with an increased risk of small bowel adenocarcinoma. Patients with HNPCC develop small bowel adenocarcinoma at a younger age, with a median age at diagnosis of 49 years. Patients with Peutz–Jeghers syndrome, an autosomal dominant polyposis disorder characterized by multiple hamartomatous polyps throughout the intestinal tract, have a markedly increased risk for small bowel adenocarcinoma.[58] Duodenal adenomas are seen in approximately 80% of patients with FAP, and these patients require regular endoscopic screening for the development of adenocarcinoma. The estimated lifetime risk for small bowel adenocarcinoma is 1–4% in patients with HNPCC, 5% in those with FAP, and 13% in those with Peutz–Jeghers syndrome.[58–61]

Pathology

Adenocarcinomas of the small bowel appear histologically similar to adenocarcinomas of colonic origin. In general, the clinical situation that presents the most diagnostic confusion occurs when transmural involvement of the small bowel is present in the context of peritoneal metastases. As small bowel adenocarcinoma is a rare disease, alternative primary cancer sites should be entertained. The presence of a precursor lesion and immunohistochemical stains can aid in the diagnosis of primary small bowel adenocarcinoma. Though the expression profile of cytokeratin 7 and cytokeratin 20 is variable, the intestinal marker CDX-2 is expressed in 70% of cases and represents the most useful marker.[50] Differentiation for small bowel adenocarcinomas is variable, though a higher rate of poor histological grade is seen for small as opposed to large bowel adenocarcinomas per the Surveillance, Epidemiology and End Results (SEER) registry: 32% versus

20%, p <0.01. The most common variants of adenocarcinoma are characterized by mucinous and signet ring cell histology. Though signet ring cell histology has been correlated with a more aggressive clinical course in other intestinal carcinomas, the impact for small bowel adenocarcinoma is not known. Additional rare subsets are adenosquamous, sarcomatoid, and pure squamous variants. In general, the approach for these rare subtypes remains unchanged from that for standard adenocarcinomas.

Clinical presentation

The incidence of small bowel adenocarcinoma peaks in the seventh and eighth decades, with a mean age at diagnosis of 65 years. The majority of tumors are localized to the duodenum. The most commonly reported symptoms are abdominal pain (45–76% of patients), nausea and vomiting (31–52%), weight loss (22–29%), and gastrointestinal bleeding (8–34%).[21,23,62–65] According to the National Cancer Database, 39% of patients present with stage I/II disease, 26% present with stage III disease, and 32% present with stage IV disease.[22]

Treatment considerations

Resectable disease

Surgery is the definitive treatment for localized small bowel adenocarcinomas (5-year survival in resected versus unresected cases is 54% versus 0%).[66,67] A wide surgical resection with negative surgical margins and local lymph node removal is critical for optimal outcome.[68–71] Based upon the proximity to the ampulla of Vater, lesions located in the duodenum, especially the second portion, may require a pancreaticoduodenectomy. For small distal lesions in the third and fourth portions of the duodenum, a wide local excision may be an option.[66,69,71–73] The only study showing survival benefit for a pancreaticoduodenectomy compared to segmental resection had a surprisingly high margin positive rate, 23%, in the limited surgery group.[69] However, recent data have suggested that duodenal adenocarcinomas are frequently understaged and that obtaining eight or more lymph nodes is strongly correlated with improved survival.[74,75] Thus, if negative resection margins and an appropriate nodal assessment (eight or more lymph nodes) can be achieved, the choice of surgical resection for distal duodenal adenocarcinomas does not appear to affect overall survival (OS). For jejunum or ileal adenocarcinomas, wide excision with a primary anastomosis is appropriate, and a right hemicolectomy is typically indicated for tumors of the distal/terminal ileum.

In multivariate analyses the factors most correlated with outcome have included lymph node involvement, tumor stage, resection margin status, and poor differentiation.[4,22,65,67,76] Moreover, in a recent SEER registry analysis, the total number of assessed lymph nodes was found to strongly correlate with cancer-specific survival (CSS) in resected stage I, II, and III adenocarcinomas of the small bowel (p <0.001).[75] For patients who had ≥8 total lymph nodes (TLNs) assessed, 5-year CSS rates for stages I, II, and III were 95%, 83%, and 56%,

respectively, while the outcome for patients with 1–7 TLNs was 93%, 69%, and 43%, respectively.[75] Stage I and II patients with no assessed lymph nodes had markedly worse outcomes with 5-year CSS rates of 70% for stage I and 44% for stage II disease.[75]

There are limited data evaluating the role of adjuvant therapy in small bowel adenocarcinoma. No prospective studies exist, and retrospective studies have demonstrated mixed results regarding the potential benefit.[67,69,71,77–80] In a subset analysis of patients ($n=30$) with high-risk disease (lymph node ratio ≥10%) treated with adjuvant systemic chemotherapy, adjuvant therapy was seen to improve median OS (>12 years versus 2 years, $p=0.04$).[77] However, a similar subset analysis in patients with positive lymph nodes ($n=105$), who had undergone complete resection, showed no benefit from the use of adjuvant chemotherapy or chemoradiation therapy (median OS 30.2 months versus 26.5 months, $p=0.36$).[78] However, over the last few decades, the use of adjuvant chemotherapy for patients with resected small bowel adenocarcinoma has increased.[4,12]

Despite the lack of conclusive data, the use of adjuvant therapy is reasonable based upon the known poor prognosis of high-risk disease, predominantly systemic relapse pattern, proven chemotherapy activity in the metastatic setting, and known benefit of adjuvant therapy in large bowel adenocarcinoma. A fluoropyrimidine with or without oxaliplatin would represent an appropriate chemotherapy choice. The use of concurrent fluoropyrimidine-based radiation therapy in either the neoadjuvant or adjuvant setting for duodenal adenocarcinomas can be considered given the known increased local recurrence risk for duodenal primaries, though data supporting this approach are limited.[81,82]

Metastatic disease

Systemic chemotherapy for patients with advanced small bowel adenocarcinoma has been shown to improve overall survival as compared with no treatment, in many retrospective reviews.[67,83,84] In the largest review of 163 patients with metastatic small bowel adenocarcinoma, patients with stage IV disease receiving chemotherapy survived longer than those without treatment (median OS 15.5 months versus 3.3 months, $p=0.001$).[78] Only two prospective phase 2 studies have been conducted in small bowel adenocarcinoma. One multicenter study conducted by the Eastern Cooperative Oncology Group using the combination of 5-fluorouracil (5-FU), doxorubicin, and mitomycin-C (FAM) in 39 patients reported an overall response rate of 18% and a median OS of 8 months.[85] A single-institution study conducted at the University of Texas MD Anderson Cancer Center evaluated the use of capecitabine and oxaliplatin (CAPOX, capecitabine 750 mg/m² twice daily on days 1 through 14, and oxaliplatin 130 mg/m² on day 1, every 21 days) in 30 patients with metastatic or locally advanced small bowel or ampullary adenocarcinomas. The overall response rate was 50%, and in the metastatic-only subset ($n=25$), the median time to progression was 6.6 months and the median OS was 15.5 months.[86] No randomized trials comparing different chemotherapy regimens have been done for adenocarcinoma of the small bowel.

However, additional retrospective studies have supported the use of a fluoropyrimidine and oxaliplatin as initial therapy.[38,87] The largest retrospective analysis ($n=93$) evaluating chemotherapy for advanced small bowel adenocarcinomas found fluorouracil and oxaliplatin (FOLFOX) to be the most active regimen, with a 34% response rate and 17.8 month median OS.[38] Several retrospective studies have confirmed the substantial activity of 5-FU combined with a platinum agent for metastatic small bowel adenocarcinoma, with response rates of 18–46%.[83,87–89] Irinotecan is also active in small bowel adenocarcinoma, with the largest reported study noting a 20% response rate and 3.5-month median progression-free survival among 25 patients treated with fluorouracil and irinotecan (FOLFIRI) in the second-line setting.[90] An additional study of irinotecan in either the first- or second-line setting reported a tumor response in five of 12 treated patients.[83] Responses to gemcitabine-based therapy have also been noted, though the number of patients treated has been small.[83,87] The role of targeted therapies against the vascular endothelial growth factor or epidermal growth factor receptors has not been studied in small bowel adenocarcinoma. Long-term survivors have been reported with the use of metastatectomy, though appropriate patient selection is critical to such an approach.[91]

Sarcoma

Gastrointestinal stromal tumor (GIST) has been discussed in detail in Chapter 33, but for completeness, we note the following key points.

Malignant mesenchymal tumors of small bowel constitute approximately 10% of all small bowel neoplasms.[22,92] Sarcomas are most common in the jejunum, 40%, followed by ileum, 33%, and duodenum, 23%.[93] They are classified broadly in two categories, namely gastrointestinal stromal tumors (GISTs) and non-GIST gastrointestinal sarcomas including leiomyosarcoma, liposarcoma, fibrosarcoma, and angiosarcoma.[4] The vast majority of small bowel sarcomas, approximately 85%, are GISTs.[94]

Non-gastrointestinal stromal tumor gastrointestinal sarcomas

Pathology
Multiple different types of non-GIST sarcomas have been identified in the small bowel. Leiomyosarcomas (LMS) represent the most common non-GIST histology. In a review of 590 small bowel sarcomas from the National Cancer Database, the other common sarcomas were Kaposi sarcoma, spindle cell sarcoma, and malignant fibrous histiocytomas.[92] Kaposi sarcoma of the small bowel is most commonly seen in the presence of the acquired immunodeficiency syndrome (AIDS), where it often presents as gastrointestinal bleeding.

Clinical presentation
The median age of presentation is 61 years, with the majority of patients, 73%, presenting with locoregional disease.[92] Desmoid tumors are a rare form of sarcoma that can occur sporadically but also in association with FAP. Approximately 10–20% of FAP will develop desmoids, which frequently occur intraabdominally at surgical resection sites. Though these tumors do not have the capacity to metastasize, they are locally invasive and have a high recurrence rate following surgical resection. In patients with FAP, desmoids are the cause of death in approximately 10% of patients.[95]

Treatment
Localized sarcomas of the small bowel are managed by *en bloc* resection of the tumor, which may include adjacent organs, in order to achieve a margin-negative resection. Tumor-free margins are essential for both local control and overall survival outcome. Sarcomas rarely metastasize to regional lymph nodes, hence dissection of lymph nodes is not required. Intraabdominal desmoids in the context of FAP are often unresectable, due to the diffuse infiltration of the surrounding mesentery. For such cases, observation in slowly growing cases or medical therapy is indicated. The role of adjuvant or neoadjuvant chemotherapy for non-GIST small bowel sarcomas is undefined.[96] Metastatic non-GIST small bowel sarcomas are managed as per therapy modeled for soft tissue sarcomas.[97] Treatment is palliative and histological subtype will guide the choice of systemic chemotherapy. Surgical resection of metastatic disease in selected settings (isolated pulmonary metastatic lesion) may extend survival and potentially even enable cure. Asymptomatic patients with low-grade sarcomas should be followed with active surveillance and treated for symptoms or progression. LMS can be treated with gemcitabine-based chemotherapy or an anthracycline/ifosfamide combination.[98] Angiosarcomas and Kaposi sarcoma should be treated with pegylated liposomal doxorubicin. Other histologies that are chemotherapy sensitive (e.g. malignant fibrous histiocytomas or high-grade pleomorphic sarcoma) can be treated with anthracyclines and ifosfamide as combination therapy or sequential agents.

Lymphoma

Biology and pathology

Gastrointestinal involvement is seen in nearly 50% of all lymphomas,[99] making the GI tract the most common extranodal site involved.[100] Lymphomas involving the GI tract can be either primary (with no peripheral lymphadenopathy, no bone marrow, and no other organ involvement) or secondary (as a manifestation of systemic lymphoma). About 12% of all primary GI lymphomas are found in the small bowel and lymphomas constitute about 15–20% of all small bowel tumors.[22,93,101] The majority of primary small bowel non-Hodgkin lymphomas (NHLs) are of B cell origin, such as diffuse large B cell lymphoma (DLBCL), mantle cell lymphoma, Burkitt and Burkitt-like lymphoma, marginal zone B cell lymphoma of mucosa-associated lymphoid tissue (MALT), small lymphocytic lymphoma, and follicular lymphoma.[100,101] Up to one-quarter of NHLs will be of T cell origin, such as peripheral enteropathy-associated T cell lymphoma.[100,101] Hodgkin lymphoma of the small bowel is extremely rare.[102,103] The etiology and pathogenesis of small bowel lymphomas are complex and partly related to chronic immune stimulation. Immunoproliferative small intestinal disease, also known as α chain disease due to the secretion of immunoglobulin α heavy chains, is a type of small intestinal MALT lymphoma that is induced by chronic antigentic stimulation from *Campylobacter jejuni* infection of the small intestine.[104] Celiac disease, an autoimmune disorder of the small bowel, increases the risk of NHLs, and in particular T cell subtype NHL.[105,106]

Clinical presentation

The incidence of lymphomas increases distally in the small bowel, with the ileum as the most common site (60%), followed by jejunum (30%) and duodenum (10%).[93] Staging for primary intestinal lymphomas is based upon the Lugano staging system in which stage I is defined as disease confined to the intestine, stage II disease involving intraabdominal lymph nodes or adjacent organs, and stage IV disseminated extranodal or supradiaphragmatic nodal involvement.[41] The most common presenting symptoms of small bowel lymphomas are pain (75%), anorexia (40%), weight loss (30%), and B-symptoms (15%).[101]

Treatment

Treatment of extranodal lymphomas involving the small bowel is similar to standard therapy for the corresponding nodal histological subtype.[107] Localized intestinal lymphomas can be managed with surgical resection, but outcomes following surgery alone are poor.[108] Systemic chemotherapy is therefore recommended after surgical removal. A recent retrospective cohort study of 250 localized intestinal DLBCL patients, in which over 90% had primary small bowel involvement, demonstrated an improvement in 3-year OS for patients treated with surgical resection and systemic chemotherapy in comparison to systemic chemotherapy alone, 91% versus 62%, $p <0.001$.[109]

Observant management for indolent lymphomas should be done unless they become symptomatic or show evidence of progression. A recent retrospective study of 63 patients with primary follicular lymphoma of the duodenum demonstrated a remarkably indolent course and rare, 3%, rate of transformation into high-grade disease.[110] Early-stage MALT lymphoma may benefit from *Helicobacter pylori* eradication as utilized for gastric MALT lymphoma, though the benefit is not known.[111] Early-stage immunoproliferative small intestinal disease responds to antibiotics for the treatment of *Campylobacter jejuni* and advanced stage disease is treated with anthracycline-based chemotherapy and antibiotics. Aggressive lymphomas and symptomatic cases of indolent lymphomas are treated with chemotherapy regimens such as R-CHOP (rituximab, cyclophosphamide, vincristine, doxorubicin and dexamethasone), Hyper-CVAD (rituximab, cyclophosphamide, vincristine, doxorubicin and dexamethasone), bendamustine, or bortezomib.[112] High-dose chemotherapy and hematopoietic stem cell transplantation may be beneficial in poor prognosis lymphomas such as mantle cell lymphoma or peripheral T cell lymphomas. Given the poor radiation tolerance of the small intestine, radiotherapy has a limited role in the curative treatment of patients with small bowel lymphoma, but can be considered as a palliative measure for management of bleeding, pain or obstruction.[113]

Uncommon neuroendocrine carcinomas

Small cell carcinomas

Poorly differentiated neuroendocrine carcinomas or small cell carcinomas represent a rare but extremely aggressive subtype of neuroendocrine carcinomas. These cancers are characterized by an aggressive natural history with early metastatic spread. In one retrospective series of small cell carcinomas of the gastrointestinal tract, small bowel represented the primary site in 3% of cases.[114] For this entire 64-patient cohort, the median OS was 11 months and did not differ by gastrointestinal location. Treatment is based upon treatment for the more common small cell lung carcinoma and should include the use of a platin and a topoisomerase inhibitor. Given the aggressive behavior, the use of adjuvant chemotherapy should be consider for resected localized disease.

Islet cell carcinomas

Islet cells of the small bowel are extremely rare and are generally limited to the presence of duodenal gastrinomas or duodenal somatostatinomas.[115,116] These cancers may be sporadic or associated with the familial cancer syndromes of multiple endocrine neoplasia (MEN) type 1 or type 2. The clinical presentation is similar to those with pancreatic primaries. Hypersecretion of gastrin results in the Zollinger–Ellison syndrome (ZES) characterized by excessive gastric acid production and recurrent or severe peptic ulcer disease. In contrast to pancreatic gastrinomas, duodenal gastrinomas are smaller, <1 cm, and localized to the first part of the duodenum.[117] In patients with MEN type 1, the majority of cases of ZES will result from one or more gastrinomas localized to the duodenum. Excess production of somatostatin results in elevated blood glucose, steatorrhea, and cholelithiasis. The treatment approach is the same as for pancreatic islet cell carcinomas with the use of medical therapy for the control of hormone-induced symptomatology and surgical resection for localized disease. For additional discussion, readers are referred to Chapter 29.

Adenocarcinoids

Adenocarcinoids or goblet cell carcinomas demonstrate features of both carcinoids and adenocarcinomas. These cancers are most commonly seen arising from the appendix, though a limited number of small bowel adenocarcinoids have been reported.[118–120] The most common small bowel subsite is the proximal jejunum. In general, these tumors demonstrate a clinical behavior more closely aligned with their adenocarcinoma component and often metastatic sites will demonstrate only the adenocarcinoma component. Small bowel adenocarcinoids should be approached as for adenocarcinomas of the small bowel.

Primary small bowel melanoma

Primary melanoma of small intestine is exceedingly rare. Some investigators feel that primary melanomas of the small bowel are in reality metastatic lesions from either an unknown or regressed primary cutaneous melanoma.[121] Primary intestinal melanomas are defined as the presence of intramucosal lesions in intestinal epithelium with no evidence of a concurrent melanoma of skin and absence of extraintestinal metastatic melanoma.[122] Distinguishing primary from metastatic disease is complex. In cases of a presumed primary small intestinal melanoma, it is imperative to exclude small bowel involvement as a component of metastatic spread from an antecedent or coexisting primary cutaneous lesion.

Treatment

Surgery is the treatment of choice in patients with primary small bowel melanomas.[123,124] A wide surgical resection with tumor-free margins and regional lymphadenectomy is preferred.[124] There are currently no standard systemic therapies for primary intestinal melanoma. The role of chemotherapy and targeted therapies in the treatment of primary melanoma of the small bowel is likely similar to that of cutaneous melanoma.[125] At present, the distribution of BRAF and c-kit mutations in primary small bowel melanoma is not known. Primary intestinal melanoma tends to be more aggressive and is associated with a worse prognosis than cutaneous melanoma.[64,125]

Metastatic disease to the small bowel

The small bowel is commonly involved by either direct invasion from a locally advanced tumor, such as a colorectal or pancreatic carcinoma, or in the setting of widespread peritoneal carcinomatosis. The areas most prone to involvement from peritoneal carcinomatosis are the ileocecal valve and small bowel loops within the cul-de-sac. Tumors arising from hematogenous spread are infrequent. The majority of these cases are associated with melanoma, lobular breast cancer, and nonsmall cell lung cancer.[126–129] Melanoma is the most common primary tumor to metastasize to the small bowel.[121,127] In particular, melanoma has a known predilection for small bowel metastases with approximately 50% of patients having gastrointestinal metastases at the time of death.[130] Expression of the chemokine receptor 9 by melanoma cells has been shown to correlate with the development of small bowel metastases.[131] Other reported primaries include renal cell, ovarian, prostate, colorectal, squamous cell carcinoma, osteosarcoma, and liposarcoma.[126] Patients with metastatic small bowel tumors present mostly in the sixth decade of life.[126] The most common presenting feature is intestinal obstruction (44%) followed by perforation (32%) and gastrointestinal bleeding (21%).[132]

Treatment

Metastatic tumors to small bowel are treated for either symptom relief (bleeding, obstruction, and perforation) or control of metastatic disease. Due to the nonspecific presentation, diagnosis of small bowel metastasis is often significantly delayed, and most often these tumors are treated with palliative intent. Limited surgical resection and intestinal bypass can result in relief of symptoms. Whenever possible, surgical resection of melanoma metastases of the small bowel should be undertaken as uncontrolled data suggest improved outcomes for such patients.[133] Systemic chemotherapy appropriate for the treatment of the primary cancer should be instituted whenever possible. Other modalities such as angiographic embolization and endoscopic laser therapy may be utilized for the control of bleeding.

References

1. Weiss NS, Yang CP. Incidence of histologic types of cancer of the small intestine. J Natl Cancer Inst 1987; 78: 653–6.
2. Jemal A, Siegel R, Xu J, et al. Cancer statistics, 2010. CA Cancer J Clin 2010; 60: 277–300.
3. Hatzaras I, Palesty JA, Abir F, et al. Small-bowel tumors: epidemiologic and clinical characteristics of 1260 cases from the connecticut tumor registry. Arch Surg 2007; 142: 229–35.
4. Bilimoria KY, Bentrem DJ, Wayne JD, et al. Small bowel cancer in the United States: changes in epidemiology, treatment, and survival over the last 20 years. Ann Surg 2009; 249: 63–71.
5. Lowenfels AB. Why are small-bowel tumours so rare? Lancet 1973; 1: 24–6.
6. Calman KC. Why are small bowel tumours rare? An experimental model. Gut 1974; 15: 552–4.
7. Blaker H, Helmchen B, Bonisch A, et al. Mutational activation of the RAS-RAF-MAPK and the Wnt pathway in small intestinal adenocarcinomas. Scand J Gastroenterol 2004; 39: 748–53.
8. Arai M, Shimizu S, Imai Y, et al. Mutations of the Ki-ras, p53 and APC genes in adenocarcinomas of the human small intestine. Int J Cancer 1997; 70: 390–5.
9. Miyaki M, Konishi M, Kikuchi-Yanoshita R, et al. Characteristics of somatic mutation of the adenomatous polyposis coli gene in colorectal tumors. Cancer Res 1994; 54: 3011–20.
10. Miyoshi Y, Nagase H, Ando H, et al. Somatic mutations of the APC gene in colorectal tumors: mutation cluster region in the APC gene. Hum Mol Genet 1992; 1: 229–33.
11. Standring S. Gray's Anatomy, The Anatomical Basis of Clinical Practice, 40th edn. Edinburgh: Churchill Livingstone, 2009.
12. Lepage C, Bouvier AM, Manfredi S, et al. Incidence and management of primary malignant small bowel cancers: a well-defined French population study. Am J Gastroenterol 2006; 101: 2826–32.
13. Haselkorn T, Whittemore AS, Lilienfeld DE. Incidence of small bowel cancer in the United States and worldwide: geographic, temporal, and racial differences. Cancer Causes Control 2005; 16: 781–7.
14. Chow JS, Chen CC, Ahsan H, et al. A population-based study of the incidence of malignant small bowel tumours: SEER, 1973–1990. Int J Epidemiol 1996; 25: 722–8.
15. Wu AH, Yu MC, Mack TM. Smoking, alcohol use, dietary factors and risk of small intestinal adenocarcinoma. Int J Cancer 1997; 70: 512–17.
16. Chow W. Risk factors for small intestine cancer. Cancer Causes Control 1993; 4: 163–9.
17. Chen CC, Neugut AI, Rotterdam H. Risk factors for adenocarcinomas and malignant carcinoids of the small intestine: preliminary findings. Cancer Epidemiol Biomarkers Prev 1994; 3: 205–7.
18. Negri E. Risk factors for adenocarcinoma of the small intestine. Int J Cancer 1999; 82: 171–4.
19. Negri E, Bosetti C, La Vecchia C, et al. Risk factors for adenocarcinoma of the small intestine. Int J Cancer 1999; 82: 171–4.
20. Ciresi DL, Scholten DJ. The continuing clinical dilemma of primary tumors of the small intestine. Am Surg 1995; 61: 698–702; discussion 702–3.

21. Talamonti MS, Goetz LH, Rao S, *et al*. Primary cancers of the small bowel: analysis of prognostic factors and results of surgical management. Arch Surg 2002; 137: 564–70; discussion 570–1.

22. Howe JR, Karnell LH, Menck HR, *et al*. The American College of Surgeons Commission on Cancer and the American Cancer Society. Adenocarcinoma of the small bowel: review of the National Cancer Data Base, 1985–1995. Cancer 1999; 86: 2693–706.

23. Cunningham JD, Aleali R, Aleali M, *et al*. Malignant small bowel neoplasms: histopathologic determinants of recurrence and survival. Ann Surg 1997; 225: 300–6.

24. Ojha A, Zacherl J, Scheuba C, *et al*. Primary small bowel malignancies: single-center results of three decades. J Clin Gastroenterol 2000; 30: 289–93.

25. Minardi AJ Jr, Zibari GB, Aultman DF, *et al*. Small-bowel tumors. J Am Coll Surg 1998; 186: 664–8.

26. Ciresi D. The continuing clinical dilemma of primary tumors of the small intestine. Am Surg 1995; 61: 698–702.

27. Minardi AJ, Zibari GB, Aultman DF, McMillan RW, McDonald JC. Small-bowel tumors. J Am Coll Surg 1998;186: 664–8.

28. Bessette JR, Maglinte DD, Kelvin FM, *et al*. Primary malignant tumors in the small bowel: a comparison of the small-bowel enema and conventional follow-through examination. Am J Roentgenol 1989; 153: 741–4.

29. Bruneton JN, Drouillard J, Bourry J, *et al*. [Adenocarcinoma of the small intestine. Current state of diagnosis and treatment. A study of 27 cases and a review of the literature]. J Radiol 1983; 64: 117–23.

30. Arslan H, Etlik O, Kayan M, *et al*. Peroral CT enterography with lactulose solution: preliminary observations. Am J Roentgenol 2005; 185: 1173–9.

31. Van Weyenberg SJ, Meijerink MR, Jacobs MA, *et al*. MR enteroclysis in the diagnosis of small-bowel neoplasms. Radiology 2010; 254: 765–73.

32. Pilleul F, Penigaud M, Milot L, *et al*. Possible small-bowel neoplasms: contrast-enhanced and water-enhanced multidetector CT enteroclysis. Radiology 2006; 241: 796–801.

33. Laurent F, Raynaud M, Biset JM, *et al*. Diagnosis and categorization of small bowel neoplasms: role of computed tomography. Gastrointest Radiol 1991; 16: 115–19.

34. Saltz J, Gollub D, Reidy DL. The role of octreotide imaging in detecting neuroendocrine tumors (NETs) in 2010. Do we still need it? Presented at the 2010 ASCO Annual Meeting, Chicago, Illinois, #4032.

35. Fry LC, Bellutti M, Neumann H, *et al*. Incidence of bleeding lesions within reach of conventional upper and lower endoscopes in patients undergoing double-balloon enteroscopy for obscure gastrointestinal bleeding. Aliment Pharmacol Ther 2009; 29: 342–9.

36. Lewis BS, Eisen GM, Friedman S. A pooled analysis to evaluate results of capsule endoscopy trials. Endoscopy 2005; 37: 960–5.

37. Eliakim R. Video capsule endoscopy of the small bowel. Curr Opin Gastroenterol 2010; 26: 129–33.

38. Zaanan A, Costes L, Gauthier M, *et al*. Chemotherapy of advanced small-bowel adenocarcinoma: a multicenter AGEO study. Ann Oncol 2010; 21: 1786–93.

39. Sjoblom S. Clinical presentation and prognosis of gastrointestinal tumors. Scand J Gastroenterol 1988; 23: 779–87.

40. Edge SB Byrd DR, Compton CC, *et al*. AJCC Cancer Staging Manual, 7th edn. New York: Springer, 2010.

41. Rohatiner A, d'Amore F, Coiffier B, *et al*. Report on a workshop convened to discuss the pathological and staging classifications of gastrointestinal tract lymphoma. Ann Oncol 1994; 5: 397–400.

42. Sellner F Investigations on the significance of the adenoma-carcinoma sequence in the small bowel. Cancer 1990; 66: 702–15.

43. Perzin KH, Bridge MF. Adenomas of the small intestine: a clinicopathologic review of 51 cases and a study of their relationship to carcinoma. Cancer 1981; 48: 799–819.

44. Blaker H, von Herbay A, Penzel R, *et al*. Genetics of adenocarcinomas of the small intestine: frequent deletions at chromosome 18q and mutations of the SMAD4 gene. Oncogene 2002; 21: 158–64.

45. Nishiyama K, Yao T, Yonemasu H, *et al*. Overexpression of p53 protein and point mutation of K-ras genes in primary carcinoma of the small intestine. Oncol Rep 2002; 9: 293–300.

46. Zhang MQ, Chen ZM, Wang HL. Immunohistochemical investigation of tumorigenic pathways in small intestinal adenocarcinoma: a comparison with colorectal adenocarcinoma. Mod Pathol 2006; 19: 573–80.

47. Rashid A, Hamilton SR. Genetic alterations in sporadic and Crohn's-associated adenocarcinomas of the small intestine. Gastroenterology 1997; 113: 127–35.

48. River L, Silverstein J, Tope JW. Benign neoplasms of the small intestine: a critical comprehensive review with reports of 20 new cases. Surg Gynecol Obstet 1956; 102: 1–38.

49. Wheeler JM, Warren BF, Mortensen NJ, *et al*. An insight into the genetic pathway of adenocarcinoma of the small intestine. Gut 2002; 50: 218–23.

50. Overman MJ, Pozadzides J, Kopetz S, *et al*. Immunophenotype and molecular characterisation of adenocarcinoma of the small intestine. Br J Cancer 2010; 102: 144–50.

51. Planck M, Ericson K, Piotrowska Z, *et al*. Microsatellite instability and expression of MLH1 and MSH2 in carcinomas of the small intestine. Cancer 2003; 97: 1551–7.

52. Diosdado B, Buffart TE, Watkins R, *et al*. High-resolution array comparative genomic hybridization in sporadic and celiac disease-related small bowel adenocarcinomas. Clin Cancer Res 2010; 16: 1391–401.

53. Potter DD, Murray JA, Donohue JH, *et al*. The role of defective mismatch repair in small bowel adenocarcinoma in celiac disease. Cancer Res 2004; 64: 7073–7.

54. Jess T, Winther KV, Munkholm P, *et al*. Intestinal and extra-intestinal cancer in Crohn's disease: follow-up of a population-based cohort in Copenhagen County, Denmark. Aliment Pharmacol Ther 2004; 19: 287–93.

55. Howdle PD, Jalal PK, Holmes GK, *et al*. Primary small-bowel malignancy in the UK and its association with coeliac disease. QJM 2003; 96: 345–53.

56. Palascak-Juif V, Bouvier AM, Cosnes J, *et al*. Small bowel adenocarcinoma in patients with Crohn's disease compared with small bowel adenocarcinoma de novo. Inflamm Bowel Dis 2005; 11: 828–32.

57. West J, Logan RF, Smith CJ, *et al*. Malignancy and mortality in people with coeliac disease: population based cohort study. BMJ 2004; 329: 716–19.

58. Giardiello FM, Brensinger JD, Tersmette AC, *et al*. Very high risk of cancer in familial Peutz–Jeghers syndrome. Gastroenterology 2000; 119: 1447–53.

59. Groves CJ, Saunders BP, Spigelman AD, *et al*. Duodenal cancer in patients with familial adenomatous polyposis (FAP): results of a 10 year prospective study. Gut 2002; 50: 636–41.

60. Aarnio M, Mecklin JP, Aaltonen LA, *et al*. Life-time risk of different cancers in hereditary non-polyposis colorectal cancer (HNPCC) syndrome. Int J Cancer 1995; 64: 430–3.

61. Vasen HF, Wijnen JT, Menko FH, *et al*. Cancer risk in families with hereditary nonpolyposis colorectal cancer diagnosed by mutation analysis. Gastroenterology 1996; 110: 1020–7.

62. Ouriel K, Adams JT. Adenocarcinoma of the small intestine. Am J Surg 1984; 147: 66–71.

63. Santoro E, Sacchi M, Scutari F, *et al*. Primary adenocarcinoma of the duodenum: treatment and survival in 89 patients. Hepatogastroenterology 1997; 44: 1157–63.

64. Wong JH, Cagle LA, Morton DL. Surgical treatment of lymph nodes with metastatic melanoma from unknown primary site. Arch Surg 1987; 122: 1380–3.

65. Wu TJ, Yeh CN, Chao TC, *et al*. Prognostic factors of primary small bowel adenocarcinoma: univariate and multivariate analysis. World J Surg 2006; 30: 391–8; discussion 399.

66. Barnes G Jr, Romero L, Hess KR, *et al*. Primary adenocarcinoma of the duodenum: management and survival in 67 patients. Ann Surg Oncol 1994; 1: 73–8.

67. Dabaja BS, Suki D, Pro B, *et al*. Adenocarcinoma of the small bowel: presentation, prognostic factors, and outcome of 217 patients. Cancer 2004; 101: 518–26.

68. Brucher BL, Stein HJ, Roder JD, *et al*. New aspects of prognostic factors in adenocarcinomas of the small bowel. Hepatogastroenterology 2001; 48: 727–32.

69. Sohn TA, Lillemoe KD, Cameron JL, et al. Adenocarcinoma of the duodenum: factors influencing long-term survival. J Gastrointest Surg 1998; 2: 79–87.

70. Abrahams NA, Halverson A, Fazio VW, et al. Adenocarcinoma of the small bowel: a study of 37 cases with emphasis on histologic prognostic factors. Dis Colon Rectum 2002; 45: 1496–502.

71. Bakaeen FG, Murr MM, Sarr MG, et al. What prognostic factors are important in duodenal adenocarcinoma? Arch Surg 2000; 135: 635–41; discussion 641–2.

72. Kaklamanos IG, Bathe OF, Franceschi D, et al. Extent of resection in the management of duodenal adenocarcinoma. Am J Surg 2000; 179: 37–41.

73. Joesting DR, Beart RW Jr, van Heerden JA, et al. Improving survival in adenocarcinoma of the duodenum. Am J Surg 1981; 141: 228–31.

74. Nicholl MB, Ahuja V, Conway WC, et al. Small bowel adenocarcinoma: understaged and undertreated? Ann Surg Oncol 2010; 17: 2728–32.

75. Overman MJ, Hu CY, Wolff RA, et al. Prognostic value of lymph node evaluation in small bowel adenocarcinoma: analysis of the surveillance, epidemiology, and end results database. Cancer 2010; 116: 5374–82.

76. Agrawal S, McCarron EC, Gibbs JF, et al. Surgical management and outcome in primary adenocarcinoma of the small bowel. Ann Surg Oncol 2007; 14: 2263–9.

77. Overman MJ, Kopetz S, Lin E, et al. Is there a role for adjuvant therapy in resected adenocarcinoma of the small intestine? Acta Oncol 2010; 49: 474–9.

78. Halfdanarson T, Quevedo F, McWilliams RR. Small bowel adenocarcinoma: a review of 491 cases (abstract). J Clin Oncol 2006; 24: 209s.

79. Struck A, Howard T, Chiorean EG, et al. Non-ampullary duodenal adenocarcinoma: factors important for relapse and survival. J Surg Oncol 2009; 100: 144–8.

80. Swartz MJ, Hughes MA, Frassica DA, et al. Adjuvant concurrent chemoradiation for node-positive adenocarcinoma of the duodenum. Arch Surg 2007; 142: 285–8.

81. Kelsey CR, Nelson JW, Willett CG, et al. Duodenal adenocarcinoma: patterns of failure after resection and the role of chemoradiotherapy. Int J Radiat Oncol Biol Phys 2007; 69: 1436–41.

82. Yeung RS, Weese JL, Hoffman JP, et al. Neoadjuvant chemoradiation in pancreatic and duodenal carcinoma. A Phase II Study . Cancer 1993; 72: 2124–33.

83. Fishman PN, Pond GR, Moore MJ, et al. Natural history and chemotherapy effectiveness for advanced adenocarcinoma of the small bowel: a retrospective review of 113 cases. Am J Clin Oncol 2006; 29: 225–31.

84. Czaykowski P, Hui D. Chemotherapy in small bowel adenocarcinoma: 10-year experience of the British Columbia Cancer Agency. Clin Oncol (R Coll Radiol) 2007; 19: 143–9.

85. Gibson MK, Holcroft CA, Kvols LK, et al. Phase II study of 5-fluorouracil, doxorubicin, and mitomycin C for metastatic small bowel adenocarcinoma. Oncologist 2005; 10: 132–7.

86. Overman MJ, Varadhachary GR, Kopetz S, et al. Phase II study of capecitabine and oxaliplatin for advanced adenocarcinoma of the small bowel and ampulla of Vater. J Clin Oncol 2009; 27: 2598–603.

87. Overman MJ, Kopetz S, Wen S, et al. Chemotherapy with 5-fluorouracil and a platinum compound improves outcomes in metastatic small bowel adenocarcinoma. Cancer 2008; 113: 2038–45.

88. Crawley C, Ross P, Norman A, et al. The Royal Marsden experience of a small bowel adenocarcinoma treated with protracted venous infusion 5-fluorouracil. Br J Cancer 1998; 78: 508–10.

89. Locher C, Malka D, Boige V, et al. Combination chemotherapy in advanced small bowel adenocarcinoma. Oncology 2005; 69: 290–4.

90. Zaanan A, Gauthier M, Malka D, et al. Second-line chemotherapy with fluorouracil, leucovorin, and irinotecan (FOLFIRI regimen) in patients with advanced small bowel adenocarcinoma after failure of first-line platinum-based chemotherapy: a multicenter AGEO study. Cancer 2011; 117: 1422–8.

91. Ercolani G, Grazi GL, Ravaioli M, et al. The role of liver resections for noncolorectal, nonneuroendocrine metastases: experience with 142 observed cases. Ann Surg Oncol 2005; 12: 459–66.

92. Howe JR, Karnell LH, Scott-Conner C. Small bowel sarcoma: analysis of survival from the National Cancer Data Base. Ann Surg Oncol 2001; 8: 496–508.

93. Schottenfeld D, Beebe-Dimmer JL, Vigneau FD. The epidemiology and pathogenesis of neoplasia in the small intestine. Ann Epidemiol 2009; 19: 58–69.

94. Miettinen M, Kopczynski J, Makhlouf HR, et al. Gastrointestinal stromal tumors, intramural leiomyomas, and leiomyosarcomas in the duodenum: a clinicopathologic, immunohistochemical, and molecular genetic study of 167 cases. Am J Surg Pathol 2003; 27: 625–41.

95. Arvanitis ML, Jagelman DG, Fazio VW, et al. Mortality in patients with familial adenomatous polyposis. Dis Colon Rectum 1990; 33: 639–42.

96. Casali PG, Picci P. Adjuvant chemotherapy for soft tissue sarcoma. Curr Opin Oncol 2005; 17: 361–5.

97. Casali PG, Jost L, Sleijfer S, et al. Soft tissue sarcomas: ESMO clinical recommendations for diagnosis, treatment and follow-up. Ann Oncol 2008; 19(Suppl 2): ii89–93.

98. Hensley ML, Maki R, Venkatraman E, et al. Gemcitabine and docetaxel in patients with unresectable leiomyosarcoma: results of a phase II trial. J Clin Oncol 2002; 20: 2824–31.

99. Dodd GD. Lymphoma of the hollow abdominal viscera. Radiol Clin North Am 1990; 28: 771–83.

100. Groves FD, Linet MS, Travis LB, et al. Cancer surveillance series: non-Hodgkin's lymphoma incidence by histologic subtype in the United States from 1978 through 1995. J Natl Cancer Inst 2000; 92: 1240–51.

101. Koch P, del Valle F, Berdel WE, et al. Primary gastrointestinal non-Hodgkin's lymphoma: I. Anatomic and histologic distribution, clinical features, and survival data of 371 patients registered in the German Multicenter Study GIT NHL 01/92. J Clin Oncol 2001; 19: 3861–73.

102. Morgan PB, Kessel IL, Xiao SY, et al. Uncommon presentations of Hodgkin's disease. Case 1. Hodgkin's disease of the jejunum. J Clin Oncol 2004; 22: 193–5.

103. Gandhi JS, Mehta A, Sharma A, et al. Primary Hodgkin lymphoma of the ileum. J Cancer Res Ther 2010; 6: 342–3.

104. Lecuit M, Abachin E, Martin A, et al. Immunoproliferative small intestinal disease associated with Campylobacter jejuni. N Engl J Med 2004; 350: 239–48.

105. Catassi C, Fabiani E, Corrao G, et al. Risk of non-Hodgkin lymphoma in celiac disease. JAMA 2002; 287: 1413–19.

106. Green PH, Fleischauer AT, Bhagat G, et al. Risk of malignancy in patients with celiac disease. Am J Med 2003; 115: 191–5.

107. Dickson BC, Serra S, Chetty R. Primary gastrointestinal tract lymphoma: diagnosis and management of common neoplasms. Expert Rev Anticancer Ther 2006; 6: 1609–28.

108. Radaszkiewicz T, Dragosics B, Bauer P. Gastrointestinal malignant lymphomas of the mucosa-associated lymphoid tissue: factors relevant to prognosis. Gastroenterology 1992; 102: 1628–38.

109. Kim SJ, Kang HJ, Kim JS, et al. Comparison of treatment strategies for patients with intestinal diffuse large B-cell lymphoma: surgical resection followed by chemotherapy versus chemotherapy alone. Blood 2011; 117: 1958–65.

110. Schmatz AI, Streubel B, Kretschmer-Chott E, et al. Primary follicular lymphoma of the duodenum is a distinct mucosal/submucosal variant of follicular lymphoma: a retrospective study of 63 cases. J Clin Oncol 2011; 29: 1445–51.

111. Park HS, Kim YJ, Yang WI, et al. Treatment outcome of localized Helicobacter pylori-negative low-grade gastric MALT lymphoma. World J Gastroenterol 2010; 16: 2158–62.

112. Ghimire P, Wu GY, Zhu L. Primary gastrointestinal lymphoma. World J Gastroenterol 2011; 17: 697–707.

113. Aleman BM, Haas RL, van der Maazen RW. Role of radiotherapy in the treatment of lymphomas of the gastrointestinal tract. Best Pract Res Clin Gastroenterol 2010; 24: 27–34.

114. Brenner B, Shah MA, Gonen M, et al. Small-cell carcinoma of the gastrointestinal tract: a retrospective study of 64 cases. Br J Cancer 2004; 90: 1720–6.

115. Jensen RT, Niederle B, Mitry E, *et al*. Gastrinoma (duodenal and pancreatic). Neuroendocrinology 2006; 84: 173–82.

116. Garbrecht N, Anlauf M, Schmitt A, *et al*. Somatostatin-producing neuroendocrine tumors of the duodenum and pancreas: incidence, types, biological behavior, association with inherited syndromes, and functional activity. Endocr Relat Cancer 2008; 15: 229–41.

117. Thom AK, Norton JA, Axiotis CA, *et al*. Location, incidence, and malignant potential of duodenal gastrinomas. Surgery 1991; 110: 1086–91; discussion 1091–3.

118. Levendoglu H, Cox CA, Nadimpalli V. Composite (adenocarcinoid) tumors of the gastrointestinal tract. Dig Dis Sci 1990; 35: 519–25.

119. Goldberg SL, Toker C. Composite tumor of small intestine. Mt Sinai J Med 1976; 43: 153–6.

120. Kochevar J. Adenocarcinoid tumor, goblet cell type, arising in a ureteroileal conduit: a case report. J Urol 1984; 131: 957–9.

121. Elsayed AM, Albahra M, Nzeako UC, *et al*. Malignant melanomas in the small intestine: a study of 103 patients. Am J Gastroenterol 1996; 91: 1001–6.

122. Blecker D, Abraham S, Furth EE, *et al*. Melanoma in the gastrointestinal tract. Am J Gastroenterol 1999; 94: 3427–33.

123. Kadivar TF, Vanek VW, Krishnan EU. Primary malignant melanoma of the small bowel: a case study. Am Surg 1992; 58: 418–22.

124. Atmatzidis KS, Pavlidis TE, Papaziogas BT, *et al*. Primary malignant melanoma of the small intestine: report of a case. Surg Today 2002; 32: 831–3.

125. Lens M, Bataille V, Krivokapic Z. Melanoma of the small intestine. Lancet Oncol 2009; 10: 516–21.

126. Idelevich E, Kashtan H, Mavor E, *et al*. Small bowel obstruction caused by secondary tumors. Surg Oncol 2006; 15: 29–32.

127. Richie RE, Reynolds VH, Sawyers JL. Tumor metastases to the small bowel from extra-abdominal sites. South Med J 1973; 66: 1383–7.

128. De Castro CA, Dockerty MB, Mayo CW. Metastatic tumors of the small intestines. Surg Gynecol Obstet 1957; 105: 159–65.

129. Kadakia SC, Parker A, Canales L. Metastatic tumors to the upper gastrointestinal tract: endoscopic experience. Am J Gastroenterol 1992; 87: 1418–23.

130. Patel JK, Didolkar MS, Pickren JW, *et al*. Metastatic pattern of malignant melanoma. A study of 216 autopsy cases. Am J Surg 1978; 135: 807–10.

131. Amersi FF, Terando AM, Goto Y, *et al*. Activation of CCR9/CCL25 in cutaneous melanoma mediates preferential metastasis to the small intestine. Clin Cancer Res 2008; 14: 638–45.

132. Catena F, Ansaloni L, Gazzotti F, *et al*. Small bowel tumours in emergency surgery: specificity of clinical presentation. ANZ J Surg 2005; 75: 997–9.

133. Agrawal S, Yao TJ, Coit DG. Surgery for melanoma metastatic to the gastrointestinal tract. Ann Surg Oncol 1999; 6: 336–44.

32 Unusual Tumors of the Colon, Rectum, and Anus

Diane Reidy-Lagunes,[1] Karyn Goodman,[2] and Leonard B. Saltz[1]

[1] Gastrointestinal Oncology Service, [2] Department of Radiation Oncology, Department of Medicine, Memorial Sloan-Kettering Cancer Center, New York, NY, USA

Introduction

Cancers of the colon, rectum, and anus account for more than 150,000 new cases in the United States each year.[1] The overwhelming majority (approximately 97%) of these are adenocarcinomas of the colon or rectum. Of the 3% that make up the uncommon tumors, approximately half, or 1.5% of the total, will be anal carcinomas (squamous and cloacogenic) and one-third of the uncommon tumors (approximately 1% of the total) will be carcinoid or neuroendocrine tumors.[2] The remaining rare tumors, together comprising about 1% of all large bowel tumors, will be primary intestinal lymphomas, sarcomas, and melanomas. Treatment and prognoses of these tumors vary greatly, and will be discussed in this chapter.

Carcinoid tumors of the colon and rectum

Carcinoid tumors (Fig. 32.1), arising from mucosal neuroendocrine cells, are rare tumors with an overall incidence estimated to be less than two cases per 100,000 people in the United States and most commonly involve the lungs/bronchi (30%) and gastrointestinal tract (55–70%).[3,4] In several series with over 10,000 cases identified from the Surveillance, Epidemiology, and End Results (SEER) Program of the National Cancer Institute between 1973 and 1999, carcinoid tumors of the colorectum were extremely rare, accounting for less than a quarter of all carcinoids.[4–6] In the last decade, the incidence of all carcinoid tumors has increased by 3% each year, likely due to improved endoscopic and diagnostic imaging with a higher detection of these indolent tumors.[6]

Gastrointestinal carcinoid tumors are classified according to their presumed derivation from different embryonic divisions of the gut, and their biological characteristics vary according to location.[3] While about half of all gastrointestinal carcinoids are functional (produce a hormone), most of these functional carcinoids arise in the small bowel or appendix (midgut). The majority of carcinoid tumors arising in colon and rectum (hindgut) are nonfunctional.[7] When carcinoid tumors do make a hormone, serotonin is by far the most common one, best detected by measuring the serotonin breakdown product, 5-hydroxyindoleacetic acid (5-HIAA), which is excreted in the urine. Elevated urinary 5-HIAA is highly specific for carcinoid tumors but is not particularly sensitive.[8] Other hormones, such as histamine, dopamine, substance P, prostaglandins, bradykinin, and corticotropin, may also be produced but are exceedingly rare.[3] Rectal carcinoids may contain glucagon and glicentin-related peptides rather than serotonin but as noted, this is rare and most are nonfunctional.[9] Thus, the carcinoid syndrome of episodic diarrhea, flushing, wheezing and eventual endomyocardial fibrosis leading to right-sided valvular heart disease is highly unusual with colorectal carcinoid.

Pathology

Neuroendocrine tumors comprise a spectrum of diseases, from well-differentiated carcinoid to poorly differentiated neuroendocrine carcinomas (NEC) (small cell or nonsmall cell carcinoma) (Fig. 32.2). NETs are classified according to their differentiation and grade. The concept of differentiation is linked to the grade of tumors, but they are different. Differentiation refers to the architecture of the tumor cells and the extent to which the cells resemble their nonneoplastic counterparts. Well-differentiated NETs have characteristic organoid arrangements of the tumor cells, with nesting, trabecular or gyriform patterns. The cells are relatively uniform and produce abundant neurosecretory granules (Fig. 32.3), reflected in the strong and diffuse immunoexpression of neuroendocrine markers such as chromogranin A and synaptophysin. Poorly differentiated NECs have a more sheet-like or diffuse architecture with irregular nuclei and less cytoplasmic granularity. Immunoexpression of neuroendocrine markers in poorly differentiated NECs is usually more limited. Grade, in contrast, refers to the biological aggressiveness of the tumor and is determined by either the proliferation marker Ki-67 or the number of mitoses per high-powered field (HPF).

Textbook of Uncommon Cancer, Fourth Edition. Edited by Derek Raghavan, Charles D. Blanke, David H. Johnson, Paul L. Moots, Gregory H. Reaman, Peter G. Rose and Mikkael A. Sekeres.
© 2012 John Wiley & Sons, Inc. Published 2012 by John Wiley & Sons, Inc.

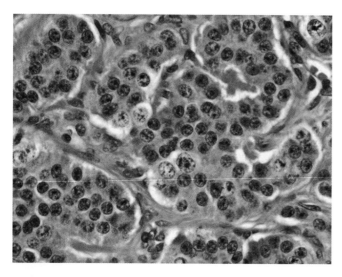

Figure 32.1 Typical carcinoid. High power showing typical neuroendocrine cytology without mitosis or necrosis. Courtesy of Dr Jinru Shia.

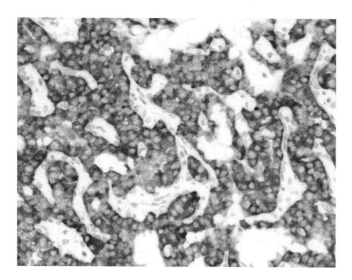

Figure 32.2 Neuroendocrine tissue markers include chromogranin, neuron-specific enolase (NSE), and synaptophysin. Synaptophysin-stained cells are seen below. Courtesy of Dr Jinru Shia.

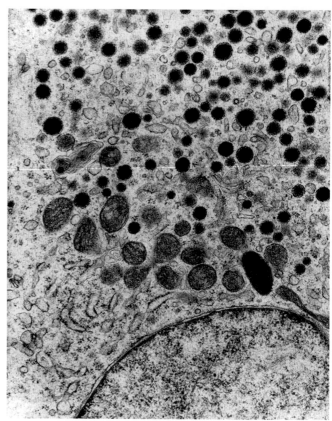

Figure 32.3 Electron microscopy of neurosecretory granules in a carcinoid tumor. Courtesy of Dr Jinru Shia.

Table 32.1 Grading of neuroendocrine tumors.

Grade	Findings
Low grade (G1) Well differentiated	<2 mitoses/10 HPF and <3% Ki-67 index
Intermediate grade (G2) Well differentiated	2–10 mitoses/10 HPF or 3–20% Ki-67 index
High grade (G3) Poorly differentiated	>20 mitoses/10 HPF or >20%

A variety of different organ-specific systems have been developed for nomenclature, grading, and staging of NETs, causing much confusion. Recently, however, a new proposal for grading and staging NETs has been published.[10] The updated WHO classification is one that proposes staging NETs as follows: well-differentiated (either low or intermediate grade) and poorly differentiated neuroendocrine carcinoma. Low grade is defined as <2 mitoses/10 HPF or a Ki-67 less than 3%. Intermediate grade is defined as 2–20 mitoses/10 HPF or a Ki-67 3–20% (Table 32.1). Poorly differentiated neuroendocrine carcinomas are aggressive and are generally managed with platinum therapy. This chapter will focus on well-differentiated neuroendocrine tumors.

Neuroendocrine tumors are of epithelial origin and thus stain positive for cytokeratins. In rare cases, colonic glands can become intermixed with carcinoid tumor cells, simulating an adenocarcinoma. Carcinoembryonic antigen (CEA) is not helpful IN distinguishing the two subtypes, since nearly a quarter of large bowel carcinoid tumors can stain positively for CEA.[11]

Clinical presentation

Within the gastrointestinal tract, the small intestine is the most common site (45%), followed by the rectum (20%), appendix (17%), colon (11%), and stomach (7%).[4] Carcinoid tumors of the colorectum and appendix often have no symptoms until and unless they become quite large, a process which can take many years.[12,13] As such, they are often incidental findings during an endoscopic, radiographic or surgical evaluation of an unrelated symptom.

Rectal carcinoids account for up to 2% of all rectal tumors, usually detected on routine endoscopy or rectal exam in the sixth decade of life. Patients who have symptoms may present with rectal bleeding, pain or constipation; carcinoid syndrome is rare.[14,15] Similarly, patients with colon carcinoids rarely (less than 5%) present with carcinoid syndrome. Patients with colon carcinoids are usually in their seventh decade of life and may have symptoms of abdominal pain, anorexia, heme-occult positive stool or weight loss, especially with larger tumors.[13] Two-thirds of colon carcinoids are found in the right side of the colon, mostly in the cecum.[13]

Appendiceal carcinoid is the most common tumor of the appendix, usually detected as an incidental finding on appendectomy. In fact, older literature suggests that about one in every 200–300 appendectomy specimens will include a carcinoid tumor.[16] Since incidental appendectomies were performed more often on women and younger patients, these studies have also shown a higher incidence of appendiceal carcinoid in women and those in the fourth or fifth decade of life.[3] In a more recent review of the SEER database analysis, however, there is no longer a significant gender difference with appendiceal carcinoids.[5] The majority of appendiceal carcinoids are asymptomatic, with less than 10% causing obstructive symptoms, since approximately 75% are located in the distal third of the appendix.[17,18] However, in a retrospective study, the rate of "incidental" carcinoid tumor was less common, with a majority of patients (54%) presenting with signs and symptoms of an acute appendicitis.[19]

Imaging

Scintigraphy was first developed in the early 1990s and octreotide labeled with indium 111 (^{111}In-pentatreotide, OctreoScan®) was successfully used to localize previously undetected primary or metastatic lesions.[20] While this approach is often used for this purpose, the incidence of tumors that are undetected by modern CT and MRI scans and then detected by ^{111}In-pentetreotide scanning, in order to change a patient's therapy, is really quite low.[21–23] Somatostatin analog scintigraphy is now used more widely to assess relevant somatostatin receptor expression *in vivo* in patient tumor samples, in order to predict who should be considered for somatostatin analog therapy. A recent report demonstrated that somatostatin receptor subtype 2 expression by ^{111}In-pentetreotide scintigraphy correlated with both tracer uptake and a better prognosis.[24] Patients with negative somatostatin scintigraphy scans and nonfunctional tumors should not be placed on somatostatin analogs.

Somatostatin analog scintigraphy has not been evaluated for assessing patients for treatment response. Computed tomography (CT) triphasic scans or magnetic resonance imaging (MRI) would be more suitable tests in this clinical situation. It is noteworthy that because NET are often isodense with normal hepatic parenchyma, routine CT scans are of somewhat less value. MRI scanning or triphasic CT scans may be more appropriate techniques for imaging.

Positron emission tomography (PET) scanning with 18-fluorodeoxyglucose (FDG) is limited, due to the low proliferative activity and high differentiation rate in carcinoid tumors. Thus, FDG-PET should not be routinely used in the management of carcinoid tumors.[25] However, from an experimental perspective, PET scans with various tracers such as 5-HTP are under investigation. Recent data suggest that PET positivity may portend a worse prognosis even in patients with low-grade tumors.[26]

Metastatic disease

Patients with nonfunctional metastatic carcinoid often present with few symptoms and an excellent clinical performance status. Intraabdominal or hepatic metastases may even present as an incidental finding of an asymptomatic mass or hepatomegaly on routine physical examination. Because of the unusually slow growth of the typical carcinoid tumor, metastatic disease *per se* does not necessarily constitute an indication for therapeutic intervention. Antineoplastic treatment need not be instituted unless there is pain or significant discomfort due to tumor bulk, uncontrollable hormonal symptoms from a functional tumor, or clear evidence of progression of disease under observation.

Management

For carcinoid tumors which are locoregionally confined at the time of diagnosis, surgery is the treatment of choice. In appendiceal carcinoid, over 95% of tumors are less than 2 cm and can be removed by simple appendectomy. Such operations are almost always curative, approaching 100% 10-year disease-free survival in one large series.[18] Lesions greater than 2 cm in diameter carry a higher risk for nodal or distant metastasis. Since the lymphatic drainage of the appendix is along the right mesocolon, a formal right hemicolectomy is required in order to accomplish an adequate regional lymphadenectomy for these larger tumors. Lesions between 1 and 2 cm in size are more controversial, with no definitive data to support a better outcome with a hemicolectomy, but with some investigators favoring this more aggressive approach. A review of the literature suggests that this aggressive approach is based on anecdotal experience of very few patients who were taken back to the operating room and found to have lymph node involvement. These patients were defined as "high risk" if they had mesoappendiceal or lymphovascular invasion (LVI).[27–29]

A similar surgical strategy is employed with rectal carcinoids. Local excision alone is adequate therapy for lesions less than 1 cm in diameter, which represent two-thirds of rectal carcinoids.[3] In lesions greater than 2 cm, spread to locoregional lymph nodes is more common, and a formal low anterior or abdominal-peritoneal resection should be considered. However, in several retrospective studies, these more aggressive surgical procedures do not appear to improve survival.[30–32] The treatment for 1–2 cm tumors is, again, somewhat controversial. Local excision may be more appropriate with tumors without muscular invasion or closer to 1 cm in size, asymptomatic or poor surgical patients, or those which would require an abdominal-peritoneal resection and thus a permanent colostomy.

Colon carcinoid tumors are treated similar to the rectal tumors. However, carcinoid tumors of the colon are more likely to present with larger tumors, with an average diameter of 5 cm at presentation. Over two-thirds of patients have either nodal or distant metastasis at time of presentation.[13] Therefore, most patients require standard hemicolectomy. For the rare patient with a tumor less than 1 cm, local excision has been reported to be effective.[12]

After surgical resection of a carcinoid tumor, patients are monitored for symptomatic recurrence of disease. Specific follow-up guidelines are not well described but given its indolent nature, routine imaging studies are often unnecessary. CT or octreotide scans may be warranted if new symptoms arise, particularly with high-risk tumors. Lastly, there is no known role for adjuvant therapy, and no evidence that any such therapy reduces the risk of recurrence.

Role of somatostatin analogs and radiolabeled somatostatin analog therapy

As noted above, carcinoid tumors typically express cell surface receptors for the regulatory hormone somatostatin. Six types of somatostatin receptors have been identified. Octreotide, which is a long-acting synthetic analog of native somatostatin, inhibits the secretion of multiple hormones, including growth hormones, insulin, glucagon, and gastrin.[33] It binds to predominantly type II somatostatin receptors, expressed on more than 80% of carcinoid tumors.[34] Both short- and long-acting formulations of octreotide, along with a related peptide lanreotide, have been shown to be effective therapeutic agents in the symptomatic control of carcinoid syndrome in up to 90% of patients. Actual radiographic tumor responses to octreotide occur anecdotally, but are extremely rare.[35,36] In addition, it has long been assumed that somatostatin analogs have moderate antiproliferative effects on tumor growth.

The first randomized data to support this hypothesis were provided by the PROMID study. In this trial, 85 patients with newly diagnosed asymptomatic midgut carcinoid tumors were randomly assigned to receive octreotide long-acting release (LAR) 30 mg intramuscularly monthly or placebo. The median time to tumor progression was 14.3 months in the octreotide arm compared to 6 months in the placebo group.[36] As would be expected in this small trial, there was no difference in overall survival. Whether the improvement in progression-free survival (PFS) would also be seen in other carcinoid tumors (i.e. outside the small bowel such as in the colon or rectum) is not directly known from the PROMID study, but most feel that extrapolation of PROMID observations to other well-differentiated NETs is reasonable.[35]

Use of radioactive-labeled somatostatin analogs (peptide receptor radiotherapy, PRRT) was developed to improve response rates. In single-center trials, PRRT for patients with advanced, indium octreotide-positive NETs has been reported to have some efficacy with acceptable toxicity. Several radioisotopes, linked to a somatostatin analog, have been used and include ^{111}In, yttrium-90 (^{90}Y), and lutetium-177 (^{177}Lu). Studies of the ^{90}Y-labeled somatostatin analog, a high-energy β-particle emitter, reported response rates of up to 27%.[37,38] A European multicenter trial known as MAURITIUS evaluated 39 patients with NET using ^{90}Y-lanreotide. Minor tumor regressions were seen in 20% of patients, with 44% of patients achieving stable disease.[39] To what degree some of these patients may have had stable disease as a consequence of the natural history of their tumor is not clear.[40]

An analysis of 504 patients with metastatic NET receiving ^{177}Lu-octreotate was also reported.[41,42] Complete remission occurred in 2% of patients, partial remission in 28%. The median time to progression was approximately 40 months overall; however, only 43% of patients had documented disease progression before therapy was initiated. Serious toxicity was seen in 3% patients who developed myelodysplastic syndrome and leukemia, and temporary nonfatal liver toxicity in two patients. Radiolabeled somatostatin analogs may hold promise as an active treatment. The degree of activity and toxicity that patients can expect from this treatment has not yet been adequately defined, and this approach remains investigational.

Interferon

Early studies on the use of interferon in patients with NET reported combined biological response (i.e. a decrease in hormone production) with objective response (i.e. tumor shrinkage), which produced very high "response" rates. In this older literature, a subjective improvement in physical exam was often accepted as satisfactory evidence of a response, a criterion which would not be accepted today. A subsequent trial from the Mayo Clinic in which patients were administered 9 million units three times per week showed a high degree of toxicity and minimal evidence of activity. The authors concluded that interferon did not have a role in the treatment of NET.[43] A recent review of the available studies by Plockinger and colleagues estimated that approximately 10% of patients achieved some degree of actual tumor regression, however modest. Major objective responses are essentially anecdotal.[44] Although interferon-α may have an antiproliferative effect, as evidenced by disease stabilization, the side-effects, including fatigue, fever and anorexia, often outweigh the benefits, and these effects should be carefully considered before using these agents.[45,46]

Cytotoxic chemotherapy

Cytotoxic chemotherapy is generally of minimal usefulness. Drugs such as doxorubicin, 5-fluorouracil with leucovorin, dacarbazine, and docetaxel have limited single-agent activity with short-lasting responses in fewer than 20% of patients.[47–49] It is noteworthy that many of these older studies accepted clinical assessment (physical exam) as the basis for declaring a "response" and as such, the true activity of these agents is likely to be lower than has been thus reported. Furthermore, in these trials, many of the "carcinoid" tumors arose from pancreatic neuroendocrine tumors, biologically different from colorectal carcinoids.

More recently, extrapolation from the 5-FU experience has led to the use of capecitabine, with some anecdotal activity. Capecitabine combined with temozolomide showed promising activity in a small study generally limited to pancreatic NETs as opposed to carcinoid tumors.[50] The dependence of temozolomide responsiveness on deficient methyl-guanine methyl transferase (MGMT) expression may explain the lack of benefit from this drug in some NETs and in carcinoids in particular. Kulke and associates retrospectively assessed 76 patients receiving temozolomide-based treatments.[51] A radiographic response (defined by RECIST criteria) was seen in approximately 33% of patients with pancreatic NETs (11/35 patients), but in 0% (0/38) of patients with carcinoid tumors (p <0.001). In 21 available specimens, complete absence of MGMT expression seemed to define patients with pancreatic NET who achieve significant benefit from temozolomide (5/8 pancreatic NET and 0/13 carcinoid tumors). These trials fail to convincingly demonstrate a meaningful benefit of combination therapy over single-agent therapy and question the utility of cytotoxic chemotherapy in carcinoid tumors.

Embolization

Because of the limited utility of chemotherapy, symptomatic hepatic carcinoid lesions may be better palliated by regional ablative therapies such as hepatic arterial embolization, which takes advantage of the dual blood supply to the liver. While the normal liver obtains approximately 75% of its blood supply from the portal vein, tumors greater than 1 cm in size obtain the majority of their blood supply through the hepatic artery. Injection of polyvinyl alcohol or other small particulate materials (so-called "bland embolization") into the angiographically located hepatic arterial blood supply to the metastasis can cause substantial tumor regressions. Thus, inducing vascular occlusion of the hepatic arterial supply can result in selective ischemia and necrosis of the tumor relative to the normal liver around it. Duration of response is highly variable and might be as brief as 4 months or as long as 2 years, again reflecting the differences in tumor biology.[52,53] Toxicities such as pain, infection, fever, nausea, and hepatorenal syndrome have been described, and treatment-related deaths have been reported.[54]

Recently, radioembolization using yttrium-90 (^{90}Y) has also been employed. ^{90}Y is a β-emitter with a very short penetrance, meaning that its radiation is delivered in close proximity to the final resting place of the carrier particle to which it is attached. The development of injectable particles conjugated to ^{90}Y permits delivery of internal radiation into the hepatic arteries that supply NET liver metastases. In the past 5 years, series reporting outcomes after radioembolization have included two in which complete responses were obtained in 12–18% of those treated, yet median survivals ranging from 22 to 36 months do not appear substantially different from those reported with either bland or chemoembolization. Both morphological and symptomatic response rates have ranged from 50% to 90%.[55–58]

To date, there are no prospective, randomized trials comparing the clinical efficacy of these embolization methods, despite apparent substantial differences in potential toxicity and cost. Therefore, there is no evidence to guide the selection of optimal arterial therapy for progressive, unresectable NET liver metastases. Patients undergoing hepatic arterial embolization should have this done by experienced physicians, and octreotide premedication should be given to patients with functional tumors to reduce the risk of carcinoid crisis.

Vascular endothelial growth factor systemic therapies

Since carcinoid is a vascular tumor that expresses vascular endothelial growth factor (VEGF),[59,60] targeted antiangiogenic drugs such as bevacizumab (Avastin™) and sunitinib have been investigated. In a phase 2 study, bevacizumab was associated with higher response rates, greater reduction in 5-hydroxyindoleacetic acid (HIAA) levels and longer 18-week progression-free survival (95% versus 67%) compared to interferon alone.[61] A phase 3 trial of bevacizumab versus interferon is now ongoing.

A phase 2 trial with sunitinib, however, did not show significant activity in carcinoid tumors. Sunitinib is an orally active, small multitargeted agent that blocks the VEGF receptor as well as platelet-derived growth factor receptor β, KIT and RET. In this phase 2 study, 109 advanced NET patients received 50 mg sunitinib for 4 weeks followed by a 2-week break. Of the patients with pancreatic NETs, 17% (11/66) achieved a confirmed partial response compared with 2% (1/41) of patients with carcinoid tumors,[62] illustrating the differences in benefit between carcinoids and pancreatic NETs. Twenty-five percent of patients had grade 3 fatigue (50 mg dose).[62] These positive results in pancreatic NETs led to a randomized phase 3 trial. One hundred and seventy-one patients with disease progression were randomly assigned to receive either 37.5 mg daily of sunitinib or a placebo.[63] The median progression-free survival was significantly longer with sunitinib (11.4 months 5.5 months) which led to its FDA approval for pancreatic NETs but not for carcinoid tumors.[63]

mTOR inhibitors

mTOR inhibitors have also been investigated. Temsirolimus was evaluated in patients with NETs and was associated with a 5.6% objective response rate (ORR) and a median time to tumor progression of 6 months and was considered negative.[64] Another mTOR inhibitor, everolimus, was evaluated in a phase 2 study and was associated with an 8% RR, a 77% clinical benefit rate, and a median PFS of 9 months.[65] Based on these positive phase 2 data, two phase 3 trials were conducted. RADIANT-2 was a randomized trial evaluating everolimus 10 mg daily versus placebo in 429 patients with progressive carcinoid tumors. Median PFS was 16.4 months versus 11.3 months. However, the PFS did not achieve its primary endpoint of PFS based on adjudicated central radiological review and the difference was not statistically different. Analyses that adjusted for imbalances in baseline characteristics, however, showed that everolimus plus octreotide LAR decreased the likelihood of disease progression.[66]

It is worth noting that, in contradistinction to the RADIANT-2 carcinoid trial, the RADIANT-3 trial, which was conducted in pancreatic neuroendocrine tumors (panNETs), had an unequivocally positive result. This phase 3 study, evaluating everolimus 10 mg/day versus best supportive care in 410 patients with progressive panNETs, demonstrated a 2.4-fold improvement in median PFS (11.0 versus 4.6 months; hazard ratio (HR) 0.35; 95% confidence interval (CI) 0.27–0.45; p <0.001) for the everolimus arm. As befit the data, everolimus has currently received FDA approval for use in panNETs, but not in carcinoid tumors.

Surgery

Surgery is generally not indicated in the management of metastatic carcinoid where an R0 resection cannot be achieved. However, in a retrospective analysis, an aggressive surgical intervention in a very selected patient cohort with small-volume bowel carcinoid and metastatic liver lesions had a sizeable number with potential cures.[67] In addition, palliative surgery may be considered in selected patients with symptomatic bulky liver metastases to try to delay the need for medical therapy, for the endocrinopathies of a functional tumor, or to alleviate pain due to tumor bulk.

Prognosis

Well-differentiated NETs pose a significant challenge because of the tumor heterogeneity, varying degree of aggressiveness, and lack of standard regimens and guidelines for treatment. The aggressiveness of a carcinoid tumor is often related to the degree of tumor grade and differentiation. The classic, well-differentiated low-grade carcinoid tumors have long survival rates, although they have poor response to chemotherapy. The tumor grade and differentiation, patient's age, size of tumor, site of primary carcinoid tumor, and presence of metastatic disease are the best predictors of prognosis.[68] According to the primary site, the 5-year survival is 71–100% (appendix), 33–75% (colon), and 62–100% (rectum).[27] Appendiceal and rectal carcinoids are usually less than 1 cm when detected and rarely metastasize. In contrast, 85–90% of colonic carcinoids are 2 cm or larger at presentation, with a high metastatic rate (60%).[27] Other indicators of a poorer prognosis are overexpression of the proliferation protein Ki-67 or the p53 tumor suppressor protein, carcinoid syndrome, carcinoid heart disease, and high concentrations of urinary 5-HIAA or plasma chromogranin A.[27]

The high-grade neuroendocrine tumors and undifferentiated small cell carcinomas are the other end of the spectrum. These tumors are very aggressive with short survival, despite high initial response rates to chemotherapy. In a retrospective analysis of 38 patients with colorectal high-grade neuroendocrine tumors or small cell carcinomas, metastatic disease was detected in up to 70% of patients at presentation. Like small cell lung cancer, these tumors had a very poor prognosis, with a median survival of 10.4 months and 3-year survival of 13%.[69]

Sarcoma of the colon and rectum

Primary colorectal sarcomas are uncommon (Table 32.2). In a retrospective review from the Memorial Sloan-Kettering Cancer Center from 1982–1991, 38 adult patients were admitted with primary gastrointestinal sarcomas, accounting for less than 2% of all adult sarcomas admissions. Only nine of these 38 patients had a large bowel sarcoma (two colon, seven rectum), mostly leiomyosarcomas (>90%).[70] In recent years, the classification and treatment options for the most common histological subtype of the bowel, leiomyosarcoma (LMS), have changed dramatically. This section will focus on the recent updates in treatment and biology of intestinal LMS and gastro-

Table 32.2 Summary of large bowel cancer (nonadenocarcinoma).

Histology	Percentage
Squamous cell carcinoma	33%
Malignant carcinoid	33%
Transitional cell like/cloacogenic	16%
Lymphoma	11%
Sarcoma	4%
Melanoma	1%

intestinal stromal cell tumors (GIST). Readers are also referred to Chapter 33 for further discussion on gastrointestinal stromal tumors.

Lymphoma of the colon and rectum

Colorectal lymphomas account for 6–14% of all gastrointestinal lymphomas, with the cecum (73%) and the rectum being the most frequently involved sites.[71] Clinical presentation of colorectal lymphoma is typically indistinguishable from colorectal adenocarcinoma. Most present with a mass, signs of intestinal obstruction, or gastrointestinal bleeding. Some patients present with pyrexia of unknown origin, or "B" symptoms with night sweats, fevers, and weight loss. Multiple polypoidal lymphoma affecting the entire colonic mucosa is an extremely rare but well-documented entity.

Primary lymphomas of the colon and rectum are believed to arise from lymphocytes associated with the bowel mucosa and may be associated with immunosuppressed states and inflammatory bowel disease.[72,73] Aggressive type histology is more frequent, with diffuse large B cell lymphoma (DLBCL) and Burkitt lymphoma accounting for up to 60% of the primary intestinal lymphomas in older retrospective reports.[74] Recent studies have reported an increase in the detection of other subtypes, including T cell lymphomas, Hodgkin disease (HD), mantle cell lymphoma (MCL) and indolent mucosa-associated lymphoid tissue (MALT) lymphoma, also known as marginal zone lymphoma (MZL). For example, investigators reported an 88% rate of colon involvement with MCL, often underreported in prior studies.[75] The use of aggressive staging with colonoscopy was found to have little impact on patient management decisions. However, for MCL and MZL, some argue for an initial evaluation of the bowel and if positive, more aggressive treatment and endoscopic follow-up.[71] To attempt to avoid frequent repeat endoscopies, 18F-FDG-PET scans are showing promise to determine response and predict recurrence.[76]

Although the role of surgery in the management of these lymphomas is debated, surgical exploration remains the initial intervention in the majority of cases, and may be life saving in the patients who present with perforation, intussusception or obstruction. Surgery also provides detailed staging and pathology. Chemotherapy, either as primary therapy or following surgery, can be curative. The choice of chemotherapy depends on the grade or aggressiveness of the lymphoma. An infectious cause for colonic MALT has not yet been discovered, although reports of response to antibiotics have also been described.[71]

Malignant melanoma

Primary malignant melanoma is an extremely rare and aggressive tumor of the anal region. Since melanocytes are absent above the pectinate line, melanoma in the colon or rectum is considered to be metastatic. As in cutaneous melanoma, depth of penetration is the most important prognostic indicator, but this can be difficult to assess in melanoma of the anal canal. Anal melanoma accounts for 24% of mucosal melanomas and less than 1% of all melanomas. Patients often present in the fifth to sixth decade of life with vague symptoms, including rectal bleeding and anal discomfort, and diagnosis is often delayed.[77]

Typically, treatment for localized disease has been complete surgical resection, ranging from a radical abdominoperineal resection (APR) with elective lymph node dissection to conservative sphincter-sparing local excision alone. Although APR has been reported to have better local control rates (70% with APR versus 35% with local excision), this surgery has high comorbidity with no improvement in overall survival (<25% 5-year survival).[78,79] Another approach is to combine sphincter-sparing local excision with adjuvant radiation (30 Gy). In a retrospective analysis of 23 patients, this combined approach appeared to be reasonably effective and well tolerated.[78] Adjuvant systemic therapy with either cytotoxic therapy or immunotherapy has been investigated, but its benefit has not been clearly defined.

Although the majority of patients (70%) present with localized disease, most will eventually succumb to systemic disease with metastases to brain, lung, and/or liver. Treatment for metastatic anal melanoma is based on available drugs for advanced cutaneous melanoma, and this field has undergone substantial recent changes. Patients whose tumor harbors a V600E BRAF mutation may be treated with the oral BRAF inhibitor vemurafinib, but BRAF mutations in melanoma of anal origin are rare. Immunotherapy with the anti-CTLA4 monoclonal antibody ipilimumab has been shown to be useful in metastatic melanoma.

Paget disease of the perianal region

Paget disease of the perianal skin is a rare intraepithelial adenocarcinoma of the dermal apocrine gland, with fewer than 200 cases reported in the literature between 1966 and 1995.[80] Extramammary Paget disease can occur in any region of skin bearing apocrine glands such as anus, axilla, scrotum, groin, eyelids, and external auditory canal. Like Paget disease of the nipple, Paget disease of the perianal skin may be associated with an underlying malignancy of the gastrointestinal tract and this should be actively looked for.

Paget disease of the perianal region usually presents as a well-demarcated, erythematous, scaly, and pruritic lesion which occasionally bleeds.[81] Diagnosis is often delayed since the lesion is confused with common conditions such as pruritus ani or bleeding hemorrhoids. Diagnosis is made with a biopsy which illustrates the classic histological finding of Paget cells: large round cells with pale vacuolated cytoplasm and reticular nucleus that stain positive for PAS, CAM5.2, CK7, and CEA.[81,82]

Paget disease of the anus appears to follow one of two clinical courses: to develop malignancy or to recur locally, often on repeated occasions. Treatment with wide local excision is recommended in the absence of underlying malignancy. Small case reports have described radiation with or without chemotherapy as a nonsurgical alternative.[81] Local recurrence with *in situ* disease is common (up to 60%), but this can be managed with repeat wide excisions with excellent long-term prognosis. In patients with an invasive component or an associated anorectal adenocarcinoma, APR is usually recommended.

Anal carcinoma

Carcinoma of the anal canal comprises 3–4% of all large bowel cancers and will account for approximately 5820 new cases and 770 deaths in 2011.[83] The median age of diagnosis in the United States is 61, with a slightly increased female prevalence. Approximately 50% of patients present with localized (stage I/II) disease, 38% with stage III, and 12% present with metastatic disease.[84] The 5-year relative survival rate for all patients is 66%, with 80% of patients with localized disease surviving 5 years.[84]

The anal canal is lined by squamous epithelium and extends proximally from the anal verge (transition to hair-bearing squamous epithelium of the perianal skin) to the dentate line (the border between the squamous mucosa and rectal glandular mucosa). Squamous cell carcinomas (SCCs) comprise between 85% and 90% of all anal canal cancers. Morphological subtypes of the SCCs include basaloid (cuboidal epithelium from the anal columns), cloacogenic (which arise from the anal columnar stratified epithelium at the dentate line), transitional, and mucoepidermoid.[85] Other histological subtypes include large cell keratinizing, large cell nonkeratinizing or adenocarcinoma, small cell carcinoma, melanoma, lymphoma, neuroendocrine tumors, or sarcomas.[85] In general, anal adenocarcinomas are treated like rectal adenocarcinoma with concurrent preoperative chemoradiation, followed by surgery and further adjuvant chemotherapy. This section will focus only on the SCCs of the anus and its subtypes.

The most important risk factor for anal SCC is infection with human papillomavirus (HPV), especially types 16 and 18. The viral proteins E6 and E7 mediate oncogenic transformation of the anal squamous epithelia. A prior history of anal condylomas and a history of immunosuppression secondary to organ transplantation, chronic steroid use, and/or the human immunodeficiency virus (HIV) are also associated with an elevated risk for anal carcinoma.[86,87]

Clinical presentation and staging work-up

Rectal bleeding is the most common presenting symptom of anal carcinoma, and patients often delay seeking medical care because symptoms simulate hemorrhoidal bleeding. Some patients present with local discomfort or pain aggravated by defecation. Change in bowel habits, presence of an anal mass, tenesmus, pruritus and foul-smelling discharge are less common presentations. Approximately 20% have no rectal symptoms at all.[87]

Staging workup should include a physical examination with careful attention to the size and location of the primary tumor on digital rectal exam, and any clinical evidence of enlarged inguinal lymph nodes. The primary tumor can be measured clinically with anoscopy and with endoscopic ultrasound, which can also visualize potentially involved perirectal lymph nodes. Biopsy of the primary tumor and/or suspicious lymph nodes should be performed to obtain the pathological diagnosis. Extent of disease workup should include a CT scan of the chest, abdomen and pelvis, and routine blood tests. Pretreatment PET-CTs have been shown to have a higher sensitivity than CT for identifying regional and distant nodal involvement and are often performed during staging or treatment planning for patients at many institutions.[88,89]

The TNM staging for anal cancers is based on tumor size, invasion of adjacent structures, nodal involvement, and distant metastases.[59] The Radiation Therapy Oncology Group (RTOG) 98-11 trial demonstrated that worse overall survival was associated with node-positive cancer, large (>5 cm) tumor diameter, and male sex.[60] Similarly, the cumulative 5-year colostomy rate was statistically significantly higher for large tumor diameter than for small tumor diameter.

Treatment

Anal SCC provides a paradigm for organ preservation in the management of cancer. Until the mid 1970s, definitive surgery with an APR was the primary therapy for anal carcinoma. The overall 5-year survival with this surgery ranged from 40% to 70%.[87] In 1974, Nigro and colleagues reported the results of a preoperative chemoradiotherapy approach for anal carcinoma.[90] Pathological complete responses were achieved with concurrent 30 Gy, mitomycin-C (MMC) and 5-FU. In a subsequent series using definitive chemoradiation as primary therapy, 38 of 45 patients were cured of disease, with a 5-year overall survival of 67% and colostomy-free survival of 59%.[91] These data suggested that definitive chemoradiation could be used to treat anal canal SCC with equivalent or better tumor control and significantly reduced morbidity and mortality compared to APR.

Combined modality therapy has been compared to radiation alone in several trials, which have all demonstrated the superiority of chemoradiation for sphincter preservation.[92-94] RTOG 87-04 was a prospective, randomized phase 3 study of 310 patients with stage I–IIIA (T1–4, N0–1) anal SCC designed to test the need for inclusion of MMC.[94] The results showed substantially greater hematological toxicity with the use of MMC, but a significant decline in local recurrence (36% versus 17%). The addition of MMC led to a statistically significantly improved colostomy-free survival at 5 years (58% versus 64%) and disease-free survival (50% versus 67%), though a significant difference in overall survival was not reached (65% versus 67%).

In the RTOG study, patients undewent a mandatory biopsy at 6 weeks post treatment. If the biopsy was positive for tumor, then salvage chemotherapy was initiated with cisplatin plus 5-FU with a concomitant dose of 9 Gy. Patients who failed to achieve a complete response to this salvage therapy and who did not have evidence of metastatic disease were treated with a salvage APR.[95] Fifty percent of the patients who underwent this salvage chemoradiation with cisplatin-based therapy were rendered disease free at 4 years.[94]

Due to the hematological toxicity reported with MMC, replacement with a less myelosuppressive chemotherapeutic agent, cisplatin, has been investigated.[95-97] In the phase 3, randomized RTOG 98-11 trial,[97] patients were randomized to the standard arm of concurrent 5-FU/MMC and pelvic radiotherapy versus two cycles of induction 5-FU and cisplatin followed by concurrent 5-FU and cisplatin with pelvic radiotherapy. Despite the enthusiasm for both induction therapy and the benefits of cisplatin in other disease sites, this study showed no benefit, and a trend towards detriment for the cisplatin-containing arm in 5-year disease-free survival (60% in the MMC group and 54% in the cisplatin arm) or overall survival (75% MMC versus 70% cisplatin).[97] Interestingly, the cisplatin arm was associated with a higher rate of locoregional recurrence (33 versus 25%; $p=0.07$) and colostomies (19 versus 10%; $p=0.02$). While the MMC arm showed a significantly increased grade 3 and above acute hematological toxicity rate as compared to cisplatin (61% versus 42%; $p <0.001$), the rate of grade 3–4 acute nonhematological toxicity was 74% in both arms (primarily dermatological for the MMC group and gastrointestinal for the cisplatin). Based on these results, 5-FU and MMC remain the standard of care for anal carcinoma. Some have speculated that the delay in definitive chemoradiation associated with induction chemotherapy on the cisplatin arm may have led to the poorer local control rates reported on this trial.[98]

The RTOG 98-11 trial has been criticized for combining two experimental questions by including the induction cisplatin/5-FU portion, thus prohibiting direct comparison of cisplatin with MMC. However, the United Kingdom Anal Cancer Trial (ACT) II also failed to confirm the superiority of cisplatin in combination with 5-FU and radiation.[99] This multicenter randomized trial used a 2×2 factorial design to examine the role of MMC versus cisplatin with 5-FU-based chemoradiation, as well as the utility of maintenance 5-FU and cisplatin chemotherapy (two cycles) following chemoradiation. Grade 3+ hematological toxicity was greater in the MMC group, but 3-year colostomy rate was similar between the two groups (13.7% MMC and 11.3% cisplatin). With regard to maintenance therapy, there was no difference in 3-year recurrence-free or overall survival rates.

Local control remains the major problem in the management of anal cancer, particularly for advanced T-stage disease.[100,101] Radiotherapy dose escalation has therefore been evaluated to determine if improved local control can be achieved with high radiation doses. The recent French Federation Nationale des Centres de Lutte Contre le Cancer ACCORD 03 trial evaluated the benefit of induction chemotherapy (two cycles of 5-FU/cisplatin) and a higher dose of radiotherapy in 307 patients in a 2×2 factorial design. Toxicities were similar in all four arms, but there was no difference in the colostomy-free, event-free, or overall survival rates at 3 years.[64]

Advances in radiotherapy techniques have allowed for more conformal pelvic radiotherapy fields, such that normal tissues can be spared from the higher radiation doses that are used to treat the primary and gross nodal disease. CT-assisted planning to define normal and target structures is now routine. A further technical innovation has been intensity-modulated radiation therapy (IMRT) which uses CT-based planning and the target volumes, and normal structures are delineated individually on axial CT imaging. The IMRT plan is developed using a computer-optimized algorithm to deliver radiation of varying intensity to the target volume via multiple beams to meet the requirements for the target volume coverage and normal tissue constraints. The overall result is a highly conformal dose distribution that is customized to the shape of the tumor.

The first study to evaluate the impact of IMRT on acute toxicity, RTOG 0529, has recently been reported.[102,103] As compared to the toxicity reported on the RTOG 98-11 5-FU/ MMC arm, there was a statistically significant reduction in ≥ grade 3 gastrointestinal (GI)/genitourinary (GU) adverse events (AE) with IMRT, 21% versus 36% 98-11, p <0.008; > grade 3 GI AEs, 21% versus 35% 98-11, p <0.012; and ≥ grade 3 dermatological AEs, 21% versus 47% 98-11, p <0.0001. Median RT duration was 42.5 days (range 32–59), as compared to 49 days (range 0–102) on the MMC arm of 98-11, p <0.0001. The local control, disease-free survival, and overall survival rates appear to be quite similar to those of the RTOG 98-11 5-FU/MMC arm.[103] Future studies incorporating new chemotherapy regimens or targeted agents will use IMRT as a standard for anal SCC radiotherapy.

In summary, concurrent 5-FU/MMC and pelvic radiotherapy is considered to be the current standard treatment for anal SCC. Many investigators favor the use of IMRT to minimize acute toxicity. In debilitated patients or patients in whom chemotherapy is contraindicated, radiation therapy alone can be offered as an alternative, but it should be recognized that this is substandard care and is being given only due to limitations imposed by a patient's medical comorbidities. HIV infection alone (CD4 count >200) does not appear to constitute a substantial contraindication to chemotherapy, but patients with clinical debilitation, clinical AIDS, and/or significant bone marrow compromise may not be appropriate candidates for full combined modality therapy due to the greatly increased risk of serious toxicities. Distant metastases ultimately develop in 10–20% of patients, with the most frequent site being the liver.[87] Palliative chemotherapy options include cisplatin and 5-FU with minimal evidence of activity for other regimens or agents.

References

1. Jemal A, *et al.* Cancer statistics, 2005. CA Cancer J Clin 2005; 55(1): 10–30.
2. DiSario JA, *et al.* Colorectal cancers of rare histologic types compared with adenocarcinomas. Dis Colon Rectum 1994; 37(12): 1277–80.
3. Kulke MH, Mayer RJ. Carcinoid tumors. N Engl J Med 1999; 340(11): 858–68.
4. Maggard MA, O'Connell JB, Ko CY. Updated population-based review of carcinoid tumors. Ann Surg 2004; 240(1): 117–22.
5. Modlin IM, Sandor A. An analysis of 8305 cases of carcinoid tumors. Cancer 1997; 79(4): 813–29.
6. Crocetti E, Paci E. Malignant carcinoids in the USA, SEER 1992–1999. An epidemiological study with 6830 cases. Eur J Cancer Prev 2003; 12(3): 191–4.
7. Spread C, *et al.* Colon carcinoid tumors. A population-based study. Dis Colon Rectum 1994; 37(5): 482–91.
8. Feldman JM. Urinary serotonin in the diagnosis of carcinoid tumors. Clin Chem 1986; 32(5): 840–4.
9. Capella C, *et al.* Revised classification of neuroendocrine tumours of the lung, pancreas and gut. Virchows Arch 1995; 425(6): 547–60.
10. Klimstra DS, *et al.* The pathologic classification of neuroendocrine tumors: a review of nomenclature, grading, and staging systems. Pancreas 2010; 39(6): 707–12.
11. Federspiel BH, *et al.* Rectal and colonic carcinoids. A clinicopathologic study of 84 cases. Cancer 1990; 65(1): 135–40.
12. Ballantyne GH, *et al.* Incidence and mortality of carcinoids of the colon. Data from the Connecticut Tumor Registry. Cancer 1992; 69(10): 2400–5.
13. Rosenberg JM, Welch JP. Carcinoid tumors of the colon. A study of 72 patients. Am J Surg 1985; 149(6): 775–9.
14. Soga J, Yakuwa Y, Osaka M. Carcinoid syndrome: a statistical evaluation of 748 reported cases. J Exp Clin Cancer Res 1999; 18(2): 133–41.
15. Jetmore AB, *et al.* Rectal carcinoids: the most frequent carcinoid tumor. Dis Colon Rectum 1992; 35(8): 717–25.
16. Moertel CG. Karnofsky memorial lecture. An odyssey in the land of small tumors. J Clin Oncol 1987; 5(10): 1502–22.
17. Moertel CG, Dockerty MB, Judd ES. Carcinoid tumors of the vermiform appendix. Cancer 1968; 21(2): 270–8.
18. Moertel CG, *et al.* Carcinoid tumor of the appendix: treatment and prognosis. N Engl J Med 1987; 317(21): 1699–701.
19. Roggo A, Wood WC, Ottinger LW. Carcinoid tumors of the appendix. Ann Surg 1993; 217(4): 385–90.
20. Lamberts S, *et al.* Somatostatin-receptor imaging in the localization of endocrine tumors. N Engl J Med 1990; 323: 1246–9.
21. Cwikla JB, *et al.* Diagnostic imaging approach to gastro-entero-pancreatic carcinomas of neuroendocrine origin – single NET center experience in Poland. Neuro Endocrinol Lett 2007; 28(6): 789–800.
22. Dromain C, *et al.* Detection of liver metastases from endocrine tumors: a prospective comparison of somatostatin receptor scintigraphy, computed tomography, and magnetic resonance imaging. J Clin Oncol 2005; 23(1): 70–8.
23. Kumbasar B, *et al.* Imaging of neuroendocrine tumors: accuracy of helical CT versus SRS. Abdom Imaging 2004; 29(6): 696–702.
24. Asnacios A, *et al.* Indium-111-pentetreotide scintigraphy and somatostatin receptor subtype 2 expression: new prognostic factors for malignant well-differentiated endocrine tumors. J Clin Oncol 2008; 26(6): 963–70.
25. Zuetenhorst JM, Taal BG. Metastatic carcinoid tumors: a clinical review. Oncologist 2005; 10(2): 123–31.
26. Oberg K. Neuroendocrine tumors of the gastrointestinal tract: recent advances in molecular genetics, diagnosis, and treatment. Curr Opin Oncol 2005; 17(4): 386–91.
27. Rorstad O. Prognostic indicators for carcinoid neuroendocrine tumors of the gastrointestinal tract. J Surg Oncol 2005; 89(3): 151–60.
28. Ponka JL. Carcinoid tumors of the appendix. Report of thirty-five cases. Am J Surg 1973; 126(1): 77–83.
29. Syracuse DC, *et al.* Carcinoid tumors of the appendix. Mesoappendiceal extension and nodal metastases. Ann Surg 1979; 190(1): 58–63.
30. Koura AN, *et al.* Carcinoid tumors of the rectum: effect of size, histopathology, and surgical treatment on metastasis free survival. Cancer 1997; 79(7): 1294–8.
31. Burke M, Shepherd N, Mann CV. Carcinoid tumours of the rectum and anus. Br J Surg 1987; 74(5): 358–61.
32. Sauven P, *et al.* Anorectal carcinoid tumors. Is aggressive surgery warranted? Ann Surg 1990; 211(1): 67–71.
33. Reichlin S. Somatostatin. N Engl J Med 1983; 309(24): 1495–501.
34. Lambert S, *et al.* Somatostatin-receptor imaging in the localization of endocrine tumors. N Engl J Med 1990; 323: 1246–9.
35. Clark OH, *et al.* NCCN Clinical Practice Guidelines in Oncology: neuroendocrine tumors. J Natl Compr Canc Netw 2009; 7(7): 712–47.
36. Rinke A, *et al.* Placebo-controlled, double-blind, prospective, randomized study on the effect of octreotide LAR in the control of tumor growth in

patients with metastatic neuroendocrine midgut tumors: a report from the PROMID Study Group. J Clin Oncol 2009; 27(28): 4656–63.

37. Walderr C, *et al.* The clinical value of [90Y-DOTA]-dPhe-Tyr-octreotide in the treatment of neuroendocrine tumours: a clinical phase II study. Ann Oncol 2001; 12: 941–5.

38. Waldherr C, *et al.* Tumor response and clinical benefit in neuroendocrine tumors after 7.4 GBq (90)Y-DOTATOC. J Nucl Med 2002; 43(5): 610–16.

39. Virgolini I, *et al.* 111In- and 90Y-DOTA-lanreotide: results and implications of the MAURITIUS trial. J Nucl Med 2002; 32(2): 148–55.

40. Valkema R, *et al.* Survival and response after peptide receptor radionuclide therapy with [90Y-DOTA0,Tyr3]octreotide in patients with advanced gastroenteropancreatic neuroendocrine tumors. Semin Nucl Med 2006; 36: 147.

41. Kwekkeboom D, *et al.* Treatment with the radiolabeled somatostatin analog [177Lu-DOTA0,Tyr3]octreotate: toxicity, efficacy, and survival. J Clin Oncol 2008; 26(13): 2124–30.

42. Kwekkeboom J, *et al.* Treatment with the radiolabeled somatostatin analogue [177Lu-DOTA°,Tyr3]octreotate in patients with gastro-enteropancreatic (GEP) tumors. J Clin Oncol 2005; 23: 2754–62.

43. Moertel C, Rubin J, Kvols L. Therapy of metastatic carcinoid tumor and the malignant carcinoid syndrome with recombinant leukocyte A interferon. J Clin Oncol 1989; 7(7): 865–88.

44. Plöckinger U, Wiedenmann B. Neuroendocrine. Biotherapy. Best Pract Res Clin Endocrinol Metab 2007; 21(1): 145–62.

45. Faiss S, *et al.* Prospective, randomized multicenter trial on the antiproliferative effect of lanreotide, interferon alpha, and their combination for therapy of metastatic neuroendocrine gastroenteropancreatic tumors – the International Lanreotided and Interferon Alpha Study Group. J Clin Oncol 2003; 21: 2689–96.

46. Välimäki M, *et al.* Is the treatment of metastatic carcinoid tumor with interferon not as successful as suggested? Cancer 1991; 67: 547–9.

47. Bukowski RM, *et al.* Phase II trial of dimethyltriazenoimidazole carboxamide in patients with metastatic carcinoid. A Southwest Oncology Group study. Cancer 1994; 73(5): 1505–8.

48. Kulke MH, *et al.* A phase II study of docetaxel in patients with metastatic carcinoid tumors. Cancer Invest 2004; 22(3): 353–9.

49. Moertel CG. Treatment of the carcinoid tumor and the malignant carcinoid syndrome. J Clin Oncol 1983; 1(11): 727–40.

50. Fine RL, Fogelman DR, Schreibman SM. Effective treatment of neuroendocrine tumors with temozolomide and capecitabine. Proc Am Soc Clin Oncol 2005; Abstr 4216.

51. Kulke M, *et al.* Prediction of response to temozolamide (TMZ)-based therapy by loss of MGMT expression in patients with advanced neuroendocrine tumors (NET). J Clin Oncol 2007; 25 (18S): 4505.

52. Gupta S, *et al.* Hepatic artery embolization and chemoembolization for treatment of patients with metastatic carcinoid tumors: the MD Anderson Experience. Cancer 2003; 9(4): 261–7.

53. Moertel C, *et al.* The management of patients with advanced carcinoid tumors and islet cell carcinomas Ann Intern Med 1994; 120(4): 302–9.

54. Gupta S, *et al.* Hepatic artery embolization and chemoembolization for treatment of patients with metastatic carcinoid tumors: the M.D. Anderson experience. Cancer J 2003; 9(4): 261–7.

55. Kennedy AS, *et al.* Radioembolization for unresectable neuroendocrine hepatic metastases using resin 90Y-microspheres: early results in 148 patients. Am J Clin Oncol 2008; 31(3): 271–9.

56. Rhee TK, *et al.* 90Y Radioembolization for metastatic neuroendocrine liver tumors: preliminary results from a multi-institutional experience. Ann Surg 2008; 247(6): 1029–35.

57. King J, *et al.* Radioembolization with selective internal radiation microspheres for neuroendocrine liver metastases. Cancer 2008; 113(5): 921–9.

58. Cao CQ, *et al.* Radioembolization with yttrium microspheres for neuroendocrine tumour liver metastases. Br J Surg 2010; 97(4): 537–43.

59. Edge S, *et al.* (eds). *AJCC Cancer Staging Manual*, 7th edn. New York: Springer, 2009.

60. Ajani JA, *et al.* US intergroup anal carcinoma trial: tumor diameter predicts for colostomy. J Clin Oncol 2009; 27(7): 1116–21.

61. Yao JC, *et al.* Improved progression free survival (PFS), and rapid, sustained decrease in tumor perfusion among patients with advanced carcinoid treated with bevacizumab. Proc Am Soc Clin Oncol 2005; Abst. 4007.

62. Kulke MH, *et al.* Activity of sunitinib in patients with advanced neuroendocrine tumors. J Clin Oncol 2008; 26(20): 3403–10.

63. Raymond E, *et al.* Sunitinib malate for the treatment of pancreatic neuroendocrine tumors. N Engl J Med 2011; 364(6): 501–13.

64. Conroy T, *et al.* Treatment intensification by induction chemotherapy (ICT) and radiation dose escalation in locally advanced squamous cell anla canal carcinoma (LAAC): definitive analysis of the intergroup ACCORD 03 trial (abstr 4033). J Clin Oncol 2009; 27: 15S.

65. Yao JC, *et al.* Efficacy of RAD001 (everolimus) and octreotide LAR in advanced low- to intermediate grade neuroendocrine tumors: results of a phase II study. J Clin Oncol 2008; 26(26): 4311–18.

66. Pavel ME, *et al.* Everolimus plus octreotide long-acting repeatable for the treatment of advanced neuroendocrine tumours associated with carcinoid syndrome (RADIANT-2): a randomised, placebo-controlled, phase 3 study. Lancet 2011; 378(9808): 2005–12.

67. McEntee GP, *et al.* Cytoreductive hepatic surgery for neuroendocrine tumors. Surgery 1990; 108(6): 1091–6.

68. Shebani KO, *et al.* Prognosis and survival in patients with gastrointestinal tract carcinoid tumors. Ann Surg 1999; 229(6): 815–21; discussion 822–3.

69. Bernick PE, *et al.* Neuroendocrine carcinomas of the colon and rectum. Dis Colon Rectum 2004; 47(2): 163–9.

70. Conlon KC, Casper ES, Brennan MF, Primary gastrointestinal sarcomas: analysis of prognostic variables. Ann Surg Oncol 1995; 2(1): 26–31.

71. Romaguera J, Hagemeister FB. Lymphoma of the colon. Curr Opin Gastroenterol 2005; 21(1): 80–4.

72. Doolabh N, *et al.* Primary colonic lymphoma. J Surg Oncol 2000; 74(4): 257–62.

73. Watanabe N, *et al.* Association of intestinal malignant lymphoma and ulcerative colitis. Intern Med 2003; 42(12): 1183–7.

74. Zighelboim J, Larson MV. Primary colonic lymphoma. Clinical presentation, histopathologic features, and outcome with combination chemotherapy. J Clin Gastroenterol 1994; 18(4): 291–7.

75. Romaguera JE, *et al.* Frequency of gastrointestinal involvement and its clinical significance in mantle cell lymphoma. Cancer 2003; 97(3): 586–91.

76. Kumar R, *et al.* 18F-FDG PET for evaluation of the treatment response in patients with gastrointestinal tract lymphomas. J Nucl Med 2004; 45(11): 1796–803.

77. Yeh JJ, *et al.* Response of stage IV anal mucosal melanoma to chemotherapy. Lancet Oncol 2005; 6(6): 438–9.

78. Ballo MT, *et al.* Sphincter-sparing local excision and adjuvant radiation for anal-rectal melanoma. J Clin Oncol 2002; 20(23): 4555–8.

79. Brady MS, Kavolius JP, Quan SH. Anorectal melanoma. A 64-year experience at Memorial Sloan-Kettering Cancer Center. Dis Colon Rectum 1995; 38(2): 146–51.

80. Beck D. Paget's disease and Bowen's disease of the anus. Semin Colon Rectal Surg 1995; 6: 143–9.

81. Moore H, Guillem J. Anal neoplasms. Surg Clin North Am 2002; 82: 1233–51.

82. Armitage NC, *et al.* Paget's disease of the anus: a clinicopathological study. Br J Surg 1989; 76(1): 60–3.

83. Siegel R, *et al.* Cancer statistics, 2011: the impact of eliminating socioeconomic and racial disparities on premature cancer deaths. CA Cancer J Clin 2011; 61(4): 212–36.

84. Horner M, *et al.* (eds). *SEER Cancer Statistics Review, 1975–2006*. Bethesda, MD: National Cancer Institute, 2009.

85. Klas JV, *et al.* Malignant tumors of the anal canal: the spectrum of disease, treatment, and outcomes. Cancer 1999; 85(8): 1686–93.

86. Daling JR, *et al.* Sexual practices, sexually transmitted diseases, and the incidence of anal cancer. N Engl J Med 1987; 317(16): 973–7.

87. Ryan DP, Compton CC, Mayer RJ. Carcinoma of the anal canal. N Engl J Med 2000; 342(11): 792–800.

88. Cotter SE, *et al.* FDG-PET/CT in the evaluation of anal carcinoma. Int J Radiat Oncol Biol Phys 2006; 65(3): 720–5.

89. Winton E, *et al*. The impact of 18-fluorodeoxyglucose positron emission tomography on the staging, management and outcome of anal cancer. Br J Cancer 2009; 100(5): 693–700.

90. Nigro ND, Vaitkevicius VK, Considine B Jr. Combined therapy for cancer of the anal canal: a preliminary report. Dis Colon Rectum 1974; 17: 354–6.

91. Leichman L, *et al*. Cancer of the anal canal. Model for preoperative adjuvant combined modality therapy. Am J Med 1985; 78(2): 211–15.

92. UKCCCR Anal Cancer Trial Working Party. Epidermoid anal cancer: results from the UKCCCR randomised trial of radiotherapy alone versus radiotherapy, 5-fluorouracil, and mitomycin. UK Co-ordinating Committee on Cancer Research. Lancet 1996; 348(9034): 1049–54.

93. Bartelink H, *et al*. Concomitant radiotherapy and chemotherapy is superior to radiotherapy alone in the treatment of locally advanced anal cancer: results of a phase III randomized trial of the European Organization for Research and Treatment of Cancer Radiotherapy and Gastrointestinal Cooperative Groups. J Clin Oncol 1997; 15(5): 2040–9.

94. Flam M, *et al*. Role of mitomycin in combination with fluorouracil and radiotherapy, and of salvage chemoradiation in the definitive nonsurgical treatment of epidermoid carcinoma of the anal canal: results of a phase III randomized intergroup study. J Clin Oncol 1996; 14(9): 2527–39.

95. Hung A, *et al*. Cisplatin-based combined modality therapy for anal carcinoma: a wider therapeutic index. Cancer 2003; 97: 1195–202.

96. Meropol NJ, *et al*. Induction therapy for poor-prognosis anal canal carcinoma: a phase II study of the cancer and Leukemia Group B (CALGB 9281). J Clin Oncol 2008; 26: 3229–34.

97. Ajani JA, *et al*. Fluorouracil, mitomycin, and radiotherapy vs fluorouracil, cisplatin, and radiotherapy for carcinoma of the anal canal: a randomized controlled trial. JAMA 2008; 299(16): 1914–21.

98. Ben-Josef E, *et al*. The impact of overall treatment time on survival and local control in anal cancer patients: a pooled data analysis of RTOG trials 8704 and 9811. Int J Radiat Oncol Biol Phys 2009; 75: S26–S27.

99. James R, *et al*. A randomized trial of chemoradiation using mitomycin or cisplatin, with or without maintenance cisplatin/5FU in squamous cell carcinoma of the anus (ACT II) (ASCO abstr LBA4009). J Clin Oncol 2009; 27: 18S.

100. Wright JL, *et al*. Squamous cell carcinoma of the anal canal: patterns and predictors of failure and implications for intensity-modulated radiation treatment planning. Int J Radiat Oncol Biol Phys 2010; 78(4): 1064–72.

101. Das P, *et al*. Predictors and patterns of recurrence after definitive chemoradiation for anal cancer. Int J Radiat Oncol Biol Phys 2007; 68: 794–800.

102. Kachnic L, *et al*. RTOG 0529: A phase II evaluation of dose-painted IMRT in combination with 5-fluorouracil and mitomycin-C for reduction of acute morbidity in carcinoma of the anal canal Int J Radiat Oncol Biol Phys 2009; 75(suppl): S5.

103. Kachnic L, *et al*. Two-year outcomes of RTOG 0529: a phase II evaluation of dose-painted IMRT in combination with 5-fluorouracil and mitomycin-C for the reduction of acute morbidity in carcinoma of the anal canal. J Clin Oncol 2011; 29(4): abstract 368.

33 Gastrointestinal Stromal Tumors

Margaret von Mehren,[1] Douglas B. Flieder,[2] and Chandrajit P. Raut[3]

[1] Department of Medical Oncology, [2] Department of Pathology, Fox Chase Cancer Center, Philadelphia, PA, USA
[3] Harvard Medical School; Division of Surgical Oncology, Brigham and Women's Hospital Center for Sarcoma and Bone Oncology; Dana-Farber Cancer Institute, Boston, MA, USA

Introduction

Gastrointestinal stromal tumors (GIST) are uncommon tumors of mesenchymal origin, arising from the intestinal tract. Prior to their recognition as a distinct biological subtype, they were termed leiomyosarcomas, leiomyomas, or leiomyoblastomas. Several findings have dramatically altered contemporary diagnostic and management strategies. First, Mazur and Clark determined that these tumors contained both smooth muscle and neural features and reclassified them as GIST.[1] Subsequently, these tumors were found to express CD34 and KIT, further aiding in their classification.[2,3] Finally, Hirota and colleagues determined that a majority of tumors contained *KIT* mutations leading to constitutive activation of the molecule.[4] These three findings aided pathologists in making the correct diagnosis and the selection of appropriate patients for KIT-targeted therapy. Since then, KIT-targeted therapy has significantly changed the management and prognosis of GIST patients.

Epidemiology

Gastrointestinal stromal tumors arise typically along the intestinal tract. The most common site of primary tumors is the stomach (39–70%), followed by the small intestine (31–45%), colon, rectum, anus (10–16%), and mesentery and peritoneum (8%), with rare cases arising in the esophagus.[5–9] Case reports in the literature also describe primary tumors of the duodenal ampulla,[10] appendix,[11] gallbladder, and urinary bladder.[12] Metastatic disease is most commonly found in the liver, as well as the peritoneum and omentum. Less common metastatic sites include lung and bone.

The true incidence of GIST is being clarified, as pathologists, surgeons, and medical oncologists become increasingly familiar with this disease entity. Pathology and autopsy studies have demonstrated that GISTs are much more common than previously recognized. In a Japanese study of 100 patients undergoing total gastrectomy for gastric adenocarcinoma, microscopic GISTs (≤5 mm) were identified in 35%.[13] In an autopsy study from Germany, 23% of adults over age 50 were found to have subcentimeter GISTs.[14]

The incidence of clinically relevant tumors has been reported to range from 1.45 to 0.65 per 100,000 people.[15–21] A population-based study of GIST analyzing tumors identified in Iceland from 1990 to 2003 estimated the annual incidence to be 1.1 per 100,000.[15] A population-based study of western Sweden, with a population of 1.3–1.6 million, identified 288 cases of primary GISTs between 1983 and 2000, with an annual incidence of 14.5 per million.[16] The authors estimated the overall prevalence to be 129 per million. Another study evaluating the Surveillance, Epidemiology and End Results (SEER) database of cases diagnosed between 1992 and 2000 determined the age-adjusted yearly incidence rate as 0.68 per 100,000.[17] In young adults, ages 20–29, the incidence has been reported to be 0.06 per 100,000, with the incidence increasing with each decade up to 2.29 per 100,000 in individuals 80 and above.[17]

The median age at diagnosis in the SEER cohorts was 63. Gender assessments have been mixed; some studies have suggested a male preponderance[16,17] while others report the disease as more common in females.[20,21] Data from SEER report a difference in the age-adjusted incidence based on ethnicity, with the highest incidence in blacks compared with other races and whites (1.16 versus 0.97 versus 0.60/100,000 population). Among the other races, the lowest incidence occurred in Native Americans and Alaskans (0.19/100,000).[17] The SEER study also identified older age, advanced stage, and lack of therapy as prognostic factors associated with a poor outcome.

Pathology

Gross features

Gastrointestinal stromal tumors can develop along any portion of the hollow viscera, within any portion of the gut wall. They are most often centered in the submucosa or muscularis propria. Some tumors are mostly extramural, while very large neoplasms can extend to or invade adjacent organs. GISTs are well circumscribed, yet may be multinodular. Overlying mucosa may be intact or ulcerated regardless of the aggressiveness of the tumor. Cut surfaces are usually tan, smooth, and lobulated with either whorled or granular appearances. Tumors may feature hemorrhage, necrosis, calcification, and/or cystic change.

Microscopic features

A diagnosis of GIST is often suspected histologically, since the majority of cases have uniform appearances falling into one of three categories: spindle cell type, epithelioid type, or mixed type. Interestingly, the majority of gastric GISTs feature an epithelioid phenotype, while small intestinal, anorectal, colonic, and esophageal tumors more often feature spindle cell morphology. GISTs with spindle cell morphology are composed of relatively uniform cells arranged in whorls or short fascicles. Individual cells have light pink (eosinophilic)

cytoplasm with indistinct cellular borders. Nuclei are uniform and spindled with open evenly distributed chromatin and inconspicuous nucleoli. Perinuclear cytoplasmic vacuoles that appear to indent the nuclei are seen in up to 5% of cases and are a characteristic feature of gastric GIST (Fig. 33.1a). These vacuoles are an artifact of fixation since they are not present in frozen section specimens. Stromal hyalinization and/or calcification are not uncommon features, and thin-walled vessels may be abundant resulting in stromal hemorrhage. Hypercellularity, tumor cell necrosis, and brisk mitotic activity may be seen.

Gastrointestinal stromal tumors of epithelioid type feature rounded cells with either pink (eosinophilic) or clear cytoplasm arranged in sheets or nests (Fig. 33.1b). In tumors with clear cytoplasm, a condensed perinuclear rim of pink cytoplasm is often observed. Nuclei are usually eccentrically placed and are round with small nucleoli and evenly distributed chromatin. While diffuse cellular pleomorphism is associated with malignant behavior, scattered bizarre cells are more commonly seen in indolent neoplasms. Mitotic counts may not be particularly helpful in discerning the aggressiveness of

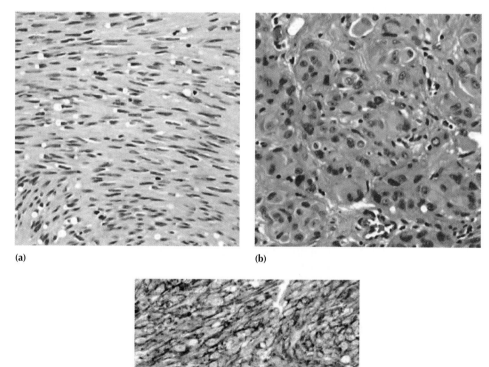

(a)

(b)

(c)

Figure 33.1 Histological sections of GISTs. (a) Spindle cell GIST. Spindle cells with inconspicuous cytoplasmic borders and bland nuclei feature scattered perinuclear vacuoles (H&E, 60× original magnification). (b) Epithelioid GIST. Clusters of neoplastic cells with round nuclei, small nucleoli, and abundant pink (eosinophilic) cytoplasm cluster in small groups (H&E, 60× original magnification). (c) CD117 immunohistochemical staining of GIST. All neoplastic cells feature cytoplasmic staining as well as membranous reactivity (H&E, 60× original magnification).

epithelioid GIST. They often have an indolent morphology with morphological heterogeneity, which upon extensive sampling will reveal malignant components within a largely "benign" tumor.

Tumors with mixed cell types may feature a comingling of spindle cell and epithelioid cells or an abrupt transition between the patterns. The recognition of this pattern simply emphasizes the unique nature of GIST and supports the distinction from smooth muscle tumors as well as neurogenic lesions of the gastrointestinal tract.

Up to 20% of GISTs, whether spindle cell or epithelioid, feature stromal hyaline or fibrillary pink material referred to as skeinoid fibers. These globular and elongated nodular tangles of collagen fibers are seen in a large percentage of small intestinal GIST and though once thought to indicate neural differentiation, are currently believed to have no histological/genetic significance.[22]

Rare morphological findings also seen in GIST include prominent myxoid stroma, nested so-called paraganglioma-like growth (especially in the small intestinal neoplasms), carcinoid-like growth pattern, signet ring cell features, granular cell changes, oncocytic cytoplasmic changes, crystalloid formation, osteoclast-like giant cells, tumor giant cells, and, although quite rare, notable cytological pleomorphism.

Immunohistochemical features

While some authorities require CD117 positivity of tumor cells in order to diagnose a tumor as a GIST, this single marker is neither required diagnostically nor pathognomonic. Rare tumors with all the morphological and phenotypic features of GIST, which do not stain for CD117, should still be diagnosed as GIST, while tumors that share few if any morphological features of GISTs should not be designated as GIST simply on account of CD117 positivity.[23] Against this background, 90–95% of GIST from all sites, regardless of their morphological features and degree of malignancy, show strong cytoplasmic CD117 staining (Fig. 33.1c).[24] Prominent membranous reactivity is the most convincing pattern of staining since other mesenchymal tumors such as fibromatosis (desmoid tumor) may stain with CD117 in a coarse granular cytoplasmic pattern. Up to 50% of GISTs show cytoplasmic dot-like (Golgi pattern) staining that often coexists with the more diffuse cytoplasmic pattern. While most GISTs show CD117 positivity in 90% or more of tumor cells, a small percentage of tumors show focal staining, that is, only 5–20% of tumor cells react with anti-CD117 antibodies. The therapeutic relevance of limited immunoreactivity appears to be unimportant; however, antigen retrieval techniques should not be performed as this increases the false-positive rate for CD117 staining. Also of note, the presence of CD117 immunoreactivity in a tumor (GIST or otherwise) does not necessarily correlate with a *KIT* gene mutation. Conversely, a *KIT* mutation can exist in the absence of CD117 immunohistochemical staining.

The immunohistochemical marker CD34 stains up to 70% of spindle cell and epithelioid GISTs, and at one time was considered a reproducible marker of GIST. Staining is most consistently seen in colorectal and esophageal primaries.

However, Schwann cell neoplasms and a proportion of true smooth muscle tumors also show CD34 positivity.

Most KIT-negative GISTs are either gastric or extravisceral tumors; however, these neoplasms are almost always positive for a *PDGFRA* mutation.[25] Interestingly, a monoclonal antibody developed against a recently identified chloride channel protein, DOG1, is immunoreactive in 95% of these tumors irrespective of mutation status.[26,27] Several studies have noted that the overall sensitivity of DOG1 and KIT in GIST is nearly identical while negativity for both DOG1 and KIT is noted in less than 3% of gastrointestinal (GI) tract GISTs. Of great value is the fact that more than one-third of KIT negative GISTs express DOG1.[28] However, DOG1 positivity is also noted in uterine type retroperitoneal leiomyomas, peritoneal leiomyomatosis, and synovial sarcomas.[29] Protein kinase C theta (PKC), once considered a promising immunohistochemical marker for GIST, has limited usefulness owing to low specificity, and low sensitivity in KIT-negative tumors.[30–32] Lastly, malignant epithelioid GISTs can feature scattered immunoreactivity with cytokeratins, but KIT positivity essentially abrogates a diagnosis of carcinoma.

Myoid marker reactivity is also seen in up to 30% of GISTs, most often in small intestinal tumors. Most of these positive reactions have been reported with smooth muscle actin, either focally or diffusely, while desmin is found in less than 5% of GIST with staining usually limited to epithelioid tumors or only scattered spindle tumor cells. Caldesmon is also detected in a significant subset of GISTs.

Neural antigens can also stain GISTs. S-100 protein may be seen focally in up to 10% of tumors yet these lesions are usually negative for neurofilament protein and glial fibrillary acidic protein.

Microscopic differential diagnosis

Given the wide morphological spectrum of GISTs, the morphological differential diagnosis includes solitary fibrous tumor, fibromatosis, inflammatory fibroid tumor, glomus tumor, schwannoma/malignant peripheral nerve sheath tumor, leiomyoma/leiomyosarcoma, and even carcinomas and lymphomas. Fibromatosis is probably the most difficult differential since it can involve the gastrointestinal wall and, as mentioned above, stains for CD117. In addition, fibromatosis can develop as a postsurgical complication of GIST resection. The distinction between GIST and leiomyoma/leiomyosarcoma along with schwannoma/malignant peripheral nerve sheath tumor is quite difficult given the smooth muscle and/or neural features of GISTs. The practical approach is to diagnose a tumor as either a smooth muscle tumor or neural tumor if the typical morphological and immunohistochemical features are seen and the neoplasm lacks CD117 immunoreactivity.

Molecular pathology

Gastrointestinal stromal tumors typically express KIT, and commonly contain mutations in the *KIT* gene. KIT is a member of the tyrosine kinase type III family that also includes the

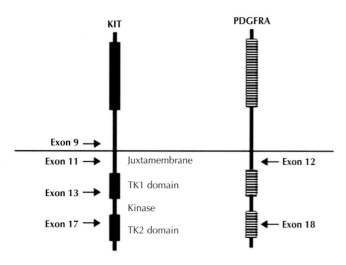

Figure 33.2 Depiction of KIT and PDGFRA tyrosine kinase receptors. The area of the receptor where the most common exon mutations occur is shown.

platelet-derived growth factor receptor (PDGFR). In the minority of tumors that are KIT negative, approximately 30% have PDGFRA mutations.[33] The protein structures of KIT and PDGFR consist of an extracellular domain with five immunoglobulin-like domains, a transmembrane domain followed by two tyrosine kinase domains. Mutations in *KIT* have been diagnosed most commonly in exon 11, followed in frequency by exons 9, 13, and 17 (Fig. 33.2). *PDGFRA* mutations are found primarily in exons 12 and 18. These mutations occur in the transmembrane domain (*KIT* exons 9 and 11 and *PDGFRA* exon 12), and tyrosine kinase domains (*KIT* exons 13 and 17 and *PDGFRA* exon 18). Mutations lead to constitutive activation of the protein and tumor formation. Tumors with *KIT* exon 11 mutations arise through the GI tract, whereas those *with KIT* exon 9 mutations predominantly arise in the small intestine.[34] Tumors with *PDGRFA* D842V mutations are most commonly found in the stomach. As discussed in the epidemiology section, pediatric GIST and GIST associated with the Carney syndrome, Carney–Stratakis syndrome and neurofibromatosis (NF)-1 typically do not carry activating mutations in *KIT* or *PDGFRA*.

Clinical presentation and diagnosis

A large fraction of patients diagnosed with GIST are asymptomatic. Occasional incidental GISTs are seen during esophagogastroduodenocopy (EGD) as submucosal lesions. Ultrasonographic criteria have been identified which increase the risk for a submucosal lesion being GIST, including irregular extraluminal margins, cystic spaces, and lymph nodes with malignant pattern.[35] However, patients can also present with a wide variety of signs and symptoms, some of which are dependent on the location of the primary tumor.[5–8] The most common are pain, a palpable mass, and bleeding, with the latter two being somewhat more common in tumors that arise in the small or large intestine. Obstructive symptoms are not often seen with gastric primaries but can be seen in patients

with tumors arising in the more distal portions of the intestinal tract. Other symptoms include nausea, vomiting, early satiety, and fever.

Patients presenting symptomatically typically undergo endoscopic evaluation and/or CT scans. Any abdominal mass is considered for resection. Preoperative biopsy of a resectable mass concerning for GIST is commonly performed, but it is not necessary and is associated with risks. GISTs may be soft and fragile, and transperitoneal biopsy risks both hemorrhage and tumor rupture. Endoscopic biopsy or fine needle aspiration (FNA), however, may be performed for diagnosis without significant risk of peritoneal seeding. Endoscopic ultrasound guidance may help access lesions for diagnosis.

On the other hand, core needle biopsies may be inconclusive if a necrotic or hemorrhagic portion of the tumor is sampled. Thus, postoperative pathology assessment is essential to confirm the diagnosis after removal of any suspected GIST. Nevertheless, if preoperative therapy is under consideration, a confirmatory biopsy may be necessary. Patients with resectable, nonmetastatic lesions, especially if not amenable to endoscopic biopsy or FNA, should undergo surgery without a definitive diagnosis.

Routine laboratory studies including a complete blood count and a complete metabolic panel are performed for staging. Radiographic studies, typically computed tomography (CT) or magnetic resonance imaging (MRI), should assess for liver and mesenteric, peritoneal, or omental metastases. Lung metastases are uncommon and generally only a very late stage event; chest x-ray is sufficient for evaluation of GIST patients. Lastly, bone metastases are seen uncommonly. Only patients with a history of bone pain or unexplained elevations in alkaline phosphatase require bone scan evaluations. Fluorodeoxyglucose positron emission tomography (FDG-PET) scans have also been shown to be highly informative, as GISTs are typically very tracer avid; some tumors, however, demonstrate minimal glucose uptake on PET scan. PET scans are not necessary for routine staging. They are useful to follow response to therapy in select individuals (see below).

Risk stratification and tumor staging

Unlike other mesenchymal tumors, GISTs are not characterized as being either benign or malignant. Instead, the risk of aggressive behavior and recurrence is based upon reproducible pathological features. A National Institutes of Health workshop on GIST proposed that tumors be described as having a very low risk, low risk, intermediate risk, or high risk of recurrence on the basis of tumor size (single largest dimension) and mitotic count (number of mitotic figures per 50 high-power fields – HPF) (Table 33.1).[23,36] Miettinen and associates subsequently revised the risk stratification to include organ site of origin as a third prognostic factor.[37] In general, patients with gastric GISTs have a lower risk of recurrence than those arising in the small bowel or colon of comparable size and mitotic count. Based on these data, a new GIST staging system was added to the 7th edition of the American Joint Committee on

Table 33.1 Risk stratification of primary GIST by mitotic index, size, and site.

Tumor parameters		Risk for progressive disease* (%)			
Mitotic index	**Size**	**Gastric**	**Jejunum/ileum**	**Duodenum**	**Rectum**
≤5 per 50 HPF	≤2 cm	None (0%)	None (0%)	None (0%)	None (0%)
	>2 ≤5 cm	Very low (1.9%)	Low (4.3%)	Low (8.3%)	Low (8.5%)
	>5 ≤10 cm	Low (3.6%)	Moderate (24%)	Insufficient data	Insufficient data
	>10 cm	Moderate (10%)	High (52%)	High (34%)	High (57%)
>5 per 50 HPF	≤2 cm	None†	High†	Insufficient data	High (52%)
	>2 ≤5 cm	Moderate (16%)	High (73%)	High (50%)	High (54%)
	>5 ≤10 cm	High (55%)	High (85%)	Insufficient data	Insufficient data
	>10 cm	High (86%)	High (90%)	High (86%)	High (71%)

Adapted from Miettinen and Lasota.[37]
Data are based on long-term follow-up of 1055 gastric, 629 small intestinal, 144 duodenal, and 111 rectal GISTs.
*Defined as metastasis or tumor-related death.
†Denotes small numbers of cases.
GIST, gastrointestinal stromal tumor; HPF, high-power field.

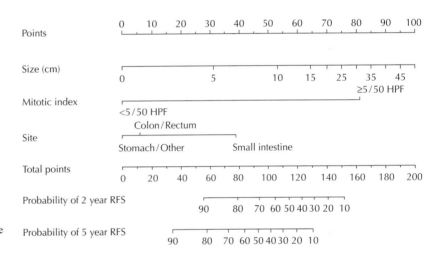

Figure 33.3 Nomogram to predict the probabilities of 2-year and 5-year recurrence-free survival. Points are assigned for size, mitotic index, and site of origin by drawing a line upward from the corresponding values to the "Points" line. The sum of these three points, plotted on the "Total points" line, corresponds to predictions of 2-year and 5-year recurrence-free survival (RFS). Data are from Gold.[39]

Cancer Staging Manual (2010). Data from American College of Surgeons Oncology Group (ACOSOG) phase 3 Z9001 trial demonstrated that tumor mitotic count is the single strongest predictor of recurrence.[38]

More recently, a GIST nomogram incorporating the three known prognostic factors was published (Fig. 33.3).[39] The validated nomogram assigns points for each of the three factors and predicts probability of the 2-year and 5-year recurrence-free survival.

Treatment

Historically, patients with GISTs could be treated with any of the three traditional cancer therapeutic modalities: surgery, chemotherapy, and radiation therapy. Surgery is potentially effective for patients with limited, resectable disease, but disease may recur in upwards of 50% of individuals treated with this single modality, based on the risk stratification described above. Standard cytotoxic chemotherapy and radiation therapy have shown remarkably little efficacy in this disease.[5,7,40,41]

General surgical principles

Surgery remains the mainstay of therapy, and the only potentially curative therapy, for patients with primary, nonmetastatic GIST. It should be the initial therapy for tumors considered technically resectable.

The goal of surgery is a macroscopically complete resection with an intact pseudocapsule and negative microscopic margins (R0 resection). At laparotomy, the abdomen should be explored thoroughly with careful inspection of the peritoneal surfaces, particularly the lesser sac in gastric GISTs, the vesicovaginal, rectovaginal, and/or rectovesical recesses as well as the liver, to identify metastasis. GISTs should be handled with care to avoid tumor rupture.

Primary gastric GISTs may be resected with a 1–2 cm margin, either as a wedge resection when feasible or a larger more anatomical resection if necessary; total gastrectomies are only rarely required. For small bowel GISTs, segmental resection of the small intestine should be performed, again with the goal of achieving negative microscopic margins. Upper rectal GISTs may require a low anterior resection (LAR) while lower-third rectal GISTs may be removed via a full-thickness transanal resection. The latter approach is associated with lower rates of R0 resections (32% versus 82%) and higher local recurrence rates (77% versus 31%) than LAR.[42–44] While abdominoperineal resections (APRs) were performed in the past for rectal GIST, it is now clear that marginal transanal resection, particularly together with neoadjuvant and/or adjuvant imatinib, is a safe alternative. Formal lymph node dissection and wider resection of uninvolved tissue are not needed, as these are not required to address the typical pattern of spread or recurrence of this disease. Lymphadenectomy is unnecessary since lymph node metastases are rare with GIST in particular and sarcomas in general.[45] Primary GISTs often arise exophytically from the stomach or intestine and, like other sarcomas, tend to displace adjacent structures. Consequently, primary GISTs can often be lifted away from surrounding organs. Some may become densely adherent to nearby structures. In this setting, an *en bloc* resection of adjacent tissue is required.

The value of negative microscopic margins is uncertain with large (>10 cm) GISTs, which may shed cells from anywhere along their surface directly into the peritoneum.[7] The management of a positive microscopic margin on final pathological analysis in a patient with a macroscopically complete resection (R1 resection) is not well defined and depends on whether the surgeon believes the finding accurately reflects the final surgical procedure. For instance, resection specimens may experience retraction of the mucosal or seromuscular edges, artificially decreasing the size of the margin. There is no evidence to suggest that patients who undergo a macroscopically complete resection but have microscopically positive margins need to undergo reexcision. Such patients should be carefully evaluated by the multidisciplinary care team to consider possible risks and benefits of reexcision, watchful waiting, or postoperative imatinib.

Some patients may require extensive surgery for a poorly situated tumor. The operative risks and anticipated postoperative recovery must be weighed against the oncological benefit of tumor resection. For instance, a tumor located near the gastroesophageal (GE) junction may require a proximal or total gastrectomy. Pancreaticoduodenectomy may be necessary to remove a duodenal GIST. Occasionally and rarely, an APR is needed for a low rectal GIST. In these situations, preoperative multidisciplinary review is critical, because such patients may be spared such a radical resection after even a partial response to preoperative imatinib.

All GISTs 2 cm or greater should be resected, though this recommendation remains somewhat arbitrary.[36] However, the management of incidentally encountered small GISTs less than 2 cm remains controversial. The natural history of such small tumors, particularly growth rate, remains unknown. As described earlier, the incidence of subclinical GIST ranges from 23% to 35%.[12,13] Thus, the percentage that may become relevant and actually require treatment remains relatively low. Endoscopic resection of small GISTs has been reported but with its inherent risks of positive margins and tumor spillage, its role remains controversial.[46] Although small GISTs may be followed endoscopically until they grow or become symptomatic,

the frequency of follow-up remains uncertain. At present, any endoscopic approach should be considered investigational, and would be best performed under the auspices of a clinical trial.

Currently, there are insufficient data to guide the management of very small GISTs (less than 2 cm) discovered incidentally during endoscopy and the usefulness of regular endoscopic ultrasound (EUS) surveillance remains unestablished. Complete surgical resection is the mainstay of treatment in symptomatic patients although, for a subset of patients with very small gastric GISTs (less than 2 cm) with no high-risk EUS features, surveillance via serial EUS examinations, at 6–12-months intervals, may be considered.[47]

The role for laparoscopy in the resection of GISTs continues to expand. The same principles of a macroscopically complete resection and avoidance of tumor rupture followed during laparotomy apply to laparoscopy.[48] Reports based on small series of patients and retrospective analyses have demonstrated that not only are laparoscopic or laparoscopy-assisted resections possible, but they are also associated with low recurrence rates, short inpatient hospital stay, and low morbidity.[48–52] Novitsky and colleagues performed 50 laparoscopic resections of gastric GISTs (mean tumor size 4.4 cm, 1.0–8.5 cm) with negative resection margins (2–45 mm).[49] At a mean follow-up of 36 months, 46 (92%) patients were disease free. Of the remaining four patients, two died of metastatic disease, one with metastases died of an unrelated event, and one was alive with recurrent disease. No local or port site recurrences were identified. Otani and colleagues removed 35 gastric GISTs measuring 2–5 cm through laparoscopic wedge resections.[48,50] No local or distant disease recurrences were noted for tumors less than 4 cm.

These data confirm that laparoscopic or laparoscopy-assisted resections can be performed safely in experienced hands. Thus, laparoscopic resection is a reasonably safe and feasible procedure for patients with low-risk smaller gastric GISTs. Larger tumors may be resected using a laparoscopic or laparoscopy-assisted technique with a hand port depending on the location and shape of the tumor. As with other laparoscopic resections for cancer, standard surgical principles should be applied, and the tumor should be removed in a protective plastic bag to minimize the risk of port site recurrence. Laparoscopic surgery could be feasible in other anatomical sites, such as small bowel GISTs. However, data on laparoscopic resection of GISTs at other sites are limited.

Early data on the efficacy of surgery for limited, resectable disease were retrospective in nature, having been collated following the identification of GIST as being distinct from leiomyosarcomas.[6,7,53,54] However, studies indicate that complete resections in all stages of disease, that is, primary presentation, locally recurrent disease and metastatic disease, lead to prolonged survival compared to patients who have incomplete resections. They also suggest that in up to 50% of patients presenting with primary disease, the tumor will eventually recur. However, when the current risk stratification system utilizing size and mitotic rate of the tumor has been applied, the risk of death is increased in patients with high-risk and metastatic disease, but not in the other risk groups (see Table 33.1).[37]

Radiation

At present, radiation therapy is not considered effective to definitively control tumor growth but it has been utilized successfully in the palliative setting, to aid in the control of pain and bleeding. A theoretic role for radiation therapy for locally advanced, symptomatic rectal GIST exists, but at this time, there are no data to support routine use of radiation for even this indication.

Systemic therapy

Chemotherapy

Standard therapy for soft tissue sarcomas utilizes doxorubicin alone or in combination with other agents, most commonly ifosfamide or dacarbazine. Review of past clinical trials in soft tissue sarcomas to determine the response rate to standard chemotherapies is confounded by the inclusion of GIST into the leiomyosarcoma subgroup or no breakdown of the histologies included. A study by Edmonson and colleagues of dacarbazine, mitomycin, doxorubicin, and cisplatin enrolled two cohorts of patients: leiomyosarcomas and GIST.[40] There was a 54% response rate in leiomyosarcomas compared with a 4.9% response rate in GIST. The reported response rates of GISTs to doxorubicin- and ifosfamide-containing regimens are 0–27%, to paclitaxel are 7%, and no responses have been seen following therapy with gemcitabine.[41] GISTs have been found to have enhanced expression of multidrug resistance proteins (compared with leiomyosarcomas), which may explain the relative chemotherapy insensitivity.[55] The limited response rate to these therapies is associated with poor survival in patients with metastatic disease, with a median overall survival of about 18 months reported.[40]

Targeted therapy: imatinib mesylate

Understanding the oncogenesis of GISTs led to a dramatically different approach to treatment. KIT and PDGFRA provided biologically meaningful targets for therapy, with imatinib mesylate (imatinib), an oral tyrosine kinase inhibitor with activity against ABL, BCR-ABL, KIT, and the PDGFR.[56,57] Preclinical data demonstrated activity against both wild type and mutant forms of KIT,[57,58] and more recently to some mutant forms of PDGFRA.[59]

Proof of the principle that inhibition of KIT by drug therapy would affect GIST growth was demonstrated by the successful imatinib treatment of one initial patient with metastatic GIST refractory to multiple types of therapies.[60] A subsequent phase 1 trial of imatinib in GIST patients tested 400 mg, 300 mg bid, 400 mg bid, and 500 mg bid, with the latter dose identified as dose limiting.[61,62] The maximum tolerated dose was 400 mg twice daily, with dose-limiting toxicities of nausea, vomiting, edema, and rash; it was noted that patients with GIST, in comparison to those receiving imatinib for chronic myelogenous leukemia (CML), experience a lower frequency of hematological toxicity.[63,64] When bleeding is noted in GIST patients, it is primarily due to responding tumors, typically bulky masses, rather than to thrombocytopenia.

The US-Finland phase 2 trial, designed and initiated in the same period as the phase 1 trial, tested 400 and 600 mg.[65–67] The study included 147 patients but was not powered to determine the superiority of one dose level over the other. The European Organization for Research and Treatment of Cancer (EORTC) performed a phase 2 trial using 400 mg bid in GIST and non-GIST soft tissue sarcomas.[68] Response rates in phase 1 and 2 trials of imatinib in GIST patients were 54–71% partial response (PR), with an additional 17–37% with stable disease (SD), with only 1% of patients achieving a complete response (CR).

The phase 1 and 2 studies of imatinib demonstrated that the drug was well tolerated at doses of 300–800 mg daily.[61,62,65,68] The most common toxicities requiring dose reduction identified in the phase 1 trial were nausea, vomiting and edema; neutropenia, rash and shortness of breath were noted less commonly.[61,62] In addition, diarrhea, anorexia, fatigue, conjunctivitis, and scleral hemorrhage were seen. The phase 2 studies reported high rates of grade 1–2 toxicities potentially related to imatinib.[65,68] The most commonly reported were edema, anemia, granulocytopenia, nausea, diarrhea, myalgias, fatigue, rash, headache, and abdominal pain in decreasing order of frequency. Toxicities were managed with symptomatic measures, temporary discontinuation of imatinib, and if recurrent, dose reductions. The factors affecting toxicity are low hemoglobin correlating with hematological toxicity, and low albumin correlating with development of edema and fatigue. Intriguingly, patients on imatinib for a prolonged period have a decline in symptoms correlated with an improvement in imatinib clearance. When serum levels on days 1 and 29 were compared to levels after more than 1 year on therapy, there was a 33% enhanced clearing of the drug between day 1 and day 29 to those drawn after 1 year.[69]

Two large international phase 3 trials assessed 400 mg daily and 400 mg bid for lack of a comparator standard therapy.[70,71] The North American phase 3 trial, S0033, was powered to determine if 400 mg twice daily versus once per day was superior in terms of overall survival, enrolling 746 patients.[71] In contrast, the EORTC-led trial had progression-free survival as its sole primary endpoint and enrolled 946 patients. The multicenter phase 3 trials demonstrated a CR rate of 3–6%, a PR rate of 45–48%, and a SD rate of 26–32%, for a total clinical benefit of 76%.[70,71] Although responses using standardized response criteria were not evident on CT scans at early time points in these studies, rapid improvement in clinical symptoms was observed. The median progression-free survival (PFS) was 84 weeks in the US-Finnish phase 2 study and survival with SD as the best response to treatment was equivalent to survival of patients who achieve partial or CRs.[70] Long-term follow-up has demonstrated that 18% of patients enrolled in the US-Finnish trial remain without disease progression on imatinib therapy at 9.4 years median follow-up.[67] The EORTC-led trial documented an advantage to the initiation of imatinib at 400 mg bid over 400 mg daily in terms of PFS, without any difference in overall survival (OS).[70] The North American trial found no statistical difference in the OS or PFS.[71] A metaanalysis combining the data from both trials confirmed a minor PFS advantage for higher dose therapy, with this advantage for the most part confined to the patients with an exon 9 mutation. There again was no overall survival advantage to higher dose therapy.[72]

Both phase 3 studies allowed patients treated with low-dose imatinib with evidence of disease progression to increase their dose up to 400 mg twice daily. This resulted in SD in 30% and PR in 2.5–6%.[73] Grades 3, 4, and 5 toxicities were noted in 23%, 7%, and 2%, with gastrointestinal and hematological toxicities being the most common. Interestingly, when compared to initial toxicities on the low-dose arm, the rate of toxicity was equivalent, with the exception of fatigue and anemia which were increased and neutropenia which was decreased. These data suggest that there may be a development of tachyphylaxis to imatinib over time or enhanced drug clearing, as was suggested in an analysis of the phase 1 and 2 trials of imatinib.[69] Although this did not meet statistical significance, the increase in clearance is intriguing as an explanation for both the restabilization of the disease as well as the apparent improvement in toxicity.

Both studies documented an increase in grade 3 and 4 toxicities in patients initially treated on the high-dose arm. Toxicities were mitigated in patients who began on the low-dose arm and then had their dose escalated to the high-dose arm with tumor progression. Neutropenia decreased in frequency, and only fatigue and anemia increased in frequency compared to what was observed at the low dose.[74]

Given the dramatic and durable responses seen with imatinib therapy, some have questioned whether the drug needs to be continued indefinitely in the metastatic setting. The French Sarcoma Group specifically designed BFR14, a phase 3 trial, to ask if imatinib can be stopped in patients with advanced disease when the disease was stabilized on imatinib after 1, 3 or 5 years.[75–77] Patients who were in CR, PR or had CD were randomized to continue on imatinib or stop therapy. The study was designed to assess the PFS, with secondary endpoints of OS and response to the reinitiation of imatinib in patients who discontinued the drug. Patients whose imatinib was discontinued had a statistically significantly shorter PFS compared to those who remained on therapy. Intriguingly, there is a suggestion that the time to progression following discontinuation of imatinib increases with longer time on imatinib before discontinuation. There has not been a difference in OS identified to date. Closer analysis of correlations

between KIT mutation and risk of secondary resistance to imatinib revealed that tumors with the 557-558 deletion of KIT exon 11 were much more likely to remain free of secondary resistance to imatinib compared with other mutations in exon 11.[78]

Determinants of imatinib therapeutic response

Studies evaluating imatinib binding to KIT have detailed important receptor structural sites for activity.[20,79] Wild-type KIT resides on the cellular membrane with the juxtamembrane portion of the molecule inserted into the kinase active site. Normally, KIT homodimerizes in the presence of its ligand, steel factor. This leads to a conformational change of the juxtamembrane domain and activation of the receptor. Imatinib binds to conserved sequences in the kinase domain, competing with adenosine triphosphate (ATP), thus inactivating the kinase activity of the molecule. Mutations in KIT lead to activation of the kinase in the absence of steel factor binding. Mutations in exon 11, in particular, disrupt the normal interactions between the juxtamembrane and kinase active site, and thus favor the active form of the kinase domain. However, these mutations do not affect the binding of imatinib, and thus the agent is effective in tumors with KIT exon 11 mutations.

In vitro, most KIT mutations appear to be sensitive to imatinib, with the exception of mutations in exon 17.[80–82] Mutations in exon 12 but not exon 18 of PDGFRA are sensitive.[80] Clinical trials have gone further, correlating tumor mutation status with efficacy.[83,84] Mutations were identified in KIT exons 8 (03.%), 11 (65.8–73.1%), 13 (0.8–1.5%), and 17 (1.1–1.5%), and PDGFRA (1.1–2.0%), with the remaining tumors without an identifiable mutation in KIT and PDGFRA (13.8–15.2%). As summarized in Table 33.2, the phase 3 trials found tumors with KIT exon 11 mutations had the highest objective response rates (64–68%), while tumors with KIT exon 9 mutations or a wild-type KIT had lower response rates of 34–37.5% and 23–37.3% respectively. In addition, PFS was also longer in the exon 11 group of tumors. There were too few patients with PGDFRA, KIT exon 13 or 17 mutations to analyze. The MetaGIST analysis found the same benefit of higher dose therapy again with no OS benefit; this benefit was observed only in the cohort of patients with mutations in exon 9.[72]

Therapy	KIT mutation status	PFS	OS
Imatinib mesylate[123]	KIT exon 11 (*n*=211)	24.7	60
	KIT exon 9 (*n*=25)	16.7	38.4
	Wild-type KIT (*n*=33)	12.8	49
Sunitinib malate[188]	Exon 9, original tumor (*n*=9)	14.3	29.2
	Exon 9, following imatinib therapy (*n*=13)	31.8	NA
	Wild type, original tumor (*n*=9)	13.8	NA
	Wild type, following imatinib therapy (*n*=8)	13.8	NA
	Exon 11, original tumor (*n*=42)	5.1	12.7
	Exon 11, following imatinib therapy (*n*=7)	3.3	NA
	Exon 11 + secondary mutations following imatinib therapy (*n*=25)	5.1	NA

NA, not available.

Table 33.2 Correlation of progression-free survival (PFS) and overall survival (OS) on kinase therapy with site of KIT mutation.

Targeted therapy: sunitinib malate

Sunitinib malate, a multitargeted tyrosine kinase inhibitor with activity against KIT, PDGFR, VEGFR, and FLT-1/KDR, is approved for the treatment of GIST patients who are refractory to or intolerant of imatinib. Phase 1 studies tested several doses and schedules and initially identified 50 mg orally for 28 days with 14 days rest as the schedule to be developed.[85] The phase 1 and 2 trials of sunitinib malate were populated mostly by patients who were refractory to imatinib of 600 mg or higher, with extensive metastatic disease. PET scans demonstrated rapid metabolic response during the 4 weeks of treatment, which became more metabolically active during the 2-week washout. Similar to imatinib, CT scan responses evolved more slowly. Response data in the early trials as well as the pivotal placebo-controlled, phase 3 trial were markedly similar, with no complete response and partial responses ranging from 7% to 13%.[85–87] Median time to tumor progression was 7.8 months and median survival 19.8 months, in the early-phase studies.

In a phase 3 trial of sunitinib compared to placebo, a statistical difference in the median time to progression was identified: 6.3 months in the patients receiving sunitinib versus 1.5 months in the patients receiving placebo (hazard ratio 0.335, $p = 0.0001$).[86] In the final analysis, the overall survival was also improved in the patients who initiated therapy on sunitinib, in spite of the cross-over design of the study (hazard ratio 0.491, $p = 0.00674$).

The tested schedule was problematic for some patients, as they noted symptoms of disease reactivation during the 2-week treatment break. However, they clearly needed a dose interruption, to manage side-effects. A phase 2 trial of continuous daily but lower dosing has now been tested in patients with GISTs.[87] The study demonstrated safety and tolerability using a starting dose of 37.5 mg daily, with similar response rates to prior studies; this regimen is preferred by most practitioners .Types of toxicities are similar with either schedule. The most common grade 3 and 4 sunitinib toxicities in GIST patients included fatigue, asymptomatic lipase and amylase increases and hypertension. Other side-effects included nausea, diarrhea, stomatitis, hand foot syndrome, anemia, and skin discoloration. Bleeding has also been described at sites of tumor biopsies when patients were on the drug. In addition, some patients with a history of coronary artery disease were found to have asymptomatic cardiac enzyme elevations. Hypothyroidism has also been observed and mandates monitoring for emergence during therapy.

Responses and clinical benefit were observed more frequently in patients with mutations that are less sensitive to imatinib such as KIT exon 9, wild-type KIT, compared to those with exon 11 mutations.[88,89] Time to progression was longest for patients whose tumors contained a KIT exon 9 mutation, followed by wild-type, exon 11, and worst for a tumor with both an exon 11 mutation and a new mutation. Patients with KIT exon 9 and wild-type mutations had the best overall survival. This does not suggest that sunitinib is inactive in exon 11 tumors; rather, it represents the fact that patients with exon 11 mutations who have progressed on imatinib have developed resistance, and typically have clones with additional mutations. Further study has shown that secondary mutations involving KIT exons 13 or 14 are sensitive to sunitinib whereas those with exon 17 and 18 secondary mutations tend to be resistant to sunitinib.

Mechanisms of resistance to imatinib and sunitinib

The initial studies of imatinib pointed to two patterns of resistance to imatinib in patients with GISTs. About 9–17% of patients who progress rapidly and have PD as their best response possess tumors with KIT or PDGFRA mutations that are less sensitive to imatinib.[61,68,70,71,80,83,84] One group of patients is those with exon 9 mutations who often achieve disease stabilization on a higher dose of imatinib.[83] Another is those with wild-type tumors who are more likely to have progressive disease on imatinib. While these tumor types are not completely resistant to imatinib, they are two cohorts of GIST patients that were the most likely to have disease stabilization or response to sunitinib.[85] Imatinib and sunitinib both are competitive inhibitors of ATP binding to the kinase. However, in the setting of KIT or PDGFRA mutations in exons 17 and 18, they are ineffective at binding and serving as competitive inhibitors.[80, 82, 85]

Resistance is also seen to develop in patients who initially respond or at least do not progress and have been maintained on imatinib for many months (defined as greater than 3 months).[62,66,70,71] The overall median time to progressive disease on imatinib is 18–24 months. Clinically, this second group contrasts with the first in that progression is more typically focal rather than involving all sites of known disease. Various mechanisms have been hypothesized but clinically, additional secondary KIT or PGFRA mutations are the most common mechanism. Sunitinib has been shown to have efficacy in tumors that have primary exon 11 mutations along with acquired mutations in exons 13 or 14, but not in the more distal portions of the KIT molecule, exons 17 or 18.[84]

Evaluation of tumors from patients with late recurrence has identified new mutations in KIT or PDGFRA in addition to the primary tumor mutation.[90–94] The sites of secondary mutations include KIT exons 1, 13, 14, and 17 or PDGFRA exon 18, and most commonly occur in tumors that have a primary KIT exon 11 mutation. Microdissection of tumor metastases from patients following progression on imatinib have shown that different sites may contain different secondary mutations.[91] This has raised the question of whether these areas represent outgrowth of preexisting clones or develop as a consequence of imatinib therapy. These additional mutations appear to overcome the KIT/PDGFRA inhibition induced by imatinib.

Medical management of gastrointestinal stromal tumors with imatinib and sunitinib resistance

Patients who have progressed following imatinib and sunitinib have no standard systemic agents available; indeed any additional approaches are experimental. If patients are poor candidates for new experimental drugs or they are not available, continuation on imatinib at a dose that is well tolerated is of modest benefit in spite of previous progression. Clinical trials that have stopped imatinib therapy prior to the initiation of alternative therapies have demonstrated rapid increases in clinical symptoms and tumor flare by PET scan.[95,96] There are anecdotal reports of doses of imatinib escalated above 400 mg bid without clear data on its benefits, and this approach cannot be recommended.[97]

Combinations of systemic and local therapies

Neoadjuvant therapy

The phase 2 RTOG 0132 trial is the only multiinstitutional, prospective study that evaluated the safety and feasibility of imatinib as a *neoadjuvant* agent.[98] In this trial, patients were treated with preoperative 600 mg of imatinib for 8–12 weeks followed by surgery and then 2 additional years of adjuvant imatinib. Fifty-two patients were entered into the trial, with 30 in a cohort with resectable, primary GIST, and 22 in a cohort with resectable recurrent or metastatic tumor. Neoadjuvant imatinib was found to be a safe and feasible treatment option for patients with primary or advanced GIST. Ninety percent of patients with primary GIST demonstrated an objective response prior to surgery, and 92% underwent R0/R1 resections. The 2-year recurrence-free survival (RFS) and OS rates among this subset were 83% and 93%, respectively. Although the study did not specifically state the type of operations performed in the recurrent/metastatic subset, 36% were multiorgan resections and seven patients underwent radiofrequency ablation

Table 33.3 Multiinstitutional trials evaluating neoadjuvant or adjuvant imatinib in the perioperative management of resected primary GIST.

Trial	Imatinib therapy	Design	Eligibility	Dose	Primary endpoint	Status
RTOG S0132	Neoadjuvant	Phase 2	Any of the following: 1. primary tumor ≥5 cm 2. recurrent tumor ≥2 cm Potentially resectable	600 mg daily × 8–10 weeks *preoperatively* + 600 mg daily × 24 months *postoperatively*	RFS	Published[98]
ACOSOG Z9000	Adjuvant	Phase 2	Any of the following: 1. tumor ≥10 cm 2. rupture/hemorrhage 3. multiple tumors (<5) Complete resection	400 mg daily × 12 months	RFS	Reported[99]
ACOSOG Z9001	Adjuvant	Phase 3	Tumor ≥3 cm Complete resection	400 mg daily v. placebo × 12 months	RFS	Published[100]
China Gastrointestinal Cooperative Group	Adjuvant	Phase 2	Any of the following: 1. tumor >5 cm 2. mitotic rate >5/50 HPF	400 mg daily × 12 months	RFS	Reported[101]
SSG XVIII	Adjuvant	Phase 3	Any of the following: 1. tumor ≥10 cm 2. rupture 3. mitotic rate >10/50 HPF 4. tumor >5 cm + mitotic rate >5/50 HPF 5. primary tumor + liver/peritoneal metastases Complete resection	400 mg daily × 12 months or 36 months	RFS	Reported[103]
EORTC 62024	Adjuvant	Phase 3	Any of the following: 1. tumor >5 cm 2. mitotic rate >10 3. tumor <5 cm + mitotic count 6–10/50 HPF Complete resection	400 mg daily v. no treatment × 24 months	Time to second-line therapy	Completed
Korea	Adjuvant	Phase 2	Any of the following: 1. tumor >5 cm + mitotic count >5/50 HPF 2. tumor >10 cm 3. mitotic count >10/50 HPF Complete resection	400 mg daily × 24 months	RFS	Reported[102]
CSIT571BUS282	Adjuvant	Phase 2	Any of the following: 1. tumor ≥2 cm + mitotic count ≥5/50 HPF 2. any nongastric tumor ≥5 cm Complete resection	400 mg daily × 5 years	RFS	Completed

ACOSOG, American College of Surgeons Oncology Group; EORTC, European Organization for the Research and Treatment of Cancer; RFS, recurrence-free survival; HPF, high power field; RTOG, Radiation Therapy Oncology Group.

(RFA) of hepatic lesions; R0 resections were performed in 58%, R1 resections were performed in 5%, and R2 resections (macroscopically incomplete resections) were performed in 32%. Three patients did not undergo surgery. There was one postoperative death in this group. The 2-year PFS and OS rates in this subset were 77.3% and 91%, respectively. Eight patients developed disease progression, including three in the first year.

In evaluating the survival data, it is important to keep in mind that this was not a strictly neoadjuvant study, as all patients were treated with 2 years of adjuvant imatinib. It is difficult to assess the independent impact of neoadjuvant imatinib on survival given the trial design. However, neoadjuvant therapy with imatinib mesylate in patients with large primary tumors that will require a procedure with excess morbidity should be considered. This setting is one in which a PET scan may be of particular utility, because of its ability to give an early indication of disease response versus progression. Patients with lack of response should be considered for early resection, before progressive disease makes such a procedure no longer feasible.[97]

Adjuvant therapy following resection of primary disease
The role of adjuvant imatinib therapy has been or is being explored in at least six prospective, multiinstitutional trials. Multiple potential imatinib durations have been assessed: 12 months (American College of Surgeons Oncology Group (ACOSOG) Z9000, ACOSOG Z9001, China Cooperative Group),[99–101] 24 months (EORTC 62024, Korean trial),[102] 12 versus 36 months (recently reported Scandinavian Sarcoma Group (SSG) XVIII trial),[103] and 5 years (recently completed phase 2 multiinstitutional trial, PERSIST-5, CSIT571BUS282) (Table 33.3). Data from the published ACOSOG Z9001 trial will be discussed in detail. In this phase 3 trial, patients with completely resected primary GISTs at least 3 cm in size were randomized to receive either placebo or imatinib postoperatively for 1 year. The trial was halted early after a planned interim analysis of 644 evaluable patients confirmed that the 1-year RFS was significantly better in the imatinib arm (97% versus 83%, $p=0.0000014$). However, the slopes of the Kaplan–Meier curves representing the two treatment arms, once recurrences were observed, were similar. Thus, the possibility that adjuvant imatinib delays recurrence without necessarily curing anyone has been raised. This theory is further supported by the observation that there was no difference in overall survival between the two treatment arms, albeit with limited follow-up. Imatinib was approved as an adjuvant agent based on the ACOSOG Z9001 data by both the Food and Drug Administration in the United States and the European Medicines Agency in Europe.

Data from the recently reported SSGXVIII trial partly address the questions about ideal adjuvant therapy duration, as well as whether postoperative tyrosine kinase treatment increases cures. This trial confirmed that 36 months of adjuvant imatinib improved both recurrence-free and, importantly, overall survival compared to 12 months. Although the optimal upper end of duration of adjuvant therapy remains unclear, it is clear that 3 years is better than 1 year. The overall survival benefit suggests adjuvant imatinib may be doing more than just

delaying recurrence. Regardless, 3 years of adjuvant imatinib following resection of at least high-risk GISTs is now the standard of care.

Special problems in patients with gastrointestinal stromal tumors

Gastrointestinal stromal tumor syndromes

KIT and PDGFRA-associated hereditary gastrointestinal stromal tumors
Although the majority of tumors are sporadic in nature, there have been reports of familial tumors associated with a germline KIT mutation.[104–112] Hereditary GIST is a rare autosomal dominant genetic disorder. Among these, the majority contain germline KIT mutations with only one demonstrating a germline mutation in PDGFRA. Patients present at an earlier age than those with sporadic GIST, also more commonly with multiple synchronous tumors, generally in the stomach and small bowel.[113] As with sporadic forms of the disease, the germline KIT mutations are gain-of-function. Mutations most commonly involve exon 11, but cases involving exons 13 and 17 have been reported. Individuals with a germline mutation may also have skin lesions such as hyperpigmentation or even melanoma. Some KIT mutant kindreds have reported multiple GISTs (3 to >100 tumors) and other types of cancer, including esophageal and breast cancers; however, it is not clear what role the inherited mutant has in the development of these additional cancers.[104,112,113]

Neurofibromatosis-associated gastrointestinal stromal tumors
In addition to primary familial GIST syndrome, GIST may also arise in the setting of NF-1 or von Recklinghausen disease. NF-1 is an autosomal dominant disorder occurring in one in 3000 individuals worldwide.[114] Clinically, patients with NF-1 are characterized by cutaneous neurofibromas, café-au-lait spots, axillary and inguinal freckling, bony lesions, as well as benign and malignant neoplasms found frequently in the nervous system and gastrointestinal tract.[115] GISTs have been reported in 5–25% of NF-1 patients; a large ($n=70$) Swedish study determined that NF-1 patients are at a 7% risk for developing GIST.[116] Sixty percent of NF-1 patients with GISTs have multiple tumors or multiple tumor sites, most frequently within the small intestine.[117] Miettinen and colleagues reported that women with NF-1 have a slightly higher incidence of GIST than men (1.4:1) with younger median age of presentation of 49 years.[118] Pathologically, NF-1-associated GISTs are similar to sporadic GIST, with rare reports of point mutations in not inactivating somatic mutations in KIT/PDGFRA or BRAF.[115–117] The inactivating somatic mutations in the NF1 gene lead to a deficiency of neurofibromin and subsequent hyperactivation of the MAP-kinase pathway.

Pediatric gastrointestinal stromal tumors
Gastrointestinal stromal tumors rarely present in children and adolescents.[119,120] The United Kingdom National Registry of Childhood Tumours reported an annual incidence of 0.02 per

million children under the age of 14. Estimates of the percentage of GIST diagnosed at 18 years of age or younger have ranged from 0.5% to 2.7%. GISTs in children have a female preponderance (70%).

Carney triad and Carney–Stratakis dyad

The Carney triad was originally described in 1977 and comprises GIST (originally called leiomyosarcoma), paraganglioma, and pulmonary chondromas.[121] Recently, esophageal leiomyomas and adrenal cortical adenomas have been added as components of the syndrome.[122,123] This is a rare presentation of GIST, with fewer than 30 complete cases (with all three tumors diagnosed in the same individual) and 100 incomplete cases (diagnoses of two of three tumors) reported. As with pediatric GISTs, there is a female preponderance in Carney triad and the majority of patients present before the age of 30. The GIST component of the triad predominantly arises in the stomach, with these tumors typically lacking detectable *KIT* and *PDGFRA* mutations.

The Carney–Stratakis syndrome is now recognized as a distinct entity. Patients with Carney–Stratakis syndrome most commonly have GISTs and paragangliomas. In addition, these patients have a germline mutation in the succinate dehydrogenase (SDH) subunits B, C, D (SDHB, SDHC, SDHD).[124] Both appear to have a chronic yet indolent course with regard to their GISTs.[122]

Local therapies for metastatic disease

Liver metastases have been managed with surgery, embolization with or without chemotherapy,[125,126] cryotherapy, RFA, and even liver transplantation. These approaches are often utilized in the palliative or refractory settings and generally tended to be more common prior to the advent of imatinib mesylate. Pawlik and colleagues reported a series of 66 patients undergoing hepatectomy with or without RFA for metastatic sarcoma, including 36 patients with metastatic GIST.[127] PFS and OS were worse in patients undergoing RFA alone or in combination with hepatectomy compared to those undergoing hepatectomy alone, perhaps not entirely surprising, since RFA is usually reserved for unresectable tumors. The authors did not separately analyze the GIST patient cohort. Liver transplantation has been reported in very few patients; in one series, patients with liver-only metastases underwent transplantation for presumed leiomyosarcoma, only to find that the diagnosis was in fact GIST after the native liver was removed.[128] All three patients recurred and were treated with imatinib; overall survival exceeded 46 months in all three. Certainly at least transplantation cannot be advocated.[129,130]

Treatment of pediatric gastrointestinal stromal tumors

The primary treatment for pediatric GIST is surgical resection of the tumor, with any involved lymph nodes. Postoperative surveillance is performed with CT alone or in conjunction with FDG-PET scans; anecdotally, PET scans may identify disease that is not measurable on CT imaging and is of unclear clinical significance. The benefit of tyrosine kinase therapy is largely

anecdotal.[131–138] A Children's Oncology Group (COG) phase 2 study in children with refractory or relapsed solid tumors showed that imatinib as a single agent ($440\,mg/m^2/day$) demonstrated no responses in children with GIST. Agaram and colleagues reported on seven pediatric GIST patients with all but one receiving therapy for metastatic disease.[131] Length of therapy ranged from 3 to 18 months (median 5 months); one patient had stable disease for 9 months and another a mixed response with some nodules stable and others that progressed albeit at a reduced rate; all others progressed. The patient in the adjuvant setting was treated for 24 months, with rapid progression at the time of imatinib discontinuation. This report also reported on sunitinib therapy in four patients, following progression on or discontinuation for intolerance to imatinib. Two patients were intolerant to sunitinib, one had stable disease after 8 months of treatment (25 mg/day), and the fourth patient received five cycles of sunitinib with dose escalation (up to 50 mg/day), before discontinuation for disease progression. Janeway and colleagues described seven imatinib-refractory pediatric patients who were placed on cycles of daily sunitinib for 4 weeks followed by 2 weeks off therapy.[139] One patient had a partial response, five had stable disease and one progressed on treatment. Mean duration of disease stabilization was 15 months, with longer time to progression on sunitinib than prior imatinib in five of six patients.

Surgical management of metastatic gastrointestinal stromal tumors

Cytoreductive surgery for resectable advanced or metastatic disease is an accepted practice for selected metastatic solid tumors including cancers of the colon, appendix, ovary, and testicle. A number of investigators have pursued a similar strategy of aggressive cytoreductive surgery in patients with metastatic GIST, with at least most disease controlled by tyrosine kinase inhibitor (TKI) therapy. The goal of cytoreductive operations is to perform a macroscopically complete (R0 or R1) resection when safely possible. However, the disease may frequently be too extensive to be removed completely, and fewer than 25% of all patients with advanced GIST on TKI therapy will be considered as surgical candidates.[140,141]

It is known that patients will experience durable periods of PR or SD on imatinib, lasting months to years. However, the overall pathological CR rate to medical therapy is less than 5% of patients.[142,143] Eventually, most patients develop TKI resistance with the median time to imatinib resistance being 18–24 months.[70,71] Once drug resistance develops, disease progression may be either limited (progression at a single site with ongoing response at all other sites of disease) or generalized (progression at more than one site).[144,145]

Several single-institution retrospective studies have documented progression-free and overall survival rates following extensive cytoreductive surgery in patients with advanced GIST treated with TKI therapy, the largest being those from Brigham and Women's Hospital/Dana-Farber Cancer Institute (BWH/DFCI), Memorial Sloan-Kettering Cancer Center (MSKCC) and Instituto Nazionale Tumori (INT).[140,141,144–146] In the experience at BWH/DFCI, the best results were generally seen in patients whose disease was still responsive to TKI therapy at the time of surgery (i.e. demonstrated ongoing PR or SD at all sites of disease). In this retrospective study of patients receiving TKI therapy (usually imatinib), a macroscopically compete resection with negative (R0) or positive (R1) microscopic margins was possible in 78%, 25%, and 7% of patients with responsive disease (CR, PR, or SD at all sites), limited progression (progressive disease [PD] at approximately one site, and CR, PR, or SD at all other sites), and generalized progression (multifocal PD), respectively ($p < 0.0001$).[144] Conversely, macroscopically incomplete (R2) resections were performed in 4%, 16%, and 43% of these patients, respectively. Thus, response to TKI therapy at the time of surgery correlated with resectability.

Furthermore, the studies from BWH/DFCI, MSKCC, and INT each demonstrated that the highest survival rates occurred when patients underwent cytoreductive surgery while still responding to TKI therapy. Progression-free survival rates for patients with PR or SD were 70–96% at 1 year after surgery and 72% at 4 years from the start of imatinib therapy, whereas those for patients with generalized progression ranged from 0% to 14%.[144,145,147] Overall survival rates approached 100% at 1 year after surgery in patients with PR/SD or limited progression, and only 0–60% at 1 year for those patients with generalized progression. Thus, response to TKI therapy at the time of surgery also correlated with both progression-free and overall survival.

In the BWH/DFCI series, approximately 40% of patients required liver resections, over 60% underwent peritonectomy and/or omentectomy, and over 60% needed multivisceral resections.[144] The MSKCC series had similar types of resection, with 43% requiring liver resection and 68% requiring resection of peritoneal metastases without major visceral involvement. Radiofrequency ablation was also employed for unresectable liver metastases. Complications rates ranged from 40% to 60% in the three large series, though the majority were minor.[145] Perioperative deaths were rare, usually occurring in the setting of emergency procedures for tumor rupture or hemorrhage, as reported in a similar French study.[140,141]

While these studies define which subset of potentially resectable patients have the best results, they do not establish whether surgery plus imatinib therapy is better than continuing imatinib alone, without surgery. Phase 3 trials attempting to answer that question under way or in development in China, Europe, and the US have all been halted due to concerns about accrual. New strategies attempting to answer this critical question are under consideration. It is clear that surgery is not a replacement for imatinib therapy. All patients should resume imatinib after surgery, as the BFR14 study has shown the high rates of relapse after imatinib interruption.[75–77] Moreover, in one of the series evaluating the role of cytoreductive surgery, relapse was noted in 80% of patients who did not resume imatinib postoperatively versus 5% for those who did (with short follow-up).[141]

Optimal timing of cytoreduction in patients receiving induction imatinib is currently unclear. From the aforementioned US-Finnish trial, the median time to a radiographic RECIST response to imatinib was 2.7 months, but more than 25% took more than 5 months to respond.[66] Thus, the practice at centers such as ours with extensive experience with cytoreductive surgery for advanced GIST is to wait a minimum of 6 months before proceeding with surgery.

Most importantly, surgery should not be the first course of therapy for first recurrence, barring an impending emergency. Elective surgery should only be entertained as a treatment option after imatinib therapy has been instituted.

Cytoreductive surgery on sunitinib

The majority of patients develop resistance to imatinib with a median of 18–24 months, and many then receive sunitinib.[148] The utility of cytoreductive surgery for patients on sunitinib is also uncertain. In a recent study, Raut and colleagues found no statistically significant difference in extent of resection based on response to sunitinib at the time of surgery.[149] R0/R1 resections occurred in 40%, 64%, and 39% of patients with responsive disease, limited progression, or progressive disease respectively. Although the progression-free and overall survival rates for the entire cohort of 50 patients are relatively high given the extensive nature of the heavily pretreated disease in these patients (15.6 months and 26 months, respectively), the authors note that the potential for bias is quite high in that surgery was only offered to a selected subset of patients. In fact, the overall mortality outcomes were not statistically significant among the different responders (responsive, limited progression, and generalized progression), which would further suggest this possibility. In general, treating physicians should carefully weigh all treatment options before recommending cytoreductive surgery for patients with drug-resistant metastatic GIST.

Experimental approaches to advanced disease

Other tyrosine kinases have been tested for therapeutic efficacy against GIST, most in the advanced disease setting. Nilotinib is a second-generation TKI, designed to optimally inhibit the ABL-kinase complex, but which retains anti-KIT and -PDGFR activity.[150,151] In contrast to imatinib, nilotinib has been shown to have increased intracellular accumulation, which may serve as a mechanism for activity in patients with imatinib-refractory disease. Phase 1 studies of nilotinib, alone and in combination with imatinib, demonstrated safety and efficacy in patients with imatinib-resistant GISTs, with no clear superiority of combination therapy.[152] Studies in patients who have progressed beyond standard therapy and treated with nilotinib at 400 mg twice daily have resulted primarily in stable disease with a median of 8–12 weeks.[153] Intriguingly, several reports have suggested potential clinical benefit in GIST with exon 11 mutations carrying secondary mutations in exon 17.[154,155] However, phase 3 studies in patients refractory to standard therapy and in the primary metastatic disease setting have been disappointing.

Nilotinib alone compared to best supportive care, including ongoing imatinib or sunitinib, did not demonstrate an improved progression-free survival based on independent radiology review.[156] A recent trial in first-line treatment for advanced

GIST (nilotinib compared with imatinib) was discontinued when superior efficacy was clearly not forthcoming.

Masitinib mesylate targets c-KIT and PDGFR, but also fibroblast growth factor receptor (FGFR) 3. *In vitro*, masitinib appears to have better activity than imatinib.[157] A phase 1 trial of masitinib showed the maximum tolerated dose [MTD] was 12 mg/kg/day, and in 5/17 imatinib-resistant patients achieved stable disease.[158] Two patients intolerant to 300 mg of imatinib daily achieved SD and PR as their best response. Toxicities appear to be similar to imatinib, except for mucosal inflammation. In the phase 2 trial in advanced previously untreated GIST, masitinib 7.5 mg/kg/day was utilized.[159] The overall response rate (CR and PR) was 53.3%, with clinical benefit (CR, PR, and SD) observed in 96.7%, and a median time to objective response of about 6 months. The median progression-free survival is estimated to be 41.3 months and a 3-year survival rate of 90%; these appear to be superior to the initial trials with imatinib, but are being tested in a noninferiority phase 3 trial comparing imatinib with masitinib in the frontline setting with PFS as the primary endpoint.

Sorafenib is a raf kinase inhibitor that also has activity against KIT, PDGFR, and VEGFR-2 and -3. *In vitro*, it has demonstrated activity against the imatinib-resistant *PDGFRA* mutation T681 and acquired imatinib-resistant *KIT* mutations, particularly those involving T670I and D820Y.[150,160,161] A phase 2 trial of sorafenib 400 mg twice daily treated 38 patients, 32 of whom were resistant to both imatinib and sunitinib; the partial response rate was 13% with an additional stable disease rate of 55%. The median progression-free survival was 5.2 months with a median overall survival of approximately 1 year.[162] Confirmatory experiences have been reported for the fourth-line setting, demonstrating partial response rates of 19–20% as well as symptomatic improvement.[163]

Regorafenib, a tyrosine kinase with a similar spectrum of activity, is currently undergoing evaluation in patients with advanced refractory GIST.[164] A phase 2 study in a group of patients with advanced disease demonstrated a partial response rate of 9% and a clinical benefit rate defined as objective response and SD lasting 16 weeks or more of 73%. The severe side-effects requiring dose reductions were anticipated for this class of drug: hand foot syndrome, hypertension, diarrhea, hypophosphatemia, bleeding, and thrombosis. A phase 3 study comparing regorafenib with placebo in patients who have progressed following imatinib and sunitinib has accrued, with results anticipated in 2012.

Dasatinib is a kinase inhibitor against BCR-ABL, SRC family (SRC, LCK, YES, FYN), c-KIT, EPHA2, and PDGFRB, and is approved for treatment of imatinib-resistant or -intolerant CML and Philadelphia chromosome-positive acute lymphoblastic leukemia. *In vitro*, this agent has activity against the kinase activity of WT KIT and juxtamembrane domain mutant KIT isoforms.[165,166] Phase 2 testing in advanced disease demonstrated a 38% response rate utilizing CHOI criteria.[167] Twenty percent of patients had SD for greater than 6 months. Notably, a response was seen in a patient with a PDGFRA D842V mutation. A phase 2 trial of dasatinib for front-line therapy in GIST is accruing.

Crenolanib is a novel PDGFR kinase inhibitor that is now in phase 2 testing for GIST patients whose tumors carry a *PDGFRA* D842V mutation that is refractory to most other kinases available.[168]

Novel therapeutic targets

In the setting of kinase-resistant disease, the benefit of targeting KIT or PDGFRA alone is limited. Additional strategies are being developed to inhibit other members of the signaling pathways associated with KIT and PDGFR or molecules important for maintaining the cell surface localization of these receptors based on preclinical data. An overview of data available is summarized below.

MEK/ERK/AKT and mTOR inhibitors

Analysis of tumor samples from GIST refractory to imatinib and sunitinib therapy have demonstrated that the MEK and AKT pathways remain active, and preclinical data suggest the benefit of targeting these pathways.[169] Testing of agents targeting these kinases and the mammalian target of rapamycin (mTOR) further downstream have started in refractory GIST patients. Everolimus (RAD001), an mTOR inhibitor, has been tested in combination with imatinib in imatinib-refractory patients and those who had progressed following imatinib and another therapy, usually sunitinib.[170] Patients received imatinib 600 mg and RAD001 2.5 mg per day. PFS at 4 months was longer in patients with more prior therapy (17.4% and 37.1%), although OS was longer in the group that received imatinib only (14.9 and 10.7 months, respectively). A second phase 2 trial tested the benefit of adding everolimus to imatinib when patients had progressed on 400 mg daily; one-third of patients achieved stable disease, but no objective responses were noted.[171] Imatinib with perifosine, an AKT inhibitor, did not lead to responses and had a median progression-free survival of 2 months.[172] The safety and potential role of other targeted agents of this pathway alone or in combinations are currently being elucidated.

HSP-90

HSP-90 is a molecular chaperone required for the stability and function of proteins involved not only in normal homeostasis but also in maintaining malignant cell pathways.[173] In particular, it stabilizes oncogenes and receptors, which become more dependent on HSP-90 as they become increasingly mutated. *In vitro*, KIT activation appears to be dependent on protein stabilization by HSP-90 and inhibition of HSP-90 leads to loss of KIT phosphorylation, degradation of wild type and an imatinib-resistant mutant KIT, as well as decreasing proliferation of imatinib-resistant cell lines *in vitro*.[174–176]

IPI-504 is a water-soluble HSP-90 inhibitor that has undergone testing in patients progressing on imatinib and sunitinib.[177,178] Initial testing in 36 patients with advanced GIST demonstrated one partial response and an additional 24 patients with stable disease. A phase 3 placebo-controlled double-blind study was subsequently initiated, but was terminated early due to increased mortality in the patients receiving IPI-504.[178]

Other HSP-90 inhibitors are also being tested alone or in combination with kinase inhibitors.

Histone deacetylyase

Preclinically, histone deacetylyase (HDAC) inhibitors have demonstrated evidence of cytotoxicity in GIST tumor cell lines and xenografts.[179,180] HDAC inhibitors *in vitro* cause downregulation of KIT protein expression associated with acetylation of its chaperone protein, HSP-90. Treatment with panobinostat leads to regression of GIST xenografts in mice and evidence of cell death, which was enhanced when combined with imatinib.[180] Early clinical trials are ongoing to test this approach.

Insulin-like growth factor type I receptor

The insulin-like growth factor type I receptor (IGF-1R) pathway has been identified as a potential pathway in the oncogenesis of GIST, particularly in those GISTs that lack *KIT* and *PDGFRA* mutations, WT-GIST, and in pediatric GIST.[181–183] WT-GIST is less responsive to imatinib-based therapies. Cell lines treated *in vitro* with an IGF-1R inhibitor or siRNA silencing of IGF-1R led to cell death and induced apoptosis.[182] OSI-906, an IGF-1R targeted tyrosine kinase inhibitor, will be tested in patients with WT-GIST.

Conclusion

The prognosis of patients diagnosed with GIST is changing in the era of targeted therapy. Prior to the development of imatinib, patients' primary treatment modality was surgery. Although patients with completely resected tumors had a median survival of 96 months, those with completely resected locally recurrent disease or metastatic disease had survivals of only 49 and 39 months respectively.[7] Patients in whom complete resection was not feasible fared worse, with survival rates of 26, 8, and 11 months following resection of primary, locally recurrent, and metastatic disease. Unfortunately, the role of other therapeutic modalities was very limited with no data to suggest an impact on survival.

Tyrosine kinase inhibitor therapy has clearly increased overall survival in patients with metastatic and unresectable disease. Prior to the development of imatinib and sunitinib, patients with metastatic disease lived approximately 12 months. With kinase inhibitors, survival has clearly been improved, with median survival of 5 years.

The role of adjuvant imatinib has been studied and has demonstrated both progression-free and overall survival benefits in patients with high-risk GIST. While 3 years of therapy are superior to 1 year of therapy in patients with high-risk disease, the optimal length of therapy in this setting is not yet clearly defined and questions remain on whether patients with lower risk tumors should be treated for 1 or 3 years, or some other interval, in the adjuvant setting. Additional data are needed to determine whether patients with specific molecular changes should receive therapy at all. Lastly, neoadjuvant imatinib with surgical resection has been shown to be feasible and safe, and has a role in the management of large marginally resectable tumors.

References

1. Mazur MT, Clark HB. Gastric stromal tumors: reappraisal of histogenesis. Am J Surg Pathol 1983; 7: 507–19.
2. Sarlomo-Rikala M, *et al.* CD117: a sensitive marker for gastrointestinal stromal tumors that is more specific than CD34. Mod Pathol 1998; 11(8): 728–34.
3. Miettinen M, Virolainen M, Maarit Sarlomo R. Gastrointestinal stromal tumors – value of CD34 antigen in their identification and separation from true leiomyomas and schwannomas. Am J Surg Pathol 1995; 19(2): 207–16.
4. Hirota S, *et al.* Gain-of-function mutations of c-kit in human gastrointestinal stromal tumors. Science 1998; 279: 577–80.
5. Crosby JA, *et al.* Malignant gastrointestinal stromal tumors of the small intestine: a review of 50 cases from a prospective database. Ann Surg Oncol 2001; 8(1): 50–9.
6. Pidhorecky I, *et al.* Gastrointestinal stromal tumors: current diagnosis, biologic behavior, and management. Ann Surg Oncol 2000; 7(9): 705–12.
7. DeMatteo RP, *et al.* Two hundred gastrointestinal stromal tumors: recurrence patterns and prognostic factors for survival. Ann Surg 2000; 231(1): 51–8.
8. Miettinen M, *et al.* Gastrointestinal stromal tumors/smooth muscle tumors (GISTs) primary in the omentum and mesentery: clinicopathologic and immunohistochemical study of 26 cases. Am J Surg Pathol 1999; 23(9): 1109–18.
9. Miettinen M, *et al.* Esophageal stromal tumors: a clinicopathologic, immunohistochemical, and molecular genetic study of 17 cases and comparison with esophageal leiomyomas and leiomyosarcomas. Am J Surg Pathol 2000; 24(2): 211–22.
10. Takahashi Y, *et al.* Gastrointestinal stromal tumor of the duodenal ampulla: report of a case. Surg Today 2001; 31(8): 722–6.
11. Miettinen M, Sobin LH. Gastrointestinal stromal tumors in the appendix: a clinicopathologic and immunohistochemical study of four cases. Am J Surg Pathol 2001; 25(11): 1433–7.
12. Lasota J, Carlson JA, Miettinen M. Spindle cell tumor of urinary bladder serosa with phenotypic and genotypic features of gastrointestinal stromal tumor. Arch Pathol Lab Med 2000; 124(6): 894–7.
13. Agaimy A, *et al.* Minute gastric sclerosing stromal tumors (GIST tumorlets) are common in adults and frequently show c-KIT mutations. Am J Surg Pathol 2007; 31(1): 113–20.
14. Kawanowa K, *et al.* High incidence of microscopic gastrointestinal stromal tumors in the stomach. Hum Pathol 2006; 37(12): 1527–35.
15. Tryggvason G, Gislason HG, Magnusson MK, Tonasson JG. Gastrointestinal stromal tumors in Iceland, 1990-2003: the Icelandic GIST Study, a population-based incidence and risk stratification study. Int J Cancer 2005; 117: 289–93.
16. Nillson B, *et al.* Gastrointestinal stromal tumors: the incidence, prevalence, clinical course and prognostication in the pre-imatinib mesylate era: a population-based study in Western Sweden. Cancer 2005; 103: 821–9.
17. Tran T, Devila JA, El-Serag HB. The epidemiology of gastrointestinal stromal tumors: an analysis of 1,458 cases from 1992–2000. Am J Gastroenterol 2005; 100: 132–68.
18. Cassier PA, *et al.* A prospective epidemiological study of new incident GISTs during two consecutive years in Rhone Alps region: incidence and molecular distribution of GIST in a European region. Br J Cancer 2010; 103: 165–70.
19. Steigen SE, Eide TJ, Wasag B, Lasota J, Miettinen M. Mutations in gastrointestinal stromal tumors: a population-based study from Northern Norway. APMIS 2007; 115: 289–98.
20. Mucciarini C, *et al.* Incidence and clinicopathologic features of gastrointestinal stromal tumors. A population-based study. BMC Cancer 2007; 7: 230.
21. Rubio J, *et al.* Population-based incidence and survival of gastrointestinal stromal tumors (GIST) in Girona, Spain. Eur J Cancer 2007; 43: 144–8.
22. Yantiss RK, *et al.* Gastrointestinal stromal tumors: an ultrastructural study. Int J Surg Pathol 2002; 10(2): 101–13.

23. Fletcher CD, *et al*. Diagnosis of gastrointestinal stromal tumors: a consensus approach. Hum Pathol 2002; 33(5): 459–65.

24. Miettinen M, Sobin LH, Sarlomo-Rikala M. Immunohistochemical spectrum of GISTs at different sites and their differential diagnosis with a reference to CD117 (KIT). Mod Pathol 2000; 13(10): 1134–42.

25. Medeiros F, *et al*. KIT-negative gastrointestinal stromal tumors: proof of concept and therapeutic implications. Am J Surg Pathol 2004; 28: 889–94.

26. Espinosa I, *et al*. A novel monoclonal antibody against DOG1 is a sensitive and specific marker for gastrointestinal stromal tumors. Am J Surg Pathol 2008; 32: 210–18.

27. Lopes LF, West RB, Bacchi LM, van de Rijn M, Bacchi CE. DOG1 for the diagnosis of gastrointestinal stromal tumor (GIST): comparison between 2 different antibodies. Appl Immunohistochem Mol Morphol 2010; 18: 333–7.

28. Liegl B, Hornick JL, Corless CL, Fletcher CD. Monoclonal antibody DOG1.1 shows higher sensitivity than KIT in the diagnosis of gastrointestinal stromal tumors, including unusual subtypes. Am J Surg Pathol 2009; 33: 437–46.

29. Miettinen M, Wang ZF, Lasota J. DOG1 antibody in the differential diagnosis of gastrointestinal stromal tumors: a study of 1840 cases. Am J Surg Pathol 2009; 33: 1401–8.

30. Blay P, *et al*. Protein kinase C theta is highly expressed in gastrointestinal stromal tumors but not in other mesenchymal neoplasias. Clin Cancer Res 2004; 10: 4089–95.

31. Lee HE, Kim MA, Lee HS, Lee BL, Kim WH. Characteristics of KIT-negative gastrointestinal stromal tumours and diagnostic utility of protein kinase C theta immunostaining. J Clin Pathol 2008; 61: 722–9.

32. Motegi A, Sakurai S, Nakayama H, Sano T, Oyama T, Nakajima T. PKC theta, a novel immunohistochemical marker for gastrointestinal stromal tumors (GIST), especially useful for identifying KIT-negative tumors. Pathol Int 2005; 55: 106–12.

33. Heinrich MC, *et al*. PDGFRA activating mutations in gastrointestinal stromal tumors. Science 2003; 299: 708–10.

34. Antonescu CR, *et al*. Association of KIT exon 9 mutations with nongastric primary site and aggressive behavior: KIT mutation analysis and clinical correlates of 120 gastrointestinal stromal tumors. Clin Cancer Res 2003; 9(9): 3329–37.

35. Palazzo L, *et al*. Endosonographic features predictive of benign and malignant gastrointestinal stromal cell tumours. Gut 2000; 46(1): 88–92.

36. Miettinen M, *et al*. Evaluation of malignancy and prognosis of gastrointestinal stromal tumors: a review. Hum Pathol 2002; 33(5): 478–83.

37. Miettinen M, Lasota J. Gastrointestinal stromal tumors: pathology and prognosis at different sites. Semin Diagn Pathol 2006; 23(2): 70–83.

38. Corless CL, *et al*. Relation of tumor pathologic and molecular features to outcome after surgical resection of localized primary gastrointestinal stromal tumor (GIST): results of the intergroup phase III trial ACOSOG Z9001. Sarcoma Oral Abstract Presentation, ASCO, 2010.

39. Gold JS, *et al*. Development and validation of a prognostic nomogram for recurrence-free survival after complete surgical resection of localised primary gastrointestinal stromal tumour: a retrospective analysis. Lancet Oncol 2009; 10(11): 1045–52.

40. Edmonson JH, *et al*. Contrast of response to dacarbazine, mitomycin, doxorubicin, and cisplatin (DMAP) plus GM-CSF between patients with advanced malignant gastrointestinal stromal tumors and patients with other advanced leiomyosarcomas. Cancer Invest 2002; 20: 605–12.

41. Dematteo RP, *et al*. Clinical management of gastrointestinal stromal tumors: before and after STI-571. Hum Pathol 2002; 33(5): 466–77.

42. Changchien CR, *et al*. Evaluation of prognosis for malignant rectal gastrointestinal stromal tumor by clinical parameters and immunohistochemical staining. Dis Colon Rectum 2004; 47(11): 1922–9.

43. Hellan M, Maker VK. Transvaginal excision of a large rectal stromal tumor: an alternative. Am J Surg 2006; 191(1): 121–3.

44. Dong C, *et al*. Gastrointestinal stromal tumors of the rectum: clinical, pathologic, immunohistochemical characteristics and prognostic analysis. Scand J Gastroenterol 2007; 42(10): 1221–9.

45. Fong Y, *et al*. Lymph node metastasis from soft tissue sarcoma in adults. Analysis of data from a prospective database of 1772 sarcoma patients. Ann Surg 1993; 217: 72–7.

46. Davila RE, Faigel DO. GI stromal tumors. Gastrointest Endosc 2003; 58: 80–8.

47. Sepe PS, Brugge WR. A guide for the diagnosis and management of gastrointestinal stromal cell tumors. Nat Rev Gastroenterol Hepatol 2009; 6(6): 363–71.

48. Otani Y, Kitajima M. Laparoscopic surgery: too soon to decide. Gastric Cancer 2005; 8: 135–6.

49. Novitsky YW, *et al*. Long-term outcomes of laparoscopic resection of gastric gastrointestinal stromal tumors. Ann Surg 2006; 243(6): 738–45; discussion 745–7.

50. Otani Y, *et al*. Operative indications for relatively small (2–5 cm) gastrointestinal stromal tumor of the stomach based on analysis of 60 operated cases. Surgery 2006; 139(4): 484–92.

51. Nishimura J, *et al*. Surgical strategy for gastric gastrointestinal stromal tumors: laparoscopic versus open resection. Surg Endosc 2007; 21(6): 875–8.

52. Nakamori M, *et al*. Laparoscopic resection for gastrointestinal stromal tumors of the stomach. Am J Surg 2008; 196(3): 425–9.

53. Clary BM, *et al*. Gastrointestinal stromal tumors and leiomyosarcoma of the abdomen and retroperitoneum: a clinical comparison. Ann Surg Oncol 2001; 8(4): 290–9.

54. Pierie JP, *et al*. The effect of surgery and grade on outcome of gastrointestinal stromal tumors. Arch Surg 2001; 136(4): 383–9.

55. Plaat BE, *et al*. Soft tissue leiomyosarcomas and malignant gastrointestinal stromal tumors: differences in clinical outcome and expression of multidrug resistance proteins. J Clin Oncol 2000; 18(18): 3211–20.

56. Buchdunger E, *et al*. Inhibition of the Abl protein-tyrosine kinase in vitro and in vivo by a 2-phenylaminopyrimidine derivative. Cancer Res 1996; 56(1): 100–4.

57. Buchdunger E, *et al*. Abl protein-tyrosine kinase inhibitor STI571 inhibits in vitro signal transduction mediated by c-kit and platelet-derived growth factor receptors. J Pharmacol Exp Ther 2000; 295(1): 139–45.

58. Heinrich MC, *et al*. Inhibition of c-kit receptor tyrosine kinase activity by STI 571, a selective tyrosine kinase inhibitor. Blood 2000; 96(3): 925–32.

59. Corless CL, *et al*. PDGFRA mutations in gastrointestinal stromal tumors: frequency, spectrum and in vitro sensitivity to imatinib. J Clin Oncol 2005; 23: 5357–64.

60. Joensuu H, *et al*. Effect of the tyrosine kinase inhibitor STI571 in a patient with a metastatic gastrointestinal stromal tumor. N Engl J Med 2001; 344(14): 1052–6.

61. Van Oosterom A, *et al*. Safety and efficacy of imatinib (STI571) in metastatic gastrointestinal stromal tumours: a phase I study. Lancet 2001; 358: 1421–3.

62. Van Oosterom A, *et al*. Update of phase I study of imatinib (STI571) in advanced soft tissue sarcomas and gastrointestinal stromal tumors: a report of the EORTC Soft Tissue and Bone Sarcoma Group. Eur J Cancer 2002; 38(Suppl 5): S83–7.

63. Druker BJ, *et al*. Efficacy and safety of a specific inhibitor of the BCR-ABL tyrosine kinase in chronic myeloid leukemia. N Engl J Med 2001; 344(14): 1031–7.

64. Druker BJ, *et al*. Activity of a specific inhibitor of the BCR-ABL tyrosine kinase in the blast crisis of chronic myeloid leukemia and acute lymphoblastic leukemia with the Philadelphia chromosome. N Engl J Med 2001; 344(14): 1038–42.

65. Demetri G, *et al*. Efficacy and safety of imatinib mesylate in advanced gastrointestinal stromal tumors. N Engl J Med 2002; 347: 472–80.

66. Blanke CD, *et al*. Long term results from a randomized phase II trial of standard versus higher dose imatinib mesylate for patients with unresectable or metastatic gastrointestinal stromal tumors expressing KIT. J Clin Oncol 2008; 16: 626–32.

67. Von Mehren M, *et al*. Follow-up results after 9 years (yrs) of the ongoing, phase II B2222 trial of imatinib mesylate (IM) in patients (pts) with metastatic or unresectable KIT+ gastrointestinal stromal tumors (GIST). J Clin Oncol 29: 2011 (Suppl): abstr 10016.

68. Verweij J, *et al*. Imatinib mesylate is an active agent for GIST but does not yield responses in other soft tissue sarcomas that are unselected for a molecular target. Eur J Cancer 2003; 39: 2006–11.

69. Judson I, *et al*. EORTC Soft Tissue and Bone Sarcoma Group. Imatinib pharmacokinetics in patients with gastrointestinal stromal tumour: a retrospective population pharmacokinetic study over time. Cancer Chemother Pharmacol 2005; 55(4): 379–86.

70. Verweij J, *et al*. Progression-free survival in gastrointestinal stromal tumours with high-dose imatinib: randomized trial. Lancet 2004; 364(9440): 1127–34.

71. Blanke CD, *et al*. Phase III randomized, intergroup trial assessing imatinib mesylate at two dose levels in patients with unresectable or metastatic gastrointestinal stromal tumors expressing the KIT receptor tyrosine kinase: S0033. J Clin Oncol 2008; 26: 620–5.

72. Gastrointestinal Stromal Tumor Meta-Analysis Group. Comparison of two doses of imatinib for the treatment of unresectable or metastatic gastrointestinal stromal tumors: a meta-analysis of 1,640 patients. J Clin Oncol 2010; 28(7):1247–53.

73. Patel S, Zalberg JR. Optimizing the dose of imatinib for treatment of gastrointestinal stromal tumours: lessons from the phase 3 trials. Eur J Cancer 2008; 44(4):501–9.

74. Van Glabbeke M, *et al*. Prognostic factors of toxicity and efficacy in patients with gastro-intestinal stromal tumors (GIST) treated with imatinib: a study of the EORTC-STBSG, ISG and AGITG. Chicago: ASCO Annual Meeting, 2003.

75. Blay J, *et al*. Prospective multicentric randomized phase III study of imatinib in patients with advanced gastrointestinal stromal tumors comparing interruption versus continuation of treatment beyond 1 year: the French Sarcoma Group. J Clin Oncol 2007; 25(9): 1107–13.

76. Le Cesne A, *et al*. Discontinuation of imatinib in patients with advanced gastrointestinal stromal tumours after 3 years of treatment: an open-label multicentre randomized phase 3 trial. Lancet Oncol 2010; 11(10): 942–9.

77. Ray-Coquard IL, *et al*. Risk of relapse with imatinib (IM) discontinuation at 5 years in advanced GIST patients: results of the prospective BFR14 randomized phase III study comparing interruption versus continuation of IM at 5 years of treatment: a French Sarcoma Group Study. J Clin Oncol 2010; 28(Suppl): abstr 10032.

78. LeCesne A, *et al*. Time to onset of progression after imatinib interruption and outcome of patients with advanced GIST: results of the BFR14 prospective French Sarcoma Group randomized phase III trial. J Clin Oncol 2010; 28(Suppl): abstr 10033.

79. Mol CD, *et al*. Structural basis for the autoinhibition and STI-571 inhibition of c-Kit tyrosine kinase. J Biol Chem 2004; 279: 31655–63.

80. Heinrich MC, *et al*. Kinase mutations and imatinib response in patients with metastatic gastrointestinal stromal tumor. J Clin Oncol 2003; 21(23): 4342–9.

81. Foster R, *et al*. Molecular basis of the constitutive activity and STI571 resistance of Asp816Val mutant KIT receptor tyrosine kinase. J Mol Graph Model 2004; 23(2): 139–52.

82. Ma Y, *et al*. The c-KIT mutation causing human mastocytosis is resistant to STI571 and other KIT kinase inhibitors; kinases with enzymatic site mutations show different inhibitor sensitivity profiles than wild-type kinases and those with regulatory-type mutations. Blood 2002; 99(5): 1741–4.

83. Debiec-Rychter M, *et al*. KIT mutations and dose selection for imatinib in patients with advanced gastrointestinal stromal tumours. Eur J Cancer 2006; 42(8): 1093–103.

84. Heinrich MC, *et al*. Correlation of kinase genotype and clinical outcome in the North American Inter-Group Phase III Trial of imatinib mesylate for treatment of advanced GI stromal tumor (CALGB 150105). J Clin Oncol 2008; 26(33): 5352–9.

85. Demetri GD, *et al*. Molecular target modulation, imaging, and clinical evaluation of gastrointestinal stromal tumor patients treated with sunitinib malate after imatinib failure. Clin Can Res 2009; 15(18): 5902–9.

86. Demetri DG, *et al*. Efficacy and safety of sunitinib in patients with advanced gastrointestinal stromal tumour after failure of imatinib: a randomized controlled trial. Lancet 2006; 368(9544): 1329–38.

87. George S, *et al*. Clinical evaluation of continuous daily dosing of sunitinib malate in patients with advanced gastrointestinal stromal tumour after imatinib failure. Eur J Cancer 2009; 45(11): 1959–68.

88. Heinrich MC, *et al*. Primary and secondary kinase genotypes correlate with the biological and clinical activity of sunitinib in imatinib-resistant gastrointestinal stromal tumor. J Clin Oncol 2008; 26(33): 5352–9.

89. Gajiwala KS, *et al*. KIT kinase mutants show unique mechanisms of drug resistance to imatinib and sunitinib in gastrointestinal stromal tumor patients. Proc Natl Acad Sci U S A 2009; 106(5): 1542–7.

90. Antonescu CR, *et al*. Acquired resistance to imatinib in gastrointestinal stromal tumor occurs through secondary gene mutation. Clin Cancer Res 2005; 11(11): 4182–90.

91. Wardelmann E, *et al*. Acquired resistance to imatinib in gastrointestinal stromal tumours caused by multiple KIT mutations. Lancet Oncol 2005; 6(4): 249–51.

92. Debiec-Rychter M, *et al*. Mechanisms of resistance to imatinib mesylate in gastrointestinal stromal tumors and activity of the PKC412 inhibitor against imatinib-resistant mutants. Gastroenterology 2005; 128(2): 270–9.

93. Chen LL, *et al*. A missense mutation in KIT kinase domain 1 correlates with imatinib resistance in gastrointestinal stromal tumors. Cancer Res 2004; 64(17): 5913–19.

94. Tamborini E, *et al*. A new mutation in the KIT ATP pocket causes acquired resistance to imatinib in a gastrointestinal stromal tumor patient. Gastroenterology 2004; 127(1): 294–9.

95. Van Oosterom A, *et al*. Combination signal transduction inhibition: a phase I/II trial of the oral mTOR-inhibitor everolimus (E, RAD001) and imatinib mesylate (IM) in patients (pts) with gastrointestinal stromal tumor (GIST) refractory to IM. New Orleans: ASCO Annual Meeting, 2004: 3002.

96. Reichardt P, *et al*. A phase I/II trial of the oral PKC inhibitor PKC412 and imatinib mesylate in patients with gastrointestinal stromal tumors (GIST) refractory to imatinib (IM). Vienna, Austria: European Society of Medical Oncology Annual Meeting, 2004.

97. Demetri G, *et al*. Optimal management of patients with gastrointestinal stromal tumor (GIST), expansion and update of NCCN clinical practice guidelines, 2004. J Natl Compr Cancer Netw 2004; 2(Suppl): S1–26.

98. Eisenberg BL, *et al*. Phase II trial of neoadjuvant/adjuvant imatinib mesylate (IM) for advanced primary and metastatic/recurrent operable gastrointestinal stromal tumor (GIST): early results of RTOG 0132/ACRIN 6665. J Surg Oncol 2009; 99(1): 42–7.

99. DeMatteo R, *et al*. Efficacy of adjuvant imatinib mesylate following complete resection of localized, primary GIST at high risk of recurrence: U.S. intergroup phase II trial ACOSOG Z9000. Orlando, FL: ASCO Gastrointestinal Cancers Symposium, 2008.

100. Dematteo RP, *et al*. Adjuvant imatinib mesylate after resection of localised, primary gastrointestinal stromal tumour: a randomised, double-blind, placebo-controlled trial. Lancet 2009; 373(9669): 1097–104.

101. Zhan WH, CGC Group. Efficacy and safety of adjuvant post-surgical therapy with imatinib in patients with high risk of relapsing GIST. Proc Am Soc Clin Oncol 2007; 25: abstract 10045.

102. Kang Y, *et al*. A phase II study of imatinib mesylate as adjuvant treatment for curatively resected high-risk localized gastrointestinal stromal tumors with c-kit exon 11 mutation. J Clin Oncol 2009; 27(Suppl): abstract e21515.

103. Joensuu H, *et al*. Twelve versus 36 months of adjuvant imatinib (IM) as treatment of operable GIST with a high risk of recurrence: final results of a randomized trial (SSGXVIII/AIO). J Clin Oncol 2011; 29(Suppl): abstract LBA1.

104. Tarn C, *et al*. Analysis of KIT mutations in sporadic and familial gastrointestinal stromal tumors: therapeutic implications through protein modeling. Clin Cancer Res 2005; 11(10): 3668–77.

105. Nishida T, *et al*. Familial gastrointestinal stromal tumours with germline mutation of the KIT gene. Nat Genet 1998; 19(4): 323–4.

106. Robson ME, *et al*. Pleomorphic characteristics of a germ-line KIT mutation in a large kindred with gastrointestinal stromal tumors, hyperpigmentation, and dysphagia. Clin Cancer Res 2004; 10(4): 1250–4.

107. Maeyama H, *et al*. Familial gastrointestinal stromal tumor with hyperpigmentation: association with a germline mutation of the c-kit gene. Gastroenterology 2001; 120(1): 210–15.

108. Isozaki K, Terris B, Belghiti J, Schiffmann S, Hirota S, Vanderwinden JM. Germline-activating mutation in the kinase domain of KIT gene in familial gastrointestinal stromal tumors. Am J Pathol 2000; 157(5): 1581–5.

109. Hirota S, et al. Familial gastrointestinal stromal tumors associated with dysphagia and novel type germline mutation of KIT gene. Gastroenterology 2002; 122(5): 1493–9.

110. Andersson J, Sihto H, Meis-Kindblom JM, Joensuu H, Nupponen N, Kindblom LG. NF1-associated gastrointestinal stromal tumors have unique clinical, phenotypic, and genotypic characteristics. Am J Surg Pathol 2005; 29(9): 1170–6.

111. Kim HJ, Lim SJ, Park K, Yuh YJ, Jang SJ, Choi J. Multiple gastrointestinal stromal tumors with a germline c-kit mutation. Pathol Int 2005; 55(10): 655–9.

112. Nishida T, et al. Familial gastrointestinal stromal tumors with germline mutation of the KIT gene. Nat Genet 1998; 19: 323–4.

113. Li FP, et al. Familial gastrointestinal stromal tumor syndrome: phenotypic and molecular features in a kindred. J Clin Oncol 2005; 23(12): 2735–43.

114. Nemoto H, et al. Novel NF1 gene mutation in a Japanese patient with neurofibromatosis type 1 and a gastrointestinal stromal tumor. J Gastroenterol 2006; 41(4): 378–82.

115. Relles D, Baek J, Witkiewicz A, Yeo CJ. Periampullary and duodenal neoplasms in neurofibromatosis type 1: two cases and an updated 20-year review of the literature yielding 76 cases. J Gastrointest Surg 2010; 14(6): 1052–61.

116. Zoller ME, Rembeck B, Oden A, Samuelsson M, Angervall L. Malignant and benign tumors in patients with neurofibromatosis type 1 in a defined Swedish population. Cancer 1997; 79(11): 2125–31.

117. Miettinen M, Fetsch JF, Sobin LH, Lasota J. Gastrointestinal stromal tumors in patients with neurofibromatosis 1: a clinicopathologic and molecular genetic study of 45 cases. Am J Surg Pathol 2006; 30(1): 90–6.

118. Maertens O, et al. Molecular pathogenesis of multiple gastrointestinal stromal tumors in NF1 patients. Hum Mol Genet 2006; 15(6): 1015–23.

119. Pappo AS, Janeway KA. Pediatric gastrointestinal stromal tumors. Hematol Oncol Clin North Am 2009; 23: 15–34.

120. Benesch M, Wardelmann E, Ferrari A, Brennan B, Verschuur A. Gastrointestinal stromal tumors (GIST) in children and adolescents: a comprehensive review. Pediatr Blood Cancer 2009; 53: 1171–9.

121. Carney JA, Sheps SG, Go VL, Gordon H. The triad of gastric leiomyosarcoma, functioning extra-adrenal paraganglioma and pulmonary chondroma. N Engl J Med 1977; 296(26): 1517–18.

122. Carney JA. Gastric stromal sarcoma, pulmonary chondroma, and extra-adrenal paraganglioma (Carney Triad): natural history, adrenocortical component, and possible familial occurrence. Mayo Clin Proc 1999; 74(6): 543–52.

123. Carney JA, Stratakis CA. Familial paraganglioma and gastric stromal sarcoma: a new syndrome distinct from the Carney triad. Am J Med Genet 2002; 108(2): 132–9.

124. McWhinney SR, Pasini B, Stratakis CA. International Carney Triad and Carney-Stratakis Syndrome Consortium. Familial gastrointestinal stromal tumors and germ-line mutations. N Engl J Med 2007; 357(10): 1054–6.

125. Rajan DK, et al. Sarcomas metastatic to the liver: response and survival after cisplatin, doxorubicin, mitomycin-C, ethiodol, and polyvinyl alcohol chemoembolization. J Vasc Interv Radiol 2001; 12(2): 187–93.

126. Mavligit GM, et al. Gastrointestinal leiomyosarcoma metastatic to the liver. Durable tumor regression by hepatic chemoembolization infusion with cisplatin and vinblastine. Cancer 1995; 75(8): 2083–8.

127. Pawlik TM, et al. Results of a single-center experience with resection and ablation for sarcoma metastatic to the liver. Arch Surg 2006; 141(6): 537–43; discussion 543–4.

128. Seralta AS, et al. Combined liver transplantation plus imatinib for unresectable metastases of gastrointestinal stromal tumours. Eur J Gastroenterol Hepatol 2004; 16(11): 1237–9.

129. DePas P, et al. Imatinib administration in two patients with liver metastases from GIST and severe jaundice. Br J Cancer 2003; 89(8): 1403–4.

130. Joensuu H. Treatment of inoperable gastrointestinal stromal tumor (GIST) with imatinib (Glivec, Gleevec). Med Klin (Munich) 2002; 97(Suppl 1): 28–30.

131. Agaram NP, et al. Novel V600E BRAF mutations in imatinib-naive and imatinib-resistant gastrointestinal stromal tumors. Genes Chromosomes Cancer 2008; 47(10): 853–9.

132. Prakash S, et al. Gastrointestinal stromal tumors in children and young adults: a clinicopathologic, molecular, and genomic study of 15 cases and review of the literature. J Pediatr Hematol Oncol 2005; 27(4): 179–87.

133. Cypriano MS, Jenkins JJ, Pappo AS, Rao BN, Daw NC. Pediatric gastrointestinal stromal tumors and leiomyosarcoma. Cancer 2004; 101(1): 39–50.

134. Sauseng W, et al. Clinical, radiological, and pathological findings in four children with gastrointestinal stromal tumors of the stomach. Pediatr Hematol Oncol 2007; 24(3): 209–19.

135. Kuroiwa M, et al. Advanced-stage gastrointestinal stromal tumor treated with imatinib in a 12-year-old girl with a unique mutation of PDGFRA. J Pediatr Surg 2005; 40(11): 1798–801.

136. Gajiwala KS, et al. KIT kinase mutants show unique mechanisms of drug resistance to imatinib and sunitinib in gastrointestinal stromal tumor patients. Proc Natl Acad Sci U S A 2009; 106(5): 1542–7.

137. Bond M, et al. A phase II study of imatinib mesylate in children with refractory or relapsed solid tumors: a Children's Oncology Group study. Pediatr Blood Cancer 2008; 50(2): 254–8.

138. Hayashi Y, et al. Gastrointestinal stromal tumor in a child and review of the literature. Pediatr Surg Int 2005; 21(11): 914–17.

139. Janeway KA, et al. Sunitinib treatment in pediatric patients with advanced GIST following failure of imatinib. Pediatr Blood Cancer 2009; 52(7): 767.

140. Bonvalot S, et al. Impact of surgery on advanced gastrointestinal stromal tumors (GIST) in the imatinib era. Ann Surg Oncol 2006; 13(12): 1596–603.

141. Rutkowski P, et al. Surgical treatment of patients with initially inoperable and/or metastatic gastrointestinal stromal tumors (GIST) during therapy with imatinib mesylate. J Surg Oncol 2006; 93(4): 304–11.

142. Scaife CL, et al. Is there a role for surgery in patients with "unresectable" cKIT+ gastrointestinal stromal tumors treated with imatinib mesylate? Am J Surg 2003; 186(6): 665–9.

143. Bauer S, et al. Resection of residual disease in patients with metastatic gastrointestinal stromal tumors responding to treatment with imatinib. Int J Cancer 2005; 117(2): 316–25.

144. Raut CP, et al. Surgical management of advanced gastrointestinal stromal tumors after treatment with targeted systemic therapy using kinase inhibitors. J Clin Oncol 2006; 24(15): 2325–31.

145. DeMatteo RP, et al. Results of tyrosine kinase inhibitor therapy followed by surgical resection for metastatic gastrointestinal stromal tumor. Ann Surg 2007; 245(3): 347–52.

146. Andtbacka RHI, et al. Surgical resection of gastrointestinal stromal tumors after treatment with imatinib. Ann Surg Oncol 2007; 14(1): 14–24.

147. Gronchi A, et al. Surgery of residual disease following molecular-targeted therapy with imatinib mesylate in advanced/metastatic GIST. Ann Surg 2007; 245(3): 341–6.

148. Braconi C, et al. Molecular targets in gastrointestinal stromal tumors (GIST) therapy. Curr Cancer Drug Targets 2008; 8(5): 359–66.

149. Raut CP, et al. Cytoreductive surgery in patients with metastatic gastrointestinal stromal tumor treated with sunitinib malate. Ann Surg Oncol 2010; 17(2): 407–15.

150. Guo T, et al. Sorafenib inhibits the imatinib-resistant KITT670I gatekeeper mutation in gastrointestinal stromal tumor. Clin Cancer Res 2007; 13: 4874–81.

151. Prenen H, et al. Cellular uptake of the tyrosine kinase inhibitors imatinib and AMN107 in gastrointestinal stromal tumor cell lines. Pharmacology 2006; 77(1): 11–16.

152. Demetri GD, *et al*. A phase I study of single-agent nilotinib or in combination with imatinib in patients with imatinib-resistant gastrointestinal stromal tumors. Clin Cancer Res 2009; 15(18): 5910–16.

153. Montemurro M, *et al*. Nilotinib in the treatment of advanced gastrointestinal stromal tumours resistant to both imatinib and sunitinib. Eur J Cancer 2009; 45(13): 2293–7.

154. Nishida T, *et al*. Phase II trial of nilotinib as third-line therapy for gastrointestinal stromal tumor (GIST) patients in Japan. J Clin Oncol 2010; 28(Suppl): abstract 10015.

155. Cauchi C, *et al*. Evaluation of nilotinib (N) in advanced GIST previously treated with imatinib mesylate (IM) and sunitinib (S). J Clin Oncol 2010; 28(Suppl): abstract 10090.

156. Reichardt P, *et al*. Phase III trial of nilotinib in patients with advanced gastrointestinal stromal tumor (GIST): first results from ENEST g3. J Clin Oncol 2010; 28(Suppl): abstract 10017.

157. Dubreil P, *et al*. Masitinib (AB1010), a potent and selective tyrosine kinase inhibitor targeting KIT. PLoS One 2009; 4(9): e7258.

158. Soria JC, *et al*. Phase 1 dose-escalation study of oral tyrosine kinase inhibitor masitinib in advanced and/or metastatic solid cancers. Eur J Cancer 2009; 45(13): 2333–41.

159. Le Cesne A, *et al*. Phase II study of oral masitinib mesilate in imatinib-naive patients with locally advanced or metastatic gastro-intestinal stromal tumour (GIST). Eur J Cancer 2010; 46(8): 1344–51.

160. Guida T, *et al*. Sorafenib inhibits imatinib-resistant KIT and platelet-derived growth factor receptor beta gatekeeper mutants. Clin Cancer Res 2007; 13: 3363–9.

161. Heinrich MC, *et al*. In vitro activity of sorafenib against imatinib-and sunitinib resistant kinase mutations associated with drug-resistant GI stromal tumors. J Clin Oncol 2010; 28(Suppl): abstract 10500.

162. Kindler HL, *et al*. Sorafenib (SOR) in patients (pts) with imatinib (IM) and sunitinib (SU)-resistant (RES) gastrointestinal stromal tumors (GIST): final results of a University of Chicago Phase II Consortium trial. J Clin Oncol 2011; 29(Suppl): abstract 10009.

163. Reichardt P, *et al*. Sorafenib fourth-line treatment in imatinib-, sunitinib-, nilotinib-resistant metastatic GIST: a retrospective analysis. J Clin Oncol 2009; 27(Suppl): abstract 10564.

164. George S, *et al*. A multi-center phase II study of regorafenib in patients (pts) with advanced gastrointestinal stromal tumor (GIST), after therapy with imatinib (IM) and sunitinib (SU). J Clin Oncol 2011; 29(Suppl): abstract 10007.

165. Agaram NP, *et al*. Novel V600E BRAF mutations in imatinib-naive and imatinib-resistant gastrointestinal stromal tumors. Genes Chromosomes Cancer 2008; 47(10): 853–9.

166. Schittenhelm MM, *et al*. Dasatinib (BMS-354825), a dual SRC/ABL kinase inhibitor, inhibits the kinase activity of wild-type, juxtamembrane, and activation loop mutant KIT isoforms associated with human malignancies. Cancer Res 2006; 66(1): 473–81.

167. Trent JC, *et al*. A phase II study of dasatinib for patients with imatinib-resistant gastrointestinal stromal tumor (GIST). J Clin Oncol 2011; 29(Suppl): abstract 10006.

168. Heinrich MC, *et al*. The effect of crenolanib (CP-868596) on phosphorylation of the imatinib-resistant D842V PDGFRA activating mutation

169. associated with advanced gastrointestinal stromal tumors. J Clin Oncol 2011; 29(Suppl): abstract 10012.

169. Bauer S, Duensing A, Demetri GD, Fletcher JA. KIT oncogenic signaling mechanisms in imatinib-resistant gastrointestinal stromal tumor: PI3-kinase/AKT is a crucial survival pathway. Oncogene 2007; 26(54): 7560–8.

170. Schoffski P, *et al*. A phase I-II study of evirolimus (RAD001) in combination with imatinib in patients with imatinib-resistant gastrointestinal stromal tumors. Ann Oncol 2010; 21: 1990–8.

171. Hohenberger P, Bauer S, Gruenwald V. Multicenter, single arm, two stage phase II trial of everolimus (RAD001) with imatinib in imatinib-resistant patients (pts) with advanced GIST. J Clin Oncol 2010; 28(Suppl): abstract 10048.

172. Conley AP, *et al*. A randomized phase II study of perifosine (P) plus imatinib for patients with imatinib-resistant gastrointestinal stromal tumor (GIST). J Clin Oncol 2009; 27(Suppl): abstract 10563.

173. Xu W, Neckers L. Targeting the molecular chaperone heat shock protein 90 provides a multifaceted effect on diverse cell signaling pathways of cancer cells. Clin Cancer Res 2007; 13: 1625–9.

174. Nakatani H, *et al*. STI571 (Glivec) inhibits the interaction between c-KIT and heat shock protein 90 of the gastrointestinal stromal tumor cell line, GIST-T1. Cancer Sci 2005; 96: 116–19.

175. Fumo G, Akins C, Metcalfe DD, Neckers L. 17-Allylamino-17-demethoxygeldanamycin (17-AAG) is effective in down-regulating mutated, constitutively activated KIT protein in human mast cells. Blood 2004; 103(3): 1078–84.

176. Bauer S, Yuk LK, Demetri GD, Fletcher JA. Heat shock protein 90 inhibition in imatinib-resistant gastrointestinal stromal tumor. Cancer Res 2006; 66: 9153–61.

177. Wagner AJ, *et al*. Results from phase 1 trial of IPI-504, a novel HSP90 inhibitor, in tyrosine kinase inhibitor-resistant GIST and other sarcomas. J Clin Oncol 2008; 26(Suppl): abstract 10503.

178. Demetri GD, *et al*. Final results form a phase III study of IPI-504 (restapimycin hydrochloride) versus placebo in patients (pts) with gastrointestinal stromal tumors (GIST) following failure of kinase inhibitor therapies. Poster presentation. ASCO Gastrointestinal Cancers Symposium, 2007; Orlando, Florida: abstract 64.

179. Muhlenberg T, *et al*. Inhibitors of deacetylases suppress oncogenic KIT signaling, acetylate HSP90, and induce apoptosis in gastrointestinal stromal tumors. Cancer Res 2009; 69: 6941–50.

180. Floris G, *et al*. High efficacy of panobinostat towards human gastrointestinal stromal tumors in a xenograft mouse model. Clin Cancer Res 2009; 15: 4066–76.

181. Agaram NP, *et al*. Molecular characterization of pediatric gastrointestinal stromal tumors. Clin Cancer Res 2008; 14(10): 3204–15.

182. Tarn C, *et al*. Insulin-like growth factor 1 receptor is a potential therapeutic target for gastrointestinal stromal tumors. Proc Natl Acad Sci U S A 2008; 105(24): 8387–92.

183. Braconi C, *et al*. Insulin-like growth factor (IGF) 1 and 2 help to predict disease outcome in GIST patients. Ann Oncol 2008; 19(7): 1293–8.

Section 7: Gynecological Cancers

34 Extraovarian Primary Peritoneal Carcinomas

Alberto E. Selman[1] and Larry J. Copeland[2]

[1] Division of Gynecologic Oncology, Department of Obstetrics and Gynecology, Clinical Hospital, Universidad de Chile, Santiago, Chile

[2] Department of Obstetrics and Gynecology, James Cancer Hospital and Solove Research Institute, The Ohio State University, Columbus, OH, USA

Introduction

Extraovarian primary peritoneal carcinoma (EOPPC) is found in 18–28% of patients with suspected epithelial ovarian carcinoma (EOC).[1–3] Basically, EOPPC is an extraovarian adenocarcinoma involving the peritoneum which spreads throughout the peritoneal cavity with minimal or no ovarian involvement, and no obvious primary site. Most EOPPC cases reported have been of serous histology, and in many cases the malignancy developed following bilateral oophorectomy for reasons other than cancer.[4] Histopathological, immunohistochemical (IHC), and clinical similarities have been observed between EOPPC and EOC, specifically the serous variety, but EOPPC involves the ovarian surface only minimally (microscopic disease) or spares the ovaries entirely.[5] On the other hand, molecular and epidemiological studies have reported some differences between the two diseases.[6,7]

Disagreement and controversy continue to exist in the literature among authorities who consider EOPPC to be a different clinical entity from EOC.[8–11] Most investigators consider these entities to be similar in clinical presentation and course, except that EOPPC patients by disease definition present at a more advanced stage.

Historical background

Numerous terms have been used to describe this entity, including serous surface carcinoma of the peritoneum, papillary tumor of the peritoneum, serous surface papillary carcinoma, serous papillary surface carcinoma of the ovary, serous borderline tumor of the peritoneum, extraovarian pelvic serous tumor, multifocal extraovarian serous carcinoma, extraovarian papillary serous carcinoma, mesothelioma, and papillary serous carcinoma of the peritoneum (PSCP).

Swerdlow, in a 1959 case report, first described malignant mesothelioma (MM) with diffuse involvement of the peritoneum, no obvious primary site, and grossly normal ovaries in a 27-year-old woman.[12] Since then, many authors have reported similar cases.[4,8,13–15] In 1977, Kannerstein pointed out the importance of distinguishing EOPPC from MM.[4] Since its first description by Swerdlow, EOPPC has been recognized in females; its histological similarities to MM and papillary serous ovarian carcinoma (PSOC) have caused difficulties in classifying it as an independent clinicopathological entity.[4] It is recognized as a distinct clinicopathological tumor that arises from mesothelial cells under müllerian influences.[16,17] Some authors have regarded the terms mesothelioma and EOPPC as synonymous.[18,19] Parmley and Woodruff have also proposed that all tumors arising from the pleural and peritoneal cavities be classified as mesotheliomas.[20]

Foyle *et al.* described 25 peritoneal tumors in women and divided them histologically into five groups: mesothelial hyperplasia, well-differentiated diffuse papillary mesothelioma, diffuse papillary mesothelioma, atypical diffuse mesothelioma, and papillary carcinoma.[13] Only three tumors closely resemble papillary or tubopapillary diffuse MM, the type associated with asbestos, which occurs in the pleural cavities in both sexes. There were eight well-differentiated mesotheliomas and these were associated with indolent behavior. However, in 10 cases, tumor resembled PSOC; these tumors were different and progressed rapidly. They concluded that EOPPC should not be merged with the general group of diffuse mesotheliomas. Other authors have also opposed the grouping of EOPPC and mesothelioma of the peritoneum because of important epidemiological, histological, ultrastructural, and biological differences.[4,8] Researches have demonstrated the link between peritoneal mesotheliomas and asbestos exposure which is not present in EOPPC.[21] Furthermore, peritoneal mesotheliomas have a male predilection and are rarely seen in women.[22]

Recent studies have examined the tubal fimbriae in women with serous ovarian carcinoma and have found serous tubal intraepithelial carcinoma (STIC) in a substantial proportion of

Textbook of Uncommon Cancer, Fourth Edition. Edited by Derek Raghavan, Charles D. Blanke, David H. Johnson, Paul L. Moots, Gregory H. Reaman, Peter G. Rose and Mikkael A. Sekeres.
© 2012 John Wiley & Sons, Inc. Published 2012 by John Wiley & Sons, Inc.

cases.[23,24] Complete examination of all fallopian tube tissue in cases of pelvic (nonuterine) serous carcinoma identifies STIC in 61% of ovarian high-grade serous carcinomas.[25] If STIC is the precursor of apparent "ovarian" serous carcinoma, then it would appear even more likely that STIC is the origin of EOPPC. Carlson *et al.* found STIC in 40% of patients with primary peritoneal serous carcinoma.[26] In a related study from the same group, patients with serous carcinoma were divided into those with or without a dominant ovarian mass and STIC was found in 45% of those without a dominant ovarian mass as compared to 11% of those with such a mass.[27] These studies suggest that cases classified as peritoneal serous carcinoma are more likely to harbor STIC.

Although preneoplastic changes such as dysplasia have so far been found almost exclusively in the fimbriated end of the fallopian tubes in surgical specimens from women undergoing prophylactic procedures because of familial predisposition to ovarian cancer, it is likely that similar dysplastic lesions would have been found within foci of endosalpingiosis if components of the secondary müllerian system had been examined in addition to the fallopian tubes in these studies.[28–31]

Biology and epidemiology

The histogenesis of this tumor is not known with certainty. The normal peritoneum is lined by a specific type of cell termed mesothelium. When mesothelial cells undergo malignant transformation, the result is a malignant mesothelioma. Malignant mesothelioma is an entirely different tumor from serous carcinoma, even though occasionally the distinction may be difficult and require special studies.

Ovarian and peritoneal epithelium share a common embryonal origin, the coelomic epithelium (mesonephric origin). In contrast, fallopian tube epithelium, endometrium, and endocervix are related to paramesonephros (müllerian duct). Surprisingly, EOC and EOPPC are histologically similar to the müllerian epithelium, not their embryonal origin, the mesonephros. Ovarian, fallopian tube, and primary peritoneal tumors are all exclusively derived from cells in which features of müllerian differentiation are already present. Either a metaplasia has occurred or müllerian remnants have been left behind in coelemic epithelium, which have turned oncogenic. The endocervix, endometrium, and fallopian tubes are not the only sites where epithelial cells derived from the müllerian ducts are found in adults. Microscopic structures lined by müllerian epithelium are very common in the paratubal and paraovarian areas and they also frequently impinge on the ovarian medulla and can even be seen within the deeper portions of the ovarian cortex. These structures are grouped under the name "secondary müllerian system."[32] They include endosalpingiosis, endometriosis, and endocervicosis. Benign serous-type epithelium on or just underneath the peritoneal surface, referred to as endosalpingiosis, is found in about 25% of women.[33] This epithelium is ciliated and is identical to that of the normal fallopian tube. Its origin is unknown and although it is possible that it is a metaplastic change of mesothelial cells, most evidence suggests that endosalpingiosis is of tubal origin. Quddus and colleagues reviewed all cases of

endosalpingiosis and endometriosis of the omentum from a single institution over a 12-year period.[34] They reported that the endosalpingiosis-to-endometriosis ratio in this cohort was similar to the ratio of primary peritoneal serous to endometrioid carcinomas, providing support for the idea that these two malignant tumor types are related to these two benign lesions, respectively.[34]

During fetal development, before the secretion of müllerian inhibiting factor (MIF) by the fetal testes, the müllerian ducts develop in male fetuses.[17] MIF subsequently inhibits their development and they degenerate and completely disappear by 9–12 weeks. This müllerian influence, however brief, may account for the rare occurrence of lesions resembling EOPPC in the male peritoneum, including rare lesions involving the tunica vaginalis testis and epididymis.[35–37]

In the absence of precursor lesions, distinct theories of carcinogenesis have been suggested: müllerian metaplasia of coelomic epithelium prior to malignant transformation, clonal origin from structures of the secondary müllerian system present in ovarian/peritoneal epithelia or development from the fallopian tube fimbriae.[38–40]

The conventional criteria that have been used to assign primary site of origin for ovarian, peritoneal, and tubal carcinomas are arbitrary and have never been validated. It now appears that the presence of a STIC is a useful criterion for establishing primary tubal versus ovarian and peritoneal origin.[15,41,42] As the presence of a STIC has not been previously used as a uniformly accepted criterion for the diagnosis of tubal carcinoma, prior data from tumor registries and clinicopathological studies have underestimated the actual frequency of primary fallopian tube carcinoma and, conversely, overestimated the frequency of primary ovarian and peritoneal carcinomas. On the basis of population-based data, the frequency distribution of primary ovarian, peritoneal, and tubal serous carcinomas is 78–90%, 8–16%, and 2–6%, respectively.[25] If STIC is used as a supplemental criterion to define tubal origin, then these figures would change to 28%, 8%, and 64%, respectively.[25] A substantial shift in the frequency distribution of primary site of origin based on the presence of STIC was also observed in another study.[43]

Initial studies focused on the epidemiological differences between MM and EOPPC. MM are particularly rare in women in whom the most common malignant peritoneal neoplasm is the EOPPC. About two-thirds of patients with MM are middle-aged or elderly men, and in more than 80% of these cases there is evidence of asbestos exposure. In addition, MM responds poorly to chemotherapy and median survival time is short.[44]

There are numerous case reports of very small series of patients with EOPPC but larger series are rare. The paper concerning the largest series (74 patients) was published in 1990.[8] This important study unveiled the characteristics of patients with EOPPC, and other studies compared the prognosis of EOPPC to that of EOC.[45–47] Studies on the molecular pathogenesis suggest some differences in the cancers affecting these two regions. While ovarian cancer appears to have a uniclonal origin, at least some of the primary peritoneal cancers have a multifocal origin.[48,49] The majority of studies have found few epidemiological differences between peritoneal and epithelial ovarian malignancies. Several studies have shown, although others have not, that women with EOPPC are older than women with ovarian cancer.[7,50] Halperin *et al.* found that women with primary peritoneal cancer had a significantly earlier menarche, a higher number of births, and a lower incidence of family history for positive gynecological malignancies, compared with women with ovarian cancer.[51] It is not known whether pregnancy and oral contraceptive use decrease the risk of peritoneal cancer, as they do for ovarian cancer. Likewise, it is unclear whether factors that increase the risk of ovarian cancer, such as infertility, also increase the risk of primary peritoneal carcinomas.

Women with deleterious mutations in the breast cancer gene 1 (BRCA1) or breast cancer gene 2 (BRCA2) have a 54–85% and 45% lifetime risk of developing breast cancer respectively and 36–63% and 10–27% lifetime risk of developing ovarian cancer respectively.[52] The mean age at diagnosis of ovarian cancer is significantly younger for BRCA1 compared to BRCA2 mutation carriers (54 versus 62 years).[53] Most BRCA-related ovarian carcinomas are of high-grade serous type.[54] The risk of ovarian/tubal/peritoneal carcinoma varies according to the type of BRCA mutation.[55] There is a 3–5% residual risk of developing EOPPC after bilateral salpingo-oophorectomy (BSO).[56,57] The published series reported an incidence of germline BRCA mutations in patients with EOPPC similar to that of patients with serous ovarian cancer (5–10%).[58]

The role of BRCA1 gene mutations in the development of EOPPC is uncertain.[29,48] Bandera *et al.* screened 17 patients with peritoneal cancer and found BRCA1 germline mutations in three (17.6%) of 17 EOPPC patients.[59] Karlan *et al.* reported that three EOPPC patients who underwent genetic testing carried BRCA1 mutations.[49] They developed the disease at the age of 38, 39, and 55 years. In one of these cases the ovaries were histologically without evidence of malignancy, while in the other two cases the two ovaries and each of the metastatic sites studied differed in their patterns of oncogene overexpression. Bandera *et al.* identified in two of 17 EOPPC patients the 185 delAG germline BRCA1 mutation described in the Ashkenazi Jewish population.[60] The family history of one patient was notable: a mother and five aunts had breast or ovarian cancer. The other patient had a personal history of breast cancer. Both patients exhibited allelic loss of the normal BRCA1 allele in their tumor. A third patient was found to have a previously undescribed exon 11 single base pair substitution at nucleotide 1239 (CAG to CAC) resulting in a missense mutation (Gln to His). The patient had no family or personal history of breast or ovarian cancer, and her tumor did not exhibit loss of heterozygosity. Halperin *et al.* found two BRCA1 mutations, but no BRCA2 mutations in 28 women with EOPPC.[51] Karlan *et al.* suggest that EOPPC may be a phenotypic variant of hereditary ovarian cancer.[49] The fact that women with BRCA1 and possibly BRCA2 mutations are at increased risk for EOPPC has implications regarding recommendations for screening and prophylactic oophorectomy. In a study of 290 Jewish women who were at risk for ovarian cancer because of their family history, intensive surveillance by use of CA-125 and ultrasound did not seem to be

an effective means of diagnosing early-stage ovarian cancer.[61] During the study, six women developed stage IIIC peritoneal cancer, and all had had normal ovaries on transvaginal ultrasound imaging. All of the primary peritoneal cancers developed in women with BRCA1 mutations.

Two studies evaluated the benefits of prophylactic oophorectomy and the potential risk of subsequent EOPPC. Kauff *et al.* studied 170 women with BRCA1 or BRCA2 mutations, 35 years of age or older, who had not undergone bilateral oophorectomy but chose to undergo either surveillance for ovarian cancer or risk-reducing salpingo-oophorectomy.[62] During a mean follow-up of 24.2 months, breast cancer was diagnosed in three of the 98 women who chose risk-reducing salpingo-oophorectomy and peritoneal cancer was diagnosed in one woman in this group. Among the 72 women who chose surveillance, breast cancer was diagnosed in eight, ovarian cancer in four, and peritoneal cancer in one. The time to breast cancer or BRCA-related gynecological cancer was longer in the salpingo-oophorectomy group, with a hazard ratio for subsequent breast cancer or BRCA-related gynecological cancer of 0.25 (95% confidence interval [CI] 0.08–0.74). In the study by Rebbeck *et al.*, there were 551 women with disease-associated germ-line BRCA1 or BRCA2 mutations (259 women who had undergone bilateral prophylactic oophorectomy and in 292 matched controls).[63] The length of postoperative follow-up for both groups was at least 8 years. Six women who underwent prophylactic oophorectomy (2.3%) received a diagnosis of stage I ovarian cancer at the time of the procedure; two women (0.8%) received a diagnosis of papillary serous peritoneal carcinoma 3.8 and 8.6 years after bilateral prophylactic oophorectomy. Among the controls, 58 women (19.9%) received a diagnosis of ovarian cancer, after a mean follow-up of 8.8 years. With the exclusion of the six women whose cancer was diagnosed at surgery, prophylactic oophorectomy significantly reduced the risk of coelomic epithelial cancer. In a subgroup of 241 women with no history of breast cancer or prophylactic mastectomy, the incidence of breast cancer was determined in 99 women who had undergone bilateral prophylactic oophorectomy and in 142 matched controls. Of the 99 women who underwent bilateral prophylactic oophorectomy, breast cancer developed in 21 (21.2%), as compared to 60 (42.3%) in the control group. Each of these studies concluded that bilateral prophylactic oophorectomy significantly reduced the risk of breast cancer and EOC. However, the risk of peritoneal cancer remains.

Risk-reducing salpingo-oophorectomy (RRSO) was shown to decrease lifetime ovarian, fallopian tube or primary peritoneal cancer risk by up to 80% and breast cancer risk by 50% in carriers of BRCA1 and BRCA2 mutations.[64,65] Furthermore, an age-matched case–control study suggests that RRSO leads to a 90% reduction in breast cancer-specific mortality, a 95% reduction in ovarian cancer-specific mortality, and a 76% reduction in overall mortality.[66]

Clinically occult carcinomas in the RRSO specimens range from 2% to 17%.[67–72] The localization of the microinvasive carcinoma in the distal part of the fallopian tube is in line with data from other studies demonstrating that clinically occult carcinomas predominantly occur in the fallopian tubes and not in the ovaries.[73,74] Combining immunohistochemistry and biomolecular studies, it becomes more and more evident that most pelvic (including tubal, ovarian, and primary peritoneal) high-grade serous carcinomas may actually have a common origin, the tubal fimbria. This fact explains the frequent difficulty in differentiating the origin of a serous carcinoma based only on anatomical and pathological criteria.[75]

Pathology

Histopathological similarities have been drawn between EOPPC and PSOC.[5] For study purposes, the Gynecologic Oncology Group (GOG) developed a set of criteria for EOPPC diagnosis.[15]

1. The ovaries are either absent or normal in size (<4 cm largest diameter).
2. The involvement in the extraovarian sites is greater than that of the surface of either ovary.
3. Microscopically, the ovaries are either not involved with tumor or exhibit only serosal or cortical implants, less than 5 mm in depth.
4. The histopathological and cytological characteristics of the tumor are predominantly of the serous type.

Other types of EOPPC have been described, including endometrioid, mucinous, clear cell, Brenner, and malignant mixed müllerian types.[76–79] Eltabbakh et al. reported that the median survival of patients who had nonserous histology was not significantly different from that of patients with serous histology.[80] Altaras et al. reported one patient with papillary clear cell EOPPC alive without evidence of disease 76 months following diagnosis.[76]

Two EOPPC variations appear less virulent.[81,82] The peritoneal serous borderline tumors (PSBTs) behave similarly to their ovarian counterparts. They have an excellent prognosis, although in rare cases transformation to carcinoma has been observed on follow-up examination.[81,83] Forty-one to ninety-nine percent of PSBTs are accompanied by endosalpingiosis, suggesting an origin therein.[81,83,84] Histologically, PSBTs are identical to the peritoneal implants found in association with ovarian serous borderline tumors. Patients with PSBTs are typically under the age of 35 years, and often infertile.[84] Malignant tumors are rare in young women.[46] The second, less virulent variety is the serous psammocarcinoma of the peritoneum. This latter group has a proportionately larger number of psammoma bodies, and less aggressive cytological appearance with absent or moderate nuclear atypicality and rare mitotic figures. Conservative management, both fertility-preserving surgery and the withholding of adjuvant chemotherapy, should be considered in the management of this disease.[85]

The presently accepted criteria for making the distinction between EOC and EOPPC are based on minimal scientific evidence. Therefore, it is likely that some tumors designated as EOPPC are actually small ovarian cancers that find the peritoneum a more hospitable site for growth than the ovary. Possible reasons why it may provide a more favorable environment are the greater density of the ovarian tissue, which may inhibit invasion of tumor cells originating within superficial layers, and the production of a tumor-inhibitory substance by

---

Box 34.1 Differential diagnosis of extraovarian primary peritoneal carcinoma.

- Variations of extraovarian primary peritoneal carcinoma:
  - Peritoneal serous borderline tumors
  - Psammocarcinomas of the peritoneum
- Endosalpingiosis
- Florid mesothelial hyperplasia
- Malignant mesotheliomas
- Metastatic adenocarcinoma

---

the ovarian stroma,[54] which has been demonstrated in vitro.[86,87] Besides separating EOPPC and EOC, there are different entities that need to be distinguished (Box 34.1). Histologically, EOPPC should be included in the differential diagnosis of all papillary serous lesions of the peritoneum, including endosalpingiosis, mesothelial hyperplasia, MM, and metastatic adenocarcinoma.[81,84]

• *Endosalpingiosis*: refers to the presence of histologically benign glands lined by tubal-type epithelium outside the confines of the fallopian tube. This disorder is often associated with chronic salpingitis and ovarian serous borderline tumors. The association with chronic salpingitis suggests that shedding of tubal epithelial cells onto the peritoneum is a route of development of endosalpingiosis. Endosalpingiosis is also a legitimate candidate, a precursor to EOPPC. In one series, two out of 14 carcinomas of this type were associated with this disorder.[83]

• *Florid mesothelial hyperplasia*: hyperplasia of mesothelial cells is a common response to inflammation and chronic effusions. Psammoma bodies may be present but rarely are as numerous as in EOPPC.[88]

• *Malignant mesotheliomas*: under light microscopy, differentiation between the two types of tumor may be difficult. Kannerstein et al. describe some morphological and histochemical differences between the mesothelioma and EOPPC.[4,22] Although not of absolute differential diagnostic value, the presence of psammoma bodies, epithelial mucin, and columnar cells, and the absence of hyaluronic acid favor the diagnosis of EOPPC over mesothelioma. Warhol et al. compared the ultrastructural features of MM and EOC, which are clinically similar to EOPPC.[89] They found that the mesotheliomas were characterized ultrastructurally by a greater content of tonofilaments, lack of mucin, fewer cilia, and dense-core granules of the neurosecretory type. Mesotheliomas may exactly mimic EOPPC, and definitive distinction requires IHC and/or electron microscopy.[90] Although the signs and symptoms of peritoneal mesothelioma and EOPPC are similar, the response to treatment and survival are generally poorer in patients with peritoneal mesothelioma. MMs of the pleura are approximately 10 times as frequent as those of the peritoneum, and MM of the peritoneum is extremely rare in the absence of pleural MM and a history of asbestos exposure.[91,92] Epidemiologically, MM is more common in older men, especially men with a history of asbestos exposure. EOPPC, an uncommon tumor in women, is likely to be overlooked in men, unless it is considered in the differential diagnosis. In males, another malignant tumor that can mimic an EOPPC is MM of the tunica vaginalis testis.[36,92]

• *Metastatic adenocarcinoma*: this is ruled out by the absence of a primary tumor elsewhere.

Moll *et al.* demonstrated p53 overexpression in 83% of 29 EOPPC patients.[93] The authors did not discuss the significance of p53 overexpression on survival. Kowalski *et al.* described p53 overexpression in 48% of 44 EOPPC patients, similar to the 59% incidence in patients with EOC.[6] The authors did not find that p53 overexpression was predictive of prognosis within the EOPPC or the EOC groups. Ben-Baruch *et al.*, using IHC of archival material, demonstrated p53 overexpression in 42.4% of 75 EOPPC patients.[47] EOPPC patients whose tumors demonstrated p53 overexpression had a shorter median survival than those whose tumors did not (11 versus 23.5 months, respectively). The difference did not achieve statistical significance.

Clinical presentation and diagnostic considerations

Although several studies have described the clinicopathological features of this tumor entity, the clinical behavior of EOPPC remains obscure.[4,8,11,14,15,22,45,46,76,80,82,94] It is not clear whether the EOPPC patients differ from PSOC patients with regard to their epidemiological characteristics. It has been suggested that biologically these tumors behave similarly to EOC of similar stage.[95] The natural history is similar to the ovarian counterpart, with the disease occurring mostly in women between 57 and 67 years and with a clinical presentation that does not differ from that of advanced stages of EOC.[76] Ben-Baruch *et al.* did not find significant differences in patient characteristics between EOPPC and EOC with regard to mean age at diagnosis, parity, and menopausal status.[47] The mean age of EOPPC diagnosis was 61.1 years, similar to that reported by Fromm *et al.*, Altaras *et al.*, Ransom *et al.*, and Fowler *et al.* and who found a mean age of 57.4, 61.2, 60, and 61.4, years, respectively.[8,76,94,96] Ben-Baruch *et al.* did not demonstrate significant differences between EOC and EOPPC in the operative findings.[47] The risk of ascites fluid volume exceeding 1000 mL and the proportion of patients with stage IV disease were the same among these two entities. The rate of stage IV disease was found to be 28%, which is similar to the rate of 29% and 32% reported by Altaras *et al.* and Killackey and Davis.[76,82] To our knowledge, there have been two reports of this tumor occurring in children. In 1983, Ulbright *et al.* described a 11-year-old girl with an extraovarian serous carcinoma of the retroperitoneum, and Wall *et al.* reported an adolescent girl with EOPPC whose tumor responded to paclitaxel after showing limited response to two other chemotherapeutic regimens, one of which included carboplatin.[97,98]

The most common symptoms are abdominal pain and distension.[5,8,11,13–15,45,46,76,80,82,94] Other EOPPC patients also presented with constipation, nausea, vomiting, loss of weight, loss of appetite, malaise, dyspareunia, and urinary symptoms.[8,22] Common presenting signs include ascites,

pelvic-abdominal mass, and peripheral edema.[8,22] The presence of psammoma bodies in the cervicovaginal smear of a EOPPC patient has also been documented.[99] The common sites of disease at the time of laparotomy are the omentum, abdominal and pelvic peritoneum, ovaries, and serosa of the bowel.[8,80,100] Eltabbakh and Piver suggested that the incidence of central nervous system metastases in EOPPC patients (1.4%) is similar to that of EOC patients.[101] A patient with inappropriate antidiuretic hormone secretion after suboptimal cytoreduction of a stage III EOPPC has also been described.[102]

Altaras *et al.* and Rose *et al.* reported the usefulness of CA-125 in diagnosis and follow-up of EOPPC patients.[76,100] In patients whose preoperative CA-125 values are known, this tumor marker was elevated in 94.4% of the cases.[80] Mills *et al.* reported elevated CA-125 values in eight EOPPC patients.[45] Altaras *et al.* described elevated CA-125 values in three EOPPC patients and found that CA-125 measurements correlated with the clinically determined status of the disease.[76] Similar to the situation in EOC patients, CA-125 values may be useful in the diagnosis of EOPPC patients and follow-up of their response to therapy.

The prognostic significance of estrogen and progesterone receptor analysis in patients with EOPPC is controversial.[103–105] A confounding problem when comparing studies on estrogen and progesterone receptors from different institutes is the different ways in which laboratories determine estrogen and progesterone receptor status. Eltabbakh *et al.* employed IHC, a technique that reduces the number of false elevated results.[80] In their study of EOPPC patients, estrogen and progesterone receptors were positive in 50% and 6.3% of the cases, respectively. Estrogen and progesterone positivity did not correlate significantly with survival. However, the median survival of EOPPC patients whose tumors were progesterone receptor positive was almost twice that of patients whose tumors were progesterone receptor negative (40 versus 21.2 months).

In practice, the difficulty is to identify EOPPC patients without subjecting patients with other less treatable malignancies to invasive procedures. In this group of patients, exhaustive investigations are usually carried out, including computed tomography (CT) of the abdomen and pelvis, barium studies, and endoscopy of the gastrointestinal tract. In patients who present ascites as the sole clinical feature (absence of a pelvic or abdominal mass), a diagnostic paracentesis is performed, and malignant cells may be seen on cytology. Some authors have suggested that the detection of signet ring cells in ascites can be taken to exclude primary ovarian or peritoneal carcinoma.[106] In the absence of these findings, all women with ascites containing adenocarcinoma cells should undergo laparoscopy and/or laparotomy as a diagnostic and potentially therapeutic debulking procedure. If during surgery no primary site is found but there are peritoneal tumor deposits, then it is recommended the patient undergo a total hysterectomy, bilateral salpingo-oophorectomy, omentectomy, and cytoreductive surgery followed by adjuvant chemotherapy (Fig. 34.1). In short, the surgical management is as for ovarian cancer.

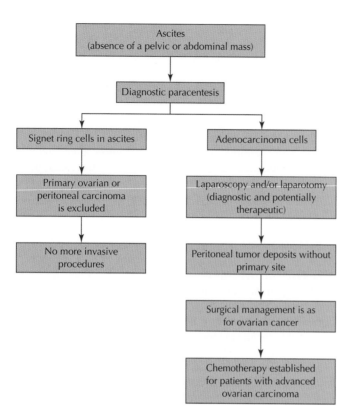

Figure 34.1 Treatment algorithm.

Table 34.1 Survival of extraovarian primary peritoneal carcinoma based on cytoreduction status.

Study	Patients	Residual disease	Median survival time (months)
Strand et al.[9]	18	<3	31
		>3	11
Fromm et al.[8]	74	<2	25
		>2	26
Fowler et al.[96]	36	<1.5	18
		>1.5	17
Ben-Baruch et al.[47]	25	<2	46
		>2	20
Eltabbakh et al.[80]	75	<1	40
		>1	18
Kennedy et al.[109]	36	<1	N/A
		>1	32.8

N/A, not available.

Treatment

There is no separate staging system for EOPPC. Most investigators have used the International Federation of Gynecology and Obstetrics (FIGO) staging system for ovarian cancer in EOPPC patients.[107] Most cases reported in the literature have been stage III or IV.

Raju et al. suggested that EOPPC should be treated as ovarian tumors of similar grade and stage.[5] Their clinical behavior, including response to treatment, is equivalent to that of EOC with a comparable extent of disease.[5,8,76] Accordingly, the standard regimen used in the treatment of EOC is generally administered to EOPPC patients.[8,94] The goal of surgical treatment is cytoreduction to no gross residual disease (Table 34.1).[94] Chemotherapy is commonly administered after cytoreductive surgery. It is generally agreed that these patients should be managed following the aggressive chemotherapeutic regimens established for patients with advanced ovarian carcinoma. However, because of the rarity of this tumor, reported experience with chemotherapeutic agents is limited (Table 34.2). Since 1979, cisplatin-based multiagent chemotherapy has been the standard treatment for patients with EOC and, consequently, for EOPPC patients. Several authors have reported that the response of EOPPC patients to platinum-based chemotherapy is similar to that of PSOC patients and have subsequently recommended treating patients with EOPPC in a fashion similar to that used in patients with EOC.[8,9,14,15,46,76,94,108] Other investigators, however, have failed to confirm these findings.[11,45] Long-term survival has been reported predominantly in patients with optimal cytoreduction and platinum-based chemotherapy.[14,94] Numerous regimens have been utilized with varying degrees of success. Recommended chemotherapy has evolved into combination treatment with taxanes and platinum.

Fromm et al. described 74 patients with primary peritoneal cancer treated with surgery and postoperative chemotherapy, of whom 29.2% received single-agent therapy while 70.8% were given a multiagent regimen.[8] Half of all patients received cisplatin, either singly or in combination with other cytotoxic drugs. An overall response rate to first-line chemotherapy (multiple regimens) of 63.6% was achieved with a median survival of 24 months. They achieved a complete response in 22.7% and a partial response in 40.9% of patients. In 31.8% cases, the disease progressed despite chemotherapy. They demonstrated that patients who received cisplatin-based regimens had a median survival of 31.5 months, whereas those who did not had a median survival of 19.5 months. This difference was not statistically significant. Survival rate was not influenced by residual tumor at primary surgery. The improved response seen with platinum-based regimens has been confirmed by other investigators.[15,46,76,82,94]

A number of authors have reported response rates of approximately 60% to platinum-based chemotherapy after cytoreduction.[15,96] These response rates were comparable to those achieved by the authors at their own institutions with similar combinations in patients with ovarian carcinomas, and who have subsequently recommended treating patients with EOPPC in a fashion similar to that used in patients with EOC.

Several case–control studies have compared the response rates of ovarian and peritoneal carcinoma to platinum-based chemotherapy. Mulhollan et al. evaluated 33 cases of EOPPC and compared them with 54 cases of EOC.[108] With at least a 4-year follow-up period, no differences in the median survival time (17 versus 18 months) were noted. Bloss et al. reported a retrospective, case–control study comparing the response and survival to cytoreductive surgery followed by cisplatin-based chemotherapy of 33 women with PSCP versus 33 cases with

Table 34.2 Response of extraovarian primary peritoneal carcinoma to first-line chemotherapy.

Study	Number of patients	Regimen	Overall response (%)
Chen and Flam[14]	3	PAC ($n=2$), DC ($n=1$)	100
Mills et al.[45]	10	PAC ($n=3$), PC ($n=4$), alkylators ($n=2$)	80
Dalrymple et al.[46]	31	Platinum based ($n=26$), chlorambucil ($n=5$)	32.3
Fromm et al.[8]	44	PC, P, M ($n=44$)	63.6
Altaras et al.[76]	7	PAC ($n=5$) PC ($n=2$)	100
Bloss et al.[15]	33	PAC ($n=29$), PC ($n=4$)	63.6
Menzin et al.[110]	4	TP ($n=4$)	100
Piver et al.[111]	46	PAC ($n=25$) TP ($n=21$)	62.5 70
Bloss et al.[112]	N/A	PC	65
Kennedy et al.[109]	38	Paclitaxel/ Ca ($n=26$) Paclitaxel/P ($n=12$)	87

Ca, carboplatin; DC, doxorubicin, cisplatin; M, melphalan; N/A, nonavailable; P, cisplatin; PAC, cisplatin, doxorubicin, cyclophosphamide; PC, cisplatin, cyclophosphamide; TP, paclitaxel, cisplatin.

EOC.[15] The authors concluded that there was no significant difference in median survival between the cases (20.8 months) and controls (27.8 months). In two other case–control studies, patients with EOPPC were reported to have reduced response rates to platinum-based chemotherapy, compared to control patients with EOC.[82,113]

The GOG conducted a prospective phase 2 trial of cisplatin and cyclophosphamide in 36 women with EOPPC.[112] Additionally, the study compares these patients with 130 women with PSOC undergoing identical therapy to determine if it may be reasonable to include EOPPC patients in future ovarian trials. After primary surgery, patients were treated with cisplatin and cyclophosphamide every 21 days for six cycles. Those women without clinical evidence of disease after study treatment then underwent a reassessment laparotomy. The clinical response rate for EOPPC to the treatment regimen was 65% compared to 59% for women with PSOC. Surgical complete responses were identical in the two groups (20%). While overall survival was not significantly different between the two groups, women with EOPPC demonstrated a greater risk of progression-free survival failure than women with PSOC. Based on this study, women with EOPPC were included in all GOG treatment studies of EOC.

In 1996, a randomized GOG trial demonstrated a significant survival advantage in patients with advanced EOC, whose residual disease was >1 cm, treated with paclitaxel plus cisplatin compared to similar patients who were treated with cisplatin plus cyclophosphamide.[114] As a result of this study, the combination of paclitaxel and cisplatin is considered first-line chemotherapy for patients with EOC. The impact on response and survival of this combination, and the relative contribution of adding a taxane to the first-line therapy in EOPPC patients, have not been thoroughly evaluated. Four EOPPC patients treated with paclitaxel (135 mg/m^{-2}) and cisplatin (50–75 mg/m^{-2}) for six cycles have been reported.[110] Reassessment surgery demonstrated complete surgical response in one and partial surgical response in three patients. Kennedy et al. treated 38 EOPPC patients (36 stage IIIC and two stage IV).[108] All patients received paclitaxel (135 mg/m^{-2} or 175 mg/m^{-2}), and cisplatin or carboplatin. Median progression-free survival was 15 months and median overall survival 40 months. Survival for optimally debulked patients was significantly better (median survival not reached) than for suboptimally debulked patients (median 32.8 months, $p=0.012$). Other authors have found that the addition of paclitaxel to cisplatin does not improve response rates for patients with EOPPC.[80]

Eltabbakh evaluated extreme drug resistance (EDR) assays among 20 consecutive women with EOPPC.[115] The results of the EDR assay and response to chemotherapy were compared with those among women with EOC. There was no significant difference in the incidence of EDR to cisplatin, carboplatin, paclitaxel, doxorubicin, cyclophosphamide, ifosfamide, etoposide, hexamethylmelamine, and topotecan among patients with EOPPC and those with EOC. The response rate of EOPPC patients to chemotherapy was 80% and unrelated to EDR to the individual drugs used in combination chemotherapy. The EDR profile and response to cisplatin-based chemotherapy among women with EOPPC were similar to those among women with EOC. These findings support treating both conditions similarly. EDR to individual drugs does not preclude response to combination chemotherapy.

The combination of paclitaxel and a platinum compound is active in the retreatment of patients with ovarian or peritoneal carcinoma who had disease recurrence >6 months following this combination.[116]

Since paclitaxel has been effective in preclinical and clinical trials in treating advanced and platinum-refractory EOC, it should be considered in the treatment of patients with platinum-resistant EOPPC.[117–119] Eltabbakh et al. reported that patients who received paclitaxel alone or in combination as second-line chemotherapy had significantly longer survival than patients who received chemotherapy without paclitaxel (median survival 23 versus 8.2 months, respectively, $p=0.026$).[80] In one report, a paclitaxel dose of 175 mg/m^2 given as 24-h continuous intravenous infusion resulted in a rapid partial response with good palliation of symptoms.[119] Another case reported a complete response after therapy with a paclitaxel dose of 420 mg/m^2 given over 24 h as a continuous intravenous infusion in a phase 1 trial.[98] The fact that paclitaxel may exhibit a dose response in the treatment of EOC can explain the presence of a complete response in the case that used 420 mg/m^2 and only a partial response when 210–250 mg/m^2 dose was used.[120,121] Further studies are required to determine the best dose schedule of paclitaxel.

Carboplatin may be active in paclitaxel-resistant EOPPC. This clinical phenomenon has been reported recently in patients treated with EOC, previously treated with paclitaxel and whose most recent platinum-based therapy was 12 months prior to carboplatin reinduction.[122] It has also been reported in patients with ovarian carcinoma whose primary treatment was single-agent paclitaxel.[123] Carboplatin therapy should be considered in patients with paclitaxel-refractory EOPPC without platinum chemotherapy for 12 months.[124]

Other forms of treatment have also been described, including radiotherapy and hormonal treatments with estrogen and progesterone preparations.[8] However, their roles in treatment are undefined.

Prognosis

The prognosis of EOPPC compared to EOC continues to be a subject of debate in the literature. Several comparative or case–control studies seem to suggest that these two tumors have a similar prognosis.[8,9,15,46,94,125] While other series suggest poorer survival in EOPPC,[11,13,45,82] some investigators have reported better prognosis in EOPPC.[14,126]

The prognostic factors in patients with EOC are better defined than those in patients with EOPPC. Multivariate analysis of 21,240 cases with primary EOC showed that stage, histology, grade, age, presence of ascites, lymph node status, and race were predictors of survival.[127] Eltabbakh et al. demonstrated that age, surgical stage, performance status, and degree of cytoreductive surgery are significant prognostic factors in EOPPC patients, and that performance status and primary debulking surgery are independent factors.[80] Mulhollan et al. investigated the significance of ovarian involvement on survival of EOPPC patients.[108] These authors demonstrated that the size of the ovarian tumor and the amount of ovarian stromal invasion had no significant effect on survival.

The amount of residual disease may be an important prognostic factor for both EOPPC and EOC patients.[9,47,128] However, controversy exits concerning the ability to perform optimal surgical debulking and its clinical significance in EOPPC. Optimal cytoreductive surgery, defined as <2 cm of residual tumor, has been accomplished in 33–69% of patients with EOPPC.[8,45,94] Strand et al. found that successful surgical cytoreduction resulted in better response to chemotherapy and prolonged survival.[9] Fromm et al. were able to accomplish optimal debulking surgery in only 41.2% of 74 patients with EOPPC.[8] They demonstrated that patients receiving multiagent chemotherapy (i.e. cisplatin and cyclophosphamide) had a statistically greater median survival rate compared to those receiving a single-agent regimen (melphalan). The median survival of EOPPC patients treated with combination chemotherapy was very similar to that of EOC patients who received the same treatment. Fromm et al. observed that neither age nor the presence of residual disease ≥2 cm after cytoreductive surgery was predictive of survival.[8] Among the pathological factors these authors examined, only the absence of mitosis was significantly predictive in survival. The presence of vascular invasion and the proportion of papillary areas in the tumor failed to predict survival.

Mills et al. as well as Fromm et al. did not find a significant prognostic value in optimal cytoreductive surgery in EOPPC

patients.[8,45] In the study by Ransom et al., only three patients who had long-term survival had optimal tumor cytoreduction.[94] Fowler et al. found that patients who underwent optimal cytoreduction had an increased survival rate, although the difference did not reach statistical significance.[96] These results are similar to those of Ben-Baruch et al.[47] In their study comparing 25 EOPPC patients with stages III–IV PSOC, the survival was significantly better in patients with optimal debulking only in the EOC group. The survival curve for patients with a residual disease ≥2 cm was almost identical for the EOPPC and EOC patients. Their rate of successful debulking and the result with platinum-based combination chemotherapy were the same in both groups. This is in contrast to a previous report of a lower rate of optimal cytoreduction and decreased response to platinum-based chemotherapy in the EOPPC group.[82] Eltabbakh et al. demonstrated that optimal cytoreductive surgery resulting in less than 1 cm residual tumor was achieved in 65.3% of their patients.[80] Optimal cytoreductive surgery was a favorable prognostic factor in both univariate and multivariate analysis. The difference in the results of these investigators could be explained by the number of patients and the definition of optimal cytoreductive surgery. Eltabbakh et al. also suggested a possible value of secondary cytoreductive surgery in EOPPC patients that was not discussed in previous reports. They found that patients who underwent cytoreductive surgery following recurrence or progression of disease had longer survival rates than patients who did not undergo secondary cytoreductive surgery (median survival 12.2 versus 3.1 months, respectively).[80]

The overall 5-year survival is about 20%, which is similar to the survival rate of patients with advanced ovarian cancer.[46,94] These results were achieved with surgery without lymphadenectomy.[130] The question remains whether retroperitoneal lymphadenectomy improves the survival rate of EOPPC patients. In addition, the inclusion of paclitaxel into adjuvant treatment protocols and/or the use of high-dose chemotherapy may improve the survival in EOPPC patients and has to be proven in clinical trials. Median survivals of 21, 17, 17.8, 19, 23, 24, and 23.5 months of EOPPC patients have been documented.[8,9,46,47,80,94,96] However, long-term survival after chemotherapy of more than 5 years has been documented in the literature.[14] Petru et al. reported a median survival of only 10 months for 14 EOPPC patients.[128] However, since seven of these patients did not undergo surgical debulking, these authors concluded that the amount of residual disease might present an important prognostic factor.[94] Foyle et al. reported that out of nine patients with documented follow-up, eight were dead 1.5 years after diagnosis.[13] In a 1985 publication of 11 cases, White et al. found that eight patients were dead within 3 years of diagnosis despite chemotherapy.[129] They reported median survival of 15 and 16 months for single (n=3) and multiple (n=8) agent chemotherapy regimens given as first line.

Conclusion

Histomorphological and molecular biological characteristics suggest that serous carcinomas, which include ovarian serous carcinoma, uterine serous carcinoma, fallopian tube serous carcinoma, cervical serous carcinoma, and primary peritoneal serous carcinoma, represent one entity. The tube and fimbrio-ovarian junction seem to be the main, but not the unique, cause of high-grade serous pelvic carcinoma. Tumors classified as primary peritoneal serous carcinoma are associated with STIC in the majority of cases in which the fallopian tubes are comprehensively examined. The absence of STIC in some cases indicates that some STICs may be extremely small and/or there are other sources of serous carcinoma, which may include the ovaries.

Determination of the primary site of pelvic high-grade serous carcinomas does not currently alter standard therapy; however, the data implicating the fallopian tube as the primary site of high-grade pelvic serous carcinoma will, in the future, have an important implication for the development of new approaches for early detection, treatment, and prevention of this lethal disease. Accordingly, screening for enlarged ovaries by any imaging modality does not target the appropriate group for a successful screening test. The possibility of bilateral salpingectomy with retention of the ovaries also merits consideration for primary prevention as it may improve both survival and quality of life.

References

1. Seidman JD, et al. The histologic type and stage distribution of ovarian carcinomas of surface epithelial origin. Int J Gynecol Pathol 2004; 23: 41–4.
2. Jaaback KS, et al. Primary peritoneal carcinoma in a UK cancer center: comparison with advanced ovarian carcinoma over a 5-year period. Int J Gynecol Cancer 2006; 16: 123–8.
3. Halperin R, et al. Primary peritoneal serous papillary carcinoma: a new epidemiologic trend? A matched-case comparison with ovarian serous papillary cancer. Int J Gynecol Cancer 2001; 11: 403–8.
4. Kannerstein M, et al. Papillary tumors of the peritoneum in women: mesothelioma or papillary carcinoma? Am J Obstet Gynecol 1977; 127: 306–14.
5. Raju U, et al. Primary papillary serous neoplasia of the peritoneum: a clinicopathological and ultrastructural study of eight cases. Hum Pathol 1989; 20: 426–36.
6. Kowalski LD, et al. A matched-case comparison of extraovarian versus primary ovarian adenocarcinoma. Cancer 1997; 79: 1587–94.
7. Eltabbakh GH, et al. Epidemiologic differences between woman with extra-ovarian primary peritoneal carcinoma and women with epithelial ovarian cancer. Obstet Gynecol 1998; 91: 254–9.
8. Fromm GL, Gershenson DM, Silva EG. Papillary serous carcinoma of the peritoneum. Obstet Gynecol 1990; 75: 89–95.
9. Strand CM, et al. Peritoneal carcinomatosis of unknown primary site in women. A distinct subset of adenocarcinoma. Ann Int Med 1989; 111: 213–17.
10. Fox H. Primary neoplasia of the female peritoneum. Histopathology 1993; 23: 103–10.
11. Gooneratne S, et al. Serous papillary carcinoma of the ovary. A clinicopathologic study of 16 cases. Int J Gynecol Pathol 1982; 1: 258–69.
12. Swerdlow M. Mesothelioma of the pelvic peritoneum resembling papillary cystadenocarcinoma of the ovary: case report. Am J Obstet Gynecol 1959; 77: 197–200.
13. Foyle A, Al-Jabi M, McCaughey WTE. Papillary peritoneal tumors in woman. Am J Surg Pathol 1981; 5: 241–9.
14. Chen KTK, Flam MS. Peritoneal papillary serous carcinoma with long-term survival. Cancer 1986; 58: 1371–3.
15. Bloss JD, et al. Extraovarian peritoneal serous papillary carcinoma: a case–control retrospective comparison to papillary adenocarcinoma of the ovary. Gynecol Oncol 1993; 50: 347–51.
16. Lauchlan SC. The secondary Müllerian system. Am J Obstet Gynecol 1972; 27: 133–46.
17. Parmley T. Embryology of the female genital tract. In: Kurman RJ (ed) Blaustein's Pathology of the Female Genital Tract, 3rd edn. New York: Springer-Verlag, 1987. pp. 1–14.
18. Hertig AT. Proceedings of Eighteenth Seminar. Chicago, IL: American Society of Clinical Pathology, 1952. p. 49.
19. Rosenbloom MA, Foster RB. Probable pelvic mesothelioma. Report of a case and review of literature. Obstet Gynecol 1961; 18: 213–22.
20. Parmley TH, Woodruff JD. The ovarian mesothelioma. Am J Obstet Gynecol 1974; 120: 234–41.
21. Selikoff IJ, Churg J, Hammond EC. Relation between exposure to asbestos and mesothelioma. N Engl J Med 1965; 272: 560–5.
22. Kannerstein M, Churg J. Peritoneal mesothelioma. Hum Pathol 1977; 8: 83–94.
23. Crum CP, et al. The distal fallopian tube: a new model for pelvic serous carcinogenesis. Curr Opin Obstet Gynecol 2007; 19: 3–9.
24. Medeiros F, et al. The tubal fimbriae is a preferred site for early adenocarcinoma in women with familial ovarian cancer syndrome. Am J Surg Pathol 2006; 30: 230–6.
25. Przybycin CG, et al. Are all pelvic (nonuterine) serous carcinomas of tubal origin? Am J Surg Pathol 2010; 34: 1407–16.
26. Carlson JW, et al. Serous tubal intraepithelial carcinoma: its potential role in primary peritoneal serous carcinoma and serous cancer prevention. J Clin Oncol 2008; 26: 4160–5.
27. Roh MH, Kindleberger D, Crum CP. Serous tubal intraepithelial carcinoma and the dominant ovarian mass: clues to serous tumor origin. Am J Surg Pathol 2009; 33: 376–83.
28. Colgan TJ, et al. Occult carcinoma in prophylactic oophorectomy specimens: prevalence and association with BRCA germline mutation status. Am J Surg Pathol 2001; 25: 1283–89.
29. Leeper K, et al. Pathologic findings in prophylactic oophorectomy specimens in high-risk women. Gynecol Oncol 2002; 87: 52–6.
30. Piek JM, et al. Dysplastic changes in prophylactically removed fallopian tubes of women predisposed to developing ovarian cancer. J Pathol 2001; 195: 451–56.
31. Tonin P, et al. Frequency of recurrent BRCA1 and BRCA2 mutations in Ashkenazi Jewish breast cancer families. Nat Med 1996; 2: 1179–83.
32. Lauchlan SC. The secondary mullerian system revisited. Int J Gynecol Pathol 1994; 13: 73–9.
33. Clement PB. Diseases of the peritoneum. In: Kurman RJ (ed) Blaustein's Pathology of the Female Genital Tract, 3rd edn. New York: Springer-Verlag, 1987. pp. 729–89.
34. Quddus MR, Sung CJ, Lauchlan SC. Benign and malignant serous and endometrioid epithelium in the omentum. Gynecol Oncol 1999; 75: 227–32.
35. Shah IA, et al. Papillary serous carcinoma of the peritoneum in a man. Cancer 1998; 82: 860–6.
36. Jones MA Young RH, Scully RE. Malignant mesothelioma of the tunica vaginalis: a clinicopathologic analysis of 11 cases with review of the literature. Am J Surg Pathol 1995; 19: 815–25.
37. Remmle W, et al. Serous papillary cystic tumor of borderline malignancy with focal carcinoma arising in testis: a case report with immunohistochemical and ultrastructural observations. Hum Pathol 1992; 23: 75–9.
38. Levanon K, Crum C, Drapkin R. New insights into the pathogenesis of serous ovarian cancer and its clinical impact. J Clin Oncol 2008; 26: 5284–93.
39. Dubeau L. The cell of origin of ovarian epithelial tumours. Lancet Oncol 2008; 9: 1191–7.
40. Piek J, Kenemans P, Verheijen R. Intraperitoneal serous adenocarcinoma: a critical appraisal of three hypotheses on its cause. Am J Obstet Gynecol 2004; 191:718–32.
41. Hu CY, Taymor ML, Hertig AT. Primary carcinoma of the fallopian tube. Am J Obstet Gynecol 1950; 59: 58–67.
42. Sedlis A. Carcinoma of the fallopian tube. Surg Clin North Am 1978; 58: 121–9.
43. Jarboe E, et al. Serous carcinogenesis in the fallopian tube: a descriptive classification. Int J Gynecol Pathol 2008; 27: 1–9.

44. Markaki S, *et al.* Primary malignant mesothelioma of the peritoneum: a clinical and immunohistochemical study. Gynecol Oncol 2005; 96: 860–4.

45. Mills SE, *et al.* Serous surface papillary carcinoma: a clinicopathologic study of 10 cases and comparison with stage III-IV ovarian serous carcinoma. Am J Surg Pathol 1988; 12: 827–34.

46. Dalrymple JC, *et al.* Extraovarian peritoneal serous papillary carcinoma. A clinicopathologic study of 31 cases. Cancer 1989; 64: 110–15.

47. Ben-Baruch G, *et al.* Primary peritoneal serous papillary carcinoma: a study of 25 cases and comparison with stage III-IV ovarian papillary serous carcinoma. Gynecol Oncol 1996; 60: 393–6.

48. Eltabbakh GH, Piver MS, Werness BA. Primary peritoneal adenocarcinoma metastatic to the brain. Gynecol Oncol 1997; 66: 160–3.

49. Karlan BY, *et al.* Secreted ovarian stromal substance inhibits ovarian epithelial cell proliferation. Gynecol Oncol 1995; 59: 67–74.

50. Chu CS, *et al.* Primary peritoneal carcinoma: a review of the literature. Obstet Gynecol Surv 1999; 54: 323–35.

51. Halperin R, *et al.* Primary peritoneal serous papillary carcinoma: a new epidemiologic trend? A matched-case comparison with ovarian serous papillary cancer. Int J Gynecol Cancer 2001; 11: 403–8.

52. Domchek SM, Stopfer JE, Rebbeck TR. Bilateral risk-reducing oophorectomy in BRCA1 and BRCA2 mutation carriers. J Natl Compr Canc Netw 2006; 4: 177–82.

53. Boyd J, *et al.* Clinicopathologic features of BRCA-linked and sporadic ovarian cancer. JAMA 2000; 283: 2260–5.

54. Prat J, Ribe A, Gallardo A. Hereditary ovarian cancer. Hum Pathol 2005; 36: 861–70.

55. Kauff ND, *et al.* Risk-reducing salpingo-oophorectomy for the prevention of BRCA1- and BRCA2- associated breast and gynecologic cancer: a multicenter, prospective study. J Clin Oncol 2008; 26: 1331–7.

56. Rebbeck TR, Kauff ND, Domchek SM. Meta-analysis of risk reduction estimates associated with risk-reducing salpingo-oophorectomy in BRCA1 or BRCA2 mutation carriers. J Natl Cancer Inst 2009; 101: 80–7.

57. Domchek SM, *et al.* Association of risk-reducing surgery in BRCA1 or BRCA2 mutation carriers with cancer risk and mortality. JAMA 2010; 304: 967–75.

58. Wang P, *et al.* BRCA1 mutations in Taiwanese with epithelial ovarian carcinoma and sporadic primary serous peritoneal carcinoma. Jpn J Clin Oncol 2000; 30: 343–8.

59. Bandera CA, *et al.* Germline BRCA1 mutations in women with papillary serous carcinoma of the peritoneum (EOPPC). Proc Am Assoc Cancer Res 1997; 38: 82.

60. Bandera CA, *et al.* BRCA1 gene mutations in women with papillary serous carcinoma of the peritoneum. Obstet Gynecol 1998; 92: 596–600.

61. Liede A, *et al.* Cancer incidence in a population of Jewish women at risk of ovarian cancer. J Clin Oncol 2002; 20: 1570–7.

62. Kauff ND, *et al.* Risk-reducing salpingo-oophorectomy in women with a BRCA1 or BRCA2 mutation. N Engl J Med 2002; 346: 1609–15.

63. Rebbeck TR, *et al.* Prophylactic oophorectomy in carriers of BRCA1 or BRCA2 mutations. N Engl J Med 2002; 346: 1616–22.

64. Rebbeck TR, Kauff ND, Domchek SM. Meta-analysis of risk reduction estimates associated with risk-reducing salpingo-oophorectomy in BRCA1 or BRCA2 mutation carriers. J Natl Cancer Inst 2009; 101: 80–7.

65. Finch A, *et al.* Salpingo-oophorectomy and the risk of ovarian, fallopian tube, and peritoneal cancers in women with a BRCA1 or BRCA2 mutation. JAMA 2006; 296: 185–92.

66. Domchek SM, *et al.* Mortality after bilateral salpingo-oophorectomy in BRCA1 and BRCA2 mutation carriers: a prospective cohort study. Lancet Oncol 2006; 7: 223–9.

67. Colgan TJ, *et al.* Occult carcinoma in prophylactic oophorectomy specimens: prevalence and association with BRCA germline mutation status. Am J Surg Pathol 2001; 25: 1283–9.

68. Kauff ND, Barakat RR. Risk-reducing salpingo-oophorectomy in patients with germline mutations in BRCA1 or BRCA2. J Clin Oncol 2007; 25: 2921–7.

69. Leeper K, *et al.* Pathologic findings in prophylactic oophorectomy specimens in high-risk women. Gynecol Oncol 2002; 87: 52–6.

70. Lu KH, *et al.* Occult ovarian tumors in women with BRCA1 or BRCA2 mutations undergoing prophylactic oophorectomy. J Clin Oncol 2000; 18: 2728–32.

71. Powell CB, *et al.* Riskreducing salpingooophorectomy in BRCA mutation carriers: role of serial sectioning in the detection of occult malignancy. J Clin Oncol 2005; 23: 127–32.

72. Rabban JT, *et al.* Transitional cell metaplasia of fallopian tube fimbriae: a potential mimic of early tubal carcinoma in risk reduction salpingo-oophorectomies from women with BRCA mutations. Am J Surg Pathol 2009; 33: 111–19.

73. Medeiros F, *et al.* The tubal fimbria is a preferred site for early adenocarcinoma in women with familial ovarian cancer syndrome. Am J Surg Pathol 2006; 30: 230–6.

74. Seidman JD, Zhao P, Yemelyanova A. "Primary peritoneal" high-grade serous carcinoma is very likely metastatic from serous tubal intraepithelial carcinoma: assessing the new paradigm of ovarian and pelvic serous carcinogenesis and its implications for screening for ovarian cancer. Gynecol Oncol 2011;120: 470–3.

75. Roh MH, Kindelberger D, Crum CP. Serous tubal intraepithelial carcinoma and the dominant ovarian mass: clues to serous tumor origin? Am J Surg Pathol 2009; 33: 376–83.

76. Altaras MM, *et al.* Primary peritoneal papillary serous adenocarcinoma: clinical and management aspects. Gynecol Oncol 1991; 40: 230–6.

77. Clark JE, *et al.* Endometrioid-type cystadenocarcinoma arising in the mesosalpinx. Obstet Gynecol 1979; 54: 656–8.

78. Lee KR, Verma U, Belinson JL. Primary clear cell carcinoma of the peritoneum. Gynecol Oncol 1991; 41: 259–62.

79. Mirc JL, Fenoglio-Preiser CM, Husseinzadeh N. Malignant mixed Müllerian tumor of extraovarian secondary Müllerian system: report of two cases and review of the literature. Arch Pathol Lab Med 1995; 119: 1044–9.

80. Eltabbakh GH, *et al.* Prognostic factors in extra-ovarian primary peritoneal carcinoma. Gynecol Oncol 1998; 71: 230–9.

81. Bell DA, Scully RE. Serous borderline tumors of the peritoneum. Am J Surg Pathol 1990; 14: 230–9.

82. Killackey MA, Davis AR. Papillary serous carcinoma of the peritoneal surface: matched-case comparison with papillary serous ovarian carcinoma. Gynecol Oncol 1993; 51: 171–4.

83. Weir MM, Bell DA, Young RH. Grade 1 peritoneal serous carcinoma: a report of 14 cases and comparison with 7 peritoneal serous psammocarcinomas and 19 peritoneal serous borderline tumors. Am J Surg Pathol 1998; 22: 849–62.

84. Biscotti CV, Hart WR. Peritoneal serous papillomatosis of low malignant potential (serous borderline tumors of the peritoneum): a clinicopathologic study of 17 cases. Am J Surg Pathol 1992; 16: 467–75.

85. Whitcomb BP, *et al.* Primary peritoneal psammocarcinoma: a case presenting with an upper abdominal mass and elevated CA-125. Gynecol Oncol 1999; 73: 331.

86. Scully RE. The Eltabbakh/Piver article reviewed. Oncology 1998; 12: 820.

87. Karlan BY, *et al.* Peritoneal serous papillary carcinoma, a phenotypic variant of familial ovarian cancer: implications for ovarian cancer screening. Am J Obstet Gynecol 1999; 180: 917–28.

88. Clement PB. Endometriosis, lesions of the secondary Müllerian system, and pelvic mesothelial proliferation. In: Kurman RJ (ed). *Blaustein's Pathology of the Female Genital Tract*, 3rd ed. New York: Springer-Verlag New York Inc., 1987: 516–59.

89. Warhol MJ, Hunter NJ, Corson JM. An ultrastructural comparison of mesotheliomas and adenocarcinomas of the ovary and endometrium. Int J Gynecol Pathol 1982; 1: 125–34.

90. Eyden BP, Banik S, Harris M. Malignant epithelial mesothelioma of the peritoneum: observation on a problem case. Ultrastruct Pathol 1996; 20: 337–44.

91. Kannerstein M, *et al.* A critique of the criteria for the diagnosis of diffuse malignant mesothelioma. Mt Sinai J Med 1977; 44: 485–94.

92. Ascoli V, *et al.* Malignant mesothelioma of the tunica vaginalis testis in a young adult. J Urol Pathol 1996; 5: 75–83.

93. Moll UM, Valea F, Chumas J. Role of p53 alteration in primary peritoneal carcinoma. Int J Gynecol Pathol 1997; 16: 156–62.

94. Ransom DT, *et al*. Papillary serous adenocarcinoma of the peritoneum: a review of 33 cases treated with platin-based chemotherapy. Cancer 1990; 66: 1091–4.

95. Khoury N, *et al*. A comparative immunohistochemical study of peritoneal and ovarian serous tumors, and mesotheliomas. Hum Pathol 1990; 21: 811–9.

96. Fowler JM, *et al*. Peritoneal adenocarcinoma (serous) of Müllerian type: a subgroup of women presenting with peritoneal carcinomatosis. Int J Gynecol Cancer 1994; 4: 43–51.

97. Ulbright TM, *et al*. Papillary serous cacinoma of the retroperitoneum. Am J Clin Pathol 1983; 79(5): 633–7.

98. Wall JE, *et al*. Effectiveness of paclitaxel in treating papillary serous carcinoma of the peritoneum in an adolescent. Am J Obstet Gynecol 1995; 172: 1049–52.

99. Shapiro SP, Nunez C. Psammoma bodies in the cervicovaginal smear in association with papillary tumor of the peritoneum. Obstet Gynecol 1983; 61: 130–4.

100. Rose PG, Reale FR. Papillary serous carcinoma of the peritoneum following endometrial cancer. Obstet Gynecol 1991; 78: 80.

101. Eltabbakh GH, Piver MS. Extraovarian primary peritoneal carcinoma. Oncology 1998; 12: 813–9.

102. Resnik E, Bender D. Syndrome of inappropriate antidiuretic hormone secretion in papillary serous surface carcinoma of the peritoneum. J Surg Oncol 1996; 61: 63–5.

103. Geisler JP, *et al*. Estrogen and progesterone receptor status as prognostic indicators in patients with optimally cytoreduced stage IIIC serous cystadenocarcinoma of the ovary. Gynecol Oncol 1996; 60: 424–7.

104. Kommos F, *et al*. Steroid receptors in ovarian carcinoma: immunohistochemical determination may lead to new aspects. Gynecol Oncol 1992; 47: 317–22.

105. Sevelda P, *et al*. Estrogen and progesterone receptor content as a prognostic factor in advanced epithelial ovarian carcinoma. Br J Obstet Gynecol 1990; 97: 706–12.

106. Della-Fiorentina SA, *et al*. Primary peritoneal carcinoma: a treatable subset of patients with adenocarcinoma of unknown primary. Aust N Z J Surg 1996; 66: 124–5.

107. Staging Announcement FIGO Cancer Committee. Cancer committee of the international federation of gynecology and obstetrics. Gynecol Oncol 1986; 25: 383–5.

108. Mulhollan TJ, *et al*. Ovarian involvement by serous surface papillary carcinoma. Int J Gynecol Pathol 1994; 13: 120–6.

109. Kennedy AW, *et al*. Experience with platinum-paclitaxel chemotherapy in the initial management of papillary serous carcinoma of the peritoneum. Gynecol Oncol 1998; 71: 288–90.

110. Menzin AW, *et al*. Surgically documented responses to paclitaxel and cisplatin in patients with primary peritoneal carcinoma. Gynecol Oncol 1996; 62: 55–8.

111. Piver MS, *et al*. Two sequential studies for primary peritoneal carcinoma: induction with weekly cisplatin followed by either cisplatindoxorubicin-cyclophosphamide or paclitaxel-cisplatin. Gynecol Oncol 1997; 67: 141–6.

112. Bloss JD, *et al*. A phase II trial cisplatin and cyclophosphamide in the treatment of extraovarian peritoneal serous papillary carcinoma with comparison to papillary serous ovarian carcinoma: a Gynecologic Oncology Group study. Gynecol Oncol 1998; 68: 109.

113. Halperin R, *et al*. Immunohistochemical comparison of primary peritoneal and primary ovarian serous papillary carcinoma. Int J Gynecol Pathol 2001; 20: 341–5.

114. McGuire WP, *et al*. Cyclophosphamide and cisplatin compared with paclitaxel plus cisplatin in patients with stage III and IV ovarian cancer. N Engl J Med 1996; 334: 1–6.

115. Eltabbakh GH. Extreme drug resistance assay and response to chemotherapy in patients with primary peritoneal carcinoma. J Surg Oncol 2000; 73: 148–52.

116. Rose PG, *et al*. Second-line therapy with paclitaxel and carboplatin for recurrent disease following first-line therapy with paclitaxel and platinum in ovarian or peritoneal carcinoma. J Clin Oncol 1998; 16: 1494–7.

117. Nicoletti MI, *et al*. Antitumor activity of taxol (NSC-125973) in human ovarian carcinomas growing in the peritoneal cavity of nude mice. Ann Oncol 1993; 4: 151.

118. Einzig AI, *et al*. Phase II study and long-term follow up of patients treated with Taxol for advanced ovarian adenocarcinoma. J Clin Oncol 1992; 10: 1748–53.

119. Wilailak S, *et al*. Peritoneal papillary serous carcinoma: response to taxol in a platinum resistant disease. Eur J Gynaecol Oncol 1995; 16: 187–9.

120. Eisenhauer EA, *et al*. European-Canadian randomized trial of paclitaxel in relapsed ovarian cancer: high-dose versus low-dose and long versus short infusion. J Clin Oncol 1994; 12: 2654–66.

121. Holmes FA, *et al*. Current status of clinical trials with paclitaxel and docetaxel. In: George GI, *et al*. (eds) *ACS Symposium. Taxane Anticancer Agent: Basic Science and Current Status*. Washington, DC: American Cancer Society, 1995: 3–31.

122. Kavanagh J, *et al*. Carboplatin reinduction after taxane in patients with platinum-refractory epithelial ovarian cancer. J Clin Oncol 1995; 13: 1584–8.

123. Thigpen T, *et al*. Cisplatin as salvage therapy in ovarian carcinoma treated initially with single agent paclitaxel: a Gynecologic Oncology Group Study. Proc Am Soc Clin Oncol 1996; 15: 778.

124. Herrada J, *et al*. Remission with carboplatin of paclitaxel resistant primary peritoneal papillary serous carcinoma: case report. Eur J Gynaecol Oncol 1997; 18: 39–41.

125. Dubernard G, *et al*. Prognosis of stage II or IV primary peritoneal serous papillary carcinoma. Eur J Surg Oncol 2004; 30: 976–81.

126. Piura B, *et al*. Peritoneal papillary serous carcinoma: study of 15 cases and comparison with stage III–IV ovarian papillary serous carcinoma. J Surg Oncol 1998; 68(3): 173–8.

127. Kosary CL. FIGO stage, histologic grade, age, and race as prognostic factors in determining survival for cancers of the female gynecological system: an analysis of 197387 SEER cases of cancers of the endometrium, cervix, ovary, vulva, and vagina. Semin Surg Oncol 1994; 10: 31–46.

128. Petru E, *et al*. Primary papillary serous carcinoma of the peritoneum: a report of experiences. Geburtsh Frauenheilk 1992; 5: 533–5.

129. White PF, Merino MJ, Barwick KW. Serous surface papillary carcinoma of the ovary: a clinical, pathological, ultrastructural, and immunohistochemical study of 11 cases. Pathol Ann 1985; 20: 403–18.

35 Borderline Tumors and Other Rare Epithelial Tumors of the Ovary

Ramez N. Eskander,[1] **Teresa P. Díaz-Montes,**[2] **Russell Vang,**[3] **Deborah K. Armstrong,**[4] **and Robert E. Bristow**[1]

[1] Division of Gynecologic Oncology, Department of Gynecology and Obstetrics, University of California Irvine, Orange, CA, USA
[2] The Kelly Gynecologic Oncology Service, Department of Gynecology and Obstetrics, [3] Division of Gynecologic Pathology, Department of Pathology, [4] Department of Medical Oncology, Johns Hopkins Medical Institutions, Baltimore, MD, USA

Introduction and historical background

In 1929, Taylor first described a subset of ovarian tumors that he termed semi-malignant, characterized by a stratified growth pattern without destructive stromal invasion.[1] These lesions had a more favorable outcome than other ovarian cancers, but they were not separately classified by the International Federation of Gynecology and Obstetrics (FIGO) and the World Health Organization (WHO) until 1971.[2,3] In 1961, the Cancer Committee of the FIGO suggested a system that subdivided the ovarian tumors into three types: benign cystadenomas, cystadenocarcinomas of low malignant potential, and cystadenocarcinomas.[2] This classification became effective in 1971. The WHO applied the designation of tumor of borderline malignancy and added the synonym of carcinoma of low malignant potential in its 1973 classification.[3]

During the past few decades, multiple terms have been applied to these neoplasms, including tumors of borderline malignancy, carcinomas of low malignant potential, borderline tumors, tumors of low malignant potential, and atypical proliferative tumors. Today no consensus has been reached on the preferred terminology of these tumors, although the most favored term is borderline ovarian tumor. The terms borderline, atypical proliferative, and low malignant potential tumors should be considered as synonymous. During the Borderline Ovarian Tumor Workshop held at Bethesda, Maryland, in 2003, a consensus was reached to not designate these tumors as carcinomas of low malignant potential or any other type of carcinoma.[4]

Biology and epidemiology

Borderline ovarian tumors are rare. The Surveillance, Epidemiology, and End Results (SEER) program indicates a United States incidence of approximately 2.5 per 100,000

women-years.[5] Approximately 3000 cases of borderline ovarian tumors are diagnosed annually in the United States.[6] The incidence rate of borderline ovarian tumors is higher among white women than black women.[5] Borderline tumors account for approximately 15% of all epithelial ovarian cancers (5% of all epithelial ovarian tumors). On average, the age at diagnosis is approximately 10 years younger than that of women with malignant ovarian cancer and ranges from 39 years to 45 years, with up to 27% of patients being younger than 40 years.[7–11]

Borderline ovarian tumors have an epidemiological risk factor profile similar to that of frankly malignant ovarian tumors, but they are associated with a significantly better prognosis and clinical outcome. In a case–control study, Harlow et al. reported that factors linked to a lower risk of (i.e. protective against) borderline ovarian tumors included the use of oral contraceptives, prior pregnancy, and lactation.[12] Use of oral contraceptives has been associated with a 60% reduction in risk. However, the magnitude of the association was independent of duration of use, age at first use, or years since last usage. Compared to nulliparous women, the relative risk of developing a borderline ovarian tumor was 0.7 for women who had given birth to one or two children and 0.4 for women with three or more children. There was no consistent influence of increasing age at first live birth. Among nulliparous women, a further increase in risk was present in those who reported a history of infertility. Adjusting for parity, a history of lactation was associated with a 50% reduction in risk. Age at menarche, menopause, or first live birth was not a significant risk factor for borderline ovarian tumor development. This study is representative of other reports and provides clear evidence that borderline ovarian tumors have a similar epidemiological and reproductive risk factor profile compared to their more malignant counterparts.

Textbook of Uncommon Cancer, Fourth Edition. Edited by Derek Raghavan, Charles D. Blanke, David H. Johnson, Paul L. Moots, Gregory H. Reaman, Peter G. Rose and Mikkael A. Sekeres.
© 2012 John Wiley & Sons, Inc. Published 2012 by John Wiley & Sons, Inc.

The majority of patients diagnosed with borderline ovarian tumors present with various nonspecific symptoms including abdominal pain, bloating or mass. In addition, nearly 16% of patients are asymptomatic at the time of diagnosis, with identification of a mass at the time of annual examination.[13]

Molecular biology and genetics of borderline tumors

It has been difficult to understand the relationship between borderline ovarian tumors (BOT) and invasive epithelial cancer. Most authors consider BOT as distinct from invasive cancer, with different epidemiological risk profiles. In order to determine if such a relationship exists, molecular abnormalities, as well as genomic instability in BOT, have been investigated.

Some authors classify epithelial ovarian tumors into two categories, "low grade" or "type I" and "high grade" or "type II" serous carcinomas.[14] The "low-grade" pathway involves serous borderline tumors identified as having *BRAF* or *K-Ras* mutations. It was reported that 88% of serous borderline ovarian tumor (SBOT) contained either *BRAF* or *K-Ras* mutations, with the same mutations present in 86% of neighboring cystadenoma epithelium. However, *BRAF* and *K-Ras* mutations are not associated with invasive cancer.[15,16] Furthermore, *p53* mutations, found in 88% of advanced serous ovarian cancers, are most often absent in serous BOT or micropapillary serous BOT.[17]

An understanding of the mechanisms underlying development of BOT and the potential associations between BOT and invasive cancers remain elusive. Continued exploration into molecular pathways and gene expression profiles of BOT may clarify this relationship.

Pathology

Serous borderline tumors

Gross

Serous borderline tumors (SBTs) are bilateral in 23–82% of cases.[18] The tumors are usually uni- or multicystic, partly solid, and in most series the reported mean/median size ranges from 7 cm to 12 cm.[19–24] The external surface may be smooth or demonstrate an exophytic tumor growth pattern (Fig. 35.1). The internal surfaces are usually lined by white to tan papillary excrescences.

Histology

Serous borderline tumors are subclassified into two forms: the typical type (atypical proliferative serous tumor) and the micropapillary type (noninvasive micropapillary serous carcinoma). Terms that have been used to classify these tumors and are considered synonymous are SBT, serous tumor of low malignant potential, and atypical proliferative serous tumor.[4,25] Both types of SBT lack destructive stromal invasion and contain papillary proliferations that are either intracystic (endophytic growth pattern) and/or exophytic on the surface of the ovary.

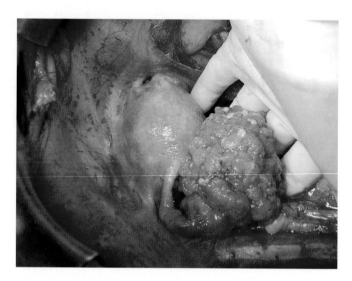

Figure 35.1 Serous borderline ovarian tumor.

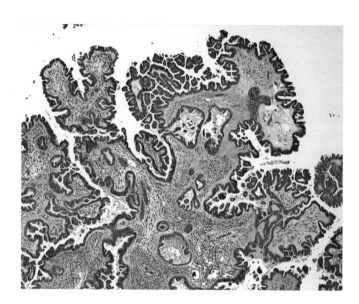

Figure 35.2 Typical serous borderline tumor.

The typical SBT is composed of broad papillary structures that progressively branch in a hierarchical fashion into smaller papillae, terminating in epithelial tufts (Fig. 35.2). The micropapillary SBTs, comprising 10% of serous tumors of low malignant potential, often arise on a background of typical SBT and contain large papillary structures in which small and elongated papillae immediately project from the underlying large papillae without the hierarchical branching of typical SBT (the so-called "Medusa appearance"). These resulting micropapillary structures lining the large papillae are generally five times longer than they are wide. Numerous detached micropapillary buds may fill the spaces between the larger papillae (Fig. 35.3). Since typical SBTs may have minor areas of micropapillary architecture, a 5 mm area of pure micropapillary/cribriform growth needs to be present in order to qualify for a diagnosis of micropapillary SBT. The cysts and papillae of SBT are lined by cuboidal or columnar serous epithelium without frankly malignant

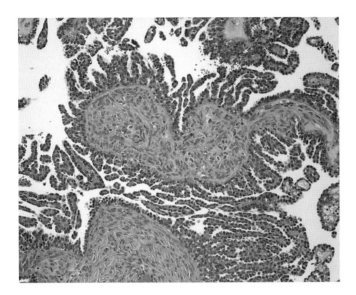

Figure 35.3 Micropapillary serous borderline tumor.

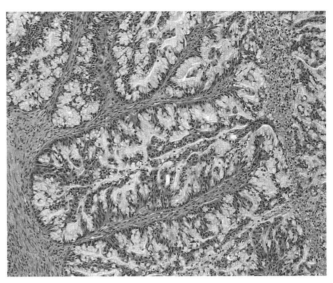

Figure 35.4 Mucinous borderline tumor, gastrointestinal type.

nuclei. These SBTs with micropapillary architecture have an increased incidence of invasive implants in extraovarian tissue.[26]

Microinvasion consists of individual cells or nests within stroma, but the size of any individual focus cannot measure greater than 3–5 mm in greatest linear extent or 10 mm^2 in overall area.[18,25] It appears more commonly in SBTs occurring in pregnancy.[27] Extraovarian disease principally exists in the form of implants, which are classified as noninvasive or invasive. Noninvasive implants are histologically classified as epithelial or desmoplastic types. Implants are considered as invasive when infiltration into underlying tissue is present,[28] although modified criteria of solid nests within clear spaces/clefts or an appearance resembling the micropapillary SBT have been used by others.[29] These invasive implants are of adverse prognostic significance.

Extraovarian disease may also be in the form of lymph node involvement (LNI) by SBT. When lymphadenectomy is performed, LNI has been reported in up to 30% of cases.[30] However, LNI did not have a significant impact on disease-free or overall survival.

Importantly, in the presence of marked nuclear atypia, a diagnosis of high-grade serous carcinoma is made, even in the absence of stromal invasion, since rare ovarian high-grade serous carcinomas may have a "borderline" growth pattern, without obvious invasion.[27]

Mucinous borderline tumors

Gastrointestinal type
Gross
These tumors are generally unilateral and have smooth external surfaces although capsular rupture may be present. The reported mean size ranges from 17 cm to 20 cm.[31–33] The cut surfaces are usually multicystic and are lined by smooth surfaces which occasionally contain papillary excrescences. On sectioning, there are multiple locules filled with mucoid material. Solid areas may be present as well.

Histology
Synonymous terms that have been used to classify these tumors are mucinous borderline tumor of the intestinal type, mucinous tumor of low malignant potential, and atypical proliferative mucinous tumor of gastrointestinal type.[4,25,34] The tumors are composed of crowded glands and cysts that are lined by stratified mucinous epithelium of gastrointestinal type with goblet cells (Fig. 35.4). Paneth cells may be present as well. Destructive stromal invasion is absent. A background of mucinous cystadenoma may be evident. As focal epithelial proliferation may be encountered in mucinous cystadenomas, it is suggested that 10% of the neoplasm contain epithelial proliferation to qualify as a borderline tumor. Intraepithelial carcinoma is diagnosed when the nuclei show marked nuclear atypia in the absence of invasion. Microinvasion consists of individual cells or nests within stroma, but the largest dimension of any individual focus is smaller than 3–5 mm in greatest linear extent or 10 mm^2 in area.[34] The distinction of the upper limit of glandular crowding in a mucinous borderline tumor from the confluent/expansile pattern of invasive mucinous carcinoma is based on the same size criteria for microinvasion.[34] Implants are generally not seen and if encountered, should suggest the possibility of a misclassified mucinous tumor secondarily involving the ovary. Occasionally a mural nodule may be identified, with a clear demarcation between the borderline tumor and a more cellular area. These mural nodules may be reactive but many are malignant and comprise anaplastic carcinoma.[35]

Endocervical type
Gross
Endocervical-type mucinous borderline tumors are much more common than the intestinal type. These lesions are bilateral in 13–40% of cases.[36–39] The reported mean size ranges from 8 cm to 13 cm.[36–39] The external surfaces may be smooth or contain exophytic tumor or capsular rupture. The cut surfaces may be uni- or multicystic, and the cysts are lined by papillary excrescences.

Histology

Terms that have been used to classify these tumors include mucinous borderline tumor of the endocervical-like or müllerian type and atypical proliferative seromucinous tumor.[37–39] The tumors lack destructive stromal invasion and have a papillary architecture as seen in SBTs. The epithelium contains mucinous columnar epithelium without goblet cells. In addition, mixtures of serous, endometrioid, squamous, and indifferent cell types may be seen. The stroma of occasional large papillae may be edematous and contain abundant neutrophils. Associated endometriosis may be present. Microinvasion, micropapillary/cribriform types of ovarian tumors, intraepithelial carcinoma, and extraovarian implants may be encountered.

Endometrioid, clear cell, and Brenner (transitional cell) borderline tumors

Gross

Endometrioid, clear cell, and Brenner borderline tumors of the ovary are almost always unilateral. The cut surfaces are usually solid, but cystic components may be present.

Histology

These tumors contain crowded glands or nests. The endometrioid and transitional cell types may show papillary architecture. The background tumor may contain adenofibroma (or benign Brenner tumor for the transitional cell type) or endometriosis (for the endometrioid or clear cell types). Intraepithelial carcinoma or microinvasion may be seen. Extraovarian implants have not been well characterized for these types of borderline tumors.

Clinical presentation and diagnostic considerations

Borderline tumors, as with other ovarian tumors, are difficult to detect clinically until they are advanced in size or stage. Like their malignant counterparts, the most common presenting symptoms are abdominal/pelvic pain or pressure, increasing abdominal girth or abdominal distension, and perception of an abdominal mass.[40] Approximately 25% of patients remain asymptomatic,[41] presenting with a mass on physical or pelvic examination, at the time of surgery, or as an incidental finding on sonography. Other symptoms reported are abnormal premenstrual bleeding, nausea, constipation,[40,41] torsion,[42] intraperitoneal hemorrhage,[41] weight loss,[43] and dyspareunia.[44]

In most cases, the diagnosis of borderline ovarian tumor is rendered during intraoperative or postoperative pathological evaluation. No preoperative tumor markers or radiological features can accurately identify a pelvic mass as a borderline ovarian tumor. Several studies have attempted to determine sonographic findings distinguishing borderline ovarian tumors from both benign and invasive malignant tumors. Exacoustos et al. reported that the presence of papillae into the cyst cavity from the cyst wall was significantly more frequent in borderline tumors (48%) than in benign (4%) and invasive tumors (4%).[45] Intracystic solid tissue was observed in 48% of invasive tumors, but in only 18% of borderline and 7% of benign

tumors.[45] Pascual et al. also reported that 63% of the cases evaluated had intracystic papillae.[46] However, neither papillae nor other sonographic features constituted highly sensitive sonographic markers of borderline ovarian tumors. In unilocular cystic tumors, the risk of neoplasia is low. McDonald et al. reported no cases of borderline tumors in 395 patients with unilocular cystic masses less than 10 cm in size.[47]

Computed tomography (CT) and magnetic resonance imaging (MRI) have also been evaluated in order to determine findings that differentiate borderline ovarian tumors from their malignant counterparts. DeSouza et al.[48] evaluated CT and MRI features and tumor marker levels that could differentiate borderline ovarian tumors from stage I ovarian tumors. They reported that borderline ovarian tumors were complex masses with imaging features similar to stage I invasive ovarian carcinoma, but the thickness of septations and the size of solid components were significantly larger in stage I ovarian cancer.[48] However, neither feature allowed for confident differentiation of borderline ovarian tumors from stage I invasive ovarian carcinoma.

CA-125 is the most useful tumor marker currently available for monitoring response to therapy among patients with epithelial ovarian cancer; however, it has not proven to be a reliable screening test because of its low specificity. The use of CA-125 has also been studied among patients diagnosed with borderline ovarian tumors. Chambers and colleagues[49] obtained CA-125 levels from 18 patients and found elevations above 35 U/mL in only four cases (22.2%). No value was noted to exceed 100 U/mL. Rice et al.[50] found that CA-125 levels were elevated in 92% of women with advanced-stage borderline ovarian tumors, but in only 40% of women with stage I. All the patients with advanced-stage disease had serous histology, compared to only 48% of those with stage I disease, leading these authors to conclude that elevated CA-125 levels correlate with advanced-stage disease in patients with serous borderline ovarian tumors.[50]

Surgical management

Early-stage disease

Surgery is the cornerstone of treatment for patients diagnosed with early-stage borderline tumors of the ovary. Apparent stage I borderline ovarian tumors diagnosed intraoperatively by frozen section should be managed, depending on the patient's child-bearing status, with bilateral salpingo-oophorectomy, hysterectomy, and staging when child bearing is completed versus conservative management, meaning ovarian cystectomy or unilateral oophorectomy, with staging, when fertility preservation is desired. In one large series of patients with borderline ovarian tumors, Lin and colleagues[51] reported that intraoperative frozen-section analysis was obtained in 196 (77%) of cases. Of the 193 cases for which the frozen-section diagnosis was known, 117 (61%) were diagnosed correctly as borderline ovarian tumors, 52 (27%) cases were interpreted as invasive ovarian cancer, and 24 (12%) cases were thought to be benign ovarian tumors intraoperatively. Overall, 66% of the patients had at least one staging biopsy performed, and 34%

had no staging biopsy. Only 12% of patients were completely staged. Among all patients, staging biopsies were positive for extraovarian disease in 37% of cases. Approximately 47% (80 of 169) of patients who underwent biopsies were upstaged as a result of positive biopsies, with 41% (70 of 169) having extrapelvic spread.

For patients with apparent stage I borderline ovarian tumors who have previously undergone a surgical procedure that did not include staging, we recommend staging/reexploration by means of a laparotomy or laparoscopy only in the presence of micropapillary serous borderline tumor histology or if there is evidence of bulky residual disease on a postoperative CT scan. If neither of the above criteria is present, reexploration for the express purpose of surgical staging is unlikely to have a meaningful impact on long-term clinical outcome and is not recommended. Rather, close clinical surveillance should be sufficient. For patients in whom an intraoperative diagnosis of mucinous borderline ovarian tumors is obtained, appendectomy and a thorough gastrointestinal evaluation should be performed to rule out a primary gastrointestinal tumor metastatic to the ovary.

Since many women affected with borderline ovarian tumors have not completed child bearing, the efficacy and safety of conservative surgery are an important concern. There is no evidence that a conservative approach has an adverse effect on survival in patients with stage I borderline ovarian tumors.[52] For this group of patients, unilateral oophorectomy or ovarian cystectomy with staging is a reasonable option. Conservative management should include visualization of the contralateral ovary, because the risk of bilateral involvement, especially in serous borderline tumors, is 40%.[53] If there is a suspicious mass or lesion, ovarian cystectomy or wedge biopsy may be performed. Random biopsies of the contralateral ovary are not recommended if no gross abnormalities are seen because of the low yield, and resultant adhesions may affect future fertility.

Several authors have reported on the safety of conservative surgery for patients with borderline ovarian tumors who desire future fertility. Although performing a unilateral oophorectomy or an ovarian cystectomy, or both, does not appear to significantly affect long-term overall survival rates, recurrence rates are higher for women who undergo conservative management. In the study of Tazelaar et al.,[54] 41 of 61 patients with stage IA borderline tumors were treated with total abdominal hysterectomy and bilateral salpingo-oophorectomy. The rest (20 patients) were treated with a variety of conservative procedures including cystectomy with (one patient) and without (three patients) a contralateral ovarian wedge biopsy, and unilateral salpingo-oophorectomy with (six patients) and without (10 patients) a contralateral wedge biopsy. After a mean follow-up of 89 months, subsequent borderline tumors had developed in three patients (15%) initially treated conservatively and in two patients (5%) initially treated with abdominal hysterectomy and bilateral salpingo-oophorectomy. In the report by Lim-Tan et al.,[55] 35 patients with serous borderline ovarian tumors underwent unilateral ovarian cystectomy, bilateral cystectomy, or unilateral cystectomy with contralateral oophorectomy or salpingo-oophorectomy. All but two of the patients had stage I disease. Tumor persisted or recurred only in the

ovary that had been subjected to cystectomy in two (6%) of 33 patients with stage I tumors, in both the ipsilateral and contralateral ovary in one patient (3%), and in the contralateral ovary only in 1 patient (3%). The authors concluded that involvement of the resection margin of the cystectomy specimen and the removal of more than one cyst from an ovary were almost always associated with persistence or recurrence of tumor.

Due to the increased risk of recurrence, ovarian cystectomy in the management of borderline ovarian tumors is not widely embraced and must be limited to exceptional cases (e.g. bilateral lesions). Morris and colleagues reported that 42% of women who underwent conservative surgery for serous borderline ovarian tumors developed a recurrence.[56] Furthermore, Cadron et al. described recurrence rates of up to 58% with cystectomy, in comparison to 5.7% with oophorectomy.[57] In view of these findings, women who undergo conservative management should be closely monitored for disease recurrence, especially if they are left with only one remaining ovary.

Women undergoing conservative surgery for child-bearing purposes should also be counseled regarding the limitations of frozen pathology evaluation relating to borderline tumors, as up to 25% of lesions may be reclassified as invasive in final pathological review.[58]

Advanced-stage and recurrent disease

Approximately 20% of patients with borderline ovarian tumors will present with advanced-stage disease at the time of diagnosis. The recommended primary surgical management of these patients is identical to that applied to patients with invasive ovarian cancer. Rates of recurrence and death for women with stage II and III disease vary from 5% to 30%.[19–23,28,29,59,60] However, even with advanced-stage borderline ovarian tumors, the long-term survival rate approaches 70%.[61] As with invasive ovarian cancer, maximal surgical cytoreduction to no gross residual disease is therefore recommended. The role of conservative surgical management, meaning unilateral oophorectomy or ovarian cystectomy, for advanced-stage disease is less well accepted than for women with early-stage borderline tumors of the ovary. Zanetta and colleagues demonstrated that 40% of the patients treated with conservative management for advanced-stage disease recurred compared to 12.9% of recurrences after nonconservative management.[60] Given these observations, conservative management (e.g. unilateral oophorectomy or ovarian cystectomy) for advanced-stage disease should be undertaken with caution.

In contrast to invasive ovarian cancer, the median time to recurrence for borderline tumors is 5–7 years, with relapses occurring as late as 39 years after initial therapy being described.[62] For patients who develop recurrent disease, secondary cytoreductive surgery is the treatment of choice. Crispens and colleagues[63] evaluated the outcome of 53 patients treated for progressive or recurrent serous borderline ovarian tumors and emphasized the importance of surgery in the management of these tumors. These authors found that patients with progressive or recurrent disease who could be optimally cytoreduced to residual disease less than or equal to 2 cm had a significantly better survival compared with patients who could not be optimally cytoreduced. The response to chemotherapy, hormonal therapy, and radiotherapy was universally poor. Among 45 patients who received nonsurgical therapy, only six patients (13%) had partial responses and six patients (13%) had complete responses. Twenty-one out of 45 patients (47%) had stabilization of disease with nonsurgical therapy. It should be noted that the clinical significance of an objective response to adjuvant therapy is unclear, given the indolent clinical course of borderline ovarian tumors.

Adjuvant therapy

For patients with disease apparently confined to the ovaries, adjuvant chemotherapy is not recommended. Barnhill et al.[52] reported a Gynecologic Oncology Group (GOG) prospective study in which 146 patients with stage I serous borderline ovarian tumors were observed without adjuvant therapy. With a median follow-up of 42.2 months, no patient developed recurrent disease. For most patients with stage I tumors, long-term disease-free survival can be expected. To underscore this point, a large metaanalysis demonstrated a disease-free survival rate of 98.2% and a disease-specific survival rate of 99.5% for women with stage I disease.[59] Four prospective randomized trials conducted in Norway showed that for stage I and II disease, the addition of adjuvant therapy did not improve survival and added toxicity, with overall survival rates of 99% and 94% for no adjuvant therapy, and adjuvant therapy respectively.[64]

Clinical significance notwithstanding, objective responses to platinum-based chemotherapy among patients with advanced-stage borderline ovarian tumors have been reported at the time of second-look surgery. Gershenson et al. reported complete responses to chemotherapy at second-look laparotomy in eight of 20 patients with macroscopic residual disease after initial cytoreductive surgery and in five of 12 patients with microscopic residual disease after initial surgery.[65] Barakat and colleagues reported that two of seven patients with macroscopic residual borderline ovarian tumors and seven of eight patients with microscopic disease had pathological complete remissions at second-look laparotomy after platinum-based chemotherapy.[66] With a mean follow-up of 64 months, only one patient had died of progressive disease. Importantly, there was no difference in survival between patients who received chemotherapy and those who did not. Sutton et al.[43] reported the GOG data using a subset of 32 women with advanced-stage borderline ovarian tumors that were optimally cytoreduced. The patients were randomized to treatment with cisplatin and cyclophosphamide with or without adriamycin. Fifteen of 32 patients underwent second-look surgery, and nine showed evidence of persistent disease. However, at a median follow-up of 31.7 months, 31 of 32 patients were alive. Only one patient died and the cause was unrelated to the ovarian disease process.

Due to the low percentage of actively dividing cells that are present in borderline ovarian tumors, these are thought to be relatively resistant to standard cytotoxic agents. Furthermore, adjuvant chemotherapy in patients with ovarian serous borderline tumors with invasive peritoneal implants showed no improvement in time to recurrence or overall survival.[67] However, given the small number of patients and variable follow-up times, it is still possible that a beneficial effect exists. As noted earlier, even patients with advanced-stage disease can be expected to have excellent overall survival rates. Therefore, patients must be counseled that the role of adjuvant chemotherapy in advanced-stage disease is still unclear. Patients should be managed with surgical debulking with the objective of removing all visible disease. Adjuvant chemotherapy is usually reserved for patients with invasive extraovarian implants, although, again, a meaningful survival benefit has been difficult to demonstrate even for this selected group of patients, as detailed above. In patients with noninvasive implants, surgical debulking should be sufficient and chemotherapy is not recommended.

The management of recurrent disease must be individualized. The decision to treat must be carefully considered, balancing the patient's symptoms, tumor growth rate, extent of disease, and overall life goals. There are no randomized or prospective studies evaluating the benefit of chemotherapy in patients with recurrent borderline ovarian tumors. As demonstrated by Crispens et al.,[63] patients with progressive or recurrent disease who could be optimally cytoreduced to less than or equal to 2 cm maximal residual disease had a significantly better survival compared with patients who could not be optimally cytoreduced (12% of optimally cytoreduced patients died of disease, in comparison to 60% of patients whose tumor was suboptimally cytoreduced). The response to chemotherapy, hormonal therapy, and radiotherapy was poor. Specifically, the authors reported only a 13% clinical complete response rate and a 13% clinical partial response rates in patients treated with platinum-based regimens. These findings did not demonstrate a significant response to nonsurgical therapy among patients with persistent or recurrent disease. In this setting, surgery should be the preferred management option for patients diagnosed with recurrent borderline ovarian tumors. Chemotherapy may be indicated if unresectable disease is present, or for tumors demonstrating a more rapid growth rate with progressive symptomatology. Ultimately, optimal cytoreduction, with no gross residual disease, should be prioritized, as the presence of macroscopic residual disease appears to be the major predictor of recurrence and survival. Kane et al. demonstrated a decline in 5-year recurrence-free survival, from 75% with no residual disease to 56% when lesions >2 cm in size remained.[68]

In summary, the recommended management of clinically apparent early-stage borderline ovarian tumors includes bilateral salpingo-oophorectomy with hysterectomy and surgical staging for women who have completed child bearing. For young patients with apparent early-stage disease who desire fertility preservation, unilateral oophorectomy or ovarian cystectomy with staging procedures is an acceptable alternative, although this approach may predispose to a higher risk of recurrence. For advanced-stage and recurrent disease, cytoreductive surgery is the cornerstone treatment, while adjuvant chemotherapy is reserved for selected cases only (e.g. unresectable disease, invasive metastatic implants, rapid growth rate with progressive symptomatology).

Stage distribution and prognosis

The surgical staging of borderline ovarian tumors is made in accordance with the same FIGO guidelines used for invasive ovarian cancer. A review of 370 patients with borderline ovarian tumors from the Norwegian Radium Institute revealed that 84% of the patients were diagnosed with stage I disease.[44] This is consistent with the review performed by Sutton of 12 published studies that revealed that 80% of the 946 patients diagnosed with borderline ovarian tumors presented with stage I disease.[69] The importance of comprehensive surgical staging in ovarian cancer also applies to borderline ovarian tumors. In a study performed by Hopkins and colleagues, 15 patients with apparent early-stage disease underwent a restaging operation and residual disease was found in seven patients.[70] One patient remained as stage IA, one patient was upstaged to stage IB, and five patients were upstaged to either FIGO stage II or III disease. The authors concluded that reexploration for staging in borderline ovarian tumors will yield a significant number of positive results.[70] Snider et al. also noted a 19% incidence of upstaging in 27 patients diagnosed with stage I disease.[71] Since the prognosis for patients with nodal involvement is similar to those without nodal involvement, it suggests that this is a metaplastic and not a metastatic process.[72,73]

Djordjevic and Malpica investigated the clinical significance of LNI in patients with serous borderline tumors. Patients with LNI had a significantly higher rate of invasive ($p=0.01$) and noninvasive ($p=0.002$) implants.[30] In 22% of the cases, LNI represented the only site of extraovarian disease. Importantly, LNI did not have a significant impact on disease-free survival or overall survival. Similarly, Fadare concluded that LNI did not adversely affect overall survival in patients with serous borderline tumors.[74]

The prognosis depends upon the stage and histological features of the tumor, but in general is good. A review of 2818 women with borderline ovarian tumors from the SEER program reported 5- and 10-year relative survival rates of 99% and 97% respectively for stage I, 98% and 90% for stage II, 96% and 88% for stage III, and 77% and 69% for stage IV.[61] Sherman et al. demonstrated that long-term survival for patients with borderline tumors staged as distant was similar to women with localized carcinoma.[75] Given the favorable long-term survival outcome of borderline ovarian tumors, the clinical significance of surgical upstaging by reexploration for apparent early-stage disease has been questioned by a number of investigators.

Other rare epithelial tumors of the ovary

Clear cell ovarian carcinoma

Epidemiology and clinical presentation

Clear cell ovarian carcinomas comprise approximately 3% of ovarian epithelial neoplasms.[76] The mean age at diagnosis is 55 years.[77] Patients usually present with symptoms related to a pelvic or abdominal mass. Clear cell carcinomas are the most common epithelial ovarian neoplasm to be associated with paraneoplastic hypercalcemia.

Pathology

About half of cases are associated with endometriosis.[78] When associated with endometriosis, mixed clear cell and endometrioid carcinoma may occur. Approximately half of patients present with stage I and 15% with stage II disease.[79] Tumors usually range up to 30 cm in diameter; with a mean of about 15 cm.[76] There are conflicting data on the behavior of these tumors. In some studies, the prognosis appears similar to that of other ovarian carcinomas[80,81] while in others, the prognosis is said to be worse.[77,79,82,83] However, when controlled by stage, the survival of patients with clear cell carcinoma may be slightly lower than that of patients with serous carcinoma. In a Gynecologic Oncology Group study, Winter et al. reported decreased progression-free survival (PFS) and overall survival (OS) amongst patients with mucinous or clear cell histologies. Specifically, patients with clear cell histology had an OS of only 24 months, in comparison to 45 and 56 months for patients with serous and endometrioid histologies, respectively.[84]

Surgical management and adjuvant therapy

The treatment of clear cell carcinoma is similar to that of other epithelial cell types of ovarian cancer and involves surgical cytoreduction followed by adjuvant chemotherapy. Clear cell carcinomas are regarded as grade III tumors. As such, the National Comprehensive Cancer Network (NCCN) Clinical Practice Guidelines recommend adjuvant chemotherapy for the tumor, even at stage IA, differentiating this histology from serous carcinoma.[85] Recio and colleagues reported that women with clear cell carcinomas treated with platinum-based chemotherapy were at significantly increased risk of thromboembolic complications compared to those with nonclear cell carcinomas, with a corresponding negative impact on survival.[86] Furthermore, clear cell ovarian carcinoma has a poor response to adjuvant chemotherapy. In a series recently published by Al-Barrak et al., benefit from chemotherapy was seen in about one-quarter of treatment courses.[87] This overall low response, and the substantial rates of progressive disease and toxicities while on treatment, lead to a low "benefit to failure" ratio, as concluded by the authors. The modest value of chemotherapy in the treatment of clear cell ovarian carcinoma is clear, and emphasizes the importance of exploration into targeted and novel therapies.

Mucinous ovarian carcinoma

Epidemiology and clinical presentation

After exclusion of metastatic tumors of the ovaries, primary ovarian mucinous carcinomas are uncommon, comprising approximately 4% of ovarian epithelial neoplasms.[76] The mean age at diagnosis is 53 years.[76] As these tumors can be quite large, the clinical presentation is generally that of a large pelvic or abdominal mass and abdominal distension. Approximately 63% of cases are stage I disease.[79] However, when stratified by stage, patients with stage III mucinous epithelial ovarian carcinoma had significantly poorer PFS and OS in comparison to serous and endometrioid histologies.[84,88–90] Advanced-stage mucinous carcinoma is uniformly fatal.

Pathology

Although identification of intracytoplasmic mucin is mandatory for pathological diagnosis, many parts of large tumors may lack apical mucin. Therefore, immunohistochemical staining can help identify primary mucinous ovarian carcinomas. Unlike many pancreatic ductal carcinomas, SMAD4 (Dpc4) expression is maintained in primary ovarian mucinous carcinomas. In addition, K-ras mutations, lack of estrogen receptor expression and lack of p16 overexpression have been described.[91]

Surgical management and adjuvant therapy

The treatment of mucinous carcinoma is similar to that of other epithelial cell types of ovarian cancer and involves surgical cytoreduction followed by chemotherapy. Traditional chemotherapeutic regimens include a platinum/taxane combination. However, mucinous epithelial ovarian cancers have shown limited response rates to platinum-based regimens. The Gynecologic Cancer Inter-Group is conducting a randomized phase 3 clinical trial evaluating carboplatin+paclitaxel +/– bevacizumab versus oxaliplatin+capecitabine +/– bevacizumab in the treatment of women with epithelial mucinous tumors of the ovary or fallopian tube. Inclusion of the oxaliplatin+capecitabine arm is based on literature illustrating up to a 50% response rate amongst patients with advanced-stage mucinous colorectal cancer.[92]

Endometrioid ovarian carcinoma

Epidemiology and clinical presentation

Endometrioid ovarian carcinomas comprise 6% of ovarian surface epithelial tumors.[76] The mean patient age at diagnosis is 56 years.[76] The most common presenting symptoms are abdominal distension and abdominal or pelvic pain. Abnormal vaginal bleeding can be a frequent symptom and could be related to the association of endometrioid ovarian carcinoma with endometrial hyperplasia and carcinoma.[93]

Pathology

The tumor size usually ranges from 12 to 20 cm with a mean of about 15 cm.[76] A high proportion of endometrioid carcinomas of the ovary are diagnosed in early stage, with 52% of cases presenting with stage I or II disease.[79] The reported association of endometrioid carcinomas with ovarian endometriosis is around 10%, although in a well-documented study of stage I cases, 40% were associated with endometriosis, one-third of which arose in the endometriosis.[94]

Surgical management and adjuvant therapy

It has been stated that these tumors have a better prognosis than serous ovarian carcinomas but this is mostly related to the fact that a great majority of the patients present with early-stage disease. Winter *et al*. described a median OS of 56 months amongst patients with epithelial ovarian carcinoma of endometrioid histology.[84] This is in comparison to 45 months amongst those with serous histology. Treatment of endometrioid carcinomas is generally the same as that of other ovarian epithelial carcinomas and involves surgical cytoreduction followed by chemotherapy.

Malignant mixed mesodermal tumor (carcinosarcoma)

Epidemiology and clinical presentation

Malignant mixed mesodermal tumors (MMMT) of the ovary comprise less than 1% of ovarian neoplasms.[76] The mean age of patients with this tumor is about 60 years.[76] Approximately 74% of patients present with advanced-stage (III or IV) disease.[93] The tumors are typically large, ranging in size from 15 cm to 20 cm in diameter.[77] Patients typically present with pelvic pain, abdominal distension/bloating, a palpable mass or symptoms of metastatic disease.

Pathology

These tumors are characterized by the presence of both carcinomatous and sarcomatous components. However, the preponderance of sarcomatous components portends a poor prognosis. The epithelial component can be classified as endometrioid, serous or undifferentiated adenocarcinoma. Homologous sarcomatous elements include endometrial stromal sarcoma, fibrosarcoma or leiomyosarcoma. Conversely, chondrosarcoma, rhabdomyosarcoma, and less commonly osteosarcoma and liposarcoma represent heterologous sarcomatous elements.

Surgical management and adjuvant therapy

The treatment of ovarian carcinosarcoma is similar to that of other epithelial cell types of ovarian cancer and involves surgical cytoreduction followed by chemotherapy. These tumors are aggressive and rapidly fatal, with a median survival of approximately 1 year[95–97] Furthermore, adjuvant chemotherapy has shown limited response rates in the treatment of carcinosarcoma of the ovary. The GOG is currently conducting a randomized phase 3 trial comparing paclitaxel plus carboplatin to ifosfamide plus paclitaxel in chemotherapy-naive patients with newly diagnosed stage I–IV, persistent or recurrent carcinosarcoma of the ovary or uterus (GOG protocol 261).

References

1. Taylor HC. Malignant and semimalignant tumors of the ovary. Surg Gynecol Obstet 1929; 48: 204–30.
2. International Federation of Gynecology and Obstetrics. Classification and staging of malignant tumors in the female pelvis. Acta Obstet Gynecol Scand 1971; 50: 1–7.
3. Serov SF, Scully RE, Sobin LH. *International Histological Classification and Staging of Tumors. No. 9 Histologic Typing of Ovarian Tumors*. Geneva: World Health Organization, 1973. pp.37–41.
4. Silverberg SG, Bell DA, Kurman RJ, *et al*. Borderline ovarian tumor workshop. Borderline ovarian tumors: key points and workshop summary. Hum Pathol 2004; 35: 910–17.
5. Mink P, Sherman ME, Devesa S. Incidence patterns of invasive and borderline ovarian tumors among white women and black women in the United States: results from the SEER program, 1978–1997. Cancer 2002; 95: 2380–9.
6. Lalwani N, Shanbhogue AK, Vikram R, *et al*. Current update on borderline ovarian neoplasms. Am J Roentgenol 2010; 194(2): 330–6.
7. Swanton A, Bankhead CR, Kehoe S. Pregnancy rates after conservative treatment for borderline ovarian tumours: a systematic review. Eur J Obstet Gynecol Reprod Biol 2007; 135(1): 3–7.
8. Nakashima N, Nagasaka T, Oiwa N, *et al*. Ovarian epithelial tumors of borderline malignancy in Japan. Gynecol Oncol 1990; 38: 90–8.

9. Barnhill D, Heller P, Brzozowski P, *et al*. Epithelial ovarian carcinoma of low malignant potential. Obstet Gynecol 1985; 65: 53–9.

10. Bostwick DG, Tazelaar HD, Ballon SC, *et al*. Ovarian epithelial tumors of borderline malignancy. A clinical and pathologic study of 109 cases. Cancer 1986; 58: 2052–65.

11. Katsube Y, Berg JW, Silverberg SG. Epidemiologic pathology of ovarian tumors: a histopathologic review of primary ovarian neoplasms diagnosed in the Denver Standard Metropolitan Statistical Area, 1 July–31 December 1969 and 1 July–31 December 1979. Int J Gynecol Pathol 1982; 1(1): 3–16.

12. Harlow BL, Weiss NS, Roth GL, *et al*. Case–control study of borderline ovarian tumors: reproductive history and exposure to exogenous female hormones. Cancer Res 1988; 48: 5849–52.

13. Webb PM, Purdie DM, Grover S, *et al*. Symptoms and diagnosis of borderline, early and advanced epithelial ovarian cancer. Gynecol Oncol 2004; 92(1): 232–9.

14. Tinelli A, Vergara D, Martignago R, *et al*. An outlook on ovarian cancer and borderline ovarian tumors: focus on genomic and proteomic findings. Curr Genom 2009; 10(4): 240–9.

15. Vergara D, Tinelli A, Martignago R, *et al*. Biomolecular pathogenesis of borderline ovarian tumors: focusing target discovery through proteogenomics. Curr Cancer Drug Targets 2010; 10(1): 107–16.

16. Mayr D, Hirschmann A, Lhrs U, *et al*. KRAS and BRAF mutations in ovarian tumors: a comprehensive study of invasive carcinomas, borderline tumors and extraovarian implants. Gynecol Oncol 2006; 103(3): 883–7.

17. Ortiz BH, Ailawadi M, Colitti C, *et al*. Second primary or recurrence? Comparative patterns of p53 and K-ras mutations suggest that serous borderline ovarian tumors and subsequent serous carcinomas are unrelated tumors. Cancer Res 2001; 61(19): 7264–7.

18. Bell DA, Longacre TA, Prat J, *et al*. Serous borderline (low malignant potential, atypical proliferative) ovarian tumors: workshop perspectives. Hum Pathol 2004; 35: 934–48.

19. Deavers MT, Gershenson DM, Tortolero-Luna G, *et al*. Micropapillary and cribriform patterns in ovarian serous tumors of low malignant potential: a study of 99 advanced stage cases. Am J Surg Pathol 2002; 26: 1129–41.

20. Eichhorn JH, Bell DA, Young RH, *et al*. Ovarian serous borderline tumors with micropapillary and cribriform patterns: a study of 40 cases and comparison with 44 cases without these patterns. Am J Surg Pathol 1999; 23: 397–409.

21. Goldstein NS, Ceniza N. Ovarian micropapillary serous borderline tumors. Clinicopathologic features and outcome of seven surgically staged patients. Am J Clin Pathol 2000; 114: 380–6.

22. Prat J, de Nictolis M. Serous borderline tumors of the ovary: a long-term follow-up study of 137 cases, including 18 with a micropapillary pattern and 20 with microinvasion. Am J Surg Pathol 2002; 26: 1111–28.

23. Seidman JD, Kurman RJ. Subclassification of serous borderline tumors of the ovary into benign and malignant types. A clinicopathologic study of 65 advanced stage cases. Am J Surg Pathol 1996; 20: 1331–45.

24. Smith Sehdev AE, Sehdev PS, Kurman RJ. Noninvasive and invasive micropapillary (low-grade) serous carcinoma of the ovary: a clinicopathologic analysis of 135 cases. Am J Surg Pathol 2003; 27: 725–36.

25. Seidman JD, Soslow RA, Vang R, *et al*. Borderline ovarian tumors: diverse contemporary viewpoints on terminology and diagnostic criteria with illustrative images. Hum Pathol 2004; 35: 918–33.

26. Kurman RJ, Seidman JD, Shih IM. Serous borderline tumours of the ovary. Histopathology 2005; 47(3): 310–15.

27. McCluggage WG. The pathology of and controversial aspects of ovarian borderline tumours. Curr Opin Oncol 2010; 22(5): 462–72.

28. Bell DA, Weinstock MA, Scully RE. Peritoneal implants of ovarian serous borderline tumors. Histologic features and prognosis. Cancer 1988; 62: 2212–22.

29. Bell KA, Smith Sehdev AE, Kurman RJ. Refined diagnostic criteria for implants associated with ovarian atypical proliferative serous tumors (borderline) and micropapillary serous carcinomas. Am J Surg Pathol 2001; 25: 419–32.

30. Djordjevic B, Malpica A. Lymph node involvement in ovarian serous tumors of low malignant potential: a clinicopathologic study of thirty-six cases. Am J Surg Pathol 2010; 34(1): 1–9.

31. Lee KR, Scully RE. Mucinous tumors of the ovary: a clinicopathologic study of 196 borderline tumors (of intestinal type) and carcinomas, including an evaluation of 11 cases with 'pseudomyxoma peritonei'. Am J Surg Pathol 2000; 24: 1447–64.

32. Riopel MA, Ronnett BM, Kurman RJ. Evaluation of diagnostic criteria and behavior of ovarian intestinal-type mucinous tumors: atypical proliferative (borderline) tumors and intraepithelial, microinvasive, invasive, and metastatic carcinomas. Am J Surg Pathol 1999; 23: 617–35.

33. Rodriguez IM, Prat J. Mucinous tumors of the ovary: a clinicopathologic analysis of 75 borderline tumors (of intestinal type) and carcinomas. Am J Surg Pathol 2002; 26: 139–52.

34. Ronnett BM, Kajdacsy-Balla A, Gilks CB, *et al*. Mucinous borderline ovarian tumors: points of general agreement and persistent controversies regarding nomenclature, diagnostic criteria, and behavior. Hum Pathol 2004; 35: 949–60.

35. Provenza C, Young RH, Prat J. Anaplastic carcinoma in mucinous ovarian tumors: a clinicopathologic study of 34 cases emphasizing the crucial impact of stage on prognosis, their histologic spectrum, and overlap with sarcomalike mural nodules. Am J Surg Pathol 2008; 32(3): 383–9.

36. Dube V, Roy M, Plante M, *et al*. Mucinous ovarian tumors of mullerian-type: an analysis of 17 cases including borderline tumors and intraepithelial, microinvasive, and invasive carcinomas. Int J Gynecol Pathol 2005; 24: 138–46.

37. Rodriguez IM, Irving JA, Prat J. Endocervical-like mucinous borderline tumors of the ovary: a clinicopathologic analysis of 31 cases. Am J Surg Pathol 2004; 28: 1311–18.

38. Rutgers JL, Scully RE. Ovarian mullerian mucinous papillary cystadenomas of borderline malignancy. A clinicopathologic analysis. Cancer 1988; 61: 340–8.

39. Shappell HW, Riopel MA, Smith Sehdev AE, *et al*. Diagnostic criteria and behavior of ovarian seromucinous (endocervical-type mucinous and mixed cell-type) tumors: atypical proliferative (borderline) tumors, intraepithelial, microinvasive, and invasive carcinomas. Am J Surg Pathol 2002; 26: 1529–41.

40. Hopkins MP, Kumar NB, Morley GW. An assessment of pathologic features and treatment modalities in ovarian tumors of low malignant potential. Obstet Gynecol 1987; 70: 923–9.

41. Hart WR, Norris HJ. Borderline and malignant mucinous tumors of the ovary. Histologic criteria and clinical behavior. Cancer 1973; 31: 1031–45.

42. Julian CG, Woodruff JD. The biologic behavior of low-grade papillary serous carcinoma of the ovary. Obstet Gynecol 1972; 40: 860–7.

43. Sutton GP, Bundy BN, Omura GA, *et al*. Stage III ovarian tumors of low malignant potential treated with cisplatin combination therapy (a Gynecologic Oncology Group study). Gynecol Oncol 1991; 41: 230–3.

44. Yazigi R, Sandstad J, Munoz AK. Primary staging in ovarian tumors of low malignant potential. Gynecol Oncol 1988; 31: 402–8.

45. Exacoustos C, Romanini ME, Rinaldo D, *et al*. Preoperative sonographic features of borderline ovarian tumors. Ultrasound Obstet Gynecol 2005; 25(1): 50–9.

46. Pascual MA, Tresserra F, Grases PJ, *et al*. Borderline cystic tumors of the ovary: gray-scale and color Doppler sonographic findings. J Clin Ultrasound 2002; 30(2): 76–82.

47. McDonald JM, Doran S, DeSimone CP, *et al*. Predicting risk of malignancy in adnexal masses. Obstet Gynecol 2010; 115(4): 687–94.

48. DeSouza NM, O'Neill R, McIndoe GA, *et al*. Borderline tumors of the ovary: CT and MRI features and tumor markers in differentiation from stage I disease. Am J Roentgenol 2005; 184(3): 999–1003.

49. Chambers JT, Merino MJ, Kohorn EI, *et al*. Borderline ovarian tumors. Am J Obstet Gynecol 1988; 159(5): 1088–94.

50. Rice LW, Lage JM, Berkowitz RS, *et al*. Preoperative serum CA-125 levels in borderline tumors of the ovary. Gynecol Oncol 1992; 46(2): 226–9.

51. Lin PS, Gershenson DM, Bevers MW, *et al*. The current status of surgical staging of ovarian serous borderline tumors. Cancer 1999; 85: 905–11.

52. Barnhill DR, Kurman RJ, Brady MF, *et al*. Preliminary analysis of the behavior of stage I ovarian serous tumors of low malignant potential: a Gynecologic Oncology Group study. J Clin Oncol 1995; 13: 2752–6.

53. Segal GH, Hart WR. Ovarian serous tumors of low malignant potential (serous borderline tumors): the relationship of exophytic surface tumor to peritoneal implants. Am J Surg Pathol 1992; 16: 577–83.

54. Tazelaar HD, Bostwick DG, Ballon SC, *et al*. Conservative treatment of borderline ovarian tumors. Obstet Gynecol 1985; 66: 417–22.

55. Lim-Tan SK, Cajigas HE, Scully RE. Ovarian cystectomy for serous borderline tumors: a follow-up study of 35 cases. Obstet Gynecol 1988; 72: 775–80.

56. Morris RT, Gershenson DM, Silva EG, *et al*. Outcome and reproductive function after conservative surgery for borderline ovarian tumors. Obstet Gynecol 2000; 95: 541–7.

57. Cadron I, Leunen K, van Gorp T, *et al*. Management of borderline ovarian neoplasms. J Clin Oncol 2007; 25(20): 2928–37.

58. Wingo SN, Knowles LM, Carrick KS, *et al*. Retrospective cohort study of surgical staging for ovarian low malignant potential tumors. Am J Obstet Gynecol 2006; 194(5): e20–2.

59. Seidman JD, Kurman RJ. Ovarian serous borderline tumors: a critical review of the literature with emphasis on prognostic indicators. Hum Pathol 2000; 31: 539–57.

60. Zanetta G, Rota S, Chiari S, *et al*. Behavior of borderline tumors with particular interest to persistence, recurrence, and progression to invasive carcinoma: a prospective study. J Clin Oncol 2001; 19: 2658–64.

61. Trimble CL, Kosary C, Trimble EL. Long-term survival and patterns of care in women with ovarian tumors of low malignant potential. Gynecol Oncol 2002; 86: 34–7.

62. Silva EG, Gershenson DM, Malpica A, *et al*. The recurrence and the overall survival rates of ovarian serous borderline neoplasms with noninvasive implants is time dependent. Am J Surg Pathol 2006; 30(11): 1367–71.

63. Crispens MA, Bodurka D, Deavers M, *et al*. Response and survival in patients with progressive or recurrent serous ovarian tumors of low malignant potential. Obstet Gynecol 2002; 99: 3–10.

64. Trope C, Kaern J, Vergote IB, *et al*. Are borderline tumors of the ovary overtreated both surgically and systemically? A review of four prospective randomized trials including 253 patients with borderline tumors. Gynecol Oncol 1993; 51(2): 236–43.

65. Gershenson DM, Silva EG. Serous ovarian tumors of low malignant potential with peritoneal implants. Cancer 1990; 65: 578–84.

66. Bakarat RR, Benjamin I, Lewis JL, *et al*. Platinum-based chemotherapy for advanced-stage serous ovarian carcinoma of low malignant potential. Gynecol Oncol 1995; 59: 390–3.

67. Gershenson DM, Silva EG, Levy L, *et al*. Ovarian serous borderline tumors with invasive peritoneal implants. Cancer 1998; 82(6): 1096–103.

68. Kane A, Uzan C, Rey A, *et al*. Prognostic factors in patients with ovarian serous low malignant potential (borderline) tumors with peritoneal implants. Oncologist 2009; 14(6): 591–600.

69. Sutton GP. Ovarian tumors of low malignant potential. In: Rubin SC, Sutton GP (eds) *Ovarian Cancer*. New York: McGraw-Hill, 1993. pp.425–49.

70. Hopkins MP, Morley GW. The second-look operation and surgical reexploration in ovarian tumor of low malignant potential. Obstet Gynecol 1989; 74: 375–8.

71. Snider DD, Stuart GCE, Nation JG, *et al*. Evaluation of surgical staging in stage I low malignant potential ovarian tumors. Gynecol Oncol 1991; 40: 129–32.

72. Shiraki M, Otis CN, Donovan JT, Powell JL. Ovarian serous borderline epithelial tumors with multiple retroperitoneal nodal involvement: metastasis or malignant transformation of epithelial glandular inclusions? Gynecol Oncol 1992; 46: 255–8.

73. Camatte S, Morice P, Atallah D, *et al*. Lymph node disorders and prognostic value of nodal involvement in patients treated for a borderline ovarian tumor: an analysis of a series of 42 lymphadenectomies. J Am Coll Surg 2002; 195: 332–8.

74. Fadare O. Recent developments on the significance and pathogenesis of lymph node involvement in ovarian serous tumors of low malignant potential (borderline tumors). Int J Gynecol Cancer 2009; 19(1): 103–8.

75. Sherman ME, Mink PJ, Curtis R, *et al*. Survival among women with borderline ovarian tumors and ovarian carcinoma: a population-based analysis. Cancer 2004; 100: 1045–52.

76. Seidman JD, Russell P, Kurman RJ. Surface epithelial tumors of the ovary. In: Kurman RJ (ed) *Blaunstein's Pathology of the Female Genital Tract*. New York: Springer-Verlag, 2002. pp.810–904.

77. O'Brien ME, Schofield JB, Tan S, *et al*. Clear cell epithelial ovarian cancer (mesonephroid): bad prognosis only in early stages. Gynecol Oncol 1993; 49: 250–4.

78. Behbakht K, Randall TC, Benjamin I, *et al*. Clinical characteristics of clear cell carcinoma of the ovary. Gynecol Oncol 1998; 70: 255–8.

79. Pecorelli S. FIGO annual report on the results of treatment in gynaecological cancer. J Epidemiol Biostat 1998; 23(3): 1–168.

80. Crozier MA, Copeland LJ, Silva EG, *et al*. Clear cell carcinoma of the ovary: a study of 59 cases. Gynecol Oncol 1989; 35: 199–203.

81. Jenison EL, Montag AG, Griffiths CT, *et al*. Clear cell adenocarcinoma of the ovary: a clinical analysis and comparison with serous carcinoma. Gynecol Oncol 1989; 32: 65–71.

82. Kennedy AW, Markman M, Biscotti CV, *et al*. Survival probability in ovarian clear cell adnocarcinoma. Gynecol Oncol 1999; 74: 108–14.

83. Tammela J, Geisler JP, Eskew PN Jr, *et al*. Clear cell carcinoma of the ovary: poor prognosis compared to serous carcinoma. Eur J Gynaecol Oncol 1998; 19: 438–40.

84. Winter WE, Maxwell GL, Tian C, *et al*. Prognostic factors for stage III epithelial ovarian cancer: a Gynecologic Oncology Group Study. J Clin Oncol 2007; 25(24): 3621–7.

85. Takano M, Sugiyama T, Yaegashi N, *et al*. Less impact of adjuvant chemotherapy for stage I clear cell carcinoma of the ovary: a retrospective Japan Clear Cell Carcinoma Study. Int J Gynecol Cancer 2010; 20(9): 1506–10.

86. Recio FO, Piver MS, Hempling RE, *et al*. Lack of improved survival plus increase in thromboembolic complications in patients with clear cell carcinoma of the ovary treated with platinum versus nonplatinum-based chemotherapy. Cancer 1996; 78: 2157–63.

87. Al Barrak J, Santos JL, Tinker A, *et al*. Exploring palliative treatment outcomes in women with advanced or recurrent ovarian clear cell carcinoma. Gynecol Oncol 2011; 122(1): 107–10.

88. Chaitin BA, Gershenson DM, Evans HL. Mucinous tumors of the ovary: a clinicopathologic study of 70 cases. Cancer 1985; 55: 1958–62.

89. Hoerl HD, Hart WR. Primary ovarian mucinous cystadenocarcinomas: a clinicopathologic study of 49 cases with long-term follow-up. Am J Surg Pathol 1998; 22: 1449–62.

90. Kikkawa F, Kawai M, Tamakoshi K, *et al*. Mucinous carcinoma of the ovary: clinicopathologic analysis. Oncology 1996; 53: 303–7.

91. Soslow RA. Mucinous ovarian carcinoma: slippery business. Cancer 2011; 117(3): 451–3.

92. Scheithauer W, Kornek GV, Raderer M, *et al*. Intermittent weekly high-dose capecitabine in combination with oxaliplatin: a phase I/II study in first-line treatment of patients with advanced colorectal cancer. Ann Oncol 2002; 13(10): 1583–9.

93. Le T, Krepart GV, Lotocki RJ, *et al*. Malignant mixed mesodermal ovarian tumor treatment and prognosis: a 20-year experience. Gynecol Oncol 1997; 65: 237–40.

94. Sainz de la Cuesta R, Eichhorn JH, Rice LW, *et al*. Histologic transformation of benign endometriosis to early epithelial ovarian cancer. Gynecol Oncol 1996; 60: 238–44.

95. Andersen WA, Young DE, Peters WA, *et al*. Platinum-based combination chemotherapy for malignant mixed mesodermal tumors of the ovary. Gynecol Oncol 1989: 32: 319–22.

96. Boucher D, Tetu B. Morphologic prognostic factors of malignant mixed mullerian tumors of the ovary: a clinicopathologic study of 15 cases. In J Gynecol Pathol 1994; 13: 22–8.

97. Dehner LP, Norris HJ, Taylor HB. Carcinosarcomas and mixed mesodermal tumors of the ovary. Cancer 1971; 27: 207–16.

36 Stromal Tumors of the Ovary

Jubilee Brown,[1] **Anuja Jhingran,**[2] **and Michael Deavers**[3]

[1] Department of Gynecologic Oncology and the Reproductive Sciences, [2] Department of Radiation Oncology,
[3] Department of Pathology, The University of Texas MD Anderson Cancer Center, Houston, TX, USA

Introduction

Stromal tumors of the ovary represent approximately 3% of ovarian neoplasms and up to 10% of all ovarian malignancies. This encompasses a diverse group of malignancies that vary in clinical presentation, natural history, prognosis, and recommended treatment. This chapter discusses the details of these rare tumors, provides a general treatment schema for such tumors, reviews details of pathological features, and provides a detailed discussion of surgical and nonsurgical treatment recommendations for patients with each specific tumor type. In addition, the issue of conservative management for preservation of fertility is discussed, and new information regarding genomics is presented.

Historical background

Sertoli stromal cell tumors, or androblastomas, were originally described in 1931 by Meyer, who theorized that they arose from the male blastema and therefore utilized the term "arrheno-blastoma" (from Greek *arrhenos*, male).[1] Terminology was changed to "Sertoli–Leydig cell tumor" in 1958 based on the recommendation of Morris and Scully, who suggested that the prior term implied masculinization, which is often absent, and was more consistent with the general classification of sex cord stromal tumors.[2]

Sex cord tumor with annular tubules (SCTAT) was first described in 1970 by Scully as a tumor associated with Peutz–Jeghers syndrome.[3] Since that time, the behavior of this tumor has become better characterized and it is now known that approximately 15% of these tumors are associated with adenoma malignum of the cervix.[4]

Steroid cell tumors, one of the rarer subtypes of stromal ovarian tumor, were historically designated as lipid cell tumors. However, it was determined that a substantial percentage of these tumors had no fatty component, so the name was changed to steroid cell tumors.[5]

In total, stromal tumors of the ovary represent a small portion of ovarian cancers, and an even smaller portion of the overall world cancer burden. However, for those women with this anomaly, many of whom are in their reproductive years, successful fertility-sparing treatment is crucial. Therefore, research has continued into the science and best management of these tumors, with continuing change and progress in the field. This chapter will present the current data with historical perspective to understand the optimal treatment for patients with stromal tumors of the ovary.

Biology and epidemiology

Specialized gonadal stromal cells and their precursors can give rise to sex cord stromal tumors of the ovary. They arise as masses in the pelvis, originating within one or both ovaries. These tumors can occur as an isolated histological subtype or in combination. The classification is presented in Box 36.1.[6] Specifically, granulosa cells and Sertoli cells arise from sex cord cells, while theca cells, Leydig cells, lipid cells, and fibroblasts arise from stromal cells and their pluripotential mesenchymal precursors. These cells are involved in the production of steroid hormones, and therefore physical manifestations of excess estrogen or androgen production are not infrequent at the time of diagnosis.[7]

The predicted incidence for all new cases of ovarian cancer in the United States is estimated to be 22,280 for 2012.[8] Ninety percent of these malignancies are epithelial in origin, with the remaining 10% comprising sex cord stromal tumors, germ cell tumors, soft tissue tumors not specific to the ovary, unclassified tumors, and metastatic tumors.[6] However, these data do not specify the exact numbers for stromal tumors of the ovary. Likewise, estimates from the Surveillance, Epidemiology, and End Results (SEER) database between 1975 and 1998 suggest that for each 5-year interval between ages 15 and 40, the incidence of nongerm cell ovarian malignancy increases from

Textbook of Uncommon Cancer, Fourth Edition. Edited by Derek Raghavan, Charles D. Blanke, David H. Johnson, Paul L. Moots, Gregory H. Reaman, Peter G. Rose and Mikkael A. Sekeres.
© 2012 John Wiley & Sons, Inc. Published 2012 by John Wiley & Sons, Inc.

eight per million to 79 per million women per year.[9] However, these data are also nonspecific for stromal ovarian tumors. In general, it has been estimated that stromal tumors of the ovary account for 3% of ovarian neoplasms and 7–10% of all ovarian malignancies,[10,11] with many of these tumors occurring in adolescent and young women.

Specific considerations with regard to pathology and prognosis of certain tumor types are noted in the following subsections of this chapter.

Molecular biology and genetics

Molecular and pathological markers have recently been evaluated as prognostic indicators for adult granulosa cell tumors. A high mitotic count appears to confer a worse prognosis, but the impact of atypia is less clear.[12–14] Aneuploidy and Ki-67 expression, markers of cellular proliferation, appear to confer a worse prognosis, but these results are somewhat controversial.[14–17] Other molecular markers

associated with poor prognosis in other tumors do not appear to play a role in granulosa cell tumors. These include p53, c-*myc*, p21, *ras*, and c-*erbB2*.[14,15,18]

Chromosomal abnormalities have also been recently evaluated in granulosa cell tumors. Detected abnormalities include trisomy 12, monosomy 22, and deletion of chromosome 6, but these studies await confirmation.[19–24] Most recently, monosomy 22, often in conjunction with trisomy 14, has been detected in these tumors, as have deletions in 22q[23] and frequent microsatellite instability.[24] In juvenile granulosa cell tumors, cytogenetic studies have identified trisomy 12[25] and a deletion in chromosome 6q.[26] Additionally, a high mitotic index may be a negative prognostic factor.[27] Although controversial, the *gsp* oncogene has been identified in advanced juvenile granulosa cell tumors of the ovary.[28]

FOXL2 is a transcription factor gene found to be important in ovarian development and function. A somatic missense point mutation in the *FOXL2* gene has recently been identified as specific for granulosa cell tumor of the ovary. This mutation involves a substitution of guanine for cytosine at the 402 locus on the *FOXL2* gene.[29]

Ovarian sex cord stromal tumors have recently been linked to pleuropulmonary blastoma, a childhood cancer associated with an inherited tumor predisposition. Germline *DICER1* mutations were identified in a majority of tested patients and kindreds, suggesting that ovarian stromal tumors may be the initial clinical presentation of patients with *DICER1* mutations in these families.[30] In contrast, there has been no association between *BRCA* mutations and ovarian sex cord stromal tumors.

Abnormalities in chromosome 12 have been described in thecomas, but these have not been specifically related to prognosis.[31]

Clinical presentation, diagnostic considerations, and techniques

The diagnosis of a stromal tumor of the ovary is based on a thorough historical and physical examination and appropriate imaging techniques. The first hint may be the age of the patient in her adolescent or young adult years. Other presenting signs and symptoms are typical for patients with a pelvic mass, with bloating, pelvic pressure or pain, increase in abdominal girth, and gastrointestinal or urinary symptoms. The physical examination, including a pelvic and rectovaginal examination, usually suggests a pelvic mass.[32] In some patients, especially those with granulosa cell tumors, evidence of hemoperitoneum can be present, with abdominal pain and tenderness, peritoneal signs, a fluid wave, and even hemodynamic instability.[33]

As noted, since stromal tumors of the ovary arise from steroid-producing cells, these tumors are often hormonally active, producing estrogen, progesterone, and androgens. Therefore, physical manifestations of excess estrogen or androgen production can be the presenting symptoms or signs of a stromal tumor.[7] If this is the case, patients may report hirsutism or virilism or, if adolescents, they may describe isosexual precocious puberty. For patients during the reproductive years, presenting signs and symptoms related to hormonal changes include menorrhagia, irregular menstrual bleeding, and amenorrhea. Postmenopausal patients may note vaginal bleeding, breast enlargement or tenderness, and vaginal cornification.[33]

During the diagnostic and/or preoperative evaluation, abnormal uterine bleeding should prompt consideration for an endometrial biopsy. Of course, in women of reproductive age, pregnancy must first be excluded. Since endometrial hyperplasia can be a secondary effect of excess estrogen production by the ovarian stromal tumor, the endometrium must be evaluated. If this is not done in the office preoperatively, it must be done in the operating room upon the diagnosis of the ovarian stromal tumor.[34]

Imaging tests which may prove useful in the diagnosis of the adnexal mass include transvaginal ultrasound, computed tomography, and magnetic resonance imaging. Of these, ultrasound is often the best for distinguishing the details of pelvic anatomy. The findings may also identify hemoperitoneum or ascites. If hemoperitoneum is present, surgery should proceed immediately, as is discussed below.

Preoperative laboratory tests which may be helpful include inhibin A and B and CA-125, in addition to the routine preoperative laboratory testing.[35,36]

Treatment

The treatment of stromal ovarian tumors is determined by many factors, including patient age, parity, desire for future fertility, extent of disease, and comorbid conditions. The surgeon may be faced with a patient with an adnexal mass, the precise histological classification of which is difficult to determine, even with the pathological evaluation of frozen tissue sections. The surgeon must then follow general guidelines for nonepithelial ovarian tumors during the initial operative management and reevaluate the need for adjuvant or additional therapy on the basis of the final pathological results. With close attention to all details, including histological type, patient characteristics, and extent of disease, the need for reexploration and more extensive surgery can be minimized.

General treatment guidelines: surgical therapy

When a pelvic mass is first diagnosed, the specific histological diagnosis is unknown. However, using patient characteristics including age, physical diagnosis, and imaging characteristics as noted above, a stromal tumor of the ovary can be suspected. A frank discussion should always be held preoperatively with any woman of child-bearing age who has an adnexal mass regarding her wishes for future fertility and her desires for maintaining ovarian and/or uterine function in light of the potential operative findings. Although this is often a difficult conversation for the physician to initiate, it is better discussed preoperatively with the patient than intraoperatively with the next of kin when a malignancy is encountered.[37]

Laparoscopy is appropriate in the occasional patient with a small solid adnexal mass or complex ovarian cyst.[38,39] However, any patient with a large, solid adnexal mass or evidence of hemodynamic instability should undergo laparotomy through a vertical skin incision to avoid morcellation and allow for appropriate surgical staging or cytoreduction.[40] Upon initial inspection, gross characteristics can suggest the diagnosis. A large,

unilateral, solid adnexal mass, often yellow and multilobulated in appearance, or hemorrhagic with hemoperitoneum evident, can suggest a granulosa cell tumor or other sex cord stromal tumor. Upon entering the peritoneal cavity, the surgeon should obtain pelvic washings and evacuate the hemoperitoneum, if present. The site of hemorrhage is most commonly the mass itself and therefore surgical removal may stop the bleeding. A unilateral mass in a patient of any age should be removed by unilateral salpingo-oophorectomy and sent for immediate histological evaluation.[37,40] Cystectomy is not appropriate in this case. Also, the mass should not be ruptured or morcellated, as this results in the disease being classified as a more advanced stage and may adversely affect survival.[41] Therefore, the tumor should not be morcellated to effect laparoscopic removal. In cases in which laparoscopy is used initially, a laparoscopic bag with an extended incision should be utilized or the procedure should be converted to a laparotomy to avoid morcellating the tumor mass.

Occasionally, to remove what is thought to be a benign dermoid cyst, an ovarian cystectomy is performed in an attempt to preserve ovarian tissue. In these cases, the tumor should be sent for immediate histological evaluation, and in the event of a sex cord stromal tumor, the entire ovary should be removed.[37,40] No support exists in the literature for ovarian cystectomy in premenopausal patients with sex cord stromal tumors. Articles that summarize "conservative management" of these tumors invariably describe unilateral salpingo-oophorectomy with conservation of the normal contralateral ovary in patients with limited disease. Therefore, unilateral salpingo-oophorectomy is the initial step in the treatment of patients with apparent limited disease.[37,40]

Once the diagnosis of a sex cord stromal tumor is made, the entire abdominopelvic cavity should be explored, with attention paid to all peritoneal surfaces and abdominopelvic organs. A complete staging procedure should be performed, including cytological evaluation of each hemidiaphragm, infracolic omentectomy, and peritoneal biopsies from each paracolic gutter, the vesicouterine fold, and the pouch of Douglas. Additionally, biopsies of any suspicious areas should be performed. Pelvic and paraaortic lymph node sampling have previously been recommended for full staging, but the incidence of primary lymphatic metastases approaches zero, so pelvic and paraaortic lymphadenectomy can be omitted from the staging procedure in patients with stromal ovarian tumors.[42–44] Any enlarged lymph nodes, however, should be removed. The bowel should be inspected from the ileocecal valve to the ligament of Treitz, with specific evaluation for tumor implants and sites of obstruction. Tumor-reductive surgery should be performed in patients with advanced disease to reduce the tumor burden as much as possible, preferably leaving the patient with no macroscopic disease.[37,40]

Patients who have completed child bearing should undergo total abdominal hysterectomy and bilateral salpingo-oophorectomy regardless of the stage of disease. However, preservation of fertility is an essential consideration in young patients.[37] If the contralateral ovary and/or uterine serosa are grossly involved by tumor, the surgeon may have no choice but to remove the uterus and both adnexae. If the contralateral ovary and uterine serosa appear normal, conservative management with preservation of the uterus and contralateral adnexa is appropriate, as 95% of sex cord stromal tumors are unilateral.

The treatment of patients who have had inadequate staging is a difficult issue. Limited information exists as to the best course of action for these patients. If the patient has documented large amounts of residual disease after a limited initial attempt at tumor reduction, repeat exploration with staging and tumor-reductive surgery would be reasonable. If the patient has had an inadequate exploration, such as through a small Pfannenstiel incision or through a limited laparoscopy, more information needs to be collected prior to making a decision about postsurgical treatment. We have recommended several options, including repeat laparoscopic or open exploration with full surgical staging or, in some circumstances, a physical examination, computed tomography (CT), and measurement of serum inhibin and CA-125 levels. If the results of all of these are negative, the decision may be made to observe the patient clinically, with or without hormonal suppression therapy using leuprolide acetate.[45]

General treatment guidelines: radiotherapy, chemotherapy, biological agents, multimodality agents

Since stromal tumors of the ovary are relatively rare, controlled clinical trials designed to determine which treatment regimens are best for certain histological subtypes are not feasible. Most published studies combine most or all subtypes of stromal ovarian tumors, and therefore treatment recommendations are based on limited data. Most data have been gathered from patients with adult granulosa cell tumors, but occasionally other tumor types are encountered, and treatment is generalized to these types as well.[11,24,37]

Most patients with surgical stage I disease do not require adjuvant treatment.[46] Patients with stage IC disease may benefit from some adjuvant therapy. Either platinum-based chemotherapy or hormonal therapy with leuprolide acetate has been recommended for this group of patients.[45]

Patients with more advanced disease are typically treated with combination chemotherapy. The data regarding platinum-based therapy originated in the 1970s and 1980s, with multiple investigators publishing anecdotal reports of several complete and partial responses to platinum-containing regimens, including vincristine, actinomycin-D, and cyclophosphamide (VAC), doxorubicin/cisplatin, cyclophosphamide, doxorubicin, cisplatin (CAP), and altretamine/cisplatin.[47-53] In 1986, Colombo investigated the combination of bleomycin, vinblastine, and cisplatin in patients treated upfront for advanced disease, and found that nine of 11 patients responded, although severe toxicity also occurred.[54] Subsequent trials used etoposide in place of vinblastine, and in 1996 Gershenson reported an 83% response rate in nine patients with advanced disease.[55] Subsequently, in 1999 Homesley reported on 57 evaluable patients with stage II–IV disease. Sixty-one percent of patients experienced grade 4 myelotoxicity, and 37% of patients had a negative second-look surgery. Thus, 69% of patients with advanced-stage primary and 51% of patients with recurrent disease remained

---

Box 36.2 Protocol for BEP (bleomycin, etoposide, and cisplatin).

Maintenance fluids of D5NS with $10\,mEq\,L^{-1}$ KCl and $8\,mEq\,L^{-1}$, magnesium sulfate at $42\,mL/h^{-1}$ are initiated on admission and continued during and for 24 h post chemotherapy.

Thirty minutes prior to cisplatin each day, prehydrate with 1 L normal saline with 20 mEq KCl and 16 mEq magnesium sulfate at $250\,mL\,h^{-1}$ for 4 h, and give:
- ondansetron 8 mg in 50 mL NS IVPB, and
- dexamethasone 20 mg in 50 mL NS IVPB, and
- diphenhydramine 50 mg in 50 mL NS.

Cisplatin $20\,mg/m^{-2}/day^{-1}$ in 1 L NS with 50 g mannitol IVPB over 4 h on days 1–5.
Etoposide $75–100\,mg/m^{-2}/day^{-1}$ in 500 mL NS IVPB over 2 h on days 1–5.
Bleomycin 10 IU in 1 L NS IVPB over 24 h on days 1–3.
Follow with:
- ondansetron 8 mg in 50 mL NS IVPB q8 h, and
- albuterol nebulizers 2.5 mg q6 h for 24 h, and
- prochlorperazine 10 mg in 50 mL NS IVPB q6 h prn nausea.

Regimen repeated every 28 days.

D5NS, 5% dextrose in normal saline; IVPB, intravenous piggyback; NS, normal saline; prn, *pro re nata*; q, every.

---

progression free. The progression-free interval was 24 months. As a result, many patients have been treated with three to four courses of bleomycin, etoposide, and cisplatin (BEP)[56] (Box 36.2). However, a recent report has shown paclitaxel and carboplatin to have good results and fewer toxic effects.[57] A randomized cooperative group trial comparing these two regimens is currently under way.

Patients with recurrent disease after a long disease-free interval may undergo secondary cytoreductive surgery, sometimes on multiple occasions.[58,59] This may require significant tumor debulking. In cases of widespread disease or disease refractory to surgery, treatment options include chemotherapy, hormonal therapy, and targeted agents. Although the response rate is higher earlier in the disease course and declines as the number of prior treatment regimens increases, paclitaxel in combination with carboplatin results in a 60% overall response rate with acceptable toxicity.[57] Other chemotherapeutic agents with demonstrated response include carboplatin; BEP; cisplatin, doxorubicin, and cyclophosphamide; etoposide and cisplatin; VAC; oral etoposide; topotecan; liposomal doxorubicin; paclitaxel; ifosfamide and etoposide.[45,58] Paclitaxel and carboplatin remain the most commonly used single agents at first and second relapse. Early in the treatment of recurrent disease, leuprolide acetate frequently results in the regression or stabilization of disease.[60] Bevacizumab has also demonstrated activity, alone and combined with cytotoxic agents, in the setting of recurrent disease.[61] Commonly used dosing schedules are listed in Table 36.1. Radiation therapy is also occasionally employed in the treatment of localized or symptomatic disease.[40,62–65]

Table 36.1 Common dosing schedules for chemotherapy, hormonal therapy, and targeted agents.

Agent	Dose	Route	Interval
Paclitaxel/carboplatin	175 mg/m^{-2}, AUC = 5	IV	Every 3 weeks
Paclitaxel	135–200 mg/m^{-2}	IV	Every 3 weeks
Paclitaxel	80–100 mg/m^{-2}	IV	Weekly
Carboplatin	AUC = 5	IV	Every 4 weeks
BEP	B 15 units day 1, E 75 mg/m^{-2} days 1–5, cisplatin 20 mg/m^{-2} days 1–5	IV	Every 3 weeks
PAC	Cisplatin 40–50 mg/m^{-2}, doxorubicin 40–50 mg/m^{-2}, cyclophosphamide 400 mg/m^{-2}	IV	Every 4 weeks
EP	Etoposide 100 mg/m^{-2}, cisplatin 75 mg/m^{-2}	IV	Every 4 weeks
VAC	Vincristine 1.5 mg/m^{-2} day 1,	IV	Every 2 weeks
	actinomycin-D 0.5 mg days 1–5,	IV	Every 4 weeks
	cyclophosphamide 150 mg/m^{-2} days 1–5	IV	Every 4 weeks
Oral etoposide	Etoposide 50 mg/m^{-2} day^{-1} × 21 days	PO	Every 21 days
Topotecan	Topotecan 1.5 mg/m^{-2} day^{-1} × 5 days	IV	Every 3 weeks
Doxil	Doxil 40 mg/m^{-2}	IV	Every 4 weeks
Ifosfamide/etoposide	Ifosfamide 1.2 g/m^{-2} day^{-1} × 5 days	IV	Every 3 weeks
	Etoposide 100 mg/m^{-2} day^{-1} × 5 days	IV	Every 3 weeks
Leuprolide acetate	7.5 mg	IM	Every 4 weeks
	or 22.5 mg	IM	Every 3 months
Bevacizumab	15 mg/kg	IV	Every 3 weeks

AUC, area under the curve; BEP, bleomycin, etoposide, and cisplatin; EP, etoposide and cisplatin; IM, intramuscular; IV, intravenous; PO, *per os*; VAC, vincristine, actinomycin-D, and cyclophosphamide.

Granulosa stromal cell tumors

Granulosa cell tumors

Granulosa cell tumors constitute between 2% and 5% of all ovarian cancers and represent 90% of stromal ovarian tumors.[40] The incidence of granulosa cell tumors varies from 0.58 to 1.6 cases per 100,000 women.[66,67] Most occur during the reproductive years, but they have been reported from infancy to the 10th decade of life. Granulosa cell tumors occur in two distinct histological varieties, adult (95%) and juvenile (5%).[32] The patient profile, histological appearance, natural history, and recommended treatment differ between these subtypes.

Adult granulosa cell tumors

Adult granulosa cell tumors represent 95% of granulosa cell tumors. They can occur at any age but are most common in perimenopausal women. Patients often present with abnormal vaginal bleeding, abdominal distension and/or pain, and occasionally signs of virilism.[11,68,69] Evaluation usually yields a solid adnexal mass. These tumors may rupture, resulting in hemoperitoneum and pain. If the patient has abnormal uterine bleeding, a preoperative endometrial biopsy or intraoperative endometrial curettage should be performed, as the excess estrogen produced by many granulosa cell tumors can lead to endometrial hyperplasia or malignancy. Up to 55% of patients have associated endometrial hyperplasia or polyps, independent of age; 4–20% of patients have a synchronous endometrial cancer, a risk identified in patients over 45 years of age.[34,70] If malignancy is encountered, the uterine cancer should also be addressed. A hysterectomy should be performed when child bearing is complete and in higher grade lesions. Hormonal therapy may be considered in the setting of low-grade endometrial cancer when fertility is desired.[71]

Occasionally, adult granulosa cell tumors are diagnosed during pregnancy.[72,73] In such patients, hormonal manifestations are less common, and the tumors are large and often complicated by rupture.[73]

The clinicopathological features of these tumors have been reported in several large series.[11,41,67,74–76] The overall 20-year survival approximates 40%. The stage at presentation is the strongest prognostic factor, with a 5–10-year survival over 90% for stage I, 55% for stage II, and 25% for stage III tumors. Two recent reviews, however, failed to identify stage as a prognostic factor in multifactorial analysis, but both reports included patients with Sertoli–Leydig cell tumors.[32,44] Adult-type granulosa cell tumors are characterized by late recurrence, and recurrence over a decade after the initial diagnosis is not unusual. The average time to recurrence is 5–10 years, but recurrence up to 30 years later has been reported.[77] A recent review of stromal ovarian tumors which included granulosa cell tumors and Sertoli–Leydig cell tumors found that important factors conferring a favorable prognosis include age less than 50 years, tumor size less than 10 cm, and absence of residual disease at the time of primary surgery.[32] Another recent report suggests that tumor size is the most important predictor of death, with no recurrences in patients with tumors less than 7 cm.[44] Other prognostic factors include tumor rupture and bilaterality. In patients with stage I disease, recurrences are rare for tumors less than 5 cm, but recurrence rates are 20% for tumors 5–15 cm in size and over 30% for tumors greater than 15 cm.[41]

Surgical recommendations are presented above. Since only 5% of adult granulosa cell tumors are bilateral, it is appropriate to conserve a normal-appearing uterus and contralateral ovary in a reproductive-age woman with apparent early-stage disease that is confirmed by frozen section analysis to be an adult granulosa cell tumor.[33,37,40,78] Surgical staging should be performed. Additionally, serum inhibin and CA-125 levels, if not obtained preoperatively, should be obtained after surgery, as they may be helpful in postoperative follow-up to confirm the resolution of disease and identify recurrence.

Even though there are no prospective randomized studies showing the value of radiotherapy in the treatment of granulosa cell tumors of the ovary, several retrospective studies have demonstrated that the use of radiation therapy may prolong disease-free survival in selected patients with advanced or recurrent disease.[40,62–65] In one study by Wolf et al.,[62] 14 patients with advanced or recurrent granulosa cell tumors were retrospectively evaluated. With a median follow-up time of 13 years, 10 patients were treated with whole abdominal/pelvic radiation therapy and four patients received only pelvic radiation therapy. Of these 14 patients, six achieved a complete clinical response and these responders were followed up for 5–12 years, and three of six patients remained in remission at the end of the study. The other three patients experienced relapse between 4 and 5 years after radiation. In another study,[63] 62 patients were evaluated, of whom eight received radiation therapy for advanced disease that was incompletely resected. Of the eight patients who received radiation therapy, four achieved a complete response, including three with disease-free intervals of at least 4 years. Even though these studies show an improvement with adjuvant radiation therapy, other studies have reported no benefit from adjuvant radiation therapy.[11,12,68]

Although adult granulosa cell tumors are indolent lesions, they can recur many years, even decades, following the initial diagnosis and treatment. Patients should be followed up at gradually increasing intervals with physical examinations and with serum inhibin A and CA-125 measurements.[24,79–81] Some have suggested that patients with granulosa cell tumors may be at increased risk for the development of breast cancer.[11,68] However, the risk has not been adequately characterized to amend screening criteria, so patients should follow routine breast screening recommendations. Additionally, one report exists of adult granulosa cell tumors of the ovary in two first-degree relatives, but this is an isolated instance and may not speak to the biology of the tumor.[82]

Recommendations for the treatment of recurrent disease are outlined above. If recurrence is diagnosed, eventual disease-related prognosis is poor, with previous statistics showing that over 70% of patients die despite treatment with chemotherapy, radiation, or both.[11] As noted above, secondary cytoreductive surgery, chemotherapy, radiation, hormonal therapy, and antiangiogenic agents all represent appropriate treatment approaches. Secondary cytoreductive surgery is most appropriate when there has been a relatively long disease-free interval and disease appears to be resectable.[83] If the patient is not a surgical candidate, or if disseminated or unresectable disease is present, or if postoperative chemotherapy is deemed appropriate, chemotherapy may be an option. Too little information exists to determine the best approach with certainty but given the largest reports, the best chemotherapeutic regimens seem to be platinum based. Either BEP, if not previously used, or a taxane-platinum combination may be the most appropriate chemotherapeutic regimen for recurrent disease, yielding similar response rates of 54% and 72%, respectively.[57]

Hormonal therapy has also been reported to be effective. Many adult granulosa cell tumors express steroid receptors, so treatment with gonadotropin-releasing hormone antagonists[45,84] and progestins[59] has been performed. Several responses to both categories of hormone have been reported. Responses to bevacizumab in patients with recurrent adult granulosa cell tumors have also been reported, and the results of a cooperative group trial are expected in the near future.[61]

The use of radiation for the treatment of recurrent disease has also been reported, with several responses noted. However, based on the small numbers of patients, the data are anecdotal, the response rates are short, and the impact on survival remains unknown.[40,47,62–65,83]

Juvenile granulosa cell tumors

Juvenile granulosa cell tumors represent only 5% of granulosa cell tumors, but are distinct from their adult counterpart in natural history and pathological characteristics. Juvenile granulosa cell tumors tend to occur in adolescents and teenagers, although most adolescents and young adults with ovarian malignancies do have germ cell tumors of the ovary. One study identified 38 cases of pediatric ovarian tumors, and 15% were stromal ovarian tumors, all of which were juvenile granulosa cell tumors.[85]

From a clinical perspective, these tumors are quite distinct from adult granulosa cell tumors. At the time of diagnosis, isosexual precocity is not unusual. They usually present with a palpable mass on pelvic or rectal examination, are unilateral in over 95% of cases, and most are diagnosed as stage IA tumors.[86,87] Even though the survival rate in patients with early-stage tumors is above 95%, patients should still be surgically staged, because advanced-stage tumors tend to be more aggressive and less responsive to treatment, with a shorter disease-free interval than adult-type tumors.

Platinum-based chemotherapy is recommended for any patient with disease over stage IA. Therefore, it is essential to stage each patient, in order not to miss any occult disease which would require treatment. Also, late relapses are unusual.

A clinical association has been described between juvenile granulosa cell tumors and Ollier disease (enchondromatosis) and Maffucci syndrome (enchondromatosis and hemangiomatosis). An increased risk for the development of breast cancer has also been reported.[88]

The gross appearance of these tumors resembles that of the adult variant. The most common presentation is a tumor with cystic and solid components. Uniformly solid tumors, uniformly cystic tumors, and hemorrhagic cysts can also occur. On microscopic examination, two cytological characteristics distinguish juvenile from adult granulosa cell tumors: the nuclei of juvenile granulosa cell tumors are rounded and hyperchromatic with moderate to abundant eosinophilic or vacuolated cytoplasm, and the cells are frequently luteinized.

Treatment of the patient with juvenile granulosa cell tumor follows the general treatment guidelines above. Over 95% of patients have unilateral disease, so conservative surgery (unilateral salpingo-oophorectomy) with preservation of fertility is almost always an option. Also, since the majority of these tumors occur in adolescent girls and young women, maintaining reproductive capacity without adversely affecting survival is of paramount importance. A complete staging procedure is a mandatory part of the procedure. In the rare patient with advanced disease, a total abdominal hysterectomy with bilateral salpingo-oophorectomy is necessary.

Again, most trials have combined adult and juvenile types, so specific treatment guidelines for the juvenile type cannot be suggested. The role of adjuvant treatment is not entirely clear, but it is recommended that all patients with over stage IA disease receive adjuvant chemotherapy, historically with BEP,[56] although a taxane/platinum combination may also be utilized as for adult granulosa cell tumors. Additionally one study has suggested that postoperative cisplatin-based chemotherapy may improve survival specifically for the juvenile granulosa cell tumor type.[27] Some have used methotrexate, dactinomycin, and cyclophosphamide with a suggested treatment benefit.[89] The role of radiation is largely unknown.

Unfortunately, when juvenile granulosa cell tumors recur, they usually do so after a shorter progression-free interval than is seen with adult granulosa cell tumors. Although many approaches to treatment have been used, including surgical cytoreduction, radiation therapy, and multiple chemotherapy regimens including high-dose chemotherapy, few sustained responses are seen in patients with recurrent juvenile granulosa cell disease. In our experience, responses have been achieved with BEP; paclitaxel and/or carboplatin; topotecan; bleomycin, vincristine, and cisplatin; etoposide and cisplatin; cisplatin, doxorubicin, and cyclophosphamide; high-dose chemotherapy; and gemcitabine.[58] According to a single report, patients with recurrent disease may benefit more from multiagent chemotherapy than single-agent chemotherapy.[27] Hormonal therapy with leuprolide acetate has resulted in several cases of stable disease.[45]

Overall, the prognosis for patients with juvenile granulosa cell tumor remains good but is related to stage. The 5-year survival for patients with stage IA disease is 99%, but this declines to 60% for patients with advanced disease.[27,87]

Thecomas/fibromas

This category of ovarian stromal tumor represents a spectrum of neoplasms with significant overlap which predominantly have clinically benign behavior and are derived from ovarian stromal cells. These tumors share many similar clinical characteristics and often cannot be assigned to either the distinct thecoma or fibroma category based on the clinical or microscopic examination.

Thecomas

Thecomas represent approximately 1% of ovarian neoplasms. Most cases occur in postmenopausal women,[11,90] and only 10% of patients are under the age of 30 years. Thecomas are often hormonally active and may cause abnormal vaginal bleeding, which is the most common presenting symptom. Additionally, 37–50% of patients with thecomas have endometrial hyperplasia and up to 27% have an associated endometrial carcinoma.[11,90,91] Therefore, just as in granulosa cell tumors, patients presenting with abnormal bleeding should always have the endometrium sampled. Thecomas may also contain a population of luteinized cells (see Box 36.1), and these luteinized thecomas may be androgenic and cause virilization.[92] Radiographically, most tumors (79%) are solid on CT and show delayed accumulation of contrast material.[93] Some have suggested that the diagnosis can be suggested by poor penetration of the mass with acoustic shadowing on ultrasound.[94] The specific radiological diagnosis, however, is nonspecific.

Histologically, thecomas are composed of lipid-laden stromal cells with abundant pale cytoplasm. Their clinical behavior is usually benign and the prognosis is excellent. Occasionally, tumors may exhibit nuclear atypia and mitoses but fibrosarcomas and luteinized granulosa cell tumors should be ruled out in these cases.[95]

Because these tumors have a benign course, surgical resection alone without staging or adjuvant treatment is the appropriate therapy. Given the age distribution for patients with this tumor, preservation of fertility is not usually an issue. Conservative management may include only removal of the ovary or ovaries, but then the endometrium should be sampled with a dilation and curettage. If the patient has associated endometrial hyperplasia or carcinoma, or if she is postmenopausal, a total hysterectomy and bilateral salpingo-oophorectomy is appropriate.[33]

Fibromas

The most common stromal tumor of the ovary is the fibroma, representing 4% of all ovarian neoplasms. These are usually benign, unilateral, and hormonally inactive tumors. The mean age at diagnosis is 48 years. Clinically, patients present with pelvic heaviness or pain and a mass. Gross examination reveals the tumors to be solid and white, although degenerative cystic cavities are not uncommon. The average size is 6 cm but size increases with the age at diagnosis.[96] The presence of ascites is not uncommon, and it tends to occur with increasing tumor size; for example, ascites is present in 30% of patients with tumors greater than 6 cm. One percent of patients will develop a hydrothorax, called Meigs syndrome.[97]

Cellular fibroma/fibrosarcoma

Approximately 10% of fibromas will show light microscope evidence of hypercellularity, as well as mitoses. Tumors of low malignant potential are designated as those with an increased cellular density, only mild nuclear atypia, and less than three mitotic figures per 10 high-power fields. Fully malignant fibrosarcomas have increased cellularity, marked pleomorphism, and frequent mitotic figures. The presence of trisomy 8 found in fibrosarcoma may be useful in distinguishing between the diagnosis of fibroma and fibrosarcoma.[98] In contrast to the benign fibroma, fibrosarcomas are highly aggressive tumors.[99] They are usually large, unilateral, and highly vascular. At the time of surgery, rupture, adhesions, hemorrhage, and necrosis are often seen.

Fibrothecoma

As noted above, fibromas and thecomas represent a spectrum of neoplasms. It is not unusual for patients to have evidence of a mixed tumor with elements of fibroma and thecoma within one ovarian tumor. These are also benign, and are treated with definitive surgery alone. They do not require adjuvant treatment and do not recur or metastasize.[33]

Sertoli stromal cell tumors

Sertoli stromal cell tumors are also known as androblastomas, and they represent a group of tumors which differentiate toward testicular structures. They are more commonly referred to as Sertoli–Leydig cell tumors, and they may contain only Sertoli cells, or both Sertoli and Leydig cells. These rare tumors represent less than 1% of all ovarian tumors. As noted in Box 36.1, they are classified into five groups: well differentiated, intermediately differentiated, poorly differentiated, retiform, and mixed. Well-differentiated tumors include Sertoli cell tumors and Sertoli–Leydig cell tumors.

Sertoli–Leydig cell tumors tend to occur in young women with a mean age of 25 years. Well-differentiated tumors tend to occur approximately 10 years later than intermediate or poorly differentiated tumors. Conversely, the retiform type is usually diagnosed at a younger age than intermediate or poorly differentiated types.[100,101] Pure Sertoli tumors are diagnosed in young women, and Sertoli–Leydig tumors tend to occur in women in their teens and 20s. Thus, fertility preservation is very important for many of these patients, and this is usually appropriate as over 95% of all tumors are unilateral with a normal uterus.[37,78]

Upon presentation, approximately 50% of patients demonstrate virilization. The differential diagnosis includes adrenal and gonadal hyperplasia and a neoplasm. The presence of a unilateral adnexal mass, however, palpated on examination or visualized on imaging, suggests an ovarian neoplasm as the source of the virilization. The size of the tumor, however, does not predict the ability to cause virilization, so a very small neoplasm can be responsible for a significant testosterone elevation and cause virilization.[101]

The evaluation of a patient with virilization, or androgen excess, includes a transvaginal pelvic ultrasound to visualize the ovaries. Also, serum dehydroepiandrostenedione sulfate (DHEA-S) and testosterone levels should be measured. An elevated DHEA-S suggests that the adrenal gland is the source of the androgen excess. Conversely, an elevated testosterone suggests an ovarian source. A CT scan may visualize an adrenal mass responsible for secretion of DHEA-S. Additional studies helpful in the workup of virilization include 17-OH progesterone (elevated in congenital adrenal hyperplasia) and cortisol (elevated in Cushing disease). Prior to surgical intervention, the offending mass should be detected by imaging or physical examination. It has been suggested that ovarian vein catheter studies can be helpful in detecting the source if the imaging and examination are unrevealing.

Gross examination shows Sertoli–Leydig cell tumors to be solid or mixed cystic and solid, with no features pathognomonic for Sertoli–Leydig cell tumors on visual inspection. The size is variable, ranging from microscopic to 25 cm.[101,102] Well-differentiated tumors tend to be smaller, and poorly differentiated tumors tend to be larger.[100] Microscopic examination shows that well-differentiated tumors, which account for 11% of cases, have a predominantly tubular pattern. The Sertoli cells are cuboidal or columnar with round nuclei, but with no prominent nucleoli. Atypical nuclei are absent or rare and few mitotic figures are seen. The stroma contains nests of Leydig cells.

As seen in Box 36.1, the most common variants are intermediate differentiation (54%) and poor differentiation (13%). These subgroups are characterized by a continuum of different patterns and combinations of cell types, with both Sertoli and Leydig components exhibiting various degrees of maturity. A retiform component is present in 15% of tumors, demonstrating tubules and cysts arranged in a pattern that resembles the rete testis. Twenty-two percent of cases contain heterologous elements, most commonly mucinous glands.

Management of patients with Sertoli Leydig cell tumors follows the guidelines above. In young patients, fertility is of course a significant issue. In young patients, a unilateral salpingo-oophorectomy and staging is usually appropriate, as 95% of lesions are unilateral.[37,78] However, in patients who have completed their child bearing, a total hysterectomy and bilateral salpingo-oophorectomy with staging procedure is the procedure of choice.[33] Patients with stage IA well-differentiated tumors do not require adjuvant therapy. Patients with stage IC disease or greater, with poorly differentiated tumors of any stage or with heterologous elements present, have a 50–60% risk of recurrence.[24] Owing to the rare nature of the disease and the lack of controlled trials, there is little scientific support for any treatment approach; however, adjuvant therapy seems reasonable given the substantial risk of recurrence. Radiation and hormone therapy have been described[100,103] but there is very limited information upon which to base treatment. Information regarding chemotherapy on these patients is available only as part of the larger, previously cited studies and therefore, it is our practice to administer adjuvant therapy in the form of 3–4 courses of BEP or six courses of paclitaxel and carboplatin to these patients.

Stage is clearly the most important prognostic factor. At the time of diagnosis, over 90% of patients have stage IA disease. This is largely dependent on grade; in one series, every patient with a well-differentiated tumor was uniformly stage IA but only 52% of patients with poorly differentiated tumors were stage IA.[104] There have been no reported patients with advanced stages or recurrence, and only one death from disease has been reported in a patient with a well-differentiated tumor. However, 10% of intermediate, 60% of poorly differentiated, and 20% of retiform and heterologous subtypes show malignant behavior, leading to the recommendation for adjuvant treatment in these groups. Other poor prognostic factors include the presence of thyroid nodules, tumor size, mitotic activity, tumor rupture, features of rhabdomyosarcoma, and other heterologous elements, especially when containing mesenchymal elements. One report of familial occurrence has been reported.[100,105,106]

Patients with Sertoli–Leydig cell tumors can be followed up with physical examination and with serum α-fetoprotein, inhibin, and testosterone level measurement. Eighteen percent of patients with Sertoli–Leydig cell tumors recur, and of those that recur, two-thirds do so within the first year. Platinum-based chemotherapy is the mainstay of treatment upon recurrence, but anecdotal reports show that outcomes are poor for patients with recurrent disease.[24]

Sex cord tumor with annular tubules

The group of tumors known as ovarian SCTAT represents a separate category of sex cord stromal tumors which was first described by Scully in 1970.[3] It is controversial whether these tumors are more closely related to granulosa cell tumors or Sertoli–Leydig cell tumors, as the cellular elements appear to be somewhat intermediate in nature, but they do seem to represent a distinct entity.

Microscopically, these tumors are characterized by either simple or complex ring-shaped tubules surrounding hyalinized basement membrane material. The clinical presentation is usually related to abnormal vaginal bleeding. Abdominal pain and intussusception have been reported but are less common. These tumors are uncommon in the adolescent population but can present with isosexual precocity.

Clinically, there appear to be two subgroups of ovarian SCTATs. The first subgroup is associated with Peutz–Jeghers syndrome and is typically multifocal, bilateral, and almost always benign. These tumors are small and rarely palpable on examination. Patients with this tumor should be carefully screened for adenoma malignum of the cervix, as up to 15% of patients may have an occult lesion.[4] Therefore, hysterectomy should be strongly considered in these patients.

The second subgroup of ovarian SCTATs occurs incidentally, independent from Peutz–Jeghers syndrome. These tumors are usually larger and have a significant potential for malignant behavior. The cornerstone of treatment remains surgical resection, following the general guidelines above.

These tumors tend to remain lateralized and have a tendency toward lymphatic spread. A percentage of these tumors recur and metastasize. Müllerian-inhibiting substance and inhibin are useful tumor markers. If the tumor recurs, repeat cytoreductive surgery is usually warranted. Chemotherapy remains unproved outside anecdotal cases.[107]

Gynandroblastoma

Gynandroblastomas are a separate, rare entity composed of granulosa cell elements and Sertoli cells. The specific cell of origin remains debated, but it may arise from undifferentiated mesenchyme.[108] Gynandroblastomas are responsible for less than 1% of all ovarian stromal tumors.

Microscopically, these combine elements of both "male and female directed cells."[109] These tumors must show unequivocal granulosa and Sertoli cell elements, must be well differentiated, and must demonstrate intimate mixing of the constituent cell types.

Clinically, signs and symptoms are related to estrogen and androgen overproduction. Most patients are in their third to fifth decades of life.[108,110,111] Androgen excess is present in 60% of patients with gynandroblastoma. Therefore, virilization is visible, but estrogenic stimulation of specific end organs still occurs, so endometrial hyperplasia is commonly noted.[112] Most of these tumors are solid and large, measuring between 7 and 10 cm in size, with yellow-white cystic areas present. Also, most gynandroblastomas are appreciated on pelvic examination because of their size.

These tumors should also be staged and aggressively cytoreduced. Since these tumors are so uncommon, a distinct preoperative diagnosis of gynandroblastoma would be uncommon. However, the workup is similar to that of other patients with androgen excess and a unilateral adnexal mass. Preoperative testing usually reveals elevated levels of testosterone[108,112,113] or urinary 17-ketosteroids.[109] Elevated androstenedione, dehydroepiandrosterone, dihydrotestosterone, and estradiol have also been variably reported.[114–116] Immunohistochemistry may demonstrate positivity for vimentin and inhibin in the granulosa cell component, with cytokeratin AE1/AE3 positive in the Sertoli component. CD99, calretinin, and reticulin may be focally positive. The tumor may be negative for epithelial membrane antigen (EMA), chromogranulin, and Melan-A.[117]

As with the other tumor types in this group, surgery is the cornerstone of therapy, and general guidelines can be followed as outlined above. In young women where reproductive function is important, a unilateral salpingo-oophorectomy and staging procedure is advocated. In postreproductive patients, hysterectomy and bilateral salpingo-oophorectomy is indicated, and in patients with advanced disease, cytoreductive surgery is appropriate. Patients with advanced disease are treated with adjuvant treatment, although the data are very limited.[112] Anecdotal reports of P32 and cyclophosphamide, actinomycin-D, and vincristine combination chemotherapy have been published. Serum estrogens or androgens can be followed as tumor markers. Recurrence is unusual but may be late, as in other stromal tumors with low-grade clinical behavior.[117]

Steroid (lipid) cell tumor

Steroid, or lipid, cell tumors consist of three lesions based on their cell of origin and microscopic features: stromal luteomas, Leydig cell tumors, and steroid cell tumors not otherwise specified (NOS). Together these three entities represent less than 0.1% of all ovarian tumors.

Stromal luteoma

Stromal luteomas are often small, with half of them being less than 5 cm.[118] Microscopically, they consist of large, rounded or polyhedral cells resembling Leydig cells, luteinized ovarian stromal cells, and adrenocortical cells. They represent approximately 25% of steroid cell tumors and have been identified during pregnancy. Most patients, however, are postmenopausal at the time of diagnosis. These tumors are benign steroid cell tumors that do not require staging or postoperative therapy. Child-bearing potential should be maintained in the occasional young patient with this diagnosis.[24]

Leydig cell tumor

Leydig cell tumors represent 15–20% of all steroid cell tumors of the ovary. They are subdivided into tumors of hilar and non-hilar type, and both are benign. Clinically, they are unilateral with a median size of less than 3 cm.[119–121] This tumor often presents in postmenopausal patients. Histologically, they consist only of Leydig cells, and crystals of Reinke are seen. These tumors are benign steroid cell tumors that do not require staging or postoperative therapy. Child-bearing potential should be maintained in the occasional young patient with this diagnosis.

Steroid cell tumors not otherwise specified

Steroid cell tumors NOS are a category of steroid cell tumor that can be malignant and aggressive. These are the most common type of steroid cell tumor and therefore, when a steroid cell tumor is diagnosed intraoperatively, it should be staged and aggressively cytoreduced. Histologically, these lipid cell tumors lack the specific characteristics of stromal luteomas or Leydig cell tumors. Clinically, they present at an earlier age, with a mean age of 43 years, and are larger than the other steroid cell tumors with an average size of 8.5 cm. Bilaterality is not infrequent. In the largest series, 43% of patients demonstrated extraovarian disease either at diagnosis or during surveillance. Negative prognostic factors included age, size, increased mitosis, and presence of necrosis.[122] The strongest prognostic factor other than stage is the number of mitotic figures, since over 90% of tumors with over two mitoses per 10 high-power fields are malignant. Stage IA tumors in women of reproductive age should be staged, and a unilateral salpingo-oophorectomy is appropriate. Patients not opting for future fertility require hysterectomy and bilateral salpingo-oophorectomy with staging, and patients with advanced disease require cytoreductive surgery. Although all reports are anecdotal, patients with tumors that are pleomorphic, have an increased mitotic count, are large, or are at an advanced stage should be treated with additional postoperative platinum-based chemotherapy.[123] Radiation, melphalan, and hormonal therapy have also been used with variable outcomes.[124–126]

Recommendations

Most ovarian stromal tumors are clinically indolent and are reported to have a good long-term prognosis. However, many occur in adolescent and reproductive-aged women, and therefore individualized treatment with consideration for fertility preservation is of great importance. Appropriate treatment guidelines based on current information have been presented in this chapter.

Since this category represents a wide range of disease entities, broad generalizations regarding prognosis and treatment recommendations cannot be made. So our approach to the management of these cases is to follow these general guidelines for appropriate treatment of patients with ovarian stromal tumors, and to undertake disease-specific therapy once the final pathology is identified.

Knowledge remains limited regarding this rare group of diseases. However, with continuing commitment from dedicated scientists and cooperative groups in order to perform high-quality research, progressively better treatment will become available and more information will be known.

References

1. Meyer R. Pathology of some special ovarian tumors and their relation to sex characteristics. Am J Obstet Gynecol 1931; 22: 697.
2. Morris JM, Scully RE. *Endocrine Pathology of the Ovary*. St Louis, MO: CV Mosby, 1958.
3. Scully RE. Sex cord tumor with annular tubules: a distinctive ovarian tumor of the Peutz–Jeghers syndrome. Cancer 1970; 25: 1107.
4. Srivasta PJ, Keeney GL, Podratz KC. Disseminated cervical adenoma malignum and bilateral ovarian sex cord tumors with annular tubules associated with Peutz–Jeghers syndrome. Gynecol Oncol 1994; 53: 256.
5. Young RH, Path FRC, Scully RE. Sex cord-stromal, steroid cell, and other ovarian tumors with endocrine, paraendocrine, and paraneoplastic manifestations. In: Kurman RJ (ed) *Blaustein's Pathology of the Female Genital Tract*. New York: Springer-Verlag, 1994. p.783.
6. World Health Organization. *International Histologic Classification of Tumors*, vol. 9. Geneva: World Health Organization, 1973.
7. Young RH, Scully RE. Endocrine tumors of the ovary. Curr Top Pathol 1992; 85: 113–64.
8. Siegel R, *et al.* Cancer statistics, 2012. CA Cancer J Clin 2012; 62: 10–29.
9. O'Leary M, *et al.* Female genital system cancers. In: Bleyer A (ed) *Adolescent and Young Adult Cancer Monograph*. New York: Springer-Verlag, 2005.
10. Koonings PP, *et al.* Relative frequency of primary ovarian neoplasms: a 10-year review. Obstet Gynecol 1989; 74: 921–6.
11. Evans AT, *et al.* Clinicopathological review of 118 granulosa and 82 thecal cell tumors. Obstet Gynecol 1980; 55: 231.
12. Malmstrom H, *et al.* Granulosa cell tumors of the ovary; prognostic factors and outcome. Gynecol Oncol 1994; 52: 50–5.
13. Miller BE, *et al.* Prognostic factors in adult granulosa cell tumor of the ovary. Cancer 1997; 79: 1951–5.
14. King LA, *et al.* Mitotic count, nuclear atypia, and immunohisto-chemical determination of Ki-67, c-myc, p21-ras, c-erbB2, and p53 expression in granulosa cell tumors of the ovary: mitotic count and Ki-67 are indicators of poor prognosis. Gynecol Oncol 1996; 61: 227–32.
15. Evans MP, *et al.* DNA ploidy of ovarian granulosa cell tumors: lack of correlation between DNA index or proliferative index and outcome in 40 patients. Cancer 1995; 75: 2295–8.
16. Costa MJ, *et al.* Transformation in recurrent ovarian granulosa cell tumors: Ki67 (MIB-1) and p53 immunohistochemistry demonstrates a possible molecular basis for the poor histologic prediction of clinical behavior. Hum Pathol 1996; 27: 274–81.

17. Roush GR, El-Naggar AK, Abdul-Karim FW. Granulosa cell tumor of ovary: a clinicopathologic and flow cytometric DNA analysis. Gynecol Oncol 1995; 56: 430–4.

18. Liu FS, et al. Overexpression of p53 is not a feature of ovarian granulosa cell tumors. Gynecol Oncol 1996; 61: 50–3.

19. Fletcher JA, et al. Ovarian granulosa-stromal cell tumors are characterized by trisomy 12. Am J Pathol 1991; 138: 515–20.

20. Persons DL, et al. Fluorescence in situ hybridization analysis of trisomy 12 in ovarian tumors. Am J Clin Pathol 1994; 102: 775–9.

21. Lindgren V, Waggoner S, Rotmensch J. Monosomy 22 in two ovarian granulosa cell tumors. Cancer Genet Cytogenet 1996; 89: 93–7.

22. Teyssier JR, et al. Chromosomal changes in an ovarian granulosa cell tumor: similarity with carcinoma. Cancer Genet Cytogenet 1985; 14: 147.

23. Lin YS, et al. Molecular cytogenetics of ovarian granulosa cell tumors by comparative genomic hybridization. Gynecol Oncol 2005; 97: 68–73.

24. Brown J, Gershenson DM. Treatment for rare ovarian malignancies. In: Eifel PJ, Gershenson DM, Kavanagh JJ, Silva EG (eds) M. D. Anderson Cancer Care Series Gynecologic Cancer. New York: Springer-Verlag, 2006.

25. Rodriguez E, Rao P, Reuter V. Cytogenetic analysis of a juvenile granulosa cell tumor. Cancer Genet Cytogenet 1992; 61: 207.

26. Zaloudek C, Norris HJ. Granulosa cell tumors of the ovary in children: a clinical and pathologic study of 32 cases. Am J Surg Pathol 1982; 6: 503.

27. Calaminus G, et al. Juvenile granulosa cell tumors of the ovary in children and adolescents: results from 33 patients registered in a prospective cooperative study. Gynecol Oncol 1997; 65: 447–52.

28. Kalfa N, et al. The new molecular biology of granulosa cell tumors of the ovary. Genome Med 2009; 1(8): 81.

29. Shah SP, et al. Mutation of FOXL2 in granulosa-cell tumors of the ovary. N Engl J Med 2009; 360: 2719–29.

30. Schultz KAP, et al. Ovarian sex cord-stromal tumors, pleuropulmonary blastoma and DICER1 mutations: a report from the International Pleuropulmonary Blastoma Registry. Gynecol Oncol 2011; 122: 246–50.

31. Izutsu T, et al. Numerical and structural chromosome abnormalities in an ovarian fibrothecoma. Cancer Genet Cytogenet 1995; 83: 84.

32. Chan JK, et al. Prognostic factors responsible for survival in sex cord stromal tumors of the ovary – a multivariate analysis. Gynecol Oncol 2005; 96: 204–9.

33. Gershenson DM, Hartmann LC, Young RH. Ovarian sex cord-stromal tumors. In: Hoskins WJ, Perez CA, Young RC (eds) Principles and Practice of Gynecologic Oncology, 4th edn. Philadelphia: Lippincott Williams and Wilkins, 2004.

34. Unkila-Kallio L, et al. Reproductive features in women developing ovarian granulosa cell tumour at a fertile age. Hum Reprod 2000; 15: 589–93.

35. Robertson DM, McNeilage J. Inhibins as biomarkers for reproductive cancers. Semin Reprod Med 2004; 22: 219–25.

36. Choi K, et al. Ovarian granulosa cell tumor presenting as Meigs' syndrome with elevated CA125. Korean J Intern Med 2005; 20: 105–9.

37. Gershenson DM. Fertility-sparing surgery for malignancies in women. J Natl Cancer Inst Monogr 2005; 34: 43–7.

38. Canis M, et al. A 12 year experience with long term follow-up. Obstet Gynecol 1994; 83: 707–12.

39. Mettler L, Semm K, Shive K. Endoscopic management of adnexal masses. J Soc Laparosc Surg 1997; 2: 103–12.

40. Schumer ST, Cannistra SA. Granulosa cell tumor of the ovary. J Clin Oncol 2003; 21: 1180–9.

41. Bjorkholm E, Silfversward C. Prognostic factors in granulosa-cell tumors. Gynecol Oncol 1981; 11: 261–74.

42. Abu-Rustum NR, et al. Retroperitoneal nodal metastasis in primary and recurrent granulosa cell tumors of the ovary. Gynecol Oncol 2006; 103: 31–4.

43. Brown J, et al. Patterns of metastasis in sex cord-stromal tumors of the ovary: can routine staging lymphadenectomy be omitted? Gynecol Oncol 2009; 113: 86–90.

44. Thrall MM, et al. Patterns of spread and recurrence of sex cord-stromal tumors of the ovary. Gynecol Oncol 2011; 122: 242–5.

45. Fishman A, et al. Leuprolide acetate for treating refractory or persistent ovarian granulosa cell tumor. J Reprod Med 1996; 41(6): 393–6.

46. Herbst AL. Neoplastic diseases of the ovary. In: Mishell DR, et al. (eds) Comprehensive Gynecology, 3rd edn. New York: Mosby-Year Book Inc., 1997.

47. Schwartz PE, Smith JP. Treatment of ovarian stromal tumors. Am J Obstet Gynecol 1976; 125: 402–11.

48. Slayton RE. Management of germ cell and stromal tumors of the ovary. Semin Oncol 1984; 11: 299–313.

49. Jacobs AJ, Deppe G, Cohen CJ. Combination chemotherapy of ovarian granulosa cell tumor with cis-platinum and doxorubicin. Gynecol Oncol 1982; 14: 294–7.

50. Camlibel FT, Caputo TA. Chemotherapy of granulosa cell tumors. Am J Obstet Gynecol 1983; 145: 763–5.

51. Neville AJ, Gilchrist KW, Davis TE. The chemotherapy of granulosa cell tumors of the ovary: experience of the Wisconsin Clinical Cancer Center. Med Pediatr Oncol 1984; 12: 397–400.

52. Kaye SB, Davies E. Cyclophosphamide, adriamycin, and cisplatinum for the treatment of advanced granulosa cell tumors, using serum estradiol as a tumor marker. Gynecol Oncol 1986; 24: 261–4.

53. Gershenson DM, et al. Treatment of metastatic stromal tumors of the ovary with cisplatin, doxorubicin, and cyclophosphamide. Obstet Gynecol 1987; 70: 765–9.

54. Colombo N, et al. Cisplatin, vinblastine, and bleomycin combination chemotherapy in metastatic granulosa cell tumor of the ovary. Obstet Gynecol 1986; 37: 265–8.

55. Gershenson DM, et al. Treatment of poor-prognosis sex cord-stromal tumors of the ovary with the combination of bleomycin, etoposide, and cisplatin. Obstet Gynecol 1996; 87: 527–31.

56. Homesley HD, et al. Bleomycin, etoposide, and cisplatin combination chemotherapy of ovarian granulosa cell tumors and other stromal malignancies: a Gynecologic Oncology Group study. Gynecol Oncol 1999; 72: 131–7.

57. Brown J, et al. The activity of taxanes compared with bleomycin, etoposide, and cisplatin in the treatment of sex cord-stromal ovarian tumors. Gynecol Oncol 2005; 97: 489–96.

58. Brown J, et al. The activity of taxanes in the treatment of sex cord-stromal ovarian tumors. J Clin Oncol 2004; 22: 3517–23.

59. Fotopoulou C, et al. Adult granulosa cell tumors of the ovary: tumor dissemination pattern at primary and recurrent situation, surgical outcome. Gynecol Oncol 2010; 119: 285–90.

60. Tresukosol D, et al. Recurrent ovarian granulosa cell tumor: a case report of a dramatic response to Taxol. Int J Gynecol Cancer 1995; 5: 156–9.

61. Tao X, et al. Anti-angiogenesis therapy with bevacizumab for patients with ovarian granulosa cell tumors. Gynecol Oncol 2009; 114: 431–6.

62. Wolf JK, et al. Radiation treatment of advanced or recurrent granulosa cell tumor of the ovary. Gynecol Oncol 1999; 73: 35–41.

63. Savage P, et al. Granulosa cell tumors of the ovary: demographics, survival, and the management of advanced disease. Clin Oncol (R Coll Radiol) 1998; 10: 242–5.

64. Lee IW, et al. Radiotherapy for the treatment of metastatic granulosa cell tumor in the mediastinum: a case report. Gynecol Oncol 1999; 73: 455–60.

65. Wessalowski R, et al. Successful liver treatment of a juvenile granulosa cell tumor in a 4-year-old child by regional deep hyperthermia, systemic chemotherapy, and irradiation. Gynecol Oncol 1995; 57: 417–22.

66. Stenwig JT, Hazekamp JT, Beecham JB. Granulosa cell tumors of the ovary: a clinicopathologic study in 118 cases with long term follow-up. Gynecol Oncol 1979; 7: 136.

67. Bjorkholm E, Silfversward C. Granulosa and theca cell tumors: incidence and occurrence of second primary tumors. Acta Radiol Oncol 1980; 19: 161.

68. Ohel G, Kaneti H, Schenker JG. Granulosa cell tumors in Israel: a study of 172 cases. Gynecol Oncol 1983; 15: 278.

69. Nakashima N, Young RH, Scully RE. Androgenic granulosa cell tumors of the ovary. Arch Pathol Lab Med 1984; 108: 786.

70. Gusberg SB, Kardon P. Proliferative endometrial response to thecagranulosa cell tumors. Am J Obstet Gynecol 1971; 111: 633.

71. Ramirez PT, et al. Hormonal therapy for the management of grade 1 endometrial adenocarcinoma: a literature review. Gynecol Oncol 2004; 95: 133–8.

72. Tanyi J, et al. Trisomy 12 in juvenile granulosa cell tumor of the ovary during pregnancy. A report of 2 cases. J Reprod Med 1999; 44: 826–32.

73. Young RH, Dudley AG, Scully RE. Granulosa cell, Sertoli–Leydig cell, and unclassified sex cord stromal tumors associated with pregnancy: a clinicopathologic analysis of thirty six cases. Gynecol Oncol 1984; 18: 181.

74. Norris HJ, Taylor HB. Prognosis of granulosa-theca cell tumors of the ovary. Cancer 1968; 21: 255.

75. Fox H, Agrawal K, Langley FA. A clinicopathologic study of 92 cases of granulosa cell tumor of the ovary with special reference to the factors influencing prognosis. Cancer 1975; 35: 231.

76. Dempster J, Geirsson RT, Duncan ID. Survival after ovarian granulosa and theca cell tumors. Scott Med J 1987; 32: 38–9.

77. Bjorkholm E. Granulosa cell tumors: a comparison of survival in patients and matched controls. Am J Obstet Gynecol 1980; 138: 329.

78. Gershenson DM. Management of early ovarian cancer: germ cell and sex cord stromal tumors. Gynecol Oncol 1994; 55(Suppl): S62–72.

79. Lappohn RE, et al. Inhibin as a marker for granulosa cell tumors. N Engl J Med 1989; 321: 790.

80. Jobling T, et al. A prospective study of inhibin in granulosa cell tumors of the ovary. Gynecol Oncol 1994; 55: 285.

81. Boggess JF, et al. Serum inhibin and disease status in women with ovarian granulosa cell tumors. Gynecol Oncol 1997; 64: 64.

82. Stevens TA, et al. Adult granulosa cell tumors of the ovary in two first-degree relatives. Gynecol Oncol 2005; 98: 502–5.

83. Pankratz E, et al. Granulosa cell tumors: a clinical review of 61 cases. Obstet Gynecol 1978; 52: 718.

84. Martikainen H, et al. Gonadotropin-releasing hormone agonist analog therapy effective in ovarian granulosa cell malignancy. Gynecol Oncol 1989; 35: 406.

85. Gribbon M, Ein SH, Mancer K. Pediatric malignant ovarian tumors: a 43-year review. J Pediatr Surg 1992; 27: 480.

86. Young RH, Dickersin GR, Scully RE. Juvenile granulosa cell tumor of the ovary. Am J Surg Pathol 1984; 8: 575.

87. Lack EE, et al. Granulosa theca cell tumors in premenarchal girls: a clinical and pathological study of ten cases. Cancer 1981; 48: 1846.

88. Schoefield DE, Fletcher JA. Trisomy 12 in pediatric granulosa-stromal cell tumors. Am J Pathol 1992; 141: 1265.

89. Vassal G, et al. Juvenile granulosa cell tumor of the ovary in children: a clinical study of 15 cases. J Clin Oncol 1988; 6: 990–5.

90. Bjorkholm E, Silfversward C. Theca cell tumors: clinical features and prognosis. Acta Radiol 1980; 19: 241.

91. Stage AH, Grafton WD. Thecomas and granulosa-theca cell tumors of the ovary: an analysis of 51 tumors. Obstet Gynecol 1977; 50: 21.

92. Zhang J, et al. Ovarian stromal tumors containing lutein or Leydig cells – a clinicopathologic analysis of fifty cases. Int J Gynecol Pathol 1982; 1: 270.

93. Bazot M, et al. Fibrothecomas of the ovary: CT and US findings. J Comput Assist Tomogr 1993; 17: 754.

94. Yaghoobian J, Pinck RL. Ultrasound findings in thecoma of the ovary. J Clin Ultrasound 1983; 11: 91.

95. Waxman M, et al. Ovarian low grade stromal sarcoma with thecomatous features. Cancer 1979; 44: 2206.

96. Dockherty MB, Masson JC. Ovarian fibromas: a clinical and pathologic study of two hundred and eighty three cases. Am J Obstet Gynecol 1944; 47: 741.

97. Meigs JV. Fibroma of the ovary with ascites and hydrothorax – Meigs syndrome. Am J Obstet Gynecol 1954; 67: 962.

98. Tsuji T, et al. Fibrosarcoma versus cellular fibroma of the ovary: a comparative study of their proliferative activity and chromosome aberrations using MIB-1 immunostaining, NDA flow cytometry, and fluorescence in situ hybridization. Am J Surg Pathol 1997; 21: 52.

99. Prat J, Scully RE. Cellular fibromas and fibrosarcomas of the ovary. Cancer 1981; 47: 2663.

100. Zaloudek C, Norris HJ. Sertoli–Leydig tumors of the ovary: a clinicopathologic study of 64 intermediate and poorly differentiated neoplasms. Am J Surg Pathol 1984; 8: 405.

101. Roth LM, et al. Sertoli–Leydig cell tumors: a clinicopathologic study of 34 cases. Cancer 1981; 48: 187.

102. O'Hern TM, Neubecker RD. Arrhenoblastoma. Obstet Gynecol 1962; 19: 758.

103. Emons G, Schally AV. The use of luteinizing hormone releasing hormone agonists and antagonists in gynaecological cancers. Hum Reprod 1994; 9: 1364.

104. Gordon MD, Ireland K. New developments in sex cord-stromal and germ cell tumors of the ovary. Clin Lab Med 1995; 15: 595.

105. O'Brien PK, Wilansky DL. Familial thyroid nodulation and arrhenoblastoma. Am J Clin Pathol 1981; 75: 578.

106. Goldstein DD, Lamb EJ. Arrhenoblastoma in first cousins: report of 2 cases. Obstet Gynecol 1970; 35: 444.

107. Puls LE, et al. Recurrent ovarian sex cord tumor with annular tubules: tumor marker and chemotherapy experience. Gynecol Oncol 1994; 54: 396.

108. Anderson MC, Rees DA. Gynandroblastoma of the ovary. Br J Obstet Gynaecol 1975; 82: 68.

109. Neubecker RD, Breen JL. Gynandroblastoma. Am J Clin Pathol 1962; 38: 60.

110. Emig OR, Hertig AT, Rowe FJ. Gynandroblastoma of the ovary. Am J Pathol 1943; 19: 633.

111. Emig OR, Hertig AT, Rowe FJ. Gynandroblastoma of the ovary. Review and report of a case. Obstet Gynecol 1959; 13: 135.

112. Novak ER. Gynandroblastoma of the ovary: review of 8 cases from the ovarian tumor registry. Obstet Gynecol 1967; 30: 709.

113. Chalvardigjian A, Derzko C. Gynandroblastoma: its ultrastructure. Cancer 1982; 50: 710.

114. Soules MR, Abraham GE, Bossen EH. The steroid profile of a virilizing ovarian tumor. Obstet Gynecol 1978; 52: 73.

115. Laatikainen T, Pelkonen R, Vihko R. Plasma steroids in two subjects with ovarian androgen producing tumors, arrhenoblastoma, gynandroblastoma. J Clin Endocrinol Metab 1972; 34: 580.

116. Luca V, et al. Gynandroblastoma of the ovary. Morphol Embryol 1983; 29: 117.

117. Chivukula M, et al. Recurrent gynandroblastoma of ovary – a case report. A molecular and immunohistochemical analysis. Int J Gynecol Pathol 2006; 26: 30–3.

118. Hayes MC, Scully RE. Stromal luteoma of the ovary: a clinicopathologic analysis of 25 cases. Int J Gynecol Pathol 1987; 6: 313.

119. Dunnihoo DR, Grieme DL, Woolf RB. Hilar cell tumors of the ovary. Obstet Gynecol 1966; 27: 713.

120. Paraskevas M, Scully RE. Hilus cell tumor of the ovary. Int J Gynecol Pathol 1989; 8: 299.

121. Roth LM, Sternberg WH. Ovarian stromal tumors containing Leydig-cells. II. Pure Leydig-cell tumor, non-hilar type. Cancer 1973; 32: 952.

122. Hayes MC, Scully RE. Ovarian steroid-cell tumors (not otherwise specified): a clinicopathological analysis of 63 cases. Am J Surg Pathol 1987; 11: 835.

123. Khoo SK, Buntine D. Malignant stromal tumor of the ovary with virilizing effects in an XXX female with streak ovaries. Aust N Z J Obstet Gynaecol 1980; 20: 123.

124. Echt GR, Hadd HE. Androgen excretion patterns in a patient with a metastatic hilus tumor of the ovary. Am J Obstet Gynecol 1968; 100: 1055.

125. Montag TW, Murphy RE, Belinson JL. Virilizing malignant lipoid cell tumor producing erythropoietin. Gynecol Oncol 1984; 19: 98.

126. Peng-Hui W, Hsiang-Tai C, Wen-Ling L. Use of a long-acting gonadotropin-releasing hormone agonist for treatment of steroid cell tumors of the ovary. Fertil Steril 1998; 69: 353.

37 Germ Cell Tumors of the Ovary

Daniela E. Matei,[1] Jeanne M. Schilder,[2] and Helen Michael[3]

[1] Department of Medicine, Hematology-Oncology, [2] Department of Obstetrics and Gynecology, Gynecology-Oncology, [3] Department of Pathology and Laboratory Medicine, Indiana University School of Medicine, Indianapolis, IN, USA

Nondysgerminomatous ovarian germ cell tumors

Epidemiology

Germ cell tumors have been described in the literature for many years, dating back at least to 1911 when Chenot described a malignant nonepithelial neoplasm of the ovary.[1] This particular tumor is now known to be the most common of the germ cell tumors, and was first termed "dysgerminoma" by Meyer in 1931.[2] Several papers over subsequent years characterized ovarian tumors with similar histological features, leading to their inclusion into a new class called germ cell tumors. Teilum first introduced this concept[3] and ovarian germ cell tumor classification was refined and formally introduced in 1973 by the World Health Organization (WHO).

Ovarian germ cell tumors (OGCT) account for 2–3% of all ovarian cancers and usually occur in young women. The peak age incidence for development of these tumors is the early 20s. In a series from the University of Texas MD Anderson Cancer Center (UTMDACC), the age of the patients ranged from 6 to 40 years, with a median age of 16–20 years.[1] Ethnic and racial differences in the incidence of germ cell tumors have been noted in an analysis based on the National Cancer Institute's Surveillance, Epidemiology, and End Results (SEER) database, with increased incidence of OGCTs being observed among pediatric black females compared to black males and among Hispanic girls aged 10–19, as compared to non-Hispanics.[4] Interestingly, a case–cohort study from the Children's Oncology Group, including 274 cases (195 OGCTs and 79 testicular cancers), showed that a family history of cancer was inversely correlated with the risk of developing germ cell tumors.[5]

Accurate diagnosis, evaluation, and treatment are essential for the cure of women diagnosed with OGCTs. Principles of diagnosis and treatment apply across all types of OGCTs, and except for a few specific characteristics, OGCTs have similar clinical presentation.

Pathology

The current WHO classification of ovarian germ cell tumors includes benign tumors, almost all of which are accounted for by dermoid cysts, malignant tumors arising from constituents of dermoid cysts, which will be discussed in a separate section, and primitive malignant germ cell tumors, which recapitulate normal embryonic and extraembryonic cells and structures. The malignant ovarian germ cell tumors account for 2–3% of all ovarian cancers and are classified as dysgerminoma, yolk sac tumor, embryonal carcinoma, polyembryoma, nongestational choriocarcinoma, mixed germ cell tumors, and teratomas (immature, mature, and monodermal types).[6] Because of its specific features, dysgerminoma will be discussed separately, while nondysgerminomatous tumors will be described together. Nondysgerminomatous tumors include yolk sac tumors, embryonal carcinoma, polyembryoma, nongestational choriocarcinoma, and mixed germ cell tumors.

Yolk sac tumor

Yolk sac tumor (endodermal sinus tumor) is the second most common ovarian germ cell tumor, accounting for 22% of the ovarian germ cell tumors studied at the Armed Forces Institute of Pathology (AFIP).[7] These tumors grow very rapidly, often becoming clinically evident in less than 1 month. Ovarian yolk sac tumors are typically large and unilateral, although metastasis to the opposite ovary may occur. On gross examination, the tumors are round, oval, or lobulated, with a smooth external surface, unless rupture or invasion into surrounding structures has occurred. On cut section, these neoplasms are tan or gray, with abundant hemorrhage and necrosis (Fig. 37.1a). They are partially solid, but they contain cysts that vary in size from a few millimeters to several centimeters in diameter. The cut surface appears mucoid, slimy, or gelatinous.

There are many histological patterns of yolk sac tumor. The most common is the reticular or microcystic pattern, in which a myxoid stroma contains a mesh-like network of flattened or

Textbook of Uncommon Cancer, Fourth Edition. Edited by Derek Raghavan, Charles D. Blanke, David H. Johnson, Paul L. Moots, Gregory H. Reaman, Peter G. Rose and Mikkael A. Sekeres.
© 2012 John Wiley & Sons, Inc. Published 2012 by John Wiley & Sons, Inc.

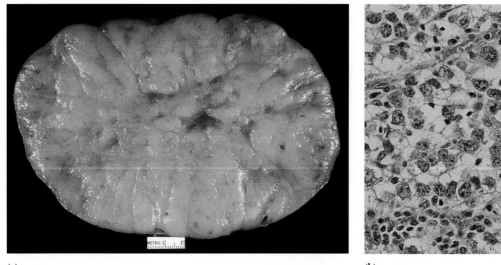

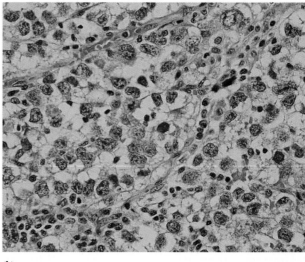

(a)   (b)

Figure 37.1 Yolk sac tumor. This neoplasm displays areas of hemorrhage and cystic degeneration (a). Both a microcystic pattern and Schiller–Duvall bodies are present (b).

cuboidal epithelial cells with varying degrees of atypia (Fig. 37.1b). The festoon pattern contains Schiller–Duvall bodies composed of a central capillary surrounded by connective tissue and a peripheral layer of columnar cells; this structure is located in a cavity lined by flattened cells (see Fig. 37.1b). When present, Schiller–Duvall bodies are diagnostic of yolk sac tumor. Other less common variants of yolk sac tumor include hepatoid, polyvesicular vitteline, enteric, endometrioid, solid, parietal, and mesenchymal patterns. Various patterns of yolk sac tumor may contain eosinophilic hyaline globules that are periodic acid-Schiff (PAS) positive and diastase resistant. These globules are not specific, do not contain α-fetoprotein (AFP), and may be seen in nongerm cell tumors. Yolk sac tumors generally display cytoplasmic staining for cytokeratin and AFP, although the parietal pattern generally does not stain for AFP. Serum AFP is a useful marker for this tumor, although a negative serum AFP does not exclude the disease. Chemotherapy has resulted in the appearance of AFP-negative parietal yolk sac tumor after eradication of AFP-positive patterns.[8] Enteric glands may be carcinoembryonic antigen (CEA) positive.

Embryonal carcinoma
Embryonal carcinoma is rarely seen in the ovary, in contrast to its frequent occurrence in the testis. Only 14 cases were identified during a 30-year period at the Armed Forces Institute of Pathology.[9] Embryonal carcinoma of the ovary is usually seen as a component of mixed germ cell tumors. It is often associated with areas of hemorrhage and necrosis on gross examination. Microscopically, this tumor is composed of very crowded cells that often display overlapping nuclei in paraffin sections. The nuclei are pleomorphic and contain large, prominent nucleoli. The mitotic rate is high. Glandular, solid, and papillary patterns may be seen. Vascular invasion is common in this tumor. Embryonal carcinoma stains positively for placenta-like alkaline phosphatase (PLAP), pancytokeratin (AE1/

AE3 and CAM 5.2), CD30, and OCT 3/4. Some embryonal carcinomas display focal AFP positivity which may represent partial transformation to yolk sac tumor. Syncytiotrophoblast cells may be present and display human chorionic gonadotropin (hCG) staining, but are not accompanied by admixed cytotrophoblast cells.

Polyembryoma
Polyembryoma is a very rare malignant ovarian tumor, typically unilateral, that displays embryoid bodies.[10] Well-developed embryoid bodies demonstrate a yolk sac and an amnionic cavity that are separated by an embryonic disk. In the few cases reported, the embryoid bodies have often coexisted with other germ cell tumor types.

Choriocarcinoma
Primary nongestational ovarian choriocarcinoma is rare.[11] It is most often seen as a component of mixed germ cell tumors of the ovary.[1,12] These tumors display abundant hemorrhage and necrosis on gross examination (Fig. 37.2a). Microscopically, they display an admixture of syncytiotrophoblast and cytotrophoblast in a haphazard, often plexiform pattern (Fig. 37.2b). Syncytiotrophoblastic giant cells have abundant eosinophilic or amphophilic cytoplasm that contains several hyperchromatic nuclei. Cytotrophoblastic and cells are round and often have fairly well-defined cell borders and clear or lightly eosinophilic, vacuolated cytoplasm with atypical nuclei. The mitotic rate may be very high. Vascular invasion is often present. Cytotrophoblast cells do not produce hCG. Syncytiotrophoblast is formed from cytotrophoblast and does produce hCG. Choriocarcinoma may also stain for PLAP, epithelial membrane antigen, and CEA. Nongestational choriocarcinoma must be distinguished from gestational choriocarcinoma because the former has a worse prognosis and requires more aggressive therapy. Identification of paternal genetic material indicates the tumor is of gestational origin.

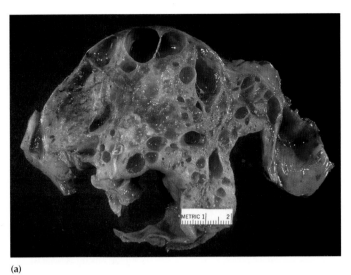

(a)

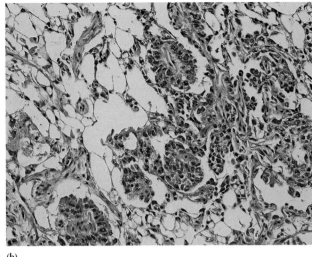

(b)

Figure 37.2 Choriocarcinoma. This tumor displays abundant hemorrhage (a). Microscopically, there is a plexiform pattern consisting of both syncytiotrophoblast and cytotrophoblast cells (b).

Mixed germ cell tumors

Mixed germ cell tumors of the ovary contain two or more different types of germ cell neoplasm, either intimately admixed or as separate foci within the tumor.[1,12] They are much less common in the ovary than in the testis, and they accounted for only 8% of malignant ovarian germ cell tumors recorded at the AFIP over a period of 30 years.[12] Malignant mixed germ cell tumors are large, unilateral neoplasms, but the gross appearance on cut surface depends on the particular types of germ cell tumor present. The most common germ cell element in the AFIP series was dysgerminoma (80%), followed by yolk sac tumor (70%), teratoma (53%), choriocarcinoma (20%), and embryonal carcinoma (13%).[12] The most frequent combination reported has been dysgerminoma and yolk sac tumor. Syncytiotrophoblast may occur either as a component of choriocarcinoma or as isolated cells in other germ cell tumor types. The diagnosis and prognosis of malignant mixed germ cell tumors depend on adequate tumor sampling in order to reveal small foci of different types of germ cell neoplasms, which may alter therapy and prognosis.

Immature teratomas

Immature teratomas are uncommon. They represent about 3% of all ovarian teratomas, but immature teratomas are the third most common form of malignant ovarian germ cell tumors. Most immature ovarian teratomas are unilateral, although they may metastasize to the opposite ovary and can be associated with mature teratoma in the opposite ovary. They are predominantly solid tumors, but they may contain scattered cystic areas. The cut surface is soft and fleshy or encephaloid in appearance, and areas of hemorrhage and necrosis are common (Fig. 37.3). Microscopically, these tumors contain a variety of mature and immature tissue elements. The immature elements almost always consist of immature neural tissue in the form of small round blue cells with rosettes and scattered tubules.

There is a correlation between prognosis and the degree of immaturity. Grade 1 neoplasms display some immaturity, but

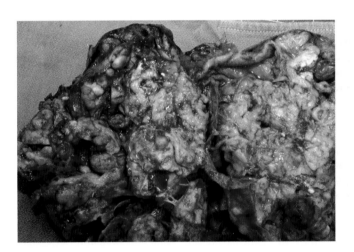

Figure 37.3 Immature teratoma. This neoplasm is largely solid and encephaloid in appearance.

immature neural tissue does not exceed in aggregate the area of one low-power field (40×) in any slide. Grade 2 teratomas display more immaturity, but immature neural tissue occupies no more than an area equal to three low-power fields in any slide. Grade 3 neoplasms have immature neural tissue occupying an area greater than three low-power fields in at least one slide.[13] Mature tissue elements are easily identified in grade 1 lesions, are present to a lesser extent in grade 2 neoplasms, and may be absent altogether in grade 3 immature teratomas. The amount of mitotic activity and immature neural tissue with rosettes also increases with increasing grade. Some authors prefer classifying immature teratomas as either low grade (grade 1) or high grade (grades 2 and 3).[14] It is clinically important to distinguish grade 1 tumors from higher-grade neoplasms, because the latter behave more aggressively and require chemotherapy. In patients whose tumors have disseminated beyond the ovary, the grade of the tumor metastases determines prognosis and guides treatment. Occasionally, patients with immature teratomas may have implants, which contain only mature tissue.

Clinical presentation

Malignant germ cell tumors of the ovary occur mainly in girls and young women. Abdominal pain associated with a palpable pelvic-abdominal mass is the presenting symptom in approximately 85% of patients with OGCTs.[1,15] Ten percent of patients present with acute abdominal pain caused by rupture, hemorrhage, or torsion of these tumors. This finding may be somewhat more common in patients with endodermal sinus tumor or mixed germ cell tumors and is frequently misdiagnosed as acute appendicitis. Less commonly, patients present with abdominal distension (35%), fever (10%), or vaginal bleeding (10%). Isosexual precocity can occur, caused by hCG production by the tumor.

Ovarian germ cell tumors can be diagnosed during pregnancy or in the immediate postpartum period.[15] As opposed to dysgerminoma, discussed in the subsequent section, nondysgerminomatous ovarian tumors occur less frequently during pregnancy.[16-19] By and large, patients with ovarian tumors diagnosed during pregnancy can be treated successfully, without compromising the health of the fetus. Surgical resection and chemotherapy have been performed safely in mid and third trimesters. However, rapid disease progression or pregnancy termination/miscarriage can occur.[20]

Germ cell tumors possess the unique property of producing biological markers. Accurate measurements of hCG and AFP in serum are useful for monitoring results of treatment and for detecting subclinical recurrences. Endodermal sinus tumor and choriocarcinoma secrete AFP and hCG, respectively. Embryonal carcinoma can secrete both hCG and AFP, but most commonly produces hCG. Mixed tumors may produce either, both, or none of the markers, depending on the type and quantity of elements present. Although immature teratomas are associated with negative markers, a few tumors can produce AFP. Levels of lactic dehydrogenase (LDH) and CA-125 can be elevated, but they are less specific than hCG or AFP.[21] Age over 45, stage greater than I, and yolk sac tumor histology have been identified as prognostic factors that affect survival.[22]

Staging

Principles for staging OGCTs follow the surgical principles applied for epithelial ovarian cancer. Table 37.1 outlines FIGO staging for germ cell tumors which is applied across all tumors, independent of histological subtype. Interestingly and in contrast to epithelial ovarian cancer, germ cell tumors are most often grossly confined to one ovary, with 60–70% of patients having stage I disease.

Treatment

Significant improvement in the management of OGCTs has been achieved during the past two decades. A combination of surgery and systemic chemotherapy often represents the backbone for therapy. The leading cause for improved outcome is

Table 37.1 FIGO staging of ovarian germ cell tumors.

Stage	Description
I	Tumor limited to ovaries
IA	Tumor limited to one ovary, no ascites, intact capsule
IB	Tumor limited to both ovaries, no ascites, intact capsule
IC	Tumor either stage IA or IB, but with ascites present containing malignant cells or with ovarian capsule involvement or rupture or with positive peritoneal washings
II	Tumor involving one or both ovaries with extension to the pelvis
IIA	Extension to uterus or tubes
IIB	Involvement of both ovaries with pelvic extension
IIC	Tumor either stage IIA or IIB, but with ascites present containing malignant cells or with ovarian capsule involvement or rupture or with positive peritoneal washings
III	Tumor involving one or both ovaries with tumor implants outside the pelvis or with positive retroperitoneal or inguinal lymph nodes. Superficial liver metastases qualify as stage III
IIIA	Tumor limited to the pelvis with negative nodes but with microscopic seeding of the abdominal peritoneal surface
IIIB	Negative nodes, tumor implants in the abdominal cavity smaller than 2 cm
IIIC	Positive nodes or tumor implants in the abdominal cavity larger than 2cm
IV	Distant metastases present

the development of more effective chemotherapy regimens, based on cisplatin. Other advances in management include a more precise surgical staging system, improved radiographic imaging, more sophisticated pathology techniques, and improved supportive care. At present, most women with ovarian germ cell tumors will become long-term survivors, suffering minimal morbidity from treatment, so strict adherence to treatment principles is critical to ensure optimal outcome.

Surgical evaluation of ovarian germ cell tumors

Once an adnexal mass is identified, other potential etiologies have been excluded, and an attempt has been made to classify the mass with tumor markers, surgical evaluation is indicated for both diagnosis and treatment. The extent of surgical extirpation and staging depends on intraoperative findings. Appropriate surgical evaluation requires an adequate vertical midline incision followed by careful inspection to determine the extent of disease. Ascites is present in 20% of patients; this should be evacuated and sent for cytological evaluation. If no ascites is present, cytological washings are obtained from the pelvis and bilateral paracolic gutters. Both ovaries should be carefully inspected. Bilaterality ranges from 5% for yolk sac tumors and immature teratomas to 10% with dysgerminomas.[23] Surgical staging is similar to that described for epithelial ovarian cancer.

In patients with apparent early-stage disease, unilateral salpingo-oophorectomy with complete surgical staging is indicated. Comprehensive surgical staging should then be undertaken as described in Box 37.1. Except for dysgerminomas, contralateral ovarian biopsy is not indicated and, in fact, is discouraged, as biopsy can result in ovarian failure or infertility as a result of adhesion formation. Approximately 10% of patients will have a mature cystic teratoma in the

Box 37.1 Comprehensive surgical staging.

- Examination under anesthesia
- Appropriate surgical incision (usually midline vertical)
- Cytological evaluation: ascites or peritoneal washings
- Pelvic cul-de-sac
- Bilateral paracolic gutters
- Left hemidiaphragm
- Comprehensive intraabdominal inspection and palpation, including:
- Small bowel: ileocecal junction to ligament of Treitz
- Large bowel: ileocecal junction to rectum
- Peritoneal surfaces and mesentery including diaphragm
- Solid organs: kidneys, liver, spleen, gallbladder, and pancreas
- Total abdominal hysterectomy*
- Unilateral or bilateral salpingo-oophorectomy*
- Infracolic omentectomy
- Appendectomy*
- Pelvic and aortic lymph node biopsies
- Resection of enlarged or suspicious nodes
- If no gross abnormalities, lymph node sampling is performed
- Peritoneal biopsies
- Pelvic cul-de-sac
- Bladder
- Bilateral sidewalls
- Bilateral paracolic gutters
- Diaphragm

_____

* Tailor to individual.

contralateral ovary. These patients can be managed with cystectomy, sparing the normal ovarian tissue.[24] Fortunately, preservation of the uterus and contralateral ovary is usually possible.[25,26] Patients with gross metastatic disease should undergo cytoreductive surgery in a fashion similar to that performed for epithelial ovarian cancer. Tumor is debulked to reduce volume to the minimal residual disease possible. The surgical approach should be tailored to the individual patient, taking operative risks into account.

While the benefit of a maximum cytoreductive surgical effort is well established for patients with epithelial ovarian cancer, such benefit remains to be proven for patients with OGCTs, as less radical surgery followed by adjuvant chemotherapy often leads to cure. If a patient has not completed child bearing, a normal ovary and/or uterus can remain _in situ_ even in the face of extensive metastatic disease elsewhere, as these tumors are typically highly sensitive to chemotherapy, and cure is often achievable.[27] An analysis of surgical trends using the SEER database showed an increase in the rates of fertility-sparing surgery during the past two decades, without altering survival.[28] In the entire cohort, fertility-sparing procedures were performed in 41% of the women. Advances in artificial reproductive techniques have made it possible for patients to conceive via donor eggs if both ovaries are involved but the uterus is preserved, or for genetic offspring to be carried by a surrogate mother if hysterectomy is necessary but one patient's ovary is retained.

Although historically, second-look laparotomy (SLL) was once implemented in the assessment of chemotherapy efficacy in patients with epithelial ovarian cancer, a benefit has not been noted in the evaluation of patients with OGCTs. In a series from UTMDACC, Gershenson reported that of 53 patients undergoing SLL, 52 were found to have no residual disease. Elevated tumor markers were present in the one patient with disease noted at SLL; furthermore, she responded well to salvage chemotherapy. Thus, SLL did not provide any clinical benefit in this study.[1] The Gynecologic Oncology Group (GOG) has determined that the only group of patients that derives a clinical benefit from SLL are those with teratoma elements who initially undergo incomplete tumor resection.[29] A well-described phenomenon noted at the time of SLL for OGCTs is called "chemotherapeutic retroconversion." Implants noted at SLL often demonstrate evidence of residual mature teratoma.[30–32] Additional chemotherapy is not indicated for this finding.

Chemotherapy for ovarian germ cell tumors

One of the great successes of cancer treatment in the 1970s and 1980s was the development of effective chemotherapy for testicular germ cell tumors.[33–35] The lessons learned from prospective, randomized trials in testis cancer have been applied to OGCTs. Currently, the majority of patients with OGCTs are long-term survivors, when treated with cisplatin-based combination chemotherapy.

Historically, the first regimen used successfully for women with OGCTs was vincristine, dactinomycin, and cyclophosphamide (VAC). Although VAC therapy had curative potential for early-stage disease, long-term survival was less than 50% in women with advanced disease. In the series from UTMDACC, 86% of patients with stage I tumors were cured with VAC[1] but only 57% of stage II patients and 50% of patients with stage III achieved long-term control. Two patients with stage IV tumors succumbed to their disease. In a GOG study, 39 of 54 patients with complete surgical resection and seven of 22 of patients with incompletely resected tumors achieved long-term disease control with VAC.[36] In this report, 11 of 15 patients with stage III and both patients with stage IV disease failed within 12 months of follow-up. These data suggested that VAC chemotherapy is insufficient for the treatment of advanced-stage and/or incompletely resected ovarian germ cell tumors.

Along with the development of cisplatin-based regimens in testes cancer, these therapies were tested in women with ovarian germ cell tumors. The vinblastin, bleomycin and cisplatin (PVB) combination was evaluated prospectively in GOG protocol 45 in patients with previously treated and untreated ovarian germ cell tumors.[37] The 4-year overall survival was 70% and 47/89 (53%) patients were disease free at 52 months. Twenty-nine percent of patients enrolled in this trial had received prior radiation or chemotherapy. Among the 30 patients with nonmeasurable disease after surgery and without prior treatment, there were eight treatment failures.

Subsequent experience in testicular cancer documented that etoposide is at least equivalent to vinblastine and induces improved outcomes in patients with high tumor volume.[34]

Table 37.2 BEP regimen.

Cisplatin	20 mg/m^2	D1–5
Etoposide (VP16)	100 mg/m^2	D1–5
Bleomycin	30 units	Weekly
Three to four courses given at 21-day interval.		

Furthermore, the use of etoposide in place of vinblastine led to decreased neurological toxicity, abdominal pain, and constipation. These observations led to the evaluation of the combination of cisplatin, etoposide and bleomycin (BEP; Table 37.2) in patients with ovarian germ cell tumors. In a series from UTMDACC, long-term remissions were recorded in 25 of 26 patients treated with BEP.[1] In a GOG protocol, 91 of 93 patients were disease free after BEP chemotherapy.[27] The inclusion of cisplatin in the treatment of ovarian tumors resulted in a significant improvement in survival and disease control.[38–40] Based on these data, although BEP and VAC have not been compared prospectively in patients with ovarian germ cell tumors, BEP emerged as the preferred regimen. Based on the experience with testicular cancer, dose intensification for patients with poor prognosis germ cell tumors has not resulted in improved outcomes compared to standard-dose BEP.[41] Thus, women with OGCT should receive 3–4 cycles of BEP chemotherapy after cytoreductive surgery.

Management of residual or recurrent disease

The large majority of patients with OGCTs are cured with surgery and platinum-based chemotherapy. However, a small percentage of patients have persistent or progressive disease during treatment or recur after completion of treatment. Most recurrences occur within 24 months from primary treatment. As in testis cancer, treatment failures are categorized as platinum resistant (progression during or within 4–6 weeks of completing treatment) or platinum sensitive (recurrence beyond 6 weeks from platinum-based therapy).[42]

Given the high curability rate of OGCTs with primary treatment, the management of recurrent disease represents a complex and often difficult issue, and should be performed in a specialized center. Data to guide the management of patients with recurrent OGCTs are scant and by and large extrapolated from the treatment of testis cancer patients. Approximately 30% of patients with recurrent platinum-sensitive testis cancer can be salvaged with second-line chemotherapy (VeIP: vinblastine, ifosfamide, platinum).[43] In patients with recurrent or persistent testicular germ cell tumors, there is evidence that high-dose therapy with carboplatin, etoposide with or without cyclophosphamide or ifosfamide and stem cell rescue is superior to standard-dose salvage therapy.[44–46] The single most important prognostic factor in patients with testis cancer is whether or not they are refractory to cisplatin. In patients who are truly cisplatin refractory, the likelihood of long-term survival and cure following high-dose therapy is low and high-dose therapy is of debatable appropriateness.[47] On the other hand, the likelihood of cure with high-dose salvage therapy in patients who relapse from a complete remission after initial

therapy is 50%. Generally, one course of standard-dose therapy, usually cisplatin, vinblastine, and ifosfamide, is given. If an initial response is seen, then patients undergo two subsequent courses of high-dose chemotherapy (carboplatin and etoposide) with stem cell rescue.[48] A recent report from Indiana University describes this approach among 184 patients with recurrent germ cell tumors. At a median follow-up of 48 months, 116 patients were in complete remission. Remarkably, of 40 patients who were platinum refractory, 18 were disease free after high-dose chemotherapy.[48]

While this approach has not been, and most probably will never be, tested prospectively in women with recurrent OGCTs, because of the small numbers of patients, the concepts are very similar and support the use of high-dose therapy in this setting. Referral to a specialized center for management of recurrent disease is desirable. Patients with platinum-refractory disease cannot be cured. Active agents in this setting include ifosfamide, taxanes, and gemcitabine,[49–51] and referral for treatment with investigational agents is appropriate.

Immediate toxicity of chemotherapy

Acute adverse effects of chemotherapy can be substantial. About 25% of patients experience febrile neutropenia and require hospitalization and broad-spectrum antibiotics.[52] Cisplatin-induced nephrotoxicity can be prevented by adequate hydration and avoidance of nephrotoxic drugs. Bleomycin can cause pulmonary fibrosis.[52] The most effective method for monitoring germ cell tumor patients for development of bleomycin-induced fibrosis is careful physical examination of the chest. Findings of early bleomycin lung disease are a lag or diminished expansion of one hemithorax or fine basilar rales that do not clear with cough. These findings can be subtle but if present, mandate discontinuation of bleomycin. As shown by randomized trials in testis cancer, bleomycin is an important component of the treatment regimen and should not be omitted in the absence of lung toxicity, particularly if only three courses of therapy are given.[53,54] Modern antiemetic therapy has greatly reduced chemotherapy-induced emesis, common in the early days of cisplatin use. Patients with advanced OGCTs should receive 3–4 courses of treatment given in full dose and on schedule. There is presumptive evidence in testis cancer that the timeliness of chemotherapy is associated with outcome. Thus, treatment is given regardless of hematological parameters on the scheduled day of treatment. By following these guidelines and by providing supportive care as indicated, virtually all patients can be treated on schedule, in full or nearly full dose. Chemotherapy-related mortality should be less than 1%.

Late sequelae of chemotherapy

Given that a high percentage of women with germ cell tumors are cured, attention should be paid to the long-term effects of treatment. A recognized late effect of chemotherapy is the risk for secondary malignancies. Etoposide is associated with the development of acute myelogenous leukemia (AML) with a characteristic chromosomal translocation at the 11q23 locus. This treatment complication occurs within 2–3 years and appears to be dose[55,56] and schedule dependent.[57] In the GOG protocol testing BEP, there was one case of AML among 91 patients.[27] An additional case of lymphoma was diagnosed, but causality remains unclear, as a correlation between chemotherapy and lymphoproliferative disorders is not established.

Chemotherapy also has long-term effects on gonadal function and leads to sterility.[58–60] Older age at initiation of therapy, greater cumulative drug dose,[61] and longer duration of therapy[60] favor premature ovarian dysfunction. However, successful pregnancies after combination chemotherapy have been documented in patients with malignant OGCTs.[1,62–65] In a review of the UTMDACC series,[1] 27 (68%) of 40 patients who had retained a normal contralateral ovary and uterus maintained regular menses consistently after completion of chemotherapy, and 33 women (83%) had regular menses at follow-up. Twelve patients had successful pregnancies. In a series from Milan, 138 of 196 patients underwent fertility-sparing surgery, and of those, 81 underwent adjuvant chemotherapy.[65] After treatment, all but one woman recovered menstrual function and 55 conceptions were recorded.

Limited reports are available concerning other late effects of chemotherapy in patients with OGCTs[66,67] but there are several articles on this topic for patients with testicular cancer.[68–73] In male patients who received cisplatin-based combination regimens, principally PVB, late toxicities included high-tone hearing loss,[68] neurotoxicity,[68,71,73] Raynaud phenomena,[69,73] ischemic heart disease,[73,74] hypertension,[73] renal dysfunction,[73] and pulmonary toxicity.[70,72] Fortunately, the majority of patients preserve an excellent overall health and functional status.[72]

The GOG recently completed an analysis evaluating the quality of life, reproductive, and psychosocial characteristics of survivors of OGCTs compared to matched controls.[67,75,76] In this analysis, the survivors appeared to be well adjusted, were able to develop strong relationships, and were free of significant depression.[77] The impact on fertility was modest or none, in those patients who underwent fertility-sparing surgeries.[76] Overall, these women appeared to be free of any major physical illnesses at a median follow-up of 10 years, compared to matched controls. The only differences consisted in higher rates of reported hypertension (17% versus 8%, $p=0.02$), hypercholesterolemia (9.8% versus 4.4%, $p=0.09$), and hearing loss (5.3% versus 1.5%, $p=0.09$) compared with controls.[75] Among chronic functional problems, numbness, tinnitus, nausea elicited by reminders of chemotherapy (versus general nausea triggers for controls), and Raynaud symptoms were reported more frequently by survivors. Despite persistence of a few sequelae of treatment, in general, OGCT survivors enjoy a healthy life comparable to that of controls, justifying administration of curative treatment in full and timely dosing.

In summary, virtually all patients with early-stage or completely resected OGCTs will be long-term survivors after careful surgical staging and three courses of adjuvant BEP. Furthermore, 70–80% of patients with incompletely resected or advanced tumors are expected to be cured. Current and future clinical trials should address the latter group of patients and those with recurrent platinum-resistant OGCT, in an effort to improve therapeutic results. Acute toxicity of treatment is relatively modest. An important but unusual late complication of treatment is etoposide-induced leukemia. Otherwise, late consequences of chemotherapy are limited. Efforts should concentrate on fertility preservation for patients who desire subsequent pregnancies.

Dysgerminoma

Epidemiology

Dysgerminoma is the female equivalent of seminoma and represents the most common of all ovarian malignant germ cell tumors.[78] Five to 10% are associated with gonadoblastomas and develop in sexually maldeveloped patients. Dysgerminoma is the most common germ cell tumor to be diagnosed during pregnancy. In a case series reported by Gordon, 20 of 158 patients with dysgerminoma were diagnosed during pregnancy or after delivery.[23]

Pathology

About 10% of dysgerminomas are bilateral on gross examination and another 10% have microscopic involvement of the contralateral ovary. On gross examination, dysgerminomas are usually large, white to gray, fleshy lobulated masses (Fig. 37.4a) with focal areas of hemorrhage or necrosis on cut section. Abundant hemorrhage, necrosis, or cystic areas should raise the question of a mixed germ cell tumor. Microscopically, dysgerminomas display nests and cords of primitive-appearing germ cells with clear to eosinophilic cytoplasm and prominent cytoplasmic borders. Nuclei are enlarged but not pleomorphic. Mitoses may be numerous. Nests of tumor cells are separated by fibrous trabeculae that contain lymphocytes (Fig. 37.4b). Syncytiotrophoblast cells are present in about 3% of dysgerminomas. Dysgerminomas contain cytoplasmic glycogen, which is seen with a PAS stain. They show diffuse staining for PLAP, usually with membrane accentuation. They stain positively the *c-kit* gene product CD117 and for OCT 3/4, a nuclear transcription factor expressed in human embryonic and stem cells. Approximately a third of dysgerminomas harbor c-kit amplifications or activating mutations and these molecular alterations correlate with advanced stage.[79] Syncytiotrophoblast cells present in dysgerminomas stain with hCG. In contrast to choriocarcinoma, the syncytiotrophoblast cells seen in dysgerminoma are not admixed with cytotrophoblast cells.

Clinical presentation

As with nondysgerminomatous tumors, the most common clinical presentation of dysgerminomas is abdominal enlargement, a mass, or pain due to torsion. Dysgerminoma is commonly devoid of hormonal production, although a small percentage of tumors produce low levels of hCG, if multinucleated syncytiotrophoblastic giant cells are present within the tumor tissue. The presence of an elevated level of AFP or high level of hCG (>100 U/mL) denotes the presence of tumor elements other than dysgerminoma and pathological review is indicated to exclude the presence of mixed elements. Therapy should be adjusted accordingly for those cases.

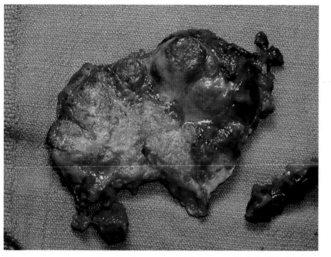

(a)

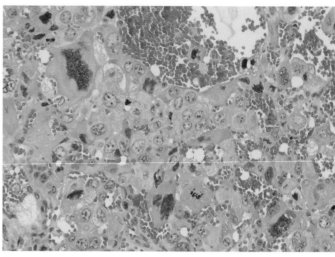

(b)

Figure 37.4 Dysgerminoma. The tumor is large, tan, and fleshy without significant hemorrhage or necrosis (a). It is composed of nests of cells with clear cytoplasm; fibrous septae separate the tumor nests (b).

Staging

Principles of FIGO staging applied to nondysgerminomatous tumors and epithelial ovarian cancer are also used for dysgerminoma (see Table 37.1). Characteristically, dysgerminomas are more likely to be localized to the ovary at the time of diagnosis (stage I) compared to nondysgerminomatous tumors. However, bilateral ovarian involvement is more common than with other OGCTs, as is dissemination to retroperitoneal lymph nodes.

Treatment

Dysgerminomas are exquisitely radiotherapy- and chemotherapy-sensitive tumors, therefore most women are cured with adequate treatment. The same principles discussed for nondysgerminomatous tumors apply for this disease, except for several specific features that are highlighted below.

Surgery for dysgerminomas

Surgical principles applied for treating nondysgerminomatous tumors apply to dysgerminomas (see Box 37.1). As most patients present with stage I disease, unilateral salpingo-oophorectomy with complete surgical staging can be considered. One notable exception is when an abnormal karyotype is identified preoperatively, or if a dysgenetic gonad is identified on frozen section, in which case bilateral salpingo-oophorectomy is indicated. However, because of potential bilateral ovarian involvement by dysgerminomas which occurs in up to 10% of patients, biopsy of a normal-appearing contralateral ovary should be considered. The postoperative approach differs from strategies pursued for nondysgerminomatous tumors.

Observation for stage I tumors

As many as two-thirds of dysgerminoma patients are stage I at diagnosis.[80,81] In the past, most of these women received postoperative radiotherapy. Given that pelvic radiotherapy

Table 37.3 Results of clinical surveillance after surgery in patients with stage IA dysgerminoma.

Institution	Period	Progression free/ total number (%)	Overall survival/ total number (%)
AFIP[15]	–1969	46/57 (80%)	52/57 (91%)
Hopkins[23]	1930–1981	58/72 (80%)	67/72 (94%)
Mayo Clinic[83]	1950–1984	9/14 (64%)	14/14 (100%)
Iowa Hospitals[81]	1935–1985	7/7 (100%)	7/7 (100%)
MD Anderson[98]	–1976	5/5 (100%)	5/5 (100%)
Mount Vernon Hospital[99]	1973–1995	6/9 (66%)	9/9 (100%)

Reproduced from Williams *et al.*[24]

leads to gonadal dysfunction and sterility, an alternative for low-risk patients is postsurgical clinical surveillance.[82] Several case series report that 80–85% of patients with stage IA dysgerminoma are cured with surgery alone (Table 37.3). Careful follow-up is required, because 15–25% of patients will recur. However, given the exquisite chemosensitivity, virtually all dysgerminoma patients can be salvaged at the time of recurrence, if adequate follow-up and early detection have been accomplished.

Radiation therapy

While less relevant currently compared to the era of modern chemotherapy, dysgerminoma is very sensitive to radiation, in contract to nondysgerminomatous tumors.[23,83,84] In the past, many stage I patients and all patients with higher stage tumors received radiotherapy. Radiation therapy was delivered to the ipsilateral hemipelvis (with shielding of the contralateral ovary and the head of the femur) and to the paraaortic nodes. A single field incorporating these areas was used. In either case, the upper limit of the field was set at T10–T11. The lower limit of the spinal field was at L4–L5. For stage III retroperitoneal

Table 37.4 Results of radiotherapy in dysgerminoma.

Institution	Period	Stage	Progression free/total number of patients (%)
AFIP[15]	–1969	I–III	12/14 (85%)
Mayo Clinic[83]	1950–1984	I–IV	16/20 (80%)
MD Anderson[98]	–1976	I–III	26/31 (84%)
Florence[86]	1960–1983	Ic–III	21/26 (80%)
NCI Milan[80]	1970–1982	I–III	21/25 (84%)
Iowa Hospitals[81]	1935–1985	I–III	12/13 (92%)
Sweden[84]	1927–1984	I–IV	49/60 (83%)
Egypt[100]	1978–1989	II–III	10/15 (66%)
Prince of Wales Hospital[85]	1969–1983	II–III	10/14 (72%)

Reprinted from Williams *et al.*[24]

disease, a prophylactic field including the mediastinum and supraclavicular nodes was included. In the presence of peritoneal involvement, the whole abdomen and pelvis, mediastinum, and supraclavicular nodes were irradiated. The usual prophylactic dose was 30 Gy (7.5–9 Gy/week). For curative irradiation, 35–40 Gy total dose was given and a boost (10 Gy) was delivered to involved nodes. Prophylactic mediastinal radiation for high-risk patients used 30 Gy given 3–6 weeks after completion of irradiation below the diaphragm.

The results of radiation therapy were reasonably favorable. DePalo reported that all 13 stage I patients (12 stage IA and one with stage IB) treated with radiation were alive and free of disease at a median follow-up of 77 months.[80] The 5-year relapse-free survival for 12 stage III patients was 61.4% and the overall survival was 89.5%. Lawson and Adler reported that 10 of 14 stage I–III patients treated with radiation were alive at a median follow-up of 54 months.[85] Others have reported similar results with overall progression-free rates varying between 70% and 90% when radiotherapy followed surgical resection[84,86] (Table 37.4). However, despite the remarkable radiosensitivity of dysgerminoma, radiotherapy is rarely performed nowadays, as chemotherapy is equally or more effective, less toxic, and allows preservation of gonadal function.

Chemotherapy

Dysgerminoma is very responsive to cisplatin-based chemotherapy, even more than nondysgerminomatous tumors.[1,87] An analysis of dysgerminoma patients treated on GOG protocols revealed that 19 of 20 patients were disease free with a median follow-up of 22 months.[88] All had stage III or IV disease and most of them had suboptimal (greater than 2 cm) residual tumor. This suggests that nearly all patients with advanced dysgerminoma treated with chemotherapy are durable complete responders. Another GOG study showed that carboplatin-etoposide is an alternative regimen for dysgerminoma patients.[89] However, at present cisplatin should not be substituted for carboplatin, given the more robust data accumulated in testis cancer, where the two approaches are not equivalent.

In summary, the majority of dysgerminoma patients have stage I disease at diagnosis. These patients can usually be treated with unilateral salpingo-oophorectomy and if fertility is an issue, they can be observed carefully with regular pelvic exams, abdominal computed tomography, and tumor markers. Fifteen to 20% of patients entering surveillance will experience a recurrence, but can be cured with chemotherapy at that time. In patients with more advanced but resected disease, the risk of recurrence is significant enough to warrant adjuvant treatment. Alternatives are chemotherapy or radiation. For the majority of patients, chemotherapy is the clear choice because of ease of administration, predictable and minimal toxicity, and fertility-sparing properties. Chemotherapy is recommended also for patients with metastatic or incompletely resected tumors, and for patients who recur after previous radiotherapy. Radiation might be considered as initial treatment in unusual circumstances, such as older patients or in those with serious concomitant illness that would preclude the use of systemic chemotherapy.

Malignant tumors associated with dermoid cysts

Epidemiology

Dermoid cysts or mature cystic teratomas account for one-quarter to one-third of all ovarian tumors. They occur most commonly in young women but are also found in children and occasionally in elderly women. Malignant tumors arising from constituents of dermoid cysts account for 2–3% of ovarian cancers and are represented mostly by squamous carcinomas. In patients older than 40, malignant transformation of dermoid cysts should always be excluded, but malignant lesions in dermoid cysts are rarely encountered before this age.

Pathology

Teratomas are neoplasms composed of tissue that is derived from two or three embryonic layers. Most often they present as cysts lined by epidermis with skin appendages. The cyst lumen contains sebaceous material and hair. In 10% of cases, dermoid cysts occur bilaterally. In two-thirds of cases, mature elements reflecting differentiation into tissues normally derived from all three embryonic germ layers (ectoderm, mesoderm, endoderm) are present. Any of these constituents has the potential for undergoing benign or malignant neoplastic transformation leading to formation of a tumor within a tumor. The malignant areas present as small nodules in the wall of the cyst and are recognized after removal of the entire content of the cyst.[90]

The most common secondary tumor associated with mature teratomas is squamous carcinoma,[91,92] which is found in about 1% of dermoid cysts. This tumor appears grossly as an eccentric solid mass in the cyst wall or as a polypoid mass within the lumen. The natural history of squamous carcinoma arising in a dermoid cyst mimics squamous carcinoma arising in other primary sites. Spread may be by direct extension or regional lymphatic metastases (paraaortic lymph nodes) and peritoneal dissemination may occur following cyst rupture.[90,93] Other tumors arising in dermoid cysts include basal cell carcinomas, sebaceous tumors, malignant melanomas, adenocarcinomas, sarcomas, and neuroectodermal tumors. Endocrine-type tumors include struma ovarii and carcinoid tumors[94]; such tumors are malignant in less than 5% of cases. The struma is rarely functional, but carcinoid tumors can induce carcinoid syndrome in one-third of cases. The syndrome is almost always curable by removal of the tumor.

Clinical presentation

Symptoms of an enlarging abdominal or pelvic mass are the most common presentations of dermoid cysts. Elevated serum markers are not observed with these tumors.

Staging

FIGO staging is not applicable to dermoid cysts, as these represent nonmalignant tumors.

Treatment

Dermoid cysts are resected surgically and extensive surgical staging is not recommended, if no malignant component is identified. For secondary squamous tumors arising from dermoid cysts, curative management can be accomplished with aggressive local therapies (surgery, radiation, chemoradiation), in a fashion analogous to the management of squamous cancer arising at other anatomical sites.

Small cell carcinoma of the ovary

Epidemiology

This represents a very rare entity, with only a few cases diagnosed annually in the United States. It is encountered in young women or girls and can be associated with malignant hypercalcemia. Systemic dissemination is common and prognosis is usually poor.

Pathology

Microscopically, the small cell carcinoma of the ovary has similar features to that of the lung. Neuroendocrine differentiation is present with typical growth pattern, evidence of secretory granules, and expression of the neuroendocrine markers synaptophysin and chromogranin.[95] A large cell variant has been described and has similar clinical features.[96] This type of tumor is poorly differentiated and carries a poor prognosis. Metastasis from another primary site (commonly lung) should be excluded. The cell of origin is not clear, but most likely this tumor originates in the epithelial layer of the ovary.

Clinical presentation

Rapidly enlarging abdominal or pelvic mass is a common manifestation. Hypercalcemia is present in two-thirds of cases and small cell carcinoma is the most common cause of ovarian tumor-associated hypercalcemia. Because of its aggressive course, some women have symptoms of overt metastatic disease at presentation.

Staging

Principles of FIGO staging used for epithelial ovarian cancer also apply to this entity (see Box 37.1).

Treatment

Stage at presentation is the most important prognostic sign. Patients with stage I disease can achieve long-term survival by employing a multimodality treatment approach.[97] However, most women who present with stage III or IV are incurable and the disease has an aggressive course. Because of its aggressive course resembling that of OGCT or of small cell carcinoma of the lung, it is frequently treated with a chemotherapy regimen analogous to that used for OGCTs (platinum, etoposide based) after surgical debulking. The role of bleomycin is not well defined, as for the treatment of other OGCTs, and platinum-etoposide is the preferred regimen. Responses to therapy in the recurrent setting are poor, and most women with relapsed small cell carcinoma succumb to disease.

Acknowledgment

This chapter is dedicated to Stephen D. Williams, MD (1947–2009), founding director of the Indiana University Simon Cancer Center, outstanding oncologist, mentor, and friend.

References

1. Gershenson DM, del Junco G, Copeland LJ, Rutledge FN. Mixed germ cell tumors of the ovary. Obstet Gynecol 1984; 64(2): 200–6.
2. Meyer R. The pathology of some special ovarian tumors and their relation to sex characteristics. Am J Obstet Gynecol 1931; 22: 697–713.
3. Teilum G. Classification of endodermal sinus tumour (mesoblatoma vitellinum) and so-called "embryonal carcinoma" of the ovary. Acta Pathol Microbiol Scand 1965; 64(4): 407–29.
4. Poynter JN, Amatruda JF, Ross JA. Trends in incidence and survival of pediatric and adolescent patients with germ cell tumors in the United States, 1975 to 2006. Cancer 2010; 116(20): 4882–91.
5. Poynter JN, *et al*. Family history of cancer and malignant germ cell tumors in children: a report from the Children's Oncology Group. Cancer Causes Control 2010; 21(2): 181–9.
6. Tavassoli FA. Pathology and genetics of tumours of the breast and female genital organs. In: *World Health Organization Classification of Tumors*. Lyon: IARC Press, 2005.
7. Kurman RJ, Norris HJ. Endodermal sinus tumor of the ovary: a clinical and pathologic analysis of 71 cases. Cancer 1976; 38(6): 2404–19.
8. Damjanov I, Amenta PS, Zarghami F. Transformation of an AFP-positive yolk sac carcinoma into an AFP-negative neoplasm. Evidence for in vivo cloning of the human parietal yolk sac carcinoma. Cancer 1984; 53(9): 1902–7.
9. Kurman RJ, Norris HJ. Embryonal carcinoma of the ovary: a clinico-pathologic entity distinct from endodermal sinus tumor resembling embryonal carcinoma of the adult testis. Cancer 1976; 38(6): 2420–33.
10. Beck JS, Fulmer HF, Lee ST. Solid malignant ovarian teratoma with "embryoid bodies" and trophoblastic differentiation. J Pathol 1969; 99(1): 67–73.
11. Vance RP, Geisinger KR. Pure nongestational choriocarcinoma of the ovary. Report of a case. Cancer 1985; 56(9): 2321–5.
12. Kurman RJ, Norris HJ. Malignant mixed germ cell tumors of the ovary. A clinical and pathologic analysis of 30 cases. Obstet Gynecol 1976; 48(5): 579–89.

13. Norris HJ, Zirkin HJ, Benson WL. Immature (malignant) teratoma of the ovary: a clinical and pathologic study of 58 cases. Cancer 1976; 37(5): 2359–72.

14. O'Connor DM, Norris HJ. The influence of grade on the outcome of stage I ovarian immature (malignant) teratomas and the reproducibility of grading. Int J Gynecol Pathol 1994; 13(4): 283–9.

15. Asadourian LA, Taylor HB. Dysgerminoma. An analysis of 105 cases. Obstet Gynecol 1969; 33(3): 370–9.

16. Christman JE, Teng NN, Lebovic GS, Sikic BI. Delivery of a normal infant following cisplatin, vinblastine, and bleomycin (PVB) chemotherapy for malignant teratoma of the ovary during pregnancy. Gynecol Oncol 1990; 37(2): 292–5.

17. Farahmand SM, Marchetti DL, Asirwatham JE, Dewey MR. Ovarian endodermal sinus tumor associated with pregnancy: review of the literature. Gynecol Oncol 1991; 41(2): 156–60.

18. Horbelt D, Delmore J, Meisel R, Cho S, Roberts D, Logan D. Mixed germ cell malignancy of the ovary concurrent with pregnancy. Obstet Gynecol 1994; 84(4 Pt 2): 662–4.

19. Rajendran S, Hollingworth J, Scudamore I. Endodermal sinus tumour of the ovary in pregnancy. Eur J Gynaecol Oncol 1999; 20(4): 272–4.

20. Bakri YN, et al. Malignant germ cell tumors of the ovary. Pregnancy considerations. Eur J Obstet Gynecol Reprod Biol 2000; 90(1): 87–91.

21. Sekiya S, Seki K, Nagai Y. Rise of serum CA 125 in patients with pure ovarian yolk sac tumors. Int J Gynaecol Obstet 1997; 58(3): 323–4.

22. Mangili G, et al. Outcome and risk factors for recurrence in malignant ovarian germ cell tumors: a MITO-9 retrospective study. Int J Gynecol Cancer 2011; 21(8): 1414–21.

23. Gordon A, Lipton D, Woodruff JD. Dysgerminoma: a review of 158 cases from the Emil Novak Ovarian Tumor Registry. Obstet Gynecol 1981; 58(4): 497–504.

24. Williams SD, et al. Ovarian germ-cell tumors. In: Hoskins WJ (ed) Principles and Practice of Gynecologic Oncology, 2nd edn. Philadelphia: Lippincot-Raven, 1997.

25. Schwartz PE. Surgery of germ cell tumours of the ovary. Forum (Genova) 2000; 10: 355–65.

26. Peccatori F, Bonazzi C, Chiari S, Landoni F, Colombo N, Mangioni C. Surgical management of malignant ovarian germ-cell tumors: 10 years' experience of 129 patients. Obstet Gynecol 1995; 86(3): 367–72.

27. Williams S, Blessing JA, Liao SY, Ball H, Hanjani P. Adjuvant therapy of ovarian germ cell tumors with cisplatin, etoposide, and bleomycin: a trial of the Gynecologic Oncology Group. J Clin Oncol 1994; 12(4): 701–6.

28. Chan JK, et al. The influence of conservative surgical practices for malignant ovarian germ cell tumors. J Surg Oncol 2008; 98(2): 111–16.

29. Williams SD, Blessing JA, DiSaia PJ, Major FJ, Ball HG, 3 rd, Liao SY. Second-look laparotomy in ovarian germ cell tumors: the gynecologic oncology group experience. Gynecol Oncol 1994; 52(3): 287–91.

30. Geisler JP, Goulet R, Foster RS, Sutton GP. Growing teratoma syndrome after chemotherapy for germ cell tumors of the ovary. Obstet Gynecol 1994; 84(4 Pt 2): 719–21.

31. Itani Y, Kawa M, Toyoda S, Yamagami K, Hiraoka K. Growing teratoma syndrome after chemotherapy for a mixed germ cell tumor of the ovary. J Obstet Gynaecol Res 2002; 28(3): 166–71.

32. Kattan J, Droz JP, Culine S, Duvillard P, Thiellet A, Peillon C. The growing teratoma syndrome: a woman with nonseminomatous germ cell tumor of the ovary. Gynecol Oncol 1993; 49(3): 395–9.

33. Einhorn LH, Donohue J. Cis-diaminedichloroplatinum, vinblastine, and bleomycin combination chemotherapy in disseminated testicular cancer. Ann Intern Med. 1977; 87(3): 293–8.

34. Williams SD, Birch R, Einhorn LH, Irwin L, Greco FA, Loehrer PJ. Treatment of disseminated germ-cell tumors with cisplatin, bleomycin, and either vinblastine or etoposide. N Engl J Med 1987; 316(23): 1435–40.

35. Einhorn LH. Curing metastatic testicular cancer. Proc Natl Acad Sci U S A 2002; 99(7): 4592–5.

36. Slayton RE, Park RC, Silverberg SG, Shingleton H, Creasman WT, Blessing JA. Vincristine, dactinomycin, and cyclophosphamide in the treatment of malignant germ cell tumors of the ovary. A Gynecologic Oncology Group Study (a final report). Cancer 1985; 56(2): 243–8.

37. Williams SD, Blessing JA, Moore DH, Homesley HD, Adcock L. Cisplatin, vinblastine, and bleomycin in advanced and recurrent ovarian germ-cell tumors. A trial of the Gynecologic Oncology Group. Ann Intern Med 1989; 111(1): 22–7.

38. Culine S, Lhomme C, Kattan J, Michel G, Duvillard P, Droz JP. Cisplatin-based chemotherapy in the management of germ cell tumors of the ovary: the Institut Gustave Roussy experience. Gynecol Oncol 1997; 64(1): 160–5.

39. Segelov E, et al. Cisplatin-based chemotherapy for ovarian germ cell malignancies: the Australian experience. J Clin Oncol 1994; 12(2): 378–84.

40. Dimopoulos MA, et al. Favorable outcome of ovarian germ cell malignancies treated with cisplatin or carboplatin-based chemotherapy: a Hellenic Cooperative Oncology Group study. Gynecol Oncol 1998; 70(1): 70–4.

41. Daugaard G, et al. A randomized phase III study comparing standard dose BEP with sequential high-dose cisplatin, etoposide, and ifosfamide (VIP) plus stem-cell support in males with poor-prognosis germ-cell cancer. An intergroup study of EORTC, GTCSG, and Grupo Germinal (EORTC 30974). Ann Oncol 2011; 22(5): 1054–61.

42. Loehrer PJ Sr, Lauer R, Roth BJ, Williams SD, Kalasinski LA, Einhorn LH. Salvage therapy in recurrent germ cell cancer: ifosfamide and cisplatin plus either vinblastine or etoposide. Ann Intern Med. 1988; 109(7): 540–6.

43. Einhorn LH. Salvage therapy for germ cell tumors. Semin Oncol 1994; 21(4 Suppl 7): 47–51.

44. Broun ER, et al. Early salvage therapy for germ cell cancer using high dose chemotherapy with autologous bone marrow support. Cancer 1994; 73(6): 1716–20.

45. Broun ER, et al. Tandem high dose chemotherapy with autologous bone marrow transplantation for initial relapse of testicular germ cell cancer. Cancer 1997; 79(8): 1605–10.

46. Lotz JP, et al. High dose chemotherapy with ifosfamide, carboplatin, and etoposide combined with autologous bone marrow transplantation for the treatment of poor-prognosis germ cell tumors and metastatic trophoblastic disease in adults. Cancer 1995; 75(3): 874–85.

47. Nichols CR, et al. Dose-intensive chemotherapy in refractory germ cell cancer – a phase I/II trial of high-dose carboplatin and etoposide with autologous bone marrow transplantation. J Clin Oncol 1989; 7(7): 932–9.

48. Enihorn L Williams SD, Chamness A. High dose chemotherapy and stem cell rescue for metastatic germ cell tumors. N Engl J Med 2007; 357(4): 340–8.

49. Loehrer PJ Sr, Gonin R, Nichols CR, Weathers T, Einhorn LH. Vinblastine plus ifosfamide plus cisplatin as initial salvage therapy in recurrent germ cell tumor. J Clin Oncol 1998; 16(7): 2500–4.

50. Hinton S, et al. Phase II study of paclitaxel plus gemcitabine in refractory germ cell tumors (E9897): a trial of the Eastern Cooperative Oncology Group. J Clin Oncol 2002; 20(7): 1859–63.

51. Nichols CR, Roth BJ, Loehrer PJ, Williams SD, Einhorn LH. Salvage chemotherapy for recurrent germ cell cancer. Semin Oncol 1994; 21(5 Suppl 12): 102–8.

52. Mann JR, et al. The United Kingdom Children's Cancer Study Group's second germ cell tumor study: carboplatin, etoposide, and bleomycin are effective treatment for children with malignant extracranial germ cell tumors, with acceptable toxicity. J Clin Oncol 2000; 18(22): 3809–18.

53. Loehrer PJ Sr, Johnson D, Elson P, Einhorn LH, Trump D. Importance of bleomycin in favorable-prognosis disseminated germ cell tumors: an Eastern Cooperative Oncology Group trial. J Clin Oncol 1995; 13(2): 470–6.

54. De Wit R, et al. Importance of bleomycin in combination chemotherapy for good-prognosis testicular nonseminoma: a randomized study of the European Organization for Research and Treatment of Cancer Genitourinary Tract Cancer Cooperative Group. J Clin Oncol 1997; 15(5): 1837–43.

55. Nichols CR, Breeden ES, Loehrer PJ, Williams SD, Einhorn LH. Secondary leukemia associated with a conventional dose of etoposide: review of serial germ cell tumor protocols. J Natl Cancer Inst 1993; 85(1): 36–40.

56. Pedersen-Bjergaard J, Daugaard G, Hansen SW, Philip P, Larsen SO, Rorth M. Increased risk of myelodysplasia and leukaemia after etoposide, cisplatin, and bleomycin for germ-cell tumours. Lancet 1991; 338(8763): 359–63.

57. Pui CH, et al. Acute myeloid leukemia in children treated with epipodophyllotoxins for acute lymphoblastic leukemia. N Engl J Med 1991; 325(24): 1682–7.

58. Horning SJ, Hoppe RT, Kaplan HS, Rosenberg SA. Female reproductive potential after treatment for Hodgkin's disease. N Engl J Med 1981; 304(23): 1377–82.

59. Byrne J, et al. Effects of treatment on fertility in long-term survivors of childhood or adolescent cancer. N Engl J Med 1987; 317(21): 1315–21.

60. Siris ES, Leventhal BG, Vaitukaitis JL. Effects of childhood leukemia and chemotherapy on puberty and reproductive function in girls. N Engl J Med 1976; 294(21): 1143–6.

61. Nicosia SV, Matus-Ridley M, Meadows AT. Gonadal effects of cancer therapy in girls. Cancer 1985; 55(10): 2364–72.

62. Brewer M, Gershenson DM, Herzog CE, Mitchell MF, Silva EG, Wharton JT. Outcome and reproductive function after chemotherapy for ovarian dysgerminoma. J Clin Oncol 1999; 17(9): 2670–75.

63. Pektasides D, Rustin GJ, Newlands ES, Begent RH, Bagshawe KD. Fertility after chemotherapy for ovarian germ cell tumours. Br J Obstet Gynaecol 1987; 94(5): 477–9.

64. Rustin GJ, Pektasides D, Bagshawe KD, Newlands ES, Begent RH. Fertility after chemotherapy for male and female germ cell tumours. Int J Androl 1987; 10(1): 389–92.

65. Zanetta G, et al. Survival and reproductive function after treatment of malignant germ cell ovarian tumors. J Clin Oncol 2001; 19(4): 1015–20.

66. Hale GA, et al. Late effects of treatment for germ cell tumors during childhood and adolescence. J Pediatr Hematol Oncol 1999; 21(2): 115–22.

67. Swenson MM, MacLeod JS, Williams SD, Miller AM, Champion VL. Quality of life after among ovarian germ cell cancer survivors: a narrative analysis. Oncol Nurs Forum 2003; 30(3): 380.

68. Hansen SW, Helweg-Larsen S, Trojaborg W. Long-term neurotoxicity in patients treated with cisplatin, vinblastine, and bleomycin for metastatic germ cell cancer. J Clin Oncol 1989; 7(10): 1457–61.

69. Hansen SW, Olsen N. Raynaud's phenomenon in patients treated with cisplatin, vinblastine, and bleomycin for germ cell cancer: measurement of vasoconstrictor response to cold. J Clin Oncol 1989; 7(7): 940–2.

70. Hansen SW, Groth S, Sorensen PG, Rossing N, Rorth M. Enhanced pulmonary toxicity in smokers with germ-cell cancer treated with cis-platinum, vinblastine and bleomycin: a long-term follow-up. Eur J Cancer Clin Oncol 1989; 25(4): 733–6.

71. Roth BJ, Greist A, Kubilis PS, Williams SD, Einhorn LH. Cisplatin-based combination chemotherapy for disseminated germ cell tumors: long-term follow-up. J Clin Oncol 1988; 6(8): 1239–47.

72. Boyer M, et al. Lack of late toxicity in patients treated with cisplatin-containing combination chemotherapy for metastatic testicular cancer. J Clin Oncol 1990; 8(1): 21–6.

73. Stoter G, et al. Ten-year survival and late sequelae in testicular cancer patients treated with cisplatin, vinblastine, and bleomycin. J Clin Oncol 1989; 7(8): 1099–104.

74. Nichols CR, et al. No evidence of acute cardiovascular complications of chemotherapy for testicular cancer: an analysis of the Testicular Cancer Intergroup Study. J Clin Oncol 1992; 10(5): 760–5.

75. Matei D, et al. Chronic physical effects and health care utilization in long-term ovarian germ cell tumor survivors: a Gynecologic Oncology Group study. J Clin Oncol 2009; 27(25): 4142–9.

76. Gershenson DM, et al. Reproductive and sexual function after platinum-based chemotherapy in long-term ovarian germ cell tumor survivors: a Gynecologic Oncology Group Study. J Clin Oncol 2007; 25(19): 2792–7.

77. Champion V, et al. Quality of life in long-term survivors of ovarian germ cell tumors: a Gynecologic Oncology Group study. Gynecol Oncol 2007; 105(3): 687–94.

78. Kurman RJ, Norris HJ. Malignant germ cell tumors of the ovary. Hum Pathol 1977; 8(5): 551–64.

79. Cheng L, et al. KIT gene mutation and amplification in dysgerminoma of the ovary. Cancer 2011; 117(10): 2096–103.

80. De Palo G, et al. Germ cell tumors of the ovary: the experience of the National Cancer Institute of Milan. I. Dysgerminoma. Int J Radiat Oncol Biol Phys 1987; 13(6): 853–60.

81. LaPolla JP, Benda J, Vigliotti AP, Anderson B. Dysgerminoma of the ovary. Obstet Gynecol 1987; 69(6): 859–64.

82. Mitchell MF, Gershenson DM, Soeters RP, Eifel PJ, Delclos L, Wharton JT. The long-term effects of radiation therapy on patients with ovarian dysgerminoma. Cancer 1991; 67(4): 1084–90.

83. Buskirk SJ, et al. Ovarian dysgerminoma: a retrospective analysis of results of treatment, sites of treatment failure, and radiosensitivity. Mayo Clin Proc 1987; 62(12): 1149–57.

84. Bjorkholm E, Lundell M, Gyftodimos A, Silfversward C. Dysgerminoma. The Radiumhemmet series 1927–1984. Cancer 1990; 65(1): 38–44.

85. Lawson AP, Adler GF. Radiotherapy in the treatment of ovarian dysgerminomas. Int J Radiat Oncol Biol Phys 1988; 14(3): 431–4.

86. Santoni R, Cionini L, D'Elia F, Scarselli GF, Branconi F, Savino L. Dysgerminoma of the ovary: a report on 29 patients. Clin Radiol 1987; 38(2): 203–6.

87. Culine S, et al. Cisplatin-based chemotherapy in dysgerminoma of the ovary: thirteen-year experience at the Institut Gustave Roussy. Gynecol Oncol 1995; 58(3): 344–8.

88. Williams SD, Blessing JA, Hatch KD, Homesley HD. Chemotherapy of advanced dysgerminoma: trials of the Gynecologic Oncology Group. J Clin Oncol 1991; 9(11): 1950–5.

89. Williams SD, Kauderer J, Burnett AF, Lentz SS, Aghajanian C, Armstrong DK. Adjuvant therapy of completely resected dysgerminoma with carboplatin and etoposide: a trial of the Gynecologic Oncology Group. Gynecol Oncol 2004; 95(3): 496–9.

90. Pins MR, Young RH, Daly WJ, Scully RE. Primary squamous cell carcinoma of the ovary. Report of 37 cases. Am J Surg Pathol 1996; 20(7): 823–33.

91. Powell JL, Stinson JA, Connor GP, Shiro BS, Mattison M. Squamous cell carcinoma arising in a dermoid cyst of the ovary. Gynecol Oncol 2003; 89(3): 526–8.

92. Mayer C, Miller DM, Ehlen TG. Peritoneal implantation of squamous cell carcinoma following rupture of a dermoid cyst during laparoscopic removal. Gynecol Oncol 2002; 84(1): 180–3.

93. Rose PG, Tak WK, Reale FR. Squamous cell carcinoma arising in a mature cystic teratoma with metastasis to the paraaortic nodes. Gynecol Oncol 1993; 50(1): 131–3.

94. Takemori M, Nishimura R, Sugimura K, Obayashi C, Yasuda D. Ovarian strumal carcinoid with markedly high serum levels of tumor markers. Gynecol Oncol 1995; 58(2): 266–9.

95. Crowder S, Tuller E. Small cell carcinoma of the female genital tract. Semin Oncol 2007; 34(1): 57–63.

96. Di Vagno G, et al. Large-cell variant of small cell carcinoma of the ovary with hypercalcaemia. Arch Gynecol Obstet 2000; 264(3): 157–8.

97. Harrison ML, et al. Small cell of the ovary, hypercalcemic type – analysis of combined experience and recommendation for management. A GCIG study. Gynecol Oncol 2006; 100(2): 233–8.

98. Krepart G, Smith JP, Rutledge F, Delclos L. The treatment for dysgerminoma of the ovary. Cancer 1978; 41(3): 986–90.

99. Dark GG, Bower M, Newlands ES, Paradinas F, Rustin GJ. Surveillance policy for stage I ovarian germ cell tumors. J Clin Oncol 1997; 15(2): 620–4.

100. Zaghloul MS, Khattab TY. Dysgerminoma of the ovary: good prognosis even in advanced stages. Int J Radiat Oncol Biol Phys 1992; 24(1): 161–5.

38 Fallopian Tube Cancer

Destin Black[1] and Richard R. Barakat[2]

[1] Division of Gynecologic Oncology, Department of Obstetrics and Gynecology, Louisiana State University Health Sciences Center, New Orleans, LA, USA
[2] Gynecology Service, Department of Surgery, Memorial Sloan-Kettering Cancer Center, New York, NY, USA

Introduction

Primary malignant tumors of the fallopian tube account for 0.3–1.0% of all gynecological cancers.[1–5] Recent reports suggest this number may be higher, based on the hypothesis that the tubal fimbria may be the source of pelvic serous carcinogenesis resulting in ovarian, primary peritoneal, or fallopian tube cancer.[6,7] The majority of patients are 40–60 years of age, with a mean age of 55,[8] although it has been reported to occur in patients as young as 18.[1] This rarity has precluded prospective randomized trials and hindered our knowledge of this disease. Our current understanding of fallopian tube cancer consists of relatively small retrospective series, with fewer than 2000 cases reported in the literature.

Anatomy

The fallopian tube extends from the posterosuperior aspect of the uterine fundus to the ovary. At the ovary, the tube is composed of approximately 25 irregular finger-like extensions called *fimbriae*. The fimbriae attach to the infundibulum, which is about 1 cm long and 1 cm in diameter. The infundibulum narrows gradually to about 4 mm in diameter and merges medially with the ampullary portion of the tube, which is the widest and longest section. At a point characterized by a thickening of the muscular wall, the isthmic portion begins and extends 2 cm to the uterus. Within the myometrium, the tube communicates with the endometrial cavity at the uterotubal junction.[9]

The fallopian tube has an internal mucosal layer, an intermediate muscular layer, and an external serosal layer. The serosa is lined by mesothelial cells that are continuous with the serosa covering the uterus. The epithelial layer of the mucosa is composed of three cell types: ciliated, secretory, and intercalary.[10]

The arterial blood supply originates from the tubal branch of the uterine artery and the tubal branch of the ovarian artery, which anastomose within the mesosalpinx. Venous drainage consists of anastomosing tubal branches of the ovarian and uterine veins. The lymphatics accompany the tubal vessels draining into the paraaortic and pelvic lymph nodes.

Staging

Because of the clinical, therapeutic, and prognostic similarities with ovarian cancer, Dodson *et al.*,[11] in 1970, proposed applying the ovarian staging system to tubal carcinoma. In 1991, the International Federation of Gynecology and Obstetrics (FIGO) Committee established an official staging system for fallopian tube cancer (Table 38.1), which is similar to that of ovarian cancer. In a review of 558 patients, 33%, 33%, and 33% were stages I, II, and III–IV, respectively.[12] These statistics are more favorable than ovarian carcinoma patient statistics; 70% of ovarian carcinoma patients have stages III and IV disease. In 1967, Erez *et al.*[13] suggested a staging system based on the Dukes colonic cancer staging, which used both depth of invasion and distant disease. This staging system would have been based on tumor penetration through the layers of the tube. In data from 18 institutions, pathological stage was closely related to survival in 76 patients with tubal cancer.[14] More recently, Peters *et al.*[8] analyzed stage I patients and found a 50% depth of tubal muscularis invasion to be the only significant prognostic variable. However, other authors have not shown the depth of tubal invasion to be prognostic of survival.[15,16]

Primary adenocarcinoma

Biology and epidemiology

There are accumulating data, based on both morphological and molecular characteristics, implicating the fallopian tube as the site of origin of a large proportion of high-grade pelvic serous carcinomas.[6,17,18] Evidence supporting this hypothesis includes the existence of tubal intraepithelial carcinoma (TIC) in fallopian tubes after risk-reducing salpingo-oophorectomy in patients who are *BRCA* mutation carriers, histological similarities between fallopian tube epithelium and disseminated papillary serous carcinoma,[6,7,17,19,20] and shared mutations in TIC and disseminated papillary serous carcinoma. A possible early precursor to TIC, the "p53 signature," commonly occurs in the same region of the tube (fimbria) as serous carcinomas and is often found to

Textbook of Uncommon Cancer, Fourth Edition. Edited by Derek Raghavan, Charles D. Blanke, David H. Johnson, Paul L. Moots, Gregory H. Reaman, Peter G. Rose and Mikkael A. Sekeres.
© 2012 John Wiley & Sons, Inc. Published 2012 by John Wiley & Sons, Inc.

Table 38.1 FIGO fallopian tube staging.

Stage	Description
Stage 0	Carcinoma *in situ* (limited to tubal mucosa)
Stage I	Growth limited to the fallopian tubes
Stage IA	Growth is limited to one tube with extension into the submucosa and/or muscularis but not penetrating the serosal surface; no ascites
Stage IB	Growth is limited to both tubes with extension into the submucosa and/or muscularis but not penetrating the serosal surface; no ascites
Stage IC	Tumor either stage IA or IB with tumor extension through or onto the tubal serosa, or with ascites present containing malignant cells or with positive peritoneal washings
Stage II	Growth involving one or both fallopian tubes with pelvic extension
Stage IIA	Extension and/or metastasis to the uterus and/or ovaries
Stage IIB	Extension to other pelvic tissues
Stage IIC	Tumor either stage IIA or IIB and with ascites present containing malignant cells or with positive peritoneal washings
Stage III	Tumor involves one or both fallopian tubes with peritoneal implants outside the pelvis and/or positive retroperitoneal or inguinal nodes. Superficial liver metastases equals stage III. Tumor appears limited to the true pelvis but with histologically proven malignant extension to the small bowel or omentum
Stage IIIA	Tumor is grossly limited to the true pelvis with negative nodes but with histologically confirmed microscopic seeding of abdominal peritoneal surfaces
Stage IIIB	Tumor involving one or both tubes with histologically confirmed implants of abdominal peritoneal surfaces, none exceeding 2 cm in diameter. Lymph nodes are negative
Stage IIIC	Abdominal implants greater than 2 cm in diameter and/or positive retroperitoneal or inguinal nodes
Stage IV	Growth involving one or both fallopian tubes with distant metastases. If pleural effusion is present, there must be positive cytology to be stage IV. Parenchymal liver metastases equals stage IV

Note: Staging for fallopian tube is by the surgical pathological system. Operative findings designating stage are determined prior to tumor debulking.

be in direct continuity with TIC. These small linear p53 foci (Fig. 38.1) harbor evidence of DNA damage, involve the tubal secretory cell, and are present more commonly in women diagnosed with serous carcinoma.[19–21] A recent study has shown that these mutations are not restricted to women with familial ovarian cancer.[20,22]

In patients diagnosed with primary fallopian tube cancer, a history of infertility is common; one study reported a 40% incidence of nulliparity in a series of 47 patients.[23] Chronic inflammation and tuberculous salpingitis have also been suggested as possible predisposing factors. Although chronic inflammation often presents with fallopian tube carcinoma, it

is doubtful that it is a causative factor. Chronic salpingitis usually involves both tubes, while the inflammatory response associated with fallopian tube cancer is usually limited to the tube involved with the carcinoma. In addition, tubal carcinoma occurs in postmenopausal women, a group with a low prevalence of chronic salpingitis. In Sedlis' review,[24] the rate of pelvic tuberculosis in patients with fallopian tube cancer was not higher than the rate of pelvic tuberculosis in the general population. The rarity of this malignancy makes any of these relatively common conditions unlikely etiological factors.

Alterations of the p53 tumor suppressor gene have been reported in 59–81% of cases.[25–28] Although p53 mutations were seen in all stages of tubal carcinoma, patients with p53 mutations had a significantly shorter survival rate compared to patients without mutations.

There is molecular and population-based evidence that fallopian tube cancer may be a component of the *BRCA*-related breast and ovarian cancer syndrome.[29–33] Aziz and colleagues reported that *BRCA* mutations accounted for 16% of fallopian tube cancers in an unselected population.[32] Levine *et al.*[34] found germline *BRCA* mutations in 17% of Ashkenazi patients with fallopian tube cancer. In addition, invasive fallopian tube carcinoma and *in situ* carcinoma have been described in approximately 2–10% of patients with *BRCA* mutations who underwent risk-reducing salpingo-oophorectomy.[35,36]

Pathology

The rarity of fallopian tube cancer occurrence is partially related to the physicians' convention of attributing tubal carcinoma involving the ovary or endometrium to an ovarian or endometrial primary.

Macroscopic appearance

The tube is usually enlarged by the growth of the intraluminal tumor and appears fusiform (Fig. 38.2). In approximately 50% of cases, the fimbriated end of the tube is occluded with the development of pyosalpinx or hematosalpinx. On opening the tube, the lumen is occupied by a solid mass, frequently with hemorrhagic and necrotic areas. The tumor may arise from any portion of the tube, but it most often originates in the ampullary portion. Fallopian tube cancer affects both the right and left tubes with similar frequency and is bilateral in 10–26% of cases.[1,14,15,24,37] In early stages, this bilaterality may represent an independent occurrence in both tubes if the intervening endometrium is free of cancer.[24] With more advanced cases, the tumor penetrates the tubal serosa and may involve the ovaries and uterus or other pelvic or abdominal organs.

Spread pattern

The disease reaches the peritoneal cavity and its viscera through the tubal fimbria or through transmural invasion of the tubal wall. The mode of metastasis according to most clinical studies is intraperitoneal via the tubal ostia. Sedlis[24] found the peritoneum to be the most frequent site of metastasis, followed by the ovaries and the uterus.

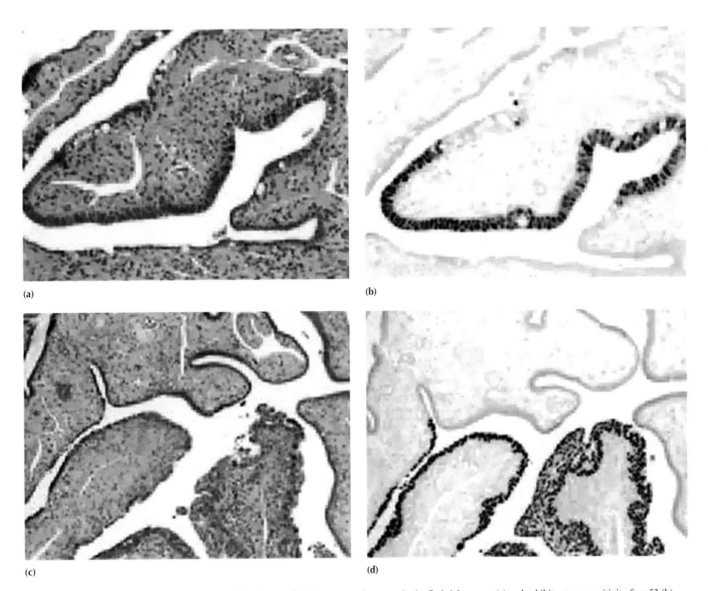

Figure 38.1 (a,b) The "p53signature" is a nonneoplastic abnormality that commonly occurs in the fimbrial mucosa (a) and exhibits strong positivity for p53 (b). The p53 signature shares several features with tubal intraepithelial carcinoma (c), including p53 staining (d) and p53 mutations. Reproduced from Crum et al.[6]

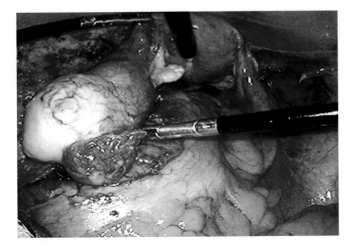

Figure 38.2 Carcinoma of the fallopian tube. This intraoperative photograph depicts the fusiform dilation of the affected tube.

Evaluation for nodal involvement has not been done routinely by most authors. Tamimi and Figge[38] reported a 33% frequency of paraaortic nodal metastasis in a series of 15 patients. Gadducci et al.[39] found histologically proven metastatic nodes in 50% of 22 patients submitted to paraaortic node dissection and in 24.2% of 33 patients submitted to pelvic node dissection. Recently, Deffieux et al.[40] reported that the left paraaortic chain above the level of the inferior mesenteric artery is the most frequently involved nodal package. In addition, nodal metastasis has been found in patients who have had no other evidence of disease.[38,41]

This potential for nodal metastasis may explain the poor survival rate even when the disease is apparently limited to the tube. Nodal involvement has been shown to negatively affect survival.[41,42] Klein et al.[43] reported improved median survival when radical lymphadenectomy was performed at the time of initial staging. Tamimi and Figge[38] and Asmussen et al.[16] found histological evidence of vascular-lymphatic space involvement to be associated with nodal metastasis and to be a poor prognostic factor in survival.

Histology

The most frequent histological type is adenocarcinoma, similar to the ovarian serous variety. Less common histological types include clear cell carcinoma, endometrioid carcinoma, adeno-squamous carcinoma, squamous cell carcinoma, sarcoma, choriocarcinoma, and malignant teratoma. The histological differential diagnosis of primary malignant tumors of the fallopian tube should include a wide variety of benign tumors and the possibility of metastasis from other primary sites. Various criteria to determine the definite diagnosis of primary fallopian tube carcinoma have been suggested. In 1949, Finn and Javert[44] proposed the following criteria, but these are currently undergoing reassessment.

Gross criteria

1. The tubes, at least in the distal portion, are abnormal. The fimbriated ends may be dilated and occluded, resembling chronic salpingitis.
2. There is a papillary growth in the endosalpinx.
3. The uterus and ovaries are either grossly normal or affected by a lesion other than cancer.

Microscopic criteria

1. The epithelium of the endosalpinx is replaced in whole or in part by adenocarcinoma, and the histological character of the cells resembles the epithelium of the endosalpinx (Fig. 38.3).
2. The endometrium and ovaries are normal or contain a malignant lesion that is secondary to a tubal primary in its size, distribution, and histological appearance.
3. Tuberculosis has been clearly excluded.

In 1950, Hu et al.[45] proposed additional criteria.

1. Grossly, the main tumor is in the tube.
2. Microscopically, the mucosa should be chiefly involved and show a papillary pattern.
3. If the tubal wall is found to be involved to a great extent, the transition between benign and malignant tubal epithelium should be demonstrable.

More recently, gynecological pathologists have thoroughly evaluated fallopian tubes removed at exploration for abdominal carcinomatosis. Some pathologists recommend the fallopian tubes be entirely sectioned using a protocol that requires amputating each fimbria at the infundibulum, longitudinal sectioning of the fimbria, and extensive cross-sectioning of the remainder of the tube at 2 mm intervals.[46,47] The transformation of in situ to invasive carcinoma in the tube has been identified and is considered diagnostic of primary fallopian tube malignancy. Numerous studies of fallopian tube cancer have also noted multifocal upper genital tract tumors.[4,8,15,48] In one study, 37% of patients (24 of 64) had multiple primary tumors occurring in the ovary (31%), uterus (11%), and cervix (3%).[15]

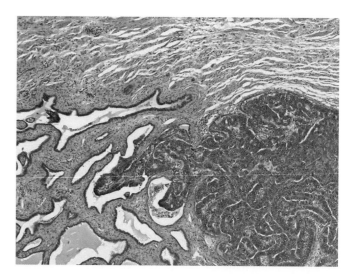

Figure 38.3 Carcinoma of the fallopian tube. In this photomicrograph, the epithelium of the endosalpinx is replaced by adenocarcinoma.

Field neoplastic changes to the müllerian epithelium were proposed to explain the existence of multiple upper genital tract neoplasias. Bannatyne and Russell[49] reported seven cases of in situ or invasive tubal carcinoma after reviewing 251 cases of epithelial ovarian cancer. These authors stress that careful sectioning of the tube may identify tubal neoplasia in 5–10% of ovarian tumors. In one series, among 1592 ovarian cancers pathologically evaluated over the study period, tubal neoplasia was present in 1.3% of cases.[15]

Adenocarcinoma in situ has been described as an entity, and some authors do not distinguish it from adenomatous hyperplasia; it is usually focal, containing abnormal mitotic figures and nuclear pleomorphism with large nucleoli.

Hu et al.[45] divided fallopian tumors into three histological classifications: grade I, papillary lesions; grade II, papillary-alveolar lesions; grade III, alveolar-medullary lesions. Most pathologists no longer use this system and the grade of the tumor is classified as well, moderately, or poorly differentiated. Uehira et al.[50] have described a transitional cell pattern. The disease-free interval was markedly improved for patients with a transitional cell pattern compared to those with a nontransitional cell pattern. The authors suggest that this may be the result of an improved response to chemotherapy, as has been demonstrated for transitional cell ovarian carcinoma.[51] Endometrioid fallopian tube carcinomas have also been identified as a less invasive and less malignant histological type.[52]

Clinical presentation and diagnostic considerations

Symptoms and signs

The most common presenting symptoms are vaginal bleeding, abdominal pain, and watery discharge. The abdominal pain is classically colicky in nature due to the peristaltic activity of the fallopian tube. A dull, constant pain may occur due to chronic distension of the tubal wall and serosa. Latzko[53] described the classic syndrome of "hydrops tubae profluens" in 1916. This is characterized by an adnexal mass and colicky lower abdominal pain that is relieved by the discharge of copious serous fluid from the vagina. Although said to be pathognomonic, it is noted in less than 15% of patients.[54] The most common finding on physical examination is an elongated pelvic mass. Ascites may also be present. Rarely, watery vaginal discharge or bleeding after hysterectomy has resulted in a diagnosis of fallopian tube carcinoma.[55,56]

Diagnostic tests

Pelvic imaging studies usually demonstrate an adnexal mass that is cystic, complex, or solid in character. No specific pattern has been defined that could differentiate a tubal neoplasm from hydrosalpinx or pyosalpinx. Additionally, this finding is usually interpreted to be an ovarian neoplasm, which is much more common. Computed tomography or magnetic resonance imaging may be helpful for evaluating spread to other intraabdominal or retroperitoneal structures. Positron emission tomography with fluorine-18-2-deoxyglucose has been reported to correlate with findings of recurrent disease.[57] Although an elevated CA-125 is not diagnostic of fallopian tube cancer, more than 80% of patients have increased CA-125 levels and 87% of tumors stain for CA-125.[58,59]

Diagnosis

Fallopian tube cancer diagnosis is seldom made prior to surgery. In one review of 780 patients, only 10 (1.3%) were diagnosed preoperatively.[60] Because of the rarity of the condition, the presence of a pelvic mass in a perimenopausal or postmenopausal woman usually suggests a primary ovarian neoplasm. Positive Papanicolaou smears have been reported in approximately 10% of cases.[37,48,61] Patients with recurrent post-menopausal vaginal bleeding or an abnormal Papanicolaou smear (and for whom cervical and endometrial cancer have been ruled out by negative dilation and curettage) should be suspected of having a tubal carcinoma. Laparoscopy may be helpful if the diagnosis is suspected and no pelvic mass is found by less invasive methods. Rarely does fallopian tube carcinoma enter the differential diagnosis of pelvic masses preoperatively. Intraoperatively, it should be distinguished from benign conditions that enlarge and affect the fallopian tubes such as endometriosis, ectopic pregnancy, hydrosalpinx, and tuboovarian abscess.

Treatment

Surgery

Surgical therapy for fallopian tube cancer should be the same as it is for ovarian cancer. In cases grossly confined to the tube, a careful staging procedure should be performed that includes peritoneal washings and systematic inspection and palpation of the peritoneal surfaces. Omentectomy, bilateral pelvic and paraaortic lymphadenectomy, and peritoneal biopsies should be performed. Maxson et al.[62] reported two of five patients who had nodal sampling at primary surgery that were positive. A limited number of patients with stage I disease have been treated with surgery alone without evidence of recurrence.[15,63] However, one study examining routine lymphadenectomy found no cases of nodal metastasis in a small series of patients with disease grossly confined to the adnexa.[64] Positive

peritoneal washings carry prognostic significance, with a 5-year survival rate of 20% compared to 67% for cases with negative peritoneal washings.[23] If extratubal spread is found at the time of surgery, a maximal tumor reductive effort should be performed with the main objective of leaving minimal (<1 cm) residual disease. Significant improvement in survival for patients with residual tumors less than 1 cm compared to those with larger residual tumor has been demonstrated.[8,23,65,66] Barakat et al.[66] evaluated 38 patients with stages II, III, or IV disease and found a 5-year survival rate of 83% for patients with no residual disease compared to 29% for those with gross residual disease.

Radiotherapy

The efficacy of radiation therapy for tubal carcinoma is difficult to determine from the current literature due to the lack of uniformity in staging criteria, treatment fields, dosage, fraction size, and type of radiation employed. A previous report[11] showed that tubal carcinoma is radiosensitive. Phelps and Chapman[3] reported survival in eight of nine stages I and II patients treated with both radioisotope and pelvic radiation ($n=5$) or pelvic radiation alone ($n=3$). Podratz et al.[23] reported four of six patients developing recurrence after pelvic radiation for stage IA, IB, and IIA disease. The use of radiation therapy directed solely to the pelvis is of doubtful benefit owing to the potential of the disease for intraperitoneal dissemination. As in ovarian cancer, the entire peritoneal cavity may be at risk, and curability is limited by our inability to deliver therapeutic doses to the entire abdomen. Brown et al.[67] reported a patient with stage III disease and long-term survival after abdominopelvic radiation. Again, in the series reported by Podratz et al.,[23] five of five patients with stages IC, IIB, or III disease who received whole-abdominal radiation recurred. Recently, Kojs et al.[68] reported 32 patients treated with whole-abdominal radiation. Five-year survival was achieved in 10 of 13 (76.9%) stage I patients, five of nine (55.6%) stage II patients, and two of 10 (20%) stage III patients. Whole-abdominal radiation was ineffective in the setting of gross (>2 cm) residual disease. Few studies have used radioisotopes alone for tubal carcinoma. In one study, four early stages I or II patients received adjuvant ^{32}P, and three patients developed recurrence.[15] Schray et al.[69] reported two patients with stages I and II disease treated with 15 mCi of ^{32}P without recurrence. As in ovarian carcinoma, a subset of surgically staged patients without metastasis may benefit from radioisotope therapy.

Chemotherapy
Hormonal therapy

The tubal epithelium is hormonally sensitive. Both estrogen and progesterone receptors have been identified in fallopian tube carcinomas.[65,70,71] Johnston[71] reported a patient with stage I disease treated by surgery and adjuvant progesterone without recurrence at 29 months. However, numerous authors have reported no response to hormonal therapy.[11,15,37,72,73] Although responses were noted with cytotoxic regimes that included progesterone,[23,37,74,75] the role of progesterone in these regimens is unclear.

Single-agent chemotherapy

A variety of alkylating agents including nitrogen mustard, thio-triethylenephosphamide (TEPA), chlorambucil, cyclo-phosphamide, and melphalan have been utilized for fallopian tube carcinoma.[74,76] Favorable responses have been seen with cisplatin or doxorubicin used as single agents.[15,72] More recently, a combination of paclitaxel and liposomal doxorubicin has demonstrated response in platinum-resistant disease.[77–80] There is modest activity using weekly docetaxel in heavily pretreated, platinum-resistant patients.[81,82]

Combination chemotherapy

Although cisplatin-based combination chemotherapy has been reported in fallopian tube cancers since 1980,[75] the cumulative experience is limited (Table 38.2).[62,66,73,80,83–87] The overall response rate is 61%, with 50% complete response rate. Peters et al.[73] reported 46 patients evaluable for chemotherapy response. The response rate for 12 patients receiving cisplatin-containing multiagent chemotherapy was 81%, 75% of which were complete responses. This was significantly different from the response rates seen with multiagent chemotherapy (29%) or single-agent therapy (9%) without cisplatin. Barakat et al. reported 38 patients treated with cisplatin, doxorubicin, and cyclophosphamide ($n = 24$) or cisplatin and cyclophosphamide ($n = 14$).[66] No difference in survival was noted, questioning the role of doxorubicin. Cormio et al.[85] also reported 38 patients treated with cisplatin, doxorubicin, and cyclophosphamide. In their study, the median survival was 38 months, with a 5-year survival rate of 35%. Pectasides et al.[86] reported 14 patients treated with platinum-based combination therapy, four of whom received carboplatin with a similar response rate. Other examples of response to carboplatin have also been reported.[87] Gemignani et al.[88] reported the use of paclitaxel-based chemotherapy after initial surgery in 24 patients with primary fallopian tube adenocarcinoma. The overall median progression-free survival was 27 months for the entire group. The 3-year progression-free survival rate was 67% for optimally cytoreduced compared with 45% for the suboptimally debulked group. Based on randomized trials in ovarian cancer, current therapy should consist of a combination of paclitaxel and a platinum compound.

Prognosis

The most important prognostic factor that correlates with survival is the stage of the disease. Most authors have found significantly different survival rates between patients with disease confined to the pelvis and those with disease beyond the pelvis.[8,23,48] Survival figures range from 40% to 60% for localized disease (stages I and II) and from 0% to 16% for more advanced disease (stages III and IV).[4,48,63,72,89] In a multicenter retrospective study of 68 patients with stages I and II fallopian tube carcinomas, patients with grade I tumors had a significantly longer survival than patients with grade II or grade III tumors.[5] Approximately 15% of patients who undergo a negative second-look laparotomy develop recurrent disease. In many cases, recurrences after negative second-look laparotomy have

Table 38.2 Platinum-based therapy for fallopian tube carcinoma.

	n	PR	CR	Total
Jacobs et al.[83]	9	–	4	4
Maxson et al.[62]	12	2	9	11
Peters et al.[73]	16	1	12	13
Rose et al.[80]	14	1	2	3
Morris et al.[84]	9*	4	1	5
Muntz et al.[87]	7	2	3	5
Barakat et al.[66]	26	–	11	11
Pectasides et al.[86]	11	2	8	10
Cormio et al.[85]	38	4	22	28
Total	144	16	72	88

* Evaluated at second-look laparotomy.
CR, complete response; PR, partial response.

been at distant sites such as the supraclavicular nodes lungs, brain, kidneys, and axilla.[63,67,90]

Response to therapy

Like ovarian cancer, in the absence of clinically evident or progressive disease, disease status is difficult to assess. Response to therapy and recurrence have been correlated with CA-125 levels.[91] Second-look laparotomy has been shown to be of prognostic importance in ovarian cancer.[92] Because of the rarity of fallopian tube cancer, second-look laparotomy was not reported in this disease until 1980.[75] Overall, 64% of patients undergoing the procedure have no evidence of disease. The likelihood of having a negative second look is related to the amount of residual tumor after initial surgery.[89,93–96] Nodal evaluation is essential, and paraaortic nodal metastases have been detected as the only evidence of persistent disease at second-look laparotomy.[38] Survival for the patients who were pathologically disease free was significantly different from those who were clinically disease free.[15,96] Second-look laparoscopy is a less invasive means to determine disease status and, if positive, may be useful. However, in ovarian carcinoma the procedure is less sensitive and, if negative, some authors recommend confirmation by second-look laparotomy.[97,98]

Sarcomas

Malignant mixed mesodermal tumors of the fallopian tube are uncommon, with slightly more than 50 cases reported.[99] Although uncommon, they comprise a greater percentage of fallopian cancers than does ovarian sarcoma compared to ovarian carcinoma. The mean age at diagnosis, clinical features, stage at presentation, and spread pattern do not appear different from the more commonly encountered adenocarcinoma. An equal number of homologous and heterologous fallopian tube tumors have been reported.[100] The diagnosis is usually not established until the final pathology is completed.

The prognosis of sarcoma patients is poor: most patients survive less than 2 years, although long-term survival has been reported.[15,101–103] Muntz et al.[102] reported improved survival when the disease is confined to the muscularis. Carlson *et al.*[103] reviewed 35 cases with sufficient treatment and follow-up data. Nine patients (26%) were disease free after 36 months. In each case, disease was limited to the pelvis, all disease was resected, and postoperative treatment was employed (chemotherapy and radiation therapy, $n=5$; chemotherapy alone, $n=2$; radiation therapy alone, $n=2$). In another review of 13 survivors, nine had stage I, one had stage II, and three had stage III disease.[100] As in ovarian carcinoma, negative second-look laparotomy has been associated with long-term survival.[15,100–102]

Trophoblastic tumors

Tubal molar pregnancy occurs in one per 5333 ectopic gestations or one per 1.6 million normal intrauterine pregnancies.[104] Primary choriocarcinoma of the tube is an even rarer entity and may be gestational or nongestational. Choriocarcinoma involving the tube should be distinguished from a primary intrauterine tumor or a malignant ovarian germ cell tumor. Preoperatively, the diagnosis mimics an ectopic pregnancy. A study from the New England Trophoblastic Disease Center reported 16 cases of tubal gestational trophoblastic disease (GTD).[105] Tubal GTD accounted for 0.8% of GTD cases managed at the referral center. The frequency rates of partial moles, complete moles, and choriocarcinoma were similar; 31%, 31%, and 38%, respectively. None of the patients presented with symptoms of hyperemesis, toxemia, theca lutein cysts, hyperthyroidism, respiratory insufficiency, or markedly elevated human chorionic gonadotropin (hCG) ($>30000\,U/mL^{-1}$).

The surgical approach may be conservative (i.e. unilateral adnexectomy). All of the partial and four of the five complete molar pregnancies reported by the New England Trophoblastic Disease Center responded to partial or complete salpingo-oophorectomy. One patient with a complete molar pregnancy developed metastatic disease requiring chemotherapy. Pregnancy after conservative therapy consisting of unilateral salpingo-oophorectomy and chemotherapy has been reported.[106]

Chemotherapy is an essential component in the management of tubal choriocarcinoma. Ober and Maier[107] reviewed 76 cases of tubal choriocarcinoma and found that of 59 patients, 46 treated in the prechemotherapy era died, in contrast to one of 17 diagnosed in the postchemotherapy era. Treatment should be monitored by serum hCG titers. Nongestational choriocarcinoma has a poorer prognosis and can be diagnosed only if germ cell elements other than choriocarcinoma are present.

Metastatic tumors

Approximately 80% of tubal malignancies are metastatic from other sites, most commonly from the ovary and endometrium.[108,109] Extragenital primary cancers metastasizing to the tube are much rarer, and other primary sites include the breast and gastrointestinal tract. With metastatic disease to the tube, the mucosa is intact. There is serosal involvement, or nests of metastatic deposits are seen in the lymphatics underneath the epithelium.

References

1. Hanton EM, *et al.* Primary carcinoma of the fallopian tube. Am J Obstet Gynecol 1966; 94(6): 832–9.
2. Momtazee S, Kempson RL. Primary adenocarcinoma of the fallopian tube. Obstet Gynecol 1968; 32(5): 649–56.
3. Phelps HM, Chapman KE. Role of radiation therapy in treatment of primary carcinoma of the uterine tube. Obstet Gynecol 1974; 43(5): 669–73.
4. Roberts JA, Lifshitz S. Primary adenocarcinoma of the fallopian tube. Gynecol Oncol 1982; 13(3): 301–8.
5. Rosen AC, *et al.* A comparative analysis of management and prognosis in stage I and II fallopian tube carcinoma and epithelial ovarian cancer. Br J Cancer 1994; 69(6): 577–9.
6. Crum CP, *et al.* The distal fallopian tube: a new model for pelvic serous carcinogenesis. Curr Opin Obstet Gynecol 2007; 19: 3–9.
7. Kindelberger DW, *et al.* Intraepithelial carcinoma of the fimbria and pelvic serous carcinoma: evidence for a causal relationship. Am J Surg Pathol 2007; 31: 161–9.
8. Peters WA III, *et al.* Prognostic features of carcinoma of the fallopian tube. Obstet Gynecol 1988; 71(5): 757–62.
9. James E, Wheeler MD. *Disease of the Fallopian Tube*, 4th edn. New York: Springer-Verlag, 1994.
10. Pauerstein CJ, Woodruff JD. The role of the "indifferent" cells of the tubal epithelium. Am J Obstet Gynecol 1967; 98: 121–5.
11. Dodson MG, Ford JH Jr, Averette HE. Clinical aspects of fallopian tube carcinoma. Obstet Gynecol 1970; 36(6): 935–9.
12. Markman M, *et al. Carcinoma of the Fallopian Tube*, 4th edn. Philadelphia: Lippincott, 2005.
13. Erez S, Kaplan AL, Wall JA. Clinical staging of carcinoma of the uterine tube. Obstet Gynecol 1967; 30(4): 547–50.
14. Schiller HM, Silverberg SG. Staging and prognosis in primary carcinoma of the fallopian tube. Cancer 1971; 28(2): 389–95.
15. Rose PG, Piver MS, Tsukada Y. Fallopian tube cancer. The Roswell Park experience. Cancer 1990; 66(12): 2661–7.
16. Asmussen M, *et al.* Primary adenocarcinoma localized to the fallopian tubes: report on 33 cases. Gynecol Oncol 1988; 30(2): 183–6.
17. Levanon K, *et al.* New insights into the pathogenesis of serous ovarian cancer and its clinical impact. J Clin Oncol 2008; 26: 5284.
18. Crum CP, *et al.* Lessons from BRCA: the tubal fimbria emerges as an origin for pelvic serous cancer. Clin Med Res 2007; 5: 35–44.
19. Piek JM, *et al.* Dysplastic changes in prophylactically removed fallopian tubes of women predisposed to developing ovarian cancer. J Pathol 2001; 195: 451–6.
20. Lee Y, *et al.* A candidate precursor to serous carcinoma that originates in the distal fallopian tube. J Pathol 2007; 211: 26–35.
21. Crum CP, *et al.* Bringing the p53 signature into focus. Cancer 2010; 116: 5119–21.
22. Shaw PA, *et al.* Candidate serous cancer precursors in fallopian tube epithelium of BRCA1/2 mutation carriers. Mod Pathol 2009; 22: 1133–8.
23. Podratz KC Jr, *et al.* Primary carcinoma of the fallopian tube. Am J Obstet Gynecol 1986; 154(6): 1319–26.
24. Sedlis A. Primary carcinoma of the fallopian tube. Obstet Gynecol Surv 1961; 16: 209–26.
25. Lacy MQ, *et al.* c-erbB-2 and p53 expression in fallopian tube carcinoma. Cancer 1995; 75(12): 2891–6.
26. Zheng W, *et al.* Early occurrence and prognostic significance of p53 alteration in primary carcinoma of the fallopian tube. Gynecol Oncol 1997; 64(1): 38–48.
27. Rosen AC, *et al.* p53 expression in fallopian tube carcinomas. Cancer Lett 2000; 156(1): 1–7.
28. Chung TK, *et al.* Overexpression of p53 and HER-2/neu and c-myc in primary fallopian tube carcinoma. Gynecol Obstet Invest 2000; 49(1): 47–51.

29. Bandera CA, *et al*. BRCA1 gene mutations in women with papillary serous carcinoma of the peritoneum. Obstet Gynecol 1998; 92(4 Pt 1): 596–600.

30. Schorge JO, *et al*. BRCA1-related papillary serous carcinoma of the peritoneum has a unique molecular pathogenesis. Cancer Res 2000; 60(5): 1361–4.

31. Zweemer RP, *et al*. Molecular evidence linking primary cancer of the fallopian tube to BRCA1 germline mutations. Gynecol Oncol 2000; 76(1): 45–50.

32. Aziz S, *et al*. A genetic epidemiological study of carcinoma of the fallopian tube. Gynecol Oncol 2001; 80(3): 341–5.

33. Menczer J, *et al*. Frequency of BRCA mutations in primary peritoneal carcinoma in Israeli Jewish women. Gynecol Oncol 2003; 88(1): 58–61.

34. Levine DA, *et al*. Fallopian tube and primary peritoneal carcinomas associated with BRCA mutations. J Clin Oncol 2003; 21(22): 4222–7.

35. Finch A, *et al*. Clinical and pathologic findings of prophylactic salpingo-oophorectomies in 159 BRCA1 and BRCA2 carriers. Gynecol Oncol 2006; 100: 58–64.

36. Powell CB, *et al*. Risk-reducing salpingo-oophorectomy in BRCA mutation carriers: role of serial sectioning in the detection of occult malignancy. J Clin Oncol 2005; 23: 127–32.

37. Yoonessi M. Carcinoma of the fallopian tube. Obstet Gynecol Surv 1979; 34(4): 257–70.

38. Tamimi HK, Figge DC. Adenocarcinoma of the uterine tube: potential for lymph node metastases. Am J Obstet Gynecol 1981; 141: 132–7.

39. Gadducci A, *et al*. Analysis of treatment failures and survival of patients with fallopian tube carcinoma: a cooperation task force (CTF) study. Gynecol Oncol 2001; 81(2): 150–9.

40. Deffieux X, *et al*. Anatomy of pelvic and para-aortic nodal spread in patients with primary fallopian tube carcinoma. J Am Coll Surg 2005; 200(1): 45–8.

41. Di Re E, *et al*. Fallopian tube cancer: incidence and role of lymphatic spread. Gynecol Oncol 1996; 62(2): 199–202.

42. Cormio G, *et al*. Primary carcinoma of the fallopian tube. A retrospective analysis of 47 patients. Ann Oncol 1996; 7(3): 271–5.

43. Klein M, *et al*. Lymphadenectomy in primary carcinoma of the fallopian tube. Cancer Lett 1999; 147(1–2): 63–6.

44. Finn WF, Javert CT. Primary and metastatic cancer of the fallopian tube. Cancer 1949; 2: 803–14.

45. Hu CY, Taymor ML, Hertig AT. Primary carcinoma of the fallopian tube. Am J Obstet Gynecol 1950; 59(1): 58–67.

46. Chang PS, *et al*. The fallopian tube and broad ligament. In: Crum CP, Lee KR (eds) *Diagnostic Gynecologic and Obstetric Pathology*. Philadelphia: Elsevier Saunders; 2006. pp.698–701.

47. Colgan TJ. Challenges in the early diagnosis and staging of Fallopian-tube carcinomas associated with BRCA mutations. Int J Gynecol Pathol 2003; 22: 109–20.

48. Eddy GL, *et al*. Fallopian tube carcinoma. Obstet Gynecol 1984; 64(4): 546–52.

49. Bannatyne P, Russell P. Early adenocarcinoma of the fallopian tubes. A case for multifocal tumorigenesis. Diagn Gynecol Obstet 1981; 3(1): 49–60.

50. Uehira K, *et al*. Transitional cell carcinoma pattern in primary carcinoma of the fallopian tube. Cancer 1993; 72(8): 2447–56.

51. Robey SS, *et al*. Transitional cell carcinoma in high-grade high-stage ovarian carcinoma. An indicator of favorable response to chemotherapy. Cancer 1989; 63(5): 839–47.

52. Navani SS, *et al*. Endometrioid carcinoma of the fallopian tube: a clinico-pathologic analysis of 26 cases. Gynecol Oncol 1996; 63(3): 371–8.

53. Latzko W. Linkseitiges Tubenkarzinom Rechtsietige Karzinomatose tuboovarial Cyste. Zentralbl Gynakol 1916; 40: 599.

54. Berek JS, Hacker NF. *Practical Gynecologic Oncology*, 4th edn. Philadelphia: Lippincott Williams and Wilkins, 2004. p.53.

55. Muntz HG, *et al*. Post-hysterectomy carcinoma of the fallopian tube mimicking a vesicovaginal fistula. Obstet Gynecol 1992; 79(5 Pt 2): 853–6.

56. Ehlen T, *et al*. Posthysterectomy carcinoma of the fallopian tube presenting as vaginal adenocarcinoma: a case report. Gynecol Oncol 1989; 33(3): 382–5.

57. Karlan BY, *et al*. Whole-body positron emission tomography with (fluorine-18)-2-deoxyglucose can detect metastatic carcinoma of the fallopian tube. Gynecol Oncol 1993; 49(3): 383–8.

58. Hefler LA, *et al*. The clinical value of serum concentrations of cancer antigen 125 in patients with primary fallopian tube carcinoma: a multi-center study. Cancer 2000; 89(7): 1555–60.

59. Puls LE, *et al*. Immunohistochemical staining for CA-125 in fallopian tube carcinomas. Gynecol Oncol 1993; 48(3): 360–3.

60. Jones OV. Primary carcinoma of the uterine tube. Obstet Gynecol 1965; 26: 122–9.

61. Takashina T, Ito E, Kudo R. Cytologic diagnosis of primary tubal cancer. Acta Cytol 1985; 29(3): 367–72.

62. Maxson WZ, *et al*. Primary carcinoma of the fallopian tube: evidence for activity of cisplatin combination therapy. Gynecol Oncol 1987; 26(3): 305–13.

63. McMurray EH, *et al*. Carcinoma of the fallopian tube. Management and sites of failure. Cancer 1986; 58(9): 2070–5.

64. Klein M, *et al*. Radical lymphadenectomy in the primary carcinoma of the fallopian tube. Arch Gynecol Obstet 1993; 253(1): 21–5.

65. Rosen A, *et al*. Primary carcinoma of the fallopian tube – a retrospective analysis of 115 patients. Austrian Cooperative Study Group for Fallopian Tube Carcinoma. Br J Cancer 1993; 68(3): 605–9.

66. Barakat RR, *et al*. Cisplatin-based combination chemotherapy in carcinoma of the fallopian tube. Gynecol Oncol 1991; 42(2): 156–60.

67. Brown MD, *et al*. Fallopian tube carcinoma. Int J Radiat Oncol Biol Phys 1985; 11(3): 583–90.

68. Kojs Z, *et al*. Whole abdominal external beam radiation in the treatment of primary carcinoma of the fallopian tube. Gynecol Oncol 1997; 65(3): 473–7.

69. Schray MF, Podratz KC, Malkasian GD. Fallopian tube cancer: the role of radiation therapy. Radiother Oncol 1987; 10(4): 267–75.

70. Rosen AC, *et al*. Prognostic factors in primary fallopian tube carcinoma. Austrian Cooperative Study Group for Fallopian Tube Carcinoma. Gynecol Oncol 1994; 53(3): 307–13.

71. Johnston GA Jr. Primary malignancy of the fallopian tube: a clinical review of 13 cases. J Surg Oncol 1983; 24(4): 304–9.

72. Denham JW, Maclennan KA. The management of primary carcinoma of the fallopian tube. Experience of 40 cases. Cancer 1984; 53(1): 166–72.

73. Peters WA III, Andersen WA, Hopkins MP. Results of chemotherapy in advanced carcinoma of the fallopian tube. Cancer 1989; 63(5): 836–8.

74. Smith JP. Chemotherapy in gynecologic cancer. Clin Obstet Gynecol 1975; 18(4): 109–24.

75. Deppe G, Bruckner HW, Cohen CJ. Combination chemotherapy for advanced carcinoma of the fallopian tube. Obstet Gynecol 1980; 56(4): 530–2.

76. Boronow RC. Chemotherapy for disseminated tubal cancer. Obstet Gynecol 1973; 42(1): 62–6.

77. Tresukosol D, *et al*. Primary fallopian tube adenocarcinoma: clinical complete response after salvage treatment with high-dose paclitaxel. Gynecol Oncol 1995; 58(2): 258–61.

78. Markman M, *et al*. Phase 2 trial of liposomal doxorubicin (40 mg/m(2)) in platinum/paclitaxel-refractory ovarian and fallopian tube cancers and primary carcinoma of the peritoneum. Gynecol Oncol 2000; 78(3 Pt 1): 369–72.

79. Markman M, *et al*. Phase II trial of weekly single-agent paclitaxel in platinum/paclitaxel-refractory ovarian cancer. J Clin Oncol 2002; 20(9): 2365–9.

80. Rose PG, *et al*. Liposomal doxorubicin in ovarian, peritoneal, and tubal carcinoma: a retrospective comparative study of single-agent dosages. Gynecol Oncol 2001; 82(2): 323–8.

81. Berkenblit A, *et al*. A phase II trial of weekly docetaxel in patients with platinum-resistant epithelial ovarian, primary peritoneal serous cancer, or fallopian tube cancer. Gynecol Oncol 2004; 95(3): 624–31.

82. Markman M, *et al.* Phase 2 trial of single agent docetaxel in platinum and paclitaxel-refractory ovarian cancer, fallopian tube cancer, and primary carcinoma of the peritoneum. Gynecol Oncol 2003; 91(3): 573–6.

83. Jacobs AJ, *et al.* Treatment of carcinoma of the fallopian tube using cisplatin, doxorubicin, and cyclophosphamide. Am J Clin Oncol 1986; 9(5): 436–9.

84. Morris M, *et al.* Treatment of fallopian tube carcinoma with cisplatin, doxorubicin, and cyclophosphamide. Obstet Gynecol 1990; 76(6): 1020–4.

85. Cormio G, *et al.* Treatment of fallopian tube carcinoma with cyclophosphamide, adriamycin, and cisplatin. Am J Clin Oncol 1997; 20(2): 143–5.

86. Pectasides D, *et al.* Treatment of primary fallopian tube carcinoma with cisplatin-containing chemotherapy. Am J Clin Oncol 1994; 17(1): 68–71.

87. Muntz HG, *et al.* Combination chemotherapy in advanced adenocarcinoma of the fallopian tube. Gynecol Oncol 1991; 40(3): 268–73.

88. Gemignani ML, *et al.* Paclitaxel-based chemotherapy in carcinoma of the fallopian tube. Gynecol Oncol 2001; 80(1): 16–20.

89. Raju KS, Barker GH, Wiltshaw E. Primary carcinoma of the fallopian tube. Report of 22 cases. Br J Obstet Gynaecol 1981; 88(11): 1124–9.

90. Semrad N, *et al.* Fallopian tube adenocarcinoma: common extraperitoneal recurrence. Gynecol Oncol 1986; 24(2): 230–5.

91. Rosen AC, *et al.* Preoperative and postoperative CA-125 serum levels in primary fallopian tube carcinoma. Arch Gynecol Obstet 1994; 255(2): 65–8.

92. Schwartz PE, Smith JP. Second-look operations in ovarian cancer. Am J Obstet Gynecol 1980; 138(8): 1124–30.

93. Guthrie D, Cohen S. Carcinoma of the Fallopian tube treated with a combination of surgery and cytotoxic chemotherapy. Br J Obstet Gynaecol 1981; 88(10): 1051–3.

94. Eddy GL, Copeland LJ, Gershenson DM. Second-look laparotomy in fallopian tube carcinoma. Gynecol Oncol 1984; 19(2): 182–6.

95. Harrison CR, *et al.* Carcinoma of the fallopian tube: clinical management. Gynecol Oncol 1989; 32(3): 357–9.

96. Barakat RR, *et al.* Second-look laparotomy in carcinoma of the fallopian tube. Obstet Gynecol 1993; 82(5): 748–51.

97. Cormio G, *et al.* Second-look laparotomy in the management of fallopian tube carcinoma. Acta Obstet Gynecol Scand 1997; 76(4): 369–72.

98. Piver MS, *et al.* Second-look laparoscopy prior to proposed second-look laparotomy. Obstet Gynecol 1980; 55(5): 571–3.

99. Weber AM, *et al.* Malignant mixed mullerian tumors of the fallopian tube. Gynecol Oncol 1993; 50(2): 239–43.

100. Imachi M, *et al.* Malignant mixed Mullerian tumor of the fallopian tube: report of two cases and review of literature. Gynecol Oncol 1992; 47(1): 114–24.

101. Kahanpaa KV, Laine R, Saksela E. Malignant mixed Mullerian tumor of the fallopian tube: report of a case with 5-year survival. Gynecol Oncol 1983; 16(1): 144–9.

102. Muntz HG, *et al.* Carcinosarcomas and mixed Mullerian tumors of the fallopian tube. Gynecol Oncol 1989; 34(1): 109–15.

103. Carlson JA Jr, Ackerman BL, Wheeler JE. Malignant mixed mullerian tumor of the fallopian tube. Cancer 1993; 71(1): 187–92.

104. Hertig AT, Gore H. *Hydatiform Mole and Choriocarcinoma*. Washington, DC: Armed Forces Institute of Pathology, 1961.

105. Muto MG, *et al.* Gestational trophoblastic disease of the fallopian tube. J Reprod Med 1991; 36(1): 57–60.

106. Dekel A, *et al.* Primary choriocarcinoma of the fallopian tube. Report of a case with survival and postoperative delivery. Review of the literature. Obstet Gynecol Surv 1986; 41(3): 142–8.

107. Ober WB, Maier RC. Gestational choriocarcinoma of the fallopian tube. Diagn Gynecol Obstet 1981; 3(3): 213–31.

108. Nordin AJ. Primary carcinoma of the fallopian tube: a 20-year literature review. Obstet Gynecol Surv 1994; 49(5): 349–61.

109. Rauthe G, Vahrson HW, Burkhardt E. Primary cancer of the fallopian tube. Treatment and results of 37 cases. Eur J Gynaecol Oncol 1998; 19(4): 356–62.

39 Nonendometrioid Endometrial Carcinomas and Uterine Sarcomas

Peter G. Rose[1] and Charles Biscotti[2]

[1] Section of Gynecologic Oncology, [2] Department of Anatomic Pathology, Cleveland Clinic, Cleveland, OH, USA

Nonendometrioid endometrial carcinomas

Endometrial carcinomas can be separated into two different pathological types as originally suggested by Bokhman et al.[1] Type I endometrial carcinomas are indolent tumors that are associated with estrogen use and obesity. Tumors are of low histological grade (grades I, II) with superficial myometrial invasion and infrequent nodal metastasis. Collectively, these tumors are of low stage and have an excellent prognosis. Conversely, type II endometrial carcinomas are not associated with estrogen use or obesity, are poorly differentiated, deeply invasive and frequently have nodal metastasis. Collectively, these tumors usually are of advanced stage and have a poor prognosis.

Since this original definition, studies on the molecular biology of endometrial carcinomas have demonstrated significant differences among type I and II tumors. Type I tumors are estrogen and progesterone receptor positive, diploid, have a low frequency of allelic imbalance and demonstrate genetic alterations in K-ras, MLH1, PTEN, and CTNNB1. Type II tumors are estrogen and progesterone receptor negative, aneuploid, have frequent allelic imbalance and demonstrate genetic alterations in p53 and erb-B2.[2,3] The risk factors for type I tumors have been identified: obesity, unopposed estrogen use, nulliparity, diabetes, and tamoxifen use. But since these tumors tend to be of low grade, cancer screening based on these risk factors would not significantly affect overall mortality from endometrial cancer. Unfortunately, the risk factors for type II tumors remain elusive. Type II endometrial carcinomas occur at a similar frequency between African-Americans and Caucasians, but due to an excess of type I carcinoma in Caucasians, an African-American with uterine cancer has a 40% chance and a Caucasian with uterine cancer has a 25% chance of having a type II carcinoma.[4]

Carcinosarcoma, which is synonymous with older terms including malignant müllerian mixed tumor, malignant mesodermal mixed tumor and metaplastic carcinoma, is the most common type of uterine sarcoma. The term carcinosarcoma was originally used to specify a tumor with a malignant epithelial element and a malignant homologous sarcomatous element. While originally believed to be the result of two separate cancers colliding (collision theory), more recent cell culture and pathological studies suggest this specific carcinoma can convert to a sarcoma (conversion theory).[5–9]

Amant et al. evaluated whether uterine carcinosarcomas have a different prognosis from other high-risk endometrial carcinomas, including serous papillary carcinoma, clear cell carcinoma, and poorly differentiated endometrioid carcinoma.[10] Carcinosarcoma and nonendometrioid carcinoma were more likely to spread to regional lymph nodes and carcinosarcomas were more likely to spread to the lungs. Among stage I–II cancers, carcinosarcomas had a poorer survival at 44% compared to 75% and 86% survival for nonendometrioid and grade III endometrioid carcinomas, respectively. However, in a subsequent study by Akahira et al., 121 patients with uterine sarcoma, including 71 with carcinosarcoma, were compared to 921 with endometrioid carcinoma.[11] For carcinosarcoma, age, treatment, and survival were different from other sarcomas and almost identical to grade III endometrioid carcinoma. More recently, with the introduction of a FIGO staging system for uterine sarcomas in 2009, carcinosarcomas are now staged as a carcinoma (Table 39.1). Controversy exists over the prognosis of patients with uterine papillary serous carcinoma, clear cell carcinoma, and poorly differentiated endometrioid carcinoma, with a poorer prognosis for uterine papillary serous carcinoma and clear cell carcinoma in some but not all series.[12–14]

The ILIADE trial comparing a more extensive modified hysterectomy (Piver-Rutledge type II) with an extrafascial hysterectomy (Piver-Rutledge type I) found no difference in locoregional control or survival.[15]

Lastly, while randomized studies have failed to demonstrate a benefit to routine lymphadenectomy in endometrial cancer, only a minority of patients in those studies had high type II tumors.[16,17] Retrospective data support the use of pelvic and paraaortic lymphadenectomy in patients with intermediate

Table 39.1 Figo staging: carcinoma of the endometrium.

Stage	Description
IA	Tumor confined to the uterus, no or < ½ myometrial invasion
IB	Tumor confined to the uterus, > ½ myometrial invasion
II	Cervical stromal invasion, but not beyond uterus
IIIA	Tumor invades serosa or adnexa
IIIB	Vaginal and/or parametrial involvement
IIIC1	Pelvic node involvement
IIIC2	Paraaortic involvement
IVA	Tumor invasion bladder and/or bowel mucosa
IVB	Distant metastases including abdominal metastases and/or inguinal lymph nodes

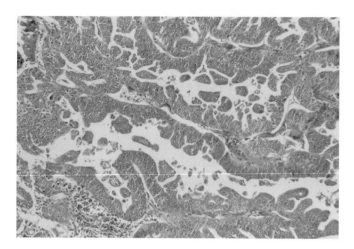

Figure 39.1 Uterine papillary serous adenocarcinomas have a complex papillary architecture with marked cellular stratification, as seen in this example.

or high risk of recurrence.[18] Models to predict the risk of recurrence based on clinical and pathological variables have been developed.[19,20]

Uterine papillary serous carcinoma

Epidemiology

Uterine papillary serous carcinoma (UPSC), resembling ovarian serous adenocarcinoma, was described independently by Hendrickson *et al.* and Christopherson *et al.* in 1982.[21,22] UPSC represents an unusual and aggressive variant, accounting for 10% of endometrial carcinomas but 39% of deaths from endometrial carcinoma.[23] Serous carcinomas affect older, usually postmenopausal patients, often arising in the setting of endometrial atrophy. Both UPSC and clear cell carcinoma are increased in African-Americans (hazard ratio [HR] 1.85, 95% confidence interval [CI] 1.61–2.12).[24]

Pathology

Microscopically, serous carcinomas usually have complex branching papillae with prominent epithelial stratification yielding epithelial tufts and apparently detached epithelial cell clusters (Fig. 39.1). The lining cells usually have marked nuclear atypia. Serous carcinomas tend to invade deeply, extending well beyond the gross extent of tumor, even in small uteri without grossly evident myometrial invasion. In one series, 40% of pathological stage I tumors involved the outer half of the myometrium.[21] Additionally, almost 50% of cases have had vascular invasion. UPSC often coexists with at least one other subtype of endometrial carcinoma. In a retrospective multiinstitutional study, classic risk factors such as age, the presence of lymph vascular space invasion (LVSI), tumor size, and percentage of serous carcinoma were not associated with the risk of recurrence or survival.[25] The adverse effect of a minor serous or clear cell component has subsequently been corroborated.[26]

The precursor lesion for UPSC is endometrial intraepithelial carcinoma (EIC).[6] This is a noninvasive glandular lesion characterized by epithelial cells with marked nuclear abnormalities, resembling nuclei seen in serous carcinoma of the endometrium. In contrast to other precursor lesions, EIC can be associated with extrauterine metastasis. More recently, a latent precursor (p53 signature) for EIC has been described.[27,28]

Molecular biology

Uterine papillary serous carcinoma is characterized by p53 mutations and HER-2/neu gene amplification. In a large cohort of 483 surgically staged endometrial cancer patients, HER-2 expression and gene amplification were seen in 43% and 29% of serous carcinomas respectively.[29] Santin *et al.* and Grushko *et al.* demonstrated HER-2/neu overexpression in 62% and 61% of UPSC tumors, respectively.[30,31] Higher overexpression has correlated with advanced disease stage. In 2007, Santin *et al.* reported the frequent expression of the *Clostridium perfringens* enterotoxin receptors claudin-3 and claudin-4 in UPSC.[32] Santin's group has also studied the expression of the epithelial cell adhesion molecule EpCAM, which has been demonstrated in 96% of UPSC tumors, and the *in vitro* response to adecatumumab (a human monoclonal antibody against EpCAM).[33] More recently, Santin's group has studied the expression of αV-integrins and human trophoblastic cell surface marker (Trop-2) and their inhibition with human monoclonal antibodies.[34,35] While p16 overexpression has been seen in both ovarian and endometrial serous carcinomas, the recent demonstration of PPP2R1A in UPSC but not high- or low-grade serous ovarian cancers provides genetic evidence that these are distinct diseases.[36,37]

Clinical presentation

Patients are evaluated for abnormal vaginal bleeding. Postmenstrual bleeding is always abnormal. Vaginal bleeding in the premenopausal patient is abnormal if increased in amount, frequency, or duration. Outpatient office endometrial biopsy is highly accurate (99%) in diagnosing type II carcinoma. However, among women with UPSC on final pathology, 25% were originally diagnosed as high-grade endometrioid carcinomas.[38] Ultrasound, commonly used to evaluate the risk of endometrial carcinoma, is less helpful with type II carcinomas where 35% measure less than 5 mm.[39]

Treatment

Surgery

One consensus regarding the management of UPSCs is that they should be very carefully staged surgically. Silva and Jenkins reported 16 patients with serous carcinoma limited to endometrial polyps.[40] Six patients had evidence of extrauterine disease at exploration. Among 10 patients with disease confined to the uterus, 60% recurred. Goff et al. demonstrated that careful staging identified metastatic disease in 72% of patients with clinical stage I UPSC.[41] Most pronounced in their study was the fact that intraperitoneal disease or nodal metastasis did not correlate with the extent of myometrial invasion. Subsequent studies of carefully staged patients demonstrated a lower risk of recurrence of 14–36%.[42–44]

For patients with advanced-stage UPSC, the prognosis is poor. However, as with ovarian cancer, numerous retrospective studies demonstrate improved survival with optimal cytoreduction (<1 cm or no residual at completion of the operation).[45–49] Following optimal cytoreduction, median survival times of 14–30.4 months have been reported.[46,48,49] In a recent study from the Mayo Clinic, patients cytoreduced to no residual disease had a median survival of 51 months.[48] In a study which utilized neoadjuvant chemotherapy and interval debulking, the median survival was 23 months and 90% of 30 patients studied had UPSC.[50]

Primary radiotherapy

The role of primary radiation therapy in high-risk cancers is limited to small case reports.[51]

Adjuvant radiotherapy

Throughout the 1980s and 1990s radiation therapy was the predominant mode of adjuvant therapy utilized for endometrial carcinoma. Discrepant results in the efficacy of adjuvant pelvic radiation therapy appear to be related to inclusion of comprehensively staged and nonstaged patients.[52] In view of the potential for peritoneal spread, a number of investigators utilized whole-abdominal radiation therapy. In the only prospective trial of whole-abdominal radiation therapy for patients with stage I–II endometrial carcinoma, the 5-year progression-free survival (PFS) for patients with UPSC was only 38%, with over half the recurrences within the radiation field.[53]

In the past, whole-abdominal radiation therapy has been advocated for advanced-stage endometrial carcinoma limited to the abdomen with less than 2 cm residual disease.[54,55] The Gynecologic Oncology Group (GOG) conducted a phase 2 trial evaluating whole-abdominal radiation therapy in stage III and IV patients with <2 cm disease limited to the abdomen.[56] Among 103 patients with uterine papillary serous carcinoma and clear cell carcinoma, the 3-year recurrence-free and overall survival rates were 27% and 35%, respectively. None of the eight patients with gross residual disease following surgery survived (median survival 11 months). The median survival for patients with completely resected gross disease was 27.4 months and for microscopic disease only was 65 months. The benefit of adjuvant radiation has been questioned by Grice et al., whose only stage I recurrence had received radiation therapy, and Huh et al. who found no difference between patients treated with radiation or observation.[42,43]

A Gynecologic Oncology Group trial (GOG 122) compared whole-abdominal radiation to chemotherapy with cisplatin and doxorubicin in advanced-stage endometrial carcinoma.[57] For all patients enrolled, an improvement in PFS (HR 0.71, $p <0.01$) and survival (HR 0.68, $p <0.01$) was seen with chemotherapy. In a review of stage III and IV patients with serous and clear cell carcinoma, local recurrence remained a concern following chemotherapy alone.[58] In view of the minimal morbidity of vaginal brachytherapy and its possible benefit, its use has been advocated.[59,60]

The GOG is currently conducting a study of high-risk stage I endometrial carcinoma that includes UPSC which involves randomization to pelvic radiation therapy versus vaginal brachytherapy and chemotherapy with paclitaxel and carboplatin (GOG 249). The use of chemotherapy and sequential radiation followed by consolidation chemotherapy, known as the sandwich approach, which allows early institution of chemotherapy and a relatively early full course of radiation without interruption, has gained popularity in high-risk endometrial cancer.[61,62] In a retrospective study of 138 stage I–IV patients with pure or mixed UPSC, radiation utilized in 80 patients reduced pelvic recurrences from 29% to 14%, $p=0.047$.[63] However, based on the results of GOG 122 and the uncertain role of radiation, the GOG is currently conducting a randomized trial of chemotherapy versus tumor-directed chemoradiation and shorter course chemotherapy for advanced-stage disease (GOG 258).

Adjuvant chemotherapy

Since UPSC resembles high-grade serous ovarian carcinoma, adjuvant chemotherapy has been advocated.[64,65] To date, all the studies have been retrospective. Longer survivals have been reported in patients who received platinum and paclitaxel combination chemotherapy compared to those treated with platinum-based chemotherapy alone.[45] In the largest retrospective study of surgically staged stage I UPSC patients, Fader et al. reported a significant decrease in recurrence and death with the use of adjuvant taxane/platinum chemotherapy +/– radiation compared to observation or radiation alone.[66] A benefit was seen with adjuvant taxane/platinum chemotherapy for patients with and without myometrial invasion. Our current practice is to utilize adjuvant paclitaxel and carboplatin for all patients with UPSC.

Chemotherapy

The Gynecologic Oncology Group has studied recurrent uterine cancers including endometrial carcinomas, carcinosarcomas, and leiomyosarcomas. All histologies of endometrial carcinoma have been combined. GOG 177 demonstrated an improvement with the addition of paclitaxel to cisplatin and doxorubicin (TAP): objective response (57% versus 34%; $p <0.01$), PFS (median 8.3 versus 5.3 months; $p <0.01$), and overall survival (OS) (median 15.3 versus 12.3 months; $p=0.037$).[67] However, the TAP combination had a significantly higher rate of neurotoxicity evident after two cycles of therapy. GOG 209, randomized 1381 women to TAP or carboplatin and paclitaxel. There were no significant differences in outcome; median progression free survival TC versus TAP, 14 versus 14 months HR=1.03, median survival 32 versus 38 months HR=1.01.[307] In an analysis of 1203 patients in

Table 39.2 Biological therapy in endometrial cancer.

Agent	Molecular target	n	Response rate	Stable disease rate	Nonendometrioid tumor histology
Tyrosine kinase inhibitors (TKI)					
Gefitinib[69]	EGFR	26	3.8%	27%	NS
Erlotinib[70]	EGFR	32	12.5%	47%	NS
Lapatinib*	EGFR+HER-2/neu				
Trastuzumab[71]	HER-2/neu	33	0%	36%	11 UPSC, 3 clear cell
Imatinib*	TKIs, Abl, c-kit, PDGFR				NS
Iressa[72]	EGFR	29	3.5%	NS	NS
mTOR inhibitors					
Temsirolimus (CCI-779)[73]	PTEN	29†	14%	69%	6 UPSC, 0 clear cell
Temsirolimus (CCI-779)[73]	PTEN	25‡	4%	48%	9 UPSC, 1 clear cell
Everolimus (RAD-001)[74]	PTEN	35	0%	43%	UPSC, clear cell excluded
Deforolimus (AP-23573)[75]	PTEN	45	7%	26%	NS
Ridaoforolimus[76]	PTEN	26	7.7%	58%	4 UPSC, 0 clear cell
Temsirolimus+megestrol acetate/tamoxifen[77]	PTEN, PR, ER	22	NS	NS	NS
Everolimus/letrozole[78]	PTEN, aromatase	28	21%	21%	NS
Other agents					
Clostridium perfringens enterotoxin*	Claudin-3 and -4				
Bevacizumab[79]	VEGF	52	13.5%	40.4%	UPSC 26.9%, clear cell 7.7%

* Not reported.
† Chemotherapy naive.
‡ Chemotherapy exposed.
EGFR, epidermal growth factor receptor; ER, estrogen receptor; *n*, number of evaluable patients; NS, not stated; PDGFR, platelet-derived growth factor receptor; PR, progesterone receptor; UPSC, uterine papillary serous carcinoma; VEGF, vascular endothelial growth factor.

GOG endometrial carcinoma trials, response rates by histology were 44%, 44%, and 32% for endometrioid, serous, and clear cell carcinoma, respectively.

Biological therapy

Numerous biological agents have been studied in endometrial cancer although the percentage of nonendometrioid tumors varied from study to study (Table 39.2). As a single agent, trastuzumab demonstrated no activity in HER-2-positive endometrial cancers, a third of which had UPSC,[71] although a randomized trial of paclitaxel/carboplatin and a HER-2-targeted agent in UPSC is planned. In chemotherapy-naïve patients, temsirolimus demonstrated a 14% response rate and stable disease in 63%[73] while ridaforolimus demonstrated a 7.7% response rate and stable disease in 58%.[76] The combination of temsirolimus with alternating megestrol acetate and tamoxifen demonstrated an unacceptable rate of venous thrombosis (32%).[77] However, the combination of everolimus and the aromatase inhibitor letrozole was associated with a high clinical benefit rate without increased thrombosis.[78] Oza *et al.* also performed a randomized phase 2 trial of ridaforolimus versus conventional therapy with progesterone or chemotherapy as second- or third-line therapy in recurrent endometrial cancer.[80] Ridaforolimus demonstrated a median survival of 10 months versus 8.9 months in the conventional therapy arm. Bevacizumab has been studied in endometrial cancer with four of 14 (29%) with UPSC responding with one response complete.[79] The GOG recently completed a three-arm phase 2 randomized trial of paclitaxel/carboplatin/bevacizumab, paclitaxel/carboplatin/ temsirolimus, and ixabepilone/carboplatin/bevacizumab as first-line therapy in patients with advanced or recurrent endometrial carcinoma (GOG 86P).

Prognosis

The prognosis of UPSC is stage dependent. Surveillance, Epidemiology, and End Results (SEER) 5-year survival rates are approximately 80%, 50%, 37%, and 15% for stages I, II, III, and IV, respectively.[81] In advanced-stage disease, survival seems to be improved with cytoreductive surgery and adjuvant chemotherapy. A retrospective review of GOG studies demonstrated that African-Americans were more likely to have a high-grade tumor, serous histology, and stage IV disease.[82] Similarly, in a review of SEER data, Wright *et al.* noted that African-American endometrial cancer patients were younger, had more advanced-stage disease and more often had type II endometrial cancers.[83] However, a recent hospital-based study of UPSC found similar survivals among African-Americans and Caucasians when a standard treatment approach was taken.[84]

Authors' recommendations

Total abdominal hysterectomy, bilateral salpingo-oophorectomy and comprehensive staging followed by vaginal radiation and platinum/taxane chemotherapy for stage I disease, sandwiched platinum/taxane chemotherapy and tumor-directed radiation for stage II, III, and IVA disease, and chemotherapy alone for stage IVB disease.

Clear cell carcinoma

Epidemiology

Although first described over 100 years ago, little attention was given to clear cell carcinoma until two papers by Silverberg and Kurman were published in the 1970s.[85,86] Clear cell adenocarcinoma accounts for approximately 3% of endometrial carcinomas but 8% of endometrial carcinoma deaths.[81] Unlike vaginal and cervical clear cell carcinomas, endometrial tumors are not related to *in utero* diethylstilbestrol (DES) exposure.

Pathology

Microscopically clear cell carcinomas appear similar regardless of site of origin in the female genital tract. Microscopically epithelial cells with vacuolated or clear cytoplasm usually predominate (Fig. 39.2). Abundant glycogen causes the cytoplasmic clearing. The carcinoma cells arrange in solid, papillary, or tubulocystic patterns, or often mixtures of these patterns. In contrast to endometrioid carcinoma and UPSC, a precursor lesion has not been identified. However, one study identified atypical glandular changes adjacent to clear cell carcinoma.[87] The immunohistochemical expression of p53, mib-1, estrogen and progesterone receptor in these putative precursor lesions was much more similar to clear cell carcinoma than normal endometrium.

Molecular biology

Clear cell carcinoma is estrogen and progesterone receptor negative.[88] p53 mutation in clear cell carcinoma is intermediate between the infrequently mutated endometrioid carcinoma and the frequently mutated UPSC. Hepatocyte nuclear factor 1β, a marker of cytoplasmic glycogen accumulation, is expressed in 100% of clear cell carcinomas.

Clinical presentation

Most patients found to have clear cell carcinoma of the endometrium are evaluated for abnormal vaginal bleeding. As in UPSC, the lack of a thickened endometrium on ultrasound should not delay endometrial sampling.[39]

Treatment

Surgery

Surgery for early-stage disease should consist of a total abdominal hysterectomy and bilateral salpingo-oophorectomy, bilateral pelvic and paraaortic lymphadenectomy and omentectomy. Cirisano *et al.* demonstrated that 39% of clinical stage I or II clear cell carcinomas were upstaged to III or IV with extended surgical staging.[12]

Radiotherapy

Abeler *et al.* reported 181 patients with clear cell carcinoma treated at the Norwegian Radium Hospital.[89] Despite adjuvant radiation in 145 of the patients, recurrences were noted in

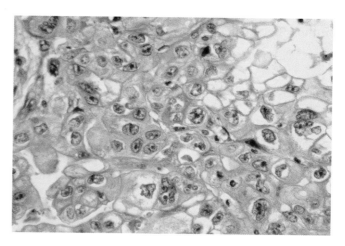

Figure 39.2 Vacuolated clear cytoplasm surrounds high-grade nucleus in this example of clear cell adenocarcinoma.

44.5% of those with stage I–II disease and 84.6% of those with stage I–II disease. Two-thirds of the relapses were extrapelvic, with the most common sites being the upper abdomen, liver, and lungs. Due to the concern about distant metastasis, a prospective study of whole-abdominal radiation was performed by the GOG.[53] Among the 13 clear cell carcinoma patients with stage I–II disease, the 5-year PFS was 54% with at least one local failure. In stage III and IV, 29 patients were studied.[56] All but one patient with gross residual disease progressed within 6 months. The recurrence-free survival of clear cell tumors at 3 years was similar across histologies, being 22.0%, 12.6%, and 11.0% for clear cell, UPSC, and endometrioid, respectively.[56] In GOG 122, 17 patients had clear cell carcinoma but a histological analysis was not performed.[57]

Chemotherapy

Among 1203 patients studied by the GOG, clear cell carcinoma comprised only 3.7% of patients.[68] Response rates were lower for clear cell carcinomas, 32% compared to 44% for either endometrioid or UPSC. In this study, patients with clear cell carcinoma had an increased risk of progression (HR 1.52) and death (HR 1.51) which were both statistically significant. Due to the rarity of clear cell carcinoma, this histology has not been studied separately.

Prognosis

In the Norwegian study of 181 patients with clear cell carcinoma of the endometrium, the 5-year survival rates for stage I, II, III, and IV were approximately 55%, 28%, 15%, and 0%, respectively.[89] In a retrospective study from Uppsala, Sweden, no difference in survival was seen between clear cell carcinoma or UPSC when patients were stratified by early- or advanced-stage disease.[90] Other studies have reported better outcomes for early-stage clear cell carcinoma which is very similar to poorly differentiated endometrial carcinoma.[91,92] In a more recent series by Murphy *et al.* of 38 patients with clear cell carcinoma, only 3.8% relapsed outside the pelvis.[93]

Authors' recommendation

These tumors are treated identically to UPSC.

Carcinosarcoma

Epidemiology

As with endometrial carcinoma, obesity, nulliparity, exogenous estrogen, and tamoxifen are associated with carcinosarcoma.[94–99] While tamoxifen is known to increase the risk of endometrial carcinoma 2.3-fold, it increases the risk of uterine carcinosarcoma eight-fold 8 years post therapy.[100] Uterine sarcomas account for a higher percentage (10%) of uterine malignancies in black women. This figure is partly explained by the fact that endometrial carcinoma is twice as frequent in the white population as in blacks. However, the incidence of mixed mesodermal tumors is higher in black women than white women (relative risk 2.33, 95% CI 1.99–2.72).[24]

Numerous authors have reported uterine sarcoma following radiation therapy for carcinoma of the cervix.[101,102] Czesnin and Wronkowski reported three uterine sarcomas developing among 8043 cervical cancer patients treated by radiation therapy, placing them at a relative risk of 5.48.[103] Mark et al. reported 13 cases of postradiation sarcoma and estimated a risk of 0.03–0.8%.[104] In a report of 23 patient who developed endometrial cancer post radiation for cervical cancer, 35% were carcinosarcomas.[105]

Pathology

Sarcomatous elements within the carcinosarcoma are further classified as homologous, containing tissue native to the uterus (e.g. smooth muscle, endometrial stroma, and blood or lymph vessels), or heterologous, with tissue foreign to the uterus (e.g. bone, cartilage, skeletal muscle, or fat) (Table 39.3, Fig. 39.3). Norris and Taylor reported that homologous carcinosarcomas had a better prognosis than heterologous tumors.[106] This suggestion, however, was not supported in a number of subsequent series.[107–109] Certain heterologous elements such as cartilage or skeletal muscle have been reported to affect survival adversely.[110] In another series, recurrence was statistically more frequent in stage I and II patients with rhabdomyosarcoma than in those with chondrosarcoma. Rhabdomyosarcomas, however, invaded deeper into the myometrium than chondrosarcomas, which may have accounted for their worse outcome.[111]

Clinical presentation

Irregular vaginal bleeding is the most common presenting symptom (80%) for all uterine sarcomas. The presence of gross tissue at the cervical os is common and in one series was present in 73% of patients with carcinosarcomas.[112] Other symptoms include pelvic or abdominal pain (16%), an enlarged uterus (12%), a pelvic or abdominal mass (9.5%), and vaginal discharge (9.5%).[113] Diagnostic techniques are identical to other high-grade uterine carcinomas.

Table 39.3 Ober classification of uterine sarcomas.

Homologous	Heterologous
Pure	
Stromal sarcoma	Rhabdomyosarcoma
Leiomyosarcoma	Chondrosarcoma
Angiosarcoma	Osteosarcoma
Liposarcoma	
Mixed	
Carcinosarcoma	Mixed müllerian tumor

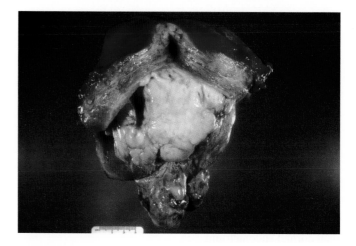

Figure 39.3 This carcinosarcoma has the characteristic bulky, polypoid, fleshy gross appearance.

Treatment

Surgery

The traditional surgical therapy for carcinosarcoma has been total abdominal hysterectomy and bilateral salpingo-oophorectomy. In a cumulative report of 90 stage I patients treated in this manner, the 2-year survival was 45%.[114] The presence of extrauterine disease significantly affected prognosis.[108–110] A number of studies have examined the role of surgical staging in carcinosarcoma.[109,115] The GOG studied 453 patients with clinical stage I and II uterine sarcoma who underwent comprehensive surgical staging.[109] Among the 287 eligible patients with carcinosarcoma, the frequency of pelvic or paraaortic node metastasis was 17.8%. Pelvic nodes were involved twice as frequently as paraaortic nodes. Factors associated with nodal involvement include adnexal metastasis, positive peritoneal cytology, outer 50% myometrial invasion, and cervical or isthmic tumor location. In a smaller single-institution study of 41 patients with apparent early carcinosarcoma, 31.7% had nodal involvement.[116] Nodal involvement was more common with greater than 50% myometrial invasion, positive peritoneal cytology, and when vascular/lymphatic invasion was present. Other sites of known intraabdominal recurrence, including the omentum, peritoneum, bowel, and liver, should be evaluated.[117]

Positive peritoneal cytology is frequently found in advanced-stage disease. Positive cytology in the absence of gross intraabdominal disease appears to be predictive of subclinical extrauterine intraperitoneal metastasis. Positive peritoneal cytology in apparent stage I mixed mesodermal tumor has a fatal prognosis, with 10 of 10 patients with positive cytology dying of disease, in contrast to six of 23 with negative cytology.[118,119] Whether lymphatic and peritoneal spread is the only mode for distant metastases is not known. In an autopsy study, a high percentage of patients had pulmonary metastasis in the absence of retroperitoneal nodal or intraperitoneal involvement.[120] This finding supports a hematogenous route of metastasis. In contrast to endometrial carcinoma, the depth of myometrial invasion in carcinosarcoma is not as prognostic of outcome, with the risk of recurrence being 40%, 50%, and 60% for patients with 0%, <50%, and >50% myometrial invasion, respectively.[109]

Adjuvant radiation therapy

Many centers have utilized adjuvant radiation therapy after primary hysterectomy to decrease recurrence as surgery alone resulted in only a 45% 2-year survival. The European Organization for Research and Treatment of Cancer (EORTC) performed a phase 3 randomized trial of adjuvant pelvic radiation versus observation for stage I and II uterine sarcomas (carcinosarcoma, leiomyosarcoma, and endometrial stromal sarcoma).[121] Among the carcinosarcoma patients, pelvic radiation decreased the local recurrence but had no effect on survival. In the large surgical randomized trial of adjuvant doxorubicin carried out by the GOG in which postoperative radiation therapy was left to the discretion of the physician, recurrences were noted in 53% of patients treated with radiation versus 57.5% of those not treated with radiation.[122,123] However, in a more recent analysis of SEER data on 2461 women with uterine carcinosarcoma, the 5-year overall survival rates (41.5% versus 33.2%, $p <0.001$) and uterine specific survival rates (56.0% versus 50.8%, $p <0.001$) were improved with the use of adjuvant pelvic radiation.[124]

Adjuvant chemotherapy

In view of frequent distant recurrence and the proved, although limited effectiveness of chemotherapy in advanced disease, there is interest in adjuvant chemotherapy for early-stage disease. The GOG performed a randomized study with 156 patients comparing doxorubicin for eight cycles to no further therapy.[122] The recurrence rate was 41% for those treated with chemotherapy compared to 53% for those not receiving chemotherapy. The progression-free interval was 73.7 months for the chemotherapy arm versus 55 months for the untreated arm. These differences were not statistically different, although the size of the trial reduced its power to detect a small, but real difference. At the time of the trial the differential response rate of leiomyosarcoma and carcinosarcomas was not known. In view of the low response rate of doxorubicin in carcinosarcomas, it is not surprising that a benefit was not seen. Furthermore, there were too few patients to allow pathology subset analysis.

Sutton *et al.* reported the largest trial of adjuvant chemotherapy for stage I and II carcinosarcomas in which patients were treated with three cycles of cisplatin and ifosfamide and no radiation therapy.[125] The 7-year disease-free survival (DFS) rate was 52%, with 10 of 19 single-site recurrences in the

pelvis. A retrospective study from the Memorial Sloan-Kettering Cancer Center of patients with stage I–IV carcinosarcoma demonstrated that adjuvant chemotherapy with or without radiation therapy improved 3-year PFS when compared to radiation alone 35% versus 9%, respectively.[126] Due to the lack of consensus regarding the adjuvant therapy for carcinosarcoma, the GOG randomized 232 patients with stage I–IV carcinosarcoma to whole-abdominal radiotherapy (WAR) versus three cycles of cisplatin, ifosfamide, and mesna (CIM).[127] The 5-year recurrence rate was 58% with WAR versus 52% with CIM. The probability of recurring within 5 years was strongly associated with disease stage, with 4-year survivals of 65%, 45%, 26%, and 26% for stage I, II, III, and IV, respectively. Similarly, age >65 had a poorer 5-year survival – 30.6% versus 50% for younger patients. After adjusting for stage and age, the risk of recurrence was reduced 21% for CIM (HR 0.789, $p=0.245$) with death reduced 29% (HR 0.712, $p=0.085$). The distant spread of uterine sarcoma particularly implies the need for adjuvant systemic therapy. Whether current agents or combinations are effective enough to result in long-term cure requires further study.

Adjuvant chemotherapy and radiation

Since the majority of first recurrences are in the pelvis, the combination of radiation therapy for local control and chemotherapy for systemic disease control might be more effective. Manolitsas *et al.* were the first to report the combined use of both localized radiation therapy and systemic chemotherapy for uterine carcinosarcoma.[128] Thirty-eight patients with clinical stage I or II disease underwent surgical staging followed by platinum/anthracycline chemotherapy for six courses with tailored radiation therapy sandwiched between cycles 2 and 3 of the chemotherapy. The entire treatment program was not completed in 17 patients due to poor performance status or patient or investigator deviations. The survival rate for those patients who completed treatment according to the multimodality protocol was 95% (20 of 21 patients) compared to a survival rate at 47% for 17 patients who did not complete the treatment protocol, with a disease-free survival rate of 90% (19 of 21 patients). Pautier *et al.* reported the use of adjuvant chemotherapy with cisplatin, ifosfamide, and doxorubicin for three cycles followed by radiotherapy in 18 patients with localized uterine sarcomas.[129] At 3 years the recurrence-free survival was 76% for those treated with both modalities versus 43% for historical controls treated with radiation therapy alone, although the 95% confidence intervals overlapped. Subsequent single-institution studies support this approach.[130,131] Further studies of radiation therapy combined with chemotherapy are needed to better determine its role.

Primary radiation therapy

DiSaia *et al.* reported 18 patients with mixed mesodermal sarcoma treated by irradiation alone.[108] For patients with disease limited of the uterus, two of five were alive and disease free at 2 years. However, if disease extended to the cervix, vagina, or parametrium ($n=6$) or outside the pelvis ($n=7$), there were no 2-year survivors. Perez *et al.* reported no 3-year survivors following irradiation alone for stage II or IV

Table 39.4 Single agents studied in uterine carcinosarcoma and leiomyosarcoma.

Agent	Complete response	Partial response	Overall response	Reference
Carcinoma				
Amonifide	0/16	1/16	6.3%	139
Cisplatin	6/91	12/91	19.8%	134, 135
Diaziquone (AZQ)	0/22	1/22	4%	140
Doxorubicin	0/56	7/56	12.5%	141, 142
Etoposide	0/31	2/31	6.5%	143
Ifosfamide	8/49	8/49	32.7%	136, 137
Paclitaxel	4/44	4/44	18.2%	138
Piperazinedione	0/6	0/6	0%	144
Trimetrexate	0/21	1/21	4.8%	145
Topotecan	5/48	0/48	10%	146
Leiomyosarcoma				
Amonifide	0/26	1/26	4%	147
Cisplatin	0/52	2/52	3.8%	134, 148
Doxorubicin		7/28*	25%	141
Etoposide	0/57	2/57	3.5%	149–151
Gemcitabine	1/44	8/44	20.5%	152
Ifosfamide	0/35	6/35	17.1%	153
Liposomal doxorubicin	1/31	4/31	16.1%	154
Paclitaxel	5/80	2/80	8.8%	155, 156
Topotecan	1/36	3/36	11%	157
Trimetrexate	1/23	0/23	4.3%	158

* Complete and partial responses not reported separately.

disease.[132] Badib *et al.* reported that only 8% of leiomyosarcoma patients and 10% of endometrial stromal sarcoma patients survived 5 years following radiation therapy compared to 17% of those with homologous carcinosarcoma and 25% of those with heterologous carcinosarcoma.[133]

Chemotherapy

In carcinosarcomas, ifosfamide, cisplatin, and paclitaxel are the most active agents, with response rates of 32%, 20%, and 18% respectively[134–138] (Table 39.4). Doxorubicin seems less active, with a 10% response rate.[141] Since those studies, the GOG has limited its studies in uterine sarcoma to either leiomyosarcoma or carcinosarcoma.

Numerous combination regimens have been studied in carcinosarcoma (Table 39.5). In the first-line setting, the combination of ifosfamide and cisplatin was studied against ifosfamide alone in a phase 3 trial in carcinosarcomas (GOG 108).[163] The response rate in the combination arm was 54% versus 36% with ifosfamide alone. However, the combination produced greater toxicity and had a small impact on progression-free survival (median 6 versus 4 months) but no difference in survival. A subsequent GOG phase 3 trial in the first-line setting compared the combination of ifosfamide, paclitaxel, and filgrastim versus ifosfamide alone (GOG 161).[170] The response rate of the paclitaxel-ifosfamide combination was 42 % versus 29% (HR 2.2, $p = 0.017$). The combination resulted in a 29% increase in PFS, 5.8 months in the combination arm versus 3.6 months for ifosfamide alone (HR 0.71, $p = 0.03$), and a 31% increase in overall survival – 13.5 months versus 8.4 months (HR 0.69, $p = 0.03$).

Because of concerns regarding the toxicity and cost of the ifosfamide, paclitaxel, and filgrastim regimen, the combination of paclitaxel and carboplatin was studied in a phase 2 GOG trial.[159] Following the initiation of that trial, a retrospective study demonstrated response rates of 60% and 55% for primary and recurrent patients, respectively. [177] In the GOG trial, a 54% response rate was seen, with a PFS of 7.6 months and overall survival of 14.7 months. This PFS and survival compares favorably to the PFS and survival of the ifosfamide, paclitaxel, and filgrastim regimen. The high response rate of the paclitaxel and carboplatin combination was confirmed by an independent phase 2 trial in which the response rate was 62%.[178] A retrospective study of paclitaxel, carboplatin, and pegylated liposomal doxorubicin produced similar response rates of 62%, PFS 8.2 months, and survival 16.4 months.[160] Based on the activity of taxanes and the synergy between docetaxel and gemcitabine, a phase 2 study of this combination as second-line therapy in uterine carcinosarcoma was performed by the GOG.[165] The combination was inactive with a response rate of 8.3%, a median PFS of 1.8 months, and median survival of 4.9 months. The GOG is currently conducting a phase 3 trial comparing paclitaxel and carboplatin with ifosfamide, paclitaxel, and filgrastim (GOG 261).

In the second-line setting, topotecan at the FDA-approved dose of 1.5 mg/m² days 1–5 every 21 days was evaluated in uterine carcinosarcoma.[146] The study population had been heavily pretreated, with 33% having prior radiation and 92% prior chemotherapy. Three of 51 patients (6%) developed neutropenic sepsis and died after the first cycle. The overall response rate was 10%, all of which were complete responses. While this dose schedule was not tolerated, it suggests that an alternative dose schedule for this active agent should be considered.

Biological therapy

Sorafenib, which inhibits the Raf-1, B-Raf, and multiple tyrosine kinases including vascular endothelial growth factor (VEGF) receptors, was studied in endometrial carcinoma and carcionsarcoma of the uterus.[179] In carcinosarcoma, there were no objective responses but 25% had stable disease. The median PFS was 1.8 months with a 6-month progression-free rate of 13%. The *Clostridium perfringens* enterotoxin receptors claudin-3 and claudin-4 are overexpressed in carcinosarcoma and therefore this may represent a promising treatment modality.[180]

Prognosis

In a retrospective study from Memorial Sloan-Kettering, the 3-year survival rate for surgically staged stage I uterine carcinosarcoma patients with heterologous elements was significantly worse compared to those with homologous elements, 45% versus 93% ($p < 0.001$).[181]

Authors' recommendation

Total abdominal hysterectomy, bilateral salpingo-oophorectomy, and comprehensive staging followed by pelvic radiation and platinum/taxane chemotherapy for stage I, II, III, and IVA disease and chemotherapy alone for stage IVB disease.

Table 39.5 Combination regimens studied in uterine carcinosarcoma and leiomyosarcoma.

Regimen	Complete response	Partial response	Overall response	Reference
Carcinosarcoma				
Carboplatin, paclitaxel	4/5	0/5	80.0%	159
Carboplatin, paclitaxel and pegylated liposomal doxorubicin			62%	160
Cisplatin, dacarbazine	1/6	1/6	16.7%	161
Cisplatin, dacarbazine, doxorubicin	1/6	1/6	16.7%	162
Cisplatin, ifosfamide	29/92	21/92	54.3%	163
Cisplatin, vincristine, doxorubicin, dacarbazine	2/13	1/13	23.1%	164
Docetaxel, gemcitabine				165
Doxorubicin, cisplatin	3/6	2/6	83.3%	166
Doxorubicin, cyclophosphamide				167
Doxorubicin, dacarbazine		7/31*	22.6%	141
Hexamethylmelamine, cyclophosphamide, doxorubicin, cisplatin	2/7	3/7	71.4%	168
Hydroxyurea, dacarbazine, etoposide	2/33	3/33	15.2%	169
Paclitaxel, ifosfamide				170
Vincristine, dactinomycin, cyclophosphamide (VAC)	0/19	3/19	15.8%	171
Leiomyosarcoma				
Cisplatin, dacarbazine	1/3	1/3	33.3%	161
Cisplatin, vincristine, doxorubicin, dacarbazine	1/3	0/3	16.7%	164
Doxorubicin, dacarbazine		6/20*	30.0%	141
Doxorubicin, ifosfamide	1/27	9/27	37.0%	172
Etoposide, cisplatin, doxorubicin	1/7	1/7	28.6%	173
Gemcitabine, docetaxel	3/29	13/29	55.2%	174
Mitomycin, cisplatin, doxorubicin	3/35	5/35	22.9%	175
Hydroxyurea, dacarbazine, etoposide	2/38	5/38	18.4%	176
Vincristine, dactinomycin, cyclophosphamide (VAC)	0/17	1/17	5.9%	171

*Complete and partial responses not reported separately.

Other rare endometrial carcinomas

Other rare endometrial carcinoma variants include small cell undifferentiated carcinoma and squamous carcinoma. Small cell undifferentiated carcinoma is a high-grade neuroendocrine carcinoma morphologically identical to those occurring in the lungs. Treatment with localized therapy and systemic therapy to prevent distant recurrence as used in lung cancer is advised.

Endometrial squamous carcinoma must be differentiated from endometrioid adenocarcinoma with extensive squamous differentiation and from cervical squamous carcinoma with extension to the uterine corpus. Limited data suggest a poor prognosis for endometrial squamous carcinoma. Forty percent of patients with pathological stage I tumors have died of disease within 3 years.[182]

Uterine sarcoma

Epidemiology

Uterine sarcomas are rare, accounting for only 3% of uterine cancers. However, their virulent course in advanced disease and high recurrence rate, even when initially limited to the uterus, make them among the most lethal of gynecological malignancies. Despite their rarity, uterine sarcomas account for 15% of uterine malignancy deaths. Even after excluding carcinosarcomas, sarcomas are more common in African-Americans (HR 1.56, 95% CI 1.31–1.86).[24] The National Cancer Institute has collected incidence data on uterine sarcoma since the 1970s, and the age-adjusted incidence has remained unchanged. Little is known about the global incidence of uterine sarcomas, as most tumor registries do not specify histological type when reporting uterine malignancy. However, in a Norwegian study the incidence and mortality of uterine sarcoma doubled from 1956 to 1992.[183] Most of this increase was due to an increase in carcinosarcoma.

Biology

Both local and distant (extrapelvic) recurrences are common with uterine sarcoma. Salazar *et al.* collected data from 235 patients with recurrent disease from the literature and noted that 85% of recurrences included extrapelvic sites.[117] Metastatic sites included the lung (69%), upper abdomen (60%), bone (24%), and brain (4%). The high recurrence rate of stage I

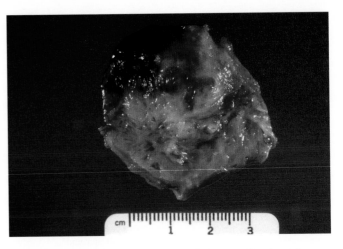

Figure 39.4 Uterine leiomyosarcomas typically have a soft variegated appearance, often containing hemorrhage and necrosis.

disease despite hysterectomy (50–80%)[94,184] implies that subclinical metastases are present.

The chemotherapy of uterine sarcoma has been integrally based on the results of other soft tissue sarcoma regimens. Because uterine sarcomas are rare they were often reported in aggregate. However, uterine sarcomas are heterogeneous with respect to their pathology, modes of metastasis, and treatment outcome. Only through recent cooperative studies by the GOG has the chemosensitivity of this heterogenous group of tumors been subdivided and studied. In view of their different response rates to chemotherapy, prior studies are difficult to interpret and not currently relevant. In view of the heterogeneity of uterine sarcoma, clinical features will be discussed based on specific pathologies separately.

Pathology

Numerous histological subtypes of uterine sarcoma have been described (Box 39.1). Ober classified these tumors as pure or mixed with either homologous or heterologous components.[185] Pure sarcomas contain a single recognizable element, whereas mixed sarcomas contain two or more elements. Kempson and Bari elaborated on this scheme, further subdividing by histological type.[186]

Leiomyosarcoma

Epidemiology

Although formerly the most frequently reported uterine sarcoma,[187] studies now report leiomyosarcoma to be second in frequency to carcinosarcoma.[94,113] Leiomyosarcoma occurs at a younger age than other uterine sarcomas.[113,188] More recent studies note a two-fold increased frequency of leiomyosarcoma in black women.[24,189] Malignant transformation of leiomyoma is rare. A review at Johns Hopkins University of 13,000 leiomyomas revealed only 38 cases with malignant change (0.29%).[190] However, this figure represented surgically treated patients and a more accurate estimate is less than 0.1%.[191] In the Mayo Clinic series, only three of 105 cases of leiomyosarcoma were thought to represent enlargement of previously diagnosed leiomyoma.[192]

Genetics

Li–Frumeni syndrome is associated with an 80% p53 mutation rate, with sarcoma the most common malignancy.[193] The type of sarcoma is age dependent, with leiomyosarcoma and liposarcoma occurring exclusively in adults. Kleinerman *et al.* analyzed soft tissue sarcomas in survivors of hereditary retinoblastoma.[194] They concluded that regardless of radiation or chemotherapy exposure, retinoblastoma survivors were at increased risk of soft tissue sarcoma. Leiomyosarcoma was the most frequent histology with four cases of uterine leiomyosarcoma reported.

Molecular biology

Arita *et al.*, studying 20 patients with uterine leiomyosarcoma, found VEGF and its receptors expressed at a significantly higher level in tumor than normal uterine smooth muscle.[195] In a study by the GOG, higher plasma VEGF expression was associated with an increased risk of progression (HR 3.5, $p = 0.003$).[196] Several studies have investigated the expression of KIT (transmembrane tyrosine kinase receptor) in leiomyosarcomas, ranging from 0% to 75%.[197–199] Although uterine sarcomas express c-kit, they lack mutations at exon 9, 11, and 17 and therefore are not expected to respond to imatinib.[200,201] Matrix metalloproteinases (MMPs) are endopeptidases, which are capable of degrading matrix proteins and play an important role in angiogenesis and tumor invasion. Bodner-Alder *et al.* analyzed the expression of MMP (MMP-1 and MMP-2) proteins in 21 patients with uterine leiomyosarcoma, with expression of MMP-1 in 86% and MMP-2 in 48% of the cases.[202] Furthermore, a statistically significant positive correlation was found between MMP-2 expression and vascular space involvement. In contrast, prolonged disease-free survival was noted in patients with no MMP-2 expression. High levels of phosphorylation of Akt and S6 ribosomal protein suggest the importance of the Akt/mTOR/S6 ribosomal protein pathway in uterine leiomyosarcoma.[203]

Pathology

Leiomyosarcoma is a pure tumor arising in the myometrium (Fig. 39.4). Approximately 70% are intramural, 20% are

Table 39.6 Hendrickson and Kempson revised classification system for uterine smooth muscle tumors.

Mitotic count per 10 HPF				
Cellular atypia	<5	5–10	11–15	>15
None	Leiomyoma	Leiomyoma	Leiomyoma	Leiomyosarcoma
Mild to moderate	Leiomyoma	Uncertain malignant potential	Leiomyosarcoma	Leiomyosarcoma
Severe	Uncertain malignant potential	Leiomyosarcoma	Leiomyosarcoma	Leiomyosarcoma

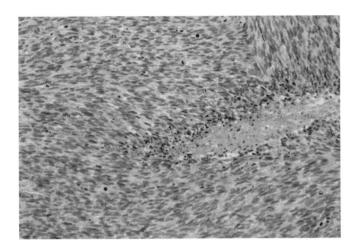

Figure 39.5 Microscopically, most leiomyosarcomas contain tumor cell necrosis (*center right*) characterized by sharp zones of necrosis lacking a healing margin.

submucosal, and 10% are subserosal.[204] A higher percentage involve the cervix than do leiomyomas.[205] The diagnosis depends on a constellation of pathological features including mitotic index, nuclear atypia, and necrosis. In one study, 90% of leiomyosarcomas had 10 or more mitoses per 10 high-power fields (HPF).[206] Mitotic count alone is not sufficient to diagnose sarcoma. Some benign, smooth muscle tumors have more than 10 mitoses per 10 HPF and some sarcomas have fewer. Among the 27 uterine smooth muscle neoplasms with 5–9 mitoses per 10 HPF, 11 (40%) recurred. Even among 42 uterine smooth muscle tumors with 1–4 mitoses per 10 HPF, five (12%) recurred.[207] However, there have been a number of favorable reports of patients with up to 15 mitoses per 10 HPF having a benign course.[208–210]

Based on this, Hendrickson and Kempson have revised the classification of smooth muscle tumors (Table 39.6). Using these criteria, Peters *et al.* reviewed the prognosis of tumors with uncertain malignant potential[211] and found that 27% of these patients developed recurrence and had a protracted course. Bell *et al.* have further identified coagulative tumor necrosis as an important criterion of malignancy[212] (Fig. 39.5). Furthermore, intraoperative frozen section evaluation for leiomyosarcoma is poor, with only three of 16 cases (18%) correctly identified.[213,214]

Myxoid leiomyosarcomas and epitheliod leiomysarcomas

Myxoid leiomyosarcomas and epitheliod leiomysarcomas have different diagnostic criteria. Myxoid smooth muscle tumors contain smooth muscle cells separated by abundant myxoid ground substance. Clinically malignant tumors can have low mitotic counts, 0–2 per 10 HPF.[215,216] An infiltrative margin with invasion of adjacent myometrium and/or vessels is a better criterion of malignancy. Predicting behavior of epithelioid smooth muscle tumors is problematic. Most are designated smooth muscle tumors of uncertain malignant potential (STUMP). Epithelioid smooth muscle tumors with significant nuclear atypia (grade 2 or 3 out of 3) and >4 mytotic figures per 10 HPF can be designated sarcoma. Most of these tumors also have tumor cell necrosis.

Clinical presentation

Leiomyosarcomas are classically felt to present as a rapidly enlarging pelvic mass. However, one review found leiomyosarcoma to occur in only 0.23% of such patients.[217] Gonadotropin-releasing hormone analogs have been used in patients with presumed leiomyoma who are subsequently found to have leiomyosarcoma.[218,219] The failure of involution or the presence of increased vaginal bleeding has been suggested as a means of identifying the leiomyosarcoma.[219,220] No imaging modality can reliably differentiate leiomyoma from leiomyosarcoma but the lack of calcification is a consistent finding in leiomyosarcoma. With magnetic resonance imaging (MRI), the lack of enhancement on T2-weighted images has correlated with malignancy.[221]

Staging

In view of the recognized discrepancies in estimated survivals of stage I–IV between the FIGO 1988 and American Joint Commission on Cancer (AJCC) staging systems,[222,223] FIGO modified the staging system in 2009 (Table 39.7). However, this staging system fails to represent other important prognostic variables, including age, mitotic index, and lymphovascular space invasion.[224,225]

Treatment
Surgery
Lymphadenectomy

In contrast to carcinosarcomas, nodal involvement was seen in only two of 57 patients (3.5%) with leiomyosarcoma.[109] This is confirmed by a large study utilizing the SEER database.[226] Among 1396 patients with leiomysarcoma, 24.9% who underwent lymphadenectomy were compared to 75% who did not, with no significant difference in the disease-specific survival at 61.9% versus 66.9%, respectively. A systematic literature review which included seven studies showed no benefit from lymphadenectomy for leiomyosarcoma.[227]

Table 39.7 FIGO staging: uterine sarcomas (leiomyosarcoma, endometrial stromal sarcoma, and adenosarcoma).

Stage	Description
IA	Tumor limited to uterus <5 cm
IB	Tumor limited to uterus >5 cm
IIA	Tumor extends to the pelvis, adnexal involvement
IIB	Tumor extends to extrauterine pelvic tissue
IIIA	Tumor invades abdominal tissues, one site
IIIB	More than one site
IIIC	Metastasis to pelvic and/or paraaortic lymph nodes
IVA	Tumor invades bladder and/or rectum
IVB	Distant metastasis
Adenosarcoma stage I differs from other uterine sarcomas	
IA	Tumor limited to endometrium/endocervix
IB	Invasion to <½ myomometrium
IC	Invasion to >½ myometrium

Source: American Joint Committee on Cancer. *Cancer Staging Handbook*, 7th edn. Chicago: Springer, 2010, p. 485.

Myomectomy

Van Dinh and Woodruff reported nine patients who were discovered to have leiomyosarcoma after myomectomy for infertility.[228] Only one patient developed a recurrence during follow-up ranging from 1 to 13 years. Three patients subsequently became pregnant. O'Connor and Norris reported 14 patients treated by myomectomy. Only one patient had a recurrence of a low-grade leiomyosarcoma, 8 years after her original surgery.[209] However, Berchuck *et al.* reported residual disease at hysterectomy in two of three patients treated originally by myomectomy.[229] Lissoni *et al.* reported eight women who following myomectomy were diagnosed with leiomyosarcoma within the myoma that were treated conservatively.[230] Only one patient was found to have recurrent cancer and died. A standard recommendation for conservative therapy cannot be made, and is largely dependent on the grade of the original histology.

Ovarian conservation

In an analysis of SEER data among 341 leiomyosarcoma patients less than 50 years of age who had stage I–II disease, there was no difference in 5-year survival for patients who did ($n=240$) or who did not ($n=101$) undergo bilateral salpingo-ooporectomy.[226] However, since 50–60% of leiomyosarcomas express estrogen and progesterone receptors and responses to hormonal therapy are documented, ovarian conservation must remain controversial.

Advanced stage disease

The role of surgery in advanced stage disease is not well documented, but isolated responses have been reported. Parente *et al.* reported a 10-month complete clinical response following primary hysterectomy and chemotherapy in a patient who had leiomyosarcoma with pulmonary metastasis.[231]

Adjuvant radiotherapy

Retrospective studies have suggested that the use of adjuvant pelvic radiation may decrease the risk of local recurrence.[232] However, as mentioned previously, the EORTC performed a phase 3 randomized trial of adjuvant pelvic radiation versus observation for stage I and II uterine sarcomas (carcinosarcoma, leiomyosarcoma, and endometrial stromal sarcoma).[121] Among leiomyosarcoma patients, adjuvant radiation failed to improve local control, progression-free or overall survival.

Adjuvant chemotherapy

The sites of first recurrence differ for leiomyosarcoma and other endometrial sarcoma histologies.[123] In leiomyosarcoma, 83% of first recurrences were at distant sites. As mentioned previously, only one randomized trial utilizing adjuvant chemotherapy in a mixture of uterine sarcoma types has been completed. Among the 48 patients with leiomyosarcoma, the recurrence rate was 61% for those assigned to observation versus 44% for those randomized to adjuvant adriamycin.[122] A metaanalysis of 14 localized resectable adult soft tissue sarcomas totaling 1568 patients demonstrated a HR of 0.75 (CI 0.64–0.87) with adjuvant doxorubicin.[233] In a retrospective of leiomyosarcoma from Chang Gung Memorial Hospital, age, stage, tumor size greater than 11 cm, and the use of adjuvant chemotherapy were predictors of survival.[234] In a prospective study from the Memorial Sloan-Kettering Cancer Center, patients with stage I–IV leiomyosarcoma received adjuvant gemcitabine-docetaxel for four cycles.[235] Among 18 patients with stage I–II disease 59% remained progression free at 2 years with a median PFS of 39 months. This appeared to be an improvement over historical controls from the Memorial Hospital 2-year PFS of 35% or other centers.

Recurrent disease: secondary cytoreduction

Most recurrences are at distant sites and require systemic therapy. Isolated late pulmonary recurrences have responded to local excision and have been associated with up to a 35% 10-year survival.[236] However, isolated pulmonary recurrences are rare, being seen in only one of 25 patients with stage I–II leiomyosarcoma in one series.[229] This patient was treated by thoracotomy but quickly recurred and died. Rarely, isolated pelvic recurrences have been treated with exenterative surgery.[237] The success of these local therapies may, in part, be due to the indolent nature of some low-grade sarcomas. The impact of secondary cytoreduction was retrospectively studied in 128 patients with recurrent leiomyosarcoma treated at Johns Hopkins and the Mayo Clinic, 80 of whom underwent surgery.[238] In 80% of the surgical cases, all disease was resected. The impact of surgery is difficult to extract because it is a marker for isolated recurrence and longer DFS at recurrence. However, the median survival was 2 years and 20% of patients achieved a 10-year survival.

Chemotherapy

In leiomyosarcoma, doxorubicin and ifosfamide had been considered the most active agents with response rates of 25% and 17%, respectively.[141,153] In combination, doxorubicin and ifosfamide has demonstrated a 37% response rate.[172] However, more recently gemcitabine has also demonstrated significant single-agent activity with a response rate of 20.9%.[152] A single-institution experience with fixed-dose rate gemcitabine and docetaxel reported a high response rate (53%) when used in either the first- or second-line setting.[174] This high response was remarkable since 50% of the patients had received prior doxorubicin.

The GOG initially studied this regimen in the second-line setting with a 28% objective response rate with disease stabilization achieved in an additional 50% of patients.[239] The same regimen as first-line therapy produced a 35.8% response rate with disease stabilization seen in 26.2%.[240] Liposomal doxorubicin is also active with a response rate of 16.1%.[154] However, cisplatin as a single agent has no significant activity (3–5%).[134,148] The combination of dacarbazine, mitomycin, doxorubicin, and cisplatin with sargramostim was studied as first-line therapy by the GOG.[241] In the first phase of accrual, the regimen was moderately active with a response rate of 27.8%. Grade 3–4 hematological toxicities were severe: leukopenia in 67%, neutropenia 78%, and thrombocytopenia 94%. Grade 3–4 sepsis occurred in five patients (26%) and the study was closed due to toxicity concerns.

Temozolomide is an orally administered alkylating prodrug with the same active metabolite as dacarbazine. Its activity in uterine leiomyosarcomas has not been extensively studied, with responses or disease stabilization reported in 5% and 47% in one study[242] and 33% and 50% in a smaller second study.[243] In the second study, progression-free survival was inversely related to the expression of O^6-methylguanine DNA methyltrasferase.

Biological therapy

Leiomyosarcomas occur at numerous sites throughout the body and many clinical trials do not restrict the site of origin for eligibility. The following discussion, however, is limited to data from uterine leiomyosarcoma alone. Leiomyosarcomas express estrogen receptor in 7–71% and progesterone receptor in 17–60%, which suggests that hormonal manipulation may have a therapeutic role.[244–247] In a retrospective study, 40 patients treated with aromatase inhibitors were included.[248] A response rate of 9% was seen, all of which were in estrogen receptor (ER)-positive tumors. Estrogen receptor-positive and progesterone receptor-positive tumors did better with a 1-year PFS of 28%. The GOG conducted a phase 2 trial of thalidomide in an effort to evaluate its activity in uterine leiomyosarcoma and its effect on angiogenic markers: VEGF, basic fibroblast growth factor, and soluble endothelial protein C receptor.[249] There were no objective responses and no effect on antiogenic markers. However, higher plasma VEGF expression was associated with an increased risk of progression (HR 3.5, $p = 0.003$). In an effort to study other antiangiogenic agents, a phase 2 trial of sunitinib malate was conducted.[250.] The regimen was inactive with an 8.7% response rate and progression-free survival at 6 months of 17%. The GOG is currently evaluating the addition of bevacizumab to gemcitabine and docetaxel in a phase 3 randomized trial (GOG 250).

Prognosis

In the SEER study by Kapp et al., 951 patients (68.1%) had stage I disease, 43 patients (3.1%) stage II disease, 99 patients (7.1%) stage III disease, and 303 patients (21.7%) stage IV disease.[226] The 5-year disease specific survival (DSS) rates for patients with stage I, II, III, and IV disease were 75.8%, 60.1%, 44.9%, and 28.7%, respectively. On multivariate analysis, older age at diagnosis, more recent year of diagnosis, African-American race, higher tumor grade, higher stage of disease, and lack of primary surgical treatment were all associated significantly with worse survival.

Authors' recommendation

Total abdominal hysterectomy followed by gemcitabine and docetaxel chemotherapy for stage I, II, III, and IVA disease and chemotherapy alone for stage IVB disease.

Endometrial stromal sarcoma: low grade

Epidemiology

In a review of SEER data from 1988 to 2005, low-grade endometrial stromal sarcoma (ESS) was the slightly more common, representing 54% of classified cases.[251] Patients with low-grade ESS were younger, with a mean age of 48.5 versus 60.5 for high-grade ESS ($p < 0.001$). Additionally, 25% of low-grade and 52.5% of high-grade tumors were stage III–IV ($p < 0.001$). Although the majority of patients (74.5%) were white, blacks were more likely to have high-grade ESS ($p = 0.014$).

In a separate SEER analysis limited to stage I disease, the new FIGO staging system which divides tumors based on size, IA <5 cm or IB >5 cm, was evaluated.[252] Among stage I patients, the percentage of low-grade tumors relative to high-grade tumors was significantly increased, at 76% versus 24%. The behavior of these two tumors in stage I disease was dramatically different with 5-year survivals of 97.2% and 45.4% for low- and high-grade ESS, respectively. The new FIGO staging system was predictive of outcome for low-grade but not high-grade ESS. The 5-year survivals for low-grade ESS were 100% and 93.5% ($p = 0.003$) for stage IA and IB, respectively, while those for high-grade ESS were 51.4% and 43.5% ($p = 0.27$) for stage IA and IB, respectively.

Biology

It has been demonstrated that low-grade ESS more commonly expresses estrogen and progesterone receptors.[244] In a recent series of 13 low-grade ESS, c-abl was universally expressed but c-Kit in only 8%.[253]

Pathology

Endometrial sarcomas are classified as low-grade endometrial stromal sarcoma or undifferentiated endometrial sarcoma (see Box 39.1).[254] Endometrial stromal nodule is a benign neoplasm of endometrial stromal cells characterized by a circumscribed margin. Stromal nodules and low-grade stromal sarcomas closely resemble proliferative endometrial stroma (Fig. 39.6). Many delicate small arterioles are characteristically present. Stromal nodules have an expansile circumscribed margin. In contrast, low-grade ESS have irregular, infiltrative margins[255] (Figs 39.7, 39.8). The definitive diagnosis of stromal nodule requires excision of the entire lesion and examination of the tumor margin. Thus, the distinction between stromal nodule and low-grade ESS is rarely possible in biopsy or curetting specimens. Low-grade ESS, previously referred to as endolymphatic

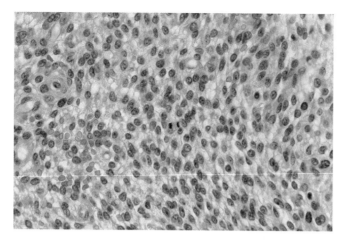

Figure 39.6 Low-grade endometrial stromal sarcomas resemble proliferative endometrial stroma. This typical example has the characteristic cellular appearance. A mitosis is present (*center*).

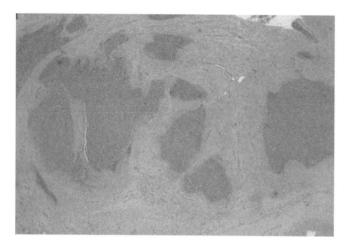

Figure 39.7 This low-grade endometrial stromal sarcoma has the characteristic pattern of myometrial infiltration.

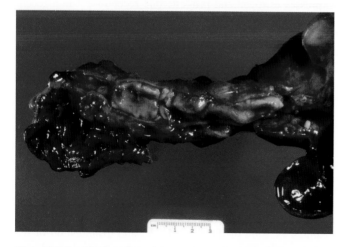

Figure 39.8 Low-grade endometrial stromal sarcomas often invade blood vessels. This example has a tumor thrombus filling the uterine vein.

stromal myosis (ESM), are indolent malignancies with a high (100%) 5-year survival. With prolonged follow-up, seven of 19 patients reported by Norris and Taylor developed recurrent disease, although it accounted for only one patient death.[256]

Clinical presentation
Vaginal bleeding is more frequent with endometrial sarcomas (94%) than with leiomyosarcomas (58%).[184] Diagnostic techniques are identical to other high-grade uterine carcinomas.

Treatment
Surgery
The surgical management of low-grade ESS involves a total abdominal hysterectomy and bilateral salpingo-oophorectomy. In cases where there is intravascular tumor extension, venotomy and careful extraction of the tumor are advised. Resection of any gross metastatic disease is also advised. In a retrospective study from Memorial Sloan-Kettering, the frequency of adnexal metastasis in 87 patients with low-grade ESS who underwent a bilateral salpingo-oophorectomy was 13%.[257] Although ovarian conservation has been reported,[258] a recent paper from MD Anderson reported a higher recurrence rate with ovarian conservation 89% versus 55%.[253] In view of the high frequency of estrogen and progesterone receptors in low-grade ESS, a bilateral salpingo-oophorectomy should be part of primary therapy. However, in the SEER data study, performance of a bilateral salpingo-oophorectomy was not an independent risk factor for survival.[252]

Regional nodal involvement is relatively uncommon (5%) and routine lymph lymphadenectomy is not commonly performed.[259] In the Memorial Sloan-Kettering study, only 36 of 94 (38%) low-grade ESS patients underwent lymphadenectomy.[257] Seven of the 36 (19%) had nodal metastasis but five were grossly positive. In the most recent SEER study, lymphadenectomy was performed in only 29% of low-grade ESS patients and was not a predictor of survival.[252] A similar lack of benefit from lymphadenectomy was seen in an earlier SEER study using data from 1983–2002.[260] In a retrospective study from the Asan Medical Center, Seoul, Korea, it was demonstrated that inadvertent uterine morcellation performed in 23 of 60 patients resulted in a decreased disease-free survival (HR 4.03, $p=0.040$).[261]

Adjuvant hormonal (low-grade endometrial stromal sarcoma) therapy
Because of the high (50%) recurrence rate for stage I low-grade ESS and objective response to progestational agents,[262–265] a number of authors have advocated adjuvant progesterone therapy.[264,266,267]

Radiotherapy
Radiation was utilized in only 14.8% of the patients with low-grade ESS in the SEER data study and was not an independent predictor of survival.[252] In a previous SEER report utilizing data from 1983–2002, adjuvant radiation did not improve overall or cause-specific survival for low-grade ESS.[260]

Chemotherapy

Consistent response to hormonal therapy has been seen with low-grade ESS and hormonal therapy is the treatment of choice for these tumors. Various hormonal therapies have been utilized, including progestational agents, most commonly medroxyprogesterone, and various aromatase inhibitors.[268–271] Cytotoxic chemotherapy regimens are only used in the rare cases of failure with hormonal therapy.

Prognosis

Among stage I low-grade ESS, age >55, HR 6.47, black race, HR 5.0, and stage IB, HR 5.4 were associated with survival.[252]

Authors' recommendation

For patients with clinical stage I, II, and III disease, total abdominal hysterectomy and bilateral salpingo-oophorectomy and adjuvant megestrol acetate or alternative hormonal therapy are recommended. For stage IV disease, megestrol acetate or alternative hormonal therapy is recommended.

Undifferentiated endometrial sarcoma

Pathology

Undifferentiated endometrial sarcoma has recently been defined as an endometrial nonepithelial neoplasm without features of endometrial stromal or other distinct sarcoma.[272] Undifferentiated endometrial sarcomas are high-grade sarcomas characterized by more nuclear pleomorphism and atypia than low-grade ESS. By definition, undifferentiated endometrial sarcoma lacks resemblance to proliferative endometrial sarcoma and heterologous differentiation. These tumors behave aggressively and have a poor prognosis.

Treatment
Surgery

In a review of the SEER data from 1988 to 2005, 96 high-grade ESS were identified. Lymphadenectomy was utilized in 60.4% and bilateral salpingo-oophorectomy was performed in 93.7%.[252] However, lymphadenectomy did not improve overall or cause-specific survival for high-grade ESS utilizing SEER data from 1983 to 2002.[260]

Radiotherapy

In the SEER report, 50.0% were treated with adjuvant radiation therapy.[252] However, in a previous SEER report utilizing data from 1983 to 2002, adjuvant radiation did not improve overall or cause-specific survival for high-grade ESS.[260] Among endometrial sarcoma histologies, 54% of patients not receiving radiation recurred in the pelvis. Radiation therapy decreased pelvic recurrences for nonleiomyosarcoma histologies from 54% to 23%.[123]

Chemotherapy

Because the clinical behavior is similar to other high-grade sarcomas, adjuvant platinum/taxane chemotherapy is advised.

Biological therapy

A case of a partial response to imatinib in a c-kit-positive tumor has been reported.[273]

Prognosis

In the most recent SEER data report, cervical involvement was common in high-grade ESS (18.8%) and associated with poorer survival.[252]

Authors' recommendation

For clinical stage I, II, and III disease, total abdominal hysterectomy, bilateral salpingo-oophorectomy, and pevic/paraaortic lymphadenectomy and adjuvant tumor-directed radiation followed by platinum/taxane chemotherapy. For stage IV disease, platinum/taxane chemotherapy.

High-grade heterologous endometrial sarcomas

These include high-grade sarcomas resembling undifferentiated endometrial sarcoma, but having heterologous differentiation. Heterologous rhabdomyosarcoma occurs most commonly, but chondrosarcoma, osteosarcoma, liposarcoma, and mixed heterologous sarcomas also occur.[274]

Treatment and prognosis

Similar to undifferentiated endometrial sarcoma.

Mixed stromal-muscle tumors

Mixed stromal-muscle tumors also occur, albeit rarely. A small amount of smooth muscle differentiation is common and irrelevant in a typical low-grade ESS.[275] Similarly, an insignificant amount of stromal differentiation has no relevance in an otherwise typical smooth muscle tumor. A minimum 30% threshold has been established for the designation of mixed stromal-muscle tumor.[276] Recently, perivascular epithelioid cell tumor has been reported in the uterus.[277] These tumors histologically resemble epithelioid smooth muscle tumors but strongly express HMB-45. These tumors should be regarded as of uncertain malignant potential based on limited experience.

Mixed epithelial and mesenchymal tumors

Adenosarcoma
Epidemiology

Based on a study from the SEER database, adenosarcomas represent approximately 10% of uterine mixed epithelial and mesenchymal tumors.[278] Compared to the more common carcinosarcomas, patients with adenosarcoma tended to be younger and more likely to have early-stage disease. The 5-year survival was significantly better for adenosarcoma than carcinosarcoma for both stage I, 79% versus 51%, and stage III, 48% versus 24%.[278]

Pathology

Adenosarcoma is composed of a sarcoma admixed with a benign epithelial component[279,280] (Figs 39.9, 39.10). Compared

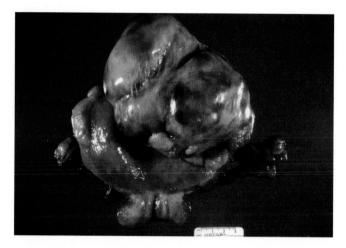

Figure 39.9 Uterine müllerian adenosarcomas usually have a polypoid gross appearance as seen in this example.

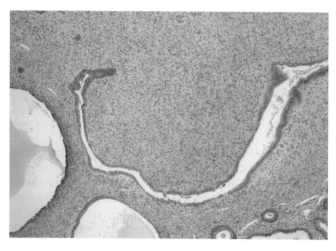

Figure 39.10 Cellular stromal papillae protrude into gland spaces, yielding a phyllodes pattern characteristic of adenosarcoma.

to carcinosarcoma, adenosarcoma has a better prognosis. Clement and Scully reported 100 patients, with long-term follow-up in 88.[279] Only 15 of the 100 patients had myometrial invasion, with only for having deep myometrial invasion Twenty-six percent of patients developed recurrent tumor, which was usually limited to the vagina, pelvis, and abdomen. Myometrial invasion was the only feature associated with recurrence. The importance of myometrial invasion is reflected in the recent FIGO staging system for adenosarcomas (see Table 39.7). The term adenosarcoma with sarcomatous overgrowth identifies a tumor in which 25% or more of the tumor is composed of a high-grade sarcomatous component.[279,280] Adenosarcomas with sarcomatous overgrowth are associated with a significantly higher risk of recurrence (44–70%) which is similar to carcinosarcoma. Rare cases of adenosarcoma recurring with heterologous sarcomatous elements have been described.[281]

Clinical presentation

There are often delays in diagnosis, especially in younger patients.[282] Patients may present with a polypoid mass coming through the cervix. In this case, the diagnosis is made following polypectomy. If a polypoid mass is not seen, outpatient endometrial office biopsy, ultrasound, and dilation and curettage may be diagnostic.

Treatment

Surgery
The standard treatment consists of total abdominal hysterectomy and bilateral salpingo-oophorectomy. However, since this is a low-grade tumor, ovarian conservation and even localized excision has been performed in a few cases.[282]

Radiotherapy and chemotherapy
These modalities are only utilized when there is sarcomatous overgrowth.

Authors' recommendation

Total abdominal hysterectomy and bilateral salpingo-oophorectomy. Adjuvant tumor-directed radiation followed by platinum/taxane chemotherapy for adenosarcoma with sarcomatous overgrowth.

Other rare tumors

Lymphomas

Primary lymphomas of the cervix and uterus are rare (see also Chapter 41). Only nine cases were reported among 9500 lymphoma patients at the Armed Forces Institute of Pathology.[283] Involvement as part of a generalized process is well recognized, and in reported series varies from 16%[284] to 40%[285] of patients. When disease is limited to the vagina, cervix or uterus, a 5-year survival of 73% is reported,[286] compared to 40% when the disease involves the ovaries.[287] If discovered at laparotomy, assessment of splenic and lymph node disease status, as well as liver biopsy, is advocated.[288] Granulocytic or myeloid sarcoma, also known as chloroma because of its green color, has been reported in the female genital tract and may precede the diagnosis of acute myelogenous leukemia.[289] Nine cases of myeloid sarcoma involving the gynecological tract, most commonly the uterus, were reported from MD Anderson over a 30-year period.[290] In their review of 76 cases in the literature, 47 patients had a history of or presented with myeloid neoplasms, while 29 did not and remained alive without evidence of leukemia. Therefore, hematological oncology consultation is essential for patients with this diagnosis.

Hemangiopericytomas

Hemangiopericytomas are a rare vascular uterine sarcoma characterized by proliferation of capillaries. These tumors are best treated surgically and respond poorly to chemotherapy or radiation therapy.[291] Gelfoam embolization preoperatively has aided in surgical excision.[292]

Benign mesenchymal tumors which mimic cancer

There are a variety of smooth mucle tumors that do not fit the criteria of leiomyosarcoma based on the presence of coagulative necrosis, high mitotic count, and cellular atypia. However, their microscopic appearance may include some of the features that suggest leiomyosarcoma. Coagulative necrosis in a "geographic" pattern best predicts malignant behavior, with one of four patients with this pathology recurring.[293] These tumors are best considered as smooth muscle tumors of uncertain malignant potential (STUMP).

The presence of some but not all the features of leiomyosarcoma, such as cellular atypia, high mitotic count, increased cellularity, or increased epithelial-like cells, results in the following diagnoses: atypical leiomyoma, mitotically active leiomyoma, celluar leiomyoma, and epithelioid leiomyoma. Atypical leiomyoma and cellular leiomyoma are best treated as STUMPs while mitotically active leiomyoma and epithelioid leiomyoma are completely benign. Epithelioid leiomyoma can be distinquished from perivascular epithelioid cell tumor (PECOMA) by the absence of CD1a expression.[294] Other benign smooth muscle variants include myxoid, plexiform or dissecting leiomyoma.

The clinical presentation and diagnostic evaluation are identical to uterine leiomyoma or leiomyosarcoma and no preoperative diagnostic test is reliable for diagnosis. The term "leiomyoblastoma" has fallen out of favor and is no longer in general use, in part because it suggests an aggressive behavior when in fact most tumors have a benign clinical course. Only three of 26 patients reported by Kurman and Norris developed recurrent disease, of whom two responded to therapy.[295] Mitotic counts correlated with outcome. Tumors previously designated as leiomyoblastoma should be included among the epithelioid smooth muscle tumors. Predicting the biological behavior is problematic and most will be regarded as of uncertain malignant potential (STUMP).

Treatment
Surgery
A total hysterectomy would be advised for STUMP but myomectomy may be adequate in selected cases, as has been reported with leiomyosarcoma.

Chemotherapy
Following hysterectomy, no additional therapy would be recommended.

Benign smooth muscle tumors with extrauterine disease

Disseminated peritoneal leiomyomatosis
Disseminated peritoneal leiomyomatosis is important in that it must be differentiated from metastatic leiomyosarcoma. This tumor is characterized by multiple peritoneal implants, generally measuring less than 1 cm in diameter, that involve the pelvic and abdominal peritoneal cavity. Leiomyosarcoma, in contrast, is characterized by fewer but larger metastatic lesions. On histological examination, the lesion appears benign with few mitotic figures and minimal nuclear atypia.[296] The lesion is generally associated with an excess of estrogen and is found in conjunction with pregnancy,[297] granulosa cell tumor,[298] and sequential oral contraceptive use.[299] Radical excision is unnecessary, as the lesion regresses following estrogen normalization. However, sarcomatous degeneration in <5% of cases has been reported.[300]

Intravenous leiomyomatosis
Intravenous leiomyomatosis is a smooth muscle tumor characterized by its direct growth into venous channels. It is believed to arise from the muscular wall of veins or from a leiomyoma with vascular invasion and subsequent extension beyond the leiomyoma from which it originated.[301]

Clinical presentation
Patients with extensive disease may present with dyspnea or symptoms of right heart failure due to the intracardiac mass. The diagnosis is suggested by CT or MR imaging demonstrating the intravascular mass.

Treatment
A hysterectomy with simultaneous extraction of the tumor from the heart and vessels is required.[302] Great care must be taken to avoid fracturing the tumor which would result in right heart and pulmonary embolization. Because of suspected estrogen dependence, oophorectomy is advocated.[302,303]

Benign metastasizing leiomyoma
Benign metastasizing leiomyoma (BML) is a smooth muscle tumor with multiple intrapulmonary nodules. It is though to arise from a cellular leiomyoma or intravenous leiomyomatosis that gains access to the vascular system and is transplanted to the lungs, where it is implanted and grows. Some authors have suggested that it arises after incomplete primary surgery such as curettage, myomectomy, or supracervical hysterostomy.[304] Hysterectomy is advised to exclude the presence of a low-grade uterine sarcoma as the primary. BML must be distinguished from lymphangioleiomyomatosis (LAM) in which the associated benign lesion is not a uterine leiomyoma. Pathologically, BML, with a well-circumscribed border with adjacent lung tissue, is distinguishable from LAM in which a diffuse interstitial infiltrate is present.

Hereditary leiomyomatosis and renal cell carcinoma syndrome
This is a rare autosomal dominant syndrome in which affected individuals have cutaneous and uterine leiomyomas and renal cell cancer. It is related to a mutation of the Krebs cycle enzyme fumarate hydrase and associated with an increased risk of uterine sarcoma in premenopausal women.[305]

Bannayan–Zonana syndrome
In this syndrome, uterine leiomyomas occur with other benign mesenchymal tumors such as lipomas and hemangiomas due to a germline mutation in the PTEN tumor suppressor gene.[306]

Conclusion

Certain nonendometrioid endometrial carcinomas, including uterine papillary serous carcinoma, clear cell carcinoma, and carcinosarcoma, are distinct in their behavior from the more common endometrioid endometrial carcinomas and warrant more aggressive treatment. Similarly, uterine sarcomas are usually virulent tumors. They have a high recurrence rate, most of which are distant recurrences. In both early- and advanced-stage disease, multimodality therapy is utilized in an effort to decrease recurrence. Significant advances in chemotherapy or biological therapy are needed to improve the current survival rates.

References

1. Bokhman JV. Two pathogenetic types of endometrial carcinoma. Gynecol Oncol 1983; 15: 10–17.
2. Sidaway MK, Silverberg SG. Endometrial carcinoma: pathologic factors of therapeutic and prognostic significance. Pathol Annu 1992; 27: 153–85.
3. An HJ, Logani S, Isacson C, Ellenson LH. Molecular characterization of uterine clear cell carcinoma. Mod Pathol 2004; 17: 530–7.
4. Plaxe SC, Saltzstein SL. Impact of ethnicity on the indidence of high-risk endometrial carcinoma. Gynecol Oncol 1997; 65(1): 8–12.
5. Silverberg SG, Major FJ, Blessing JA, et al. Carcinosarcoma (malignant mixed mesodermal tumor) of the uterus. Int J Gynecol Pathol 1990; 9: 1–19.
6. Sherman ME, Bitterman P, Rosenshein NB, et al. Uterine serous carcinoma. A morphologically diverse neoplasm with unifying clinico-pathologic features. Am J Surg Pathol 1992; 16: 600–10.
7. Sreenan JJ, Hart WR. Carcinosarcomas of the female genital tract. Am J Surg Pathol 1995; 19: 666–74.
8. Itsuo G, Chie D, Minaguchi H. Establishment and characterization of carcinosarcoma cell line of the human uterus. Cancer 1993; 71: 775–86.
9. Kernochan LE, Garcia RL. Carcinosarcomas (malignant mixed Mullerian tumor) of the uterus: advances in elucidation of biologic and clinical characteristics. J Natl Comp Canc Netw 2009; 7: 550–6.
10. Amant F, Cadron I, Fuso L, et al. Endometrial carcinosarcomas have a different prognosis and pattern of spread compared to high risk epithelial endometrial cancer. Gynecol Oncol 2005; 98: 274–80.
11. Akahira J, Tokunaga H, Toyoshima M, et al. Prognoses and prognostic factors of carcinosarcoma, endometrial stromal sarcoma and uterine leiomyosarcoma: a comparison with uterine endometrial adenocarcinoma. Oncology 2006; 71: 333–40.
12. Cirisano FD Jr, Robboy SJ, Dodge RK, et al. The outcome of stage I–II clinically and surgically staged papillary serous and clear cell endometrial cancers when compared with endometrioid carcinoma. Gynecol Oncol 2000; 77: 55–65.
13. Creasman WT, Kohler MF, Odicino F, et al. Prognosis of papillary serous, clear cell, and grade 3 stage I carcinoma of the endometrium. Gynecol Oncol 2004; 95: 593–6.
14. Alektiar KM, McKee A, Lin O, et al. Is there a difference in outcome between stage I–II endometrial cancer of papillary serous/clear cell and endometrioid FIGO Grade 3 cancer? Int J Radiat Oncol Biol Phys 2002; 54: 79–85.
15. Signorelli M, Lissoni AA, Cormio G, et al. Modified radical hysterectomy versus extrafascial hysterectomy in the treatment of stage I endometrial cancer: resuls from the ILIADE randomized study. Ann Sug Oncol 2009; 16: 3431–41.
16. Benedini-Panici P, Basile S, Maneschi F, et al. Systematic pelvic lymphadenectomy vs no lymphadenectomy in early-staged endometrial carcinoma: randomized clinical trial. J Natl Cancer Inst 2008; 100(23): 1707–16.
17. ASTEC Study Group, Kitchener H, Swart AM, et al. Efficacy of systematic pelvic lyphadenectomy in endometrial cancer (MRC ASTEC trial): a randomised study. Lancet 2009; 373(9658): 125–36.
18. Todo Y, Kato H, Kaneuchi M, et al. Survival effect of para-aortic lymphadenectomy in endometrial cancer (SEPAL study): a retrospective cohort analysis. Lancet 2010; 375: 1165–72.
19. Zaino RJ, Jurman RJ, Diana KL, et al. Pathologic models to predict outcome for women with endometrial adenocarcinoma: the importance of the distinction between surgical stage and clinical stage. A Gynecologic Oncology Group study. Cancer 1996; 77(6): 1151–21.
20. Abu-Rustum NR, Zhou Q, Gomez JD, et al. A nomogram for predicting overall survival of women with endometrial cancer following primary therapy: toward improving individualized cancer care. Gynecol Oncol 2010; 116: 399–403.
21. Hendrickson M, Ross J, Eifel P, et al. Uterine papillary serous carcinoma: a highly malignant form of endometrial adenocarcinoma. Am J Surg Pathol 1982; 6: 93–108.
22. Christopherson WM, Alberhasky RC, Connely PJ. Carcinoma of the endometrium II. Papillary adenocarcinoma: a clinical pathological study of 46 cases. Am J Clin Pathol 1982; 77: 534–40.
23. Hamilton CA, Cheung MK, Osann K, et al. Uterine papillary serous and clear cell carcinomas predict for poorer survival compared to grade 3 endometrioid corpus cancers. Br J Cancer 2006; 94: 642–6.
24. Sherman ME, Devesa SS. Analysis of racial differences in incidence, survival, and mortality for malignant tumors of the uterine corpus. Cancer 2003; 98: 176.
25. Nickles Fader A, Starks D, Gehrig PA, et al. An updated clinicopathologic study of early-stage uterine papillary serous carcinoma (UPSC). Gynecol Oncol 2009; 115: 244–8.
26. Quddus MR, Sung CJ, Zhang C, et al. Minor serous and clear cell components adversely affect prognosis in "Mixed-Type" endometrial carcinomas: a clinicopathologic study of 36 stage-I cases. Reprod Sci 2010; 17: 673–8.
27. Jarboe EA, Pizer ES, Miron A, et al. Evidence for a latent precursor (P53 signature) that may precede serous endometrial intraepithelial carcinoma. Mod Pathol 2009; 22(3); 345–50.
28. Zhang X, Liang SX, Jia L, et al. Molecular identification of "Latent precancers" for endometrial serous carcinoma in benign-appearing endometrium. Am J Pathol 2009; 174(6); 2000–6.
29. Morrison C, Zanagnolo V, Ramirez N, et al. HER-2 is an independent prognostic factor in endometrial cancer: association with outcome in a large cohort of surgically staged patients. J Clin Oncol 2006; 24: 2376–85.
30. Santin AD, Bellone S, Gokden M, et al. Overexpression of HER-2/neu in uterine serous papillary cancer. Clin Cancer Res 2002; 8: 1271–9.
31. Grushko TA, Filiaci VL, Mundt AJ, et al. An exploratory analysis of HER-2 amplification and overexpression in advanced endometrial carcinoma: a Gynecologic Oncology Group study. Gynecol Oncol 2009; 108(1): 3–9.
32. Santin AD, Bellone S, Marizzoni M, et al. Overexpression of claudin-3 and claudin-4 receptors in uterine serous papillary carcinoma: novel targets for a type-specific therapy using clostridium prefingess enterotoxin (CPE). Cancer 2007; 109: 1312–22.
33. El-Sahwi K, Bellone S, Cocco E, et al. Overexpression of EpCAM in uterine serous papillary carcinoma: implications for EpCam-specific immunotherapy with human monoclonal antibody adecatumumab (MT201). Mol Cancer Ther 2010; 9: 57–66.
34. Bellone M, Cocco E, Varughese J, et al. Expression of αV-integrins in uterine serous papillary carcinomas; implications for targeted therapy with Intetumumab (CNTO95), a fully human antagonist anti-αV-integrin antibody. Int J Gynecol Cancer 2011; 21: 1084–90.
35. Varughese J, Cocco E, Bellone S, et al. Uterine serous papillary carcinomas overexpress human trophoblast-cell-surface marker (Trop-2) and are highly sensitive to immunotherapy with hRS7, a humanized anti-Trop-2 monoclonal antibody. Cancer 2011; 117: 3163–72.
36. Armes JE, Lourie R, deSilva M, et al. Abnormalities of the RB1 pathway in ovarian serous papillary carcinoma as determined by overexpression of the p 16 (INK4A) protein. Int J Gynecol Pathol 2005; 24: 363–8.
37. McConechy MK, Anglesio MS, Kalloger SE, et al. Subtype-specific mutation of PPP2R1A in endometrial and ovarian carcinomas. J Pathol 2011; 223: 567–73.

38. Huang GS, Gebb JS, Einstein MH, *et al.* Accuracy of preoperative endometrial sampling for the detection of high-grade endometrial tumors. Am J Obstet Gynecol 2007; 196: 243.

39. Wang J, Wieslander C, Hansen G, *et al.* Thin endometrial echo complex on ultrasound does not reliably exclude type 2 endometrial cancers. Gynecol Oncol 2006; 101: 120–5.

40. Silva EG, Jenkins R. Serous carcinoma in endometrial polyps. Mod Pathol 1990; 3: 120–8.

41. Goff BA, Kato D, Schmidt RA, *et al.* Uterine papillary serous carcinoma: patterns of metastatic spread. Gynecol Oncol 1994; 54: 264–8.

42. Grice J, Ek M, Greer B, *et al.* Uterine papillary serous carcinoma: evaluation of long-term survival in surgically staged patients. Gynecol Oncol 1998; 69: 69–73.

43. Huh WK, Leath III CA, Straughn JM Jr, *et al.* Uterine papillary serous carcinoma: comparisons of outcomes of surgical stage I patients with and without adjuvant therapy. Gynecol Oncol 2003; 88: 209 (abstract 110).

44. Kelly MG, O'Malley DM, Hui P, *et al.* Improved survival in surgical stage I patients with uterine papillary serous carcinoma (UPSC) treated with adjuvant platinum-based chemotherapy. Gynecol Oncol 2005; 98: 353–9.

45. Bristow RE, Duska LR, Montz JF. The role of cytoreductive surgery in the management of stage IV uterine papillary serous carcinoma. Gynecol Oncol 2001; 81: 92–9.

46. Moller KA, Gehrig PA, van Le L, *et al.* The role of optimal debulking in advanced stage serous carcinoma of the uterus. Gynecol Oncol 2004; 94: 170–4.

47. Memarzadeh S, Holschneider CH, Bristow RE, *et al.* FIGO stage III and IV uterine papillary serous carcinoma: impact of residual disease on survival. Int J Gynecol Cancer 2002; 12: 454–8.

48. Thomas MB, Mariani A, Cliby WA, *et al.* Role of cytoreduction in stage III and IV uterine papillary serous carcinoma. Gynecol Oncol 2007; 107: 190–3.

49. Patsavas K, Woessner J, Gielda B, *et al.* Optimal surgical debulking in uterine papillary serous carcinoma affects survival. Gynecol Oncol 2011; 121: 581–5.

50. Vandenput I, van Calster B, Capoen A, *et al.* Neoadjuvant chemotherapy followed by interval debulking surgery in patients with serous endometrial cancer with transperitoneal spread (Stage IV): a new preferred treatment. Br J Cancer 2009; 101: 244–9.

51. Bachelor EC, Watkins JM, Jenrette JM. Definitive radiotherapy for medically inoperable early-stage serous and clear cell uterine carcinoma. Radiat Med 2007; 25: 536–40.

52. Goff BA. Uterine papillary serous carcinoma: what have we learned over the past quarter century? Gynecol Oncol 2005; 98: 341–3.

53. Sutton G, Axelrod JH, Bundy BN, *et al.* Adjuvant whole abdominal irradiation in clinical stages I and II papillary serous or clear cell carcinoma of the endometrium: a phase I study of the Gynecologic Oncology Group. Gynecol Oncol 2006; 100: 349–54.

54. Greer BE, Hamburger AD. Treatment of intraperitoneal metastatic adenocarcinoma of the endometrium by whole-abdominal moving strip technique and pelvic boost irradiation. Gynecol Oncol 1983 16: 365–73.

55. Martinez AA, Weiner S, Podratz K, *et al.* Improved outcome at 10 years for serous-papillary/clear cell or high-risk endometrial cancer patients treated with adjuvant high-dose abdomino-pelvic irradiation. Gynecol Oncol 2003; 90: 537–46.

56. Sutton G, Axelrod JH, Bundy BN, *et al.* Whole abdominal radiotherapy in the adjuvant treatment of patients with stage III and IV endometrial cancer: a Gynecologic Oncology Group study. Gynecol Oncol 2005; 97: 755–63.

57. Randall ME, Filiaci VL, Muss H, *et al.* Randomized phase III trial of whole-abdominal irradiation versus doxorubicin and cisplatin chemotherapy in advanced endometrial carcinoma: a Gynecologic Oncology Group Study. J Clin Oncol 2006; 24: 36–44.

58. Murphy KT, Rotmensch J, Yamada SD, Mundt AJ. Outcome and patterns of failure in pathologic stages I–IV clear-cell carcinoma of the endometrium: implications for adjuvant radiation therapy. Int J Radiat Oncol Biol Phys 2003; 55: 1272–6.

59. Kelly MG, O'Malley DM, Hui P, *et al.* Improved survival in surgical stage I patients with uterine papillary serous carcinoma (UPSC) treated with adjuvant platinum-based chemotherapy. Gynecol Oncol 2005; 98: 353–9.

60. DuBeshter B, Estler K, Altobelli K, *et al.* High-dose rate brachytherapy for stage I/II papillary serous or clear cell endometrial cancer. Gynecol Oncol 2004; 94: 383–6.

61. Geller MA, Ivy J, Dusenbery KE, *et al.* A single institution experience using sequential multi-modality adjuvant chemotherapy and radiation in the "sandwich" method for high risk endometrial carcinoma. Gynecol Oncol 2010; 118: 19–23.

62. Lupe K, D'Souza DP, Kwon JS, *et al.* Adjuvant carboplatin and paclitaxel chemotherapy interposed with involved field radiation for advanced endometrial cancer. Gynecol Oncol 2009; 114(1): 94–8.

63. Goldberg H, Miller RC, Abdah-Bortnyak R, *et al.* Outcome after combined modality treatment for uterine papillary serous carcinoma: a study by the Rare Cancer Network (RCN). Gynecol Oncol 2008; 108(2): 398–405.

64. Zanotti KM, Belinson JL, Kennedy AW, *et al.* The use of paclitaxel and platinum-based chemotherapy in uterine papillary serous carcinoma. Gynecol Oncol 1999; 74: 272–7.

65. Low JS, Wong EH, Tan HS, *et al.* Adjuvant sequential chemotherapy and radiotherapy in uterine papillary serous carcinoma. Gynecol Oncol 2005; 97: 171–7.

66. Fader AN, Drake RD, O'Malley DM, *et al.* Platinum/taxane-based chemotherapy with or without radiotherapy favorably impacts survival outcomes in stage I uterine papillary serous carcinoma. Cancer 2009; 115: 2119–27.

67. Flemming GF, Brunetto VL, Cella D, *et al.* Phase III trial of doxorubicin plus cisplatin with or without paclitaxel plus filgrastim in advanced endometrial carcinoma: a Gynecologic Oncology Group study. J Clin Oncol 2004; 22(11): 2159–66.

68. McMeekin DS, Filiaci VL, Thigpen JT, *et al.* Gynecologic Onocology Group study: the relationship between histology and outcome in advanced and recurrent endometrial cancer patients participating in first-line chemotherapy trials. Gynecol Oncol 2007; 106: 16–22.

69. Leslie KK, Sill MW, Darcy KM, *et al.* Efficacy and safety of gefitinib and potential prognostic value of soluble EGFR, EGFR mutations, and tumor markers in a Gynecologic Oncology Group phase II trial of persistent or recurrent endometrial cancer. J Clin Oncol 2009; 27(Suppl); abstract e16542.

70. Oza AM, Eisenhauer EA, Elit L, *et al.* Phase II study of erlotinib in recurrent or metastatic endometrial cancer: NCIC IND-148. J Clin Oncol 2008: 26: 4319–25.

71. Fleming GF, Sill MW, Darcy KM, *et al.* Phase II trial of trastuzumab in women with advanced or recurrent, HER2-positive endometrial carcinoma: a Gynecologic Oncology Group study. Gynecol Oncol 2010; 116: 15–20.

72. Broaddus RR, Lu KH. Future challenges in clinical and translational research for endometrial cancer. Int J Gynecol Cancer 2005; 15: 398–411.

73. Oza AM, Elit L, Tsao MS, *et al.* A phase II study of temsirolimus in women with recurrent or metastatic endometrial cancer: a trial of the NCIC Clinical Trials Group. J Clin Oncol 2011; 29: 3278–85.

74. Slomovitz BM, Lu KH, Johnston T, *et al.* A phase 2 study of the oral mammalian target of rapamycin inhibitor, everolimus in patients with recurrent endometrial carcinoma. Cancer 2010; 116: 5415–19.

75. Colombo N, McMeekin S, Schwartz P, *et al.* A phase II trial of the mTOR inhibitor AP23573 as a single agent in advanced endometrial cancer. J Clin Oncol 2007; 25: abstract 5516.

76. Mackay H, Welch S, Tsao MS, *et al.* Phase II study of oral ridaforolimus in patients with metastatic and/or locally advanced recurrent endometrial cancer: NCIC CTG IND 192. Proc ASCO 2011; 29(15 S): abstract 5013.

77. Fleming GF, Filiaci VL, Hanjani P, *et al.* Hormone therapy plus temsirolimus for endometrial carcinoma (EC): Gynecologic Oncology Group trial #248. J Clin Oncol 2011; 29(Suppl): abstract 5014.

78. Slomovitz BM, Brown J, Johnston TA, *et al.* A phase II study of everolimus and letrozole in patients with recurrent endometrial carcinoma. Proc ASCO 2011; 29(15 S): abstract 5012.

79. Aghajanian C, Sill MW, Darcy KM, *et al*. Phase II trial of bevacizumab in recurrent or persistent endometrial cancer: a Gynecologic Oncology Group study. J Clin Oncol 2011; 29: 2259–65.

80. Oza AM, Poveda A, Clamp AR, *et al*. A randomized phase II (RP2) trial of ridaforolimus (R) compared with progestin (P) or chemotherapy (C) in female adult patients with advanced endometrial carcinoma. Proc ASCO 2011; 29(15 S): abstract 5009.

81. Hamilton CA, Cheung MK, Osann K, *et al*. Uterine papillary serous and clear cell carcinomas predict for poorer survival compared to grade 3 endometrioid corpus cancers. Br J Cancer 2006; 94: 642–6.

82. Maxwell GL, Tian C, Risinger J, *et al*. Racial disparity in survival among patients with advanced/recurrent endometrial adenocarcinoma. A Gynecologic Oncology Group study. Cancer 2006; 107: 2197–205.

83. Wright JD, Fiorelli J, Schiff PB, *et al*. Racial disparities for uterine corpus tumors: changes in clinical characteristics and treatment over time. Cancer 2009; 115: 1276–85.

84. Al-Wahab Z, Ali-Fehmi R, Cote ML, *et al*. The impact of race on survival in uterine serous carcinoma: a hospital-based study. Gynecol Oncol 2011; 121: 577–80.

85. Silverberg SG, DeGiorgi LS. Clear cell carcinoma of the endometrium. Clinical, pathologic, and ultrastructural findings. Cancer 1973; 31: 1127–40.

86. Kurman RJ, Scully RE. Clear cell carcinoma of the endometrium: an analysis of 21 cases. Cancer 1976; 37: 872–82.

87. Fadare O, Liang SX, Ulukus EC, *et al*. Precursors of endometrial clear cell carcinoma. Am J Surg Pathol 2006; 30: 1519–30.

88. Gadducci A, Cosio S, Spirito N, *et al*. Clear cell carcinoma of the endometrium: a biological and clinical enigma. Anticancer Res 2010; 30: 1327–34.

89. Abeler VM, Vergote IB, Kjørstad KE, Tropé CG. Clear cell carcinoma of the endometrium: prognosis and metastatic pattern. Cancer 1996; 78: 1740–7.

90. Lindahl B, Persson J, Ranstam J, *et al*. Long-term survival in uterine clear cell carcinoma and uterine papillary serous carcinoma. Anticancer Res 2010; 30: 3727–30.

91. Malpica An, Tornos C, Burke TW, Silva EG. Low-stage clear-cell carcinoma of the endometrium. Am J Surg Pathol 1995; 19: 769–74.

92. Carcangiu ML, Chambers JT. Early pathologic stage clear cell carcinoma and uterine papillary serous carcinoma of the endometrium: comparison of clinicopathologic features and survival. Int J Gynceol Pathol 1995; 14: 30–8.

93. Murphy KT, Rotmensch J, Yamada SD, Mundt AJ. Outcome and patterns of failure in pathologic stages I–IV clear-cell carcinoma of the endometrium: implications for adjuvant radiation therapy. Int J Radiat Oncol Biol Phys 2003; 55(5): 1272–6.

94. Marchese JM, Liskow LS, Crum CP, *et al*. Uterine sarcomas: a clinicopathologic study, 1965–1981. Gynecol Oncol 1984; 18: 299–312.

95. Schwartz SM, Weiss NS. Martial status and the incidence of sarcomas of the uterus. Cancer Res 1990; 50: 1886–9.

96. Press MF, Scully RE. Endometrial sarcomas complicating ovarian thecoma, polycystic ovarian disease and estrogen therapy. Gynecol Oncol 1985; 21: 135–54.

97. Altaras MM, Jaffe R, Cohen I, *et al*. Role of prolonged excessive estrogen stimulation in the pathogenesis of endometrial sarcomas: two cases and a review of the literature. Gynecol Oncol 1990; 38: 273–7.

98. Altaras MM, Aviram R, Cohen I, *et al*. Role of prolonged stimulation of tamoxifen therapy in the etiology of endometrial sarcomas. Gynecol Oncol 1993; 49: 255–8.

99. Schwartz SM, Wisss NS, Daling JR, *et al*. Exogenous sex hormone use, correlates of endogenous hormone levels and the incidence of histologic types of sarcoma of the uterus. Cancer 1996; 77: 717–24.

100. Curtis RE, Freedman DM, Sherman ME, *et al*. Risk of malignant mixed mullerian tumors after tamoxifen therapy for breast cancer. J Natl Cancer Inst 2004; 96: 70–4.

101. Thomas WO, Harris HH, Enden JA. Postirradiation malignant neoplasms of the uterine fundus. Am J Obstet Gynecol 1969; 104: 209–19.

102. Fehr PE, Prem KA. Malignancy of the uterine corpus following irradiation therapy for squamous cell carcinoma of the cervix. Am J Obstet Gynecol 1974; 119: 685–92.

103. Czesnin K, Wronkowski Z. Second malignancies of the irradiated area in patients treated for uterine cervix cancer. Gynecol Oncol 1978; 6: 309–15.

104. Mark RJ, Poen J, Tran LM, *et al*. Positrradiation sarcoma of the gynecologic tract. A report of 13 cases and a discussion of the risk of radiation-induced gynecologic malignancies. Am J Clin Oncol 1996; 19: 59–64.

105. Pothuri B, Ramondetta L, Eifel P, *et al*. Radiation-associated endometrial cancers are prognostically unfavorable tumors: a clinicopathologic comparison with 527 sporadic endometrial cancers. Gynecol Oncol 2006; 103: 948–51.

106. Norris HJ, Taylor HB. Mesenchymal tumors of the uterus: a clinical and pathological study of 53 endometrial stromal tumors. Cancer 1966; 19: 755–66.

107. Chuang JT, van Velden DJJ, Graham JB. Carcinosarcoma and mixed mesodermal tumor of the uterine corpus: a review of 49 cases. Obstet Gynecol 1970; 35: 769–79.

108. DiSaia PJ, Castro JR, Rutledge FN. Mixed mesodermal sarcoma of the uterus. Am J Roentgenol 1973; 117: 632–6.

109. Major FJ, Blessing JA, Silverberg SG, *et al*. Prognostic factors in early-stage uterine sarcoma. A Gynecologic Oncology Group study. Cancer 1993; 71(4 Suppl): 1702–9.

110. Norris HJ, Roth E, Taylor HB. Mesenchymal tumors of the uterus: a clinical and pathologic study of 31 mixed mesodermal tumors. Obstet Gynecol 1966; 28: 57–63.

111. Peters WA, Kumar NB, Fleming WP, Morely GW. Prognostic features of sarcomas and mixed tumors of the endometrium. Obstet Gynecol 1984; 63: 550–6.

112. Doss LL, Llorens AS, Hernandez EM, Carcinosarcoma of the uterus: a 40 year experience from the state of Missouri. Gynecol Oncol 1984; 18: 43–53.

113. Covens AL, Nisker JA, Chapman WB, *et al*. Uterine sarcoma: an analysis of 74 cases. Am J Obstet Gynecol 1987; 156: 370–4.

114. Belgrad R, Elbadawi N, Rubin P. Uterine sarcoma. Radiology 1975; 114: 181–8.

115. Chen SS. Propensity of retroperitoneal lymph node metastasis in patients with stage I sarcoma of the uterus. Gynecol Oncol 1989; 32: 215–17.

116. Park JY, Kim DY, Kim JH, *et al*. The role of pelvic and paraaortic lymphadenectomy in surgical management of apparent early carcinosarcoma of the uterus. Ann Surg Oncol 2010; 17: 861–8.

117. Salazar OM, Bonfiglio TA, Pattern SF, *et al*. Uterine sarcomas: analysis of failures with special emphasis on the use of adjuvant radiation therapy. Cancer 1978; 42: 1161–70.

118. Geszler G, Szpak CA, Harris RE, *et al*. Prognostic value of peritoneal washings in patients with malignant mixed mullerian tumors of the uterus. Am J Obstet Gynecol 1986; 155: 83–9.

119. Kanbour AI, Buchsbaum HJ, Hall A, *et al*. Peritoneal cytology in malignant mixed mullerian tumors of the uterus. Gynecol Oncol 1989; 33: 91–5.

120. Rose PG, Piver MS, Tsukada Y, *et al*. Patterns of metastasis in uterine sarcoma: an autopsy study. Cancer 1989; 63: 935–8.

121. Reed NS, Mangioni C, Malmstom H, *et al*. Phase III randomized study to evaluate the role of adjuvant pelvic radiotherapy in the treatment of uterine sarcomas stage I and II: a European Organization for Research and Treatment of Cancer Gynecologic Cancer Group study (protocol 55874). Eur J Cancer 2008; 44: 808–18.

122. Omura GA, Blessing JA, Major F, *et al*. A randomized clinical trial of adjuvant Adriamycin in uterine sarcomas: a Gynecologic Oncology Group study. J Clin Oncol 1985; 9: 1240–5.

123. Hornback NB, Omura G, Major FJ. Observations on the use of adjuvant radiation therapy in patients with stage I and II uterine sarcoma. Int J Radiat Oncol Biol Phys 1986; 12: 2127–30.

124. Smith DC, Macdonald OK, Gaffney DK. The impact of adjuvant radiation therapy on survival in women with uterine carcinosarcoma. Radiother Oncol 2008; 88: 227–32.

125. Sutton G, Kauderer J, Carson LF, *et al.* Adjuvant ifosfamide and cisplatin in patients with completely resected stage I or II carcinosarcomas (mixed mesodermal tumors) of the uterus: a Gynecologic Oncology Group study. Gynecol Oncol 2005; 96: 630–4.

126. Makker V, Abu-Rustum NR, Alektiar KM, *et al.* A retrospective assessment of outcomes of chemotherapy-based versus radiation-only adjuvant treatment for completely resected stage I–IV uterine carcinosarcoma. Gynecol Oncol 2008; 111: 249–54.

127. Wolfson AH, Brady MF, Rocereto T, *et al.* A Gynecologic Oncology Group randomized phase III trial of whole abdominal irradiation (WAI) vs cisplatin-ifosfamide and mesna (CIM) as post-surgical therapy in stage I–IV carcinosarcoma (CS) of the uterus. Gynecol Oncol 2007; 107: 177–85.

128. Manolitsas TP, Wain GV, Williams KE, *et al.* Multimodality therapy for patients with clinical stage I and II malignant mixed Müllerian tumors of the uterus. Cancer 2001; 91: 1437–43.

129. Pautier P, Rey A, Haie-Meder C, *et al.* Adjuvant chemotherapy with cisplatin, ifosfamide, and doxorubicin followed by radiotherapy in localized uterine sarcomas: results of a case–control study with radiotherapy alone. Int J Gynecol Cancer 2004; 14: 1112–17.

130. Menczer J, Levy T, Piura B, *et al.* A comparison between different postoperative treatment modalities of uterine carcinosarcoma. Gynecol Oncol 2005; 97: 166.

131. Wong L, See HT, Khoo-Tan HS, *et al.* Combined adjuvant cisplatin and ifosfamide chemotherapy and radiotherapy for malignant mixed mullerian tumors of the uterus. Int J Gynecol Cancer 2006; 16: 1364.

132. Perez CA, Askin F, Baglan RJ. Effects of irradiation on mixed mullerian tumors of the uterus. Cancer 1979; 43: 1274–84.

133. Badib AO, Vongtama V, Kurohara SS, Webster JH. Radiotherapy in the treatment of sarcomas of the corpus uteri. Cancer 1969; 24: 724–9.

134. Thigpen JT, Blessing JA, Beecham J, *et al.* Phase II trial of cisplatin as first-line chemotherapy in patients with advanced or recurrent uterine sarcomas: a Gynecologic Oncology Group study. J Clin Oncol 1991; 9: 1962–6.

135. Thigpen JT, Blessing JA, Orr JW, DiSai PJ. Phase II trial of cisplatin in the treatment of patients with advanced or recurrent mixed mesodermal tumor of the uterus: a Gynecologic Oncology Group study. Cancer Treat Rep 1986; 70: 271–4.

136. Sutton GP, Blessing JA, Rosenshein N, *et al.* Phase II trial of ifosfamide and mesna in mixed mesodermal tumors of the uterus (a Gynecologic Oncology Group study). Am J Obstet Gynecol 1989; 161: 309–12.

137. Sutton GP, Blessing JA, Homesley HD, Malfetano JH. A phase II trial of ifosfamide and mesna in patients with advanced or recurrent mixed mesodermal tumors of the ovary previously treated with platinum-based chemotherapy: a Gynecologic Oncology Group study. Gynecol Oncol 1994; 53: 24–6.

138. Curtin JP, Blessing JA, Soper JT, DeGreest K. Paclitaxel in the treatment of carcinosarcoma of the uterus: a Gynecologic Oncology Group study. Gynecol Oncol 2001; 83: 268–70.

139. Asbury R, Blessing JA, Podczaski E, Ball H. A phase II trial of amonafide in patients with mixed mesodermal tumors of the uterus: a Gynecologic Oncology Group study. Am J Clin Oncol 1998; 21: 306–7.

140. Slayton RE, Blessing JA, Clarke-Pearson D. A phase II trial of diaziquone (AZQ) in mixed mesodermal sarcomas of the uterus: a Gynecologic Oncology Group study. Invest New Drugs 1991; 9: 93–4.

141. Omura GA, Major FJ, Blessing JA, *et al.* A randomized study of adriamycin with and without dimethyl triazenoimidazole carboxamide in advanced uterine sarcomas. Cancer 1983; 52: 626–32.

142. Gershenson DM, Karanagh JJ, Copeland J, *et al.* High-dose doxorubicin infusion therapy for disseminated mixed mesodermal sarcoma of the uterus. Cancer 1987; 59: 1264–7.

143. Slayton RE, Blessing JA, DiSaia PJ, *et al.* Phase II trial of etoposide in the management of advanced or recurrent mixed mesodermal sarcomas

of the uterus: a Gynecologic Oncology Group study. Cancer Treat Rep 1987; 71: 661–2.

144. Thigpen JT, Blessing JA, Hommesley HD, *et al.* Phase II trial of piperazinedione with advanced or recurrent mixed mesodermal uterine sarcoma. Am J Clin Oncol 1985; 8: 350–2.

145. Fowler JM, Blessing JA, Burger RA, Malfetano JH. Phase II evaluation of oral trimetrexate in mixed mesodermal tumors of the uterus: a Gynecologic Oncology Group study. Gynecol Oncol 2002; 85: 311–14.

146. Miller DS, Blessing JA, Schilder J, *et al.* Phase II evaluation of topotecan in carcinosarcoma of the uterus: a Gynecologic Oncology Group study. Gynecol Oncol 2005 98: 217–21.

147. Asbury R, Blessing JA, Buller R, *et al.* Amonafide in patients with leiomyosarcoma of the uterus: a phase II Gynecologic Oncology Group study. Am J Clin Oncol 1998; 21: 145–6.

148. Thigpen JT, Blessing JA, Willbanks GD. Cisplatin as second line chemotherapy in the treatment of advanced or recurrent leiomyosarcoma of the uterus. Am J Clin Oncol 1986; 9: 18–20.

149. Slayton R, Blessing J, Angel C, *et al.* Phase II trial of etoposide in the management of advanced and recurrent leiomyosarcoma of the uterus: a Gynecologic Oncology Group study. Cancer Treat Rep 1987; 71: 1303–4.

150. Rose PG, Blessing JA, Soper JT, Barter JF. Prolonged oral etoposide in recurrent or advanced leiomyosarcoma of the uterus: a Gynecologic Oncology Group study. Gynecol Oncol 1998; 70: 267–71.

151. Thigpen T, Blessing JA, Yordan E, *et al.* Phase II trial of etoposide in leiomyosarcoma of the uterus: a Gynecologic Oncology Group study. Gynecol Oncol 1996; 63: 120–2.

152. Look KY, Sandler A, Blessing JA, *et al.* Phase II trial of gemcitabine as second-line chemotherapy of uterine leiomyosarcoma: a Gynecologic Oncology Group (GOG) study. Gynecol Oncol 2004; 92: 644–7.

153. Sutton GP, Blessing JA, Barrett RJ, McGehee R. Phase II trial of ifosfamide and mesna in leiomyosarcoma of the uterus: a Gynecologic Oncology Group study. Am J Obstet Gynecol 1992; 166: 556–9.

154. Sutton G, Blessing J, Hanjani P, Kramer P. Phase II evaluation of liposomal doxorubicin (DOXIL) in recurrent or advanced leiomyosarcoma of the uterus: a Gynecologic Oncology Group study. Gynecol Oncol 2005; 96: 749–52.

155. Gallup DG, Blessing JA, Andersen W, Morgan MA. Evaluation of zpaclitaxel in previously treated leiomyosarcoma of the uterus: a Gynecologic Oncology Group study. Gynecol Oncol 2003; 89: 48–51.

156. Sutton G, Blessing JA, Ball H. Phase II trial of paclitaxel in leiomyosarcoma of the uterus: a Gynecologic Oncology Group study. Gynecol Oncol 1999; 74: 346–9.

157. Miller DS, Blessing JA, Kilgore LC, *et al.* Phase II trial of topotecan in patients with advanced, persistent or recurrent uterine leiomyosarcomas: a Gynecologic Oncology Group study. Am J Clin Oncol 2000; 23: 355–7.

158. Smith HO, Blessing JA, Vacarello L. Trimetrexate in the treatment of recurrent or advanced leiomyosarcoma of the uterus: a Phase II study of the Gynecologic Oncology Group. Gynecol Oncol 2002; 84: 140–4.

159. Powell MA, Filiaci VL, Rose PG, *et al.* Phase II evaluation of paclitaxel and carboplatin in the treatment of carcinosarcoma of the uterus: a Gynecologic Oncology Group study. J Clin Oncol 2010; 28: 2727–31.

160. Pectasides D, Pectasides E, Papaxoinis G, *et al.* Combination chemotherapy with carboplatin, paclitaxel and pegylated liposomal doxorubicin for advanced and recurrent carcinosarcoma of the uterus: clinical experience of a single institution. Gynecol Oncol 2008; 110: 299–303.

161. Piver MS, Lele SB, Patsner B, Cisdiamminedichloroplatinum plus dimethyl-triazeno imidazole carboximide as second and third line chemotherapy for sarcomas of the female pelvis. Gynecol Oncol 1986; 23: 371–5.

162. Baker TR, Piver MS, Caglar H, Piedmonte M. Prospective trial of cisplatin adriamycin and dacarbazine in the metastatic mixed mesodermal sarcomas of the uterus and ovary. Am J Clin Oncol 1991; 14: 246–50.

163. Sutton G, Brunetto VL, Kilgore L, *et al.* A phase III trial of ifosfamide with or without cisplatin in carcinosarcoma of the uterus: a Gynecologic Oncology Group study. Gynecol Oncol 2000; 79: 147–53.

164. Piver MS, DeEulis TG, Lele SB, Barlow JJ. Cyclophosphamide, vincristine, adriamycin and dimethyl-triazeno imidazole carboxamide (CYVADIC) for sarcomas of the female genital tract. Gynecol Oncol 1982; 14: 319–23.

165. Miller BE, Blessing JA, Stehman FB, et al A phase II evaluation of weekly gemcitabine and docetaxel for second-line treatment of recurrent carcinosarcoma of the uterus: a Gynecologic Oncology Group study. Gynecol Oncol 2010; 118: 139–44.

166. Seltzer V, Kaplan B, Vogl S, Spitzer M. Doxorubicin and cisplatin in the treatment of advanced mixed mesodermal uterine sarcoma. Cancer Treat Rep 1984; 68: 1389–90.

167. Muss HB, Bundy B, DiSaia PJ, et al. Treatment of recurrent or advanced uterine sarcoma. A randomized trial of doxorubicin versus doxorubicin and cyclophosphamide (a phase III trial of the Gynecologic Oncology Group). Cancer 1985; 55: 1648–53.

168. Jansen RL, van der Burg ME, Verweij J, Stoter G. Cyclophosphamide, hexamethylmelamine, adriamycin and cisplatin combination chemotherapy in mixed mesodermal sarcoma of the female genital tract. Eur J Cancer Clin Oncol 1987; 23: 1131–3.

169. Curry JL, Blessing JA, McGehee R, et al. Phase II trial of hydroxyurea, dacarbazine (DTIC), and etoposide (VP-16) in mixed mesodermal tumors of the uterus: a Gynecologic Oncology Group study. Gynecol Oncol 1996; 61: 94–6.

170. Homesley HD, Filiaci VL, Markman M, et al. Phase III trial of ifosfamide with or without paclitaxel in advanced uterine carcinosarcoma: a Gynecologic Oncology Group study. J Clin Oncol 2007; 25: 526–31.

171. Hannigan EV, Freedman RS, Elder KW, Rutledge FN. Treatment of advanced uterine sarcoma with vincristine, actinomycin-D and cyclophosphamide. Gynecol Oncol 1983; 115: 224–9.

172. Sutton G, Blessing JA, Malfetano JH. Ifosfamide and doxorubicin in the treatment of advanced leiomyosarcomas of the uterus: a Gynecologic Oncology Group study. Gynecol Oncol 1996; 62: 226–9.

173. Resnik E, Chambers SK, Carcangiu ML, et al. Malignant uterine smooth muscle tumors: role of etoposide, cisplatin, and doxorubicin (EPA) chemotherapy. J Surg Oncol 1996; 63: 145–7.

174. Hensley ML, Maki R, Venkatraman E, et al. Gemcitabine and docetaxel in patients with unresectable leiomyosarcoma: results of a phase II trial. J Clin Oncol 2002; 20: 2824–31.

175. Edmonson JH, Blessing JA, Cosin JA, et al. Phase II study of mitomycin, doxorubicin, and cisplatin in the treatment of advanced uterine leiomyosarcoma: a Gynecologic Oncology Group study. Gynecol Oncol 2002; 85: 507–10.

176. Currie J, Blessing JA, Muss HB, et al. Combination chemotherapy with hydroxyurea, dacarbazine (DTIC), and etoposide in the treatment of uterine leiomyosarcoma: a Gynecologic Oncology Group study. Gynecol Oncol 1996; 61: 27–30.

177. Hoskins PJ, Le N, Ellard S, et al. Carboplatin plus paclitaxel for advanced or recurrent uterine malignant mixed mullerian tumors. The British Columbia Cancer Agency experience. Gynecol Oncol 2008; 108: 58.

178. Lacour RA, Euscher E, Atkinson EN, et al. A phase II trial of paclitaxel and carboplatin in women with advanced and recurrent uterine carcinosarcoma. Int J Gynecol Cancer 2011; 21: 517–22.

179. Nimeiri HS, Oza AO, Morgan RJ, et al. A phase II study of sorafenib in advanced uterine carcinoma/carcinosarcoma: a trial of Chicago, PMH, and California phase II consortia. Gynecol Oncol 2010; 117: 37–40.

180. Santin AD, Bellone S, Siegal ER, et al. Overexpression of clostridium prefingess enterotoxin receptors claudin-3 and claudin-4 in uterine carcinosarcomas. Clin Cancer Res 2007; 13: 3339–46.

181. Ferguson SE, Tornos C, Hummer A, et al. Prognostic features of surgical stage I uterine carcinosarcoma. Am J Surg Pathol 2007; 31: 1653–61.

182. Clement PB, Scully RE. Endometrial hyperplasia and carcinoma. In: Clement PB, Young RH (eds) Contemporary Issues in Surgical Pathology. New York: Churchill Livingstone, 1993. pp.181–264.

183. Nordal RR, Thoresen SO. Uterine sarcomas in Norway 1956–1992: incidence, survival and mortality. Eur J Cancer 1997; 33: 907–11.

184. Wheelock JB, Krebs HB, Schneider V, et al. Uterine sarcoma: analysis of prognostic variables in 71 cases. Am J Obstet Gynecol 1987; 151: 1016–22.

185. Ober WB. Uterine sarcomas: histogenesis and taxonomy. Ann N Y Acad Sci 1959; 75: 568–85.

186. Kempson RL, Bari W. Uterine sarcomas: classification, diagnosis and prognosis. Hum Pathol 1970; 1: 331–49.

187. Silverberg SG. Leiomyosarcoma of the uterus: a clinicopathologic study. Obstet Gynecol 1971; 38: 613–28.

188. Schwartz Z, Dgani R, Lancet M, Kessler I. Uterine sarcoma in Israel: a study of 104 cases. Gynecol Oncol 1985; 20: 354–63.

189. Brooks SE, Zhan M, Cote T, Baquet CR. Surveillance, epidemiology, and end results analysis of 2677 cases of uterine sarcoma 1989–1999. Gynecol Oncol 2004; 93: 204–8.

190. Montague AC, Swartz DP, Woodruff JD. Sarcoma arising in a leiomyoma of the uterus. Am J Obstet Gynecol 1965; 92: 421–7.

191. Torpin R, Pund E, Peeples WJ. The etiologic and pathologic factors in a series of 1,741 fibromyomas of the uterus. Am J Obstet Gynecol 1942; 44: 569–74.

192. Aaro LA, Symmonds RE, Dockerty MB. Sarcoma of the uterus: a clinical and pathologic study of 177 cases. Am J Obstet Gynecol 1966; 94: 101–9.

193. Ognjanovic S, Oliver M, Bergemann TL, Hainaut P. Sarcomas in TP53 germline mutation carriers: a review of the IARC TP53 database. Cancer 2012; 118(5): 1387–96.

194. Kleinerman RA, Tucker MA, Abramson DH, et al. Risk of soft tissue sarcomas by individual subtype in survivors of hereditary retinoblastoma. J Natl Cancer Inst 2007; 99: 24–31.

195. Arita S, Kikkawa F, Kajiyama H, et al. Prognostic importance of vascular endothelial growth factor and its receptors in uterine sarcoma. Int J Gynecol Cancer 2005; 15: 329–36.

196. McMeekin DS, Filiaci VL, Thigpen JT, et al. The relationship between histology and outcome in advanced and recurrent endometrial cancer patients participating in first-line chemotherapy trials: a Gynecologic Oncology Group study. Gynecol Oncol 2007; 106(1): 16–22.

197. Wang L, Felix JC, Lee JL, et al. The proto-oncogene c-kit is expressed in leiomyosarcomas of the uterus. Gynecol Oncol 2003; 90: 402–6.

198. Winter WE 3rd, Seidman JD, Krivak TC, et al. Clinicopathological analysis of c-kit expression in carcinosarcomas and leiomyosarcomas of the uterine corpus. Gynecol Oncol 2003; 91: 3–8.

199. Klein WM, Kurman RJ. Lack of expression of c-kit protein (CD117) in mesenchymal tumors of the uterus and ovary. Int J Gynecol Pathol 2003; 22: 181–4.

200. Rushing RS, Shajahan S, Chendil D, et al. Uterine sarcomas express KIT protein but lack mutation(s) in exon 11 or 17 of c-KIT. Gynecol Oncol 2003; 91: 9–14.

201. Raspollini MR, Pinzani P, Simi L, et al. Uterine leiomyosarcomas express KIT protein but lack mutation(s) in exon 9 of c-KIT. Gynecol Oncol 2005; 98: 334–5.

202. Bodner-Adler B, Bodner K, Kimberger O, et al. MMP-1 and MMP-2 expression in uterine leiomyosarcoma and correlation with different clinicopathologic parameters. J Soc Gynecol Invest 2003; 10: 443–6.

203. Garg G, Short A, Liu JR, et al. Akt-mTOR pathway in uterine leiomyosarcoma. Proc ASCO 2011; 15 S: abstract 5040.

204. Taylor HB, Norris HJ. Mesenchymal tumors of the uterus. Arch Pathol 1966; 82: 40–4.

205. Leibsohn S, d'Ablaing G, Mishell DR, Schlaerth JB. Leiomyosarcoma in a series of hysterectomies performed for presumed uterine leiomyomas. Am J Obstet Gynecol 1990; 162: 968–76.

206. Barter JF, Smith EB, Szpak CA, et al. Leiomyosarcoma of the uterus: clinicopathologic study of 21 cases. Gynecol Oncol 1985; 21: 220–7.

207. Hannigan EV, Gomez LG. Uterine leiomyosarcoma: a review of prognostic clinical and pathologic features. Am J Obstet Gynecol 1979; 134: 557–64.

208. Perrone T, Dehner LP. Prognostically favorable 'mitotically active' smooth-muscle tumors of the uterus. Am J Surg Pathol 1988; 12: 1–8.

209. O'Connor DM, Norris HJ. Mitotically active leiomyomas of the uterus. Hum Pathol 1990; 21: 223–7.

210. Prayson RA, Hart WR. Mitotically active leiomyomas of the uterus. Am J Clin Pathol 1992; 97: 14–20.

211. Peters WA, Howard DR, Andersen WA, Figge DC. Uterine smooth-muscle tumors of uncertain malignant potential. Obstet Gynecol 1994; 83: 1015–20.

212. Bell SW, Kempson RL, Hendrickson MR. Problematic uterine smooth muscle neoplasms: a clinicopathologic study of 213 cases. Am J Surg Pathol 1994; 18: 535–58.

213. Schwartz LB, Diamond MP, Schwartz PE. Leiomyosarcomas: clinical presentation. Am J Obstet Gynecol 1993; 168: 180–3.

214. Barter JF, Smith EB, Szpak CA, et al. Leiomyosarcoma of the uterus: clinicopathologic study of 21 cases. Gynecol Oncol 1985; 21: 220–7.

215. King ME, Dickersin GR, Scully RE. Myxoid leiomyosarcoma of the uterus: a report of six cases. Am J Surg Pathol 1982; 6: 589–98.

216. Chen KTK. Myxoid leiomyosarcoma of the uterus. Int J Gynecol Pathol 1984; 3: 389–92.

217. Parker WH, Fu Yao S, Berek JS. Uterine sarcoma in patients operated on for presumed leiomyoma and rapidly growing leiomyoma. Obstet Gynecol 1994; 83: 414–18.

218. Meyer WR, Mayer AR, Diamond MP, et al. Unsuspected leiomyosarcoma: treatment with a gonadotropin-releasing hormone analogue. Obstet Gynecol 1990; 75: 529–31.

219. Hitti IF, Glasberg SS, McKenzie C, Meltzer BA. Uterine leiomyosarcoma with massive necrosis diagnosed during gonadotropin-releasing hormone analog therapy for presumed uterine fibroid. Fertil Steril 1991; 56: 779–80.

220. Schwartz LB, Diamond MP, Schwartz PE. Leiomyosarcomas: clinical presentation. Am J Obstet Gynecol 1993; 168: 180–3.

221. Tanaka YO, Nishida M, Tsunoda H, et al. Smooth muscle tumors of uncertain malignant potential and leiomyosarcomas of the uterus: MR findings. J Magn Reson Imaging 2004; 20: 998–1007.

222. Zivanovic O, Leitao MM, Iasonas A, et al. Stage-specific outcomes of patients with uterine leiomyosarcoma: a comparison of the International Federation of Gynecology and Obstetrics and American Joint Committee on Cancer staging systems. J Clin Oncol 2009; 27: 2066–72.

223. Raut CP, Nucci MR, Wang Q, et al. Predictive value of the FIGO and AJCC staging systems in patients with uterine leiomyosarcoma. Eur J Cancer 2009; 45: 2818–24.

224. Pelmus M, Penault-Llorca F, Guillou L, et al. Prognostic factors in early leiomyosarcoma of the uterus. Int J Gynecol Cancer 2009; 19: 385–90.

225. Zivanovic O, Jacks LM, Iasonas A, et al. A normogram to predict postresection 5-year overall survival for patients with uterine leiomyosarcoma. Cancer 2012; 118(3): 660–9.

226. Kapp D, Shin J, Chan J. Prognostic factors and survival in 1396 patients with uterine leiomyosarcomas. Emphasis on impact of lymphadenectomy and oophorectomy. Cancer 2008; 112: 820–30.

227. Dafopoulos A, Tsikouras P, Dimitraki M, et al. The role of lymphadenectomy in uterine leiomyosarcoma: review of the literature and recommendations for the standard surgical procedure. Arch Gynecol Obstet 2010; 282: 293–300.

228. Van Dinh T, Woodruff JD. Leiomyosarcoma of the uterus. Am J Obstet Gynecol 1982; 144: 817–23.

229. Berchuck A, Rubin SC, Hoskins WJ, et al. Treatment of uterine leiomyosarcoma. Obstet Gynecol 1988; 71: 845–50.

230. Lissoni A, Cormio G, Bonazzi C, et al. Fertility-sparing surgery in uterine leiomyosarcoma. Gynecol Oncol 1998; 70: 348.

231. Parente JT, Axelrod MR, Levy JL, Chiang CE. Leiomyosarcoma of the uterus with pulmonary metastases: a favorable response to operation and chemotherapy in a patient monitored with serial carcinoembryonic antigen. Am J Obstet Gynecol 1978; 131: 812–15.

232. Mahdavi A, Monk BJ, Ragazzo J, et al. Pelvic radiation improves local control after hysterectomy for uterine leiomyosarcoma: a 20 year experience. Int J Gynecol Cancer 2009; 19: 1080–4.

233. Tierney JF, Stewart LA, Parmar MKB, et al. Adjuvant chemotherapy for localized resectable soft-tissue sarcoma of adults: meta-analysis of individual data. Lancet 1997; 350 (ii): 1647–54.

234. Wu TI, Chang TC, Hsueh S, et al. Prognostic factors and impact of adjuvant chemotherapy for uterine leiomyosarcoma. Gynecol Oncol 2006; 100: 166–72.

235. Hensley ML, Ishill N, Soslow R, et al. Adjuvant gemcitabine plus docetaxel for completely resected stages I–IV high grade uterine leiomyosarcoma: results of a prospective study. Gynecol Oncol 2009; 112: 563–7.

236. Levenback C, Rubin SC, McCormack PM, et al. Resection of pulmonary metastases from uterine sarcomas. Gynecol Oncol 1992; 45: 202–5.

237. Reid GC, Morley GW, Schmidt RW, Hopkins MP. The role of pelvic exenteration for sarcomatous malignancies. Obstet Gynecol 1989; 74: 80–4.

238. Giuntoli RL, Garrett-Mayer E, Bristow RE, et al. Secondary cytoreduction in the management of recurrent uterine leiomyosarcoma. Gynecol Oncol 2007; 107: 82–8.

239. Hensley ML, Blessing J, DeGeest K, et al. Fixed-dose rate gemcitabine plus docetaxel as second-line therapy for metastatic uterine leiomyosarcoma. A Gynecologic Oncology Group phase II study. Gynecol Oncol 2008; 109: 323–8.

240. Hensley ML, Blessing JA, Mannel R, Rose PG. Fixed-dose rate gemcitabine plus docetaxel as first-line therapy for metastatic uterine leiomyosarcoma: a Gynecologic Oncology Group phase II trial. Gynecol Oncol 2008; 109: 329–34.

241. Long HJ, Blessing JA, Sorosky J. Phase II trial of dacarbazine, mitomycin, doxorubicin, and cisplatin with sargramostimin uterine leiomyosarcoma: a Gynecologic Oncology Group study. Gynecol Oncol 2005; 99: 339–42.

242. Anderson S, Aghajanian C. Temozolomide in uterine leiomyosarcomas. Gynecol Oncol 2005; 98: 99–103.

243. Ferriss JS, Atkins KA, Lachance JA, et al. Temozolomide in advanced and recurrent uterine leiomyosarcomas and correlation wuith O[6]-methylguanine DNA methyltrasferase expression: a case series. Int J Gynecol Cancer 2010; 20: 120–5.

244. Sutton GP, Stehman FB, Michael H, et al. Estrogen and progesterone receptors in uterine sarcomas. Obstet Gynecol 1986; 68: 709–14.

245. Wade K, Quinn MA, Hammond I, et al. Uterine sarcoma: steroid receptors and response to hormonal therapy. Gynecol Oncol 1990; 39: 364.

246. Zhai YL, Kobayashi Y, Mori A, et al. Expression of steroid receptors, Ki-67, and p53 in uterine leiomyosarcomas. Int J Gynecol Pathol 1999; 18: 20.

247. Bodner K, Bodner-Adler B, Kimberger O, et al. Estrogen and progesterone receptor expression in patients with uterine leiomyosarcoma and correlation with different clinicopathological parameters. Anticancer Res 2003; 23: 729.

248. O'Cearbhaill R, Zhou Q, Iasonas A, et al. Treatment of uterine leiomyosarcoma with aromatase inhibitors. Gynecol Oncol 2010; 116: 424–9.

249. McMeekin DS, Sill MW, Darcy KM, et al. A phase II trial of thalidomide in patients with refractory leiomyosarcoma of the uterus and correlation with biomarkers of angiogenesis: a Gynecologic Oncology Group study. Gynecol Oncol 2007; 106: 596–603.

250. Hensley ML, Sill MW, Scribner DR, et al. Sunitinib malate in the treatment of recurrent or persistent uterine leiomyosarcoma: a Gynecologic Oncology Group study. Gynecol Oncol 2009; 115: 460–5.

251. Shah JP, Bryant CS, Kumar S, et al. Lymphadenectomy and ovarian preservation in low-grade endometrial stromal sarcoma. Obstet Gynecol 2008; 112: 1102–8.

252. Garg G, Shah JP, Toy EP, et al. Stage IA vs IB endometrial stromal sarcoma: does the new staging system predict survival? Gynecol Oncol 2010; 118: 8–13.

253. Cheng X, Yang G, Schmeler KM, et al. Recurrence patterns and prognosis of endometrial stromal sarcoma and the potential of tyrosine kinase-inhibiting therapy. Gynecol Oncol 2011; 121: 323–7.

254. Tavassoli FA, Devilee P. *World Health Organization Classification of Tumors. Pathology and Genetics. Tumors of the Breast and Female Genital Organs*. Lyon, France: IARC Press, 2003.

255. Chang KL, Crabtree GS, Lim-Tan SK, *et al*. Primary uterine endometrial stromal neoplasms. Am J Surg Pathol 1990; 14: 415–38.

256. Norris HJ, Taylor HB. Mesenchymal tumors of the uterus: a clinical and pathologic study of 31 carcinosarcomas. Cancer 1966; 19: 1459–65.

257. Dos Santos LA, Garg K, Diaz JP, *et al*. Incidence of lymph node and adnexal metastasis in endometrial stromal sarcoma. Gynecol Oncol 2011; 121: 319–22.

258. Michener CM, Simon NL. Ovarian conservation in a woman of reproductive age with Mullerian adenosarcoma. Gynecol Oncol 2001; 83: 424–7.

259. Signorelli M, Fruscio R, Dell'Anna T, *et al*. Lymphadenectomy in uterine low-grade endometrial stromal sarcoma: an analysis of 19 cases and a literature review. Int J Gynecol Cancer 2010; 20: 1363–6.

260. Barney B, Tward JD, Skidmore T, *et al*. Does radiotherapy or lymphadenectomy improve survival in endometrial stromal sarcoma? Int J Gynecol Cancer 2009; 19: 1232–8.

261. Park JY, Kim DY, Kim JH, *et al*. The impact of tumor morcellation during surgery on the outcomes of patients with apparent early low-grade endometrial stromal sarcoma of the uterus. Ann Surg Oncol 2011; 18(12): 3453–61.

262. Baggish MS, Woodruff JD. Uterine stomatosis: clinicopathologic features and hormone dependency. Obstet Gynecol 1972; 40: 487–90.

263. Krumholts BA, Lobovsky FYI, Halitsky V. Endolymphatic stromal myosis with pulmonary metastasis, remission with progestin therapy: report of a case. J Reprod Med 1973; 10: 85–9.

264. Thatcher SS, Woodruff JD. Uterine stromatosis: a report of 33 cases. Obstet Gynecol 1982; 59: 428–34.

265. Gloor E, Schnyder P, Cikes M. Endolymphatic stromal myosis: surgical and hormonal treatment of extensive abdominal recurrence 20 years after hysterectomy. Cancer 1982; 50: 1888–93.

266. Piver MS, Rutledge FN, Copeland L, *et al*. Uterine endolymphatic stromal myosis: a collaborative study. Obstet Gynecol 1984; 64: 173–8.

267. Tsukamoti N, Kamura T, Matsukuma K, *et al*. Endolymphatic stromal myosis: a case with positive estrogen and progesterone receptors and good response to progestins. Gynecol Oncol 1985; 20: 120–8.

268. Tzakas E, Liu S, Todd W, *et al*. Hormonal therapy with letrozole prior to surgical management of recurrent metastatic low-grade endometrial stromal sarcoma (LGESS). J Obstet Gynaecol 2009; 29(8): 778–9.

269. Dahhan T, Fons G, Buist MR, *et al*. The efficacy of hormonal treatment for residual or recurrent low-grade endometrial stromal sarcoma. A retrospective study. Eur J Obstet Gynecol Reprod Biol 2009; 144: 80–4.

270. Nakayama K, Ishikawa M, Nagai Y, *et al*. Prolonged long-term survival of low-grade endometrial stromal sarcoma patients with lung metastasis following treatment with medroxyprogesterone acetate. Int J Clin Oncol 2010; 15: 179–83.

271. Shoji K, Oda K, Nakagawa S, *et al*. Aromatase inhibitor anastrozole as a second-line hormonal treatment to a recurrent low-grade endometrial stromal sarcoma: a case report. Med Oncol 2011; 28: 771–4.

272. Altrabulsi B, Malpica A, Deavers MT, *et al*. Undifferentiated carcinoma of the endometrium. Am J Surg Pathol 2005; 29: 1316–21.

273. Salvatierra A, Tarrats A, Gomez C, *et al*. A case of c-kit positive high-grade stromal endometrial sarcoma responding to imatinib mesylate. Gynecol Oncol 2006; 101(3): 545–7.

274. August CZ, Bauer KD, Lurain J, Murad T. Neoplasms of endometrial stroma: histopathologic and flow cytometric analysis with clinical correlation. Hum Pathol 1989; 20: 232–7.

275. Zoloudek C, Norris HJ. Mesenchymal tumors of the uterus. In: Kurman RJ (ed) *Blaustein's Pathology of the Female Genital Tract*, 4th edn. New York: Springer, 1994. p.519.

276. Oliva E, Clement PB, Young RH, Skully RE. Mixed endometrial stromal and smooth muscle tumors of the uterus: a clinicopathologic study of 15 cases. Am J Surg Path 1998; 22: 997–1005.

277. Vang R, Kempson RL. Perivascular epithelioid cell tumor (PEComa) of the uterus: a subset of HMB-45-positive epithelioid mesenchymal neoplasms with an uncertain relationship to pure smooth muscle tumors. Am J Surg Path 2002; 26: 1–13.

278. Arend R, Bagaria M, Lewin SN, *et al*. Long-term outcome and natural history of uterine adenosarcomas. Gynecol Oncol 2010; 119: 305–8.

279. Clement PB, Scully RE. Mullerian adenosarcoma of the uterus: a clinicopathologic analysis of 100 cases with a review of the literature. Hum Pathol 1990; 21: 363–81.

280. Krivak TC, Seidman JD, McBroom JW, *et al*. Uterine adenosarcoma with sarcomatous overgrowth versus uterine carcinosarcoma: comparison of treatment and survival. Gynecol Oncol 2001; 83: 89–94.

281. Taskin S, Bozaci EA, Sonmezer M, *et al*. Late recurrence of uterine mullerian adenosarcoma as heterologous sarcoma: three recurrences in 8 months increasing in number and grade of sarcomatous components. Gynecol Oncol 2006; 101: 179–82.

282. Shi Y, Liu Z, Peng Z, *et al*. The diagnosis and treatment of mullerian adenosarcoma of the uterus. Aust N Z J Obstet Gynaecol 2008; 48(6): 596–600.

283. Chorlton I, Karnei RF, Norris HJ. Primary malignant reticuloendothelial disease involving the vagina, cervix and corpus uteri. Obstet Gynecol 1974; 44: 735–48.

284. Lathrop JC. Malignant pelvic lymphomas. Obstet Gynecol 1967; 30: 137–45.

285. Rosenberg SA, Diamond HD, Jaslowitz B, Craver LF. Lymphosarcoma: a review of 1269 cases. Medicine 1961; 40: 31–76.

286. Harris NL, Scully RE. Malignant lymphoma and granulocytic sarcoma of the uterus and vagina. Cancer 1984; 53: 2530–45.

287. Osborne BM, Robboy SJ. Lymphomas or leukemia presenting as ovarian tumors: an analysis of 42 cases. Cancer 1983; 52: 1933–43.

288. Crisp WE, Surwit EA, Grogan TM, Freedman MF. Malignant pelvic lymphoma. Am J Obstet Gynecol 1982; 143: 69–74.

289. Friedman HD, Adelson MD, Elder RC, Lemke SM. Granulocytic sarcoma of the uterine cervix – literature review of granulocytic sarcoma of the female genital tract. Gynceol Oncol 1992; 46: 128–37.

290. Garcia M, Deavers MT, Knoblock RJ, *et al*. Myeloid sarcoma involving the gynecologic tract. Am J Clin Pathol 2006; 125: 783–90.

291. Wilbanks GD, Szymanska Z, Miller AW. Pelvic hemangiopericytoma: report of 4 patients and review of the literature. Am J Obstet Gynecol 1975; 123: 555–69.

292. Smullens SN, Scotti DJ, Osterholm JL, Weiss AJ. Preoperative embolization of retroperitoneal hemangiopericytomas as an aid to their removal. Cancer 1982; 50: 1870–5.

293. Bell SW, Kempson RL, Hendrickson MR. Problematic uterine smooth muscle neoplasms. A clinicopathologic study of 213 cases. Am J Surg Pathol 1994; 18: 535.

294. Fadare O, Liang SX. Epithelioid smooth muscle tumors of the uterus do not express CD1a: a potential immunohistochemical adjunct in their distinction from uterine perivascular epithelioid cell tumors. Ann Diagn Pathol 2008; 12: 401–5.

295. Kurman RJ, Norris HJ, Mesenchymal tumors of the uterus: epithelioid smooth muscle tumors including leiomyoblastoma and clear cell leiomyoma. Cancer 1976; 37: 1853–65.

296. Goldberg MF, Hurt WG, Frable WJ. Leiomyomatosis peritonealis disseminata: report of a case and review of the literature. Obstet Gynecol 1977; 49: 46S–52S.

297. Williams LJ, Pavlick FJ. Leiomyomatosis peritonealis disseminata: two case reports and a review of the medical literature. Cancer 1980; 45: 1726–33.

298. Wilson JR, Peale AR. Multiple peritoneal leiomyomas associated with a granulosa-cell tumor of the ovary. Am J Obstet Gynecol 1952; 64: 204–8.

299. Tavassoli FA, Norris HJ. Peritoneal leiomyomatosis (leiomyomatosis peritonealis disseminata): a clinicopathologic study of 20 cases with ultrastructural observations. Int J Gynecol Pathol 1982; 1: 59–74.

300. Akkersdijk GJM, Flu PK, Giard RWM, *et al*. Malignant leiomyomatosis peritonealis disseminata. Am J Obstet Gynecol 1990; 163: 591–3.

301. Norris HJ, Parmley T. Mesenchymal tumors of the uterus: intravenous leiomyomatosis. Cancer 1975; 36: 2164–78.

302. Tierney WM, Ehrlich CE, Bailey JC, *et al*. Intravenous leiomyomatosis of the uterus with extension into the heart. Am J Med 1980; 69: 471–5.

303. Evans AT, Symmonds RE, Gaffey TA. Recurrent pelvic intravenous leiomyomatosis. Obstet Gynecol 1981; 57: 260–4.

304. Abell MR, Littler ER. Benign metastasizing uterine leiomyoma: multiple lymph node metastases. Cancer 1975; 36: 2206–13.

305. Lehtonen HJ, Kiuru M, Ylisaukko-Oja SK, *et al*. Increased risk of cancer in patients with fumarate hydratase germline mutation. J Med Genet 2006; 43: 523.

306. Stratakis CA, Kirschner LS, Taymans SE, *et al*. Carney complex, Peutz–Jeghers syndrome, Cowden disease, and Bannayan–Zonana syndrome share cutaneous and endocrine manifestations, but not genetic loci. J Clin Endocrinol Metab 1998; 83: 2972.

307. Miller D, Filiaci V, Fleming G, *et al*. Randomized phase III noninferiority trial of first line chemotherapy for metastatic or recurrent endometrial carcinoma: A Gynecologic Oncology Group study. Late-Breaking Abstract 1, Society of Gynecologic Oncology Annual Meeting, March 25, 2012.

40 Tumors of the Cervix

Krishnansu S. Tewari[1] and Bradley J. Monk[2]

[1] Division of Gynecologic Oncology, Department of Obstetrics and Gynecology, University of California, Irvine Medical Center, Orange, CA, USA
[2] Division of Gynecologic Oncology, Department of Obstetrics and Gynecology, Creighton University School of Medicine at St Joseph's Hospital and Medical Center, Phoenix, AZ, USA

Historical notes

In January 1878, Freund of Germany "extirpated a cancerous uterus through an abdominal incision" but limited the procedure to removal of the parametrial tissues only as far lateral as the ureteral tunnel, without removal of lymph nodes.[1] John Goodrich Clark (1927), a resident under Howard Atwood Kelly at the Johns Hopkins Hospital, studied 20 autopsy cases of cervical cancer and in April 1895, performed what is considered to be the first true radical hysterectomy in which he removed all of the parametria to the lateral pelvic wall. His paper included illustrations by the eminent artist Max Brödel and was published in the July–August 1895 issue of *The Bulletin of the Johns Hopkins Hospital*.[2] Clark credited Freund with the earliest attempt at an abdominal approach to cervical cancer and noted that because of the high primary mortality associated with abdominal hysterectomy for cancer, most gynecologists during Freund's era moved to vaginal hysterectomy.

Because the Americans would eventually recognize the need for a formal lymphadenectomy, the vaginal radical hysterectomy, commonly called the Schauta operation after the Austrian surgeon Friedrich Shauta (1849–1919), never became popular in the United States.[3] Ernst Wertheim (1864–1920), a student of Shauta's, developed an abdominal version of Shauta's radical vaginal operation but during his early experience from 1900 to 1912, he had sepsis to contend with.[4] Of those who survived the operation, many would go on to fail at the pelvic sidewall, where the lymph nodes reside.

While studying the refraction of light from a cathode tube, Wilhelm Konrad von Röentgen (1845–1923) accidentally discovered x-rays and went on to win the first Nobel Prize in Physics in 1901 for this achievement and the era of diagnostic radiology commenced.[5] Next, Madame Marie Sklowdowska Curie (1867–1934), from a French family of scientists, discovered radium while working with an extract from pitchblende and was given the Nobel Prize in Physics in 1903.[6] However, it was the Scottish-American inventor, Alexander Graham Bell, who suggested the vaginal insertion of radium to treat a patient with cervical cancer, in 1908 nearly three decades after having demonstrated the first telephone apparatus.[7] Thus, radiotherapeutics found a role in the management of cervical cancer through the transvaginal insertion of long radium needles. Only after World War II did particle accelerators powerful enough to generate a therapeutic beam of radiation become available.

Meanwhile, surgeons continued to refine their approach toward cervical tumors. Frederick Taussig (1891–1943) developed the technique of transperitoneal pelvic lymphadenectomy,[8] which was later combined with the Wertheim operation by Joseph Vincent Meigs (1892–1963) of the Massachusetts General Hospital in Boston. From 1940 to 1951, Meigs performed 100 consecutive, personalized radical hysterectomies without a single perioperative mortality.[9] In Japan, Shuichi Okabayashi (1884–1953) pioneered the Japanese radical abdominal hysterectomy[10] and later, Alexander Brunschwig (1901–1974) in the United States became the architect of pelvic exenterative surgery for centrally recurrent disease.[11]

On the preventive front, George Nicolas Papanicoloau (1883–1962), working first with the hamster cervix, invented the screening procedure that bears his name.[12] The widespread implementation of the Papanicoloau test has resulted in a substantial decrease in the incidence of and mortality from cervical cancer in developed countries.

Henrietta Lacks (1920–1951) died of cervical cancer at Johns Hopkins University. The cells of her cancer, known as *HeLa cells*, were the first human cells discovered to thrive and multiply outside the body, seemingly indefinitely, allowing investigators to create the polio vaccine, unravel the mechanistics of malignant transformation, and study molecular therapeutics.[13] Finally, during the 1980s Henrich zur Hausen performed cross-hybridization studies and identified two new human papillomavirus (HPV) subtypes, designated HPV subtypes 16 and 18, both of which have been implicated separately (i.e. one or the other) in the pathogenesis of the majority of cervical cancers.[14,15]

Textbook of Uncommon Cancer, Fourth Edition. Edited by Derek Raghavan, Charles D. Blanke, David H. Johnson, Paul L. Moots, Gregory H. Reaman, Peter G. Rose and Mikkael A. Sekeres.
© 2012 John Wiley & Sons, Inc. Published 2012 by John Wiley & Sons, Inc.

Epidemiology

In 2011 there were 12,710 new cases of invasive cervical cancer and 4290 deaths from this disease in the United States.[16] It is particularly distressing that more than one-third of women diagnosed will die from a disease that is largely preventable by vaccination and screening. Epidemiological surveillance studies performed in the United States during the past two decades have documented decreased incidence rates for invasive cervical cancer. Ethnic and racial disparities, however, still exist. In a Surveillance, Epidemiology, and End Results (SEER) analysis of 13 US cancer registries containing cases from 1992 to 2003,[17] Hispanic whites had the highest incidence rate of cervical cancer overall (24 per 100,000), squamous cell carcinoma (18 per 100,000), and adenocarcinoma (5 per 10,000). Non-Hispanic whites had the lowest rates of cervical cancer overall (11 per 100,000) and squamous cell carcinoma (7 per 100,000), while African-Americans had the lowest rate of adenocarcinoma (2 per 100,000). In a recent study using data obtained from the Cancer in North America (CINA) deluxe 1995–2004 database created by the North American Association of Central Cancer Registries (NAACCR), African-American and Hispanic US populations continue to have the highest rates of invasive cervical cancer compared to non-Hispanic whites.[18] Variations in screening utilization and socioeconomic status are thought to account for the majority of the racial/ethnic disparities.

Staging of cervical cancer

Cervical cancer is staged clinically. In addition to a medical and gynecological history and physical examination, a comprehensive review of systems is mandatory. Common procedures endorsed by the International Federation of Gynecology and Obstetrics (FIGO) include cervical biopsy, endocervical curretage, and cervical conization.[19,20] A complete blood count, serum chemistries and urinalysis should also be obtained. Patients with locally advanced disease should also undergo pelvic examination under anesthesia as indicated, with or without urethrocystoscopy and/or proctoscopy. Finally, an intravenous pyelogram, lymphangiogram, and chest radiograph can be scheduled to evaluate for hydronephrosis, retroperitoneal adenopathy, and pulmonary metastases, respectively.[19] Although not officially endorsed by FIGO, many patients in the United States undergo computed tomography (CT) imaging of the chest, abdomen, and pelvis to determine whether regional and distant metastases are present. Magnetic resonance imaging (MRI) of the pelvis may be of some value when a pelvic examination under anesthesia is inconclusive regarding parametrial involvement in a patient being considered for radical surgery. Positron emission tomography (PET) is more sensitive than CT or MRI in the evaluation of metastatic spread of cervical cancer.[19]

In 2009, FIGO updated the staging classification for invasive cervical cancer with the addition of FIGO stages IIA_1 and IIA_2. The 2009 FIGO staging of cervical cancer appears in Box 40.1.[20]

Clinical presentation

Oncogenic (high risk) HPV infection is a necessary cause (99.7%) of cervical cancer; worldwide, approximately 70% of all cervical cancer cases are attributable to types 16 and 18; the next two most prevalent oncogenic types are 45 and 31, which together account for an additional 10% of all cervical cancer cases.[19] The disease spreads locally into the surrounding tissues (vagina, uterine corpus, parametrium, bladder, and

---

Box 40.1 Carcinoma of the cervix uteri.

Stage 1	The carcinoma is strictly confined to the cervix (extension to the corpus would be disregarded)
IA	Invasive carcinoma which can be diagnosed only by microscopy, with deepest invasion ≤ 5 mm and largest extension ≤ 7 mm
IA1	Measured stromal invasion of ≤ 3.0 mm in depth and extension of ≤ 7.0 mm
IA2	Measured stromal invasion of > 3.0 mm and not > 5.0 mm with an extension of not > 7.0 mm
IB	Clinically visible lesions limited to the cervix uteri or pre-clinical cancers greater than stage IA*
IB1	Clinically visible lesion ≤ 4.0 cm in greatest dimension
IB2	Clinically visible lesion > 4.0 cm in greatest dimension
Stage II	Cervical carcinoma invades beyond the uterus, but not to the pelvic wall or to the lower third of the vagina
IIA	Without parametrial invastion
IIA1	Clinically visible lesion ≤ 4.0 cm in greatest dimension
IIA2	Clinically visible lesion > 4.0 cm in greatest dimension
IIB	With obvious parametrial invasion
Stage III	The tumor extends to the pelvic wall and/or involves lower third of the vagina and/or causes hydronephrosis or non-functioning kidney**
IIIA	Tumor involves lower third of the vagina, with no extension to the pelvic wall
IIIB	Extension to the pelvic wall and/or hydronephrosis or non-functioning kidney
Stage IV	The carcinoma has extended beyond the true pelvis or has involved (biopsy proven) the mucosa of the bladder or rectum. A bullous edema, as such, does not permit a case to be allotted to Stage IV
IVA	Spread of the growth to adjacent organs
IVB	Spread to distant organs

---

* All macroscopically visible lesions–even with superficial invasion–are allotted to stage IB carcinomas. Invasion is limited to a measured stromal invasion with a maximal depth of 5.00 mm and a horizontal extension of not > 7.00 mm. Depth of invasion should not be > 5.00 mm taken from the base of the epithelium of the original tissue–superficial or glandular. The depth of invasion should always be reported in mm, even in those cases with "early (minimal) stromal invasion" (-1 mm). The involvement of vascular/lymphatic spaces should not change the stage allotment.
** On rectal examination, there is no cancer-free space between the tumor and the pelvic wall. All cases with hydronephrosis or non-functioning kidney are included, unless they are known to be due to another cause.

rectum) and metastasizes into the lymphatics (pelvic then aortic); hematogenous spread is less common. The most common symptom is bleeding although pain as well as intestinal or urinary symptoms can be associated with advanced disease.[19] Most lesions are exophytic; a second type of cervical carcinoma is created by an infiltrating tumor that tends to show little visible ulceration or exophytic mass but is initially seen as a stone-hard cervix; a third category of lesion is the ulcerative tumor, which usually erodes a portion of the cervix.[19]

The presenting symptoms depend on the extent of disease. Microinvasive carcinomas may be asymptomatic and only detected by high-risk HPV DNA testing and/or cytological screening. Early-stage tumors (FIGO stage IB$_1$) may present with abnormal vaginal bleeding, vaginal discharge, dyspareunia, and occasionally vaginal pressure.[19] Locally advanced cancers (FIGO IB$_2$–IVA) may present with the same signs and symptoms of early-stage disease but in addition may be associated with pelvic pain, flank pain, lower extremity lymphedema and paresthesia, as well as vulvovaginal involvement and vesicovaginal and rectovaginal fistula formation.[19] In addition to all of the above, women with metastatic (FIGO IVB) and recurrent disease may experience gastric outlet obstruction, hemoptysis, bony fractures, and neck swelling.[19]

Uncommon histologies and prognosis

Cervical cancer is a disease of epidemic proportions. It is the third most common cancer diagnosis in women worldwide, with 480,000 new cases diagnosed annually, but is probably underreported.[19] In developed nations, there has been a dramatic decrease in the incidence and death rates because of screening. The median age at diagnosis for preinvasive disease of the cervix is 29 years, and 47 years for invasive carcinoma.[19] This section focuses on many of the uncommon and scarce tumors of the cervix (see Table 40.1). Because of the rarity of many of these lesions, their real nature and clinical course have not been fully clarified. Importantly, some tumors have a highly aggressive course (e.g. adenoid cystic carcinoma [ACC] and small cell carcinoma), while others actually have a better prognosis when they arise in the cervix as opposed to other sites (e.g. embryonal rhabdomyosarcoma, E-RMS). For many of these entities, arriving at the correct diagnosis may be a complex process and immunohistochemical studies may be required. The differential diagnosis can become frustrating for the pathologist. In some cases (e.g. warty carcinoma), careful cytological examination may hint at the diagnosis when histological material is equivocal. Finally, some tumor types may be indicative of systemic disease (e.g. granulocytic sarcoma [GS] and lymphoepithelioma-like carcinoma [LELC]).

Squamous cell carcinomas

Verrucous carcinoma

Pipe smoking, chewing tobacco, dipping snuff, and poor oral hygiene and dentures have been cited as etiological factors for verrucous carcinoma of the oral cavity. Ackerman described the first case in 1948. Preexisting condyloma acuminata, poor hygiene, and an infected prepuce has been linked with the development of penile verrucous carcinoma. The first case of verrucous carcinoma of the cervix was reported by Jennings and Barclay in 1972. An intranuclear virus-like particle measuring 45–50 nm in diameter has been identified in some cases of female genital verrucous carcinomas, suggesting that perhaps the human papillomavirus may play a role. Among 29

Table 40.1 Histological classification of cervical cancer.

Nonglandular	Glandular	Other, including mixed
Epithelial tumors		
Squamous cell carcinoma	Adenocarcinoma, usual endocervical type	Adenosquamous
Verrucous carcinoma	Mucinous adenocarcinoma	Glassy cell carcinoma
Warty (condylomatous) carcinoma	Endometrioid adenocarcinoma	Mucoepidermoid carcinoma
Papillary squamotransitional carcinoma	Well-differentiated villoglandular adenocarcinoma	Adenoid cystic carcinoma
Lymphoepithelioma-like carcinoma	Adenoma malignum (minimal deviation)	Adenoid basal carcinoma
Sarcomatoid carcinoma	Intestinal-like adenocarcinoma	Small cell carcinoma
	Signet ring cell adenocarcinoma	Classic carcinoid tumor
	Colloid adenocarcinoma	Gestational choriocarcinoma
	Clear cell adenocarcinoma	
	Serous papillary adenocarcinoma	
	Mesonephric adenocarcinoma	
	Germ cell tumors	**Miscellaneous**
Mesenchymal tumors		
Carcinosarcoma	Mature teratoma	Melanoma
Leiomyosarcoma	Immature teratoma	Lymphoma
Epithelioid leiomyosarcoma	Yolk sac tumor	Primitive neuroectodermal tumor
Extrauterine endometrial stromal sarcoma	Nongestational choriocarcinoma	
Adenosarcoma		
Embryonal rhabdomyosarcoma		
Granulocytic sarcoma (chloroma)		

patients with verrucous carcinoma of the cervix reported by Degefu *et al.*, the mean age was 51 years at diagnosis (range, 30–84 years). Most often, patients presented with persistent vaginal discharge and bleeding.[21] Frega *et al.* identified high-risk HPV DNA using hybrid capture technology in three cases of FIGO stage IB verrucous carcinoma, suggesting that viral infection may be associated with this lesion.[22]

Grossly, verrucous carcinoma of the cervix appears as cauliflower-like, exophytic, and warty, with a grayish-white to brick-red color. Because cellular differentiation appears to proceed in a normal pattern throughout the thickened layer of the epidermis, dysplastic cells are not usually evident, and cytology does not alert the clinician to the lesion. Additionally, histopathological misinterpretation was identified by Degefu *et al.* as a second factor leading to a delay in diagnosis and treatment, with 12 of the lesions in their report being originally assigned a diagnosis of benign squamous papilloma of the cervix resembling condyloma acuminata.[21] Patients who were initially treated with podophyllin, cautery, or trachelectomy generally had a shortened survival following accurate diagnosis and further therapy.

Histologically, the lesions manifest as well-differentiated squamous epithelium with benign-appearing cells and an intact basement membrane. Nuclear atypia may be present, and the parabasal and prickle cell nuclei tend to be enlarged and pleomorphic. The rete ridges undergo cystic dilation, forming epithelial fronds, and contain flakes of keratin. Unlike condyloma acuminata, the fibrovascular core is usually absent and the epithelium consists of bulbous fronds compressing the surrounding tissue and underlying stroma. In addition, while the deeper portions of condyloma acuminata are papillary, the deeper portions of verrucous carcinoma form a solid nest of epithelial cells with a wide base. A biopsy should incorporate the base of the tumor and underlying stroma since it is in the depths of these lesions that distinguishing characteristics of an infiltrating growth pattern extending into the stroma are found.

The importance of direct communication to the pathologist about the clinical appearance and extent of the lesion cannot be overemphasized.

The traditional view has held verrucous carcinomas to have an indolent course with little invasive potential, but in the advanced stages or in the recurrent setting, this tumor may be aggressive. Primary radical excision is recommended for both primary and recurrent disease. Inadequate resection at the outset has resulted in rapid (i.e. within 1 year) central pelvic or vaginal recurrence. Although the incidence of nodal metastases is very low, pelvic lymphadenectomy may identify the occasional high-risk patient who may benefit from closer surveillance or some form of adjuvant therapy. Radiotherapy adds little to the treatment program, and among patients with verrucous carcinomas of the larynx and of the oral cavity, this treatment modality has been associated with prompt and explosive anaplastic transformation of the tumor in 30% of cases.

Although several previous reviews of female genital verrucous carcinoma have considered the cervical cases and vulvar cases collectively, it is interesting that there is a distinct difference in the uncorrected 2-year survival for verrucous carcinoma of the cervix (40%) compared with that for vulvar lesions (75%). In both diseases, histologically confirmed pulmonary metastases have been observed.

Warty (condylomatous) carcinoma

This tumor is characterized by marked condylomatous changes. It is a recently described variant of squamous cell carcinoma (SCC) of the cervix, and is histologically identical to warty carcinoma of the vulva. Unlike its homolog in the vulva, these cervical cancers exhibit evidence of SCC at the deep margin. Multiple subtypes of HPV (including low-risk strains) can be detected in the majority of tumors. Ng *et al.* have performed thin-layer cytological preparations on three cases and noted small, cohesive clusters and syncytial sheets of tumor cells, with necrotic tumor debris (diathesis) in the background.[23] The tumor cells were polygonal to elongated and contained oval nuclei, coarse chromatin, and sometimes distinct nuclei. Dyskeratotic tumor cells with bizarre shapes were also noted. These three lesions were also characterized by having many koilocytic cells possessed of pleomorphic nuclei, distinct nucleoli, and perinuclear cytoplasmic halos. Because koilocytes are rarely found in cervical cytology specimens of conventional SCC, the authors emphasize that a correct cytological diagnosis is possible if one pays attention to extreme koilocytotic atypia when present. Although experience has been slow to accumulate, some authors have noted a less aggressive clinical behavior when these tumors are compared to the more common well-differentiated SCCs of the cervix.

Papillary squamotransitional carcinoma

Papillary squamous carcinomas were initially described in 1986 by Randall *et al.* who noted a histological resemblance to transitional cell carcinoma of the bladder. The tumors are composed of papillary projections that are covered by several layers of atypical epithelial cells. Because they demonstrate a spectrum of histological appearances, these tumors have been referred to as papillary squamotransitional carcinomas (PSTCs). Unlike transitional cell tumors of the urinary tract, PSTCs are typically positive for cytokeratin 7 and negative for cytokeratin 20. Koenig *et al.* have subdivided the tumors into three histological groups: predominantly squamous, predominantly transitional, and mixed squamous and transitional. In cases that appear more transitional, the cells are oval with their long axis oriented perpendicular to the surface with minimal flattening.[24] An inverted endophytic pattern similar to that of transitional cell carcinoma of the urothelium can also be present. In cases with more squamous differentiation, the cells are more basaloid and resemble those of a high-grade squamous intraepithelial lesion devoid of frank keratinization and koilocytic change. Typical invasive SCC can often be identified at the base of the tumor, appearing as well-circumscribed nests of epithelium in continuity with papillae that extend deeply into the stroma. Focal invasion of the papillae themselves has also been reported. Microscopically, the tumor can be misinterpreted as a cervical intraepithelial neoplasia grade 3 with a papillary configuration or as a squamous papilloma. The tumor must also be differentiated from other rare variants of SCC, including verrucous and condylomatous carcinoma.

Papillary squamotransitional carcinomas are potentially aggressive, with many lesions presenting at a more advanced stage than would be expected based on a histological appearance reminiscent of a superficial or early invasive lesion. In the report by Koenig et al. containing 32 cases, the mean age at diagnosis was 50 years (range, 22–93 years).[24] Three of the 12 patients with follow-up information died of disease at a mean of 13 months following diagnosis. In a case series by Ortega-Gonzalez et al., all six of their patients presented at an advanced clinical stage, two had recurrences and one metastasized.[25]

Lymphoepithelioma-like carcinoma

Lymphoepithelioma-like carcinoma of the cervix is a distinct variant of SCC, in which the tumor cells are well circumscribed and composed of undifferentiated cells surrounded by a marked stromal inflammatory infiltrate. The tumor may confer a more favorable prognosis than conventional SCC. Typically, it is found in a population of younger women and is more prevalent in non-Caucasian populations, especially those of Asian descent. LELC of the cervix also lacks a clearly defined association with HPV infection.[26] The Epstein–Barr virus (EBV) has been postulated to play an etiological role in LELC in diverse anatomical locations. Tseng et al. studied 15 cervical LELC tumors and 15 SCC controls and detected EBV genomes more frequently in LELC than in conventional SCC (73.3 versus 26.7%, $p = 0.01$).[27] The detection rate of HPV-16 and HPV-18 DNA was significantly lower in patients with LELC tumors than in patients with conventional SCC (20 versus 80%, $p = 0.001$). After a median follow-up of 3.9 years (range, 1.8–5.3 years), all 15 patients with cervical LELC were disease free following radical hysterectomy or radiotherapy. Three cases were recently reported by Takai et al., all of which were negative for EBV and HPV using in situ hybridization and immunohistochemistry.[28] The inflammatory background in this series contained many CD3+ and CD8+ cells but very few CD4+, CD20+, and CD79a+ cells.[28]

Sarcomatoid carcinoma

Sarcomatoid carcinomas are uncommon variants of epithelial carcinoma. The diagnosis is based on histological, immuno-histochemical, and ultrastructural features. A recognizable SCC typically merges with a spindle cell component. The spindle cell component characterizes this tumor by its prominence, and bizarre, multinucleated tumor giant cells may also be present. The lesion is distinguished from a sarcoma by immunostaining, through which both the spindled component and the multinucleated tumor cells are positive for the epithelial marker, cytokeratin. Thus, unlike true sarcomas or malignant mixed mesodermal tumors, sarcomatoid carcinomas lack a malignant stromal or mesenchymal component.

Sarcomatoid carcinomas have been identified in the oral cavity, pharynx, esophagus, and larynx. There have been less

than 20 reported cases of sarcomatoid SCC of the cervix. Most patients have presented with abnormal vaginal bleeding, and all have had a visible cervical lesion amenable to biopsy. Of 10 patients for whom detailed clinical information was available, six were diagnosed with locally advanced disease (FIGO stages IB$_2$–IVA), and two presented with metastatic disease. Eight of nine patients reported by Brown et al. were treated with primary or adjuvant pelvic irradiation, and five suffered a recurrence with a median disease-free interval of 4.9 months (range, 2–9.5 months).[29] Only three patients in the literature have remained disease free following primary therapy for 22, 40, and 42 months as well as one additional patient successfully treated by Kong et al. with laparoscopic radical hysterectomy for whom follow-up has been short.[30] Although the data are limited, it appears that the disease is aggressive as evidenced by an advanced stage at presentation and early recurrence following therapy. Pelvic irradiation can salvage approximately 25% of patients.

Glandular tumors

Adenocarcinoma, usual endocervical type

The relative proportions and absolute incidences of SCCs and adenocarcinomas (ACs) of the cervix have been changing in industrialized nations during the preceding 40 years since the implementation of cytological screening. Endocervical AC and its variants now account for approximately 20–25% of cervical cancers.[31] The percentage of women younger than 35 years with AC has increased from 16% in 1964 to 25% in the 1990s. Historically, cervical AC has often been referred to as mucinous AC. Although a subset of endocervical AC are overtly mucinous (see following section), the usual endocervical type of AC most often shows no mucin or no greater amount than can be seen in nonmucinous tumors. The cell of origin is likely a pluripotential subcolumnar reserve cell of the columnar endocervical epithelium, with adenocarcinoma in situ (AIS) regarded as an immediate precursor to invasive endocervical AC. Recent studies that have controlled for HPV and sexual behavior have not found oral contraceptive usage to be a significant risk factor in this disease.

The differential diagnosis of the usual endocervical type of AC includes other forms of primary and secondary AC, AIS, and benign lesions such as normal endocervical glands and Nabothian cysts that extend deeply into the cervical wall. Early invasion may be appreciated when irregularly arranged glands, small clusters of cells, or single cells are clearly seen to infiltrate from a parent gland showing in situ AC, especially when there is an associated stromal response and inflammation. Nevertheless, because of the difficulty in interpreting the irregular distribution and complex architecture of the normal endocervical crypts in the cervical stroma, microinvasive AC (i.e. stage IA) as a histologically recognizable entity has been the subject of much debate.

Because of the varied morphology of these tumors, the glandular lesions account for many problematic issues in cervical pathology. The ACs of usual endocervical type account for 80% of cervical ACs, and are characterized by moderate differentiation and glands of medium size. The cells have eosinophilic cytoplasm and brisk mitotic activity with frequent apoptotic bodies.

Abnormal vaginal bleeding occurs in 75% of patients. Fifty percent of cases are characterized by a fungating, polypoid, or papillary mass. In 15% of patients, the cervix is diffusely enlarged or nodular, and in 15% no gross lesion is visible. Eighty percent of patients present with stage I or stage II disease. Deep invasion is common, even with early-stage tumors, because the carcinoma can arise deep within the endocervical canal.

Mucinous adenocarcinoma

These tumors are characterized by easily identifiable mucin-rich cells that predominate over any other cell type that may be present. The tumors may be graded on the basis of the proportion of solid and glandular areas (akin to what is done for endometrial cancers) or on the basis of nuclear grade. The majority of glands are frankly malignant on a combined architectural and cytological analysis.

The differentiation of a primary cervical mucinous or endometrioid AC from an endometrioid AC of the endometrium with cervical extension can be problematic. In some cases, an endometrial lesion will be demonstrable on pelvic ultrasonography, while a primary cervical tumor may result in cervical expansion in the absence of uterine enlargement. Immunostaining can be used as a diagnostic adjunct, with carcinoembryonic antigen (CEA) and mucus antigen positivity being observed in 59–80% and 56% of endocervical tumors, respectively, compared to 8–50% and 0% of endometrial carcinomas, respectively. In contrast, 0% of endocervical lesions will stain for vimentin, while 66% of endometrial cancers will be positive.

In 1990, Konishi et al. investigated the clinical significance of mucin leakage into the cervical stroma in 35 cases of cervical AC.[32] Histological evidence of mucin leakage was identified in 14 cases (40%) as amorphous materials dissecting the connective tissues and permeating the lymphatic channels, associated with and without tumor cells. The cases with mucin leakage showed a significantly higher incidence of lymph node involvement than those without mucin leakage (71.4 versus 23.8%, $p < 0.01$). In addition, when the mucin leakage was immunohistochemically positive for CEA or CA19-9, elevated serum levels of these antigens were frequently observed. The investigators suggest that mucin leakage into the cervical stroma is not only indicative of stromal invasion but also allows for the conduct of tumor cells into the lymphatic channels.

Recently, Togami et al. studied mucin expression in 52 patients with mucinous adenocarcinoma of the endocervical type and reported that overexpression of both MUC1 and MUC16 was associated with lower survival rates and that absence of expression of these antigens was associated with longer overall and disease-free survival.[33] For the 35 women with FIGO stage IB disease, MUC1 and/or MUC16 was an independent prognostic factor for overall survival (hazard ratio [HR] 6.16, 95% confidence interval [CI] 1.01–118.5, $p < 0.05$).

Their work suggests that MUC1 and MUC16 may be used as prognostic markers in this disease.[33]

Endometrioid adenocarcinoma

True endometrioid carcinomas of the cervix are rare, with the characteristic histology of tubular glands, sometimes with villous papillae, and ciliated cells. The cells tend to be stratified and have oval nuclei arranged with their long axis perpendicular to the basement membrane of the gland. The cells do not contain mucin and have less cytoplasm than do the cells of a mucinous AC. Interestingly, endometrioid ACs frequently contain small foci of squamous epithelium. There have been scattered cases of endometrioid endocervical AC arising from cervical endometriosis.

An important consideration in the management of this disease is to recognize that although the majority of endometrial endometrioid adenocarcinomas and cervical endometrioid adenocarcinomas have similar tumor morphology, there are some cases in which the morphology may be different. For example, in some cases with disease coexisting in the endometrium and in the endocervix, invasion may be deeper in the endocervical component or invasion may occur only in the endocervical stroma with no concurrent myometrial invasion. In a study of 14 cases of endometrioid adenocarcinoma involving the cervix and endometrium, Jiang et al. suggest that clonality tests, receptor expression analyses, and high-risk HPV DNA testing may help determine where the primary has arisen.[34]

In 1997, Fujiwara et al. investigated the expression and clinical significance of estrogen receptor (ER) and progesterone receptor (PR) in 84 cervical ACs.[35] ER was identified in 17 cases (20%) and PR in 23 cases (27%). ER positivity was most frequently detected in mucinous AC of the endocervical type ($n = 11$ of 48 cases) and endometrioid AC ($n = 4$ of 10 cases). PR positivity was also most frequently detected in mucinous AC of the endocervical type ($n = 15$ of 48 cases) and endometrioid AC ($n = 6$ of 10 cases). Mucinous AC of the intestinal type ($n = 5$), glassy cell carcinoma (GCC) ($n = 2$), and clear cell AC ($n = 2$) were uniformly negative for both ER and PR. No association was detected between FIGO stage and receptor status but there was a somewhat lower frequency of ER positivity in poorly differentiated tumors ($p = 0.07$). Receptor status was not significantly associated with either overall survival or disease-free survival.

Comment on the clinical profile of the adenocarcinomas

It is a complex task to extract clinical information from the literature specific for each of the three tumor types discussed above because in many reports concerning endocervical ACs, investigators have not made distinctions between the usual type, the mucinous AC, and the endometrioid AC, oftentimes lumping them together. The problem is compounded by the tendency of many pathologists to regard mucinous AC as the most common form of endocervical AC and either relegate those tumors that demonstrate minimal to no mucin staining (i.e. the usual type) to a subset of mucinous AC or to incorrectly characterize them as endometrioid ACs. This last detail has resulted in a relative increase in the proportion of endometrioid ACs that have been reported in some series, with several authorities suggesting that endometrioid ACs account for up to 30% of endocervical ACs. True endometrioid ACs are exceedingly rare. Therefore, in the paragraph that follows, the term "ACs" is used to represent the usual type of endocervical AC as well as the mucinous and endometrioid subtypes of endocervical AC.

The management of ACs follows that which has been outlined for SCC. In 1991, Hopkins and Morley performed a survival analysis of 203 patients (21%) with adenocarcinoma and 756 (79%) with SCC treated from 1970 to 1985.[36] Survival by stage was significantly influenced by the cell type, with 90% 5-year survival observed for patients with SCC as compared to 60% 5-year survival among patients with adenocarcinoma ($p < 0.001$). Patients with stage II SCC had a 62% survival, compared with 47% for adenocarcinoma ($p = 0.01$); patients with stage III squamous cell disease had a 36% survival, compared with 8% for adenocarcinoma ($p = 0.002$). Other features that influenced survival included node status ($p = 0.001$), poor differentiation of tumor histology ($p = 0.001$), diabetes ($p = 0.001$), and Pap smear interval ($p = 0.001$). Other studies, including population-based reports, have failed to confirm that prognosis is affected by histological type. In 2002, Lea et al. identified 83 patients with stage IIB–IVB tumors, and during a median follow-up period of 33 months, 66 (80%) died of disease.[37] Stage IIB disease, young patient age, and grade 1 histology were independent variables having a favorable impact on survival.

Villoglandular papillary adenocarcinoma

Although approximately 10–15% of cervical adenocarcinomas have a papillary pattern, villoglandular papillary adenocarcinoma (VGPA) constitutes only a small proportion of these tumors. Young and Scully first established VGPA of the cervix as a distinct histological entity and a subtype of well-differentiated adenocarcinoma in 1989.[38] It has been further subclassified into endocervical, endometrioid, and intestinal types. Approximately 90 cases have been reported in the English medical literature.

Compared with the common types of cervical adenocarcinomas, VGPA is morphologically characterized by extremely villous and papillary growth. Specifically, the cardinal feature of the VGPA is a surface papillary component of variable thickness with papillae that are usually tall and thin with a fibrous, stromal core (Fig. 40.1). Small cellular budding may be present but to a lesser extent than is seen in serous papillary carcinomas. The invasive portion of the tumor has a pushing border and is composed of elongated branching glands separated by a fibrous stroma; the stroma may be desmoplastic or myxoid at the advancing margin of the tumor. The papillae and glands are lined by stratified nonmucinous columnar cells, and only mild to moderate nuclear atypicality and scattered mitotic figures (MFs) are present in the tumor cells. The adjacent cervical glandular epithelium often contains an AIS.

In 2004, Utsugi et al. published a series of 13 patients.[39] The median age was 45 years (range, 36–64 years). Interestingly, the Pap test was positive for adenocarcinoma in all patients,

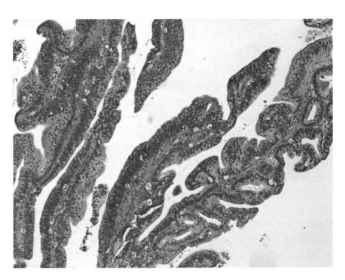

Figure 40.1 Well-differentiated villoglandular adenocarcinoma of the cervix.

with tall and thin papillae present in 10 patients allowing the investigators to predict VGPA cytologically. In contrast to earlier reports, these investigators encountered high mitotic counts, lymphovascular space invasion, and lymph node metastases in several of their patients. As of December 2002, all patients were alive and without recurrence during 3–19 years of follow-up. Indeed, the prognosis has been reported to be more favorable in patients with VGPA when compared with the common types of cervical adenocarcinomas, with only one of 85 patients appearing in the English literature having developed recurrence. This patient originally underwent radical hysterectomy with lymphadenectomy for a stage IIB lesion, and received adjuvant pelvic radiotherapy due to lymphatic metastases; she developed a vaginal recurrence at 30 months and died of disease at 46 months. Four other patients with lymph node metastases who received postsurgical pelvic irradiation have remained without evidence of disease for 10–220 months.

Young and Clement caution that a tumor should not be placed in this group if any ominous pathological feature is present, as that may lead to undertreatment of a potentially fatal lesion.[40] It must be emphasized that adenocarcinomas of the usual type, including deeply invasive tumors, may have a papillary component, and the diagnosis of VGPA should be reserved for lesions that are exclusively grade I and unassociated with an underlying component of conventional adenocarcinoma. The diagnosis of VGPA should only be suggested upon small biopsy material, with a requirement for a cone biopsy or hysterectomy specimen before the term can be used definitively. Making the diagnosis with limited clinical material may result in overly conservative treatment of a lesion with a prognosis worse than that of VGPA. The successful management of VGPA in pregnancy was recently reported by Takai et al., further underscoring the relatively favorable prognosis of this lesion.[41] There has, however, been one report of an extremely aggressive case of VGPA in a 22-year-old woman, underscoring the need for careful pathological review, clinical staging, and timely therapeutic intervention.[42]

Adenoma malignum (minimal deviation adenocarcinoma)

Adenoma malignum of the uterine cervix was first described by Gusserow in 1987. The term is often considered to be synonymous with "minimal deviation adenocarcinoma," which was proposed by Silverberg and Hurt in 1975.[43] The tumor accounts for only 1–3% of adenocarcinomas of the cervix. It is considered a variant of mucinous adenocarcinoma. In the case series by Hirai *et al.*, the mean age was 53.3 years (range, 38–70 years), and presenting symptoms often include both watery or mucoid discharge and atypical vaginal bleeding.[44] Peutz–Jeghers syndrome (PJS) is a rare genetic disorder characterized by melanotic macules, gastrointestinal polyps and increased cancer risks. Female patients with PJS are at risk not only for adenoma malignum but also ovarian sex cord tumors with annular tubules.[45]

It is difficult to correctly diagnose adenoma malignum because the cytological deviation from the normal glandular cells is considered to be too small, and the histological deviation is minimal (Fig. 40.2). Hirai *et al.* have identified four common characteristic cytological features in a review of Papanicoloau smears associated with this lesion.
• Large sheets of tumor cells are apparent. The tumor cells have abundant mucin and are arranged in palisades at the circumferences of the sheets.
• In the area with a palisading arrangement, nuclei are constantly positioned in the cytoplasm and overlap side by side.
• Nuclei are tensile and some are irregular in shape. The nuclear chromatin is fine granular and reveals frequent nuclear clearing, which is suggestive of increased euchromatins.
• The ordinary form of adenocarcinoma cells in clusters is occasionally present.[44]
Since most of the tumor glands are highly differentiated, Hirai *et al.* emphasize that it is exceedingly difficult to histologically differentiate these tumor glands from normal endocervical glands, particularly in specimens taken from cervical punch biopsies.[44] Thus, since the ability to make a preoperative diagnosis of adenoma malignum is limited, the disease is often undertreated initially, and the final diagnosis assigned only after a comprehensive review of the surgical specimens. Therefore, when the preoperative punch biopsy leads to the diagnosis of typical endocervical adenocarcinoma, it is expected that the disease will be treated correctly. However, when the punch biopsy reveals no sign of malignancy, the possibility of having the disease undertreated exists.

Because cytological examination is a potent aid to detect this tumor, for those cases with negative punch biopsy having cytological features that suggest the presence of adenoma malignum, it is important to obtain a sample of the deeply positioned tumor glands preoperatively through a deep biopsy or cervical conization. The combination of clinical understaging and undertreatment has resulted in the majority of the early reports suggesting an unfavorable prognosis for this disease. Recent studies suggest that the survival of adenoma malignum is consistent with that of other forms of well-differentiated adenocarcinoma of the cervix.

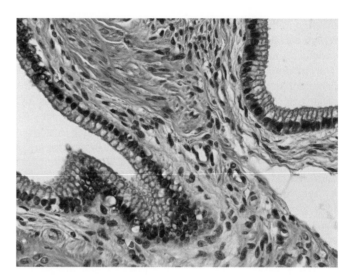

Figure 40.2 Minimal deviation adenocarcinoma of the cervix (adenoma malignum).

Intestinal-type, signet ring cell, and colloid adenocarcinomas

The intestinal type of mucinous adenocarcinoma is composed of cells similar to those present in adenocarcinomas of the large intestine. Goblet cells are common, and are occasionally admixed with argentaffin cells and Paneth cells. There may also be pseudostratification, and only small amounts of intracellular mucin present.[40] Signet ring cells may also be found within cervical adenocarcinomas, and also in some cervical adenosquamous carcinomas (ASC). Pure signet ring cell adenocarcinomas and colloid adenocarcinomas are both extraordinarily rare. Shintaku *et al.* recently reported a 4 cm colloid carcinoma in a 69 year old in which intracytoplasmic sequestration of mucus was evident on immunohistochemistry.[46] The cytoplasm of neoplastic cells was immunoreactive for cytokeratins 7 and 20, and the intracytoplasmic mucus was immunoreactive for MUC2 but negative for MUC5AC and MUC6. Nuclei of tumor cells were immunoreactive for CDX2.[46]

Clear cell adenocarcinoma

Clear cell carcinomas (CCAs) of the cervix account for 4–9% of adenocarcinomas of the cervix. They are cytologically, histologically, and ultrastructurally identical to their counterparts at other sites of the female genital tract such as the vagina, endometrium, and ovary. It has been suggested that this tumor arises from pluripotent reserve cells of the cervix that through faulty differentiation remain at an intermediate stage of development between keratinization and mucin secretion. In addition to *in utero* exposure to diethylstilbestrol (DES), genetic factors, microsatellite instability, HPV infection, Bcl-2 protein overexpression, p53 mutation, and other exogenous risk factors are likely to play an etiological role in this disease. Importantly, these tumors can develop in the absence of DES exposure. A bimodal age distribution among patients without DES exposure has been detected, with one peak at 26 years and a second peak at 71 years.

Clear cell carcinomas are predominantly endophytic and tend toward deep infiltration with creation of a barrel-shaped cervix. They are more likely to extend to the lower uterine segment and uterine endometrium more often than SCCs and non-CCA adenocarcinomas. When this occurs, the tumor may be distinguished from a primary endometrial CCA with cervical extension on the basis of the pattern of invasion. Histologically, the neoplastic cells have abundant clear or vacuolated cytoplasm that can contain glycogen. The growth pattern can be classified as solid, tubulocystic, or papillary, with flat, cuboidal, and hobnail cells being prominent in the tubular and tubulocystic patterns.

Several commentators have speculated that CCAs of the cervix are associated with a poorer prognosis than SCCs and non-CCA adenocarcinoma. In 1979, Herbst *et al.* collected 145 cervical CCAs in women with and without *in utero* exposure to DES and with a median follow-up of 4 years, reported 5-year survival rates of 91% (stage I), 77% (stage IIA), and 60% (stage IIB).[47] In a contemporary series of 15 patients reported by Reich *et al.*,[48] the 5-year survival rate of 67% in patients with stages IB–IIB disease was consistent with the results reported by Herbst *et al.*,[47] and although the CCAs tended to have a slightly worse 5-year survival rate than SCCAs and other cervical adenocarcinomas, this observation was not statistically significant. In a multiinstitutional review of 34 patients diagnosed and treated in the post-DES era, Thomas *et al.* reported 25% nodal metastases and also noted that for those with low-risk early-stage disease, radical surgery without adjuvant chemotherapy can be curative.[49]

Serous papillary adenocarcinoma

Serous papillary carcinoma of the cervix (SPCC) is a recently described variant of cervical adenocarcinoma that is morphologically similar to serous papillary adenocarcinoma of the ovary, endometrium, fallopian tube, and peritoneum. Rose and Reale provided the first detailed description of this tumor in 1993.[50] Among the first several reports, angiolymphatic space invasion, lymph node metastases, or extracervical spread or both were common. In point of fact, in a review of 67 cases of cervical adenocarcinoma and ASC, Costa *et al.* determined that the presence of serous differentiation in the glandular component was associated with an increased risk of recurrence.[51] Similar to what has been observed among women with clear cell adenocarcinoma of the cervix not associated with *in utero* DES exposure, some studies on SPCC of the cervix have detected a bimodal age distribution with one peak occurring before 40 years and the second peak after the age of 65. This represents a distinguishing clinical feature of SPCC when compared to the more common variants of cervical adenocarcinoma.

The differential diagnosis of clinical stage I SPCC includes cervical involvement of a uterine papillary serous carcinoma (UPSC) of the endometrium, as well as well-differentiated villoglandular adenocarcinoma and papillary clear cell adenocarcinoma arising in the cervix. A stage II UPSC may be excluded by a fractional dilation and curettage or examination of a hysterectomy specimen. The distinction between SPCC and well-differentiated villoglandular adenocarcinoma (see preceding section) is critical because the latter almost always has an excellent prognosis and some cases have been successfully treated with cone biopsy. Although papillary clear cell adenocarcinoma and SPCC share the histological features of papillae covered by round to oval cells with round nuclei and prominent nucleoli, the former typically has a hyalinized papillary core and a majority of epithelial cells with clear cytoplasm or a hobnail appearance, as well as the tubular, cystic, and solid patterns that are uncommon or absent in SPCCs.

Immunohistochemistry studies have demonstrated frequent CA-125 positivity among SPCC. Interestingly, however, in noncervical sites, serous papillary carcinomas are typically CEA negative, but SPCC is frequently CEA positive (although not as consistently as mucinous adenocarcinoma of the cervix). The serum CA-125 has also been reported to be increased in some cases of SPCC, with some patients presenting with carcinomatosis, ascites, or subdiaphragmatic metastases. Nofech-Mozes *et al.* reported that when compared to other more common tumors of the cervix, serous papillary endocervical lesions exhibit significantly higher p53 and lower CEA reactivity.[52]

Zhou *et al.* have published a series of 17 cases in which 11 patients presented with abnormal vaginal bleeding, four with abnormal exfoliative cervical cytology, and two with a watery vaginal discharge.[35] Eight of the women had a polypoid or exophytic cervical mass, two had an ulcerated or indurated cervix, and no gross abnormality was detected in seven patients. In their report, the stage distribution included stage IA ($n=1$), stage IB ($n=12$), stage II ($n=2$), and stage III ($n=1$). On low-power microscopic examination, all the tumors had a complex papillary pattern with epithelial stratification and tufting with the formation of cellular buds. The papillary nature of the tumors was most striking in the exophytic portions of the tumors. In nonpapillary areas, the tumors exhibited a predominantly glandular growth pattern, with elongated and slit-like spaces. In the invasive areas, nests of tumor cells infiltrated the cervical stroma in an irregular pattern, with clefts around the tumor cell nests. An intense acute and chronic inflammatory infiltrate was typically present within the core of the papillae and in areas of stromal invasion. All of the tumors had >10 mitotic figures per 10 high-power fields (MFs/10 HPF), with most showing >30 MFs/HPF. Only three tumors had psammoma bodies.

In the study by Zhou *et al.*, all three patients with stage II and III tumors experienced metastases.[53] Three of the 12 patients with stage IB lesions received primary radiotherapy with ($n=1$) and without ($n=2$) chemotherapy, and all died of disease. Among the eight patients with stage IB tumors who survived without disease, six had undergone radical hysterectomy (with adjuvant radiotherapy given to three), and one was treated with simple hysterectomy and adjuvant radiation. Although the numbers are very small, the authors suggest that primary surgical therapy may be preferable to primary radiotherapy in early-stage SPCC. Although the tumors can behave aggressively and be associated with a rapidly fatal course, the outcome for patients with stage I disease is similar to that of patients with cervical adenocarcinoma of the usual type. The impact of concurrent radiosensitizing chemotherapy for locally advanced disease and the efficacy of platinum-based combination chemotherapy for metastatic disease have not been studied.

Mesonephric carcinoma

Pathologists have been fascinated by the embryology and pathology of the paired mesonephric ducts for decades. The distal portion of each duct courses through the parametrial tissues and enters the lateral wall of the cervix at the isthmus where it dilates to form an ampulla from which numerous tubules ramify. It then extends to the lateral walls of the vagina where it is referred to as Gartner's duct. Remnants of the mesonephric duct and its tubules can be found in up to 22% of adult uterine cervices. In 1990, Ferry and Scully identified several cases of lobular mesonephric hyperplasia, diffuse mesonephric hyperplasia, mesonephric ductal hyperplasia, and mesonephric carcinoma from a batch of 49 cervixes containing mesonephric remnants.[54] The mean age of patients with mesonephric carcinoma is 52–55 years (range, 34–72 years), and most present with abnormal bleeding, often with a visible cervical lesion.

Mesonephric carcinomas typically exhibit morphological diversity, with considerable variability within a tumor, including ductal, tubular, retiform, solid, and sex cord-like patterns. One pattern usually predominates, with the ductal and tubular pattern being most commonly encountered. In the tubular pattern, the tumor consists of large sheets of closely packed small round tubules, often with dense intraluminal eosinophilic secretions that resemble the malignant counterpart of mesonephric remnants (Fig. 40.3). The ductal pattern consists of larger glands, often with intraglandular villous papillae that may simulate endometrioid carcinoma. Many tumors are found adjacent to hyperplastic mesonephric remnants. Most are pure adenocarcinomas, although half of the tumors in one series were biphasic with a sarcomatoid component (the so-called "malignant mesonephric mixed tumor"). The spindle cell component generally resembles endometrial stromal sarcoma (ESS) or a nonspecific spindle cell sarcoma. Fukunaga et al. reported a mesonephric cervical carcinoma with lobular mesonephric hyperplasia in a 46 year old.[55] The tumor was positive for CAM5.2, CK7, epithelial membrane antigen, calretinin, and chromogranin A, and negative for vimentin, CEA, estrogen and progesterone receptors, and CD10.[55] An ultrastructural analysis showed telolysomes, which are characteristic of mesonephric epithelium.[55]

In a comprehensive review, Hart noted that while most reported cases had been confined to the cervix at diagnosis and exhibited a more indolent behavior than their müllerian counterparts, a few had been accompanied by extrauterine spread, including lymph node metastases.[56] Among those tumors with a malignant spindle cell component, several had metastasized. There was an apparent tendency for late recurrences, and a few higher stage tumors had taken an aggressive course. In 2001, Silver et al. presented follow-up

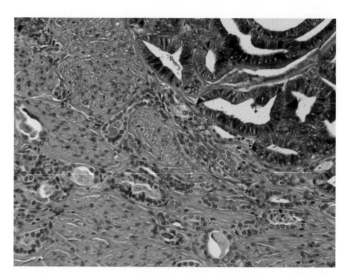

Figure 40.3 Mesonephric adenocarcinoma of the cervix.

data on 10 cases and found six of eight patients with stage IB tumors to be alive without disease after a mean of 4.8 years.[57] Whenever possible, radical surgery with lymphadenectomy appears to be the preferred treatment modality.

Other epithelial tumors

Adenosquamous carcinomas

Adenosquamous carcinomas account for 5–6% of all cervical cancers, occurring in both young and old women, and occasionally associated with pregnancy. The epidemiological risk factors are more similar to those with SCC than adenocarcinoma. The diagnosis is confined to those tumors that contain malignant glandular and squamous elements that are recognizable without the use of special stains. The squamous component is well differentiated and can contain keratin pearls and may be glycogenated. The glandular component is commonly the usual endocervical type but may also be mucinous, including signet ring cell, or mixed endocervical and mucinous, endometrioid, or clear cell.

In a novel study involving separate microdissection of the squamous and glandular components, Yoshida et al. studied the prevalence, physical status, and viral load of HPV-16 and -18 in 20 cases of adenosquamous carcinoma.[58] The percentages of HPV-16- and -18-positive cases among all the HPV-positive cases were 36.8% (7/19) and 57.9% (11/19) in the squamous epithelial elements and 33.3% (6/18) and 61.1% (11/18) in the glandular elements, respectively.[58] The mean HPV-16 DNA copy numbers/cell was 7.22 in the squamous elements and 1.33 in the glandular elements ($p = 0.04$) while the corresponding mean HPV-18 DNA copy numbers/cell were 1.50 and 0.89, respectively.[58] The investigators speculate that the more aggressive transformation with early integration of HPV-18 results in cases with greater chromosomal instabilities, higher growth rates, and rapid progression.

As discussed earlier, several studies have suggested that cervical ACs have a poorer prognosis than SCC, while other investigations have found no difference. Most comparison studies have not separated ACs from those tumors with ASC histology. In a prospective study by the Gynecologic Oncology Group (GOG) examining stage IB cervical cancer, Look et al. observed that patients with ASC histology had a worse prognosis than patients with SCC or other AC.[59]

Farley et al. compared the survival rates between patients with endocervical AC (n = 185) and ASC (n = 88).[60] Although 66% of ASC tumors were poorly differentiated, there was no difference in the incidence of positive lymph nodes associated with the two histological types. Patients with ASC had a significantly decreased 5-year survival rate compared with those with AC (65 versus 83%, p < 0.002); however, this decrease in survival was observed only in patients with stage II–IV disease (p = 0.01). The 5-year survival rate for patients with grade I AC was 93%, compared with 50% for patients with grade I ASC (p < 0.01). The investigators concluded that ASC histology is an independent predictor of poor outcome among women with cervical cancer.

Using the surgicopathological risk factors employed in GOG protocols 92 and 109, Lea et al. studied 230 patients with stage IB_1 endocervical AC, for whom the overall 5-year survival rate was 89%.[61] Among those patients with low-risk tumors (n = 178), ASC histology was the only independent risk factor of disease recurrence (p < 0.01), with a 5-year disease-free survival of 79% compared to that of 96% for other histological subtypes (p < 0.01).

Glassy cell carcinoma

Glassy cell carcinoma (GCC) accounts for only 1–5% of all cervical cancers. It was first described in 1956 by Glucksman and Cherry who considered the disease to be very aggressive because there were no survivors among the 41 cases they reported. Histologically, the tumor cells have moderate ground glass cytoplasm, large nuclei, prominent nucleoli with background eosinophilia, and distinct cell membranes that stain positively with periodic acid-Schiff (PAS). In one series, the tumor was diagnosed among patients with a mean age of 44 (range, 12–69 years). Some authors have associated this tumor type with pregnancy. Kuroda et al. studied 11 cases of which five (45.4%) over expressed HER-2/neu, a finding that may potentially correlate with aggressive behavior and worse clinical outcome.[62]

In 1976, Littman et al. cited a survival rate of 31% among a series of 13 patients with GCC. In 1988 Tamimi et al. reported on 29 patients with stage I disease for whom overall survival was only 55%. Gray et al. have collected approximately 103 cases from the literature and calculated the overall survival for all patients to be approximately 50%; for patients with stage I tumors, overall survival is still diminished at 64%.[63] These investigators provided details on an additional 22 patients and demonstrated improved prognosis with a disease-free survival of 64% and an overall survival of 73%.

Hopkins and Morley have conducted an extensive review of the literature and have added 21 of their own cases to the analysis.[64] If the original report by Glucksman and Cherry is excluded, there are approximately 100 patients available for analysis. Thus, Hopkins and Morley emphasize that conclusions made for this cell type's influence on survival must be drawn with caution. If the original report is excluded, the overall survival is 47% (48 of 107); if the original report is included, the overall survival is decreased to 33% (48 of 148). Survival for this tumor is influenced markedly by the stage of the disease. In the original report by Glucksman and Cherry, the stage of disease was not available. Thus, for those cases in which clinical stage has been reported, the overall survival for stage I disease is approximately 60%.

Of particular interest was the observation that in the report by Gray et al., the overall survival for the 14 patients with stage I disease was 86%, comparable to what is reported in the literature for stage I SCC.[63] Importantly, Gray et al. found that intermediate-risk histopathological features known to predict a higher rate of relapse after radical surgery in SCC patients (lymphovascular space involvement, deep stromal invasion, and large tumor diameter) appear to be predictive of relapse in GCC as well.[63] Because the tumor has a propensity for pelvic and vaginal failure, Gray et al. advocate adjuvant pelvic irradiation in patients with these tumor-related poor prognostic findings.[63]

Mucoepidermoid carcinoma

Mucoepidermoid carcinoma (MEC) is defined as a tumor with the appearance of SCC but lacks a recognizable glandular pattern and demonstrates intracellular mucin. The squamous component is usually large cell nonkeratinizing or focally keratinizing, and the mucin-producing cells are frequently localized in the center of nests of SCC. These tumors can account for up to 36% of cervical carcinomas in some series. The mucinous component includes goblet or signet ring type cells. The mucin may extrude into the intercellular spaces where it may collect in lakes. The mucin is best demonstrated by alcian blue and PAS diastase. Lennerz et al. identified seven cases and demonstrated a CRTC1-MAML2 fusion in one case, rearrangements of CRTC1 in four cases, and aberrations of MAML2 in five cases (rearrangements in two cases, amplification in three cases). None of the 14 adenosquamous controls harbored rearrangements or amplifications at either the CRTC1 or MAML2 loci.[65] These are genes typically rearranged in mucoepidermoid carcinomas of the salivary gland.

In some series, MEC has been found more commonly among younger patients. Thelmo et al. noted that while the overall rate of lymph node metastases was 14% among 265 cases of stage IB SCC of the cervix, those cases that were classified as MEC had a 33% incidence of nodal metastases.[66] Because MEC may be more aggressive than conventional SCC, several authorities have advised staining all cervical SCCs if they demonstrate finely vacuolated cytoplasm and lack peripheral palisading. The detection of CEA (by immunostaining or serum measurement) may also be of clinical utility in establishing the diagnosis.

Adenoid cystic carcinoma

Adenoid cystic carcinomas (ACCs) may arise in diverse anatomical sites, including the salivary glands, tracheobronchial tree, and breast, and were first described by Billroth in 1859. In the female genital tract, ACC occurs in Bartholin's gland, the endometrium, and the uterine cervix. ACCs represent less than 1% of cervical adenocarcinomas. The first example of this tumor was reported by Paalman and Counsellor in 1949 as "cylindroma" of the cervix because of the highly characteristic cytoarchitectural features. More than 150 cases have been reported since McGee et al. introduced the currently accepted designation of "adenoid cystic" carcinoma.

The only lesion in the differential diagnosis is the adenoid basal carcinoma (ABC). Indeed, as has been observed with ABC, ACC has a predilection for the postmenopausal, black patient, with a mean age of 63 (range, 31–99 years) in one literature review containing 59 cases. Grayson et al. have demonstrated that there are no significant differences in mucin staining between ACC and ABC, and, with the exception of type IV collagen and laminin staining found exclusively in ACC, the immunohistochemical profiles are similar.[67] Both tumors can be S-100 positive, and both are associated with integration of high-risk HPV DNA.

Young and Clement have observed that unlike ABC, patients with ACC usually have an obvious exophytic or endophytic cervical mass that can vary greatly in size.[40] Microscopic examination shows nests of cells often with a focal cribriform pattern resembling that seen in ACC of the salivary glands, as well as sheets, trabeculae, and cords. The glandular lumens may contain hyaline or mucinous material, and there is usually focal palisading of cells at the periphery of tumor nests. The neoplastic cells are larger than those of ABC, and more pleomorphic nuclei are present. The mitotic rate is high and necrosis can be extensive. Unlike ABC, there is a stromal response that may be myxoid, fibroblastic, or hyaline.

Whereas ABC has an excellent prognosis, that of ACC is poor. Survival for all stages is approximately 32.5%. In a review of 43 cases, Prempree et al. noted a 56.2% 3–5-year survival for stage I disease, regardless of treatment modality.[68] The optimal primary treatment for early-stage lesions is unknown. Because of the high incidence of lymphatic metastases, vascular space involvement, and distant metastases, most treatment programs include adjuvant cisplatin-based chemotherapy. King et al. reported a survivorship of 12 and 64 months for two patients with stage IB disease who were treated with primary radical hysterectomy with lymphadenectomy, and adjuvant cisplatin at 100 mg/m².[69] In both patients, vascular space permeation was extensive and the long-term survivor had a positive obturator node and bilateral parametrial extension. Elhassani et al. recently reported the successful management of a patient with FIGO stage IIIB disease with concurrent chemoradiation and upon reviewing the literature, concluded that multimodality therapy may offer patients with locally advanced disease an opportunity for long-term durable remission.[70]

Adenoid basal carcinoma

Baggish and Woodruff introduced the concept of ABC of the cervix in 1966. The lesion accounts for less than 1% of cervical adenocarcinomas, with approximately 50 examples appearing in the literature. The tumor has a striking propensity to occur in postmenopausal black women, and the integration of high-risk HPV DNA, particularly HPV-16, has recently been implicated in its pathogenesis. The rarity of ABC has been attributed to an unidentified cofactor. Although Russell and Fadare have presented a strong argument to discard the term ABC and substitute the term adenoid basal epithelioma,[71] for the purposes of this text we will continue to use ABC as the proposed replacement has not been uniformly adopted among pathologists.

Adenoid basal carcinoma shares some characteristics with ACC with which it often has been confused. An accurate distinction between the two is best made morphologically. Numerous widely separated, small, round to oval nests of variable size composed of uniform, cytologically bland basaloid cells with peripheral palisading is often present in ABC (Fig. 40.4). Some of the neoplastic islands can be closely packed, exhibiting a minor degree of lobulation. Stromal reaction is absent. Divergent epithelial differentiation can occur in both ABC and ACC, and the occurrence of ABC areas in some ACCs and vice versa suggests that these tumors may share a common histogenesis from pluripotent reserve cells. Circumstantial evidence even suggests that ABC may be a precursor of cervical ACC. Both ABC-like and ACC-like areas have been reported in or adjacent to some malignant müllerian mixed tumors (MMMT) of the cervix.

Brainard et al. reported 12 cases of ABC in 1998.[72] The mean age was 71 years (range, 30–91 years), and all were asymptomatic. Almost all presented with an abnormal Pap smear that usually showed a squamous epithelial abnormality. None of the patients had a clinically or grossly recognizable cervical lesion. The depth of stromal invasion ranged from 2 to 10 mm (mean, 4.3 mm), exceeding 3 mm in six tumors. Treatment was predominantly surgical, with conization alone being employed in three patients. One hundred and four lymph nodes were removed from five patients, none of which contained metastases. At the time of publication, nine patients were alive without disease at a mean follow-up period of

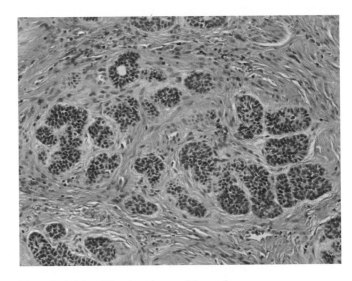

Figure 40.4 Adenoid basal carcinoma of the cervix.

30 months (range, 4–82 months), and three had died without disease after 24, 63, and 87 months.

The prognosis of ABC is excellent, with few clinical features of an invasive cervical carcinoma.

Small cell carcinoma

Small cell carcinoma of the cervix (SCCC) was first described in 1957 and accounts for 3% of all cervical neoplasms. On the basis of contemporary series, the median age is 43 years at diagnosis (range, 23–75 years). Histologically, these tumors are indistinguishable from small cell carcinoma in other sites, with small cells containing scant cytoplasm, hyperchromatic nuclei, and a high nuclear:cytoplasmic ratio. Electron microscopy often reveals dense-core, membrane-bound, neurosecretory granules. Neuroendocrine markers are commonly used to assist in classification, with up to 80% of tumors staining for synaptophysin, chromogranin, or CD56 (neural cell adhesion molecule) or all three.

Similar to what has been observed among patients with small cell lung cancer, SCCC is characterized by frequent and early nodal metastases (50–60%), vascular invasion, and a relapse pattern consistent with hematogenous dissemination. For example, Viswanathan et al. observed a 66% relapse rate, with a course frequently characterized by the development of widespread distant metastases.[73] Locoregional recurrence outside irradiated fields was also frequently observed. In the group studied, the overall survival rate at 5 years was only 29%, with none of the patients who had disease more extensive than FIGO stage IB$_1$ or clinical evidence of lymph node metastases surviving their disease.

In a multivariate analysis of different prognostic factors among 34 patients, Chan et al. documented that only those with early lesions amenable to extirpation were curable.[74] Chang et al. have evaluated the role of adjuvant chemotherapy in patients who underwent primary radical hysterectomy for SCCC.[75] From 1988 to 1996, 14 women received a combination of vincristine, doxorubicin, and cyclophosphamide alternating with cisplatin and etoposide (VAC/PE). Their outcomes were compared with those of nine patients treated from 1984 to 1988, eight of whom received a combination of cisplatin, vinblastine, and bleomycin (PVB) in the adjuvant setting. The stage distribution included 19 patients with stage IB tumors and four with stage II tumors. Ten of the 14 patients (68%) who received VAC/PE had no evidence of disease during a median follow-up of 41 months, whereas only three of the nine (33%) who received PVB or another regimen survived. All 10 women who died failed at distant sites. Seventy percent of patients without nodal involvement at the time of surgery and 35% of those with lymphatic metastases survived.

Cisplatin plus etoposide with the early use of irradiation is generally regarded as the standard regimen for small cell lung cancer and, by extrapolation, may have some activity in SCCC. Hoskins et al. have reported a 14-year institutional experience involving 31 patients with SCCC.[76] The clinical stage distribution included stage I (n = 16), stage IIA (n = 3), stage IIB (n = 3), stage III (n = 6), stage IVB (n = 1), and unknown (n = 2). Importantly, clinical staging significantly underestimated the true disease extent, with 38% of patients (n = 13) upstaged on the basis of further imaging studies. Seventeen patients were treated from 1988 to 1995 on protocol SMCC, which included cisplatin, etoposide, and involved-field irradiation with concurrent chemotherapy; 14 women treated from 1996 to 2002 also received carboplatin and paclitaxel, along with para-aortic irradiation (protocol SMCC2). None of the patients underwent radical surgery. The 3-year overall and failure-free survival rates for the study group were 60% and 57%, respectively. The survival results were equivalent between SMCC and SMCC2, with the latter regimen associated with increased hematological toxicity and decreased hospital admissions for emesis and dehydration.

In an extensive review of the literature to which 52 additional patients were added from four medical centers, Cohen et al. described the treatment and survival outcomes for 188 women with small cell carcinoma of the cervix (FIGO I–IIA, n = 135; FIGO IIB–IVA, n = 45; FIGO IVB, n = 8).[77] The 5-year disease-specific survival in stage I–IIA, IIB–IVA, and IVB disease was 36.8%, 9.8%, and 0%, respectively (p < 0.001).[77] On multivariable analysis, early-stage disease and use of chemotherapy or chemoradiation were independent prognostic factors for improved survival.[77]

Carcinoid tumors

Well-differentiated carcinoid tumors of the cervix were originally described by Albores-Saavedra et al.[78] Histologically, they are similar to intestinal carcinoid tumors and contain neurosecretory granules that can be observed by electron microscopy. The tumors grow in a trabecular, nodular, or cord-like pattern, and rosette-like structures are common. The classic carcinoid has neoplastic cells with finely granular cytoplasm and oval spindle-shaped nuclei. Mitoses are infrequently observed. Greater than 70% are argyrophilic and stain with synaptophysin, chromogranin A, and neuron-specific enolase.

Syndrome X and elevated serum serotonin levels have been associated with cervical carcinoid tumors. Although there has been one report of carcinoid syndrome occurring in a patient with an atypical carcinoid tumor of the cervix, there have been no cases of carcinoid syndrome associated with the classic cervical carcinoid. While the growth pattern has been previously described as indolent, some reports have been notable for a malignant course, with both local and distant metastases. For example, Seidel and Steinfeld reported brain metastases manifesting 4 years after the diagnosis and primary treatment of a stage IB tumor.[79] In their review of reported cases, they found that even patients with early-stage lesions may die of disseminated disease.

Sarcomas

A variety of sarcomas can arise from the cervix, including carcinosarcoma, leiomyosarcoma, epithelioid leiomyosarcoma, müllerian adenosarcoma (MA), and extrauterine ESS. Granulocytic sarcoma (also known as chloroma) and embryonal rhabdomyosarcoma, along with its variant, sarcoma botryoides (SB), will be discussed separately. Sarcomatoid carcinomas, which lack a malignant stromal or mesenchymal component, were described in an earlier section. Bansal et al. recently published a SEER database analysis that included 323 sarcomas of the cervix (1% of the total cervical cancers identified).[80] Carcinosarcoma was the most common and accounted for 40% ($n = 128$) of the cases while adenosarcomas and leiomyosarcomas each accounted for 21% ($n = 67$).[80] Compared to women with squamous cell and adenocarcinomas, patients with cervical sarcomas tended to be younger, diagnosed in the later years of the study, have larger tumors, and have more advanced stage disease ($p < 0.05$ for all).[80] After adjusting for other known prognostic factors, patients with cervical sarcomas were 60% more likely to die from their tumors (cancer-specific survival HR 1.60, 95% CI 1.30–1.96; overall survival HR 1.60, 95% CI 1.36–1.89) than patients with squamous cell carcinomas.[80]

Wright et al. conducted a single-institution review spanning nearly two decades, which included 1583 cervical neoplasms and found only eight sarcomas (0.005%), five of which were carcinosarcomas.[81] Five of their patients (62.5%) were alive without evidence of disease and one patient (12.5%) was alive with disease at a median follow-up of 2.2 years. Among the disease-free survivors, two had been diagnosed with carcinosarcoma, and one each with a leiomyosarcoma, unspecified sarcoma, and extrauterine ESS.

Approximately 50 cases of *cervical carcinosarcoma* have been reported. The largest review was conducted by Clement et al. who noted that most patients present with vaginal bleeding and a cervical mass.[82] Disease is confined to the cervix in the majority of patients, although in the series by Wright et al.,[81] four of five patients with cervical carcinosarcoma had bulky stage IB$_2$ tumors and one had a large stage IIIA tumor. Histologically, the tumors exhibit a malignant epithelial component in conjunction with a malignant stromal component. Both homologous and heterologous sarcomatous elements have been reported in cervical carcinosarcomas. Interestingly, integrated HPV DNA has been detected not only in the epithelial components but also in the sarcomatous elements of some tumors. Radical abdominal hysterectomy with bilateral salpingo-oophorectomy and lymphadenectomy is a reasonable approach for tumors confined to the cervix.

Less than 25 cases of *primary cervical leiomyosarcoma* have appeared in the literature. Most afflicted patients are perimenopausal and present with vaginal bleeding and a cervical mass. Diagnostic criteria have been outlined by Bell et al. and include a combination of high mitotic rate, coagulative tumor cell necrosis, or high-grade cytological atypia.[83] Treatment recommendations have been extrapolated from the soft tissue sarcoma and uterine sarcoma literatures. When disease is confined to the cervix, radical abdominal hysterectomy with bilateral salpingo-oophorectomy may be considered. Because of the low incidences of nodal spread in uterine leiomyosarcoma (3.5%) and in soft tissue sarcoma (5.8%), the value of routine lymphadenectomy has been questioned for primary cervical leiomyosarcomas.

Müllerian adenosarcoma is a variant of the mixed mesodermal tumor of the uterus. It is composed of benign epithelial (glandular) and malignant stromal components. The tumor most commonly occurs within the uterine body in postmenopausal women, sometimes in association with tamoxifen therapy. Roth et al. first described its location in the cervix and the presence of heterologous elements (i.e. cartilage, bone, skeletal muscle, etc.) in 1976. Only 14 reports have been published subsequently. Ramos et al. have noted that an interesting feature of cervical müllerian adenosarcoma with heterologous elements is the age of clinical presentation, with five postmenarchal patients and eight young women (range, 18–45 years) diagnosed with this unusual neoplasm.[84] Many had a history of recurrent polyps. Cartilage and striated muscle were the most common heterologous elements encountered in 13 of the reported cases, and crossed cytoplasmic striations were observed in half of the study population. Many authors have recommended radical or extrafascial hysterectomy and bilateral salpingo-oophorectomy, with adjuvant radiation therapy reserved for deeply infiltrating tumors. Ten of the 15 patients (66%) reviewed by Ramos et al. were known to be alive without disease at 2.5–7 years of follow-up.[84] Because the lesion seems to appear in the earliest stages of the reproductive lifespan in women, local excision may be curative in rare cases when a pedunculated cervical tumor and uninvolved stalk are encountered, thereby allowing conservation of reproductive function.

Epithelioid leiomyosarcoma is a rare variant characterized by a proliferation of predominantly round and polygonal epithelioid cells with eosinophilic cytoplasm in a malignant tumor component of smooth muscle cells. Most tumors have occurred in the uterine body, with only four reported cases having arisen from the uterine cervix. The age distribution ranged from 47 to 72 years, and initial treatment included total abdominal hysterectomy and bilateral salpingo-oophorectomy in all cases.[85] Three patients received adjuvant therapy, and all three of these patients were alive without disease at 4, 10, and 20 months of follow-up.

Finally, *extrauterine emdometrial stromal sarcoma* (ESS) histologically resembles ESS and commonly arises within foci of endometriosis. The tumors have been found in the peritoneum, omentum, ovary, and cervix. In two of the three cases of primary cervical extrauterine ESS, the tumor appeared to arise from an endocervical polyp. This rare entity is included in this chapter only for the sake of completeness.

Embryonal rhabdomyosarcoma

Embryonal rhabdomyosarcoma (E-RMS) is a highly malignant tumor that accounts for 4–6% of all malignancies in childhood and young adults. It is the most common soft tissue sarcoma in this age group and occurs primarily in the head and neck region, the genitourinary tract, and the extremities. The Intergroup Rhabdomyosarcoma Study (IRS) Group recognizes three major histological subtypes: embryonal, alveolar, and undifferentiated.

Sarcoma botryoides (SB) is a variant of E-RMS and manifests with a "grape-like" appearance due to a layer of spindle cells pushing up beneath the mucosa in polypoid masses. Although SB is usually found in the infantile vagina, it can also arise from the vulva, the uterus, and the cervix. Histologically, SB contains malignant rhabdomyoblasts within a loose, myxoid stroma. Unlike alveolar E-RMS, SB is not associated with a unique genetic translocation. Interestingly, while vaginal RMS manifests normally before the age of 4 (mean age, 23.5 months), cervical RMS usually presents during the second decade of life (mean age, 14 years). Brand et al. published the first comprehensive review of cervical SB, adding four of their own cases to the 17 that had appeared in the literature up to 1987.[86] After 68 months of follow-up, 80% of the patients were alive. Among five patients (24%) with recurrent disease, three had died of disease.

The treatment of SB has undergone rigorous scrutiny and dramatic changes over the decades. Traditionally, treatment included ultraradical or radical fertility-compromising surgery. For example, during the 1960s pelvic exenteration was the treatment of choice but a comprehensive review showed that the results were unsatisfactory. Multiagent chemotherapy or pelvic irradiation with limited surgery or both resulted in a considerable improvement in survival during the 1970s. The 1980s were dominated by combined treatment options including radical hysterectomy; however, during the 1990s there was a gradual shift toward less invasive and more organ-sparing procedures such as local excision, polypectomy, trachelectomy, or conization with or without adjuvant chemotherapy. Importantly, in recent years it has been recognized that cervical SB behaves less aggressively than vaginal or uterine SB.

Given the predilection of this tumor to afflict young children and adolescents, functional preservation of the bladder and reproductive organs is implicit when considering long-term quality of life. Fertility-sparing surgery appears to be appropriate in IRS clinical classification group I patients (i.e. those with localized disease, completely resected, with no regional nodes involved). The most widely used chemotherapy regimen includes vincristine, dactinomycin, and cyclophosphamide (VAC), and 6–12 cycles should permit a resumption of menstrual function and preservation of reproductive capacity.

In 2003, Behtash et al. reviewed the literature and identified 17 additional cases since 1987, and added two of their own.[87] All 19 patients survived beyond 24 months (range, 24–96 months). Eleven patients underwent conservative surgery, including polypectomy, dilation and curettage, trachelectomy, partial excision and local excisions, three of whom did not receive adjuvant chemotherapy. Two additional reports of cervical SB in patients treated with fertility-sparing surgery and adjuvant chemotherapy appeared in 2004.[88,89] Karaman et al. recently reported successful fertility-sparing surgery and adjuvant chemotherapy in a 22-year-old nulliparous woman.[90] The authors recommend a minimally invasive (i.e. conservative fertility-sparing surgical approach) for those patients with favorable prognostic factors such as localized disease, single polyp and embryonal histological subtype, and without deep invasion.[90]

Granulocytic sarcoma

Granulocytic sarcoma (GS) is an extramedullary tumor of malignant granulocytic progenitor cells that heralds, accompanies, or signals relapse of acute myelogenous leukemia (AML). GS has been reported in 3–5% of AML patients and because it can precede other manifestations of leukemia, misdiagnosis often occurs. A conclusive diagnosis of GS requires demonstration of granulocytic differentiation of the tumor cells, for which the Leder stain and the antilysozyme immunoperoxidase stain are particularly useful.[91]

Granulocytic sarcoma of the cervix is very rare and is also called chloroma because of its greenish appearance. The majority of patients with cervical GS present with vaginal bleeding and abdominal pain and may also have other systemic symptoms. Chemotherapy has been the mainstay of treatment for GS. Unfortunately, the overall 2-year survival rates for all patients with GS in the literature is 6%, and none of the reported patients lived 5 years. In a recent review of the literature to which the authors added their own case, Chiang and Chen have noted that survival is improved with multimodality therapy and in patients without leukemia.[92]

Miscellaneous

Melanoma

Only 5% of melanoma in women are located in the genitalia, with the vast majority occurring in the vulva. Rarely, the ovary, uterus, or uterine cervix may be the primary site of origin. Historically, the lack of melanocytes in the vaginal and cervical mucous membranes has deterred the acceptance of primary melanomas in these areas; however, in 1959, Cid reported the presence of melanin-containing cells in 3.5% of cervices. The principal requirement is the evidence of junctional activity of the cervical epithelium along with the absence of any demonstrable skin, vaginal, or retinal lesion.

In a review of the published literature, Cantuaria et al. have identified 27 cases of primary malignant melanoma of the cervix.[93] The mean age at diagnosis was 55 years (range, 26–78 years), and 83% presented with abnormal vaginal bleeding. In the majority of cases, an exophytic cervical lesion was encountered, varying in color, which included red, brown, gray, black, and blue. The tumor was typically fragile and easily bled to touch. Because of the extreme rarity of this lesion, the FIGO clinical staging system is recommended rather than one of the microstaging systems of Clark et al., Breslow et al., or Chung et al. Importantly, 88% of the patients identified by Cantuaria et al. presented with stage I (n = 12) and stage II (n = 9) disease.[93]

Treatment of melanoma is primarily surgical, and a variety of procedures have been applied to this disease when it originates in the cervix. When there is only clinical involvement of the cervix, we recommend a radical abdominal hysterectomy with the performance of a concomitant upper vaginectomy as needed to obtain satisfactory margins of at least 2 cm. Because the presence of lymphatic metastases is negligible in patients with melanomas <1 mm thick, we do not advocate elective lymphadenectomy for such lesions. The management of clinically negative regional lymph nodes for thicker tumors, and especially for those >4 mm thick, is controversial. Randomized trials by the Mayo Clinic have not demonstrated enhanced survival among patients with melanoma of the extremities who underwent elective lymphadenectomy when compared with similar patients treated with wide excision alone. For these reasons, unless a patient is interested in investigational adjuvant therapy that may require lymph node biopsy as part of the protocol eligibility criteria, we do not recommend elective lymphadenectomy for this disease. Pelvic and para-aortic lymphadenectomy for grossly enlarged lymph nodes may have a palliative role.

Radiation therapy has not been studied in the adjuvant setting for this disease, and may be employed for palliation of unresectable, advanced tumors and possibly in the setting when satisfactory surgical resection has not been accomplished. The role of adjuvant chemotherapy and biological modifiers such as interferon is also a topic of debate, with disappointing results when chemotherapy has been used for metastatic cutaneous melanomas. Response rates for dacarbazine have ranged between 15% and 20%.

Many of the 27 patients reported by Cantuaria et al. lack follow-up data.[93] For five patients with stage I disease and for six with stage II disease, the mean survival was 49 and 41 months, respectively. Despite the majority of patients having been diagnosed with early-stage tumors, only two have survived beyond 5 years. It appears that the prognosis is unfavorable when compared with SCCs and typical endocervical adenocarcinomas of the cervix. Extrapolating from the cutaneous melanoma literature, even long disease-free intervals are no guarantee against recurrent disease with this unpredictable tumor. Fortunately, because most patients present with early-stage disease, many are candidates for surgical therapy, at least initially.

Recently, Pusceddu et al. reviewed all 78 published reports from 1889 to 2011.[94] The authors noted that a feature further supporting the poor prognosis lies in the observation that, despite the fact that 50% of patients had been diagnosed as stage I, only a small percentage survived more than 5 years.[94] Globally, the 5-year survival rate observed in the evaluated patients accounted for 18.8% for stage I, 11.1% for stage II, and 0% for stages III–IV. The clinical impression derived from the analysis of their century-plus case list is that melanoma of the cervix does not substantially differ from most frequent cutaneous melanomas; in fact, it can have a very rapid evolution with development of distant metastases, or may remain dormant for a few years. Furthermore, cervical melanoma is characterized by a greater tendency to relapse locally rather than developing distant metastases, the most frequent sites being vagina, vulva, or labia and alongside suture line.[94]

Lymphoma

Lymphomas account for 3.5% of all cancers in women. Twenty-five percent arise in extragonadal tissues, with the gastrointestinal tract and skin being most common. Secondary involvement of the genital tract may occur in up to 40% of disseminated lymphomas. Primary genital tract lymphomas, however, account for only 1.5% of extranodal lymphomas, of which 0.6% are of cervical origin. Primary cervical lymphomas are defined as lymphomas that originate and localize from the uterine cervix without any myometrial involvement and without any evidence of leukemia at the time of diagnosis. They were first reported by Freeman et al. in 1972.

The etiology and pathogenesis of cervical lymphomas are perplexing, with some authorities attributing the increase in incidence of extranodal lymphomas during the preceding two decades to be secondary to the increase in immunosuppressive therapies, human immunodeficiency virus (HIV) infections, environmental toxins, and even chronic inflammatory conditions. Approximately 80% of patients with cervical lymphoma are premenopausal (range, 20–80 years), and when compared to other non-Hodgkin lymphomas (NHLs), there is a tendency to occur in younger age groups. Although some reports claim that patients with systemic lymphoma have more abnormal Pap smears than controls, primary cervical lymphomas are rarely diagnosed by screening cytology because they originate from the cervical stroma, and the overlying squamous epithelium is generally preserved. Up to 67% of these tumors may present with a subepithelial mass without obvious ulceration. In a review from 1983 to 2003, Dursun et al. identified 31 patients (including two of their own) for whom abnormal lymphoid cells were present in the cervical smears of only 6.5% of cases.[95]

Patients typically present with abnormal vaginal bleeding or discharge, although pelvic pain and dyspareunia may also occur. Interestingly, fever, night sweats, and weight loss, which are common among patients with systemic lymphomas, are rarely reported in women with primary cervical lymphoma. On examination, there is cervical-uterine enlargement with fixation, and vaginal or parametrial infiltration or both may be palpable. The differential diagnosis of cervical lymphomas includes benign chronic inflammation, poorly differentiated and small cell cervical carcinomas, sarcomas, and lymphoma-like lesions. Because therapy for cervical lymphomas differs from that of other cervical cancers, it is imperative that the correct diagnosis is made. Histological analysis of a deep cervical biopsy is diagnostic, with the appearance being similar to lymphomas from other sites. Occasionally, immunophenotypings may be required as diagnostic adjuncts.

Although the World Health Organization classification scheme has replaced the Ann Arbor staging system (which includes stages IE, IIE, IIIE, and IVE), it must be recognized that most reports from the literature have used the latter system. The histological classification is according to the International Working Formulation for NHLs and includes low grade (A–C), intermediate grade (D–G), and high grade (H–J).

Treatment modalities employed in the management of cervical lymphoma have included chemotherapy alone, neoadjuvant chemotherapy followed by surgery, radiotherapy alone, or radiotherapy combined with either chemotherapy or surgery. The most commonly used chemotherapy regimen is CHOP (cyclophosphamide, doxorubicin, vincristine, and prednisone). Recently, a group of investigators reported the successful treatment of primary NHL of the cervix with the chimeric anti-CD20 antibody, rituximab.[96]

Some authorities have advocated surgical resection in localized lymphoma (e.g. large loop excision of the transformation zone, trachelectomy, or hysterectomy), and in well-selected cases this may be a reasonable approach. There is no clear evidence, however, that hysterectomy improves survival for this group of patients. Chan *et al.* have conducted an extensive review of the literature and identified 64 patients (including six of their own).[97] The disease-free survival rate among the 39 patients with stage IE disease (i.e. involvement of a single extralymphatic organ or site) was 87%. While patients with localized stage IE disease with nonbulky lesions will often respond to primary surgery, chemotherapy, or radiotherapy alone, combined therapy seems to be preferred in most centers. Since the survival rates in patients with early-stage cervical lymphomas are excellent, young women who desire future child bearing will benefit from combination chemotherapy. For patients with more advanced disease, combination chemotherapy with tailored radiotherapy appears to be favored.

Curiosities

There have been at least 10 reports of a peripheral primitive neuroectodermal tumor of the cervix.[98] These tumors should be treated in accordance with the protocol for bony Ewing sarcoma with induction chemotherapy, surgery, and consolidation chemotherapy. Gestational choriocarcinoma has also been reported, most possibly arising from a preexisting cervical pregnancy or displaced intrauterine molar tissue.[99] Finally, primary tumors of germ cell origin have arisen from the cervix. These include cases of mature teratomas with lymphoid hyperplasia[100] or pulmonary differentiation,[101] as well as malignant germ cell tumors, including an immature teratoma,[102] yolk sac tumor,[103] and choriocarcinoma.[104] Dysgerminoma has not yet been reported to originate in the cervix.

Treatment

In the vast majority of cases, treatment of cervical cancer is dependent on stage. Early-stage disease (FIGO stage I) is often treated surgically, although chemoradiation plus brachytherapy is equally curative in most cases when significant medical comorbidities or other concerns preclude a surgical approach.[19] Many microinvasive carcinomas (FIGO IA$_1$) can be treated safely by simple hysterectomy, while FIGO IA$_2$ disease is best treated with modified radical hysterectomy plus pelvic lymphadenectomy.[19] FIGO IB$_1$ and selected cases of FIGO IB$_2$–IIA$_1$ may be cured with radical hysterectomy plus bilateral pelvic lymphadenectomy.[19] In contrast to extrafascial (i.e. simple) hysterectomy, radical surgery for cervical cancer involves removal of the cardinal and uterosacral ligaments and the proximal vagina.[19] Postoperative adjuvant pelvic radiotherapy with or without radiosensitizing chemotherapy may be prescribed depending on the presence of intermediate-risk (lymphovascular space invasion, large tumor diameter, deep stromal invasion) or high-risk (positive vaginal margin, occult parametrial extension, lymph node metastases) factors.[19]

In young women desirous of future child bearing, microinvasive disease can be excised by conization and for those with early-stage disease (<2 cm maximal tumor diameter), a simple or radical trachelectomy with or without lymph node dissection can be accomplished to preserve fertility.[19] Many of the surgical procedures for cervical cancer can be performed via minimally invasive approaches using either straight-stick laparoscopic or robotic-assisted technology.

Locally advanced disease (FIGO IB$_2$–IVA) can be successfully treated using chemoradiation plus high-dose rate intracavitary brachytherapy. Typically, 50.4 Gy is administered in 1.8 Gy daily fractions with weekly cisplatin (40 mg/m^2). Brachytherapy brings the total dose to point A (location of the parametria) to approximately 85 Gy.[19] The Australia New Zealand Gynaecological Oncology Group (ANZGOG), the Gynecologic Oncology Group (GOG), and the Radiation Therapy Oncology Group (RTOG) are currently studying the efficacy and tolerability of additional systemic chemotherapy following completion of radiation therapy in the OUTBACK trial.

Patients diagnosed with metastatic disease (FIGO IVB) as well as those with persistent disease following definitive locoregional therapy and recurrent disease should be diverted to clinical trials employing novel targeted agents (e.g. antiangiogenesis therapy) and nonplatinum chemotherapy doublets, as most of these patients have platinum-resistant disease for which the prognosis is very poor. Patients with isolated central pelvic recurrences without evidence of hydronephrosis may be salvaged through pelvic exenteration with urinary diversion.[19]

Although FIGO stage determines treatment in most cases of cervical cancer, in some instances histology may dictate the therapeutic program. For example, bulky FIGO stage IB$_2$ adenocarcinomas may be relatively radioresistant when compared to their squamous counterparts, and therefore some oncologists favor a primary surgical approach. Similarly, neuroendocrine (small) cell carcinomas have a predilection for hematogenous metastases and therefore following surgical resection, adjuvant systemic chemotherapy is administered without pelvic radiotherapy. Finally, primary cervical lymphomas are often treated with primary combination chemotherapy exclusively.

References

1. Freund AW. Zu meiner methode der total uterus extirpation. Zbl Gynaek 1878; 2: 265.
2. Clark JG. A more radical method for performing hysterectomy for cancer of the uterus. Bull Johns Hopkins Hosp 1895; 6: 120.
3. Schauta F. Die *Erweiterte Vaginale Totalexstirpation des Uterus bei Kollumkarzinom*. Wien, Leipzig, Germany: Josef Safar, 1908.
4. Wertheim E. The extended abdominal operation for carcinoma uteri (based on 500 operative cases). Am J Obstet Gynecol 1912; 66: 169.
5. Roentgen WC. On a new kind of rays. Nature 1896; 53: 274–6.
6. Curie P, Curie MS, Bémont G. On a new, strongly radioactive substance, contained in pitchblende. C R Acad Sci Paris 1898; 127: 1215–17.
7. Pasteau O, Degrais P. The radium treatment of cancer of the prostate. Rev Mal Nutr 1911; 10: 363–7.
8. Taussig FJ. Iliac lymphadenectomy with irradiation in the treatment of cancer of the cervix. Am J Obstet Gynecol 1934; 28: 650–2.
9. Meigs JV. Radical hysterectomy with bilateral node dissection. A report of 100 patients operated five or more years ago. Am J Obstet Gynecol 1951; 62: 854.

10. Okabayashi H. Radical abdominal hysterectomy for cancer of the cervix uteri. Surg Gynecol Obstet 1921; 33: 335–41.

11. Brunschwig A. Complete excision of pelvic viscera for advanced cancer. Cancer 1948; 1: 177.

12. Papanicoloau GN, Trout HF. *Diagnosis of Uterine Cancer by Vaginal Smears*. New York: The Commonwealth Fund, 1943.

13. Gey GO, Coffman WD, Kubicek MT. Tissue culture studies of the proliferative capacity of cervical carcinoma and normal epithelium. Cancer Res 1952; 12: 264–5.

14. Durst M, *et al*. A papillomavirus DNA from a cervical carcinoma and its prevalence in cancer biopsy samples from different geographic regions. Proc Natl Acad Sci USA 1983; 80: 3812–15.

15. Boshart M, *et al*. A new type of papillomavirus DNA, its presence in genital cancer biopsies and in cell lines derived from cervical cancer. EMBO J 1984; 3: 1151–7.

16. Siegel R, Ward E, Brawley O, Jemal A. Cancer statistics, 2011: the impact of eliminating socioeconomic and racial disparities on premature cancer deaths. CA Cancer J Clin 2011;61:212–36.

17. McDougall JA, Madeleine MM, Daling JR, Li CI. Racial and ethnic disparities in cervical cancer incidence rates in the United States, 1992–2003. Cancer Causes Control 2007;18:1175–86.

18. Horner MJ, *et al*. U.S. geographical distribution of prevaccine era cervical cancer screening, incidence, stage, and mortality. Cancer Epidemol Biomarkers Prev 2011; 20: 591–9.

19. Tewari KS, Monk BJ. Invasive cervical cancer. In: DiSaia P, Creasman W (eds) *Clinical Gynecologic Oncology*, 8th edn. Philadelphia, PA: Elsevier, 2012.

20. Pecorelli S. Revised FIGO staging for carcinoma of the vulva, cervix, and endometrium. Int J Gynaecol Obstet 2009; 105: 103–4.

21. Degefu S, *et al*. Verrucous carcinoma of the cervix: a report of two cases and literature review. Gynecol Oncol 1986; 25: 37–47.

22. Frega A, *et al*. Verrucous carcinoma of the cervix: detection of carcinogenetic human papillomavirus types and their role during follow-up. Anticancer Res 2007; 27: 4491–4.

23. Ng WK, Cheung LK, Li AS. Warty (condylomatous) carcinoma of the cervix. A review of 3 cases with emphasis on thin-layer cytology and molecular analysis for HPV. Acta Cytol 2003; 47: 159–66.

24. Koenig C, *et al*. Papillary squamotransitional cell carcinoma of the cervix: a report of 32 cases. Am J Surg Pathol 1997; 21: 915–21.

25. Ortega-Gonzalez P, Chanona-Vilchis J, Dominguez-Malagon H. Transitional cell carcinoma of the uterine cervix. A report of six cases with clinical, histologic and cytologic findings. Acta Cytol 2002; 46: 585–90.

26. Bais AG, *et al*. Lymphoepithelioma-like carcinoma of the uterine cervix: absence of Epstein–Barr virus, but presence of multiple human papillomavirus infection. Gynecol Oncol 2005; 97: 716–18.

27. Tseng CJ, *et al*. Lymphoepithelioma-like carcinoma of the uterine cervix: association with Epstein–Barr virus and human papillomavirus. Cancer 1997; 80: 91–7.

28. Takai N, *et al*. Lymphoepithelioma-like carcinoma of the uterine cervix. Acta Gynecol Obstet 2009; 280: 725–7.

29. Brown J, *et al*. Sarcomatoid carcinoma of the cervix. Gynecol Oncol 2003; 90: 23–8.

30. Kong TW, *et al*. Sarcomatoid squamous cell carcinoma of the uterine cervix successfully treated by laparoscopic radical hysterectomy: a case report. J Reprod Med 2010; 55: 445–8.

31. Wright TC, Ferenczy A, Kurman RJ. Carcinoma and other tumors of the cervix. In: Kurman RJ (ed) *Blaustein's Pathology of the Female Genital Tract*, 5th edn. New York: Springer-Verlag, 2002.

32. Konishi I, *et al*. Mucin leakage into the cervical stroma may increase lymph node metastasis in mucin-producing cervical adenocarcinomas. Cancer 1990; 65: 229–37.

33. Togami S, *et al*. Expression of mucin antigens (MUC1 and MUC16) as a prognostic factor for mucinous adenocarcinoma of the uterine cervix. J Obstet Gynaecol Res 2010; 36: 588–97.

34. Jiang L, *et al*. Endometrial endometrioid adenocarcinoma of the uterine corpus involving the cervix: some cases probably represent independent primaries. Int J Gynecol Pathol 2010; 29: 146–56.

35. Fujiwara H, *et al*. Adenocarcinoma of the cervix. Expression and clinical significance of estrogen and progesterone receptors. Cancer 1997; 79: 505–12.

36. Hopkins MP, Morley GW. A comparison of adenocarcinoma and squamous cell carcinoma of the cervix. Obstet Gynecol 1991; 77: 912–17.

37. Lea JS, *et al*. Stage IIB–IVB cervical adenocarcinoma: prognostic factors and survival. Gynecol Oncol 2002; 84: 115–19.

38. Young RH, Scully RE. Villoglandular papillary adenocarcinoma of the uterine cervix. A clinicopathologic analysis of 13 cases. Cancer 1989; 63: 1773–9.

39. Utsugi K, *et al*. Clinicopathologic features of villoglandular papillary adenocarcinoma of the uterine cervix. Gynecol Oncol 2004; 92: 64–70.

40. Young RH, Clement PB. Endocervical adenocarcinoma and its variants: their morphology and differential diagnosis. Histopathology 2002; 41: 185–207.

41. Takai N, *et al*. Villoglandular papillary adenocarcinoma of the uterine cervix diagnosed during pregnancy. Eur J Gynaecol Oncol 2010; 31: 573–4.

42. Rubesa-Mihaljevic R, *et al*. Villoglandular papillary adenocarcinoma of the uterine cervix with aggressive clinical course – a case report. Coll Anthropol 2010; 34: 291–4.

43. Silverberg SG, Hurt WG. Minimal deviation adenocarcinoma ("adenoma malignum") of the cervix: a reappraisal. Am J Obstet Gynecol 1975; 121: 971–5.

44. Hirai Y, *et al*. A clinicocytopathologic study of adenoma malignum of the uterine cervix. Gynecol Oncol 1998; 70: 219–23.

45. Riegert-Johnson D, *et al*. Case studies in the diagnosis and management of Peutz–Jeghers syndrome. Fam Cancer 2011; 10(3): 463–8.

46. Shintaku M, *et al*. Colloid carcinoma of the intestinal type I the uterine cervix: mucin immunohistochemistry. Pathol Int 2010; 60: 119–24.

47. Herbst AL, Anderson D. Clear cell adenocarcinoma of the vagina and cervix secondary to intrauterine exposure to diethylstilbestrol. Semin Surg Oncol 1990; 6: 343–6.

48. Reich O, *et al*. Clear cell carcinoma of the uterine cervix: pathology and prognosis in surgically treated stage IB–IIB disease in women not exposed in utero to diethylstilbestrol. Gynecol Oncol 2000; 76: 331–5.

49. Thomas MB *et al*. Clear cell carcinoma of the cervix: a multi-institutional review in the post-DES era. Gynecol Oncol 2008; 109: 335–9.

50. Rose PG, Reale FR. Serous papillary carcinoma of the cervix. Gynecol Oncol 1993; 50: 361–4.

51. Costa MJ, McIlnay KR, Trelford J. Cervical carcinoma with glandular differentiation: histological evaluation predicts disease recurrence in clinical stage I or II patients. Hum Pathol 1995; 26: 829–37.

52. Nofech-Mozes S, *et al*. Immunohistochemical characterization of endocervical papillary serous carcinoma. Int J Gynecol Cancer 2006; 16(Suppl 1): 286–92.

53. Zhou C, *et al*. Papillary serous carcinoma of the uterine cervix: a clinicopathologic study of 17 cases. Am J Surg Pathol 1998; 22: 113–20.

54. Ferry JA, Scully RE. Mesonephric remnants, hyperplasia, and neoplasia in the uterine cervix. A study of 49 cases. Am J Surg Pathol 1990; 14: 1100–11.

55. Fukunaga M, Takahashi H, Yasuda M. Mesonephric adenocarcnioma of the uterine cervix: a case report with immunohistochemical and ultrastructural studies. Pathol Res Pract 2008; 204: 671–8.

56. Hart WR. Symposium part II: special types of adenocarcinoma of the uterine cervix. Int J Gynecol Pathol 2002; 21: 327–46.

57. Silver SA, *et al*. Mesonephric adenocarcinomas of the uterine cervix: a study of 11 cases with immunohistochemical findings. Am J Surg Pathol 2001; 25: 379–87.

58. Yoshida T, *et al*. Prevalence, viral load, and physical status of HPV 16 and 18 in cervical adenosquamous carcinoma. Virchows Arch 2009; 455: 253–9.

59. Look KY, *et al*. An analysis of cell type in patients with surgically staged stage IB carcinoma of the cervix: a Gynecologic Oncology Group study. Gynecol Oncol 1996; 63: 304–11.

60. Farley JH, *et al*. Adenosquamous histology predicts a poor outcome for patients with advanced-stage, but not early-stage, cervical carcinoma. Cancer 2003; 97: 2196–202.

61. Lea JS, *et al*. Adenosquamous histology predicts poor outcome in low-risk stage IB1 cervical adenocarcinoma. Gynecol Oncol 2003; 91: 558–62.

62. Kuroda H, *et al*. Glassy cell carcinoma of the cervix: cytologic features and expression of estrogen receptor, progesterone receptor and Her2/neu protein. Acta Cytol 2006; 50: 418–22.

63. Gray HJ, *et al*. Glassy cell carcinoma of the cervix revisited. Gynecol Oncol 2002; 85: 274–7.

64. Hopkins MP, Morely GW. Glass cell adenocarcinoma of the uterine cervix. Am J Obstet Gynecol 2004; 190: 67–70.

65. Lennerz JK, *et al*. Mucoepidermoid carcinoma of the cervix: another tumor with the t(11;19)-associated CRTC1-MAML2 gene fusion. Am J Surg Pathol 2009; 33: 835–43.

66. Thelmo WL, *et al*. Mucoepidermoid carcinoma of uterine cervix stage IB. Long-term follow-up, histochemical and immunohistochemical study. Int J Gynecol Pathol 1990; 9: 316–24.

67. Grayson W, Taylor LF, Cooper K. Adenoid cystic and adenoid basal carcinoma of the uterine cervix: comparative morphologic, mucin, and immunohistochemical profile of two rare neoplasms of putative 'reserve cell' origin. Am J Surg Pathol 1999; 23: 448–58.

68. Prempree T, Villasanta U, Tang CK. Management of adenoid cystic carcinoma of the uterine cervix (cylindroma): report of six cases and reappraisal of all cases reported in the medical literature. Cancer 1980; 46: 1631–5.

69. King LA, *et al*. Adenoid cystic carcinoma of the cervix in women under age 40. Gynecol Oncol 1989; 32: 26–30.

70. Elhassani LK *et al*. Advanced adenoid cystic carcnoma of the cervix: a case report and review of the literature. Cases J 2009; 2: 6634.

71. Russell MJ, Fadare O. Adenoid basal lesions of the uterine cervix: evolving terminology and clinicopathological concepts. Diagn Pathol 2006; 1: 18.

72. Brainard JA, Hart WR. Adenoid basal epitheliomas of the uterine cervix: a reevaluation of distinctive cervical basaloid lesions currently classified as adenoid basal carcinoma and adenoid basal hyperplasia. Am J Surg Pathol 1998; 22: 965–75.

73. Viswanathan AN, *et al*. Small cell neuroendocrine carcinoma of the cervix: outcome and patterns of recurrence. Gynecol Oncol 2004; 93: 27–33.

74. Chan JK, *et al*. Prognostic factors in neuroendocrine small cell cervical carcinoma: a multivariate analysis. Cancer 2003; 97: 568–74.

75. Chang TC, *et al*. Prognostic factors in surgically treated small cell cervical carcinoma followed by adjuvant chemotherapy. Cancer 1998; 83: 712–18.

76. Hoskins PJ, *et al*. Small-cell carcinoma of the cervix: fourteen years of experience at a single institution using a combined-modality regimen of involved-field irradiation and platinum-based combination chemotherapy. J Clin Oncol 2003; 21: 3495–501.

77. Cohen JG, *et al*. Small cell carcinoma of the cervix: treatment and survival outcomes of 188 patients. Am J Obstet Gynecol 2010; 203: 347.

78. Albores-Saavedra J, *et al*. Carcinoid tumors of the uterine cervix. Cancer 1976; 38: 2328–42.

79. Seidel RJ, Steinfeld A. Carcinoid of the cervix: natural history and implications for therapy. Gynecol Oncol 1988; 30: 114–19.

80. Bansal S *et al*. Sarcma of the cervix: natural history and outcomes. Gynecol Oncol 2010; 118: 134–8.

81. Wright JD, *et al*. Cervical sarcomas: an analysis of incidence and outcome. Gynecol Oncol 2005; 99: 348–51.

82. Clement PB, *et al*. Malignant mullerian mixed tumors of the uterine cervix: a report of nine cases of a neoplasm with morphology often different from its counterpart in the corpus. Int J Gynecol Pathol 1998; 17: 211–22.

83. Bell SW, Kempson RL, Hendrickson MR. Problematic uterine smooth muscle neoplasms. A clinicopathologic study of 213 cases. Am J Surg Pathol 1994; 18: 535–8.

84. Ramos P, *et al*. Mullerian adenosarcoma of the cervix with heterologous elements: report of a case and review of the literature. Gynecol Oncol 2002; 84: 161–6.

85. Toyoshima M, *et al*. Epithelioid leiomyosarcoma of the uterine cervix: a case report and review of the literature. Gynecol Oncol 2005; 97: 957–60.

86. Brand E, *et al*. Rhabdomyosarcoma of the uterine cervix. Sarcoma botryoides. Cancer 1987; 60: 1552–60.

87. Behtash N, *et al*. Embryonal rhabdomyosarcoma of the uterine cervix: case report and review of the literature. Gynecol Oncol 2003; 91: 452–5.

88. Gruessner SE, *et al*. Management of stage I cervical sarcoma botryoides in childhood and adolescence. Eur J Pediatr 2004; 163: 452–6.

89. Bernak KL, *et al*. Embryonal rhabdomyosarcoma (sarcoma botryoides) of the cervix presenting as a cervical polyp treated with fertility-sparing surgery and adjuvant chemotherapy. Gynecol Oncol 2004; 95: 243–6.

90. Karaman E, *et al*. Successful treatment of a very rare case: locally treated cervical rhabdomyosarcoma. Arch Gynecol Obstet 2011; 284(4): 1019–22.

91. Pathak B, *et al*. Granulocytic sarcoma presenting as tumors of the cervix. Gynecol Oncol 2005; 98: 493–7.

92. Chiang YC, Chen CH. Cervical granulocytic sarcoma: report of one case and review of the literaure. Eur J Gynaecol Oncol 2010; 31: 697–700.

93. Cantuaria G, *et al*. Primary malignant melanoma of the uterine cervix: case report and review of the literature. Gynecol Oncol 1999; 75: 170–4.

94. Pusceddu S, *et al*. A literature overview of primary cervical malignant melanoma: an exceedingly rare cancer. Crit Rev Oncol Hematol 2012; 81(2): 185–95.

95. Dursun P, *et al*. Primary cervical lymphoma: report of two cases and review of the literature. Gynecol Oncol 2005; 98: 484–9.

96. Ustaalioglu BB, *et al*. Primary non-Hodgkin lymphoma of cervix successfully treated with rituximab: positron emission tomography images before and after therapy: a case report. Leuk Res 2010; 34: e108–10.

97. Chan JK, *et al*. Clinicopathologic features of six cases primary cervical lymphoma. Am J Obstet Gynecol 2005; 193: 866–72.

98. Snijders-Keilholz A, *et al*. Primitive neuroectodermal tumor of the cervix uteri: a case report – changing concepts of therapy. Gynecol Oncol 2005; 98: 516–19.

99. Roopnarinesingh R, Igoe S, Gillan JE. Choriocarcinoma presenting as a primary lesion of the cervix. Ir Med J 2004; 97: 147–8.

100. Lim SC, *et al*. Mature teratoma of the uterine cervix with lymphoid hyperplasia. Pathol Int 2003; 53: 327–31.

101. Khoor A, *et al*. Mature teratoma of the uterine cervix with pulmonary differentiation. Arch Pathol Lab Med 1995; 119: 848–50.

102. Cortes J, *et al*. Immature teratoma primary of the uterine cervix. First case report. Eur J Gynaecol Oncol 1990; 11: 37–42.

103. Yadav K, *et al*. Endodermal sinus tumor of cervix – case report. Indian J Cancer 1996; 33: 43–5.

104. Maesta I, *et al*. Primary non-gestational choriocarcinoma of the uterine cervix: a case report. Gynecol Oncol 2005; 98: 146–50.

41 Tumors of the Vulva and Vagina

Joshua P. Kesterson[1] and Shashikant B. Lele[2]

[1] Division of Gynecologic Oncology, Penn State Milton S. Hershey Medical Center, Hershey, PA, USA
[2] Division of Gynecologic Oncology, Roswell Park Cancer Institute, Buffalo, NY, USA

Vulvar cancer

Introduction

Cancers of the vulva and vagina are relatively rare, with an estimated 3900 and 2300 cases, respectively, diagnosed in the United States in 2010. These cancers result in approximately 1700 deaths each year.[1] In this chapter we discuss the histological subtypes, clinical presentation, diagnosis, and treatment of these uncommon tumors, with a focus on recent developments (sentinel lymph node [LN] mapping, novel therapeutic agents, etc). As squamous cell carcinoma is the most common type of vulvar and vaginal tumor, the bulk of the chapter will be dedicated to discussion of it. We do not discuss the management of recurrent disease as that is often individualized based on the patient's overall condition, site of recurrence, previous therapy, and expected efficacy of available therapies, resulting in multiple considerations and permutations which are beyond the scope of this chapter.

Squamous cell cancer of the vulva

Epidemiology and pathogenesis

In the United States, there were almost 4000 new cases of vulvar cancer diagnosed in 2010.[1] This is primarily a disease of postmenopausal women but there is a trend toward an earlier age at presentation. One study noted a decrease in the average age at presentation from 69 years to 55 years from 1979 to 1993.[2] Risk factors for developing vulvar cancer include vulvar dystrophy, human papillomavirus (HPV) infection, cigarette smoking, cervical dysplasia and/or cancer, and an immuno-compromised condition.[3] The variety of risk factors highlights the existence of two distinct pathways for the development of vulvar cancer.[4,5] One pathway involves chronic inflammation while the other is related to an infectious etiology, specifically human papillomavirus.[3,4] In fact, a majority of vulvar cancers in younger women contain HPV DNA,[6] with types 16 and 33[5] being most prevalent. Patients with non-HPV-associated

lesions tend to be older nonsmokers, in contrast to their HPV-associated vulvar cancer counterparts. The exact inciting agent, dystrophy or inflammation, in this older patient population is still uncertain. Lichen sclerosus has been implicated in the genesis of non-HPV-associated vulvar cancer. However, in a large pathological review, Hart et al. were unable to identify a transition from lichen sclerosus to vulvar cancer.[7] In contrast, Hording et al. did note a higher incidence of adjacent dystrophic lesions, including lichen sclerosus, in patients with non-HPV keratinizing squamous cell cancer.[4] Regardless, the overall risk of progressing from lichen sclerosus to cancer is thought to be quite low.[8]

Pathology

Squamous cell carcinoma (SCC) is the most common type of vulvar cancer, accounting for over 90% of all vulvar cancer cases. SCC is classically divided into two subtypes: keratinizing type and warty type. The keratinizing type is most often found in elderly women and is not HPV associated. The warty type is predominantly found in younger women and is associated with HPV infection.[2,3] Verrucous carcinoma is a variant of SCC. Grossly, it has a cauliflower-like appearance and is distinguished histologically by papillary fronds at its base without a central connective core. Clinically, it grows slowly and rarely metastasizes.

Clinical presentation

Pruritus and the presence of a mass are the most common presenting symptoms.[6,9] Other frequently described symptoms are bleeding and pain. Less commonly, patients experience dysuria, discharge, or ulceration. Most patients have more than one symptom. Unfortunately, for diverse reasons, there is frequently a delay between the onset of symptoms and diagnosis, often due to a significant interval between the appearance of symptoms and the seeking of medical attention or a delay secondary to medical management for an unbiopsied, presumed benign vulvar lesion. In one series, 18% of patients had

Textbook of Uncommon Cancer, Fourth Edition. Edited by Derek Raghavan, Charles D. Blanke, David H. Johnson, Paul L. Moots, Gregory H. Reaman, Peter G. Rose and Mikkael A. Sekeres.
© 2012 John Wiley & Sons, Inc. Published 2012 by John Wiley & Sons, Inc.

experienced symptoms for over 6 months.[10] More significant is the delay in diagnosis. In this same series, the mean time to diagnosis was 3.9 months.

Vulvar carcinomas are usually unifocal. The lesion can be ulcerative, infiltrative, or exophytic. Therefore it can resemble several benign lesions such as condyloma accuminata, vulvar dystrophy, and Bartholin duct cyst. For these reasons it is recommended that patients who have a vulvar lesion should undergo colposcopy and/or a directed biopsy. It is important to thoroughly examine the vagina, cervix, and anus in addition to the vulva, as other anogenital neoplasms can occur simultaneously.[11]

Staging

Vulvar cancer is surgically staged. Recently, the International Federation of Gynecology and Obstetrics (FIGO) changed the staging system for vulvar cancer.[12] This change was incorporated in order to better reflect prognostic factors. The following changes have been made to the FIGO 1988 staging (Tables 41.1, 41.2):

- tumors involving the vagina and/or urethra with negative lymph node involvement are now stage II
- size of vulvar lesion is omitted for stage II
- the number and morphology of positive lymph nodes are accounted for in the stage III substages
- bilaterality of positive lymph nodes is not mentioned.

This new staging system incorporates the major prognostic factors in vulvar cancer: depth of invasion, number and morphology of nodal involvement, and distant metastasis.[13] The vulvar lesion size is not a part of the staging, in the absence of positive nodes, as the lesion size is of no prognostic significance if lymph nodes are negative for metastasis. In a recent comparison of outcomes based on FIGO 2009 versus FIGO 1988 staging system, Tan et al. demonstrated a difference in survival between those with FIGO 2009 stage IIIA, IIIB, and IIIC, reinforcing the prognostic value of number and morphology of lymph nodes metastases, as incorporated into the FIGO 2009 staging system.[14] Similarly, in a retrospective study of 269 patients with vulvar cancer, van der Steen et al. also found the new 2009 FIGO staging system to be a better indicator of prognosis.[15]

Treatment

The standard initial management of vulvar SCC is surgical. The extent of surgery is dependent upon the size of the lesion, its location, depth of invasion, and risk for lymph node metastasis.

The surgical management has gone through several variations since Basset first proposed an *en bloc* dissection of the vulva and ingino-femoral lymph nodes a century ago.[16] Subsequently, Taussig[17] and Way[18] reported their experiences with a more radical *en bloc* approach. While these methods conferred an improved survival, complications included wound breakdown requiring prolonged hospitalization. Byron et al.,[19] subsequently Ballon and Lamb,[20] reported on their experience performing radical vulvectomies with bilateral inguinal lymphadenectomies via three separate incisions. The three-incision technique resulted in less post-operative

Table 41.1 FIGO 2009 staging of vulvar cancer.

Stage	Description
Stage I	Tumor confined to the vulva
IA	Lesions ≤2 cm in size, confined to the vulva or perineum and with stromal invasion ≤1 mm,* no nodal metastasis
IB	Lesion >2 cm in size or with stromal invasion >1 mm,* confined to the vulva or perineum, with negative nodes
Stage II	Tumor of any size with extension to adjacent perineal structures (lower 1/3 of urethra, lower 1/3 of vagina, anus) with negative nodes
Stage III	Tumor of any size with or without extension to adjacent perineal structures with positive inguinofemoral lymph nodes
IIIA	i. With 1 lymph node metastasis (≥5 mm), or ii. 1–2 lymph node metastases (<5 mm)
IIIB	i. With 2 or more lymph node metastases (≥5 mm), or ii. Three or more lymph node metastases (>5 mm)
IIIC	With positive nodes with extracapsular spread
Stage IV	Tumor invades other regional (upper 2/3 of urethra, upper 2/3 of vagina) or distant structures
IVA	Tumor invades any of the following: i. upper urethral and/or vaginal mucosa, bladder mucosa, rectal mucosa, or fixed to pelvic bone, or ii. fixed or ulcerated inguinofemoral lymph nodes
IVB	Any distant metastasis including pelvic lymph nodes

* The depth of invasion is defined as the measurement of the tumor from the epithelial-stromal junction of the adjacent most superficial dermal papilla to the deepest point of invasion.
Reproduced from Pecorelli et al.[12]

Table 41.2 FIGO 1988 staging of vulvar cancer.

Stage	Description
Stage I	Lesions <2 cm in size confined to the vulva or perineum, no nodal metastasis
IA	Lesions ≤2 cm in size, confined to the vulva or perineum with stromal invasion ≤1 mm,[3] no nodal metastasis
IB	Lesions ≤2 cm in size confined to the vulva or perineum with stromal invasion >1 mm,* no nodal metastasis
Stage II	Tumor >2 cm in largest dimension confined to the vulva or perineum, no nodal metastasis
Stage III	Tumor of any size with adjacent spread to the lower urethra, the vagina, or the anus or with unilateral regional lymph node metastasis
Stage IV	
IVA	Tumor invading any of the following: upper urethra, bladder mucosa, rectal mucosa, pelvic bone or bilateral regional lymph nodes
IVB	Any distant metastasis including pelvic lymph nodes

* The depth of invasion is defined as the measurement of the tumor from the epithelial-stromal junction of the adjacent most superficial dermal papilla to the deepest point of invasion.

morbidity. This approach was further validated in a large series by Hacker et al. where they demonstrated improved wound healing and decreased hospitalization time without compromising survival.[21] The three-incision technique is now standard of care for those with a vulvar lesion warranting a bilateral lymphadenectomy. The necessity of an inguino-femoral lymphadenectomy, ipsilateral or bilateral, is tailored based on the primary vulvar lesion's depth of invasion and location as well as the presence or suggestion of ipsilateral lymph node metastasis.

Surgical management and staging

Patients with lesions with ≤1 mm stromal invasion have a negligible risk of lymph node metastases, and thus do not require a lymphadenectomy and can be cured with wide local excision (WLE) with the goal of a 1.5 cm tumor-free margin.[22–28] Microinvasive tumors are more common in young women with multifocal preinvasive disease, and are frequently associated with HPV infections. Therefore the entire vulva and lower genital tract should be evaluated with colposcopy prior to surgical resection.

For patients with stromal invasion >1 mm, the risk of lymph node metastasis is great enough to warrant an inguinofemoral lymphadenectomy. The risk of lymph node metastasis progressively increases with depth of invasion, from 11% for 1.1–2 mm stromal invasion to 43% with >5 mm stromal invasion.[29] The decision to perform a unilateral versus a bilateral lymphadenectomy is based on results from the Gynecologic Oncologic Group (GOG) study 74 which demonstrated a <1% risk of contralateral node metastasis if the following criteria were met: unifocal lesion more than 1 cm from midline, lesion is not periclitoral, no palpable groin lymphadenopathy bilaterally, and no evidence of lymph node metastases at unilateral lymph node dissection.[30] A vulvar tumor-free margin of at least 1.5 cm should be obtained, as the risk of local recurrence is markedly increased for margins ≤8 mm.[26] The 1.5 cm margin allows for contraction of the surgical specimen following fixation.[23]

The presence of metastatic disease within the lymph nodes is a significant prognostic indicator and dictates adjuvant therapy, however only a minority of patients undergoing an inguinofemoral lymphadenectomy will have positive lymph nodes.[24,31] Considering the lack of benefit from an inguinal lymphadenectomy, with its associated morbidity,[32,33] in women without lymph node metastasis, efforts have been undertaken to both predict the risk of metastatic spread to the draining lymph nodes and to minimize the extent of the lymphadenectomy (e.g. superficial lymphadenectomy, identification of sentinel lymph nodes). Physical examination with palpation of the inguinal area is neither specific nor sensitive.[30,34,35] Similarly, ultrasound-guided fine needle aspiration (FNA) cytology has a high false-negative rate.[36,37]

Investigators from the United Kingdom assessed the accuracy of magnetic resonance imaging (MRI) to predict inguinofemoral lymph node metastasis and concluded that it was accurate in predicting negative nodal status and can be used to identify those who can be spared inguinofemoral lymphadenectomy.[38] However, we would caution against MRI acting as a surrogate for staging surgery. Considering the reported sensitivity of 86%, this would mean that a significant proportion of women with metastatic spread would go undetected by MRI and thus not be offered nodal resection, the most effective modality for staging and possible cure. The role of positron emission tomography (PET) scan is undetermined. In a study of 15 patients from Washington University, the

sensitivity and specificity were not high enough to obviate a nodal dissection.[39] Whilst PET, with its ability to identify hypermetabolic lesions, may be difficult to interpret in vulvar cancer, in that any prior vulvar biopsy may increase metabolic activity in the area, in addition to the fact that completely necrotic tumors may be metabolically inactive.

In the absence of sensitive noninvasive imaging techniques to detect groin metastases and considering the morbidity of an extensive inguinofemoral lymphadenectomy, including alteration in cosmetic and sexual function, local inguinal complications, lymphocyst formation and lower extremity lymphedema,[33,40] investigators have proposed lessening the extent of nodal dissection. In 1979, DiSaia et al. were the first to suggest that a selected superficial groin node dissection would be an adequate assessment of the deeper lymph nodes.[41] Support for this was based on the assumption that lymphatic spread from vulvar carcinomas is first to the superficial inguinal nodes and then to the deep femoral nodes. However, this approach resulted in undertreatment of the nodal disease as 5% of patients experienced a nodal recurrence prior to a central failure. This is likely a product of nonuniform lymphatic spread, whereby femoral node metastases are present in the absence of superficial nodal metastases.[42]

Several subsequent studies have borne out a high rate of groin relapse (5–9%) when only a superficial dissection is employed.[30,43–45] Most impressive is the failure rate of almost 9% presented in the retrospective review of 104 patients treated at MD Anderson.[44] Of these 104 patients who underwent a superficial groin node dissection with negative pathology, nine recurred in one or both groins. Groin recurrences are often fatal.[30,43,44] These high rates of groin recurrence are in stark contrast to the groin recurrence rates of <1% when a full inguinofemoral lymphadenectomy is performed.[28,46,47] The potential for a reduction in postsurgical complication with a less complete nodal dissection cannot be justified in light of an increased risk of the often fatal nodal recurrence.

Sentinal lymph node mapping

Considering the absence of an imaging technique capable of effectively predicting lymph node metastasis, a sentinel lymph node biopsy has been proposed as an alternative to the full inguinofemoral lymph node dissection and its attendant morbidity. The sentinel lymph node is the first node in the lymphatic chain that receives primary lymphatic flow. Sentinel lymph node biopsy has been used with success in patients with breast cancer and melanoma.[48,49] There are two different methods by which to identify the sentinel lymph node, injection of either a blue dye (isosulfan blue or methylene blue) or a radioactive tracer (technetium-99 sulfur colloid).[50–53]

For sentinel lymph node biopsy to be a viable alternative to full lymphadenectomy, the false-negative rate must approach zero so as to avoid the failure to recognize metastatic disease and then unknowingly not treat it. A recent multiinstitutional study from Germany reported a high false-negative rate of 7.7%.[54] All patients with a false-negative sentinel lymph node biopsy had midline vulvar lesions and two of the three patients had lesions ≥4 cm. Also, there were no experience criteria required of the surgeons in the study. Based on this study, the authors concluded that sentinel lymph node biopsy should be performed by experienced teams and limited to women with smaller lesions, not encroaching upon the midline.

While initial studies investigating the safety of sentinel lymph node biopsy incorporated a full inguinofemoral lymphadenectomy immediately following sentinel node assessment, a recent observational trial followed patients with a negative sentinel lymph node study after foregoing a full lymphadenectomy.[31] Two hundred and seventy six patients with vulvar cancers less than 4 cm (a majority unifocal) with negative sentinel lymph node biopsy after identification with blue dye and radioactive tracer were followed every 3 months. At a median follow-up of 35 months, there were eight groin recurrences. Upon review of those recurrences, two patients had only one sentinel lymph node removed when the lymphoscintigram showed two sentinel lymph nodes, two patients had positive lymph nodes at ultrastaging only detected at pathology review, and the other four recurrences were unexplainable. Morbidity, including wound breakdown and cellulitis, was significantly decreased when compared to those with a positive sentinel lymph node who underwent an inguinofemoral lymphadenectomy.

These studies highlight several important points regarding sentinel lymph node detection. First and foremost, patient selection is critical. Ideal candidates are those with unifocal lesions less than 4 cm with clinically negative inguinal lymph nodes. Second, a team skilled in the techniques of sentinel lymph node detection as well as experienced pathologists are necessary. These factors must be considered in the context of the relative rarity of vulvar cancer in the United States, thus making it difficult for many gynecological oncologists to acquire enough experience. The stakes are high in that a groin failure is often fatal.

Radiotherapy

Postoperative radiation therapy (RT) has a role for patients with certain risk factors. We do not advocate primary radiation therapy for the treatment of vulvar cancer, except in rare cases where the patient is not a candidate for surgery and/or anesthesia. Consideration should be given to radiation for close or positive surgical margins, if surgical reexcision is not possible, secondary to the risk of local recurrence. The role of adjuvant RT for patients with high-risk lesions, with nodes negative for metastatic disease, is not known as results from the GOG trial 145 are pending. Enthusiasm for any expected beneficial effect from radiation in this particular population may be tempered by a recent trial from The Netherlands which failed to show a benefit for adjuvant radiotherapy in patients with one intracapsular nodal metastasis.[55] Of note, that trial contained patients with high-risk characteristics (i.e. tumor size >4 cm and lymphvascular space invasion).

For patients who have received an adequate lymphadenectomy with only one positive lymph node, adjuvant RT can be omitted as its addition does not improve survival.[55,56] While this remains the accepted standard, one might exercise caution extrapolating from these data to include patients who receive

only a superficial lymphadenectomy. As discussed previously, even with a negative nodal assessment, these patients have a high groin failure rate likely due to unresected deeper positive groin nodes. Denying adjuvant radiation to patients with one pelvic lymph node positive after a superficial dissection based on data obtained from a full inguinal pelvic lymphadenectomy may lead to undertreatment. Adjuvant RT is generally recommended for patients with ≥ 2 microscopically positive lymph nodes, ≥ 1 macroscopically involved lymph node, extracapsular spread or a limited lymph node sampling.[57] A smaller lymph node yield may be an inverse marker for residual positive nodal tissue. This is in part supported by a recent analysis by Parthasarathy *et al.* using the Surveillance, Epidemiology, and End Results (SEER) database, in which they demonstrated that women with ≤ 12 lymph nodes removed showed a survival benefit for RT (77% vs. 55%).[56] The implication is that there was residual disease unresected which benefited from further therapy.

Chemoradiation

Chemoradiation has been proposed in the neoadjuvant setting as a means by which to lessen the extent of surgery for those with locally advanced or inoperable patients. The efficacy of radiation sensitizers (cisplatin, 5-fluorouracil [FU] used in cervical cancer treatment has influenced the choice of agents used in vulvar cancer. The GOG conducted a trial in which women with stage III and IV SCC of the vulva were initially treated with cisplatin and 5-FU with concurrent radiation therapy, followed by surgical resection plus bilateral inguinofemoral lymph node dissection.[58] The efficacy of this regimen is demonstrated by the complete clinical response in 47% of patients, with only two of 71 (2.8%) patients having residual, unresectable disease. Urine and stool continence was maintained in a majority of patients. This approach is not without complications, including moist desquamation, wound complications, sepsis, fistulas, and death. In a Cochrane review of five studies in which patients were treated with neoadjuvant chemotherapy followed by surgical resection, the authors noted the lack of uniformity with regard to chemoradiation schedules, the significant side-effects, including almost universal skin toxicity, as well as wound breakdown, infection, and lymphedema.[59] They concluded that "with the current knowledge neoadjuvant chemotherapy is not justified in patients with tumours that can be adequately treated with radical vulvectomy and bilateral groin node dissection alone."

Chemotherapy

The lack of effective chemotherapy for patients with either unresectable recurrent disease or widespread metastases is borne out in their dismal 5-year overall survival. Historically, these tumors have been considered chemoresistant. However, more recently, large European Organization for Research and Treatment of Cancer (EORTC) trials have revealed encouraging response rates of 64% and 56% in patients with advanced or recurrent disease using bleomycin, methotrexate, and CCNU.[60,61] The combination therapy resulted in a median progression-free survival (PFS) of almost 5 months.[25] In another EORTC study with the Gynecologic Cancer Society, of patients with advanced vulvar cancer treated with paclitaxel, they noted only a 14% overall response rate, for a median PFS of 2.6 months.[62] This is similar to the 3.2-month median PFS seen with single-agent mitoxantrone.[63] It appears that combination chemotherapy results in improved response rates but overall survival is still poor. Newer agents are desperately needed. There are case reports of clinical responses with erlotinib[64] and cetuximab.[65]

Melanoma of the vulva

Melanoma constitutes the second most common malignant tumor of the vulva. It represents 5–10% of all malignant vulvar tumors.[66,67] This tumor frequently affects postmenopausal white women. The median age at diagnosis is 68–70 years of age.[68] Vulvar melanomas are classified into three categories: superficial spreading melanoma, nodular melanoma, and acral lentiginous melanoma. Acral lentiginous melanoma is the most common histological type.

Clinical presentation

Presenting symptoms for vulvar melanoma include pruritus, bleeding, and ulceration.[67] A majority of lesions originate on the labia minora, clitoris, or inner portion of the labia majora. Vulvar melanomas are characterized by a clinically aggressive course with a tendency for local recurrence and distant metastases. This may be due in part to the prominent lymphatic and vascular network of the vulva, delay in diagnosis, and subsequent poor outcome due to ineffective therapies. In fact, malignant melanoma of the urogenital tract is associated with the lowest five year survival (11%) of all malignant melanomas.[69]

Staging

There are several staging systems for vulvar melanomas, including those based on tumor depth of invasion as proposed by Clark et al.,[70] Chung et al.,[71] and Breslow.[72] Alternatively, there are the classic FIGO vulvar staging criteria which take into account lesion size, regional, and metastatic spread. However, the system most predictive of disease-free survival appears to be the American Joint Committee on Cancer (AJCC) melanoma staging system. The AJCC system (Table 41.3) takes into account tumor size, presence of ulceration, depth of invasion, lymph node status, and distant metastases, as well as serum lactic dehydrogenase (LDH) level.[73]

Surgical management

Historically, the initial surgical management for vulvar melanoma has been a radical *en bloc* resection with inguinofemoral lymphadenectomy. However, as radical surgery has failed to improve survival,[74] the goal now is to individualize therapy with a focus on more conservative surgery,[67] including avoidance of routine lymphadenectomy as several trials have shown no survival benefit with lymph node dissection in cutaneous melanoma.[75–78] Treatment should be dictated by depth of primary tumor invasion and lymph node status. Thin tumors (less than 1 mm) rarely involve regional lymph nodes and have an excellent prognosis. Therefore, for tumors ≤1 mm thick, a WLE with a 1 cm circumferential and 1 cm deep margin is recommended[79] with sentinel lymph node (SLN) biopsy if there are any suspicious lesions on clinical exam or imaging. For deeper lesions with or without ulceration, a 2 cm surgical margin should be obtained with bilateral SLN sampling.[75] For patients with positive sentinel lymph nodes, a complete groin lymphadenectomy is warranted. If sentinel lymph nodes are positive for metastatic disease bilaterally or if the vulvar lesion is centrally located, then a bilateral lymphadenectomy is warranted. For patients with lymph node metastases, adjuvant therapy is warranted. For patients with metastatic disease, a wide local resection should be attempted for the primary vulvar tumor, with further therapy, including the aggressiveness of surgery, lymphadenectomy, resection of metastatic lesions, and addition of individualized adjuvant therapies.

Immunotherapy
Interferon-α

Interferon (IFN)-α is a cytokine with immunomodulating effects. In prior clinical trials it has shown improvement in PFS in patients with metastatic cutaneous melanoma.[80,81] IFN-α has been used in patients with vulvovaginal melanoma. Harting and Kim examined the clinical efficacy of biochemotherapy, including IFN-α, in women with advanced vulvovaginal melanoma.[82] They reported a 36% overall response rate, with a median overall survival of 10 months from the start of therapy. Adverse effects of IFN-α include myelosuppression, fatigue, depression, and thyroid dysfunction. The decision to use IFN-α must be individualized with consideration given to the risk:benefit ratio, considering its toxicity and expected 20–30% improvement in overall survival in cutaneous melanoma trials, but limited testing in vulvar melanoma.[83,84]

Interleukin-2

Interleukin (IL)-2 is a T cell growth factor and a potent inducer of cytokines IL-1, tumor necrosis factor (TNF), and IFN-α. It has been used on a small scale in patients with metastatic melanoma and while response rates have been poor overall (<20%), those who have responded have experienced prolonged periods of remission.[85,86] Toxic effects include hypotension, cardiac dysrhythmias, pulmonary edema, fever, sepsis, and death.[87] The significant toxicity has limited the use of IL-2 on a widespread basis.

Ipilimumab

Ipilimumab is a monoclonal antibody against CTLA-4, which acts as an inhibitor of an activated immune response. By blocking CTLA-4, ipilimumab allows for a robust, uninhibited immune response against tumor. The responses seen with this monoclonal antibody are different from those seen with cytotoxic therapy in that initially, there may be a worsening of disease before tumor response, responses may take longer to achieve, and responses, although clinically significant, may not be classified as a response by Response Evaluation Solid Tumors (RECIST) criteria.[88] Recently, investigators reported on 676 HLA-specific patients with unresectable stage II or IV melanoma who had received prior cytotoxic chemotherapy or IL-2, who were randomized to receive ipilimumab or a vaccine.[89] They noted an overall survival of 10 months for the group receiving ipilimumab which was almost 4 months

Table 41.3 TNM staging categories for cutaneous melanoma.

Classification

T	Thickness (mm)	Ulceration status/mitoses
Tis	NA	NA
T1	≤1.00	a: Without ulceration and mitosis $<1/mm^2$
		b: With ulceration or mitoses $\geq 1/mm^2$
T2	1.01–2.00	a: Without ulceration
		b: With ulceration
T3	2.01–4.00	a: Without ulceration
		b: With ulceration
T4	>4.00	a: Without ulceration
		b: With ulceration
N	**No. of metastatic nodes**	**Nodal metastatic burden**
N0	0	NA
N1	1	a: Micrometatasis*
		b: Macrometasis†
N2	2–3	a: Micrometatasis*
		b: Macrometasis†
		c: In transit metasteses/satellites without metastatic nodes
N3	4+ metastatic nodes, or matted nodes, or in transit metastases/satellites with metastatic nodes	
M	**Site**	**Serum LDH**
M0	No distant metastases	NA
M1a	Distant skin, subcutaneous, or nodal metastases	Normal
M1b	Lung metastases	Normal
M1c	All other visceral metastases	Normal
	Any distant metastases	Elevated

NA, not applicable; LDH, lactate dehydrogenase.

* Micrometastases are diagnosed after sentinel lymph node biopsy

† Macrometastases are defined as clinically detectable nodal metastases confirmed pathologically.

Anatomic stage groupings for cutaneous melanoma

	Clinical staging*				Pathologic staging‡		
	T	N	M		T	N	M
0	Tis	N0	M0	0	Tis	N0	M0
IA	T1a	N0	M0	IA	T1a	N0	M0
IB	T1b	N0	M0	IB	T1b	N0	M0
	T2a	N0	M0		T2a	N0	M0
IIA	T2a	N0	M0	IIA	T2b	N0	M0
	T3a	N0	M0		T3a	N0	M0
IIB	T3b	N0	M0	IIB	T3b	N0	M0
	T4a	N0	M0		T4a	N0	M0
IIC	T4b	N0	M0	IIC	T4b	N0	M0
III	Any T	N>N0	M0	IIIA	T1-4a	N1a	M0
					T1-4a	N2a	M0
				IIIB	T1-4b	N1a	M0
					T1-4b	N2a	M0
					T1-4a	N1b	M0
					T1-4a	N2b	M0
					T1-4a	N2c	M0
				IIIC	T1-4b	N1b	M0
					T1-4b	N2b	M0
					T1-4b	N2c	M0
					Any T	N3	M0
IV	Any T	Any N	M1	IV	Any T	Any N	M1

* Clinical staging includes microstaging of the primary melanoma and clinical/radiographic evaluation for metastases.

‡ Pathologic staging includes microstaging of the primary melanoma and pathologic information about the regional lymph nodes after partial or complete lymphadenectomy. Pathologic stage 0 or IA patients do not require pathologic evaluation of their lymph nodes.

Source: Balch *et al.* J Clin Oncol 2009: 27: 6199–6206.

longer than for patients treated with the vaccine against the melanosomal protein, glycoprotein 100 (gp100). Grade 3 or 4 immune-related toxicity was experienced by 10–15% of patients treated with ipilimumab, including several resultant deaths. The long-term survival rates for ipilimumab monotherapy are encouraging, with 1- and 2-year survival rates of 46% and 24%, respectively, which compares favorably to the survival rates from prior trials with similar patient populations treated with various agents. Ipilimumab does appear to have a role in the treatment of chemotherapy-refractory malignant melanoma, although the side-effects may be limiting.

Targeted therapies

Secondary to the rarity of vulvar melanoma, most of the data concerning targeted therapies are based on cutaneous melanoma. Several agents show promise. Imatinib and sunitinib, tyrosine kinase inhibitors (TKI), have shown clinical activity in patients with metastatic mucosal melanoma who had c-kit mutations.[88,90] All TKIs may not have similar applicability. For example, sorafenib, which targets the RAS-RAF pathway, may not be effective in vulvar melanomas as they have a lower frequency of NRAS and BRAF mutations, in contrast to their sun-exposed cutaneous melanoma counterparts.[91,92] Other targeted agents such as temsirolimus (mTOR inhibitor), thalidomide (antiangiogenic, immunomodulator), and bortezomib (proteasome inhibitor) have not shown activity in metastatic melanoma.[93–95] More recently, the combination of bevacizumab with paclitaxel and carboplatin has shown promising response rates.[96] Bcl-2 antisense (oblimersen) with dacarbazine resulted in a small but statistically significant improvement in PFS when compared to dacarbazine alone (2.6 versus 1.6 months, $p < 0.001$).[97]

Basal cell carcinoma

Basal cell carcinoma (BCC) is the most common malignant neoplasm in humans,[98] but BCC of the vulva is relatively uncommon, accounting for approximately 2–4% of vulvar malignancies.[99–101] Exposure to ultraviolet light is the main risk factor for sun-exposed BCCs, but the exact etiology of BCC in nonsun-exposed areas such as the vulva is unknown. These patients may have genetic predispositions, similar to that seen in basal cell nevus syndrome patients who have increased susceptibility to BCC.[102] Most tumors are diagnosed in the postmenopausal woman. While often asymptomatic, frequent symptoms include pruritus or a palpable nodule. Lesions may be ulcerated and their color may range from darkly pigmented to gray to pearly. Lesions are often misdiagnosed, including as eczema, psoriasis, vascular lesions, and melanocytic nevi. A delay in diagnosis, secondary to being asymptomatic, nonvisualization of the area, patient hesitation to consult a healthcare provider or misdiagnosis with subsequent mistreatment with medical therapy, allows the neoplasm to grow (average size 2.1 cm) and frequently ulcerate.[103] Treatment of BCC of the vulva is WLE, with care taken to ensure negative resection margins. Metastases are very rare, thus obviating the need for a lymphadenectomy.

Bartholin gland carcinoma

The Bartholin glands drain mucin, via two small ducts located at the 4 and 8 o'clock positions of the vaginal orifice, just below the hymenal ring. Cancers arising in the Bartholin gland are rare, accounting for 4–7% of all vulvar cancers.[104–106] Cancer may arise within the gland itself or within the duct. The most common histological subtypes are adenocarcinoma and squamous cell carcinoma. Patients usually present with a painless vulvar mass. The median age at diagnosis is 50 years.[105] As cancers of the Bartholin gland are more common in postmenopausal women,[106] women more than 40 years of age presenting with a Bartholin cyst should have it biopsied. Initial management consists of WLE of the primary tumor with ipsilateral lymphadenectomy with selective adjuvant radiation therapy, for positive margins or lymphatic involvement. Bilateral inguinofemoral lymph node dissection may be warranted for larger lesions, encroaching on the midline.[104,105] Five-year survival ranges from 56% to 84%, with survival being stage dependent.[104,105,107,108]

Sarcomas of the vulva

Sarcomas of the vulva are exceptionally rare, accounting for only 1–2% of all vulvar malignancies. Different subtypes include leiomyosarcoma, rhabdomyosarcoma, liposarcoma, angiosarcoma, neurofibrosarcoma, fibrous histiocytoma, and epithelioid sarcoma. Leiomyosarcoma is the most common sarcoma of the vulva. Information regarding the more rare subtypes of vulvar sarcoma is limited to case reports and small case series. Most patients present with a painful mass in the labia majora or Bartholin gland area.

Leiomyosarcoma

Leiomyosarcoma is the most common sarcoma of the vulva. These tumors are frequently larger than 5 cm. Histologically, they are composed of interlacing spindle-shaped cells; epithelioid cells can also be present. Diagnostic criteria include three or more of the following: mitotic count of ≥5 mitoses per 10 high-power fields, infiltrating border, cytological atypia, and size ≥5 cm in greatest diameter.[109] Initial treatment includes surgical resection with adjuvant radiation for high-grade tumors or for positive surgical margins.[110] There is no indication for lymph node dissection. The role of adjuvant therapy is unclear. It has not been shown to improve survival. In advanced or recurrent disease the response rate to systemic chemotherapy is low.

Rare types of vulvar carcinoma

Other histological vulvar types include verrucous, Kaposi sarcoma, metastatic disease (endometrium, ovary, cervix, breast, kidney, urethra, and lymphoma), lymphoma, and Merckel cell carcinoma. The evidence base in these tumors is limited and the basis for treatment decisions is often anecdotal. In general, these lesions are excised with wide margins. The role of lymphadenectomy is undefined.

Vaginal cancer

Squamous cell cancer

Primary tumors of the vagina are the least common gynecological malignancy, accounting for approximately 2300 new cases annually in the United States, with 780 resultant deaths.[1] SCC is the most common subtype. The risk factors for SCC of the vagina are the same as for SCC of the cervix, including multiple lifetime sexual partners, early age at sexual debut, and tobacco smoking. The etiology for most cases of vaginal cancer is HPV infection.[111] However, the risk of progression from HPV infection to malignancy is less than that of cervical cancer, secondary to the cervix's persistent metaplasia, in marked excess of the relatively stable vaginal epithelium.[112]

Most patients present with vaginal bleeding. A fifth of patients will be asymptomatic, with their disease detected via exam and/or Pap smear.[113,114] A large percentage of women have undergone a prior hysterectomy.[113] The mean age at diagnosis is 60–65 years.[115] Most tumors arise within the posterior, upper third of the vagina. Diagnosis is by biopsy of the suspicious lesion, found at routine exam or identified during colposcopic evaluation, with care taken to exam the entire vagina, including the posterior portion, which is often obscured by the speculum blades. Lesions may be an exophytic mass, plaque-like, or ulcerative. Consideration must be given to ruling out a coexisting or recurrent malignancy as gynecological malignancies are common in this patient population, including cervical cancer.

Vaginal cancer, like cervical cancer, is staged clinically using the FIGO staging system[116] (Table 41.4). Disease confined to the vagina is stage I, disease beyond the vagina but not to the pelvic sidewall is stage II, tumor extending to the sidewall is classified as stage III, while tumor extending to the bladder or rectum, or the presence of distant metastases is stage IV.[116] A quarter of patients will present with disease confined to the vagina, while almost 40% of cases will have spread to the paravaginal tissues at diagnosis. The remaining cases will either be regionally advanced or metastatic (stage III [24%], stage IV [13%]). The FIGO staging system is an accurate predictor of survival, with 5-year survival ranging from 78% for those with stage I disease to 13% for those with distant metastases (Table 41.5).[117] Vaginal cancer spreads via several routes: contiguous extension, hematogenous spread, lymphatic spread. Secondary to the rich lymphatic drainage of the vagina, nodal sites at greatest risk for metastasis vary with the site of primary tumor. Lesions at the upper portion of the vagina most often metastasize to the pelvic and paraaortic lymph nodes, while lesions located at the distal portion of the vagina preferentially metastasize initially to the inguinofemoral lymph nodes.

Treatment
Early and regional disease
Secondary to its rarity and the lack of randomized controlled trials, there is no standard therapy for SCC of the vagina. Treatment should be individualized based on stage, tumor size, and tumor location, all of prognostic significance,[118] as well as

Table 41.4 FIGO staging of vaginal cancer.

Stage	Description
Stage I	Tumor confined to vagina
Stage II	Tumor invades paravaginal tissues but not to pelvic wall
Stage III	Tumor extends to pelvic wall and/or pelvic or inguinal lymph node metastasis
Stage IVA	Tumor invades mucosa of the bladder or rectum and/or extends beyond the true pelvis
Stage IVB	Distant metastasis

Reproduced from Benedet et al.[116]

Table 41.5 Five-year survival per FIGO stage for women with vaginal cancer.

Stage	Five-year survival
I	77.6%
II	52.2%
III	42.5%
IVA	20.5%
IVB	13%

Reproduced from Beller et al.[117]

any antecedent pelvic radiation. Patients with stage I disease, with small lesions in the upper third of the vagina, can be treated with either surgery (radical hysterectomy, upper vaginectomy, and bilateral pelvic lymph node dissection) or intracavitary radiation therapy.[119] In their review of 84 patients with vaginal cancer, a majority treated with initial surgical resection with selected radiation, Tjalma et al. reported a 5-year survival of 91% for patients with stage I disease.[118] In a report of 89 patients with early-stage vaginal cancer treated at the Mayo Clinic, the 5-year survival for patients with stage I disease was 82%, with no difference in survival based on treatment with surgery, surgery plus radiation, or radiation alone.[120] Lesions located in the lower third of the vagina are often treated with radiation therapy to the lesion as well as the inguinal lymph nodes,[121] although radical vulvectomy with lymphadenectomy may be similarly efficacious.[120,122]

Recent evidence suggests that neoadjuvant chemotherapy may have a role in the treatment of early-stage vaginal cancer. Investigators from Italy, in a treatment approach extrapolated from the cervical cancer literature, reported their experience with 11 patients with stage II vaginal cancer, who were treated with three cycles of cisplatin and paclitaxel followed by a radical hysterectomy with vaginectomy.[123] At a median follow-up of 75 months, nine patients were alive without evidence of disease. While encouraging, these results are still considered preliminary and this approach has not been compared to other treatment modalities. However, the use of neoadjuvant chemotherapy may be another treatment option in certain vaginal cancer patients with paravaginal involvement. At present, we recommend initial surgical management of early-stage SCC of the vagina, with selective adjuvant therapy for high-risk features. While there are no prospective trials comparing adjuvant radiation versus radiation plus cisplatin, based on the similar cell type and etiology of vaginal cancer and cervical cancer, we recommend the addition of cisplatin to radiation therapy.[124,125]

Metastatic vaginal squamous cell cancer

Therapy for women with widespread metastatic vaginal cancer is inadequate, with disappointing results. Experience with chemotherapy regimens is limited to case series and phase 2 trials. Eligible patients should be offered enrolment in clinical trials investigating novel agents. Radiation therapy can be utilized for symptom palliation.

Adenocarcinoma

Primary vaginal adenocarcinoma is an uncommon neoplasm, representing less than 5% of vaginal cancers. However, a variant, clear cell adenocarcinoma (CCA) of the vagina, warrants special attention. A majority of cases of CCA of the vagina are linked to maternal diethylstibestrol (DES) ingestion during pregnancy.

Diethylstilbestrol is a nonsteroidal estrogen, which readily crosses the placenta. It was initially used in the treatment of postmenopausal symptoms and then as a means to prevent spontaneous abortions and preterm birth. Subsequently, it was found to be a transplacental carcinogen after it was linked to vaginal clear cell carcinoma in female offspring exposed *in utero*, prompting the FDA to issue a bulletin in 1971 warning against its use.[126]

The absolute risk of developing vaginal CCA after DES exposure is quite small, approximately one in 1000,[127] but this does represent an increased relative risk compared to the general population.[128] The greatest risk is seen in women exposed to DES in the first trimester. CCA is thought to arise within vaginal adenosis, present in a third of women exposed to DES *in utero*. The peak incidence of CCA secondary to DES exposure occurred in the late 1970s.[127] Since then there has been a decrease in its incidence, with 33 and 23 cases new cases diagnosed in the United States in 1990 and 1991, respectively.[129]

Clinical presentation

Grossly, the lesions have a polypoid appearance, most commonly on the anterior vaginal wall. A majority of cases are stage I at presentation. Most cases occur between 15 to 27 years of age, with a median of 19 years.[127] However, recent reports suggest that non-CCA can occur also in older DES-exposed patients.[130] Some authors have identified a second peak during the eighth decade of life.[131] In addition, late recurrences of CCA have been reported.[132] For this reason long-term surveillance of DES-exposed women is warranted.

Treatment

Any treatment needs to take into account the tumor size and location, patient's age, desire for fertility, implications of potentially disfiguring surgery, site of potential metastatic spread, and historical outcomes. In a review of 219 cases of stage I vaginal CCA, Senekjian *et al.* reported a 5-year survival of 92%. They compared outcomes for different therapy modalities, including "conventional therapy" which consisted of (1) total vaginectomy, radical hysterectomy, pelvic lymphadenectomy, (2) radiation therapy, or (3) a combination thereof, with those for "local therapy" which included local excision with or without radiation.[133] There was no difference in overall survival between the two groups. There also was no difference in the risk of recurrence between those treated with conventional therapy and those treated with local therapy. However, there was a statistically significant reduction in recurrence for those treated with local excision with radiation therapy, compared to those treated with local excision only. Eight of 41 patients treated with localized therapy became pregnant.

Vaginal melanoma

Primary vaginal melanoma is remarkably rare, accounting for 4–5% of all vaginal cancers. Considering that there were an estimated 2300 new cases of vaginal cancer diagnosed in 2010, this would mean that there are only around 100 cases of vaginal melanoma diagnosed in the United States each year.[1,134] These cancers are thought to arise from vaginal melanocytes, present in 3% of adult females.[135] Vaginal melanoma occurs primarily in postmenopausal white women.[134,136–138] Most women present with vaginal bleeding.[137] On examination, the lesion is most often in the distal third of the vagina[139] and may appear as a darkly pigmented mass or ulceration. It is important to realize that a vaginal melanoma may also be nonpigmented.

Outcomes for vaginal melanoma are significantly worse than those of their squamous cell counterparts, with 5-year survival rates less than 20%.[137,139–143] Tumor size appears to predict survival. In a metaanalysis of patients with vaginal melanoma, those with tumor size <3 cm survived 41 months, compared to 12 months for those with tumors ≥3 cm.[144] Interestingly, tumor thickness did not predict survival.

While surgery continues to be the mainstay of initial therapy, the extent of that surgery is a source of debate. In their review of long-term survivors, Buchanan *et al.* did not demonstrate any difference in survival between those undergoing wide excision, radical surgery, radiation therapy, and wide excision with radiation therapy.[144] This is in contrast to a recent study by Frumovitz *et al.* which reported a significantly longer survival for those treated surgically.[137] However, 5-year recurrence-free survival and overall survival rates were only 9.5% and 20%, respectively. The role of surgery and/or radiation needs to be appreciated in the context of their both being localized therapies, effective for unifocal, confined disease; however, vaginal melanomas recur distally most of the time, most often in the lungs and liver.

Considering its inherent morbidity and disfigurement, without a proven survival benefit, we do not advocate radical surgery for the treatment of vaginal melanoma, but rather local excision. The dismal survival rates and propensity for distal recurrence highlight the need for targeted therapies for this rare disease, including tyrosine kinase inhibitors, antiangiogenics, and monoclonal antibodies.[145,146]

Vaginal sarcoma

There are four major types of rhabdomyosarcoma (RMS): leiomyomatous, embryonal, alveolar, and undifferentiated.

Embryonal rhabdomyosarcoma is the most common malignant tumor of the vagina in the pediatric population. Most tumors are diagnosed before the age of 5 but adult cases have been reported.[147] The botryoid variant, as its name implies, presents with an appearance similar to a bunch of grapes. Sarcoma botryoides presents almost exclusively in infants. Other common symptoms of vaginal RMS are vaginal bleeding and discharge.

The genesis of embryonal rhabdomyosarcoma may be a loss of heterozygosity at the 11p15 chromosome locus, which is the site of the insulin-like growth factor (IGF) II gene.[148,149] IGF-II has been shown to stimulate tumor growth *in vitro*.[150] Additionally, several metabolic pathway aberrations have been implicated in the development of rhabdomyoscarcoma.[151]

Treatment for vaginal RMS is extrapolated from the trials conducted by the Intergroup Rhabdomyosarcoma Study Group (IRSG). Vaginal RMS is treated with multimodality therapy, including surgery, chemotherapy, and RT. Vaginal RMS responds well to initial multiagent chemotherapy.[152,153] The need for adjuvant surgery is dictated by residual disease.

Conclusion

Primary tumors of the vulva and vagina are rare entities with varied histological subtypes, with similarities limited only to their pattern of presentation and spread pattern, thus limiting our ability to broadly categorize them and make generalized statements. Treatment for these uncommon malignancies is predicated on histological cell type and presence of tumor spread beyond the site of origin. In general, surgical excision is the mainstay of initial therapy, with surgical staging performed based on the risk of metastatic spread and any therapeutic benefit it may tender. Optimal therapy for some of the more common tumors, e.g. squamous cell cancer, is based on Level I evidence generated from large, prospective clinical trials, whereby therapy for relatively rarer tumors must be extrapolated from historical case series, phase 1 and 2 trials, and expert opinion. Future research is needed to identify novel agents capable of generating clinically meaningful responses for chemotherapy-refractory and/or recurrent disease.

References

1. Jemal A, Siegel R, Xu J, Ward E. Cancer statistics, 2010. CA Cancer J Clin 2010; 60: 277–300.
2. Messing MJ, Gallup DG. Carcinoma of the vulva in young women. Obstet Gynecol 1995; 86: 51–4.
3. Madsen BS, Jensen HL, van den Brule AJ, Wohlfahrt J, Frisch M. Risk factors for invasive squamous cell carcinoma of the vulva and vagina – population-based case–control study in Denmark. Int J Cancer 2008; 122: 2827–34.
4. Hording U, Junge J, Daugaard S, Lundvall F, Poulsen H, Bock JE. Vulvar squamous cell carcinoma and papillomaviruses: indications for two different etiologies. Gynecol Oncol 1994; 52: 241–6.
5. Kurman RJ, Trimble CL, Shah KV. Human papillomavirus and the pathogenesis of vulvar carcinoma. Curr Opin Obstet Gynecol 1992; 4: 582–5.
6. Trimble CL, Hildesheim A, Brinton LA, Shah KV, Kurman RJ. Heterogeneous etiology of squamous carcinoma of the vulva. Obstet Gynecol 1996; 87: 59–64.
7. Hart WR, Norris HJ, Helwig EB. Relation of lichen sclerosus et atrophicus of the vulva to development of carcinoma. Obstet Gynecol 1975; 45: 369–77.
8. Carlson JA, *et al.* Vulvar lichen sclerosus and squamous cell carcinoma: a cohort, case control, and investigational study with historical perspective; implications for chronic inflammation and sclerosis in the development of neoplasia. Hum Pathol 1998; 29: 932–48.
9. Rosen C, Malmstrom H. Invasive cancer of the vulva. Gynecol Oncol 1997; 65: 213–7.
10. Rhodes CA, Cummins C, Shafi MI. The management of squamous cell vulval cancer: a population based retrospective study of 411 cases. Br J Obstet Gynaecol 1998; 105: 200–5.
11. Mitchell MF, Prasad CJ, Silva EG, Rutledge FN, McArthur MC, Crum CP. Second genital primary squamous neoplasms in vulvar carcinoma: viral and histopathologic correlates. Obstet Gynecol 1993; 81: 13–8.
12. Pecorelli S. Revised FIGO staging for carcinoma of the vulva, cervix, and endometrium. Int J Gynaecol Obstet 2009; 105: 103–4.
13. Mutch DG. The new FIGO staging system for cancers of the vulva, cervix, endometriuma and sarcomas. Gynecol Oncol 2009; 115: 325–8.
14. Tan J CN, *et al.* Applying the FIGO 2009 staging system for carcinoma of the vulva to patients previously staged with the FIGO 1988 staging system. Gynecol Oncol 2010; 116: S21–22.
15. Van der Steen S, de Nieuwenhof HP, Massuger L, Bulten J, de Hullu JA. New FIGO staging system of vulvar cancer indeed provides a better reflection of prognosis. Gynecol Oncol 2010; 119: 520–5.
16. A B. Traitement chirurgical operatoire de l'epithelioma primitif du clitoris indications-technique-resultats. Rev Chir 1912; 46: 645.
17. Taussig F. Cancer of the vulva. An analysis of 155 cases. Am J Obstet Gynecol 1940; 40: 764.
18. Way S. The anatomy of the lymphatic drainage of the vulva and its influence on the radical operation for carcinoma. Ann R Coll Surg Engl 1948; 3: 187–209.
19. Byron RL, Jr., Mishell DR, Jr., Yonemoto RH. The surgical treatment of invasive carcinoma of the vulva. Surg Gynecol Obstet 1965; 121: 1243–51.
20. Ballon SC, Lamb EJ. Separate inguinal incisions in the treatment of carcinoma of the vulva. Surg Gynecol Obstet 1975; 140: 81–4.
21. Hacker NF, Leuchter RS, Berek JS, Castaldo TW, Lagasse LD. Radical vulvectomy and bilateral inguinal lymphadenectomy through separate groin incisions. Obstet Gynecol 1981; 58: 574–9.
22. Farias-Eisner R, *et al.* Conservative and individualized surgery for early squamous carcinoma of the vulva: the treatment of choice for stage I and II (T1-2 N0-1 M0) disease. Gynecol Oncol 1994; 53: 55–8.
23. Gotlieb WH. The assessment and surgical management of early-stage vulvar cancer. Best Pract Res Clin Obstet Gynaecol 2003; 17: 557–69.
24. Hacker NF, Berek JS, Lagasse LD, Leuchter RS, Moore JG. Management of regional lymph nodes and their prognostic influence in vulvar cancer. Obstet Gynecol 1983; 61: 408–12.
25. Magrina JF, *et al.* Squamous cell carcinoma of the vulva stage IA: long-term results. Gynecol Oncol 2000; 76: 24–7.
26. Heaps JM, Fu YS, Montz FJ, Hacker NF, Berek JS. Surgical-pathologic variables predictive of local recurrence in squamous cell carcinoma of the vulva. Gynecol Oncol 1990; 38: 309–14.
27. Oonk MH, Hollema H, de Hullu JA, van der Zee AG. Prediction of lymph node metastases in vulvar cancer: a review. Int J Gynecol Cancer 2006; 16: 963–71.
28. Sedlis A, *et al.* Positive groin lymph nodes in superficial squamous cell vulvar cancer. A Gynecologic Oncology Group Study. Am J Obstet Gynecol 1987; 156: 1159–64.
29. Hacker NF, Berek JS, Lagasse LD, Nieberg RK, Leuchter RS. Individualization of treatment for stage I squamous cell vulvar carcinoma. Obstet Gynecol 1984; 63: 155–62.
30. Stehman FB, Bundy BN, Dvoretsky PM, Creasman WT. Early stage I carcinoma of the vulva treated with ipsilateral superficial inguinal lymphadenectomy and modified radical hemivulvectomy: a prospective study of the Gynecologic Oncology Group. Obstet Gynecol 1992; 79: 490–7.
31. Van der Zee AG, *et al.* Sentinel node dissection is safe in the treatment of early-stage vulvar cancer. J Clin Oncol 2008; 26: 884–9.
32. Gaarenstroom KN, *et al.* Postoperative complications after vulvectomy and inguinofemoral lymphadenectomy using separate groin incisions. Int J Gynecol Cancer 2003; 13: 522–7.

33. Rouzier R, Haddad B, Dubernard G, Dubois P, Paniel BJ. Inguinofemoral dissection for carcinoma of the vulva: effect of modifications of extent and technique on morbidity and survival. J Am Coll Surg 2003; 196: 442–50.

34. Gonzalez Bosquet J, Kinney WK, Russell AH, Gaffey TA, Magrina JF, Podratz KC. Risk of occult inguinofemoral lymph node metastasis from squamous carcinoma of the vulva. Int J Radiat Oncol Biol Phys 2003; 57: 419–24.

35. Gonzalez Bosquet J, et al. Patterns of inguinal groin metastases in squamous cell carcinoma of the vulva. Gynecol Oncol 2007; 105: 742–6.

36. Hall TB, et al. The role of ultrasound-guided cytology of groin lymph nodes in the management of squamous cell carcinoma of the vulva: 5-year experience in 44 patients. Clin Radiol 2003; 58: 367–71.

37. Moskovic EC, Shepherd JH, Barton DP, Trott PA, Nasiri N, Thomas JM. The role of high resolution ultrasound with guided cytology of groin lymph nodes in the management of squamous cell carcinoma of the vulva: a pilot study. Br J Obstet Gynaecol 1999; 106: 863–7.

38. Hawnaur JM, Reynolds K, Wilson G, Hillier V, Kitchener HC. Identification of inguinal lymph node metastases from vulval carcinoma by magnetic resonance imaging: an initial report. Clin Radiol 2002; 57: 995–1000.

39. Cohn DE, et al. Prospective evaluation of positron emission tomography for the detection of groin node metastases from vulvar cancer. Gynecol Oncol 2002; 85: 179–84.

40. Rutledge F, Smith JP, Franklin EW. Carcinoma of the vulva. Am J Obstet Gynecol 1970; 106: 1117–30 .

41. DiSaia PJ, Creasman WT, Rich WM. An alternate approach to early cancer of the vulva. Am J Obstet Gynecol 1979; 133: 825–32.

42. Hudson CN, Shulver H, Lowe DC. The surgery of 'inguino-femoral' lymph nodes: is it adequate or excessive? Int J Gynecol Cancer 2004; 14: 841–5.

43. Burke TW, Levenback C, Coleman RL, Morris M, Silva EG, Gershenson DM. Surgical therapy of T1 and T2 vulvar carcinoma: further experience with radical wide excision and selective inguinal lymphadenectomy. Gynecol Oncol 1995; 57: 215–20.

44. Gordinier ME, et al. Groin recurrence in patients with vulvar cancer with negative nodes on superficial inguinal lymphadenectomy. Gynecol Oncol 2003; 90: 625–8.

45. Kirby TO, et al. Outcomes of Stage I/II vulvar cancer patients after negative superficial inguinal lymphadenectomy. Gynecol Oncol 2005; 98: 309–12.

46. Homesley HD, Bundy BN, Sedlis A, Adcock L. Radiation therapy versus pelvic node resection for carcinoma of the vulva with positive groin nodes. Obstet Gynecol 1986; 68: 733–40.

47. Homesley HD, et al. Assessment of current International Federation of Gynecology and Obstetrics staging of vulvar carcinoma relative to prognostic factors for survival (a Gynecologic Oncology Group study). Am J Obstet Gynecol 1991; 164: 997–1003; discussion 1003–4.

48. Morton DL, et al. Sentinel-node biopsy or nodal observation in melanoma. N Engl J Med 2006; 355: 1307–17.

49. Veronesi U, et al. A randomized comparison of sentinel-node biopsy with routine axillary dissection in breast cancer. N Engl J Med 2003; 349: 546–53.

50. Levenback C, Coleman RL, Burke TW, Bodurka-Bevers D, Wolf JK, Gershenson DM. Intraoperative lymphatic mapping and sentinel node identification with blue dye in patients with vulvar cancer. Gynecol Oncol 2001; 83: 276–81.

51. Oonk MH, van de Nieuwenhof HP, de Hullu JA, van der Zee AG. The role of sentinel node biopsy in gynecological cancer: a review. Curr Opin Oncol 2009; 21: 425–32.

52. Alex JC, Weaver DL, Fairbank JT, Rankin BS, Krag DN. Gamma-probe-guided lymph node localization in malignant melanoma. Surg Oncol 1993; 2: 303–8.

53. Morton DL, Wen DR, Wong JH, Economou JS, Cagle LA, Storm FK, Foshag LJ, Cochran AJ. Technical details of intraoperative lymphatic mapping for early stage melanoma. Arch Surg 1992; 127: 392–9.

54. Hampl M, Hantschmann P, Michels W, Hillemanns P. Validation of the accuracy of the sentinel lymph node procedure in patients with vulvar cancer: results of a multicenter study in Germany. Gynecol Oncol 2008; 111: 282–8.

55. Fons G, et al. Adjuvant radiotherapy in patients with vulvar cancer and one intra capsular lymph node metastasis is not beneficial. Gynecol Oncol 2009; 114: 343–5.

56. Parthasarathy A, et al. The benefit of adjuvant radiation therapy in single-node-positive squamous cell vulvar carcinoma. Gynecol Oncol 2006; 103: 1095–9.

57. Kunos C, Simpkins F, Gibbons H, Tian C, Homesley H. Radiation therapy compared with pelvic node resection for node-positive vulvar cancer: a randomized controlled trial. Obstet Gynecol 2009; 114: 537–46.

58. Moore DH, Thomas GM, Montana GS, Saxer A, Gallup DG, Olt G. Preoperative chemoradiation for advanced vulvar cancer: a phase II study of the Gynecologic Oncology Group. Int J Radiat Oncol Biol Phys 1998; 42: 79–85.

59. Van Doorn HC, Ansink A, Verhaar-Langereis M, Stalpers L. Neoadjuvant chemoradiation for advanced primary vulvar cancer. Cochrane Database Syst Rev 2006; 3: CD003752.

60. Durrant KR, et al. Bleomycin, methotrexate, and CCNU in advanced inoperable squamous cell carcinoma of the vulva: a phase II study of the EORTC Gynaecological Cancer Cooperative Group (GCCG). Gynecol Oncol 1990; 37: 359–62.

61. Wagenaar HC, et al. Bleomycin, methotrexate, and CCNU in locally advanced or recurrent, inoperable, squamous-cell carcinoma of the vulva: an EORTC Gynaecological Cancer Cooperative Group Study. European Organization for Research and Treatment of Cancer. Gynecol Oncol 2001; 81: 348–54.

62. Witteveen PO, et al. Phase II study on paclitaxel in patients with recurrent, metastatic or locally advanced vulvar cancer not amenable to surgery or radiotherapy: a study of the EORTC-GCG (European Organisation for Research and Treatment of Cancer-Gynaecological Cancer Group). Ann Oncol 2009; 20: 1511–16.

63. Muss HB, Bundy BN, Christopherson WA. Mitoxantrone in the treatment of advanced vulvar and vaginal carcinoma. A Gynecologic Oncology Group study. Am J Clin Oncol 1989; 12: 142–4.

64. Olawaiye A, Lee LM, Krasner C, Horowitz N. Treatment of squamous cell vulvar cancer with the anti-EGFR tyrosine kinase inhibitor Tarceva. Gynecol Oncol 2007; 106: 628–30.

65. Richard SD, Krivak TC, Beriwal S, Zorn KK. Recurrent metastatic vulvar carcinoma treated with cisplatin plus cetuximab. Int J Gynecol Cancer 2008; 18: 1132–5.

66. Panizzon RG. Vulvar melanoma. Semin Dermatol 1996; 15: 67–70.

67. Piura B. Management of primary melanoma of the female urogenital tract. Lancet Oncol 2008; 9: 973–81.

68. Sugiyama VE, Chan JK, Shin JY, Berek JS, Osann K, Kapp DS. Vulvar melanoma: a multivariable analysis of 644 patients. Obstet Gynecol 2007; 110: 296–301.

69. Chang AE, Karnell LH, Menck HR. The National Cancer Data Base report on cutaneous and noncutaneous melanoma: a summary of 84,836 cases from the past decade. The American College of Surgeons Commission on Cancer and the American Cancer Society. Cancer 1998; 83: 1664–78.

70. Clark WH Jr, From L, Bernardino EA, Mihm MC. The histogenesis and biologic behavior of primary human malignant melanomas of the skin. Cancer Res 1969; 29: 705–27.

71. Chung AF, Woodruff JM, Lewis JL Jr. Malignant melanoma of the vulva: a report of 44 cases. Obstet Gynecol 1975; 45: 638–46.

72. Breslow A. Thickness, cross-sectional areas and depth of invasion in the prognosis of cutaneous melanoma. Ann Surg 1970; 172: 902–8.

73. Balch CM, Gershenwald JE, Soong SJ, Thompson JF, Atkins MB, Byrd DR, Buzaid AC, Cochran AJ, Coit DG, Ding S, Eggermont AM, Flaherty KT, Gimotty PA, Kirkwood JM, McMasters KM, Mihm MC, Jr., Morton DL, Ross MI, Sober AJ, Sondak VK. Final version of 2009 AJCC melanoma staging and classification. J Clin Oncol 2009; 27: 6199–206.

74. Trimble EL, et al. Management of vulvar melanoma. Gynecol Oncol 1992; 45: 254–8.

75. Balch CM, et al. Efficacy of 2-cm surgical margins for intermediate-thickness melanomas (1 to 4 mm). Results of a multi-institutional randomized surgical trial. Ann Surg 1993; 218: 262–7; discussion 267–9.

76. Cascinelli N, Morabito A, Santinami M, MacKie RM, Belli F. Immediate or delayed dissection of regional nodes in patients with melanoma of the trunk: a randomised trial. WHO Melanoma Programme. Lancet 1998; 351: 793–6.

77. Veronesi U, et al. Inefficacy of immediate node dissection in stage 1 melanoma of the limbs. N Engl J Med 1977; 297: 627–30.

78. Veronesi U, et al. Delayed regional lymph node dissection in stage I melanoma of the skin of the lower extremities. Cancer 1982; 49: 2420–30.

79. Veronesi U, et al. Thin stage I primary cutaneous malignant melanoma. Comparison of excision with margins of 1 or 3 cm. N Engl J Med 1988; 318: 1159–62.

80. Eggermont AM, et al. Adjuvant therapy with pegylated interferon alfa-2b versus observation alone in resected stage III melanoma: final results of EORTC 18991, a randomised phase III trial. Lancet 2008; 372: 117–26.

81. Kirkwood JM, Strawderman MH, Ernstoff MS, Smith TJ, Borden EC, Blum RH. Interferon alfa-2b adjuvant therapy of high-risk resected cutaneous melanoma: the Eastern Cooperative Oncology Group Trial EST 1684. J Clin Oncol 1996; 14: 7–17.

82. Harting MS, Kim K. Biochemotherapy in patients with advanced vulvo-vaginal mucosal melanoma. Melanoma Res 2004; 14: 517–20.

83. Cole BF, Gelber RD, Kirkwood JM, Goldhirsch A, Barylak E, Borden E. Quality-of-life-adjusted survival analysis of interferon alfa-2b adjuvant treatment of high-risk resected cutaneous melanoma: an Eastern Cooperative Oncology Group study. J Clin Oncol 1996; 14: 2666–73.

84. Sabel MS, Sondak VK. Point: Interferon-alpha for adjuvant therapy for melanoma patients. J Natl Compr Canc Netw 2004; 2: 61–8.

85. Dutcher JP, et al. A phase II study of interleukin-2 and lymphokine-activated killer cells in patients with metastatic malignant melanoma. J Clin Oncol 1989; 7: 477–85.

86. Rosenberg SA, et al. Treatment of 283 consecutive patients with metastatic melanoma or renal cell cancer using high-dose bolus interleukin 2. JAMA 1994; 271: 907–13.

87. Atkins MB, et al. High-dose recombinant interleukin 2 therapy for patients with metastatic melanoma: analysis of 270 patients treated between 1985 and 1993. J Clin Oncol 1999; 17: 2105–16.

88. Eisenhauer EA, et al. New response evaluation criteria in solid tumours: revised RECIST guideline (version 1.1). Eur J Cancer 2009; 45: 228–47.

89. Hodi FS, et al. Major response to imatinib mesylate in KIT-mutated melanoma. J Clin Oncol 2008; 26: 2046–51.

90. Quintas-Cardama A, Lazar AJ, Woodman SE, Kim K, Ross M, Hwu P. Complete response of stage IV anal mucosal melanoma expressing KIT Val560Asp to the multikinase inhibitor sorafenib. Nat Clin Pract Oncol 2008; 5: 737–40.

91. Haluska F, Pemberton T, Ibrahim N, Kalinsky K. The RTK/RAS/BRAF/PI3K pathways in melanoma: biology, small molecule inhibitors, and potential applications. Semin Oncol 2007; 34: 546–54.

92. Omholt K, Grafstrom E, Kanter-Lewensohn L, Hansson J, Ragnarsson-Olding BK. KIT pathway alterations in mucosal melanomas of the vulva and other sites. Clin Cancer Res 2011; 17: 3933–42.

93. Margolin K, et al. CCI-779 in metastatic melanoma: a phase II trial of the California Cancer Consortium. Cancer 2005; 104: 1045–8.

94. Markovic SN, et al. A phase II study of bortezomib in the treatment of metastatic malignant melanoma. Cancer 2005; 103: 2584–9.

95. Pawlak WZ, Legha SS. Phase II study of thalidomide in patients with metastatic melanoma. Melanoma Res 2004; 14: 57–62.

96. Perez DG, et al. Phase 2 trial of carboplatin, weekly paclitaxel, and biweekly bevacizumab in patients with unresectable stage IV melanoma: a North Central Cancer Treatment Group study, N047A. Cancer 2009; 115: 119–27.

97. Bedikian AY, et al. Bcl-2 antisense (oblimersen sodium) plus dacarbazine in patients with advanced melanoma: the Oblimersen Melanoma Study Group. J Clin Oncol 2006; 24: 4738–45.

98. Miller DL, Weinstock MA. Nonmelanoma skin cancer in the United States: incidence. J Am Acad Dermatol 1994; 30: 774–8.

99. Benedet JL, Miller DM, Ehlen TG, Bertrand MA. Basal cell carcinoma of the vulva: clinical features and treatment results in 28 patients. Obstet Gynecol 1997; 90: 765–8.

100. Feakins RM, Lowe DG. Basal cell carcinoma of the vulva: a clinico-pathologic study of 45 cases. Int J Gynecol Pathol 1997; 16: 319–24.

101. Hoffman MS, Roberts WS, Ruffolo EH. Basal cell carcinoma of the vulva with inguinal lymph node metastases. Gynecol Oncol 1988; 29: 113–9.

102. Susong CR, Ratz JL. Basal-cell carcinoma occurring in an axilla: a case presentation and a review of factors related to tumor development. J Dermatol Surg Oncol 1985; 11: 526–30.

103. De Giorgi V, Salvini C, Massi D, Raspollini MR, Carli P. Vulvar basal cell carcinoma: retrospective study and review of literature. Gynecol Oncol 2005; 97: 192–4.

104. Copeland LJ, Sneige N, Gershenson DM, McGuffee VB, Abdul-Karim F, Rutledge FN. Bartholin gland carcinoma. Obstet Gynecol 1986; 67: 794–801.

105. Leuchter RS, Hacker NF, Voet RL, Berek JS, Townsend DE, Lagasse LD. Primary carcinoma of the Bartholin gland: a report of 14 cases and review of the literature. Obstet Gynecol 1982; 60: 361–8.

106. Visco AG, del Priore G. Postmenopausal bartholin gland enlargement: a hospital-based cancer risk assessment. Obstet Gynecol 1996; 87: 286–90.

107. Cardosi RJ, Speights A, Fiorica JV, Grendys EC Jr, Hakam A, Hoffman MS. Bartholin's gland carcinoma: a 15-year experience. Gynecol Oncol 2001; 82: 247–51.

108. Wheelock JB, Goplerud DR, Dunn LJ, Oates JF 3rd. Primary carcinoma of the Bartholin gland: a report of ten cases. Obstet Gynecol 1984; 63: 820–4.

109. Nielsen GP, Rosenberg AE, Koerner FC, Young RH, Scully RE. Smooth-muscle tumors of the vulva. A clinicopathological study of 25 cases and review of the literature. Am J Surg Pathol 1996; 20: 779–93.

110. Hensley ML. Uterine/female genital sarcomas. Curr Treat Options Oncol 2000; 1: 161–8.

111. Daling JR, et al. A population-based study of squamous cell vaginal cancer: HPV and cofactors. Gynecol Oncol 2002; 84: 263–70.

112. Ikenberg H, Runge M, Goppinger A, Pfleiderer A. Human papillomavirus DNA in invasive carcinoma of the vagina. Obstet Gynecol 1990; 76: 432–8.

113. Gallup DG, Talledo OE, Shah KJ, Hayes C. Invasive squamous cell carcinoma of the vagina: a 14-year study. Obstet Gynecol 1987; 69: 782–5.

114. Pride GL, Schultz AE, Chuprevich TW, Buchler DA. Primary invasive squamous carcinoma of the vagina. Obstet Gynecol 1979; 53: 218–25.

115. Herbst AL, Green TH Jr, Ulfelder H. Primary carcinoma of the vagina. An analysis of 68 cases. Am J Obstet Gynecol 1970; 106: 210–18.

116. Benedet JL, Bender H, Jones H 3rd, Ngan HY, Pecorelli S. FIGO staging classifications and clinical practice guidelines in the management of gynecologic cancers. FIGO Committee on Gynecologic Oncology. Int J Gynaecol Obstet 2000; 70: 209–62.

117. Beller U, et al. Carcinoma of the vagina. FIGO 26th Annual Report on the Results of Treatment in Gynecological Cancer. Int J Gynaecol Obstet 2006; 95(Suppl 1): S29–42.

118. Tjalma WA, Monaghan JM, de Barros Lopes A, Naik R, Nordin AJ, Weyler JJ. The role of surgery in invasive squamous carcinoma of the vagina. Gynecol Oncol 2001; 81: 360–5.

119. Perez CA, et al. Definitive irradiation in carcinoma of the vagina: long-term evaluation of results. Int J Radiat Oncol Biol Phys 1988; 15: 1283–90.

120. Davis KP, Stanhope CR, Garton GR, Atkinson EJ, O'Brien PC. Invasive vaginal carcinoma: analysis of early-stage disease. Gynecol Oncol 1991; 42: 131–6.

121. Chyle V, Zagars GK, Wheeler JA, Wharton JT, Delclos L. Definitive radiotherapy for carcinoma of the vagina: outcome and prognostic factors. Int J Radiat Oncol Biol Phys 1996; 35: 891–905.

122. Rubin SC, Young J, Mikuta JJ. Squamous carcinoma of the vagina: treatment, complications, and long-term follow-up. Gynecol Oncol 1985; 20: 346–53.

123. Benedetti Panici P, et al. Neoadjuvant chemotherapy followed by radical surgery in patients affected by vaginal carcinoma. Gynecol Oncol 2008; 111: 307–11.

124. Dalrymple JL, *et al*. Chemoradiation for primary invasive squamous carcinoma of the vagina. Int J Gynecol Cancer 2004; 14: 110–17.

125. Grigsby PW. Vaginal cancer. Curr Treat Options Oncol 2002; 3: 125–30.

126. Food and Drug Administration. *Drug Bulletin: Diethylstilbestrol contraindicated in pregnancy*. Washington, DC: US Department of Health, 1971.

127. Melnick S, Cole P, Anderson D, Herbst A. Rates and risks of diethylstilbestrol-related clear-cell adenocarcinoma of the vagina and cervix. An update. N Engl J Med 1987; 316: 514–16.

128. Troisi R, *et al*. Cancer risk in women prenatally exposed to diethylstilbestrol. Int J Cancer 2007; 121: 356–60.

129. Trimble EL, Rubinstein LV, Menck HR, Hankey BF, Kosary C, Giusti RM. Vaginal clear cell adenocarcinoma in the United States. Gynecol Oncol 1996; 61: 113–15.

130. DeMars LR, van Le L, Huang I, Fowler WC. Primary non-clear-cell adenocarcinomas of the vagina in older DES-exposed women. Gynecol Oncol 1995; 58: 389–92.

131. Hanselaar A, van Loosbroek M, Schuurbiers O, Helmerhorst T, Bulten J, Bernhelm J. Clear cell adenocarcinoma of the vagina and cervix. An update of the central Netherlands registry showing twin age incidence peaks. Cancer 1997; 79: 2229–36.

132. Fishman DA, *et al*. Late recurrences of vaginal clear cell adenocarcinoma. Gynecol Oncol 1996; 62: 128–32.

133. Senekjian EK, Frey KW, Anderson D, Herbst AL. Local therapy in stage I clear cell adenocarcinoma of the vagina. Cancer 1987; 60: 1319–24.

134. Sugiyama VE, Chan JK, Kapp DS. Management of melanomas of the female genital tract. Curr Opin Oncol 2008; 20: 565–9.

135. Nigogosyan G, Delapava S, Pickren JW. Melanoblasts in vaginal mucosa. Origin for primary malignant melanoma. Cancer 1964; 17: 912–13.

136. DeMatos P, Tyler D, Seigler HF. Mucosal melanoma of the female genitalia: a clinicopathologic study of forty-three cases at Duke University Medical Center. Surgery 1998; 124: 38–48.

137. Frumovitz M, *et al*. Primary malignant melanoma of the vagina. Obstet Gynecol 116: 1358–65.

138. Gupta D, Malpica A, Deavers MT, Silva EG. Vaginal melanoma: a clinicopathologic and immunohistochemical study of 26 cases. Am J Surg Pathol 2002; 26: 1450–7.

139. Reid GC, Schmidt RW, Roberts JA, Hopkins MP, Barrett RJ, Morley GW. Primary melanoma of the vagina: a clinicopathologic analysis. Obstet Gynecol 1989; 74: 190–9.

140. Creasman WT, Phillips JL, Menck HR. The National Cancer Data Base report on cancer of the vagina. Cancer 1998; 83: 1033–40.

141. Irvin WP Jr, Bliss SA, Rice LW, Taylor PT Jr, Andersen WA. Malignant melanoma of the vagina and locoregional control: radical surgery revisited. Gynecol Oncol 1998; 71: 476–80.

142. Pandey M, Mathew A, Abraham EK, Ahamed IM, Nair KM. Primary malignant melanoma of the mucous membranes. Eur J Surg Oncol 1998; 24: 303–7.

143. Weinstock MA. Malignant melanoma of the vulva and vagina in the United States: patterns of incidence and population-based estimates of survival. Am J Obstet Gynecol 1994; 171: 1225–30.

144. Buchanan DJ, Schlaerth J, Kurosaki T. Primary vaginal melanoma: thirteen-year disease-free survival after wide local excision and review of recent literature. Am J Obstet Gynecol 1998; 178: 1177–84.

145. Manchana T, Ittiwut C, Mutirangura A, Kavanagh JJ. Targeted therapies for rare gynaecological cancers. Lancet Oncol 2010; 11: 685–93.

146. Robert C, *et al*. Ipilimumab plus dacarbazine for previously untreated metastatic melanoma. N Engl J Med 2011; 364: 2517–26.

147. Shy SW, Lee WH, Chen D, Ho SY. Rhabdomyosarcoma of the vagina in a postmenopausal woman: report of a case and review of the literature. Gynecol Oncol 1995; 58: 395–9.

148. Scrable H, *et al*. Molecular differential pathology of rhabdomyosarcoma. Genes Chromosomes Cancer 1989; 1: 23–35.

149. Scrable HJ, Witte DP, Lampkin BC, Cavenee WK. Chromosomal localization of the human rhabdomyosarcoma locus by mitotic recombination mapping. Nature 1987; 329: 645–7.

150. El-Badry OM, Minniti C, Kohn EC, Houghton PJ, Daughaday WH, Helman LJ. Insulin-like growth factor II acts as an autocrine growth and motility factor in human rhabdomyosarcoma tumors. Cell Growth Differ 1990; 1: 325–31.

151. Mercado GE, Barr FG. Fusions involving PAX and FOX genes in the molecular pathogenesis of alveolar rhabdomyosarcoma: recent advances. Curr Mol Med 2007; 7: 47–61.

152. Flamant F, Gerbaulet A, Nihoul-Fekete C, Valteau-Couanet D, Chassagne D, Lemerle J. Long-term sequelae of conservative treatment by surgery, brachytherapy, and chemotherapy for vulval and vaginal rhabdomyosarcoma in children. J Clin Oncol 1990; 8: 1847–53.

153. Martelli H, *et al*. Conservative treatment for girls with nonmetastatic rhabdomyosarcoma of the genital tract: A report from the Study Committee of the International Society of Pediatric Oncology. J Clin Oncol 1999; 17: 2117–22.

Section 8: Hematological Malignancies

42 Rare Acute Leukemias

B. Douglas Smith[1] and Eunpi Cho[2]

[1] Division of Hematologic Malignancies, Sidney Kimmel Comprehensive Cancer Center at Johns Hopkins, Baltimore, MD, USA
[2] Department of Internal Medicine, Johns Hopkins University School of Medicine, Baltimore, MD, USA

Introduction

While all acute leukemias are considered rare malignancies, the six acute leukemias discussed in this chapter are seen infrequently even in tertiary referral centers with large leukemia-focused programs. Three are rare leukemias associated with myeloproliferative neoplasms (MPN), two are rare subtypes of acute myeloid leukemia (AML), and the last is a stem cell leukemia (Table 42.1). These leukemias are often hard to accurately diagnose and all are considered difficult to treat. The following pages will highlight these rare leukemias and their associated diagnostic and therapeutic challenges.

Rare leukemias associated with myeloproliferative neoplasms

Chronic myeloid leukemia in blast crisis

Chronic myeloid leukemia (CML) is a myeloproliferative neoplasm that is defined by the presence of the Philadelphia chromosome and characterized by a triphasic progression from chronic phase (CP) to advanced or accelerated phase (AP) and eventually to blast crisis (BC). In its most advanced phase, CML in blast crisis (CML-BC) is considered an acute leukemia representing either an acute lymphoblastic leukemia (ALL)-like disorder with lymphoblasts or an AML-like disease when defined by myeloblasts. Like other acute leukemias, the diagnosis is confirmed by review of the peripheral smear and bone marrow, with ≥20% blasts present. Patients often present with anemia and thrombocytopenia and commonly have B symptoms associated with CML-BC.

The biological basis of CML-BC is poorly understood. In general, this disorder behaves as a fundamentally different disease from CP CML due to the marked changes in proliferation, differentiation, apoptosis, and cellular adhesion.[1,2] Unfortunately, it also differs in its response to tyrosine kinase inhibitor (TKI) therapy, which is significantly diminished

compared to response in chronic phase: only 20% of patients will achieve a complete cytogenetic response (CCR) to imatinib (compared to ~80% in chronic phase).[3] Long-term, disease-free survival after allogeneic transplant is also dramatically reduced, from about 50–70% for patients transplanted in CP to 20–30% in patients transplanted after they have progressed to AP/BC in the pre-TKI era.[4] Patients transplanted in active blast crisis experience <10% long-term disease-free survival.[5]

The exact role of *BCR/ABL* in CML progression has not been completely elucidated but the dramatic lowering of BC events seen since the introduction of successful TKI therapy certainly suggests that *BCR/ABL*-dependent mechanisms are involved.[6] It is known that *BCR/ABL* expression shifts cellular regulation toward antiapoptosis,[7] which aids in the accumulation of mutations.[8] Numerous studies have implicated *BCR/ABL* in providing a milieu favorable for the generation and maintenance of secondary DNA alterations.[9–12] This is further enhanced as *BCR/ABL* promotes various mechanisms of DNA repair, though the repair is unfaithful, leading to defects in S phase[13] and G2/M checkpoint.[14] *BCR/ABL* kinase activity also increases reactive oxygen species, which are thought to induce DNA damage.[12] Taken together, unopposed *BCR/ABL* kinase activity promotes a DNA damage-friendly milieu. Clinically, patients who achieve complete cytogenetic remission in CML-CP are less likely to progress to blast crisis. Those who had a suboptimal response to imatinib at 12 months had a reduced 5-year progression-free survival of 76% (versus 90% in those with CCR).[15] There is also a progression-free survival benefit for those who achieved a major molecular response (MMR) to dasatinib versus those who did not, of 96% versus 82% at 24 months of follow-up.[16]

However, *BCR/ABL* activity may not explain all the changes involved in transformation to BC. CML stem cells are less dependent on *BCR/ABL* kinase activity than later progenitors,[17] and CML stem cells continue to proliferate in the presence of

Table 42.1 Characteristics of six rare acute leukemias.

	Category	Diagnostic testing	Diagnostic marker	Other markers
Chronic myeloid leukemia in blast crisis	MPD	Cytogenetic and molecular	Ph chromosome, *BCR/ABL*	Dup Ph, trisomy 8, p53 mutation
Chronic neutrophilic leukemia	MPD	Bone marrow appearance	None	Inc LAP, dec G-CSF
Chronic eosinophilic leukemia, *PDGFR/FGF1*	MPD	Molecular testing	*FIL1P1/PDGFRA*	Responsiveness to imatinib
Chronic eosinophilic leukemia, lymphocytic	MPD	Flow cytometry	CD3-/CD4+ clonal population	Inc TARC, inc IgE, TCR gene rearrangement
Acute erythroid leukemia	AML	Immuno-phenotype	Glycoprotein A	ABH antigen or carbonic anhydrase positivity
Acute megaloblastic leukemia	AML	Immuno-phenotype	Glycoprotein IIb/IIIa	Glycoprotein IIIa, factor VIII positivity
Bilineage AML	MPAL	Flow cytometry	MPO, CD3, CD19	*BCR/ABL, MLL* rearrangement

AML, acute myeloid leukemia; G-CSF, granulocyte colony stimulating factor; LAP, leukocyte alkaline phosphatase; MPD, myeloproliferative disorder; MPO, myeloperoxidase; Ph, Philadelphia chromosome; TARC, thymus and activation-regulated chemokine; TCR, T cell receptor.

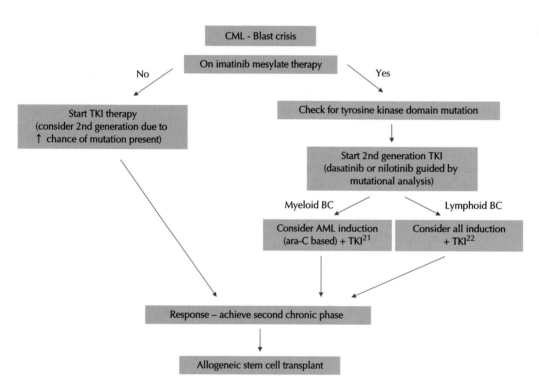

Figure 42.1 Treatment approach for CML-BC.

numerous cytokines, including SCF, FLT3 ligand, GSCF, IL-3, and IL-6, even with effective *BCR-ABL* inhibition.[18] It is likely that CML stem cells use additional survival signals, in part provided by the microenvironment, to maintain their viability in the presence of TKIs. A recent mathematical analysis of blast crises by Sachs *et al.* based on the 1987 data set presented by Sokal[19] concluded that cooperation between leukemic and normal cells is the indicated mechanism for the origination of blast crisis, rather than a single cell model of leukemogenesis.[20]

The treatment approach to CML-BC is based on the introduction of TKI therapy, with or without traditional cytotoxic drugs. As there is an increase in the number of *BCR/ABL* mutations, many that confer resistance to imatinib mesylate (IM), clinicians often opt to start even TKI-naive patients on one of the second-generation TKIs that are generally more active against most of the common *BCR/ABL* mutations. Figure 42.1

represents a proposed treatment schema for patients presenting with or progressing to CML-BC. The ultimate goal is to stabilize the advancing CML and to arrange for eligible patients who achieve a second CP to have an allogeneic transplant, the only potential cure of CML-BC.

Chronic neutrophilic leukemia

Chronic neutrophilic leukemia (CNL) is characterized by a peripheral leukocytosis exceeding ≥25,000/μL, of which segmented neutrophils and band forms constitute more than 80% of white blood cells (WBCs).[23] Making the diagnosis of CNL is often a clinical challenge, as it is necessary to differentiate CNL from other conditions with marked neutrophilia, including true leukemoid reactions to occult infections or malignancies, and a "neutrophilic" form of CML (CML-n)

Table 42.2 Clinical features of chronic neutrophilic leukemia versus similar disorders.

	Leukemoid reaction	CNL	CML-n
Molecular markers	None	None	*BCR/ABL* p230
Peripheral blood	Left shift, mainly myelocytes and metamyelocytes	↑ % of Mature PMN (no ↑ in basophils or eosinophils)	Left shift, ↑ eosinophils and ↑basophils
Bone marrow fibrosis	No	Mild to none	Often ↑ fibrosis, dysplasia and maturation arrest
Bone marrow cellularity	Myeloid proliferation, orderly maturation	Myeloid proliferation, no ↑ in blasts	Left shift, with ↑ basophilia, eosinophilia, monocytosis, dysplasia and maturation arrest
Leukocyte alkaline phosphase level	High	High	Low
G-CSF level	High	Low	Low
Karyotype	Normal	Most frequently normal	t(9;22)
B12, uric acid	Normal	High	High

CML, chronic myeloid leukemia; G-CSF, granulocyte colony-stimulating factor; PMN, polymorphologic neutrophils.

which resembles CNL but is characterized by the presence of the *BCR/ABL* p230 transcript. Table 42.2 helps differentiate the characteristics of chronic neutrophilic leukemia, chronic myeloid leukemia with neutrophilia, and leukemoid reactions. A critical review of case reports published through the year 2001 found only 33 cases of true CNL,[24] which highlights its rare nature.

Chronic neutrophilic leukemia appears to arise in a granulocyte-committed progenitor population that is capable of spontaneous proliferation.[25] It is proposed that resistance of CNL neutrophils to apoptosis[26] results in the accumulation of cells. The bone marrow is hypercellular because of infiltration by neutrophils, ranging from metamyelocytes to mature segmented cells, without increased blasts. Other lineages appear normal. This contrasts the expansion of all three lineages and of all levels of granulocytes seen in Ph+CML. Dysplasia, maturation arrest, and significant marrow fibrosis are notably absent in CNL but a mild degree of reticulin fibrosis may be present, and may help differentiate CNL from leukemoid reaction.[27] Ultimately, these cells infiltrate the bone marrow and other tissues, resulting in end-organ dysfunction. The median survival time for CNL is 30 months, and the 5-year survival rate is 28%.[24]

The median age at diagnosis in an adult series from the Mayo Clinic was 66 years (range 54–86),[27] and a separate case series review by Reilly suggested a male preponderance of 2:1.[24] In the Mayo Clinic series, the median leukocyte and absolute neutrophil counts were 67,900/μL and 62,200/μL, respectively.[27] The peripheral blood smear in CNL shows mature neutrophils, few immature cells, and no blasts, eosinophilia, or basophilia. This is in contrast to the "left shift" seen in both CML and leukemoid reactions. The neutrophils often contain toxic granules and/or Dohle bodies, while erythrocytes and platelets are morphologically normal. The leukocyte alkaline phosphatase (LAP) score is increased in CNL, in contrast to the low score in CML. Abnormalities in other laboratory values include elevated uric acid and serum vitamin B12 levels, as seen in other MPNs, and a low granulocyte colony-stimulating factor (G-CSF) level, in contrast to the elevated levels seen in leukemoid reactions.

Cytogenetic and molecular studies must confirm the absence of the t(9;22) and the *BCR/ABL* gene rearrangement that define Ph+CML. A normal karyotype is most commonly found in CNL but clonal chromosome abnormalities can include +8, +9, del (20q), and del(11q), all of which are also found in other myeloid neoplasms and thus are not disease-defining lesions in CNL. Cytogenetic abnormalities occur in 37% of patients and most frequently involve chromosome 20.[24,28] CNL has also been associated with plasma cell dyscrasias such as monoclonal gammopathy of unknown significance and multiple myeloma.[29] However, it is still unclear if the neutrophilia in these cases can be classified as CNL or would be better considered a leukemoid reaction to the plasma cell dyscrasia.

Common presenting symptoms include weight loss, fatigue, splenomegaly, and pruritus. Interestingly, patients do not generally present with fever, and most have normal hemoglobin and platelet counts.[24] Treatment has generally focused on lowering counts in the hope of reducing tissue infiltration and damage. Hydroxyurea is often used to accomplish these goals. Splenectomy is indicated for symptomatic resistant splenomegaly but may worsen neutrophilia. The disease commonly progresses despite these measures, requiring second-line therapy with agents that include low-dose cytarabine, 2-chlorodeoxyadenosine (cladribine), 6-thioguanine (6-TG), and interferon-α (IFN-α), all of which have produced responses. The standard AML induction has not been traditionally successful and may result in prolonged cytopenias and poor outcomes, including death.[24,27,30] Allogeneic hematopoietic stem cell transplantation following myeloablative therapy has been successful in patients of appropriate age with suitable donors[30,31] and is indicated due to the high incidence of secondary refractory disease, the progression to AML in 20%, and short median survival.

Chronic eosinophilic leukemia and hypereosinophilic syndrome

Chronic eosinophilic leukemia (CEL) and hypereosinophilic syndrome (HES) comprise a heterogeneous spectrum of indolent to aggressive diseases characterized by peripheral blood

Table 42.3 Characteristics of chronic eosinophilic leukemia (CEL), hypereosinophilic syndrome disorders (HES).

	PDGRFA/B or FGFR1	HES, leukocytic variant	CEL, NOS
Pathophysiology	Tyrosine kinase dysregulation	Increased IL-5 and cytokine release	Unknown
Diagnosis	FIP1L1-PDGRFA mutation, ↑ tryptase	Flow, clonal TCR rearrangement, ↑ TARC	Diagnosis of exclusion
First-line treatment	Imatinib mesylate	Glucocorticoids	Glucocorticoids
Second-line treatment	Nilotinib, sorafenib	Interferon α	Hydroxyurea? Alemtuzumab? Mepolizumab?

IL, interleukin; NOS, not otherwise specified; TARC, thymus and activation-regulated chemokine; TCR, T cell receptor.

eosinophilia of >1500/μL and signs or symptoms of eosinophil-mediated end-organ dysfunction. Making the diagnosis involves exclusion of other hematological disorders associated with eosinophilia, either as part of the malignant clone (as in CML, systemic mastocytosis, other MPNs, and some subtypes of AML) or as a reactive component because of cytokine production (as in Hodgkin lymphoma, T cell non-Hodgkin lymphoma [NHL], and ALL).[32]

Patients with these disorders are often discovered due to symptoms of eosinophilic infiltration of organs and/or effects of cytokines and humoral factors released from eosinophilic granules. End-organ involvement has been described in the heart (Loeffler endomyocarditis, endomyocardial fibrosis, restrictive cardiomyopathy, mural thrombosis), lungs (pulmonary infiltrates, emboli, fibrosis, effusions), liver, spleen, skin (urticaria, angioedema, papules/nodules), gastrointestinal tract, and the central and peripheral nervous systems (peripheral neuropathy, eosinophilic meningitis).[32,33]

Molecular characterization of these disorders has allowed for further separation into subgroups based on the mechanisms driving the eosinophilia. For the purposes of this chapter, we will use the following subdivisions: PDGFR/FGFR1-related eosinophilia, lymphocytic variant HES, and chronic eosinophilic leukemia, not otherwise specified (Table 42.3). The distinctions carry significance for prognosis and treatment options.

PDGFR/FGFR1-related eosinophilic disorders

The 2008 World Health Organization (WHO) classification of hematopoietic and lymphoid tissues includes a special category for myeloid and lymphoid disorders with eosinophilia and abnormalities in one of the following: PDGFRA (platelet-derived growth factor receptor α), PDGFRB (platelet-derived growth factor receptor β), and FGFR1 (fibroblast growth factor receptor 1).[23] These patients display features more typical of MPNs, including increased serum vitamin B12 levels (>2000 pg/mL), chromosomal abnormalities, anemia and/or thrombocytopenia, hepatomegaly, splenomegaly, and circulating leukocyte precursors.[34] (See Chapter 47 for more extensive discussion on MPNs.) Serum tryptase is often elevated.[35] The most frequently observed chromosomal aberration in this subgroup is an interstitial deletion on chromosome 4q12 resulting in the fusion of two genes, Fip1-like1 (FIP1L1) and PDGFRA, estimated to be present in 10–14% of patients.[35,36] Like other genetic findings seen in MPNs, the FIP1L1/PDGRFA fusion gene displays constitutive tyrosine kinase activity.[34,37,38]

The identification of a PDGFR or FGFR1 mutation is a critical component of determining treatment. The first-line therapy for all patients with FIP1L1- and PDGFRA-positive disease is the TKI imatinib mesylate (IM); treatment should begin as soon as the diagnosis is established, with a goal of stabilizing the eosinophilia and ultimately preventing progression of cardiac disease and other severe end-organ damage. IM can produce clinical, hematological, and molecular remission in the majority of patients with FIP1L1/PDGFRA-associated HES.[37,39] Clinical symptom improvement and normalization of eosinophil counts begin within 1–2 weeks of starting therapy, and treatment is continued indefinitely. Interestingly, FIP1L1/PDGFRA-driven disorders are particularly sensitive to IM, with doses as low as 100 mg daily controlling eosinophilia in most patients; however, higher doses (400 mg/day) may be more effective at eliminating molecular evidence of the disease. The clinical significance of complete molecular remissions is not yet known.[40,41] Ultimately, the therapeutic goal is to decrease residual disease, based on data from CML patients in whom there is a clear correlation between residual disease and risk of progression to blast crisis. Patients who present with or have evidence of cardiac involvement should also be started on concomitant treatment with glucocorticoids for 1–2 weeks to decrease risk of myocardial damage.[42]

Primary resistance to imatinib is uncommon but has been reported.[43] Secondary resistance has been associated with a single base (T6741) substitution in the imatinib-binding portion of the kinase.[44] The best approach to managing imatinib-resistant disease is unknown but there are some data to suggest efficacy of other tyrosine kinase inhibitors such as nilotinib and sorafenib in these patients.[40]

Lymphocytic-variant hypereosinophilic syndrome

Lymphocytic-variant HES is characterized by abnormal T cell subsets that produce increased levels of interleukin (IL)-5[45] as well as increased levels of Th2 cytokines that stimulate B cell production of IgE synthesis.[46] Phenotypically, the T cells involved in this disorder are commonly CD3 negative and CD4 positive. The clinical presentation of lymphocytic-variant HES includes cutaneous symptoms such as erythroderma, urticaria, and plaques. Typically the disease is indolent, though rare patients have progressed to T cell lymphoma or Sézary syndrome, indicating the malignant potential of this condition.[47]

Diagnostic testing for this disorder usually involves the discovery of an abnormal population of T cells on flow cytometry,

T cell clonality (T cell receptor gene rearrangement), increased levels of serum thymus and activation-regulated chemokine (TARC), and elevated serum IgE. Consensus criteria for the diagnosis of lymphocytic-variant HES have not yet been established, and although no one test is specific for this disorder, elevated TARC levels serve as a helpful marker.[48]

Prior to initiating therapy for lymphocytic-variant HES, one must rule out infections associated with eosinophilia, including strongyloides.[35] Glucocorticoids are the initial therapy of choice for patients with organ involvement who do not have the *FIP1L1-PDGFRA* fusion or another IM-sensitive tyrosine kinase mutation. Prednisone at doses of 1 mg/kg or 60 mg daily for 1–2 weeks is considered first-line therapy. Once blood eosinophilia is suppressed, daily doses can be reduced to the lowest that maintains control of the eosinophil count and clinical manifestations. Interferon (IFN)-α can be used as adjunctive therapy in patients who do not respond to glucocorticoids alone, or who require excessive doses to keep their disease under control.[49]

Chronic eosinophilic leukemia, not otherwise specified

By definition, patients in this group do not demonstrate the Philadelphia chromosome, the *BCR/ABL* fusion gene, or a rearrangement involving *PDGFRA/B* and *FGFR1*. The peripheral blood demonstrates mature eosinophils and only a small number of eosinophilic myelocytes or promyelocytes. There may be a variety of morphological abnormalities, including sparse granulation, cytoplasmic vacuolization or hyper/hyposegmentation, but none of these is specific for CEL. Additional clonal abnormalities and/or a population of blasts in the peripheral blood (>2%) or marrow (>5% but <20%) differentiate CEL from HES.[23] Human androgen receptor analysis (HUMARA) is one study that can show clonal populations of mature eosinophils in these patients, though these X-linked analyses can only be performed on women.[50]

As with HES, glucocorticoids are the mainstay of therapy for patients with CEL-NOS and are effective in rapidly reducing the eosinophil count.[35] However, treatment success may be short-lived or incomplete with recrudescence of symptoms, signs of organ damage, and/or worsening eosinophilia common. If progression occurs at doses of prednisone >10 mg daily, additional agents are generally indicated. Hydroxyurea can be used in conjunction with steroids or in steroid non-responders.[51] Interferon-α is another agent that can be used in patients with steroid-refractory CEL-NOS.[35] The optimal dose and duration of therapy with IFN-α are unknown. Newer agents, including mepolizumab (anti-IL-5 antibody) and alemtuzumab (anti-CD52 antibody), have shown some promise in investigational studies,[52,53] though long-term safety and efficacy data are lacking.

Rare subtypes of acute myeloid leukemia

Acute erythroblastic leukemia

Acute erythroblastic leukemia (AEL), previously denoted as M6 AML by the FAB classification, is characterized by the expansion of morphologically abnormal and malignant erythroid cells in the bone marrow. AEL has two recognized subtypes: *erythroleukemia*, which is defined by ≥50% erythroid precursors in marrow nucleated cells and ≥20% myeloblasts in nonerythroid cells, and *pure erythroid leukemia (Di Gulielmo disease)*, which is defined by ≥80% immature erythroid cells in the marrow nucleated cell population without a significant myeloblastic component.[54] Studies suggest that erythroleukemia likely arises in a multipotent stem cell and accounts for the varying degrees of erythroid and myeloid maturation whereas pure erythroid leukemia likely arises in a stem cell line committed to the erythroid lineage.

The incidence of AEL peaks in younger (<20 years) and older (>50 years) patients and accounts for only 3–5% of all AML cases.[55] A previous diagnosis of myelodysplastic syndrome (MDS) or unexplained cytopenias is seen in approximately 32% of patients diagnosed with AEL according to the 2008 WHO classification.[56] Most patients present with profound anemia, thrombocytopenia, and varying degrees of neutropenia along with signs of hepatomegaly and/or splenomegaly.[57–59]

Review of the peripheral blood smear reveals numerous dysplastic erythroblasts, nucleated red blood cells, schistocytes, teardrop and pincered red cells, basophilic stippling, as well as myeloblasts, pseudo-Pelger–Huet cells, hypogranular neutrophils, and giant and hypogranular platelets.[57,58,60,61] The bone marrow aspirate and biopsy in patients usually reveals a hypercellular marrow with an increased number of erythroid cells.[56] In erythroleukemia, erythroid cells are comprised mainly of proerythroblasts and basophilic erythroblasts, while in pure erythroleukemia, marrow findings reveal sheets of immature proerythroblasts.[62] Patients with erythroleukemia also have elevated myeloid blasts, which may or may not contain Auer rods and often show signs of myeloid and/or megakaryocytic dysplasia.[63] The immunophenotype of leukemic cells in AEL can be distinct, with antiglycophorin A antibody widely used for flow cytometric diagnosis.[64] Carbonic anhydrase I and ABH antigens aid in diagnosis when there is an immature phenotype of minimally differentiated AEL which does not express glycophorin A.[65]

Chromosomal abnormalities are common and detected in over three-quarters of cases of acute erythroblastic leukemia, often showing a complex karyotype. Chromosomes 5 and/or 7 are involved in two-thirds of cases.[66]

Traditionally, both subtypes of acute erythroid leukemia have carried a poor prognosis, with a median survival reported as low as 36 weeks.[55] Adverse prognostic factors include a high proerythroblast-to-myeloblast ratio in the bone marrow, a high proliferative index, unfavorable karyotypes, expression of the multidrug resistance (MDR) protein P-glycoprotein (Pgp) and FAB M6b disease.[67,68] A morphological diagnosis of pure erythroleukemia is associated with a poorer prognosis than erythroleukemia.[59,68] Patients with normal versus abnormal karyotypes had complete remission (CR) rates of 73% versus 42%,[66] and patients with chromosomes 5 and/or 7 abnormalities had median survivals of 16 weeks versus 77 weeks for those without these chromosome abnormalities.[58]

Treatment of erythroleukemia is similar to that of other AML subtypes. No specific chemotherapeutic regimen has been identified for treating this disorder.[55,56] Based on published data, the rate of CR after conventional induction chemotherapy ("7 + 3") in patients with this disease is approximately 50%[55]; allogeneic stem cell transplantation (SCT) is recommended for patients with a poor-risk karyotype.[56] However, patients with pure erythroleukemia respond poorly to conventional agents, with reported CR rates <25%[59] and median survival of 1.8–4 months.[59,68] Patients with pure erythroleukemias should ideally be enrolled into prospective clinical trials and/or considered for allogeneic SCT when feasible.

Acute megakaryoblastic leukemia

Acute megakaryoblastic leukemia (AMKL) is diagnosed when ≥50% of marrow blasts (which make up >20% of cells) are megakaryoblasts.[54] This leukemia, like AEL, has a bimodal age distribution, with incidence peaks in very young children and in older adults.[69–71] The disorder is extremely rare in adults, with only 20 (1.2%) of 1649 patients enrolled in Eastern Cooperative Oncology Group (ECOG) AML trials between 1984 and 1997 carrying the diagnosis of AMKL.[72] The incidence was even lower, at 0.6%, among the 3606 patients enrolled in GIMEMA trials over an 18-year period.[73] Adult patients will present with cytopenias and circulating megakaryoblasts, and often have dysplastic neutrophils, thrombocytosis, and giant platelets with hypogranulation on blood smear. The reported median leukocyte count at the time of presentation is often low[70] and hepatosplenomegaly is uncommon in adults.

Morphological review of the bone marrow includes blasts that are generally 12–18 μ in size, have distinct basophilic cytoplasm, and often have cellular blebs and pseudopods. The blasts also typically show fine nuclear chromatin, with 1–3 nucleoli. Extensive marrow fibrosis is typically present, which can be confirmed by a positive reticulin stain. In addition to megakaryoblasts, fragments and micromegakaryocytes may be detected. The blasts do not stain with Sudan Black B or myeloperoxidase but may stain with periodic acid-Schiff (PAS), acid phosphatase, or nonspecific esterase. Electron microscopy demonstrates platelet peroxidase in nuclear membranes and endoplasmic reticulum. The diagnosis can also be established with a positive immunocytochemistry stain for factor VIII, glycoprotein IIb/IIIa (CD41), or glycoprotein IIIa (CD61) on bone marrow biopsy.[74,75]

In children, the disease is often associated with either Down syndrome or the t(1;22)(p13;p13) translocation (which is associated with the *OTT-MAL* fusion gene). The first group has a better prognosis, with a favorable 2-year event-free survival

estimate of 83%, compared to other patients with *de novo* AMKL (14%) or secondary AMKL (20%).[76] The latter group with the presence of an *OTT-MAL* fusion gene often presents with hepatosplenomegaly and aggressive disease that is refractory to induction chemotherapy. Further investigations into patients with Down syndrome and AMKL have revealed a specific molecular mutation involving *GATA1*, an erythroid transcription factor, which is found in virtually all such patients.[77–79]

Cytogenetic abnormalities are less well characterized in adults with AMKL. Of the 20 patients with AMKL in the ECOG series, only eight had cytogenetic studies. Abnormalities in chromosome 3 were the most frequent in this small series.[72] Eleven of the 24 patients in the GIMEMA group with AMKL had cytogenetic testing. Two patients had a normal karyotype, two had a chromosome 3 abnormality, two had complex cytogenetics, and five patients had no metaphases. Another series of 30 children and 23 adults by Dastugue *et al.* showed that 58.5% of adults had complex cytogenetics, and the most common recurrent abnormalities in this series also involved chromosome 3.[70]

Treatment outcome is poor in adults, with a reported CR rate of 33–50% to AML-based regimens and a median duration of remission of 8–10 months.[70–73] Given the poor response to standard AML therapies, experimental therapies are justified, and enrollment on clinical trials is strongly encouraged. Aggressive approaches using allogeneic SCT are also appropriate in eligible patients.

Rare stem cell leukemias

Bilineal leukemia (mixed phenotype acute leukemia)

Bilineal leukemia is defined by the presence of two or more morphologically and phenotypically distinct populations of blasts. Historically, this entity has been differentiated from biphenotypic leukemia, which is characterized by a single blast population that expresses mixed phenotypic markers. The 2001 WHO classification highlighted this morphological difference within the family of "acute leukemia of ambiguous lineage." However, bilineal and biphenotypic leukemias are no longer cataloged into different disorders (Fig. 42.2), as the 2008 changes to the WHO classification renamed this family of disorders as mixed phenotype acute leukemia (MPAL) and shifted the focus to separating disorders by cytogenetic abnormalities, namely the presence of t(9;22) or t(v;11q23).[23] More specifically, inclusion in the family of MPAL requires that the leukemia cannot be classified in another category, by either genetic or clinical features.[23]

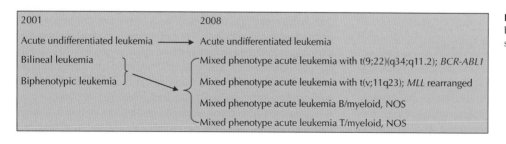

Figure 42.2 2001 versus 2008 criteria for bilineal leukemias. NOS, not otherwise specified.

For cases of bilineal leukemia, one population of blasts should meet the immunophenotypic criteria for AML; however, the presence of ≥20% myeloblasts in the peripheral blood or bone marrow is not required when the total number of leukemic blasts, including nonmyelobasts, is ≥20%. If there is only a single population of blasts present that otherwise meets the criteria for B cell acute lymphoblastic leukemia (B-ALL) and T cell acute lymphoblastic leukemia (T-ALL), myeloid lineage is defined by the presence of myeloperoxidase (MPO) positivity using flow cytometry, immunohistochemistry, or cytochemistry. The prevalence and clinical significance of MPAL using the new 2008 WHO definition remain to be determined, yet the focus on defining disorders based on their genetic basis may ultimately lead to improvements in making the diagnosis and more successful treatment paradigms.

There are two possible biological explanations for the occurrence of a bilineal leukemia: the malignant transformation of a myeloid or lymphoid stem cell with the potential to differentiate into other lineages, or the clonal evolution of a common stem cell that can generate both myeloid and lymphoid progeny. That T lymphoid/myeloid and B lymphoid/myeloid leukemias are seen in about equal frequencies, while T lymphoid/B lymphoid leukemias rarely occur, is consistent with findings documented in fetal mouse hematopoiesis, where early B and T lymphoid precursors retain myeloid potential.[80–82] The lack of MPALs that involve erythroid/megakaryoblastic phenotype supports the existence of a multipotent progenitor with B cell, T cell, and granulocyte/macrophage but no or little erythroid/megakaryoblastic potential.[83]

A review of 1477 cases of acute leukemia processed by the Johns Hopkins Hospital Clinical Flow Cytometry Laboratory over a 10-year period identified 19 cases of acute bilineage leukemia by the 2001 WHO criteria.[84] Seventeen cases represented de novo acute leukemia, one represented transformation of a myelodysplastic syndrome, and another represented relapse in a patient originally diagnosed as T-ALL. Peripheral white blood cell count at presentation ranged from 1800 to 522,500/μL. While all cases included a myeloid component, 10 were characterized by a T lymphoid component and nine by a B lymphoid component; no cases comprised a combination of B and T lymphoid blast populations. There were frequent but nonrecurring abnormalities in the T lymphoid/myeloid series. The only abnormality seen in more than one case was a translocation involving chromosome 2p13. In the B lymphoid/myeloid leukemias, karyotypic analysis revealed t(9;22) and 11q23 abnormalities as relatively common recurring translocations – the two genetic lesions that have now been reported frequently enough in MPAL to be considered separate entities by the 2008 WHO criteria.

Matutes et al. recently published a retrospective case series of 100 MPALs that meet the WHO 2008 criteria.[85] These cases were chosen from archives of acute leukemias over a 15-year period in seven countries. The frequency of MPAL in these countries was 0.5–1%, and of the 100 cases, 59 were B lymphoid/myeloid, 35% were lymphoid/myeloid, 4% were B/T lymphoid, and 2% were trilineage. The following cytogenetic abnormalities were observed: t(9;22)/Ph+(20%), 11q23/MLL rearrangements (8%), complex (32%), aberrant (27%), and normal karotype (13%). Information on response to first-line treatment was available for 67 patients: 27 received therapy for ALL, 34 were treated for AML, five received a combination of chemotherapy for ALL and AML, and one received imatinib monotherapy. Twenty patients underwent transplant. A CR was seen in 23/27 patients who received ALL-based chemotherapy, compared to 13/34 of those receiving AML-based therapy and 3/5 receiving combination therapy. Imatinib monotherapy did not result in a response. Overall median survival was 18 months and 37% of patients were alive at 5 years. Age, Ph+, and AML therapy appeared to be predictors for poor outcome, though the study was limited by its small patient numbers and retrospective nature. These results suggest a potential benefit of using an ALL-based regimen for induction and noting the overall poor outcome, allogeneic SCT should be considered for eligible patients.

References

1. Calabretta B, Perrotti D. The biology of CML blast crisis. Blood 2004; 103: 4010–22.

2. Shet AS, Jahagirdar BN, Verfaillie CM. Chronic myelogenous leukemia: mechanisms underlying disease progression. Leukemia 2002; 16: 1402–11.

3. Druker BJ, Talpaz M, Resta DJ, et al. Efficacy and safety of a specific inhibitor of the BCR-ABL tyrosine kinase in chronic myeloid leukemia. N Engl J Med 2001; 344: 1031–7.

4. Weisdorf DJ, Anasetti C, Antin JH, et al. Allogeneic bone marrow transplantation for chronic myelogenous leukemia: comparative analysis of unrelated versus matched sibling donor transplant. Blood 2002; 99: 1971–7.

5. Gratwohl A, Hermans J, Niederwieser D, et al. Bone-marrow transplantation for chronic myeloid-leukemia – long-term results. Bone Marrow Transplant 1993; 12: 509–16.

6. O'Brien SG, Guilhot F, Larson RA, et al. Imatinib compared with interferon and low-dose cytarabine for newly diagnosed chronic-phase chronic myeloid leukemia. N Engl J Med 2003; 348: 994–1004.

7. Amarante-Mendes GP, Kim CN, Liu L, et al. Bcr-Abl exerts its antiapoptotic effect against diverse apoptotic stimuli through blockage of mitochondrial release of cytochrome c and activation of caspase-3. Blood 1998; 91: 1700–5.

8. Skorski T. BCR/ABL regulates response to DNA damage: the role in resistance to genotoxic treatment and in genomic instability. Oncogene 2002; 21: 8591–604.

9. Salloukh HF, Laneuville P. Increase in mutant frequencies in mice expressing the BCR-ABL activated tyrosine kinase. Leukemia 2000; 14: 1401–4.

10. Canitrot Y, Falinski R, Louat T, et al. p210 BCR/ABL kinase regulates nucleotide excision repair NER and resistance to UV radiation. Blood 2003; 102: 2632–7.

11. Deutsch E, Dugray A, AbdulKarim B, et al. BCR-ABL down-regulates the DNA repair protein DNA-PKcs. Blood 2001; 97: 2084–90.

12. Sattler M, Verma S, Shrikhande G, et al. The BCR/ABL tyrosine kinase induces production of reactive oxygen species in hematopoietic cells. J Biol Chem 2000; 275: 24273–8.

13. Dierov J, Dierova R, Carroll M. BCR/ABL translocates to the nucleus and disrupts an ATR-dependent intra-S phase checkpoint. Cancer Cell 2004; 5: 275–85.

14. Bedi A, Barber JP, Bedi GC, et al. Bcr-Abl-mediated inhibition of apoptosis with delay of G2/M transition after DNA damage – a mechanism of resistance to multiple anticancer agents. Blood 1995; 86: 1148–58.

15. Quintas-Cardama A, Kantarjian H, Jones D, et al. Delayed achievement of cytogenetic and molecular response is associated with increased risk of progression among patients with chronic myeloid leukemia in early

chronic phase receiving high-dose or standard-dose imatinib therapy. Blood 2009; 113: 6315–21.

16. Hochhaus A, Muller MC, Radich J, et al. Dasatinib-associated major molecular responses are rapidly achieved in patients with chronic myeloid leukemia in chronic phase CML-CP following resistance, suboptimal response, or intolerance on imatinib. Blood 2008; 112: 400.

17. Bueno-da-Silva AEB, Brumatti G, Russo FO, Green DR, Amarante-Mendes GP. Bcr-Abl-mediated resistance to apoptosis is independent of constant tyrosine-kinase activity. Cell Death Different 2003; 10: 592–8.

18. Corbin AS, Agarwal A, Loriaux M, et al. Human chronic myeloid leukemia stem cells are insensitive to imatinib despite inhibition of BCR-ABL activity. J Clin Invest 2011; 121: 396–409.

19. Sokal JE. Prognosis in chronic myeloid leukaemia: biology of the disease vs. treatment. Baillière's Clin Haematol 1987; 1: 907–29.

20. Sachs RS, Johnsson K, Hahnfeldt P, et al. A multicellular basis for the origination of blast crisis in chronic myeloid leukemia. Cancer Res 2011; 71: 2838–47.

21. Barone S, Baer MR, Sait SNJ, et al. High-dose cytosine arabinoside and idarubicin treatment of chronic myeloid leukemia in myeloid blast crisis. Am J Hematol 2001; 67: 119–24.

22. Verma D, Kantarjian HM, Jones D, et al. Chronic myeloid leukemia CML with P190BCR-ABL: analysis of characteristics, outcomes, and prognostic significance. Blood 2009; 114: 2232–5.

23. Swerdlow SH, Campo E, Harris NL, et al. WHO Classification of Tumours of Haematopoietic and Lymphoid Tissues. Lyon: IARC Press, 2008.

24. Reilly JT. Chronic neutrophilic leukaemia: a distinct clinical entity? Br J Haematol 2002; 116: 10–18.

25. Yanagisawa K, Ohminami H, Sato V, et al. Neoplastic involvement of granulocytic lineage, not granulocytic-monocytic, monocytic, or erythrocytic lineage, in a patient with chronic neutrophilic leukemia. Am J Hematol 1998; 57: 221–4.

26. Hara K, Abe Y, Hirase N, et al. Apoptosis resistance of mature neutrophils in a case of chronic neutrophilic leukaemia. Eur J Haematol 2001; 66: 70–1.

27. Elliott MA, Dewald GW, Tefferi A, Hanson CA. Chronic neutrophilic leukemia CNL: a clinical, pathologic and cytogenetic study. Leukemia 2001; 15: 35–40.

28. Verstovsek S, Lin H, Kantarjian H, et al. Neutrophilic-chronic myeloid leukemia – low levels of p230 BCR/ABL mRNA and undetectable p230 BCR/ABL protein may predict an indolent course. Cancer 2002; 94: 2416–25.

29. Bohm J, Schaefer HE. Chronic neutrophilic leukaemia: 14 new cases of an uncommon myeloproliferative disease. J Clin Pathol 2002; 55: 862–4.

30. Piliotis E, Kutas G, Lipton JH. Allogeneic bone marrow transplantation in the management of chronic neutrophilic leukemia. Leukemia Lymphoma 2002; 43: 2051–4.

31. Hasle H, Olesen G, Kerndrup G, Philip P, Jacobsen N. Chronic neutrophil leukaemia in adolescence and young adulthood. Br J Haematol 1996; 94: 628–30.

32. Gotlib J, Cools J, Malone JM, et al. Practical caveats to the classification of chronic eosinophilic leukemia and idiopathic hypereosinophilic syndrome as mutually exclusive diagnoses. Blood 2004; 104: 3836–7.

33. Brito-Babapulle F. The eosinophilias, including the idiopathic hypereosinophilic syndrome. Br J Haematol 2003; 121: 203–23.

34. Bain BJ, Fletcher SH. Chronic eosinophilic leukemias and the myeloproliferative variant of the hypereosinophilic syndrome. Immunol Allergy Clin North Am 2007; 27: 377.

35. Ogbogu PU, Bochner BS, Butterfield JH, et al. Hypereosinophilic syndrome: a multicenter, retrospective analysis of clinical characteristics and response to therapy. J Allergy Clin Immunol 2009; 124: 1319–25.

36. Pardanani A, Brockman SR, Paternoster SF, et al. FIP1L1-PDGFRA fusion: prevalence and clinicopathologic correlates in 89 consecutive patients with moderate to severe eosinophilia. Blood 2004; 104: 3038–45.

37. Cools J, DeAngelo DJ, Gotlib J, et al. A tyrosine kinase created by fusion of the PDGFRA and FIP1L1 genes as a therapeutic target of imatinib in idiopathic hypereosinophilic syndrome. N Engl J Med 2003; 348: 1201–14.

38. Griffin JH, Leung J, Bruner RJ, Caligiuri MA, Briesewitz R. Discovery of a fusion kinase in EOL-1 cells and idiopathic hypereosinophilic syndrome. Proc Natl Acad Sci USA 2003; 100: 7830–5.

39. Baccarani M, Cilloni D, Rondoni M, et al. The efficacy of imatinib mesylate in patients with FIP1L1-PDGFR alpha-positive hypereosinophilic syndrome. Results of a multicenter prospective study. Haematologica 2007; 92: 1173–9.

40. Metzgeroth G, Walz C, Erben P, et al. Safety and efficacy of imatinib in chronic eosinophilic leukaemia and hypereosinophilic syndrome – a phase II study. Br J Haematol 2008; 143: 707–15.

41. Klion AD. How I treat hypereosinophilic syndromes. Blood 2009; 114: 3736–41.

42. Pitini V, Arrigo C, Azzarello D, et al. Serum concentration of cardiac troponin T in patients with hypereosinophilic syndrome treated with imatinib is predictive of adverse outcomes. Blood 2003; 102: 3456–7.

43. Simon D, Salemi S, Yousefi S, Simon HU. Primary resistance to imatinib in Fip1-like 1-platelet-derived growth factor receptor alpha – positive eosinophilic leukemia. J Allergy Clin Immunol 2008; 121: 1054–6.

44. Von Bubnoff N, Sandherr M, Schlimok G, et al. Myeloid blast crisis evolving during imatinib treatment of an FIP1L1-PDGFR alpha-positive chronic myeloproliferative disease with prominent eosinophilia. Leukemia 2005; 19: 286–7.

45. Roufosse F, Cogan E, Goldman M. Lymphocytic variant hypereosinophilic syndromes. Immunol Allergy Clin North Am 2007; 27: 389.

46. Roufosse F, Schandene L, Sibille C, et al. Clonal Th2 lymphocytes in patients with the idiopathic hypereosinophilic syndrome. Br J Haematol 2000; 109: 540–8.

47. Simon HU, Plotz SG, Dummer R, Blaser K. Abnormal clones of T cells producing interleukin-5 in idiopathic eosinophilia. N Engl J Med 1999; 341: 1112–20.

48. De Lavallade H, Apperley JF, Khorashad JS, et al. Imatinib for newly diagnosed patients with chronic myeloid leukemia: incidence of sustained responses in an intention-to-treat analysis. J Clin Oncol 2008; 26: 3358–63.

49. Roufosse F, Cogan E, Goldman M. Recent advances in pathogenesis and management of hypereosinophilic syndromes. Allergy 2004; 59: 673–89.

50. Chang HW, Leong KH, Koh DR, Lee SH. Clonality of isolated eosinophils in the hypereosinophilic syndrome. Blood 1999; 93: 1651–7.

51. Weller PF, Bubley GJ. The idiopathic hypereosinophilic syndrome. Blood 1994; 83: 2759–79.

52. Rothenberg ME, Klion AD, Roufosse FE, et al. Treatment of patients with the hypereosinophilic syndrome with mepolizumab. N Engl J Med 2008; 358: 1215–28.

53. Verstovsek S, Tefferi A, Kantarjian H, et al. Alemtuzumab therapy for hypereosinophilic syndrome and chronic eosinophilic leukemia. Clin Cancer Res 2009; 15: 368–73.

54. Jaffee ES, Harris NL, Stein H. Pathology and Genetics of Tumours of Haematopoietic and Lymphoid Tissues. Lyon: IARC Press, 2001.

55. Santos FPS, Faderl S, Garcia-Manero G, et al. Adult acute erythroleukemia: an analysis of 91 patients treated at a single institution. Leukemia 2009; 23: 2275–80.

56. Hasserjian RP, Zuo Z, Garcia C, et al. Acute erythroid leukemia: a reassessment using criteria refined in the 2008 WHO classification. Blood 2010; 115: 1985–92.

57. Park S, Picard F, Dreyfus F. Erythroleukemia: a need for a new definition. Leukemia 2002; 16: 1399–401.

58. Olopade OI, Thangavelu M, Larson RA, et al. Clinical, morphologic, and cytogenetic characteristics of 26 patients with acute erythroblastic leukemia. Blood 1992; 80: 2873–82.

59. Goldberg SL, Noel P, Klumpp TR, Dewald GW. The erythroid leukemias – a comparative study of erythroleukemia FAB M6 and Di Guglielmo disease. Am J Clin Oncol Cancer Clin Trials 1998; 21: 42–7.

60. Mazzella FM, Kowal-Vern A, Shrit MA, et al. Acute erythroleukemia – evaluation of 48 cases with reference to classification, cell proliferation, cytogenetics, and prognosis. Am J Clin Pathol 1998; 110: 590–8.

61. Jaffee EM, Hruban RH, Biedrzycki B, et al. Novel allogeneic granulocyte-macrophage colony-stimulating factor-secreting tumor vaccine for pancreatic

cancer: a phase I trial of safety and immune activation. J Clin Oncol 2001; 19: 145–56.

62. Hasserjian RP, Howard J, Wood A, Henry K, Bain B. Acute erythremic myelosis true erythroleukaemia: a variant of AML FAB-M6. J Clin Pathol 2001; 54: 205–9.

63. Domingo-Claros A, Larriba I, Rozman M, et al. Acute erythroid neoplastic proliferations. A biological study based on 62 patients. Haematologica 2002; 87: 148–53.

64. Chasis JA, Mohandas N. Red-blood-cell glycophorins. Blood 1992; 80: 1869–79.

65. Villeval JL, Cramer P, Lemoine F, et al. Phenotype of early erythroblastic leukemias. Blood 1986; 68: 1167–74.

66. Davey FR, Abraham N, Brunetto VL, et al. Morphologic characteristics of erythroleukemia (acute myeloid-leukemia Fab-M6): a CALGB study. Am J Hematol 1995; 49: 29–38.

67. Mazzella FM, Alvares C, Kowal-Vern A, Schumacher HR. The acute erythroleukemias. Clin Lab Med 2000; 20: 119.

68. Kowal-Vern A, Mazzella FM, Cotelingam JD, et al. Diagnosis and characterization of acute erythroleukemia subsets by determining the percentages of myeloblasts and proerythroblasts in 69 cases. Am J Hematol 2000; 65: 5–13.

69. Gassmann W, Loffler H. Acute megakaryoblastic leukemia. Leukemia Lymphoma 1995; 18: 69–73.

70. Dastugue N, Lafage-Pochitaloff M, Pages MP, et al. Cytogenetic profile of childhood and adult megakaryoblastic leukemia M7: a study of the Groupe Francais de Cytogenetique Hematologique (GFCH). Blood 2002; 100: 618–26.

71. Oki Y, Kantarjian HM, Zhou X, et al. Adult acute megakaryocytic leukemia: an analysis of 37 patients treated at MD Anderson Cancer Center. Blood 2006; 107: 880–4.

72. Tallman MS, Neuberg D, Bennett JM, et al. Acute megakaryocytic leukemia: the Eastern Cooperative Oncology Group experience. Blood 2000; 96: 2405–11.

73. Pagano L, Pulsoni A, Vignetti M, et al. Acute megakaryoblastic leukemia: experience of GIMEMA trials. Leukemia 2002; 16: 1622–6.

74. Innes DJ, Mills SE, Walker GK. Megakaryocytic leukemia – identification utilizing anti-factor-Viii immunoperoxidase. Am J Clin Pathol 1982; 77: 107–10.

75. Ruizarguelles GJ, Marinlopez A, Lobatomendizabal E, et al. Acute megakaryoblastic leukemia – a prospective study of its identification and treatment. Br J Haematol 1986; 62: 55–63.

76. Athale UH, Razzouk BI, Raimondi SC, et al. Biology and outcome of childhood acute megakaryoblastic leukemia: a single institution's experience. Blood 2001; 97: 3727–32.

77. Wechsler J, Greene M, McDevitt M, et al. Acquired mutations in GATA1 in the megakaryoblastic leukemia of Down syndrome. Exper Hematol 2002; 30: 109.

78. Stachura DL, Chou ST, Weiss MJ. An early block to erythro-megakaryocytic development conferred by loss of transcription factor GATA-1. Blood 2005; 106: 493A.

79. Rainis L, Toki T, Pimanda JE, et al. The proto-oncogene ERG in megakaryoblastic leukemias. Cancer Res 2005; 65: 7596–602.

80. Blom B, Spits H. Development of human lymphoid cells. Annu Rev Immunol 2006; 24: 287–320.

81. Wada H, Masuda K, Satoh R, et al. Adult T-cell progenitors retain myeloid potential. Nature 2008; 452: 768–72.

82. Bell JJ, Bhandoola A. The earliest thymic progenitors for T cells possess myeloid lineage potential. Nature 2008; 452: 764–7.

83. Luc S, Buza-Vidas N, Jacobsen SEW. Delineating the cellular pathways of hematopoietic lineage commitment. Semin Immunol 2008; 20: 213–20.

84. Weir EG, Ansari-Lari MA, Batista DAS, et al. Acute bilineal leukemia: a rare disease with poor outcome. Leukemia 2007; 21: 2264–70.

85. Matutes E, Pickl WF, van't Veer M, et al. Mixed-phenotype acute leukemia: clinical and laboratory features and outcome in 100 patients defined according to the WHO 2008 classification. Blood 2011; 117: 3163–71.

43 Unusual Myelodysplastic Syndromes and Myeloproliferative Neoplasms

Eric Padron and Rami Komrokji

Moffitt Cancer Center and Research Institute, Tampa, FL, USA

Introduction

The World Health Organization (WHO) current classification of myeloid neoplasms includes three major categories in addition to acute myeloid leukemia (AML) (Fig. 43.1). The myelodysplastic syndromes (MDS) and myeloproliferative neoplasms (MPN) constitute two distinct and rare hematological malignancies. See Chapters 42 and 47 for more information on acute leukemias and myeloproliferative neoplasms, respectively. They are recognized as separate entities by the WHO and each have designated subdiagnoses that are highly relevant to the natural history and treatment of individual patients[1] (see Fig. 43.1). The age-adjusted yearly incidence rate in the United States for MDS is 3.42 per 100,000.[2] The myelodysplastic syndromes are clinically characterized by cytopenias secondary to ineffective hematopoiesis and the propensity to transform to AML. As MDS carries significant clinical heterogeneity (Table 43.1), the disease is further stratified by using independently validated prognosis scoring tools, such as the International Prognostic Scoring System (IPSS), to predict the natural history of individual patients.[3,4] Most simply, patients are divided into lower- and higher-risk disease. The median survival of lower-risk patients is measured in years (although still inferior to their age-matched population), and they are only treated to ameliorate the symptoms secondary to cytopenias and to decrease the need for transfusions.[4] Higher-risk patient have a short overall survival, and the standard of care is to treat initially with hypomethylating agents, with consideration of allogeneic stem cell transplantation in eligible patients.[5]

The most common morphological subtypes of MDS from the North American Association of Central Cancer Registries (NAACCR) and Surveillance, Epidemiology, and End Results (SEER) registries between 2001 and 2003 were refractory anemia (RA), refractory anemia with excess blasts (RAEB), refractory anemia with ring sideroblasts (RARS), and refractory cytopenia with multilineage dysplasia (RCMD).[2] A large number of patients were coded MDS not otherwise specified (NOS), bringing into question the accuracy of the registry data.

The last 10 years have resulted in an exponential increase in the discovery of genetic mutations for MDS. These mutations span a wide array of biological processes, though they are not disease defining or necessarily disease initiating.[6] They represent yet another level of heterogeneity whose clinical significance and epidemiology are under intense investigation.

The WHO also identifies a third group known as the myelodysplastic/myeloproliferative neoplasms (MDS/MPN).[1] This group is molecularly distinct and has a natural history that is different from MDS or MPN but includes clinical features of both. Chronic myelomonocytic leukemia (CMML) is the most common subtype of the MDS/MPN (Table 43.2).

In this chapter we will discuss the epidemiologically uncommon diagnoses of MDS and the MDS/MPN overlap syndrome. We will briefly review the presentation, treatment, and molecular pathogenesis (if known) of these uncommon malignancies.

Rare myelodysplastic syndromes

The 5q- syndrome

Van den Berghe and colleges first described the 5q- syndrome as a disease characterized by anemia, a normal to elevated platelet count, and an indolent course with only 10% of patients transforming to AML.[7] The bone marrow examination is characterized by profound erythroid hypoplasia, small hypolobated megakaryocytes, and a deletion of the long arm of chromosome 5. The SEER database estimates the age-adjusted incidence rate of MDS with the 5q deletion to be 0.06 per 100,000 in the United States.[2] However, this is likely an overestimate, because having the 5q deletion is not sufficient to diagnose the 5q- syndrome.[8] The 5q- syndrome specifically refers to the above clinical characteristics along with a myeloblast percentage of <5% in the bone marrow aspirate and no other karyotypic abnormalities. Despite the rarity of this disease, our understanding of its molecular pathobiology is quickly growing.

Textbook of Uncommon Cancer, Fourth Edition. Edited by Derek Raghavan, Charles D. Blanke, David H. Johnson, Paul L. Moots, Gregory H. Reaman, Peter G. Rose and Mikkael A. Sekeres.
© 2012 John Wiley & Sons, Inc. Published 2012 by John Wiley & Sons, Inc.

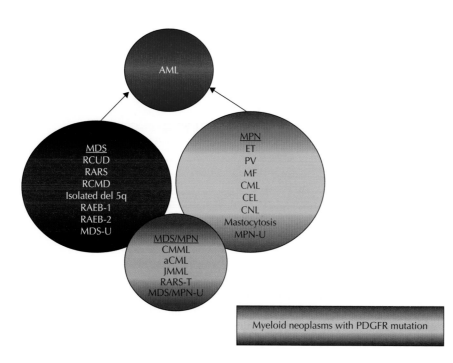

Figure 43.1 World Health Organization (WHO) classification of myeloid neoplasms. AML, acute myeloid leukemia; CEL, chronic eosinophilic leukemia; (a) CML, (atypical) chronic myeloid leukemia; CNL, chronic neutrophilic leukemia; CMML, chronic myelomonocytic leukemia; ET, essential thrombocytosis; JMML, juvenile myelomonocytic leukemia; MDS, myelodysplastic syndromes; MF, myelofibrosis; MPN, myeloproliferative neoplasms; PDGFR, platelet-derived growth factor receptor; PV, polycythemia vera; RAEB, refractory anemia with excess blasts; RARS, refractory anemia with ring sideroblasts; RARS-T, RARS with thrombocytosis; RCMD, refractory cytopenia with multilineage dysplasia; RCUD, refractory cytopenia with unilineage dysplasia; U, unclassified.

Table 43.1 Myelodysplastic syndromes (MDS).

WHO subtype	Peripheral blood	Bone marrow
Refractory anemia with unilineage dysplasia • Refractory anemia • Refractory neutropenia • Refractory thrombocytopenia	≤1% blasts Hemoglobin <10 g/dL or ANC <100,000/μL or platelet count <100,000/μL No monocytosis	<5% myeloblast >10% dysplasia in affected lineage <15% ringed sideroblasts
Refractory anemia with ringed sideroblasts	Cytopenias as above ≤1% blasts No monocytosis	<5% myeloblast >10% dysplasia in erythroid lineage >15% ringed sideroblasts
Refractory cytopenia with multilineage dysplasia	≤1% blasts Hemoglobin <10 g/dL and/or ANC <100,000/μL and/or platelet count <100,000/μL No monocytosis	<5% myeloblast >10% dysplasia in 2 or more lineages No Auer rods
Refractory anemia with excess blasts – 1	<5% blasts, no Auer rods Hemoglobin <10 g/dL and/or ANC <100,000/μL and/or platelet count <100,000/μL No monocytosis	5–9% myeloblast >10% dysplasia in 2 or more lineages No Auer rods
Refractory anemia with excess blasts – 2	5–19% blasts, +/– Auer rods Hemoglobin <10 g/dL and/or ANC <100,000/μL and/or platelet count <100,000/μL No monocytosis	5–9% myeloblast >10% dysplasia in 2 or more lineages +/– Auer rods
Myelodysplastic syndrome with isolated del (5q)	≤1% blasts Hemoglobin <10 g/dL or ANC <100,000/μL or platelet count typically normal to elevated No monocytosis	<5% myeloblast >10% dysplasia in affected lineage <15% ringed sideroblasts Del(5q) only
Myelodysplastic syndrome unclassifiable	≤1% blasts Hemoglobin <10 g/dL and/or ANC <100,000/μL and/or platelet count <100,000/μL No monocytosis	<10% dysplasia in one or more lineage with accompanying cytogenetic findings <5% blasts

Table 43.2 Chronic myelomonocytic leukemia (CMML).

WHO subtype	Peripheral blood	Bone marrow
Chronic myelomonocytic leukemia *CMML-1 †CMML-2	*<5% blasts †<19% blasts Persistent monocytosis >1000/μL +/− cytopenias Leukocytosis frequent	*<10% myeloblast †<19% blasts >10% dysplasia in affected lineage †Auer rods

The starting point began with the pathognomonic deletion of chromosome 5. Efforts by Boultwood and others have identified two distinct common deleted regions on chromosome 5, and further work using models of haploinsufficiency have narrowed these deletions to a series of specific candidate genes.[9] The haploinsufficiency of one such candidate gene, RPS14, has provided a molecular explanation for the erythroid hypoplasia seen in the 5q- syndrome.[10,11] RPS14 is a component of the structural framework of the 40s ribosomal subunit. Haploinsufficiency of RPS14 leads to free ribosomal proteins that inhibit the action of a key negative regulator of p53 (MDM2) and consequent p53 stabilization.[10] This discovery has led to grouping of the 5q- syndrome with other "ribosomopathies" such as Diamond–Blackfan anemia (DBA), Schwachman–Diamond syndrome (SDS), cartilage hair hypoplasia (CHH), and Treacher Collins syndrome.[12]

Despite its benign course, patients with the 5q- syndrome can experience significant morbidity as a result of transfusion-dependent anemia. Lenalidomide, an immunomodulatory drug, can reduce this impact, as has been shown in three independent clinical trials.[13–15] Approximately 70% of patients experience an erythroid response, with a significant proportion of patients experiencing a cytogenetic response. However, relapse is universally seen. The mechanism of sensitivity to lenalidomide is not completely understood, though sensitivity to lenalidomide appears to be mediated by the haploinsufficiency of PP2A, a tyrosine phosphatase.[16] Lenalidomide is a weak inhibitor of PP2A, resulting in the aberrant phosphorylation of MDM2, driving degradation of p53 and preventing premature apoptosis and erythroid hypoplasia.[17] Current therapeutic research is focused on potent inhibitors of p53 and disruption of the MDM2/P53 axis.

Familial myelodysplastic syndrome

The vast majority of MDS cases occur sporadically in older adults. In exceedingly rare circumstances, suspicion is raised for a hereditary cause when the age at diagnosis is young and MDS is identified in more than one first-degree relative. To date, three inherited genetic lesions have been associated with myelodysplastic syndrome.[18] These are distinct from syndromes in which the risk of MDS is elevated, as these occur more frequently compared to the above inherited lesions. Bone marrow failure syndromes, defects in DNA repair, and defects in p53 have all been associated with an increased risk of MDS in the context of a broader syndrome.[19]

The most well-described familial disease is the familial platelet disorder caused by mutations in RUNX1. RUNX1 is an important member of the core binding factor (CBF) complex, located on chromosome 21q22. It contains a DNA binding domain and protein interaction domain that allow it to partner with other members of the CBF.[20,21] Heterogeneous, inactivating mutations in RUNX1 have been reported in sporadic cases of MDS and in translocations seen in AML. Patients with the familial platelet syndrome typically present with a bleeding tendency at a young age. The platelet count is mild to moderately decreased, with measurable platelet dysfunction by epinephrine aggregation studies in the absence of platelet morphology abnormalities. Approximately 50% of these patients progress to MDS. Of over a dozen pedigrees described, mutations in RUNX1 are heterogeneous.[22–25] Point mutations in the DNA binding and noncoding regions can result in both haploinsufficiency and dominant-negative models of genetic pathogenesis.[22,24] The inheritance is usually autosomal dominant, and the risk of malignancy is usually restricted to abnormalities in the myeloid lineage.

Defined as the sole cytogenetic abnormality in the bone marrow in two or more siblings, the familial monosomy 7 syndrome is another inherited form of MDS.[26] Monosomy 7 is associated with a series of syndromes, but 14 families have been described with monosomy 7 and MDS/AML alone.[26–28] As the most common abnormality seen in familial MDS, pancytopenia appears to be the first presenting symptom, occurring at a median age of 10 years.[26] The inheritance pattern is autosomal dominant.[29] Without allogeneic transplant, the prognosis appears to be as poor as adult MDS with the monosomy 7 abnormality.[30] In adult MDS, monosomy is thought to be a secondary event associated with leukemogenesis. In the familial monosomy 7, the precise genetic lesion remains unknown. Interestingly, because of the inheritance pattern and nature of monosomy 7 in sporadic MDS, many have postulated that the genetic lesion may not reside on chromosome 7.[27] Rather, an occult "mutator" lesion may be responsible for the MDS/AML phenotype and the universally apparent monosomy karyotype.

More recently, three families with multiple cases of MDS or AML over consecutive generations have been found to have point mutations in GATA2.[31] GATA2 is a transcription factor with a zinc finger DNA binding domain critical for hematopoiesis in a murine model.[32,33] A recurrent point mutation in threonine 354 within the zinc finger domain was conserved in all affected families. In a fourth family, a microdeletion at threonine 355 was detected. These families did not have a mutation in RUNX1 or CEPB-α (associated with familial AML but not MDS) and did not have a predisposition to other malignancies outside AML/MDS.

Refractory neutropenia and refractory thrombocytopenia

In 2008, the WHO introduced a new subclassification of MDS that requires unilineage dysplasia and a solitary cytopenia within the same myeloid lineage, termed "refractory cytopenia with unilineage dysplasia" (RCUD), that includes RA, refractory neutropenia (RN), and refractory thrombocytopenia (RT).

These patients must also have <1% blasts in the peripheral blood and <5% blasts in the marrow.[1] While it is common for MDS patients to have solitary anemia and erythroid dysplasia (i.e. RA), it is much more uncommon to see solitary dysplasia/cytopenias of the other myeloid lineages. In a single-institution review of 126 of 650 patients with RCUD, 18% and 19% of these patients had refractory neutropenia and refractory thrombocytopenia, respectively.[34] The natural history of this subclassification is unknown. However, most patients in this category will be at lower risk for AML transformation, and thus treatment will focus on symptomatic cytopenias.[35]

Therapy-related myelodysplastic syndrome

Therapy-related MDS (t-MDS) is a subclassification of MDS that the 2008 WHO classification includes in the category of therapy-related neoplasms.[1] In a large Japanese registry, it is responsible for approximately 10–20% of all MDS diagnoses captured.[36] The diagnosis of this disease requires the pathological diagnosis of MDS along with a history of previous exposure to cytotoxic agents implicated in the pathogenesis of t-MDS.[37] As a class, alkylating agents, topoisomerase II inhibitors, nucleoside analogs, ionizing radiation, and others have been associated with t-MDS (Table 43.3). The time to diagnosis after exposure is varied, though the latency period after treatment with alkylating agents is typically 5–7 years and is associated with an unfavorable karyotype, including complex cytogenetics and, more frequently, monosomy 7 in over 90% of cases.[38] With exposure to topoisomerase II inhibitors, the latency period is much shorter, estimated to be 1–3 years. The cytogenetic lesions usually involve abnormalities of the long arms of chromosomes 11 and 21.[39–41] Most patients present with frank treatment-related AML, with t-MDS being a much rarer initial presentation. The prognosis of t-MDS is generally poor compared to *de novo* MDS but whether this is independent of the complex cytogenetics remains unclear.[39–41] Allogeneic stem cell transplant remains the only curative option.

In the case of cytotoxic therapy and ionizing radiation, the etiology of t-MDS is thought to initiate secondary to bystander DNA damage of normal hematopoietic precursors. However, polymorphisms in NQO1, GST-M1, GST-T1, and CYP3A4

have been associated with patients who had t-MDS/t-AML.[42–44] t-MDS has also been associated with stem cell transplantation. The incidence of t-MDS after autologous stem cell transplant for lymphomas, for example, is reported to be 1–20% at 20 years, with a median latency period of 1–2 years.[45] In addition to the cytotoxic therapy in the induction and conditioning regimens, strain on normal telomere dynamics has been implicated in the pathogenesis of t-MDS following stem cell transplant. After the engraftment period, supraphysiological strain is placed on the transplanted stem cells to repopulate the entire bone marrow. This places strain on the machinery responsible for regenerating telomeres. This and telomere shortening have been associated with genomic instability[46,47] and, in the context of t-MDS, with the development of secondary malignancies.[48] In rare cases in which induction therapy is used to treat *de novo* MDS, t-MDS can arise and be distinguished from relapse by cytogenetic differences between the *de novo* and t-MDS within the same patient.[37]

Rare myelodysplastic syndrome/myeloproliferative neoplasms

Atypical chronic myeloid leukemia

Atypical chronic myeloid leukemia (aCML) refers to patients whose disease is morphologically consistent with CML but who lack evidence of the BCR-Abl fusion protein. See Chapter 47 for a discussion of CML. Approximately 90% of patients who meet morphological criteria for CML harbor the Philadelphia chromosome by conventional G-banding cytogenetics. Of those who do not, 25–50% of cases have the BCR-Abl fusion protein detected by the polymerase chain reaction (PCR) assay.[49] The natural history and response to imatinib between those who have the Philadelphia chromosome and those who have the BCR-Abl transcript detected by PCR are essentially identical. However, the very small proportion of cases that do not have either cytogenetic or molecular abnormalities detected represent a distinctly different disease. They do not respond to imatinib, carry an aggressive course with a median survival of 11–18 months, and can transform to AML.[50] The WHO diagnosis of this subtype is classified under the MDS/MPNs and recognizes that aCML carries similar morphological criteria to CML, but is also characterized by granulocytic dysplasia, a feature not seen in CML.[1] The treatment of aCML is not standardized, and both cytotoxic induction and interferon have had reported responses.[51] Allogeneic stem cell transplant has also been reported, with success rates similar to that of BCR-Abl-positive CML.[52]

Refractory anemia with ring sideroblasts and thrombocytosis

Refractory anemia with ring sideroblasts and thrombocytosis (RARS-T) is a rare disease that includes features of RARS, a common subtype of MDS, and essential thrombocytosis (ET), a classic MPN subtype. While debate exists as to whether RARS-T represents a distinct disease or is an ET variant,[53] the WHO does endorse RARS-T as a unique provisional entity

Table 43.3 Therapy-related myelodysplastic syndromes.

Feature	Class I	Class II
Chemotherapy	Alkylating agent	Topoisomerase II
Patient age	Older	Younger
Cytogenetics	Unbalanced (monosomy 5 or 7)	Balanced (11q23 or band 21q22)
MDS phase	Yes	No
Length of latency period	Long (usually >5 years)	Short (2–5 years)
Response to therapy	CR ±	CR likely

Modified from Bennett J, *et al*. The myelodysplastic syndromes. In: Abeloff MD, Armitage JO, Niederhuber JE (eds) *Clinical Oncology*. New York: Churchill Livingstone, 2004. pp. 2849–81.
CR, complete response.

classified under the MDS/MPNs. The diagnosis of RARS-T requires greater than 15% ring sideroblasts in the bone marrow along with a platelet count of greater than 450×10^9/L. The megakaryocytes are typically large and resemble those seen in ET.[1] Anemia may be present, and the prognosis is usually indolent, with overall survival rates similar to that of patients with ET, and better than that of RARS.[54] However, the thrombotic risk associated with RARS-T is unknown and thus recommendations regarding antiplatelet or cytoreductive therapy cannot be made.

The molecular genetics of RARS-T is interesting and supports the notion that RARS-T is distinct from ET and RARS. The frequency of the JAK2V617F mutation in RARS-T has been reported to be approximately 50–67%, similar to that of ET.[54] However, exciting new work has found mutations in SF3B1, a critical component of the splicing machinery, in up to 68% of patients with RARS-T, which may be associated with a favorable outcome.[55,56] Further, ring sideroblasts alone have been highly associated with SF3B1 mutations but, to our knowledge, ET does not. Coexistence of JAK2V617F and SF3B1 in the same patient with RARS-T has also been reported. The treatment of RARS-T should focus on treating the anemia, similar to RARS in MDS.

Conclusion

Classification of myeloid neoplasms based on further understanding of the biology of the disease has resulted in a more complex categorization. We have focused our discussion here on the rarely encountered MDS or MDS/MPN disorders. Recognition of these disorders and the underlying molecular biology can significantly influence treatment choices.

References

1. Vardiman JW, Thiele J, Arber DA, et al. The 2008 revision of the World Health Organization (WHO) classification of myeloid neoplasms and acute leukemia: rationale and important changes. Blood 2009; 114: 937–51.

2. Rollison DE, Howlader N, Smith MT, et al. Epidemiology of myelodysplastic syndromes and chronic myeloproliferative disorders in the United States, 2001–2004, using data from the NAACCR and SEER programs. Blood 2008; 112: 45–52.

3. Greenberg P, Cox C, LeBeau M, et al. International scoring system for evaluating prognosis in myelodysplastic syndromes. Blood 1997; 89: 2079.

4. Kantarjian H, O'Brien S, Ravandi F, et al. Proposal for a new risk model in myelodysplastic syndrome that accounts for events not considered in the original International Prognostic Scoring System. Cancer 2008; 113: 1351–61.

5. Fenaux P, Mufti G, Hellstrom-Lindberg E, et al. Efficacy of azacitidine compared with that of conventional care regimens in the treatment of higher-risk myelodysplastic syndromes: a randomised, open-label, phase III study. Lancet Oncol 2009; 10: 223–32.

6. Bejar R, Stevenson K, Abdel-Wahab O, et al. Clinical effect of point mutations in myelodysplastic syndromes. N Engl J Med 2011; 364: 2496–506.

7. Van den Berghe H, Cassiman JJ, David G, Fryns JP, Michaux JL, Sokal G. Distinct haematological disorder with deletion of long arm of No. 5 chromosome. Nature 1974; 251: 437–8.

8. Kantarjian H, O'Brien S, Ravandi F, et al. The heterogeneous prognosis of patients with myelodysplastic syndrome and chromosome 5 abnormalities: how does it relate to the original lenalidomide experience in MDS? Cancer 2009; 115: 5202–9.

9. Boultwood J, Fidler C, Strickson AJ, et al. Narrowing and genomic annotation of the commonly deleted region of the 5q- syndrome. Blood 2002; 99: 4638–41.

10. Barlow JL, Drynan LF, Hewett DR, et al. A p53-dependent mechanism underlies macrocytic anemia in a mouse model of human 5q- syndrome. Nat Med 2010; 16: 59–66.

11. Ebert BL, Pretz J, Bosco J, et al. Identification of RPS14 as a 5q- syndrome gene by RNA interference screen. Nature 2008; 451: 335–9.

12. Narla A, Ebert BL. Ribosomopathies: human disorders of ribosome dysfunction. Blood 2010; 115: 3196–205.

13. Fenaux P, Giagounidis A, Selleslag DL, et al. Safety of lenalidomide (LEN) from a randomized phase III trial (MDS-004) in low-/int-1-risk myelodysplastic syndromes (MDS) with a del(5q) abnormality. J Clin Oncol (Meeting Abstracts) 2010; 28: 6598.

14. List A, Dewald G, Bennett J, et al. Lenalidomide in the myelodysplastic syndrome with chromosome 5q deletion. N Engl J Med 2006; 355: 1456–65.

15. List A, Kurtin S, Roe DJ, et al. Efficacy of lenalidomide in myelodysplastic syndromes. N Engl J Med 2005; 352: 549–57.

16. Wei S, Chen X, Rocha K, et al. A critical role for phosphatase haplodeficiency in the selective suppression of deletion 5q MDS by lenalidomide. Proc Natl Acad Sci U S A 2009; 106: 12974–9.

17. Momand J, Zambetti GP, Olson DC, George D, Levine AJ. The mdm-2 oncogene product forms a complex with the p53 protein and inhibits p53-mediated transactivation. Cell 1992; 69: 1237–45.

18. Owen C, Barnett M, Fitzgibbon J. Familial myelodysplasia and acute myeloid leukaemia – a review. Br J Haematol 2007; 140: 123–32.

19. Liew E, Owen C. Familial myelodysplastic syndromes: a review of the literature. Haematologica 2011; 96: 1536–42.

20. Ho CY, Otterud B, Legare RD, et al. Linkage of a familial platelet disorder with a propensity to develop myeloid malignancies to human chromosome 21q22.1-22.2. Blood 1996; 87: 5218–24.

21. Cleary ML. A new angle on a pervasive oncogene. Nat Genet 1999; 23: 134–5.

22. Song WJ, Sullivan MG, Legare RD, et al. Haploinsufficiency of CBFA2 causes familial thrombocytopenia with propensity to develop acute myelogenous leukaemia. Nat Genet 1999; 23: 166–75.

23. Heller PG, Glembotsky AC, Gandhi MJ, et al. Low Mpl receptor expression in a pedigree with familial platelet disorder with predisposition to acute myelogenous leukemia and a novel AML1 mutation. Blood 2005; 105: 4664–70.

24. Michaud J, Wu F, Osato M, et al. In vitro analyses of known and novel RUNX1/AML1 mutations in dominant familial platelet disorder with predisposition to acute myelogenous leukemia: implications for mechanisms of pathogenesis. Blood 2002; 99: 1364–72.

25. Dowton SB, Beardsley D, Jamison D, Blattner S, Li FP. Studies of a familial platelet disorder. Blood 1985; 65: 557–63.

26. Gaitonde S, Boumendjel R, Angeles R, Rondelli D. Familial childhood monosomy 7 and associated myelodysplasia. J Pediatr Hematol Oncol 2010; 32: e236–7.

27. Minelli A, Maserati E, Giudici G, et al. Familial partial monosomy 7 and myelodysplasia: different parental origin of the monosomy 7 suggests action of a mutator gene. Cancer Genet Cytogenet 2001; 124: 147–51.

28. Kwong YL, Ng MH, Ma SK. Familial acute myeloid leukemia with monosomy 7: late onset and involvement of a multipotential progenitor cell. Cancer Genet Cytogenet 2000; 116: 170–3.

29. Porta G, Maserati E, Mattarucchi E, et al. Monosomy 7 in myeloid malignancies: parental origin and monitoring by real-time quantitative PCR. Leukemia 2007; 21: 1833–5.

30. Patnaik MM, Hanson CA, Hodnefield JM, Knudson R, van Dyke DL, Tefferi A. Monosomal karyotype in myelodysplastic syndromes, with or without monosomy 7 or 5, is prognostically worse than an otherwise complex karyotype. Leukemia 2011; 25: 266–70.

31. Hahn CN, Chong CE, Carmichael CL, et al. Heritable GATA2 mutations associated with familial myelodysplastic syndrome and acute myeloid leukemia. Nat Genet 2011; 43: 1012–17.

32. Dorfman DM, Wilson DB, Bruns GA, Orkin SH. Human transcription factor GATA-2. Evidence for regulation of preproendothelin-1 gene expression in endothelial cells. J Biol Chem 1992; 267: 1279–85.

33. Tsai FY, Keller G, Kuo FC, *et al.* An early haematopoietic defect in mice lacking the transcription factor GATA-2. Nature 1994; 371: 221–6.

34. Breccia M, Latagliata R, Cannella L, *et al.* Refractory cytopenia with unilineage dysplasia: analysis of prognostic factors and survival in 126 patients. Leuk Lymphoma 2010; 51: 783–8.

35. Steensma DP. Hematopoietic growth factors in myelodysplastic syndromes. Semin Oncol 2011; 38: 635–47.

36. Takeyama K, Seto M, Uike N, *et al.* Therapy-related leukemia and myelo-dysplastic syndrome: a large-scale Japanese study of clinical and cytoge-netic features as well as prognostic factors. Int J Hematol 2000; 71: 144–52.

37. Larson RA. Etiology and management of therapy-related myeloid leuke-mia. Hematol Am Soc Hematol Educ Program 2007: 453–9.

38. Pedersen-Bjergaard J, Andersen MK, Andersen MT, Christiansen DH. Genetics of therapy-related myelodysplasia and acute myeloid leukemia. Leukemia 2008; 22: 240–8.

39. Rowley JD, Golomb HM, Vardiman JW. Nonrandom chromosome abnor-malities in acute leukemia and dysmyelopoietic syndromes in patients with previously treated malignant disease. Blood 1981; 58: 759–67.

40. Traweek ST, Slovak ML, Nademanee AP, Brynes RK, Niland JC, Forman SJ. Clonal karyotypic hematopoietic cell abnormalities occurring after autologous bone marrow transplantation for Hodgkin's disease and non-Hodgkin's lymphoma. Blood 1994; 84: 957–63.

41. Kantarjian HM, Keating MJ, Walters RS, *et al.* Therapy-related leukemia and myelodysplastic syndrome: clinical, cytogenetic, and prognostic fea-tures. J Clin Oncol 1986; 4: 1748–57.

42. Larson RA, Wang Y, Banerjee M, *et al.* Prevalence of the inactivating 609C ->T polymorphism in the NAD(P)H: quinone oxidoreductase (NQO1) gene in patients with primary and therapy-related myeloid leuke-mia. Blood 1999; 94: 803–7.

43. Allan JM, Wild CP, Rollinson S, *et al.* Polymorphism in glutathione S-transferase P1 is associated with susceptibility to chemotherapy-induced leukemia. Proc Natl Acad Sci U S A 2001; 98: 11592–7.

44. Naoe T, Takeyama K, Yokozawa T, *et al.* Analysis of genetic polymor-phism in NQO1, GST-M1, GST-T1, and CYP3A4 in 469 Japanese patients with therapy-related leukemia/ myelodysplastic syndrome and de novo acute myeloid leukemia. Clin Cancer Res 2000; 6: 4091–5.

45. Stone RM, Neuberg D, Soiffer R, *et al.* Myelodysplastic syndrome as a late complication following autologous bone marrow transplantation for non-Hodgkin's lymphoma. J Clin Oncol 1994; 12: 2535–42.

46. Ly H, Calado RT, Allard P, *et al.* Functional characterization of telomerase RNA variants found in patients with hematologic disorders. Blood 2005; 105: 2332–9.

47. Savage SA, Calado RT, Xin ZT, Ly H, Young NS, Chanock SJ. Genetic variation in telomeric repeat binding factors 1 and 2 in aplastic anemia. Exp Hematol 2006; 34: 664–71.

48. Chakraborty S, Sun CL, Francisco L, *et al.* Accelerated telomere shorten-ing precedes development of therapy-related myelodysplasia or acute myelogenous leukemia after autologous transplantation for lymphoma. J Clin Oncol 2009; 27: 791–8.

49. Van der Plas DC, Grosveld G, Hagemeijer A. Review of clinical, cytoge-netic, and molecular aspects of Ph-negative CML. Cancer Genet Cytogenet 1991; 52: 143–56.

50. Onida F, Ball G, Kantarjian HM, *et al.* Characteristics and outcome of patients with Philadelphia chromosome negative, bcr/abl negative chronic myelogenous leukemia. Cancer 2002; 95: 1673–84.

51. Kurzrock R, Bueso-Ramos CE, Kantarjian H, *et al.* BCR rearrangement-negative chronic myelogenous leukemia revisited. J Clin Oncol 2001; 19: 2915–26.

52. Koldehoff M, Beelen DW, Trenschel R, *et al.* Outcome of hematopoietic stem cell transplantation in patients with atypical chronic myeloid leuke-mia. Bone Marrow Transplant 2004; 34: 1047–50.

53. Bang SM. Is RARS-T a new disease entity or a subtype of RARS or ET? Korean J Hematol 2010; 45: 139–40.

54. Schmitt-Graeff AH, Teo SS, Olschewski M, *et al.* JAK2V617F mutation status identifies subtypes of refractory anemia with ringed sideroblasts associated with marked thrombocytosis. Haematologica 2008; 93: 34–40.

55. Malcovati L, Papaemmanuil E, Bowen DT, *et al.* Clinical significance of SF3B1 mutations in myelodysplastic syndromes and myelodysplastic/ myeloproliferative neoplasms. Blood 2011; 118: 6239–46.

56. Papaemmanuil E, Cazzola M, Boultwood J, *et al.* Somatic SF3B1 muta-tion in myelodysplasia with ring sideroblasts. N Engl J Med 2011; 365: 1384–95.

44 Rare B Cell Lymphoproliferative Disorders

Paul M. Barr and Jonathan W. Friedberg

Department of Medicine, James P. Wilmot Cancer Center, University of Rochester, Rochester, NY, USA

Introduction

This chapter focuses on the rarest of the mature B cell neoplasms as defined in the current World Health Organization (WHO) classification, the current reference for classification of hematological malignancies.[1] As with any classification system, it is constantly evolving based on available technology and data, and periodically updated reflecting this rapidly evolving field. As such, this chapter provides a "snapshot" of these uncommon diagnoses. The summarized data can assist in guiding the diagnosis and management in certain cases, while in others, the data only highlight our lack of knowledge. To better inform the practicing oncologist, we focus on entities for which large prospective studies are not available. As they are covered elsewhere, we will not include plasma cell neoplasms (see Chapter 45) or cutaneous diseases (see Chapter 49).

Box 44.1 lists the current mature B cell neoplasms according to the WHO classification. Diseases are defined primarily by morphology and immunophenotype, at times considering clinical features. In the current era, genetic abnormalities now define certain entities, or assist in making a diagnosis. Therefore, there is no "gold standard" by which all diseases are defined. Some provisional categories are included to preserve the homogeneity of well-defined categories; these are likely to change or to be further divided in future classification iterations.

B cell prolymphocytic leukemia

Accounting for <1% of mature B cell neoplasms and <1% of B cell leukemias, B prolymphocytic leukemia (PLL) is a neoplasm of mature activated B cells primarily affecting the peripheral blood, bone marrow, and spleen.[2] Of all PLL diagnoses, 80% are of B cell etiology with the remaining being T cell in origin. The diagnosis requires that malignant prolymphocytes constitute >55% of circulating lymphocytes, and that transformed chronic lymphocytic leukemia (CLL) be excluded. Cases harboring a t(11;14), though previously included in this cateory, have been subsequently reclassified as mantle cell lymphoma.

Primarily a disease of the elderly, patients present with a progressive lymphocytosis, splenomegaly and often anemia, thrombocytopenia, and systemic symptoms.[3] The medium sized prolymphocyte (Fig. 44.1) expresses B cell antigens, including CD19, CD20, and CD79a. Most cases are negative for CD5 and CD23, while half of cases are positive for CD38 and ZAP-70.[4] As opposed to CLL, it is not clear if these markers are predictive of outcome. Deletion of chromosome 17p was detected in half of studied cases, likely accounting for the aggressive nature of the disease observed in certain patients. With this in mind, the median overall survival has been estimated at 3–5 years based on small patient cohorts.[5]

Treatment options are similar to those for CLL. Small series have demonstrated a complete remission rate of less than 20% when purine analogs are administered as single agents.[6,7] A 7-day course of cladribine may provide somewhat better activity, as five of eight patients achieved complete remission in one small series.[8] Studies of purine analog-based combinations are lacking. As in other B cell lymphoproliferative disorders, monoclonal antibodies have been evaluated in PLL. While several studies have investigated the humanized anti-CD52 antibody alemtuzumab in T cell PLL, outcomes of B cell PLL patients treated with alemtuzumab are rare.[9] Case reports have documented the activity of the anti-CD20 antibody rituximab, albeit with modest response durations.[10,11]

Hairy cell leukemia

Also a rare B cell leukemia, hairy cell leukemia (HCL) accounts for <1% of mature B cell neoplasms and 2% of B cell leukemias.[12] It is an indolent lymphoproliferative disorder predominantly affecting middle-aged Caucasian males. Patients present commonly with weakness and fatigue, but also may have fevers, pancytopenia and abdominal fullness from hepatosplenomegaly. Rarely, vasculitis or other autoimmune disorders are observed.[13] The disease is characterized by mature-appearing B cells with abundant cytoplasm and

Textbook of Uncommon Cancer, Fourth Edition. Edited by Derek Raghavan, Charles D. Blanke, David H. Johnson, Paul L. Moots, Gregory H. Reaman, Peter G. Rose and Mikkael A. Sekeres.
© 2012 John Wiley & Sons, Inc. Published 2012 by John Wiley & Sons, Inc.

Box 44.1 Mature B cell neoplasms.

- Chronic lymphocytic leukemia/small lymphocytic lymphoma
- B cell prolymphocytic leukemia
- Splenic marginal zone lymphoma
- Hairy cell leukemia
- Splenic B cell lymphoma/leukemia, unclassifiable
  - Splenic diffuse red pulp small B cell lymphoma
  - Hairy cell leukemia variant
- Lymphoplasmacytic lymphoma
- Heavy chain diseases
  - γ Heavy chain disease
  - μ Heavy chain disease
  - α Heavy chain disease
- Plasma cell neoplasms
  - Monoclonal gammopathy of undetermined significance
  - Plasma cell myeloma
  - Solitary plasmacytoma of bone
  - Extraosseous plasmacytoma
  - Monoclonal immunoglobulin deposition disease
- Extranodal marginal zone lymphoma of mucosa-associated lymphoid tissue
- Nodal marginal zone lymphoma
- Follicular lymphoma
- Primary cutaneous follicular center lymphoma
- Mantle cell lymphoma
- Diffuse large B cell lymphoma, not otherwise specified
  - T cell/histiocyte-rich large B cell lymphoma
  - Primary diffuse large B cell lymphoma of the central nervous system
  - Primary cutaneous diffuse large B cell lymphoma, leg type
  - Epstein–Barr virus-positive diffuse large B cell lymphoma of the elderly
- Diffuse large B cell lymphoma associated with chronic inflammation
- Lymphomatoid granulomatosis
- Primary mediastinal (thymic) large B cell lymphoma
- Intravascular large B cell lymphoma
- ALK-positive large B cell lymphoma
- Plasmablastic lymphoma
- Large B cell lymphoma arising in human herpesvirus-8-associated multicentric Castleman disease
- Primary effusion lymphoma
- Burkitt lymphoma
- B cell lymphoma, unclassifiable, with features intermediate between diffuse large B cell lymphoma and Burkitt lymphoma
- B cell lymphoma, unclassifiable, with features intermediate between diffuse large B cell lymphoma and classic Hodgkin lymphoma

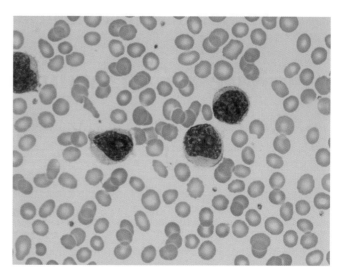

Figure 44.1 B cell prolymphocytic leukemia peripheral blood smear. The cells are medium to large with prominent vesicular nucleoli.

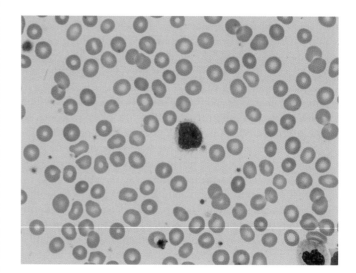

Figure 44.2 Hairy cell leukemia as seen on peripheral blood smear demonstrating a "fried egg" appearance.

circumferential projections found predominantly in the bone marrow and spleen, which are responsible for a classic "fried egg" appearance microscopically (Fig. 44.2). The malignant cell immunophenotype includes the pan B cell antigens, CD19, CD20, and CD22, in addition to CD11c, CD25, and CD103.[14] Annexin A1 positivity is specific to HCL and is not expressed on other B cell neoplasms. Positivity for the *VH4-34* gene may predict for an inferior response to purine analogs and a shorter

overall survival.[15] The diagnosis is typically made by identifying the characteristic cells on bone marrow biopsy, replacing the technically challenging tartrate-resistant acid phosphatase stain. Most cases of HCL demonstrate mutation of immunoglobulin heavy chain genes, consistent with a postgerminal center cell of origin.[16]

Despite the rarity of HCL, multicenter studies have significantly advanced the treatment paradigm, providing many patients with a lifespan comparable to age-matched controls. While HCL was initially managed with splenectomy in the 1960s and 1970s, treatment with interferon-α in the early 1980s induced complete remissions. At nearly the same time, the first report of the effectiveness of the purine analog pentostatin was published,[17] with activity ultimately confirmed in a randomized trial.[18] Subsequent studies demonstrated that 76–95% of patients could achieve complete remissions with a first-line, single 7-day continuous infusion of cladribine, another purine analog.[19–21]

Median progression-free survival is in excess of a decade, and durable complete remissions can be reinduced upon retreatment with purine analogs. Additional studies focused on subcutaneous use of cladribine, as well as a weekly schedule of administration,[22–24] which confirmed the efficacy of cladribine, though with continued myelosuppression and infectious complications. Preliminary data from the Italian Cooperative Group suggest that the reduced-dose 5-day subcutaneous administration may be less toxic compared to 7-day administration.[25]

In spite of the dramatic responses observed in the above studies, prolonged follow-up suggests a pattern of continuous relapse, consistent with disease control rather than cure.[26] A recombinant immunotoxin, BL22, combining the variable domains of an anti-CD22 monoclonal antibody with a *Pseudomonas* exotoxin, has been tested in a phase 2 trial.[27] In patients with relative refractoriness to purine analogs, 47% achieved a complete remission and 11% achieved a partial response. In patients achieving a complete remission, the median response duration had not been reached at 22 months. Toxicities to the immunotoxin were largely grade 1 or 2 in severity. Eight percent of patients did develop hemolytic uremic syndrome, none requiring plasma exchange. Rituximab has been shown to be efficacious in relapsed as well as in treatment-naïve patients, converting incomplete responders to complete remissions.[28–30] Combination purine analog and rituximab therapy has been shown to be effective in relapsed patients, and an ongoing trial will attempt to determine if combination or sequential treatment will offer the best long-term outcomes in the newly diagnosed setting.[31]

Lymphomatoid granulomatosis

Lymphomatoid granulomatosis (LG) affects mainly middle-aged adults, with a median age at diagnosis of 48 years, and men twice as often as women. Predominantly involving the lungs (with bilateral pulmonary nodular infiltrates often observed on imaging studies), the most common initial complaints are fever and cough, with other constitutional symptoms including weight loss.[32] Extrapulmonary involvement most often occurs in the skin as well as the central and peripheral nervous system. While the Epstein–Barr virus (EBV) is involved in the pathogenesis of LG,[33–35] significant variability of immunohistochemical EBV-related staining and initial false-negative results have been reported. Histologically, the mixed mononuclear cell infiltrate includes large CD20+ B lymphocytes in a background of T lymphocytes, histiocytes, and plasma cells.[36] Prominent vascular invasion led to previous descriptions of "angiocentric lymphoma." The grading system for LG is based on the proportion of large cell involvement, similar to that for follicular lymphoma, and on the proportion of EBV-positive B cells in the current WHO classification.[1]

Consistent with its relationship to EBV, several investigators have reported LG in association with inherited and acquired immunodeficiency states. However, given the histological similarity of LG to posttransplant lymphoproliferative disorder, it has been suggested that the diagnosis of LG should not be made in the setting of a previous solid organ or stem cell transplant.[37]

Limited data are available to guide the management of LG. Treatment with chemotherapeutics has resulted in poor outcomes, with median survivals reported at 1–2 years.[36,38,39] Anecdotal reports have suggested improved outcomes with rituximab.[40,41] Interferon-α2b treatment provided a prolonged disease-free interval in three patients and a partial response in another.[42] Further, a preliminary study of interferon-α treatment in 31 patients with polyclonal or oligoclonal disease reported a complete remission rate of 60%, with a progression-free survival of 56% at 5 years.[43] Complete remission following high-dose chemotherapy and autologous stem cell rescue has also been reported in a patient with otherwise refractory disease.

Intravascular large B cell lymphoma

Identified by various names over recent decades, this rare variant of extranodal diffuse large B cell non-Hodgkin lymphoma (NHL) is characterized by tumor involvement within the lumina of small to intermediate sized vessels, resulting in insults to nearly all organ systems and a notable absence of lymphadenopathy. As a large cell lymphoma variant, malignant lymphocytes are typically described as being large, having prominent nucleoli and frequent mitoses, and expressing common B cell antigens including CD20.[44] Primarily a disease of the elderly, intravascular large B cell lymphoma (IVLBL) can affect any organ, resulting in a variety of presentations, with geographical differences in clinicopathological characteristics. Individuals in Asian countries often present with fever, universal elevation of lactate dehydrogenase (LDH), laboratory findings suggestive of disseminated intravascular coagulation (DIC), frequent bone marrow involvement, and hemophagocytic syndrome in 59% of patients.[45] European patients had a higher incidence of cutaneous eruptions, potentially suggesting a cutaneous variant.[46] Between 25% and 34% of patients demonstrate neurological symptoms at presentation, including cognitive deficits, gait impairment, seizures, and sensory/motor deficits. Laboratory abnormalities may suggest hepatic and renal dysfunction; pulmonary symptoms occur frequently.

Astute clinical suspicion is needed to make a timely diagnosis given the nonspecific presentation, lack of lymphadenopathy, and often rapidly progressive nature of the disease. The diagnosis is made by biopsy of involved organs, demonstrating the monoclonal B cell population. Notably, reports of random skin biopsies suggest that this practice may aid in confirming the diagnosis.[47,48] Largely due to difficulties in diagnosis leading to delayed therapy, early reports of clinical outcomes suggested dismal results,[49] which have improved in more contemporary studies. One retrospective comparison demonstrated an advantage for regimens containing rituximab in Asian patients.[45] Two-year overall survival was reported as 66% in those who received rituximab, compared to 46% in those only receiving chemotherapy. A cohort of European patients treated with combination immunochemotherapy had an overall survival (OS) of 81% at 3 years.[50] Given the predominant intravascular involvement, a notable incidence of infusion reactions has accompanied these reports, leading some investigators to suggest that initial administration of rituximab should be delayed until after the first course of chemotherapy.

Primary effusion lymphoma

First described in 1989, primary effusion lymphoma (PEL) occurs in the setting of immunodeficiency, most commonly the human immunodeficiency virus (HIV).[51] As indicated by its name, PEL uniquely presents with lymphomatous pleural, peritoneal and pericardial effusions, causing the presenting symptoms of dyspnea and abdominal distension. PEL is exceedingly rare, accounting for <1% of NHLs and only 3% of NHL in the setting of HIV.[52] More than 90% of reports involve men, with a mean age of 62 years.[53]

While the oncogenic mechanisms are not completely understood, PEL is further related to human herpesvirus-8 (HHV-8) infection. The prevalence of this double-stranded DNA virus is high in sub-Saharan Africa (>50%), intermediate in Mediterranean areas (20–30%) and very low in northern Europe and the United States (<3%).[54] Incorporation of the HHV-8 genome appears to result in the production of the gene products: latency-associated nuclear antigen-1, viral cyclins and viral FLICE inhibitory protein, acting to promote viral replication, inhibit tumor suppressor genes, promote cell cycle progression, and inhibit apoptosis, ultimately promoting neoplastic transformation.[55–59] Evidence of concurrent EBV infection in PEL suggests a supportive, albeit poorly understood, role.[60]

The B cell lineage derivation of PEL cells is based on clonal rearrangements of the heavy immunoglobulin genes and preferential expression of λ light chain genes by polymerase chain reaction, suggesting clonal proliferation by an antigen selection process.[61] Despite this, it is most commonly of a null phenotype, although cases expressing B and T cell antigens have been reported. Based on frequent expression of activation and plasma cell markers, the cell of origin is thought to be a post-germinal center B cell approaching plasma cell differentiation.[62,63] Given its varying phenotype, it may be difficult to differentiate from other lymphomas, namely anaplastic large T cell lymphoma or the immunoblastic phenotype of diffuse large B cell lymphoma (DLBCL). The diagnosis may be confirmed by HHV-8 positivity.

Most cases of PEL behave in a highly aggressive fashion, with a median survival of less than 6 months despite multiagent chemotherapy and antiretroviral therapy in HIV-related cases.[64] In addition to lymphoma progression, death is often due to opportunistic infection and other HIV-related complications, secondary to these patients' profound immunosuppression. Antiviral therapy with intracavitary cidofovir led to sustained remissions in a few patients.[65,66] In the rare case expressing CD20, rituximab may be of benefit.[67]

Castleman disease

Also associated with HHV-8 and most frequently occurring in the setting of concomitant HIV infection is Castleman disease. Rarely, it is localized, presenting without systemic symptoms and termed *unicentric* Castleman disease. Somewhat more common is multicentric Castleman disease (MCD), a rare lymphoproliferative disorder related to an aggressive immunoresponse to HHV-8, causing systemic symptoms and diffuse lymphadenopathy.[68] Hepatosplenomegaly, respiratory symptoms, and edema, along with hypoalbuminemia and pancytopenia are frequently observed.[69] The development of NHL has been documented in the setting of MCD and is now recognized as a separate pathological entity in the current WHO classification.[70,71] Concurrent polyneuropathy and myasthenia gravis have been reported, as well as the constellation of signs making up POEMS (polyneuropathy, organomegaly, endocrinopathy, monoclonal gammopathy, and skin changes) syndrome[72,73] – see Chapter 45.

As a result of HHV-8 infection, involved cells produce interleukin (IL)-6, partly accounting for the systemic manifestations in MCD.[74] Histological types include hyaline-vascular, plasmacytic, mixed cellularity, and plasmablastic, the plasma cell variants being most commonly encountered in HIV.[75] It has been hypothesized that activation of IL-6 signaling, acting as an autocrine and paracrine growth factor, transforms naïve B cells into plasmablasts, leading to MCD and subsequent cases of plasmablastic large cell lymphoma.[76] Similar to PEL, the diagnosis is made based on histology in the setting of HHV-8 positive plasmablasts, occasionally being EBV positive as well.

While surgery can definitively address unicentric Castleman disease, it is not commonly indicated for MCD. Previously reported treatment options include single and multiagent chemotherapy, corticosteroids, antiviral agents, immunotherapy, and monoclonal antibodies. Chemotherapeutic approaches can control symptoms and induce objective responses. However, these are usually short-lived, resulting in the need for repeated treatments.[69] Responses to anti-herpesvirus therapies have also been transient.[77] Disease control with the immunomodulatory agent thalidomide has been reported.[78] Based on retrospective analyses and small prospective trials, monoclonal antibodies have provided the most encouraging responses. Twenty-two of 24 patients treated with weekly rituximab for four infusions achieved remissions for a median of 60 days, maintained in 17 patients at 1 year.[79] A separate investigation in 21 patients demonstrated 2-year overall and disease-free survivals of 95% and 79%, respectively, after four infusions of rituximab.[80] The main adverse event in these patients was reactivation of Kaposi sarcoma. Siltuximab, a chimeric, monoclonal antibody to IL-6, was prospectively evaluated in a phase 1 trial.[81] Twenty-three patients with MCD were enrolled, with 52% responding in the absence of dose-limiting toxicities. Consistent with the proposed growth factor properties of IL-6, the median time to response was 6 months.

B cell lymphoma, unclassifiable, with features intermediate between diffuse large B cell lymphoma and Burkitt lymphoma

At either end of the spectrum between DLBCL and Burkitt lymphoma (BL) are the homogenous entities with typical morphology, immunophenotype and gene expression patterns defining DLBCL and BL. In the middle of this spectrum lies a

Table 44.1 Summary of features differentiating diffuse large B cell lymphoma, Burkitt lymphoma, and intermediate DLBCL/BL according to the WHO classification.

	DLBCL	Intermediate DLBCL/BL	Sporadic BL
Demographics			
Median age	70s	Undefined	30s (adult patients)
Male:female ratio	M = F	M > F	M > F
Morphology	Large cells	Mixture	Small to medium cells
Proliferation (Ki-67)	40–90%	Variable	~100%
Genotype*			
MYC	<10%	35–60%	95%
BCL2	20–30%	15%	0
BCL6	25–40%	~5%	0

* Percentage of cases having abnormalities or translocations involving the indicated genes.
BL, Burkitt lymphoma; DLBCL, diffuse large B cell lymphoma; WHO, World Health Organization.
Reproduced with permission from Swerdlow et al.[1]

heterogeneous group of aggressive lymphomas, also described as "gray zone lymphomas," defined somewhat differently based on histology or gene expression. As the disease incidence is difficult to detemine, its rarity can be questioned. However, as these gray zone lymphomas are further defined, specific genetic patterns are being recognized, suggesting that within this heterogeneous group there are distinct entities, albeit rare.

This diagnostic category in the WHO classification was created to classify aggressive NHLs with features of both DLBCL and BL that did not definitively fit into either (Table 44.1). Primarily a morphological definition, these intermediate cases are typically composed of a diffuse proliferation of medium to large transformed cells, displaying a germinal center phenotype (cell surface expression of CD10 and BCL6 and lack of MUM1) and a high proliferation rate. Many harbor a translocation affecting the MYC/8q24 locus, present in 58% of patients in one series.[82] Further, many cases can be further defined as "double hit lymphomas," whereby recurrent chromosomal breakpoints activate multiple oncogenes.[1] As expected, the most common chromosomal breakpoint affects MYC, representing a secondary event rather than a primary oncogenic stimulus. This abnormality is observed in combination with another recurrent breakpoint, including BCL2/18q21 or more rarely BCL6/3q27, CCND1/11q13 or BCL3/19q13.[83] In contrast to BL, these cases frequently carry highly complex karyotypes.

Gene expression analyses support the distinct classification of these gray zone lymphomas. While subgroups of DLBCL, including germinal center B cell-like and activated B cell-like, have been defined by gene expression,[84] and patients with "molecular Burkitt lymphoma" have a fairly specific gene signature (suggesting that sporadic BL is a biologically homogenous group),[85,86] the gray zone lymphomas displayed molecularly indeterminate gene signatures, different from either category. Further, those demonstrating a pattern between that of DLBCL and BL were enriched for cases harboring a MYC translocation along with a second BCL2 or BCL6

translocation. Patients with double hit lymphomas have a poor survival, with a median of less than 1.5 years irrespective of the therapeutic approach.[87–91]

Other gray zone lymphomas included in the intermediate DLBCL/BL category, in addition to double hit lymphomas, include pediatric aggressive lymphomas not fitting into either DLBCL or BL but genetically most similar to BL.[92] Consistent with this, therapeutic outcomes do not appear worse for these patients compared to BL. Currently, cases with a Burkitt morphology and phenotype but otherwise without a MYC translocation are classified as BL. However, genetic differences have been identified, questioning whether these cases truly represent BL.[93,94] Aggressive lymphomas having intermediate morphology with a MYC translocation as the sole cytogenetic abnormality are included in the intermediate category. Cases with the morphological and phenotypic characteristics of DLBCL but having a MYC break continue to be classified as DLBCL. However, substantial evidence suggests the MYC break point predicts for a poor outcome, questioning whether all MYC positive lymphomas should be categorized separately.[95,96] Aggressive lymphomas having MYC recombinations with non-immunoglobulin partners have been described.[97,98] Most are likely secondary events as part of disease transformation from a more indolent lymphoma subtype. As mentioned, outcomes in MYC-positive aggressive lymphomas or those having complex karyotypes including a double hit are resistant to standard treatment regimens, with patients having short survivals. No standard therapy exists. Investigations testing genetically based therapeutic approaches are needed.

B cell lymphoma, unclassifiable, with features intermediate between diffuse large B cell lymphoma and classic Hodgkin lymphoma

This provisional category for borderline cases may represent a smaller number of diagnoses compared to those intermediate to DLBCL and BL. It defines lymphomas with overlapping clinical, morphological, and immunophenotypic features between classic Hodgkin lymphoma (HL) and DLBCL, especially primary mediastinal large B cell lymphoma (PMBL).[1] Table 44.2 lists the demographic and immunophenotype differences between these entities. Composed of more pleomorphic cells compared to typical PMBL, large cells with Reed Sternberg-like morphology may be observed. Originating from the thymic B cell, the tumor cell immunophenotype displays B cell-associated antigens often intermediate between HL and PMBL, being positive for CD20, CD79a, CD30, and CD15. Individual tumors may have separate areas, each resembling HL, DLBCL, and PBML. While HL and PMBL display additional genetic similarities,[99,100] gene expression analyses of the intermediate cases have not yet been performed. Further, altered signaling through the JAK/STAT pathway, in addition to activation of the NFκB and PI3K/AKT pathways, has been demonstrated in both HL and PMBL.[101–104] While these data suggest a continuum between the two entities, recent work by Eberle and colleagues suggests important differences for the intermediate DLBCL/HL cases.[105] The gray zone lymphomas varied in their resemblance to PMBL and HL but had a similar methylation profile, also

Table 44.2 Summary of features differentiating mediastinal lymphomas according to the WHO classification.

	PMBL	Intermediate DLBCL/HL	Classic HL
Demographics			
Age	35 year median	20–40 years	Bimodal; 15–35 and >50 years
Male:female ratio	M<F	M>F	M=F
Immunophenotype			
CD20	+	+	+/–
CD79a	+	+	–
PAX5	+	+	+
BOB.1	+	+	–
OCT2	+	+	–
CD45	+	+	–
CD15	–	+	+
CD30	Weak	+	+
EBER/LMP1	–	+/–	+/–

DLBCL, diffuse large B cell lymphoma; HL, Hodgkin lymphoma; PMBL, primary mediastinal B cell lymphoma; WHO, World Health Organization. Reproduced with permission from Swerdlow et al.[1]

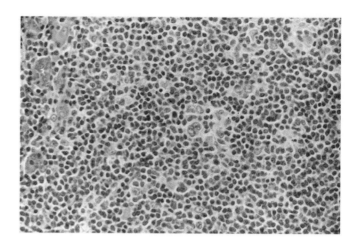

Figure 44.3 Nodular lymphocyte-predominant Hodgkin lymphoma. Note LP or "popcorn" cells with lobated nuclei visible in a background of small lymphoid cells.

found to be separate from HL and PMBL. The authors further developed a prediction model able to distinguish between nodular sclerosing HL, PBML, and gray zone lymphomas.

More commonly reported in western countries, gray zone lymphomas typically present in young men with a large anterior mediastinal mass.[106] These tumors tend to be highly aggressive, causing symptoms of respiratory distress or superior vena cava syndrome, and have been associated with a worse outcome than HL or PMBL.[107] Supporting this is the observation that CD20 positivity has been recognized as a poor prognostic factor in classic HL.[108,109] While these studies predate the current WHO classification, some individual cases may be better classified in the intermediate category. There is no consensus as to the optimal treatment, though some series suggest that therapy developed for large B cell lymphoma may be most effective.[110]

Nodular lymphocyte-predominant Hodgkin lymphoma

Nodular lymphocyte-predominant Hodgkin lymphoma (NLPHL) represents only 5% of Hodgkin lymphoma. As the name implies, a nodular or nodular and diffuse infiltrate replaces the lymph node architecture. Variants of the typical Reed Sternberg cells, known as LP cells (Fig. 44.3), are positive for CD20 and CD79a, negative for CD15 and CD30, and are typically observed in a mesh-like background of follicular dendritic cells filled with normal B cells, histiocytes, and CD4+ T cells.[1] Rearranged immunoglobulin genes have been demonstrated in LP cells consistent with their germinal center derivation.[111]

The condition predominantly affects males aged 30–50 years and patients present with localized disease 70–80% of the time. Mediastinal involvement, B symptoms, and bulky disease are rare.[112,113] Peripheral lymphadenopathy involving the neck or axilla is more common compared to central nodes.

While classic HL tends to spread to contiguous lymph nodes, spread in NLPHL is discontiguous and extranodal involvement is rare.[114]

The correlation of survival and lymphocyte infiltration in HL was documented in 1936.[115] Two large retrospective studies led by the European Task Force on Lymphoma (ETFL) and the German Hodgkin Study Group (GHSG), along with numerous smaller publications, provide important findings regarding NLPHL. The GHSG reported a 50-month freedom from treatment failure and overall survival of 88% and 96% among 394 patients, highlighting the indolent nature of NLPHL.[113] Responses to initial therapy are high, with more than 90% of patients achieving a complete response (CR). However, long-term follow-up has demonstrated a pattern of continuous relapse, with prolonged times to subsequent treatment. Reports on smaller cohorts have documented a 10-year overall survival of 71–85% and a 15-year overall survival of 63–80%.[116–118] One recently reported 30-year follow-up on 88 patients demonstrated a 44% relapse rate for the entire cohort.[119]

For treatment, complete surgical excision of limited-stage disease has provided long-term survival in children.[120, 121] As the majority of patients present with stage Ia and IIa involvement, long-term data, primarily in adults, suggest that the disease can be managed effectively with involved field radiation therapy. The ETFL included 219 patients with NLPHL, making it possible to analyze patient outcomes by stage.[112] With the majority of stage I and II patients being treated with radiation therapy alone, 8-year freedom from treatment failure and overall survival were 85% and 99%, respectively, for stage I disease and 71% and 94%, respectively, for stage II disease. Given the above long-term outcomes and the predisposition for peripheral lymph node involvement, most groups recommend that stage Ia and IIa disease be treated with 30–35 Gy of involved field radiation therapy.

As patients tend to be young at presentation of NLPHL with long median survivals, therapy-related toxicities are of concern, similar to patients with classic HL. While some studies report the majority of deaths as being disease related,[112,116] others have reported a higher rate of secondary malignancies in patients treated with radiation therapy alone.[122,123]

Combined modality therapy is often used for patients with B symptoms. However, data supporting this practice in NLPHL are limited. Similarly, limited studies are available to guide recommendations for advanced-stage patients. Given their previous inclusion in trials focused on classic HL, treatment recommendations are largely similar to those for these patients. Primarily treated with chemotherapy with or without radiation, single-institution reports have demonstrated no decrement in survival for advanced-stage disease.[124] However, larger cohorts may suggest otherwise. From the ETFL report, 59 patients with stage III disease and 19 patients with stage IV disease were included. Primarily receiving MOPP-like based chemotherapy protocols, the 8-year freedom from treatment failure and overall survival were 62% and 94%, respectively, for stage III disease and 24% and 41%, respectively, for stage IV disease.

For patients who relapse after initial therapy, the antibody rituximab represents an important treatment option, given the CD20 positivity of the LP cell. Encouraging results, including a median time to progression of 33 months, were reported by the GHSG in a small number of relapsed patients.[125] A subsequent GHSG trial in 28 previously untreated patients reported a progression-free survival and overall survival of 81% and 100%, respectively, at 3 years.[126] Despite an excellent response rate, conflicting data from another small trial suggested a much shorter time to progression with rituximab in a cohort of untreated and relapsed patients.[127]

Conclusion

With further characterizations of B cell lymphoproliferative disorders at the genetic and molecular levels, an increasing number of distinct pathological entities are being recognized. As a result, further classification systems will include an increasing number of diagnoses. With further divisions, we may one day recognize all lymphoproliferative disorders to be rare. It is to be hoped that accompanying these investigations will be an improved understanding of the disease biology, translating into targeted and individualized therapeutic approaches.

Acknowledgment

Drs Barr and Friedberg are supported in part by the University of Rochester SPORE in lymphoma, P50 CA13080503. Dr Barr is supported in part by the Wilmot Cancer Research Foundation. Dr Friedberg is a Scholar in Clinical Research of the Leukemia and Lymphoma Society.

References

1. Swerdlow SH, *et al*. (eds). *WHO Classification of Tumours of Haematopoietic and Lymphoid Tissues*. Lyon: International Agency for Research on Cancer, 2008.

2. Yamamoto JF, Goodman MT. Patterns of leukemia incidence in the United States by subtype and demographic characteristics, 1997–2002. Cancer Causes Control 2008; 19(4): 379–90.

3. Krishnan B, *et al*. Prolymphocytic leukemias. Semin Oncol 2006; 33(2): 257–63.

4. Del Giudice I, *et al*. IgVH genes mutation and usage, ZAP-70 and CD38 expression provide new insights on B-cell prolymphocytic leukemia (B-PLL). Leukemia 2006; 20(7): 1231–7.

5. Hercher C, *et al*. A multicentric study of 41 cases of B-prolymphocytic leukemia: two evolutive forms. Leuk Lymphoma 2001; 42(5): 981–7.

6. Kantarjian HM, *et al*. Efficacy of fludarabine, a new adenine nucleoside analogue, in patients with prolymphocytic leukemia and the prolymphocytoid variant of chronic lymphocytic leukemia. Am J Med 1991; 90(2): 223–8.

7. Dohner H, *et al*. Pentostatin in prolymphocytic leukemia: phase II trial of the European Organization for Research and Treatment of Cancer Leukemia Cooperative Study Group. J Natl Cancer Inst 1993; 85(8): 658–62.

8. Saven A, *et al*. Major activity of cladribine in patients with de novo B-cell prolymphocytic leukemia. J Clin Oncol 1997; 15(1): 37–43.

9. Bowen AL, *et al*. Subcutaneous CAMPATH-1H in fludarabine-resistant/relapsed chronic lymphocytic and B-prolymphocytic leukaemia. Br J Haematol 1997; 96(3): 617–19.

10. Vartholomatos G, *et al*. Rituximab (anti-CD20 monoclonal antibody) administration in a young patient with resistant B-prolymphocytic leukemia. Acta Haematol 1999; 102(2): 94–8.

11. Mourad YA, *et al*. Successful treatment of B-cell prolymphocytic leukemia with monoclonal anti-CD20 antibody. Ann Hematol 2004; 83(5): 319–21.

12. Dores GM, *et al*. Hairy cell leukaemia: a heterogeneous disease? Br J Haematol 2008; 142(1): 45–51.

13. Hoffman MA. Clinical presentations and complications of hairy cell leukemia. Hematol Oncol Clin North Am 2006; 20(5): 1065–73.

14. Sharpe RW, Bethel KJ. Hairy cell leukemia: diagnostic pathology. Hematol Oncol Clin North Am 2006; 20(5): 1023–49.

15. Arons E, *et al*. VH4-34+ hairy cell leukemia, a new variant with poor prognosis despite standard therapy. Blood 2009; 114(21): 4687–95.

16. Arons E, *et al*. Somatic hypermutation and VH gene usage in hairy cell leukaemia. Br J Haematol 2006; 133(5): 504–12.

17. Spiers AS, *et al*. Hairy-cell leukemia: induction of complete remission with pentostatin (2′-deoxycoformycin). J Clin Oncol 1984; 2(12): 1336–42.

18. Grever M, *et al*. Randomized comparison of pentostatin versus interferon alfa-2a in previously untreated patients with hairy cell leukemia: an intergroup study. J Clin Oncol 1995; 13(4): 974–82.

19. Goodman GR, *et al*. Extended follow-up of patients with hairy cell leukemia after treatment with cladribine. J Clin Oncol 2003; 21(5): 891–6.

20. Chadha P, *et al*. Treatment of hairy cell leukemia with 2-chlorodeoxyadenosine (2-CdA): long-term follow-up of the Northwestern University experience. Blood 2005; 106(1): 241–6.

21. Else M, *et al*. Long-term follow-up of 233 patients with hairy cell leukaemia, treated initially with pentostatin or cladribine, at a median of 16 years from diagnosis. Br J Haematol 2009; 145(6): 733–40.

22. Juliusson G, *et al*. Subcutaneous injections of 2-chlorodeoxyadenosine for symptomatic hairy cell leukemia. J Clin Oncol 1995; 13(4): 989–95.

23. Robak T, *et al*. Cladribine in a weekly versus daily schedule for untreated active hairy cell leukemia: final report from the Polish Adult Leukemia Group (PALG) of a prospective, randomized, multicenter trial. Blood 2007; 109(9): 3672–5.

24. Zenhausern R, *et al*. Randomized trial of daily versus weekly administration of 2-chlorodeoxyadenosine in patients with hairy cell leukemia: a multicenter phase III trial (SAKK 32/98). Leuk Lymphoma 2009; 50(9): 1501–11.

25. Forconi F, *et al*. (2010). Analysis of toxicity and efficacy of subcutaneous cladribine at reduced or standard doses (five versus seven consecutive days) in patients with hairy cell leukemia (HCL) in the ICGHCL2004 protocol by the Italian Cooperative Group on Hcl. ASH Annual Meeting Abstracts. Blood 2010; 116(21): 309–10.

26. Grever MR, Lozanski G. Modern strategies for hairy cell leukemia. J Clin Oncol 2011; 29(5): 583–90.

27. Kreitman RJ, *et al*. Phase II trial of recombinant immunotoxin RFB4(dsFv)-PE38 (BL22) in patients with hairy cell leukemia. J Clin Oncol 2009; 27(18): 2983–90.

28. Nieva J, *et al*. Phase 2 study of rituximab in the treatment of cladribine-failed patients with hairy cell leukemia. Blood 2003; 102(3): 810–13.

29. Thomas DA, *et al*. Rituximab in relapsed or refractory hairy cell leukemia. Blood 2003; 102(12): 3906–11.

30. Cervetti G, *et al*. Rituximab as treatment for minimal residual disease in hairy cell leukaemia. Eur J Haematol 2004; 73(6): 412–17.

31. Kreitman RJ, *et al*. Approach to the patient after relapse of hairy cell leukemia. Leuk Lymphoma 2009; 50(Suppl 1): 32–7.

32. McCloskey M, *et al*. A case of lymphomatoid granulomatosis masquerading as a lung abscess. Thorax 2004; 59(9): 818–19.

33. Guinee D Jr, *et al*. Pulmonary lymphomatoid granulomatosis. Evidence for a proliferation of Epstein–Barr virus infected B-lymphocytes with a prominent T-cell component and vasculitis. Am J Surg Pathol 1994; 18(8): 753–64.

34. Myers JL, *et al*. Lymphomatoid granulomatosis. Evidence of immunophenotypic diversity and relationship to Epstein–Barr virus infection. Am J Surg Pathol 1995; 19(11): 1300–12.

35. Nicholson AG, *et al*. Lymphomatoid granulomatosis: evidence that some cases represent Epstein–Barr virus-associated B-cell lymphoma. Histopathology 1996; 29(4): 317–24.

36. Liebow AA, *et al*. Lymphomatoid granulomatosis. Hum Pathol 1972; 3(4): 457–558.

37. Katzenstein AA, *et al*. Lymphomatoid granulomatosis: insights gained over 4 decades. Am J Surg Pathol 2010; 34(12): e35–e48.

38. Saldana MJ, *et al*. Pulmonary angiitis and granulomatosis. The relationship between histological features, organ involvement, and response to treatment. Hum Pathol 1977; 8(4): 391–409.

39. Koss MN, *et al*. Lymphomatoid granulomatosis: a clinicopathologic study of 42 patients. Pathology 1986; 18(3): 283–8.

40. Jordan K, *et al*. Successful treatment of mediastinal lymphomatoid granulomatosis with rituximab monotherapy. Eur J Haematol 2005; 74(3): 263–6.

41. Ishiura H, *et al*. Lymphomatoid granulomatosis involving central nervous system successfully treated with rituximab alone. Arch Neurol 2008; 65(5): 662–5.

42. Wilson W, *et al*. Association of lymphomatoid granulomatosis with Epstein–Barr viral infection of B lymphocytes and response to interferon-alpha 2b. Blood 1996; 87(11): 4531–7.

43. Dunleavy K, *et al*. Immune Characteristics associated with lymphomatoid granulomatosis and outcome following treatment with interferon-alpha. ASH Annual Meeting Abstracts. Blood 2010; 116(21): 424.

44. Ponzoni M, *et al*. Definition, diagnosis, and management of intravascular large B-cell lymphoma: proposals and perspectives from an international consensus meeting. J Clin Oncol 2007; 25(21): 3168–73.

45. Shimada K, *et al*. Retrospective analysis of intravascular large B-cell lymphoma treated with rituximab-containing chemotherapy as reported by the IVL Study Group in Japan. J Clin Oncol 2008; 26(19): 3189–95.

46. Yegappan S, *et al*. Angiotropic lymphoma: an immunophenotypically and clinically heterogeneous lymphoma. Mod Pathol 2001; 14(11): 1147–56.

47. Gill S, *et al*. Use of random skin biopsy to diagnose intravascular lymphoma presenting as fever of unknown origin. Am J Med 2003; 114(1): 56–8.

48. Le EN, *et al*. The use of blind skin biopsy in the diagnosis of intravascular B-cell lymphoma. J Am Acad Dermatol 2008; 59(1): 148–51.

49. Domizio P, *et al*. Angiotropic large cell lymphoma (ALCL): morphological, immunohistochemical and genotypic studies with analysis of previous reports. Hematol Oncol 1989; 7(3): 195–206.

50. Ferreri AJ, *et al*. Can rituximab change the usually dismal prognosis of patients with intravascular large B-cell lymphoma? J Clin Oncol 2008; 26(31): 5134–6.

51. Knowles DM, *et al*. Molecular genetic analysis of three AIDS-associated neoplasms of uncertain lineage demonstrates their B-cell derivation and the possible pathogenetic role of the Epstein–Barr virus. Blood 1989; 73(3): 792–9.

52. Gaidano G, Carbone A. Primary effusion lymphoma: a liquid phase lymphoma of fluid-filled body cavities. Adv Cancer Res 2001; 80: 115–46.

53. Brimo F, *et al*. Primary effusion lymphoma: a series of 4 cases and review of the literature with emphasis on cytomorphologic and immunocytochemical differential diagnosis. Cancer 2007; 111(4): 224–33.

54. Dukers NH, Rezza G. Human herpesvirus 8 epidemiology: what we do and do not know. AIDS 2003; 17(12): 1717–30.

55. Swanton C, *et al*. Herpes viral cyclin/Cdk6 complexes evade inhibition by CDK inhibitor proteins. Nature 1997; 390(6656): 184–7.

56. Thome M, *et al*. Viral FLICE-inhibitory proteins (FLIPs) prevent apoptosis induced by death receptors. Nature 1997; 386(6624): 517–21.

57. Ballestas ME, *et al*. Efficient persistence of extrachromosomal KSHV DNA mediated by latency-associated nuclear antigen. Science 1999; 284(5414): 641–4.

58. Friborg J Jr, *et al*. p53 inhibition by the LANA protein of KSHV protects against cell death. Nature 1999; 402(6764): 889–94.

59. Matta H, Chaudhary PM. Activation of alternative NF-kappa B pathway by human herpes virus 8-encoded Fas-associated death domain-like IL-1 beta-converting enzyme inhibitory protein (vFLIP). Proc Natl Acad Sci USA 2004; 101(25): 9399–404.

60. Horenstein MG, *et al*. Epstein–Barr virus latent gene expression in primary effusion lymphomas containing Kaposi's sarcoma-associated herpesvirus/human herpesvirus-8. Blood 1997; 90(3): 1186–91.

61. Fais F, *et al*. Immunoglobulin V region gene use and structure suggest antigen selection in AIDS-related primary effusion lymphomas. Leukemia 1999; 13(7): 1093–9.

62. Carbone A, *et al*. Expression profile of MUM1/IRF4, BCL-6, and CD138/syndecan-1 defines novel histogenetic subsets of human immunodeficiency virus-related lymphomas. Blood 2001; 97(3): 744–51.

63. Klein U, *et al*. Gene expression profile analysis of AIDS-related primary effusion lymphoma (PEL) suggests a plasmablastic derivation and identifies PEL-specific transcripts. Blood 2003; 101(10): 4115–21.

64. Ascoli V, *et al*. Human herpesvirus 8-associated primary effusion lymphoma in HIV-patients: a clinicopidemiologic variant resembling classic Kaposi's sarcoma. Haematologica 2002; 87(4): 339–43.

65. Halfdanarson TR, *et al*. A non-chemotherapy treatment of a primary effusion lymphoma: durable remission after intracavitary cidofovir in HIV negative PEL refractory to chemotherapy. Ann Oncol 2006; 17(12): 1849–50.

66. Moyo TK, *et al*. Use of cidofovir for the treatment of HIV-negative human herpes virus-8-associated primary effusion lymphoma. Clin Adv Hematol Oncol 2010; 8(5): 372–4.

67. Matsumoto Y, *et al*. Human herpesvirus 8-negative malignant effusion lymphoma: a distinct clinical entity and successful treatment with rituximab. Leuk Lymphoma 2005; 46(3): 415–19.

68. Soulier J, *et al*. Kaposi's sarcoma-associated herpesvirus-like DNA sequences in multicentric Castleman's disease. Blood 1995; 86(4): 1276–80.

69. Oksenhendler E, *et al*. Multicentric Castleman's disease in HIV infection: a clinical and pathological study of 20 patients. AIDS 1996; 10(1): 61–7.

70. Kojima M, *et al*. Nodal marginal zone B-cell lymphoma resembling plasmacytoma arising from a plasma cell variant of localized Castleman's disease: a case report. APMIS 2002; 110(7–8): 523–7.

71. Venizelos I, *et al*. Diffuse large B-cell lymphoma arising from a multicentric mixed variant of Castleman's disease. Indian J Cancer 2004; 41(3): 135–7.

72. Papo T, *et al*. Human herpesvirus 8 infection, Castleman's disease and POEMS syndrome. Br J Haematol 1999; 104(4): 932–3.

73. Day JR, *et al*. Castleman's disease associated with myasthenia gravis. Ann Thorac Surg 2003; 75(5): 1648–50.

74. Deng H, *et al*. Transcriptional regulation of the interleukin-6 gene of human herpesvirus 8 (Kaposi's sarcoma-associated herpesvirus). J Virol 2002; 76(16): 8252–64.

75. Waterston A, Bower M. Fifty years of multicentric Castleman's disease. Acta Oncol 2004; 43(8): 698–704.

76. Dupin N, *et al*. HHV-8 is associated with a plasmablastic variant of Castleman disease that is linked to HHV-8-positive plasmablastic lymphoma. Blood 2000; 95(4): 1406–12.

77. Casper C, *et al*. Remission of HHV-8 and HIV-associated multicentric Castleman disease with ganciclovir treatment. Blood 2004; 103(5): 1632–4.

78. Starkey CR, *et al*. Near-total resolution of multicentric Castleman disease by prolonged treatment with thalidomide. Am J Hematol 2006; 81(4): 303–4.

79. Gerard L, *et al*. Prospective study of rituximab in chemotherapy-dependent human immunodeficiency virus associated multicentric Castleman's disease: ANRS 117 CastlemaB Trial. J Clin Oncol 2007; 25(22): 3350–6.

80. Bower M, *et al*. Brief communication: rituximab in HIV-associated multicentric Castleman disease. Ann Intern Med 2007; 147(12): 836–9.

81. Van Rhee F, *et al*. Siltuximab, a novel anti-interleukin-6 monoclonal antibody, for Castleman's disease. J Clin Oncol 2010; 28(23): 3701–8.

82. Lin P, *et al*. Prognostic value of MYC rearrangement in cases of B-cell lymphoma, unclassifiable, with features intermediate between diffuse large B-cell lymphoma and Burkitt lymphoma. Cancer 2012; 118: 1566–73.

83. Aukema SM, *et al*. Double-hit B-cell lymphomas. Blood 2011; 117(8): 2319–31.

84. Alizadeh AA, *et al*. Distinct types of diffuse large B-cell lymphoma identified by gene expression profiling. Nature 2000; 403(6769): 503–11.

85. Dave SS, *et al*. Molecular diagnosis of Burkitt's lymphoma. N Engl J Med 2006; 354(23): 2431–42.

86. Hummel M, *et al*. A biologic definition of Burkitt's lymphoma from transcriptional and genomic profiling. N Engl J Med 2006; 354(23): 2419–30.

87. Kanungo A, *et al*. Lymphoid neoplasms associated with concurrent t(14;18) and 8q24/c-MYC translocation generally have a poor prognosis. Mod Pathol 2006; 19(1): 25–33.

88. Le Gouill S, *et al*. The clinical presentation and prognosis of diffuse large B-cell lymphoma with t(14;18) and 8q24/c-MYC rearrangement. Haematologica 2007; 92(10): 1335–42.

89. Johnson NA, *et al*. Lymphomas with concurrent BCL2 and MYC translocations: the critical factors associated with survival. Blood 2009; 114(11): 2273–9.

90. Niitsu N, *et al*. Clinical features and prognosis of de novo diffuse large B-cell lymphoma with t(14;18) and 8q24/c-MYC translocations. Leukemia 2009; 23(4): 777–83.

91. Tomita N, *et al*. Clinicopathological features of lymphoma/leukemia patients carrying both BCL2 and MYC translocations. Haematologica 2009; 94(7): 935–43.

92. Bentink S, *et al*. Pathway activation patterns in diffuse large B-cell lymphomas. Leukemia 2008; 22(9): 1746–54.

93. Pienkowska-Grela B, *et al*. Frequent aberrations of chromosome 8 in aggressive B-cell non-Hodgkin lymphoma. Cancer Genet Cytogenet 2005; 156(2): 114–21.

94. Leucci E, *et al*. MYC translocation-negative classical Burkitt lymphoma cases: an alternative pathogenetic mechanism involving miRNA deregulation. J Pathol 2008; 216(4): 440–50.

95. Klapper W, *et al*. Structural aberrations affecting the MYC locus indicate a poor prognosis independent of clinical risk factors in diffuse large B-cell lymphomas treated within randomized trials of the German High-Grade Non-Hodgkin's Lymphoma Study Group (DSHNHL). Leukemia 2008; 22(12): 2226–9.

96. Savage KJ, *et al*. MYC gene rearrangements are associated with a poor prognosis in diffuse large B-cell lymphoma patients treated with R-CHOP chemotherapy. Blood 2009; 114(17): 3533–7.

97. Bertrand P, *et al*. Mapping of MYC breakpoints in 8q24 rearrangements involving non-immunoglobulin partners in B-cell lymphomas. Leukemia 2007; 21(3): 515–23.

98. Bertrand P, *et al*. Characterization of three t(3;8)(q27;q24) translocations from diffuse large B-cell lymphomas. Leukemia 2008; 22(5): 1064–7.

99. Rosenwald A, *et al*. Molecular diagnosis of primary mediastinal B cell lymphoma identifies a clinically favorable subgroup of diffuse large B cell lymphoma related to Hodgkin lymphoma. J Exp Med 2003; 198(6): 851–62.

100. Savage KJ, *et al*. The molecular signature of mediastinal large B-cell lymphoma differs from that of other diffuse large B-cell lymphomas and shares features with classical Hodgkin lymphoma. Blood 2003; 102(12): 3871–9.

101. Guiter C, *et al*. Constitutive STAT6 activation in primary mediastinal large B-cell lymphoma. Blood 2004; 104(2): 543–9.

102. Feuerhake F, *et al*. NFkappaB activity, function, and target-gene signatures in primary mediastinal large B-cell lymphoma and diffuse large B-cell lymphoma subtypes. Blood 2005; 106(4): 1392–9.

103. Weniger MA, *et al*. Mutations of the tumor suppressor gene SOCS-1 in classical Hodgkin lymphoma are frequent and associated with nuclear phospho-STAT5 accumulation. Oncogene 2006; 25(18): 2679–84.

104. Renne C, *et al*. High expression of several tyrosine kinases and activation of the PI3K/AKT pathway in mediastinal large B cell lymphoma reveals further similarities to Hodgkin lymphoma. Leukemia 2007; 21(4): 780–7.

105. Eberle FC, *et al*. Methylation profiling of mediastinal gray zone lymphoma reveals a distinctive signature with elements shared by classical Hodgkin's lymphoma and primary mediastinal large B-cell lymphoma. Haematologica 2011; 96(4): 558–66.

106. Traverse-Glehen A, *et al*. Mediastinal gray zone lymphoma: the missing link between classic Hodgkin's lymphoma and mediastinal large B-cell lymphoma. Am J Surg Pathol 2005; 29(11): 1411–21.

107. Quintanilla-Martinez L, *et al*. Gray zones around diffuse large B cell lymphoma. Conclusions based on the workshop of the XIV meeting of the European Association for Hematopathology and the Society of Hematopathology in Bordeaux, France. J Hematopathol 2009; 2(4): 211–36.

108. Von Wasielewski R, *et al*. Classical Hodgkin's disease. Clinical impact of the immunophenotype. Am J Pathol 1997; 151(4): 1123–30.

109. Portlock CS, *et al*. Adverse prognostic significance of CD20 positive Reed–Sternberg cells in classical Hodgkin's disease. Br J Haematol 2004; 125(6): 701–8.

110. Zinzani PL, *et al*. Anaplastic large cell lymphoma Hodgkin's-like: a randomized trial of ABVD versus MACOP-B with and without radiation therapy. Blood 1998; 92(3): 790–4.

111. Marafioti T, *et al*. Origin of nodular lymphocyte-predominant Hodgkin's disease from a clonal expansion of highly mutated germinal-center B cells. N Engl J Med 1997; 337(7): 453–8.

112. Diehl V, *et al*. Clinical presentation, course, and prognostic factors in lymphocyte-predominant Hodgkin's disease and lymphocyte-rich classical Hodgkin's disease: report from the European Task Force on Lymphoma Project on Lymphocyte-Predominant Hodgkin's Disease. J Clin Oncol 1999; 17(3): 776–83.

113. Nogova L, *et al*. Lymphocyte-predominant and classical Hodgkin's lymphoma: a comprehensive analysis from the German Hodgkin Study Group. J Clin Oncol 2008; 26(3): 434–9.

114. Mauch PM, *et al*. Patterns of presentation of Hodgkin disease. Implications for etiology and pathogenesis. Cancer 1993; 71(6): 2062–71.

115. Rosenthal SR. Significance of tissue lymphocytes in prognosis of lymphogranulomatosis. Arch Pathol 1936; 21: 628–31.

116. Orlandi E, *et al*. Nodular lymphocyte predominance Hodgkin's disease: long-term observation reveals a continuous pattern of recurrence. Leuk Lymphoma 1997; 26(3–4): 359–68.

117. Ha CS, *et al*. Hodgkin's disease with lymphocyte predominance: long-term results based on current histopathologic criteria. Int J Radiat Oncol Biol Phys 1999; 43(2): 329–34.

118. Chera BS, *et al*. Clinical presentation and outcomes of lymphocyte-predominant Hodgkin disease at the University of Florida. Am J Clin Oncol 2007; 30(6): 601–6.

119. Jackson C, *et al*. Lymphocyte-predominant Hodgkin lymphoma – clinical features and treatment outcomes from a 30-year experience. Ann Oncol 2010; 21(10): 2061–8.

120. Pellegrino B, *et al*. Lymphocyte-predominant Hodgkin's lymphoma in children: therapeutic abstention after initial lymph node resection – a Study of the French Society of Pediatric Oncology. J Clin Oncol 2003; 21(15): 2948–52.

121. Mauz-Korholz C, *et al*. Resection alone in 58 children with limited stage, lymphocyte-predominant Hodgkin lymphoma – experience from the European Network Group on pediatric Hodgkin lymphoma. Cancer 2007; 110(1): 179–85.

122. Bodis S, *et al*. Clinical presentation and outcome in lymphocyte-predominant Hodgkin's disease. J Clin Oncol 1997; 15(9): 3060–6.

123. Wirth A, *et al*. Long-term outcome after radiotherapy alone for lymphocyte-predominant Hodgkin lymphoma: a retrospective multicenter study of the Australasian Radiation Oncology Lymphoma Group. Cancer 2005; 104(6): 1221–9.

124. Pappa VI, *et al*. Nodular type of lymphocyte predominant Hodgkin's disease. A clinical study of 50 cases. Ann Oncol 1995; 6(6): 559–65.

125. Schulz H, *et al*. Rituximab in relapsed lymphocyte-predominant Hodgkin lymphoma: long-term results of a phase 2 trial by the German Hodgkin Lymphoma Study Group (GHSG). Blood 2008; 111(1): 109–11.

126. Eichenauer DA, *et al*. (2011). Phase II study of rituximab in newly diagnosed stage IA nodular lymphocyte-predominant Hodgkin lymphoma: a report from the German Hodgkin Study Group. Blood 2011; 118(16): 4363–5.

127. Ekstrand BC, *et al*. Rituximab in lymphocyte-predominant Hodgkin disease: results of a phase 2 trial. Blood 2003; 101(11): 4285–9.

45 Uncommon Presentations of Plasma Cell Dyscrasias

Rachid Baz[1] and Mohamad A. Hussein[2]

[1] Department of Malignant Hematology, H. Lee Moffitt Cancer Center and Research Institute; Department of Oncologic Sciences and Medicine, University of South Florida, Tampa, FL, USA
[2] Division of Medicine, University of South Florida, Tampa, FL, USA

Plasma cell leukemia

Biology

Primary plasma cell leukemia (PCL) refers to the *de novo* presence of greater than 20% plasma cells in the peripheral blood and/or an absolute plasma cell count of greater than 2000/μL.[1–3] Secondary plasma cell leukemia is thought to represent leukemic transformation of a patient's known multiple myeloma, which is thought to be a terminal event and implies a median survival of about 2–3 months, compared to 11 months for the primary type.[4] While about 40% of plasma cell leukemia is secondary, only 1% of patients with multiple myeloma develop the disease.

Presentation

Patients with primary PCL present on average 10 years younger than patients developing secondary PCL, or their myeloma counterpart. Overall, PCL has a more aggressive clinical behavior than multiple myeloma. Accordingly, extramedullary involvement, renal dysfunction, severe anemia, and thrombocytopenia are more common at presentation. Conversely, bony involvement is less likely than with multiple myeloma.[2,4,5] Deletion of *17p* is more prevalent among patients with PCL (56%) than in patients with multiple myeloma.[6]

The surface phenotype of plasma cells in plasma cell leukemia is different from that of bone marrow plasma cells in patients with multiple myeloma, as CD9, HLADR, CD117, and CD20 are differentially expressed in circulating plasma cells compared with expression on bone marrow plasma cells seen in myeloma patients. The plasma cells that circulate do not appear to express CD56. The lack of (or weak) expression of CD56 is a characteristic feature of plasma cell leukemia, and delineates this special subset of myeloma patients at diagnosis.[7]

Management and prognosis

Consistent with the more aggressive behavior, primary PCL implies a poor prognosis with lower response rates to chemotherapy compared to myeloma patients and median survivals of 8–10 months.[2,4,5] The treatment of PCL has traditionally been similar to the treatment of multiple myeloma. The more aggressive course often implies a more intensive chemotherapy regimen often with multiagent chemotherapy including bortezomib and immunomodulatory agents as well as alkylating agents (for example, VDT-PACE in fitter patients). Nonrandomized retrospective studies suggest an improved outcome with autologous stem cell transplantation and novel agents.[8,9]

Nonsecretory multiple myeloma

Biology

Nonsecretory multiple myeloma accounts for 1–5% of patients with multiple myeloma.[4] Differences in its prevalence likely relate to referral biases and differences in the diagnostic evaluations among different series.[10–12] Diagnostic and therapeutic challenges in the management of patients with nonsecretory multiple myeloma are mainly related to the absence of a clear disease parameter to follow. Nonsecretory myeloma is commonly defined as patients who do not have an adequate amount of monoclonal protein to follow, i.e. those who demonstrate positive monoclonal protein by immunofixation, yet lack any significant M-protein as measured by serum protein electrophoresis or 24-h urine. Yet, in truth, these conditions are better termed oligosecretory myeloma. True nonsecretory multiple myeloma is defined by the absence of monoclonal protein in the serum or urine in patients with other characteristic signs and symptoms of multiple myeloma (including increased plasma cells in the bone marrow or lytic bone lesions).[4]

Immunofluorescence studies must be performed in all patients in whom this diagnosis is suspected; in a large subset of patients, a cytoplasmic immunoglobulin often is identified, indicating oligosecretory disease. Patients who lack cytoplasmic immunoglobulin are defined as having truly nonproducer multiple myeloma. More recently, the use of the serum free light chain test has helped identify a tumor marker to follow in a substantial number of patients with nonsecretory myeloma. Several hypotheses have been proposed for the lack of an M-protein in patients with nonsecretory multiple myeloma, including the inability to excrete the immunoglobulin by the plasma cell, production of a rapidly degradable immunoglobulin, and low synthetic capability of the plasma cell clone.[4]

Presentation

Dreicer and Alexanian reported on the presenting feature of 29 patients with nonsecretory multiple myeloma.[12] They noted a lower age at diagnosis compared to patients with a measurable monoclonal protein. Patients were also less likely to have anemia, renal dysfunction, or hypercalcemia at presentation.[12] Other smaller series did not identify differences in the presentation of patients with nonsecretory myeloma compared to patients with an M-protein, with the exception of the lack of renal dysfunction at the time of presentation.[10,11] Unpublished Southwest Oncology Group (SWOG) data show that approximately 5% of multiple myeloma patients will have monoclonal proteins detected mostly by immunofixation, with the main presenting feature being skeletal disease. In a more recent report from the Center for International Blood and Marrow Transplant Research (CIBMTR), the progression-free survival post transplant of patients with nonsecretory myeloma was statistically better than patients with secretory disease while there was only a trend towards an improved overall survival for patients with nonsecretory disease.[13]

Management and prognosis

The natural history of patients with nonsecretory multiple myeloma is not thought to be different from that of other patients with multiple myeloma. Treatment of nonsecretory multiple myeloma does not differ from the treatment of multiple myeloma with a measurable M-protein. Specifically, patients are generally treated with a combination of a novel agent (lenalidomide or bortezomib) and a corticosteroid followed by consideration for high-dose therapy in first or subsequent remission.

Patients who have a measurable involved serum free light chain greater than 100 mg/L, as well as an abnormal serum free κ to λ ratio, can have their disease monitored using this test based on the uniform response criteria of the International Myeloma Working Group.[14] For the remainder of patients who have no measurable tumor marker, a response to treatment is defined as improvement in the signs and symptoms of bone pains, anemia, hypercalcemia, and the absence of new lytic bone lesions. A decrease in bone marrow plasmacytosis is thought to be an objective marker of response as well. Conversely, progressive disease is characterized by progressive bony disease, hypercalcemia or an increase in bone marrow plasmacytosis.[4]

Immunoglobulin D myeloma

Biology and presentation

Within multiple myeloma, immunoglobulin (Ig) G or A is commonly secreted (in about 60% and 20% respectively). Secretion of immunoglobulin D as the monoclonal protein occurs in only approximately 2% of patients.[15,16]

The presenting clinical features of IgD myeloma are similar to those in myeloma patients with other immunoglobulin secretion, with the exception of a few noted associations. As compared to patients with the more common myelomas, patients with IgD myeloma are on average younger at diagnosis (about 54 years compared to a median age of about 69 years of age).[15–18] Lymph node enlargement, an unusual sign in patients with classic multiple myeloma, is noted in approximately 10% of patients with IgD myeloma.[15,16] The prevalence of extramedullary plasmacytomas in patients with IgD myeloma is about 15–20%.[15,16] The electrophoretic pattern of the serum and urine of patients with IgD myeloma is not different from that of patients with light chain multiple myeloma: usually an M-spike of less than 2 g/dL and light chain proteinuria.[15,17]

The detection of an immunoglobulin D monoclonal protein in the serum or urine does not in itself make the diagnosis of IgD myeloma; rare cases of monoclonal gammopathy of undetermined significance (MGUS) with IgD productions have been described.[19]

λ Light chains are thought to be more commonly associated with IgD myeloma than κ. Hence, patients with λ light chain myeloma with a discrete M-spike on serum electrophoresis should have immunofixation for immunoglobulin D.[4]

Wechalekar et al. reported that monoclonal IgD was detectable by immunofluorescence in 25 of 26 patients with IgD myeloma, with only one patient having measurable serum IgD.[18] The same authors noted several associated hematological disorders in their cohort of patients (total 26 patients) with IgD myeloma: one patient with chronic lymphocytic leukemia, one patient with hairy cell leukemia, and three patients with increased bone marrow reticulin stains. They noted chromosome 13q (a poor prognostic factor in patients with classic multiple myeloma) deletions in three of the nine tested patients. Other series did not report on the frequency of chromosome 13q deletions.[18]

Prognosis and management

The survival of patients with IgD multiple myeloma is thought to be less than that in their counterparts with classic multiple myeloma. This observation may be biased by the difference in the dates of diagnosis in different series, with more contemporary series describing a similar survival.[15–18,20]

Chemotherapeutic regimens used for the treatment of patients with classic multiple myeloma are thought to have efficacy in the treatment of IgD myeloma. Wechalekar et al.

suggest a possible benefit from autologous stem cell transplantation when compared to conventional chemotherapy.[18] A more recent study noted similar outcomes for patients with IgD myeloma undergoing high-dose therapy compared to patients with other myeloma subtypes.[21] However, the retrospective, nonrandomized study design and the small sample size may have biased the findings.

Immunoglobulin E myeloma

Less than 50 cases of IgE myeloma have been reported in the literature, and many of these reports suggest an aggressive presentation with rapid progression to plasma cell leukemia or extramedullary involvement. Given the rare nature of this entity, definitive conclusions about distinctive therapy or management cannot be drawn, and therapy for IgE myeloma is generally similar to that of other myeloma subtypes.

Immunoglobulin M myeloma

Biology and presentation

Immunoglobulin M myeloma is a rare entity that is characterized by an IgM monoclonal protein, and greater than 10% bone marrow plasmacytosis with either lytic bone lesions or the chromosomal translocation (11;14).[22] The last two criteria are important in distinguishing this entity from Waldenström macroglobulinemia, in which bone lesions are very uncommon and the t(11;14) abnormality is not present. Hyperviscosity can be present, and again does not imply a diagnosis of Waldenström macroglobulinemia. In one study of 15 IgM myeloma cases with known immunophenotype analysis, plasma cells from 10 patients were CD20 negative.[22] Generally plasma cells from patients with IgM myeloma express CD138, CD38, and frequently CD56.

Prognosis and management

The median overall survival of patients in this series was no different from non-IgM myeloma patients, and therapeutic options are generally similar to those for other myeloma subtypes.[21,22]

Waldenström macroglobulinemia

Biology and presentation

Waldenström macroglobulinemia (WM) is a B cell lymphoproliferative disorder characterized by the production of a monoclonal immunoglobulin of the IgM subtype and by intertrabecular bone marrow infiltration with a lymphoplasmacytic infiltrate.[23] The second international workshop on WM proposed the following diagnostic criteria[24]:
• an IgM monoclonal protein of any concentration
• bone marrow infiltration with small lymphocytes exhibiting plasmacytoid differentiation
• a suggestive immunophenotype (expression of surface IgM, CD19, CD20, CD25, CD27, FMC7, and CD138 without the expression of CD5, CD10, CD23, and CD103).[24]

Symptoms attributable to WM are related to tumor infiltration and/or to the monoclonal protein. The former results in constitutional symptoms (fevers, sweats, and weight loss), cytopenias (secondary to bone marrow involvement), lymphadenopathy, and hepatosplenomegaly.[23,25] Symptoms related to the monoclonal protein are associated with hyperviscosity, cryoglobulinemia, cold agglutinin, neuropathy, and amyloidosis. Hyperviscosity develops because the IgM molecules are large intravascular structures with carbohydrate content that tend to bind to water and increase the resistance to blood flow in the microcirculation.[26,27] The Bing–Neel syndrome, rarely reported in patients with WM, refers to confusion, memory loss, and eventual coma secondary to long-standing hyperviscosity with resultant increase in vascular permeability and deposition of lymphoplasmacytic cells.[28] Increase in cryoglobulins is noted in 20% of patients with WM; however, clinical signs of cryoglobulinemia (skin ulcerations, Raynaud phenomenon) occur in only 5% of patients.[29,30] Depositions of the M-protein in tissues may result in organ dysfunction; such deposits have been described in glomerular loops in the kidneys and may result in proteinuria and uremia, which may be reversed with apheresis of the monoclonal protein; deposition into the skin results in flesh-colored skin papules called *macroglobulinemia cutis*; and deposits in the gastrointestinal tract may result in malabsorption and diarrhea.[23,26,31] Less commonly, amyloidosis may result from deposition of the M-protein in tissues and can cause cardiac dysfunction, neuropathy, and renal dysfunction.[32] Autoantibodies to the glycolipid on nerve sheets can cause a distal, symmetrical, peripheral neuropathy. In this case, antimyelin-associated glycoprotein (MAG) IgM antibodies are noted.[33] Occasional patients are diagnosed incidentally, and are asymptomatic at presentation.[34]

Prognosis and management

The median survival of patients with WM ranges from 5 to 10 years, with improved outcomes noted in more recent reports.[23] Adverse prognostic factors identified in several series of patients include the following: age greater than 65, the presence of anemia, thrombocytopenia, serum β2-microglobulin, and the level of the monoclonal protein.[35–39] The presence of one or more of these risks factors is the basis of the Waldenstrom Macroglobulinemia International Prognostic Scoring System (WM IPSS, Table 45.1).[40]

Table 45.1 Waldenström macroglobulinemia International Prognostic Scoring System.[40]

Risk factors	5-year overall survival
0–1 risk factor and younger than 65 years	87%
Two risk factors or older than 65 years	68%
More than two risk factors	36%

Risk factors: hemoglobin ≤11.5 g/dL, platelet count ≤100×10⁹/L, serum β2-microglobulin >3 mg/L, monoclonal protein concentration >7 g/dL.

Treatment should be instituted in symptomatic patients and considered in those with cytopenias, bulky adenopathy, or organomegaly. The level of the monoclonal protein should not be used as an indication for treatment. Treatment responses for comparison of clinical trials have been defined by the third international workshop on WM.[41] A complete response is defined as the disappearance of the monoclonal protein, and by resolution of infiltration of lymph node and visceral organs confirmed on two separate evaluations 6 weeks apart. A partial response is defined as greater than 50% reduction in the monoclonal protein, and greater than 50% reduction in lymphadenopathy with the resolution of symptoms related to WM. Progressive disease is defined as a greater than 25% increase in the monoclonal protein, worsening of cytopenias, organ infiltration or disease-related symptoms.[42]

The data supporting treatment recommendations are mostly based on case series, phase 2 trials, and only two randomized controlled trials. Accordingly, the following guidelines for treatment should be viewed as recommendations and treatment should be individualized whenever possible according to patient presentation and preference. Referral to an academic center experienced in the treatment of patients with WM or enrollment in clinical trials should be sought. In addition, the fourth international workshop on WM has reviewed treatment recommendations.[43]

Plasmapheresis is an effective method for the rapid reduction of the monoclonal protein when it causes hyperviscosity, peripheral neuropathy or cryoglobulinemia. A single session will often result in greater than 50% reduction in serum viscosity.[44,45] The benefits of plasmapheresis are unfortunately short-lived and it is only indicated for chronic management in patients with hyperviscosity who are resistant to systemic treatment.

Splenectomy may result in durable remissions in case reports of patients resistant to systemic treatment.[46] The beneficial effects of splenectomy have been attributed to cytoreduction of T cells necessary for the B lymphocyte differentiation into IgM-producing cells.[23] Splenectomy cannot be routinely recommended in the management of patients with WM but may be considered in selected situations.

Systemic therapies are reviewed in Table 45.2 and high-dose therapy trials in Table 45.3. Traditionally, oral alkylating agents were used for the systemic control of WM. A prospective randomized trial comparing low-dose daily chlorambucil to high intermittent dosing did not identify a survival advantage to either approach, with patients having a median overall survival of approximately 5 years.[47] While complete responses are rare with the use of alkylating agents, partial responses approach 50% in some series. The time to response has been slow with alkylating agents.[47] The duration of treatment has not been defined, but it is generally recommended to withhold treatment after best response.[23] The use of alkylating agents should be considered in older patients in whom rapid control of the disease is not necessary.

Numerous nonrandomized studies have reported on the efficacy of nucleoside analogs (fludarabine or cladribine), with response rates ranging from 30% to 70%.[48–50] A randomized controlled trial compared fludarabine treatment with treatment with the combination of cyclophosphamide, adriamycin, and prednisone in patients who had failed

Table 45.2 Overview of systemic therapies for Waldenström macroglobulinemia.

Therapy	n	ND ORR, %	RR ORR, %	CR, %	TTR, mo	TTP, mo	OS, mo
Nucleoside analogs							
Fludarabine[51]	182	38	33	3	3–6	36	60
2CDA[96]	46	–	43	–	–	18	28
2CDA[50]	16	94	–	20	1	23	73
Alkylators							
Chlorambucil/pred[97]	110	31	–	NR	NR	NR	60
Monoclonal antibodies							
Rituximab[36]	69	35	20	0	NR	27	NR
Combination therapy							
CAP[51]	45	–	11	0	NR	3*	45
CHOP[98]	20	65	–	NR	NR	NR	87
CHOP-R[99]	16	91	–	NR	1.6	NR	NR
RCD[100]	72	74	–	7	4	NR	NR
2CDACR[50]	27	94	–	–	1	60	NR
FC[101]	49	85	70	0	NR	27	NR
Novel agents							
Bortezomib[58]	27	–	48	0	1.4	6.6	NR
BDR[102,103]	26/37	66	51	4–5	NR	16.4	NR
Thalidomide[60]	20	33	20	NR	0.8–2.8	NR	NR
Thalidomide rituximab[61]	25	80	40	2.5	NR	36/15	NR

* in patients who had failed alkylating agents.
2CDA, cladribine; 2CDACR, cladribine cyclophosphamide rituximab; BDR, bortezomib dexamethasone; CAP, cyclophosphamide adriamycin prednisone; CHOP, cyclophosphamide adriamycin vincristine prednisone; CR, complete remission, rituximab; mo, months; ND, newly diagnosed; NR, not reported; ORR, overall response rate; OS, overall survival; Pred, prednisone; R, rituximab; RCD, rituximab cyclophosphamide dexamethasone; RR, relapsed or refractory; TTP, time to progression; TTR, time to response.

Table 45.3 Trials of high-dose therapy for Waldenström macroglobulinemia.

Study	n	Regimen	TRM	ORR	CR	PFS	OS
Autologous							
Anagnostopoulos[104]	22	BuCy+other	11%	58%*	29%*	65% @ 3y	70% @ 3y
Dreger[105]	12	Cy+TBI	0%	100%	17%	75% @ 3y	100% @ 5y
Munshi[106]	8	MEL200/TBI	0%	100%	12%	NR	NR
Tournilhac[57]	19	Various	6%	95%	NR	NR	NR
Allogeneic							
Anagnostopoulos[104]	35	20% NMA	40%	58%*	29%*	21% @ 3y	46% @ 3y
Tournilhac[57]	10	10% NMA	40%	80%	NR	NR	NR

* in patients who had failed alkylating agents.
Bu, busulfan; CR, complete remission; Cy, cyclophosphamide; ORR, overall response rate; OS, overall survival; MEL200, melphalan at $200\,mg/m^2$; NMA, nonmyeloablative; NR, not reported; PFS, progression-free survival; TBI, total body irradiation; TRM, transplant-related mortality.

alkylating agents. Fludarabine was associated with responses in 28% of patients, compared to only 11% of patients treated with combination chemotherapy. Survival was similar, as nonresponders were allowed to cross over.[51] The faster time to response is a major advantage to treatment with nucleoside analogs, and these agents are generally indicated in patients when rapid responses are needed.[52] Long-term toxicity to stem cells limits the use of this class of agents in younger patients who may be candidates for high-dose therapy and stem cell transplant.

Rituximab, a monoclonal anti-CD20 antibody, has been used in newly diagnosed and previously treated patients in phase 2 trials; response rates are 20–70% in the former and around 30% in the latter group of patients. Time to response in rituximab-treated patients is approximately 3 months.[36,52,53] A flare reaction to rituximab has been well characterized and is manifest by increasing IgM levels 1–4 months after initiation of treatment. In some instances, this flare reaction can result in symptoms of hyperviscosity among patients with a high tumor burden or high baseline IgM levels.[54] Accordingly, rituximab is often used as a first-line agent in patients who may be candidates for autologous stem cell transplantation, and in whom a longer time to response is acceptable, especially with low tumor burden. In addition, patients with peripheral neuropathy associated with IgM antibodies to myelin-associated glycoprotein will often respond to rituximab therapy.[55]

High-dose therapy and autologous stem cell transplantation have resulted in high response rates (approaching 90%), that may be durable (progression-free survival approaching 70 months) in small series of patients.[56,57] The small number of patients, the nonrandomized nature of the studies, and the potential for treatment-related morbidity make it difficult to routinely recommend this approach to all patients. It should, however, be considered in younger patients after cytoreductive treatment with rituximab. Treatment with alkylating agents and nucleoside analogs may impair the ability to collect stem cells and should be used judiciously in younger patients.

Bortezomib, a first in class proteasome inhibitor, approved for the treatment of multiple myeloma and mantle cell lymphoma, is also active in WM. Bortezomib results in a response rate of 48% as a single agent, and 83% in combination with rituximab and dexamethasone.[58,59] A bortezomib-based regimen can be considered in younger individuals with a high tumor burden and/or renal insufficiency, in whom a rapid response is needed.

Thalidomide, an immunomodulatory agent with antiangiogenic properties, is approved for the treatment of multiple myeloma and has activity in WM. As a single agent, a response rate of 25% was noted in one study and therapy was limited due to neuropathy.[60] It has also been combined with rituximab in one report as well.[61]

Novel therapies including but not restricted to everolimus, alemtuzumab, pomalidomide, and bendamustine are the subjects of ongoing research.

Heavy chain disease

Biology

Heavy chain diseases (HCD) are characterized by the production of an abnormal truncated immunoglobulin heavy chain, with no associated light chain, by monoclonal plasma cells.[62] The three types of HCD refer to the heavy chain produced: α, γ, and μ. The diagnosis of HCD often requires serum immunofixation, as protein electrophoresis often does not detect the monoclonal protein, but may occasionally detect depressed or increased immunoglobulins.[62]

Presentation

α HCD is an enteric disease and usually involves secretory IgA. A geographic clustering of reports in the Mediterranean basin has been noted, as has an association with lower socioeconomic status and poor hygiene in immigrants to developed countries.[63] Affected patients tend to be males in their second or third decades of life who present with diarrhea, malabsorption, and abdominal pain. The diagnosis often requires endoscopy with biopsy. Different stages may coexist in a particular patient. The presentation of γ HCD is one of a lymphoproliferative disorder with lymphadenopathy and constitutional symptoms, but without a specific histopathological pattern (often lymphoplasmacytic infiltration).[64] The diagnosis requires a consistent immunofixation pattern. An association with autoimmune conditions has been described.[65]

μ HCD is a very rare disorder of adults and often coexists with a chronic lymphocytic leukemia. While lymphadenopathy is less common, hepatosplenomegaly often is present. This diagnosis also requires a consistent immunofixation. The course is of a slowly progressive disease.

Treatment and prognosis

For α HCD, stage A involves the presence of a mature plasmacytic infiltrate in the intestinal mucosa, and usually responds to long-term antimicrobial treatment. Stage B is characterized by involvement of the submucosa, while stage C involves extensive involvement of the bowels.

Treatment recommendations for γ HCD vary according to the course of the disease; some patients have an indolent course and even spontaneous regression, while others have aggressive disease requiring treatment with systemic chemotherapy (often melphalan and prednisone).[62,65] Treatment of μ HCD involves the treatment of the underlying lymphoproliferative disorder.[62]

Osteosclerotic myeloma

Presentation

Osteosclerotic myeloma, also known as POEMS syndrome, Crow–Fukase syndrome, PEP syndrome or Takatsuki syndrome, represents a constellation of findings including the following: polyneuropathy, organomegaly, endocrinopathy, the presence of a monoclonal protein, and a variety of dermatological findings.[66,67] Other associated findings include sclerotic bony lesions, Castleman disease (see Chapter 45), papilledema, erythrocytosis, and thrombocytosis.[66,68,69]

Patients frequently present in the fifth decade of life, often with signs and symptoms of polyneuropathy.[66] Sensory deficits in the lower extremities occur early and are followed by motor deficits, which may result in significant disabilities. While no characteristic electromyographic findings have been identified, slowing of nerve conduction velocity and decreased muscle action potentials have been associated with the polyneuropathy.[70,71] An increase in the cerebrospinal fluid protein is seen in the overwhelming majority of patients.[33,70] Hepatosplenomegaly or lymphadenopathy is found in about half the patients.

Frequently, Castleman disease and reactive lymphadenopathy were the diagnoses rendered on lymph node biopsies in patients with POEMS syndrome.[72] Endocrinopathies associated with the diagnosis of POEMS syndrome include hypogonadism, hypothyroidism, and dysfunction of the pituitary adrenal axis.[66] Evidence of a monoclonal plasma cell dyscrasia was noted in all patients within one series, approximately 90% of whom had evidence of a monoclonal protein in the serum or urine, while the remainder had evidence of monoclonal plasmacytosis on biopsy specimen.[66] Reported skin changes associated with the diagnosis of POEMS syndrome include hyperpigmentation, acrocyanosis, hypertrichosis, angiomas, and plethora.[73] Most patients with POEMS syndrome have demonstrable bony lesions on x-rays,

---

Box 45.1 Criteria for the diagnosis of POEMS.[66]

Patients must have evidence of polyneuropathy, and
A monoclonal plasma cell dyscrasia and
One of the following findings:
- sclerotic bone lesions
- evidence of Castleman disease on a lymph node biopsy
- organomegaly
- endocrinopathy (with the exception of diabetes or hypothyroidism)
- evidence of volume overload
- papilledema or consistent skin changes
- thrombocytosis

---

a mixture of sclerotic and lytic lesions, or only sclerotic lesions.[66] About half the patients present with a single lesion, while others have multiple lesions. Hypercalcemia was not associated with bony lesions. Renal dysfunction occasionally requiring dialysis has been described at diagnosis or during the course of the disease.[74] Arterial or venous thrombotic events (including myocardial infarction, strokes, Budd–Chiari syndrome) have been described in a number of series, which suggests a greater prevalence than expected by chance.[66] Pulmonary arterial hypertension has been observed in a small series of patients.[75] Erythrocytosis was more common than anemia in one series of patients, and leukocytosis and thrombocytosis have also been reported. Only about 30% of patients with osteosclerotic myeloma present with the five findings of the POEMS acronym.[66]

Dispenzieri et al. have proposed diagnostic criteria for the diagnosis of POEMS syndrome (Box 45.1).[66]

Because of the protean nature of the findings in patients with osteosclerotic myeloma and the independent multidisciplinary evaluation, the clinician must have a high index of suspicion in patients presenting with unexplained polyneuropathy and evidence of a monoclonal plasma cell disorder.

Prognosis and management

The natural history of patients with POEMS syndrome is frequently one of progressive neurological deterioration. The median survival of patients exceeds a decade in many series.[66,68,69] Adverse prognostic factors include evidence of volume overload or clubbing.[66] Patients with single or multiple localized osteosclerotic lesions benefit from radiation therapy to the area (often 40–50 Gy of radiation are delivered). Improvement in the neuropathy is often slow after radiation therapy. Patients with widespread lesions require systemic therapy.[66] Therapeutic agents that have been used in this setting include melphalan and prednisone, combination chemotherapy such as CHOP or VAD, as well as corticosteroids as single agents.[66,69,76] Responses to autologous stem cell transplantation have been described.[77] More recently, therapy with lenalidomide or bortezomib has been successful in case reports.[78–81] An evidence-based approach for the choice of systemic therapy cannot be recommended with the available data.

Solitary plasmacytomas

Presentation

Plasmacytomas have been described in virtually every organ in multiple myeloma patients. Solitary plasmacytoma of bone (SPB) refers to a single bony lesion composed of monoclonal plasma cells without evidence of a systemic multiple myeloma. SPB accounts for about 5% of patients with plasma cell dyscrasias.[82] Patients present in their fifth decade of life, with a male predominance. Patients with SPB usually present with bony pain related to the skeletal lesion.[83] Vertebral involvement is most common and occasionally patients have frank spinal cord compression. Appearance on plain radiograph is that of a lytic lesion.

Solitary extramedullary plasmacytoma (EMP) refers to involvement of a nonmarrow-containing organ by monoclonal plasma cells[83] and is seen in fewer than 3% of patients with plasma cell dyscrasias.[84] Most lesions have been reported in the head and neck, but any organ may be affected.[85] The presenting symptoms are mostly related to the site of involvement; for example, submucosal nasal involvement may results in nasal discharge, epistaxis, or nasal obstruction.[85] Occasionally, plasmacytomas are asymptomatic and detected on imaging studies for other conditions, as may be seen with plasmacytoma of the lungs. Involvement of adjacent lymph nodes and bone is still consistent with the localized nature of the disease.[86]

To make the diagnosis, a skeletal survey must not reveal involvement of other bony structure, while a serum protein electrophoresis may show a low concentration of a monoclonal protein with preservation of the uninvolved immunoglobulins.[87] A bone marrow biopsy should be performed to rule out a systemic myeloma. In addition, the patient must not have evidence of anemia, hypercalcemia, or renal dysfunction related to the monoclonal protein.[87] While magnetic resonance imaging has been used to identify additional skeletal abnormalities, it is not an integral part of the workup.[87] Positron emission tomography (PET) is increasingly being used as part of the diagnostic workup to exclude additional areas of involvement, and in one study PET imaging detected additional bone lesions in 27% of patients imaged.[88]

Prognosis and management

The median survival of patients with SPB is approximately 10 years; almost half of the patients eventually develop multiple myeloma after a median time of 2 years.[89–91] The development of multiple myeloma has been described as late as 15 years after radiotherapy. Several series have attempted to identify predictors of progression to multiple myeloma, but results have been difficult to duplicate because of limited patient numbers and due to differences in diagnostic criteria. That being said, some predictors of progression include advanced age, axial lesions, larger lesions, and the lack of resolution of the monoclonal protein following radiotherapy.[84,90,92] For EMP, treatment involves definitive radiotherapy and is associated with excellent local control rates.[93] Progression to multiple myeloma occurs in about 15% of patients.[86]

The treatment of SPB and EMP has been definitive local radiotherapy. Local control rates exceed 90% with this modality alone.[89–91,94,95] Recurrences tend to cluster in the first 3 years after the original diagnosis. The use of surgery followed by radiotherapy is occasionally needed for patients who present with acute neurological dysfunction or who require prophylactic internal fixation. Radiotherapy often results in the disappearance of the monoclonal protein from the serum of patients. There is no role for systemic therapy.[83]

References

1. Costello R, et al. Primary plasma cell leukaemia: a report of 18 cases. Leuk Res 2001; 25(2): 103–7.
2. Dimopoulos MA, Palumbo A, Delasalle KB, Alexanian R. Primary plasma cell leukaemia. Br J Haematol 1994; 88(4): 754–9.
3. Swerdlow S, et al. (eds). WHO Classification of Tumours of Haematopoietic and Lymphoid Tissues, 4th edn. Lyon: International Agency for Research on Cancer, 2008.
4. Garcia-Sanz R, et al. Primary plasma cell leukemia: clinical, immunophenotypic, DNA ploidy, and cytogenetic characteristics. Blood 1999; 93(3): 1032–7.
5. Noel P, Kyle RA. Plasma cell leukemia: an evaluation of response to therapy. Am J Med 1987; 83(6): 1062–8.
6. Tiedemann RE, et al. Genetic aberrations and survival in plasma cell leukemia. Leukemia 2008; 22(5): 1044–52.
7. Pellat-Deceunynck C, et al. The absence of CD56 (NCAM) on malignant plasma cells is a hallmark of plasma cell leukemia and of a special subset of multiple myeloma. Leukemia 1998; 12(12): 1977–82.
8. Hovenga S, de Wolf JT, Klip H, Vellenga E. Consolidation therapy with autologous stem cell transplantation in plasma cell leukemia after VAD, high-dose cyclophosphamide and EDAP courses: a report of three cases and a review of the literature. Bone Marrow Transplant 1997; 20(10): 901–4.
9. Saccaro S, et al. Primary plasma cell leukemia: report of 17 new cases treated with autologous or allogeneic stem-cell transplantation and review of the literature. Am J Hematol 2005; 78(4): 288–94.
10. Bourantas K. Nonsecretory multiple myeloma. Eur J Haematol 1996; 56(1–2): 109–11.
11. Cavo M, et al. Nonsecretory multiple myeloma. Presenting findings, clinical course and prognosis. Acta Haematol 1985; 74(1): 27–30.
12. Dreicer R, Alexanian R. Nonsecretory multiple myeloma. Am J Hematol 1982; 13(4): 313–18.
13. Kumar S, et al. Comparable outcomes in nonsecretory and secretory multiple myeloma after autologous stem cell transplantation. Biol Blood Marrow Transplant 2008; 14(10): 1134–40.
14. Durie BG, et al. International uniform response criteria for multiple myeloma. Leukemia 2006; 20(9): 1467–73.
15. Blade J, Lust JA, Kyle RA. Immunoglobulin D multiple myeloma: presenting features, response to therapy, and survival in a series of 53 cases. J Clin Oncol 1994; 12(11): 2398–404.
16. Jancelewicz Z, Takatsuki K, Sugai S, Pruzanski W. IgD multiple myeloma. Review of 133 cases. Arch Intern Med 1975; 135(1): 87–93.
17. Sinclair D. IgD myeloma: clinical, biological and laboratory features. Clin Lab 2002; 48(11–12): 617–22.
18. Wechalekar A, Amato D, Chen C, Keith Stewart A, Reece D. IgD multiple myeloma – a clinical profile and outcome with chemotherapy and autologous stem cell transplantation. Ann Hematol 2005; 84(2): 115–17.
19. Blade J, Kyle RA. IgD monoclonal gammopathy with long-term follow-up. Br J Haematol 1994; 88(2): 395–6.
20. Fibbe WE, Jansen J. Prognostic factors in IgD myeloma: a study of 21 cases. Scand J Haematol 1984; 33(5): 471–5.
21. Reece DE, et al. Outcome of patients with IgD and IgM multiple myeloma undergoing autologous hematopoietic stem cell transplantation: a retrospective CIBMTR study. Clin Lymphoma Myeloma Leuk 2010; 10(6): 458–63.

22. Schuster SR, *et al*. IgM multiple myeloma: disease definition, prognosis, and differentiation from Waldenstrom's macroglobulinemia. Am J Hematol 2010; 85(11): 853–5.

23. Dimopoulos MA, Kyle RA, Anagnostopoulos A, Treon SP. Diagnosis and management of Waldenstrom's macroglobulinemia. J Clin Oncol 2005; 23(7): 1564–77.

24. Owen RG, *et al*. Clinicopathological definition of Waldenstrom's macroglobulinemia: consensus panel recommendations from the Second International Workshop on Waldenstrom's Macroglobulinemia. Semin Oncol 2003; 30(2): 110–15.

25. Dimopoulos MA, Panayiotidis P, Moulopoulos LA, Sfikakis P, Dalakas M. Waldenstrom's macroglobulinemia: clinical features, complications, and management. J Clin Oncol 2000; 18(1): 214–26.

26. Fudenberg HH, Virella G. Multiple myeloma and Waldenstrom macroglobulinemia: unusual presentations. Semin Hematol 1980; 17(1): 63–79.

27. Kwaan HC, Bongu A. The hyperviscosity syndromes. Semin Thromb Hemost 1999; 25(2): 199–208.

28. Civit T, Coulbois S, Baylac F, Taillandier L, Auque J. [Waldenstrom's macroglobulinemia and cerebral lymphoplasmocytic proliferation: Bing and Neel syndrome. Apropos of a new case]. Neurochirurgie 1997; 43(4): 245–9.

29. Dispenzieri A. Symptomatic cryoglobulinemia. Curr Treat Options Oncol 2000; 1(2): 105–18.

30. Farhangi M, Merlini G. The clinical implications of monoclonal immunoglobulins. Semin Oncol 1986; 13(3): 366–79.

31. Daoud MS, Lust JA, Kyle RA, Pittelkow MR. Monoclonal gammopathies and associated skin disorders. J Am Acad Dermatol 1999; 40(4): 507–35; quiz 36–8.

32. Gertz MA, Kyle RA, Noel P. Primary systemic amyloidosis: a rare complication of immunoglobulin M monoclonal gammopathies and Waldenstrom's macroglobulinemia. J Clin Oncol 1993; 11(5): 914–20.

33. Ropper AH, Gorson KC. Neuropathies associated with paraproteinemia. N Engl J Med 1998; 338(22): 1601–7.

34. Alexanian R, Weber D, Delasalle K, Cabanillas F, Dimopoulos M. Asymptomatic Waldenstrom's macroglobulinemia. Semin Oncol 2003; 30(2): 206–10.

35. Dimopoulos M, *et al*. The international staging system for multiple myeloma is applicable in symptomatic Waldenstrom's macroglobulinemia. Leuk Lymphoma 2004; 45(9): 1809–13.

36. Dimopoulos MA, *et al*. Treatment of Waldenstrom's macroglobulinemia with rituximab: prognostic factors for response and progression. Leuk Lymphoma 2004; 45(10): 2057–61.

37. Garcia-Sanz R, *et al*. Waldenstrom macroglobulinaemia: presenting features and outcome in a series with 217 cases. Br J Haematol 2001; 115(3): 575–82.

38. Morel P, *et al*. Prognostic factors in Waldenstrom macroglobulineamia: a report on 232 patients with the description of a new scoring system and its validation on 253 other patients. Blood 2000; 96(3): 852–8.

39. Dimopoulos MA, *et al*. Survival and prognostic factors after initiation of treatment in Waldenstrom's macroglobulinemia. Ann Oncol 2003; 14(8): 1299–305.

40. Morel P, *et al*. International Prognostic Scoring System (IPSS) for Waldenstrom's Macroglobulinemia (WM). ASH Annual Meeting Abstracts, November 16, 2006; 108(11): 127.

41. Kimby E, *et al*. Update on recommendations for assessing response from the Third International Workshop on Waldenstrom's Macroglobulinemia. Clin Lymphoma Myeloma 2006; 6(5): 380–3.

42. Weber D, *et al*. Uniform response criteria in Waldenstrom's macroglobulinemia: consensus panel recommendations from the Second International Workshop on Waldenstrom's Macroglobulinemia. Semin Oncol 2003; 30(2): 127–31.

43. Dimopoulos MA, *et al*. Update on treatment recommendations from the Fourth International Workshop on Waldenstrom's Macroglobulinemia. J Clin Oncol 2009; 27(1): 120–6.

44. Zarkovic M, Kwaan HC. Correction of hyperviscosity by apheresis. Semin Thromb Hemost 2003; 29(5): 535–42.

45. Drew MJ. Plasmapheresis in the dysproteinemias. Ther Apher 2002; 6(1): 45–52.

46. Cavanna L, Berte R, Lazzaro A, Vallisa D, Moroni CF, Civardi G. Advanced Waldenstrom's macroglobulinemia: a case of possible cure after systemic chemotherapy, splenic radiation and splenectomy. Acta Haematol 2002; 108(2): 97–101.

47. Kyle RA, *et al*. Waldenstrom's macroglobulinaemia: a prospective study comparing daily with intermittent oral chlorambucil. Br J Haematol 2000; 108(4): 737–42.

48. Dimopoulos MA, O'Brien S, Kantarjian H, Estey EE, Keating MJ, Alexanian R. Treatment of Waldenstrom's macroglobulinemia with nucleoside analogues. Leuk Lymphoma 1993; 11(Suppl 2): 105–8.

49. Dimopoulos MA, *et al*. Treatment of Waldenstrom's macroglobulinemia with the combination of fludarabine and cyclophosphamide. Leuk Lymphoma 2003; 44(6): 993–6.

50. Weber DM, Dimopoulos MA, Delasalle K, Rankin K, Gavino M, Alexanian R. 2-Chlorodeoxyadenosine alone and in combination for previously untreated Waldenstrom's macroglobulinemia. Semin Oncol 2003; 30(2): 243–7.

51. Leblond V, *et al*. Multicenter, randomized comparative trial of fludarabine and the combination of cyclophosphamide-doxorubicin-prednisone in 92 patients with Waldenstrom macroglobulinemia in first relapse or with primary refractory disease. Blood 2001; 98(9): 2640–4.

52. Gertz MA, *et al*. Treatment recommendations in Waldenstrom's macroglobulinemia: consensus panel recommendations from the Second International Workshop on Waldenstrom's Macroglobulinemia. Semin Oncol 2003; 30(2): 121–6.

53. Dimopoulos MA, *et al*. Predictive factors for response to rituximab in Waldenstrom's macroglobulinemia. Clin Lymphoma 2005; 5(4): 270–2.

54. Ghobrial IM, *et al*. Initial immunoglobulin M 'flare' after rituximab therapy in patients diagnosed with Waldenstrom macroglobulinemia: an Eastern Cooperative Oncology Group Study. Cancer 2004; 101(11): 2593–8.

55. Dalakas MC, *et al*. Placebo-controlled trial of rituximab in IgM anti-myelin-associated glycoprotein antibody demyelinating neuropathy. Ann Neurol 2009; 65(3): 286–93.

56. Anagnostopoulos A, *et al*. High-dose chemotherapy followed by stem cell transplantation in patients with resistant Waldenstrom's macroglobulinemia. Bone Marrow Transplant 2001; 27(10): 1027–9.

57. Tournilhac O, *et al*. Transplantation in Waldenstrom's macroglobulinemia – the French experience. Semin Oncol 2003; 30(2): 291–6.

58. Treon SP, *et al*. Multicenter clinical trial of bortezomib in relapsed/refractory Waldenstrom's macroglobulinemia: results of WMCTG Trial 03-248. Clin Cancer Res 2007; 13(11): 3320–5.

59. Treon SP, *et al*. Primary therapy of Waldenstrom macroglobulinemia with bortezomib, dexamethasone, and rituximab: WMCTG clinical trial 05-180. J Clin Oncol 2009; 27(23): 3830–5.

60. Dimopoulos MA, *et al*. Treatment of Waldenstrom's macroglobulinemia with thalidomide. J Clin Oncol 2001; 19(16): 3596–601.

61. Treon SP, *et al*. Thalidomide and rituximab in Waldenstrom macroglobulinemia. Blood 2008; 112(12): 4452–7.

62. Fermand JP, Brouet JC. Heavy-chain diseases. Hematol Oncol Clin North Am 1999; 13(6): 1281–94.

63. Ben-Ayed F, *et al*. Treatment of alpha chain disease. Results of a prospective study in 21 Tunisian patients by the Tunisian-French intestinal Lymphoma Study Group. Cancer 1989; 63(7): 1251–6.

64. Wester SM, Banks PM, Li CY. The histopathology of gamma heavy-chain disease. Am J Clin Pathol 1982; 78(4): 427–36.

65. Kyle RA, Greipp PR, Banks PM. The diverse picture of gamma heavy-chain disease. Report of seven cases and review of literature. Mayo Clin Proc 1981; 56(7): 439–51.

66. Dispenzieri A, *et al*. POEMS syndrome: definitions and long-term outcome. Blood 2003; 101(7): 2496–506.

67. Nakanishi T, *et al*. The Crow–Fukase syndrome: a study of 102 cases in Japan. Neurology 1984; 34(6): 712–20.

68. Perniciaro C. POEMS syndrome. Semin Dermatol 1995; 14(2): 162–5.

69. Soubrier MJ, Dubost JJ, Sauvezie BJ. POEMS syndrome: a study of 25 cases and a review of the literature. French Study Group on POEMS Syndrome. Am J Med 1994; 97(6): 543–53.

70. Min JH, Hong YH, Lee KW. Electrophysiological features of patients with POEMS syndrome. Clin Neurophysiol 2005; 116(4): 965–8.

71. Sung JY, Kuwabara S, Ogawara K, Kanai K, Hattori T. Patterns of nerve conduction abnormalities in POEMS syndrome. Muscle Nerve 2002; 26(2): 189–93.

72. Papo T, *et al*. Human herpesvirus 8 infection, Castleman's disease and POEMS syndrome. Br J Haematol 1999; 104(4): 932–3.

73. Kanitakis J, Roger H, Soubrier M, Dubost JJ, Chouvet B, Souteyrand P. Cutaneous angiomas in POEMS syndrome. An ultrastructural and immunohistochemical study. Arch Dermatol 1988; 124(5): 695–8.

74. Modesto-Segonds A, Rey JP, Orfila C, Huchard G, Suc JM. Renal involvement in POEMS syndrome. Clin Nephrol 1995; 43(5): 342–5.

75. Lesprit P, *et al*. Pulmonary hypertension in POEMS syndrome: a new feature mediated by cytokines. Am J Respir Crit Care Med 1998; 157(3 Pt 1): 907–11.

76. Kuwabara S, Hattori T, Shimoe Y, Kamitsukasa I. Long term melphalan-prednisolone chemotherapy for POEMS syndrome. J Neurol Neurosurg Psychiatry 1997; 63(3): 385–7.

77. Soubrier M, Ruivard M, Dubost JJ, Sauvezie B, Philippe P. Successful use of autologous bone marrow transplantation in treating a patient with POEMS syndrome. Bone Marrow Transplant 2002; 30(1): 61–2.

78. Sethi S, Tageja N, Arabi H, Penumetcha R. Lenalidomide therapy in a rare case of POEMS syndrome with kappa restriction. South Med J 2009; 102(10): 1092–3.

79. Dispenzieri A, Klein CJ, Mauermann ML. Lenalidomide therapy in a patient with POEMS syndrome. Blood 2007; 110(3): 1075–6.

80. Ohguchi H, *et al*. Successful treatment with bortezomib and thalidomide for POEMS syndrome. Ann Hematol 2011; 90(9): 1113–14.

81. Tang X, *et al*. Successful bortezomib-based treatment in POEMS syndrome. Eur J Haematol 2009; 83(6): 609–10.

82. Hjorth M, Holmberg E, Rodjer S, Westin J. Impact of active and passive exclusions on the results of a clinical trial in multiple myeloma. The Myeloma Group of Western Sweden. Br J Haematol 1992; 80(1): 55–61.

83. Dimopoulos MA, Kiamouris C, Moulopoulos LA. Solitary plasmacytoma of bone and extramedullary plasmacytoma. Hematol Oncol Clin North Am 1999; 13(6): 1249–57.

84. Knowling MA, Harwood AR, Bergsagel DE. Comparison of extramedullary plasmacytomas with solitary and multiple plasma cell tumors of bone. J Clin Oncol 1983; 1(4): 255–62.

85. Miller FR, Lavertu P, Wanamaker JR, Bonafede J, Wood BG. Plasmacytomas of the head and neck. Otolaryngol Head Neck Surg 1998; 119(6): 614–18.

86. Galieni P, *et al*. Clinical outcome of extramedullary plasmacytoma. Haematologica 2000; 85(1): 47–51.

87. Soutar R, *et al*. Guidelines on the diagnosis and management of solitary plasmacytoma of bone and solitary extramedullary plasmacytoma. Clin Oncol (R Coll Radiol) 2004; 16(6): 405–13.

88. Schirrmeister H, Buck AK, Bergmann L, Reske SN, Bommer M. Positron emission tomography (PET) for staging of solitary plasmacytoma. Cancer Biother Radiopharm 2003; 18(5): 841–5.

89. Frassica DA, Frassica FJ, Schray MF, Sim FH, Kyle RA. Solitary plasmacytoma of bone: Mayo Clinic experience. Int J Radiat Oncol Biol Phys 1989; 16(1): 43–8.

90. Holland J, Trenkner DA, Wasserman TH, Fineberg B. Plasmacytoma. Treatment results and conversion to myeloma. Cancer 1992; 69(6): 1513–17.

91. Galieni P, *et al*. Solitary plasmacytoma of bone and extramedullary plasmacytoma: two different entities? Ann Oncol 1995; 6(7): 687–91.

92. Chak LY, Cox RS, Bostwick DG, Hoppe RT. Solitary plasmacytoma of bone: treatment, progression, and survival. J Clin Oncol 1987; 5(11): 1811–15.

93. Harwood AR, Knowling MA, Bergsagel DE. Radiotherapy of extramedullary plasmacytoma of the head and neck. Clin Radiol 1981; 32(1): 31–6.

94. Dimopoulos MA, Goldstein J, Fuller L, Delasalle K, Alexanian R. Curability of solitary bone plasmacytoma. J Clin Oncol 1992; 10(4): 587–90.

95. Liebross RH, Ha CS, Cox JD, Weber D, Delasalle K, Alexanian R. Solitary bone plasmacytoma: outcome and prognostic factors following radiotherapy. Int J Radiat Oncol Biol Phys 1998; 41(5): 1063–7.

96. Dimopoulos MA, Weber D, Delasalle KB, Keating M, Alexanian R. Treatment of Waldenstrom's macroglobulinemia resistant to standard therapy with 2-chlorodeoxyadenosine: identification of prognostic factors. Ann Oncol 1995; 6(1): 49–52.

97. Facon T, *et al*. Prognostic factors in Waldenstrom's macroglobulinemia: a report of 167 cases. J Clin Oncol 1993; 11(8): 1553–8.

98. Dimopoulos MA, Alexanian R. Waldenstrom's macroglobulinemia. Blood 1994; 83(6): 1452–9.

99. Abonour R, *et al*. Phase II pilot study of rituximab + CHOP in patients with newly diagnosed Waldenstrom's macroglobulinemia, an Eastern Cooperative Oncology Group Trial (Study E1A02). ASH Annual Meeting Abstracts, November 16, 2007; 110(11): 3616.

100. Dimopoulos MA, *et al*. Primary treatment of Waldenstrom macroglobulinemia with dexamethasone, rituximab, and cyclophosphamide. J Clin Oncol 2007; 25(22): 3344–9.

101. Tamburini J, *et al*. Fludarabine plus cyclophosphamide in Waldenstrom's macroglobulinemia: results in 49 patients. Leukemia 2005; 19(10): 1831–4.

102. Ghobrial IM, *et al*. Phase II trial of weekly bortezomib in combination with rituximab in untreated patients with Waldenstrom macroglobulinemia. Am J Hematol 2010; 85(9): 670–4.

103. Ghobrial IM, *et al*. Phase II trial of weekly bortezomib in combination with rituximab in relapsed or relapsed and refractory Waldenstrom macroglobulinemia. J Clin Oncol 2010; 28(8): 1422–8.

104. Anagnostopoulos A, *et al*. Autologous or allogeneic stem cell transplantation in patients with Waldenstrom's macroglobulinemia. Biol Blood Marrow Transplant 2006; 12(8): 845–54.

105. Dreger P, Schmitz N. Autologous stem cell transplantation as part of first-line treatment of Waldenstrom's macroglobulinemia. Biol Blood Marrow Transplant 2007; 13(5): 623–4.

106. Munshi NC, Barlogie B. Role for high-dose therapy with autologous hematopoietic stem cell support in Waldenstrom's macroglobulinemia. Semin Oncol 2003; 30(2): 282–5.

46 Rare Bone Marrow Failure Conditions

Valeria Visconte[1] and Ramon V. Tiu[1,2]

[1] Department of Translational Hematology and Oncology Research, [2] Department of Hematologic Oncology and Blood Disorders, Taussig Cancer Institute, Cleveland Clinic, OH, USA

Introduction

The bone marrow failure (BMF) syndromes encompass diseases characterized by a failure of hematopoietic stem cells (HSC) to sustain normal blood cell production. The impairment can affect all hematopoietic lineages, leading to cytopenia. The incidence of BMF in the general population is from 1 in 250,000 individuals per year for idiopathic aplastic anemia (AA) to 1 in 1,000,000 per year for rare inherited forms of aplastic anemia like dyskeratosis congenita (DKC). BMF syndromes can be either inherited or acquired. Inherited BMF syndromes include Fanconi anemia (FA), DKC, and Diamond–Blackfan anemia (DBA), while acquired conditions include idiopathic AA, paroxysmal nocturnal hemoglobinuria (PNH) and T cell large granular lymphocyte leukemia (T-LGL). Their pathogenesis is diverse and includes immune dysregulation, as seen in AA and T-LGL, and genetic defects, as in PNH (Fig. 46.1). Although clinical and pathogenetic heterogeneity is common within each disease, it is not uncommon to see overlap between these diseases at first diagnosis and during the disease course. This chapter will focus on the biology, clinical features, epidemiology, and management of several rare BMF disorders (Table 46.1).

Acquired bone marrow failure syndromes

Idiopathic aplastic anemia

Epidemiology

The incidence of AA is higher in Asia than in western countries. Several epidemiological studies have determined an incidence of 3.9 cases per million in Bangkok, six cases per million in rural areas of Thailand, and 14 cases per million in Japan.[1,2] The higher incidence in Asian countries has been linked to environmental factors, such as exposure to chemicals like benzene, more than genetic factors. In Europe, the incidence has been estimated at two cases per million by the International Agranulocytosis Study.[3] AA shows two peaks of incidence, the first between 15 and 25 years and the second at 60 years of age. It is possible that the second peak includes patients with myelodysplastic syndromes (MDS). Both males and females are equally affected.

Etiology/clinical features

Aplastic anemia is characterized by cytopenias, typically pancytopenia with hypocellular bone marrow (<25%) (Fig. 46.2). Historically, chemicals, pesticides, and environmental exposure have been identified as causes of AA, chiefly in Thailand.[4,5] Most cases of acquired AA are idiopathic, characterized by an aberrant immunological process leading to the destruction of HSC mediated by cytotoxic T lymphocytes and cytokines such as interferon-γ (IFN-γ) and tumor necrosis factor (TFN-α) (see Fig. 46.1a).[6–8] More recently, acquired AA has been associated with telomere dysfunction. Indeed, 10% of patients with acquired AA have mutations in *TERT* (the telomerase gene) or *TERC* (the telomerase RNA template gene). All *TERT* and *TERC* mutations cause short telomeres.[9,10] Approximately one-third of patients with acquired AA have short telomeres at the time of initial presentation. Aside from being a treatment response biomarker, short telomere length (TL) may be predictive of a higher relapse rate compared to patients with normal TL, and is a risk factor for clonal evolution.[11] The association of TL and cancer reinforces the concept to use the measurement of TL as a diagnostic screening test.[12,13]

Clinically, at presentation, patients manifest with fatigue, weakness, pallor, and headaches due to anemia. The criteria to discriminate between severe or moderate patients are based on two out of three blood parameters: absolute neutrophil count <500/μL, platelet count <20,000/μL, and reticulocyte count <60,000/μL. Often, patients may also present with petechiae of the skin and mucous membranes, epistaxis, and gum bleeding usually related to severe thrombocytopenia. Similarly, patients may present with fever and infections related to low white blood cell counts. Sometimes, dark-colored urine, referred to

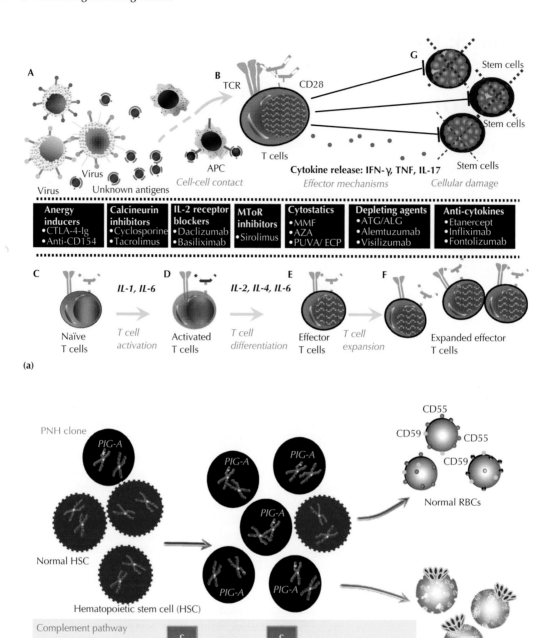

Figure 46.1 Pathogenesis of selected bone marrow failure (BMF) syndromes. Defects in specific genes and immune dysregulation explain the disease pathogenesis in some BMF conditions, including aplastic anemia (AA), paroxysmal nocturnal hemoglobinuria (PNH), and T cell large granular lymphocyte leukemia (T-LGL). (a) Immune pathogenesis in AA. In AA, a cryptic antigenic stimulus (possibly a virus) leads to subsequent T cell activation, differentiation, and expansion of a cytotoxic T cell clone that causes stem cell killing by several effector mechanisms. The various stages of T cell development leading to the final effector phase can serve as targets for immunosuppression. (b) Complement mediated intravascular hemolysis in PNH. In PNH, a somatic mutation in the *phosphatidylinositol glycan-A* gene (*PIG-A*) on the X chromosome leads to absence of GPI-linked proteins on the surface of the cell, including CD55 and CD59 which are necessary to prevent complement-mediated destruction of red blood cells. This subsequently leads to the chronic, ongoing intravascular hemolysis observed in PNH. (c) Immune mediated destruction in T-LGL leukemia. In T-LGL, little is known about its true pathogenesis but two prevailing hypotheses are chronic antigenic stimulation and decreased apoptosis of T-LGL clones. Illustrations by Ramon V. Tiu, MD.

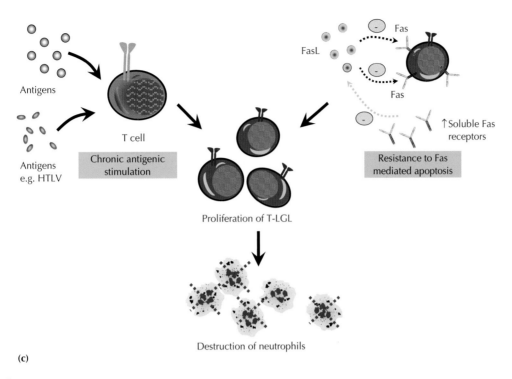

(c)

Figure 46.1 (*Cont'd*)

Table 46.1 Distribution, clinical/genetic features, and management of bone marrow failure syndromes.

Syndrome	Incidence	Clinical features	Genetic defects	Treatments
Inherited				
Fanconi anemia	1:350,000	Skin hyperpigmentation, short stature, skeletal abnormalities, malformation of the eyes and ears, mental retardation, renal insufficiency, hypogenitalia	*FANCA, FANCB, FANCC, FANCD1/BRCA2, FANCD2, FANCE, FANCF, FANCG/XRCC9, FANCI, FANCJ/BACH1/BRIP1, FANCL, FANCM, FANCN/PALB2*	HSCT Androgens G-CSF
Diamond–Blackfan anemia	1:100,000–1:200,000	Thumb anomalies, short stature, cardiac dysfunction, facies anomalies	*RPS19, RPS17, RPS24, RPL5, RPL11, RPL35A*	Corticosteroids Transfusion HSCT
Dyskeratosis congenita	1:1000000	Nail dystrophy, reticular pigmentation, leukoplakia, retardation, eye and dental anomalies, short stature, microcephaly, cardiopulmonary dysfunction	*DKC1, TINF2, TERC, TERT, NOP10/NOLA3, NH2/NOLA2*	SCT Androgens EPO/G-CSF
Acquired				
Aplastic anemia	1:250,000	Fatigue, weakness, headaches, anemia, petechiae of the skin, gum bleeding, hemoglobinuria	10% have defects in *TERT* and *TERC**	ATG/CsA HSCT Androgens Alemtuzumab
Paroxysmal nocturnal hemoglobinuria	1:100,000–1:1000000	Intravascular hemolysis, venous thrombosis (intraabdominal, arterial, and cerebral), bone marrow failure, pulmonary hypertension, and chronic kidney disease, neutropenia and thrombocytopenia	*PIG-A*	Eculizumab Transfusions HSCT
T cell large granular lymphocyte leukemia	1:10,000,000	Neutropenia, anemia, splenomegaly	None*	Methotrexate Cyclophosphamide Alemtuzumab CsA

*Mostly due to immune dysregulation.
ATG, antithymocyte globulin; CsA, cyclosporine; EPO, erythropoietin; G-CSF, granulocyte colony-stimulating factor; HSCT, hematopoietic stem cell transplantation; SCT, stem cell transplantation.

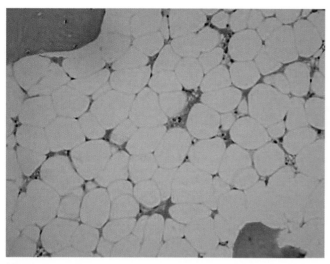

(a)

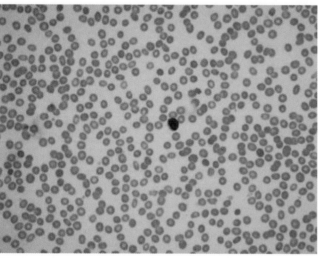

(b)

Figure 46.2 Photomicrograph of bone marrow and peripheral blood smear of a patient with aplastic anemia. (a) Bone marrow core biopsy shows hypocellular bone marrow (less than 5%) with reduced hematopoiesis. Increased fat spaces fill the bone marrow cavities. (b) Peripheral blood smear shows pancytopenia.

as hemoglobinuria, may be seen and may suggest the presence of underlying PNH.

Management

The decision to treat patients with AA is mainly based on disease severity. Definitive treatment with either immunosuppressive therapy or allogeneic hematopoietic stem cell transplantation (HSCT) is necessary for patients with severe AA, while no standard of care exists for moderate AA. Once severity criteria are fulfilled, the type of treatment used is mainly influenced by the patient's age and the availability of a matched sibling donor (MSD). A younger age (typically <30–40 years of age) and the presence of a MSD favor the use of allogeneic HSCT, while older age (>40 years old) and absence of a MSD favor the use of immunosuppressive therapy. Immunosuppression using a combination of antithymocyte

globulin (ATG) and cyclosporine (CsA) represents the standard therapy in AA.[14–16] A long-term study (11-year follow-up) showing overall response rates (ORR) of 60–80%, overall survival (OS) of 58%, relapse rate of ~35% and risk of clonal evolution of 6–15% was reported in AA patients treated with ATG and CsA.[17] Biomarkers predictive of good response to ATG and CsA include younger age (<18 years) and higher absolute reticulocyte count ($\geq 25 \times 10^9$/L), while a higher absolute lymphocyte count ($\geq 1 \times 10^9$/L) correlates with response to ATG.[18]

Two ATG preparations are commonly used in clinical practice: horse (hATG) and rabbit ATG (rATG). Recent data show that hATG is superior to rATG in the frontline treatment of severe AA.[16] The standard protocol uses a dose of 40 mg/kg/day of hATG for 4 days while rATG is given at a dose of 3.5 mg/kg/day for 5 days. CsA is given at 12–15 mg/kg in divided doses twice daily. Corticosteroids are also administered during the first 2 weeks to prevent serum sickness. A second course of ATG can be given to patients who do not respond to the first cycle or who relapse. Approximately 30% of nonresponders and 65% of relapsing patients achieve hematological response to a second ATG course.[18] Attempts to improve clinical and response duration using less toxic drugs in AA have led to the development and testing of novel therapeutics, including a phase 1/2 study of alefacept, a CD2 receptor antagonist for relapsed/refractory AA patients. Alefacept is a human recombinant protein composed of the terminal portion of leukocyte functioning antigen-3 (LFA3/CD58) and the human IgG1 Fc portion. Alefacept inhibits the activation of CD4$^+$ and CD8$^+$ T cells by blocking LFA-3/CD2 interaction and induces apoptosis of CD4$^+$ and CD8$^+$ memory effector T cells.

The definitive therapy for AA is HSCT. Overall survival is around 70% in patients over 16 years of age.[19] HSCT using a MSD is indicated as frontline approach in children and patients up to 20 years. However, ~70% of patients do not have a MSD. Further, clonal evolution often occurs in patients with AA. About 15% of patients with AA evolve to MDS with cytogenetic abnormalities, most commonly trisomy 8 and monosomy 7.[20,21] Based on marrow morphology, the distinction between AA and hypocellular MDS is generally difficult. Thus, some patients classified as MDS have refractory anemia, hypocellular marrow, normal cytogenetics, and a favorable response to immunosuppressive therapy. These patients most likely have moderate AA rather than MDS.[22] See Chapter 43 for a more complete discussion of MDS.

Paroxysmal nocturnal hemoglobinuria

Epidemiology

Paroxysmal nocturnal hemoglobinuria is a rare hematological disorder with a prevalence estimated at 1–1.5 cases per million. The epidemiology is often similar to AA, especially in Thailand. The disease usually affects younger adults and individuals around 60 years of age. Males and females are equally affected. The occurrence of thrombotic events, a cardinal feature of the disease, seems to be higher in European compared to East Asian populations (30–40% versus 5–10%). In the US, the prevalence is around 900–1800 cases.

Etiology/clinical features

Paroxysmal nocturnal hemoglobinuria is a consequence of the nonmalignant expansion of HSC that acquire a somatic mutation in the phosphatidylinositol glycan anchor biosynthesis, class A gene, *PIG-A*.[23,24] The *PIG-A* product is required for the adequate biosynthesis of glycosylphosphatidylinositol (GPI) anchors. Due to this intrinsic genetic defect, GPI-anchored proteins are partially or totally absent on the plasma membrane of PNH cells.

The absence of two proteins, CD59 (MIRL or membrane inhibitor of reactive lysis) and CD55 (DAF or decay accelerating factor), is fundamental in the pathophysiology of PNH. Physiologically, CD55 inhibits C3 convertases and CD59 blocks C9 incorporation in the membrane attack complex. The lack of both proteins on the surface of red blood cells (RBC) leads to complement-induced intravascular hemolysis (see Fig. 46.1b).[25,26] The mechanism by which PNH clones become dominant and expand also remains an open question. Three leading hypotheses explaining this expansion have been proposed. The first is the "two-step model" which proposes that HSCs that harbor *PIG-A* mutations undergo clonal expansion when an immune selection mechanism spares the PNH stem cells but targets the normal HSC.[27,28] A second hypothesis postulates that PNH cells need to acquire a second mutational event to elicit a survival advantage or that PNH cells manifest a reduced tendency to apoptosis, particularly in the setting of a bone marrow injury.[29–31] The third hypothesis proposes that PNH cells have no survival advantage but that expansion may be favorable when PNH cells are few and highly replicating.[32]

Clinically, PNH is classified into three categories:
• classic PNH: evidence of PNH clones above 50% associated with intravascular hemolysis and without any other sign of BMF
• PNH in the setting of another BMF disorder: AA/PNH and MDS/PNH syndromes
• subclinical PNH: small clones without sign of intravascular hemolysis.

Paroxysmal nocturnal hemoglobinuria can coexist with other BMF disorders. About 50% of patients with AA at presentation have PNH clones, which may be stable for years or increase in size with time. The proportion of PNH clones is much lower than in classic hemolytic PNH. PNH clones often appear in AA patients after immunosuppression, leading to the possible association between the presence of a PNH clone and response to ATG.[33] Minor PNH clones (<0.1%) can also occur in about 20% of patients with MDS and BMF at the time of presentation.[34,35]

Clinical features are mainly intravascular hemolysis (intermittent episodes of dark urine in the morning with persistent RBC destruction), venous thrombosis (intraabdominal, arterial, and cerebral veins), marrow failure (frank or reduced marrow function despite a relatively normal cellularity), pulmonary hypertension, and chronic kidney disease. Patients with PNH may present with a history of hemoglobinuria, increased lactate dehydrogenase (LDH) levels, sometimes concomitant neutropenia and thrombocytopenia, and abdominal pain related to the development of Budd–Chiari syndrome.

Key laboratory tests include complete blood and reticulocyte counts, LDH levels, iron studies, and high-sensitivity PNH flow cytometry. Although historically the Ham and sucrose hemolysis tests were used for PNH diagnosis, both have been widely replaced by the more sensitive and reliable PNH flow cytometry. Flow cytometric analysis uses labeled antibodies directed against GPI-anchored proteins (CD55, CD59, CD24, CD16, CD66b). Typically, the diagnosis of PNH is reached by the assessment of at least two different GPI-anchored proteins on granulocytes/monocytes and RBC. Frequently the estimation is based mostly on granulocytes, since transfusions and ongoing hemolysis may underestimate the true PNH clone size if solely assessed in erythrocytes.[36] Recently, fluorescent labeled aerolysin (FLAER) has also been used successfully in routine screening for PNH.[37]

Management

The median OS in patients who do not receive treatment is about 10–20 years. The most common cause of morbidity in patients with PNH is thrombosis, which occurs in about 40–50% of patients and accounts for one-third of deaths.[38] The probability of developing thrombosis correlates with PNH clone size. Patients with <50% clone size have a lower but not negligible risk of developing thrombosis. The risk increases about 1.64 times for each 10% increase in the PNH size clone.[39,40]

Supportive treatments for PNH include RBC transfusions, androgen derivates, and steroids. In 2007, a major breakthrough in PNH treatment came with the development and subsequent FDA approval of eculizumab.[41,42] Eculizumab is a humanized monoclonal antibody directed against C5 that prevents terminal complement activation. Since C5 deficiency is associated with increased risk of *Neisseria* meningitides infection, all patients on eculizumab treatment must be vaccinated before treatment. Eculizumab abrogates the intravascular hemolysis and reduces transfusion requirements and life-threatening thrombotic events in PNH.[43]

Allogeneic HSCT from unrelated and related donors is the only potential curative option for PNH and should be considered in patients with severe marrow failure, refractory/recurrent thrombotic events, and refractory transfusion dependency.[40] The rationale for the success of HSCT in PNH is most likely due to restoration of normal hematopoiesis, previously damaged by an active immune process. Recent discoveries of novel therapeutic fusion proteins, such as TT30 which modulates the complement alternative pathway, might also have a future role in PNH.[44]

T cell large granular lymphocyte leukemia

Epidemiology

T cell large granular lymphocyte leukemia (T-LGL) is a rare lymphoid neoplasm characterized by a chronic elevation (>6 months) of large granular lymphocytes (LGL) in the peripheral blood ($2–20 \times 10^9$/L) not attributable to any other cause.[45] Males and females are equally affected. The median age at diagnosis is 60 years (range 12–87 years).[46] It is estimated that the incidence of T-LGL in the US is 1 in 10,000,000 individuals.[47] It rarely occurs in children.

Etiology/clinical features

The exact pathophysiological mechanism underlying T-LGL is not well understood. However, T-LGL cells share many features of normal cytotoxic effector cells. Several theories have been proposed regarding disease pathogenesis.

• T-LGL is a result of persistent and prolonged immune stimulation. This theory is supported by common association with other autoimmune diseases like rheumatoid arthritis.

• T-LGL occurs because there is a lack of physiological apoptosis, leading to the theory that it is related to activation of prosurvival pathways. T-LGL cells express high levels of FAS (CD95, APO) (see Fig. 46.1c). The interaction of FAS with its ligand FASL can induce death in FAS-expressing cells. Signaling through FAS has previously been shown to induce apoptosis of CD34$^+$ human hematopoietic progenitor cells after exposure to IFN-γ or TNF-α. In contrast, FASL promoted a significantly increased viability of primitive CD34$^+$CD38$^-$ cells.[48]

• Clonal expansions are also seen after HSCT, usually reflecting a restricted T cell repertoire.

Most cases of T-LGL follow a chronic course. The most frequent hematological findings are either isolated neutropenia or neutropenia with concomitant anemia. Splenomegaly is a common physical examination finding seen in 25–50% of cases while the hepatomegaly and lymphadenopathy observed with other lymphoid neoplasms are uncommon.[46] The presence of persistently elevated LGL levels in the peripheral blood accompanied by neutropenia and other commonly observed clinical findings in T-LGL is what prompts the subsequent workup. Bone marrow is usually hypercellular (Fig. 46.3). Flow cytometry is an important diagnostic tool. Most T-LGL show an immunophenotypic profile that is indicative of a constitutively activated T cell phenotype: CD3$^+$, T cell receptor (TCR)-$\alpha\beta^+$, CD45R0$^-$, CD57$^+$, CD4$^-$, CD5^{dim}, CD8$^+$, CD16$^+$, CD27$^-$, CD28$^-$.[49] Some cases express CD4 antigen with or without coexpression of CD8. FAS (CD95) and FASL (CD178) are expressed in the majority of cases.[50] Diagnostic tools utilized to assess clonality in T-LGL include TCR-γ polymerase chain reaction (PCR) and Vβ TCR gene repertoire analysis by flow cytometry.[51] The presence of a TCR-γ gene rearrangement allows for differentiation between clonal T-LGL from LGL generated from a reactive processes. The current Vβ monoclonal antibody panel covers 75% of the Vβ spectrum and in some studies shows a very high correlation with TCR-γ PCR results.

Management

Treatment is indicated in T-LGL if patients are symptomatic from their disease, including the presence of severe cytopenias, recurrent infections, constitutional and symptomatic splenomegaly. Asymptomatic patients are best observed with routine blood counts and clinical follow-up. Although effective therapies are available for patients with symptomatic T-LGL, treatment practices are strongly influenced and driven by retrospective and small prospective case studies. Therapies commonly used include methotrexate (MTX), cyclophosphamide, CsA and more recently alemtuzumab. Low-dose MTX at 10 mg/m^2 per week can produce durable responses with ~50% of cases achieving complete response with single-agent MTX.

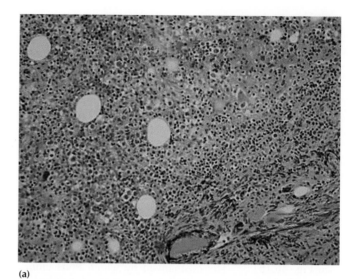

(a)

(b)

Figure 46.3 Photomicrograph of bone marrow and peripheral blood smear of a patient with T cell large granular lymphocyte leukemia. (a) Bone marrow core biopsy shows hypercellularity (90%). Myeloid/erythroid ratio is normal. Panhyperplasia and increases in lymphocytes are present (CD20, CD2, CD3, CD5, CD7, CD8, TIA-I, and granzyme were increased by flow cytometry analysis). (b) Characteristic large granular lymphocytes with abundant cytoplasm and azurophilic granules are noted with TIA-I staining.

However, long-term treatment is necessary to maintain prolonged durable responses.[52] Cyclophosphamide at 50–100 mg daily and CsA at 5–10 mg/kg daily are also effective alternatives.[52] Other supportive agents include alemtuzumab and steroids. The response duration to steroids is typically brief and less frequent compared to patients treated with MTX, CsA, or cyclophosphamide.[53]

Hematopoietic growth factors, like erythropoietin and granulocyte-stimulating factor, have also been used to support anemia and neutropenia in T-LGL. Given the limited data on using allogeneic HSCT for T-LGL, it is not common practice to manage patients using this therapeutic approach.[46] Ongoing studies for the management of T-LGL include tipifarnib (a farnesyltransferase inhibitor) and siplizumab (a humanized anti-CD2 monoclonal antibody).

Inherited bone marrow failure syndromes

Fanconi anemia

Epidemiology

Fanconi anemia (FA) is a genetic disease with an autosomal recessive or X-linked inheritance. The incidence is approximately one per 350,000 births. The age at diagnosis is usually the first decade of life although rare cases presenting during young adulthood (17–21 years of age) have been reported.

Etiology/clinical features

Fanconi anemia is a very heterogeneous disease in terms of its clinical manifestations, since many systems of the body can be affected.[54] Patients may present with congenital malformations, hematological abnormalities, and increased predisposition to acute myeloid leukemia (AML) and solid tumors. The genetic defects causing FA affect a cluster of genes necessary for DNA repair. As an autosomal recessive disorder, one gene from each parent has to be mutated to cause the disease. About 2% of FA cases are X-linked recessive disorders. The FA pathway includes 13 disease-causing genes involved in the surveillance of genomic instability: FANCA, FANCB, FANCC, FANCD1/BRCA2, FANCD2, FANCE, FANCF, FANCG, FANCI, FANCJ/BACH1/BRIP1, FANCL, FANCM, and FANCN/PALB2. Several FA proteins act as signal transducers and scaffolding proteins in the homologous recombination-mediated DNA repair.

Initially, patients with FA may present with unusual macrocytosis. Over 50% of patients later develop pancytopenia, thrombocytopenia, and ultimately BMF. Indeed, FA accounts for 25% of the AA cases, which sometimes makes distinction difficult between the two diseases. About 10% of FA patients develop AML by the age of 25 years and 5% develop MDS, often associated with a poor prognosis. Cytogenetic abnormalities, such as chromosome 3q gains, are associated with poor prognosis. Due to the nature of the disease, a breakdown in genome maintenance is highly associated with cancer predisposition. Squamous cell cancer of head and neck is observed in 5–10% of FA patients. Other evident signs include hyperpigmentation, malformation of the ears and eyes, small stature, hypogonadism, abnormalities of the gastrointestinal and genitourinary tracts, and cardiopulmonary and central nervous systems issues. Genetic screenings are suggested for suspected parents and siblings who may be carriers of FA, independent of the presence of physical signs, in addition to a complete family history, physical examination, complementation group assignment, and mutational analysis. Diagnostic tests are based on chromosomal fragility in blood lymphocytes, especially exposure to alkylating agents, diepoxybutane or mitomycin C. Skin fibroblasts are often required for conclusive diagnosis.

Management

Approximately 50% of patients with FA initially respond to androgens, even though androgen therapy has side-effects, such as liver toxicity, acne, and behavioral anomalies. Growth factors also seem to benefit some patients.[55] Allogeneic HSCT represents the best option for a potential cure of the bone marrow aplasia and the preexisting MDS and AML in FA, especially when patients become refractory to supportive therapies. Low doses of radiation are usually safe preparative regimens for HSCT.

Diamond–Blackfan anemia

Epidemiology

Diamond–Blackfan anemia (DBA) is a congenital hypoplastic anemia condition that can present in the first decades of life.[56] The median age of diagnosis is 12 weeks. It was first described in 1936 by Josephs but more extensively characterized by Diamond and Blackfan in 1938.[57] The pattern of inheritance is generally autosomal dominant.

Etiology/clinical features

Diamond–Blackfan anemia is considered a ribosomopathy, caused by defects in the ribosomal machinery leading to dysfunctional assembly of ribosomal subunits.[58,59] Haploinsufficiency for a given ribosomal protein gives rise to the disease. The genetic basis for DBA is known in 50% of cases and the genes affected include RPS7, RPS10, RPS17, RPS19, RPS24, RPS26, RPL5, RPL11, and RPL35A. The most frequently mutated gene is RPS19, accounting for 25% of DBA cases.[60] Knockdown of RPS19 in zebrafish models using antisense oligonucleotides resulted in a DBA hematological phenotype with concomitant structural malformations.[61,62] Hypoproliferative anemias and growth retardation as observed in DBA were also observed when RPS19 transgenic mice were studied.[63] Recent studies in DBA show that the patency of TP53 is necessary for proapoptosis and subsequently mutations of TP53 can result in a partial or complete rescue.[64] Polymorphisms in RPS15, RPS27, and RPL36 have also been reported but have not been conclusively linked to DBA.[65,66] A majority of the evidence points toward an intrinsic defect in erythropoiesis, with few cases showing decreased numbers of erythroid colony-forming units while in some there is a defect in maturation.[67]

Very young patients presenting with severely reduced erythroid precursors, anemia, and reticulocytopenia, especially when accompanied by a significant family history and skeletal deformities, must raise the suspicion of DBA.[55] Musculoskeletal malformations are common in patients with DBA and include facial deformities (Cathie facies – short nose with a broad nasal bridge, widely spaced eyes, and thick upper lip), triphalangeal thumbs, microcephaly, and congenital cataracts. Genitourinary and cardiac defects are also common. Diagnosis is suspected based on the presence of typical clinical and laboratory features and ultimately confirmed by mutational analysis. In children, a frequent differential diagnosis is transient erythroblastopenia of childhood (TEC), which can be differentiated from DBA based on its transient nature and other clinical and laboratory grounds. Patients with TEC do not have congenital abnormalities and generally have normal mean corpuscular volume, fetal hemoglobin levels, and erythrocyte adenosine deaminase activity.[68]

Management

Supportive therapies in the form of corticosteroids and RBC transfusions are the main therapies for DBA. Corticosteroids can produce responses of 79% while steroid-refractory patients may benefit from RBC transfusions.[55] Prednisone is started at a dose of 2 mg/kg/day. Patients who do not respond within a month after steroid therapy are considered steroid refractory and must receive RBC transfusions.[55] In general, a corticosteroid dose equivalent of 0.5 mg/kg/day is suggested as a maximum maintenance dose.[69] HSCT is a treatment option for DBA patients. A large study involving 61 patients (41 HLA identical sibling donor, eight nonsibling family donor, and 12 unrelated donors) with DBA conducted by the International Bone Marrow Transplant Registry showed 1-year and 3-year actuarial survivals of 67% and 63% respectively. Patients who received a MSD have better 1-year (78% versus 45%) and 3-year survival (76% versus 39%) compared to their unrelated counterparts.[70]

The outcomes with MSD are excellent, in particular for patients <10 years of age. Although outcomes using unrelated donors have improved, given the low incidence of AA, MDS and other hematological malignancy associated with DBA, matched unrelated HSCT are best reserved for steroid-refractory patients under transfusion.

Dyskeratosis congenita

Epidemiology

An association between the constellation of clinical symptoms in dyskeratosis congenita (DKC) was first reported in 1910.[71] The median age at diagnosis is around 15 years old (range 0–75). There is a higher male preponderance for DKC compared to females (3:1).[72]

Etiology/clinical features

The exact etiology of DKC is incompletely understood. However, similar to FA, defects in the telomere maintenance machinery seem to be important. The maturation and stability of TERC are dependent on several components. One of the most important TERC components is the H/ACA box domain which is composed of several subunits including dyskerin1, GAR1, NHP2, and NOP10. Mutations involving genes that code for dyskerin1, NHP2, and NOP10 can produce diseases resembling DKC. Polymorphisms and mutations involving *DKC1* are inherited as X-linked recessive while *NHP2* and *NOP10* are inherited in an autosomal recessive manner. Intracellular TERC levels are reduced in patients who harbor these mutations and consequently have shorter telomeres.

The initial diagnosis of DKC is mainly based on clinical findings. However, unlike other forms of inherited BMF disorders, almost all cases of DKC are diagnosed later on in adult life since the classic clinical triad of oral leukoplakia, nail dystrophy, and lacy reticulated skin changes develops later. Patients suspected of having DKC must subsequently undergo genetic testing for disease confirmation. TL measurement using Southern blots, fluorescence *in situ* hybridization (FISH), and flow cytometry with FISH is helpful in the management of DKC.[73]

Management

Similar to other rare inherited BMF conditions, randomized trials are not available for patients with DKC. The guidelines for treatment of the concomitant BMF are based on the presence of the following counts: platelet counts $<30 \times 10^9$/L, absolute neutrophil count $<1 \times 10^9$/L, and hemoglobin <8 g/dL. Allogeneic HSCT remains the only curative option and should be the foremost therapeutic consideration for patients with BMF and a MSD. In the absence of a suitable MSD, androgens may be used and alternative sources of donors for HSCT must be considered. Oxymetholone can be started at 0.5–1 mg/kg/day and response may take as long as 2–3 months. Close monitoring for androgen-related side-effects like liver transaminitis and liver adenomas must be undertaken.[74] Other agents that have been found to be useful are the combination of granulocyte colony-stimulating factor (G-CSF) and erythropoietin agonists, but their combination with androgens should be avoided as cases of splenic peliosis have been encountered.[75]

Conclusion

Bone marrow failure syndromes are a very heterogeneous group of diseases both clinically and biologically. The complex nature of these diseases coupled with their overlapping features can pose a challenge for diagnosis and identification of appropriate therapies. Improvement in diagnostic tests, molecular screening, alternative treatments, and cooperation between expert physicians has significantly increased our understanding of these diseases, leading to improvement in patient survival in some diseases. The identification of novel molecular targets using new technologies and development of targeted therapies may further improve outcomes.

References

1. Issaragrisil S, *et al*. The epidemiology of aplastic anemia in Thailand. Blood 2006; 107: 1299–307.
2. Young NS, Kaufman DW. The epidemiology of acquired aplastic anemia. Haematologica 2008; 93: 489–92.
3. Young NS. Acquired aplastic anemia. Ann Intern Med 2002; 136: 534–46.
4. Issaragrisil S, *et al*. Low drug attributability of aplastic anemia in Thailand. The Aplastic Anemia Study Group. Blood 1997; 89: 4034–9.
5. Issaragrisil S, Chansung K, Kaufman DW, Sirijirachai J, Thamprasit T, Young NS. Aplastic anemia in rural Thailand: its association with grain farming and agricultural pesticide exposure. Aplastic Anemia Study Group. Am J Public Health 1997; 87: 1551–4.
6. Sloand E, Kim S, Maciejewski JP, Tisdale J, Follmann D, Young NS. Intracellular interferon-gamma in circulating and marrow T cells detected by flow cytometry and the response to immunosuppressive therapy in patients with aplastic anemia. Blood 2002; 100: 1185–91.
7. Risitano AM, Maciejewski JP, Green S, Plasilova M, Zeng W, Young NS. In-vivo dominant immune responses in aplastic anaemia: molecular tracking of putatively pathogenetic T-cell clones by TCR beta-CDR3 sequencing. Lancet 2004; 364: 355–64.
8. De Latour RP, *et al*. Th17 immune responses contribute to the pathophysiology of aplastic anemia. Blood 2010; 116: 4175–84.
9. Yamaguchi H, *et al*. Mutations in TERT, the gene for telomerase reverse transcriptase, in aplastic anemia. N Engl J Med 2005; 352: 1413–24.
10. Calado RT, Young NS. Telomere maintenance and human bone marrow failure. Blood 2008; 111: 4446–55.

11. Scheinberg P, Cooper JN, Sloand EM, Wu CO, Calado RT, Young NS. Association of telomere length of peripheral blood leukocytes with hematopoietic relapse, malignant transformation, and survival in severe aplastic anemia. JAMA 2010; 304: 1358–64.

12. Savage SA, Bertuch AA. The genetics and clinical manifestations of telomere biology disorders. Genet Med 12: 753–64.

13. Hampton T. Studies probe role of telomere length in predicting, modulating cancer risk. JAMA 305: 2278–9.

14. Maciejewski JP, Risitano AM. Aplastic anemia: management of adult patients. Hematol Am Soc Hematol Educ Program 2005: 110–17.

15. Afable MG 2nd, et al. Efficacy of rabbit anti-thymocyte globulin in severe aplastic anemia. Haematologica 2011; 96: 1269–75.

16. Scheinberg P, Nunez O, Weinstein B, Biancotto A, Wu CO, Young NS. Horse versus rabbit antithymocyte globulin in acquired aplastic anemia. N Engl J Med 2011; 365: 430–8.

17. Frickhofen N, Heimpel H, Kaltwasser JP, Schrezenmeier H. Antithymocyte globulin with or without cyclosporin A: 11-year follow-up of a randomized trial comparing treatments of aplastic anemia. Blood 2003; 101: 1236–42.

18. Scheinberg P, Wu CO, Nunez O, Young NS. Predicting response to immunosuppressive therapy and survival in severe aplastic anaemia. Br J Haematol 2009; 144: 206–16.

19. Locasciulli A, et al. Outcome of patients with acquired aplastic anemia given first line bone marrow transplantation or immunosuppressive treatment in the last decade: a report from the European Group for Blood and Marrow Transplantation (EBMT). Haematologica 2007; 92: 11–18.

20. Maciejewski JP, Selleri C. Evolution of clonal cytogenetic abnormalities in aplastic anemia. Leuk Lymphoma 2004; 45: 433–40.

21. Maciejewski JP, Risitano A, Sloand EM, Nunez O, Young NS. Distinct clinical outcomes for cytogenetic abnormalities evolving from aplastic anemia. Blood 2002; 99: 3129–35.

22. Afable MG 2nd, et al. SNP array-based karyotyping: differences and similarities between aplastic anemia and hypocellular myelodysplastic syndromes. Blood 2011; 117: 6876–84.

23. Takeda J, et al. Deficiency of the GPI anchor caused by a somatic mutation of the PIG-A gene in paroxysmal nocturnal hemoglobinuria. Cell 1993; 73: 703–11.

24. Bessler M, et al. Paroxysmal nocturnal haemoglobinuria (PNH) is caused by somatic mutations in the PIG-A gene. EMBO J 1994; 13: 110–17.

25. Lewis SM, Dacie JV. The aplastic anaemia–paroxysmal nocturnal haemoglobinuria syndrome. Br J Haematol 1967; 13: 236–51.

26. Parker C, et al. Diagnosis and management of paroxysmal nocturnal hemoglobinuria. Blood 2005; 106: 3699–709.

27. Rotoli B, Luzzatto L. Paroxysmal nocturnal haemoglobinuria. Baillière's Clin Haematol 1989; 2: 113–38.

28. Gargiulo L, et al. Highly homologous T-cell receptor beta sequences support a common target for autoreactive T cells in most patients with paroxysmal nocturnal hemoglobinuria. Blood 2007; 109: 5036–42.

29. Inoue N, et al. Molecular basis of clonal expansion of hematopoiesis in 2 patients with paroxysmal nocturnal hemoglobinuria (PNH). Blood 2006; 108: 4232–6.

30. Brodsky RA, Vala MS, Barber JP, Medof ME, Jones RJ. Resistance to apoptosis caused by PIG-A gene mutations in paroxysmal nocturnal hemoglobinuria. Proc Natl Acad Sci USA 1997; 94: 8756–60.

31. Hanaoka N, Kawaguchi T, Horikawa K, Nagakura S, Mitsuya H, Nakakuma H. Immunoselection by natural killer cells of PIGA mutant cells missing stress-inducible ULBP. Blood 2006; 107: 1184–91.

32. Dingli D, Luzzatto L, Pacheco JM. Neutral evolution in paroxysmal nocturnal hemoglobinuria. Proc Natl Acad Sci USA 2008; 105: 18496–500.

33. Sugimori C, et al. Minor population of CD55-CD59- blood cells predicts response to immunosuppressive therapy and prognosis in patients with aplastic anemia. Blood 2006; 107: 1308–14.

34. Iwanaga M, et al. Paroxysmal nocturnal haemoglobinuria clones in patients with myelodysplastic syndromes. Br J Haematol 1998; 102: 465–74.

35. Maciejewski JP, Rivera C, Kook H, Dunn D, Young NS. Relationship between bone marrow failure syndromes and the presence of glycophosphatidyl inositol-anchored protein-deficient clones. Br J Haematol 2001; 115: 1015–22.

36. Hochsmann B, Rojewski M, Schrezenmeier H. Paroxysmal nocturnal hemoglobinuria (PNH): higher sensitivity and validity in diagnosis and serial monitoring by flow cytometric analysis of reticulocytes. Ann Hematol 90: 887–99.

37. Brodsky RA, et al. Improved detection and characterization of paroxysmal nocturnal hemoglobinuria using fluorescent aerolysin. Am J Clin Pathol 2000; 114: 459–66.

38. Hillmen P, Lewis SM, Bessler M, Luzzatto L, Dacie JV. Natural history of paroxysmal nocturnal hemoglobinuria. N Engl J Med 1995; 333: 1253–8.

39. Hall C, Richards S, Hillmen P. Primary prophylaxis with warfarin prevents thrombosis in paroxysmal nocturnal hemoglobinuria (PNH). Blood 2003; 102: 3587–91.

40. Young NS, Meyers G, Schrezenmeier H, Hillmen P, Hill A. The management of paroxysmal nocturnal hemoglobinuria: recent advances in diagnosis and treatment and new hope for patients. Semin Hematol 2009; 46: S1–S16.

41. Hillmen P, et al. The complement inhibitor eculizumab in paroxysmal nocturnal hemoglobinuria. N Engl J Med 2006; 355: 1233–43.

42. Hillmen P. The role of complement inhibition in PNH. Hematol Am Soc Hematol Educ Program 2008: 116–23.

43. Hillmen P, et al. Effect of the complement inhibitor eculizumab on thromboembolism in patients with paroxysmal nocturnal hemoglobinuria. Blood 2007; 110: 4123–8.

44. Fridkis-Hareli M, et al. Design and development of TT30, a novel C3d-targeted C3/C5 convertase inhibitor for treatment of the human complement alternative pathway-mediated diseases. Blood 2011; 118(17): 4705–13.

45. Swerdlow SH, et al. (eds). WHO Classification of Tumours of Haematopoietic and Lymphoid Tissues: T-Cell Large Granular Lymphocytic Leukaemia. Lyon: IARC Press, 2008.

46. Lamy T, Loughran TP Jr. How I treat LGL leukemia. Blood 2011; 117: 2764–74.

47. Yamamoto JF, Goodman MT. Patterns of leukemia incidence in the United States by subtype and demographic characteristics, 1997–2002. Cancer Causes Control 2008; 19: 379–90.

48. Josefsen D, Myklebust JH, Lynch DH, Stokke T, Blomhoff HK, Smeland EB. Fas ligand promotes cell survival of immature human bone marrow CD34+CD38- hematopoietic progenitor cells by suppressing apoptosis. Exp Hematol 1999; 27: 1451–9.

49. Lundell R, Hartung L, Hill S, Perkins SL, Bahler DW. T-cell large granular lymphocyte leukemias have multiple phenotypic abnormalities involving pan-T-cell antigens and receptors for MHC molecules. Am J Clin Pathol 2005; 124: 937–46.

50. Lamy T, Liu JH, Landowski TH, Dalton WS, Loughran TP Jr. Dysregulation of CD95/CD95 ligand-apoptotic pathway in CD3(+) large granular lymphocyte leukemia. Blood 1998; 92: 4771–7.

51. Lima M, et al. Immunophenotypic analysis of the TCR-Vbeta repertoire in 98 persistent expansions of CD3(+)/TCR–alphabeta(+) large granular lymphocytes: utility in assessing clonality and insights into the pathogenesis of the disease. Am J Pathol 2001; 159: 1861–8.

52. Epling-Burnette PK, et al. Inhibition of STAT3 signaling leads to apoptosis of leukemic large granular lymphocytes and decreased Mcl-1 expression. J Clin Invest 2001; 107: 351–62.

53. Loughran TP Jr. Clonal diseases of large granular lymphocytes. Blood 1993; 82: 1–14.

54. Bagby GC, Alter BP. Fanconi anemia. Semin Hematol 2006; 43: 147–56.

55. Shimamura A, Alter BP. Pathophysiology and management of inherited bone marrow failure syndromes. Blood Rev 2010; 24: 101–22.

56. Ito E, Konno Y, Toki T, Terui K. Molecular pathogenesis in Diamond–Blackfan anemia. Int J Hematol 2010; 92: 413–18.

57. Josephs HW. Anaemia of infancy, early childhood. Medicine 1936; 15: 307.

58. Flygare J, et al. Human RPS19, the gene mutated in Diamond–Blackfan anemia, encodes a ribosomal protein required for the maturation of 40S ribosomal subunits. Blood 2007; 109: 980–6.

59. Doherty L, *et al*. Ribosomal protein genes RPS10 and RPS26 are commonly mutated in Diamond–Blackfan anemia. Am J Hum Genet 2010; 86: 222–8.

60. Ellis SR, Gleizes PE. Diamond Blackfan anemia: ribosomal proteins going rogue. Semin Hematol 2011; 48: 89–96.

61. Danilova N, Sakamoto KM, Lin S. Ribosomal protein S19 deficiency in zebrafish leads to developmental abnormalities and defective erythropoiesis through activation of p53 protein family. Blood 2008; 112: 5228–37.

62. Uechi T, Nakajima Y, Chakraborty A, Torihara H, Higa S, Kenmochi N. Deficiency of ribosomal protein S19 during early embryogenesis leads to reduction of erythrocytes in a zebrafish model of Diamond–Blackfan anemia. Hum Mol Genet 2008; 17: 3204–11.

63. Jaako P, *et al*. Mice with ribosomal protein S19 deficiency develop bone marrow failure and symptoms like patients with Diamond–Blackfan anemia. Blood 2011; 118(23): 6087–96.

64. Dutt S, *et al*. Haploinsufficiency for ribosomal protein genes causes selective activation of p53 in human erythroid progenitor cells. Blood 2011; 117: 2567–76.

65. Gazda HT, *et al*. Ribosomal protein L5 and L11 mutations are associated with cleft palate and abnormal thumbs in Diamond–Blackfan anemia patients. Am J Hum Genet 2008; 83: 769–80.

66. Cmejla R, *et al*. Identification of mutations in the ribosomal protein L5 (RPL5) and ribosomal protein L11 (RPL11) genes in Czech patients with Diamond–Blackfan anemia. Hum Mutat 2009; 30: 321–7.

67. Da Costa L, Moniz H, Simansour M, Tchernia G, Mohandas N, Leblanc T. Diamond–Blackfan anemia, ribosome and erythropoiesis. Transfus Clin Biol 2010; 17: 112–19.

68. Lipton JM, Kudisch M, Gross R, Nathan DG. Defective erythroid progenitor differentiation system in congenital hypoplastic (Diamond–Blackfan) anemia. Blood 1986; 67: 962–8.

69. Tsakiri KD, *et al*. Adult-onset pulmonary fibrosis caused by mutations in telomerase. Proc Natl Acad Sci USA 2007; 104: 7552–7.

70. Narla A, Vlachos A, Nathan DG. Diamond Blackfan anemia treatment: past, present, and future. Semin Hematol 2011; 48: 117–23.

71. Walne AJ, Dokal I. Dyskeratosis congenita: a historical perspective. Mech Ageing Dev 2008; 129: 48–59.

72. Dokal I. Dyskeratosis congenita in all its forms. Br J Haematol 2000; 110: 768–79.

73. Lin KW, Yan J. The telomere length dynamic and methods of its assessment. J Cell Mol Med 2005; 9: 977–89.

74. Velazquez I, Alter BP. Androgens and liver tumors: Fanconi's anemia and non-Fanconi's conditions. Am J Hematol 2004; 77: 257–67.

75. Giri N, Pitel PA, Green D, Alter BP. Splenic peliosis and rupture in patients with dyskeratosis congenita on androgens and granulocyte colony-stimulating factor. Br J Haematol 2007; 138: 815–17.

Section 8: Hematological Malignancies

47 Myeloproliferative Neoplasms: Chronic Myelogenous Leukemia, Polycythemia Vera, Essential Thrombocythemia, and Primary Myelofibrosis

Raoul Tibes,[1] Gurcharan Singh Khera,[2] and Ruben A. Mesa[1]

[1] Division of Hematology and Medical Oncology, Mayo Clinic, Scottsdale, AZ, USA
[2] Maricopa Integrated Health Trust, Phoenix, AZ, USA

Introduction and classification of myeloproliferative neoplasm

The myeloproliferative neoplasms (MPNs) are a group of clonal hematological (stem cell) disorders with terminal myeloid cell expansion in the peripheral blood. Originally described by William Dameshek in 1951,[1] based on clinical and bone marrow similarities, in 2001 MPNs were classified by the World Health Organization (WHO) Classification which was updated in 2008.[2] Myeloproliferative neoplasms are classified into five major entities summarized in Box 47.1 (acute myeloid and lymphoid leukemias are separate entities) (see Chapter 43). MPNs can be divided into "classic" MPNs, which are chronic myeloid leukemia (CML), polycythemia vera (PV), essential thrombocythemia (ET), and primary myelofibrosis (PMF), and "atypical" MPNs, consisting of chronic neutrophilic leukemia (CNL), chronic eosinophilic leukemia not otherwise specified (CEL-NOS), mastocytosis (MS), and MPN unclassifiable.[2,3] The four "classic" MPNs will be discussed in this chapter, along with the "atypical" MPNs, given their rarity.

The discovery of the Philadelphia (Ph) chromosome and the (9:22) chromosomal translocation, that uniquely distinguish CML, was a benchmark for the molecular understanding of cancer in general.[4] It was the first description of a chromosomal translocation, that resulted in the BCR-ABL 1 fusion gene and protein that constitutively activates the ABL1 kinase with subsequent cellular myeloid cell proliferation.[4] The BCR-ABL1 translocation defines CML and it is almost obligatory to confirm the diagnosis. CML also brought a profound understanding of how receptor and intracellular tyrosine kinases (ABL1 is a nonreceptor [=intracellular] tyrosine kinase)

stimulate growth and lead to downstream signal transduction pathway activation.[4] The discovery of mutant alleles (mutations) in various other myeloid (proliferative) diseases, such as chronic myelomonocytic leukemia (CMML), CEL and systemic mastocytosis (SM) leading to constitutive activation of tyrosine kinase signaling,[5] indicates that tyrosine kinase activation is a common pathogenetic mechanism in MPN and other hematopoietic neoplasms. Importantly, positivity for JAK2V617F and other genes/kinases (see the section on "Mutations and pathogenesis in polycythemia vera, essential thrombocythemia, and primary myelofibrosis") can confirm the clonality of a disease process (versus reactive), and the presence of disease-defining mutations, like JAK2V617F, has now been incorporated into the WHO 2008 diagnostic criteria for MPNs (see Box 47.1). Finally, these mutated kinases and genes can serve as validated targets for the design of molecularly directed therapies, and possibly as prognostic and predictive markers in the future.

Chronic myeloid leukemia: prevalence and molecular background

Chronic myeloid leukemia (CML) accounts for approximately 15% of adult leukemias or ~5000 cases per year in the United States.[6] The age-adjusted annual incidence is approximately 1.5 per 100,000 persons, with a male predominance of 1.5:1.[1] The median age at presentation is around 67 years.

Chronic myeloid leukemia arises from translocation of the *ABL* gene (able murine leukemia) on chromosome 9 and the *BCR* gene (breakpoint cluster region) on chromosome 22, producing a reciprocal balanced translocation termed the

Textbook of Uncommon Cancer, Fourth Edition. Edited by Derek Raghavan, Charles D. Blanke, David H. Johnson, Paul L. Moots, Gregory H. Reaman, Peter G. Rose and Mikkael A. Sekeres.
© 2012 John Wiley & Sons, Inc. Published 2012 by John Wiley & Sons, Inc.

Philadelphia (Ph) chromosome.[7,8] The cell of origin of CML is a pluripotent hematopoietic stem cell. The resulting *BCR-ABL* fusion gene (oncoprotein) codes for a constitutively active tyrosine kinase that drives proliferation and impedes differentiation and apoptosis, leading to malignant transformation of myeloid cells.[9] The BCR-ABL fusion gene/protein appears to be the initial event in the pathogenesis of CML, as opposed to JAK2V617F in MPNs, which may be a later acquired event.

Presentation and diagnosis of chronic myeloid leukemia

The natural history of untreated CML is typically biphasic or triphasic: an initial indolent chronic phase (CP) followed by an accelerated phase (AP) and blast phase (BP). The course of CML is variable, and untreated CML commonly advances in 3–7 years (median time of 4 years) without treatment.[6]

Many patients (~20–50%) are asymptomatic, with CML being discovered via routine laboratory assessment for other reasons. Symptomatic patients commonly present with fatigue/

malaise, weight loss, early satiety, excessive sweating, and abdominal pain from splenomegaly. Lymph node, skin, and soft tissue involvement is uncommonly seen. The diagnosis of CML is first suspected on a peripheral blood smear demonstrating leukocytosis with a left shift encompassing the complete spectrum of myeloid differentiation (i.e. myelocytes, metamyelocytes, neutrophils). Absolute basophilia is a hallmark feature of CML, and platelets are often elevated (thus CML is a rule out and differential diagnosis for MPNs and ET); a normochromic, normocytic anemia is seen in half of the patients. Confirmation of CML is established by demonstrating the Philadelphia chromosome by conventional cytogenetics, fluorescence *in situ* hybridization (FISH) or molecular tests for the BCR-ABL fusion gene/mRNA by polymerase chain reaction (RT-PCR).[10] It should be noted that FISH or PCR is not a substitute for conventional karyotyping, because additional clonal events or rare translocations cannot be detected, and a marrow aspirate and biopsy are essential at diagnosis to distinguish chronic phase from more advanced subtypes.[11]

Treatment evolution in chronic myeloid leukemia

In the pre-tyrosine kinase inhibitor (TKI) era, hydroxyurea, busulphan or interferon (IFN) was used therapeutically. Single-agent IFN-α2a produced complete cytogenetic remissions in up to 25–30% of patients[12] while the combination of IFN-α2 with cytarabine was the gold standard for chemotherapy approaches. Allogeneic hematopoietic stem cell transplant (allo-HSCT) was indicated for young patients with CML.[13,14]

Linking the molecular pathogenesis of the BCR-ABL translocation with kinase activation and inhibition of its kinase activity by imatinib mesylate (formerly STI571) was a hallmark of molecular targeted cancer therapy.[15] This discovery and rapid clinical translation have dramatically changed CML from a fatal disease to a chronic one that can be controlled in most cases, with remarkable improvement in long-term progression-free survival (PFS) and overall survival (OS).[16]

The first large multicenter trial of imatinib, the International Randomized Study of Interferon and ST1571 (IRIS), randomized 1106 patients with newly diagnosed Ph+CML-CP to either imatinib 400 mg/d or gradually escalating doses of IFN-α plus subcutaneous low-dose cytarabine. All study endpoints, including hematological and cytogenetic responses, were significantly improved with imatinib compared to IFN+cytarabine; at 18 months, major cytogenetic responses (MCyR) were 87.1% versus 34.7% ($p<0.001$); complete cytogenetic responses (CCyR) were 76.2% and 14.5% ($p<0.001$) and major molecular responses (MMR; defined as ≥3-log reduction in *BCR-ABL1* transcript level, at 12 months) were 57% versus 24% ($p=0.003$), respectively.[16,17] Subsequent analyses demonstrated that deeper molecular (and cytogenetic) responses achieved faster are associated with better long-term outcome.[18] Thus, CCyR and MMR have become endpoints in trials for second-generation BCR-ABL TKIs.[19,20] In follow-up analyses, patients who had MMR at 12 or 18 months exhibited significantly superior event-free survival (EFS) rates at 84 months of 91% versus 79.4%, $p=0.001$ (MMR at 12 months) or 94.9% versus 75.3%, $p<0.001$ (MMR at 18 months).

Progression to AP/BP at 84 months was also reduced if a MMR was achieved at 12 (99% versus 89.9%, $p=0.0004$) and 18 months (99.1% versus 90.1%, $p<0.001$), compared to patients without MMR. The value of achieving a MMR early during therapy (12–18 months) was associated with an improved outcome at 60 months, with estimated rates of progression to AP/BC of 0%, 2%, and 13% for patients achieving CCyR and MMR, CCyR without MMR, and no CCyR, respectively. Improved outcome with greater depth of MMR was confirmed in other trials.[18,21] From these data, guidelines for optimal, suboptimal, and failure of response have been developed.[11] Clinicians can now routinely monitor BCR-ABL transcript load by PCR from blood (or marrow) to determine the depth and quality of response, allowing for early therapy changes in the setting of suboptimal responses.

With improved molecular understanding of CML, second-generation TKIs were developed that either are more specific for BCR-ABL (i.e. nilotinib) and/or target additional kinases downstream or parallel to imatinib (i.e. dasitinib).[22] Both nilotinib (ENESTnd Trial)[20] and dasatinib (DASISION Trial)[19] have completed large randomized trials in which they were compared to therapy with imatinib in first-line CML-CP. Both agents were superior to imatinib in achieving either MMR or CCyR. In the ENESTnd Trial, the rate of MMR for patients with CML-CP at 12 months was 71% for nilotinib 300 mg twice daily and 67% for nilotinib 400 mg twice daily versus 44% for imatinib ($p<0.0001$ for both comparisons). Complete molecular responses (CMRs) were significantly better as well: 26% and 21% with nilotinib at 300 and 400 mg versus 10% with imatinib.[20] Survival was comparable in all treatment groups, but fewer CML-related deaths occurred in both nilotinib groups compared to what occurred in the imatinib group.[20] The 18-month follow-up data for the DASISION Trial were similarly consistent, with superiority of dasatinib versus imatinib in terms of MMR rate ($p=0.0002$)[19,23]; CMR was reported in 13% of dasatinib-treated and 7% of imatinib-treated patients at 18 months of follow-up.[23] As a result of these studies, many consider nilotinib and dasatinib to be the preferred upfront treatment choices for CML-CP.

Other BCR-ABL TKIs in clinical trials include bosutinib, a dual Src/Abl TKI, and ponatinib, with activity against the T315I mutation (see below).[24]

Progression of disease and role of allogeneic hematopoietic stem cell transplant in chronic myeloid leukemia

Progression of disease can be defined by advancing to the accelerated or blastic phase of CML or molecularly defined by losing a CCyR or MMR. Blast crisis results in a myelogenous leukemic phenotype in ~75% and a lymphoblastic leukemic phenotype in ~25% of cases.[25] TKIs have reduced the progression to AP/BP significantly when compared to the historical IFN-α/cytarabine combination, while second-generation TKIs reduce progression to AP and BP compared to imatinib. Molecular relapse or progression is defined as a 10-fold increase of PCR positivity without signs of cytogenetic relapse.[11] In addition, mutations in BCR-ABL tyrosine kinase

were detected in ~50% of patients who become resistant to imatinib or other TKIs.[26] A third-generation TKI, ponatinib, appears to be promising against the most resistant T315I mutation.[24] Thus, mutation testing at progression and tailoring TKI therapy has become an essential workup, and switching to a nonresistant TKI may be effective.[27] Allo-HSCT at progression should be considered, especially for younger patients, particularly as it is the only curative treatment modality.[28]

Tyrosine kinase inhibitors should be considered lifelong therapy in a responding patient. In one small study (Stop Imatinib – STIM) with short follow-up, 59% of patients who discontinued imatinib only after multiple CMR assessments experienced a molecular relapse at 12 months. Of relapsed patients, 62% achieved another CMR with reinstitution of TKI therapy.[29]

Mutations and pathogenesis in polycythemia vera, essential thrombocythemia, and primary myelofibrosis

Activation of the JAK-STAT signaling pathway has been recognized as a hallmark of Ph(-) MPNs.[30–34] This cytokine-activated pathway drives proliferation and differentiation of hematopoietic progenitor cells to mature leukocytes, erythrocytes, thrombocytes, and monocytes.[35,36] The detailed pathophysiology underlying these events was unclear until the discovery of mutations in JAK2.[30,32,33,37] The JAK2V617F mutation results in constitutive activation of downstream signaling pathways, including the STATs (signal transducer and activator of transcription) which are the main transcription factors regulating a host of genes involved in driving proliferation and preventing apoptotic (cell death) processes.[32]

The incidence of JAK2V617F mutations is close to 100% (>95–97%) in PV, approximately 50–60% in ET, and 50–60% in PMF.[30,32,33,37] In contrast, the frequency is lower at ~3–13% in chronic myelomonocytic leukemia (CMML), 3–5% in myelodysplastic syndromes (MDS), and less than 5% in acute myeloid leukemia (AML), mostly arising from MPNs.[38,39] Unexplained to date is how a single gene mutation (JAK2) is involved in different phenotypic presentations of PV, ET, and PMF.[40] Despite the significant contribution to the development and maintenance of a myeloproliferative state, whether JAK2V617F is indeed the major underlying transforming event is still controversial,[41] as other genetic events may occur earlier in the disease.

Other frequent genetic alterations in MPNs affect the JAK-STAT pathway directly, i.e. mutations in JAK2 exon 12 or the thrombopoietin receptor MPL; in adaptor proteins (LNK) or genes downregulating activated signaling (C-CBL); or in genes involved in epigenetic control of transcription (TET2, ASXL1/2, IDH1/2) or in transcription factors themselves (IKZF1).[41,42] TET2 mutations, which can be found early in the disease course, may occur prior to acquisition of JAK2V617F mutations.[43] JAK2 exon 12 mutations are important, as these are found in a majority of JAK2V617F-negative PV patients (~50–80%).[44] Thus, almost all PV patients harbor some form of JAK2 mutational event[45,46] and testing for exon 12 mutations is recommended for JAK2V617F-negative PV.

Mutations in the MPL gene are absent in PV and occur in ~1% of ET and 5–10% of PMF patients,[47,48] often in JAK2V617F-negative MPNs.[49] The various mutations alone and in combination influence clinical disease manifestations, and bear different risk for disease complications and progression, a field currently under active investigation.[50,51]

Clinical presentation, diagnosis and treatment of polycythemia vera, essential thrombocythemia, and primary myelofibrosis

The incidence rates for PV, ET, and PMF are 1.9, 2.5, and 1.5[52] per 100,000 per year, respectively.[52–54] Men have a higher incidence rate of PV, whereas in ET the incidence rate is higher in women (~1.5–2:1-fold).[54,55] Although all diseases can occur at any age, the median age upon presentation is around 60, 60, and 67 years for PV, ET, and PMF, respectively.[52–54] Approximately 20% of PV and ET and 5% of PMF patients are below age 40 years.[52,54,55] The natural history of PV shows a variable course: median survival of untreated symptomatic patients according to historic data was estimated at 6–18 months from diagnosis. In treated patients, recent publications report median survival approaching or exceeding 20 years for PV and ET and 10 years for PMF patients.[56–58] Many studies report close to normal life expectancies in treated patients with ET and PV,[59,60] resulting in a high prevalence rate of 22 and 24 patients per 100,000, with an estimated total number of 65,243 and 71,078 patients living with PV and ET respectively, in the United States in 2003.[61] Familial clustering of all three disease entities is documented and family members were afflicted in 8.7%, 6.0%, and 8.2% of PV, ET, and PMF cases, respectively.[62,63]

From a practical management aspect and clinical presentation, patients fall into two groups. The first group includes patients with ET or PV who, early in their disease course, are predisposed to developing thromboembolic events. Microvascular symptoms such as headache, light-headedness, acral paresthesias, erythromelalgia, atypical chest pain, and, in PV, pruritus are common.[64,65] A small number of PV and ET patients, over decades, transform to either a myelofibrosis (MF) stage/phase (post-ET/PV MF) or a blast phase resembling acute myeloid leukemia (MPN-BP).[66]

The second group of MPN patients, mainly those with PMF, have a life-threatening illness, presenting with more severe constitutional symptoms and faster progression. Patients with overt primary myelofibrosis (PMF) or with secondary post-ET/PV-associated MF are often clinically indistinguishable.[67] Patients suffer from significant disease-associated symptoms such as fatigue, night sweats, bone pain, fevers and chills, splenomegaly, and anemia of multifactorial origin[66,68] as well as slow, progressive marrow fibrosis with a predisposition to transform into AML.

The diagnostic criteria for MPNs have evolved and are summarized in Table 47.1. From a practical perspective, a JAK2V617F mutation analysis should first be undertaken if an MPN is suspected. If a patient does not have the mutation, JAK2 exon 12 mutations should be evaluated in PV, and a MPL mutation tested for in ET and PMF patients. Lower than normal erythropoietin levels are found in ~85% of PV patients.

The diagnosis of ET and PMF requires the exclusion of PV and of BCR-ABL-positive CML.

Risk stratification and prognosis of myeloproliferative neoplasms

The most important risk factors for both PV and ET are age older than 60 years and a previous history of thrombosis. Either criterion places PV and ET patients in the high-risk category and constitutes an indication for treatment. In PV the low-risk category is age <60 years and absence of thrombosis and cardiovascular risk factors; presence of one or more cardiovascular risk factors constitutes intermediate risk. In ET, the low-risk category is age <40 years without history of thrombosis or hemorrhage; intermediate risk in ET is age 40–60 years and/or presence of cardiovascular risk factors. Leukocytosis (white blood count (WBC) >15000 × 10^9/L) and extreme thrombocytosis (platelets >1000–1500 × 10^9/L) have been suggested as possible adverse risk factors in PV[69] and ET.[70]

Risk in PMF is assessed according to the Dynamic International Prognostic Scoring System (DIPSS). Points are assigned based on age >65 years, hemoglobin <10 g/dL, leukocyte count >25 × 10^9/L, circulating blasts >1%, and presence of constitutional symptoms. The overall score predicts progression and survival and can direct choice of therapy.[67] The DIPPS was recently expanded (DIPPS-Plus; Table 47.2) to include the previous criteria and platelets <100 × 10^9/L, red cell transfusions, and unfavorable karyotype. DIPPS-plus can be used at baseline and over time to assess risk of progression. Survival ranges from ~16 months in high-risk to ~185 months in low-risk PMF patients depending on DIPPS score.[71,72]

Despite the JAK2 mutation being a well-accepted diagnostic criterion for MPNs, the prognostic relevance for survival of patients is not fully established. As a general tendency, JAK2V617F mutated MPNs have a more advanced and more progressive clinical presentation (erythrocytosis, leukocytosis, and thrombocytosis)[46,73,74] and can be associated with an increased risk of thrombosis.[45,46,75] Some studies also found an association with leukemic transformation in PMF patients.[44,76,77] The data with respect to survival and JAK2V617F mutational status remain controversial.

Treatment of polycythemia vera and essential thrombocythemia

The primary goal of treatment is the prevention of primary and recurrent thromboembolic and thrombohemorrhagic complications (Table 47.3). Cardiovascular risk factors should be managed aggressively in all patients (low and high risk)[78]; low-dose aspirin (40 or 75 to 100 mg daily, i.e. 81 mg in US) is recommended for all PV and ET patients and can alleviate vasomotor/microvascular symptoms as well as reducing the risk of thromboembolic events.[79] Aspirin showed superiority over placebo in a large randomized study in PV patients with a significant reduction in cardiovascular death, thrombosis, strokes, and in overall mortality by 46%.[80] Caution should be exercised in patients with previous hemorrhagic complication and platelet counts >1000– 1500 × 10^9/L (ET and PV), as very

Table 47.1 WHO 2008 diagnostic criteria for polycythemia vera (PV), essential thrombocythemia (ET), and primary myelofibrosis (PMF).

	PV	ET	PMF
Major criteria	1. Hemoglobin >18.5 g/dL in men, 16.5 g/dL in women or other evidence of increased red cell volume* 2. Presence of *JAK2V617F* or other functionally similar mutation (i.e. JAK2 exon 12 mutation)	1. Sustained platelet count >450 × 10⁹/L 2. Marrow biopsy proliferation mainly of megakaryocytic lineage with increased numbers of enlarged, mature megakaryocytes; no significant increase or left shift of granulopoiesis or erythropoiesis 3. Not meeting WHO criteria for PV,[†] PMF,[‡] CML,[§] MDS,[¶] or other myeloid neoplasm 4. Demonstration of JAK2617V617F or other clonal marker, or in the absence of a clonal marker, no evidence for reactive thrombocytosis^	1. Presence of megakaryocyte proliferation and atypia,** accompanied by reticulin and/or collagen fibrosis, or, in the absence of significant reticulin fibrosis, megakaryocyte changes accompanied by increased bone marrow cellularity with granulocytic proliferation, often decreased erythropoiesis (i.e. prefibrotic cellular-phase disease) 2. Not meeting WHO criteria for PV,[††] CML,[‡‡] MDS,[§§] or other myeloid neoplasm 3. Demonstration of JAK2617V617F or other clonal marker (e.g. MPL515W > L/K), or in absence of clonal marker, no evidence of bone marrow fibrosis due to inflammatory or other neoplastic diseases[¶¶]
Minor criteria	1. Bone marrow biopsy with hypercellularity for age with trilineage myeloproliferation (panmyelosis) 2. Serum erythropoietin level below the reference range for normal 3. Endogenous erythroid colony formation *in vitro*		1. Leukoerythroblastosis 2. Increase in serum lactate dehydrogenase (LDH) 3. Anemia 4. Palpable splenomegaly
Diagnostic comment	Diagnosis requires the presence of both major criteria and 1 minor criterion or the presence of the first major criterion together with 2 minor criteria	Diagnosis requires meeting all 3 major criteria and 2 minor criteria	Diagnosis requires meeting all 3 major criteria and 2 minor criteria

* Hemoglobin or hematocrit greater than 99th percentile of method-specific reference range for age, sex, altitude of residence or hemoglobin greater than 17 g/dL in men, 15 g/dL in women if associated with a documented and sustained increase of at least 2 g/dL from an individual's baseline value that cannot be attributed to correction of iron deficiency, or elevated red cell mass greater than 25% above mean normal predicted value.

[†] Failure of iron replacement to increase hemoglobin to PV range if decreased serum ferritin. Exclusion of PV based on hemoglobin and hematocrit, red cell mass not required.

[‡] Requires absence of reticulin or collagen fibrosis, peripheral blood leukoerythroblastosis, or hypercellular marrow for age with megakaryocyte morphology typical for PMF.

[§] Requires the absence of BCR-ABL.

[¶] Requires absence of dyserythropoiesis and dysgranulopoiesis.

^ Causes of reactive thrombocytosis (i.e. iron deficiency, splenectomy, surgery, infection, inflammation, connective tissue disease, metastatic cancer, and lymphoproliferative disorders) to be excluded.

** Small to large megakaryocytes with aberrant nuclear:cytoplasmic ratio and hyperchromatic, bulbous, or irregularly folded nuclei and dense clustering.

[††] Requires failure of iron replacement therapy to increase hemoglobin level to PV range in if decreased serum ferritin. Exclusion of PV based on hemoglobin and hematocrit levels. Red cell mass measurement is not required.

[‡‡] Requires the absence of BCR-ABL.

[§§] Requires the absence of dyserythropoiesis and dysgranulopoiesis.

[¶¶] Secondary to infection, autoimmune disorder, chronic inflammatory condition, hairy cell leukemia, lymphoid neoplasm, metastatic malignancy, toxic (chronic) myelopathies.

CML, chronic myeloid leukemia; MDS, myelodysplastic syndromes.

Reproduced with permission from Tefferi and Vardiman.[3]

high platelets paradoxically increase the risk of bleeding, due to acquired von Willebrand factor diseases/deficiency; ristocetin cofactor activity can help assess bleeding risk.[79] For low-risk PV patients, in addition to aspirin, phlebotomy to keep the hematocrit (HCT) in the range of 0.40–0.55 (40–55%) is recommended.[81]

For high-risk patients with PV and ET and those requiring cytoreduction, hydroxycarbamide (hydroxyurea, HU) is the preferred initial treatment, although PEG-IFN-α2a shows promising activity. Cytotoxics/alkylating agents (i.e. busulfan, chlorambucil, pipobroman) are generally not recommended for upfront therapy. Overall, HU is superior to anagrelide in first-line therapy for ET if platelet lowering is indicated, as demonstrated in a large randomized trial[82] in which HU had less risk of arterial thrombosis, major hemorrhage, and fibrotic transformation (see Table 47.3).

Second-line management

Patients with PV intolerant or resistant to hydroxyurea can be managed with PEG-INF-α2a, which is often chosen for

Table 47.2 DIPPS-Plus.

Criteria	Score	Outcome (median survival)
Hemoglobin <10 g/dL	Low risk: 0 adverse points	~185 months
Circulating blasts ≥1%	Intermediate-1 risk: 1 adverse points	~78 months
White blood cells >25 K		
Constitutional symptoms	Intermediate-2 risk: 2 or 3 adverse points	~35 months
Age >65 years	High risk: 4 or more adverse points	~16 months
Transfusion need		
Platelets <100 K		
Unfavorable karyotype (monosomal or complex karyotype, +8, −7/del(7q), del(5q), inv(3), isochromosome 17q/17p−, 12p,11q23)		

Reproduced from Gangat et al.[71]

younger patients (i.e. <60–65 years), or with cytotoxic agents like busulfan or pipobroman, often given to older patients (>65 years).[83,84] For ET patients intolerant to or failing HU, anagrelide or PEG-IFN-α2a are effective second-line choices for younger patients (<60–65 years); in older patients either anagrelide or cytoreduction with busulfan, pipobroman or radioactive phosphorus may be effective in lowering platelets.

Data on PEG- IFN-α2a are encouraging, with 95% of PV patients achieving lasting complete hematological remission (CHR).[81] A second study demonstrated similar results, with complete hematological remissions of 70% and 76% in advanced PV and ET patients, respectively. Molecular responses were seen in 38% and 54% of patients, with complete molecular response observed in 6% and 14% of ET and PV patients, respectively. Constitutional symptoms resolved in 57%, hemoglobin and WBC normalized in 47% and 59%, and a number of patients became transfusion independent.[85] Platelet normalization was achieved in 52% of patients.[86] A first-line trial comparing PEG- IFN-α2a with HU is ongoing and will clarify which of these agents is superior for upfront treatment.

Treatment of primary myelofibrosis and post-polycythemia vera/essential thrombocythemia myelofibrosis

In PMF and post-PV/ET MF, alleviation of anemia, splenomegaly, and constitutional symptoms as well as delay in progression to MPN-BC are primary treatment goals. There is no curative treatment for MPNs except for allo-HSCT.

Low-risk PMF patients (DIPPS or DIPPS-plus) are often followed by observation. Therapy for intermediate-1 risk patients may include observation or the conventional treatment options outlined under PV and ET (i.e. HU). Therapy for high- or intermediate-2 risk PMF patients depends on clinical symptoms: for anemia, androgens (i.e. danazol) or steroids

(prednisone) may be given. The immunomodulatory drugs lenalidomide and thalidomide, widely used in multiple myeloma and myelodysplastic syndromes, can improve anemia in roughly 20–30% of patients, with best responses achieved in combination with steroids.[87–89] Platelet responses were observed and splenomegaly improved in 10% and 42% of patients, respectively, in two independent studies.[87–89] For symptomatic splenomegaly, HU may improve symptoms and reduce spleen size. Splenectomy can be effective or rarely splenic radiation can be used for symptom control as a palliative option.

To date, there is no conclusive evidence and no larger comparative studies to show that HU increases the risk of leukemic transformation in ET and PV patients,[90,91] except in patients treated with alkylating agents (i.e. busulfan, pipobroman, chlorambucil or radioactive phosphorus) prior to receiving HU.[90] This topic is an ongoing controversy and we refer the reader to detailed reviews and the primary literature. Anagrelide does not seem to increase leukemic transformation, but may accelerate marrow fibrosis.[83,92]

Leukemic transformation of myeloproliferative neoplasms

After many years, a small fraction of PV and ET[90,93] patients (less than 1–4%)[91] and somewhat more patients with PMF (~5–10% at 10 years)[90,93] progress to more aggressive stages of MPN, including a blastic phase (MPN-BP) that resembles AML, defined by >20% blasts in the marrow or blood. Clinically, patients present with decreased intramedullary hematopoiesis manifested by worsening cytopenias and constitutional symptoms. The molecular events leading to leukemic transformation have not been well defined. Several mutations occur at higher frequency in MPN-BP (i.e. IDH and EZH2).[94] The JAK2V617F mutation can be lost at leukemic transformation, suggesting that it is not obligatory for disease progression.[95] Response to induction therapy and outcome are dismal, with a median overall survival of ~2–3 months in one study,[93] though several studies report encouraging outcomes with allo-HSCT at disease acceleration and transformation. Using reduced-intensity conditioning regimens, overall survival rates range from 43% to >90%, depending on study and length of follow-up.[96] Best results for allo-HSCT are achieved if patients are transplanted before frank leukemic transformation.

Data for other therapies are limited. A recent study of low-intensity treatment with azacitidine[97] in 54 patients with advanced PMF and post-PV/ET MF showed an overall response rate of 52%; 24% of patients achieved a CR, with a median response duration of 9 months. In MPN-BP, the response was 38%.[97] In early-stage PV and ET, azacitidine is not as active.[98]

The discovery of JAK2 mutations paved the way for clinical development of JAK2 inhibitors,[94,99] with more than 10 JAK2 inhibitors being investigated in clinical trials.[56,94] Most are not specific for the mutant JAK2V617F and inhibit wild-type JAK2, as well as other kinases, possibly explaining the varying response rates and side-effect profiles.[100] An emerging body of clinical data published in abstract and manuscript form supports the activity of JAK2 inhibitors in advanced and early-stage MPNs. Patients experience improvement in constitutional disease-associated symptoms in greater than 90%,

Table 47.3 Treatment options for MPNs. Listed are selected drugs with clinical trial data available in MPNs. Examples of representative studies are provided in the table, *not* a complete assembly of data. Experimental agents are not listed or discussed.

Drug and target	Disease	Efficacy	Toxicity	Reference
Hydroxyurea	PV ET PMF/MF	Very effective in lowering counts in most patients (>50%); trial endpoints often assessed reduction in risk (RR) of thrombosis and PV/ET typical symptoms; large trials showed benefit, i.e. in ET HU versus no treatment reduced vascular events from 10.7% to 1.6%. In PMF/MF mainly for symptomatic control of counts and splenomegaly	Skin and mucosal ulcers; cytopenias (incl. macrocytic anemia)	82, 130
Anagrelide	ET	Platelet reduction by 50% or <6 × 10⁹/L in 93% patients	Cardiovascular/vasodilatory effects, headache, skin	131
Pegylated IFN-α2a	PV, ET	PV: CHR 70%, MR 54%, CMR 14% ET: CHR 76%, MR 38%, CMR 6% PV: CHR 95%, any MR 90%, CMR 18%	Musculoskeletal pain, skin toxicity, asthenia, gastrointestinal symptoms	85, 132
Aspirin	PV, ET	PV: RR 0.4 versus placebo; total and cardiovascular mortality reduced by 46% and 59% ET:	Increased bleeding risk; especially in ET platelets >1–1.5 × 10⁹/L	80
Androgens (i.e. danazol)	MF	Anemia ~20–44%		133, 134
JAK2 Inhibitors immunomodulatory drugs in PMF/MF				
Ruxolitinib	MF/PMF	HB: 14% (became transfusion independent) PLAT: 58% (normalized thrombocytosis) SPLN: 44% (reduction size) Improvement in constitutional symptoms	Diarrhea, fatigue, myelosuppression	101
Thalidomide (THAL)	MF/PMF	HB: 29% PLAT: 38% SPLN: 41%	Neurotoxicity, myelosupression, thrombovascular events	135
THAL-PRED (prednisone)	MF/PMF	HB: 62% PLAT: 75% SPLN: 19%	Constipation, leukocytosis, neuropathy, sedation, hyperglycemia, visual changes, anxiety	87
Lenalidomide (LEN)	MF/PMF	HB: 22% PLAT: 50% SPLN: 33%	Neutropenia, thrombocytopenia	136
LEN-PRED	MF/PMF	HB: 19% PLAT: n/a SPLN: 10% HB: 30% PLAT: n/a SPLN: 42%	Neutropenia, thrombocytopenia, anemia	88 89

CHR, complete hematological response; CMR, complete molecular response; HB, hemoglobin; MR, molecular response; PLT, platelet; SPLN, spleen;

with pruritus improving or resolving in 50–90% of patients. Spleen responses are seen in around 40–60% of patients, leukocytosis is reduced or normalized in 50–60%, and thrombocytosis improves in greater than 90%, especially in early-stage MPNs. The only JAK2 inhibitor approved by the US Food and Drug Administration is ruxolitinib. In a randomized phase 1/2 trial of 153 patients with PMF and post-PV/ET MF treated with ruxolitinib, 71–78% of patients responded.[101] In the first of two large randomized phase 3 trials in a similar patient population, in which patients treated with ruxolitinib were compared to those treated with placebo, 42% versus 0.7% ($p < 0.0001$) achieved a ≥35% reduction in spleen volume; in a validated symptom burden score (SS), 46% versus 5.3% ($p < 0.0001$) of patients also reported improvement.[102] In the second phase 3 trial, spleen response was 28.5% versus

0% with ruxolitinib versus best available therapy ($p < 0.0001$).[103] Adverse events included thrombocytopenia (44.5% versus 9.6%), anemia (40.4% versus 12.3%), diarrhea (24.0% versus 11.0%), and peripheral edema (21.9% versus 26.0%). hile these clinical responses are compelling, no data exist to suggest that these inhibitors lead to either molecular remissions or improvement of marrow histological features, or alter the natural history of these disorders.

Several other JAK2 inhibitors are in preclinical or clinical development. For example, the investigational JAK2 targeting agent CYT387[104] led to anemia responses in ~50% of patients, while 57–69% of patients became transfusion independent depending on drug dose.[105] LY2784544,[106] AZD-1480, R723,[107] NS-018,[108] and BMS-911543[106] are other investigational agents with early clinical trial data, though responses to most JAK2 inhibitors have been independent of underlying disease, i.e. PMF, post-PV or post-ET MF, or JAK2V617F mutation status, an observation not understood to date.

Other experimental therapies, such as mTor or HDAC inhibitors, have been investigated in small studies and show activity reducing constitutional symptoms and splenomegaly, and improving cytopenias.[109–111]

In summary, research into and molecular understanding of PV, ET, and PMF have rapidly increased over the last years. The discovery of the JAK2V617F mutation led to accelerated development of JAK2 inhibitors, which have shown clinical benefit in patients with MPNs. Early-stage PV and ET can be indolent for decades. The overall role of JAK2 inhibitors needs to be assessed in the context of durable benefit and modification of the natural history of MPNs.

Chronic neutrophilic leukemia

Chronic neutrophilic leukemia (CNL) is a myeloproliferative neoplasm characterized by mature neutrophilic differentiation. The diagnostic criteria established by the WHO[3] are a peripheral blood WBC >25,000/μL, segmented neutrophils and bands >80%, immature granulocytes <10 and myeloblasts <1% of the WBC, no evidence of dysplasia and monocytes <1000/μL. Bone marrow diagnostic criteria are hypercellularity, increased neutrophilic granulocytes, myeloblasts <5% and no evidence of dysplastic changes. CNL is a diagnosis of exclusion especially for other MPNs, negativity for the Philadelphia chromosome and/or BCR-ABL fusion gene(s) as well as secondary causes of neutrophilia. A distinct entity to be differentiated from CNL is atypical, Ph chromosome-negative CML (aCML)[112] and neutrophilic CML (n-CML), the latter with a mostly benign course.[113]

Chronic neutrophilic leukemia appears to arise in granulocyte-committed progenitors that are capable of spontaneous proliferation.[114] There is an equal sex distribution, median age is 66 years, with a wide range of age groups reported (range 54–86 years).[115] Presenting symptoms included weight loss, fatigue, and pruritus and symptoms associated with hyperproliferation of WBC, but not fever. The peripheral blood smear in CNL shows mature neutrophils, few immature cells, and no blasts. Neither basophilia nor eosinophilia is present. The neutrophils often contain toxic granules and/or Döhle bodies, while erythrocytes and platelets are morphologically normal. The leukocyte alkaline phosphatase (LAP) score is increased in CNL, in contrast to the low score in CML. Elevated levels of uric acid and serum vitamin B_{12} may be noted. Karyotype is commonly normal in CNL, but recurrent myeloid-specific translocations can be found at diagnosis or progression.[116,117] In contrast to leukemoid reactions, CNL is associated with low granulocyte colony-stimulating factor (G-CSF) level and the presence of reticulin fibrosis or cytogenetic abnormalities can distinguish CNL from reactive leukocytosis.

The disease course of CNL is highly variable from 1 to >20 years and up to 20% of cases progress to a blast phase resembling AML and rarely to myelodysplasias. Although no treatment has been effective in altering the natural history of CNL, hydroxyurea is the usual first-line treatment and is effective in controlling neutrophilia, organ infiltration, and associated symptoms. However, reduction of high neutrophil counts may not be indicated because neutrophils in CNL are not invasive and unlikely to cause leukostasis. Second-line treatments including cytarabine, cladribine, 6-thioguanine, and interferon result in short-lived responses. There is no role for splenectomy. Isolated cases of JAK2V617F-positive CNL have been reported.[118]

Chronic eosinophilic leukemia

Chronic eosinophilic leukemia not otherwise specified (CEL-NOS) is a clonal autonomous proliferation of eosinophil precursors. This diagnosis of CEL requires demonstration of clonality (i.e. cytogenetic aberration) and exclusion of reactive/secondary eosinophilia per WHO criteria. Dysplasia can be found in CEL. Peripheral blood blasts (>2%) or increased blasts in the bone marrow (>5 to <19% blasts) in addition or alternatively to clonal markers may indicate the leukemic phenotype of CEL. Whereas idiopathic hypereosinophilic syndrome (HES) is a diagnosis of exclusion: in HES eosinophils are elevated to $\geq 1.5 \times 10^9$/L for >6 months and end-organ damage is often present, but clonal and leukemia markers are not found.[119] Interestingly, the presence of very high levels of serum vitamin B_{12} (>2000 pg/mL) and tryptase is suggestive of the presence of the fusion gene. Ninety percent are symptomatic with clinical manifestations reflecting the effects of eosinophilic infiltration and of cytokines and humoral factors released from eosinophilic granules on diverse organs, including the heart (Loeffler endomyocarditis, endomyocardial fibrosis, restrictive cardiomyopathy, mural thrombosis), lungs (pulmonary infiltrates, emboli, fibrosis, effusions), liver, spleen, skin (urticaria, angioedema, papules/nodules), gastrointestinal tract, and nervous system (thromboemboli, peripheral neuropathy, eosinophilic meningitis).[120] Causes of death include organ failure and transformation into more aggressive malignancies.

A subset of CEL (and encountered in HES as well) is caused by an interstitial deletion in chromosome 4q12 leading to the formation of fusion gene Fip1-like1-platelet-derived growth factor (FIP1L1-PDGFRA), which results in constitutive activation of the tyrosine kinase activity of the platelet-derived growth factor receptor α.[121] This fusion gene can be routinely tested for by FISH to detect a deletion of the CHIC2 locus at 4q12 as a surrogate for the FIP1L1-PDGFRA fusion. FIP1L1-PDGFRA fusion gene-positive CEL and HES patients dramatically respond to low doses of imatinib (100 mg daily), although patients without the rearrangement can respond as well. Imatinib is currently the first-line treatment for patients with and without FIP1L1-PDGFRA disease, with or without increased serum tryptase levels. For patients whose disease is resistant to imatinib, sorafenib or experimental tyrokinase kinase inhibitors (i.e. PKC412, also with activity against D816V KIT mutation) have shown activity. Other agents used include hydroxyurea, IFN-α, cladribine, and cyclosporine. Allogeneic transplantation should be considered for patients with aggressive disease.

Systemic mastocytosis

Systemic mastocytosis (SM) is characterized by mast cell infiltrates in extracutaneous organs, most commonly the bone marrow. It has equal sex incidence. To establish a diagnosis, the major criteria (multifocal dense infiltrates of 15 or more mast cells in bone marrow and/or other extracutaneous organ sections) plus one minor criterion (25% of mast cells in tissue sections or bone marrow aspirate smear, c-kit point mutation at codon 816, expression of CD2 and/or CD25 by mast cells, baseline serum tryptase persistently >20 ng/mL or three minor criteria are required. SM can be categorized into different types based on organ involvement and clinical behavior. The most common type is indolent systemic mastocytosis (ISM), which progresses slowly and has good prognosis but can transform to more severe forms in up to 5% of cases, especially those with elevated β2-microglobulin and positive c-kit mutations.[122] Smoldering systemic mastocytosis (SSM) is associated with B symptoms, >30% marrow infiltration, hepatosplenomegaly and high tryptase levels >200 ng/mL. Isolated bone marrow mastocytosis (BMM) is confined to marrow infiltration without skin involvement. Systemic mastocytosis with an associated hematological nonmast cell lineage disorder (SM-AHNMD) (i.e. myeloproliferative, myelodysplastic, or lymphoproliferative disorder) is a distinct entity. Aggressive systemic mastocytosis (ASM) is uncommon and is associated with evidence of tissue and organ dysfunction from mast cell infiltration. The clinical course is highly variable and survival ranges from 12 months to several years. Mast cell leukemia (MCL) is very rare and is characterized by presence of >10% immature mast cells in the peripheral blood or >20% immature mast cells.

The receptor for stem cell factor (SCF) on mast cells is called the receptor tyrosine kinase c-kit (CD 117 or c-kit receptor). Mutations of the c-kit receptor allow constitutive activation of SCF, leading to clonal proliferation of mast cells in tissues.[123,124] More than 90% of c-kit mutations involve the codon 816 comprising substitution of valine for aspartate (Asp816Val). This mutation is significant for resistance to imatinib.[125] Mutations in TET2, a tumor suppressor gene, is the second most common identified mutation.[126]

Commonly used therapies include IFN-α2b (for rapid response), cladribine, glucocorticoids, and hydroxyurea. Imatinib is indicated for patients with wild-type c-kit mutation (negative for D816V KIT mutation) or whose mutational status is unknown. Patients with D816V KIT mutation can be treated with cladribine, prednisone or IFN-α. Upon progression, patients can be enrolled in clinical trials investigating tyrosine kinase inhibitors such as PKC412 (midostaurin).[127] Results with other tyrosine kinase inhibitors like dasatinib have not been as good.[128] Splenectomy may be considered for hypersplenism-related refractory cytopenias. Allogeneic hematopoietic cell transplantation has not demonstrated significant survival benefit, although remissions have been reported.[129] Treatment of mast cell leukemia with cladribine, chemotherapy, and marrow transplantation yields short-lived and low response rates, death usually occurring within 1–2 years. Mast cell sarcomas and extracutaneous mastocytomas may progress to mast cell leukemia. Selection of treatment options including local (surgery, radiation) and systemic (chemotherapy or TKI therapy) is based on the location of the sarcoma and presence or absence of D816V KIT mutation.

References

1. Dameshek W. Some speculations on the myeloproliferative syndromes. Blood 1951; 6(4): 372–5.
2. Tefferi A, Vardiman JW. Classification and diagnosis of myeloproliferative neoplasms: the 2008 World Health Organization criteria and point-of-care diagnostic algorithms. Leukemia 2008; 22(1): 14–22.
3. Vardiman JW, Thiele J, Arber DA, et al. The 2008 revision of the World Health Organization (WHO) classification of myeloid neoplasms and acute leukemia: rationale and important changes. Blood 2009; 114(5): 937–51.
4. Tibes R, Trent J, Kurzrock R. Tyrosine kinase inhibitors and the dawn of molecular cancer therapeutics. Annu Rev Pharmacol Toxicol 2005; 45: 357–84.
5. Levine RL, Pardanani A, Tefferi A, Gilliland DG. Role of JAK2 in the pathogenesis and therapy of myeloproliferative disorders. Nat Rev Cancer 2007; 7(9): 673–83.
6. Randolph TR. Chronic myelocytic leukemia – Part I: History, clinical presentation, and molecular biology. Clin Lab Sci 2005; 18(1): 38–48.
7. Nowell PC, Hungerford DA. Chromosome studies on normal and leukemic human leukocytes. J Natl Cancer Inst 1960; 25: 85–109.
8. Rowley JD. Letter: a new consistent chromosomal abnormality in chronic myelogenous leukaemia identified by quinacrine fluorescence and Giemsa staining. Nature 1973; 243(5405): 290–3.
9. Daley GQ, van Etten RA, Baltimore D. Induction of chronic myelogenous leukemia in mice by the P210bcr/abl gene of the Philadelphia chromosome. Science 1990; 247(4944): 824–30.
10. Haferlach T, Bacher U, Kern W, Schnittger S, Haferlach C. The diagnosis of BCR/ABL-negative chronic myeloproliferative diseases (CMPD): a comprehensive approach based on morphology, cytogenetics, and molecular markers. Ann Hematol 2008; 87(1): 1–10.
11. Baccarani M, Cortes J, Pane F, et al. Chronic myeloid leukemia: an update of concepts and management recommendations of European Leukemia Net. J Clin Oncol 2009; 27(35): 6041–51.
12. Talpaz M, Kantarjian HM, McCredie KB, Keating MJ, Trujillo J, Gutterman J. Clinical investigation of human alpha interferon in chronic myelogenous leukemia. Blood 1987; 69(5): 1280–8.
13. Thomas ED, Clift RA, Fefer A, et al. Marrow transplantation for the treatment of chronic myelogenous leukemia. Ann Intern Med 1986; 104(2): 155–63.
14. Radich JP, Gooley T, Bensinger W, et al. HLA-matched related hematopoietic cell transplantation for chronic-phase CML using a targeted busulfan and cyclophosphamide preparative regimen. Blood 2003; 102(1): 31–5.
15. Druker BJ. Translation of the Philadelphia chromosome into therapy for CML. Blood 2008; 112(13): 4808–17.
16. Druker BJ, Guilhot F, O'Brien SG, et al. Five-year follow-up of patients receiving imatinib for chronic myeloid leukemia. N Engl J Med 2006; 355(23): 2408–17.
17. Druker BJ, Talpaz M, Resta DJ, et al. Efficacy and safety of a specific inhibitor of the BCR-ABL tyrosine kinase in chronic myeloid leukemia. N Engl J Med 2001; 344(14): 1031–7.
18. Hughes TP, Hochhaus A, Branford S, et al. Long-term prognostic significance of early molecular response to imatinib in newly diagnosed chronic myeloid leukemia: an analysis from the International Randomized Study of Interferon and STI571 (IRIS). Blood 2010; 116(19): 3758–65.
19. Kantarjian H, Shah NP, Hochhaus A, et al. Dasatinib versus imatinib in newly diagnosed chronic-phase chronic myeloid leukemia. N Engl J Med 2010; 362(24): 2260–70.
20. Saglio G, Kim DW, Issaragrisil S, et al. Nilotinib versus imatinib for newly diagnosed chronic myeloid leukemia. N Engl J Med 2010; 362(24): 2251–9.
21. Hochhaus A, Druker B, Sawyers C, et al. Favorable long-term follow-up results over 6 years for response, survival, and safety with imatinib mesylate therapy in chronic-phase chronic myeloid leukemia after failure of interferon-alpha treatment. Blood 2008; 111(3): 1039–43.
22. Kantarjian HM, Baccarani M, Jabbour E, Saglio G, Cortes JE. Second-generation tyrosine kinase inhibitors: the future of frontline CML therapy. Clin Cancer Res 2011; 17(7): 1674–83.

23. Shah N, Kantarjian H, Hochhaus A, *et al*. Dasatinib versus imatinib in patients with newly diagnosed chronic myeloid leukemia in chronic phase (CML-CP) in the DASISION trial: 18-month follow-up. Blood (ASH Annual Meeting Abstracts) 2010; 116(21): 206.

24. O'Hare T, Shakespeare WC, Zhu X, *et al*. AP24534, a pan-BCR-ABL inhibitor for chronic myeloid leukemia, potently inhibits the T315I mutant and overcomes mutation-based resistance. Cancer Cell 2009; 16(5): 401–12.

25. Druker BJ, Sawyers CL, Kantarjian H, *et al*. Activity of a specific inhibitor of the BCR-ABL tyrosine kinase in the blast crisis of chronic myeloid leukemia and acute lymphoblastic leukemia with the Philadelphia chromosome. N Engl J Med 2001; 344(14): 1038–42.

26. Bixby D, Talpaz M. Mechanisms of resistance to tyrosine kinase inhibitors in chronic myeloid leukemia and recent therapeutic strategies to overcome resistance. Hematology Am Soc Hematol Educ Program 2009: 461–76.

27. Cortes J, Hochhaus A, Hughes T, Kantarjian H. Front-line and salvage therapies with tyrosine kinase inhibitors and other treatments in chronic myeloid leukemia. J Clin Oncol 2011; 29(5): 524–31.

28. Radich J. Stem cell transplant for chronic myeloid leukemia in the imatinib era. Semin Hematol 2010; 47(4): 354–61.

29. Mahon FX, Rea D, Guilhot J, *et al*. Discontinuation of imatinib in patients with chronic myeloid leukaemia who have maintained complete molecular remission for at least 2 years: the prospective, multicentre Stop Imatinib (STIM) trial. Lancet Oncol 2010; 11(11): 1029–35.

30. Baxter EJ, Scott LM, Campbell PJ, *et al*. Acquired mutation of the tyrosine kinase JAK2 in human myeloproliferative disorders. Lancet 2005; 365(9464): 1054–61.

31. James C, Ugo V, Le Couedic JP, *et al*. A unique clonal JAK2 mutation leading to constitutive signalling causes polycythaemia vera. Nature 2005; 434(7037): 1144–8.

32. Levine RL, Wadleigh M, Cools J, *et al*. Activating mutation in the tyrosine kinase JAK2 in polycythemia vera, essential thrombocythemia, and myeloid metaplasia with myelofibrosis. Cancer Cell 2005; 7(4): 387–97.

33. Zhao R, Xing S, Li Z, *et al*. Identification of an acquired JAK2 mutation in polycythemia vera. J Biol Chem 2005; 280(24): 22788–92.

34. Kralovics R, Passamonti F, Buser AS, *et al*. A gain-of-function mutation of JAK2 in myeloproliferative disorders. N Engl J Med 2005; 352(17): 1779–90.

35. Wolanskyj AP, Lasho TL, Schwager SM, *et al*. JAK2 mutation in essential thrombocythaemia: clinical associations and long-term prognostic relevance. Br J Haematol 2005; 131(2): 208–13.

36. Trelinski J, Wierzbowska A, Krawczynska A, *et al*. Circulating endothelial cells in essential thrombocythemia and polycythemia vera: correlation with JAK2-V617F mutational status, angiogenic factors and coagulation activation markers. Int J Hematol 2010; 91(5): 792–8.

37. Ugo V, James C, Vainchenker W. [A unique clonal JAK2 mutation leading to constitutive signalling causes polycythaemia vera]. Med Sci (Paris) 2005; 21(6–7): 669–70.

38. Steensma DP, Dewald GW, Lasho TL, *et al*. The JAK2 V617F activating tyrosine kinase mutation is an infrequent event in both "atypical" myeloproliferative disorders and myelodysplastic syndromes. Blood 2005; 106(4): 1207–9.

39. Jelinek J, Oki Y, Gharibyan V, *et al*. JAK2 mutation 1849G>T is rare in acute leukemias but can be found in CMML, Philadelphia chromosome-negative CML, and megakaryocytic leukemia. Blood 2005; 106(10): 3370–3.

40. Larsen TS, Pallisgaard N, Moller MB, Hasselbalch HC. The JAK2 V617F allele burden in essential thrombocythemia, polycythemia vera and primary myelofibrosis – impact on disease phenotype. Eur J Haematol 2007; 79(6): 508–15.

41. Van Etten RA, Koschmieder S, Delhommeau F, *et al*. The Ph-positive and Ph-negative myeloproliferative neoplasms: some topical pre-clinical and clinical issues. Haematologica 2011; 96(4): 590–601.

42. Tefferi A. Novel mutations and their functional and clinical relevance in myeloproliferative neoplasms: JAK2, MPL, TET2, ASXL1, CBL, IDH and IKZF1. Leukemia 2010; 24(6): 1128–38.

43. Delhommeau F, Dupont S, Della Valle V, *et al*. Mutation in TET2 in myeloid cancers. N Engl J Med 2009; 360(22): 2289–301.

44. Pardanani A, Lasho TL, Finke C, Hanson CA, Tefferi A. Prevalence and clinicopathologic correlates of JAK2 exon 12 mutations in JAK2V617F-negative polycythemia vera. Leukemia 2007; 21(9): 1960–3.

45. Figueroa ME, Abdel-Wahab O, Lu C, *et al*. Leukemic IDH1 and IDH2 mutations result in a hypermethylation phenotype, disrupt TET2 function, and impair hematopoietic differentiation. Cancer Cell 2010; 18(6): 553–67.

46. Vannucchi AM, Antonioli E, Guglielmelli P, *et al*. Prospective identification of high-risk polycythemia vera patients based on JAK2(V617F) allele burden. Leukemia 2007; 21(9): 1952–9.

47. Pardanani AD, Levine RL, Lasho T, *et al*. MPL515 mutations in myeloproliferative and other myeloid disorders: a study of 1182 patients. Blood 2006; 108(10): 3472–6.

48. Pikman Y, Lee BH, Mercher T, *et al*. MPLW515L is a novel somatic activating mutation in myelofibrosis with myeloid metaplasia. PLoS Med 2006; 3(7): e270.

49. Lasho TL, Pardanani A, McClure RF, *et al*. Concurrent MPL515 and JAK2V617F mutations in myelofibrosis: chronology of clonal emergence and changes in mutant allele burden over time. Br J Haematol 2006; 135(5): 683–7.

50. Vannucchi AM, Antonioli E, Guglielmelli P, *et al*. Characteristics and clinical correlates of MPL 515W>L/K mutation in essential thrombocythemia. Blood 2008; 112(3): 844–7.

51. Vannucchi AM, Pieri L, Bogani C, *et al*. Constitutively activated and hyper-sensitive basophils in patients with polycythemia vera: role of JAK2V617F mutation and correlation with pruritus. ASH Annual Meeting Abstracts, November 16, 2008; 112(11): 3714.

52. Mesa RA, Silverstein MN, Jacobsen SJ, Wollan PC, Tefferi A. Population-based incidence and survival figures in essential thrombocythemia and agnogenic myeloid metaplasia: an Olmsted County Study, 1976–1995. Am J Hematol 1999; 61(1): 10–15.

53. Berk PD, Goldberg JD, Donovan PB, Fruchtman SM, Berlin NI, Wasserman LR. Therapeutic recommendations in polycythemia vera based on Polycythemia Vera Study Group protocols. Semin Hematol 1986; 23(2): 132–43.

54. Fenaux P, Simon M, Caulier MT, Lai JL, Goudemand J, Bauters F. Clinical course of essential thrombocythemia in 147 cases. Cancer 1990; 66(3): 549–56.

55. Cortelazzo S, Viero P, Finazzi G, d'Emilio A, Rodeghiero F, Barbui T. Incidence and risk factors for thrombotic complications in a historical cohort of 100 patients with essential thrombocythemia. J Clin Oncol 1990; 8(3): 556–62.

56. Barbui T, Barosi G, Birgegard G, *et al*. Philadelphia-negative classical myeloproliferative neoplasms: critical concepts and management recommendations from European LeukemiaNet. J Clin Oncol 2011; 29(6): 761–70.

57. Crisa E, Venturino E, Passera R, *et al*. A retrospective study on 226 polycythemia vera patients: impact of median hematocrit value on clinical outcomes and survival improvement with anti-thrombotic prophylaxis and non-alkylating drugs. Ann Hematol 2010; 89(7): 691–9.

58. Vaidya R, Siragusa S, Huang J, *et al*. Mature survival data for 176 patients younger than 60 years with primary myelofibrosis diagnosed between 1976 and 2005: evidence for survival gains in recent years. Mayo Clin Proc 2009; 84(12): 1114–19.

59. Rozman C, Giralt M, Feliu E, Rubio D, Cortes MT. Life expectancy of patients with chronic nonleukemic myeloproliferative disorders. Cancer 1991; 67(10): 2658–63.

60. Tefferi A, Fonseca R, Pereira DL, Hoagland HC. A long-term retrospective study of young women with essential thrombocythemia. Mayo Clin Proc 2001; 76(1): 22–8.

61. Ma X, Vanasse G, Cartmel B, Wang Y, Selinger HA. Prevalence of polycythemia vera and essential thrombocythemia. Am J Hematol 2008; 83(5): 359–62.

62. Rumi E, Passamonti F, Della Porta MG, *et al*. Familial chronic myeloproliferative disorders: clinical phenotype and evidence of disease anticipation. J Clin Oncol 2007; 25(35): 5630–5.

63. Landgren O, Goldin LR, Kristinsson SY, Helgadottir EA, Samuelsson J, Bjorkholm M. Increased risks of polycythemia vera, essential thrombocythemia, and myelofibrosis among 24,577 first-degree relatives of 11,039 patients with myeloproliferative neoplasms in Sweden. Blood 2008; 112(6): 2199–204.

64. Tefferi A, Vainchenker W. Myeloproliferative neoplasms: molecular pathophysiology, essential clinical understanding, and treatment strategies. J Clin Oncol 2011; 29(5): 573–82.

65. Vannucchi AM, Guglielmelli P, Tefferi A. Advances in understanding and management of myeloproliferative neoplasms. CA Cancer J Clin 2009; 59(3): 171–91.

66. Passamonti F, Rumi E, Arcaini L, et al. Prognostic factors for thrombosis, myelofibrosis, and leukemia in essential thrombocythemia: a study of 605 patients. Haematologica 2008; 93(11): 1645–51.

67. Cervantes F, Dupriez B, Pereira A, et al. New prognostic scoring system for primary myelofibrosis based on a study of the International Working Group for Myelofibrosis Research and Treatment. Blood 2009; 113(13): 2895–901.

68. Mesa RA, Niblack J, Wadleigh M, et al. The burden of fatigue and quality of life in myeloproliferative disorders (MPDs): an international Internet-based survey of 1179 MPD patients. Cancer 2007; 109(1): 68–76.

69. Landolfi R, di Gennaro L, Barbui T, et al. Leukocytosis as a major thrombotic risk factor in patients with polycythemia vera. Blood 2007; 109(6): 2446–52.

70. Carobbio A, Finazzi G, Antonioli E, et al. Thrombocytosis and leukocytosis interaction in vascular complications of essential thrombocythemia. Blood 2008; 112(8): 3135–7.

71. Gangat N, Caramazza D, Vaidya R, et al. DIPSS plus: a refined Dynamic International Prognostic Scoring System for primary myelofibrosis that incorporates prognostic information from karyotype, platelet count, and transfusion status. J Clin Oncol 2011; 29(4): 392–7.

72. Passamonti F, Cervantes F, Vannucchi AM, et al. A dynamic prognostic model to predict survival in primary myelofibrosis: a study by the IWG-MRT (International Working Group for Myeloproliferative Neoplasms Research and Treatment). Blood 2010; 115(9): 1703–8.

73. Mesa RA, Tefferi A. Emerging drugs for the therapy of primary and post essential thrombocythemia, post polycythemia vera myelofibrosis. Expert Opin Emerg Drugs 2009; 14(3): 471–9.

74. Pietra D, Li S, Brisci A, et al. Somatic mutations of JAK2 exon 12 in patients with JAK2 (V617F)-negative myeloproliferative disorders. Blood 2008; 111(3): 1686–9.

75. Kosmider O, Gelsi-Boyer V, Cheok M, et al. TET2 mutation is an independent favorable prognostic factor in myelodysplastic syndromes (MDSs). Blood 2009; 114(15): 3285–91.

76. Scott LM, Tong W, Levine RL, et al. JAK2 exon 12 mutations in polycythemia vera and idiopathic erythrocytosis. N Engl J Med 2007; 356(5): 459–68.

77. Barosi G, Mesa RA, Thiele J, et al. Proposed criteria for the diagnosis of post-polycythemia vera and post-essential thrombocythemia myelofibrosis: a consensus statement from the International Working Group for Myelofibrosis Research and Treatment. Leukemia 2008; 22(2): 437–8.

78. McMullin MF, Bareford D, Campbell P, et al. Guidelines for the diagnosis, investigation and management of polycythaemia/erythrocytosis. Br J Haematol 2005; 130(2): 174–95.

79. Alvarez-Larran A, Cervantes F, Pereira A, et al. Observation versus antiplatelet therapy as primary prophylaxis for thrombosis in low-risk essential thrombocythemia. Blood 2010; 116(8): 1205–10; quiz 1387.

80. Landolfi R, Marchioli R, Kutti J, et al. Efficacy and safety of low-dose aspirin in polycythemia vera. N Engl J Med 2004; 350(2): 114–24.

81. Di Nisio M, Barbui T, di Gennaro L, et al. The haematocrit and platelet target in polycythemia vera. Br J Haematol 2007; 136(2): 249–59.

82. Harrison CN, Campbell PJ, Buck G, et al. Hydroxyurea compared with anagrelide in high-risk essential thrombocythemia. N Engl J Med 2005; 353(1): 33–45.

83. Beer PA, Erber WN, Campbell PJ, Green AR. How I treat essential thrombocythemia. Blood 2011; 117(5): 1472–82.

84. Kiladjian JJ, Chevret S, Dosquet C, Chomienne C, Rain JD. Treatment of polycythemia vera with hydroxyurea and pipobroman: final results of a randomized trial initiated in 1980. J Clin Oncol 2011; 29(29): 3907–13.

85. Quintas-Cardama A, Kantarjian H, Manshouri T, et al. Pegylated interferon alfa-2a yields high rates of hematologic and molecular response in patients with advanced essential thrombocythemia and polycythemia vera. J Clin Oncol 2009; 27(32): 5418–24.

86. Ianotto JC, Boyer-Perrard F, Demory JL, et al. Efficacy and safety of Peg-Interferon-{alpha}2a In myelofibrosis: a study of the FIM and GEM French Cooperative Groups. ASH Annual Meeting Abstracts, November 19, 2010; 116(21): 4103.

87. Mesa RA, Steensma DP, Pardanani A, et al. A phase 2 trial of combination low-dose thalidomide and prednisone for the treatment of myelofibrosis with myeloid metaplasia. Blood 2003; 101(7): 2534–41.

88. Mesa RA, Yao X, Cripe LD, et al. Lenalidomide and prednisone for myelofibrosis: Eastern Cooperative Oncology Group (ECOG) phase 2 trial E4903. Blood 2010; 116(22): 4436–8.

89. Quintas-Cardama A, Kantarjian HM, Manshouri T, et al. Lenalidomide plus prednisone results in durable clinical, histopathologic, and molecular responses in patients with myelofibrosis. J Clin Oncol 2009; 27(28): 4760–6.

90. Finazzi G, Caruso V, Marchioli R, et al. Acute leukemia in polycythemia vera: an analysis of 1638 patients enrolled in a prospective observational study. Blood 2005; 105(7): 2664–70.

91. Gangat N, Wolanskyj AP, McClure RF, et al. Risk stratification for survival and leukemic transformation in essential thrombocythemia: a single institutional study of 605 patients. Leukemia 2007; 21(2): 270–6.

92. Campbell PJ, Bareford D, Erber WN, et al. Reticulin accumulation in essential thrombocythemia: prognostic significance and relationship to therapy. J Clin Oncol 2009; 27(18): 2991–9.

93. Mesa RA, Li CY, Ketterling RP, Schroeder GS, Knudson RA, Tefferi A. Leukemic transformation in myelofibrosis with myeloid metaplasia: a single-institution experience with 91 cases. Blood 2005; 105(3): 973–7.

94. Tibes R, Mesa RA. Myeloproliferative neoplasms 5 years after discovery of JAK2V617F: what is the impact of JAK2 inhibitor therapy? Leuk Lymphoma 2011; 52(7): 1178–87.

95. Schaub FX, Looser R, Li S, et al. Clonal analysis of TET2 and JAK2 mutations suggests that TET2 can be a late event in the progression of myeloproliferative neoplasms. Blood 2010; 115(10): 2003–7.

96. Kroger N, Mesa RA. Choosing between stem cell therapy and drugs in myelofibrosis. Leukemia 2008; 22(3): 474–86.

97. Thepot S, Itzykson R, Seegers V, et al. Treatment of progression of Philadelphia-negative myeloproliferative neoplasms to myelodysplastic syndrome or acute myeloid leukemia by azacitidine: a report on 54 cases on the behalf of the Groupe Francophone des Myelodysplasies (GFM). Blood 2010; 116(19): 3735–42.

98. Mesa RA, Verstovsek S, Rivera C, et al. 5-Azacitidine has limited therapeutic activity in myelofibrosis. Leukemia 2009; 23(1): 180–2.

99. Quintas-Cardama A, Kantarjian H, Cortes J, Verstovsek S. Janus kinase inhibitors for the treatment of myeloproliferative neoplasias and beyond. Nat Rev Drug Discov 2011; 10(2): 127–40.

100. Wernig G, Kharas MG, Okabe R, et al. Efficacy of TG101348, a selective JAK2 inhibitor, in treatment of a murine model of JAK2V617F-induced polycythemia vera. Cancer Cell 2008; 13(4): 311–20.

101. Verstovsek S, Kantarjian H, Mesa RA, et al. Safety and efficacy of INCB018424, a JAK1 and JAK2 inhibitor, in myelofibrosis. N Engl J Med 2010; 363(12): 1117–27.

102. Verstovsek S, Mesa R, Gotlib JR, et al. Results of COMFORT-I, a randomized double-blind phase III trial of JAK 1/2 inhibitor INCB18424 (424) versus placebo (PB) for patients with myelofibrosis (MF). J Clin Oncol 2011; 29(Suppl): abstr 6500.

103. Harrison CN, Kiladjian J, Al-Ali HK, et al. Results of a randomized study of the JAK inhibitor ruxolitinib (INC424) versus best available therapy (BAT) in primary myelofibrosis (PMF), post-polycythemia vera-myelofibrosis (PPV-MF) or post-essential thrombocythemia-myelofibrosis (PET-MF). J Clin Oncol 2011; 29(Suppl): abstr LBA6501.

104. Tyner JW, Bumm TG, Deininger J, *et al*. CYT387, a novel JAK2 inhibitor, induces hematologic responses and normalizes inflammatory cytokines in murine myeloproliferative neoplasms. Blood 2010; 115(25): 5232–40.

105. Pardanani A, George G, Lasho T, *et al*. A phase I/II study of CYT387, an oral JAK-1/2 inhibitor, in myelofibrosis: significant response rates in anemia, splenomegaly, and constitutional symptoms. ASH Annual Meeting Abstracts, November 19, 2010; 116(21): 460.

106. Ma L, Zhao B, Walgren R, *et al*. Efficacy of LY2784544, a small molecule inhibitor selective for mutant JAK2 kinase, in JAK2 V617F-induced hematologic malignancy models. ASH Annual Meeting Abstracts, November 19, 2010; 116(21): 4087.

107. Shide K, Kameda T, Markovtsov V, *et al*. Efficacy of R723, a potent and selective JAK2 inhibitor, in JAK2V617F-induced murine MPD model. ASH Annual Meeting Abstracts, November 20, 2009; 114(22): 3897.

108. Shide K, Nakaya Y, Kameda T, *et al*. NS-018, a potent novel JAK2 inhibitor, effectively treats murine MPN induced by the janus kinase 2 (JAK2) V617F mutant. ASH Annual Meeting Abstracts, November 19, 2010; 116(21): 4106.

109. Mascarenhas J, Wang X, Rodriguez A, *et al*. A Phase I study of LBH589, a novel histone deacetylase inhibitor in patients with primary myelofibrosis (PMF) and post-polycythemia/essential thrombocythemia myelofibrosis (Post–PV/ET MF). ASH Annual Meeting Abstracts, November 20, 2009; 114(22): 308.

110. Rambaldi A, Dellacasa CM, Salmoiraghi S, *et al*. A phase 2A study of the histone-deacetylase inhibitor ITF2357 in patients with Jak2V617F positive chronic myeloproliferative neoplasms. ASH Annual Meeting Abstracts, November 16, 2008; 112(11): 100.

111. Vannucchi AM, Guglielmelli P, Lupo L, *et al*. A phase 1/2 study of RAD001, a mTOR Inhibitor, in patients with myelofibrosis: final results. ASH Annual Meeting Abstracts, November 19, 2010; 116(21): 314.

112. Kurzrock R, Bueso-Ramos CE, Kantarjian H, *et al*. BCR rearrangement-negative chronic myelogenous leukemia revisited. J Clin Oncol 2001; 19(11): 2915–26.

113. Verstovsek S, Lin H, Kantarjian H, *et al*. Neutrophilic-chronic myeloid leukemia: low levels of p230 BCR/ABL mRNA and undetectable BCR/ABL protein may predict an indolent course. Cancer 2002; 94(9): 2416–25.

114. Yanagisawa K, Ohminami H, Sato M, *et al*. Neoplastic involvement of granulocytic lineage, not granulocytic-monocytic, monocytic, or erythrocytic lineage, in a patient with chronic neutrophilic leukemia. Am J Hematol 1998; 57(3): 221–4.

115. Elliott MA, Dewald GW, Tefferi A, Hanson CA. Chronic neutrophilic leukemia (CNL): a clinical, pathologic and cytogenetic study. Leukemia 2001; 15(1): 35–40.

116. Elliott MA, Hanson CA, Dewald GW, Smoley SA, Lasho TL, Tefferi A. WHO-defined chronic neutrophilic leukemia: a long-term analysis of 12 cases and a critical review of the literature. Leukemia 2005; 19(2): 313–17.

117. Reilly JT. Chronic neutrophilic leukaemia: a distinct clinical entity? Br J Haematol 2002; 116(1): 10–18.

118. Lea NC, Lim Z, Westwood NB, *et al*. Presence of JAK2 V617F tyrosine kinase mutation as a myeloid-lineage-specific mutation in chronic neutrophilic leukaemia. Leukemia 2006; 20(7): 1324–6.

119. Gotlib J. World Health Organization-defined eosinophilic disorders: 2011 update on diagnosis, risk stratification, and management. Am J Hematol 2011; 86(8): 677–88.

120. Gotlib J, Cools J, Malone JM 3rd, Schrier SL, Gilliland DG, Coutre SE. The FIP1L1-PDGFRalpha fusion tyrosine kinase in hypereosinophilic syndrome and chronic eosinophilic leukemia: implications for diagnosis, classification, and management. Blood 2004; 103(8): 2879–91.

121. Cools J, DeAngelo DJ, Gotlib J, *et al*. A tyrosine kinase created by fusion of the PDGFRA and FIP1L1 genes as a therapeutic target of imatinib in idiopathic hypereosinophilic syndrome. N Engl J Med 2003; 348(13): 1201–14.

122. Lim KH, Tefferi A, Lasho TL, *et al*. Systemic mastocytosis in 342 consecutive adults: survival studies and prognostic factors. Blood 2009; 113(23): 5727–36.

123. Longley BJ, Tyrrell L, Lu SZ, *et al*. Somatic c-KIT activating mutation in urticaria pigmentosa and aggressive mastocytosis: establishment of clonality in a human mast cell neoplasm. Nat Genet 1996; 12(3): 312–14.

124. Akin C, Fumo G, Yavuz AS, Lipsky PE, Neckers L, Metcalfe DD. A novel form of mastocytosis associated with a transmembrane c-kit mutation and response to imatinib. Blood 2004; 103(8): 3222–5.

125. Ma Y, Zeng S, Metcalfe DD, *et al*. The c-KIT mutation causing human mastocytosis is resistant to STI571 and other KIT kinase inhibitors; kinases with enzymatic site mutations show different inhibitor sensitivity profiles than wild-type kinases and those with regulatory-type mutations. Blood 2002; 99(5): 1741–4.

126. Tefferi A, Levine RL, Lim KH, *et al*. Frequent TET2 mutations in systemic mastocytosis: clinical, KITD816V and FIP1L1-PDGFRA correlates. Leukemia 2009; 23(5): 900–4.

127. Gotlib J, Berube C, Growney JD, *et al*. Activity of the tyrosine kinase inhibitor PKC412 in a patient with mast cell leukemia with the D816V KIT mutation. Blood 2005; 106(8): 2865–70.

128. Verstovsek S, Tefferi A, Cortes J, *et al*. Phase II study of dasatinib in Philadelphia chromosome-negative acute and chronic myeloid diseases, including systemic mastocytosis. Clin Cancer Res 2008; 14(12): 3906–15.

129. Nakamura R, Chakrabarti S, Akin C, *et al*. A pilot study of nonmyeloablative allogeneic hematopoietic stem cell transplant for advanced systemic mastocytosis. Bone Marrow Transplant 2006; 37(4): 353–8.

130. Cortelazzo S, Finazzi G, Ruggeri M, *et al*. Hydroxyurea for patients with essential thrombocythemia and a high risk of thrombosis. N Engl J Med 1995; 332(17): 1132–6.

131. Anagrelide Study Group. Anagrelide, a therapy for thrombocythemic states: experience in 577 patients. Am J Med 1992; 92(1): 69–76.

132. Kiladjian JJ, Cassinat B, Chevret S, *et al*. Pegylated interferon-alfa-2a induces complete hematologic and molecular responses with low toxicity in polycythemia vera. Blood 2008; 112(8): 3065–72.

133. Cervantes F, Alvarez-Larran A, Domingo A, Arellano-Rodrigo E, Montserrat E. Efficacy and tolerability of danazol as a treatment for the anaemia of myelofibrosis with myeloid metaplasia: long-term results in 30 patients. Br J Haematol 2005; 129(6): 771–5.

134. Shimoda K, Shide K, Kamezaki K, *et al*. The effect of anabolic steroids on anemia in myelofibrosis with myeloid metaplasia: retrospective analysis of 39 patients in Japan. Int J Hematol 2007; 85(4): 338–43.

135. Barosi G, Elliott M, Canepa L, *et al*. Thalidomide in myelofibrosis with myeloid metaplasia: a pooled analysis of individual patient data from five studies. Leuk Lymphoma 2002; 43(12): 2301–7.

136. Tefferi A, Cortes J, Verstovsek S, *et al*. Lenalidomide therapy in myelofibrosis with myeloid metaplasia. Blood 2006; 108(4): 1158–64.

48 Rare T Cell Lymphomas

Aleksandr Lazaryan and John Sweetenham

Department of Hematologic Oncology and Blood Disorders, Taussig Cancer Institute, Cleveland Clinic, Cleveland, OH, USA

Introduction

This chapter contains up-to-date information on rare precursor and mature T cell lymphomas according to the 2008 World Health Organization (WHO) Classification of Tumours of the Haematopoietic and Lymphoid Tissues.[1] We have specifically focused on T cell lymphoblastic lymphoma, representing the minority of adult precursor T cell neoplasms, as well as on the rare mature T cell lymphomas such as hepatosplenic T cell lymphoma (HSTCL), enteropathy-associated T cell lymphoma (EATL), and subcutaneous panniculitis-like T cell lymphoma (SPTL), accounting individually for less than 5% of all the cases in the landmark International Peripheral T cell and Natural Killer/T cell Lymphoma Study[2] (Fig. 48.1).

The clinical course of these rare T cell malignancies can be quite aggressive, leading to poor overall survival, particularly for HSTCL, EATL, and SPTL in association with hemophagocytic syndrome (Fig. 48.2). Therefore, early clinical recognition of these unique T cell lymphomas is essential in avoiding diagnostic delays and initiating appropriate therapy. The chapter is structured to provide the reader with a clinician's perspective on the individual disease epidemiology, diagnostic workup, clinicopathological/molecular prognostic factors, and evidence-based therapy.

T cell lymphoblastic lymphoma

T cell lymphoblastic lymphoma (T-LBL) is a rare malignancy, accounting for 1.7% of all non-Hodgkin lymphomas (NHL) and about 14% of all T cell NHLs.[3] The disease has a male predominance (70%) and its incidence rates follow a bimodal pattern, peaking below age 20 years and above 50 years.[4]

Like T cell lymphoblastic leukemia (T-ALL), T-LBL arises from immature T lymphoblasts and it is therefore classified as a precursor T cell lymphoid neoplasm according to the recent WHO nomenclature.[1] Despite morphological and immunophenotypic similarities between these two entities, T-LBL has a distinct pattern of bone marrow involvement,

anatomical localization, and gene expression signature.[5] Conventional separation between T-LBL and T-ALL has been largely based on the degree of bone marrow involvement, defined as below 25% for T-LBL. In 80–90% of cases, T-LBL manifests as an anterior mediastinal tumor, with simultaneous pleural effusions in 40–60% of patients.[6,7] Thus, patients with T-LBL often present with cough, dyspnea and occasionally with superior vena cava syndrome. About 70% of patients have stage III or IV disease at the time of diagnosis, with elevated lactate dehydrogenase in about a third of the cases.[7] Involvement of the central nervous system (CNS) has been described in up to 10% of cases.

Compared to T-ALL, the immunophenotypic features of T-LBL have been less well characterized. T-lymphoblasts are usually TdT positive (Fig. 48.3) and the expression of other T cell markers, such as CD1a, CD2, CD3, CD7, CD4, and CD8, varies according to the degree of T cell maturation. In children with T-LBL, a cortical/thymic immunophenotype has been reported in 70% of cases. Although T-LBL is often thought to have a more mature immunophenotype (i.e. CD1a$^+$, CD3$^+$) compared to T-ALL, a significant overlap exists between these two entities. Recent microarray studies, however, revealed complete genetic separation between T-LBL and T-ALL, with overexpression of *MLL1* in the former and CD47 in the latter.[5]

Factors shown to have prognostic significance for clinical outcomes in T-LBL have varied across published series. Elevated serum lactate dehydrogenase (LDH) levels and CNS involvement portended poor overall and progression-free survival (PFS), respectively,[7–9] in contrast to age, stage, and immunophenotype, which appeared to have no prognostic significance. Time to complete remission has also been correlated with better outcomes for patients with mediastinal tumors at diagnosis[10] whereas achieving partial response or less by the end of therapy appears disadvantageous.[7]

The therapeutic management of T-LBL has gradually evolved from less successful NHL-type therapy with cyclophosphamide, doxorubicin, vincristine, and prednisone (CHOP)-based

Textbook of Uncommon Cancer, Fourth Edition. Edited by Derek Raghavan, Charles D. Blanke, David H. Johnson, Paul L. Moots, Gregory H. Reaman, Peter G. Rose and Mikkael A. Sekeres.
© 2012 John Wiley & Sons, Inc. Published 2012 by John Wiley & Sons, Inc.

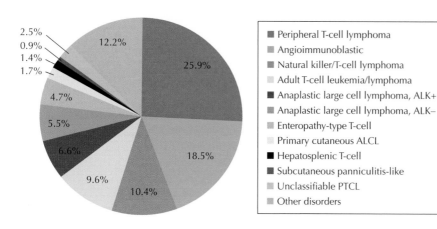

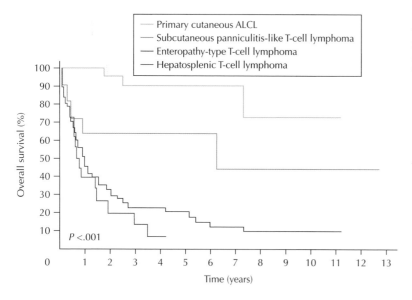

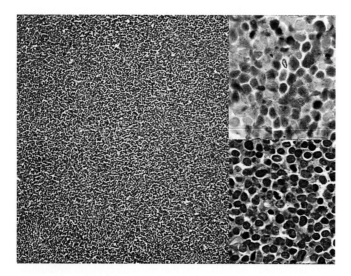

Figure 48.3 T cell lymphoblastic lymphoma. Numerous lymphoblasts in biopsy sample (*low magnification, left image*). Immunohistochemical detection of nuclear antigen terminal deoxynucleotidyl transferase (TdT) within neoplastic T lymphoblasts (*high magnification, upper right image*). Lymphoblasts with round to oval to irregularly shaped nuclei with dispersed chromatin. Images courtesy of Dr Eric Hsi.

regimen(s) to more intense and effective protocols for aggressive NHLs or ALL-type regimens. Although early data on standard CHOP-based chemotherapy did not differentiate between B or T cell lymphoblastic lymphomas, an overall complete remission was attained in approximately 50–80% of cases across all published series.[11–14] Early CNS relapses were observed in 40% of patients who did not receive intrathecal CNS prophylaxis with either methotrexate or cytarabine, resulting in similarly unsatisfactory long-term disease-free survival (DFS) rates of 20–50% with CHOP-like therapy. Addition of L-asparaginase to CHOP along with CNS prophylaxis and maintenance therapy with 6-mercaptopurine combined with methotrexate (Stanford/NCOG data[15]) significantly improved complete response (CR) rates to 95%, with an overall survival of 56% after a median of 26 months of follow-up in the seminal study of 44 patients. Estimates for 5-year DFS varied from 19% to 94% depending on risk stratification by advanced stage, bone marrow involvement, and elevated LDH level. Altogether, Stanford data justified the clinical benefit of using CNS prophylaxis and maintenance chemotherapy in improving outcomes in patients with lymphoblastic lymphoma. French investigators used the LNH-84 protocol (adriamycin, cyclophosphamide, vindesine, bleomycin, prednisone for four cycles with six cycles of intrathecal methotrexate followed by sequential courses of high-dose methotrexate (MTX), ifosfamide, etoposide, L-asparaginase, and cytarabine for 4 months) to treat 30 patients, most of whom had T-LBL.[12] Although 25 (83%) out of 30 patients achieved a CR by the end of therapy, 14 patients relapsed (56%) within 2 years of follow-up.

Given the many similarities between ALL and LBL, ALL-like treatment protocols (L2, L10, L17) for LBL were initially popularized by the Memorial Sloan-Kettering Cancer Center based on overall CR rates of 80% and 5-year survival rates of 45%.[16] Other studies employing ALL-type regimens yielded 55–100% CR rates and 45–67% DFS rates.[17] The Hyper-CVAD (8–9 alternating cycles of fractionated cyclophosphamide, vincristine, adriamycin, dexamethasone) regimen popularized by the MD Anderson Cancer Center (MDACC)[18] produced 91% CR and 9% partial response (PR) rates with a 30% relapse rate within approximately 1 year of follow-up in 33 patients with LBL (80% with T-LBL).[9] All patients received CNS prophylaxis (6–8 cycles of intrathecal alternating MTX and cytarabine) and maintenance chemotherapy with 6-mercaptopurine, MTX, vincristine, and prednisone (POMP). Seventy percent of patients had mediastinal disease for which they received consolidative radiation therapy (30–39 Gy). Three-year PFS and OS rates were 62% and 67%, respectively. CNS involvement at diagnosis (9% of patients) was the sole predictor of relapse in that study.

Similarly, the German Multicenter Study Group for adult ALL (GMALL) reported a 93% CR rate after remission induction therapy, 36% relapse within a year and close to 60% OS at 3-year follow-up in the cohort of 45 patients with T-LGL who were treated with ALL protocols (04/89 and 05/93).[7] The total duration of therapy was 6–12 months, and treatments did not contain maintenance therapy. Although the majority of patients received cranial and mediastinal radiation (24 Gy), nearly all of the relapses occurred within a year and half of those relapses were localized to the mediastinum, with only a single CNS relapse. The rates of mediastinal relapse have been lower (~20%) in pediatric T-LBL, either due to more intense pediatric regimens (including ara-C or high-dose MTX) and/or different disease biology. In fact, mediastinal relapse was limited to 20% in a study of 27 T-LBL patients who similarly experienced 63% OS at 3 years when treated with a modified pediatric ALL protocol, LMT-89.[19] It remains unclear if the higher rate of mediastinal recurrence in GMALL was related to the lower dose of consolidative mediastinal radiation as compared to the above mentioned MDACC study (30–39 Gy) and/or to the differences in administered chemotherapy including absence of maintenance therapy in GMALL. The former assumption is supported by interim data from recent GMALL protocols using 36 Gy of radiation, resulting in lower mediastinal relapse rates (30%). However, the analysis from MDACC is confounded by the fact that most of the patients who received mediastinal irradiation had also received chemotherapy with the Hyper-CVAD regimen. The relative contributions of chemotherapy and radiation therapy to the improved local control in the mediastinum are therefore unclear.

Given the relatively high relapse rate after initial induction therapy, high-dose chemotherapy followed by autologous stem cell transplantation has been used as a consolidation strategy in the first complete remission (CR1). A number of retrospective studies produced estimates of DFS ranging from 40% to 70%.[6,20–24] Although limited by poor accrual, a randomized multicenter European trial[25] did not demonstrate clinical superiority of autologous stem cell transplantation (ASCT) as compared to conventional maintenance therapy on LSA$_2$L$_2$[26] or Stanford[15] protocols. In that study, 31 patients randomized to high-dose chemotherapy with ASCT had a 50% DFS and 57% OS with 2-year follow-up. Of note, 12 patients with HLA-matched donors underwent allogeneic stem cell transplantation (allo-SCT) in CR1, resulting in a 59% 3-year OS. A retrospective comparison between ASCT and allo-SCT among 204 LBL patients from the IBMTR/ABMTR registries demonstrated comparable 5-year OS estimates (44% versus 39%) with more treatment-related morbidity and mortality for allo-SCT and more relapses for ASCT.[27] Patients with relapsed or primary refractory disease who were salvaged with high-dose chemotherapy followed by ASCT had significantly lower OS (~15–25%) compared to recipients of ASCT in CR1 (63% 6-year OS).[28] The precise role of the SCT for T-LBL in CR1 and in the relapsed/refractory settings remains uncertain and will need to be defined in randomized clinical trials.

In summary, even though no single standard approach to treating T-LBL has been established, the use of ALL-type multiagent upfront chemotherapy ± CNS prophylaxis ± maintenance chemotherapy ± mediastinal radiation has been associated with improved clinical outcomes. Future insights into molecular subtypes of T-LBL may guide development of better therapies.

Hepatosplenic T cell lymphoma

Hepatosplenic T cell lymphoma (HSTCL) is a rare type of peripheral T cell lymphoma (PTCL) that predominantly affects adult males in their 30s–40s, who often present with hepatosplenomegaly, cytopenia(s), and significant constitutional symptoms in the absence of lymphadenopathy.[29] The pathological hallmarks of HSTCL include sinusoidal involvement of liver, bone marrow, and red pulp of the spleen by clonal cytotoxic T cells that express γδ T cell receptors (TCR) (with occasional αβ TCR expression).[1]

Up to 20% of patients with HSTCL have a history of long-term exposure to immunosuppressive medications in the setting of previous autoimmune disease or solid organ transplantation.[30] Some patients undergo exhaustive initial workup for fever of unknown origin, with hematology consultation initiated upon detection of cytopenias and/or massive splenomegaly. In one of the largest published series of 21 patients with γδ HSTCL, thrombocytopenia, anemia, neutropenia, and elevated LDH were found in 95%, 70%, 50%, and 55% of cases, respectively.[31] Involvement of the bone marrow at diagnosis may account for cytopenias, though these may occur in the presence of a normal bone marrow exam. Detection of neoplastic T cells in the biopsy specimen is enhanced by specific immunohistochemical stains for T cells, and can be missed by initial hematoxylin and eosin (H&E) staining.

Common immunophenotype consists of CD2$^+$, CD3$^+$, CD4$^-$, CD5$^-$, CD7$^{+/-}$, CD8$^-$, CD16$^{+/-}$, CD25$^-$, CD30$^-$, CD38$^+$, CD56$^+$,

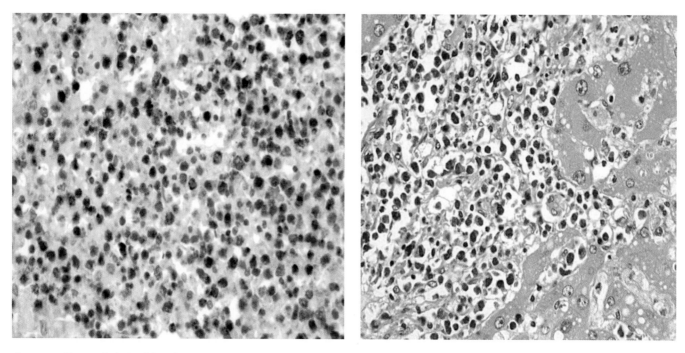

Figure 48.4 Hepatosplenic T cell lymphoma (HSTCL): morphological and immunophenotypic features. Expansion of hepatic sinusoids by neoplastic T cells (*left*). The neoplastic cells are positive for TIA-1, a cytotoxic T cell marker (*right*). All images courtesy of Dr Eric Hsi.

and CD57⁻ cytotoxic T cells, which demonstrate excessive production of TIA1 (Fig. 48.4), while lacking expression of other cytotoxic molecules such as granzyme B and perforin.[29] In addition to flow cytometry and immunohistochemistry, TCR gene rearrangement studies are also helpful to prove the clonal origin of neoplastic T cells and to differentiate HSTCL into γδ or αβ subtypes.[1] The clinical relevance of γδ and αβ subtyping, however, remains unclear. Typical patterns of sinusoidal infiltration of the bone marrow, liver, and splenic red pulp by small, monotonous T cells in the early stages of disease may occasionally transform to interstitial infiltration by larger cells of blastoid morphology with disease progression.[29] Hemophagocytosis can be present in the pathological specimen, and may portend a fulminant clinical course.[32] Isochromosome 7q is the most frequent cytogenetic abnormality detected in HSTCL, whereas trisomy 8 and loss of chromosome Y are less common findings.[33]

With rare exceptions, HSTCL has an aggressive clinical course with poor responsiveness to conventional treatment strategies, and high disease-related mortality with a median OS of approximately 1 year (see Fig. 48.2). Even though initial responses among patients treated with CHOP or CHOP-like chemotherapy range from 33%[34] to 63%,[31] response duration is short-lived and survival rates are poor. Only four out of 15 patients in the US series from MD Anderson remained alive by the end of follow-up. Three of those survivors received intense frontline treatment with hyperfractionated cyclophosphamide, vincristine, liposomal doxorubicine, dexamathasone, methotrexate, and cytarabine (Hyper-CVIDD/MTX/Ara-C) followed by allogeneic or autologous stem cell transplantation in two cases. Another survivor achieved complete response with the combination of pentostatin and alemtuzumab followed by consolidative allogeneic

stem cell transplantation.[34] In a similar case series, only two out of 21 patients remained alive beyond 3 years of follow up; both received platinum- and cytarabine-based regimens and consolidation with autologous stem cell transplantation.[31] The use of pentostatin has resulted in complete responses in several case reports,[35,36] though more systematic data are needed to establish its role in HSTCL.

In the absence of effective standard treatment approaches, patients with HSTCL can potentially benefit from the use of novel investigational drugs in clinical trials. Outside clinical trials, all responders to intensive, upfront combination chemotherapy should be considered for immediate consolidative high-dose chemotherapy followed by stem cell transplantation.

Enteropathy-associated T cell lymphoma

Enteropathy-associated T cell lymphoma (EATL) is an aggressive type of NHL with an estimated annual incidence of 0.5–1.4 per million in the western world.[37–39] EATL accounts for 1–2% of all NHLs in population-based studies from Europe, and up to 9.1% of all peripheral T cell or NK cell lymphomas among Europeans in the International Peripheral T Cell Lymphoma Project. This contrasts with rates of 1.9% in Asia and 5.8% in the US.[38–40] Relatively higher rates of EATL among patients of northern European ancestry are attributed to well-known epidemiological associations between EATL and celiac disease (CD)[1,41–44] and the incidence rate of EATL has been estimated to approach 10% among patients with long-standing history of CD,[45] emphasizing the role of chronic inflammation in gastrointestinal lymphomagenesis. Furthermore, concurrent CD has been reported in 50–90% of newly diagnosed EATL patients.[38,39,46]

Table 48.1 EATL subtypes.

Characteristics	Type I	Type II
Geographic distribution	West > East	East > West
Gender	M > F	M > F
Histology	Variable	Monomorphic
Immunophenotype		
CD3	+	+
CD8	+/−	+
CD30	+/−	−
CD56	−	+
Genetic signatures		
9q+	+	+
16q−	+	+
1q+/5q+	+	Rare
8q+(myc)	−	+
HLA DQ2/DQ8	+	−

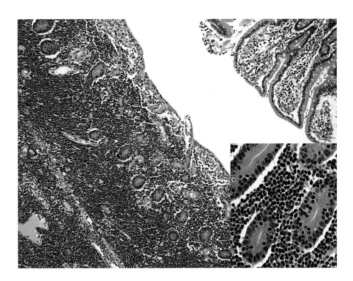

Figure 48.5 Enteropathy-associated T cell lymphoma (EATL) type II. A diffuse infiltrate of the mucosa by monomorphous small to medium-sized lymphocytes. The inset demonstrates the tropism for intestinal crypt epithelium. All images courtesy of Dr Eric Hsi.

Enteropathy-associated T cell lymphoma tends to arise in the jejunum and less frequently the ileum, with both anatomical sites accounting for over >90% of cases. In rare cases, the disease may involve stomach, duodenum, or colon. EATL affects patients in their fifth and sixth decades of life and appears to have a male predominance. According to the 2008 WHO classification,[1] EATL is divided into two subtypes based on morphological, immunophenotypic, and genetic features (Table 48.1). Type I EATL accounts for approximately 80% of all cases in western populations and has the strongest association with CD. Variable histology is seen in EATL type I, ranging from monotonous appearing, small to medium-sized to large anaplastic or immunoblastic T cells infiltrating the intestinal wall beneath impaired mucosa. Both villous atrophy and intraepithelial lymphocytosis in neighboring gut epithelium accompany these intestinal lesions in over 80% of cases. Typical immunohistochemical markers of type I EATL include expression of CD3, CD7, CD103, and TIA1 in the absence of CD4, CD5, CD56, variable expression of CD30 and less frequent expression of CD8 (~20%). Common gains of chromosomes 1q and 5q have been described for EATL type I.[47] In contrast, EATL type II is more prevalent in Asia and accounts for almost half of all cases in North America, and for a minority (~20%) of all EATL cases in Europe.[2] Association of EATL type II with CD appears to be weaker.[2] Histological features of EATL type II include florid infiltration of intestinal crypts by monomorphic, small to medium-sized T lymphocytes (Fig. 48.5).[1] Expression of CD3, CD8, CD56, and TCRβ represents a distinct immunophenotype of EATL type II, and its most common genetic aberration involves gain of chromosome 8q containing the *myc* oncogene locus. Recent whole-genome analysis has demonstrated chromosome 9q gain in over 80% of all EATL cases, whereas a mutually exclusive loss of chromosome 16q is usually detected in the absence of 9q gain.[47]

Abdominal pain (>80%), weight loss, fatigue, nausea/vomiting, anorexia, small bowel obstruction, and bowel perforation are common presenting symptoms of EATL, and prompt emergency therapeutic and diagnostic laparotomy in over 80% of

cases.[38,46] The majority of patients are diagnosed with an advanced stage of disease,[38,40] even though involvement of bone marrow (~3%) or CNS is extremely rare.[2] While the applicability of Ann Arbor staging to gastrointestinal lymphomas remains questionable, alternative staging classifications (such as Lugano[48] or Manchester stages) have been used for EATL.[38]

The prognosis of patients with EATL remains poor. Early mortality from EATL can be over 40%, secondary to intestinal perforation and/or sepsis.[49] In major retrospective studies, approximately one-third of patients with EATL were treated with surgery alone, as poor performance status precluded subsequent chemotherapy.[38,46,50] Among the rest of patients treated with chemotherapy (mainly anthracycline based) with or without surgery, only about half were able to complete their scheduled treatment because of disease progression or treatment-related complications. Median progression-free and overall survival are less than 6 and 10 months, respectively, with sobering 5-year OS of approximately 20% with conventional chemotherapy regimens such as CHOP.[2] Patients with a history of celiac disease, poor performance status, high LDH, and large tumor mass (≥5 cm) have worse outcomes[2] whereas those receiving anthracycline-based chemotherapy (versus surgery alone or nonanthracycline based) have better survival. A high prognostic index for peripheral T cell lymphoma, which includes age, performance status, bone marrow involvement, and LDH, may be a better predictor of survival, compared to the International Prognostic Index (IPI) in patients with EATL.[2] There is no difference in survival between EATL types I and II.

Given the poor results with conventional anthracycline-based chemotherapy, a more intense upfront regimen with ifosfamide, etoposide, and epirubicin alternating with methotrexate (IVE/MTX) followed by high-dose chemotherapy and ASCT has been recently reported to produce a higher overall survival rate of 60%,[38] although it is not clear whether this represents an improvement in therapy or reflects selection bias. Similar results have been reported in a recent phase 2 study by the Nordic Lymphoma Group with upfront dose-intense CHOEP followed by high-dose chemotherapy and ASCT in 160 patients with PTCL, including 21 patients with EATL, about half of whom were alive and free of disease after 3 years.[51]

Subcutaneous panniculitis-like T cell lymphoma

Subcutaneous panniculitis-like T cell lymphoma (SPTL) is an extremely rare subtype of extranodal NHL which accounts for 0.9% of all peripheral T cell lymphomas around the world.[2] Preferentially multifocal nodular skin involvement and infiltration of subcutaneous tissue by neoplastic T lymphocytes in SPTL may mimic benign lobular panniculitis, or the spectrum of cutaneous manifestations of autoimmune conditions, making the diagnosis of SPTL particularly challenging. Until recently, SPTL has been divided into αβ (75%) and γδ (25%) subtypes based on clonal T cell receptor gene rearrangement.[52] Growing evidence has led to reclassification[1] of the SPTL-γδ subtype into cutaneous γδ T cell lymphoma (CGD-TCL) based on striking clinicopathological and prognostic differences between SPTL-αβ and -γδ phenotypes (Table 48.2). Patients with γδ phenotype tend to express CD56 (~60%) and to follow a more aggressive clinical course frequently associated (up to 45% of cases) with hemophagocytic syndrome (HPS), high case fatality (~80%), and a median overall survival slightly over a year from the time of diagnosis.[53,54]

In contrast, patients with SPTL-αβ phenotype tend to exhibit an indolent clinical course with overall favorable prognosis, unless they too develop HPS (<20%), which is associated with a two-fold decline in their 5-year survival, from 91% to 46%.[53] According to the most recent WHO-EORTC classification, the diagnosis of SPTL is restricted to SPTL-αβ phenotype.[1] Skin ulcerations in SPTL are rare and spontaneous regressions of typical nodular or deeply seated plaque-type lesions may leave areas of lipoatrophy. Approximately half of patients with SPTL have B symptoms and/or laboratory abnormalities including cytopenia(s) or elevated liver function tests.[53] Up to 20% of cases have an associated autoimmune disorder (e.g. systemic lupus erythematosus, rheumatoid arthritis, Sjögren disease, juvenile rheumatoid arthritis.[53] Tissue diagnosis of SPTL is based on characteristic infiltration of subcutaneous fat by CD3[+], CD4[-], CD56[-], βF1[+], and CD8[+] cytotoxic αβ T lymphocytes, which surround adipocytes in a "wreath-like" fashion (Fig. 48.6). Positive staining for βF1 confirms the αβ phenotype of SPTL.[55] Strong expression of granzyme B, perforin, and T cell intracellular antigen-1 (TIA-1) by lymphoma cells may be responsible for commonly observed subcutaneous tissue necrosis and karyorrhexis. Epstein-Barr virus (EBV) tissue assay is routinely negative in SPTL. A recent analysis of genetic aberrations among patients with SPTL demonstrated deletion of the *NAV3* (neuron navigator 3) tumor suppression gene in about half of cases.[56] While *NAV3* deletion and other genetic abnormalities such as gains in chromosomes 2q and 4q or losses in 10p, 17p, or chromosome 19 can be also found in mycosis fungoides and Sézary syndrome,[56–59] it appears that 5q and 13q chromosomal gains are SPTL specific.[56]

Table 48.2 Comparison between former subtypes of SPTL: αβ (currently SPTL) and γδ (currently within CGD-TCL).

Characteristics	αβ	γδ
Gender	Female>Male	Female>Male
Median age (range)	36 (9–79)	59 (13–79)
T cell receptors	TCRδ1[-], βF1[+]	TCRδ1[+], βF1[-]
Cytotoxic proteins	Granzyme B, perforin, TIA-1	Granzyme B, perforin, TIA-1
Tissue infiltration	Subcutaneous Adipocyte rimming Fat necrosis, karyorrhexis	Subcutaneous ± dermal/ epidermal Adipocyte rimming Angiocentric, hemorrhagic, necrotic
Skin ulceration	Rare	Common
B-symptoms	Variable	Common
Immunophenotype	CD3[+], CD4[-], CD8[+], CD56[-], CD30[-]	CD3[+], CD4[-], CD8[-], CD56[+] (60%), CD30[+/-]
Genetic associations	*NAV3* gene deletion Chromosome 5q or 13q gains	
Hemophagocytic syndrome	Uncommon (lowers survival)	Common (no impact on survival)
Prognosis	Good (5-yr OS ~70–80%)	Poor (5-yr OS ~10%)
Treatment	Systemic corticosteroids Radiation therapy CHOP-like chemotherapy	Multiagent chemotherapy Stem cell transplantation

CGD-TCL, cutaneous γδ T cell lymphoma; OS, overall survival; SPTL, subcutaneous panniculitis-like T cell lymphoma; TCR, T cell receptor.

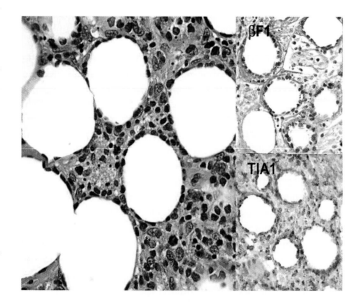

Figure 48.6 Subcutaneous panniculitis-like T cell lymphoma (SPTL). H&E stain shows tight rimming of lymphoma cells around individual adipocytes (*left*). Positive βF1 staining confirms SPTL-αβ phenotype (*upper right*). A TIA-1 stain demonstrates that the atypical lymphocytes are cytotoxic T cells (*lower right*). All images courtesy of Dr Eric Hsi.

Given the rarity of SPTL, most of the available data on treatment are based on individual case reports and case series with a mixture of indolent αβ and more aggressive γδ subtypes of SPTL.[54] While radiotherapy, immunosuppressive therapy (steroids, cyclosporine A), or single-agent chemotherapy (cyclophosphamide, methotrexate, cladribine, fludarabine) have been historically reserved for upfront use in more indolent cases, anthracycline-containing combination chemotherapy was associated with long-lasting remissions in about a third of patients, most of whom required a more aggressive upfront approach.[54] One of the largest series of patients with SPTL demonstrated refractoriness of γδ subtype to upfront combination chemotherapy. Only two out of four long-term survivors in that study received high-dose chemotherapy with either autologous or allogeneic stem cell transplantation.[53] In contrast, excellent outcomes of patients with the αβ subtype, particularly in the absence of HPS, have called into question the routine upfront use of anthracycline-based multiagent chemotherapy. Based on limited retrospective data, it appears that equally favorable long-term results in management of SPTL-αβ may be achieved with the use of systemic corticosteroids or immunosuppressive agents.[53,60]

References

1. Swerdlow SH, *et al*. *WHO Classification of Tumours: Tumours of Haematopoietic and Lymphoid Tissues.* Lyon: IARC Press, 2008.
2. Vose J, Armitage J, Weisenburger D. International Peripheral T Cell and Natural Killer/T Cell Lymphoma Study: pathology findings and clinical outcomes. J Clin Oncol 2008; 26(25): 4124–30.
3. Non-Hodgkin's Lymphoma Classification Project. A clinical evaluation of the International Lymphoma Study Group classification of non-Hodgkin's lymphoma. Blood 1997; 89(11): 3909–18.
4. Groves FD, Linet MS, Travis LB, Devesa SS. Cancer surveillance series: non-Hodgkin's lymphoma incidence by histologic subtype in the United States from 1978 through 1995. J Natl Cancer Inst 2000; 92(15): 1240–51.
5. Raetz EA, *et al*. Gene expression profiling reveals intrinsic differences between T cell acute lymphoblastic leukemia and T cell lymphoblastic lymphoma. Pediatr Blood Cancer 2006; 47(2): 130–40.
6. Song KW, *et al*. Primary therapy for adults with T cell lymphoblastic lymphoma with hematopoietic stem-cell transplantation results in favorable outcomes. Ann Oncol 2007; 18(3): 535–40.
7. Hoelzer D, *et al*. Outcome of adult patients with T-lymphoblastic lymphoma treated according to protocols for acute lymphoblastic leukemia. Blood 2002; 99(12): 4379–85.
8. Thomas DA, Kantarjian HM. Lymphoblastic lymphoma. Hematol Oncol Clin North Am 2001; 15(1): 51–95, vi.
9. Thomas DA, *et al*. Outcome with the hyper-CVAD regimens in lymphoblastic lymphoma. Blood 2004; 104(6): 1624–30.
10. Reiter A, *et al*. Intensive ALL-type therapy without local radiotherapy provides a 90% event-free survival for children with T cell lymphoblastic lymphoma: a BFM group report. Blood 2000; 95(2): 416–21.
11. Salloum E, *et al*. Lymphoblastic lymphoma in adults: a clinicopathological study of 34 cases treated at the Institut Gustave-Roussy. Eur J Cancer Clin Oncol 1988; 24(10): 1609–16.
12. Morel P, *et al*. Prognosis and treatment of lymphoblastic lymphoma in adults: a report on 80 patients. J Clin Oncol 1992; 10(7): 1078–85.
13. Kaiser U, Uebelacker I, Havemann K. Non-Hodgkin's lymphoma protocols in the treatment of patients with Burkitt's lymphoma and lymphoblastic lymphoma: a report on 58 patients. Leuk Lymphoma 1999; 36(1–2): 101–8.
14. Voakes JB, Jones SE, McKelvey EM. The chemotherapy of lymphoblastic lymphoma. Blood 1981; 57(1): 186–8.
15. Coleman CN, Cohen JR, Burke JS, Rosenberg SA. Lymphoblastic lymphoma in adults: results of a pilot protocol. Blood 1981; 57(4): 679–84.
16. Slater DE, *et al*. Lymphoblastic lymphoma in adults. J Clin Oncol 1986; 4(1): 57–67.
17. Hoelzer D, Gokbuget N. T cell lymphoblastic lymphoma and T cell acute lymphoblastic leukemia: a separate entity? Clin Lymphoma Myeloma 2009; 9(Suppl 3): S214–21.
18. Kantarjian HM, *et al*. Results of treatment with hyper-CVAD, a dose-intensive regimen, in adult acute lymphocytic leukemia. J Clin Oncol 2000; 18(3): 547–61.
19. Jabbour E, *et al*. High survival rate with the LMT-89 regimen in lymphoblastic lymphoma (LL), but not in T cell acute lymphoblastic leukemia (T-ALL). Leukemia 2006; 20(5): 814–19.
20. Milpied N, *et al*. Bone marrow transplantation for adult poor prognosis lymphoblastic lymphoma in first complete remission. Br J Haematol 1989; 73(1): 82–7.
21. Santini G, *et al*. Autologous bone marrow transplantation for adult advanced stage lymphoblastic lymphoma in first CR. A study of the NHLCSG. Leukemia 1991; 5(Suppl 1): 42–5.
22. Baro J, *et al*. Autologous bone marrow transplantation in 22 adult patients with lymphoblastic lymphoma responsive to conventional dose chemotherapy. Bone Marrow Transplant 1992; 10(1): 33–8.
23. Verdonck LF, Dekker AW, de Gast GC, Lokhorst HM, Nieuwenhuis HK. Autologous bone marrow transplantation for adult poor-risk lymphoblastic lymphoma in first remission. J Clin Oncol 1992; 10(4): 644–6.
24. Bouabdallah R, *et al*. Role of induction chemotherapy and bone marrow transplantation in adult lymphoblastic lymphoma: a report on 62 patients from a single center. Ann Oncol 1998; 9(6): 619–25.
25. Sweetenham JW, *et al*. High-dose therapy and autologous stem-cell transplantation versus conventional-dose consolidation/maintenance therapy as postremission therapy for adult patients with lymphoblastic lymphoma: results of a randomized trial of the European Group for Blood and Marrow Transplantation and the United Kingdom Lymphoma Group. J Clin Oncol 2001; 19(11): 2927–36.
26. Sullivan MP, *et al*. Pediatric Oncology Group experience with modified LSA2-L2 therapy in 107 children with non-Hodgkin's lymphoma (Burkitt's lymphoma excluded). Cancer 1985; 55(2): 323–36.
27. Peniket A, Ruiz de Elvira M, Taghipour G. Allogeneic transplantation for lymphoma produces a lower relapse rate than autologous transplantation but survival is worse because of higher treatment related mortality – a report of 764 cases from the EBMT lymphoma registry. Blood 1997; 90(Suppl): 225a.
28. Sweetenham JW, Liberti G, Pearce R, Taghipour G, Santini G, Goldstone AH. High-dose therapy and autologous bone marrow transplantation for adult patients with lymphoblastic lymphoma: results of the European Group for Bone Marrow Transplantation. J Clin Oncol 1994; 12(7): 1358–65.
29. Vega F, Medeiros LJ, Gaulard P. Hepatosplenic and other gammadelta T cell lymphomas. Am J Clin Pathol 2007; 127(6): 869–80.
30. Hanson MN, *et al*. Posttransplant T cell lymphoproliferative disorders – an aggressive, late complication of solid-organ transplantation. Blood 1996; 88(9): 3626–33.
31. Belhadj K, *et al*. Hepatosplenic gammadelta T cell lymphoma is a rare clinicopathologic entity with poor outcome: report on a series of 21 patients. Blood 2003; 102(13): 4261–9.
32. Allory Y, *et al*. Bone marrow involvement in lymphomas with hemophagocytic syndrome at presentation: a clinicopathologic study of 11 patients in a Western institution. Am J Surg Pathol 2001; 25(7): 865–74.
33. Alonsozana EL, *et al*. Isochromosome 7q: the primary cytogenetic abnormality in hepatosplenic gammadelta T cell lymphoma. Leukemia 1997; 11(8): 1367–72.
34. Falchook GS, *et al*. Hepatosplenic gamma-delta T cell lymphoma: clinicopathological features and treatment. Ann Oncol 2009; 20(6): 1080–5.
35. Bennett M, Matutes E, Gaulard P. Hepatosplenic T cell lymphoma responsive to 2'-deoxycoformycin therapy. Am J Hematol 2010; 85(9): 727–9.

36. Grigg AP. 2'-Deoxycoformycin for hepatosplenic gammadelta T cell lymphoma. Leuk Lymphoma 2001; 42(4): 797–9.

37. Catassi C, Bearzi I, Holmes GK. Association of celiac disease and intestinal lymphomas and other cancers. Gastroenterology 2005; 128(4 Suppl 1): S79–86.

38. Sieniawski M, et al. Evaluation of enteropathy-associated T cell lymphoma comparing standard therapies with a novel regimen including autologous stem cell transplantation. Blood 2010; 115(18): 3664–70.

39. Verbeek WH, van de Water JM, Al-Toma A, Oudejans JJ, Mulder CJ, Coupe VM. Incidence of enteropathy-associated T cell lymphoma: a nation-wide study of a population-based registry in The Netherlands. Scand J Gastroenterol 2008; 43(11): 1322–8.

40. Delabie J, et al. Enteropathy-associated T cell lymphoma: clinical and histological findings from the international peripheral T cell lymphoma project. Blood 2011; 118(1): 148–55.

41. Van de Water JM, Cillessen SA, Visser OJ, Verbeek WH, Meijer CJ, Mulder CJ. Enteropathy associated T cell lymphoma and its precursor lesions. Best Pract Res Clin Gastroenterol 2010; 24(1): 43–56.

42. Green PH, Cellier C. Celiac disease. N Engl J Med 2007; 357(17): 1731–43.

43. Cellier C, et al. Refractory sprue, coeliac disease, and enteropathy-associated T cell lymphoma. French Coeliac Disease Study Group. Lancet 2000; 356(9225): 203–8.

44. Howdle PD, Jalal PK, Holmes GK, Houlston RS. Primary small-bowel malignancy in the UK and its association with coeliac disease. QJM 2003; 96(5): 345–53.

45. Holmes GK, Prior P, Lane MR, Pope D, Allan RN. Malignancy in coeliac disease – effect of a gluten free diet. Gut 1989; 30(3): 333–8.

46. Gale J, Simmonds PD, Mead GM, Sweetenham JW, Wright DH. Enteropathy-type intestinal T cell lymphoma: clinical features and treatment of 31 patients in a single center. J Clin Oncol 2000; 18(4): 795–803.

47. Deleeuw RJ, et al. Whole-genome analysis and HLA genotyping of enteropathy-type T cell lymphoma reveals 2 distinct lymphoma subtypes. Gastroenterology 2007; 132(5): 1902–11.

48. Rohatiner A, et al. Report on a workshop convened to discuss the pathological and staging classifications of gastrointestinal tract lymphoma. Ann Oncol 1994; 5(5): 397–400.

49. Zettl A, deLeeuw R, Haralambieva E, Mueller-Hermelink HK. Enteropathy-type T cell lymphoma. Am J Clin Pathol 2007; 127(5): 701–6.

50. Daum S, et al. Intestinal non-Hodgkin's lymphoma: a multicenter prospective clinical study from the German Study Group on Intestinal non-Hodgkin's Lymphoma. J Clin Oncol 2003; 21(14): 2740–6.

51. D'Amore F, Relander T, Lauritzen G, et al. Dose-dense induction followed by autologous stem cell transplant (ASCT) leads to sustained remissions in a large fraction of patients with previously untreated peripheral T cell lymphomas (PTCLs) – overall and subtype specific results of a phase II study from the Nordic Lymphoma Group. Haematologica 2009; 94[suppl.2]:437 abs. 1082.

52. Willemze R, Meijer CJ. Classification of cutaneous T cell lymphoma: from Alibert to WHO-EORTC. J Cutan Pathol 2006; 33(Suppl 1): 18–26.

53. Willemze R, et al. Subcutaneous panniculitis-like T cell lymphoma: definition, classification, and prognostic factors: an EORTC Cutaneous Lymphoma Group Study of 83 cases. Blood 2008; 111(2): 838–45.

54. Go RS, Wester SM. Immunophenotypic and molecular features, clinical outcomes, treatments, and prognostic factors associated with subcutaneous panniculitis-like T cell lymphoma: a systematic analysis of 156 patients reported in the literature. Cancer 2004; 101(6): 1404–13.

55. Koh MJ, et al. Aggressive subcutaneous panniculitis-like T cell lymphoma with hemophagocytosis in two children (subcutaneous panniculitis-like T cell lymphoma). J Am Acad Dermatol 2009; 61(5): 875–81.

56. Hahtola S, et al. Clinicopathological characterization and genomic aberrations in subcutaneous panniculitis-like T cell lymphoma. J Invest Dermatol 2008; 128(9): 2304–9.

57. Hahtola S, et al. Th1 response and cytotoxicity genes are down-regulated in cutaneous T cell lymphoma. Clin Cancer Res 2006; 12(16): 4812–21.

58. Mao X, et al. Molecular cytogenetic analysis of cutaneous T cell lymphomas: identification of common genetic alterations in Sezary syndrome and mycosis fungoides. Br J Dermatol 2002; 147(3): 464–75.

59. Karenko L, Kahkonen M, Hyytinen ER, Lindlof M, Ranki A. Notable losses at specific regions of chromosomes 10q and 13q in the Sezary syndrome detected by comparative genomic hybridization. J Invest Dermatol 1999; 112(3): 392–5.

60. Massone C, et al. Subcutaneous, blastic natural killer (NK), NK/T cell, and other cytotoxic lymphomas of the skin: a morphologic, immunophenotypic, and molecular study of 50 patients. Am J Surg Pathol 2004; 28.

49 Unusual Cutaneous Malignancies

Sara Peters[1] and Thomas Olencki[2]

[1] Department of Pathology, [2] Department of Internal Medicine, The Ohio State University, Columbus, OH, USA

Introduction

In this chapter, we have attempted to review the patterns of presentation of a protean group of tumors, linked by their initial presentation within the skin but representing a range of different embryological and histogenetic origins, patterns of presentation, and approaches to treatment. As will be seen, we have attempted to cover what is known about each tumor, and have been careful to try to identify the benefits and drawbacks of different diagnostic and therapeutic approaches, focusing wherever possible on evidence-based medicine. As there is a paucity of large series and level 1–2 evidence regarding management, we have attempted to avoid spurious recommendations based only on anecdotal evidence.

Tumors of the epidermis and epidermal appendages

Hair follicle and hair matrix tumors

Trichilemmal carcinoma

This extremely rare tumor arises from the external root sheet of the hair follicle and characteristically presents as a solitary ulcerating lesion on sun-exposed skin of the elderly; however, it can rarely present as multiple tumors.[1] Clinically it has been misdiagnosed as a basal cell carcinoma. The lesion is composed of large cells with periodic acid-Schiff (PAS)-positive, diastase-sensitive clear cytoplasm with central trichilemmal keratinization invading downward from the epidermis or from the external root sheath in a multilobular, trabecular of diffuse pattern of growth.[2] Most lesions have an indolent clinical course but perineural invasion, recurrence and metastases, although uncommon, have been described.[3,4]

Wide surgical excision with clear margins is the current treatment of choice. However, as the margins of the tumor may extend beyond what is clinically detectable, Mohs micrographic surgery has also been used without signs of recurrence.[5,6] Recently, there has been a report on the use of imiquimod 5% cream as sole therapy with complete pathological response.[7]

Pilomatrix carcinoma (pilomatricarcinoma)

This rare follicular tumor presents a rapidly growing, firm nodule that usually arises *de novo* but in some cases may arise in a pilomatrixoma or at the site of a previously excised pilomatrixoma.[8] The cancer commonly arises on the scalp and face of elderly males and has a propensity for recurrence. Distant metastases can occur.[9]

Histological examination shows a poorly circumscribed neoplasm composed of pleomorphic basaloid cells. Mitotic figures and atypical mitotic figures are common. Anucleate "shadow" cells are present within nests of basaloid cells.[10] Mutations in the *CTNNB1* gene that encodes β-catenin have been reported in most cases of pilomatrix carcinoma and in pilomatrixomas. Both entities are frequently found in Gardner syndrome because they have a similar pathogenesis.[11]

Wide local excision is required with regular follow-up because of concerns for local and distant recurrence.[11] However, because local recurrence can be devastating, Mohs micrographic surgery has been proposed as the new standard of care for primary excision.[11] Adjuvant radiation therapy may be considered when surgical margins are equivocal[11] and there are several case reports indicating the local activity of radiotherapy, including electron beam therapy, in locally recurrent cases. Chemotherapy is inactive and has no defined therapeutic role; the anecdotal case literature is replete with single cases showing resistance to a range of chemotherapy options.

Sebaceous gland tumors

Sebaceous carcinoma

Sebaceous carcinomas are rare neoplasms that most commonly arise in ocular and extraocular adnexal structures including meibomian glands and glands of Zeiss; however, extraocular sebaceous carcinomas also occur, especially in the head and

Textbook of Uncommon Cancer, Fourth Edition. Edited by Derek Raghavan, Charles D. Blanke, David H. Johnson, Paul L. Moots, Gregory H. Reaman, Peter G. Rose and Mikkael A. Sekeres.

neck areas of the elderly.[12] Although extraocular sebaceous carcinomas were thought to be less aggressive than the ocular variant, more recent studies have concluded that extraocular tumors are also associated with metastasis and significant mortality.[12] Ocular sebaceous carcinoma most commonly arises in meibomian glands of the tarsus and less commonly in the glands of Zeis, lacrimal glands or the lacrimal caruncle. Lesions are commonly firm and solitary with a nonspecific clinical appearance and occur in older patients, especially women. Ocular sebaceous carcinoma is frequently mistaken for a chalazion or an inflammatory disorder such as blepharitis or keratoconjunctivitis, and delayed diagnosis is not uncommon.[12]

Approximately 20% of sebaceous carcinomas occur in extraocular sites, with most presenting on the head and neck of the elderly. Less common sites of presentation include leg, foot, vulva, salivary glands, and bronchus.[13,14] Sebaceous carcinomas have been associated with prior radiation exposure to the face, immunosuppressive therapy after renal transplantation and with Muir–Torre syndrome, an autosomal dominant syndrome characterized by the presence of sebaceous gland neoplasms and visceral malignancies.[15–18] It has also been more broadly associated with Lynch syndrome, characterized by a variety of tumors occurring before age 44.[19] These include carcinomas of the right colon, endometrium, ovary, breast, stomach, small bowel, pancreas, hepatobiliary structures, ureter, and renal pelvis. Studies of DNA mismatch repair gene abnormalities associated with Lynch syndrome in sebaceous carcinomas have been inconclusive. Nevertheless, diagnosis of sebaceous gland carcinoma should prompt a consideration of these syndromes and an investigation for an internal malignancy.

Sebaceous carcinoma consists of lobules of small epithelioid cells with variable sebaceous differentiation in a fibrovascular stroma. Infiltrative nests and cords of lesional cells are present often at the periphery of the lesion. Mitoses and areas of necrosis may be present. Periocular sebaceous carcinomas often extend into the overlying epidermis or into conjunctival epithelium. Lesional cells are positive for epithelial membrane antigen (EMA) and androgen receptor (AR) and are negative for S-100, carcinoembryonic antigen (CEA), and gross cystic disease fluid protein 15 (GCDFP-15). In some reports tumor cells have been positive for Cam 5.2 and BRST-1. Ocular sebaceous carcinomas are positive for cytokeratin 7 (CK7). Negative histological prognostic factors include pagetoid extension into the epidermis, lymphatic and/or vascular invasion, poorly differentiated lesional cells, and an infiltrative pattern of growth.[12]

Sebaceous carcinoma is characterized by frequent recurrences (40% of patients) and a tendency to metastasize (18–25% of cases).[12,20] Long-term survival is reported in approximately 30% of patients. Poor outcome is associated with involvement of both upper and lower eyelids, orbital extension, duration of symptoms greater than 6 months, and tumor diameter exceeding 10 mm.[12]

Complete excision remains the treatment of choice because many of the tumors are periocular and clear margins are critical; Mohs micrographic surgery has become the modality of choice.[12,21] The benefit of radiation therapy as adjuvant or for unresectable disease remains uncertain. No chemotherapy has been shown to be reliably effective for regional or metastatic disease, and the majority of published case reports relate to neoadjuvant or adjuvant use in unstructured and uninterpretable settings.

Sweat gland carcinomas with apocrine differentiation

Apocrine carcinoma (apocrine adenocarcinoma)

Apocrine carcinoma is a rare sweat gland neoplasm that occurs most commonly in the axilla, usually in middle-aged to older women. Other sites of involvement include the anogenital region, scalp, eyelid, ear, chest, wrist, lip, foot, toe, and finger.[22] These lesions classically present as slow-growing, painless, colorless to reddish firm nodules. More than 50% of patients with apocrine carcinoma have lymph node metastasis at the time of diagnosis. Death has been reported in approximately 40% of cases, usually from visceral metastases.

Histological examination reveals a nonencapsulated tumor composed of solid, ductal, cord-like and glandular areas composed of epithelioid cells with eosinophilic cytoplasm. Some of the lesional cells may demonstrate decapitation secretion. Cellular and nuclear atypia are variable. The cells are immunohistochemically positive for Cam 5.2, CKAE1/AE3, EMA, CK15, and GCDFP-15. CEA expression is variable.

Therapy is discussed under the heading of eccrine porocarcinoma.

Sweat gland carcinomas with eccrine differentiation

Eccrine ductal carcinoma

Eccrine ductal carcinomas are rare neoplasms that occur as firm nodules primarily on the head and neck and extremities of middle-aged to elderly patients. Recurrences are common and metastases occur in a high percentage of patients (57% in one study), with an overall mortality rate of 70%.[23,24]

Microscopically eccrine ductal carcinomas are composed of nests and cords of small epithelioid cells in the dermis in a background of fibrosis. Lesional cells exhibit extensive ductal differentiation. Perineural and lymphovascular invasion are common. Tumor cells are positive for CAM 5.2 and CEA. Variable positivity for S-100, GCDFP-15, estrogen receptor (ER), progesterone receptor (PR) and Her-2-neu has been reported. Microscopically and immunohistochemically, it is not possible to distinguish eccrine ductal carcinoma from metastatic breast carcinoma and metastatic carcinoma from the large bowel involving skin. Before a diagnosis of eccrine ductal carcinoma can be made, it is necessary to exclude a visceral adenocarcinoma metastatic to skin.

Therapy is discussed under the heading of eccrine porocarcinoma.

Eccrine porocarcinoma (malignant eccrine poroma)

Eccrine porocarcinoma arises from the intraepidermal component of the eccrine duct or, less commonly, from an underlying eccrine poroma.[24] The tumor presents as an exophytic growth, most commonly on the lower extremities, trunk, head, and upper extremities of elderly patients. There is a slight female predilection. Local recurrence and metastatic spread to regional lymph nodes are not uncommon. Distant metastases have been reported in approximately 11% of cases studied.[25,26]

Histologically porocarcinoma is characterized by nests of characteristic small poromatous basaloid epithelial cells displaying foci of ductal differentiation in the epidermis. Nests and cords of lesional cells extend into the dermis. Areas of clear cell change, ductal differentiation, and squamous differentiation can be present in the dermis. Mature, well-formed eccrine ducts having an eosinophilic luminal cuticle are found in more than two-thirds of cases. The remaining lesions contain intracytoplasmic lumina and/or small, ill-formed ducts.[27] Lesional cells express pancytokeratin, CEA, CK5/6, and EMA. Most porocarcinomas express p16. Unfavorable histological prognostic features include mitotic activity, lymphovascular and/or perineural invasion, and depth of invasion.

Therapy for apocrine carcinoma, eccrine ductal carcinoma, and eccrine porocarcinoma is surgical excision with clear margins. Both wide surgical excision and Mohs micrographic surgery have been used with success.[28–30] One surgical oncology group has advocated use of lymphoscintigraphy and sentinel lymph node biopsy in most patients with these subtypes, especially those with angiolymphatic invasion in the primary.[30] There are rare single case reports of response to chemotherapy. Overall, there is no evidence that chemotherapy has any reproducible or definitive role in treatment of this cancer. One interesting case report indicated a sustained remission from single-agent docetaxel in a patient previously resistant to anthracycline therapy,[31] but again this was simply anecdotal information.

Malignant hidradenoma (hidradenocarcinoma, clear cell hidradenocarcinoma, malignant acrospiroma)

Malignant hidradenoma is a rare sweat gland neoplasm that usually presents as an ulcerated nodule on the face and extremities of older patients, although the age range is wide. Hidradenocarcinoma rarely arises from a preexisting hidradenoma.[32]

On histological examination, the lesion is composed of lobules and sheets of glycogen-rich cells in the dermis. Areas of basaloid or squamous differentiation can be prominent. Nuclear pleomorphism, mitotic activity and necrosis are variable. Cytoplasmic vacuoles that in areas coalesce to form ductal structures are characteristic. Some lesions demonstrate deceptively bland cytological features while others demonstrate nuclear pleomorphism. Lesional cells are positive for AE1/AE3, CK5/6, and Ki-67 and some lesions express nuclear p53. Staining for CEA, S-100 protein, and EMA has been inconsistent. Because some lesions are composed of small bland-appearing cells, a careful search for lymphovascular and perineural invasion characteristic of malignancy is necessary.

Malignant hidradenomas can be aggressive, and recurrence and lymph node, bone, and pulmonary metastases have been reported.[33] Treatment recommendations of this entity are identical to those for the eccrine carcinomas.

Aggressive digital papillary adenocarcinoma

Aggressive digital papillary adenocarcinoma (ADPA) is a rare sweat gland carcinoma of the digits with high local recurrence rates and the potential for highly aggressive biological behavior. Aggressive digital papillary adenocarcinoma characteristically occurs as a solitary, rubbery, painless mass on the fingers and toes and adjacent skin of the palms and soles. This presentation often leads to diagnostic delay. The most common site of occurrence is the volar aspect of the tip of the digit between the nail bed and distal interphalangeal joint.[34,35] Metastases, even from low-grade lesions, have been documented.[35] Both sexes, at any age, are affected.

Histopathology reveals a poorly circumscribed lesion in the dermis with frequent extension into the subcutis composed of multiple cystic nodules made up of cuboidal and columnar cells. Papillary structures lined by multiple layers of basaloid epithelioid cells project into the cystic cavities. Ductal and cribriform structures are present and in some areas solid nodules of lesional cells may be present. Nuclear pleomorphism, mitotic activity, and necrosis can be variable.[34] Lesional cells are strongly positive for cytokeratins and S-100 protein. Lesional cells are also positive for CEA, especially for the luminal cells in the cystic areas.

Aggressive primary surgical treatment is advised. Usually amputation of the involved digit with prior lymphoscintigraphy and sentinel lymph node biopsy has been suggested.[36] However, in those patients with long-standing low-grade disease, wide excision may be all that is necessary.[37] There are no definitive data regarding adjuvant chemotherapy or radiation therapy, nor is there level 1–2 information regarding optimal management of metastatic and recurrent disease.

Malignant cylindroma

Malignant cylindroma is a very rare, focally aggressive tumor that commonly arises from a preexisting cylindroma on the head and neck, particularly the scalp, in elderly patients. Malignant cylindromas are slightly more common in females than males. Malignant cylindromas can arise in lesions of familial cylindromatosis (Brooke–Spiegler syndrome), a rare autosomal dominant disease characterized by multiple cylindromas, trichoepitheliomas, and spiradenomas.[38] Malignant cylindromas are high-grade, aggressive neoplasms with a recurrence rate of approximately 40% and a metastatic rate up to 70%.[39]

Histologically, the tumors usually exhibit a transitional zone between benign cylindroma and areas of clear malignant transformation. Mitotic activity, cytological atypia, loss of mosaic appearance, and an invasive pattern of growth are identified in malignant foci.[38] Lymphovascular and/or perineural invasion are histological features associated with an aggressive clinical course. Lesional cells are positive for Cam 5.2, EMA, and CEA. Lesional cells variably express S-100 protein and GCDFP-15.[40,41] Recommendations for therapy include wide excision or Mohs micrographic surgery. Because of the high rate of local recurrence, initial complete resection is extremely important.[39] Use of radiation therapy may occasionally address local recurrence, although the role for adjuvant therapy remains unclear. Similarly, there is no definitive literature on the use of systemic chemotherapy for this condition.. The low number of reported cases (less than 100) explains the lack of specific recommendations.[39]

For patients with unresectable disease, treatment on an investigational protocol is recommended.

Eccrine spiradenocarcinoma (malignant eccrine spiradenoma)

Eccrine spiradenocarcinomas are very rare sweat gland neoplasms that arise from a preexisting eccrine spiradenoma. A relatively large series reported 12 cases with equal sex distribution and a mean age of 62 years. Large nodular lesions, some of which had been present for months to years, were noted on the trunk and occasionally on the extremities and head and neck regions.[42] Lesions are reportedly aggressive, with a metastatic rate of approximately 30–40%.[43–46]

Histologically, areas of malignant change are present in a benign spiradenoma. Features of malignancy include nuclear pleomorphism, increased mitotic activity, necrosis, infiltrating pattern of growth, lymphovascular and perineural invasion and loss of two distinct populations of tumor cells. Some lesions are characterized by an abrupt transition between benign spiradenoma and frank malignancy. Other lesions, however, show minimal cytological and architectural atypia. Areas of spiradenoma express S-100 protein and Cam 5.2 while areas of ductal differentiation express CEA and EMA.[47] Malignant cells are positive for p53.

Therapy for this rare entity is identical to that for eccrine porocarcinoma, including strong consideration of lymphoscintigraphy and sentinel lymph node biopsy. As noted above, no definitive recommendations for systemic chemotherapy can be made, despite a profusion of isolated case reports that are difficult to interpret.

Microcystic adnexal carcinoma (sclerosing sweat duct carcinoma)

Microcystic adnexal carcinoma is a rare, locally aggressive sweat gland neoplasm that predominantly affects the cheek and upper lip of young and middle-aged adults. Occurrences at a wide variety of other sites have been reported. Histology shows small, usually superficial keratocysts, small ductal structures and infiltrative cords composed of small epithelial cells. Lesional cells stain positive for CKAE1/AE3. Ductal differentiation is highlighted by CEA and /or EMA. Lesional cells are negative for S-100 protein. Biopsy should include a deep specimen since clues to the diagnoses reside in identifying an infiltrative growth pattern, variable ductal differentiation, and prominent perineural invasion. Although microcystic adnexal carcinomas rarely metastasize, aggressive local growth and recurrence are not uncommon.

The management of these tumors is primarily surgical resection. Because the margins often extend beyond what is clinically appreciated, aggressive treatment by Mohs micrographic surgery appears to offer the greatest likelihood of cure while providing conservation of normal tissues.[48] It has been suggested that postoperative radiotherapy may improve local control for patients with high-risk tumors who have undergone surgical resection or Mohs surgery,[49] although this has not been

proven in randomized trials. For patients with unresectable disease, treatment on an investigational protocol is recommended as there are no definitive series indicating specific roles for radiotherapy or chemotherapy.

Primary mucinous carcinoma

Primary mucinous carcinoma is a slow-growing, flesh-colored erythematous or blue mucin-producing tumor arising as a painless nodule in the head and neck region, particularly in the eyelids.[50] Histology reveals clusters of tumor cells within abundant pools of mucin separated by thin fibrous septae.[51] Lesional cells are positive for CKAE1/AE3, CEA, EMA and CK7 and are negative for CK20. Cam 5.2 expression is variable.[52] Immunohistochemistry is necessary to distinguish primary cutaneous mucinous adenocarcinoma from metastatic adenocarcinomas, especially of breast or gastrointestinal origin to skin.[53]

Once again, the key to therapy is surgical resection. The low rate of metastatic disease and the tendency to affect the face have led many to recommend Mohs micrographic surgery as the best primary therapy for this skin cancer. For patients with unresectable disease, treatment on an investigational protocol is recommended.

Syringoid eccrine carcinoma (eccrine epithelioma)

This lesion was originally considered to be a basal cell carcinoma with eccrine differentiation.[54] It is an extremely rare, locally aggressive tumor commonly found on the scalp as a large, tender, and ulcerated plaque or nodule. Fewer than 20 cases have been reported in the literature. Histologically, the tumor consists of many small nests and cords of small basaloid epithelial cells with ductal differentiation reminiscent of syringoma in a prominent fibrous stroma. Lesional cells extend from the reticular dermis into subcutaneous tissue. Tumor cells are positive for high and low molecular weight cytokeratins and ductal structures are highlighted by CEA and EMA.[55]

As for the other skin cancers, the key to successful therapy is local surgical resection. Wide local excision with regular follow-up is required because there is chance of recurrence.[56] These tumors are uncommon and we know of no large radiotherapy or chemotherapy series to inform on the management of locally extensive or unresectable tumors.

Adenoid cystic carcinoma

Adenoid cystic carcinoma or primary cutaneous adenocystic carcinoma presents as a slow-growing painful nodule on the scalp and neck, and frequently in the oral cavity. Pathology shows large masses of cells with cytological atypia, arranged in a distinct adenoidal or cribriform pattern.[57] Lesional cells are positive for high and low molecular weight cytokeratins and S-100 protein. CEA and EMA highlight ductal structures. Perineural invasion is common and is associated with pain and an increased recurrence rate.[58] Metastases to local lymph nodes or lungs have been recorded.[59]

Combination treatment with initial wide resection followed by definitive radiation therapy is commonly used to control the subclinical perineural and perivascular infiltration. Chemotherapy is of uncertain benefit in the setting of metastatic disease. Perhaps the most useful analysis of systemic chemotherapy for adenoid cystic carcinomas is a metaanalysis, focused predominantly on tumors of the head and neck, performed by Laurie *et al.*[60] This analysis noted response rates in the range of 30–50% for several single agents, including cisplatin, carboplatin, doxorubicin, epirubicin, and mitoxantrone, but with generally short duration and median survival figures (where stated) of less than a year. Of an extensive range of combination regimens, the combination of a platinum complex with an anthracycline appeared to give the most consistent pattern of sustained response, but usually not longer than 1–2 years.[60] Although adenoid cystic carcinomas express c-kit, imatinib did not prove to be a reliably useful agent, despite occasional short-term responses.[60] Recently a single case report of disease control with sorafenib has been presented.[61]

Lymphoepithelioma-like carcinoma

Lymphoepithelioma (LE)-like carcinomas are characteristically seen in the nasopharynx, but a rare subtype originates in the skin as a nodule in the head and neck area of older individuals. Approximately 40 cases of cutaneous LE-like carcinoma have been reported. These are Epstein–Barr virus (EBV) negative and exhibit less aggressive behavior than those originating in the nasopharynx.[62]

Microscopic examination shows a lesion in the dermis and subcutis composed of nests, cords and strands of large epithelioid cells with vesicular nuclei and prominent nucleoli with an associated dense lymphoplasmacytic infiltrate. Lesional cells stain positive for cytokeratin and EMA. Negativity for EBV distinguishes LE-like carcinoma from metastatic undifferentiated carcinoma and metastatic LE-like carcinomas from other primary sites. Mitotic figures are found easily. Local recurrence and distant metastases are possible.

Treatment consists of wide total resection and adjuvant radiotherapy (RT).[63] In the uncommon situation of recurrent or metastatic disease, protocols adapted from the management of progressive pulmonary lymphoepitheliomas may have some utility, although there is no significant published experience in the setting of cutaneous disease.

Extramammary Paget disease

Extramammary Paget disease was originally described in 1889 by Crocker, who reported lesions on the scrotum and penis with histological features similar to those originally described by James Paget on the areola.[64] Extramammary Paget disease is a rare neoplasm that arises in areas of the body with prominent apocrine sweat glands. Extramammary Paget (EP) disease characteristically presents as slow-growing pruritic erythematous to red scaly plaques primarily in women in the sixth to eighth decades.[65] Repeated excoriations or superimposed infection can result in misdiagnosis of an inflammatory or infectious skin condition.

Histological examination shows large epithelioid cells with abundant (eosinophilic) cytoplasm and prominent vesicular nuclei in the epidermis, individually and in clusters. Primary extramammary Paget cells are usually positive for CK7 and negative for CK20, All extramammary Paget cells are negative for melanoma markers and *in situ* squamous cell cancer of the skin markers (p63). Primary extramammary Paget is thought to arise as an *in situ* cancer derived from the intraepithelial portion of apocrine ducts. Primary EP has a poor prognosis in the presence of dermal invasion because clear surgical margins, regardless of technique, are difficult to obtain.[66]

Mohs micrographic surgery, with a recurrence rate less than seen with standard surgery, may have evolved to be the resection method of choice.[67] In rare instances of confined disease, radical surgical resection may be considered. Imiquimod cream and photodynamic therapy have been used individually in limited *in situ* disease.[68,69] Radiation therapy may be effective in select cases of perineal disease.[70] For patients with unresectable disease, treatment on an investigational protocol is recommended whenever feasible.

Soft tissue tumors

Fibrous and myofibroblastic tumors

Dermatofibrosarcoma protuberans (see also Chapter 50)
Dermatofibrosarcoma protuberans (DFSP) is a rare cutaneous/subcutaneous soft tissue sarcoma. It characteristically develops on the trunk and extremities, with about 15% on the head and neck region. While predominantly found in young adults, occurrence in infants and young children has been reported. DFSP arises from a chromosomal translocation of chromosomes 17 and 22 t(17;22) that results in fusion of the platelet-derived growth factor β (PDGFβ) gene with the promoter collagen Type *1A1* gene.[71] This results in constitutive activation of the PDGF tyrosine kinase receptor, PDGFβ.[72] Early in the course of the tumor, there may be a narrow tumor-free, "Grenz zone" between the tumor and epidermis. Later DFSP is frequently fixed to underlying structures.

Uncommon variants include pigmented DFSP (Bednar tumor) with melanin-containing dendritic cells in between spindled lesional cells and myxoid DFSP with mucin between the spindled cells. Approximately 10–15% of DFSP contains elements of fibrosarcoma (DFSP-FS), a finding which increases the grade from low to intermediate and suggests a worse prognosis.[73]

Histologically, DFSP is composed of diffuse infiltration of the dermis and/or subcutis by monomorphic benign-appearing spindle cells arranged in a characteristic storiform pattern, sometimes around small vascular structures. It usually stains positive for CD34 and vimentin and negative for factor XIIIa, S-100 protein, smooth muscle actin (SMA), and desmin. In contradistinction, dermatofibroma usually stains positive for factor XIIIa and stromolysin and negative for CD34 and vimentin.[74,75]

Preoperative staging consists primarily of magnetic resonance imaging (MRI) of the affected area. A chest computed tomography (CT) scan may be considered if the patient has fibrosarcomatous elements or has had long-standing disease. In practice, the American Musculoskeletal Tumor Society (MSTS) staging system is often used: DFSP/DFSP-FS within a compartment that may be managed by wide excision alone is stage 1A. The same tumor that extends beyond a tissue compartment requiring extensive surgical resection is stage 1B.[76]

Definitive therapy for DFSP is surgical resection with pathologically negative margins. Size and location of the tumor determine whether traditional surgical resection or Mohs micrographic surgery (MMS) is most appropriate in a given patient.[74] Over time MMS, often with immunohistochemical stains, has evolved to become the mainstay of surgical resection. Use of this technique may also be integrated into the wide surgical resection approach to ensure good margin control. Because of undetectable subcutaneous migration of tumor, wide surgical margins of 2–4 cm are suggested by the National Comprehensive Cancer Network (NCCN). With MMS more tissue sparing can be accomplished with a more cosmetic closure. The accuracy of margin determination can be increased further with "slow Mohs" with final sections evaluated by fresh frozen paraffin embedded tissues stained with H&E and immunohistochemistry.[77–80] Clear margins are critical in this disease. Recurrent disease is more likely with microscopically positive or narrow margins of less than 1 mm.

Recurrent disease is an ominous event because it increases the likelihood of deep invasion, making resection even more difficult, as well as increasing the likelihood of metastasis. Recurrence is greater for DFSP-FS than DFSP. Most recurrences develop with 3 years of initial excision. In the setting of postsurgical narrow or positive margins, and when re-resection is not feasible to achieve negative margins, definitive adjuvant radiation therapy (doses of 50–64 Gy) is indicated.[74,81] Lymph node involvement is rare. Metastasis, primarily to the lungs, may occur in those individuals with multiple recurrent disease or individuals with DFSP-FS. Aggressive surgical resection of metastatic disease should be considered in those individuals with adequate performance status and when the likelihood of obtaining a clear margin is high.

For individuals with regionally advanced or metastatic disease, chemotherapy is no longer considered mainstream. Rather, therapy has now targeted the tyrosine kinase receptor PDGFβ. The constitutively activated PDGFβ tyrosine kinase receptor, secondary to the t(17;22) translocation, serves as a marker for those patients who may benefit from imatinib (Gleevec®). Imatinib, which inhibits PDGFβ, has been administered by mouth at 400 mg daily with variable success.[82,83] All reports have been small retrospective case series. No prospective studies documenting reproducible benefit in this disease have been published. The drug has been used in the neoadjuvant manner for 3–6 months to "debulk" regional advanced disease prior to possible resection and to treat metastatic disease.[74,84] Sunitinib and dasatininb have also been used in this setting.

Giant cell fibroblastoma

This locally recurrent fibroblastic tumor closely resembles DFSP and is even considered by some authorities to be the juvenile form of DFSP.[85] It usually presents as a slow-growing nodule or subcutaneous mass on the thumb or proximal extremities of male children under the age of 10.

Pathology reveals a lesion composed of bland to moderately atypical spindle and giant cells in a loose fibromyxoid stroma with variable collagen deposition, and dilated pseudovascular spaces irregularly lined by hyperchromatic spindle and/or multinucleated tumor cells.[86] Lesional cells stain positive for CD34 and CD99.

There is a close relationship between DFSP and giant cell fibroblastoma clinically, histologically, and molecularly.[87] Treatment of this entity should be identical to that for DFSP.

Epithelioid sarcoma

This tumor usually presents in young adults as a small, ulcerated, cutaneous nodule on the extremities, referred to as conventional type, and in the inguinal and pelvic regions, referred to as proximal type.[88] This sarcoma is unique in that it has no normal precursor counterpart. In greater than 90% of cases there is a characteristic loss of INI1 expression, a finding which is useful in making the diagnosis.[88]

Histologically, lesions consist of multiple nodules composed of epithelioid or spindle cells, often with central necrosis. Because lesion resemble granulomas, immunohistochemical staining is usually necessary. Immunohistochemical staining is commonly positive for INI1, vimentin, cytokeratin, EMA, and CA-125 and negative for S-100, actin, and CK5/6. Epithelioid sarcoma tends to grow along fascial planes, making resection difficult. Because of growth along fascial planes and because at least 35% of patients are found to have involved regional lymph nodes, this tumor has been associated with a high rate of local and regional recurrence.[89] Sentinel lymph node evaluation at presentation has been proposed to select patients who may benefit from complete lymph node dissection.

There is optimism that this aggressive surgical approach may decrease the high incidence of lung metastases seen with this tumor. Adjuvant radiation therapy has been suggested by some, but even retrospective data are sparse. Chemotherapy has been of minimal benefit for metastatic disease, and the role of imatinib and similar agents appears undefined.

Fibrohistiocytic tumors

Undifferentiated pleomorphic sarcoma (malignant fibrous histiocytoma)

Undifferentiated pleomorphic sarcoma (UPS)/malignant fibrous histiocytoma (MFH) is an anaplastic sarcoma composed of pleomorphic spindle and epithelioid cells derived from progenitor cells capable of fibroblastic or myofibroblastic differentiation.[90] It is a common sarcoma that occurs as an enlarging deep soft tissue mass, most often on the lower extremities, in middle-aged to older adults.[91] A few lesions occur superficially and are often initially diagnosed as atypical fibroxanthoma. Lesions are usually high grade and because the histological features of UPS/MFH can be found in many lesions of different lineage, diagnosis is one of exclusion.

Treatment consists of wide resection. Adjuvant radiation therapy is recommended if the tumor is greater than 5 cm in diameter, clear margins are less than 1 cm or microscopic positive margins are seen on pathological evaluation. Treatment of unresectable disease consists of appropriate chemotherapy regimens for soft tissue sarcoma. As for the ensuing variants of soft tissue sarcoma (below), there are no specific tailored chemotherapy regimens for any of these subtypes, and we believe it appropriate to approach such cases with relatively conventional sarcoma chemotherapy regimens or, if feasible, to enter patients into clinical trials. The role of imatinib and similar agents has not yet been defined.

Myxofibrosarcoma (myxoid malignant fibrous histiocytoma)

Myxofibrosarcoma is a relatively common neoplasm of dermal and subcutaneous tissues that presents as an asymptomatic growth in middle-aged or older adults on the extremities or the trunk.[91]

Distinctive histological features include a multinodular neoplasm composed of atypical fusiform, round, or stellate fibroblastic cells with indistinct cell margins in a myxoid stroma with characteristics of curvilinear vascular channels. Cells are positive for vimentin and some lesions demonstrate equivocal positivity for CD34 or SMA. Myxoid change should be seen in 10% or more of the tumor before a lesion can be classified as myxofibrosarcoma.[92] The grading of the tumor is particularly important because low-grade lesions typically recur while intermediate and high-grade lesions metastasize in 30–35% of cases.[93]

As with MFH, treatment consists of wide resection. Adjuvant radiation therapy is recommended if the tumor is greater than 5 cm in diameter, clear margins are less than 1 cm or microscopic positive margins are seen on pathological evaluation. Treatment of unresectable disease consists of appropriate sarcoma chemotherapy.

Angiomatoid fibrous histiocytoma

This rare low-grade tumor presents on the limbs or trunk of children and young adults as a slow-growing asymptomatic, blue or skin-colored, subcutaneous nodule. Some patients present with fever, malaise, and generalized lymphadenopathy, weight loss, paraproteinemia, and anemia.

On low-power examination, the tumor has sinusoidal spaces filled with red blood cells surrounded by nodules of spindle and round cells with ovoid vesicular nuclei. Approximately 50% of the lesional cells stain positive for desmin and msuscle-specific actin (MSA) (HHF35) but are negative for SMA. Variable staining for EMA, CD99, and CD68 has been reported.[94] A fusion of the *ATF1* gene on chromosome 12q13 with the FUS on chromosome 16p11 or EWSR1 gene on chromosome 22q12 has been reported and may be useful as a diagnostic tool.[95]

Treatment consists of surgery to achieve clear margins. The use of radiation therapy has been suggested, as presurgical or postsurgical therapy, to maximize margin control.[96] Treatment of unresectable disease consists of appropriate sarcoma chemotherapy.

Plexiform fibrohistiocytic tumor (plexiform fibrous histiocytoma)

This rare asymptomatic, indurated, solitary lesion occurs on the upper limbs of children and young adults with a slight female predominance. Lesions are usually poorly defined subcutaneous nodules or plaques although some lesions are dermal based.

Histopathology reveals two components, either of which can predominate in a given lesion: fascicles of bland, spindle-shaped fibroblastic/myofibroblastic cells and nodules of histiocyte-like cells with focal hemorrhage and hemosiderin deposition. The spindle-shaped cells stain focally for smooth muscle actin and calponin and the epithelioid and giant cells in the nodules are at least focally positive for CD68.[97,98] Therapy is complete surgical excision.[99] Treatment of unresectable disease consists of appropriate sarcoma chemotherapy.

Atypical fibroxanthoma

Atypical fibroxanthoma occurs as a frequently ulcerated firm nodule on sun-damaged skin of the head and neck of elderly patients, with a male predominance. Ultraviolet light-induced mutations of the *p53* gene, local skin trauma, and prior radiation exposure have all been implicated as possible causes.[100] If the lesion does not invade the muscle or the fascia, its clinical course is relatively benign.[101] Deeper, large lesions carry a worse prognosis with a 10% recurrence rate and a 1% distant metastasis rate.[102] A recent report concluded that the metastatic potential of atypical fibroxanthoma may be underestimated.[98,103]

Histologically, the tumor is composed of dense spindle-shaped cells, histiocytoid cells, xanthomatous cells, and multi-nucleated giant cells. Any or all of the cells may show marked pleomorphism, atypical mitoses, and nuclear hyperchromasia. A patchy chronic inflammatory infiltrate may be found, usually at the border of the lesion. Necrosis, perineural invasion or lymphovascular invasion is almost never present. The diagnosis can be confirmed with immunohistochemical studies that show that the spindle cells are positive for SMA and calponin and the multinucleate cells are variably positive for CD68. A number of other immuno stains have been reported as being focally positive for lesional cells. A minority of the lesional cells are positive for CD10. Atypical fibroxanthoma remains a diagnosis of exclusion. Spindle cell squamous cell carcinoma, malignant melanoma, and other spindle cell neoplasms must be excluded.[103]

Mohs micrographic surgery has evolved to be the therapy of choice.[103] Radiation therapy is used in the setting of locally recurrent disease.[103] We know of no published level 1–2 information regarding treatment of metastatic disease. Given that these tumors have relatively low metastatic potential, we believe it important to confirm the histology of lesions that might represent recurrence or metastasis before embarking on treatment.

Vascular tumors

Angiosarcoma

Angiosarcoma has also been referred to as hemangiosarcoma, malignant hemangioendothelioma, and hemangioblastoma. It is a malignant neoplasm composed of mesenchymal cells recapitulating vascular and lymphatic endothelial cells. This aggressive tumor tends to develop in three situations: as an idiopathic angiosarcoma of the head and neck in elderly individuals, as a lymphedema-associated angiosarcoma (Stewart–Treves syndrome), and as a postirradiation angiosarcoma.[104] Stewart–Treves syndrome was originally described in patients with iatrogenic lymphedema after radical mastectomy and axillary lymph node dissection for breast cancer.[104] However, it has also been observed in cases of lymphedema not associated with mastectomy, suggesting that it is chronic lymph stasis which in fact predisposes to the onset of angiosarcoma.[105] Postirradiation angiosarcoma primarily affects women with breast carcinoma who have undergone breast-sparing surgery. Lymphedema does not seem to contribute to the pathogenesis of this subtype, which is associated with chronic radiation dermatitis.[106]

Skin changes usually precede the diagnosis of angiosarcoma. The tumor occurs as bluish or purple nodules with purple discoloration of the skin, or as erythematous macules, frequently in combination with diffuse erythema.

The most common histological pattern is characterized by irregular anastomosing vascular channels lined by atypical endothelial cells, with some cases showing solid areas of lesional cells. The majority of lesional cells express CD34, CD31, FLI-1, and D2-40 and are negative for pancytokeratin and S-100. Expression of Ki-67 and cyclin-D1, markers of proliferative potential, is also elevated.

Advanced age, delay in diagnosis, and comorbid issues all contribute to the overall poor prognosis of this cancer.[107,108] Positive surgical margins and lack of adjuvant radiation therapy administration correlate with an adverse outcome. Size greater than 5 cm is another poor prognostic variable but is very hard to quantify.[107,108] Local recurrence and distant metastasis are major problems. Overall 5-year survival is around 30%.[105]

Chemotherapy may increase progression-free survival but not overall survival. The three most active regimens include weekly paclitaxel, doxorubicin, ifosfamide and mesna (AIM), and doxil with a median progression-free survival of 4.0–5.4 months.[108] Median survival for metastatic disease is 8.5 months.[108] Recently, in a phase 3 trial for soft tissue sarcoma failing at least one anthracycline regimen, patients were treated with a tyrosine kinase inhibitor and a progression-free survival of 13 months was seen.[109] It remains to be determined whether this class of drugs may have utility in this specific sarcoma.

Epithelioid angiosarcoma

Epithelioid angiosarcoma is an aggressive variant of angiosarcoma that is composed of large epithelioid cells that can mimic carcinoma on low-power histological examination. Epithelioid angiosarcoma develops in the deep dermis and occasionally in the skin. Unlike classic angiosarcoma, it can present as an asymptomatic hemorrhagic papule or nodule on the extremities of young to middle-aged males.[110] Rare cases associated with radiation or foreign bodies have been reported.[111]

Histological examination reveals atypical epithelioid cells with eosinophilic cytoplasm, intracytoplasmic vacuoles, vesicular nuclei, and prominent eosinophilic nucleoli.[112] Lesional cells are positive for CD31 while 50–60% stain positive for cytokeratin.

Therapy is the same as for angiosarcoma.

Malignant glomus tumor (glomangiosarcoma)

Malignant glomus tumor presents in older individuals as a painful mass, most frequently on the distal extremities.[113,114] These tumors have a considerable potential for metastasis,

with 12 of the reported 45 cases in one series having metastatic involvement.[114]

Histologically, it is composed of spindle or round cells, and numerous vascular components. The tumor cells are pleomorphic with large perivascular myoid cells with marked cytological atypia. Mitotic figures and necrosis are common. Lesional cells are positive for SMA, HCAD, and type IV collagen and are negative for CD34, desmin, pancytokeratin, and S-100.

Treatment recommendations are limited by the low number of recorded patients (less than 50). At this time primary therapy consists of complete resection by wide resection or Mohs micrographic surgery. No other treatment modality has been described to have a high level of anticancer activity.[113] For patients with unresectable disease, treatment on an investigational protocol is recommended when feasible.

Epithelioid hemangioendothelioma

Epithelioid hemangioendothelioma is an extremely rare vascular malignancy that rarely presents in the skin. The few reported cases of cutaneous epithelioid hemangioendothelioma in the literature describe a solitary, slightly raised, erythematous and sometimes painful dermal nodule. Sex distribution seems to be equal, with an age range of 21–84 years.[115] Approximately half of all lesions arise in or are associated with preexisting blood vessels.

Histologically, nodules composed of cords, strands or nests of rounded or slightly spindled epithelioid endothelial cells with eosinophilic cytoplasm are found embedded in a hyalinized or myxoid stroma.[116] Lesional cells often contain cytoplasmic vacuoles that may contain red blood cells. Obvious vascular channels are rare. Lesional cells are positive for CD31, CD34, D2-40, and FL-1 and are often positive for CD10. In up to 25% of cases, lesional cells express cytokeratin.

Treatment consists of resection with negative margins. For patients with unresectable or metastatic disease, treatment on an investigational protocol is recommended when feasible. Epithelioid hemangiomas occasionally metastasize from sites in the liver or lung, but there is a paucity of structured information about management, although there have been isolated case reports of the use of anthracylines, interferon-β, and recent use of tyrosine kinase inhibitors in view of the vascularity of the tumors.

Retiform hemangioendothelioma (hobnail hemangioendothelioma)

This locally aggressive neoplasm typically occurs in middle-aged adults and is more common in women than men; however, lesions have been reported in children.[117] Human herpesvirus-8 (HHV-8) was described in one case of retiform hemangioendothelioma but it does not appear to have an etiological role.[118] Microscopically, a diffuse and infiltrative lesion composed of long, arborizing blood vessels arranged in a retiform pattern lined by flattened endothelial cells with occasional hobnail appearance resembling rete testis is present in the dermis and is associated with a prominent lymphocytic infiltrate.[119] Lesional cells stain positive for CD31 and CD34.

Treatment consists of surgical resection to achieve negative margins. For patients with unresectable disease, there is no standard of care and we recommend treatment on a protocol if feasible. As these tumors are so rarely metastatic, the emphasis should be on local control.

Giant cell angioblastoma

This very rare pediatric tumor may be congenital or may present shortly after birth. Three case reports describe tumors arising on the hand, the palate, and the scalp. All tumors were ulcerated; lesions on the hand and palate also infiltrated soft tissue and bone.[120] Histologically, a concentric proliferation of oval to spindle-shaped cells around vascular channels is present. The oval to spindle cells are differentiated along the lines of pericytes and express smooth muscle actin while the cells lining the vascular channels express CD31 and factor VIII-related antigen. Commingled with these cells are large mononuclear and multinucleate giant cells with histiocytic features.[121]

Treatment consists of resection with negative margins. For patients with unresectable disease, treatment on a protocol is recommended.

Kaposiform hemangioendothelioma

Kaposiform hemangioendothelioma, also known as Kaposi-like infantile hemangioendothelioma, is a locally aggressive vascular neoplasm that normally occurs in the abdominal cavity but can affect the skin and the soft tissues.[122] Its name has been derived from features common to both hemangiomas and Kaposi sarcoma. Cutaneous lesions typically present as violaceous plaques in children and teenagers on the extremities and head and neck. More than half of the patients present with Kasabach–Merritt syndrome, a condition characterized by consumptive coagulopathy, profound thrombocytopenia, and life-threatening hemorrhage. This tumor is not associated with HHV-8, a finding which helps distinguish it from Kaposi sarcoma.[123]

Histologically, tumors consist of irregular nodules of compressed vascular channels resembling capillary hemangioma and areas of spindle cells resembling Kaposi sarcoma. Lymphatic channels occur frequently and are typically seen adjacent or deep to the main tumor mass. Lesional cells are positive for CD31, CD34, FLI-1, and D2-40 and are negative for GLUT-1. Regional lymph node metastases are rare and distant metastases have not been reported. Mortality is approximately 10% and is due to local tumor effects or to Kasabach–Merritt syndrome.[124]

Due to its rarity, therapy has been empiric and included complete excision by wide resection or Mohs micrographic surgery. A wide variety of ineffective medical therapy has been explored as well.[125]

Muscle tumors

Superficial leiomyosarcoma

Superficial leiomyosarcoma is a rare neoplasm of smooth muscle derivation that is subdivided into cutaneous and subcutaneous types because of their different prognostic implications.[122] The cutaneous form is believed to derive from the erector pili muscle of the hair follicle or genital dartos muscle, whereas the subcutaneous type is thought to arise from the smooth muscle wall of blood vessels.[126] Although this tumor is most frequent in middle-aged adults, it can develop in infants and the elderly.[127] The lesions are usually solitary, but may occasionally appear as grouped nodules. Overlying skin discoloration and pain with pressure are reported in the majority of cases.[128]

Histologically, superficial leiomyosarcomas are large, poorly circumscribed dermal proliferations composed of fascicles of elongated spindle cells with eosinophilic cytoplasm and elongated blunt-ended nuclei. Lesional cells are positive for desmin, SMA, and MSA. Nuclear pleomorphism, mitotic activity greater than that allowable in leiomyomas and necrosis may be present.[127] The histological differential diagnosis must take into account the possibility of a metastasis from an extracutaneous site, such as the uterus.

The local recurrence rate for cutaneous leiomyosarcoma in the current literature is low. Mohs micrographic surgery and definitive margin determination appear to have made a significant contribution to this low rate.[129] This subtype is thought to rarely if ever metastasize. Because some authors claim that metastases do not occur and others report rare metastases, it has been suggested that these lesions be termed "atypical smooth muscle tumors."[94] Subcutaneous leiomyosarcomas, on the other hand, recur locally in 70% of cases, with metastases occurring in about 30–40%.

Surgical resection of this subtype may be with wide resection or MMS. Uncertainty remains regarding the optimal margin width. Adjuvant external beam radiation therapy has been recommended for high-grade variants of either subtype.[129] Recurrences most frequently develop in a 1–5-year period after initial surgery, and positive margins are the most important risk factor for recurrence.[126] Treatment of unresectable disease consists of appropriate sarcoma chemotherapy.

Cutaneous rhabdomyosarcoma

Only few cases of primary cutaneous rhabdomyosarcoma have been reported in the literature.[130] The lesion is found most commonly in neonates and children and presents as a solitary skin lesion on the face[131] (see also Chapter 70). Histology shows a diffuse dermal infiltrate composed of poorly differentiated cells, with foci of confluent aggregates in a vague alveolar pattern. Lesional cells are small and round with hyperchromatic nuclei and pale cytoplasm. Tumor cells are positive for desmin, CD56, myo-D1 and myogenin and are focally positive for smooth muscle actin.[130] Treatment of this tumor is highly complex and specifics need to be discussed with physicians who specialize in sarcoma therapy.

Fat cell tumors

Liposarcoma

Primary liposarcoma of the skin is extremely uncommon.[132] In the largest series to date involving seven patients, the tumor occurred in patients ranging in age from 39 to 95 years (median 72 years) with an equal sex distribution. The scalp and the extremities were the most common sites of involvement.[133] Clinically the tumor presents as a polypoid nodule.

Histology is characterized by a proliferation of relatively mature adipocytes with variation in cell size and shape, with scattered vacuolated lipoblasts.[134] Lesional cells usually stain positive for CDK4 and MDM2. Primary myxoid and pleomorphic variants of liposarcoma rarely involve skin. Soft tissue pathology texts should be consulted when the differential diagnosis includes these variants.

Treatment consists of wide resection. Adjuvant radiation therapy is recommended if the tumor is greater than 5 cm in diameter, clear margins are less than 1 cm or microscopic positive margins are seen on pathological evaluation. Treatment of unresectable disease consists of appropriate sarcoma chemotherapy.

Merkel cell carcinoma

Merkel cell carcinoma (MCC) is an aggressive cutaneous small cell undifferentiated neuroendocrine carcinoma of neural crest origin that usually presents as a small painless nodule on sun-damaged skin (Fig. 49.1). The cancer cells were originally described by Toker in 1972, and in 1978 Tang and Toker detected neurosecretory granules within the cells.[135,136] In 1980, the term Merkel cell cancer was proposed because of the similarity of the tumor cells to normal Merkel cells.[137] Normal Merkel cells function to transduce the mechanical function of touch to electrical stimuli traveling to sensory organs. Approximately 1500 new patients are diagnosed yearly. Since the 1990s, the incidence appears to be increasing yearly for an as yet unknown reason. The availability of more accurate immunohistochemistry has been considered as one possibility.

Risk factors for the development of the disease include age greater than 65 years, significant ultraviolet light exposure from sun or PUVA (psoralen and ultraviolet light A), prior radiation therapy or thermal burns, prior diagnosis of skin malignancy or immunosuppression including HIV (8× risk), solid organ transplant (10× risk) or chronic lymphocyte lymphoma (34–48× risk).[138] A recently discovered polyoma virus termed Merkel cell virus (MCV) has been found integrated into the DNA of Merkel cell cancer, in both primary and metastatic lesions.[139–141] It is a circular double-stranded DNA virus found in 80% of Merkel cancers. The viral load is 60 times greater in Merkel cell cancer than the normal host cells. Interestingly, the specific DNA composition and viral load have not changed significantly over the past 26 years. Uncertainty remains as to what, if any, role the virus has in the development and maintenance of the cancer. Eighty-eight percent of the general population has been exposed to the virus and it is also found in other cancers such as small cell of the lung (40%) and squamous cell carcinoma of the skin (20%) and adjacent normal skin. Those patients with viral integration in their Merkel cell carcinoma appear to have a better prognosis. Currently, the virus is a topic of research but has no role in the diagnosis or treatment of Merkel cell cancer.

Given the predilection for development on sun-exposed sites, Merkel cell carcinoma is most commonly found on the face, scalp, and neck followed by the upper extremities and shoulder, then lower extremities and buttocks and finally trunk. Ten percent of cases have no known primary. The mnemonic "A, E, I, O, U" (Asymptomatic, Expanding rapidly, Immune suppression, Older than 50, and UV light/fair skin) has been proposed as a clinical diagnostic aid.[142]

Pathological diagnosis is made on hematoxylin and eosin-stained sections as well as on immunoperoxidase-stained slides (Fig. 49.2). The lesion consists of nests and sheets and/or trabeculae composed of basaloid epithelioid cells with scant cytoplasm and nuclei with "watery" to punctate chromatin. A perinuclear dot-like positivity for CK20 is often the histological hallmark of diagnosis.[141] However, a minority of Merkel cell cancers may be CK20 negative, and chromogranin, neuron-specific enolase, and synaptophysin may be variably present.[143] In many cases CKAE1/AE3 is positive in a perinuclear dot-like pattern. Neural cell adhesion molecule (CD56) and c-kit (CD117) are sensitive but not specific markers. Markers for melanoma and lymphoma must be negative (Table 49.1).

Merkel cell cancer must be distinguished from metastatic neuroendocrine carcinoma from other primary sites. Negative

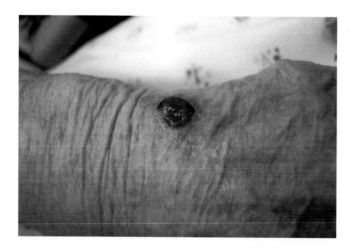

Figure 49.1 Appearance of an ulcerated 1 cm Merkel cell carcinoma on the wrist of an 83-year-old woman.

Table 49.1 Immunohistochemistry of Merkel cell cancer.

Tumor	AE1/AE3	CK20	NEM*	CK7	TTF-1	CD45	S-100/HMB-45
MCC	+	+	+/–	–	–		
SCLC	+	+/–	+	+	+		
Lymphoma						+	
Melanoma							+

*Neuroendocrine markers: chromogranin, neuron-specific enolase, synaptophysin.
MCC, Merkel cell carcinoma; SCLC, small cell lung cancer.
Adapted from MCC-Seattle Cancer Care Alliance: www.merkelcell.org.

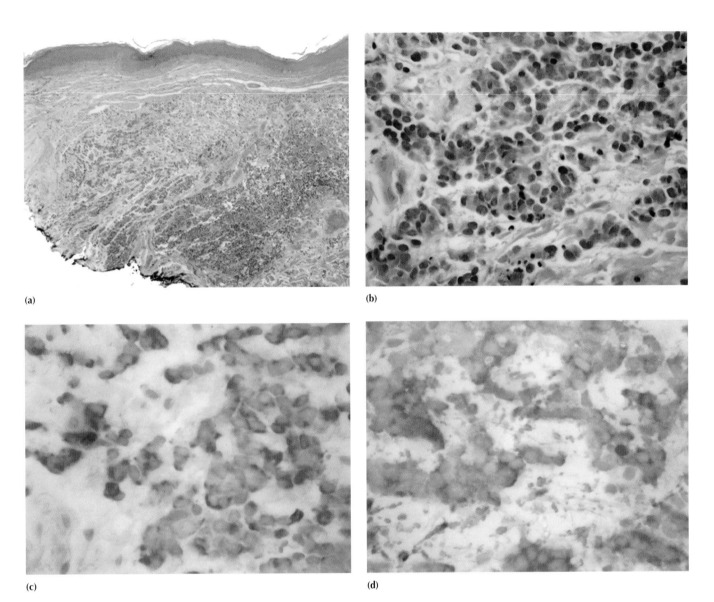

(a)

(b)

(c)

(d)

Figure 49.2 Histology of Merkel cell carcinoma. An 85-year-old man presented with a papule on the scalp, with a clinical impression of basal cell carcinoma. (a) Within the dermis are infiltrative aggregates and (b) strands of neoplastic small blue cells with a high nuclear:cytoplasmic ratio, "salt and pepper" chromatin pattern, and nuclear molding. Scattered apoptotic bodies are seen. (c) Tumor cells demonstrate strong perinuclear "dot" and cytoplasmic immunoreactivity with CK20 and (d) cytoplasmic immunoreactivity with CD117. The tumor cells showed no immunoreactivity with thyroid transcription factor-1 (*not shown*).

staining for TTF-1 distinguishes Merkel cell carcinoma from metastatic small cell lung cancer.

Staging has been updated and simplified.[144] A prospective evaluation of 5823 patients with a mean follow-up of 64 months led to the current system. The larger the diameter of the primary, the worse the prognosis. Lymph node status is prefixed by "c," meaning after clinical evaluation/palpation, and "p," meaning after surgery and pathological review. Suffixes of "a" and "b" imply, respectively, after surgical/pathological review and after clinical evaluation. Unlike the situation in melanoma, metastatic subset staging has no prognostic significance. Overall survival is measured at 5 years, instead of 10 years as with melanoma, as Merkel cell has more than twice the mortality of melanoma (Tables 49.2, 49.3).

Mostly due to the low incidence, definitive prospective randomized trials have not been conducted in Merkel cell carcinoma as they have for other more common tumor types. Consequently, there is wide variability in therapy. Treatment of the primary site is surgical resection. Some physicians use MMS and others rely on traditional surgical resection. Clear margin width has varied from margin negative to 2 cm (cm).[145,146]

Adjuvant RT to the primary has been reported, but extraordinary variability occurs in actual practice. Some centers recommend no adjuvant RT, whereas others recommend RT to all except for those situations where the primary is less than 1 cm diameter and margins are negative. Another center suggests RT if the primary is greater than 2 cm, margins are positive or if the primary is less than 2 cm and angiolymphatic invasion is seen. Finally another center recommends RT to 50–54 Gy if margins are negative, 54–60 Gy if margins are microscopically positive and 60–66 Gy if margins are grossly positive.[145–147]

As with melanoma, the pathological status of the regional lymph nodes is the most significant prognostic factor of overall survival by multivariate analysis. It is widely agreed that the sentinel lymph node biopsy (SLNBx) will not increase overall survival but it will give prognostic information that will help patients plan for their future. Sentinel lymph node biopsy status will help physicians treat patients with minimal toxicity and maximal benefit and facilitate the development of trials which will yield meaningful information for care of

future patients. Five-year overall survival of patients with a negative sentinel lymph node biopsy is close to 97% whereas with a positive biopsy it is close to 52%.[146]

Data are being accumulated to correlate tumor diameter with sentinel lymph node recovery but at this time, there is no size below which a SLNBx is not recommended (personal communication with Chris Bichakjian MD, Director, Multidisciplinary Merkel Cell Carcinoma Program, University of Michigan, Ann Arbor, Michigan). If a SLNBx is negative, the regional lymph node basin requires no further therapy (a minority of clinicians will recommend bilateral head and neck radiation in the setting of a negative SLNBx in the head and neck region). If the SLNBx is positive, a completion lymph node dissection is recommended.

Adjuvant RT may be considered to the regional lymph node basin instead of surgery if the patient is too frail or refuses to undergo SLNBx. Doses recommended by the NCCN include 46–50 Gy if the basin is clinically negative. If the basin has palpable lymph nodes or they are seen on CT scan, then 60–66 Gy is suggested. One center suggests RT to all patients except those with a primary smaller than 1 cm, negative margins, and negative SLNBx.

The administration of adjuvant chemotherapy remains controversial as no well-powered prospective randomized studies have been completed. While toxicity has been minimized in the current era, the lack of efficacy data predominates. Some medical oncologists will consider 4–6 cycles of cisplatin and etoposide in younger patients with resected high-risk disease. The rationale is that in the setting of inadvertently resected small cell lung cancer (which has histological resemblance to Merkel cell cancer), the same chemotherapy would be considered the standard of care.

Therapy for metastatic Merkel cell cancer remains poorly defined and investigational. Traditionally first-line therapy has consisted of cisplatin and etoposide for 4–6 cycles. Responses, however, have been poorly characterized and of brief duration. Use of imatinib has been attempted but patients were not selected for mutated c-kit and the response rate and duration were poor.[148] Because many of the patients who develop metastatic Merkel cell cancer are elderly and of borderline performance status, new effective agents are sorely needed. Ideally patients with metastatic disease should be treated on clinical trials.

Table 49.2 Merkel cell cancer AJCC staging system.

Tumor classification	Based on tumor diameter
T1	≤2.0 cm
T2	>2.0 but ≤5 cm
T3	>5.0 cm
T4	Directly invades adjacent organ(s)

Lymph node classification		
N0 → 0 LN	cN0	By clinical exam
	pN0	By SLNBx
N1 → ≥1 LN	cN1	Nodes clinically detectable
	N1a	Micrometastasis by SLNBx
	N1b	Micrometastasis by clinical then surgery
N2	N2	In transit metastasis

Metastasis classification	
M1a	Distant skin, SQ or LN
M1b	Lung metastasis
M1c	Visceral/distant LN

Terms M1a–c are descriptive only with no survival difference.
Adapted from the *American Joint Committee on Cancer Staging Manual*, 7th edn, 2010.
LN, lymph node; SLNBx, sentinal lymph node biopsy; SQ, subcutaneous tissue.
Reproduced from Edge *et al.*[164] Used with the permission of the American Joint Committee on Cancer (AJCC), Chicago, Illinois. The original source for this material is the AJCC Cancer Staging Manual, 7th edn (2010) published by Springer Science and Business Media LLC, www.springer.com.

Table 49.3 Merkel cell cancer AJCC staging and survival.

Stage	T Classification	N Classification	M Classification	Merkel cell 5-yr survival
Stage I A	T1	pN0	M 0	80 (2010)
Stage I B	T1	cN0	M 0	60
Stage II A	T2/T3	pN0	M 0	58
Stage II B	T2/T3	cN0	M 0	49
Stage III C	T4	N0	M 0	47
Stage III A	Any T	N1a	M 0	42
Stage III B	Any T	N1b/N2	M 0	26
Stage IV	Any T	Any N	M 1	18

Adapted from the *American Joint Committee on Cancer Staging Manual*, 7th edn, 2010, and Lemos *et al.* J Am Acad Dermatol 2010; 63: 751.

Other tumors

Malignant peripheral nerve sheath tumor

This very rare tumor usually arises from malignant change in a neurofibroma in approximately 2–3% of adults with neurofibromatosis type 1. However, the lesions can develop following radiation therapy or from dermal extension from a soft tissue malignant peripheral nerve sheath tumor (MPNST).[149,150] It grows as a nodular or polypoid lesion of the skin with the overlying epidermis often demonstrating epidermal hyperpigmentation. The majority of tumors are large and located on the flexor aspects of the limbs.

Histologically, MPNSTs are composed of fascicles of hyperchromatic spindle cells in alternating cellular and myxoid areas. Perivascular whorls of tumor cells are also characteristic. Degree of pleomorphism and mitotic activity correlate with tumor grade. Low-grade tumors account for only about 10–15% of cases. Twenty percent of cases have unusual and potentially misleading histological features, such as epithelioid cells and divergent mesenchymal or glandular differentiation.[151]

Loss of *NF1* tumor suppressor gene function in schwannoma cells is a key step in progression from neurofibroma to MPNST. Additional abnormalities of tumor suppressor genes, including *p53* and *INK4a*, contribute to the malignant growth.[152] Lesional cells are positive for nestin and are focally positive for S-100 protein in the majority of cases.

High-grade status, truncal location, and size greater than 5 cm predict poor overall survival.[153] Prognosis is poor with a high incidence of relapse and distant metastases, particularly to the lungs. Long-term survival is 20–30%.

Aggressive surgical resection should be performed. Use of radiation pre- or postoperatively has been evaluated. Despite the absence of level 1 randomized data, many agree on using adjuvant radiation therapy for all patients even if the surgical margins are negative.[154] Although commonly administered, no studies have shown a consistent benefit with chemotherapy in the adjuvant setting. However, recently the combination of doxorubicin and ifosfamide has demonstrated activity comparable to other soft tissue sarcomas.[155]

Peripheral primitive neuroectodermal tumor

Also known as extraosseous Ewing sarcoma or peripheral neuroepithelioma, the occurrence of extraosseous disease in deep soft tissues has been well described but primary cutaneous lesions are rare. In a review of cutaneous Ewing sarcoma, the median age at presentation was 16 years (range 7–21 years).[156] The tumor presents as nonspecific solitary nodules on the trunk and extremities with a median size of 3 cm (range 1–12 cm).[157]

The lesion is composed of masses of small blue cells, with perilobular fibrosis, focal hemorrhage, and ill-defined pale cytoplasm containing glycogen, and absent pericellular reticulin. An ultrastructural study shows a monotonous cell population, with focal thickening of membranes and high nuclear:cytoplasmic ratio. A reciprocal translocation t(11,22) (q24;q12) can help establish the diagnosis.[158] Fluorescence

in situ hybridization (FISH) with a break-apart probe for the *EWSR1* gene (at 22q12) can demonstrate this arrangement.

Wide resection to achieve negative microscopic margins is standard. Adjuvant radiation therapy should be given if microscopic margins are positive. Its role in the setting of negative margins remains uncertain. The potential benefits of adjuvant chemotherapy need to be weighed against the potential long-term complications. The prognosis of the cutaneous presentation of this tumor is uncertain because of the small number of patients in the literature and very late recurrence has been documented. Consultation with physicians specializing in the treatment of peripheral primitive neuroectodermal tumor/ Ewing sarcoma is recommended prior to possible adjuvant chemotherapy in this setting.[157,158]

Malignant granular cell tumor

Malignant granular cell tumor is a rare neoplasm thought to be of neural crest origin. Very few have been reported in skin. Most cases of malignant granular cell tumor (MGCT) develop in mucosa (mainly the tongue), or in cutaneous or subcutaneous tissue.[159] The tumor appears clinically as a rapidly enlarging small firm nodule, with occasional ulceration. Individuals between 30 and 60 years of age are frequently affected with a significant female predominance.

Histologically, the lesion is composed of large sheets of polygonal cells infiltrating dermal and subcutaneous tissue. Cytoplasm of tumor cells is pale, with acidophilic granules, and nuclei are vesicular. Originally described as myoblasts, these cells are now believed to be of neuroectodermal origin.[160] Malignant granular cell tumors demonstrate three or more atypical features including >2 mitosis per 10 high-power field, prominent nucleoli, high nuclear:cytoplasmic ratio, pleomorphism, necrosis, and spindled cells.[94]

The prognosis of MGCT is dismal, with extensive local and distant metastases reported. Specific therapy guidelines do not exist as too few patients have been diagnosed with the tumor. However, early aggressive surgical resection with wide margins has been advocated.[161] Adjuvant radiation therapy (60 Gy) may possibly have a useful role.[161] For patients with unresectable disease, treatment on a sarcoma-based protocol is recommended.

Clear cell sarcoma (malignant melanoma of soft parts)

Primary clear cell sarcoma of soft tissue is a very rare, distinctive mesenchymal neoplasm with melanocytic differentiation. It usually presents as a slow-growing and frequently painful soft tissue mass, occurring primarily in young adults. It has a predilection for the lower extremities, especially around the ankle and knee.[162] The tumor is usually associated with tendons and aponeuroses structures, but may regularly involve the subcutaneous tissue and dermis by direct extension.

Histology demonstrates nests of monomorphic epithelioid and/or spindle cells with clear to eosinophilic cytoplasm, vesicular nuclei, and prominent nucleoli. Melanin synthesis and expression of Mart-1, HMB-45, and S-100 protein are usually present, as well as vimentin and occasionally minimal levels of low molecular weight CKs.[162] Many lesions are also positive for MITF, CD117, CD57, and BCL2. Melanocytic differentiation and cytoplasmic premelanosomes in various stages of maturation are seen.[162] A balanced translocation, t(12;22)(q13;q12), has been identified in 50–75% of clear cell sarcomas but not in melanoma.[162]

Treatment consists of complete surgical excision with margins as wide as possible. Because of early lymph node involvement, sentinel lymph node biopsy should be considered. Radiation therapy and/or chemotherapy have demonstrated no benefit at this time in the adjuvant or metastatic setting.[162,163] Late recurrences have been recorded.

References

1. Reis JP, *et al*. Trichilemmal carcinoma: review of 8 cases. J Cutan Pathol 1993; 20(1): 44–9.
2. Waibel M, *et al*. Tumors of the pilosebaceous unit. Skin Pharmacol 1994; 7(1–2): 90–3.
3. Knoeller SM, *et al*. Skeletal metastasis in trichilemmal carcinoma. Clin Orthop Relat Res 2004; 423: 213–16.
4. Amaral AL, Nascimento AG, Goellner JR. Proliferating pilar (trichilemmal) cyst. Report of two cases, one with carcinomatous transformation and one with distant metastases. Arch Pathol Lab Med 1984; 108(10): 808–10.
5. Elder D, Elenitsas R, Ragsdale BD. Tumors of the epidermal appendages. In: Elder D, Elenitsas R, Jaworsky C (eds) *Histopathology of the Skin*. Philadelphia: Lippincott-Raven, 1997. p.763.
6. Satyaprakash AK, Sheehan DJ, Sangueza OP. Proliferating trichilemmal tumors: a review of the literature. Dermatol Surg 2007; 33(9): 1102–8.
7. Jo J, Ko HC, Jang HS. Infiltrative trichilemmal carcinoma treated with 5% imiquimod cream. Dermatol Surg 2005; 31(8): 973–6.
8. Hardisson D, *et al*. Pilomatrix carcinoma: a clinicopathologic study of six cases and review of the literature. Am J Dermatopathol 2001; 23(5): 394–401.
9. Bremnes RM, *et al*. Pilomatrix carcinoma with multiple metastases: report of a case and review of the literature. Eur J Cancer 1999; 35(3): 433–7.
10. Dutta R, Boadle R, Ng T. Pilomatrix carcinoma: case report and review of literature. Pathology 2001; 33(2): 248–51.
11. Melancon JM, Tom WL, Lee RA. Management of pilomatrix carcinoma: a case report of successful treatment with Mohs micrographic surgery and review of the literature. Dermatol Surg 2011; 37(12): 1798–805.
12. Shields JA, Demirci H, Marr H. Sebaceous carcinoma of the ocular region: a review. Surv Ophthalmol 2005; 50(2): 103–22.
13. Escalonilla P, *et al*. Sebaceous carcinoma of the vulva. Am J Dermatopathol 1999; 21(5): 468–72.
14. Borczuk AC, *et al*. Sebaceous carcinoma of the lung: histologic and immunohistochemical characterization of an unusual pulmonary neoplasm: report of a case and review of the literature. Am J Surg Pathol 2002; 26(6): 795–8.
15. Rumelt S, *et al*. Four-eyelid sebaceous cell carcinoma following irradiation. Arch Ophthalmol 1998; 116(12): 1670–2.
16. Harwood CA, *et al*. An association between sebaceous carcinoma and microsatellite instability in immunosuppressed organ transplant recipients. J Invest Dermatol 2001; 116(2): 246–53.
17. Ponti G, *et al*. Identification of Muir–Torre syndrome among patients with sebaceous tumors and keratoacanthomas: role of clinical features, microsatellite instability, and immunohistochemistry. Cancer 2005; 103(5): 1018–25.
18. Dores GM, Curtis RE, Toro JR. Incidence of cutaneous sebaceous carcinoma and risk of associated neoplasms. Cancer 2008; 113: 3372–81.
19. Lynch HT, Lynch J. Lynch syndrome: genetics, natural history, genetic counseling, and prevention. J Clin Oncol 2000; 18(21 Suppl): 19S–31S.
20. Rao NA, *et al*. Sebaceous carcinomas of the ocular adnexa: a clinicopathologic study of 104 cases, with five-year follow-up data. Hum Pathol 1982; 13(2): 113–22.
21. Snow SN, *et al*. Sebaceous carcinoma of the eyelids treated by Mohs micrographic surgery: report of nine cases with review of the literature. Dermatol Surg 2002; 28(7): 623–31.
22. Paties C, *et al*. Apocrine carcinoma of the skin. A clinicopathologic, immunocytochemical and ultrastructural study. Cancer 1993; 71(2): 375–81.
23. Wick MR, *et al*. Adnexal carcinoma of the skin. I. Eccrine carcinomas. Cancer 1985; 56: 1147–62.
24. Robson A, *et al*. Eccrine porocarcinoma (malignant eccrine poroma): a clinicopathologic study of 69 cases. Am J Surg Pathol 2001; 25(6): 710–20.
25. Goldner R. Eccrine poromatosis. Arch Dermatol 1970; 101: 606–8.
26. Roaf V, Chin N, Lynfield Y. Pigmented sweat gland tumor mimicking melanoma. Cutis 1970; 59: 43–6.
27. Robson A, *et al*. Eccrine porocarcinoma (malignant eccrine poroma): a clinicopathologic study of 69 cases. Am J Surg Pathol 2001; 25(6): 710–20.
28. Wildemore JK, Lee JB, Humphreys TR. Mohs surgery for malignant eccrine neoplasms. Dermatol Surg 2004; 30(12 Pt 2): 1574–9.
29. Halachmi S, Lapidoth M. Approach to the rare eccrine tumors. Dermatol Surg 2011; 37: 1194–5.
30. Delgado R, *et al*. Sentinel lymph node analysis in patients with sweat gland carcinoma. Cancer 2003; 97(9): 2279–84.
31. Plunkett TA, Hanby AM, Miles DW, Rubens RD. Metastatic eccrine porocarcinoma: response to docetaxel (Taxotere) chemotherapy. Ann Oncol 2001; 12: 411–14.
32. Ohta M, *et al*. Nodular hidradenocarcinoma on the scalp of a young woman: case report and review of literature. Dermatol Surg 2004; 30(9): 1265–8
33. Gortler I, *et al*. Metastatic malignant acrospiroma of the hand. Eur J Surg Oncol 2001; 27(4): 431–5.
34. Kao GF, Helwig EB, Graham JH. Aggressive digital papillary adenoma and adenocarcinoma. A clinicopathological study of 57 patients, with histochemical, immunopathological, and ultrastructural observations. J Cutan Pathol 1987; 14(3): 129–46.
35. Duke WH, Sherrod TT, Lupton GP. Aggressive digital papillary adenocarcinoma (aggressive digital papillary adenoma and adenocarcinoma revisited). Am J Surg Pathol 2000; 24(6): 775–84.
36. Frey J, Shimek C, Woodmansee C. Aggressive digital papillary adenocarcinoma: a report of two diseases and review of the literature. J Am Acad Dermatol 2009; 60(2): 331–9.
37. Hsu HC, Ho CY, Chen CH. Aggressive digital papillary adenocarcinoma: a review. Clin Exper Dermatol 2009; 35: 113–19.
38. De Francesco V, *et al*. Carcinosarcoma arising in a patient with multiple cylindromas. Am J Dermatopathol 2005; 27(1): 21–6.
39. Kuklani RM, Glavin FL. Malignant cylindroma of the scalp arising in a setting of multiple cylindromatosis: a case report. Head Neck Pathol 2009; 3: 315–19.
40. Durani BK, *et al*. Malignant transformation of multiple dermal cylindromas. Br J Dermatol 2001; 145(4): 653–6.
41. Lin PY, Fatteh SM, Lloyd SM. Malignant transformation in a solitary dermal cylindroma. Arch Pathol Lab Med 1987; 111: 765–7.
42. Granter SR, *et al*. Malignant eccrine spiradenoma (spiradenocarcinoma): a clinicopathologic study of 12 cases. Am J Dermatopathol 2000; 22(2): 97–103.
43. Santa Cruz DJ, Sweat gland carcinoma: a comprehensive review. Semin Diagn Pathol 1987; 4: 38–74.
44. Beekley AC, Brown TA, Porter C. Malignant eccrine spiradenoma: a previously unreported presentation and review of the literature. Am Surg 1999; 65: 236–40.
45. Huerre M, *et al*. Carcinosarcoma arising in eccrine spiradenoma: a morphologic and immunohistochemical study. Ann Pathol 1994; 14: 168–73.
46. Abbate M, *et al*. Clinical course, risk factors, and treatment of microcystic adnexal carcinoma: a short series report. Dermatol Surg 2003; 29(10): 1035–8.
47. Argenyi ZB, *et al*. malignant eccrine spiradenoma: a clinicopathologic study. Am Dermatopathol 1992; 14: 381–2.

48. Friedman PM, *et al*. Microcystic adnexal carcinoma: collaborative series review and update. J Am Acad Dermatol 1999; 41(2 Pt1): 225–31.

49. Pugh TJ, Lee NY, Pacheco T, Raben D. Microcystic adnexal carcinoma of the face treated with radiation therapy. A case report and review of the literature. Head Neck 2011; Mar 7 [Epub ahead of print].

50. Cabell CE, *et al*. Primary mucinous carcinoma in a 54-year-old man. J Am Acad Dermatol 2003; 49(5): 941–3.

51. Santa-Cruz DJ, *et al*. Primary mucinous carcinoma of the skin. Br J Dermatol 1978; 98(6): 645–53.

52. Eckert F, *et al*. Cytokeratin expression in mucinous sweat gland carcinomas: an immunohistochemical analysis of four cases. Histopathology 1992; 21(2): 161–5.

53. Marra DE, Schanbacher CF, Torres A. Mohs micrographic surgery of primary cutaneous mucinous carcinoma using immunohistochemistry for margin control. Dermatol Surg 2004; 30(5): 799–802.

54. Freeman RG, Winkelmann RK. Basal cell tumor with eccrine differentiation (eccrine epithelioma). Arch Dermatol 1969; 100(2): 234–42.

55. Ohnishi T, *et al*. Syringoid eccrine carcinoma: report of a case with immunohistochemical analysis of cytokeratin expression. Am J Dermatopathol 2002; 24(5): 409–13.

56. Malmusi M, Collina G. Syringoid eccrine carcinoma: a case report. Am J Dermatopathol 1997; 19(5): 533–5.

57. Urso C, *et al*. Adenoid cystic carcinoma of sweat glands: report of two cases. Tumori 1991; 77(3): 264–7.

58. Salzman MJ, Eades E. Primary cutaneous adenoid cystic carcinoma: a case report and review of the literature. Plast Reconstr Surg 1991; 88(1): 140–4.

59. Chang SE, *et al*. Primary adenoid cystic carcinoma of skin with lung metastasis. J Am Acad Dermatol 1999; 40(4): 640–2.

60. Laurie SA, Ho AL, Fury MG, Sherman E, Pfister DG. Systemic therapy in the management of metastatic or locally recurrent adenoid cystic carcinoma of the salivary glands: a systematic review. Lancet Oncol 2011; 12: 815–24.

61. Dammrich DJ, Santos ES, Raez LE. Efficacy of sorafenib, a multi-tyrosine kinase inhibitor, in an adenoid cystic carcinoma metastatic to the lung: case report and review of the literature. J Med Case Rep 2011; 5: 483–6.

62. Ferlicot S, *et al*. Lymphoepithelioma-like carcinoma of the skin: a report of 3 Epstein–Barr Virus (EBV)-negative additional cases. Immunohistochemical study of the stroma reaction. J Cutan Pathol 2000; 27(6): 306–11.

63. Takayasu S, *et al*. Lymphoepithelioma-like carcinoma of the skin. J Dermatol 1996; 23(7): 472–5.

64. Crocker H. Paget's disease affecting the scrotum and penis. Trans Pathol Soc London 1888–1889; 40: 187–91.

65. Goldblum JR, Hart WR. Vulvar Paget's disease: a clinicopathologic and immunohistochemical study of 19 cases. Am J Surg Pathol 1997; 21(10): 1178–87.

66. Lai YL, *et al*. Penoscrotal extramammary Paget's disease: a review of 33 cases in a 20-year experience. Plast Reconstr Surg 2003; 112(4): 1017–23.

67. Hendi A, Brodland DG, Zitelli JA. Extramammary Paget's disease: surgical treatment with Mohs micrographic surgery. J Am Acad Dermatol 2004; 51(5): 767–73.

68. Cohen PR, *et al*. Treatment of extramammary Paget disease with topical imiquimod cream: case report and literature review. South Med J 2006; 99(4): 396–402.

69. Nardelli AA, Stafinski T, Menon D. Effectiveness of photodynamic therapy for mammary and extra mammary Paget's disease: a state of the scientific review. BMC Dermatol 2011; 11: 13.

70. Moreno-Arias GA, *et al*. Radiotherapy for in situ extramammary Paget disease of the vulva. J Dermatolog Treat 2003; 14(2): 119–23.

71. Simon MP, *et al*. Deregulation of the platelet derived growth factor β chain via fusion with collagen gene COL1A1 in dermatofibrosarcoma protuberans and giant cell fibroblastoma. Nat Genet 1997; 15: 95–8.

72. Patel KU, *et al*. Dermatofibrosarcoma protuberans COL1A1-PDGFB fusion is identified in virtually all dermatofibrosarcoma protuberans cases when investigated by newly developed multiplex reverse transcription polymerase chain reaction and fluorescence in situ hybridization assays. Hum Pathol 2008; 39(2): 184.

73. Minter RM, Reith JD, Hochwald SN. Metastatic potential of dermatofibrosarcoma protuberans with fibrosarcomatous change. J Surg Oncol 2003; 82(3): 201–8.

74. Mattox AK, *et al*. Response of malignant scalp dermatofibrosarcoma to presurgical targeted growth factor inhibition: a case report. J Neurosurg 2010; 112(5): 965–77.

75. Calikoglu E, *et al*. CD44 and hyaluronate in the differential diagnosis of dermatofibroma and dermatofibrosarcoma protuberans. J Cutan Pathol 2003; 30(3): 185–9.

76. Enneking WF, Spanier SS, Goodman MA. A system for the surgical staging of musculoskeletal sarcoma. Clin Orthop Relat Res 1980; 153: 106–20.

77. DuBay D, *et al*. Low recurrence rate after surgery for dermatofibrosarcoma protuberans: a multidisciplinary approach from a single institution. Cancer 2004; 100: 1008–16.

78. Snow SN, *et al*. Dermatofibrosarcoma portuberans: a report on 29 patients treated by Mohs micrographic surgery with long term follow up and review of the literature. Cancer 2004; 101: 28–38.

79. Wacker J, Khan-Durani B, Hartschuh W. Modified Mohs micrographic surgery in the therapy of dermatofibrosarcoma protuberans: analysis of 22 patients. Ann Surg Oncol 2004; 11: 438–44.

80. Nouri K, *et al*. Mohs micrographic surgery for dermatofibrosarcoma protuberans: University of Miami and NYU experience. Dermatol Surg 2002; 28(11): 1060–4; discussion 4.

81. Mendenhall WM, Zlotecki RA, Scarborough MT. Dermatofibrosarcoma protuberans. Cancer 2004; 101(11): 2503–8.

82. Labropoulos SV, *et al*. Sustained complete remission of metastatic dermatofibrosarcoma protuberans with imatinib mesylate. Anticancer Drugs 2005; 16(4): 461–6.

83. McArthur GA, *et al*. Molecular and clinical analysis of locally advanced dermatofibrosarcoma protuberans treated with imatinib: imatinib target expiration consortium study B 2225. J Clin Oncol 2005; 23: 866–73.

84. Kerob D, *et al*. Imatinib mesylate as a preoperative therapy in dermatofibrosarcoma: results of a multicenter phase II study on 25 patients. Clin Cancer Res 2010; 16(12): 3285–95.

85. Layfield LJ, Gopez EV. Fine-needle aspiration cytology of giant cell fibroblastoma: case report and review of the literature. Diagn Cytopathol 2002; 26(6): 398–403.

86. Billings SD, Folpe AL. Cutaneous and subcutaneous fibrohistiocytic tumors of intermediate malignancy: an update. Am J Dermatopathol 2004; 26(2): 141–55.

87. Sandberg AA, Bridge JA. Updates on the cytogenetics and molecular genetics of bone and soft tissue tumors. Dermatofibrosarcoma protuberans and giant cell fibroblastoma. Cancer Genet Cytogenet 2003; 140(1): 1–12.

88. Hornick JL, *et al*. Loss of INI1 expression is characteristic of both conventional and proximal-type epithelioid sarcoma. Am J Surg Pathol 2009; 33(4): 542–50.

89. Sakharpe A, *et al*. Epithelioid sarcoma and unclassified sarcoma with epithelioid features: clinicopathological variables, molecular markers and a new experimental model. Oncologist 2011; 16: 512–22.

90. Erlandson RA, Antonescu CR. The rise and fall of malignant fibrous histiocytoma. Ultrastruct Pathol 2004; 28(5–6): 283–9.

91. Love WE, Schmitt AR, Bordeax JS. Management of unusual cutaneous malignancies: atypical fibroxanthoma, malignant fibrous histiocytoma, sebaceous carcinoma, extramammary Paget disease. Dermatol Clin 2011; 29(2): 210–16.

92. Mentzel T, *et al*. Myxofibrosarcoma. Clinicopathologic analysis of 75 cases with emphasis on the low-grade variant. Am J Surg Pathol 1996; 20(4): 391–405.

93. Merck C, *et al*. Myxofibrosarcoma. A malignant soft tissue tumor of fibroblastic-histiocytic origin. A clinicopathologic and prognostic study of 110 cases using multivariate analysis. Acta Pathol Microbiol Immunol Scand Suppl 1983; 282: 1–40.

94. Fisher C, *et al*. Soft tissue tumors. Manitoba, Canada: Amirsys 2011, 15.24-1529.

95. Thway K. Angiomatoid fibrous histiocytoma. Arch Pathol Lab Med 2008; 321(2): 273–7.

96. Mansfield A, et al. Angiomatoid fibrous histiocytoma in a 25 year old male. Rare Tumors 2010; 2(2): 54–6.

97. Mori O, Hashimoto T. Plexiform fibrohistiocytic tumor. Eur J Dermatol 2004; 14(2): 118–20.

98. Luzar B, Calonie E. Cutaneous fibrohistiocytic tumours – an update. Histopathology 2010; 56(1): 148–65.

99. Rahimi AD, et al. Mohs micrographic surgery of a plexiform fibrohistiocytic tumor. Dermatol Surg 2001; 27(8): 768–71.

100. Giuffrida TJ, Kligora CJ, Goldstein GD. Localized cutaneous metastases from an atypical fibroxanthoma. Dermatol Surg 2004; 30(12 Pt 2): 1561–4.

101. Fish FS. Soft tissue sarcomas in dermatology. Dermatol Surg 1996; 22(3): 268–73.

102. Davis JL, et al. A comparison of Mohs micrographic surgery and wide excision for the treatment of atypical fibroxanthoma. Dermatol Surg 1997; 23(2): 105–10.

103. Iorizzo LJ, Brown MD. Atypical fibroxanthoma: a review of the literature. Dermatol Surg 2011; 37(2): 146–57.

104. Ruocco V, Schwartz RA, Ruocco E. Lymphedema: an immunologically vulnerable site for development of neoplasms. J Am Acad Dermatol 2002; 47(1): 124–7.

105. Komorowski AL, Wysocki WM, Mitus J. Angiosarcoma in a chronically lymphedematous leg: an unusual presentation of Stewart–Treves syndrome. South Med J 2003; 96(8): 807–8.

106. Tomasini C, Grassi M, Pippione M. Cutaneous angiosarcoma arising in an irradiated breast. Case report and review of the literature. Dermatology 2004; 209(3): 208–14.

107. Pawlik TM, et al. Cutaneous angiosarcoma of the scalp. Cancer 2003; 98: 1716–26.

108. Fury MG, et al. A 14 year retrospective review of angiosarcoma: clinical characteristics, prognostic factors and treatment outcomes with surgery and chemotherapy. Cancer J 2005; 11(3): 241–7.

109. Van der Graaf W, et al. Palette: A randomized double blind phase III trial of pazopanib versus placebo in patients (pts) with soft tissue sarcoma (STS) whose disease has progressed during or following priory chemotherapy. An EORTC STBSG Global Network Study (EORTC 62072). J Clin Oncol 2011; 29: abstract LBA 10002.

110. Farina MC, et al. Epithelioid angiosarcoma of the breast involving the skin: a highly aggressive neoplasm readily mistaken for mammary carcinoma. J Cutan Pathol 2003; 30(2): 152–6.

111. Enzinger FM, Weiss WS. Malignant Soft Tissue Tumors of Unknown Type. St Louis, MO: CV Mosby, 1995.

112. Prescott RJ, et al. Cutaneous epithelioid angiosarcoma: a clinicopathological study of four cases. Histopathology 1994; 25(5): 421–9.

113. Kayal JD, et al. Malignant glomus tumor: a case report and review of the literature. Dermatol Surg 2001; 27(9): 837–40.

114. Khoury T, et al. Malignant glomus tumor: a case report and review of literature, focusing on its clinicopathologic features and immunohistochemical profile. Am J Dermatopathol 2005; 27: 428–31.

115. Quante M, et al. Epithelioid hemangioendothelioma presenting in the skin: a clinicopathologic study of eight cases. Am J Dermatopathol 1998; 20(6): 541–6.

116. Tyring S, et al. Epithelioid hemangioendothelioma of the skin and femur. J Am Acad Dermatol 1989; 20(2 Pt 2): 362–6.

117. Calonje E, et al. Retiform hemangioendothelioma. A distinctive form of low-grade angiosarcoma delineated in a series of 15 cases. Am J Surg Pathol 1994; 18(2): 115–25.

118. Gutzmer R, et al. Absence of HHV-8 DNA in hobnail hemangiomas. J Cutan Pathol 2002; 29(3): 154–8.

119. Fukunaga M, et al. Retiform haemangioendothelioma. Virchows Arch 1996; 428(4–5): 301–4.

120. Marler JJ, et al. Successful antiangiogenic therapy of giant cell angioblastoma with interferon alfa 2b: report of 2 cases. Pediatrics 2002; 109(2): E37.

121. Vargas SO, et al. Giant cell angioblastoma: three additional occurrences of a distinct pathologic entity. Am J Surg Pathol 2001; 25(2): 185–96.

122. Lyons LL, et al. Kaposiform hemangioendothelioma: a study of 33 cases emphasizing its pathologic, immunophenotypic, and biologic uniqueness from juvenile hemangioma. Am J Surg Pathol 2004; 28(5): 559–68.

123. Cheuk W, et al. Immunostaining for human herpesvirus 8 latent nuclear antigen-1 helps distinguish Kaposi sarcoma from its mimickers. Am J Clin Pathol 2004; 121(3): 335–42.

124. Hu B, et al. Kasabach–Merritt syndrome-associated kaposiform hemangioendothelioma successfully treated with cyclophosphamide, vincristine, and actinomycin D. J Pediatr Hematol Oncol 1998; 20(6): 567–9.

125. Fernandez Y, Bernabeu-Wittel M, Garcia-Morillo JS. Kaposiform hemangioendothelioma. Eur J Intern Med 2009; 20: 106–13.

126. Holst VA, Junkins-Hopkins JM, Elenitsas R. Cutaneous smooth muscle neoplasms: clinical features, histologic findings, and treatment options. J Am Acad Dermatol 2002; 46(4): 477–90; quiz, 91–4.

127. Jensen ML, et al. Intradermal and subcutaneous leiomyosarcoma: a clinicopathological and immunohistochemical study of 41 cases. J Cutan Pathol 1996; 23(5): 458–63.

128. Fields JP, Helwig EB. Leiomyosarcoma of the skin and subcutaneous tissue. Cancer 1981; 47(1): 156–69.

129. Annest NM, et al. Cutaneous leiomyosarcoma: a tumor of the head and neck. Dermatol Surg 2007; 33: 628–33.

130. Wong TY, Suster S. Primary cutaneous sarcomas showing rhabdomyoblastic differentiation. Histopathology 1995; 26(1): 25–32.

131. Brecher AR, et al. Congenital primary cutaneous rhabdomyosarcoma in a neonate. Pediatr Dermatol 2003; 20(4): 335–8.

132. Dei Tos AP. Liposarcoma: new entities and evolving concepts. Ann Diagn Pathol 2000; 4(4): 252–66.

133. Dei Tos AP, Mentzel T, Fletcher CD. Primary liposarcoma of the skin: a rare neoplasm with unusual high grade features. Am J Dermatopathol 1998; 20(4): 332–8.

134. Val-Bernal JF, Gonzalez-Vela MC, Cuevas J. Primary purely intradermal pleomorphic liposarcoma. J Cutan Pathol 2003; 30(8): 516–20.

135. Toker C. Trabecular carcinoma of the skin. Arch Derm 1972; 105(1): 107–10.

136. Tang CK, Toker C. Trabecular carcinoma of the skin: an ultrastructural study. Cancer 1978; 42(5): 2311–21.

137. Johannessen JV, Gould VE. Neuroendocrine skin carcinoma associated with calcitonin production: a Merkel cell carcinoma? Hum Pathol 1980; 11(5 Suppl): 586–8.

138. Agelli M, Clegg LX. Epidemiology of primary Merkel cell carcinoma in the United States. J Am Acad Dermatol 2003; 49: 832–41.

139. Feng, H, Shuda M, Chang Y, Moore PS. Clonal integration of a polyomavirus in human Merkel cell carcinoma. Science 2008; 319: 1096–100.

140. Touze A, et al. High levels of antibodies against Merkel cell polyomavirus identify a subset of patients with Merkel cell carcinoma with better outcome. J Clin Oncol 2011; 29(12): 1612–19.

141. Koljonen V. Merkel cell carcinoma: what we know now. Expert Rev Dermatol 2010; 5(3): 345–55.

142. Adapted from the Merkel Cell Carcinoma – Seattle Cancer Care Alliance: www.merkelcell.org.

143. Calder KB, Coplowitz S, Schlauder S, Morgan MB. A case series and immunophenotypic analysis of CK20-/CK7+ primary neuroendocrine carcinoma of the skin. J Cutan Pathol 2007; 34(12): 918–23.

144. Lemos BD, et al. Pathologic nodal evaluation improves prognostic accuracy in Merkel cell carcinoma: analysis of 5823 cases as the basis of the first consensus staging system. J Am Acad Dermatol 2010; 63: 751–61.

145. Bichakjian CK, et al. Merkel cell carcinoma: critical review with guidelines for multidisciplinary management. Cancer 2007; 110: 1–12.

146. Allen PJ, et al. Merkel cell carcinoma: prognosis and treatment of patients from a single institution. J Clin Oncol 2005; 23: 2300–9.

147. National Comprehensive Cancer Network. Guidelines in Oncology, Merkel Cell Carcinoma, Version 1.2012. www.NCCN.org.

148. Samlowski W, et al. A phase II trial of imatinib mesylate in Merkel cell carcinoma (neuroendocrine carcinoma of the skin). Am J Clin Oncol 2010; 33(5): 495–9.

149. Brooks DG. The neurofibromatoses: hereditary predisposition to multiple peripheral nerve tumors. Neurosurg Clin North Am 2004; 15(2): 145–55.

150. Kourea HP, *et al*. Subdiaphragmatic and intrathoracic paraspinal malignant peripheral nerve sheath tumors: a clinicopathologic study of 25 patients and 26 tumors. Cancer 1998; 82(11): 2191–203.

151. Ducatman BS, *et al*. Malignant peripheral nerve sheath tumors. A clinicopathologic study of 120 cases. Cancer 1986; 57(10): 2006–21.

152. Carroll SL, Stonecypher MS. Tumor suppressor mutations and growth factor signaling in the pathogenesis of NF1-associated peripheral nerve sheath tumors: II. The role of dysregulated growth factor signaling. J Neuropathol Exp Neurol 2005; 64(1): 1–9.

153. Stucky CC, *et al*. Malignant peripheral nerve sheath tumors (MPNST): the Mayo Clinic experience. Ann Surg Oncol 2012; 19(3): 878–85.

154. Vauthey JN, Woodruff JM, Brennan MF. Extremity malignant peripheral nerve sheath tumors (neurogenic sarcomas): a 10-year experience. Ann Surg Oncol 1995; 2(2): 126–31.

155. Kroep JR, *et al*. First line chemotherapy for malignant peripheral nerve sheath tumors (MPNST) versus other histological soft tissue sarcoma subtypes and as a prognostic factor for MPNST: an EORTC soft tissue and bone sarcoma group study. Ann Oncol 2011; 22(1): 207–14.

156. Perrin RG, Guha A. Malignant peripheral nerve sheath tumors. Neurosurg Clin North Am 2004; 15(2): 203–16.

157. Chow E, *et al*. Cutaneous and subcutaneous Ewing's sarcoma: an indolent disease. Int J Radiat Oncol Biol Phys 2000; 46(2): 433–8.

158. Banerjee SS, *et al*. Clinicopathological characteristics of peripheral primitive neuroectodermal tumour of skin and subcutaneous tissue. Histopathology 1997; 31(4): 355–66.

159. Kershisnik M, Batsakis JG, Mackay B. Granular cell tumors. Ann Otol Rhinol Laryngol 1994; 103(5 Pt 1): 416–19.

160. Becelli R, *et al*. Abrikossoff's tumor. J Craniofac Surg 2001; 12(1): 78–81.

161. Ramos PC, *et al*. Malignant granular cell tumor of the vulva in a 17 year old: case report and literature review. Int J Gyn Cancer 2001; 10(5): 429–34.

162. Dim DC, *et al*. Clear cell sarcoma of tendons and aponeuroses. Arch Pathol Lab Med 2007; 131: 152–6.

163. Malchau SS, *et al*. Clear cell sarcoma of soft tissues. J Surg Oncol 2007; 95: 519–22.

164. Edge SB, Byrd DR, Compton CC, (eds). *AJCC Cancer Staging Manual*, 7th edn. New York, NY: Springer, 2010.

50 Dermatofibrosarcoma Protuberans

Michael Alvarado,[1] Jane L. Messina,[2,4] Rahel Mathew,[2,4] and Vernon K. Sondak[3,4]

[1] Department of Surgery, University of California San Francisco; Helen Diller Family Comprehensive Cancer Center, San Francisco, CA, USA
[2] Departments of Pathology & Cell Biology and Dermatology, [3] Departments of Oncologic Sciences and Surgery, University of South Florida College of Medicine, Tampa, FL, USA
[4] Department of Cutaneous Oncology, H. Lee Moffitt Cancer Center, Tampa, FL, USA

Introduction

Dermatofibrosarcoma protuberans (DFSP) is an uncommon low-grade cutaneous sarcoma that typically has an indolent clinical course with a propensity for locally aggressive and infiltrative behavior. Although first described by Taylor in 1890,[1] it was not until 1924 that Darier and Ferrand recorded a detailed clinical and pathological description.[2] Finally, 1 year later, Hoffman gave the disease process its current name, dermatofibrosarcoma protuberans.[3]

Biology

Dermatofibrosarcoma protuberans tumorigenesis is almost always attributed to rearrangements involving chromosomes 17 and 22, leading to the fusion of *collagen type 1α1* and *platelet-derived growth factor (PDGF)-β* genes.[4] The resulting fusion protein causes the continuous activation of the tyrosine kinase receptor PDGF-β. The *PDGF-β* gene is the cellular homolog of the v-*sis* oncogene, implicated in causing simian sarcoma.[5,6] *PDGF-β* has been associated with several other tumors as well as DFSP, and the consequence of the t(17;22) translocation is activation of the PDGFB receptor via autocrine and paracrine production of its functional ligand.[7,8]

Pathology

Microscopi examination reveals a spindle cell proliferation of uncertain histogenesis arranged in a "cartwheel" or storiform pattern, often surrounding and trapping subcutaneous fat to produce a "honeycomb" appearance (Fig. 50.1). The fibroblast appearing cells tend to be uniform with hyperchromatic and elongated nuclei.[9] The spindle cell tumor may contain melanin pigment; this uncommon pigmented variant is known as the "Bednar tumor" (Fig. 50.2).[10] Immunohistochemical staining will identify the cells of a DFSP as being CD34 negative and vimentin positive, which helps distinguish this lesion from benign dermatofibromas.[11] However, the significant overlap with other spindle cell neoplasms poses a challenge in terms of differential diagnosis. Other immunohistochemical markers which have been proposed to assist in the differentiation of DFSP from dermatofibroma or other cutaneous neoplasms include D2-40[12] (an antibody recognizing a marker on lymphatic endothelium) and apolipoprotein D.[13] More recently, cDNA microarrays have been used to profile gene expression of these mesenchymal tumors to help with histological diagnosis.[14] Linn *et al.* were able to distinguish DFSP from other soft tissue tumors based on their gene expression pattern.[15] By combining morphology, immunohistochemistry and when necessary genetic profiling, pathologists can correctly identify DFSP and allow for appropriate surgical treatment.

Dermatofibrosarcoma protuberans has characteristic finger-like projections that infiltrate either laterally or deep, and can be found to extend far from the main tumor in a very asymmetrical fashion.[16–18] If not completely resected, these projections lead to local recurrence, placing a significant burden on the pathologist to thoroughly evaluate the peripheral and deep margins of resection specimens.

Sarcomatous transformation of DFSP is recognized in up to 10–15% of all cases; usually the transformation is to a low-grade fibrosarcoma (Fig. 50.3), but other and higher-grade transformants are seen on occasion.[19,20] Histologically, the transformed lesion has areas with a more fascicular or herring-bone pattern of growth, an increased mitotic rate and greater nuclear pleomorphism.[21] These features along with increased cellularity have been associated with an increased risk of local recurrence.[20] The fibrosarcomatous areas are typically CD34 negative.[22] Rarely, areas of malignant fibrous histiocytoma may be identified within a DFSP.[23] There is evidence that recurrent DFSPs, particularly multiply recurrent lesions, are more prone to sarcomatous transformation, which in turn may increase the risk for the rare metastatic DFSP tumor.[20,24]

Textbook of Uncommon Cancer, Fourth Edition. Edited by Derek Raghavan, Charles D. Blanke, David H. Johnson, Paul L. Moots, Gregory H. Reaman, Peter G. Rose and Mikkael A. Sekeres.
© 2012 John Wiley & Sons, Inc. Published 2012 by John Wiley & Sons, Inc.

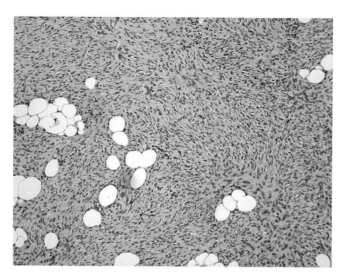

Figure 50.1 Dermatofibrosarcoma protuberans demonstrating typical storiform pattern of proliferation with extension into subcutaneous fat and a honeycomb pattern of infiltration. H&E, 200×.

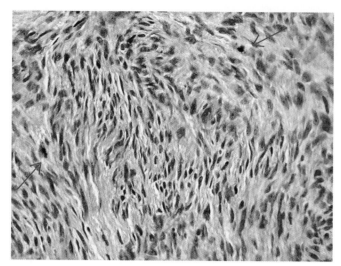

Figure 50.3 Fibrosarcomatous transformation of dermatofibrosarcoma protuberans. There is increased tumor cellularity, and mitoses are readily visible. H&E, 400×.

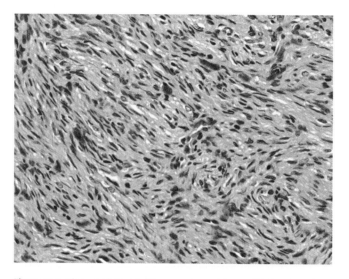

Figure 50.2 Pigmented dermatofibrosarcoma protuberans (Bednar tumor), demonstrating melanin within lesional spindle cells. H&E, 400×.

Presentation

Dermatofibrosarcoma protuberans classically presents as a slowly progressive, painless cutaneous lesion. It begins as a flat, violet or pink plaque, but usually progresses to incorporate a nodular component. It is not uncommon for the lesion to ulcerate or bleed. The history is usually described as slow growing, often with long periods of time with apparent stability in size. Most often, there is a delay in diagnosis secondary to patient and even physician neglect, and a history of the lesion being present for multiple years is more the rule than the exception.

Dermatofibrosarcoma protuberans is found on all areas of the skin, roughly in proportion to the surface area involved. There is no apparent predilection for sun-exposed skin. Accordingly, DFSP is most commonly located on the trunk (roughly 50–60% of cases), followed by the extremities

(20–30%), and head and neck (10–15%).[25,26] Most reports state that men tend to be affected slightly more often than women, and the age at presentation is most often between the second and fifth decades of life. Although uncommon, there are cases of DFSP in infants and children. There are over 180 published childhood cases, 21 of which were described as congenital.[27–29]

Treatment

Wide excision with histologically negative margins is the mainstay of treatment for DFSP. Historically, high recurrence rates have been described in the literature, particularly when conservative resection is employed (Table 50.1). Likely due to the difficulty in achieving wide margins of resection, the highest rate of recurrence is usually reported on the head and neck. Adequate primary resection is important because persistent lesions tend to be more invasive at re-resection with invasion into underlying fascia, muscle and even bone, along with the possibility of sarcomatous transformation that markedly increases the risk of distant metastasis.[30] An extensive review of literature published in 1996 found a mean local recurrence rate of 43% (range 26–60%) for 317 patients who underwent "conservative" excision. The authors tabulated another 489 patients with wide excision (greater than 2 cm resection margin) with an aggregate recurrence rate of 20% (range 0–60%).[31]

Mohs micrographic surgery (MMS) represents an alternative to wide excision. It was first reported in 1978 for seven patients with DFSP (six of whom had been previously treated surgically) treated with no local recurrences; five of the patients had >5 years of follow-up at the time of the report.[32] Since that initial report, Mohs surgery has been widely utilized for DFSP. Snow *et al.* reported on 29 patients from their institution who underwent MMS for DFSP and had at least 5 years of follow-up.[33] Their 29 patients had tumors located in the head and neck (45%) and the trunk and extremities (55%). Of these lesions, 21 were primary and eight were recurrent after previous

Table 50.1 Literature review of surgical management and outcomes for DFSP.

Author	Year	Number of patients	Type of excision	Margin size	Positive margins (%)	Recurrence (%)	Median Follow up (months)
Cai et al.	2011	260 (overall)	LE	<1 cm	50	45	
		236	WLE	1.5–2.5 cm	Not reported	13.6	85 (overall)
			WLE	>3.0 cm	Not reported	5.7	
Fields et al.	2011	244	WLE	2–3 cm	14.6	6.5	50
Farma et al.	2010	206	WLE	2 cm	3	1	64
Heuvel et al.	2009	38	WLE	2–3 cm	5	7	89
Love et al.	2009	11 (congential)	MMS	1.7	Not available	0	51.6
		46 (congential)	WLE	2.8	Not available	11	22.8
Meguerditchian et al.	2009	28	WLE	2 cm	22	3.6	49.9
		20	MMS	0.5–1 cm/stage	0	0	40.4
Yu et al.	2008	14	WLE	3 cm	0	0	
		4	Modified WLE#	3 cm	0	0	68 (overall)
		7	MMS	2–5 mm/stage	86*	0	
Monnier et al.	2006	4		<0.9 cm		50	
		31	WLE	1–2.9 cm	Not reported	46	115
		31		>3.0 cm		7	
Fiore et al.	2005	136 primary	WLE	Not reported	12	4	
							78
		88 recurrence	WLE	Not reported	15	5	
Dubay et al.	2003	11	MMS	5.3 cm	15	0	62.4
		43	WLE	14.8 cm	5	0	48
		9	Combination**	10.7 cm	22	0	64.8
Chang et al.	2003	60	WLE	3.1 cm	2–3	16	59
Bowne et al.	2000	159	Not available	Not available	32	21	57

LE, local excision; MMS, Mohs micrographic surgery; WLE, wide local excision.

3 cm margins with Mohs-like processing.

* 6 of 7 patients had modified WLE.

** 3 patients underwent margin removal "square technique" with permanent histology analysis.

non-MMS resection. There were no local recurrences or metastases during the follow-up period (mean 10.6 years, range 5–20 years). They also reviewed the literature for DFSP patients who underwent MMS and had at least 5 years of follow-up; their review identified 136 additional patients. Again, tumor sites were located throughout the body (25% head and neck, 62% trunk, and 13% extremities). The local recurrence rate was 6.6% (nine patients). In 2007, Kimmel et al. performed a metaanalysis of pathological data from 98 cases collected from four studies of DFSP in the literature. They concluded that a surgical margin of 4 cm would be required for margin clearance in 95% of cases. They caution that such large margins may result in unnecessary removal of normal skin.[34] The methodology they used, however, has not been substantiated and could well be associated with significant overestimation of the width of excision required to achieve a histologically negative margin for most patients.

Parker and Zitelli used MMS in an attempt to define margins needed for complete tumor removal.[35] The authors found that a margin of 2.5 cm cleared all the tumors in 20 patients analyzed. Dividing the tumors by size revealed that tumors measuring less than 2 cm were completely cleared with a 1.5 cm margin. Ratner et al. used MMS to analyze the extent of microscopic spread in 58 patients with primary and recurrent DFSP.[18] Using a concentric tumor growth model, the authors estimated the potential for inadequate resection using various margins. For example, a 3 cm margin was estimated to have resulted in an inadequate resection in 15.5% of 58 patients analyzed. The authors stress that positive margins likely go undetected secondary to sampling error with standard pathological examination.

Mohs surgery is a labor-intensive technique that most likely does have significant value for tumors in locations where wide excision would be difficult or particularly deforming. More importantly, MMS has helped to define the extent for wide local excision and solidify the need for more exhaustive pathological examination of the margins of resection. However, more recent results of standard surgical resection have shown recurrence rates that compare favorably with MMS. Wide excision with careful pathological examination of resection margins has lead to recurrence rates under 5% at 10 years.[26] Khatri et al. reported on 24 patients (with 11 primary and 13 recurrent tumors) who underwent wide excision for DFSP.[36] Resection margins ranged from 2.5 to 3 cm. At a median follow-up of 54 months, there were no recurrences. Stojadinovic et al. reviewed 33 patients with histologically proven DFSP of the head and neck.[37] Gross surgical margin ≥2 cm (17 patients) was predictive of negative histological margin. Eleven of 16 patients with less than a 2 cm gross margin had positive microscopic margins. At median follow-up of 82 months, no local recurrences occurred in the ≥2 cm excision group, while the <2 cm group had three local failures. The authors also performed an extensive literature search that revealed two series with no reported local recurrences, as well as a series with a 6% recurrence rate when surgical margins were ≥2 cm. Dubay et al. reported their experience of 62 patients with DFSP and stressed not only the need for wide excision, but also the importance of careful pathological analysis of surgical margins based on knowledge gained from Mohs surgery.[38] Forty-two patients underwent definitive surgical therapy by wide excision alone, with no local or distant recurrences at a median follow-up of 4.4 years. The authors described a diamond-shaped surgical specimen, which facilitates a more complete peripheral margin assessment of each diamond edge.

Farma et al. published combined results from two large tertiary centers involving a total of 206 DFSP lesions in 204 patients.[39] Based on the approach first described by Dubay et al.,[38] surgeons at both institutions carefully marked out the excision in a diamond shape and resected the tumors with measured margins of 1–2 cm. If positive margins were found at final pathology, reexcision was undertaken with additional 1 cm margins. If the wound could not be closed primarily, temporary skin coverage was used until final margins were deemed negative. The authors stressed the need for meticulous analysis of all margins, including immunohistochemistry when necessary (Fig. 50.4). The median number of excisions required to achieve negative margins was one (range 1–4) and the median margin width was 2 cm (range 0.5–3 cm). Eighty-one percent of patients required one resection, 16% required two resections and 3.5% required either three or four resections to achieve negative margins at final pathology. Primary closure was utilized in 69% of patients, skin graft in 25% and local tissue flap in the remaining 5%. Only two patients (1%) recurred locally at a median follow-up of 64 months. The authors concluded that a single wide excision with 1–2 cm margins is an adequate approach, with only 4% requiring more than two resections to achieve final negative margins. This allows the majority of patients to have primary wound closure with a very

low rate of recurrence, in contrast to earlier reports suggesting that a skin graft should be used "in nearly every instance."[40]

Fields et al. analyzed 244 patients with primary or recurrent DFSP treated over a 27-year period at a single institution.[41] At a median follow-up of 50 months, there were 14 local recurrences (5.7%) and two distant metastases (0.8%). Twenty-two of their patients received only nonsurgical therapy. On multivariate analysis, only tumor depth (superficial versus deep) and margin status (for patients with locally recurrent disease only) were associated with disease-free survival. There were no tumor-related deaths among their patients presenting with primary DFSP, and only one tumor-related death among patients presenting with recurrent disease.

Adjuvant radiation therapy

The use of radiation in combination with surgical resection has been employed when wide surgical margins are not achievable, due to either anatomical constraints or to widespread local extension of tumor. Historically, it had been thought that DFSP was resistant to radiotherapy.[16,42] However, there have been multiple reports of using radiation as the only therapy in isolated cases with adequate local control.[43,44] Subsequently, radiation was proposed as an adjunct to surgery when close or positive margins were left behind. A study of 18 patients who received either radiation alone (three patients) or radiation in combination with surgery (15 patients) revealed a 10-year actuarial local control rate of 88%.[1] There were three local failures, each of which underwent successful salvage procedures. The three patients who were treated with radiation alone (one primary, two recurrent) were followed for 85–108 months with no evidence of disease recurrence. Ballo et al. reviewed 19 consecutive patients treated with radiation as an adjuvant to surgical therapy, six of whom had positive margins.[45] They observed only one recurrence in the 19 patients. Sun et al. evaluated the treatment results of 34 evaluable patients undergoing surgery either alone or in conjunction with radiation.[46] Ten patients received postoperative radiation. Of the 24 patients who underwent surgery alone, nine had local recurrence (37.5%). Only one of the 10 patients (10%) who received both radiation and surgery recurred.

With current surgical techniques, local recurrence rates should be low after complete excision to histologically negative margins, and adjuvant radiation therapy is not indicated. If, however, a maximal effort at resecting a DFSP results in persistently positive margins, radiation therapy should be considered and is associated with good long-term control rates. In patients with sarcomatous transformation of their DFSP, particularly if there are areas of high-grade sarcoma apparent, adjuvant radiation should be considered on a routine basis.

Systemic therapy

Systemic therapy for DFSP has historically had a limited role, in view of the extremely low rate of metastasis. However, because large lesions in "precarious" locations can be difficult to excise with adequate margins without causing significant deformity, recent investigations have examined the potential

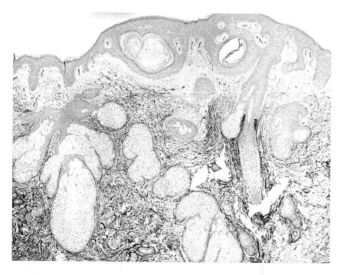

Figure 50.4 CD34 immunostaining performed on a tangential section of the peripheral margin of an excision, demonstrating strong positivity of tumor cells and establishing the presence of tumor at the margin. 100×.

role of systemic therapy in large primary tumors as well as in the rare case of metastatic disease. The recognition of the central role of deregulation of PDGFR-β and its activation by autocrine and paracrine pathways[4] has led to investigations of receptor inhibition using imatinib mesylate (Gleevec©, Novartis).[47,48] Imatinib is known to be a selective inhibitor of PDGFRα, PDGFRβ, BCR-ABL, and KIT receptor tyrosine kinases.[49] One of the first clinical experiences with imatinib for DFSP was in two patients with metastatic DFSP.[50] The first patient responded after 4 weeks of treatment, but died soon after from aggressive pulmonary metastases. The second patient experienced a partial response within 2 months of treatment, lasting at least 6 months. Evidence of successful treatment was seen in the reduction volume of lung metastases as well as the disappearance of a paratracheal mass, and was accompanied by symptomatic relief.

In another study, a patient with an unresectable paravertebral metastasis of DFSP was treated for 4 months with 400 mg imatinib twice daily.[51] The authors used fluordeoxyglucose positron emission tomography (FDG-PET) and magnetic resonance imaging (MRI) to document response to therapy. Within 2 weeks of initiating therapy, the FDG-PET uptake decreased to background levels. Tumor volume was reduced by 75% by the end of 4 months. This dramatic response to treatment allowed for the surgical resection of the mass. Final pathology revealed no viable tumor in the resected specimen.

Labropoulos *et al.* treated a patient with locally recurrent and metastatic DFSP refractory to systemic chemotherapy with 400 mg of imatinib once daily.[52] Pretreatment physical exam demonstrated a recurrent nodule on the right upper back as well as three lung nodules seen on computed tomography (CT) scan. Following 1 month of treatment, the patient experienced a dramatic response to therapy with disappearance of the upper back recurrent nodule. Three months after starting therapy, CT scan showed resolution of the pulmonary nodules. The patient remained in sustained complete remission for at least 20 months with minimal toxicity.

These earlier case reports and small series were followed by the Imatinib Target Exploration Consortium Study B2225.[53] Ten patients with advanced primary or metastatic DFSP were treated with 400 mg of imatinib twice daily. The tumors underwent molecular analysis to identify the classic translocation, t(17;22), leading to the continuous activation of PDGFRβ. Eight of the patients had locally advanced disease and the t(17;22) translocation. The two patients with metastatic disease had complex karyotypes, lacking the typical t(17;22) translocation, and did not respond to therapy. Of the eight patients with locally advanced DFSP, four had complete clinical responses. The remaining four had partial responses and went on to surgery for complete excision, rendering them disease free.

A recent combined analysis of two phase 2 trials showed a 46% response rate and a 1-year progression-free survival rate of 56%.[54] The EORTC and SWOG trials had small differences in trial design, but showed that a daily dose of 400 mg was as effective as 800 mg, resulting in a median time to progression of 1.7 years. This combined effort was similar to that of Rutkowski *et al.*, in which 15 patients were treated off

protocol.[55] Treatment with imatinib mesylate resulted in a 2-year progression-free survival rate of 60% and a 2-year overall survival rate of 78%. Partial response was seen in 67% of patients, and 47% of patients underwent surgical resection of residual disease with long-term disease-free survival, emphasizing imatinib's success in allowing for potentially less radical surgery.

Recommendations

For localized DFSP, complete resection with histologically confirmed negative margins should be the goal of treatment. No specific recommendation for a minimum margin of excision can be made on the basis of available data, but we begin with a margin width of 1 cm – carefully defined from the visible and palpable edge of the tumor – for smaller lesions or in tight anatomical confines. We design a diamond-shaped incision that encompasses at least the minimum measured margin. Any questionable or obviously positive margins are further excised with an additional centimeter of normal-appearing tissue. The same margin taken at the skin surface is taken full thickness down to and including the underlying muscular fascia. If the wound cannot be closed primarily or would require extensive undermining to achieve a primary closure, a staged approach is taken. The surgical wound is covered with a homograft, biological dressing or other skin substitute, and definitive closure deferred until the final pathology has returned, the options then being primary closure with significant undermining, split- or full-thickness skin graft or myocutaneous flap reconstruction. When margins are found to be positive at permanent pathological analysis, reexcision of the positive margins is performed and reconstruction is deferred again, if necessary. In the rare case where anatomical constraints do not allow for further surgical treatment despite a positive margin, radiation should be employed as adjuvant therapy.

In cosmetically sensitive situations or where tissue conservation is critical, such as the face or ears, Mohs surgery is an appropriate option. Locally advanced cases of DFSP, or those which are identified as metastatic and cannot be treated surgically, should be considered for imatinib treatment. Patients with sarcomatous transformation of the tumor should be treated in a manner consistent with the treatment of the highest grade sarcoma found in the specimen.

References

1. Suit H, *et al.* Radiation in management of patients with dermatofibrosarcoma protuberans. J Clin Oncol 1996; 14: 2365–9.
2. Darier J, Ferrand M. Dermatofibromas progressifs et recidivants ou fibrosarcomas de la peau. Ann Dermatol Syphiligr 1924; 5: 545–62.
3. Hoffman E. Uber das krollentreibende fibrosarkom der haut (dermatofibrosarkoma protuberans). Dermat Zeitschr 1925; 43: 1–28.
4. Shimizu A, *et al.* The dermatofibrosarcoma protuberans-associated collagen type I alpha1/platelet-derived growth factor (PDGF) B-chain fusion gene generates a transforming protein that is processed to functional PDGF-BB. Cancer Res 1999; 59: 3719–23.
5. Doolittle RF, *et al.* Simian sarcoma virus onc gene, v-sis, derived from the gene (or genes) encoding platelet-derived growth factor. Science 1983; 221: 275–7.

6. Waterfield MD, *et al*. Platelet-derived growth factor is structurally related to the putative transforming protein p28sis of simian sarcoma virus. Nature 1983; 304: 35–9.

7. Smits A, *et al*. Expression of platelet-derived growth factor and its receptors in proliferative disorders of fibroblastic origin. Am J Pathol 1992; 140: 639–48.

8. Llombart B, *et al*. Dermatofibrosarcoma protuberans: clinical, pathological, and genetic (COL1A1-PDGFB) study with therapeutic implications. Histopathology 2009; 54: 860–72.

9. Weiss SW, Goldblum JR. *Enzinger and Weiss's Soft Tissue Tumors*, 5th edn. St. Louis, MO: Mosby, 2008. pp.371–82.

10. Dupress WB, *et al*. Pigmented dermatofibrosarcoma protuberans (Bednar tumor). A pathologic, ultrastructural, and immunohistochemical study. Am J Surg Pathol 1985; 9: 630–9.

11. Mendenhall WM, *et al*. Dermatofibrosarcoma protuberans. Cancer 2004; 101: 2503–8.

12. Bandarchi B, *et al*. D2-40, a novel immunohistochemical marker in differentiating dermatofibroma from dermatofibrosarcoma protuberans. Mod Pathol 2010; 23: 434–8.

13. Lisovsky M, *et al*. Apolipoprotein D in CD34-positive and CD34-negative cutaneous neoplasms: a useful marker in differentiating superficial acral fibromyxoma from dermatofibrosarcoma protuberans. Mod Pathol 2008; 21: 31–8.

14. Sandberg AA, Bridge JA. Updates on the cytogenetics and molecular genetics of bone and soft tissue tumors: dermatofibrosarcoma protuberans and giant cell fibroblastoma. Cancer Genet Cytogenet 2003; 140: 1–12.

15. Linn SC, *et al*. Gene expression patterns and gene copy number changes in dermatofibrosarcoma protuberans. Am J Pathol 2003; 163: 2383–95.

16. Taylor HB, Helwig EB. Dermatofibrosarcoma protuberans: a study of 115 cases. Cancer 1962; 15: 717–25.

17. Hobbs ER, Wheeland RG. Treatment of dermatofibrosarcoma protuberans with Mohs micrographic surgery. Ann Surg Oncol 1988; 207: 102–7.

18. Ratner D, *et al*. Mohs micrographic surgery for the treatment of dermatofibrosarcoma protuberans. Results of a multiinstitutional series with an analysis of the extent of microscopic spread. J Am Acad Dermatol 1997; 37: 600–13.

19. Szollosi Z, Nemes Z. Transformed dermatofibrosarcoma protuberans: a clinicopathological study of eight cases. J Clin Pathol 2005; 58: 751–6.

20. Bowne WB, *et al*. Dermatofibrosarcoma protuberans: a clinicopathologic analysis of patients treated and followed at a single institution. Cancer 2000; 88: 2711–20.

21. Connelly JH, Evans HL. Dermatofibrosarcoma protuberans. A clinicopathologic review with emphasis on fibrosarcomatous areas. Am J Surg Pathol 1992; 16: 921–5.

22. Goldblum JR. CD34 positivity in fibrosarcomas which arise in dermatofibrosarcoma protuberans. Arch Pathol Lab Med 1995; 119: 238–4.

23. O'Dowd J, Laidler P. Progression of dermatofibrosarcoma protuberans to malignant fibrous histiocytoma: report of a case with implications for tumor histogenesis. Hum Pathol 1988; 19: 368–70.

24. Bennabeau RC Jr, *et al*. Dermatofibrosarcoma protuberans. Report of a case with pulmonary metastasis and multiple intrathoracic recurrences. Oncology 1974; 29: 1–12.

25. Gloster HM. Dermatofibrosarcoma protuberans. J Am Acad Dermatol 1996; 35: 335–74.

26. Fiore M, *et al*. Dermatofibrosarcoma protuberans treated at a single institution: a surgical disease with a high cure rate. J Clin Oncol 2005; 23: 7669–75.

27. Checketts SR, Hamilton TK, Baughman RD. Congenital and childhood dermatofibrosarcoma protuberans: a case report and review of the literature. J Am Acad Dermatol 2000; 42: 907–13.

28. Thornton SL, *et al*. Childhood sermatofibrosarcoma protuberans: role of preoperative imaging. J Am Acad Dermatol 2005; 53: 76–83.

29. Weinstein JM, *et al*. Congenital dermatofibrosarcoma protuberans: variability in presentation. Arch Dermatol 2003; 139: 207–11.

30. Rutgers EJ, Kroon BB, Albus-Lutter CE, Gortzak E. Dermatofibrosarcoma protuberans: treatment and prognosis. Eur J Surg Oncol 1992; 18: 241–8.

31. Gloster HM Jr, Harris KR, Roenigk RK. A comparison between Mohs micrographic surgery and wide surgical excision for the treatment of dermatofibrosarcoma protuberans. J Am Acad Dermatol 1996; 35: 82–7.

32. Mohs FE. *Chemosurgery: Microscopically Controlled Surgery for Skin Cancer*. Springfield, IL: Charles C Thomas, 1978. pp. 249–55.

33. Snow SN, *et al*. Dermatofibrosarcoma protuberans: a report on 29 patients treated by Mohs micrographic surgery with long-term follow-up and review of the literature. Cancer 2004; 101: 28–38.

34. Kimmel Z, *et al*. Peripheral excision margins for dermatofibrosarcoma protuberans: a meta-analysis of spatial data. Ann Surg Oncol 2007; 14: 2113–20.

35. Parker TL, Zitelli JA. Surgical margins for excision of dermatofibrosarcoma protuberans. J Am Acad Dermatol 1995; 32(2 Pt 1): 233–6.

36. Khatri VP, *et al*. Dermatofibrosarcoma protuberans: reappraisal of wide local excision and impact of inadequate initial treatment. Ann Surg Oncol 2003; 10: 1118–22.

37. Stojadinovic A, *et al*. Dermatofibrosarcoma protuberans of the head and neck. Ann Surg Oncol 2000; 7: 696–704.

38. Dubay D, *et al*. Low recurrence rate after surgery for dermatofibrosarcoma protuberans. A multidisciplinary approach from a single institution. Cancer 2004; 100: 1008–16.

39. Farma JM, *et al*. Dermatofibrosarcoma protuberans: how wide should we resect? Ann Surg Oncol 2010; 17: 2112–18.

40. Bendix-Hansen K, Myhre-Jensen O, Kaae S. Dermatofibrosarcoma protuberans. A clinico-pathological study of nineteen cases and review of world literature. Scand J Plast Reconstr Surg 1983; 17: 247–52.

41. Fields RC, *et al*. Dermatofibrosarcoma protuberans (DFSP): predictors of recurrence and use of systemic therapy. Ann Surg Oncol 2011; 18: 328–36.

42. Burkhardt BR, *et al*. Dermatofibrosarcoma protuberans. Study of fifty-six cases. Am J Surg 1966; 111: 638–44.

43. Mark RJ, *et al*. Dermatofibrosarcoma protuberans of the head and neck. A report of 16 cases. Arch Otolaryngol Head Neck Surg 1993; 119: 891–6.

44. Marks LB, *et al*. Dermatofibrosarcoma protuberans treated with radiation therapy. Int J Radiat Oncol Biol Phys 1989; 17: 379–84.

45. Ballo MT, *et al*. The role of radiation therapy in the management of dermatofibrosarcoma protuberans. Int J Radiat Oncol Biol Phys 1998; 40: 823–7.

46. Sun LM, *et al*. Dermatofibrosarcoma protuberans: treatment results of 35 cases. Radiother Oncol 2000; 57: 175–81.

47. Sjoblom T, *et al*. Growth inhibition of dermatofibrosarcoma protuberans tumors by the platelet-derived growth factor receptor antagonist STI571 through induction of apoptosis. Cancer Res 2001; 61: 5778–83.

48. Stacchiotti S, *et al*. Dermatofibrosarcoma protuberans-derived fibrosarcoma: clinical history, biological profile and sensitivity to imatinib. Int J Cancer 2011; 129: 1761–72.

49. Zhang J, Yang PL, Gray NS. Targeting cancer with small molecule kinase inhibitors. Nat Rev Cancer 2009; 9: 28–39.

50. Maki RG, *et al*. Differential sensitivity to imatinib of 2 patients with metastatic sarcoma arising from dermatofibrosarcoma protuberans. Int J Cancer 2002; 100: 623–6.

51. Rubin BP, *et al*. Molecular targeting of platelet-derived growth factor B by imatinib mesylate in a patient with metastatic dermatofibrosarcoma protuberans. J Clin Oncol 2002; 20: 3586–91.

52. Labropoulos S, *et al*. Sustained complete remission of metastatic dermatofibrosarcoma protuberans with imatinib mesylate. Anticancer Drugs 2005; 16: 461–6.

53. McArthur GA, *et al*. Molecular and clinical analysis of locally advanced dermatofibrosarcoma protuberans treated with imatinib: Imatinib Target Exploration Consortium Study B2225. J Clin Oncol 2005; 23: 866–73.

54. Rutkowski P, *et al*. Imatinib mesylate in advanced dermatofibrosarcoma protuberans: pooled analysis of two phase II clinical trials. J Clin Oncol 2010; 28: 1772–9.

55. Rutkowski P, *et al*. Treatment of advanced dermatofibrosarcoma protuberans with imatinib mesylate with or without surgical resection. J Eur Acad Dermatol Venereol 2011; 25: 264–70.

Section 9: Cutaneous Malignancies

51 Unusual Melanomas

Omid Hamid,[1] Richard D. Carvajal,[2] Donald L. Morton,[3] and Mark Faries[3]

[1] Melanoma Center, The Angeles Clinic and Research Institute, Santa Monica, CA, USA
[2] Melanoma/Sarcoma and Developmental Therapeutics Services, Memorial Sloan-Kettering Cancer Center, New York, NY, USA
[3] John Wayne Cancer Institute, Santa Monica, CA, USA

Introduction

Malignant melanoma is a malignant neoplasm that arises from melanocytes and accounts for 1–2% of all malignancies. Despite public health measures regarding sun exposure, its incidence is rising rapidly, and there has been a 300% increase in its incidence over the last four decades, with this statistic continuing to rise. In 5–10% of cases, melanoma arises from sites not originating in the skin. These sites can comprise the oral cavities, nasal sinuses, genital tract, and rectum which have mucosa leading to mucosal melanomas. Melanoma may also occur on the retina of the eye or in the uveal tract, commonly referred to as uveal melanoma.

The paradigm of therapy for cutaneous melanoma has experienced tremendous change recently. Immunotherapeutic options have diversified to include immunomodulatory antibodies with randomized trials showing survival advantage. The rebirth of immunotherapy has created therapeutic opportunities not limited strictly to the inpatient setting. This progress, combined with the effective translation of therapies targeting pathways known to be important in oncogenic transformation, has created a renaissance in melanoma care. The wealth of novel therapeutic options available to patients has changed the landscape of melanoma therapy. Several rational targets have been elucidated and are being interrogated in large-scale trials for cutaneous melanoma. In view of the dramatic progress in this field, there is now a mandate for physicians to become versed not only in the molecular oncology but also the basis of immunotherapy in this disease. Unfortunately, the majority of these trials have excluded rare variants of malignant melanoma, such as mucosal melanoma and uveal melanoma. While melanoma of the mucosal tract has been included in the evaluation of therapeutics, their outcomes have never been presented separately. Uveal melanomas, conversely, have been excluded from participation and evaluation. The divergence in therapeutic information for these variants has created a dearth of clinical pathways for these rare tumors. Given the recent success with personalized therapeutics in cancer care, it becomes even more important to recognize these melanoma variants and their potential therapeutic similarities and differences.

Mucosal melanoma

Overview

Although melanoma is a relatively common malignancy, the vast majority of cases arise in the skin, and most may be related to ultraviolet radiation exposure. Mucosal melanoma does not conform to this pattern as it arises in areas with mucosal epithelium and in regions of the body that are largely shielded from ultraviolet radiation. Mucosal melanomas are distinct from cutaneous melanoma in their affected population, their clinical presentation, and their prognosis. In the United States, where cutaneous melanoma is relatively common, mucosal melanoma makes up only 1.3% of all cases (Fig. 51.1a).[1] However, mucosal primary sites may account for over 10% of melanoma among African-Americans and about a third of cases in China.[2] It appears that, even though the proportion of mucosal primaries is higher, the absolute incidence of mucosal melanoma does not vary markedly among different populations[3] and is approximately 0.15/100,000.[4] In contrast to cutaneous melanoma, which has increased dramatically in incidence, with the exceptions noted below, the rate of mucosal melanoma has not changed substantially over time.

Although the absolute incidence of melanoma in mucosal sites is low, an interesting examination of spatial density of melanoma in "sun-shielded" sites has been performed.[5] In this analysis, the frequency of melanomas in the vulvar, subungual, palmar, and volar skin as well as mucosal sites (anal canal and vagina) was reviewed and was actually quite high relative to the small amount of body surface area occupied by those sites.

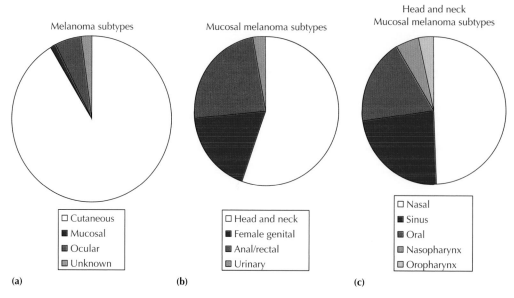

Figure 51.1 (a) Proportions of several melanoma subtypes as described by the National Cancer Database. (b) Proportions of subtypes of mucosal melanoma. (c) Proportions of subtypes of head and neck mucosal melanoma.

For example, anal canal melanomas demonstrated almost twice the average density of cutaneous melanoma, and vaginal melanomas occurred in a density roughly equal to that of typical cutaneous primaries. The chronically sun-exposed skin of the face has twice the average cutaneous melanoma density but interestingly, the vulva has almost the same density. This suggests that while the *absolute* incidence of melanoma in these regions is quite low, the high frequency relative to surface area may be due to a specific vulnerability to melanocytic malignant transformation in those regions.

The adverse clinical behavior of mucosal melanoma has been attributed to late diagnosis, due to the relatively hidden anatomical sites, or to the rich network of blood and lymphatic vessels that invest their mucosal locations. These may well play a role but recent research into the biology of these tumors has revealed a different genetic basis for these melanomas. These differences may begin to explain the differences in behavior and may also open new avenues for treatment.

The age of diagnosis of mucosal melanomas is approximately 10 years more than that of cutaneous melanoma, with peak age in the seventh decade. Mucosal melanomas are most common in the head and neck (55.4%), followed by the ano-rectum (23.8%), female genital tract (18%), and urinary tract (2.8%) (Fig. 51.1b).[1] Overall, there is a female predominance, due to the much greater frequency of the disease in the vulva or vagina relative to the penis. These different sites have largely been studied separately because in most centers, the primary treatment of different sites is provided by different disciplines, and this chapter will consider each anatomical site individually. This class of melanoma overall has recently been the subject of intense research due to the specific genetic abnormalities found in these lesions, which have opened new avenues for potential treatment for a disease that has proved resistant to most therapies to date.

Head and neck

Presentation and prognosis

First described by Weber in 1859, head and neck mucosa melanoma is the most common mucosal subtype.[6] A population-based evaluation of these tumors found the most common primary site to be the nasal cavity (49.1%) followed by paranasal sinuses (23.1%), the oral cavity (18.8%), the nasopharynx (5.5%), and the oropharynx (3.2%) (Fig. 51.1c).[7] The larynx and middle ear have also been reported as primary sites, although only very rarely.[8] This pattern of presentation mimics the migration of melanocytes from the neural crest during development, leading to much less frequent melanoma in mucosa derived from endoderm such as in the oropharynx or below. This distribution following developmental patterns has led some to suggest embryonic abnormalities as an etiological factor. Other possible etiologies include tobacco and other environmental factors, including exposure to formaldehyde.[6] Several reports have suggested a slight male predominance, but the same population-based study found a slight female predominance (53.9%).[7] There may be regional variation in the epidemiology of head and neck mucosal melanoma as a relatively large series from Shanghai found a 2:1 male predominance and a much younger age of onset (54.1 years).

The presenting signs and symptoms of head and neck mucosal melanoma are largely location dependent and may be present for 3–8 months prior to diagnosis.[6] For lesions in the nasal cavity, the most common symptoms are epistaxis (72%) and unilateral nasal obstruction (53.5%), but pain, facial deformity or blindness may occur with more advanced lesions.[9] Oral melanomas are frequently discovered due to a pigmented lesion (62%), ill-fitting dentures (25%) or bleeding (13%) (Fig. 51.2).[6] Areas of pigmentation in the oral cavity are common and are most frequently benign. A common cause is tattooing due to leaching of dental amalgam.[10] Oral melanosis,

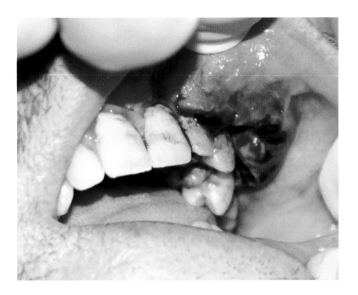

Figure 51.2 Oral mucosal melanoma arising on the gingiva. The advanced nature of the lesion is clearly visible and is typical.

a generally benign proliferation of melanocytes in the mucosa, may precede melanoma in up to one-third of cases.[3] Most lesions present while still clinically localized (60–88%), with a minority having evident nodal (10–30%) or distant (<15%) metastases.[9,11–13]

Despite this localized presentation, the prognosis is poor. As is the case with many mucosal sites, prognostic factors are difficult to determine due to the poor outcomes of these patients overall and the small numbers of cases. As a result, staging has been inconsistent over time. The most commonly employed staging system has been that proposed by Ballantyne in 1970,[14] utilizing three stages: I localized, II regional metastases, III distant metastases. This has generally been found to be prognostic, but since the vast majority of patients present with localized disease, its ability to provide useful information is limited. Some have employed the American Joint Commission on Cancer (AJCC) staging system for head and neck epithelial tumors and found it to be prognostic in melanoma as well. In the most recent AJCC staging manual (7th edition), head and neck mucosal melanoma was given its own classification.[15] This system is interesting in that the tumor staging begins with T3 as the lowest tumor stage, which is considered stage III disease. T4a tumors are moderately advanced disease involving deep soft tissue, cartilage, bone or overlying skin. This, or any nodal involvement, is categorized as stage IVA. T4b tumors are "very advanced" and involve brain, dura, skull base, lower cranial nerves, masticator space, carotid artery, prevertebral space, or mediastinum. As with the earlier staging system, the relatively small number of categories may limit the ability of this system to provide prognostic discrimination.

Additional prognostic factors have been proposed. Tumor size,[6,7,16] thickness,[17] and level of invasion[18] have been found by some to be prognostic, but not by others.[19] Possibly due to ease of diagnosis, primary site appears to affect outcome, with nasal lesions being most favorable (5-year survival 15–30%) followed by oral (5-year survival 12%), and sinus (5-year survival 0–5%).[6] Increased age,[12] increased mitoses,[9] increased

Ki-67,[20] absence of p53,[13] margin-positive resection,[12] and vascular invasion[6] are also potential prognostic variables. Pseudopapillomatous growth has been associated with a markedly higher local recurrence rate in one large series, but this was not confirmed in a subsequent study.[9,12]

Treatment

Treatment of head and neck mucosal melanoma is challenging. The modalities available include surgery, radiotherapy, and medical therapy. Surgical resection remains the main modality, but the possibility of radical resection is limited due to the frequently advanced nature of the primary lesion and the close proximity of vital structures. In addition, in mucosal melanomas of the head and neck and other sites, the microscopic extent of the tumor frequently exceeds the visible area of involvement. This characteristic makes clear margins even more difficult to achieve and local recurrence is a frequent problem.

When the lesion is relatively small, which is most common with nasal or oral melanomas, surgical resection may be considered as a sole therapy. This is dependent on securing negative margins. Negative margins have been associated with better overall survival and may be achieved in a repeated resection with equally favorable outcomes.[12] An *en bloc* resection has been associated with improved prognosis, but it is not clear from the retrospective data available whether this association was due to the surgical technique or to the size and location of tumors that could be successfully excised in this fashion.[21] In recent series, several authors have recommended consideration of endoscopic resection. This generally precludes the possibility of an *en bloc* resection, but a complete resection may be possible. One endoscopic series reported that 70% of endoscopic resections were complete, which was similar to the 80% rate recorded with the conventional approach.[22] It should be noted, however, that a functional and cosmetically acceptable result can be obtained in many radical, open resections through the use of prosthodontic obturators, which play an important role in preserving quality of life for these patients.[23]

Regional lymph nodes are a frequent site of early metastasis. The pathological status of these nodes may impact prognosis. However, not all series have found prognostic significance of nodal involvement. This is likely due to the advanced nature of the most primary lesions and the likelihood of hematogenous dissemination in many patients at presentation. Thus, an elective complete lymph node dissection is not indicated. However, some have proposed the use of lymphatic mapping and sentinel lymph node biopsy in selected patients with no clinically involved regional lymph nodes.[6] This may be of particular use in patients with oral and possibly nasal primary lesions.

Since the anatomical location and pathological nature of head and neck mucosal melanoma are associated with high local recurrence rates (>50%), even with radical approaches, the addition of other modalities to surgery may be advisable in many cases. Melanoma has traditionally been considered a radioresistant tumor. In addition to their role in skin protection against ultraviolet radiation, melanocytes are thought to play a role in detoxifying reactive compounds. This ability has suggested the possibility of a more extensive mechanism for repairing radiation-induced damage in melanocytes and melanoma cells, limiting the potential therapeutic impact of radiation therapy. However, both the preclinical and clinical data regarding this subject are mixed.

A review of 160 patients at several institutions in France demonstrated that there was a substantial improvement (55.6% versus 29.9%, *p* <0.01) in local recurrence when radiotherapy was used as a postsurgical adjuvant. The multivariate hazard ratio for local recurrence was 0.31 (95% confidence interval (CI) 0.15–0.61, *p* <0.01) in favor of radiation.[24] Although the multivariate analysis did not indicate an overall survival benefit, given the morbidity of recurrence in these locations, improvement in local control alone is sufficient to justify recommending radiation for many of these patients. Other reports demonstrate similar findings.[9] Radiotherapy has also been used as a definitive therapy without surgery in a few small series. Some have suggested that it is not an adequate option, but others have reported patients with sustained periods of remission using definitive radiotherapy, particularly for sinonasal primaries.[25]

Due to these biological concerns, hypofractionated radiotherapy consisting of larger fractions of radiation given at each treatment was suggested in melanoma.[26] This approach is often used in adjuvant radiotherapy of metastatic cutaneous melanoma. In head and neck mucosal melanoma, hypofractionation has been reported to induce higher response rates and better outcomes in some series.[27] However, a relatively recent report from the MD Anderson Cancer Center, an early proponent of hypofractionation, suggested that standard fractionation regimens were associated with better outcomes.[22] Toxicity, manifested by mucositis, has been associated with more favorable responses, but managing such toxicity is difficult because treatment breaks due to toxicity have been associated with compromised local control.[21,22]

Cutaneous melanoma has not responded well to systemic, cytotoxic chemotherapy and there is little evidence of efficacy in mucosal head and neck melanoma. However, some centers commonly use chemotherapy consisting of dacarbazine and cisplatin as a postsurgical adjuvant and have reported favorable outcomes in those patients compared to those who did not receive chemotherapy.[28] No randomized comparisons have been possible. A series of 15 patients receiving biochemotherapy demonstrated a remarkably high rate of objective response (47%) and complete response (27%).[11] Several of those

responses were durable up to 49 months. Biochemotherapy is used in metastatic cutaneous melanoma only in highly selected cases at most institutions currently, but may be a reasonable option in these highly aggressive mucosal lesions.

Anorectal melanoma
Presentation and prognosis

Anorectal melanoma was first described by Moore in 1857.[29] It constitutes approximately 0.31% of melanomas in the United States, and 1–5% of anal canal tumors.[1,30,31] In Sweden, the rates are similar with anal primaries representing 0.4% of melanomas and having an incidence of 1.0/million in women and 0.7/million in men.[32] The incidence appears to have been stable over time,[17] although a surge in incidence was reported among young men in San Francsiso in the late 1980s.[33] This led to speculation that the human immunodeficiency virus was a risk factor for the disease. However, there have not been further data to substantiate this theory. The disease has a female predominance (1.5–2:1).[34–36] As with head and neck melanoma, it occurs in an older age group than cutaneous melanoma with a mean age of onset in the late seventh or eighth decade and is extremely rare in the pediatric age group.[37] There does not appear to be a relationship with environmental ultraviolet radiation exposure.[38]

Anorectal melanoma is thought to originate from the region of the anal canal. Clemmensen and colleagues examined the epithelial zones of this area and found melanocytes to be frequently present in the anal squamous zone, sporadically in the transitional zone and not at all in the colorectal zone (Fig. 51.3).[39] This largely parallels the location of anorectal melanomas, with the majority of lesions arising at or near the dentate line. The possibility of a true rectal primary melanoma has been disputed, although some evidence of this as a very rare occurrence exists.[40] Baskies *et al.*[41] reported that 90% in their series arose at or near the dentate line, and Cooper *et al.* reported two-thirds of their cases from the proximal pectin (distal portion of the anal canal, covered by stratified squamous epithelium) at or near the anal valves.[42] In a review of a large number of cases from the Swedish National Cancer Registry, Ragnarsson-Olding *et al.* found that 54% of tumors arose in the anal canal, and 10% from the anal verge.[32] Highlighting the difficulty in making a meaningful distinction of the site of origin of these

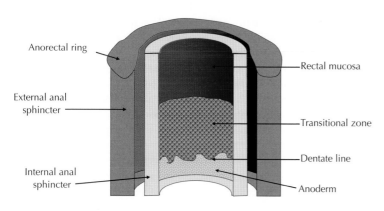

Figure 51.3 Anatomical structure of the anal canal. The canal is bordered by the intersphincteric groove at the distal aspect and by the anorectal ring at the proximal point. It is surrounded by the internal anal sphincter. The epithelium transitions from squamous anoderm into the mucosal rectum. The dentate line marks the distal end of the transitional mucosa. Most anal melanomas arise from this transitional area but due to the size of lesions, it is often difficult to determine the exact site of origin.

frequently advanced tumors, they found that 24% of tumors encompassed the entire anorectal unit.

Most patients present with bleeding (45–78%). Other common symptoms include pain (13–27%), mass (16–34%), change in bowel habits (10–22%), and pruritus (3–8%).[31,43–48] Anorectal melanoma is also commonly diagnosed as a "hemorrhoid" (8–16%), frequently considered thrombosed due to dark coloration and pain. Symptoms are typically present for a number of months (mean 3–5 months) before a diagnosis is made.[49] A longer symptom duration has been associated with worse outcomes[50] but the diagnosis is frequently made at a late stage because of the relatively hidden nature of the anatomical location, the lack of apparent pigment in approximately one-third of tumors and a low index of suspicion. At the time of biopsy, only a minority of cases are clinically suspected to be melanoma. In a review of several studies, 40% of melanomas were thought to be carcinoma, 17% hemorrhoid, and 14% polyp, and only 23% were thought to be melanoma.[42] Melanoma may also be confused with anaplastic squamous cell carcinoma, and immunohistochemical staining with S-100, Melan-A, and HMB-45 is helpful in establishing the diagnosis.[50]

Staging in anorectal melanoma has followed the Ballantyne three-stage classification described above (I localized, II regional, III distant). Stage is the most significant prognostic variable. Survival at 5 years is 27–32% for stage I, 10–17% for stage II, and 0% for stage III. Median survivals are 24 months, 17 months and 8 months, respectively.[34,51] Thin lesions (<2 mm[52] or <4 mm[53]) have better survival. Other potential prognostic factors include tumor size,[43] ulceration,[54] anatomical invasion,[30] age,[32] perineural invasion,[54] and Ki-67 expression.[55]

Tumor sizes are large, compared to cutaneous melanoma. Mean tumor diameter is between 2 and 5 cm, and tumors can preferentially spread radially or form nodules, leading to a polypoid configuration.[43,45,54,56,57] Mean depth is between 3.7 and 8 mm.[58] Most anorectal melanomas present with clinically localized disease, but a substantial fraction demonstrate either regional or distant metastasis at presentation. Iddings *et al.* examined the Surveillance, Epidemiology, and End Results (SEER) database in which 60% of anorectal melanomas were localized, but 19% had lymph node metastases and 21% had distant metastases.[34] Presentation stage is similar in the Swedish National Registry with one-third of patients presenting with metastases.[31] Fourteen percent of patients reported palpable metastatic lymph nodes. Data over time are mixed with regard to whether anorectal melanomas are being detected at an earlier point. In some series in recent years, the mean tumor thickness appears to be decreasing[51,54] but in a population-based evaluation, either the same or a greater number of tumors were diagnosed with lymph node metastases.[1,51] The continued poor prognosis for these patients demonstrates that if progress has been made in detection, it has been inadequate.

The workup of a patient with anorectal melanoma should include a thorough history and physical examination with careful attention to potential involvement of the anal sphincter and regional lymph nodes. Due to the high likelihood of metastases, radiographic staging should usually be performed as well to assess for regional and distant spread. Evaluation of the primary tumor may be facilitated in some cases by the use of endorectal ultrasound to provide a more detailed assessment of the potential for involvement of the sphincter.[59] Magnetic resonance imagng (MRI) may also be useful, particularly in pigmented melanomas as the melanin in these tumors exhibits specific characteristics on MR imaging.[60] Such involvement of the sphincter would alter possible local surgical therapy.

Treatment

Surgery is an important component of therapy for most patients with anorectal melanoma. For those with localized or regional disease, resection is performed with potential curative intent, and for those with metastases, surgery may play a role to control pain, bleeding or obstruction (Fig. 51.4). With involvement of the anal sphincter, the choice of surgical approach is clear and requires abdominoperineal resection (APR). For those without such involvement, it has been highly controversial whether APR or wide local excision (WLE) should be preferred. Data to inform a comparison of APR and WLE are difficult to obtain and rely on retrospective series. These are uniformly hampered by small numbers, case selection biases, and unmeasured covariates, which are likely to have a marked impact on outcome. Furthermore, even when experts agree on basic findings with regard to outcomes with each surgical approach, the implications of these data and treatment recommendations that result are often very different.

There is now general agreement that APR, the more radical procedure, does not improve overall survival for patients with this disease. Many series also conclude that local disease control rates are higher with APR compared to WLE.[30,50,61,62] While this is not universal, and a few reports show equivalent or improved rates of local control with WLE,[54,63] even those authors who assume that APR improves local recurrence rates do not conclude that it is the more favored procedure. This is due to the adverse effects of APR on quality of life, the possibility of salvage APR if local recurrence does occur, and the poor survival of these patients overall. The experience of the Memorial Sloan-Kettering Cancer Center is illustrative in this regard. An initial report from that institution found that 90% of long-term survivors were treated by APR. Given the high risk of systemic disease in locally advanced tumors, their recommendation at the time was for APR in relatively early cases in which long-term survival might be achieved.[43] A more recent analysis from the same institution demonstrated a marked change in the practice pattern that occurred in approximately 1997, with most patients now being treated by WLE.[54] In this recent report the authors conclude, "There is no convincing evidence to indicate that radical resection of primary anorectal melanoma is associated with improvement in local control or survival. Patients should undergo [local excision] whenever technically feasible." This evolution mirrors that at many melanoma centers.[64] However, on a population basis, SEER data reveal that the rate of APR, which was 27% between 1973 and 1996, actually increased to 43.2% between 1997 and 2003.[34] The reason for this trend is unknown, but it indicates that many physicians treating anorectal

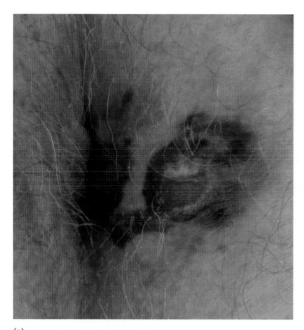
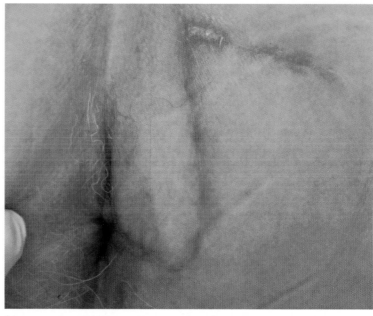

(a)   (b)

Figure 51.4 Anal melanoma. (a) As is evident, the lesion is quite broad at presentation. (b) Despite its size, it is possible to perform a sphincter-preserving wide local excision with flap reconstruction. Although there has been considerable debate regarding optimal surgical management, most melanoma centers now recommend this approach if it is technically possible.

melanoma remain unfamiliar with current expert recommendations or are uncertain about the interpretation of available data.

Regional nodal evaluation has historically also been the subject of some controversy. Since the anus is a lymphatic watershed area, anorectal melanoma may spread to either inguinal or perirectal/mesenteric lymph nodes. Series vary considerably in reporting frequency of metastatic nodes in each location. Brady *et al.* reported involvement of mesenteric lymph nodes in 42% of cases, and Cooper *et al.* 69%.[42,43] However, the rate of involvement of these nodes is likely to be dependent on the size of the primary tumor and the extent to which it has grown cephalad. Small series of lymphatic mapping and sentinel node biopsy have also been reported, indicating more common primary inguinal drainage.[65–67]

Due to the difficulty in imaging this anatomical area by planar lymphoscintigraphy, axial imaging using single photon emission computed tomography (SPECT) may be helpful in determining the likelihood of mesenteric nodal involvement.[68] Radiation therapy may also be employed as a postsurgical adjuvant. The utility of this therapy is not clearly established, and some nonrandomized comparisons have failed to show a benefit for radiation.[51] However, a report from Ballo and colleagues in which 23 patients with anorectal melanoma underwent sphincter sparing surgery followed by hypofractionated radiotherapy demonstrated favorable local and nodal control rates of 74% and 84%, respectively, at 5 years.[53]

Radiation is also one of the modalities that has been used for local palliation in cases of unresectable disease. Unfortunately, disease control rates with gross disease are not favorable, with some series reporting a majority of patients progressing despite radiation.[30] Other local palliative treatments have been reported

including electrochemotherapy[69] and local injection of interferon-β.[70]

Success in systemic therapy of anal melanoma has been limited. One series has examined the use of biochemotherapy in 18 patients with metastatic anorectal melanoma.[71] In this series, 44% of patients had major responses, two (11%) of which were complete, and the median overall survival was 12.2. months. As discussed below, there is currently a significant interest in targeted therapies for these tumors, which may harbor specific mutations making them potentially sensitive to such therapies.

Genitourinary tract

The female genitourinary tract is the site of 18% of mucosal melanomas, and the urinary tract constitutes just over 2%.[1] Since vulvar and vaginal melanomas are so much more common than melanoma of the penis, the ratio of female to male is more than 10:1. Vaginal melanoma has no predilection for populations based upon ethnic differences, and any difference in incidence in vulvar melanomas is much less than that of cutaneous melanoma. This suggests that there is little or no influence of ultraviolet radiation in its etiology.[72]

Vulvar melanoma is much more common than vaginal melanoma. Most primary lesions are pigmented and the most common primary site is the labia minora. The labia majora and clitoris are less common sites, and lesions frequently extend to the mucocutaneous junction with the vagina.[17] Early reports recommended radical vulvectomy with concomitant inguinal node dissection. More recent recommendations follow those for cutaneous melanoma sites and lymphatic mapping with sentinel lymph node biopsy has been employed in place of elective lymph node dissection. Overall, the prognosis for vulvar melanoma remains poor, although it is significantly better than that of vaginal melanoma. Vaginal melanomas most commonly occur in the lower third of the vagina. Rarely melanoma can develop in the cervix, representing less than 5% of mucosal primaries. Melanoma of the penis is equally rare at 2.5% of mucosal melanomas.[73] Urethral melanomas are also more common in women by nearly 2:1.

Esophagus

Esophageal melanoma is quite rare. It presents at a similar, later age as other mucosal melanomas, but is frequently more advanced at presentation due to its internal location. Presenting symptoms include dysphagia, weight loss, and anemia due to gastrointestinal bleeding. The primary sites appear to be fairly evenly distributed through the esophagus, extending down to the gastroesophageal junction. Some have recommended radical excision as the best treatment[74] but given the poor prognosis of these lesions related to the high rate of systemic spread, and the advanced age of many of the patients, treatment decisions should be individualized.

Etiology/genetic basis

Unlike cutaneous melanoma, mucosal melanoma does not appear to be related to ultraviolet radiation exposure. This is suggested by the sun-protected sites of most of these lesions, the lack of increase with decreasing latitude, and the relatively similar incidences among ethnic groups with different pigmentation. In addition, mutations that are common in cutaneous melanoma and genetic changes consistent with ultraviolet damage are almost never found in mucosal melanomas. Various alternative etiologies, including viral causes such as human herpesvirus-8 and human papillomavirus-16, have been examined but no evidence for these as causative agents has been found.[75] There has also been speculation that environmental factors, related to the potential role of melanocytes in detoxifying polycyclic hydrocarbons, including those in tobacco, may play a role in mucosal melanoma, but firm evidence is still lacking.[17]

Curtin et al. examined genetic changes found in melanomas from various body sites including melanomas from chronically sun-damaged skin, intermittently exposed skin, acral skin and from mucosal sites.[76] This important study evaluated specimens from the following sites: chronically sun-damaged skin ($n=30$), intermittently sun-exposed skin ($n=40$), palmar/volar/subungual sites ($n=36$), and mucosal sites ($n=20$). The specimens were examined for genome-wide alterations in copy number and mutations in BRAF and N-RAS. Specimens derived from mucosal or acral sites demonstrated a much greater degree of chromosomal aberrations than those from chronically or intermittently sun-exposed skin. In particular, amplifications were much more frequent (85%) in mucosal melanoma than in the chronic or intermittent sun-exposed sites. Whereas mutations in specific components of the mitogen-activated protein kinase (MAPK) pathway were common in intermittently sun-exposed areas (BRAF 59%,

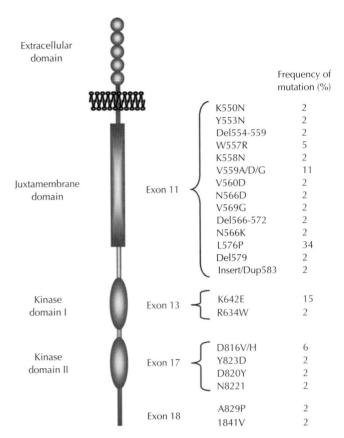

Figure 51.5 Schematic representation of the KIT tyrosine kinase receptor mutation frequency. Five immunoglobulin-like regions are located in the extracellular domain and serve as the binding site for the KIT ligand, stem cell factor. The juxtamembrane autoinhibitory domain serves to maintain the kinase domains in an inhibited state unless the receptor is bound by ligand. KIT mutations occur with highest frequency (~70%) in exon 11 of the juxtamembrane domain. Mutations also occur in the kinase domain I, exon 13 (~13%), and kinase domain II, exon 17 (~9%). All percentages are rounded to the nearest whole number. Reproduced with permission from Woodman and Davies.[80]

N-RAS 22%), they were very uncommon in mucosal sites (BRAF 11%, N-RAS 5%). This demonstrates that the genetic alterations that lead to malignancy for each of these subtypes of melanoma are different, and raises the possibility that other mechanisms of transformation could be identified and might lead to targeted therapeutic interventions for mucosal melanoma.

N-RAS mutations are of particular interest in esophageal melanoma, with 6/16 cases (37.5%) mutated in one series.[77] A separate series found N-RAS mutations in 2/3 esophageal melanoma patients.[78] It may also be a relatively common finding in vaginal primary melanomas, with one series finding N-RAS mutations in 43% of those lesions (3/7).[79]

In this regard, KIT has been a particular gene of interest for mucosal melanoma (Fig. 51.5).[80] The KIT gene was identified in 1987 and codes for CD117, a type III receptor tyrosine kinase, the ligand of which is stem cell factor.[81] Activation of CD117 leads to signaling through several downstream pathways, including the MAPK and PI3kinase pathways, both of which, as noted above, are involved in melanoma development.

It is also involved in the normal melanocyte migration during development.[82,83]

Paradoxically, although CD117 is commonly expressed in normal melanocytes and benign nevi, it is frequently lost in dysplastic nevi and is not commonly seen in nodular melanomas or superficial spreading melanomas.[84] In addition, expression of CD117 has been associated with a loss of malignant behavior in some experiments, and loss of the protein is associated with melanoma progression.[85] These findings did not suggest that KIT would play a significant role in melanoma, but screens by immunohistochemistry of some melanoma subtypes demonstrated expression of the protein, and follow-up genetic studies found mutation or amplification of the gene to be present in some patients. Several series have now examined the frequency of CD117 expression and KIT aberration in melanoma. Mutations in KIT in melanoma have been identified in exons 11, 13, 17, and 18. In contrast with gastrointestinal stromal tumors, mutations in melanoma have not been found in exon 9.

These changes are relatively common in melanomas arising in chronically sun-damaged, acral or mucosal sites. Curtin et al. reported a frequency of 21% (8/38) of KIT mutations and 26% (10/38) of amplifications in mucosal melanoma.[76] Very similar mutation frequencies (15–38%) and amplification frequencies (20–33%) have been reported in several subsequent series.[86–91] There may be some regional variation, as a large study of 167 tumors among Chinese patients found a KIT mutation rate of only 9.6% and an amplification rate of 10.2%, and less than 6% of mucosal melanomas in a Korean series demonstrated mutations[2,92] There is also some variability in the specific mutations noted among different world regions. While it is clear that the majority of even mucosal melanomas do not harbor KIT mutations, the proportion of mutated cases is sufficient to justify testing in this subgroup.

In an effort to facilitate evaluation of mutation status, immunohistochemical (IHC) staining for CD117 has been proposed as a screening tool. If mutation or amplification status, which are likely to be predictive markers for sensitivity to targeted therapies, is correlated with staining for CD117, the simpler, faster, and less expensive IHC test could be used to select patients for genetic evaluation. There appears to be some correlation between the two modalities, but controversy remains as to whether CD117 staining is adequately sensitive to serve as a reliable screening method. Some have found that nearly all patients with KIT mutations have very strong CD117 expression. For example, Torres-Cabala et al. found that 82% of KIT mutant tumors stained positive in >50% of tumor cells.[90]

However, in a study of gastrointestinal stromal tumor (GIST), KIT mutations were found in 4/25 CD117 negative cases, including mutations that predict sensitivity to targeted therapy.[93] Furthermore, the degree of CD117 staining in GIST does not appear to be correlated with benefit from therapy.[94] In melanoma, Kong et al. reported that CD117 expression was positively correlated with KIT gene copy number, though not with mutation status.[2] In fact, CD117 was positive in only 44% of their tumors with KIT mutations. Beadling et al. reported that CD117 staining was absent in 50% of their patients with KIT mutation, while one-third did not have an increased KIT copy number.[88] Overall, it appears that CD117 staining may not be sufficiently sensitive as a screening tool to identify KIT mutations, and that among patients with mucosal melanoma, mutational analysis may be required.

The object of identifying KIT abnormalities in mucosal melanomas is to be able to select those patients who may benefit from targeted tyrosine kinase inhibitors such as imatinib, dasatinib, or sorafenib. Such inhibitors have demonstrated dramatic effectiveness in GIST and it is hoped they may be similarly beneficial in selected melanoma patients. However, initial clinical results were disappointing. In several trials of unselected melanoma patients, the agents led to no detectible benefit.[95–98] When it became evident that KIT abnormalities were only present in a relatively small subset of melanoma patients, interest in the therapeutic potential of these inhibitors was focused on identifying the subgroup that might benefit. Several striking case reports documented remarkable responses in a handful of patients who harbored KIT aberrations.[91,99–101] These were then followed by larger clinical trials examining selected patient populations.

Two such trials have been reported to date. One trial conducted by Fisher et al. has only been reported in abstract form.[102] The trial enrolled 20 patients with acral melanoma, mucosal melanoma or melanoma arising in chronically sun-damaged sites. No responses were seen in KIT wild-type patients but among patients with KIT mutations, 5/10 had partial responses. The second trial was recently reported by Carvajal and colleagues.[103] This multicenter phase 2 study screened 295 patients for KIT mutation or amplification. Among 51 patients with genetic aberrations, 28 were treated with imatinib 400 mg twice daily. The overall durable response rate was 16% and median overall survival was 46.3 weeks. Responses tended to occur in patients with mutations at certain hot spots (e.g. exon 11 L576P, exon 13 K642E) and in tumors with a high mutant to wild-type allele ratio. As more clinical experience with the use of these inhibitors in mucosal melanoma patients is acquired, better methods of predicting clinical benefit will likely be developed.

Summary

Mucosal melanoma is a rare disease typified by late presentation and often rapid progression. It appears to arise in populations that are distinct from those of cutaneous melanoma and to stem from different etiological factors. Recent data suggest that specific genetic alterations occur in mucosal melanoma and these may make the disease amenable to treatment with new or emerging targeted therapies.

Uveal melanoma

Uveal melanomas (UM) arise from melanocytes within the uveal tract, which consists of the iris, ciliary body, and choroid of the eye, and account for 70% of all primary eye malignancies, making them the most common primary intraocular malignancy in adults.[104] Despite this fact, uveal melanoma constitutes about only 5% of all melanoma. Its incidence is 4.3 individuals per million per year with 1500 cases diagnosed in the United

States yearly.[1,105-107] There is a higher rate in men (4.9 per million) than women (3.7 cases per million). Incidence is higher in older age. Current understanding of the biology of UM proposes that it is biologically distinct from cutaneous melanomas.[1,105] Development of metastasis is common and occurs in approximately 50% of patients within two decades of diagnosis. Median survival from the time of diagnosis of distant disease is 6–12 months.

Despite good local tumor control, the survival rate for uveal melanoma has not improved for decades. It remains unclear if early local intervention improves survival. Eskelin *et al.* stipulated that micrometastases can develop as long as 5 years before the local ocular therapy, when the tumor size is as small as 3 mm in largest basal diameter and 1.5 mm in thickness.[108] Only 2% of patients present with clinically evident metastatic disease at the time of initial diagnosis. The liver is the predominant site of metastasis involved in 70–90% of all patients with metastatic disease. Given the failures of therapy in the past coupled with the high risk for distant spread, uveal melanoma is a rare tumor with many questions still left unanswered.

Staging

Melanoma of the uvea is been classified as small (less than 3 mm in thickness), medium (3–10 mm in thickness or less than 15 mm in largest basal diameter), and large (more than 10 mm in thickness or more than 15 mm in largest basal diameter). A strong correlation between tumor size and mortality has been described. The 5-year mortality rate is 16% for small tumors, 32% for medium size tumors, and 53% for large tumors.[109]

The Collaborative Ocular Melanoma Study (COMS), a multicenter investigation designed to evaluate therapeutic interventions for patients who have choroidal melanoma, sought to elucidate the appropriate therapy for newly diagnosed uveal mealnaoma. Begun in 1986, the COMS' primary objective was to identify patients who could be treated with radiation therapy in place of enucleation in order to avoid enucleation and preserve vision. Evaluations conducted in the COMS aimed at determining which of two alternative therapies better prolongs the remaining lifetime of individuals diagnosed as having choroidal melanoma. Freedom from recurrence and vision preservation were secondary endpoints. Two randomized controlled trials are being conducted as separate substudies: (a) comparison of enucleation versus radiation for tumors at least 2.5 mm but no more than 10 mm in height and no more than 16 mm in basal diameter, referred to as medium-sized tumors; (b) comparison of standard enucleation versus enucleation preceded by external beam radiation for tumors greater than 10 mm in height or greater than 2 mm in height and greater than 16 mm in basal diameter or greater than 8 mm in height if there is optic nerve involvement (large tumors). In addition to the two randomized trials, a number of pilot studies and ancillary studies have been and continue to be conducted by COMS investigators.

Patient enrollment in the COMS randomized trial of ^{125}I brachytherapy for medium choroidal melanoma began in February 1987 and was completed in July 1998. To be eligible for this trial, a patient had to have choroidal melanoma from 2.5 to 10.0 mm in apical height and no more than 16.0 mm in longest basal diameter. Eligible patients were at least 21 years old, had no other primary tumor, and had no other disease that threatened their lives within the next 5 years. Previous treatment related to eye cancer rendered a patient ineligible. Eligible patients enrolled and received treatment at 43 clinical centers located in major population areas of the United States and Canada.

The first study enrolled 1317 patients with medium-sized choroidal melanoma. About 98% were non-Hispanic whites. The group was evenly divided by gender and the mean age was approximately 60 years. Patients were assigned to one of two treatment groups by randomization. One group, 660 patients, was assigned to have enucleation. The other group, 657 patients, was assigned to radiation treatment. Radiation was delivered via an iodine-125 episcleral plaque. Prior to the treatment, the dimensions of the tumor were measured.

In the study of large-sized choroidal melanoma, two groups of patients with tumors large enough to require removal of the eye were followed. One group received radiation treatment to the affected eye before it was removed. The other group had the eye removed without the radiation treatment. Researchers found that, after 5 years of follow-up study, the radiation treatment had no effect on survival rates.

Prognosis

Features of the primary tumor associated with poor prognosis, include location in the ciliary body or choroid (as opposed to the iris), diffuse configuration, and larger size. Uveal melanomas with epithelioid morphology fare worse than those with spindle cells,[110] as do those with higher mitotic activity, extrascleral invasion, or the presence of microvascular networks.[111-113]

There is no clear procedure for screening for metastatic disease in patients. No clear systemic treatment options exist for UM, and outcomes are dreadful once metastatic disease is diagnosed, with patients progressing through multiple deficient lines of therapy. The most common site of metastatic disease with uveal melanoma is the liver. A comprehensive review of the experience at the Memorial Sloan-Kettering Cancer Center by Rietschel *et al.* noted that 89% of all patients had single organ involvement at the time of first evidence of metastatic disease, 68% of the time involving the liver. Almost 40% of patients presented with nonhepatic involvement as first site of disease with the most common site being the lung. Twenty percent of patients underwent complete surgical metastatectomy. Factors relating to improved outcomes included female gender, age younger than 60, longer time from treatment for the primary uveal melanoma to the development of metastases, surgical resection of metastases, and lung or soft tissue as sole site of metastasis. This fact underlines the inefficacy of liver-only imaging as a screening procedure which would miss a substantial number of patients. Nevertheless, the liver remains the main battlefield for patient mortality, with a total of 77.3% of patients ultimately developing hepatic involvement and 42.9% of patients never manifesting extrahepatic disease. About 10% of patients eventually develop metastasis to the brain with 17% of patients developing metastasis to bone. Analyses have suggested that survival correlates with female sex, age under 60 at diagnosis, metastasis to lung and soft tissue sites only, prolonged interval between initial diagnosis and metastatic disease, and surgical or intrahepatic therapy for disease.[114]

Genetic features of UM are rapidly clarifying prognostic importance. Monosomy of chromosome 3 and amplification of chromosome 8q have recently been identified as poor prognostic indicators.[115] Damato *et al.* reported that metastatic death occurs almost exclusively in patients with monosomy 3 melanoma; almost 85% of these patients had enucleation as primary treatment.[116] Chromosome 6 may also play a role in uveal melanoma; amplification of 6p seems to have a protective role for systemic metastases, to the point of being mutually exclusive with monosomy 3. The combination of monosomy 3 with trisomy 8 seems to almost always result in demise from metastatic disease. Uveal melanomas cluster into two molecular groups based on their gene expression profile. Zuidervaart *et al.* have recently shown a dichotomy in uveal melanomas based on these two distinct classes on a three gene expression profile.[117] This molecular classification strongly predicts metastatic death and lends credence to the existence of a subpopulation of uveal melanoma with an indolent course.[118] Tumors with the class 1 signature rarely metastasize, whereas those with the class 2 signature have a very high rate of metastasis and are associated with increased mortality. However, the biological basis for this metastatic propensity of class 2 tumors remains unclear. On average, class 2 uveal melanomas have a higher proliferative rate than class 1 tumors. It remains to be seen whether loss of chromosome 3,[119] increased aneuploidy, or other factors are the determinants for the increased proliferation.[118,120]

Cutaneous and uveal melanoma exhibit different patterns of metastatic spread. Cutaneous melanomas metastasize either through the lymphatic system or hematogenously or both. Uveal melanomas, due to the lack of lymphatic drainage in the eye, spread hematogenously. Sites of hematogenous spread between the two diseases differ, with the most common sites of metastatic dissemination in cutaneous melanoma being the skin, soft tissue, lymph nodes, lung and brain, while the most common distant site of disease involvement in ocular melanoma is the liver. Central nervous system metastases are rare. This divergence reflects differences in tumor biology between these two melanoma types.[121]

Survival

There exists no effective adjuvant therapy for ocular melanoma post definitive local therapy. Over 50% of patients develop metastasis, which can happen up to several decades later.[105,122,123] There are no effective long-term treatments for the majority of patients with metastatic ocular melanoma, perhaps because metastases are found in the liver and other visceral organs in the vast number of cases. The prognosis is poor, with reported median survivals ranging from 2 to 12 months.[124] The Collaborative Ocular Melanoma Study was the largest published experience with uveal melanoma. Median survival after diagnosis was 3.6 months and 5-year survival was less than 1%. Retrospective analyses report survival from time of

diagnosis from metastasis to be 6 months or less.[125,126] Overall 1-year survival rate is 13% and 2-year survival is 5%. This survival rate of uveal melanoma has not changed over a 25-year period. The Collaborative Ocular Melanoma Study Group reported a 1-year survival in patients who develop hepatic metastasis of only 20%.

Follow-up

Regardless of the lack of efficacious therapy and the controversy over lead-time bias, frequent imaging may lead to the discovery of hepatic metastasis and so lead to patient benefit. [Editorial note: the preceding issue remains quite controversial, and the potential benefit from frequent imaging may simply represent lead-time bias.] Benefit related to the ability to see multiple treatment options before progression may exist. There does not exist a clear follow-up regimen and no set definition of high-risk patients. Clinicopathological features are utilized to identify these high-risk patients. These features include most importantly size, location, tumor cell type, mitotic activity, vascular architecture, tumor infiltrating lymphocytes, and presence of extrascleral extension.[127] A specific modality of choice does not exist amongst physicians: CT, ultrasound, or MRI. With the significant disease appearing in the liver, most physicians agree that serial evaluation of this organ is necessary at 3–6-month intervals. Reports of the utility of hepatic function tests and transaminases revealed surprising ineffectiveness in identifying early-stage disease with sensitivities noted (0.27–0.67). Serum lactate dehydrogenase (LDH) showed the highest sensitivity, mimicking its role with cutaneous melanoma therapy.[108,128] While MRI of the abdomen may demonstrate hepatic metastasis at an earlier time, this has not become a standard in the United States.

Therapy

There are no standard long-term treatments for the majority of patients with metastatic ocular melanoma. When aggressive local management with radiotherapy or surgical enucleation ultimately fails, the armamentarium left to combat progressive disease is meager. This area continues to remain largely investigational with the majority of these patients excluded from clinical trials due to their perceived differences in epidemiology, molecular biology, pathogenesis, and metastatic pattern from cutaneous melanoma. Controversy exists about their ability to respond to conventional chemotherapy and immunotherapies and therefore they are mainly excluded from clinical trials for malignant cutaneous melanoma.[129] There are preliminary data suggesting that uveal melanoma has a biological and a molecular basis that can be characterized and exploited therapeutically, but this will require further study.

Conventional chemotherapy has historically been ineffective in therapy for metastatic disease. In the COMS study, only 39% of patients received therapy for metastatic disease. In the Memorial Sloan-Kettering experience, 81% of patients received treatment for stage IV disease with similar outcomes. This negative experience has been repeatedly presented. Cooperative groups reviewing their experience have emphasized these failures through the Eastern Cooperative Oncology Group (ECOG) and the South Western Oncology Group (SWOG).[130,131] A phase 2 study of temozolomide (TMZ) demonstrated a response rate of 0%, a median time to progression of 1.8 months, and median survival of 6.7 months.[132] The MD Anderson Cancer Center experience of 143 treated patients reported a single objective response.[133] The Collaborative Ocular Melanoma Study was the largest published experience with uveal melanoma. Median survival after diagnosis was 3.6 months and 5-year survival was less than 1%. Currently there is no significant chemotherapy that lends to clinical benefit for patients with metastatic UM. With the lack of efficacy or benefit with systemic therapy and an urgent mandate to control local progression of life-threatening disease, locoregional therapy is tantamount to control of UM.

Surgical resection of metastatic uveal melanoma is rare, with only 9% of patients eligible for curative resection. In a review of 75 patients with uveal melanoma metastatic to the liver, 74 of 75 patients were found to have metastatic disease in both lobes of the liver. Macroscopic resection of tumor was possible in 28.5% of patients. Significant debulking was possible in another 49% of patients. A majority of patients were able to tolerate subsequent intraarterial therapy. When curative resection was possible, survival increased from median survival of 10 months to 22 months ($p < 0.001$). Complete resection provided survival advantage. These data presented a basis for adjuvant intraarterial therapy that will need to be reviewed through clinical trials.[134] Local ablative procedures without surgical intervention involve the use of radiofrequency ablation or cryoablation. This process would be applicable to patients with few hepatic metastases or excessive risk of surgical morbidity.

Given the fact that approximately 90% of patients with metastatic uveal melanoma die from the sequelae of diffuse hepatic disease,[135] intrahepatic therapy has been investigated as a possible route for improving survival. Historical series note that only 9% of patients with intrahepatic involvement are eligible for resection due to the extent of involvement when a patient comes to physician care. Many more patients are taken to the operating room for failed resection upon the discovery of micrometastatic disease that is not observed with conventional imaging techniques.[136]

Direct treatment of the liver through a number of different strategies has been evaluated for the treatment of metastatic uveal melanoma. Such liver-directed therapies appear rational for several reasons: (1) the liver is the first site of metastasis in greater than 60% of cases of uveal melanoma and may be the dominant site of disease; (2) currently available systemic treatments for metastatic disease have limited effectiveness; (3) the application of regional therapy allows for dose escalation to the cancer-bearing organ while minimizing systemic exposure and toxicity via separation of the regional and systemic circulation; and (4) based on its unique vascular anatomy, the liver is a favorable site for regional therapy, as established tumors in the liver derive the majority of their blood flow from the arterial tree[137] while normal liver derives approximately 50% of its oxygen supply from the portal system.[138,139]

Multiple techniques have been developed with the intention of extending survival through control of the life-threatening portion of this disease process, including transarterial catheter-directed liver therapies, such as hepatic arterial chemoinfusion, transarterial chemoembolization (TACE), immunoembolization, and isolated hepatic perfusion (Table 51.1). Despite this, most patients with hepatic metastasis from uveal melanoma eventually progress through these approaches. Subsequent salvage therapy is needed to lengthen the survival of patients with hepatic metastasis of uveal melanoma. Salvage therapy with radioembolization of yttrium 90 microspheres, trans-arterial immunoembolization with granulocyte-macrophage colony-stimulating factor, and chemoembolization with 1,3-bis(2-chloroethyl) -1-nitrosurea has achieved partial and complete responses. Extended survival has been reported, with overall survival that was apparently longer among responding patients than in patients achieving only stable disease.[140] However, in most cases, this approach has not been validated in well-powered, randomized controlled trials.

Although a number of various liver-directed strategies have been utilized, including surgery, bland embolization, chemoembolization, immunoembolization, radioembolization, hepatic intraarterial chemotherapy, and hepatic arterial perfusion, percutaneous hepatic perfusion (PHP) with melphalan using a Delcath double-balloon inferior vena cava catheter (Delcath Systems, New York, NY) is the only system to have been tested in a phase 3 randomized fashion.[141–143] This trial randomized 93 patients with melanoma metastatic to the liver to either PHP ($n = 44$) or best alternative care ($n = 49$). Patients initially randomized to best alternative care were allowed to receive PHP at the time of progression. The primary endpoint of this study was hepatic progression-free survival, with secondary endpoints including overall progression-free survival and overall survival. Of the 93 patients randomized, 82 had disease arising from the eye. Hematological toxicity due to PHP was significant in this trial, with 61.2% developing grade 3–4 neutropenia, 74.1% developing grade 3–4 thrombocytopenia, and 46.6% developing grade 3–4 anemia. Two deaths occurred associated with severe neutropenia.

Table 51.1 Localized therapies for metastatic uveal melanoma.

Modality	Agents utilized
Immunoembolization	GM-CSF, IL-2
Internal radiation therapy	Yttrium
Hepatic intraarterial chemotherapy	Adriamycin, BCNU, cisplatin, carboplatin, fotemustine,
Chemoembolization	mitomycin
Hepatic arterial perfusion	Melphalan, tissue necrosis factor
Radiation	Cyberknife radiotherapy
Radiofrequency ablation (RFA)	
Cryoablation	
Drug-eluting beads	Irinotecan, doxorubicin
Radiosphere	
Surgical resection	

BCNU, carmustine; GM-CSF, granulocyte macrophage colony-stimulating factor; IL, interleukin.
Reproduced with permission from Miller *et al.*[38]

The study met its primary endpoint of hepatic progression-free survival, with a hazard ratio of 0.301 ($p < 0.001$), as well as the secondary endpoint of overall progression-free survival ($p < 0.001$), both in favor of PHP. However, no impact upon overall survival in the intention-to-treat population was observed (hazard ratio 0.920; $p = 0.78$). Interestingly, survival was improved for those initially randomized to best alternative care if they subsequently received PHP when compared to those who did not (124 versus 398 days; $p = 0.01$); however, this finding is likely heavily influenced by selection bias.

Despite the benefit with liver-directed therapies, major advancements in therapy have yet to be made. Fortunately, the advent of immune manipulative and targeted therapies has brought newfound hope to therapy of UM (Table 51.2). Melanoma is one of the first examples where significant progress has been made based on identification of prognostic, predictive, and diagnostic biomarkers. Progress in effectively blocking the B-RAF mutation has produced clear survival benefit in metastatic melanoma, leading to the FDA approval of vemurafenib in August 2011. With the identification of other genetic mutations in this system, the use of multiple drug targets in this tumor system may lead to additive increase in survival. Conversely, in patients not harboring the BRAF mutation, identification and targeting of distinct oncogenes can lead to long-term clinical benefits.

Given its promising results in cutaneous melanoma, ipilimumab may have clinical activity in metastatic ocular melanoma. Effective antitumor responses are being observed in metastatic melanoma patients with this anti-CTLA-4 antibody[144] in clinical trials but no data currently support the feasibility and clinical utility of ipilimumab use in ocular melanoma. Ipilimumab may result in a long-term survival benefit in patients with advanced melanoma. Currently 2-year survival rates for cutaneous melanoma across three phase 2 (CA184022, CA184008, and CA184007) studies range from 29% to 41%. These results indicate that more than one-third of ipilimumab-treated patients with advanced melanoma experience a long-term survival benefit, including some patients characterized as

having progressive disease by modified World Health Organization criteria. Immunotherapy may provide long-term disease control and survival for ocular melanoma patients in the same manner as it has for mucosal and cutaneous melanomas.

Despite the clinical benefits seen in personalized medicine with cutaneous melanoma, UM is not characterized by the presence of activating mutations. Activating mutations in the BRAF[145] and N-RAS pathways do not exist in UM. There is a belief that despite the absence of these mutations, activation of the MAPK pathway remains important in UM to the development and progression of metastatic disease. Deletion mutations in the tumor suppressor gene PTEN have been described in approximately 15% of uveal melanomas in small cohort studies.[146,147] Additional studies have shown amplification (but not mutation) of a number of genes in high percentages of uveal melanoma samples, including NBS1, MYC, DDEF1, CCND1, HDM2, and Bcl-2, as reviewed. Unlike cutaneous melanoma, uveal melanoma has been noted to lack mutations in BRAF, N-RAS, or KIT.[148] BRAF mutations have been found in 10% of conjunctival melanomas and 50% of conjunctival nevi.[149] However, Malaponte et al. described a case with uveal melanoma harboring a BRAF mutation (V600E).[150] Investigators have also detected BRAF mutations in melanomas of the conjunctiva and iris but mutations have not been noted in uveal melanoma of other locations.[151,152] However, 86% of uveal melanomas express activation of the MAPK pathway as evidenced by activation of phospho-ERK.

Studies have identified G-proteins as potential drivers of MAPK activation in uveal melanoma (Fig. 51.6). Genetic screens have shown that 46–53% of uveal melanoma exhibit mutations in GNAQ. Data suggest that over half of uveal melanomas lacking a mutation in GNAQ exhibit a mutation in GNA11.[153] Examination of overall survival and disease-free survival for 81 patients did not reveal a significant difference between those with tumors bearing a GNAQ mutation and those with tumors bearing a GNA11 mutation. A trend toward increased survival among patients with tumors carrying a

Table 51.2 Open clinical trials for uveal melanoma.

Clinical trials #	Agent	Phase	Mechanism
6 NCT01430416	Safety and efficacy of AEB071 in metastatic uveal melanoma patients	I	Protein kinase C inhibitor
5 NCT01377025	Sorafenib in patients with chemonaive metastatic uveal melanoma (STREAM)	II	b-Raf and Raf-1, VEGFR, PDGFR
7 NCT01034787	Anti-CTLA4 in patients with unresectable or metastatic uveal melanoma	II	Immunomodulatory
2 NCT00506142	Safety and efficacy of Marqibo in metastatic malignant uveal melanoma	II	Liposomal vincristine
8 NCT01100528	Dacarbazine and recombinant interferon-α2b in treating patients with primary uveal melanoma with genetic imbalance	II	Biochemotherapy
2 NCT01200342	Genasense, carboplatin, paclitaxel (GCP) combination in uveal melanoma	II	Bcl-2 target
1 NCT01252251	RAD001 (everolimus) and pasireotide (SOM230) LAR in patients with advanced uveal melanoma	II	mTOR inhibitor, multigland somatostain analog
1 NCT01413191	Cixutumumab in treating patients with metastatic melanoma of the eye	II	Insulin-like growth factor-1 receptor antibody
2 NCT01143402	Temozolomide or MEK inhibitor AZD6244 in treating patients with metastatic melanoma of the eye	II	MEK inhibition
8 NCT01217398	Temozolomide and bevacizumab in treating patients with metastatic melanoma of the eye	II	VEGF

LAR, long-acting release; PDGFR, platelet-derived growth factor receptor; VEGF, vascular endothelial growth factor; VEGFR, VEGF receptor.

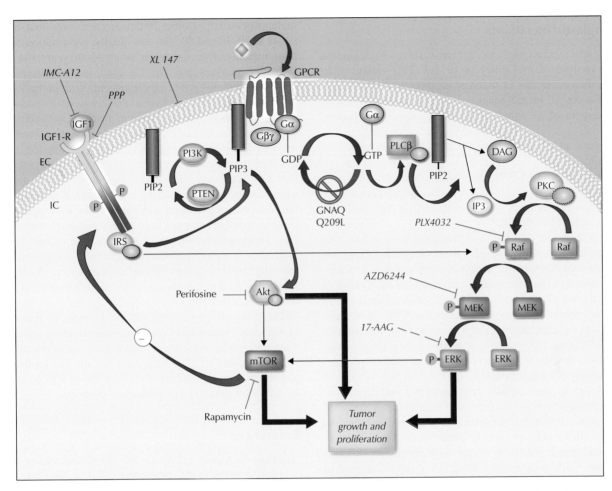

Figure 51.6 Major signaling pathways in uveal melanoma. The MAPK, PI3K (phosphatidylinositol-3-kinase), mTOR, and IGF-1R pathways intersect significantly in uveal melanoma pathogenesis. These signalling pathways can be manipulated and inhibited with current therapeutics in an effort to control metastatic disease. Adapted and reprinted with permission from the American Association for Cancer Research: Patel *et al*. Therapeutic Implications of the Emerging Molecular Biology of Uveal Melanoma. Clin Cancer Res 2011; 17: 2087–2100.

GNA11 mutation, as compared with those carrying a GNAQ mutation or those not carrying either a GNA11 or a GNAQ mutation, was seen.[154,155] An activating mutation in codon 209 at Q209L of guanine nucleotide-binding protein Q polypeptide (Gnaq), a heterotrimeric protein that couples cell surface 7-transmembrane domain receptors to intracellular signaling pathways such as the MAPK pathway, was seen in 45–50% of primary UMs.[153,155] *In vitro* analysis of UM cell lines harboring a mutation in GNAQ or GNA11 with two pharmacological inhibitors of MEK showed suppression of tumor growth. Subgroup analysis of outcomes of patients with UM treated on clinical trials of a MEK inhibitor AZD6244 demonstrated a increase of time to progression greater than twice that achieved with the use of standard chemotherapy. Although all patients with UM appeared to derive a greater benefit from treatment with AZD6244 when compared with temozolomide, patients with UM characterized by a GNAQ mutation achieve a median time to progression more than double that achieved in patients with wild-type GNAQ.

These findings indicate a potential predictive biomarker that indicates response for patients harboring this mutation when treated with MEK inhibitor. GNAQ and GNA11 share overlapping functions in melanocytes, and both activate the MAPK pathway when constitutively active. MEK inhibition in both GNAQ and GNA11 mutant cells may result in similar biological effects.

A search for metastasis-related mutations in highly metastatic uveal melanomas of the eye identified inactivating somatic mutations in the gene encoding BRCA1-associated protein 1 (BAP1) on chromosome 3p21.1. BAP1 is vital in the assembly of multiprotein complexes containing numerous transcription factors and cofactors, and activates transcription and therefore regulates the expression of a variety of genes involved in cellular processes. In 26 of 31 (84%) metastasizing tumors, including 15 mutations causing premature protein termination and five affecting its ubiquitin carboxyl-terminal hydrolase domain, knock-down of BAP1 in cell lines resulted in a more aggressive phenotype and shifts in gene expression patterns consistent with poor prognosis tumors. BAP1 encodes a deubiquinating enzyme and has binding domains for the tumor suppressors BRCA1 and BARD1 and has a role in histone modification during cell division, stem cell pluripotency, and other developmental processes. These findings implicate loss of BAP1 in uveal melanoma metastasis and suggest that the BAP1 pathway may be a valuable therapeutic target.[156]

Desmoplastic melanoma

Desmoplastic melanomas are a rare variant of melanoma initially recognized by Conley in 1971.[157] This variant often presents as a cutaneous or mucosal pigmentation overlying a detectable dermal or submucosal nodule. Often these lesions are misdiagnosed as scar, basal cell carcinoma, or fibroma. Their misdiagnosis is compounded by the fact that only half of desmoplastic melanomas are pigmented.[158] Desmoplastic carcinomas have a predeliction for the head, neck, upper back and often mucosal areas. In direct contrast to cutaneous melanoma which has a younger incidence, desmoplastic melanomas have a mean age of incidence of 60–80 years old with increased incidence in males of 1.75 to 1.[159]

Early lesions are difficult to differentiate from a Sitz type nevus, and thus expert histological evaluation is needed. Prognosis differs between desmoplastic melanoma and traditional cutaneous melanomas, with desmoplastic melanomas of equal depth of invasion having a significantly smaller risk of dissemination than their conventional melanoma counterparts.[160-162] Conversely, these tumors are associated with high recurrence rate. Recurrences can be amelanotic and present in an area of prior scar with invasion of local structures. Neurotropism in these tumors increases the probability of local recurrence.

Histologically, desmoplastic melanoma is a vertical growth phase melanoma with invasive cells exhibiting a spindled morphology. Surrounding these cells is a desmoplastic stromal response. Tumor cells are poorly circumscribed with reactive fibroblasts found within a tumor with abundant collagen deposition. Cells may be positioned in a fascicular pattern surrounded by a mucinous matrix, leading to misdiagnosis as a form of peripheral nerve sheath tumor such as schwannoma, neuroma, or neurofibroma.

Desmoplastic melanoma exhibits up to a three-fold greater thickness at presentation with better survivorship than conventional melanomas of similar thickness.

Therapy for desmoplatic melanoma may at times entail deep excision to encompass fascia due to the invasive nature of neurotropism of this tumor and the delays in initial therapy due to prior misdiagnosis. Perineural invasion remaining at the margins should be avoided as this is a cause for rapid local recurrence. Five-year survival is approximately 75%, and, 90% in thinner lesions of less than 2 mm thickness.[163] Desmoplastic melanomas with foci of conventional vertical growth phase melanoma manifest significantly worse prognosis, with regional lymph node metastases in 10% of cases as opposed to only 1% of pure desmoplastic melanoma.[164] Disease-specific 5-year mortality differed from 11% for pure desmoplastic vertical growth phase tumors, compared to 31% for those neoplasms with hybrid morphology.

Testicular melanoma

Malignant melanoma metastasizing to the testes is rare. It represents an aggressive variant with poor prognosis and high mortality.[165] This may simulate primary testicular neoplasm and is most often found during autopsy.[166,167] It presents as a rapidly growing testicular mass and, less frequently, as melanospermia.[168] Unlike testicular carcinoma that has incidence at 20–30 and 50–70 years old, the presentation of malignant melanoma to the testis is at 43–80 years old. Serum testicular markers are not elevated in this disease state. Prognosis remains poor in these patients with mortality within 12 months in most cases.[169,170]

The existence of a diagnosis of primary melanoma of the testis is currently disputed. Like other cases of widespread melanoma where a primary site cannot be located, they are ascribed to melanomas in which the initial cutaneous or other site has regressed due to autoimmunity. This dispute is supported by the idea that the embryological development of the testis stems from a mesodermal origin, making it unlikely that a melanoma can arise from type of tissue. However, others cite nonneoplastic melanoblasts that can result from the migration of melanin-producing cells from the neural crest to mesodermal derivatives during embryological development, which can lead to the possibility of transformation to primary melanoma at this site.[171]

There are no particularly unique features of management of testicular melanoma, with surgery being the mainstay of treatment, including assessment of draining nodal status. As with melanoma at other sites, radiotherapy has limited value, and the systemic therapies discussed above will occasionally be useful for patients with metastatic disease.

References

1. Chang AE, Karnell LH, Menck HR. The National Cancer Data Base report on cutaneous and noncutaneous melanoma: a summary of 84,836 cases from the past decade. The American College of Surgeons Commission on Cancer and the American Cancer Society. Cancer 1998; 83: 1664–78.
2. Kong Y, Si L, Zhu Y, et al. Large-scale analysis of KIT aberrations in Chinese patients with melanoma. Clin Cancer Res 2011; 17: 1684–91.
3. Seetharamu N, Ott PA, Pavlick AC. Mucosal melanomas: a case-based review of the literature. Oncologist 2010; 15: 772–81.
4. Scotto J, Fraumeni JF Jr, Lee JA. Melanomas of the eye and other noncutaneous sites: epidemiologic aspects. J Natl Cancer Inst 1976; 56: 489–91.
5. Ragnarsson-Olding BK. Spatial density of primary malignant melanoma in sun-shielded body sites: a potential guide to melanoma genesis. Acta Oncol 2011; 50: 323–8.
6. Gavriel H, McArthur G, Sizeland A, et al. Review: mucosal melanoma of the head and neck. Melanoma Res 2011; 21: 257–66.
7. Jethanamest D, Vila PM, Sikora AG, et al. Predictors of survival in mucosal melanoma of the head and neck. Ann Surg Oncol 2011; 18: 2748–56.
8. Sherman IW, Swift AC, Haqqani MT. Primary mucosal malignant melanoma of the middle ear. J Laryngol Otol 1991; 105: 1061–4.
9. Moreno MA, Roberts DB, Kupferman ME, et al. Mucosal melanoma of the nose and paranasal sinuses, a contemporary experience from the M. D. Anderson Cancer Center. Cancer 2010; 116: 2215–23.
10. Amano H, Tamura A, Yasuda M, et al. Amalgam tattoo of the oral mucosa mimics malignant melanoma. J Dermatol 2011; 38: 101–3.
11. Bartell HL, Bedikian AY, Papadopoulos NE, et al. Biochemotherapy in patients with advanced head and neck mucosal melanoma. Head Neck 2008; 30: 1592–8.
12. Shuman AG, Light E, Olsen SH, et al. Mucosal melanoma of the head and neck: predictors of prognosis. Arch Otolaryngol Head Neck Surg 2011; 137: 331–7.
13. Ahn HJ, Na, II, Park YH, et al. Role of adjuvant chemotherapy in malignant mucosal melanoma of the head and neck. Oral Oncol 2010; 46: 607–11.

14. Ballantyne AJ. Malignant melanoma of the skin of the head and neck. An analysis of 405 cases. Am J Surg 1970; 120: 425–31.

15. Edge SB, Byrd DR, Compton CC, et al. AJCC Cancer Staging Manual, 7th edn. New York: Springer, 2010.

16. Wang X, Wu HM, Ren GX, et al. Primary oral mucosal melanoma: advocate a wait-and-see policy in the clinically no patient. J Oral Maxillofac Surg 2011; Jul 23 [Epub ahead of print].

17. Patrick RJ, Fenske NA, Messina JL. Primary mucosal melanoma. J Am Acad Dermatol 2007; 56: 828–34.

18. Prasad ML, Patel SG, Huvos AG, et al. Primary mucosal melanoma of the head and neck: a proposal for microstaging localized, Stage I (lymph node-negative) tumors. Cancer 2004; 100: 1657–64.

19. Clifton N, Harrison L, Bradley PJ, et al. Malignant melanoma of nasal cavity and paranasal sinuses: report of 24 patients and literature review. J Laryngol Otol 2011; 125: 479–85.

20. Kim DK, Kim DW, Kim SW, et al. Ki67 antigen as a predictive factor for prognosis of sinonasal mucosal melanoma. Clin Exp Otorhinolaryngol 2008; 1: 206–10.

21. Thariat J, Poissonnet G, Marcy PY, et al. Effect of surgical modality and hypofractionated split-course radiotherapy on local control and survival from sinonasal mucosal melanoma. Clin Oncol (R Coll Radiol) 2011; 23: 579–86.

22. Moreno MA, Hanna EY. Management of mucosal melanomas of the head and neck: did we make any progress? Curr Opin Otolaryngol Head Neck Surg 2010; 18: 101–6.

23. Marunick M, Oh WS. Prosthodontic treatment considerations for patients with oral sinonasal mucosal malignant melanoma: a clinical report. J Prosthet Dent 2009; 101: 85–91.

24. Benlyazid A, Thariat J, Temam S, et al. Postoperative radiotherapy in head and neck mucosal melanoma: a GETTEC study. Arch Otolaryngol Head Neck Surg 2010; 136: 1219–25.

25. Douglas CM, Malik T, Swindell R, et al. Mucosal melanoma of the head and neck: radiotherapy or surgery? J Otolaryngol Head Neck Surg 2010; 39: 385–92.

26. Bentzen SM, Overgaard J, Thames HD, et al. Clinical radiobiology of malignant melanoma. Radiother Oncol 1989; 16: 169–82.

27. Harwood AR, Dancuart F, Fitzpatrick PJ, et al. Radiotherapy in nonlentiginous melanoma of the head and neck. Cancer 1981; 48: 2599–605.

28. Yang X, Ren GX, Zhang CP, et al. Neck dissection and postoperative chemotherapy with dimethyl triazeno imidazole carboxamide and cisplatin protocol are useful for oral mucosal melanoma. BMC Cancer 2010; 10: 623.

29. Moore W. Recurrent melanoma of the rectum, after previous removal from the anal verge in a man aged sixty-five. Lancet Oncol 1857; 1: 290.

30. Ramakrishnan AS, Mahajan V, Kannan R. Optimizing local control in anorectal melanoma. Indian J Cancer 2008; 45: 13–19.

31. Goldman S, Glimelius B, Pahlman L. Anorectal malignant melanoma in Sweden. Report of 49 patients. Dis Colon Rectum 1990; 33: 874–7.

32. Ragnarsson-Olding BK, Nilsson PJ, Olding LB, et al. Primary anorectal malignant melanomas within a population-based national patient series in Sweden during 40 years. Acta Oncol 2009; 48: 125–31.

33. Cagir B, Whiteford MH, Topham A, et al. Changing epidemiology of anorectal melanoma. Dis Colon Rectum 1999; 42: 1203–8.

34. Iddings DM, Fleisig AJ, Chen SL, et al. Practice patterns and outcomes for anorectal melanoma in the USA, reviewing three decades of treatment: is more extensive surgical resection beneficial in all patients? Ann Surg Oncol 2010; 17: 40–4.

35. Kiran RP, Rottoli M, Pokala N, et al. Long-term outcomes after local excision and radical surgery for anal melanoma: data from a population database. Dis Colon Rectum 2010; 53: 402–8.

36. Kim HS, Kim EK, Jun HJ, et al. Noncutaneous malignant melanoma: a prognostic model from a retrospective multicenter study. BMC Cancer 2010; 10: 167.

37. Ellis ZM, Jassim AD, Wick MR. Anorectal melanoma in childhood and adolescence. Ann Diagn Pathol 2010; 14: 69–73.

38. Miller BJ, Rutherford LF, McLeod GR, et al. Where the sun never shines: anorectal melanoma. Aust N Z J Surg 1997; 67: 846–8.

39. Clemmensen OJ, Fenger C. Melanocytes in the anal canal epithelium. Histopathology 1991; 18: 237–41.

40. Werdin C, Limas C, Knodell RG. Primary malignant melanoma of the rectum. Evidence for origination from rectal mucosal melanocytes. Cancer 1988; 61: 1364–70.

41. Baskies AM, Sugarbaker EV, Chretien PB, et al. Anorectal melanoma. The role of posterior pelvic exenteration. Dis Colon Rectum 1982; 25: 772–7.

42. Cooper PH, Mills SE, Allen MS Jr. Malignant melanoma of the anus: report of 12 patients and analysis of 255 additional cases. Dis Colon Rectum 1982; 25: 693–703.

43. Brady MS, Kavolius JP, Quan SH. Anorectal melanoma. A 64-year experience at Memorial Sloan-Kettering Cancer Center. Dis Colon Rectum 1995; 38: 146–51.

44. Che X, Zhao DB, Wu YK, et al. Anorectal malignant melanomas: retrospective experience with surgical management. World J Gastroenterol 2011; 17: 534–9.

45. Droesch JT, Flum DR, Mann GN. Wide local excision or abdominoperineal resection as the initial treatment for anorectal melanoma? Am J Surg 2005; 189: 446–9.

46. Nilsson PJ, Ragnarsson-Olding BK. Importance of clear resection margins in anorectal malignant melanoma. Br J Surg 2010; 97: 98–103.

47. Thibault C, Sagar P, Nivatvongs S, et al. Anorectal melanoma – an incurable disease? Dis Colon Rectum 1997; 40: 661–8.

48. Wanebo HJ, Woodruff JM, Farr GH, et al. Anorectal melanoma. Cancer 1981; 47: 1891–900.

49. Homsi J, Garrett C. Melanoma of the anal canal: a case series. Dis Colon Rectum 2007; 50: 1004–10.

50. Pessaux P, Pocard M, Elias D, et al. Surgical management of primary anorectal melanoma. Br J Surg 2004; 91: 1183–7.

51. Podnos YD, Tsai NC, Smith D, et al. Factors affecting survival in patients with anal melanoma. Am Surg 2006; 72: 917–20.

52. Roumen RM. Anorectal melanoma in The Netherlands: a report of 63 patients. Eur J Surg Oncol 1996; 22: 598–601.

53. Ballo MT, Gershenwald JE, Zagars GK, et al. Sphincter-sparing local excision and adjuvant radiation for anal-rectal melanoma. J Clin Oncol 2002; 20: 4555–8.

54. Yeh JJ, Shia J, Hwu WJ, et al. The role of abdominoperineal resection as surgical therapy for anorectal melanoma. Ann Surg 2006; 244: 1012–17.

55. Ben-Izhak O, Bar-Chana M, Sussman L, et al. Ki67 antigen and PCNA proliferation markers predict survival in anorectal malignant melanoma. Histopathology 2002; 41: 519–25.

56. Luna-Perez P, Rodriguez DF, Macouzet JG, et al. Anorectal malignant melanoma. Surg Oncol 1996; 5: 165–8.

57. Zhang S, Gao F, Wan D. Abdominoperineal resection or local excision? A survival analysis of anorectal malignant melanoma with surgical management. Melanoma Res 2010; 20: 338–41.

58. Wong JH, Cagle LA, Storm FK, et al. Natural history of surgically treated mucosal melanoma. Am J Surg 1987; 154: 54–7.

59. Malik A, Hull TL, Floruta C. What is the best surgical treatment for anorectal melanoma? Int J Colorectal Dis 2004; 19: 121–3.

60. Ishida J, Sugimura K, Okizuka H, et al. Malignant anorectal melanoma: usefulness of fat saturation MR imaging. Eur J Radiol 1993; 16: 195–7.

61. Weyandt GH, Eggert AO, Houf M, et al. Anorectal melanoma: surgical management guidelines according to tumour thickness. Br J Cancer 2003; 89: 2019–22.

62. Moozar KL, Wong CS, Couture J. Anorectal malignant melanoma: treatment with surgery or radiation therapy, or both. Can J Surg 2003; 46: 345–9.

63. Bullard KM, Tuttle TM, Rothenberger DA, et al. Surgical therapy for anorectal melanoma. J Am Coll Surg 2003; 196: 206–11.

64. Yap LB, Neary P. A comparison of wide local excision with abdominoperineal resection in anorectal melanoma. Melanoma Res 2004; 14: 147–50.

65. Tien HY, McMasters KM, Edwards MJ, et al. Sentinel lymph node metastasis in anal melanoma: a case report. Int J Gastrointest Cancer 2002; 32: 53–6.

66. Damin DC, Rosito MA, Spiro BL. Long-term survival data on sentinel lymph node biopsy in anorectal melanoma. Tech Coloproctol 2010; 14: 367–8.

67. Iddings DM, Chen SL, Faries MB, *et al*. *A New Paradigm in the Management of Anorectal Melanoma: Trans-Anal Excision with Sphincter Preservation and Sentinel Node Biopsy*. Chicago: American Society of Clinical Oncology, 2007. pp.851–3.

68. Vermeeren L, van der Ploeg IM, Olmos RA, *et al*. SPECT/CT for preoperative sentinel node localization. J Surg Oncol 2010; 101: 184–90.

69. Snoj M, Rudolf Z, Cemazar M, *et al*. Successful sphincter-saving treatment of anorectal malignant melanoma with electrochemotherapy, local excision and adjuvant brachytherapy. Anticancer Drugs 2005; 16: 345–8.

70. Ulmer A, Metzger S, Fierlbeck G. Successful palliation of stenosing anorectal melanoma by intratumoral injections with natural interferon-beta. Melanoma Res 2002; 12: 395–8.

71. Kim KB, Sanguino AM, Hodges C, *et al*. Biochemotherapy in patients with metastatic anorectal mucosal melanoma. Cancer 2004; 100: 1478–83.

72. Hu DN, Yu GP, McCormick SA. Population-based incidence of vulvar and vaginal melanoma in various races and ethnic groups with comparisons to other site-specific melanomas. Melanoma Res 2010; 20: 153–8.

73. DeMatos P, Tyler D, Seigler HF. Mucosal melanoma of the female genitalia: a clinicopathologic study of forty-three cases at Duke University Medical Center. Surgery 1998; 124: 38–48.

74. Sabanathan S, Eng J. Primary malignant melanoma of the esophagus. Scand J Thorac Cardiovasc Surg 1990; 24: 83–5.

75. Heyn J, Placzek M, Ozimek A, *et al*. Malignant melanoma of the anal region. Clin Exp Dermatol 2007; 32: 603–7.

76. Curtin JA, Fridlyand J, Kageshita T, *et al*. Distinct sets of genetic alterations in melanoma. N Engl J Med 2005; 353: 2135–47.

77. Sekine S, Nakanishi Y, Ogawa R, *et al*. Esophageal melanomas harbor frequent NRAS mutations unlike melanomas of other mucosal sites. Virchows Arch 2009; 454: 513–1.

78. Wong CW, Fan YS, Chan TL, *et al*. BRAF and NRAS mutations are uncommon in melanomas arising in diverse internal organs. J Clin Pathol 2005; 58: 640–4.

79. Omholt K, Grafstrom E, Kanter-Lewensohn L, *et al*. KIT pathway alterations in mucosal melanomas of the vulva and other sites. Clin Cancer Res 2011; 17: 3933–42.

80. Woodman SE, Davies MA. Targeting KIT in melanoma: a paradigm of molecular medicine and targeted therapeutics. Biochem Pharmacol 2010; 80: 568–74.

81. Yarden Y, Kuang WJ, Yang-Feng T, *et al*. Human proto-oncogene c-kit: a new cell surface receptor tyrosine kinase for an unidentified ligand. EMBO J 1987; 6: 3341–51.

82. Geissler EN, Ryan MA, Housman DE. The dominant-white spotting (W) locus of the mouse encodes the c-kit proto-oncogene. Cell 1988; 55: 185–92.

83. Fleischman RA. From white spots to stem cells: the role of the Kit receptor in mammalian development. Trends Genet 1993; 9: 285–90.

84. Ohashi A, Funasaka Y, Ueda M, *et al*. c-KIT receptor expression in cutaneous malignant melanoma and benign melanotic naevi. Melanoma Res 1996; 6: 25–30.

85. Montone KT, van Belle P, Elenitsas R, *et al*. Proto-oncogene c-kit expression in malignant melanoma: protein loss with tumor progression. Mod Pathol 1997; 10: 939–44.

86. Antonescu CR, Busam KJ, Francone TD, *et al*. L576P KIT mutation in anal melanomas correlates with KIT protein expression and is sensitive to specific kinase inhibition. Int J Cancer 2007; 121: 257–64.

87. Rivera RS, Nagatsuka H, Gunduz M, *et al*. C-kit protein expression correlated with activating mutations in KIT gene in oral mucosal melanoma. Virchows Arch 2008; 452: 27–32.

88. Beadling C, Jacobson-Dunlop E, Hodi FS, *et al*. KIT gene mutations and copy number in melanoma subtypes. Clin Cancer Res 2008; 14: 6821–8.

89. Satzger I, Schaefer T, Kuettler U, *et al*. Analysis of c-KIT expression and KIT gene mutation in human mucosal melanomas. Br J Cancer 2008; 99: 2065–9.

90. Torres-Cabala CA, Wang WL, Trent J, *et al*. Correlation between KIT expression and KIT mutation in melanoma: a study of 173 cases with emphasis on the acral-lentiginous/mucosal type. Mod Pathol 2009; 22: 1446–56.

91. Handolias D, Hamilton AL, Salemi R, *et al*. Clinical responses observed with imatinib or sorafenib in melanoma patients expressing mutations in KIT. Br J Cancer 2010; 102: 1219–23.

92. Yun J, Lee J, Jang J, *et al*. KIT amplification and gene mutations in acral/mucosal melanoma in Korea. APMIS 2011; 119: 330–5.

93. Medeiros F, Corless CL, Duensing A, *et al*. KIT-negative gastrointestinal stromal tumors: proof of concept and therapeutic implications. Am J Surg Pathol 2004; 28: 889–94.

94. Chirieac LR, Trent JC, Steinert DM, *et al*. Correlation of immunophenotype with progression-free survival in patients with gastrointestinal stromal tumors treated with imatinib mesylate. Cancer 2006; 107: 2237–44.

95. Kim KB, Eton O, Davis DW, *et al*. Phase II trial of imatinib mesylate in patients with metastatic melanoma. Br J Cancer 2008; 99: 734–40.

96. Ugurel S, Hildenbrand R, Zimpfer A, *et al*. Lack of clinical efficacy of imatinib in metastatic melanoma. Br J Cancer 2005; 92: 1398–405.

97. Wyman K, Atkins MB, Prieto V, *et al*. Multicenter phase II trial of high-dose imatinib mesylate in metastatic melanoma: significant toxicity with no clinical efficacy. Cancer 2006; 106: 2005–11.

98. Kluger HM, Dudek AZ, McCann C, *et al*. A phase 2 trial of dasatinib in advanced melanoma. Cancer 2011; 117(10): 2202–8.

99. Hodi FS, Friedlander P, Corless CL, *et al*. Major response to imatinib mesylate in KIT-mutated melanoma. J Clin Oncol 2008; 26: 2046–51.

100. Woodman SE, Trent JC, Stemke-Hale K, *et al*. Activity of dasatinib against L576P KIT mutant melanoma: molecular, cellular, and clinical correlates. Mol Cancer Ther 2009; 8: 2079–85.

101. Satzger I, Kuttler U, Volker B, *et al*. Anal mucosal melanoma with KIT-activating mutation and response to imatinib therapy – case report and review of the literature. Dermatology 2010; 220: 77–81.

102. Fisher DE, Barnhill R, Hodi FS, *et al*. Melanoma from bench to bedside: meeting report from the 6th International Melanoma Congress. Pigment Cell Melanoma Res 2010; 23: 14–26.

103. Carvajal RD, Antonescu CR, Wolchok JD, *et al*. KIT as a therapeutic target in metastatic melanoma. JAMA 2011; 305: 2327–34.

104. Strickland D, Lee JA. Melanomas of eye: stability of rates. Am J Epidemiol 1981; 113: 700–2.

105. Singh AD, Topham A. Incidence of uveal melanoma in the United States: 1973–1997. Ophthalmology 2003; 110: 956–61.

106. Abramson D, Dunkel I, McCormick B. Neoplasms of the eye. In: Bast R Jr, Kufe D, Pollock R, *et al*. (eds) *Cancer Medicine*, 5th edn. Hamilton, Ontario, Canada: BC Decker Inc, 2000.

107. Singh AD, Bergman L, Seregard S. Uveal melanoma: epidemiologic aspects. Ophthalmol Clin North Am 2005; 18: 75–84.

108. Eskelin S, Pyrhonen S, Summanen P, Prause JU, Kivela T. Screening for metastatic malignant melanoma of the uvea revisited. Cancer 1999; 85: 1151–9.

109. Margo CE. The Collaborative Ocular Melanoma Study: an overview. Cancer Control 2004; 11: 304–9.

110. McLean IW, Foster WD, Zimmerman LE. Uveal melanoma: location, size, cell type, and enucleation as risk factors in metastasis. Hum Pathol 1982; 13: 123–32.

111. Seddon JM, Albert DM, Lavin PT, Robinson N. A prognostic factor study of disease-free interval and survival following enucleation for uveal melanoma. Arch Ophthalmol 1983; 101: 1894–9.

112. Folberg R, Rummelt V, Parys-van Ginderderen R, *et al*. The prognostic value of tumor blood vessel morphology in primary uveal melanoma. Ophthalmology 1993; 100: 1389–98.

113. McLean MJ, Foster WD, Zimmerman LE. Prognostic factors in small malignant melanomas of choroid and ciliary body. Arch Ophthalmol 1977; 95: 48–58.

114. Rietschel P, Panageas KS, Hanlon C, Patel A, Abramson DH, Chapman PB. Variates of survival in metastatic uveal melanoma. J Clin Oncol 2005; 23: 8076–80.

115. Prescher G, Bornfeld N, Hirche H, Horsthemke B, Jockel KH, Becher R. Prognostic implications of monosomy 3 in uveal melanoma. Lancet 1996; 347: 1222–5.

116. Damato B, Duke C, Coupland SE, et al. Cytogenetics of uveal melanoma: a 7-year clinical experience. Ophthalmology 2007; 114: 1925–31.

117. Zuidervaart W, van der Velden PA, Hurks MH, et al. Gene expression profiling identifies tumour markers potentially playing a role in uveal melanoma development. Br J Cancer 2003; 89: 1914–19.

118. Onken MD, Worley LA, Ehlers JP, et al. Gene expression profiling in uveal melanoma reveals two molecular classes and predicts metastatic death. Cancer Res 2004; 64: 7205–9.

119. Tschentscher F, Husing J, Holter T, et al. Tumor classification based on gene expression profiling shows that uveal melanomas with and without monosomy 3 represent two distinct entities. Cancer Res 2003; 63: 2578–84.

120. Onken MD, Worley LA, Harbour JW. Association between gene expression profile, proliferation and metastasis in uveal melanoma. Curr Eye Res 2010; 35(9): 857–63.

121. Van den Bosch T, Kilic E, Paridaens D, de Klein A. Genetics of uveal melanoma and cutaneous melanoma: two of a kind? Dermatol Res Pract 2010; 2010: 360136.

122. Diener-West M, Reynolds SM, Agugliaro DJ, et al. Development of metastatic disease after enrollment in the COMS trials for treatment of choroidal melanoma: Collaborative Ocular Melanoma Study Group Report No. 26. Arch Ophthalmol 2005; 123: 1639–43.

123. Lorigan JG, Wallace S, Mavligit GM. The prevalence and location of metastases from ocular melanoma: imaging study in 110 patients. Am J Roentgenol 1991; 157: 1279–81.

124. Char DH. Ocular melanoma. Surg Clin North Am 2003; 83: 253–74, vii.

125. Gragoudas ES, Egan KM, Seddon JM, et al. Survival of patients with metastases from uveal melanoma. Ophthalmology 1991; 98: 383–90.

126. Singh AD, Shields CL, Shields JA. Prognostic factors inuveal melanoma. Melanoma Res 2001; 11: 255–63.

127. Diener-West M, Reynolds SM, Agugliaro DJ, et al. Screening for metastasis from choroidal melanoma: the Collaborative Ocular Melanoma Study Group Report 23. J Clin Oncol 2004; 22: 2438–44.

128. Brownstein S. Malignant melanoma of the conjunctiva. Cancer Control 2004; 11: 310–16.

129. Albert DM, Ryan LM, Borden EC. Metastatic ocular and cutaneous melanoma: a comparison of patient characteristics and prognosis. Arch Ophthalmol 1996; 114: 107–8.

130. Nathan F, Sato T, Hart E, et al. Response to combination chemotherapy of liver metastasis from chorhoidal melanoma compared with cutaneous melanoma. Proc Am Soc Clin Oncol 1994; 13: 394.

131. Bedikian AY, Papadopoulos N, Plager C, Eton O, Ring S. Phase II evaluation of temozolomide in metastatic choroidal melanoma. Melanoma Res 2003; 13: 303–6.

132. Bedikian AY, Legha SS, Mavligit G, et al. Treatment of uveal melanoma metastatic to the liver: a review of the M. D. Anderson Cancer Center experience and prognostic factors. Cancer 1995; 76: 1665–70.

133. Salmon RJ, Levy C, Plancher C, et al. Treatment of liver metastases from uveal melanoma by combined surgerychemotherapy. Eur J Surg Oncol 1998; 24: 127–30.

134. Char DH. Metastatic choroidal melanoma. Am J Ophthalmol 1978; 86: 76–80.

135. Mavligit GM, Charnsangavej C, Carrasco CH, Patt YZ, Benjamin RS, Wallace S. Regression of ocular melanoma metastatic to the liver after hepatic arterial chemoembolization with cisplatin and polyvinyl sponge. JAMA 1988; 260: 974–6.

136. Gonsalves CF, Eschelman DJ, Sullivan KL, Anne PR, Doyle L, Sato T. Radioembolization as salvage therapy for hepatic metastasis of uveal melanoma: a single institution experience. Am J Roentgenol 2011; 196: 1–6.

137. Breedis C, Young G. The blood supply of neoplasms in the liver. Am J Pathol 1954; 30: 969–77.

138. Lien WM, Ackerman NB. The blood supply of experimental liver metastases. II. A microcirculatory study of the normal and tumor vessels of the liver with the use of perfused silicone rubber. Surgery 1970; 68: 334–40.

139. Ackerman NB, Lien WM, Silverman NA. The blood supply of experimental liver metastases. III. The effects of acute ligation of the hepatic artery or portal vein. Surgery 1972; 71: 636–41.

140. Sato T. Locoregional management of hepatic metastasis from primary uveal melanoma. Semin Oncol 2010; 37: 127–38.

141. Miao N, Pingpank JF, Alexander HR, Steinberg SM, Beresneva T, Quezado ZM. Percutaneous hepatic perfusion in patients with metastatic liver cancer: anesthetic, hemodynamic, and metabolic considerations. Ann Surg Oncol 2008; 15: 815–23.

142. Pingpank JF. Hyperthermic isolated hepatic perfusion (IHP) using melphalan for patients with ocular melanoma metastatic to the liver. Proceedings of Perspectives in Melanoma VII Meeting, 2004, pp. 117–25.

143. Pingpank JF, Hughes MS, Faries MB, et al. A phase III random assignment trial comparing percutaneous hepatic perfusion with melphalan (PHP-mel) to standard of care for patients with hepatic metastases from metastatic ocular or cutaneous melanoma. J Clin Oncol 2010; 28: 18 s (abstr LBA8512).

144. Hodi FS, O'Day SJ, McDermott DF, et al. Improved survival with ipilimumab in patients with metastatic melanoma. N Engl J Med 2010; 363: 711–23.

145. Chapman PB, Hauschild A, Robert C, et al. Improved survival with vemurafenib in melanoma with BRAF V600E mutation. N Engl J Med 2011; 364(26): 2507–16.

146. Abdel-Rahman MH, Yang Y, Zhou XP, Craig EL, Davidorf FH, Eng C. High frequency of submicroscopic hemizygous deletion is a major mechanism of loss of expression of PTEN in uveal melanoma. J Clin Oncol 2006; 24: 288–95.

147. Ehlers JP, Worley L, Onken MD, Harbour JW. Integrative genomic analysis of aneuploidy in uveal melanoma. Clin Cancer Res 2008; 14: 115–22.

148. Zuidervaart W, van Nieuwpoort F, Stark M, et al. Activation of the MAPK pathway is a common event in uveal melanomas although it rarely occurs through mutation of BRAF or RAS. Br J Cancer 2005; 92: 2032–8.

149. Thomas NE. BRAF somatic mutations in malignant melanoma and melanocytic naevi. Melanoma Res 2006; 16: 97–103.

150. Malaponte G, Libra M, Gangemi P, et al. Detection of BRAF gene mutation in primary choroidal melanoma tissue. Cancer Biol Ther 2006; 5: 225–7.

151. Spendlove HE, Damato BE, Humphreys J, Barker KT, Hiscott PS, Houlston RS. BRAF mutations are detectable in conjunctival but not uveal melanomas. Melanoma Res 2004; 14: 449–52.

152. Henriquez F, Janssen C, Kemp EG, Roberts F. The T1799A BRAF mutation is present in iris melanoma. Invest Ophthalmol Vis Sci 2007; 48: 4897–900.

153. Onken MD, Worley LA, Long MD, et al. Oncogenic mutations in GNAQ occur early in uveal melanoma. Invest Ophthalmol Vis Sci 2008; 49: 5230–4.

154. Van Raamsdonk CD, Griewank KG, Crosby MB, et al. Mutations in GNA11 in uveal melanoma. N Engl J Med 2010; 363: 2191–9.

155. Van Raamsdonk CD, Bezrookove V, Green G, et al. Frequent somatic mutations of GNAQ in uveal melanoma and blue naevi. Nature 2009; 457: 599–602.

156. Harbour JW, Onken MD, Roberson ED, Duan S, Cao L. Frequent mutation of BAP1 in metastasizing uveal melanomas. Science 2010: 330(6009): 1410–13.

157. Conley J, Lattes R, Orr W. Desmoplastic malignant melanoma (a rare variant of spindle cell melanoma). Cancer 1971; 28: 914–36.

158. Wharton JM, Carlson JA, Mihm MC Jr. Desmoplastic malignant melanoma: diagnosis of early clinical lesions. Hum Pathol 1999; 30: 537–42.

159. Quinn MJ, Crotty KA, Thompson JF, et al. Desmoplastic and desmoplastic neurotropic melanoma: experience with 280 patients. Cancer 1998; 83: 1128–35.

160. Magro C, Crowson AN, Mihm MC Jr. Unusual variants of malignant melanoma. Mod Pathol 2006; 19: S41–S70.

161. Tsao H, Sober AJ, Barnhill RL. Desmoplastic neurotropic melanoma. Semin Cutan Med Surg 1997; 16: 131–6.

162. Carlson JA, Dickersin GR, Sober AJ, *et al*. Desmoplastic neurotropic melanoma. A clinicopathologic analysis of 28 cases. Cancer 1995; 75: 478–94.

163. Sagebiel RW. Unusual variants of melanoma: fact or fictioin? Semin Oncol 1996; 23: 703–8.

164. Hawkins WG, Busam KJ, Ben-Porat L, *et al*. Desmoplastic melanoma: a pathologically and clinically distinct form of cutaneous melanoma. Ann Surg Oncol 2005; 12: 197–9.

165. Aslam MZ, Ahmed MS, Nagarajan S, Rizvi ST. Malignant melanoma representing with testicular metastasis: a case report and review of the literature. Can Urol Assoc J 2010; 4(4): E103–4.

166. Price EB, Mostoffi FK. Secondary carcinoma of the testis. Cancer 1957; 10: 592–5.

167. Johnson DE, Jackson L, Ayala AG. Secondary carcinoma of the testis. South Med J 1971; 64: 1128–30.

168. Lowell DM, Lewis EL. Melanospermia: a hitherto undescribed entity. J Urol 1966; 95: 407–11.

169. Hida T, Saga K, Ogino J, *et al*. Testicular swelling as the presenting sign of cutaneous malignant melanoma. J Eur Acad Dermatol Venereol 2006; 20: 351–3.

170. Datta MW, Young RH. Malignant melanoma metastatic to the testis: a report of 3 cases with clinically significant manifestations. Int J Surg Pathol 2008; 8: 49–57.

171. Katiyar RK, Singh A, Kumar D. Primary melanoma of the testis. J Cancer Res Ther 2008; 4(2): 97–8.

52 Primary Melanotic Tumors of the Central Nervous System

L. Burt Nabors,[1] Rong Li,[2] Cheryl A. Palmer,[2] and Philip R. Chapman[3]

[1] Division of Neuro-Oncology, Department of Neurology, [2] Division of Neuropathology, Department of Pathology, [3] Neuroradiology Section, Department of Radiology, University of Alabama, Birmingham, AL, USA

Introduction

Primary melanotic tumors of the central nervous system (CNS) encompass a wide variety of lesions with clear differences in features and treatment options. The cellular origin of pigmentation and pigmented lesions is melanocytes. These normal cells are derived from the neural crest and are dispersed in the leptomeninges with a concentration in the posterior fossa and upper spinal cord locations. Melanotic tumors of the CNS can be considered as primary or secondary. The majority of secondary tumors result from metastasis of systemic melanoma. Primary melanotic tumors include melanocytomas and primary melanomas which range in behavior from benign to malignant. A subset of meningiomas, medulloblastomas, and schwannomas may also be pigmented and considered as melanotic. In this review, we present clinical, radiographic, pathological, and treatment considerations for these rare tumors.

The incidence of primary melanotic tumors of the CNS is extremely rare. Tumors may occur at any level of the neural axis. A comprehensive pathological analysis reported a distribution of primary melanomas as 38% in the spinal cord, 38% in the posterior fossa, and 23% supratentorial. For melanocytomas, the distribution was weighted far more commonly in the spinal cord (65%).[1] These tumors may occur at any age from children to older adults. Melanocytomas are typically considered benign but case reports exist of those that transformed with dissemination and/or metastasis.[2–4] A widely disseminated form termed melanomatosis occurs in the setting of dermatological syndromes such as neurocutaneous melanosis syndrome and nevus of Ota.[5–7] Melanoma may either metastasize from systemic melanoma or occur as a primary CNS melanoma.

The differentiation of pigmented lesions of the CNS can be very important as those derived from systemic metastasis would require a different workup and treatment considerations. The unique aspects of primary pigmented lesions likewise are important to recognize as behavior, treatment, and prognosis may be affected.

Clinical presentation

The clinical presentation of pigmented lesions of the CNS is influenced by the location and pattern of tumor. The more disseminated lesions such as primary leptomeningeal melanomatosis may present diffusely throughout the CNS and leptomeninges or concentrated in the posterior fossa with symptoms consistent with such a location, including seizure, hydrocephalus, mental status change, cranial nerve palsies, or myelopathy. Neurocutaneous melanosis is considered when an infant presents with large or multiple congenital nevi associated with meningeal melanosis or CNS melanoma.[6,8] Melanocytoma and primary CNS melanoma are typically solitary lesions with symptoms dependent upon tumor location.

Neuroimaging features

The melanin-containing tumors of the CNS are rare and comprise a heterogeneous group of lesions, ranging from benign to malignant, focal to diffuse, and from leptomeningeal to intraparenchymal. Melanin-containing lesions can affect the intracranial or spinal compartments. As expected, the radiological features are highly variable and nonspecific, making preoperative diagnosis difficult.

Melanin has a unique chemical structure and offers a potential radiological signature on magnetic resonance imaging (MRI). Melanin contains two unpaired electrons which can react with water in a dipole–dipole interaction. This causes paramagnetic effects and on MRI produces T1 and T2 shortening.[9] Classically, melanin-containing lesions demonstrate T1 hyperintensity and T2 hypointensity[10] but these signal characteristics are not always present and are ultimately

Textbook of Uncommon Cancer, Fourth Edition. Edited by Derek Raghavan, Charles D. Blanke, David H. Johnson, Paul L. Moots, Gregory H. Reaman, Peter G. Rose and Mikkael A. Sekeres.
© 2012 John Wiley & Sons, Inc. Published 2012 by John Wiley & Sons, Inc.

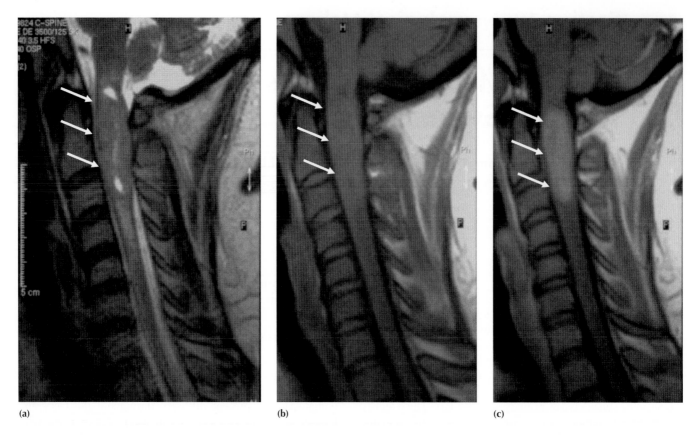

Figure 52.1 This series of sagital images through the cervical spine demonstrates a melanocytoma. The tumor is demonstrated as an expansile intrinsic cervical cord mass that is hyperintense on T2 (a), isointense on T1 (b), and enhances homogeneously with contrast (c). The white arrows localize the mass.

nonspecific. Subacute hemorrhage can produce a similar MRI appearance and intratumoral hemorrhage invariably contributes to the "classic" appearance in many of these tumors.[11] A melanocytoma of the cervical cord is illustrated on MRI in Figure 52.1.

Neurocutaneous melanosis

In neurocutaneous melanosis, there is proliferation of melanin-producing cells within the leptomeninges with predilection for the posterior fossa. There is relative sparing of the dura. Intraparenchymal lesions can occur, presumably via migration of the melanocytes along the perivascular spaces. Unenhanced computed tomography (CT) is relatively insensitive but may demonstrate leptomeningeal isodensity or hyperdensity. Associated findings can include obstructive hydrocephalus or Dandy–Walker complex. Postcontrast CT images demonstrate variable leptomeningeal enhancement mimicking meningitis or carcinomatosis. With MRI, lesions may reveal typical hyperintensity on unenhanced T1-weighted MR images with associated T2 hypointensity secondary to paramagnetic properties of melanin. Intraparenchymal foci most commonly occur in the temporal lobes and cerebellum. Variable leptomeningeal gadolinium enhancement has been reported. Focal nodular or thick plaque-like enhancement is suggestive of the malignant degeneration to malignant melanoma that occurs in 40–60% of patients.[12]

Meningeal melanocytoma

Meningeal melanocytoma, historically referred to as melanotic meningioma, arises from melanocytic cells that normally occur in the leptomeninges, and subsequently occurs predominantly in the posterior fossa, Meckel's cave, and cervical spinal canal. On CT, these lesions present as unifocal isodense or hyperdense extraaxial lesions that enhance following contrast administration. The imaging appearance is nonspecific and suggestive of meningioma, but calcification and hyperostosis are generally not present. MRI demonstrates an extraaxial enhancing lesion that is variably hyperintense on precontrast T1-weighted images. Serial imaging demonstrates a slow, benign growth pattern.[13]

Primary leptomeningeal melanomatosis

Primary leptomeningeal melanomatosis is an aggressive neoplasm arising from the primary melanocytes of the meninges. There is typically diffuse involvement of the leptomeninges as malignant melanocytes disseminate into the cerebrospinal fluid (CSF) pathways and along the perivascular spaces with invasion of the brain parenchyma. Unenhanced CT images may demonstrate isodensity or hyperdensity within the subarachnoid spaces, effacing the basilar cisterns.[14] Postcontrast images demonstrate diffuse nodular enhancement. MRI reveals extensive leptomeningeal contrast

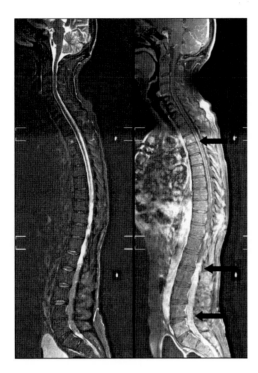

Figure 52.2 A total spine localizer study demonstrates the diffuse thickening with areas of nodular disease formation in a patient with leptomeningeal melanomatosis. After the administration of contrast, the leptomeninges enhance diffusely from the structures of the posterior fossa to the thecal sac which has been filled with tumor (*arrows*).

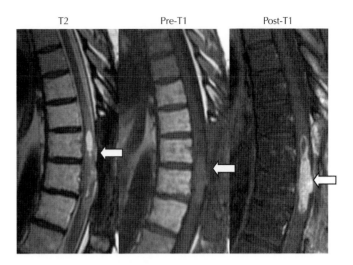

Figure 52.3 A sagittal series through the thoracic spine demonstrates an intraparenchymal mass in the thoracic cord. The mass is isointense to cord on T2 with a bright cyst on the superior aspect. There is T1 shortening (bright) prior to the administration of contrast on the pre-T1 with intense enhancement after contrast administration (post-T1). The mass is a primary CNS melanoma localized by the arrows.

enhancement with obliteration of normal CSF signal in the affected cisterns of the brain or spinal canal. The total spine images in Figure 52.2 demonstrate the extensive leptomeningeal involvement with filling of the thecal sac inferiorly in a patient with melanomatosis. The appearance mimics leptomeningeal carcinomatosis (including metastatic melanoma), infectious meningitis, or granulomatous meningitis.[12,15]

Melanotic schwannoma

Melanotic schwannomas of CNS are of Schwann cell origin and thus occur in typical schwannoma locations, along the cranial or spinal nerves, and present as well-marginated extraaxial masses on CT and MRI, indistinguishable from typical schwannoma. Rarely, intramedullary spinal cord lesions can occur. MRI findings are nonspecific but T1 and T2 shortening may be present to suggest the diagnosis.[12]

Melanoma metastases and primary central nervous system melanoma

Melanoma commonly metastasizes to the brain. Typically, metastatic melanoma affects the brain parenchyma but can result in leptomeningeal dissemination as well. In addition, melanoma can occur as a primary CNS neoplasm. The spinal cord is a common site. In Figure 52.3, a parencyhmal cord mass is shown. It has T1 shortening as seen by the bright signal prior to the administration of contrast on the pre-T1 image. Lesions are typically hyperdense on precontrast CT images

and show some degree of focal enhancement following contrast administration. On MRI, metastatic melanoma classically exhibits T1 shortening and T2 hypointensity secondary to intrinsic melanin and/or hemorrhage. These lesions typically enhance with gadolinium contrast.[16] Gradient echo images reveal focal hypointensity related to susceptibility effects of melanin and/or hemorrhage.[15]

Neuropathological features

Gross neuropathology

Central nervous system melanocytomas and melanomas usually arise from the leptomeninges and present as extraaxial masses. They are grossly gray, brown or black due to variable pigment production. However, primary CNS melanomas can rarely appear as intraaxial masses and most commonly involve the spinal cord or posterior fossa. Melanocytomas are relatively well-circumscribed, unilocular or nodular lesions attached to the dura. Multifocal meningeal melanocytoma is rare.[17] They tend to compress rather than infiltrate the surrounding structures. Occasional cases of parenchymal invasion and malignant transformation have been reported.[1,18–20]

Histopathology

Melanocytoma

The most common histological pattern of melanocytoma consists of nests of spindle-shaped melanin-containing cells surrounded by a fine network of reticulin fibers. To some extent, this pattern resembles the whorls of meningioma. Heavily pigmented melanocytes are frequently located peripherally. Tumor cells arranged around blood vessels or in patternless sheets can be seen in other variants. In some

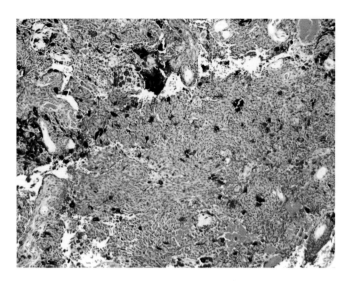

Figure 52.4 Melanocytoma consists of monomorphic-appearing spindle-shaped cells with melanin deposition. H&E, 100×.

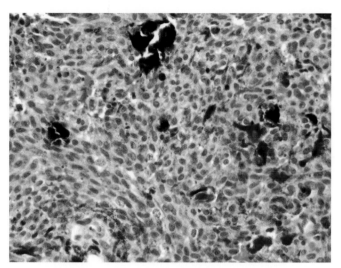

Figure 52.5 Melanocytoma consists of monomorphic-appearing spindle-shaped cells with melanin deposition. H&E, 400×.

melanocytomas, epithelioid pigmented tumor cells comprise the majority of the tumor. The tumor cells have low-grade nuclear features with no significant cytological atypia. They have oval to reniform nuclei, small round nucleoli, and abundant eosinophilic cytoplasm. Mitotic figures are rarely seen – less than 1 per 10 high power fields. The MIB proliferation index is usually less than 2%. Most melanocytomas contain a number of melanophages admixed with melanocytes. Psammoma bodies and calcifications have also occasionally been reported[21,22] but necrosis or hemorrhage is not seen.[21,23] Amelanocytic melanocytoma can rarely occur as well. Their recognition requires a panel of histological, immunohistochemical, or ultrastructural studies. An intermediate-grade melanocytoma with no cytological atypia but an increased MIB proliferation index has been proposed by some authors.[24] These may have more progressive clinical behavior and/or malignant progression (Figs 52.4–52.6).

Melanoma

Malignant leptomeningeal melanomas are histologically similar to their systemic counterparts. The tumor cells are arranged in loose nests, fascicles or sheets and contain variable amounts of melanin.[1] Unlike melanocytomas, tight nests or a whorl-like architecture are not commonly seen. Melanomas have high-grade nuclear features characterized by significant pleomorphism and atypia. Cellularity and mitotic activity are also greatly increased. In addition, they tend to invade adjacent tissue and may demonstrate necrosis. Similar to melanomas arising from other sites of the body, the histology of primary CNS melanomas can vary substantially. In some melanomas, tumor cells have enlarged bizarre nuclei, prominent eosinophilic nucleoli, abundant cytoplasm, and frequent atypical mitotic figures. However, some melanomas demonstrate hypercellularity and are composed of relatively uniform spindle cells having oval nuclei with fine chromatin and prominent round nucleoli (Fig. 52.7).

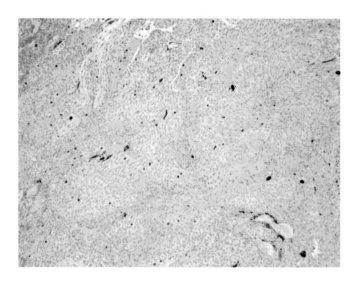

Figure 52.6 MIB proliferation index is low in a melanocytoma. Ki-67 stain, 100×.

The histological differentiation between malignant melanoma and melanocytoma is critical as primary CNS melanoma has an extremely poor prognosis.[25] A diagnosis of melanocytoma is favored when the tumor lacks mitotic activity, nuclear pleomorphism, hyperchromasia, and indolent tumor growth spanning more than 4 years.[26]

Ancillary diagnostic studies

Immunohistochemical analysis demonstrates the expression of melanocytic marker proteins, such as S-100, Melan A, and HMB-45, but an absence of meningothelial cell markers (such as epithelial membrane antigen).[27,28] Microophthalmia transcription factor (MTF) can be used as a marker for melanocytic origin, especially when other commonly used melanocytic markers are negative or equivocal. Immunoreaction to cytokeratin, glial fibrillary acidic protein, neuron-specific enolase, and Leu-7 is usually negative.[22,27]

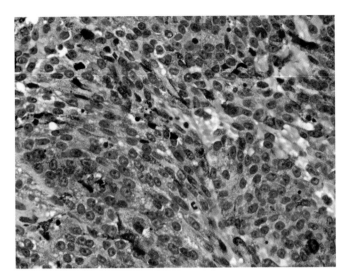
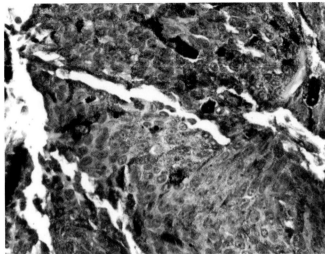

Figure 52.7 Malignant melanoma demonstrates pleomorphic tumor cells with prominent nucleoli and scattered mitotic figures. H&E, 400×.

Electron microscopy demonstrates an absence of desmosomes and interdigitating cellular processes that are found in meningiomas. Instead, melanomas and melanocytomas have intracytoplasmic melanosomes.

Treatment

The modalities available for the treatment of patients with primary melanotic tumors of the CNS include surgery, radiation therapy, and chemotherapy. There are no clinical trials to offer suggestions on treatment role and benefit. The majority of treatment decisions are based on case reports and small, single-institution experiences. Factors to consider in the treatment planning for patients include age, functional status, neurological deficits related to disease, and pathological features.

Neurocutaneous melanosis patients are typically young, develop symptoms related to CSF flow obstruction, and surgical management of hydrocephalus is often the primary goal of treatment. Through life, patients may develop benign proliferation or transformation to malignant melanoma.[6,29,30] These tumors have shown little response to radiation or chemotherapy and prognosis is poor.

Melanocytomas are typically solitary and histologically benign lesions. Complete surgical resection should be the goal for such patients and typically is associated with a good prognosis.[31] In cases where complete surgical resection is not possible or practical, adjuvant radiation therapy has been utilized with a suggestion of reasonable local control.[32]

Primary CNS malignant melanomas are thought to have a better prognosis than systemic disease but remain an aggressive cancer with a high tendency for recurrence and spread. Surgical resection is the initial goal and this may be followed by radiation therapy to the resection cavity or residual disease. At present, chemotherapy has a limited role. CNS permeable agents such as temozolomide may be considered. The use of molecularly targeted agents is emerging as a therapeutic option in patients with melanoma. Approximately, 66%

of malignant melanoma have a *BRAF* somatic missense mutation. The majority of these are within the kinase domain resulting in elevated kinase activity and transformation.[33] The suppression of BRAF expression in melanoma inhibits the mitogen-activated kinase cascade with growth arrest and apoptosis.[34] Clinical trials in metastatic systemic melanoma with the *BRAF* kinase inhibitor vemurafenib (PLX4032) have shown high response rates (>50%) and improved survival in patients with the *BRAF* V600E mutation.[35,36] At present, there are no case reports of vemurafenib for primary CNS melanoma.

Conclusion

Primary melanotic tumors of the CNS are extremely rare pigmented lesions that may occur in a widespread, diffuse way or as focal, solitary lesions. The determination of a primary CNS process versus metastasis from a systemic source is of high clinical importance. The treatment of primary melanotic CNS lesions is determined by patient features such as age, functional status, tumor location, and pathological features. The modalities that appear to offer the most benefit are surgical resection and focal radiation therapy. At present, the role of chemotherapy is not defined. Targeted molecular therapeutics may be considered for patients with melanoma demonstrating a mutation of *BRAF*.

References

1. Brat DJ, Giannini C, Scheithauer BW, Burger PC. Primary melanocytic neoplasms of the central nervous systems. Am J Surg Pathol 1999; 23(7): 745–54.
2. Uozumi Y, Kawano T, Kawaguchi T, et al. Malignant transformation of meningeal melanocytoma: a case report. Brain Tumor Pathol 2003; 20(1): 21–5.
3. Wang F, Qiao G, Lou X, Song X, Chen W. Malignant transformation of intracranial meningeal melanocytoma. Case report and review of the literature. Neuropathology 2007; 31(4): 414–20.

4. Perrini P, Caniglia M, Pieroni M, Castagna M, Parenti GF. Malignant transformation of intramedullary melanocytoma: case report. Neurosurgery 2010; 67(3): E867–9; discussion E869.

5. Balmaceda CM, Fetell MR, O'Brien JL, Housepian EH. Nevus of Ota and leptomeningeal melanocytic lesions. Neurology 1993; 43(2): 381–6.

6. Kadonaga JN, Frieden IJ. Neurocutaneous melanosis: definition and review of the literature. J Am Acad Dermatol 1991; 24(5 Pt 1): 747–55.

7. Kadonaga JN, Barkovich AJ, Edwards MS, Frieden IJ. Neurocutaneous melanosis in association with the Dandy–Walker complex. Pediatr Dermatol 1992; 9(1): 37–43.

8. Fox H. Neurocutaneous melanosis. In: Viriken PI, Bruyn GW (eds) *Handbook of Clinical Neurology.* Amsterdam: Elsevier, 1972. pp.414–28.

9. Atlas SW, Grossman RI, Gomori JM, *et al*. MR imaging of intracranial metastatic melanoma. J Comput Assist Tomogr 1987; 11(4): 577–82.

10. Isiklar I, Leeds NE, Fuller GN, Kumar AJ. Intracranial metastatic melanoma: correlation between MR imaging characteristics and melanin content. Am J Roentgenol 1995; 165(6): 1503–12.

11. Woodruff WW Jr, Djang WT, McLendon RE, Heinz ER, Voorhees DR. Intracerebral malignant melanoma: high-field-strength MR imaging. Radiology 1987; 165(1): 209–13.

12. Smith AB, Rushing EJ, Smirniotopoulos JG. Pigmented lesions of the central nervous system: radiologic-pathologic correlation. Radiographics 2009; 29(5): 1503–24.

13. Jaiswal S, Vij M, Tungria A, Jaiswal AK, Srivastava AK, Behari S. Primary melanocytic tumors of the central nervous system: a neuroradiological and clinicopathological study of five cases and brief review of literature. Neurol India 2011; 59(3): 413–19.

14. Demir MK, Aker FV, Akinci O, Ozgultekin A. Case 134: primary leptomeningeal melanomatosis. Radiology 2008; 247(3): 905–9.

15. Gaviani P, Mullins ME, Braga TA, *et al*. Improved detection of metastatic melanoma by T2*-weighted imaging. Am J Neuroradiol 2006; 27(3): 605–8.

16. Berman C, Reintgen D. Radiologic imaging in malignant melanoma: a review. Semin Surg Oncol 1993; 9(3): 232–8.

17. Ali Y, Rahme R, Moussa R, Abadjian G, Menassa-Moussa L, Samaha E. Multifocal meningeal melanocytoma: a new pathological entity or the result of leptomeningeal seeding? J Neurosurg 2009; 111(3): 488–91.

18. Bydon A, Gutierrez JA, Mahmood A. Meningeal melanocytoma: an aggressive course for a benign tumor. J Neurooncol 2003; 64(3): 259–63.

19. Gempt J, Buchmann N, Grams AE, *et al*. Black brain: transformation of a melanocytoma with diffuse melanocytosis into a primary cerebral melanoma. J Neurooncol 2011; 102(2): 323–8.

20. Wang F, Qiao G, Lou X, Song X, Chen W. Malignant transformation of intracranial meningeal melanocytoma. Case report and review of the literature. Neuropathology 2011; 31(4): 414–20.

21. Ibanez J, Weil B, Ayala A, Jimenez A, Acedo C, Rodrigo I. Meningeal melanocytoma: case report and review of the literature. Histopathology 1997; 30(6): 576–81.

22. Winston KR, Sotrel A, Schnitt SJ. Meningeal melanocytoma. Case report and review of the clinical and histological features. J Neurosurg 1987; 66(1): 50–7.

23. Clarke DB, Leblanc R, Bertrand G, Quartey GR, Snipes GJ. Meningeal melanocytoma. Report of a case and a historical comparison. J Neurosurg 1998; 88(1): 116–21.

24. Navas M, Pascual JM, Fraga J, *et al*. Intracranial intermediate-grade meningeal melanocytoma with increased cellular proliferative index: an illustrative case associated with a nevus of Ota. J Neurooncol 2009; 95(1): 105–15.

25. Larson TC 3rd, Houser OW, Onofrio BM, Piepgras DG. Primary spinal melanoma. J Neurosurg 1987; 66(1): 47–9.

26. Painter TJ, Chaljub G, Sethi R, Singh H, Gelman B. Intracranial and intraspinal meningeal melanocytosis. Am J Neuroradiol 2000; 21(7): 1349–53.

27. Uematsu Y, Yukawa S, Yokote H, Itakura T, Hayashi S, Komai N. Meningeal melanocytoma: magnetic resonance imaging characteristics and pathological features. Case report. J Neurosurg 1992; 76(4): 705–9.

28. Beseoglu K, Knobbe CB, Reifenberger G, Steiger HJ, Stummer W. Supratentorial meningeal melanocytoma mimicking a convexity meningioma. Acta Neurochir (Wien) 2006; 148(4): 485–90.

29. Di Rocco F, Sabatino G, Koutzoglou M, Battaglia D, Caldarelli M, Tamburrini G. Neurocutaneous melanosis. Childs Nerv Syst 2004; 20(1): 23–8.

30. Caldarelli M, Tamburrini G, Di Rocco F. Neurocutaneous melanosis. J Neurosurg 2005; 103(4 Suppl): 382.

31. Rades D, Heidenreich F, Tatagiba M, Brandis A, Karstens JH. Therapeutic options for meningeal melanocytoma. Case report. J Neurosurg 2001; 95(2 Suppl): 225–31.

32. Rades D, Schild SE. Dose–response relationship for fractionated irradiation in the treatment of spinal meningeal melanocytomas: a review of the literature. J Neurooncol 2006; 77(3): 311–14.

33. Davies H, Bignell GR, Cox C, *et al*. Mutations of the BRAF gene in human cancer. Nature 2002; 417(6892): 949–54.

34. Hingorani SR, Jacobetz MA, Robertson GP, Herlyn M, Tuveson DA. Suppression of BRAF(V599E) in human melanoma abrogates transformation. Cancer Res 2003; 63(17): 5198–202.

35. Chapman PB, Hauschild A, Robert C, *et al*. Improved survival with vemurafenib in melanoma with BRAF V600E mutation. N Engl J Med 2011; 364(26): 2507–16.

36. Vultur A, Villanueva J, Herlyn M. Targeting BRAF in advanced melanoma: a first step toward manageable disease. Clin Cancer Res 2011; 17(7): 1658–63.

53 Langerhans Cell Histiocytosis of the Central Nervous System

Rima F. Jubran[1] and Jonathan L. Finlay[1,2]

[1]Division of Pediatric Hematology/Oncology, Department of Pediatrics, Keck School of Medicine at USC, University of Southern California, Los Angeles, CA, USA

[2]Children's Center for Cancer and Blood Diseases, Children's Hospital Los Angeles, Los Angeles, CA, USA

Introduction

Over a century has passed since Langerhans cell histiocytosis (LCH) or histiocytosis X was first described by Hand in 1893, yet central nervous system (CNS) involvement remains a poorly understood entity. This chapter attempts to assemble the available information on CNS involvement in LCH in a comprehensive fashion, based on a literature review.

Epidemiology

The true incidence of this disease is not known because many patients are undiagnosed. Nevertheless, in children 15 years old or younger, the incidence rate is estimated to be between 2–10 cases per million with an equal distribution between males and females.[1–3] The median age of presentation has been reported to be 30 months, with younger children more likely to develop systemic disease and older children more likely to have isolated bone involvement. In adults, incidence rates have been reported at 1–2 cases per million with a predominance of lung involvement that is closely related to smoking.[4] Gotz and Fichter reported results from 55 adults with LCH in Germany and found that the mean age of presentation was 43.5 years and that there was a female predominance (66%).[5] As for CNS involvement, it is known that the hypothalamic-pituitary axis is the most common site of CNS disease and estimates for children approximate 30%.[6–8] Frequencies for neurodegenerative disease, however, vary between 2% and 4% and are mainly in children who had high-risk multisystem disease or those diagnosed with maxillofacial involvement.

Biology

The etiology of LCH remains unknown. Much debate has revolved around whether it is a malignant disease or a proliferative response to external stimuli.[9–12] Regardless, the LCH cells from these lesions require interaction with lymphocytes, eosinophils, and macrophages.[13] Together, these cells form granulomas in a variety of affected tissues. These granulomas are characterized by a "cytokine storm." The predominant source of these cytokines is the CD4[+] T helper cells, with LCH cells and macrophages being additional producers.[14,15]

Central nervous system involvement has been recognized since the earliest descriptions of LCH.[16,17] However, the prevalence of such involvement among patients with LCH is not known and the pathogenesis of CNS LCH remains a matter of speculation.[18]

The writing committee of the Histiocyte Society at its annual meeting in 1996 tried to explain the pathogenesis.[19] They described a histochemical entity of neuronal injury and astrocytosis mediated by neuroexcitatory transmitters, glutamate, and N-methyl-D-aspartate, by a similar mechanism as described by Lipton and Gendelman[20,21] to explain the mechanism of neuronal death in dementia associated with acquired immunodeficiency syndrome (AIDS). They reported that the human immunodeficiency virus (HIV) glycoprotein (gp) 120 coat stimulates brain macrophages and microglial cells, causing them to secrete neurotoxins and cytokines. This leads to neuronal death through cytotoxic calcium influx.

As LCH cells exhibit characteristics of activated macrophages in other organs, it is likely that similar mechanisms may play a pivotal role in the CNS as well. The local production of cytokines may recruit inflammatory cells into the brain, creating the inflammatory lesions seen within and surrounding LCH granulomas. On the other hand, some authors have also described autoantibodies to neuronal tissue in LCH.[22,23] It is possible that LCH granulomas could harvest neuronal antigens and stimulate an autoimmune destruction of brain tissue. This would explain the neurodegenerative lesions that lack LCH cells.

Pathology

On light microscopy of typical LCH granulomas, Langerhans cells are characterized as large mononucleated cells with abundant eosinophilic cytoplasm and "coffee bean" nuclei.[13]

Textbook of Uncommon Cancer, Fourth Edition. Edited by Derek Raghavan, Charles D. Blanke, David H. Johnson, Paul L. Moots, Gregory H. Reaman, Peter G. Rose and Mikkael A. Sekeres.

Electron microscopy reveals the diagnostic Birbeck bodies or granules, which are rigid tubular structures with an average diameter of 34 nm and a tennis racket shape. They can easily be identified by the immunochemical staining of Langerin (CD207). This transmembrane c-type lectin was recently identified and found to be specific to the cytoplasm and cell surface of immature Langerhans cells and is associated with Birbeck granule formation.[24,25] The presence of Birbeck granules/CD207 or immune-histochemical staining for CD1a positivity[26] is required for the definitive diagnosis of LCH.

A report by Grois et al.[27] represents a comprehensive study of the histopathology of CNS lesions in LCH. They presented material from 12 CNS biopsy specimens and one autopsy. These investigators identified three discrete pathological lesions of LCH in the CNS. The first were well-circumscribed granulomas within the brain connective tissue space (meninges and choroid plexus). The second were granulomas within the brain connective tissues with partial infiltration of the surrounding parenchyma. The third were neurodegenerative lesions in the cerebellum and the brainstem.

Histopathology of granulomas in the brain connective tissue showed them to be discretely separate from the CNS tissue. They consisted of histiocytes, foamy macrophages, lymphocytes, plasma cells, multinucleated giant cells, and eosinophils. This is very similar to the composition of LCH granulomas in other organs, with the exception of the CD8+ T cells in the CNS lesions outnumbering the CD3+/CD8− cells. The presence of CD1a+ cells was variable, being more abundant in newly diagnosed lesions when compared with material from a patient diagnosed 5 years earlier.

Granulomas with partial infiltration into CNS tissue were found in patients with infundibular lesions infiltrating into the hypothalamus. This is the most common site of CNS involvement with LCH. Histopathology of the granuloma was the same as described above but the adjacent tissue was found to be infiltrated by CD1a+ cells, CD68+ macrophages, and lymphocytes with nearly complete loss of neurons and axons. In addition, a much larger area of inflammation dominated by CD8+ lymphocytes surrounded these lesions.

Finally, autopsy of a patient with neurodegenerative lesions demonstrated the full spectrum of this disease. There was diffuse inflammation in the brain dominated by CD8+ lymphocytes, as well as microglial activation and tissue degeneration. No focal granulomas or CD1a+ cells were found. Tissue degeneration was most profound in the cerebellum, brainstem, infundibulum, optic chiasm, and basal ganglia. In the cerebellum, the deep white matter was atrophic with loss of neurons and myelin and reactive glial scar formation. The Virchow–Robin spaces were enlarged and contained macrophages and T lymphocytes. Atrophy was also found in the cerebellar cortex. Other lesions throughout the brain showed similar histopathological changes, but were less extensive.

Clinical features

The clinical spectrum shows that all regions of the CNS can be involved in this disease. CNS disease, in order of frequency, involves the hypothalamic–pituitary axis, cerebellum, pons,

and cerebral hemispheres. However, a small number of other cases involving the basal ganglia, spinal cord, and optic nerves and tracts have also been reported. Involvement of the choroid plexus has been reported in exceedingly rare cases. Signs and symptoms of CNS lesions can occur years before presentation of any other manifestations.[6] Some patients have presented with acute signs of intracranial hypertension or with focal neurological symptoms.

Neurodegenerative disease has been described in 2–4% of patients with LCH. Risk factors include multisystem disease at diagnosis, involvement of maxillofacial bone lesions with soft tissue extension and history of pituitary involvement.[7,8] Neurodegenerative disease (NDD) can manifest with radiographic changes on magnetic resonance imaging (MRI) and/or clinical symptoms.[28] Various signs and symptoms include, but are not limited to, ataxia, dysarthria, tremors, dysdiadochokinesis, and hyperreflexia.[29] Eventually, the disease can progress, leading to marked neurological disability ranging from spastic diplegia and quadriplegia, to discrete intellectual and behavioral changes.[30] Studies on cerebrospinal fluid of patients with neurodegenerative disease have not been performed in a standardized fashion and the few reported show no typical pattern.[31] The hallmark of neuroendocrine manifestations of CNS LCH is diabetes insipidus.[19] Growth hormone deficiency is the second most common manifestation of pituitary involvement.[8]

Radiographic features

Magnetic resonance imaging remains the technique of choice for demonstrating CNS lesions. In 1996, the writing committee of the Histiocyte Society proposed the following classification based on MRI to illustrate the spectrum of lesions. MRI and the pattern of gadolinium contrast enhancement suggest the correct diagnosis in any given clinical setting.[32]

• *Type Ia*: white matter lesions without enhancement. These lesions were predominantly located in the pons, cerebellar peduncles, and cerebellar white matter. They presented as poorly defined areas of low signal intensity on T1-weighted images and high signal intensity on T2-weighted and proton density-weighted images. Multiple sclerosis, acute disseminated encephalomyelitis (ADEM), leukodystrophies, and infections have to be considered among alternative possible diagnoses.

• *Type Ib*: white matter lesions with enhancement. As with type Ia, there was a striking infratentorial location. The lesions presented as poorly to well-defined areas of prolonged T1 and T2 relaxation times, that is, low signal intensity on T1-weighted images and high signal intensity on T2-weighted and proton density-weighted images, without mass effect and with strong gadolinium enhancement. The differential diagnoses to be considered include multiple sclerosis, ADEM, metastases, and sarcoidosis.

• *Type IIa*: gray matter lesions without enhancement. Changes of this type were mostly seen in the dentate nucleus with bilateral involvement, as areas of low signal intensity on T1-weighted images and high signal intensity on T2-weighted and proton density-weighted images. These lesions showed no mass effect. However, calcifications were occasionally present.

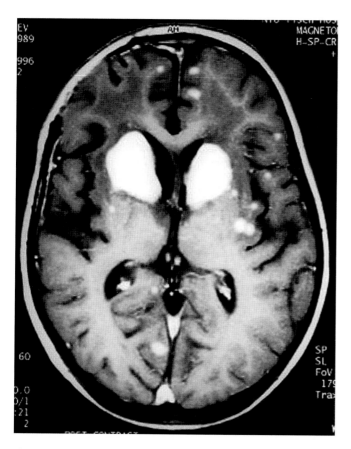

Figure 53.1 Axial contrast-enhanced T1-weighted section through the basal ganglia shows several bilateral enhancing brain lesions, the largest at the heads of the caudate nuclei.

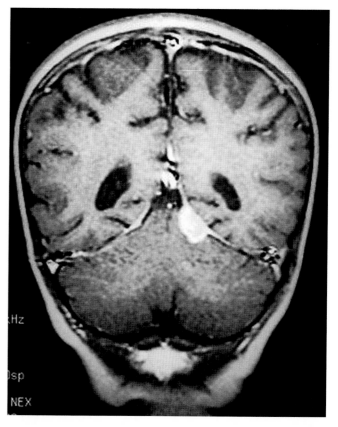

Figure 53.2 Coronal contrast-enhanced T1-weighted image shows enhancing dural mass arising from the edge of the tentorium.

These lesions must be distinguished from Fahr disease (if calcified), ADEM, glioma, and infarction.

• *Type IIb*: gray matter lesions with enhancement. These lesions were predominantly located in the cerebellar gray matter and basal ganglia (Fig. 53.1). Well-defined areas of low signal intensity on T1-weighted images and high signal intensity on T2-weighted and proton density-weighted images showed mass effect and strong gadolinium enhancement, and were sometimes surrounded by edema. Such lesions can be mistaken for low-grade glial tumors.

• *Type III*: extraparenchymal lesions. These masses were (i) dural based (Fig. 53.2), (ii) arachnoid based, or (iii) choroid plexus based, and appeared iso- to hypointense to brain on T1-weighted images, hypointense on T2-weighted images, and showed uniform contrast enhancement. Alternative diagnoses for meningeal-based lesions include leukemia, lymphoma, and carcinomatous masses, and, for type IIIc lesions, choroid plexus tumors have to be considered.

• *Type IV*: lesions of the hypothalamic–pituitary axis. These lesions include (i) type IVa, infundibular thickening, (ii) type IVb, a partially or completely empty sella, and (iii) type IVc, lack of the posterior pituitary bright signals on T1-weighted MR images and hypothalamic mass lesions (Fig. 53.3). Alternative diagnoses of infundibular thickening include sarcoidosis, posttraumatic states, and rare neoplasm; those for

hypothalamic mass lesions include malignant germ cell tumors, glioma, lymphoma, hamartoma, and sarcoidosis.

• *Type V*: atrophy. Local or diffuse atrophy was the nonspecific finding with a multifactorial etiology.

• *Type VI*: therapy-related white matter changes with/without contrast enhancement and specific high signal intensity changes. These can be seen bilaterally within the deep gray matter as foci of calcification. These changes are not entirely specific but are characteristic sequelae of irradiation and chemotherapy damage to the CNS. They have to be considered in patients who are treated with these modalities for LCH at an early age.

Treatment

There are no standard recommendations concerning the choice of treatment of CNS LCH; the individual strategy is based on type, site, and extra-CNS involvement.[33] Therapy in patients with types I and II MRI changes remains controversial. These patients may or may not have clinical signs of ataxia and neurological dysfunction. Several agents have been tried in an effort to reverse or stop the progression of these changes but the numbers are small and the follow-up too short to make definitive recommendations.

Idbaih *et al.* reported on 10 patients with clinical and radiological neurodegeneration whom they treated with 13-cis-retinoic acid.[34] All patients remained clinically stable but the follow-up was only for 1 year. Imashuku *et al.* reported on

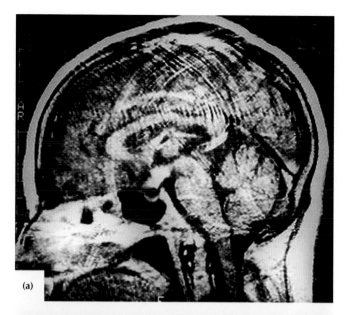

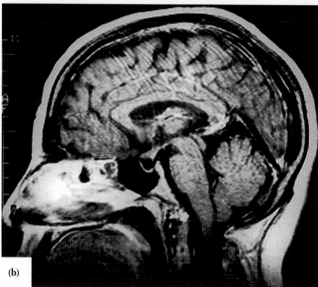

Figure 53.3 Sagittal contrast-enhanced T1-weighted images of the brain at midline (a) pretreatment and (b) post treatment show enhancing hypothalamic lesion (a) that resolves on follow-up treatment (b).

11 patients with NDD. They treated four patients with intravenously administered immune globulin (IVIG) for greater than 12 months and compared them to eight who did not receive IVIG. They found a possible delay in clinical neurological deterioration in the IVIG-treated group.[35] Allen *et al.* described eight patients with clinical NDD and changes on brain MRI, who were treated with either cytosine arabinoside and vincristine or cytosine arabinoside alone. Five of the eight patients demonstrated improvement in both clinical and radiological findings after a follow-up period of 2 months to 7 years.[36]

Therapy for mass lesions includes surgical resection or systemic chemotherapy. Endoscopic surgical techniques may be used in choroid plexus lesions. Chemotherapeutic agents with documented efficacy in systemic LCH have been employed

to treat LCH in the CNS.[37] Etoposide, cyclosporine A,[38] vinblastine, methotrexate, chlorambucil, corticosteroids, and 2-chlorodeoxyadenosine (2-CDA) have produced responses in individual cases. 2-CDA is a purine analog with potent toxicity to monocytes *in vitro*. As tissue histiocytes are derived from the same marrow precursors as monocytes, it has been employed to treat patients with LCH. This drug has shown encouraging results and is especially useful in treating refractory LCH in patients without liver, spleen, lung, or hematological involvement.[39–41] Other therapeutic agents in combination are recommended if treatment with a single agent fails.

Systemic chemotherapy is the treatment of choice for patients with hypothalamic/pituitary involvement. Ideally, the patient is diagnosed with LCH because of another lesion elsewhere that has been biopsied. However, if pituitary stalk thickening is the only manifestation, a biopsy is necessary to establish the diagnosis prior to the initiation of chemotherapy. External beam irradiation is not recommended for the treatment of any CNS lesions since the presence of CNS involvement predisposes patients to the development of neurodegenerative lesions that may be prevented if systemic chemotherapy is administered.[42] In addition, irradiation will affect the more normal brain tissue and cause additional deficits.

Prognosis

The prognosis for patients with LCH depends on the degree of "risk organ" involvement. The Histiocyte Society defines "risk organs" as liver, spleen, lung, or hematological involvement. In addition, early response to chemotherapy is a good prognostic indicator in patients with systemic disease. Patients who have a poor response have a 65% mortality rate compared with 20% in responders.

Recent reports show that patients with head and neck lesions are at increased risk of developing CNS involvement – 30% will develop pituitary involvement.[7] D'Ambrosio *et al.* reviewed the brain MRIs of 100 patients with LCH and found that 50% of them had lesions in the craniofacial bones.[43] Patients with lesions involving the orbit, sphenoid, ethmoid, mastoid, and temporal bones are at higher risk for the development of diabetes insipidus and other CNS disease.[8,27,44] Once patients develop complete diabetes insipidus, it is only rarely reversible despite systemic chemotherapy.[45] In addition, 2–4% of patients with multiple organ involvement or maxillofacial lesions will develop irreversible neurodegenerative changes.

The optimal time to initiate therapy for patients with neurodegenerative disease is not known. Studies in other CNS degenerative diseases recommend early therapy to prevent further neuronal loss.[46,47] Unfortunately, there is no definitive evidence at this time that any intervention will affect the course of this disease, making recommendations premature. Further study in this area is needed.

Recommendations

There are no standardized treatment approaches for children or adults with CNS disease. The standard initial approach for children who require treatment for systemic disease is a combination of prednisone and vinblastine for 6–12 months. 2-CDA has also been shown to be effective for patients with pituitary involvement and may be used upfront if the patient is an adult or in a child with a reactivation involving the pituitary. Unfortunately, the optimal therapy to prevent permanent sequelae of endocrine dysfunction and neurodegenerative disease is still not known.

References

1. Stålemark H, Laurencikas E, Karis J, Gavhed D, Fadeel B, Henter JI. Incidence of Langerhans cell histiocytosis in children: A population based study. Pediatr Blood Cancer 2008; 51(1): 76–81.

2. Salotti JA, Nanduri V, Pearce MS, et al. Incidence and clinical features of Langerhans cell histiocytosis in the UK and Ireland. Arch Dis Child 2009; 94: 376–80.

3. Guyot-Goubin A, Donadieu J, Barkaoui M, et al. Descriptive epidemiology of childhood Langerhans cell histiocytosis. Br J Haematol 1999; 107(4): 883–8.

4. Baumgartner I, von Hochstetter A, Baumert B, et al. Langerhans cell histiocytosis in adults. Med Pediatr Oncol 1997; 28(1): 9–14.

5. Gotz G, Fichter J. Langerhans cell histiocytosis in 58 adults. Am J Med Res 2004; 9(11): 510–14.

6. Grois N, Barkovich AJ, Rosenau W, Ablin AR. Central nervous system disease associated with Langerhan's cell histiocytosis. Am J Pediatr Hematol Oncol 1993; 15: 245–54.

7. Donadieu J, Rolon MA, Thomas C, et al., French LCH Study Group. Endocrine involvement in pediatric-onset Langerhans' cell histiocytosis: a population-based study. J Pediatr 2004; 144(3): 344–50.

8. Haupt R, Nanduri V, Calevo MG, et al. Permanent consequences in Langerhans cell histiocytosis patients: a pilot study from the Histiocyte Society–Late Effects Study Group. Pediatr Blood Cancer 2004; 42(5): 438–44.

9. Egeler RM, van Halteren AG, Hogendoorn PC, Laman JD, Leenen PJ. Langerhans' cell histiocytosis: fascinating dynamics of the dendritic cell-macrophage lineage. Immunol Rev 2010; 234(1): 213–32.

10. Coppes-Zantinga A, Egeler RM. The Langerhans' cell histiocytosis X files revealed. Br J Haematol 2002; 116(1): 3–9.

11. Nezelof C, Basset F, Rousseau MF. Histiocytosis X histiogenetic arguments for a Langerhans cell origin. Biomedicine 1973; 18(5): 365–71.

12. Laman JD, Leenen PJ, Annels NE, Hogendoorn PC, Egeler RM. Langerhans cell histiocytosis "insight into DC biology." Trends Immunol 2003; 24: 190–6.

13. Favara BE, Jaffe R. Pathology of Langerhans cell histiocytosis. Hematol Oncol Clin North Am 1987; 1: 75–97.

14. Senechal B, Elain G, Jeziorski E, et al. Expansion of regulatory T cells in patients with LCH. PLoS Med 2007; 4(8): e253.

15. Egeler RM, Favara BE, van Meurs M, Laman JD, Claassen E. Differential in situ cytokine profiles of Langerhans-like cells and T cells in Langerhans cell histiocytosis: abundant expression of cytokines relevant to disease and treatment. Blood 1999; 94: 4195–201.

16. Schuller A. Uber eigenartige Shandeldefekte im Jugendalter. Fortschr Rontgenstr 1915; 23: 12.

17. Christian HA. Defects in membranous bones, exophthalmos and diabetes insipidus. Med Clin North Am 1920; 3: 849.

18. Hamre M, Hedberg J, Buckley J, et al. Langerhans cell histiocytosis: an explanatory epidemiology study of 177 cases. Med Pediatr Oncol 1997; 28: 92–7.

19. Report of Histiocyte Society workshops on 'central nervous system disease in Langerhans cell histiocytosis'. Med Pediatr Oncol 1997; 29(2): 73–8.

20. Lipton SA, Rosenberg PA. Mechanism of disease: excitatory amino acids as a final common pathway for neurologic disorders. N Engl J Med 1994; 330: 613–22.

21. Lipton SA, Gendelman HE. Seminars in medicine of the Beth Israel Hospital, Boston: dementia associated with the acquired immunodeficiency syndrome. N Engl J Med 1995; 332: 934–40.

22. Greenlee JE, Brashear HR. Antibodies to cerebellar Purkinje cells in patients with paraneoplastic cerebellar degeneration and ovarian carcinoma. Ann Neurol 1983; 14: 609–13.

23. Brashear H, Caccamo D, Heck A, Keeney P. Localization of antibody in the central nervous system of a patient with paraneoplastic encephalomyelitis. Neurology 1991; 41: 1583–7.

24. Mizumoto N, Takashima A. CD1a and Langerin: acting more than Langerhans' cell markers. J Clin Invest 2004; 113: 658–60.

25. Valladeau J, Ravel O, Dezutter-Dambuyant C, et al. Langerin, a novel C-type lectin specific to Langerhans cells is an endocytic receptor that induces the formation of Birbeck granules. Immunity 2000; 12 :71–81.

26. Emile J, Wechsler J, Brousse N, et al. Langerhans' cell histiocytosis: definitive diagnosis in the use of monoclonal antibody 010 on routinely paraffin embedded samples. Am J Surg Pathol 1995; 19: 636–41.

27. Grois N, Prayer D, Prosch H, Lassman H, CNS LCH Cooperative Group. Neuropathology of CNS disease in Langerhans' cell histiocytosis. Brain 2005; 128(Pt 4): 829–38.

28. Wnorowski M, Prosch H, Prayer D, Janssen D, Gadner H, Grois N. Pattern and course of neurodegeneration in Langerhans cell histiocytosis. J Pediatr 2008; 153: 127–32.

29. Vaquero J, Leunda G, Cabezudo JM, e Juan M, Herrero J, Bravo G. Posterior fossa xanthogranuloma. Case report. J Neurosurg 1979; 51: 718–22.

30. Vrijmoet-Wiersma CM, Kooloos VM, Koopman HM, et al. Health-related quality of life, cognitive functioning and behavior problems in children with Langerhans cell histiocytosis. Pediatr Blood Cancer 2009; 52: 116–22.

31. Gavhed D, Akefeldt SO, Osterlundh G, et al. Biomarkers in the cerebrospinal fluid and neurodegeneration in Langerhans' cell histiocytosis. Pediatr Blood Cancer 2009; 53: 1264–70.

32. Prayer D, Grois N, Prosch H, et al. MR imaging presentation of intracranial disease associated with LCH. Am J Neuroradiol 2004; 25: 880–91.

33. Grois N, Fahrner B, Arceci RJ, et al. Central nervous system disease in Langerhans' cell histiocytosis. J Pediatr 2010; 156: 873–81.

34. Idbaih A, Donadieu J Barthez MA, et al. Retinoic acid therapy in "degenerative-like" neuroLangerhans cell histiocytosis: a prospective pilot study. Pediatr Blood Cancer 2004; 43: 55–8.

35. Imashuku S, Shoida Y, Kaboyashi R, et al. Neurodegenerative central nervous sytem disease as a late sequelae of Langerhans cell histiocytosis. Report from the Japan LCH Study Group. Haematologica 2008; 93: 615–18.

36. Allen CE, Flores R, Rauch R, et al. Neurodegenerative central nervous system Langerhans cell histiocytosis and coincident hydrocephalus treated with vincristine/arabinoside. Pediatr Blood Cancer 2009; 11: 416–23.

37. Hayward J, Packer R, Finlay J. Central nervous system and Langerhans' cell histiocytosis. Med Pediatr Oncol 1990; 18: 325–8.

38. Aricò M, Colella R, Conter V, et al. Cyclosporine therapy for refractory Langerhans cell histiocytosis. Med Pediatr Oncol 1995; 25: 12–16.

39. Stine KC, Saylors RL, Saccent S, McClain KL, Becton DL. Efficacy of continuous infusion 2CDA (cladrabine) in pediatric patients with Langerhans cell histiocytosis. Pediatr Blood Cancer 2004; 43: 81–4.

40. Saven A, Foon KS, Piro LD. 2 Chlorodeoxyadenosine induced complete remissions in Langerhans cell histiocytosis. Ann Intern Med 1994; 121: 430–2.

41. Dhall G, Finlay JL, Ettinger LJ, et al. Treatment of patients with Langerhans cell histiocytosis and central nervous system involvement with 2-chlorodeoxyadenosine. Pediatr Blood Cancer 2008; 50: 72–9.

42. Grois N, Favara BE, Mostbeck GH, Prayer D. Central nervous system disease in Langerhans cell histiocytosis. Br J Cancer 1994; 70: S24–8.

43. D'Ambrosio N, Soohoo S, Warshall C, Johnson A, Karimi S. Craniofacial and intracranial manifestations of Langerhans cell histiocytosis: report of findings in 100 patients. Am J Roentgenol 2008; 191: 589–97.

44. Dunger DB, Broadbent V, Yeoman E, *et al*. The frequency and natural history of diabetes insipidus in children with Langerhans cell histiocytosis. N Engl J Med 1989; 321: 1157–62.

45. Ottaviano F, Finlay JL. Diabetes insipidus and Langerhans' cell histiocytosis: a case report of reversibility with 2-chlorodeoxyadenosine. J Pediatr Hematol Oncol 2003; 25: 575–7.

46. Bjartmar C, Kidd G, Mork S, Rudick R, Trapp BD. Neurological disability correlates with spinal cord axonal loss and reduced N-acetyl aspartate in chronic multiple sclerosis patients. Ann Neurol 2000; 48: 893–901.

47. Bradley WG. Recent views on amyotrophic lateral sclerosis with emphasis on electrophysiological studies. Muscle Nerve 1987; 10: 490–502.

54 Chordomas

Herbert B. Newton

Division of Neuro-Oncology, Dardinger Neuro-Oncology Center, Ohio State University Medical Center and James Cancer Hospital, Columbus, OH, USA

Introduction

Chordomas are rare, histologically benign, but clinically aggressive tumors of the axial skeleton first described in 1856 by both Virchow and Luschka.[1,2] The tumor discovered by Virchow was found within the clivus during a routine autopsy, prompting the theory that the tumor had arisen from cartilage. In 1858, Muller was the first to suggest that chordomas may originate from embryonic rests of the primitive notochord, the "chorda dorsalis."[3] The first description of a symptomatic chordoma was made in 1864 by Klebs, in a patient with a tumor of the sphenooccipital region.[4] In 1894, Ribbert was the first to use the term "chordoma" and further characterized Muller's theory by producing experimental chordomas after releasing tissue of notochordal origin from the nucleus pulposus of rabbits.[5,6] The tumors produced in these experiments were histologically similar to *de novo* chordomas. The experiments of Ribbert were replicated by Congdon in 1952 using a similar rabbit model.[7]

The modern theory of the origin of chordomas proposes that the tumors derive from embryonic rests of the primitive notochord that persist within the axial skeleton.[8–11] The notochord forms from ectodermal cells during the third or fourth week of development and is believed to act as an embryonic organizer.[12] During the fourth to sixth week of development, mesenchymal cells from adjacent sclerotomes envelop the notochord as they merge to form the spinal vertebral bodies.[8,12] The notochord degenerates during this process and by the seventh week remains only between the vertebral bodies as the nucleus pulposus of the intervertebral disks. Pathological studies of tissue using both light and electron microscopic techniques have demonstrated similarities between chordoma and human intervertebral disk.[8,12] It is postulated that incomplete degeneration of residual notochord may occur within the vertebral body at the junction of the adjacent sclerotomal regions. These incompletely degenerated rests can potentially undergo malignant transformation and develop into a chordoma. Investigations of the persistence and regression of the human notochord in fetuses of 4–18 weeks' gestation suggest that there is great variation in this process and that the presence of aberrant notochordal tissue is not uncommon.[13] Furthermore, the topographical distribution of these heterotopic notochordal rests corresponds closely to the common sites of chordoma in the adult (i.e. sacrococcygeal, clivus).[12,14] Autopsy studies reveal rests of presumed notochordal tissue anterior to the clivus and around the sacrum in up to 2% of cases.[10,11]

Finally, a shared immunophenotype is noted between notochordal and chordoma cells, with both types of cells containing S-100 protein, cytokeratins, and human epithelial polymorphic mucin.[14]

Tumor epidemiology

Chordomas are rare neoplasms, representing only 0.1–0.2% of all intracranial tumors, 6.15% of all primitive skull base tumors, and 1–4% of primary malignant bone tumors.[8–11,15] They can arise anywhere within the midline axial skeleton where the notochord existed (i.e. clivus, sellar and parasellar region, nasopharynx, foramen magnum, vertebrae, and sacrococcygeal region), but have a predilection for the sacrum and clivus. In adults, approximately 50% of chordomas arise in the sacrum, 35–40% within the base of skull and clivus, and 10–15% throughout the true vertebrae.[8,15–17] When chordomas affect the vertebral column, more than half will occur in the lumbar region, 25–30% in the cervical vertebrae, and 10–15% in the thoracic spine.[16] In children, chordomas most often involve the skull base.[18,19] On rare occasions, chordomas can arise in extraosseous or off-the-midline sites such as the transverse process of a vertebra, skin, paranasal sinuses, sella turcica, hypothalamus, or foramen magnum.[8–11,15,20–23]

Chordomas can occur at any age but are most common between the fourth and sixth decades of life.[8–11,15] Although these tumors can arise in children, less than 5% of all cases develop before 20 years of age.[18,19] There is a male predominance in some series, especially for tumors of the sacrum, with

Textbook of Uncommon Cancer, Fourth Edition. Edited by Derek Raghavan, Charles D. Blanke, David H. Johnson, Paul L. Moots, Gregory H. Reaman, Peter G. Rose and Mikkael A. Sekeres.

a ratio ranging from 2:1 to 3:1.[8–11,15] In other series, especially chordomas of the skull base, the male to female frequency is equal.[8]

Pathology

Chordomas are generally slow-growing, unencapsulated neoplasms that are locally invasive within bone and soft tissues.[8–11,24–26] A pseudocapsule may be noted around tumors that grow into soft tissues or the dura mater. As the tumors enlarge, they often stretch cranial nerves and displace structures such as blood vessels and the brainstem. Grossly, the tumors are usually reddish or purple in color, with a nodular appearance to the surface. Internally, the mass is frequently gelatinous and soft; regions that contain cartilage or calcium are firmer. Foci of hemorrhage may be present and can be small or extensive. The size of the lesion can be quite variable, with sacral tumors often becoming very large. In one series of cranial base chordomas, average tumor volume was 58 cm.[3,8]

On microscopic examination, chordomas can be grouped into several different histological categories, including a typical pattern, a chondroid pattern, and tumors with features of malignant degeneration.[8–11,24–30] The typical or classic pattern of chordoma (65–80% of all cases) is distinguished by a lobular arrangement, with the neoplastic cells disposed in solid sheets or irregular intersecting cords (Fig. 54.1). The sheets and cords of cells are set in a stroma that contains an abundant mucinous matrix. The individual cells are large, often with vacuolated eosinophilic cytoplasm, and contain variable amounts of mucin. The cell type considered diagnostic for chordomas is called physaliphorous (i.e. bubble-bearing). These cells are distinctively large and vacuolated, with eccentric nuclei (see Fig. 54.1). Nuclei tend to be hyperchromatic, with prominent nucleoli, and rarely demonstrate atypia. Potentially aggressive features such as mitoses, necrosis, hypervascularity, and spindle cells (i.e. sarcomatous degeneration) are typically absent or rare.[24–31] DNA ploidy analysis of typical chordomas demonstrates aneuploidy in 15–40% of cases.[8–11,25] There is a trend for tumors with aneuploid DNA content to behave more aggressively and for patients with these tumors to have shorter survival.[25] Other authors have not found a correlation between DNA ploidy status and tumor behavior, in terms of overall survival and tendency for local recurrence or distant metastases.[32]

Many authors contend that the chondroid pattern (15–30% of all cases) is a separate histological variant of chordoma, although this is controversial.[8–11,24–31,33] The chondroid pattern has been associated with a more favorable prognosis, as originally described by Heffelfinger and colleagues.[31] However, other authors contend that chondroid chordomas are a subgroup of low-grade chondrosarcoma and are not related to chordomas.[34,35] By definition, chondroid chordomas contain regions of typical chordoma with physaliphorous cells, against a background of areas characterized by cartilaginous matrix that have stellate tumor cells occupying lacunar spaces (resembling chondrocytes; Fig. 54.2).[31,33] As in typical chordoma, anaplastic or aggressive features such as mitoses, necrosis, hypervascularity, and spindle cells are typically

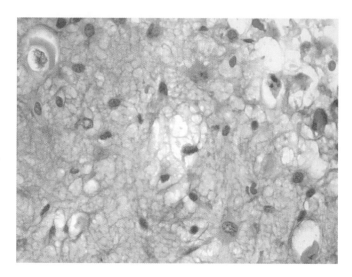

Figure 54.1 High-power view (600×) of classic or typical chordoma, demonstrating physaliphorous (bubble-bearing) cells. Note the large size, vacuolization, and eccentric nuclei. Several cells have hyperchromatic nuclei and prominent nucleoli. Mitoses, spindle cells, and regions of necrosis are absent.

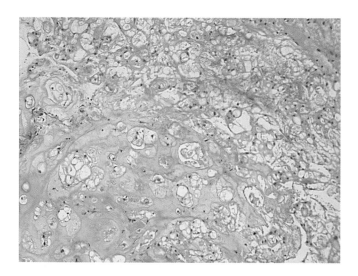

Figure 54.2 Low-power view (100×) of chondroid chordoma, demonstrating an area of classic chordoma with physaliphorous cells in the upper portion of the field, with a chondroid region that demonstrates cartilaginous metaplasia in the lower portions of the field. No anaplastic or malignant features are present.

absent or rare.[24–31,33] Electron microscopic studies support the dual nature (i.e. epithelial–mesenchymal) of these neoplasms by identifying cells with epithelial features and other cells consistent with chondrocytes.[36]

Chordomas with malignant degeneration (less than 5% of all nonirradiated cases) typically demonstrate sarcomatous features (i.e. spindle cells).[8–11,37–40] These tumors will contain areas of classic chordoma admixed with regions characterized by the presence of atypical spindle cells. The spindle cell component demonstrates high cellularity, marked nuclear pleomorphism, and a high mitotic rate. Within the malignant spindle cell zones, regions of cartilaginous or osseous differentiation may be noted. In many tumors, a transitional zone may be present between the regions of typical chordoma and regions containing the malignant spindle cells. This transitional zone may contain an intermediate, stellate type of cell. DNA ploidy analysis of chordomas with sarcomatous degeneration usually demonstrates aneuploid cell populations with a high proliferating fraction.[37,40] The mean proliferating fraction (%S + G2M) of a series of spindle cell chordomas was 34.1%.[37] In comparison to the mean proliferating fraction of a series of typical chordomas (20.2%), the growth fraction of spindle cell chordomas was significantly larger (p <0.01).

In addition to the diagnostic information obtained from the histological evaluation of chordomas, immunohistochemical analysis may also be helpful in clarifying the pathological differential diagnosis.[8,11,28,33,34,37,40–45] Other tumor types to be considered are ependymoma, schwannoma, neurofibroma, metastasis (e.g. clear cell type), chondrosarcoma, and fibrous histiocytoma. The immunohistochemical profile of typical chordomas illustrates the dual epithelial–mesenchymal nature of these tumors and consists of frequent positivity to cytokeratin and epithelial membrane antigen (EMA) and less consistent staining for S-100 protein and vimentin.[8,12,33,37,42] Variable staining has also been noted with α1-antichymotrypsin and tissue polypeptide antigen.[41,42] Chondroid chordomas with a small cartilaginous component may have variable staining of S-100, with preserved positivity to cytokeratin and EMA.[33] When the cartilaginous component is more robust (20–50%), the staining within the chondroid regions for cytokeratin and EMA may become variable, with persistent positivity for S-100.[33] Chondrosarcomas stain consistently negative for cytokeratin and EMA since there is no epithelial component to these tumors. Chordomas with sarcomatous degeneration have an alteration of the immunohistochemical profile in the malignant regions containing spindle cells.[37,38,40] The staining for vimentin becomes more prominent, while staining for cytokeratin and EMA is markedly decreased. In some tumors, staining for S-100 may also be reduced.[40]

Other immunohistochemical studies of chordomas have evaluated the expression of cell adhesion molecules (CAMs), including E-, P-, and N-cadherin, CD44, β-catenin, intercellular CAM, neural CAM, and vascular CAM.[46,47] Overall, chordomas were shown to frequently demonstrate expression of N-CAM, VCAM-1, CD44, N-cadherin, and E-cadherin. The expression of E-cadherin, in particular, was very prominent and ubiquitous, and was noted in all histological variants of chordoma.

Preliminary data from studies using cytogenetic and molecular techniques are beginning to elucidate the mechanisms of transformation of chordomas.[48–57] No specific or characteristic chromosomal abnormalities have been described thus far. Many of the cases have shown hypodiploidy or near-diploidy, which is in contrast to the DNA flow cytometry data. Several tumors have shown structural anomalies of chromosomes 1 and 21, while others have alterations (usually elongation) of the telomere.[52,53] A loss of heterozygosity (LOH) analysis by Riva *et al.* suggests that the 1p36.13 region is abnormal in up to 85% of chordomas.[55] Candidate tumor suppressor genes in this region with a potential role in oncogenesis include *CASP9*, *EPH2A*, and *DVL1*. LOH at 1p36.13 appeared to be an early

event in the transformation process, since it was present in tumors of all grades and locations.

Using immunohistochemical techniques, Matsuno *et al.* found that p53 protein was present in chordomas that had a high proliferative index (as determined by MIB-1 staining) and in recurrent tumors.[56] Furthermore, a significant correlation was noted between cyclin D1 staining and MIB-1 proliferative index or tumor recurrence. Interestingly, none of the tumors evaluated for bcl-2 were immunopositive, suggesting that apoptosis may not contribute to the recurrence of chordomas.

Eisenberg *et al.* studied seven skull base chordomas and found that, in two very aggressive cases, there was LOH for the *Rb* tumor suppressor gene on chromosome 13, suggesting that alterations or loss of *Rb* may play a role in the transformation of chordomas.[57] A study of skull base chordomas evaluated the expression of growth factors and structural proteins in good prognosis versus poor prognosis patient cohorts.[58] The mean expression of transforming growth factor-α and basic fibroblast growth factor was elevated in the patients with a poor prognosis and more rapid tumor progression. A similar, but not as pronounced, difference was noted for fibronectin.

Several authors have attempted to correlate pathological features of chordomas with prognosis.[24,28,29] In a series of 48 mixed chordomas, Rich *et al.* were unable to detect a correlation between cellular pleomorphism, mitotic figures, or hyperchromatic nuclei with survival.[24] The only histological variable to correlate with survival was the presence of chondroid elements. Chondroid chordomas had a more indolent course, longer duration of symptoms, and increased survival. Forsyth *et al.* evaluated 51 intracranial chordomas and were unable to detect a correlation between mitosis, chondroid elements, and survival.[28] In a series of 62 skull base chordomas, O'Connell *et al.* found that tumors with greater than 10% necrosis were associated with shorter patient survival.[29] The presence of chondroid elements, mitoses, pleomorphism, nucleolar prominence, and vascular invasion was not correlated with overall survival.

A molecular evaluation of a similar series of skull base tumors revealed that the expression of human telomerase reverse transcriptase (*hTERT*) messenger RNA was frequently associated with faster rates of tumor growth and an increased risk of recurrence.[59] The expression of *hTERT* was also associated with the presence of mutated p53 protein and an increased doubling time for residual tumor following surgical resection. Naka *et al.* performed a clinicopathological comparison of skull base and nonskull base chordomas in a series of 122 patients.[60] Skull base tumors were noted to have a higher MIB-1 labeling index than nonskull base tumors. The higher MIB-1 labeling index was often associated with older age, greater risk of recurrence, and nuclear pleomorphism. In contrast, for patients with nonskull base chordomas, only nuclear pleomorphism was noted to be a significant negative prognostic factor. A similar study by Horbinski *et al.* evaluated the prognostic value of Ki-67, p53, epidermal growth factor receptor (EGFR), and various chromosomal deletions in a series of 28 patients with skull base chordomas.[61] Tumors with a Ki-67 labeling index of 5% or higher (69.2 months versus 159.3 months; p =0.005) and deletion at 9p21 (71.7 months versus 146.2 months; $p = 0.03$) were noted to have a more aggressive course and shorter overall survival. Expression of EGFR, accumulation of p53, and loss of chromosomes 1p36, 10q23, and 17p13 did not correlate with survival.

Another molecular target under consideration is c-Met, a receptor tyrosine kinase that binds hepatocyte growth factor/scatter factor (HGF), is localized to chromosome 7, and is known to function as an oncogene in other solid tumors.[62–64] In a series of 22 chordoma samples, Walter and colleagues evaluated for changes in copy number of chromosome 7 and correlated it with EGFR and C-Met protein expression.[62] Aneusomy of chromosome 7 was noted in 73% of all samples, including 100% of the recurrent tumors. In addition, there was a significant correlation between chromosome 7 aneusomy and C-Met expression ($p = 0.001$). In a human sacral chordoma cell line, it has also been shown that C-Met and HGF are often coexpressed in the same cells, and that aberrations of chromosome 7 may be involved in altered tyrosine kinase signaling.[63] Using micro-RNA (miRNA) microarray techniques, Duan et al. evaluated the miRNA expression profiles of a series of chordoma cell lines and tissue samples.[64] They noted that the expression of miRNA-1 and miRNA-206 was markedly reduced in chordoma cell lines and samples. When miRNA-1 was transfected back into chordoma cell lines, the expression of C-Met was downregulated. These results suggest that the reduced level of miRNA-1 in chordoma tissue may be related to the frequent finding of overexpression of C-Met, and could be a contributing factor to the transformation process in these tumors.

Clinical features and presentation

Approximately 50% of chordomas arise in the sacrum, 35–40% within the skull base and clivus, and 10–15% throughout the vertebral column.[8–11,15–17] In general, chordomas are relatively slow growing and often have a prolonged duration of symptoms before diagnosis. The specific symptoms and neurological findings noted at presentation will vary according to the location of the tumor. Although these tumors are often benign histologically, systemic metastases have been noted in 10–40% of cases.[8–11,65,66] The most frequent sites for metastases are the lungs, regional lymph nodes, liver, bone, and skin.

Chordomas of the sacrum

Chordomas represent the most common primary neoplasm of the sacrum.[10,11,67–70] They often reach substantial size prior to diagnosis because of the ample room for tumor growth before critical structures are disturbed. The median age of patients in the majority of series is approximately 60 years; males are affected more often than females. The most common symptom (60–70% of patients) consists of persistent low back pain, which is slowly progressive and is often present for 12–18 months before diagnosis (Table 54.1).[10,11,67–70] Patients occasionally complain of more specific locations of the pain, such as the coccygeal, buttock, or anal regions. The pain may have a radicular component to it, with radiation down one of the legs. This presentation often leads to the erroneous

Table 54.1 Symptoms and signs in patients with chordoma of the sacral region.

Symptoms and signs	Percentage of patients
General low back pain	60–70
Rectal dysfunction	40–45
Constipation	30–35
Sciatica	25–30
Coccygeal pain	20
Sacral pain	15
Urinary incontinence	10–15
Buttock pain	5–7
Anal pain	5–7
Perianal numbness	5
Impotence	5
Fecal incontinence	5

Data compiled from Sundaresan,[10] Healey and Lane,[11] Bethke et al.,[67] Lybeert and Meerwaldt,[68] Schoenthaler et al.[69]

diagnosis of nonspecific "sciatica," delaying discovery of the tumor by many months. Rectal dysfunction consisting of alteration of bowel habits (i.e. constipation), tenesmus, or bleeding is common (approximately 40% of patients).

As the tumor continues to enlarge, it usually grows ventrally and may encroach on the sacral foramina and nerve roots, causing neurological dysfunction. Symptoms from sacral nerve root compression are variable and include perianal numbness, urinary hesitancy or retention, urinary incontinence, impotence, and rectal incontinence. The general physical examination is typically benign, except for the rectal examination, which often demonstrates a presacral mass.[10,67] The neurological examination may be normal or show evidence of sacral root dysfunction (e.g. perianal numbness, loss of anal sphincter tone).

Chordomas of the skull base, clivus, and intracranial cavity

Chordomas comprise 6.15% of all skull base tumors and 0.1–0.2% of all intracranial tumors.[8–11,15] They occur most often in the clivus but can arise in other areas such as the sphenoid sinus, cavernous sinus, occipital condyle, and sella.[8–11,18,22,28,29,71–74] Depending on the primary site of tumor involvement and direction of growth (e.g. anterior, lateral, posterior), symptoms and signs may vary considerably. The mean age of patients with skull base chordomas is in the range of 38–45 years.[68,69,71] In the majority of series, the most common symptoms are either diplopia or headache (Table 54.2).[8,9,24,28,71–74] Diplopia is the initial symptom in 50–90% of patients. The diplopia is usually horizontal and exacerbated by attempts at lateral gaze. Headache is noted at presentation in 25–60% of patients. In many patients, headache and diplopia develop simultaneously. Symptoms such as facial pain, vertigo, tinnitus, dysphagia, hoarseness, alterations of vision, and gait disturbance are present in 12–15% of patients.[71–74] Infrequent complaints include hearing loss, dizziness, unilateral weakness, facial dysesthesias, and neck pain.

On neurological examination, the most common findings are cranial nerve palsies (see Table 54.2).[8,9,24,28,71–74] The VIth

Table 54.2 Symptoms and signs in patients with chordoma of the skull base, clivus, and intracranial cavity.

Symptoms and signs	Percentage of patients
Diplopia	50–90
Cranial nerve VI palsy	45–75
Headache	25–60
Cranial nerve IX, X, XI, XII palsy	25–40
Cranial nerve II, III, IV, V$_1$, VII palsy	15–25
Diplopia and headache	15–20
Pyramidal tract dysfunction	15–20
Facial pain	12–15
Vertigo/tinnitus	12–15
Dysphagia/hoarseness	12–15
Alterations of vision	12–15
Gait disturbance	12–15

Data compiled from Gay et al.,[8] Miller,[9] Rich et al.,[24] Forsyth et al.,[28] Yoneoka et al.,[71] Al-Mefty and Borba,[72] Volpe et al.[73]

cranial nerve is involved most frequently, with abnormal function noted in 45–75% of patients. The deficit is usually unilateral but can be bilateral in some cases. Abducens palsy can be associated with dysfunction of cranial nerves II, III, IV, V[1], and VII in 15–25% of patients.[28,73,74] Although uncommon, isolated palsy of cranial nerves II, III, or IV is seen in some patients. Abnormalities of the lower cranial nerves (i.e. IX, X, XI, XII) are noted in 25–40% of patients.[28,71–74] Similar to abducens palsy, the deficits are usually unilateral but can be bilateral in some cases. Cranial nerves of the cerebellopontine angle (i.e. VII, VIII) are rarely affected on examination at presentation, but can develop in patients with large tumors. Pyramidal tract dysfunction is present in 15–20% of patients and develops from tumors that compress the ventral surface of the brainstem.[8,9,28] The findings may be unilateral or bilateral and in some cases are associated with ataxia. Furthermore, patients with brainstem compression by tumor may manifest inappropriate laughing or crying. The emotional lability is thought to occur from disturbance of ventral pontine tegmental pathways.[9]

Chordomas of the true vertebrae

Chordomas are uncommon tumors of the vertebral column (usually the vertebral body), representing less than 5% of all tumors in this region.[16,17] Approximately 60% of vertebral chordomas arise in the lumbar region, 10–15% develop in the thoracic area, and 25–30% in the cervical spine. Ventral tumor growth will cause bone destruction and infiltration into paraspinal soft tissues, while dorsal expansion may cause nerve root displacement or spinal cord compression. The mean age of patients with spinal chordomas ranges from 45 to 50 years. Patients with these tumors often have a shorter duration of symptoms before diagnosis than patients with tumors of the sacrum, due to the smaller volume of bone in proximity to sensitive neural structures.[70] In one series, the mean duration of symptoms prior to diagnosis was 7 months.[16] In the majority of cases (>90%), the initial symptom is localized pain in and around the involved vertebral body. There

may be a radicular component to the pain from displacement or compression of nerve roots, with lancinating pain in a limb or anteriorly around the thorax. Other alterations of sensation, such as dysesthesias or sensory deficits, may occur. Cervical chordomas that grow ventrally and compress the esophagus may cause dysphagia.[17] Occasionally, tumors can cause myelopathic weakness, gait ataxia, or sphincter dysfunction.

Several authors have attempted to correlate various clinical parameters with overall survival and prognosis.[28,29] Patients less than 40 years appear to have improved survival and a better prognosis. Forsyth et al. noted a significant difference in survival (5-year survival of 75% versus 30%) for patients less than 40 years ($p < 0.0001$).[28] The presence of diplopia was also suggestive of a better prognosis and improved survival, especially when correlated with patient age.[28] Female sex was associated with improved survival (median 158 months versus 86 months; $p < 0.004$) and a better prognosis in both univariate and multivariate analyses by O'Connell et al.[29] For patients with sacral and spinal chordomas, negative prognostic factors included larger tumor size, inadequate surgical margins, the presence of necrosis, a labeling index of greater than 5%, and local recurrence.[70]

Radiological diagnosis

Patients with a history and neurological examination suspicious for a chordoma of the skull base, vertebral column, or sacrum require a radiological evaluation with either computed tomography (CT) or magnetic resonance imaging (MRI).[8,75–84] CT and MRI are equivalent in their ability to delineate the presence of a tumor. Both modalities clearly demonstrate the mass within bone, bone erosion or destruction, and extension into soft tissues.[75–78,82–84] Rarely, MRI may have trouble detecting small tumors confined within the margins of the clivus.[76] On noncontrast CT, the tumor usually appears as a soft tissue mass, isodense or hyperdense with neural tissues, causing destruction of the adjacent bone (Fig. 54.3). Bone-windowed CT scans demonstrate the precise amount of bone destruction caused by the tumor, with sharp margins (see Fig. 54.3). Calcification is noted in 40–70% of chordomas (especially clival) with CT imaging. Small regions of sequestered bone can also be noted in approximately 15–20% of cases. MRI is inferior to CT in its ability to delineate the exact margins of bone destruction or the presence of calcification.[75,76] With the administration of contrast, chordomas always demonstrate contrast enhancement. The amount of enhancement may vary but is often quite dense and homogeneous. Sagittal and coronal reconstruction of CT images is sometimes helpful to better delineate the extent of skull base and sacral tumors. However, the ability of CT to evaluate tumors in the sagittal and coronal planes is inferior to MRI.

In general, MRI with sagittal, coronal, and axial sections clearly defines the margins of chordomas of the skull base, vertebral column, and sacrum.[8,75–84] On T1-weighted images, 75% of tumors appear isointense, while 25% appear hypointense, compared to surrounding neural tissues (Fig. 54.4).[8,76,84] With administration of gadolinium, chordomas usually enhance. As with CT, the degree of enhancement is variable; in most

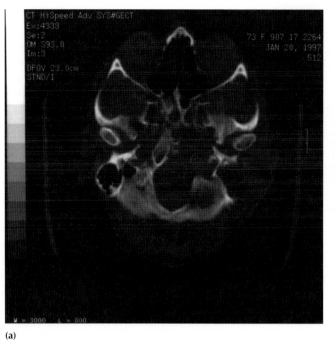
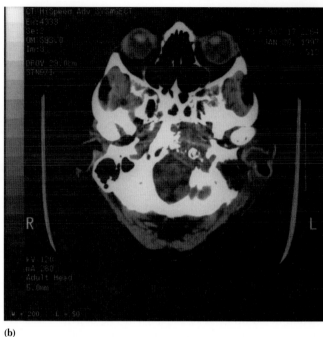

(a)   (b)

Figure 54.3 (a) Bone-windowed CT of the skull base demonstrating a large, eccentric chordoma of the clivus on the left side, which is causing severe erosion and destruction of surrounding bone. (b) Noncontrast CT of the skull base at the same level as Fig. 54.3(a), demonstrating the clival chordoma as a mass with soft tissue density within the region of eroded bone.

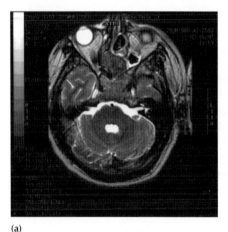
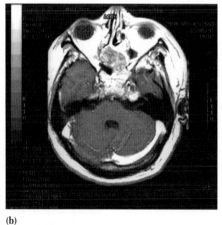
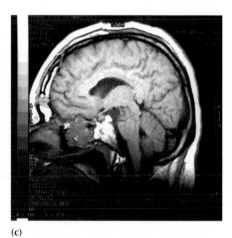

(a)   (b)   (c)

Figure 54.4 (a) Noncontrast MRI (TR 7500, TE 102) of the brain, at the level of the upper clivus and orbits, demonstrating an isointense chordoma within the clivus that extends into the sphenoid sinus region and tracks along both optic nerves. (b) Gadolinium-enhanced MRI (TR 600, TE 23) of the brain, at the same level as Fig. 54.4(a), demonstrating heterogeneous enhancement of the chordoma within the clivus and sphenoid sinus. (c) Midsagittal, noncontrast MRI (TR 500, TE 16) of the brain, demonstrating the chordoma anterior to the brainstem within the clivus and extending into the sphenoid sinus region. The signal intensity of the mass is heterogeneous: hyperintense within the bone of the clivus and more isointense in the sinus.

tumors, the pattern is heterogeneous. On T2-weighted images, chordomas are always hyperintense to all surrounding structures. The pattern of hyperintensity is homogeneous in 20% of cases and heterogeneous in the remaining 80% (mild in 30%, marked in 50%).[76–78] Tumor calcification, exact margins of eroded bone, and the presence of sequestered bone are noted in some tumors, but these are not demonstrated as well as with CT. However, the multiplanar capability of MRI allows for better visualization of the extent of tumor margins and infiltration into soft tissues than is possible on CT.

Sagittal MRI clearly shows the anterior–posterior margins of tumor involvement. For chordomas of the skull base, MRI is helpful for determining the anterior extension of tumor into the sinuses or nasopharynx and posterior extension toward the brainstem.[77,78] The posterior fossa is affected by tumor (e.g. brainstem compression, cranial nerve displacement) in approximately 80% of skull base tumors.[78] Sagittal MRI is essential for tumors of the sacrum to determine the extent of the lesion anteriorly into the rectum and other soft tissues.[82] Coronal MRI images are useful for assessing lateral extension of skull base tumors toward the cavernous sinuses. The cavernous sinuses are infiltrated by tumor in approximately 65% of skull base chordomas.[78] Furthermore, with sacral chordomas, coronal MRI can determine involvement of sacral nerve roots within the neural foramina.

Magnetic resonance imaging is far superior to CT in demonstrating the relationship of tumor to cranial nerves and vascular structures.[75–78,84] The carotid and basilar arteries are delineated clearly on T2-weighted images because of the contrast between the flow void inside the vessels and surrounding high signal tumor. Meyer *et al.* noted displacement of the carotid or basilar arteries in 57% of skull base chordomas.[78] Furthermore, in 36% of their cohort, vascular encasement was present. Encasement of vessels by chordomas has also been reported by other authors.[75–78,84] Universally, the lumen of encased vessels is not compromised by tumor and they continue to have normal blood flow.

Most authors do not report any MRI signal characteristics that can be used to differentiate between typical chordomas and those with chondroid regions.[78] However, Sze *et al.* noted that chondroid chordomas were less intense on T2-weighted images than were conventional chordomas.[76] Assessment of mean quantitative T1 and T2 relaxation values (msec) has shown that chondroid tumors often have shorter times than conventional chordomas. The use of MR angiography can further delineate the presence of arterial vascular encasement and luminal narrowing.[84] In addition, MR venography can also clearly demonstrate any venous involvement by tumor (e.g. narrowing, occlusion).

Treatment

The treatment of many chordomas is limited by the invasive and infiltrative nature of these tumors. The tumor is often too extensive at diagnosis for a complete, curative resection.[8,69,72] Even when the lesion is small and radical surgery is attempted, local recurrence rates remain high (i.e. 50–100%). Therefore, the therapeutic approach for chordomas is primarily to maintain local control and minimize regional damage to neural structures.[8,69,72] Despite the emphasis on local disease, systemic metastases can occur and are noted in 10–30% of patients.[8,66,67] The most common sites for metastases are the lungs, regional lymph nodes, liver, bone, and skin. Infrequent sites include cardiac muscle, brain, adrenal glands, pancreas, pituitary gland, and eyelid.[66,67] In the majority of patients, recurrence at the local site is most likely to affect morbidity and survival.

Surgical resection

Most authors agree that surgical resection is an important aspect of the initial treatment of patients with chordoma.[8,10,11,28,67,72,74,84–88] The most aggressive resection possible should be attempted after initial diagnosis, depending on the location (e.g. clivus, vertebral body, sacrum) and the extent of the tumor. It appears that the aggressiveness of resection has a critical impact on local control rates and may correlate with overall survival.[8,28,72,74] In a review of 51 patients with intracranial chordomas, Forsyth *et al.* found that the extent of resection

affected survival.[28] In a univariate analysis, the extent of resection was significantly ($p=0.02$) associated with survival. For patients receiving only biopsy, the 5- and 10-year survival rates were 36% and 0%, respectively. In the cohort of patients undergoing subtotal resections, the 5- and 10-year survival rates were 55% and 45%, respectively. This effect of resection on survival was most apparent in younger patients.

Chordomas of the skull base and clivus can be grouped according to their size and extension into contiguous areas.[72] Type I tumors are small and restricted to one compartment of the skull base (e.g. clivus or sphenoid sinus). Type II tumors are larger and extend to two or more contiguous areas of the skull base. Type III lesions are very extensive and involve several contiguous compartments of the skull base (e.g. clivus, sphenoid sinus, and middle fossa). In most series type I chordomas are rare and usually amenable to radical resection using a single skull base approach.[8,72] Type II tumors are most common (50–65%) and in many cases can also be radically resected using a single skull base procedure.[72] The type III chordomas develop in 10–20% of patients and require two or more surgical procedures to attempt radical removal.

There are numerous surgical approaches and techniques available for resection of skull base and clivus chordomas.[8,72,74,85,86,89–98] The approach will depend on the location of the tumor and the degree of extension from the primary site. Most often, tumors are centered within the lower, middle, or upper clivus and extend into the cavernous sinus or petrous apex.[72,85,86] The four most common approaches allow for an extensive resection of tumor either extradurally or intradurally. The subtemporal, transcavernous, transpetrous apex approach is used most often (30–35%) and provides access to the clivus, cavernous sinus, sella turcica, and petrous apex.[8,72,94] The extended frontal approach is used in 25–30% of patients and is advantageous for tumors with extension into the orbits, ethmoid sinus, and anterior skull base.[8,85] The subtemporal–infratemporal approach is utilized in approximately 20% of patients and offers excellent exposure of the middle fossa, clivus, and lateral skull base.[8,85] For chordomas of the lower clivus, temporal bone, and occiput, the extreme lateral transcondyle and transjugular approach is used (approximately 15% of patients).[8,85]

Uncommon surgical approaches include the transoral, transmaxillary, transcervical–transclival, anterior cervical, and transsphenoidal procedures.[8,74,86,89–95,97] Recent reports suggest that the transsphenoidal approach can even be used in combination with endoscopy for removal of clival chordomas in selected cases.[98] In general, most authors would agree that the choice of surgical approach is less important than the expertise of the surgical team and its ability to perform an extensive resection of the tumor.[74]

Studies using the most advanced skull base approaches for removal of chordomas report various results. Radical or total resection of tumor is achieved in 43.5–55% of patients, near-total or subtotal resection is noted in 40–47%, and partial resection is attained in 8–10%.[8,72,74,85,86] In a series of patients with chordomas and chondrosarcomas involving the skull base and cavernous sinus, after a median follow-up of 24 months, Lanzino *et al.* noted three recurrences in 14 patients with subtotal or partial removal of tumor.[85] No recurrences were observed in the group of patients that had undergone radical resections. In a study of skull base chordomas by Gay et al., there was a statistically significant difference ($p < 0.05$) between the risk of recurrence in patients with radical or near-total resections and patients with subtotal or partial resections.[86] The overall recurrence-free survival estimates were 80% at 3 years and 76% at 5 years. In contrast, the survival estimates for patients who had recurrence of disease were 52% at 2 years and 26% at 3 years. Previous surgery or radiation therapy was associated with an increased risk of recurrence and surgical complications. Similar survival rates are described by Crockard et al. in a series of 42 patients with skull base chordomas, with 5- and 10-year rates of 77% and 69%, respectively.[74] Overall, an aggressive surgical resection at the time of tumor diagnosis, regardless of the approach and technique used, has the most impact on subsequent local tumor control and survival.

Sacral chordomas are often very large at diagnosis but most authors advise radical resection whenever possible.[10,11,67,88,99] Similar to the experience with skull base tumors, recurrence-free survival is improved after radical or near-total resection. For tumors of the lower sacrum and coccygeal region, many authors recommend a posterior approach.[11,88] Other investigators argue that a combined anterior–posterior approach is preferable.[67] Tumors of the upper sacrum are resected most efficiently with a staged, combined anterior–posterior approach.[10,11,67,88,99] Regardless of the approach used to resect the tumor, it is important to attempt preservation of the upper sacral nerve roots and the pudendal nerve. If the bilateral S2 nerve roots are sectioned during surgery, urogenital and rectal function will be lost or impaired. If both S2 nerve roots are preserved, 50% of patients will retain at least partial bladder and bowel control.[87,95] To maintain normal bowel continence, preservation of at least one set of ipsilateral S1, S2, and S3 nerve roots is recommended. The local recurrence rates are approximately 25–30% for tumors removed en bloc by radical resection.[10,11,67] If the tumor is removed by subtotal or partial resection, local recurrence rates increase to approximately 60–65%.

It is also recommended that chordomas of the true vertebrae be radically resected whenever feasible.[11,17,87] For tumors of the cervical vertebrae, most authors recommend an anterior approach to perform a corporectomy, followed by bone grafting, if necessary.[16] Thoracic tumors are best approached by thoracotomy or a staged procedure that combines a laminectomy and thoracotomy.[11] Lumbar chordomas will usually require an anterior approach; on occasion, a posterolateral approach may be necessary.[11]

Radiation therapy

Although radical resection is considered in each patient with a chordoma of the skull base, vertebrae, or sacrum, it is often impossible due to the invasive nature of these tumors. Therefore, radiation therapy to eradicate residual or recurrent disease is an important therapeutic consideration in many patients.[8,10,11,28,69] Unfortunately, chordomas have proved to be

relatively radioresistant tumors. The clinical results in most radiation therapy trials of chordomas have demonstrated only modest improvements in local control, recurrence-free survival, and overall survival.[8,10,11,28,69,100–106] Early reports in the radiation oncology literature using photon-based megavoltage therapy suggested a dose–response relationship for chordoma.[105,106] It was recommended that patients received at least 6000–7000 cGy to the tumor bed for optimal response. However, more recent studies have been unable to document a consistent dose–response relationship for chordoma using conventional photon techniques.[8,106–108] In the reports by Cummings et al. and Saxton, doses of 2500–7000 cGy were used for patients with chordomas of various sites after surgical resection.[107,108] Palliation of symptoms and improvement of relapse-free survival were as likely to occur with doses of 4000–5500 cGy as with higher doses.

In an extensive review of reported dose–response data for photon techniques in treatment of cranial chordoma, Tai et al. concluded that no dose–response relationship was evident.[106] Administration of doses in the range of 4500–5500 cGy were as effective as higher doses. In addition, the authors state that surgical resection in combination with irradiation significantly prolongs survival when compared to either modality used alone. In a study of 21 patients with chordomas of various sites, Keisch et al. concluded that irradiation prolonged the time to first relapse for tumors of the lower spine and sacrum, but not for tumors of the skull base.[103] The overall 5- and 10-year actuarial survival rates were 74% and 46%, respectively. Forsyth et al. evaluated the results of 51 patients with intracranial chordomas and determined that conventional irradiation did not affect the overall survival of the cohort, but did prolong disease-free survival, especially in younger patients.[28] The 5- and 10-year disease-free survival rates in irradiated patients were 39% and 31%, respectively. A similar improvement of progression-free survival, without a change in overall survival, has been reported by Thieblemont et al. in 26 patients with chordomas of various sites.[105]

Newer radiation therapy techniques currently being applied to patients with chordomas include intensity-modulated radiation therapy (IMRT) and conformal techniques. Several case studies have reported using IMRT for chordomas of the sacrum and spine.[109,110] IMRT was well tolerated and appeared to offer a more homogeneous radiation distribution pattern within the planning target volume. Conformal radiotherapy approaches have also been reported and have similar radiation distribution patterns to IMRT.[111]

Irradiation of chordomas with charged particles (i.e. protons, carbon, helium, neon) has shown promise as a more efficacious therapeutic option.[8,69,100–102,106,112–116] There are several radiobiological advantages of charged particles over photons. The high linear energy transfer (LET) of charged particles allows for a more defined and superior dose distribution (i.e. steeper fall-off in dose). Higher doses can be prescribed to the tumor volume with minimal risk of augmented toxicity to surrounding normal structures. Austin-Seymour et al. have used fractionated proton irradiation for skull base chordomas and chondrosarcomas, administering a mean total dose of 69 GyE (gray equivalent).[101,102,106] The 5- and 10-year local control rates were 82% and 58% respectively, while the 5- and 10-year disease-free survival rates were 76% and 53%, respectively. The median time to local failure was 53 months. In their opinion, these results represent a significant improvement over the results of conventional radiation techniques. A similar study in a series of 34 patients with skull base chordomas used a combination of high-energy photons and protons, in a two-thirds to one-third ratio of the total dose, respectively.[117] The 3-year local control rate was 83.1%, with a 3-year overall survival rate of 91%.

The superiority of proton therapy in comparison to photon irradiation techniques has been corroborated by a recent metaanalysis of more than 200 studies and a total of 416 patients with skull base chordoma.[113] In a study using helium and neon particles, Berson et al. treated 25 patients with chordomas of the skull base and cervical spine and reported a 5-year local control rate of 55%.[100,106] Recent experience with carbon ion radiotherapy after surgical resection from Takahashi et al. suggests improved efficacy over photon irradiation or untreated follow-up, with a 3-year recurrence-free survival rate of 70% versus 57.1% and 7.1% ($p = 0.001$), respectively.[114] In a review of 14 patients with sacral chordomas treated with charged helium and neon particles, Schoenthaler et al. reported a 5-year local control rate of 55%.[69] The 5- and 10-year survival rates were 85% and 22%, respectively, with an overall median survival of 77 months.

Several authors have reported their experience with carbon ion radiotherapy in chordomas.[116,118,119] Schulz-Ertner et al. evaluated a series of 24 patients with skull base chordoma, using a median tumor dose of 60 GyE.[118] With a mean follow-up of 13 months, the 2-year local control and progression-free survival rates were 83% and 83%, respectively. A similar study in 30 patients with unresectable sacral chordomas used carbon ion radiotherapy at a median dose of 70.4 GyE.[119] At a median follow-up of 30 months, the 5-year local control and overall survival rates were 96% and 52%, respectively. A recent summary of phase 1/2 and phase 2 trials of carbon ion radiotherapy in 38 patients with inoperable sacral chordoma demonstrated a 5-year overall survival rate of 86% and a 5-year local control rate of 89%.[116]

Other methods of irradiation of chordoma include brachytherapy with radioactive seeds (e.g. iodine-125) and radiosurgery.[8,101,120–124] It is difficult to evaluate the efficacy of these modalities because of the small number of patients that have been treated and the limited follow-up intervals reported.[8,101,120–124] There may be a role for brachytherapy and radiosurgery in the palliation of residual and recurrent disease in carefully selected patients. One recent approach that has been applied to a small group of patients with skull base chordomas involves the combination of maximal tumor resection and gamma-knife radiosurgery, with a mean treatment dose of 17 Gy.[122] Although follow-up was limited, the local tumor control rate of 93.3% and mean tumor-free survival of 17 months were encouraging. In a similar and more recent study of 19 patients with clival chordomas, Ito and co-workers noted 2- and 5-year progression-free survival rates of 77.9% and 47.9%, respectively.[123] Another group has reported the use of the CyberKnife for adjuvant therapy in a series of 18 patients

with chordomas of the cranium, mobile spine, and sacrum.[124] Treatment was administered over five sessions, with a median dose of 35 Gy (range 24.0–40.0 Gy). The overall survival rate at 65 months was 74.3%, with a local control rate of 88.9%.

Chemotherapy

The role of chemotherapy in the treatment of chordomas remains limited.[8,11,87,105,125,126] The main indication for chemotherapy has been in patients with recurrent or widespread disease not amenable to further surgery or radiation therapy. In most cases, the regimens have been designed to resemble protocols used for soft tissue sarcomas. Unfortunately, very few patients have responded to this approach. Chemotherapeutic agents that have been used (as single agents or in combination) without success include methotrexate, vincristine, cisplatin, doxorubicin, etoposide, actinomycin-D, and cyclophosphamide.[11,87,105,125]

Fleming et al. report two patients with malignant sacral chordomas and lung metastases in whom chemotherapy produced objective responses.[125] One patient responded to a multiagent regimen consisting of etoposide, cisplatin, vincristine, dacarbazine, cyclophosphamide, and doxorubicin administered intravenously over 3 days every 4–5 weeks. The second patient responded to this multiagent regimen for five cycles and then progressed. A second regimen of single-agent continuous infusion ifosfamide was initiated, which produced dramatic shrinkage of the lung lesion.

In recent years, many investigators have been attempting to treat chordomas with molecular treatment approaches, as the molecular biology of these tumors has been elucidated.[126,127] One report evaluated the efficacy of imatinib mesylate, a tyrosine kinase inhibitor with activity against c-KIT, BCR-ABL, and platelet-derived growth factor receptors (PDGFR) that has been previously utilized for gastrointestinal stromal tumors (GIST) and high-grade gliomas.[128] Six patients with advanced chordoma (five sacral, one skull base) were treated with imatinib mesylate (800 mg/day). Pathologically, all the tumors were noted to be positive for expression of PDGFR. Several of the patients had evidence of liquefaction on CT and MRI scans, as well as reduced glucose uptake on positron emission tomography scans. Four of five symptomatic patients also reported subjective improvement, usually early in the course of treatment. A phase 2 trial with a larger cohort of patients has been initiated and remains open to further accrual.

A case report by Singhal et al. demonstrated tumor shrinkage in a patient with a progressive sacral chordoma after treatment with erlotinib, a tyrosine kinase inhibitor with specificity for EGFR.[129] The tumor was positive for EGFR and responded to erlotinib (150 mg/day) after 3 months of treatment, with a partial reponse and improvement of symptoms. Stacchiotti et al. treated a series of 10 patients with advanced and progressive chordoma using a combination molecular therapeutic approach of imatinib and sirolimus.[130] Sirolimus (rapamycin) is an inhibitor of the mammalian target of rapamycin (mTOR), which is often upregulated in solid tumors.[131] Treatment consisted of imatinib (400 mg/day) and sirolimus (2 mg/day), with a mean treatment duration of 9 months.

On follow-up imaging, there was one partial response and seven tumors with stable disease. Molecular therapy directed at inhibiting the PI3Kinase/mTOR signaling pathway has also been supported by *in vitro* studies from Schwab *et al.*[132] Activation of the PI3K/mTOR pathway was first verified in 13 chordoma tumor resection specimens. Then they used a dual kinase inhibitor, PI-103, to treat a chordoma cell line (UCH-1), and noted reduced activation of the Akt and mTOR pathways. In addition, cell proliferation of the cultures was inhibited and apoptosis was induced in over 50% of cells.

Conclusion

Chordomas are rare, locally invasive tumors that arise from embryonic rests of the primitive notochord, with the potential to develop anywhere along the midline of the axial skeleton. Patients with chordomas of the skull base, true vertebrae, or sacrum in whom a gross total resection has been performed can be followed closely with serial contrast-enhanced MR imaging, without further treatment. For the more typical patient, with significant residual disease after surgery, some form of irradiation should be considered. The most effective radiotherapy techniques use charged particles (e.g. protons, carbon), which allow for higher doses to the tumor bed in a more well-defined dose distribution. However, access to facilities which can offer charged particle radiotherapy remains somewhat limited. If charged particle radiation therapy is not available, aggressive photon-based irradiation is still strongly recommended. Chemotherapy has a limited role in the treatment of chordoma, but should be considered for patients with recurrent or progressive disease that is refractory to further surgical intervention or irradiation.

Acknowledgments

Dr Newton was supported in part by grant P30CA16058, National Cancer Institute, Bethesda, MD, and the Esther Dardinger Neuro-Oncology Center Endowment Fund. The author would like to thank Ray Chaudhury MD for assistance with the neuropathological materials, and Jamie Zeal and Sheheryar Jamali for research assistance.

References

1. Virchow R. *Untersuchungen Uber die Entwickelung des Schadelgrundes.* Berlin: George Reimer, 1857.
2. Luschka H. Die altersveranderungen der zwischen-wirbelknorpel. Virchows Arch Pathol Anat Physiol Klin Med 1864; 31: 396–9.
3. Muller H. Ueber das vorkommen von resten der chorda dorsalis bei menschen nach der geburt und uber ihr verhaltnis zu den gallertgeschwulsten am clivus. Ztschr Rat Med 1858; 2: 202.
4. Klebs E. Ein fall von ecchondrosis spheno-occipitalis amylacea. Virchows Arch Pathol Anat 1864; 31: 396.
5. Ribbert H. Ueber die echondrosis physalifora spheno-occipitalis. Centralbl Allg Pathol Pathol Anat 1894; 5: 457.
6. Ribbert H. Ueber die experimentelle erzeugung einer ecchondrosis physalifora. Verh Dtsch Kong Inn Med 1895; 13: 455.
7. Congdon CC. Proliferative lesions resembling chordoma following puncture of nucleus pulposus in rabbits. J Natl Cancer Inst 1952; 12: 893.
8. Gay E, Sekhar LN, Wright DC. Chordomas and chondrosarcomas of the cranial base. In: Kaye H, Laws ER (eds) *Brain Tumors. An Encyclopedic Approach.* New York: Churchill Livingstone, 1995. pp. 777–94.
9. Miller NR. Secondary tumors of the central nervous system. In: Miller NR (eds) *Walsh and Hoyt's Clinical Neuro-Ophthalmology*, 4th edn. Baltimore, MD: Williams and Wilkins, 1988. pp. 1662–709.
10. Sundaresan N. Chordomas. Clin Orthop Relat Res 1986; 204: 135–42.
11. Healey JH, Lane JM. Chordoma: a critical review of diagnosis and treatment. Orthop Clin North Am 1989; 20: 417–26.
12. Salisbury JR. The pathology of the human notochord. J Pathol 1993; 171: 253–5.
13. Horwitz T. Chordal ectopia and its possible relation to chordoma. Arch Pathol 1941; 31: 354–62.
14. Salisbury JR, *et al.* Three-dimensional reconstruction of human embryonic notochords: clue to the pathogenesis of chordoma. J Pathol 1993; 171: 59–62.
15. McMaster ML, *et al.* Chordoma: incidence and survival patterns in the United States, 1973–1995. Cancer Causes Control 2001; 12: 1–11.
16. Klekamp J, Samii M. Spinal chordomas – results of treatment over a 17-year period. Acta Neurochir 1996; 138: 514–19.
17. D'Haen B, *et al.* Chordoma of the lower cervical spine. Clin Neurol Neurosurg 1995; 97: 245–8.
18. Yadav YR, *et al.* Cranial chordoma in the first decade. Clin Neurol Neurosurg 1992; 94: 241–6.
19. Coffin CM, *et al.* Chordoma in childhood and adolescence. A clinicopathologic analysis of 12 cases. Arch Pathol Lab Med 1993; 117: 927–33.
20. Katayama Y, *et al.* Intradural extraosseous chordoma of the foramen magnum region. Case report. J Neurosurg 1991; 75: 976–9.
21. Commins D, *et al.* Hypothalamic chordoma. Case report. J Neurosurg 1994; 81: 130–2.
22. Elias Z, Powers LK. Intrasellar chordoma and hyperprolactinemia. Surg Neurol 1985; 23: 173–6.
23. Kakuno Y, *et al.* Chordoma in the sella turcica. Neurol Med Chir 2002; 42: 305–8.
24. Rich TA, *et al.* Clinical and pathologic review of 48 cases of chordoma. Cancer 1985; 56: 182–7.
25. Schoedel KE, *et al.* Chordomas: pathological features; ploidy and silver nucleolar organizing region analysis. A study of 36 cases. Acta Neuropathol 1995; 89: 139–43.
26. Crapanzano JP, *et al.* Chordoma. A cytologic study with histologic and radiologic correlation. Cancer 2001; 93: 40–51.
27. Chetty R, Levin CV, Kalan MR. Chordoma: a 20-year clinicopathologic review of the experience at Groote Schuur Hospital, Cape Town. J Surg Oncol 1991; 46: 261–4.
28. Forsyth PA, *et al.* Intracranial chordomas: a clinicopathological and prognostic study of 51 cases. J Neurosurg 1993; 78: 741–7.
29. O'Connell JX, *et al.* Base of skull chordoma. A correlative study of histologic and clinical features of 62 cases. Cancer 1994; 74: 2261–7.
30. Kay PA, *et al.* Chordoma. Cytomorphologic findings in 14 cases diagnosed by fine needle aspiration. Acta Cytol 2003; 47: 202–20.
31. Heffelfinger MJ, *et al.* Chordomas and cartilaginous tumours at the skull base. Cancer 1973; 32: 410–20.
32. Berven S, *et al.* Clinical outcome in chordoma. Utility of flow cytometry in DNA determination. Spine 2002; 27: 374–9.
33. Ishida T, Dorfman HD. Chondroid chordoma versus low-grade chondrosarcoma of the base of the skull: can immunohistochemistry resolve the controversy? J Neurooncol 1994; 18: 199–206.
34. Bottles K, Beckstead JH. Enzyme histochemical characterization of chordomas. Am J Surg Pathol 1984; 8: 443–7.
35. Brooks JJ, LiVolsi VA, Trojanowski JQ. Does chondroid chordoma exist? Acta Neuropathol 1987; 72: 229–35.
36. Valderrama E, *et al.* Chondroid chordoma: electron-microscopic study of two cases. Am J Surg Pathol 1983; 7: 625–32.
37. Hruban RH, *et al.* Chordomas with malignant spindle cell components. A DNA flow cytometric and immunohistochemical study with histogenetic implications. Am J Pathol 1990; 137: 435–47.

38. Hruban RH, *et al*. Lumbo-sacral chordoma with high-grade malignant cartilaginous and spindle cell components. Am J Surg Pathol 1990; 14: 384–9.

39. Fukuda T, *et al*. Sacrococcygeal chordoma with a malignant spindle cell component. A report of two autopsy cases with a review of the literature. Acta Pathol Jpn 1992; 42: 448–53.

40. Tomlinson FH, *et al*. Sarcomatous transformation in cranial chordoma. Neurosurgery 1992; 31: 13–18.

41. Burger PC, Makek M, Kleihues P. Tissue polypeptide antigen staining of the chordoma and notochordal remnants. Acta Neuropathol 1986; 70: 269–72.

42. Meis JM, Giraldo AA. Chordoma. An immunohistochemical study of 20 cases. Arch Pathol Lab Med 1988; 112: 553–6.

43. Bouropoulou V, *et al*. Immunohistochemical investigation of chordomas: histogenetic and differential diagnostic aspects. Curr Top Pathol 1989; 80: 183–203.

44. Maiorano E, *et al*. Expression of intermediate filaments in chordomas. An immunocytochemical study of five cases. Pathol Res Pract 1992; 188: 901–7.

45. Plate KH, Bittenger A. Value of immunocytochemistry in aspiration cytology of sacrococcygeal chordoma. A report of two cases. Acta Cytol 1992; 36: 87–90.

46. Mori K, *et al*. Expression of E-cadherin in chordomas: diagnostic marker and possible role in tumor cell affinity. Virchows Arch 2002; 440: 123–7.

47. Hiroguchi H, *et al*. Expression of cell adhesion molecules in chordomas: an immunohistochemical study of 16 cases. Acta Neuropathol 2004; 107: 91–6.

48. Persons DL, Bridge JA, Neff JR. Cytogenetic analysis of two sacral chordomas. Cancer Genet Cytogenet 1991; 56: 197–201.

49. Gibas Z, Miettinen M, Sandberg AA. Chromosomal abnormalities in two chordomas. Cancer Genet Cytogenet 1992; 58: 169–73.

50. DeBoer JM, Neff JR, Bridge JA. Cytogenetics of sacral chordoma. Cancer Genet Cytogenet 1992; 64: 95–6.

51. Mertens F, *et al*. Clonal chromosome aberrations in three sacral chordomas. Cancer Genet Cytogenet 1994; 73: 147–51.

52. Bridge JA, Pickering D, Neff JR. Cytogenetic and molecular cytogenetic analysis of sacral chordoma. Cancer Genet Cytogenet 1994; 75: 23–5.

53. Butler MG, *et al*. Cytogenetic, telomere, and telomerase studies in five surgically managed lumbosacral chordomas. Cancer Genet Cytogenet 1995; 85: 51–7.

54. Gil Z, *et al*. Cytogenetic analysis of three variants of clival chordoma. Cancer Genet Cytogenet 2004; 154: 124–30.

55. Riva P, *et al*. Mapping of candidate region for chordoma development to 1p36.13 by LOH analysis. Int J Cancer 2003; 107: 493–7.

56. Matsuno A, *et al*. Immunohistochemical examination of proliferative potentials and the expression of cell cycle-related proteins of intracranial chordomas. Hum Pathol 1997; 28: 714–19.

57. Eisenberg MB, *et al*. Loss of heterozygosity in the retinoblastoma tumor suppressor gene in skull base chordomas and chondrosarcomas. Surg Neurol 1997; 47: 156–61.

58. Deniz ML, *et al*. Expression of growth factors and structural proteins in chordomas: basic fibroblast growth factor, transforming growth factor α, and fibronectin are correlated with recurrence. Neurosurgery 2002; 51: 753–60.

59. Pallini R, *et al*. Chordoma of the skull base: predictors of tumor recurrence. J Neurosurg 2003; 98: 812–22.

60. Naka T, *et al*. Skull base and nonskull base chordomas. Clinicopathologic and immunohistochemical study with special reference to nuclear pleomorphism and proliferative activity. Cancer 2003; 98: 1934–41.

61. Horbinski C, *et al*. The prognostic value of Ki-67, p53, epidermal growth factor receptor, 1p36, 9p21, 10q23, and 17p13 in skull base chordomas. Arch Pathol Lab Med 2010; 134: 1170–6.

62. Walter BA, Begnami M, Valera VA, Santi M, Rushing EJ, Quezado M. Gain of chromosome 7 by chromogenic in situ hybridization (CISH) in chordomas is correlated to c-MET expression. J Neurooncol 2011; 101: 199–206.

63. Ostroumov E, Hunter CJ. Identifying mechanisms for therapeutic intervention in chordoma: c-Met oncoprotein. Spine 2008; 33: 2774–80.

64. Duan Z, *et al*. Differential expression of microRNA (miRNA) in chordoma reveals a role for miRNA-1 in Met expression. J Orthop Res 2010; 28: 746–52.

65. Ogi H, *et al*. Cutaneous metastasis of CNS chordoma. Am J Dermatol 1995; 17: 599–602.

66. Hall WA, Clark HB. Sacrococcygeal chordoma metastatic to the brain with review of the literature. J Neurooncol 1995; 25: 155–9.

67. Bethke KP, Neifeld JP, Lawrence W. Diagnosis and management of sacrococcygeal chordoma. J Surg Oncol 1991; 48: 232–8.

68. Lybeert MLM, Meerwaldt JH. Chordoma. Report on treatment results in eighteen cases. Acta Radiol Oncol 1986; 25: 41–3.

69. Schoenthaler R, *et al*. Charged particle irradiation of sacral chordomas. Int J Radiat Oncol Biol Phys 1993; 26: 291–8.

70. Bergh P, *et al*. Prognostic factors in chordoma of the sacrum and mobile spine. A study of 39 patients. Cancer 2000; 88: 2122–34.

71. Yoneoka Y, *et al*. Cranial base chordoma – long term outcome and review of the literature. Acta Neurochir (Wien) 2008; 150: 773–8.

72. Al-Mefty O, Borba LAB. Skull base chordomas: a management challenge. J Neurosurg 1997; 86: 182–289.

73. Volpe NJ, *et al*. Neuro-ophthalmologic findings in chordoma and chondrosarcoma of the skull base. Am J Ophthalmol 1993; 115: 97–104.

74. Crockard HA, *et al*. A multidisciplinary team approach to skull base chordomas. J Neurosurg 2001; 95: 175–83.

75. Oot RF, *et al*. The role of MR and CT in evaluating clival chordomas and chondrosarcomas. Am J Roentgenol 1988; 151: 567–75.

76. Sze G, *et al*. Chordomas: MR imaging. Radiology 1988; 166: 187–91.

77. Larson TC, Houser OW, Laws ER. Imaging of cranial chordomas. Mayo Clin Proc 1987; 62: 886–93.

78. Meyer SP, *et al*. Chordomas of the skull base: MR features. Am J Neuroradiol 1992; 13: 1627–36.

79. Leproux F, *et al*. MRI of cranial chordomas: the value of gadolinium. Neuroradiology 1993; 35: 543–5.

80. Kumar AJ, *et al*. Imaging features of skull base tumors. Neuroimag Clin North Am 1993; 3: 715–34.

81. Ikushima I, *et al*. Chordomas of the skull base: dynamic MRI. J Comp Ass Tomogr 1996; 20: 547–50.

82. Rosenthal DI, *et al*. Sacrococcygeal chordoma: magnetic resonance imaging and computed tomography. Am J Roentgenol 1985; 145: 143–7.

83. De Bruïne FT, Kroon HM. Spinal chordoma: radiologic features in 14 cases. Am J Roentgenol 1988; 150: 861–3.

84. Erdem E, *et al*. Comprehensive review of intracranial chordoma. Radiographica 2003; 23: 995–1009.

85. Lanzino G, *et al*. Chordomas and chondrosarcomas involving the cavernous sinus: review of surgical treatment and outcome in 31 patients. Surg Neurol 1993; 40: 359–71.

86. Gay E, *et al*. Chordomas and chondrosarcomas of the cranial base: results and follow-up of 60 patients. Neurosurgery 1995; 36: 887–97.

87. Sciubba DM, Chi JH, Rhines LD, Gokaslan ZL. Chordoma of the spinal column. Neurosurg Clin North Am 2008; 19: 5–15.

88. Ozaki T, Hillmann A, Winkelmann W. Surgical treatment of sacrococcygeal chordoma. J Surg Oncol 1997; 64: 274–9.

89. Arnold H, Herrmann HD. Skull base chordoma with cavernous sinus involvement. Partial or radical tumour-removal? Acta Neurochir 1986; 83: 31–7.

90. Crumley RL, Gutin PH. Surgical access for clivus chordoma. The University of California, San Francisco, experience. Arch Otolaryngol Head Neck Surg 1989; 115: 295–300.

91. Sen CN, *et al*. Chordoma and chondrosarcoma of the cranial base: an 8-year experience. Neurosurgery 1989; 25: 931–41.

92. Goel A. Middle fossa sub-gasserian ganglion approach to clivus chordomas. Acta Neurochir 1995; 136: 212–16.

93. Maira G, *et al*. Surgical treatment of clival chordomas: the transsphenoidal approach revisited. J Neurosurg 1996; 85: 784–92.

94. Megerian CA, *et al*. The subtemporal-transpetrous approach for excision of petroclival tumors. Am J Otol 1996; 17: 773–9.

95. Jho HD, *et al*. Endoscopic transsphenoidal resection of a large chordoma in the posterior fossa. Acta Neurochir 1997; 139: 343–8.

96. Samii A, *et al*. Chordomas of the skull base: surgical management and outcome. J Neurosurg 2007; 107: 319–24.

97. Al-Mefty O, Kadri PAS, Hasan DM, Isolan GR, Pravdendova S. Anterior clivectomy: surgical technique and clinical applications. J Neurosurg 2008; 109: 783–93.

98. Dehdashti AR, Karabatsou K, Ganna A, Witterick I, Gentili F. Expanded endoscopic endonasal approach for treatment of clival chordomas: early results in 12 patients. Neurosurgery 2008; 63: 299–309.

99. Samson IR, *et al*. Operative treatment of sacrococcygeal chordoma. A review of twenty-one cases. J Bone Joint Surg 1993; 75: 1476–84.

100. Berson AM, *et al*. Charged particle irradiation of chordoma and chondrosarcoma of the base of skull and cervical spine: the Lawrence Berkeley laboratory experience. Int J Radiat Oncol Biol Phys 1988; 15: 559–65.

101. Austin-Seymour M, *et al*. Fractionated proton radiation therapy of chordoma and low-grade chondrosarcoma of the base of skull. J Neurosurg 1989; 70: 13–17.

102. Austin-Seymour M, *et al*. Fractionated proton radiation therapy of cranial and intracranial tumors. Am J Clin Oncol 1990; 13: 327–30.

103. Keisch ME, Garcia DM, Shibuya RB. Retrospective long-term follow-up analysis in 21 patients with chordomas of various sites treated at a single institution. J Neurosurg 1991; 75: 374–7.

104. Austin JP, *et al*. Probable causes of recurrence in patients with chordoma and chondrosarcoma of the base of skull and cervical spine. Int J Radiat Oncol Biol Phys 1993; 25: 439–44.

105. Thieblemont C, *et al*. Prognostic factors in chordoma: role of postoperative radiotherapy. Eur J Cancer 1995; 31: 2255–9.

106. Tai PTH, Craighead P, Bagdon F. Optimization of radiotherapy for patients with cranial chordoma. A review of dose-response ratios for photon techniques. Cancer 1995; 75: 749–56.

107. Saxton JP. Chordoma. Int J Radiat Oncol Biol Phys 1981; 7: 913–15.

108. Cummings BJ, Hodson DI, Bush RS. Chordoma: the results of megavoltage radiation therapy. Int J Radiat Oncol Biol Phys 1983; 9: 633–42.

109. Thilmann C, *et al*. Intensity-modulated radiotherapy of sacral chordoma. A case report and a comparison with stereotactic conformal radiotherapy. Acta Oncol 2002; 41: 395–9.

110. Gabriele P, *et al*. Feasibility of intensity-modulated radiation therapy in the treatment of advanced cervical chordoma. Tumori 2003; 89: 298–304.

111. Jena R, *et al*. Conformal rotation therapy with central axis beam block is a feasible alternative to intensity-modulated radiotherapy for chordomas of the cervical spine. Clin Oncol 2004; 16: 449–56.

112. Taylor RE, *et al*. Proton therapy for base of skull chordoma: a report of the Royal College of Radiologists. The proton therapy working party. Clin Oncol 2000; 12: 75–9.

113. Amichetti M, Cianchetti M, Amelio D, Enrici RM, Minniti G. Proton therapy in chordoma of the base of the skull: a systematic review. Neurosurg Rev 2009; 32: 403–16.

114. Takahashi S, Kawase T, Yoshida K, Hasegawa A, Mizoe J. Skull base chordomas: efficacy of surgery followed by carbon ion radiotherapy. Acta Neurochir 2009; 151: 759–69.

115. DeLaney TF, Liebsch NJ, Pedlow FX, *et al*. Phase II study of high-dose photon/proton radiotherapy in the management of spine sarcomas. Int J Rad Oncol Biol Phys 2009; 74: 732–9.

116. Imai R, *et al*. Effect of carbon ion radiotherapy for sacral chordoma: results of phase I-II and phase II clinical trials. Int J Rad Oncol Biol Phys 2010; 77: 1470–6.

117. Noël G, *et al*. Combination of photon and proton radiation therapy for chordomas and chondrosarcomas of the skull base: the Centre de Protontherapie D'Orsay experience. Int J Rad Oncol Biol Phys 2001; 51: 392–8.

118. Schulz-Ertner D, *et al*. Radiotherapy for chordomas and low-grade chondrosarcomas of the skull base with carbon ions. Int J Rad Oncol Biol Phys 2002; 53: 36–42.

119. Imai R, *et al*. Carbon ion radiotherapy for unresectable sacral chordomas. Clin Cancer Res 2004; 10: 5741–6.

120. Kumar PP, *et al*. Local control of recurrent clival and sacral chordoma after interstitial irradiation with iodine-125: new techniques for treatment of recurrent or unresectable chordomas. Neurosurgery 1988; 22: 479–83.

121. Kondziolka D, Lunsford LD, Flickinger JC. The role of radiosurgery in the management of chordoma and chondrosarcoma of the cranial base. Neurosurgery 1991; 29: 38–46.

122. Feigl GC, Bundschuh O, Gharabachi A. *et al*. Evaluation of a new concept for the management of skull base chordomas and chondrosarcomas. J Neurosurg 2005; 102: 165–70.

123. Ito E, Saito K, Okada T, Nagatani T, Nagasaka T. Long-term control of clival chordoma with initial aggressive surgical resection and gamma knife radiosurgery for recurrence. Acta Neurochir (Wien) 2010; 152: 57–67.

124. Henderson FC, McCool K, Seigle J, Walter J, Harter W, Gagnon GJ. Treatment of chordomas with cyberknife: Georgetown University experience and treatment recommendations. Neurosurgery 2009; 64: A44–A53.

125. Fleming GF, *et al*. Dedifferentiated chordoma. Response to aggressive chemotherapy in two cases. Cancer 1993; 72: 714–18.

126. Newton HB. Molecular neuro-oncology and the development of "targeted" therapeutic strategies for brain tumors. Part 1 – growth factor and ras signaling pathways. Expert Rev Anticancer Ther 2003; 3: 595–614.

127. Barry JJ, *et al*. The next step: innovative molecular targeted therapies for treatment of intracranial chordoma patients. Neurosurgery 2011; 68: 231–40.

128. Casali PG, *et al*. Imatinib mesylate in chordoma. Cancer 2004; 101: 2086–97.

129. Singhal N, Kotasek D, Parnis FX. Response to erlotinib in a patient with treatment refractory chordoma. Anti-Cancer Drugs 2009; 20: 953–5.

130. Stacchiotti S, Marrari A, Tamborini E, *et al*. Response to imatinib plus sieolimus in advanced chordoma. Ann Oncol 2009; 20: 1886–94.

131. Newton HB. Molecular neuro-oncology and the development of "targeted" therapeutic strategies for brain tumors. Part 2 – PI3K/Akt/PTEN, mTOR, SHH/PTCH, and angiogenesis. Expert Rev Anticancer Ther 2004; 4: 105–28.

132. Schwab J, *et al*. Combination of PI3K/mTOR inhibition demonstrates efficacy in human chordoma. Anticancer Res 2009; 29: 1867–72.

55 Atypical and Malignant Meningiomas

George A. Alexiou,[1] Samer E. Kaba,[2] and Athanassios P. Kyritsis[3]

[1] Department of Neurosurgery, [3] Department of Neurology, University Hospital of Ioannina, Ioannina, Greece
[2] Clinical Research and Medical Management, Scirex Corporation, Horsham, PA, USA

Introduction and definition

Meningioma is the most common intracranial tumor. It originates from the meninges of the skull or spinal canal and compresses the adjacent neural tissues, causing several symptoms and signs, depending on the tumor location. Larger tumors can produce a remarkable degree of disability and even mortality.

Most meningiomas are histologically benign and potentially curable with surgical resection. However, about 6% of meningiomas are classified as atypical or anaplastic tumors because they display malignant histological features and are associated with increased risk of recurrence. Most authors reserve the term "malignant meningioma" to describe tumors infiltrating the brain parenchyma. Brain invasion by itself, however, is not enough to classify the tumor as malignant unless it is associated with other cellular and structural features of malignancy. In this chapter we will use the World Health Organization (WHO) classification of meningiomas, which recognizes benign meningiomas (grade I), atypical meningiomas (grade II), and anaplastic meningiomas (grade III). Also we will use the term "malignant meningioma" interchangeably with "anaplastic meningioma" and refer to atypical and anaplastic meningiomas combined as "nonbenign meningiomas."

Surgery is the treatment of choice for symptomatic meningiomas. In benign meningiomas gross total resection is associated with a high cure rate. Recurrence is very common in nonbenign meningiomas, even after total resection. In addition, total resection cannot be achieved in a large number of aggressive nonbenign meningiomas, where the recurrence rate reaches 100%. Radiation therapy was shown to be effective in delaying the recurrence in malignant meningiomas. Medical treatments such as hormonal therapy, mifepristone, and hydroxyurea may have some role in the future management of recurrent or unresectable meningiomas.

Anatomy

Meningiomas can be intracranial or spinal. Intracranial meningiomas are much more common and more likely to be atypical or malignant than spinal ones. The most common locations of intracranial meningiomas are cerebral convexity, parasagittal, sphenoid wing, lateral ventricle, tentorium, and tuberculum sellae. Other less common locations include optic nerve sheath, cerebellopontine angle, olfactory groove and intraventricular. In children, a high proportion of meningiomas are multiple or intraventricular and may be associated with neurofibromatosis type II or previous cranial irradiation.[1] Meningiomas in general are well-circumscribed spherical tumors attached to the dura. They compress the adjacent brain but are usually separated from the underlying parenchyma, except for highly malignant tumors that invade the brain. Meningiomas of the skull base, especially the sphenoid wing, tend to grow in what is called *en plaque* pattern. These tumors grow within and expand the meninges without forming an exophytic mass pattern.[2] The surface of these tumors can be smooth or nodular, depending on their location. Hyperostosis or erosion of the bone can be seen adjacent to meningiomas. This can cause a growing mass on the skull. While benign meningiomas can excavate and compress surrounding tissue, actual invasion of neural and vascular structure is associated with atypical and malignant variants.

Epidemiology

Meningiomas are common tumors of the central nervous system, and the vast majority are histologically benign. Intracranial meningiomas constitute 18–29% of all primary brain tumors.[3,4] The annual incidence per 100,000 people is 2–7 for females and 1–5 for males, while it reaches 10 per 100,000 in people older than 65 years of age.[4,5] In the pediatric population, meningiomas are uncommon, accounting for approximately 1.7%

of intracranial tumors.[6] Spinal meningiomas are relatively rare but constitute one of the most common spinal tumors. They are usually localized lateral to the spinal cord and in the thoracic region.[7]

In a large series of 936 cases of intracranial meningiomas, 94.3% were histologically benign, 4.7% atypical, and 1% anaplastic (malignant).[8] Similar figures were reported in another series of meningioma patients, where 6.2% had atypical and 1.7% malignant tumors.[9] Atypical and anaplastic meningiomas are more common in the sixth and seventh decades and slightly more common in males.[10]

Molecular biology

Meningiomas express a complex of active molecules, including sex hormone receptors and a variety of growth factors.[11] It was noted for a long time that meningiomas are more common in women and they tend to grow faster during pregnancy. They were also associated with breast cancer in many cases but recent studies have not found an increased prevalence of meningioma in breast cancer survivors.[12] These observations prompted the investigation of the role of sex hormones in the development of meningioma and the possible prognostic significance of sex hormone receptors.

Initially, the interest was focused on estrogen receptors (ER) but they are not consistently found in meningiomas.[13] Progesterone receptors (PR) are expressed in 40–100% of meningiomas, are localized to the nuclei and are transcriptionally active.[14] Expression of PR is associated with lower frequency of recurrence and overall favorable prognosis, since they tend to decrease during malignant progression. PR-negative meningiomas tend to be larger than PR-positive, and atypical and malignant meningiomas are more often PR negative.[15–17] A recent report showed that over half of meningiomas are regulated by the expression of gonadotropin-releasing hormone and its receptor in an autocrine fashion.[18] This may also have therapeutic implications.[19]

Meningiomas vary in expression of receptors for other hormones. Epidermal growth factor receptor (EGFR) and its ligands, EGF and transforming growth factor-α (TGF-a) can be found and may promote tumor growth.[20] The EGFR inhibitors gefitinib and erlotinib have been evaluated for treatment of recurrent meningioma but no significant effect was observed.[21] Platelet-derived growth factor (PDGF) may act as a stimulator of meningioma growth. Expression levels of PDGF were higher in atypical and malignant meningiomas than benign.[22] Wen *et al.* evaluated the therapeutic potential of imatinib mesylate, a PDGFR inhibitor, in patients with recurrent meningiomas but no significant benefit was found.[23] High levels of basic fibroblast growth factor (bFGF) are found in meningioma cells.[24] This growth factor is a potent mitogen and angiogenic agent and it is highly likely that it plays an important role in the development of meningioma.[25] FGF receptor-3 activation has been found to stimulate meningioma cell proliferation.[26] Vascular endothelial growth factor (VEGF) expression has also been studied in meningiomas. Lamszus *et al.* reported a two-fold higher VEGF expression in atypical than in benign meningiomas and 10-fold higher in malignant than in benign

meningiomas.[27] Recent reports suggested that VEGF may play a critical role in formation of peritumoral brain edema associated with meningiomas.[28] VEGF inhibitors are currently being tested for use against meningiomas.[29]

Somatostatin receptors, predominantly type 2a, are usually found in the same tumors expressing EGF receptors but their role in the development of meningioma is not clearly defined. Their activation has been associated with an antiproliferative effect. Somatostatin receptors were frequently expressed in high-grade meningiomas in accordance with higher microvessel density.[30] Recent studies showed that somatostatin analogs may have a potential role in meningioma treatment.[31]

Pathology and classifications

Based on WHO classification, meningiomas are graded as grade I, grade II, and grade III.[32] The WHO classification distinguishes neoplasms from meningothelial origin, or meningiomas *per se*, from other nonmeningothelial tumors originating in the meninges (Box 55.1). Meningothelial tumors include several benign variants, papillary meningioma, atypical meningioma,

Box 55.1 The WHO classification of tumors associated with the meninges.

Tumors of meningothelial cells	Meningioma	a. Meningothelia (syncytial)
		b. Transitional/mixed
		c. Fibrous (fibroblastic)
		d. Psammomatous
		e. Angiomatous
		f. Microcystic
		g. Secretory
		h. Lymphoplasmacyte rich
		i. Metaplastic variant (xanthomatous, myxoid, osseous, and so on)
	Atypical meningioma	a. Variants of 1 a–i (above)
		b. Clear cell
		c. Chordoid
	Anaplastic (malignant) meningioma	a. Variants of 1 a–i (above)
		b. Papillary
		c. Rhabdoid
Nonmeningothelial tumors of the meninges	Mesenchymal tumors	Benign neoplasms:
		a. Osteocartilaginous tumors
		b. Lipoma
		c. Fibrous histiocytoma
		Malignant neoplasms:
		a. Hemangiopericytoma
		b. Chondrosarcoma
		c. Mesenchymal chondrosarcoma
		d. Malignant fibrous histiocytoma
		e. Rhabdomyosarcoma
		f. Meningeal sarcomatosis
	Tumors of uncertain origin	Hemangioblastoma

and anaplastic meningioma. Meningeal sarcomas and hemangiopericytoma, once classified as meningiomas, are now considered mesenchymal nonmeningothelial tumors.

Pathology

Many different variants of meningiomas exist, with each variant having a distinguishing architecture and cellular appearance (see Box 55.1). Multiple types can coexist in the same tumor. Benign meningiomas, in general, display a uniform cellular appearance, whorling structures, and calcification. They have normal blood vessels and no mitotic activity. A group of meningiomas display variable degrees of malignant features, including loss of architecture, increased cellularity, nuclear pleomorphism, mitotic figures, focal necrosis, and brain invasion. Depending on the abundance of malignant features, this group of tumors is further classified into atypical and anaplastic (malignant) meningiomas. From the above features, brain invasion has been recognized as a criterion for atypia.[32] Invasion of bone, dura, or dural sinuses can be seen in benign meningiomas and is not by itself a marker of malignancy. It is noteworthy that the clinical and biological behavior of the tumor does not always correlate with the histological appearance, and seemingly less malignant tumors can progress more rapidly and invade surrounding tissues more aggressively than expected.

Atypical meningioma (WHO grade 2)

This tumor is constituted of a patternless, sheet-like growth of an increased number of small cells with a high nuclear:cytoplasmic ratio and prominent nucleoli.[9] A fair amount of mitotic activity can be seen. Focal necrosis and brain invasion are not usually seen in atypical meningioma.

Anaplastic (malignant) meningioma (WHO grade 3)

This tumor is highly malignant, exhibiting cellular anaplasia, frequent mitotic figures, and striking necrosis, on a patternless background. Frank extensive invasion of the brain is frequently seen. Proliferation markers, such as bromodeoxyuridine (BrdU), Ki-67, and proliferating cell nuclear antigen (PCNA), are usually markedly elevated in atypical and malignant meningiomas compared with their benign counterpart, and can help in establishing the diagnosis (see further discussion under "General considerations" below).[33–35]

Papillary meningioma

This is a group of meningiomas characterized by a papillary pattern intermixed with other more usual meningiomatous areas. The cells are usually uniform, long or tapered, and radiate toward blood vessels forming pseudorosettes. Although this tumor may not have the typical malignant features, it corresponds to WHO grade 2 or 3. Clinically, papillary meningiomas are usually aggressive and have the tendency to recur, invade the brain, and metastasize.[36,37] These tumors are rare and, unlike other meningiomas, can occur in young adults and children.

Rhabdoid meningioma

This is a grade 3 meningioma and in most cases it exhibits histological features of malignancy and follows an aggressive course. However, if the rhabdoid histological subtype is the only feature of the tumor without other signs of malignancy such as brain invasion and high proliferation rate, the expected behavior of the rhabdoid meningioma cannot be predicted.

Etiology

Radiation

The occurrence of meningioma following low-dose, medium-dose, and high-dose radiation therapy is well documented in the literature and it is the most common brain tumor that develops after radiation exposure.[38] For a tumor to be considered secondary to radiation, it has to fulfill three criteria: (i) arise in the radiation field, (ii) develop many years after radiation, and (iii) appear histologically different from any primary tumor that existed before radiation. The overwhelming majority of radiation-induced meningiomas occurred after low-dose irradiation, less than 10 Gy, as had been used for treatment of tinea capitis.[38] Childhood leukemia survivors who received cranial irradiation have an increased risk of developing secondary brain tumors.[39] High incidence of meningioma has been observed in these patients and they usually have long latency periods.[40,41] Radiation-induced meningiomas have the tendency to occur in younger patients, be atypical histologically, have a high proliferative index, and to recur after resection. The latency between radiation and the development of these tumors ranges from 19.5 to 35 years, depending on the patient's age and radiation dose.[42]

Trauma

Head trauma has been advocated as a possible etiological factor for meningioma development. Posttraumatic meningiomas have been suggested to be frequently atypical or anaplastic and to have a poor outcome.[43] Nevertheless, the issue of meningioma development after head trauma remains controversial. A large prospective study on patients with head trauma found no increased incidence of brain tumors after long periods of follow-up.[44]

Cytogenetics

Both chromosomal loss and structural rearrangement are found in meningiomas.[45] The most frequent chromosomal abnormality is chromosome 22 monosomy, which occurs in 70–85% of all meningiomas.[11,46] Less often, a deletion of 22q occurs instead.[47] Transitional and fibrous meningiomas exhibit the above abnormalities more frequently than the meningothelial variant. Trisomy and tetrasomy 22 are usually related to younger patients, aggressive histopathological features, a greater incidence of DNA aneuploidy, and higher proportion of S-phase tumor cells.[48] Other frequent genetic abnormalities that have been reported are the 1p and 14q deletions.[11] In fact, loss of chromosome 14 is the most common chromosomal abnormality encountered in atypical and malignant meningiomas, suggesting loss of a tumor suppressor gene located on the long arm of this chromosome.[49]

All the above suggest that the progression of normal meningeal cells to a malignant phenotype is characterized genetically by early loss of a tumor suppressor gene on chromosome 22 followed by alterations of chromosomes 10 and 14, and other less common changes. Both 1p and 14q deletions are highly associated with increasing histological grade and play an important role in meningioma tumor progression.[50] Monosomy 14 has an adverse prognostic impact and these patients have an increased risk for tumor recurrence.[51] Furthermore, chromosome 1p was found to have frequent deletions of up to 17 possible tumor suppression genes, especially at 1p34 and 1p36.[52] Recently, genes located at 1p, 6q, and 14q were found to be underexpressed in meningioma recurrences. Thus, at these locations, there may be novel candidate genes that could be involved in meningioma recurrence.[53]

While histologically benign meningiomas show a normal karyotype or 22 monosomy, atypical and anaplastic meningiomas display more complex structural and numerical chromosomal abnormalities.[54] Loss of heterozygosity (LOH) of chromosome 10 was found in one of two atypical, four of 13 malignant, and 0 of 20 benign meningiomas. This loss of heterozygosity was not observed in tumors classified as malignant by invasive criteria only.[55] These changes were shown to correlate with shorter time to recurrence and shorter survival. Also, there was a significant correlation between tumor location, grade, recurrence, and patient's age with LOH of chromosome 10.[56] Adverse prognostic factors and shorter relapse-free survival were associated with abnormalities in chromosomes 9, 11, 15, 17 and the sex chromosomes.[57] Chromosome 7p loss is seen only in a small group of meningiomas in general, but is seen in the majority of radiation-induced meningiomas.[58]

Specific gene abnormalities in meningiomas

The analysis of meningiomas associated with neurofibromatosis type 2 (NF-2) revealed loss of genetic information in the same region of chromosome 22 involved in sporadic meningiomas. Up to 60% of meningiomas show a somatic mutation of the NF2 tumor suppressor gene, resulting in a nonfunctional merlin or schwannomin protein.[11] An association has been reported between the histological variant and the frequency of NF-2 mutations. Nearly 70–80% of fibroblastic and transitional meningiomas carry NF-2 mutations, compared with only 25% of meningoepithelial meningiomas, suggesting the presence of different molecular subgroups of meningiomas.[59]

The product of the DAL-1 gene, protein 4.1B, which has a homology with merlin, has been observed in 60% of meningiomas regardless of the histological grade and has been implicated in familial meningiomas and meningioma evolution.[60] Loss of expression of this protein is an early event in tumorigenesis.[61]

A 6–8-fold increase in expression of the k-ras oncogene was observed in meningiomas with normal karyotypes of 22 monosomy.[62] This increase in the expression of k-ras is probably secondary to the lack of activity of a tumor suppressor gene because it is not associated with any changes in the k-ras gene itself. On the other hand, the locus of the c-sis gene lies in the region of the putative meningioma locus of chromosome 22, and it was implicated in the pathogenesis of meningiomas but no relation to meningioma malignancy was found.[22,63]

A 5–20-fold increase in the expression of c-myc has been observed in 63% of meningiomas, without amplification or rearrangement of its gene. Malignant meningiomas have been shown to be positive for c-myc.[22] The level of expression of c-myc was higher in cases with loss of heterozygosity of chromosome 22 than in those without, suggesting again the loss of a tumor suppressor gene on chromosome 22.[64]

Mutations of the p53 gene are rare in benign meningiomas but were found in malignant meningiomas, suggesting that p53 may be considered a marker for malignant transformation in meningiomas.[65] In addition, the inactivation of p53 by p14ARF loss and MDM2-mediated degradation of p53 may contribute to meningioma progression.[66] The bcl-2 protooncogene is also correlated with higher-grade meningiomas.[67]

Phosphatase and tensin homolog deleted on chromosome 10 (10q23.3) (PTEN) was identified in 1997 as a tumor suppressor gene.[68] PTEN has been reported to contribute to the malignant progression in a fraction of anaplastic meningiomas.[69] The phosphatidylinositol 3-kinase (PI3K)/Akt signaling contributes to the aggressive behavior of malignant meningiomas.[70] PTEN is the sole central negative regulator of PI3K signaling because no other protein compensates if there is a loss of its function.

Other changes in genes or gene products have been reported recently in meningioma cells, including increased activity of telomerase (human telomerase reverse transcriptase [hTERT]), amplification of chromosome 17q23, and modulation of meningioma cell growth in vitro by somatostatin and TGF-β.[71] Atypical and anaplastic meningiomas had increased telomerase activity compared to benign tumors. Telomerase activity has also been associated with poor outcome.[72] Maes et al. reported that hTERT expression is an early event in carcinogenesis in contrast to telomerase activity.[73] Telomere shortening was shown to be a critical step in pathogenesis of atypical and malignant meningiomas.[74]

Epigenetic changes may also be involved in malignant progression of meningiomas by altering gene expression and protein function. Aberrant methylation of the promoter is an epigenetic change that can lead to tumor suppressor gene inactivation. TP53 Pro47Ser and Arg72Pro polymorphisms and DNA hypermethylation may promote the development of extraaxial brain tumors.[75] Furthermore, aberrant CpG island hypermethylation has been associated with the malignant progression of meningiomas.[76]

Clinical presentation

The presenting symptoms of meningioma depend on the tumor's location, size, and rate of growth. Small convexity meningiomas can be found incidentally on brain imaging studies, while those in the base of the skull tend to be symptomatic early in their course. The most common symptoms include headache, focal motor deficit, seizures, personality changes, and visual impairments. The common presenting symptoms of meningiomas are summarized in Table 55.1. Specific syndromes can result from tumors in certain locations, making the diagnosis easier on a clinical basis. The most common examples are tuberculum sellae, olfactory groove, and cavernous

Table 55.1 The most common presenting symptoms of meningiomas ($n=193$).

Symptoms	Malignant meningioma (%)	Benign meningioma (%)
Paresis	43	19
Headache	36	36
Visual impairment	29	16
Personality change/mental decline	21	22
Ataxia	21	15
Decreased level of consciousness	14	7
Aphasia	14	10
Focal seizure	14	15
Generalized seizures	7	19

Reproduced from Jun *et al.*[76] by permission of Oxford University Press.

Table 55.2 Specific neurological syndromes associated with meningiomas.

Tumor location	Syndrome	Findings
Tuberculum sellae	Chiasmal syndrome	Visual field defects (bitemporal hemianopia, altitudinal hemianopia, homonymous hemi- or quadrantanopia), ± pituitary insufficiency
Cavernous sinus	Cavernous syndrome	Cranial nerves III, IV, VI, and V^1 deficits ± Horner syndrome
Sphenoidal wing	Superior orbital fissure syndrome	Ophthalmoplegia, exophthalmos, pain behind the eye
Olfactory groove	Foster Kennedy syndrome	Ipsilateral optic atrophy + contralateral papilledema, mental and personality changes, anosmia
Cerebellopontine angle		Cranial nerves VI, VII, and VIII deficits. Less commonly IX, X, and brainstem deficits

meningiomas. The symptoms and signs of these syndromes, and the corresponding tumors, are illustrated in Table 55.2.

No clinical features are specific for atypical or anaplastic meningiomas but rapid progression of symptoms in the absence of intratumoral hemorrhage can suggest the malignant nature of the tumor.[77]

Diagnosis and neuroimaging

Computed tomography and magnetic resonance imaging

Atypical and anaplastic meningiomas can look identical to benign meningiomas on brain imaging. On nonenhanced computed tomography (CT) scan, meningioma appears as an isodense, well-demarcated mass. Magnetic resonance imaging (MRI) allows a more accurate evaluation of the size, location, and invasiveness of meningiomas, especially in the base of the skull. Meningiomas are usually isointense on both T1- and T2-weighted images. Occasionally they can be hypointense on

T1 and hyperintense on T2.[78] After the injection of contrast material, these tumors enhance homogeneously and intensely in most cases. Atypical and malignant meningiomas are most commonly not located at the skull base.[79] They can be multiple in about 20% of cases.[78]

Some imaging features suggest an atypical or anaplastic histology of the tumor. A nodular growth pattern, or what is called mushrooming, is seen in 67% of cases of atypical/anaplastic meningiomas.[80–82] Indistinct margins and areas of hyperintensity on MRI were also reported.[82,83] Heterogeneous enhancement on CT and MRI is a common feature in atypical/anaplastic meningiomas, seen in 40–50% of these tumors.[82,83] Recently, intratumoral cystic change and extracranial tumor extension through the skull base foramina were found to be more prevalent in atypical/malignant meningiomas.[84] Reactive vasogenic edema in the adjacent brain can be seen with all meningiomas but is more common with higher grade meningiomas, where it is noted in up to 50% of tumors.[81] Multiplicity, osteolysis, and soft tissue invasion are less consistent features of atypical and malignant meningiomas. These features may make the differentiation of nonbenign meningiomas and dural metastases difficult in some cases. Finally, metastatic disease is a clear indication of malignancy.

Nevertheless, none of the above imaging features is unique and reliable for diagnosing atypical/malignant meningiomas. The latest MR techniques such as diffusion, perfusion and MR spectroscopy have also been evaluated for the noninvasive differentiation of atypical/malignant from benign meningiomas. Diffusion MRI allows evaluation of the rate of microscopic diffusion of free water molecules within tissues. The magnitude of diffusion is quantified by the apparent diffusion coefficient (ADC) and mean diffusivity (MD) indices.[85] Atypical/malignant meningiomas have lower intratumoral ADC values than typical meningiomas.[86] A more sophisticated extension of diffusion MRI is diffusion tensor imaging (DTI), measuring the magnitude and directionality of water diffusion in tissues. DTI has shown that intratumoral microscopic water motion is less organized in classic than in atypical meningiomas.[87]

Perfusion MRI measures the vascularity within brain lesions and is an indirect measure of tissue metabolic activity. The assessment of the maximal relative cerebral blood volume and the corresponding relative mean time to enhance in the peritumural edema allowed differentiation between benign and malignant meningiomas.[88] MR spectroscopy is able to depict noninvasively the metabolic composition of the tissue under investigation. Recent reports suggest that MR spectroscopy can noninvasively evaluate meningioma's aggressiveness but its efficacy in the assessment of tumor grade has yet to be established.[89]

Angiography

The angiographic appearance of atypical and anaplastic meningiomas is similar to that of their benign counterpart. Most of these tumors derive their blood supply from a meningeal arterial branch.[5] The need for standard angiography has declined rapidly with the availability of MR angiography. However, angiography is still a useful tool when preoperative embolization of the tumor is planned.

Positron emission tomography

Brain PET has been introduced as a method of intracranial lesion metabolic imaging. The glucose analog $2[^{18}F]$ fluorodeoxy-D-glucose (FDG) was the first radiotracer used.[90,91] Lippitz et al. in a series of 62 meningiomas reported that ^{18}F-FDG is suitable as a noninvasive predictor of tumor growth characteristics.[92] Furthermore, ^{18}F-FDG uptake in meningioma was a significant predictive factor of tumor recurrence and significantly correlated with the meningioma's proliferative potential.[93] Recently, 1-(11)C-acetate, another PET tracer, was found to be useful for detecting meningiomas and evaluating the extent of meningiomas and potentially useful for monitoring tumor response to radiosurgery. However, ^{18}F-FDG proved to be superior to 1-(11)C-acetate for the evaluation of tumor grade.[94] Other PET tracers such as [18]F-3′-deoxy-3′-fluoro-thymidine (^{18}F-FLT), that has been found useful for glioma assessment, have not been evaluated yet in meningiomas. Nevertheless, nuclear medicine techniques have a relative lack of specificity in differentiating meningiomas from other lesions.

Single photon emission computed tomography

Single photo emission computed tomography (SPECT) compared to PET has the advantage of lower cost and wider availability but its main disadvantages are lower sensitivity and the ability to provide quantitative measurements of physiological parameters. Various SPECT radiotracers have been evaluated. Thallium-201 (^{201}Tl) was one of the first tracers extensively applied for studies of brain tumors and proved useful in evaluating the aggressiveness and level of malignancy of meningioma.[95,96] Furthermore, ^{201}Tl uptake index correlated with Ki-67 index and VEGF.[97] Technetium-99m-labeled compounds, mainly ^{99m}Tc-hexakis-2-methoxyisobutylisonitrile (^{99m}Tc-MIBI) and ^{99m}Tc-tetrofos-min (^{99m}Tc-TF), have also been studied. They were proven advantageous over ^{201}Tl, due to 140 keV γ-ray energy, high photon flux, higher spatial resolution, less radiation burden to the patient, and excellent availability.[98] ^{99m}Tc-TF is not influenced by tumor multidrug resistance phenotype and thus may be superior to ^{99m}Tc-MIBI for brain tumor imaging.[99] This tracer proved to accurately differentiate malignant from benign meningiomas. A lesion to normal uptake value of 9.6 was proposed as the optimal cut-off value, discriminating between the two groups with 96% sensitivity and 100% specificity.[100] Furthermore, the intensity of ^{99m}Tc-TF uptake correlated significantly with meningioma aggressiveness as assessed by Ki-67 index and number of cells in S-phase. A positive correlation between ^{99m}Tc-TF uptake and progression-free survival was also reported.[101,102] A plausible interesting field would be the evaluation of imaging protein synthesis by means of SPECT. Labeled amino acid tracers have been used with promising results mostly in glioma studies. The greatest advantage lies in their low uptake in normal brain, thus amino acids provide better contrast between tumor and normal brain.

Initial management of atypical and malignant meningioma

Surgical resection is the mainstay of management, because total resection produces a high cure rate in benign meningiomas.[78] Total resection, however, is not always possible and residual tumors almost always recur. Atypical and anaplastic meningiomas have the tendency to recur even after gross total resection and require close follow-up.

Surgery

The goal of surgery in meningioma is to remove all the tumor mass and any dural attachment. This goal cannot be achieved in all cases of atypical and anaplastic meningioma.[78] The latest imaging techniques have allowed better preoperative planning, and advances in skull base surgery have greatly improved patient outcome for tumors in precarious locations once thought to be inoperable.[103,104] Nevertheless, tumors located at the tuberculum sellae, cavernous sinus, and superior sagittal sinus are particularly difficult to resect completely because of their proximity to cranial nerves and major blood supply to the brain.[105] The histological nature of the tumor cannot be predicted from the gross appearance during surgery but atypical and anaplastic meningiomas are more likely to be soft and adherent to the cortex. Intraoperative bleeding and duration of surgery are not different between benign and malignant meningiomas.

The extent of surgical resection has been identified as one of the most important factors affecting the rate of recurrence and time to progression in meningioma. Simpson's scale of surgical resection in meningioma is widely used because it correlates with clinical outcome (Box 55.2). Younis et al.[81] reported a median time to progression (MTP) of 35 and 5 months in totally and partially resected aggressive meningiomas, respectively. None of the patients who had partial resection was recurrence free after 2 years. Jaaskelainen et al.[8] reported recurrence rates of 38%, 49%, and 54% at 5, 10, and 15 years, respectively, in completely resected atypical meningiomas. The median time to recurrence was 2.4 years. Anaplastic meningioma recurred in 78% of the patients within 5 years, with a median time to recurrence of 3.5 years. In the same study, the recurrence rates of histologically benign meningioma at 5, 10,

---

Box 55.2 Simpson's grading of surgical resection in meningiomas.

Grade 1	Gross-total resection of tumor, with dural attachments and abnormal bone
Grade 2	Gross-total resection of tumor, coagulation of dural attachments
Grade 3	Gross-total resection of tumor, without resection or coagulation of dural attachments, or alternatively of its extradural extensions
Grade 4	Partial resection of tumor
Grade 5	Simple decompression or biopsy

Reproduced from Jun et al.[76] by permission of Oxford University Press.

and 15 years were 3%, 9%, and 15%, respectively.[8] Palma et al.[106] reported median times to recurrence of 5 and 2 years in atypical and malignant meningiomas. In this series, radical resection (Simpson grade 1) was correlated with a better clinical course, longer time to progression, and longer survival. In a more recent study, Aghi et al. reported that 28% of atypical meningioma recurred 3–144 months after gross total resection. The 10-year recurrence rate was 48%. These recurrences required several surgical interventions and shortened patient survival.[107] Sughrue et al. reported that in malignant meningioma, the patients who were treated with near-total resection experienced improved overall survival compared to patients with gross-total resection and repeat operations. Furthermore, the risk for postoperative neurological deficits is high when gross-total resection is attempted.[108]

Tumor location is another major factor in predicting tumor recurrence, with base of skull meningiomas being the most commonly recurring tumors, followed by sagittal and falx meningiomas, and finally convexity meningiomas.[80] The high rate of recurrence in malignant meningiomas can be explained at least partially by the microscopic infiltration of tumor cells in the dura and cerebral cortex.

Radiation therapy

The role of radiation therapy in the treatment of meningiomas in general has been under intense discussion over the past decade. Nowadays radiotherapy has been used as an adjunct to surgery following subtotal resection, as treatment for recurrent meningiomas, or as primary therapy. A longer time to progression was documented in patients treated with radiation.[109,110]

Milosevic et al.[111] reported the outcome of 59 cases of non-benign meningiomas treated between 1966 and 1990 with adjuvant radiotherapy. This series included tumors designated as malignant meningioma based solely on brain invasion and/or hemangiopericytic features. The actuarial 5-year survival rate was 28%, and radiation doses higher than 50 Gy produced significantly longer survival. Similar observations were reported by Shimizu et al.,[112] who found no difference between giving radiation as part of the initial therapy or at the time of recurrence. In a large series of radiotherapy-treated meningiomas, 23 patients had malignant meningiomas. The 5-year progression-free survival rate of these patients was 48% and the overall 5-year survival rate was 58%. Chamberlain[113] reported the results of a prospective study using adjuvant radiotherapy and chemotherapy in 14 patients with malignant meningiomas. Gross-total resection was achieved in only four patients, and a radiation dose of 59–60 Gy was given to all patients. In addition, all patients received CAV (cyclophosphamide, adriamycin, and vincristine) chemotherapy. The MTP was 4.6 years and median survival was 5.3 years. Because the MTP reported in this study is comparable to what was achieved by radiation alone, it is unlikely that chemotherapy had a major impact on the outcome.

Aghi et al studied retrospectively 108 cases of atypical meningiomas that were gross totally resected and reported that the 5-year recurrence rate was 28%. Eight patients who received postoperative radiation had no recurrence.[107] Another study showed that in patients with atypical meningiomas, adjuvant radiotherapy improved patient survival only if there was brain invasion.[114] For atypical meningiomas, a recent study suggested that radiotherapy should not be administered if gross-total resection has been performed. For any postoperative tumor remnant, radiosurgery should be administered. For those remnants too large for radiosurgery or if another operation is not planned, radiotherapy should be administered.[115]

Stereotactic radiosurgery (SRS) delivered via gamma-knife or linear accelerator is an alternative to surgery and conventional radiotherapy in patients with brain tumors. Its main advantage is that it allows for a more accurate and focused treatment, because it not only limits the amount of radiation to the healthy tissues but it allows larger doses of radiation to be delivered with great precision. Local control rates following SRS have been reported to be as high as 75–100% at 5–10 years.[116,117] Apart from SRS, stereotactic fractionated radiotherapy (SFRT) spares the normal tissues that are sensitive to hypofractionation. This technique is mainly used in optic nerve sheath meningioma.[118] For irregularly shaped tumors and those too large for stereotactic radiotherapy, intensity-modulated radiotherapy (IMRT) is a viable alternative.[119]

Chemotherapy

Although meningiomas were found to be sensitive to cytotoxic agents in vitro,[120,121] few attempts have been made to evaluate the efficacy of adjuvant chemotherapy in high-grade malignant meningiomas. A report showed a relatively long progression-free survival in malignant meningioma patients treated with CAV after surgical resection and radiotherapy.[122] Similar results, however, were observed when radiation was used alone. Hydroxyurea is well tolerated and has modest activity against meningiomas. It has been used for unresectable tumors and large residual tumors but its efficacy in atypical or malignant meningiom has yet to be established.[123,124] Based on the available evidence, chemotherapy cannot be recommended in the initial treatment of atypical and malignant meningiomas.

Management of recurrent atypical and malignant meningiomas

General considerations

Recurrence is still the rule in atypical and malignant meningiomas. Recurrence can be recognized clinically, by the appearance of new symptoms and signs or the worsening of preexisting ones, or it can be seen on brain imaging before it produces clinical symptoms. In the latter case, definite tumor progression should be documented on serial studies before therapeutic intervention is planned, because the growth rate of meningiomas can vary over time. Recurrence is local in the vast majority of patients but multiple intracranial lesions and even extracranial metastases have been reported.[125,126] Fourteen percent of benign meningiomas transform into atypical or anaplastic histology upon recurrence, and 26% of atypical tumors.

Certain factors are very important in determining the likelihood, and the time, of recurrence of a given tumor. The most important factors are the extent of surgical resection, male gender, and the location of the tumor, as mentioned above. Proliferation labeling indices have been used to predict recurrence in meningiomas. Various methods employing tissue samples and immunohistological markers have been proposed to estimate proliferation, namely flow cytometry, BrdU labeling index (LI), MIB-1 antibody staining to nuclear antigen Ki-67 and staining to PCNA.[127,128] Meningiomas with a BrdU LI >5% had a 100% recurrence rate, while tumors with an LI of 3–5% had a 55.6% recurrence rate.[129] Increasing BrdU LI in consecutive recurrences of a malignant meningioma has also been reported.[130] Ki-67 index over 4% has been associated with repeated recurrences.[131] Furthemore, high Ki-67 index indicates higher grade of meningioma.[132]

Surgery

Surgical resection is still the most effective treatment of recurrent meningiomas. With the availability of advanced brain imaging techniques, recurrences are diagnosed relatively early. Multiple surgical resections are not an unusual occurrence in patients with malignant meningiomas, especially those located at the base of the skull. Subsequent surgical resections are less likely to be more radical than the first one, because of the relentless infiltration of recurrent tumors into the surrounding neural and vascular structures. In addition, surgery produces fibrosis and other changes in the anatomy of the region, rendering subsequent surgeries technically more difficult. Typically, the time to next recurrence becomes shorter after each resection. In a large series of meningiomas, the mean interval between the first and second operations was 6 years, between second and third operations it was 3.4 years, and between fourth and fifth operations it was 1.6 years.[133] Further surgery may not be feasible in a significant portion of cases because of the location of the tumor or the poor general medical condition of the patient.

Radiation therapy

Considering currently available data, radiation therapy should be used after the first recurrence if it was not given initially. A recent study suggested that for any postoperative tumor remnant, radiosurgery can be administered. For those remnants too large for radiosurgery or if another operation is not planned, radiotherapy should be administered.[115] Stafford *et al.* in a series of 206 recurrent or residual meningiomas treated with stereotactic radiosurgery reported a 93% 5-year local control rate in benign and 68% in atypical meningiomas.[134] For parasagittal meningioma, radiosurgery resulted in 60% 5-year control rates for recurrent and 93% for residual disease.[135] A recent metaanalysis revealed that with SRS, the overall disease stabilization rate was 89.0%, while the overall complication rate was 7.0%.[136] Brachytherapy was also used in the treatment of meningiomas, with good results.[137] For meningiomas that are not suitable candidates for radiosurgery, resection followed by permanent brachytherapy has been

employed as a potential salvage treatment. However, the complication rate was high.[138]

Chemotherapy

Treatment with various chemotherapeutic agents has been tried for patients with recurrent, unresectable, previously irradiated meningiomas but has been largely ineffective.[139] Scattered reports are available, however, on the efficacy of chemotherapy in individual cases.[140] The experience of the MD Anderson Cancer Center using ifosfamide/mesna or dacarbazine/adriamycin regimens was not rewarding.[15] Early reports suggested that hydroxyurea may have some efficacy against meningioma cells *in vitro* and in clinical settings.[141–143] Larger subsequent studies suggested that although oral hydroxyurea has a stabilizing effect on recurrent or progressive meningiomas, it does not seem to be very effective against atypical meningiomas.[144–146] Temozolomide failed to show any efficacy in a series of 16 patients with refractory recurrent meningiomas.[147]

Hormonal therapy

Several factors suggest that sex hormones, that is, progesterone, estrogen, and androgen, may play a role in stimulating the growth of meningiomas, as mentioned above.[148] Mifepristone (RU 486), an antiprogesterone agent, was shown to inhibit the growth of meningioma cells *in vitro*.[149] In the clinical setting, mifepristone resulted in minor meningioma regression, especially in male and premenopausal female patients.[150] Although the expression of ERs is less consistent, tamoxifen, an antiestrogen agent, induced transient stabilization or minor response in nine of 10 patients with recurrent unresectable meningiomas.[151] Somatostatin analogs arrested the progression of unresectable or recurrent benign meningiomas of the skull base in some patients but their efficacy in atypical or malignant meningiomas has not yet been established.[152]

Interferon-α

There has been *in vitro* and *in vivo* evidence suggesting that IFN-α may be active against meningiomas. Koper *et al.*[153] reported that adding low concentrations of IFN-α to meningioma cell cultures produced a 70–100% inhibition of thymidine DNA incorporation. Bergstrom *et al.*[154] observed an inhibitory effect of IFN-α on the metabolism of meningiomas as measured by PET, which was associated with decreased tumor growth rate in some patients. In addition, IFN-α has been shown to have a moderate antiangiogenic activity, which may be important in highly vascular tumors such as meningioma.[155,156] Wober-Bingol *et al.*[157] reported a marked effect of IFN-α2b on one patient with meningioma. We reported a positive response in five of six patients with recurrent unresectable meningiomas who were treated with recombinant IFN-α2b. Two of these meningiomas were histologically benign, one was atypical, and three were malignant.[158]

More patients have been treated with IFN since this publication, eight of them with atypical or malignant tumors. Five of the eight patients experienced remissions lasting 6–14 months,

Table 55.3 The effects of interferon (IFN)-α2b on atypical and malignant meningiomas.

		Previous therapy				IFN-α treatment history			
Case	Histology	Number of surgical resections	Radiation therapy	Chemotherapy	RU 486	IFN daily dose (MU/m⁻²) (per week)	Persistent side-effects	Outcome	Duration of therapy (months)
1	Atypical	2	Yes	No	No	4 × 5	None	Lost to follow-up	14+
2	Atypical	2	Yes	No	No	4 × 5	None	Progressed	2
3	Malignant	4	Yes	Yes	No	4 × 5	Fatigue	Progressed*	12 + 12
4	Malignant	1	Yes	No	No	4 × 5	None	Progressed	N/A
5	Malignant	3	Yes	No	Yes	4 × 5	Leukopenia	Progressed	12
6	Malignant	1	No	No	No	4 × 5	Fatigue	Stable	13+
7	Malignant	2	Yes	No	No	5 × 3	Fatigue	Stable†	2+
8	Malignant	5	Yes	No	No	4 × 5	None	Stable	6+

* Tumor recurred only after stopping interferon, and was stable for another year after resuming IFN postoperatively.
† Interferon therapy stopped because of toxicity despite stable tumor; MU, million units.

and two are still on therapy. In two patients, the tumor continued to grow despite therapy, and one patient elected to stop the treatment after 2 months despite the observed stabilization of the tumor. The toxicity associated with prolonged use of IFN-α was moderate and generally well tolerated (Yung et al., personal communication). These results are illustrated in Table 55.3. Other similar studies confirmed these findings. Muhr et al. reported stabilization in the size of the tumor in nine of 12 patients. Three of the nine patients were followed for relatively long times (8, 8, and 4.5 years). Two of these patients are still stable on therapy.[159] Furthermore, [¹¹C]-L-methionine PET scans done on these patients were able to predict responses and the suitability of patient for long-term treatment.

These results suggest that IFN-α can produce long-lasting remissions in rapidly progressing atypical and malignant meningioma, and may represent a valid therapeutic option for patients with recurrent or unresectable tumors.

Extracranial metastases of meningioma

Extracranial metastases of meningiomas are well documented, occurring usually with local recurrence of the tumor.[160] Metastases to all organ systems have been reported but the most common sites are lung (35%), bone (17%), liver (13%), and lymph nodes (11%).[161] Dissemination of the tumor through the cerebrospinal fluid (CSF) can also occur, producing tumor depositions in the spinal cord and other cerebral locations.[162] Although most metastases are associated with histologically malignant meningiomas, occasional cases have been reported with atypical or even "benign" meningiomas.[163,164] The rate of distant metastases ranged between 3% and 16% of atypical and malignant meningiomas and 13–41% of papillary meningiomas.[165] There are no clear guidelines for the treatment of metastatic meningiomas. Radiotherapy, chemotherapy, and biological therapy can be used in different combinations depending on the individual circumstances. Long-term survival after distant metastases has been reported but is not the rule.

Prognosis

Five-year survival for typical meningiomas exceeds 80% but is poorer (<60%) in malignant and atypical meningiomas.[166] As discussed earlier in this chapter, most patients with high-grade meningiomas will experience multiple recurrences and death as a result of local invasion. The 5-year recurrence rates are 38% and 78% and median time to first recurrence is 2.4 and 3.5 years in atypical and malignant meningiomas, respectively.[5] The recurrence rate in papillary meningioma is 59%.[12] Most patients undergo multiple surgical resections and sustain variable degrees of neurological dysfunction. Loss of vision in one eye, ophthalmoplegia, seizures, and hemiparesis are a few of the common sequelae of tumor invasion and repeated craniotomies. Durand et al. reported that in grade II meningiomas, the 5- and 10-year overall survival rates were 78.4% and 53.3%, respectively, while for patients with malignant meningiomas, the corresponding values were 44.0% and 14.2%.[167] With the advent of new radiation techniques and medical treatments, it is our hope that long-term control, and even cure, will be possible.

Hemangiopericytoma

The term "angioblastic meningioma" was widely used in the 1940s to describe a meningeal tumor that is highly vascularized and has a malignant aggressive course. Around the same time, a malignant and vascular soft tissue sarcoma, composed of cells resembling capillary pericytes, was described and called hemangiopericytoma. Later it was recognized that angioblastic meningiomas are simply hemangiopericytomas originating from the meninges.[168,169] In the WHO classification, meningeal hemangiopericytomas are classified as mesenchymal nonmeningothelial tumors.

Hemangiopericytomas are usually attached to the dura, not encapsulated, and sometimes invade the brain parenchyma. Histologically, they are composed of uniform polygonal cells with large hyperchromatic nuclei. These cells are arranged in sheets around abundant branching blood vessels. These tumors are highly vascular and often hemorrhagic. Mitotic figures, anaplastic cells, and focal necrosis are common features, while the typical meningothelial features are usually absent. Strong immunohistochemical staining for reticulin helps distinguish these tumors from meningiomas.

Meningeal hemangiopericytomas are rare, with an incidence of 2–4% of meningiomas.[32] They occur more commonly in males in the third or fourth decade of life.[170] These tumors occur in the convexity, tentorium, posterior fossa, and spine, mimicking meningiomas in appearance and presentation. The period between presenting symptoms and diagnosis is typically shorter than for meningiomas.

Radical surgical resection with amputation of all meningeal attachments is the treatment of choice. Recently a systematic review showed that the overall median survival was 13 years, with 1-, 5-, 10-, and 20-year survival rates of 95%, 82%, 60%, and 23%, respectively. Gross-total resection was associated with superior survival rates. Postoperative adjuvant radiation does not confer a survival benefit. Patients receiving over 50 Gy of radiation had worse survival outcomes. Furthermore, patients with posterior fossa tumors had a median survival of 10.75 versus 15.6 years for those with tumors located elsewhere.[171] At recurrence, further surgical resection or stereotactic radiosurgery can be offered. Chemotherapy was not effective in most reported cases.[172]

Recommendations

Patients of advanced age or poor surgical candidates with asymptomatic small benign meningiomas should be followed without therapy. In symptomatic patients complete surgical resection should be attempted, which is often curative. For incompletely resected benign tumors, radiosurgery or close follow-up is recommended. Radiosurgery or external radiotherapy should be considered in unresectable tumors. For recurrent, previously completely or incompletely resected tumors, re-resection is recommended followed by radiosurgery or external radiotherapy. Atypical and malignant meningiomas should be maximally resected followed by radiosurgery if there is residual tumor and must be carefully observed for early signs of recurrence. In malignant meningiomas, postoperative adjuvant radiotherapy is effective in decreasing recurrence rates and may be considered in addition to surgery and radiosurgery. The management of recurrent atypical and malignant meningiomas should be individualized and apart from surgery, may include either radiosurgery or limited field external radiotherapy if it was not given initially. Chemotherapy should be reserved for selected cases.

References

1. Alexiou GA, *et al*. Intracranial meningiomas in children: report of 8 cases. Pediatr Neurosurg 2008; 44: 373.
2. Lantos PL, Vandenberg SR, Kleihues P. Tumors of the nervous system. In: Graham DI, Lantos PL (eds) *Greenfield's Neuropathology*, 6th edn. London: Arnold, 1997. p.583.
3. Rigau V, *et al*. French brain tumor database: 5-year histological results on 25,756 cases. Brain Pathol. 2011; 21(6): 633.
4. Central Brain Tumor Registry of the United States. CBTRUS First Annual Report. Chicago: Central Brain Tumor Registry of the United States, 1995.
5. Longstreth WT Jr, *et al*. Epidemiology of intracranial meningioma. Cancer 1993; 72: 639.
6. Alexiou GA, *et al*. Epidemiology of pediatric brain tumors in Greece (1991–2008). Experience from the Agia Sofia Children's Hospital. Cen Eur Neurosurg. 2011; 72: 1.
7. Voulgaris S, *et al*. Posterior approach to ventrally located spinal meningiomas. Eur Spine J 2010; 19: 1195.
8. Jaaskelainen J, Haltia M, Servo A. Atypical and anaplastic meningiomas: radiology, surgery, radiotherapy, and outcome. Surg Neurol 1986; 25: 233.
9. Mahmood A, *et al*. Atypical and malignant meningiomas: a clinicopathological review. Neurosurgery 1993; 33: 955.
10. Bondy M, Ligon BL. Epidemiology and etiology of intracranial meningiomas: a review. J Neurooncol 1996; 29: 197.
11. Alexiou GA, *et al*. Genetic and molecular alterations in meningiomas. Clin Neurol Neurosurg 2011; 113: 261.
12. Koppelmans V, *et al*. Incidental findings on brain magnetic resonance imaging in long-term survivors of breast cancer treated with adjuvant chemotherapy. Eur J Cancer 2011; 47(17): 2531.
13. Koehorst SG, *et al*. Detection of an oestrogen receptor-like protein in human meningiomas by band shift assay using a synthetic oestrogen responsive element (ERE). Br J Cancer 1993; 68: 290.
14. Carroll RS, *et al*. Progesterone and glucocorticoid receptor activation in meningiomas. Neurosurgery 1995; 37: 92.
15. Kyritsis AP. Chemotherapy for meningiomas. J Neurooncol 1996; 29: 269.
16. Custer B, *et al*. Hormonal exposures and the risk of intracranial meningioma in women: a population-based case-control study. BMC Cancer 2006; 6: 152.
17. Pravdenkova S, *et al*. Progesterone and estrogen receptors: opposing prognostic indicators in meningiomas. J Neurosurg 2006; 105: 163.
18. Hirota Y, *et al*. Gonadotropin-releasing hormone (GnRH) and its receptor in human meningiomas. Clin Neurol Neurosurg 2009; 111: 127.
19. Lee G, Ge B. Growth inhibition of tumor cells in vitro by using monoclonal antibodies against gonadotropin-releasing hormone receptor. Cancer Immunol Immunother 2010; 59: 1011–19.
20. Andersson U, *et al*. Epidermal growth factor receptor family (EGFR, ErbB2-4) in gliomas and meningiomas. Acta Neuropathol 2004; 108: 135–42.
21. Norden AD, *et al*. Phase II trials of erlotinib or gefitinib in patients with recurrent meningioma. J Neurooncol 2010; 96: 211–17.
22. Nagashima G, *et al*. Involvement of disregulated c-myc but not c-sis/PDGF at atypical and anaplastic meningiomas. Clin Neurol Neurosurg 2001; 103: 13–18.
23. Wen PY, *et al*. Phase II study of imatinib mesylate for recurrent meningiomas (North American Brain Tumor Consortium study 01-08). Neuro Oncol 2009; 11: 853–60.
24. Takahashi JA, *et al*. Gene expression of fibroblast growth factors in human gliomas and meningiomas: demonstration of cellular source of basic fibroblast growth factor mRNA and peptide in tumor tissues. Proc Nat Acad Sci USA 1990; 87: 5710.
25. Jensen RL, *et al*. In vitro growth inhibition of growth factor-stimulated meningioma cells by calcium channel antagonists. Neurosurgery 1995; 36: 365.
26. Johnson MD, *et al*. Fibroblast growth factor receptor-3 expression in meningiomas with stimulation of proliferation by the phosphoinositide 3 kinase-Akt pathway. J Neurosurg 2010; 112: 934–9.
27. Lamszus K, *et al*. Vascular endothelial growth factor, hepatocyte growth factor/scatter factor, basic fibroblast growth factor, and placenta growth factor in human meningiomas and their relation to angiogenesis and malignancy. Neurosurgery 2000; 46: 938–47.
28. Ding YS, *et al*. Expression of vascular endothelial growth factor in human meningiomas and peritumoral brain areas. Ann Clin Lab Sci 2008; 38: 344–51.
29. Puchner MJ, *et al*. Bevacizumab-induced regression of anaplastic meningioma. Ann Oncol 2010; 21: 2445–6.
30. Arena S, *et al*. Expression of somatostatin receptor mRNA in human meningiomas and their implication in in vitro antiproliferative activity. J Neurooncol 2004; 66: 155–66.
31. Chamberlain MC, Glantz MJ, Fadul CE. Recurrent meningioma: salvage therapy with long-acting somatostatin analogue. Neurology 2007; 69: 969–73.

32. Louis DN, *et al.* The 2007 WHO classification of tumours of the central nervous system. Acta Neuropathol 2007; 114: 97–109.

33. Hoshino T, *et al.* S-phase fraction of human brain tumors in situ measured by uptake of bromodeoxyuridine. Int J Cancer 1986; 38: 369.

34. Miyagami M, *et al.* Analysis of the proliferative potential of meningiomas with MIB-1 monoclonal antibodies. No to Shinkei 1996; 48: 39.

35. Cobb MA, *et al.* Significance of proliferating cell nuclear antigen in predicting recurrence of intracranial meningioma. J Neurosurg 1996; 84: 85.

36. Ludwin SK, Rubinstein LJ, Russell DS. Papillary meningioma: a malignant variant of meningioma. Cancer 1975; 36: 1363.

37. Pasquier B, *et al.* Papillary meningioma. Clinicopathologic study of seven cases and review of the literature. Cancer 1986; 58: 299.

38. Umansky F, *et al.* Radiation-induced meningioma. Neurosurg Focus 2008; 24: E7.

39. Alexiou GA, *et al.* Anaplastic oligodendrogliomas after treatment of acute lymphoblastic leukemia in children: report of 2 cases. J Neurosurg Pediatr 2010; 5: 179–83.

40. Banerjee J, *et al.* Radiation-induced meningiomas: a shadow in the success story of childhood leukemia. Neuro Oncol. 2009; 11: 543–9.

41. Goshen Y, *et al.* High incidence of meningioma in cranial irradiated survivors of childhood acute lymphoblastic leukemia. Pediatr Blood Cancer 2007; 49: 294–7.

42. Ghim TT, *et al.* Childhood intracranial meningiomas after high-dose irradiation. Cancer 1993; 71: 4091.

43. François P, *et al.* Post-traumatic meningioma: three case reports of this rare condition and a review of the literature. Acta Neurochir (Wien) 2010; 152: 1755–60.

44. Annegers JF, *et al.* Head trauma and subsequent brain tumors. Neurosurgery 1979; 4: 203.

45. Lee Y, *et al.* Genomic landscape of meningiomas. Brain Pathol 2010; 20: 751–62.

46. Gabeau-Lacet D, *et al.* Genomic profiling of atypical meningiomas associates gain of 1q with poor clinical outcome. J Neuropathol Exp Neurol 2009; 68: 1155–65.

47. Poulsgard L, Schroder HD, Ronne M. Cytogenetic studies of 11 meningiomas and their clinical significance. II. Anticancer Res 1990; 10: 535.

48. Maillo A, *et al.* Gains of chromosome 22 by fluorescence in situ hybridization in the context of an hyperdiploid karyotype are associated with aggressive clinical features in meningioma patients. Cancer 2001; 92: 377–85.

49. Menon AG, *et al.* Frequent loss of chromosome 14 in atypical and malignant meningioma: identification of a putative 'tumor progression' locus. Oncogene 1997; 14: 611.

50. Cai DX, *et al.* Chromosome 1p and 14q FISH analysis in clinicopathologic subsets of meningioma: diagnostic and prognostic implications. J Neuropathol Exp Neurol 2001; 60: 628–36.

51. Tabernero MD, *et al.* Characterization of chromosome 14 abnormalities by interphase in situ hybridization and comparative genomic hybridization in 124 meningiomas: correlation with clinical, histopathologic, and prognostic features. Am J Clin Pathol 2005; 123: 744–51.

52. Lomas J, *et al.* Methylation status of TP73 in meningiomas. Cancer Genet Cytogenet 2004; 148: 148–51.

53. Pérez-Magán E, *et al.* Differential expression profiling analyses identifies downregulation of 1p, 6q, and 14q genes and overexpression of 6p histone cluster 1 genes as markers of recurrence in meningiomas. Neuro Oncol 2010; 12: 1278–90.

54. Vagner-Capodano AM, *et al.* Correlation between cytogenetic and histopathological findings in 75 human meningiomas. Neurosurgery 1993; 32: 892.

55. Rempel SA, *et al.* Loss of heterozygosity for loci on chromosome 10 is associated with morphologically malignant meningioma progression. Cancer Res 1993; 53: 2386.

56. Mihaila D, *et al.* Meningiomas: loss of heterozygosity on chromosome 10 and marker-specific correlations with grade, recurrence, and survival. Clin Cancer Res 2003; 9: 4443–51.

57. Maillo A, *et al.* New classification scheme for the prognostic stratification of meningioma on the basis of chromosome 14 abnormalities, patient age, and tumor histopathology. J Clin Oncol 2003; 21: 3285–95.

58. Rajcan-Separovic E, *et al.* Loss of 1p and 7p in radiation-induced meningiomas identified by comparative genomic hybridization. Cancer Genet Cytogenet 2003; 144: 6–11.

59. Hartmann C, *et al.* NF2 mutations in secretory and other rare variants of meningiomas. Brain Pathol 2006; 16: 15–19.

60. Gutmann DH, *et al.* Loss of DAL-1, a protein 4.1-related tumor suppressor, is an important early event in the pathogenesis of meningiomas. Hum Mol Genet 2000; 9: 1495–500.

61. Perry A, *et al.* Merlin, DAL-1, and progesterone receptor expression in clinicopathologic subsets of meningioma: a correlative immunohistochemical study of 175 cases. J Neuropathol Exp Neurol 2000; 59: 872–9.

62. Carstens C, *et al.* Human KRAS oncogene expression in meningioma. Cancer Lett 1988; 43: 37.

63. Smidt M, Kirsch I, Ratner L. Deletion of Alu sequences in the fifth c-sis intron in individuals with meningiomas. J Clin Invest 1990; 86: 1151.

64. Kazumoto K, *et al.* Enhanced expression of the sis and c-myc oncogenes in human meningiomas. J Neurosurg 1990; 72: 786.

65. Mashiyama S, *et al.* Detection of p53 gene mutations in human brain tumors by single-strand conformation polymorphism analysis of polymerase chain reaction products. Oncogene 1991; 6: 1313.

66. Amatya VJ, Takeshima Y, Inai K. Methylation of p14(ARF) gene in meningiomas and its correlation to the p53 expression and mutation. Mod Pathol 2004; 17: 705–10.

67. Abramovich CM, Prayson RA. Apoptotic activity and bcl-2 immunoreactivity in meningiomas. Association with grade and outcome. Am J Clin Pathol 2000; 114: 84–92.

68. Li J, *et al.* The PTEN/MMAC1 tumor suppressor induces cell death that is rescued by the AKT/protein kinase B oncogene. Cancer Res 1998; 58: 5667–72.

69. Peters N, *et al* . Analysis of the PTEN gene in human meningiomas. Neuropathol Appl Neurobiol 1998; 24: 3–8.

70. Mawrin C, *et al.* Different activation of mitogen-activated protein kinase and Akt signaling is associated with aggressive phenotype of human meningiomas. Clin Cancer Res 2005; 11: 4074–82.

71. Lusis E, Gutmann D. Meningioma: an update. Curr Opin Neurol 2004; 17: 687–92.

72. Chen HJ, *et al.* Implication of telomerase activity and alternations of telomere length in the histologic characteristics of intracranial meningiomas. Cancer 2000; 89: 2092–8.

73. Maes L, *et al.* Telomerase activity and hTERT protein expression in meningiomas: an analysis in vivo versus in vitro. Anticancer Res 2006; 26: 2295–300.

74. Maes L, *et al.* Progression of astrocytomas and meningiomas: an evaluation in vitro. Cell Prolif 2007; 40: 14–23.

75. Almeida LO, *et al.* Polymorphisms and DNA methylation of gene TP53 associated with extra-axial brain tumors. Genet Mol Res 2009; 8: 8–18.

76. Jun P, *et al.* Epigenetic silencing of the kinase tumor suppressor WNK2 is tumor-type and tumor-grade specific. Neuro Oncol 2009; 11: 414–22.

77. Rohringer M, *et al.* Incidence and clinicopathological features of meningioma. J Neurosurg 1989; 71: 665.

78. Alexiou GA, *et al.* Management of meningiomas. Clin Neurol Neurosurg 2010; 112: 177–82.

79. Kane AJ, *et al.* Anatomic location is a risk factor for atypical and malignant meningiomas. Cancer 2011; 117: 1272–8.

80. DeMonte F, al-Mefty O. Meningiomas. In: Kaye AH, Laws ER (eds) *Brain Tumors*. New York: Churchill Livingstone, 1995. p. 675.

81. Younis GA, *et al.* Aggressive meningeal tumors: review of a series. J Neurosurg 1995; 82: 17.

82. Zee CS, *et al.* Magnetic resonance imaging of meningiomas. Semin Ultrasound CT MR 1992; 13: 154–69.

83. Modha A, Gutin PH. Diagnosis and treatment of atypical and anaplastic meningiomas: a review. Neurosurgery 2005; 57: 538–50

84. Hsu CC, *et al.* Do aggressive imaging features correlate with advanced histopathological grade in meningiomas? J Clin Neurosci 2010; 17: 584–7.

85. Alexiou GA, *et al.* Assessment of glioma proliferation using imaging modalities. J Clin Neurosci 2010; 17: 1233–8.

86. Hakyemez B, *et al*. The contribution of diffusion-weighted MR imaging to distinguishing typical from atypical meningiomas. Neuroradiology 2006; 48: 513–20.

87. Toh CH, *et al*. Differentiation between classic and atypical meningiomas with use of diffusion tensor imaging. Am J Neuroradiol 2008; 29: 1630–5.

88. Zhang H, *et al*. Perfusion MR imaging for differentiation of benign and malignant meningiomas. Neuroradiology 2008; 50: 525–30.

89. Chernov MF, *et al*. ¹H-MRS of intracranial meningiomas: what can it add to known clinical and MRI predictors of the histopathological and biological characteristics of the tumor? Clin Neurol Neurosurg 2011; 113: 202–12.

90. Di Chiro G, *et al*. Glucose utilization by intracranial meningiomas as an index of tumor aggressivity and probability of recurrence: a PET study. Radiology 1987; 164: 521.

91. Cremerius U, *et al*. Fasting improves discrimination of grade 1 and atypical or malignant meningioma in FDG-PET. J Nucl Med 1997; 38: 26.

92. Lippitz B, *et al*. PET-study of intracranial meningiomas: correlation with histopathology, cellularity and proliferation rate. Acta Neurochir 1996; 65(Suppl): 108–11.

93. Lee JW, *et al*. 18F-FDG PET in the assessment of tumor grade and prediction of tumor recurrence in intracranial meningioma. Eur J Nucl Med Mol Imaging 2009; 36: 1574–82.

94. Liu RS, *et al*. 1-11C-acetate versus 18F-FDG PET in detection of meningioma and monitoring the effect of gamma-knife radiosurgery. J Nucl Med 2010; 51: 883–91.

95. Tedeschi E, *et al*. Different thallium-201 single-photon emission tomographic patterns in benign and aggressive meningiomas. Eur J Nucl Med 1996; 23: 1478–84.

96. Kinuya K, *et al*. Thallium-201 brain SPECT to diagnose aggressiveness of meningiomas. Ann Nucl Med 2003; 17: 463–7.

97. Takeda T, *et al*. Usefulness of thallium-201 SPECT in the evaluation of tumor natures in intracranial meningiomas. Neuroradiology 2011; 53(11): 867–73.

98. Alexiou G, *et al*. Single-photon emission computed tomography in the evaluation of brain tumors and the diagnosis of relapse vs radiation necrosis. Hell J Nucl Med 2007; 10: 205–8.

99. Alexiou GA, *et al*. Influence of glioma's multidrug resistance phenotype on (99m)Tc-tetrofosmin uptake. Mol Imaging Biol 2011; 13(2): 348–52.

100. Fotopoulos AD, *et al*. Characterization of intracranial space-occupying lesions by (99m)Tc-tetrofosmin SPECT. J Neurooncol 2011; 101(1): 83–9.

101. Fotopoulos AD, *et al*. (99m)Tc-tetrofosmin brain SPECT in the assessment of meningiomas – correlation with histological grade and proliferation index. J Neurooncol 2008; 89: 225–30.

102. Alexiou GA, *et al*. Correlation of glioma proliferation assessed by flow cytometry with (99m)Tc-tetrofosmin SPECT uptake. Clin Neurol Neurosurg 2009; 111: 808–11.

103. Gardner PA, *et al*. Endoscopic endonasal resection of anterior cranial base meningiomas. Neurosurgery 2008; 63: 36–52.

104. Dehdashti AR, *et al*. Expanded endoscopic endonasal approach for anterior cranial base and suprasellar lesions: indications and limitations. Neurosurgery 2009; 64: 677–87.

105. Philippon J, Cornu P. The recurrence of meningiomas. In: al-Mefty O (ed) *Meningiomas*. New York: Raven Press, 1991. p.87.

106. Palma L, *et al*. Long-term prognosis for atypical and malignant meningiomas: a study of 71 surgical cases. J Neurosurg 1997; 86: 793

107. Aghi MK, *et al*. Long-term recurrence rates of atypical meningiomas after gross total resection with or without postoperative adjuvant radiation. Neurosurgery 2009; 64: 56–60.

108. Sughrue ME, *et al*. Outcome and survival following primary and repeat surgery for World Health Organization Grade III meningiomas. J Neurosurg 2010; 113: 202–9.

109. Barbaro NM, *et al*. Radiation therapy in the treatment of partially resected meningiomas. Neurosurgery 1987; 20: 525.

110. Chan MD, *et al*. Radiation oncology in brain tumors: current approaches and clinical trials in progress. Neuroimaging Clin North Am 2010; 20: 401–8.

111. Milosevic MF, *et al*. Radiotherapy for atypical or malignant intracranial meningioma. Int J Radiat Oncol Biol Phys 1996; 34: 817.

112. Shimizu T, Iijima M, Tanaka Y. Radiotherapy for intracranial meningioma: special reference to malignant and high risk benign meningioma. Nippon Igaku Hoshaen Gakkai Zasshi 1995; 55: 1047.

113. Chamberlain MC. Adjuvant combined modality therapy for malignant meningiomas. J Neurosurg 1996; 84: 753.

114. Yang SY, *et al*. Atypical and anaplastic meningiomas: prognostic implications of clinicopathological features. J Neurol Neurosurg Psychiatry 2008; 79: 574–80.

115. Mair R, *et al*. Radiotherapy for atypical meningiomas. J Neurosurg 2011; 115(4): 811–819.

116. Pollock BE, *et al*. Stereotactic radiosurgery provides equivalent tumor control to Simpson Grade 1 resection for patients with small-to medium size meningiomas. Int J Radiat Oncol Biol Phys 2003; 55: 1000–5.

117. Santacroce A, *et al*. Long term tumor control of benign intracranial meningiomas after radiosurgery in a series of 4565 patients. Neurosurgery 2012; 70(1): 32–9.

118. Adler JR Jr, *et al*. Visual field preservation after multisession cyberknife radiosurgery for perioptic lesions. Neurosurgery 2006; 59: 244–54.

119. Milker-Zabel S, Zabel-du Bois A, Huber P, Schlegel W, Debus J. Intensity-modulated radiotherapy for complex-shaped meningioma of the skull base: long-term experience of a single institution. Int J Radiat Oncol Biol Phys 2007; 68: 858–63.

120. Taut FJ, Zeller WJ. In vitro chemotherapy of steroid receptor positive human meningioma low-passage primary cultures with nitrosoureamethionine-steroid conjugates. Clin Neuropharmacol 1996; 19: 520.

121. Tsuchida T, *et al*. Chemosensitivity of cultured meningiomas. Hum Cell 1995; 8: 155.

122. Lunsford DL. Contemporary management of meningiomas: radiation therapy as an adjuvant and radiosurgery as an alternative to surgical removal? J Neurosurg 1994; 80: 187–90.

123. Mason WP, *et al*. Stabilization of disease progression by hydroxyurea in patients with recurrent or unresectable meningioma. J Neurosurg 2002; 97: 341–6.

124. Weston GJ, *et al*. Hydroxyurea treatment of meningiomas: a pilot study. Skull Base 2006; 16: 157–60.

125. Russell T, Moss T. Metastasizing meningioma. Neurosurgery 1986; 19: 1028.

126. Philippon J, *et al*. Recurrent meningioma. Neurochirurgie 1986; 32: 1.

127. Quiñones-Hinojosa A, *et al*. Techniques to assess the proliferative potential of brain tumors. J Neurooncol 2005; 74: 19–30.

128. Prayson R. The utility of MIB-1/Ki-67 immunostaining in the evaluation of central nervous system neoplasms. Adv Anat Pathol 2005; 12: 144–8.

129. Hoshino T, *et al*. Proliferative potential of human meningiomas of the brain. A cell kinetics study with bromodeoxyuridine. Cancer 1986; 58: 1466.

130. Kakinuma K, *et al*. Proliferative potential of recurrent intracranial meningiomas as evaluated by labelling indices of BUdR and Ki-67, and tumour doubling time. Acta Neurochir (Wien) 1998; 140: 26–31.

131. Abry E, *et al*. The significance of Ki-67/MIB-1 labeling index in man meningiomas: a literature study. Pathol Res Pract 2010; 206: 810–15.

132. Babu S, *et al*. Meningiomas: correlation of Ki67 with histological grade. Neurol India 2011; 59: 204–7.

133. Boker DK, Meurer H, Gullotta F. Recurring intracranial meningiomas. Evaluation of some factors predisposing for tumor recurrence. J Neurosurg Sci 1985; 29: 11.

134. Stafford SL, *et al*. Meningioma radiosurgery: tumor control, outcomes, and complications among 190 consecutive patients. Neurosurgery 2001; 49: 1029–37.

135. Kondziolka D, Flickinger JC, Perez B. Judicious resection and/or radiosurgery for parasagittal meningiomas: outcomes from a multicenter review. Gamma Knife Meningioma Study Group. Neurosurgery 1998; 43: 405–13.

136. Pannullo SC, *et al*. Stereotactic radiosurgery: a meta-analysis of current therapeutic applications in neuro-oncologic disease. J Neurooncol 2011; 103: 1–17.

137. Vuorinen V, *et al*. Interstitial radiotherapy of 25 parasellar/clival meningiomas and 19 meningiomas in the elderly. Analysis of short-term tolerance and responses. Acta Neurochir 1996; 138: 495.

138. Ware ML, *et al*. Surgical resection and permanent brachytherapy for recurrent atypical and malignant meningioma. Neurosurgery 2004; 54: 55–63.

139. Stewart DJ, *et al*. Intraarterial cisplatin plus intravenous doxorubicin for inoperable recurrent meningiomas. J Neurooncol 1995; 24: 189.

140. Bernstein M, *et al*. Necrosis in a meningioma following systemic chemotherapy. Case report. J Neuro-surg 1994; 81: 284.

141. Dashti SR, *et al*. Nonsurgical treatment options in the management of intracranial meningiomas. Front Biosci (Elite Ed) 2009; 1: 494–500.

142. Schrell UM, *et al*. Hydroxyurea for treatment of unresectable and recurrent meningiomas. I. Inhibition of primary human meningioma cells in culture and in meningioma transplants by induction of the apoptotic pathway. J Neurosurg 1997; 86: 845.

143. Schrell UM, *et al*. Hydroxyurea for treatment of unresectable and recurrent meningiomas. II. Decrease in the size of meningiomas in patients treated with hydroxyurea. J Neurosurg 1997; 86: 840.

144. Mason WP, *et al*. Stabilization of disease progression by hydroxyurea in patients with recurrent or unresectable meningioma. J Neurosurg 2002; 97: 341–6.

145. Newton HB, Slivka MA, Stevens C. Hydroxyurea chemotherapy for unresectable or residual meningioma. J Neurooncol 2000; 49: 165–70.

146. Chamberlain MC, Johnston SK. Hydroxyurea for recurrent surgery and radiation refractory meningioma: a retrospective case series. J Neurooncol 2011; 104(3): 765–71.

147. Chamberlain MC, Tsao-Wei DD, Groshen S. Temozolomide for treatment-resistant recurrent meningioma. Neurology 2004; 62: 1210–12.

148. Sioka C, Kyritsis AP. Chemotherapy, hormonal therapy, and immunotherapy for recurrent meningiomas. J Neurooncol 2009; 92: 1–6.

149. Grunberg SM. Role of antiprogestational therapy for meningiomas. Hum Reprod 1994; 9: 202.

150. Grunberg SM, *et al*. Long-term administration of mifepristone (RU486): clinical tolerance during extended treatment of meningioma. Cancer Invest 2006; 24: 727–33.

151. Goodwin JW, *et al*. A phase II evaluation of tamoxifen in unresectable or refractory meningiomas: a Southwest Oncology Group study. JNO 1993; 15: 75.

152. Schulz C, *et al*. Treatment of unresectable skull base meningiomas with somatostatin analogs. Neurosurg Focus 2011; 30: E11.

153. Koper JW, *et al*. Inhibition of the growth of cultured human meningioma cells by recombinant interferon-alpha. Eur J Cancer 1991; 27: 416.

154. Bergstrom M, *et al*. Modulation of tumor metabolism using hormonally acting drugs in patients with meningioma. J Endocrinol Invest 1989; 12(Suppl 2): 91.

155. Li VW, *et al*. Microvessel count and cerebral fluid basic fibroblast growth factor in children with brain tumours. Lancet 1994; 344: 82.

156. Folkman J, Klagsburn M. Angiogenic factors. Science 1987; 235: 442.

157. Wober-Bingol C, *et al*. Interferon-alfa-2b for meningioma. Lancet 1995; 345: 331.

158. Kaba SE, *et al*. The treatment of recurrent unresectable and malignant meningiomas with interferon alpha-2B. Neurosurgery 1997; 40: 271–5.

159. Muhr C, *et al*. Meningioma treated with interferon-alpha, evaluated with [(11)C]-L-methionine positron emission tomography. Clin Cancer Res 2001; 7: 2269–76.

160. Salcman M. Malignant meningiomas. In: al-Mefty O (ed) *Meningiomas*. New York: Raven Press, 1991. p.75.

161. Teague SD, Conces DJ Jr. Metastatic meningioma to the lungs. J Thorac Imaging 2005; 20: 58–60.

162. Kleinschmidt-DeMasters BK, Avakian JJ. Wallenberg syndrome caused by CSF metastasis from malignant intraventricular meningioma. Clin Neuropathol 1985; 4: 214.

163. Som PM, *et al*. 'Benign' metastasizing meningiomas. Am J Neuroradiol 1987; 8: 127.

164. Miller DC, *et al*. Benign metastasizing meningioma. Case report. J Neurosurg 1985; 62: 763.

165. Fukushima T, *et al*. Papillary meningioma with pulmonary metastasis. Case report. J Neurosurg 1989; 70: 478.

166. Marosi C, *et al*. Meningioma. Crit Rev Oncol Hematol 2008; 67: 153–71.

167. Durand A, *et al*. WHO grade II and III meningiomas: a study of prognostic factors. J Neurooncol 2009; 95: 367–75.

168. Guthrie BL. Meningeal hemangiopericytomas. In: Kaye AH, Laws ER (eds) *Brain Tumors*. New York: Churchill Livingstone, 1995. p.705.

169. Begg CF, Garret R. Hemangiopericytoma occurring in the meninges. Cancer 1954; 7: 602.

170. Guthrie BL, *et al*. Meningeal hemangiopericytoma: histopathological features, treatment, and long-term follow-up of 44 cases. Neurosurgery 1989; 25: 514.

171. Rutkowski MJ, *et al*. Predictors of mortality following treatment of intracranial hemangiopericytoma. J Neurosurg 2010; 113: 333–9.

172. Borg MF, Benjamin CS. Haemangiopericytoma of the central nervous system. Australas Radiol 1995; 39: 36.

56 Primary Central Nervous System Lymphoma

Lisa M. DeAngelis

Department of Neurology, Memorial Sloan-Kettering Cancer Center; Department of Neurology and Neuroscience, Weill Cornell Medical College of Cornell University, New York, NY, USA

Introduction

Primary central nervous system lymphoma (PCNSL) was first described as perithelial sarcoma by Bailey.[1] It was subsequently classified as reticulum cell sarcoma because of the characteristic reticulum it deposited around blood vessels.[2] Later, it was described as a microglioma after the presumed cell of origin, the microglia.[3] Henry et al.[4] classified these tumors as primary malignant lymphomas of the central nervous system (CNS) because of their histological similarities to extraneural malignant lymphoma. The lymphoid nature of PCNSL was established unequivocally by modern immunohistochemical techniques.[5–8]

Epidemiology

Primary central nervous system lymphoma accounts for 1–2% of non-Hodgkin lymphoma (NHL) and at least 0.5–1.2% of all primary brain tumors.[9,10] The National Cancer Institute Surveillance, Epidemiology, and End Results (SEER) database revealed a three-fold increase in the incidence of PCNSL between 1973–1984 and 1985–1997 among presumed immunocompetent patients.[11] This increase reflected an overall increase in all extranodal lymphomas but the rise was proportionately greatest in the CNS. However, the rate of increase slowed after 1985. A second study demonstrated a decreased rate in patients over the age of 60 after 1995, although the rate remained elevated in younger patients.[12] The increased incidence has not been seen worldwide. Data from Denmark, Scotland, and Alberta, Canada, failed to show a significant change in the incidence of PCNSL in immunocompetent individuals,[13–15] raising the question of an environmental contribution to tumorigenesis. The reason for the apparent increased incidence in immunocompetent patients in the United States cannot be explained by better ascertainment or changes in tumor nosology.

Primary central nervous system lymphoma has been associated with a variety of congenital (Wiskott–Aldrich syndrome, ataxia-telangiectasia) and acquired (human immunodeficiency virus [HIV], renal transplant recipients) immunodeficiency states.[9,10,16] It is particularly common in HIV-infected individuals, where the incidence is 1.6–9.0%.[17,18] After toxoplasmosis, PCNSL is the second most common intracranial mass lesion found in HIV-infected patients. Prior to the introduction of the new anti-HIV agents, there was growing evidence that PCNSL was rising in the acquired immunodeficiency syndrome (AIDS) population.[19] However, the incidence of PCNSL in AIDS patients has fallen significantly since the introduction of highly active antiretroviral therapy (HAART) which helps restore immune function.[20]

Primary central nervous system lymphoma can also occur as a secondary malignancy in 7.9–13% of patients.[21,22] Median latency from initial tumor to diagnosis of PCNSL was 8 years.[22] Whether PCNSL develops as a consequence of genetic predisposition or prior antineoplastic treatment is not clear, although no patient received prior cranial radiotherapy (RT). Nonetheless, it is important to keep PCNSL in mind as a possible cause of an intracranial mass lesion in patients with a history of systemic cancer because treatment for brain metastasis differs markedly from treatment for PCNSL.

Pathology

Primary central nervous system lymphomas are usually diffuse intermediate or high-grade NHLs, the majority of which are diffuse large cell, large cell immunoblastic or lymphoblastic subtypes. Phenotypically, more than 95% are of B-cell origin, CD20+ (Fig. 56.1),[5–8,23] but T-cell tumors, CD3+ or CD45RO+, are occasionally reported.[24] Cytogenetic abnormalities in PCNSL have been reported involving chromosomes 1, 6, 7, and 14.[25] These abnormalities are similar to those seen in nodal B-cell lymphomas. Kumanishi et al.[26] reported p15 and p16 deletions on chromosome 9 by Southern blot analysis in four out of five PCNSL tumors.

Because PCNSL is confined to the nervous system, a single extranodal site, it is classified as a stage IE NHL; however, it

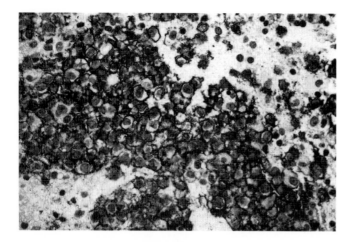

Figure 56.1 Immunohistochemistry of PCNSL showing CD20 positivity.

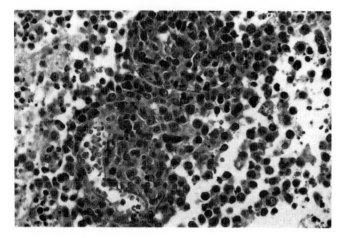

Figure 56.2 PCNSL hematoxylin and eosin stain showing angiocentricity.

can be disseminated throughout the nervous system, involving the brain, leptomeninges, spinal cord, or eyes.[5,16] There may be involvement of one or all of these structures, but PCNSL is usually manifest as a brain tumor. There is a single brain lesion in approximately 70% of immunocompetent individuals[8,27] but multifocal lesions are almost always seen in immunocompromised individuals.[27] PCNSL usually involves deep structures, frequently periventricular in location and often abutting the ventricles. Grossly, it is a soft, gray, ill-defined solid lesion. In immunocompetent patients, hemorrhage, cysts, and necrosis are rare but necrosis is frequently seen in AIDS-related PCNSL. Occasionally, extensive subependymal spread is seen. Microscopically, PCNSL is composed of large cells with round nuclei, vesicular chromatin, and prominent nucleoli; mitoses are frequently seen.[28] PCNSL is highly infiltrative, poorly demarcated, and angiocentric.[28] The latter is a characteristic feature where aggregates of cells surround blood vessels and infiltrate vessel walls without endothelial reaction or thrombosis (Fig. 56.2). Vascular proliferation is not seen. Small reactive T-lymphocytes, histiocytes, and reactive astrocytes are seen frequently.[28] PCNSL is usually leukocyte common antigen positive, which helps distinguish it from gliomas or carcinomas.[28] Ultrastructurally,

PCNSL lacks intermediate filaments, specific organelles, and intracellular junctions.[28]

Leptomeningeal infiltration is present in nearly all cases of parenchymal involvement[29] but is usually patchy. Cerebrospinal fluid (CSF) cytology is positive in 26% of patients, but 42% have demonstrable leptomeningeal involvement when pathological and radiographic examinations of the meninges are combined.[30] Primary leptomeningeal lymphoma is rare, accounting for only 7% of all PCNSL cases[31]; isolated dural-based lesions have also been reported.[32]

Ocular lymphoma typically involves the retina, choroid, or vitreous. Large gray patches of subretinal and retinal infiltrates or thickened choroid are seen on examination. Lymphoma cells are found between Bruch's membrane and the retinal pigment epithelium. Evaluation of vitreal specimens may show malignant lymphocytes along with reactive lymphocytes, histiocytes, necrotic debris, and fibrous material. Immuno-histochemistry for B-cell markers or identification of a monoclonal κ or λ light chain may be needed to make the diagnosis if standard cytology is inconclusive.[33]

The origin of the malignant lymphocytes in PCNSL is unknown because the tumor develops in an environment normally devoid of lymphoid tissue. There are several theoretical mechanisms.[5] The first suggests that a normal but reactive population of lymphocytes is attracted into the CNS where a second event then transforms a clone of the inflammatory cell population into neoplastic cells. However, the reactive lymphocytes that ordinarily traffic through the CNS are overwhelmingly T-cells, which does not explain this predominantly B-cell tumor. The second possibility is that extranodal B-lymphocytes, with a propensity for the CNS because of a CNS-specific binding marker, are activated; they then proliferate and transform into neoplastic cells. These cells migrate through the bloodstream into the CNS where they multiply and become tumors, with the original site of disease remaining obscure. There is no identifiable difference in the adhesion molecules and the integrins seen in PCNSL and systemic NHL, but there may be a CNS signature of upregulated genes that control the extracellular matrix and adhesion pathways.[34,35] A third possibility is that neoplastic lymphocytes in the periphery are eradicated but persist in the CNS because of poor immune surveillance.[27] There are no data to support any of these hypotheses and the pathogenesis of PCNSL remains unknown.

The pathogenesis of PCNSL in immunodeficient patients is better understood. The Epstein–Barr virus (EBV) plays an important role in initiating the development of PCNSL in immunocompromised patients. The EBV genome was found in 91% of AIDS-related PCNSLs and 100% of post-organ transplant patients; alternatively, EBV has been found in only 17% of PCNSL in immunocompetent patients.[36] In the normal host, EBV-driven B-cell lymphoproliferation is inhibited by T-cells. This control is absent in immunocompromised patients, thereby facilitating B-cell proliferation that can lead to an individual clone evolving into a malignancy. The CNS is a preferred site for EBV-driven lymphomas, presumably because of decreased immune surveillance. Some allogeneic bone marrow transplant recipients have had regression of their tumor when treated with donor cytotoxic T-lymphocytes, which reconstitutes T-cell control over the EBV-driven B-cells.[37]

Human herpesvirus-6 (HHV-6) has been suggested as an etiological agent, but confirmatory studies have been negative thus far.[38] HHV-8 has been studied as a potential source of chronic antigenic stimulation leading to PCNSL but no association with AIDS or non-AIDS patients was found.[39] Data suggest that Bcl-6 expression, indicating a germinal center phenotype, predicts improved survival in PCNSL patients treated with high-dose methotrexate (MTX).[40] Proto-oncogenes Bcl-1 and Bcl-2 have no detectable rearrangement in PCNSL.[38]

Clinical presentation

Primary central nervous system lymphoma occurs in all age groups, with a peak in the sixth and seventh decades for immunocompetent individuals (mean age 55 years) and in the third to fourth decades in immunocompromised individuals (mean age 30 years). There is a 3:2 male-to-female ratio among immunocompetent patients but in those with AIDS more than 90% are men. Symptom duration prior to diagnosis averages 2.8 months for immunocompetent patients and 1.8 months for immunocompromised patients.[27]

The clinical presentation of PCNSL is similar to other intracranial mass lesions (Box 56.1). Cognitive and personality changes, reflecting frontal lobe predilection, are the most common symptoms but patients frequently have lateralizing signs as well. Seizures occur in 10% of patients at presentation, a lower percentage than seen with gliomas or brain metastases, due to the subcortical location of most PCNSL lesions. In AIDS patients, however, seizures occur in 25% at presentation.[27] Headache is common but other symptoms of raised intracranial pressure are rare.

More than 40% of patients have dissemination of PCNSL to the leptomeninges, yet symptoms of leptomeningeal involvement are rare.[30] This is in contradistinction to systemic NHL where CNS metastasis primarily affects the leptomeninges, causing multifocal neurological symptoms. Patients with primary leptomeningeal lymphoma present with symptoms of increased intracranial pressure along with multifocal signs indicating cranial nerve or multilevel root involvement. These patients do not develop parenchymal or systemic lymphoma.[31]

Ocular lymphoma can occur in isolation or concomitant with brain lymphoma. It can originate in the eye but 50–80% of these patients subsequently relapse a median of 19 months from ocular diagnosis.[41] Relapse primarily affects the brain but can also occur in the eyes and CSF. Alternatively, 20–25% of patients with brain lymphoma have ocular involvement at diagnosis. Symptoms are usually "floaters", blurred or cloudy vision, and diminished visual acuity but approximately 50% of patients are asymptomatic. Eye pain and conjunctival hyperemia are rare. Involvement may be unilateral or bilateral but is usually asymmetrical. Mean time from symptom onset to diagnosis of intraocular lymphoma is 21.4 months[33] because ocular lymphoma is frequently mistaken for chronic vitreitis or uveitis.

Fewer than 1% of PCNSL patients present with spinal cord involvement; they may have back pain and symptoms and

signs of myelopathy. Lesions are usually seen in the lower cervical or upper thoracic region.[42]

Diagnostic considerations

Primary central nervous system lymphoma is confined to the CNS and does not represent metastatic disease. Therefore, an extent of disease evaluation at diagnosis should focus on the nervous system (Box 56.2). All patients should have enhanced cranial magnetic resonance imaging (MRI). Every patient

---

Box 56.1 Symptoms and signs of primary central nervous system lymphoma.

Cerebral

- Personality/cognitive changes
- Lateralizing, i.e. hemiparesis, aphasia
- Seizures
- Headache

Ocular

- Floaters
- Blurred or cloudy vision
- Decreased visual acuity

Leptomeningeal

- Headache
- Cranial neuropathy
- Radiculopathy

Spinal cord

- Back pain
- Limb paresis
- Sensory level or paresthesias
- Bowel or bladder dysfunction

Box 56.2 Evaluation of patients with primary central nervous system lymphoma.

- Enhanced brain magnetic resonance imaging*
- Ophthalmological and slit-lamp examination
- Cerebrospinal fluid analysis
- Human immunodeficiency virus test
- Enhanced spinal magnetic resonance imaging if clinically indicated
- Chest, abdomen, pelvic computed tomography scan
- Consider body positron emission tomography scan
- Bone marrow

---

* CT scan only if MRI contraindicated.

should have an ophthalmological examination, including slit lamp. MRI of the spine should be performed in patients with signs or symptoms of back pain, myelopathy, or radiculopathy. CSF should be obtained from all patients and analyzed for cell count, protein, glucose, cytology, and tumor markers (lactate dehydrogenase [LDH] isoenzymes, β-glucuronidase, and β2-microglobulin).

Immunocytochemical analysis[43] and polymerase chain reaction (PCR) for detection of immunoglobulin gene rearrangements[44] may be a useful adjunct in the diagnosis of lymphomatous meningitis. An association between interleukin (IL)-10 and PCNSL has been reported. Patients with ocular lymphoma have an elevated IL-10 to IL-6 ratio in the vitreal fluid, and those with brain or ocular lymphoma have an elevated IL-10 to IL-6 ratio in the CSF.[45] Elevated IL-10 levels correlate with the presence of malignant cells.

In patients with AIDS, examination of the CSF for EBV by PCR may establish the diagnosis of PCNSL.[46] Demonstrating hypermetabolic lesions on single photon emission computed tomography (SPECT) or positron emission tomographic (PET) scans differentiate PCNSL from infection in AIDS patients with an intracranial mass. When SPECT or PET is positive in combination with identification of EBV in the CSF of an AIDS patient, the diagnosis of PCNSL can be established with accuracy, thus avoiding a brain biopsy.[47]

Systemic evaluation occasionally identifies another site of disease in PCNSL patients. Comprehensive testing for sites of systemic NHL in 128 patients with PCNSL yielded evidence of systemic disease in only five patients (4%).[48] All sites of disease were identified by abdominal CT scan or bone marrow biopsy,[48] thereby excluding the need for additional testing. Our own experience confirms the relatively low yield of systemic evaluation in patients with PCNSL; however, body PET may reveal a site of disease not appreciated on other imaging studies.[49] In older series, when patients did not undergo systemic workup, only 7% of PCNSL patients ever developed autopsy-proven systemic disease, demonstrating the rarity of multiorgan involvement even late in the course of the illness.[4,50]

Imaging

Magnetic resonance imaging is the optimal imaging technique. CT scan should be used only if MRI is unavailable or contraindicated, such as in patients with pacemakers. On MRI, PCNSL lesions are typically isointense to hypointense on T1-weighted images and bright on diffusion sequences. Enhancement tends to be solid and homogeneous in immunocompetent patients (Fig. 56.3) but irregular and heterogeneous, often with a ring-like pattern, in immunodeficient patients. This ring enhancement is due to central necrosis of the tumor, which makes radiographic distinction from CNS infections difficult. On T2-weighted images, PCNSL is usually diffusely hyperintense but may also be hypointense to isointense. Hypointensity on T2 may help differentiate this lesion from gliomas or demyelinating lesions. Peritumoral edema is variable and may be less than seen in gliomas or metastases of comparable size. Also, the amount of mass effect is less than expected given the size of the lesion. Calcification, hemorrhage, and cyst formation are rare

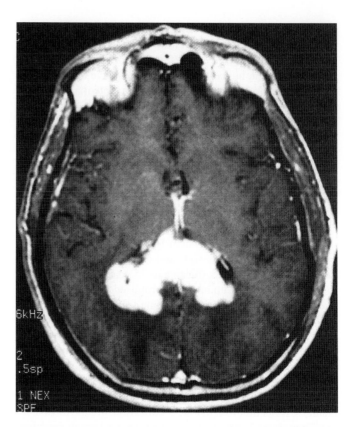

Figure 56.3 Typical contrast-enhanced MRI showing involvement of the splenium of the corpus callosum. Note the diffuse, homogeneous enhancement pattern.

and should raise the suspicion of an alternative pathological process. Nonenhancing tumors have been reported in approximately 10% of PCNSL patients, both immunocompetent and immunodeficient.[27,51] This can present as a focal lesion(s) or as a diffuse infiltrative process, lymphomatosis cerebri.

Primary central nervous system lymphoma tends to be supratentorial, periventricular, and involve the deep structures such as the basal ganglia.[27] Ependymal contact is seen in approximately 50% of patients.[8] The frontal lobe is the most commonly involved region of the brain, followed in decreasing order by the temporal, parietal, and occipital lobes.[8] Other areas of involvement include the corpus callosum, hypothalamus and septum, brainstem, and cerebellum.[8]

On magnetic resonance spectroscopy (MRS), PCNSL has a higher choline:creatinine ratio than all grades of glioma.[52] In addition, PCNSL often has marked elevation of lipid and lactate, which may identify patients with a worse prognosis.[52,53] On PET, PCNSL is hypermetabolic with a high fluorodeoxyglucose (FDG) uptake. With methionine PET,[54] there is increased lesional uptake and this tracer may be better at delineating lesion size when compared to CT or MRI.

Treatment

Prognostic factors

Although patient numbers are small, several authors have attempted to define prognostic factors that influence survival.

Age and performance status are consistently recognized as influential prognostic factors, with patients younger than 60 and those with a Karnofsky performance status (KPS) greater than 70 surviving longer.[13,16,49] A prognostic index has been proposed incorporating age, performance status, CSF protein concentration, serum LDH level and tumor involving deep structures on a five-point scale predicting outcome, but this has not been validated.[55] A three-tiered prognostic model has been validated and adopted by multiple groups in which patients in class 1 (≤50 years old) have a median overall survival (OS) of 8.5 years, those in class 2 (age >50 and KPS ≥70) had a median OS of 3.2 years and those in class 3 (age >50 and KPS <70) had a median OS of 1.1 years.[56]

Supportive care

Untreated, PCNSL is rapidly fatal (Table 56.1). Henry et al.[4] found a median survival of 3.3 months for patients treated with supportive care only. An analysis of 50 English-language papers between 1980 and 1995 found a median survival of 2 months for patients who underwent a biopsy only and received no treatment.[57]

Surgery

Surgical resection does not prolong survival (see Table 56.1) as median survival ranges from only 1 to 6 months after resection.[4] Furthermore, resection may worsen a patient's neurologic function due to the deep location of most PCNSL lesions. In a patient with acute neurological deterioration due to herniation, a resection may be indicated for immediate decompression; however, biopsy is the preferred method for tissue diagnosis and is usually safe regardless of tumor site. A frozen section could be performed intraoperatively and if consistent with PCNSL, the neurosurgeon should proceed no further.

Radiation therapy

Primary central nervous system lymphoma is an exquisitely radiosensitive tumor and RT prolongs survival (see Table 56.1). In a large multicenter Radiation Therapy Oncology Group (RTOG) trial, Nelson et al.[50] found a median survival of 11.6 months from the onset of treatment and 12.6 months from the time of diagnosis. Of the 41 patients, 21 failed locally at the original site of disease, four failed locally and had distant CNS or extraneural disease, and three had only distant extraneural disease, despite the RTOG's use of high-dose and large-volume RT. These data are identical to historical series of whole-brain radiation therapy (WBRT). Despite CSF dissemination in many patients, craniospinal (CS) RT does not improve survival, as seen in a report by Reni et al.[57] where median survival for patients treated with WBRT was 17 months but only 14 months for those receiving CS RT. Brada et al.[61] also found no survival advantage to CS versus cranial radiotherapy alone. In addition, CS RT irradiates a large volume of bone marrow, compromising subsequent administration of chemotherapy.

Whole brain is the recommended RT port because of the multifocal and infiltrative nature of PCNSL and the wide-

Table 56.1 Therapeutic outcomes for patients with non-AIDS primary central nervous system lymphoma.

Reference	Therapy	Median survival (months)
Supportive care		
Reni et al.[57]	None	2.0
Surgery alone		
Reni et al.[57]	Surgery	1.5
Radiotherapy alone		
Nelson et al.[50]	RT	12.0
Standard lymphoma regimens		
Lachance et al.[58]	CHOP/RT	16.5
O'Neill et al.[59]	CHOP/RT	10.4
Schultz et al.[60]	CHOD/RT	16.0
Brada et al.[61]	MACOP-B/RT	14.0
Methotrexate-based regimens		
O'Brien[62]	M/RT	36
Glass et al.[63]	M/RT	33.0
Poortmans et al.[64]	MVBP	46
DeAngelis et al.[74]	M/RT/A	42.5
Abrey et al.[65]	MVP/RT/A	60.0
Chemotherapy only		
McAllister et al.[66]	BBBD/M	40.7
Batchelor et al.[67]	M (8 g/m²)	23+
Herrlinger et al.[68]	M (8 g/m²)	25
Randomized trials		
Ferreri et al.[69]	M	"10"*
	M+A	"31"*
Thiel et al.[70]	M±I/RT	32.4
	M±I	37.1
HDCT and ASCT±RT		
Abrey et al.[85]	M+A/BEAM	NR (median f/u 28 mo)
Colombat et al.[71]	MVBP, I+A/BEAM+RT	NR (median f/u 34 mo)
Illerhaus et al.[72]	M+A/B+T±RT	NR (median f/u 25 mo)

A, cytarabine; BEAM, carmustine, etoposide, cytarabine, melphalan; ASCT, autologous stem cell transplant; B, carmustine; BBBD, blood–brain barrier disruption; CHOD, cyclophosphamide, doxorubicin, vincristine, and dexamethasone; CHOP, cyclophosphamide, doxorubicin, vincristine, and prednisone; f/u, follow-up; HDCT, high-dose chemotherapy; I, ifosfamide; M, methotrexate; MACOP-B, methotrexate, doxorubicin, cyclophosphamide, vincristine, prednisone, and bleomycin; MCHOD, methotrexate, cyclophosphamide, doxorubicin, vincrisitine and dexamethasone; mo, months; MVBP, methotrexate, etoposide, carmustine, methylprednisolone; MVP, methotrexate, vincristine, and procarbazine; NR, no response; RT, radiation therapy; T, thiotepa; *, read off survival curve but not reported.

spread microscopic disease seen in patients at autopsy. Shibamoto et al. reviewed patients with PCNSL treated with focal RT using margins <4 cm compared to those treated with margins ≥4 cm.[73] Patients treated with the smaller margins had a significantly higher incidence (83%) of outfield recurrences than patients with larger margins (22%).[73] These data support the decision to use WBRT to achieve local control. The optimal dose of WBRT has not been defined, but most data indicate the need for at least 4000 cGy. In the RTOG study, 4000 cGy WBRT and a 2000 cGy boost to the tumor did not result in improved disease control since most patients relapsed within the boosted field.[50] These data confirm our own experience using 4000 cGy WBRT and a 1440 cGy boost.[74] Therefore, patients do not appear to benefit from doses greater than 5000 cGy. Furthermore, patients radiated with greater than 5000 cGy may experience increased neurotoxicity. Currently, when using RT, we treat patients with 4500 cGy WBRT and no boost.

Efforts to reduce the dose of WBRT to decrease the incidence of neurotoxicity have produced mixed results. The RTOG conducted a study using a high-dose MTX-based regimen plus 4500 cGy WBRT.[75] Patients who achieved a complete response (CR) from chemotherapy received only 3600 cGy WBRT. Survival, disease control, and neurotoxicity were identical regardless of WBRT dose. However, Bessell et al. used a different preradiation chemotherapy protocol and reduced the WBRT dose from 4500 cGy to 3060 cGy in those who achieved a CR.[76] No difference in outcome was seen in patients older than 60 years, but younger patients had significantly longer survival if the full dose of WBRT was used. There was no information concerning neurotoxicity. More recently, preliminary data on reducing the dose of WBRT to 2340 cGy after a CR was obtained using rituximab, MTX, vincristine, and procarbazine showed excellent results but a final report from this study is needed.[77] These data are inconclusive regarding the ability of chemotherapy to permit safe dose reduction of WBRT.

In patients with ocular lymphoma, RT should include the posterior two-thirds of the globe to a dose of 3000–4000 cGy.[41] At these doses, improvements in visual acuity are seen but frequently patients relapse within the brain, and this is the ultimate cause of death. Ocular toxicities include epithelioid keratopathy, posterior subcapsular cataracts, and radiation retinopathy or optic neuropathy. If cerebral involvement is present at the same time and cranial irradiation is being performed, the treatment plan should include both regions simultaneously to eliminate overlapping fields and minimize toxicity to the optic nerve and retina.

Chemotherapy

Like systemic NHL, PCNSL is highly sensitive to glucocorticoids and has been called a "ghost tumor" because the lesion may vanish with steroid use. About 40% of patients treated with steroids will have tumor shrinkage but the tumor usually recurs within a short period. Half of 20 patients treated with steroids had an evaluable response ranging from complete to minor, with two having a CR lasting 6 and 15 months prior to needing further therapy.[64] There are other reports of long-term remissions in patients treated with glucocorticoids lasting from 6 to 60 months but this is rare.[78] Some patients may have repeated responses to steroids.[79] Corticosteroids are chemotherapeutic agents for PCNSL and lesion disappearance is due to cell lysis, not reconstitution of the blood–brain barrier (BBB). Because steroids are oncolytic, they should be withheld until a tissue diagnosis is established. Furthermore, steroid response should not be used as a diagnostic test for PCNSL because other CNS processes, such as multiple sclerosis or sarcoidosis, can have a similar radiographic appearance and regress after steroid administration.

The standard chemotherapeutic regimen for systemic NHL is cyclophosphamide, doxorubicin, vincristine, and prednisone (CHOP); rituximab is now added to CHOP.[80] Lachance et al.[58] treated six PCNSL patients with pre-RT CHOP (see Table 56.1). All responded initially but developed progressive disease, frequently between the second and third cycle of chemotherapy. Median survival was 8.5 months for the group but 16.5 months for the four patients who were able to receive RT after chemotherapy. The authors terminated the trial early because patients did so poorly. O'Neill et al.[59] completed a multicenter trial using preirradiation CHOP. The median survival for the 46 patients was 41.7 weeks but survival was better for patients younger than 60 years of age (47.4 weeks) than for those older than 60 (32.9 weeks). In addition, significant chemotherapy-related toxicities were seen and only 54% of patients ever proceeded to RT in this study. The RTOG[60] used preirradiation CHOD (substituting dexamethasone for prednisone) and found a median survival of 16 months and a median disease-free survival of 9.2 months. In a randomized control trial that was terminated before completion because of poor accrual, the addition of CHOP to RT did not prolong survival over WBRT alone.[81] Brada et al.[61] used MACOP-B (methotrexate [0.4 g/m²], doxorubicin, cyclophosphamide, vincristine, prednisone, and bleomycin) followed by whole-brain or CS RT in 10 patients. There was a median survival of only 14 months compared to those treated with RT only who had a median survival of 16 months.

These studies demonstrate that chemotherapy regimens efficacious for systemic NHL have no role in the treatment of PCNSL and should not be used. These regimens use anthracyclines and cyclophosphamide, neither of which effectively penetrates the intact BBB. Patients may have an initial response because of BBB disruption in areas of bulky disease but recurrence is seen, often in areas remote from the initial tumor site, where lymphoma was present behind a relatively intact BBB.

There have been numerous phase II trials all consistently indicating that high-dose MTX is the single most important chemotherapeutic agent to treat PCNSL. Initial studies focused on adding MTX-based regimens to WBRT. Glass et al.[63] used 3.5 g/m² MTX prior to RT in 25 patients, of whom 14 had a CR to chemotherapy and eight had a partial response (PR); 20 of the 25 had a CR after RT. Median survival for the group was 33 months and for responders, 42.5 months. In 1992, DeAngelis et al.[74] reported results using MTX (1 g/m²), WBRT, and then high-dose cytarabine (3 g/m²) to treat 31 patients. They found a median disease-free survival of 41 months and a median overall survival of 42.5 months. In long-term follow-up, seven of the original 31 patients were still alive (47–126 plus months), six of whom were less than 50 years of age at diagnosis.[82] The 5-year survival rate was 22%, markedly better than the 3–4% rate with RT alone.[50]

The use of single-agent, very high-dose MTX (8 g/m²) with the intention of deferring radiotherapy has produced conflicting results. Batchelor et al. treated 25 patients with MTX alone for over a year and reported a 74% response rate and median progression-free survival of 12.8 months with OS not reached at 23 months follow-up.[67] In a similar study, Herrlinger et al. had a comparable relapse-free survival of 13.7 months in patients with a CR but 38% of patients progressed and OS was only 25 months.[68,83] They abandoned the study early because of patients' poor response.

An alternative approach has been promoted by Angelov et al.[66] They treated patients with intraarterial (IA) mannitol for BBB disruption followed by IA MTX. In a multicenter study, 149 patients were treated and the median survival was 3.1 years. These results are better than WBRT alone but not superior to standard systemic high-dose MTX regimens. Furthermore, this technique is invasive and has acute morbidity, such as acute arterial injuries, stroke, and seizures.

Multidrug regimens including MTX have been used to treat PCNSL. MTX (3.5 g/m^2), procarbazine, and vincristine is an effective combination given prior to WBRT, achieving a median survival of 60 months.[65] A large multicenter trial using a comparable regimen, but with a lower dose of MTX (2.5 g/m^2), achieved a median survival of 37 months, which was an improvement over WBRT alone but a decrease from the single institutional experience achieving a median survival of 60 months with a similar regimen.[65,75] A randomized phase II study examined the role of single-agent MTX versus a combination of MTX plus cytarabine with both groups receiving WBRT. The combination was significantly superior in response rate and gave a 3-year failure-free survival of 21% for MTX alone compared to 38% for MTX plus cytarabine ($p=0.01$).[69]

The only randomized phase III trial completed in PCNSL examined the role of WBRT. Patients received MTX ± ifosfamide and those who achieved a CR were randomized to receive 4500 cGy WBRT or not.[70] The authors did not meet their primary endpoint for a noninferiority trial design but their data strongly suggest that WBRT significantly prolonged progression-free survival but not OS. They concluded that RT has no role in initial treatment of PCNSL, but the study was hampered by a number of controversial analyses.

Immunotherapy

Rituximab, an anti-CD20 monoclonal antibody that targets B-cells, is highly effective in the treatment of comparable systemic NHLs. It has been incorporated into some chemotherapeutic regimens for PNCSL. A study of 12 patients examined its efficacy as a single agent in relapsed disease. Confirmed responses were seen in 36% and median progression-free survival was 57 days but median OS was 21 months.[84] There is a suggestion that combining it with chemotherapy may enhance disease response, but its role remains to be defined.[77]

High-dose chemotherapy with autologous stem cell transplantation

Several recent studies examined the potential role for high-dose chemotherapy followed by autologous stem cell rescue without cranial RT. Overall event-free survival was only 5.6 months for all patients and 9.3 months for patients who underwent transplantation.[85] However, OS had not been reached with a median follow-up of 28 months. Other studies have achieved superior results but have often included WBRT into the regimen with its attendant risk of neurotoxicity (see below) or the patient number has been small and highly selected with short follow-up.[71,72] The role of transplantation as part of initial therapy is being subjected to two randomized trials which should clarify its value in the coming years.

Transplantation for primary refractory or relapsed disease appears promising.[86] Using an induction regimen of high-dose cytarabine and etoposide, 20 of 43 patients achieved a response. A total of 27 patients (15 responders and 12 nonresponders) proceeded to intensive thiotepa, busulfan, and cyclophosphamide followed by autologous stem cell transplantation. The median OS was 18.3 months for all 43 patients and 58.6 months for those who completed the transplant regimen. This is an excellent outcome for patients with recurrent disease but was limited to those aged 65 or younger.

Recurrent disease

Despite initial high response rates using any high-dose MTX-based regimen, some patients will have primary progression and many will relapse. There is no standard therapeutic approach at recurrence, and prior treatment and location of relapse, e.g. isolated ocular relapse, determine the choice of therapy. However, most relapses occur within the brain and within the first 2 years of diagnosis. Some chemotherapeutic regimens that are reportedly useful include rituximab and temozolomide,[87] topotecan,[88] and repeating MTX. RT is an option if not previously administered.[89]

Neurotoxicity

Leukoencephalopathy is a serious complication of effective PCNSL treatment, but apparent only when the patient is in a durable remission.[83] Therefore, it is rarely observed in patients treated with WBRT alone because they die of tumor progression, but it has been seen in patients treated with combined modality therapy, especially high-dose MTX-based regimens. There is synergistic toxicity when methotrexate is combined with WBRT, which can be minimized when the MTX is administered prior to RT. However, it has also been observed in patients treated with MTX and no cranial irradiation.[68,70]

Treatment-related leukoencephalopathy occurs primarily in patients older than 60 years of age. These patients present with a syndrome similar to normal pressure hydrocephalus with significant cognitive impairment, gait ataxia, and incontinence; some improve with ventriculoperitoneal shunting. Given the high incidence of this treatment complication in older patients, we treat these patients with chemotherapy alone (Fig. 56.4) and avoid WBRT. In older patients, eliminating WBRT does not compromise outcome.[65]

Ocular lymphoma

Ocular lymphoma is uncommon, so defining an optimal therapy is difficult. Grimm et al.[41] reported 83 patients with ocular lymphoma who were treated with a variety of regimens including topical or systemic steroids, WBRT, ocular RT, and chemotherapy. Most of the patients had improvement in their symptoms but relapse was common in both the brain and the eyes.

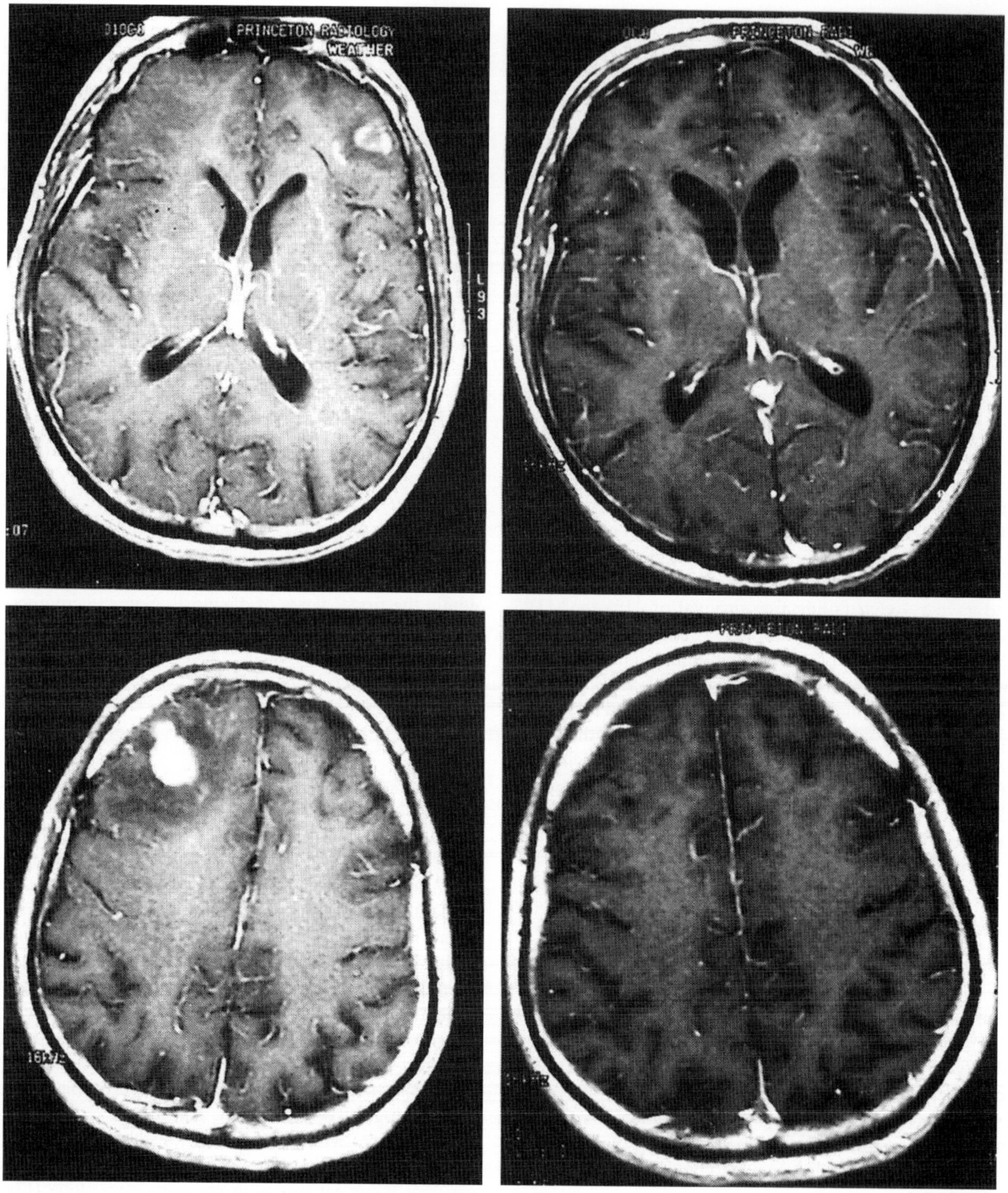

Figure 56.4 Patient with multifocal PCNSL before (*left*) and after (*right*) chemotherapy with high-dose methotrexate, procarbazine, and vincristine, and no radiation therapy. There is a complete regression of all lesions. The patient was off corticosteroids when response was assessed.

Treatment type did not affect the pattern of relapse and, most importantly, systemic chemotherapy did not reduce subsequent CNS recurrences. Baumann *et al.*[90] reported a patient with ocular lymphoma who responded to high-dose cytarabine and had therapeutic drug levels measured in intraocular fluid. Cytarabine was then used as sole treatment in six patients with ocular lymphoma; one complete and four partial responses were achieved prior to RT.[91] Batchelor *et al.* treated nine patients with ocular lymphoma using single-agent high-dose MTX ($8\,g/m^2$). All patients achieved a therapeutic concentration of drug in both the aqueous and vitreous humor 4 h after completion of the infusion. Seven patients had an ocular response but three relapsed, requiring orbital RT.[92] Recently, patients with ocular lymphoma have been treated successfully with intravitreal MTX or rituximab, which has the advantage of requiring fewer injections.[93,94] Response is usual and adverse reactions are rare.

Approach

Our approach to patients with newly diagnosed PCNSL is to perform complete neurological staging with cranial MRI, CSF, and ophthalmological examinations. We usually perform body CT and PET but do not always do a bone marrow examination. From a therapeutic perspective, we always try to enroll a patient onto a clinical trial if available as there are so many unanswered questions regarding PCNSL. However, if that is not feasible or the patient refuses, we initiate treatment with a combination of MTX (3.5 g/m²), vincristine, and procarbazine. We use intrathecal MTX only if the CSF cytology shows malignant cells.

We assess response after five cycles of MTX and if a complete response is achieved, we consolidate with two cycles of high-dose cytarabine (3 g/m²). If only a partial response is attained, we continue with at least two more cycles of MTX-based therapy and reassess. We seek to avoid WBRT in all patients as part of initial therapy to avoid the long-term cognitive complications that may be associated with combined modality therapy.

References

1. Bailey P. Intracranial sarcomatous tumors of leptomeningeal origin. Arch Surg 1929; 18: 1359–402.
2. Yuile CL. Case of primary reticulum cell sarcoma of the brain. Relationship of microglia cells to histiocytes. Arch Pathol 1938; 26: 1037–44.
3. Russell DS, Marshall AHE, Smith FB. Microgliomatosis. A form of reticulosis affecting the brain. Brain 1948; 71: 1–15.
4. Henry JM, et al. Primary malignant lymphomas of the central nervous system. Cancer 1974; 34: 1293–302.
5. Deckert M, et al. Modern concepts in the biology, diagnosis, differential diagnosis and treatment of primary central nervous system lymphoma. Leukemia 2011; 25(12): 1797–807.
6. Nakhleh RE, et al. Central nervous system lymphomas. Immunohistochemical and clinicopathologic study of 26 autopsy cases. Arch Pathol Lab Med 1989; 113: 1050–6.
7. Taylor CR, et al. An immunohistological study of immunoglobulin content of primary central nervous system lymphomas. Cancer 1978; 41: 2197–205.
8. Tomlinson FH, et al. Primary intracerebral lymphoma: a clinicopathological study of 89 patients. J Neurosurg 1995; 82: 558–66.
9. Jellinger KA, Radaskiewicz TH, Slowik F. Primary malignant lymphomas of the central nervous system in man. Acta Neuropathol 1975; 6(Suppl): 95–102.
10. Zimmerman HM. Malignant lymphomas of the nervous system. Acta Neuropathol 1975; 6(Suppl): 69–74.
11. Olson JE, et al. The continuing increase of primary central nervous system non-Hodgkins lymphoma. A surveillance, epidemiology, and end results analysis. Cancer 2002; 95: 1504–10.
12. Kadan-Lottick NS, Skluzacek MC, Gurney JG. Decreasing incidence rates of primary central nervous system lymphoma. Cancer 2002; 95: 193–202.
13. Krogh-Jensen M, et al. Clinicopathological features, survival, and prognostic factors of primary central nervous system lymphomas: trends in incidence of primary central nervous system lymphomas and primary malignant brain tumors in a well-defined geographic area. Leuk Lymphoma 1995; 19: 223–33.
14. Yau Y, et al. Primary lymphoma of the central nervous system in immunocompetent patients in south-east Scotland. Lancet 1996; 348: 890.
15. Hao D, et al. Is the incidence of primary CNS lymphoma increasing? A population-based study of incidence, clinicopathological features, and outcomes in Alberta from 1975 to 1996. Ann Neurol 1997; 42: 537.
16. DeAngelis LM, Yahalom J. Primary central nervous system lymphoma. In: DeVita VTJ, Lawrence TS, Rosenberg SA (eds) Principles and Practice of Oncology Updates, 9th edn. Philadelphia: JB Lippincott, 2011. p.1908.
17. Rosenblum ML, et al. Primary central nervous system lymphomas in patients with AIDS. Ann Neurol 1988; 23(Suppl): S13–16.
18. Welch K, et al. Autopsy findings in the acquired immune deficiency syndrome. JAMA 1984; 252: 1152–9.
19. Ling SM, et al. Radiotherapy of primary central nervous system lymphoma in patients with and without human immunodeficiency virus. Ten years of treatment experience at the University of California San Francisco. Cancer 1994; 73: 2570–82.
20. Wolf T, et al. Changing incidence and prognostic factors of survival in AIDS-related non-Hodgkin's lymphoma in the era of highly active antiretroviral therapy (HAART). Leuk Lymphoma 2005; 467: 207–15.
21. DeAngelis LM. Primary central nervous system lymphoma as a secondary malignancy. Cancer 1991; 67: 1431–5.
22. Reni M, et al. Primary brain lymphomas in patients with a prior or concomitant malignancy. J Neurooncol 1997; 32: 135–42.
23. Bashir R, et al. Immunophenotypic profile of CNS lymphoma: a review of eighteen cases. J Neurooncol 1989; 7: 249–54.
24. Gijtenbeek JM, Rosenblum MK, DeAngelis LM. Primary central nervous system T-cell lymphoma. Neurology 2001; 57(4): 716–18.
25. Itoyama T, et al. Primary central nervous system lymphomas. Cancer 1994; 73: 455–63.
26. Kumanishi T, et al. Primary malignant lymphoma of the brain: demonstration of frequent p16 and p15 gene deletions. Jpn J Cancer Res 1996; 87: 691–5.
27. Fine HA, Mayer RJ. Primary central nervous system lymphoma. Ann Intern Med 1993; 119: 1093–104.
28. Paulus W, et al. Malignant lymphomas In: Kleihues P Cavenee WK (eds) World Health Organization Classification of Tumours, Pathology and Genetics. Tumours of the Nervous System. Lyon, France: IARC Press, 2000. pp.198–203.
29. Schaumberg HH, Plank CR, Adams RD. The reticulum cell sarcomamicroglioma group of brain tumors. A consideration of their clinical features and therapy. Brain 1972; 95: 199–212.
30. Balmaceda C, et al. Leptomeningeal tumor in primary central nervous system lymphoma: recognition, significance, and implications. Ann Neurol 1995; 38: 202–9.
31. Lachance DH, et al. Primary leptomeningeal lymphoma: report of 9 cases, diagnosis with immunocytochemical analysis, and review of the literature. Neurology 1991; 41: 95–100.
32. Miranda RN, et al. Stage 1E non-Hodgkin's lymphoma involving the dura. A clinicopathologic study of five cases. Arch Pathol Lab Med 1996; 120: 254–60.
33. Whitcup SM, et al. Intraocular lymphoma: clinical and histopathologic diagnosis. Ophthalmology 1993; 100: 1399–406.
34. Paulus W, Jellinger K. Comparison of integrin adhesion molecules expressed by primary brain lymphomas and nodal lymphomas. Acta Neuropathol 1993; 86: 360–4.
35. Tun HW, et al. Pathway analysis of primary central nervous system lymphoma. Blood 2008; 111: 3200–10.
36. Morgello S. Pathogenesis and classification of primary central nervous system lymphoma: an update. Brain Pathol 1995; 5: 383–93.
37. Papadopoulos EB, et al. Infusions of donor leukocytes to treat Epstein–Barr virus-associated lymphoproliferative disorders after allogeneic bone marrow transplantation. N Engl J Med 1994; 330: 1185–91.
38. Jellinger KA, Paulus W. Primary central nervous system lymphomas – new pathological developments. J Neurooncol 1995; 24: 33–6.
39. Montesinos-Rongen M, et al. Human herpes virus-8 is not associated with primary central nervous system lymphoma in HIV-negative patients. Acta Neuropathol 2001; 102: 489–95.
40. Levy O, et al. Bcl-6 predicts improved prognosis in primary central nervous system lymphoma. Cancer 2008; 112: 151–6.
41. Grimm SA, et al. Primary intraocular lymphoma: an International Primary Central Nervous System Lymphoma Collaborative Group Report. Ann Oncol 2007; 18(11): 1851–5.

42. Schild SE, *et al*. Primary lymphoma of the spinal cord. Mayo Clin Proc 1995; 70: 256–60.

43. Li CY, *et al*. Diagnosis of B-cell non-Hodgkin's lymphoma of the central nervous system by immunocytochemical analysis of cerebrospinal fluid lymphocytes. Cancer 1986; 57: 737–44.

44. Gleissner B, *et al*. CSF evaluation in primary CNS lymphoma patients by PCR of the CDR III IgH genes. Neurology 2002; 58: 390–6.

45. Whitcup SM, *et al*. Association of interleukin 10 in the vitreous and cerebrospinal fluid and primary central nervous system lymphoma. Arch Ophthalmol 1997; 115: 1157–60.

46. Arribas JR, *et al*. Detection of Epstein–Barr virus DNA in cerebrospinal fluid for diagnosis of AIDS-related central nervous system lymphoma. J Clin Microbiol 1995; 33: 1580–3.

47. Antinori A, *et al*. Value of combined approach with thallium-201 single-photon emission computed tomography and Epstein-Barr virus DNA polymerase chain reaction in CSF for the diagnosis of AIDS-related primary CNS lymphoma. J Clin Oncol 1999; 17: 554–60.

48. O'Neill BP, *et al*. Occult systemic non-Hodgkin's lymphoma (NHL) in patients initially diagnosed as primary central nervous system lymphoma (PCNSL): how much staging is enough? J Neurooncol 1995; 25: 67–71.

49. Mohile NA, DeAngelis LM, Abrey LE. The utility of body PDG PET in staging primary central nervous system lymphoma. Neuro Oncol 2008; 10: 223–8.

50. Nelson DF, *et al*. Non-Hodgkin's lymphoma of the brain: can high dose, large volume radiation therapy improve survival? Report on a prospective trial by the Radiation Therapy Oncology Group (RTOG): RTOG 8315. Int J Radiat Oncol Biol Phys 1992; 23: 9–17.

51. DeAngelis LM. Cerebral lymphoma presenting as a nonenhancing lesion on computed tomographic/magnetic resonance scan. Ann Neurol 1993; 33: 308–11.

52. Harting I, *et al*. Differentiating primary central nervous system lymphoma from glioma in humans using localized proton magnetic resonance spectroscopy. Neurosci Lett 2003; 342: 163–6.

53. Raizer JJ, *et al*. Proton magnetic resonance spectroscopy in immunocompetent patients with primary central nervous system lymphoma. J Neurooncol 2005; 71(2): 173–80.

54. Ogawa T, *et al*. Methionine PET for follow-up of radiation therapy of primary lymphoma of the brain. Radiographics 1994; 14: 101–10.

55. Ferreri AJ, *et al*. Prognostic scoring system for primary CNS lymphomas: the International Extranodal Lymphoma Study Group experience. J Clin Oncol 2003; 21: 266–72.

56. Abrey LE, *et al*. Primary central nervous system lymphoma: the Memorial Sloan-Kettering Cancer Center prognostic model. J Clin Oncol 2006; 24: 5711–15.

57. Reni M, *et al*. Therapeutic management of primary central nervous system lymphoma in immunocompetent patients: results of a critical review of the literature. Ann Oncol 1997; 8: 227–34.

58. Lachance DH, *et al*. Cyclophosphamide, doxorubicin, vincristine, and prednisone for primary central nervous system lymphoma: short-duration response and multifocal intracerebral recurrence preceding radiotherapy. Neurology 1994; 44: 1721–7.

59. O'Neill BP, *et al*. Primary central nervous system non-Hodgkin's lymphoma: survival advantages with combined initial therapy? Int J Radiat Oncol Biol Phys 1995; 33: 663–73.

60. Schultz C, *et al*. Preirradiation chemotherapy with cyclophosphamide, doxorubicin, vincristine, and dexamethasone for primary CNS lymphomas: initial report of Radiation Therapy Oncology Group protocol 88-06. J Clin Oncol 1996; 14: 556–64.

61. Brada M, *et al*. Management of primary cerebral lymphoma with initial chemotherapy: preliminary results and comparison with patients treated with radiotherapy alone. Int J Radiat Oncol Biol Phys 1990; 18: 787–92.

62. O'Brien PC, *et al*. Combined-modality therapy for primary central nervous system lymphoma: long-term data from a Phase II multicenter study (Trans-Tasman Radiation Oncology Group). Int J Radiat Oncol Biol Phys 2006; 64: 408–13.

63. Glass J, *et al*. Preirradiation methotrexate chemotherapy of primary central nervous system lymphoma: long-term outcome. J Neurosurg 1994; 81: 188–95.

64. Poortmans PM, *et al*. High-dose methotrexate-based chemotherapy followed by consolidation radiotherapy in non-AIDS-related primary central nervous system lymphoma: European Organization for Research and Treatment of Cancer Lymphoma Group Phase II Trial 20962. J Clin Oncol 2003; 21: 4483–8.

65. Abrey LE, Yahalom J, DeAngelis LM. Treatment for primary CNS lymphoma: the next step. J Clin Oncol 2000; 18: 3144–50.

66. Angelov L, *et al*. Blood-brain barrier disruption and intra-arterial methotrexate-based therapy for newly diagnosed primary CNS lymphoma: a multi-institutional experience. J Clin Oncol 2009; 27: 3503–9.

67. Batchelor T, *et al*. Treatment of primary CNS lymphoma with methotrexate and deferred radiotherapy: a report of NABTT 96-07. J Clin Oncol 2003; 21(6): 1044–9.

68. Herrlinger U, *et al*. Neuro-Oncology Working Group of the German Society. NOA-03 trial of high-dose methotrexate in primary central nervous system lymphoma: final report. Ann Neurol 2005; 57(6): 843–7.

69. Ferreri AJ, *et al*. High-dose cytarabine plus high-dose methotrexate versus high-dose methotrexate alone in patients with primary CNS lymphoma: a randomized phase 2 trial. Lancet 2009; 374(9700): 1512–20.

70. Thiel E, *et al*. High-dose methotrexate with or without whole brain radiotherapy for primary CNS lymphoma (G-PCNSL-SG-1); a phase 3, randomized, non-inferiority trial. Lancet Oncol 2010; 11(11): 1036–47.

71. Colombat P, *et al*. High-dose chemotherapy with autologous stem cell transplantation as first-line therapy for primary CNS lymphoma in patients younger than 60 years: a multicenter phase II study of the GOELAMS group. Bone Marrow Transplant 2006; 38(6): 417–20.

72. Illerhaus G, *et al*. High-dose chemotherapy and autologous stem-cell transplantation without consolidating radiotherapy as first-line treatment for primary lymphoma of the central nervous system. Haematologica 2008; 93(1): 147–8.

73. Shibamoto Y, *et al*. Is whole-brain irradiation necessary for primary central nervous system lymphoma? Patterns of recurrence after partial-brain irradiation. Cancer 2003; 97: 128–33.

74. DeAngelis LM, *et al*. Combined modality therapy for primary CNS lymphoma. J Clin Oncol 1992; 10: 635–43.

75. DeAngelis LM, Seiferheld W, Schold SC. Combination chemotherapy and radiotherapy for primary central nervous system lymphoma: Radiation Therapy Oncology Group Study 93-10. J Clin Oncol 2002; 20: 4643–8.

76. Bessell EM, *et al*. Importance of radiotherapy in the outcome of patients with primary CNS lymphoma: an analysis of the CHOD/BVAM regimen followed by two different radiotherapy treatments. J Clin Oncol 2002; 20: 231–6.

77. Shah GD, *et al*. Combined immunochemotherapy with reduced whole-brain radiotherapy for newly diagnosed primary CNS lymphoma. J Clin Oncol 2007; 25: 4730–5.

78. Pirotte B, *et al*. Glucocorticoid-induced long-term remission in primary cerebral lymphoma: case report and review of the literature. J Neurooncol 1997; 32: 63–9.

79. Singh A, *et al*. Steroid-induced remissions in CNS lymphoma. Neurology 1982; 32: 1267–71.

80. Coiffier B, *et al*. CHOP chemotherapy plus rituximab compared with CHOP alone in elderly patients with diffuse large-B-cell lymphoma. N Engl J Med 2002; 346: 235–42.

81. Mead GM, *et al*. A medical research council randomized trial in patients with primary central non-Hodgkin lymphoma. Cerebral radiotherapy with and without cyclophosphamide, doxorubicin, vincristine, and prednisone chemotherapy. Cancer 2000; 89: 1359–70.

82. Abrey LE, DeAngelis LM, Yahalom J. Long-term survival in primary central nervous system lymphoma. J Clin Oncol 1998; 16: 1–6.

83. Herrlinger U, *et al*. German Cancer Society Neuro-Oncology Working Group NOA-03 multicenter trial of single-agent high-dose methotrexate for primary central nervous system lymphoma. Ann Neurol 2002; 51(2): 247–52.

84. Batchelor TT, *et al*. Rituximab monotherapy for patients with recurrent primary CNS lymphoma. Neurology 2011; 76(10): 929–30.

85. Abrey LE, *et al*. Intensive methotrexate and cytarabine followed by high-dose chemotherapy with autologous stem cell rescue in patients with newly diagnosed primary CNS lymphoma: an intent-to-treat analysis. J Clin Oncol 2005; 21: 4151–6.

86. Soussain C, *et al*. Intensive chemotherapy followed by hematopoietic stem-cell rescue for refractory and recurrent primary CNS and intraocular lymphoma: Société Française de Greffe de Moëlle Osseuse-Thérapie Cellulaire. J Clin Oncol 2008; 26(15): 2512–18.

87. Enting RH, *et al*. Salvage therapy for primary CNS lymphoma with a combination of rituximab and temozolomide. Neurology 2004; 63(5): 901–3.

88. Fischer L, *et al*. Response of relapsed or refractory primary central nervous system lymphoma (PCNSL) to topotecan. Neurology 2004; 62(10): 1885–7.

89. Hottinger AF, *et al*. Salvage whole brain radiotherapy for recurrent or refractory primary CNS lymphoma. Neurology 2007; 69(11): 1178–82.

90. Baumann MA, *et al*. Treatment of intraocular lymphoma with high dose Ara-C. Cancer 1986; 57: 1273–5.

91. Strauchen JA, Dalton J, Friedman AH. Chemotherapy in the management of intraocular lymphoma. Cancer 1989; 63: 1918–21.

92. Batchelor TT, *et al*. High-dose methotrexate for intraocular lymphoma. Clin Cancer Res 2003; 9(2): 711–15.

93. Frenkel S, *et al*. Intravitreal methotrexate for treating vitreoretinal lymphoma: 10 years of experience. Br J Ophthalmol 2008; 92(3): 383–8.

94. Ohguro N, Hashida N, Tano Y. Effect of intravitreous rituximab injections in patients with recurrent ocular lesions associated with central nervous system lymphoma. Arch Opthalmol 2008; 126(7): 1002–3.

Section 10: Neurological Malignancies

57 Choroid Plexus Papilloma and Carcinoma

Derek R. Johnson and Julie E. Hammack

Department of Neurology, Mayo Clinic, Rochester, MN, USA

Introduction

Choroid plexus tumors are rare intraventricular neoplasms derived from choroid plexus epithelium. These tumors can occur at any age but are most frequent in children and often present with symptoms of hydrocephalus. The first choroid plexus papilloma (CPP) was described in 1833 by Guerard.[1] In 1840, Rokitansky described a supposed primary choroid plexus carcinoma (CPC)[2] and in 1868, LeBlanc is credited with reporting the first case of distant seeding of a choroid plexus tumor (CPT).[3] The first surgical attempt at treatment, although unsuccessful due to resulting death, was reported by Bielschowsky and Unger in 1902.[4] This was followed by the first successful surgical resection by Perthes in 1919.[5] Despite the work of these pioneering surgeons, antemortem diagnosis of choroid plexus tumors was relatively rare until the advent of modern imaging techniques such as computed tomography (CT) and ultimately magnetic resonance imaging (MRI).

Aggressive surgical resection is the cornerstone of therapy for CPP and CPC. Patients with CPP can often be surgically cured and even in the case of subtotal resection, other treatments such as radiation and chemotherapy are generally reserved for progressive disease. CPC is a significantly more aggressive tumor than CPP and some data support the use of adjuvant therapies following surgery regardless of extent of resection. In the near future, molecular diagnostic testing is likely to yield improved choroid plexus tumor risk stratification, which will help clinicians to rationally treat patients with aggressive tumors and spare those patients with indolent tumors from treatment-related side-effects.

Biology and epidemiology

Choroid plexus tumors are epithelial neoplasms arising from the choroid plexus. Given that CP epithelial cells are glial cells, CPTs are classified as gliomas but they share little with other gliomas in terms of behavior, appearance, and treatment.

Intuitively, choroid plexus tumors are almost always intraventricular in location. Most pediatric CPP and CPC arise from the choroid plexus of the lateral ventricle (usually near the trigone). The left lateral ventricle appears to be more likely to be involved than the right, and occasionally the tumor may be bilateral.[6–10] Most adult tumors arise from the fourth ventricle or cerebello-pontine angle (CPA). Those tumors arising in the CPA presumably originate from the tuft of choroid within the foramen of Luschka. Origin of the tumor within the third ventricle is rare[11–13] but is occasionally seen in both adult and pediatric patients. Bilateral ventricular involvement has been reported[14,15] and there is also one case report of a CPC arising in the left frontal lobe without ventricular system involvement.[16]

Choroid plexus papillomas usually cause morbidity and mortality via progressive local growth. Rarely, CPP can metastasize to the leptomeninges and extraneural metastasis is exceedingly rare.[17] When CPP recurs after initial treatment, it typically returns as CPP but progression into CPC at time of recurrence following gross total resection (GTR) has been reported.[18] CPC are significantly more aggressive than CPP and can grow locally within the ventricles, invade the parenchyma of the brain, spread through the cerebrospinal fluid (CSF) to the leptomeninges of the brain or spine or, rarely, spread outside the nervous system.[19]

Choroid plexus papillomas and CPC are rare neoplasms that account for 0.4–0.6% of all brain tumors.[20,21] These tumors are more common in the pediatric age group, in which they account for between 2% and 4% of all intracranial tumors, depending on the series.[22–26] The vast majority of choroid plexus neoplasms occur in children less than 2 years of age.[23,27] These tumors have even been diagnosed *in utero* via fetal ultrasound.[28] CPPs are considerably more common than CPCs by a factor of about 5:1 in most series[29,30] and it has been estimated that fewer than 20 CPCs are diagnosed in the United States each year.[31] These tumors are equally distributed among males and females, although a slight male predominance has been reported.[7,31,32]

Textbook of Uncommon Cancer, Fourth Edition. Edited by Derek Raghavan, Charles D. Blanke, David H. Johnson, Paul L. Moots, Gregory H. Reaman, Peter G. Rose and Mikkael A. Sekeres.
© 2012 John Wiley & Sons, Inc. Published 2012 by John Wiley & Sons, Inc.

Molecular biology and genetics

Choroid plexus tumors are typically sporadic. The most important heritable syndrome associated with CPT is Li–Fraumeni syndrome.[33] There have also been a few case reports of these tumors occurring in patients with Aicardi syndrome,[34,35] von Hippel–Lindau disease,[36] and other rare genetic diseases.[37] Li–Fraumeni syndrome, the familial cancer syndrome most closely associated with CPT, is caused by a germline mutation in the *TP53* tumor suppressor gene. Germline mutations in *TP53* have also been described in the familes of patients with CPT who do not meet the criteria for Li–Fraumeni syndrome.[38] Somatic mutations of *TP53* are important in CPT and occur significantly more frequently in CPC than in CPP. Highlighting the importance of this tumor suppressor pathway in CPC tumorigenesis, many CPCs with wild-type *TP53* contain multiple polymorphisms known to confer *TP53* dysfunction.[39] Further, somatic *TP53* status may be an important predictor of tumor behavior, with tumors with wild-type *TP53* following a more indolent course.

Given that most CPT are not associated with familial cancer predisposition syndromes, other risk factors for these tumors have been sought. There is some evidence that simian virus 40 (SV40), a polyomavirus, may play an etiological role in the development of CPT.[40,41] Expression of the T antigen of SV40 leads to the development of CPT in transgenic mice[42] and DNA sequences similar to SV40 have been found within human choroid plexus tumors.[40] To date, a causative role for SV40 in CPT tumorigenesis has not been proven.

Pathology

Macroscopically and microscopically, these tumors resemble the choroid epithelial tissue from which they are derived. Traditionally, primary tumors of the choroid plexus were divided into CPP, classified as a World Health Organization (WHO) grade 1 tumor, and CPC, classified as a WHO grade 3 tumor.[43] Recently, the existence of atypical choroid plexus papilloma, classified as WHO grade 2, has been recognized.

On gross examination, CPP are typically well-circumscribed, globular lesions arising from the choroidal tissue to fill and/or expand the involved ventricle (Fig. 57.1). Microscopically, CPP display a single layer of columnar epithelium well organized along a continuous basement membrane in a papillary pattern (Fig. 57.2). When cut in cross-section, these papillae have a "cobblestone" appearance. Mitoses are rare. Necrosis may be present but it usually is not extensive. Calcification is common in both CPP and CPC[23] but actual bone formation within these tumors is rare.[44] Focal glial differentiation is common.[45]

Atypical choroid plexus papilloma (APP), WHO grade 2, was first formally recognized in the 2007 edition of the WHO central nervous system tumor classification guidelines.[43] In a report that provided much of the rationale for the recognition of APP, a large series of choroid plexus tumors was evaluated for atypical features, including mitotic activity, increased cellularity, nuclear pleomorphism, blurring of papillary growth pattern, and necrosis.[46] Of these features, only elevated mitotic activity was associated with an increased risk of tumor

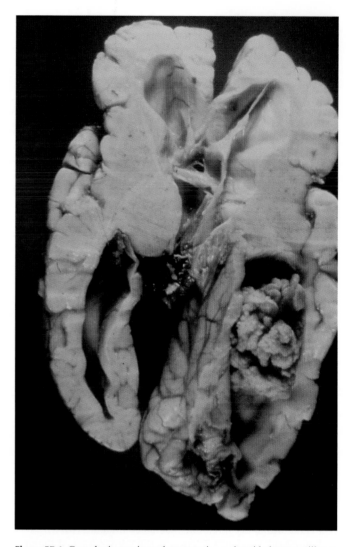

Figure 57.1 Gross brain specimen demonstrating a choroid plexus papilloma within the left lateral ventricle near the atrium. This patient also has associated hydrocephalus.

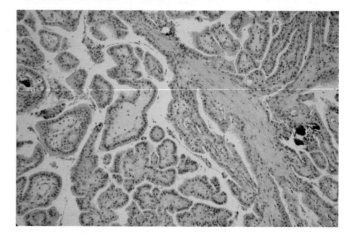

Figure 57.2 Choroid plexus papilloma. H&E stained section.

recurrence. Thus, the primary feature that distinguishes APP from CPP is level of mitotic activity, with APP containing >2 mitoses per 10 high-power fields.

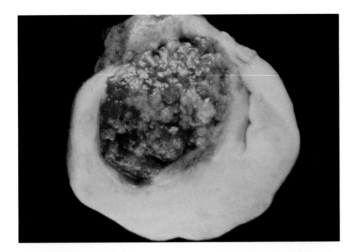

Figure 57.3 Gross specimen of the brainstem demonstrating a choroid plexus carcinoma of the fourth ventricle. Note the invasion of the pons and marked tumor vascularity.

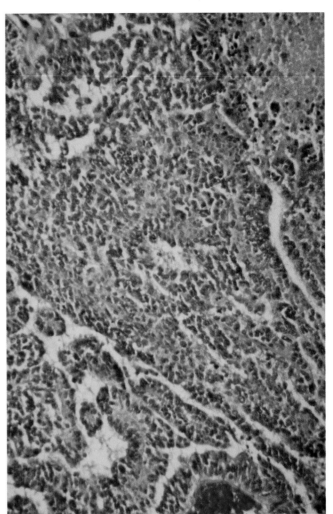

Figure 57.5 Choroid plexus carcinoma showing sheets of undifferentiated cells. H&E stained section.

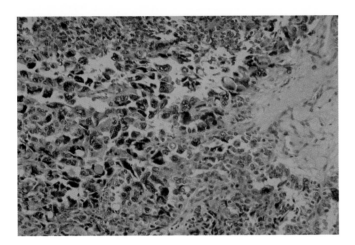

Figure 57.4 Choroid plexus carcinoma. H&E stained section.

Choroid plexus carcinomas are WHO grade 3 tumors and resemble their benign counterparts but are grossly and microscopically invasive (Fig. 57.3). Histologically, the epithelial cells are poorly differentiated, pleomorphic, and actively mitotic (Fig. 57.4). Well-formed papillae are typically not seen and the papillary arrangement may give way altogether to form sheets of undifferentiated cells (Fig. 57.5). Necrosis may be extensive. In some cases the pathology may be difficult to distinguish from a metastatic epithelial neoplasm, especially if the tumor lacks areas of more organized papillae. Electron microscopy demonstrating a basement membrane and cilia may be helpful in differentiating difficult cases.[47]

Immunohistochemically, CPP, APP, and CPC tumors will demonstrate immunoreactivity for S-100 protein, cytokeratins, and vimentin.[47] Glial fibrillary acidic protein (GFAP) immunopositivity is found in 25–55% of CPP and 20% of CPC and is usually restricted to a small subset of cells. Transthyretin immunoreactivity is seen in normal choroid plexus cells, CPP, and CPC but does not reliably differentiate these tumors from metastatic carcinomas.[48] Synaptophysin is also immunopositive in normal and neoplastic choroid plexus but negative in metastatic carcinomas with the exception of neuroendocrine carcinomas.[49,50] A high Ki-67/MIB-1 labeling index is also indicative of a more aggressive tumor, with a mean of 1.9% for CPP and 13.8% for CPC.[30,51]

Clinical aspects

The clinical presentation of choroid plexus tumors depends on the age of the patient and the location and size of the tumor. Most commonly, signs and symptoms include those of increased intracranial pressure with or without focal neurological deficit due to hydrocephalus. Hydrocephalus may be caused by mechanical obstruction of the ventricular system, CSF overproduction by the tumor, reduced CSF resorption, or a combination of all these factors.[22,45,52–55]

In infants and very young children, the presentation may be quite nonspecific, with somnolence, apnea, vomiting, weight loss, ataxia, and loss of developmental milestones. A rapidly increasing head circumference may be seen in young children in whom the cranial sutures have not yet fused. Older children and adults usually present with progressive headache and

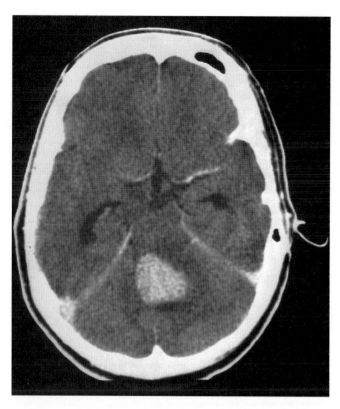

Figure 57.6 Contrasted CT of the brain in an adult patient with a fourth ventricular choroid plexus papilloma. Note also the enlargement of the temporal horns of the lateral ventricles from associated hydrocephalus.

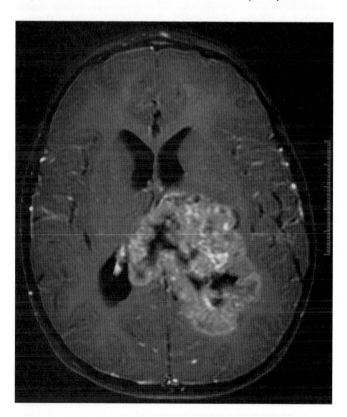

Figure 57.7 Axial T1-weighted MRI of the brain with gadolinium contrast in a child with a large left ventricular choroid plexus carcinoma. Note the intense contrast enhancement and central necrosis within the tumor.

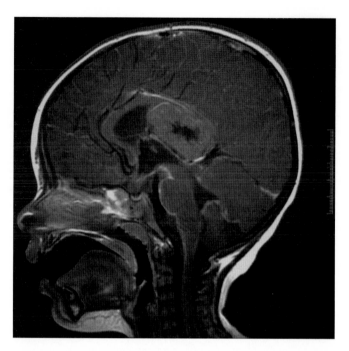

Figure 57.8 Sagittal T1-weighted MRI of the brain with gadolinium contrast in a child with left ventricular choroid plexus carcinoma and leptomeningeal spread of tumor. Note the intense leptomeningeal enhancement.

vomiting with or without complaints of a focal neurological deficit. Seizures may occur. Cerebellar signs may predominate in adults, reflecting the tumor's propensity for the fourth ventricle in older patients. Papilledema is common. Focal neurological signs including hemiparesis, aphasia, visual field defect, reduced vertical gaze, and sixth cranial nerve weakness may occur. A few patients have presented with signs and symptoms of acute intracranial hemorrhage.[31]

Due to the nonspecific symptoms associated with CPT, imaging is important in the early recognition of these tumors. CT and MRI typically demonstrate a large, intraventricular, well-delineated, lobulated mass with robust, homogeneous enhancement (Figs 57.6, 57.7). Both CPC and CPP may have cysts or small foci of necrosis. Calcification is seen in approximately 25% of the cases. T2-weighted MRI sequences may reveal vascular flow voids. Transependymal resorption of CSF is common when hydrocephalus is present, and peritumoral edema may be seen in CPC. Ependymal or leptomeningeal spread of tumor is best appreciated by gadolinium-enhanced MRI and is more common in CPC than CPP (Fig. 57.8).

There is no radiographic feature that reliably distinguishes between CPP and CPC. Moreover, this CT and MRI appearance is not unique to these tumors. Glial-derived tumors (especially ependymomas and subependymomas), primitive neuroectodermal tumors, central neurocytomas, and metastatic carcinomas may arise or appear to arise from within the ventricular system and have similar radiographic characteristics. MR spectroscopy may be helpful in differentiating CPP from CPC.[56] In addition, MRI evaluation of the total spine should be part of the routine evaluation in patients with CPC.

Cerebrospinal fluid examination may be useful in some cases. Dissemination of tumor via ventricular and subarachnoid space is far more common in CPC than in CPP, and tumor cells can be identified by cytological examination.[57] In practice, as most patients have significantly raised intracranial pressure, a CSF examination to look for neoplastic cells is usually contraindicated prior to tumor removal.

Treatment

Surgery

Numerous studies suggest that the extent of surgical resection is the single most important treatment variable predicting disease-free survival, regardless of age or histology.[27,29,31,32,53,58,59] Unfortunately, a GTR may be difficult to achieve due to the often large and highly vascularized nature of CPT. Futher, many patients require pre- or postoperative ventriculoperitoneal shunting of their hydrocephalus. Subdural hematomas and hygromas are a frequent complication as a result of brain collapse following shunting of the hydrocephalus or resection of the large mass.[7,60,61] A series of 41 surgically treated patients found a 22% incidence of temporary swallowing dysfunction, which often led to placement of a percutaneous endoscopic gastrostomy tube or tracheostomy.[58]

In the absence of leptomeningeal metastases, GTR is often curative for CPP. Most deaths from CPP have been in the early perioperative period and survival in CPP significantly improved in publications after 1970, likely owing to improved surgical techniques.[32] Even in cases when GTR is not possible, patients with nonmetastatic CPP or APP are often observed following surgery, with further treatment deferred until the time of progression.

For CPC, the degree of surgical resection is still the best predictor of outcome; nevertheless, CPC tends to recur even in those that are completely resected. This is due to their propensity to invade the brain and spread to transependymal or leptomeningeal locations. GTR is achieved in only 40–57% of patients in the literature.[62] Given the importance ascribed to GTR as a predictor of long-term outcome in CPC, neoadjuvant chemotherapy to treat residual tumor followed by second surgery is sometimes employed. This strategy is associated with a high rate of GRT or extensive subtotal resection at the time of second surgery[63] and metaanalysis suggests that patients with incompletely resected CPC who undergo second surgery have a higher rate of 10-year survival than patients who do not.[64]

Radiotherapy

Radiotherapy for CPT has been used since at least 1929 when van Wagenen reported size reduction of a CPP using radiation therapy (RT) allowing for GTR at a second-stage operation.[9] Because of the rarity of these tumors, no prospective randomized trials of radiotherapy exist. Instead, the data on radiation consist largely of case series and metaanalyses.

There appears to be no rationale for the use of radiation in patients who have had a GTR of a CPP. Even patients with subtotal resections (STR) have had prolonged survivals without receiving RT.[53] A review of 41 patients treated at the Mayo Clinic found that only half of the patients who received an STR required a reoperation for recurrence and that RT after initial STR did not appear to influence outcome.[58] Thus, radiation is often reserved for the treatment of recurrent CPP when GTR is not feasible. Successful treatment of CPP with stereotactic radiosurgery has been reported.[12,65]

The role of RT in the treatment of CPC varies with patient age. RT is generally avoided in patients younger than 3 years of age due to adverse sequelae. In patients older than 3 years, postoperative RT is often recommended, especially in the setting of residual or recurrent disease. One report showed improved survival regardless of the degree of resection.[66] Although no prospective systematic comparison of local versus craniospinal axis radiation (CSI) in CPC has been performed, a comprehensive literature review found that patients who underwent CSI had higher rates of 5-year progression-free survival than patients receiving less than CSI.[67] However, given the increased toxicity of CSI, it may reasonably be reserved for patients with leptomeningeal spread of tumor. There is no report in the literature on the use of radiosurgery for CPC.

Chemotherapy

There is currently no proven role for chemotherapy in the treatment of nonmetastatic CPP. Numerous reports of giving chemotherapy for the treatment of CPC exist in the literature but the usefulness of this is uncertain.[7,19,27,29,68–70] These patients have received a variety of chemotherapy agents in various combinations but VP16, vincristine, cyclophosphamide, and the platinum drugs are the agents with the best evidence of efficacy. Of note, most of these studies were performed prior to the recognition of APP as an entity distinct from CPP, so they contain a mixture of both tumor types under the heading of CPP. Treatment with chemotherapy is often employed in patients with metastatic CPP, due to the paucity of other treatment options.

As in CPP, the treatment of APP begins with surgery. In contrast to CPP, the greater aggressiveness of APP prompts many physicians to treat subtotally resected CPP with chemotherapy immediately after surgery, rather than waiting for tumor progression. Currently, no randomized trials are ongoing to compare chemotherapy with observation in patients with APP but patients with APP are included in an ongoing trial evaluating etoposide and vincristine given in combination with either carboplatin or cyclophosphamide for CPT.

The optimum role of chemotherapy for CPC remains undetermined. The use of neoadjuvant chemotherapy with the goal of reducing the vascularity of residual tumor, allowing for a second more extensive resection, has been described but this approach is not widely used in clinical practice.[63,71] Following an initial GTR, studies evaluating the use of adjuvant chemotherapy to reduce the risk of tumor recurrence in patients too young to tolerate radiation therapy have reached differing conclusions.[29,62,69,70] Proponents of adjuvant chemotherapy after GTR note the high rate of tumor recurrence after resection alone, while opponents emphasize that a number of patients who receive no adjuvant chemotherapy or RT following GTR of CPC enjoy many years of disease-free survival.[31,72] In patients with an initial subtotal resection, no published randomized trials have demonstrated the benefit of early chemotherapy but metaanalysis of the published literature suggests that chemotherapy improves survival.[73]

Ongoing and planned trials will help refine the treatment of CPT in the future. The largest such trial, the Choroid Plexus Tumor (CPT)-SIOP-2000 study, has been active for over a decade.[74] In this collaborative trial, including over 100 institutions from more than 20 countries, patients with low-risk CPT (i.e. nonmetastatic CPP and totally resected nonmetastatic APP) are observed, and patients with high-risk CPT (i.e. metastatic CPP, subtotally resected or metastatic APP, and all CPC) are randomized between two chemotherapy regimens containing etoposide and vincristine in combination with either carboplatin or cyclophosphamide. Radiotherapy is given to patients older than 3 years of age following the second of the six cycles of chemotherapy. Craniospinal radiation is utilized in patients with metastatic CPP or APP, as well as patients with CPC without a radiographic response to chemotherapy. All other patients are treated with local radiation. A follow-up study, CPT-SIOP-2009, will treat high-risk patients (defined as in CPT-SIOP-2009) with radiation therapy, intrathecal cytarabine, and one of four intravenous chemotherapy regimens.[75]

Prognosis

In a metaanalysis of 217 publications and 566 patients, the 1-, 5-, and 10-year projected survival rates were 90%, 81%, and 77% in CPP compared to 71%, 41%, and 35% in CPC.[32] Metastases at presentation and/or age over 40 were poor prognostic indicators. As noted above, the extent of surgical resection is the best predictor of long-term survival. CPP patients with GTR had an 85% 10-year survival rate compared with 56% in those with STR. The 2-year survival in CPC was 72% and 34% for patients with GTR and STR, respectively.

Only one prospective study, that of Wrede *et al.*, reports survival of patients classified by the latest WHO criteria including APP.[74] In the 39 patients with CPP, the 5-year overall survival (OS) probability was 100% and 5-year event-free survival (EFS) probability was 92%. In 24 patients with APP, OS and EFS probabilities were 89% and 83%, respectively. The 29 patients with CPC had the worst outcomes, with a 5-year OS of 36% and EFS of 28%.

As previously noted, some patients with CPC have good outcomes even in the absence of treatment with radiation or chemotherapy. The ability to identify these patients at time of diagnosis would be of great utility, as it could allow potentially morbid treatments such as radiation to be deferred or omitted altogether. Tumor *TP53* status, as measured by immunostaining or mutation analysis, may be one such useful prognostic marker. Tabori and colleagues report that in a series of 26 patients with CPC, 5-year overall survival was 82±9% for the 16 *TP53* immunonegative tumors and 0% for 10 *TP53* immunopositive tumors.[39] These results await prospective confirmation within the framework of a clinical trial but raise the possibility of a personalized medicine approach to CPT in the future.

Recommendations

In summary, aggressive surgical resection is the treatment of choice and best prognostic indicator for patients with CPP, APP, and CPC. Postoperative management of nonmetastatic CPP should generally be a conservative "wait and see" approach, even in the presence of residual disease. Given the potential for long-term adverse sequelae (especially in young children), it is probably best to reserve RT for patients 3 years of age and older with symptomatic disease not amenable to surgical resection. Radiosurgery might be a consideration for symptomatic, residual disease, although very few data exist on its use in this setting. If CPP recurs, consideration should again be given to surgical resection prior to use of chemotherapy or RT.

Patients with nonmetastatic APP can be closely observed if GTR is achieved. In patients with metastatic disease or residual tumor after surgery, adjuvant treatment is a reasonable option. Again, chemotherapy is preferred in young children, and radiation alone or in combination with chemotherapy can be used in older children and adults. Whenever possible, APP patients requiring adjuvant therapy should be enrolled in prospective clinical trials.

Regarding CPC, the question of adjuvant treatment versus observation following GTR remains open and as ongoing large prospective trials treat all CPC patients with adjuvant therapy regardless of extent of resection, it is unlikely to be settled in the foreseeable future. Patients with CPC should be entered into clinical trials or enrolled in the CPT-SIOP registry if trial treatment is not possible. In patients with recurrent or residual inoperative disease, adjuvant treatment is recommended. Children less than 3 years of age should be treated with chemotherapy alone, and radiation should be reserved for patients over 3 years of age. Radiosurgery might also be an option in this setting; however, there are no data available to support a recommendation. Despite chemotherapy and/or radiotherapy, there are few long-term survivors among those who had not also received aggressive surgical resections. These data appear to underscore the importance of extent of resection on prognosis in CPC.

References

1. Guerard M. Tumeur fongueuse dans le ventricule droit du cerveau chez une petite fille de trois ans. Bull Soc Anat 1833; 8: 211.
2. Rokitansky C. *Handbuch der Specieleen Pathologischen Anatomie.* Vienna, Austria: Braumüller and Seidel, 1844.
3. LeBlanc C. *Papilloma myxomatodes*, Beitr. z. path. Anat. d. Gehirn Tumoren. Inaug Dissert. Bonn, Germany,1868.
4. Bielschowsky M, Unger E. Zur kenntnis der primaren epithelgeschwulste der adergeflechte des gehirns. Arch Klin Chir 1902; 81: 61–82.
5. Perthes GC. Gluckliche entfernung eines tumors des plexus choriodeus an dem seitenventrikel des cerebrum. Munch Med Wochenschr 1919; 66: 677–8.
6. Di Rocco C, Iannelli A. Poor outcome of bilateral congenital choroid plexus papillomas with extreme hydrocephalus. Eur Neurol 1997; 37(1): 33–7.

7. Ellenbogen RG, Winston KR, Kupsky WJ. Tumors of the choroid plexus in children. Neurosurgery 1989; 25(3): 327–35.

8. Gudeman SK, Sullivan HG, Rosner MJ, Becker DP. Surgical removal of bilateral papillomas of the choroid plexus of the lateral ventricles with resolution of hydrocephalus. Case report. J Neurosurg 1979; 50(5): 677–81.

9. Van Wagenen WP. Papillomas of the choroid plexus: report of two cases, one with removal of tumor at operation and one with "seeding" of the tumor in the ventricular system. Arch Surg 1930; 20: 199–231.

10. Yoshino A, Katayama Y, Watanabe T, Kurihara J, Kimura S. Multiple choroid plexus papillomas of the lateral ventricle distinct from villous hypertrophy. Case report. J Neurosurg 1998; 88(3): 581–5.

11. Carson BS, Weingart JD, Guarnieri M, Fisher PG. Third ventricular choroid plexus papilloma with psychosis. Case report. J Neurosurg 1997; 87(1): 103–5.

12. Duke BJ, Kindt GW, Breeze RE. Pineal region choroid plexus papilloma treated with stereotactic radiosurgery: a case study. Comput Aided Surg 1997; 2(2): 135–8.

13. Nakano I, Kondo A, Iwasaki K. Choroid plexus papilloma in the posterior third ventricle: case report. Neurosurgery 1997; 40(6): 1279–82.

14. Erman T, Gocer AI, Erdogan S, Tuna M, Ildan F, Zorludemir S. Choroid plexus papilloma of bilateral lateral ventricle. Acta Neurochir (Wien) 2003; 145(2): 139–43; discussion 43.

15. Fujimura M, Onuma T, Kameyama M, et al. Hydrocephalus due to cerebrospinal fluid overproduction by bilateral choroid plexus papillomas. Childs Nerv Syst 2004; 20(7): 485–8.

16. Carter AB, Price DL Jr, Tucci KA, Lewis GK, Mewborne J, Singh HK. Choroid plexus carcinoma presenting as an intraparenchymal mass. J Neurosurg 2001; 95(6): 1040–4.

17. Valladares JB, Perry RH, Kalbag RM. Malignant choroid plexus papilloma with extraneural metastasis. Case report. J Neurosurg 1980; 52(2): 251–5.

18. Jeibmann A, Wrede B, Peters O, Wolff JE, Paulus W, Hasselblatt M. Malignant progression in choroid plexus papillomas. J Neurosurg 2007; 107(3 Suppl): 199–202.

19. St Clair SK, Humphreys RP, Pillay PK, Hoffman HJ, Blaser SI, Becker LE. Current management of choroid plexus carcinoma in children. Pediatr Neurosurg 1991; 17(5): 225–33.

20. Matson DD, Crofton FD. Papilloma of the choroid plexus in childhood. J Neurosurg 1960; 17: 1002–27.

21. Peschgens T, Stollbrink-Peschgens C, Mertens R, Volker A, Thron A, Heimann G. [Therapy of choroid plexus carcinoma in childhood. Case report and review of the literature]. Klin Paediatr 1995; 207(2): 52–8.

22. Boyd MC, Steinbok P. Choroid plexus tumors: problems in diagnosis and management. J Neurosurg 1987; 66(6): 800–5.

23. Ho DM, Wong TT, Liu HC. Choroid plexus tumors in childhood. Histopathologic study and clinico-pathological correlation. Childs Nerv Syst 1991; 7(8): 437–41.

24. Pollack IF. Brain tumors in children. N Engl J Med 1994; 331(22): 1500–7.

25. Rovit RL, Schechter MM, Chodroff P. Choroid plexus paillomas. Observations on radiographic diagnosis. Am J Roentgenol Radium Ther Nucl Med 1970; 110(3): 608–17.

26. Sharma R, Rout D, Gupta AK, Radhakrishnan VV. Choroid plexus papillomas. Br J Neurosurg 1994; 8(2): 169–77.

27. Allen J, Wisoff J, Helson L, Pearce J, Arenson E. Choroid plexus carcinoma – responses to chemotherapy alone in newly diagnosed young children. J Neurooncol 1992; 12(1): 69–74.

28. Romano F, Bratta FG, Caruso G, et al. Prenatal diagnosis of choroid plexus papillomas of the lateral ventricle. A report of two cases. Prenat Diagn 1996; 16(6): 567–71.

29. Pierga JY, Kalifa C, Terrier-Lacombe MJ, Habrand JL, Lemerle J. Carcinoma of the choroid plexus: a pediatric experience. Med Pediatr Oncol 1993; 21(7): 480–7.

30. Rickert CH, Paulus W. Tumors of the choroid plexus. Microsc Res Tech 2001; 52(1): 104–11.

31. Packer RJ, Perilongo G, Johnson D, et al. Choroid plexus carcinoma of childhood. Cancer 1992; 69(2): 580–5.

32. Wolff JE, Sajedi M, Brant R, Coppes MJ, Egeler RM. Choroid plexus tumours. Br J Cancer 2002; 87(10): 1086–91.

33. Yuasa H, Tokito S, Tokunaga M. Primary carcinoma of the choroid plexus in Li–Fraumeni syndrome: case report. Neurosurgery 1993; 32(1): 131–3; discussion 3–4.

34. Trifiletti RR, Incorpora G, Polizzi A, Cocuzza MD, Bolan EA, Parano E. Aicardi syndrome with multiple tumors: a case report with literature review. Brain Dev 1995; 17(4): 283–5.

35. Uchiyama CM, Carey CM, Cherny WB, et al. Choroid plexus papilloma and cysts in the Aicardi syndrome: case reports. Pediatr Neurosurg 1997; 27(2): 100–4.

36. Blamires TL, Maher ER. Choroid plexus papilloma. A new presentation of von Hippel–Lindau (VHL) disease. Eye (Lond) 1992; 6(Pt 1): 90–2.

37. Steichen-Gersdorf E, Trawoger R, Duba HC, Mayr U, Felber S, Utermann G. Hypomelanosis of Ito in a girl with plexus papilloma and translocation (X; 17). Hum Genet 1993; 90(6): 611–13.

38. Krutilkova V, Trkova M, Fleitz J, et al. Identification of five new families strengthens the link between childhood choroid plexus carcinoma and germline TP53 mutations. Eur J Cancer 2005; 41(11): 1597–603.

39. Tabori U, Shlien A, Baskin B, et al. TP53 alterations determine clinical subgroups and survival of patients with choroid plexus tumors. J Clin Oncol 2010; 28(12): 1995–2001.

40. Bergsagel DJ, Finegold MJ, Butel JS, Kupsky WJ, Garcea RL. DNA sequences similar to those of simian virus 40 in ependymomas and choroid plexus tumors of childhood. N Engl J Med.1992; 326(15): 988–93.

41. Martini F, Iaccheri L, Lazzarin L, et al. SV40 early region and large T antigen in human brain tumors, peripheral blood cells, and sperm fluids from healthy individuals. Cancer Res 1996; 56(20): 4820–5.

42. Brinster RL, Chen HY, Messing A, van Dyke T, Levine AJ, Palmiter RD. Transgenic mice harboring SV40 T-antigen genes develop characteristic brain tumors. Cell 1984; 37(2): 367–79.

43. Louis DN, Ohgaki H, Wiestler OD, Cavenee WK (eds). WHO Classification of Tumours of the Central Nervous System, 4th edn. Geneva: World Health Organization, 2007.

44. Doran SE, Blaivas M, Dauser RC. Bone formation within a choroid plexus papilloma. Pediatr Neurosurg 1995; 23(4): 216–18.

45. Buxton N, Punt J. Choroid plexus papilloma producing symptoms by secretion of cerebrospinal fluid. Pediatr Neurosurg 1997; 27(2): 108–11.

46. Jeibmann A, Hasselblatt M, Gerss J, et al. Prognostic implications of atypical histologic features in choroid plexus papilloma. J Neuropathol Exp Neurol 2006; 65(11): 1069–73.

47. Gaudio RM, Tacconi L, Rossi ML. Pathology of choroid plexus papillomas: a review. Clin Neurol Neurosurg 1998; 100(3): 165–86.

48. Albrecht S, Rouah E, Becker LE, Bruner J. Transthyretin immunoreactivity in choroid plexus neoplasms and brain metastases. Mod Pathol 1991; 4(5): 610–14.

49. Kepes JJ, Collins J. Choroid plexus epithelium (normal and neoplastic) expresses synaptophysin. A potentially useful aid in differentiating carcinoma of the choroid plexus from metastatic papillary carcinomas. J Neuropathol Exp Neurol 1999; 58(4): 398–401.

50. Kohmura E, Maruno M, Sawada K, Arita N, Yoshimine T. Usefulness of synaptophysin immunohistochemistry in an adult case of choroid plexus carcinoma. Neurol Res 2000; 22(5): 478–80.

51. Vajtai I, Varga Z, Aguzzi A. MIB-1 immunoreactivity reveals different labelling in low-grade and in malignant epithelial neoplasms of the choroid plexus. Histopathology 1996; 29(2): 147–51.

52. Eisenberg HM, McComb JG, Lorenzo AV. Cerebrospinal fluid overproduction and hydrocephalus associated with choroid plexus papilloma. J Neurosurg 1974; 40(3): 381–5.

53. McGirr SJ, Ebersold MJ, Scheithauer BW, Quast LM, Shaw EG. Choroid plexus papillomas: long-term follow-up results in a surgically treated series. J Neurosurg 1988; 69(6): 843–9.

54. Milhorat TH, Hammock MK, Davis DA, Fenstermacher JD. Choroid plexus papilloma. I. Proof of cerebrospinal fluid overproduction. Childs Brain 1976; 2(5): 273–89.

55. Smith JF. Hydrocephalus associated with choroid plexus papillomas. J europathol Exp Neurol 1955; 14(4): 442–9.

56. Horska A, Ulug AM, Melhem ER, *et al.* Proton magnetic resonance spectroscopy of choroid plexus tumors in children. J Magn Reson Imaging 2001; 14(1): 78–82.

57. Savage NM, Crosby JH, Reid-Nicholson MD. The cytologic findings in choroid plexus carcinoma: report of a case with differential diagnosis. Diagn Cytopathol 2012; 40(1): 1–6.

58. Krishnan S, Brown PD, Scheithauer BW, Ebersold MJ, Hammack JE, Buckner JC. Choroid plexus papillomas: a single institutional experience. J Neurooncol 2004; 68(1): 49–55.

59. McEvoy AW, Harding BN, Phipps KP, *et al.* Management of choroid plexus tumours in children: 20 years experience at a single neurosurgical centre. Pediatr Neurosurg 2000; 32(4): 192–9.

60. Knierim DS. Choroid plexus tumors in infants. Pediatr Neurosurg 1990; 16(4–5): 276–80.

61. Pencalet P, Sainte-Rose C, Lellouch-Tubiana A, *et al.* Papillomas and carcinomas of the choroid plexus in children. J Neurosurg 1998; 88(3): 521–8.

62. Berger C, Thiesse P, Lellouch-Tubiana A, Kalifa C, Pierre-Kahn A, Bouffet E. Choroid plexus carcinomas in childhood: clinical features and prognostic factors. Neurosurgery 1998; 42(3): 470–5.

63. Lafay-Cousin L, Mabbott DJ, Halliday W, *et al.* Use of ifosfamide, carboplatin, and etoposide chemotherapy in choroid plexus carcinoma. J Neurosurg Pediatr 2010; 5(6): 615–21.

64. Wrede B, Liu P, Ater J, Wolff JE. Second surgery and the prognosis of choroid plexus carcinoma – results of a meta-analysis of individual cases. Anticancer Res 2005; 25(6C): 4429–33.

65. Eder HG, Leber KA, Eustacchio S, Pendl G. The role of gamma knife radiosurgery in children. Childs Nerv Syst 2001; 17(6): 341–6; discussion 7.

66. Wolff JE, Sajedi M, Coppes MJ, Anderson RA, Egeler RM. Radiation therapy and survival in choroid plexus carcinoma. Lancet 1999; 353(9170): 2126.

67. Mazloom A, Wolff JE, Paulino AC. The impact of radiotherapy fields in the treatment of patients with choroid plexus carcinoma. Int J Radiat Oncol Biol Phys 2010; 78(1): 79–84.

68. Arico M, Raiteri E, Bossi G, *et al.* Choroid plexus carcinoma: report of one case with favourable response to treatment. Med Pediatr Oncol 1994; 22(4): 274–8.

69. Duffner PK, Kun LE, Burger PC, *et al.* Postoperative chemotherapy and delayed radiation in infants and very young children with choroid plexus carcinomas. The Pediatric Oncology Group. Pediatr Neurosurg 1995; 22(4): 189–96.

70. Gianella-Borradori A, Zeltzer PM, Bodey B, Nelson M, Britton H, Marlin A. Choroid plexus tumors in childhood. Response to chemotherapy, and immunophenotypic profile using a panel of monoclonal antibodies. Cancer 1992; 69(3): 809–16.

71. Souweidane MM, Johnson JH Jr, Lis E. Volumetric reduction of a choroid plexus carcinoma using preoperative chemotherapy. J Neurooncol 1999; 43(2): 167–71.

72. Fitzpatrick LK, Aronson LJ, Cohen KJ. Is there a requirement for adjuvant therapy for choroid plexus carcinoma that has been completely resected? J Neurooncol 2002; 57(2): 123–6.

73. Wrede B, Liu P, Wolff JE. Chemotherapy improves the survival of patients with choroid plexus carcinoma: a meta-analysis of individual cases with choroid plexus tumors. J Neurooncol 2007; 85(3): 345–51.

74. Wrede B, Hasselblatt M, Peters O, *et al.* Atypical choroid plexus papilloma: clinical experience in the CPT-SIOP-2000 study. J Neurooncol 2009; 95(3): 383–92.

75. Intercontinental Multidisciplinary Registry and Treatment Optimization Study for Choroid Plexus Tumors. US National Institutes of Health. Available from: http://clinicaltrials.gov/ct2/show/NCT01014767.

58 Glioma and Other Neuroepithelial Neoplasms

Kevin T. Palka,[1,6,7] **Brett Mobley,**[2] **Stephanie Perkins,**[3] **Michael Cooper,**[4,6] **Allen K. Sills,**[5] **and Paul L. Moots**[1,4,6]

[1] Department of Medicine, [2] Department of Pathology, Microbiology and Immunology (Neuropathology), [3] Department of Radiation Oncology, [4] Department of Neurology, [5] Department of Neurosurgery, Vanderbilt-Ingram Cancer Center, Vanderbilt University Medical Center, Nashville, TN, USA
[6] Tennessee Valley Healthcare Systems, Veterans Administration Medical Center, Nashville, TN, USA
[7] Department of Medicine, Meharry Medical College, Nashville, TN, USA

Introduction

As a group, neuroepithelial neoplasms are uncommon cancers but by no means rare ones. Primary central nervous system (CNS) neoplasms account for 1.3% of all cancers and are about one-fifth as common as metastatic neoplasms involving the CNS. The frequency with which various neuroepithelial neoplasms are encountered changes considerably with age. This chapter will focus predominantly on adult gliomas. However, many of the rare forms occur more frequently in the pediatric population. In recent years, the classification of neuroepithelial neoplasms has evolved considerably.[1] Aside from the astrocytic neoplasms (i.e. glioblastoma, anaplastic astrocytoma, and low-grade astrocytoma) and the oligodendrogliomas, the remainder of the neuroepithelial neoplasms constitute rare entities. Most of the treatment plans used for the rarer forms of glioma are derived from the knowledge of treatment for the more common forms, and some of the recent developments regarding the treatment of those neoplasms will be reviewed.

The primary neuroepithelial neoplasms share similar growth patterns, with a high propensity for local invasion and little likelihood of systemic dissemination. The clinical symptomatology, largely reflecting local cerebral dysfunction, at times combined with altered intracranial pressure, is similar among the various types of CNS neoplasms. The principles of therapy, in respect of both neurological and oncological management, also share many similarities among the various gliomas, and will be reviewed.

The development of therapies specific to a given histological type of glioma is apparent in the evolution of clinical trials over the past 30 years. The tendency to include all high-grade gliomas in the same treatment protocol was common through the 1980s but has since been supplanted by protocols specific to particular glioma histologies and tumor grades. In current practice, the histological distinctions remain the primary piece of information upon which prognosis and treatment planning are based. Increasingly, the molecular analysis of individual tumors is being used to develop predictive and prognostic information for a variety of CNS malignancies. For example, assessment of O^6-methylguanine-DNA methyltransferase (MGMT) promoter methylation in glioblastomas and assessment of loss of heterozygosity on chromosomes 1 and 19 in oligodendrogliomas have added refinements in stratification for clinical trials and in treatment planning.

Epidemiology

As a group, primary CNS tumors of neuroepithelial origin are not uncommon entities. Using the National Program of Cancer Registries (NPCR) and Surveillance, Epidemiology and End Results (SEER) databases, an estimated 95,945 cases of neuroepithelial and spinal cord tumors were reported in the US between 2004 and 2008 (Table 58.1). In 2011, an estimated 22,340 cases will be diagnosed. The overall age-adjusted incidence rates for neuroepithelial CNS tumors between 2004 and 2007 is 8.21 per 100,000 person-years. The incidence rate for malignant pediatric CNS tumors was much lower (3.2 per 100,000 person-years, for patients less than 20 years) than the adult rates (8.9 per 100,000 person-years for patients over 20 years of age). However, it should be noted that CNS tumors are the second most common type of childhood cancers, second only to the leukemias. In general, the incidence rates for neuroepithelial CNS tumors are higher among males (9.38 per 100,000 person-years) than females (7.21 per 100,000 person-years). These tumors are also more common in Caucasian patients compared to African-American and Hispanic patients. The prevalence rate for neuroepithelial CNS tumors in the US was estimated to be 42 per 100,000 person-years in 2004,

Table 58.1 The incidence of primary CNS neoplasms of various histologies.

Histology	Rate*
Neuroepithelial	5.9
Glioblastoma	2.6
Anaplastic astrocytoma	0.5
Astrocytoma (including variants)	1.6v
Oligodendroglioma	0.3
Anaplastic oligodendroglioma	0.1
Ependymoma	0.2
Medulloblastoma	0.2
Benign mixed neuroglial	0.1
Other	0.3
Cranial/spinal nerve sheath	0.9
Meningeal	3.0
Lymphoma	0.4
Germ cell tumors	0.1
Sellar/pituitary	1.2

Source: CBTRUS.[2]
* Rates are per 100,000 person-years.

Box 58.1 Hereditary cancer syndromes associated with primary neuroepithelial neoplasms.

- Neurofibromatosis type I
- Neurofibromatosis type II
- Tuberous sclerosis
- Nevoid basal cell syndrome
- Li–Fraumeni syndrome
- Turcot syndrome
- Hereditary retinoblastoma
- Von Hippel–Lindau syndrome
- Multiple endocrine neoplasia type IIa

representing 124,000 patients living with the diagnosis of a neuroepithelial CNS tumor.[2,3]

To consider gliomas in the context of all CNS primaries, meningiomas and glioblastoma (GBM) are the most common CNS tumors. Meningiomas account for approximately 34% of CNS tumors, while 17% are classified as glioblastoma. The vast majority of patients diagnosed with a meningioma or glioblastoma are older, with a peak incidence rate in the 84+ age group for meningioma (38.5 cases per 100,000 person-years) and the 75–84 year old age group for glioblastomas (14.49 cases per 100,000 person-years). In children under the age of 14, pilocytic astrocytoma (19%), malignant glioma not otherwise specified (NOS) (14%), and embryonal cancers, such as medulloblastoma (13%), comprise the most common histologies. The most common histologies in the 15–19-year-old age group include pituitary tumors (22%) and pilocytic astrocytomas (12%). Pituitary tumors (13.1%), primary CNS lymphomas (2.4%) and CNS germ cell tumors (0.5%) constitute a minority of CNS tumors.

Epidemiological studies have provided some information regarding the causes of primary neuroepithelial neoplasms. A small percentage of patients, 5% at most, have defined hereditary predispositions to cancer that generally include non-CNS as well as CNS malignancies (Box 58.1). In addition, a few families have been described in which multiple individuals have had only neuroepithelial neoplasms, although these are rare. A positive family history of cancer (all types) is noted in about 20% of patients with primary CNS neoplasms. However, case–control studies do not indicate an increased risk of brain tumors in patients with a family history of non-CNS cancers. Aside from defined familial cancer syndromes such as neurofibromatosis, a family history of a brain tumor is associated with a modestly increased risk of a primary CNS neoplasm (odds ratio 2.3).[4]

Exposure to therapeutic radiation is the only environmental factor which is unequivocally associated with an increased risk of CNS neoplasms. This link is particularly strong in children who receive prophylactic cranial irradiation for acute lymphoblastic leukemia (ALL), in whom tumors may develop as early as 7–9 years after treatment. A few other environmental factors have been weakly associated with an increased risk of CNS neoplasms.[5] These include exposure to chlorinated aliphatic hydrocarbons (e.g. carbon tetrachloride), lead, polyvinyl chloride, and organic solvents used in synthetic rubber production. Exposure to electromagnetic fields does not appear to be related to the incidence of CNS tumors in adults, nor does the use of cellular telephones, although active research in this area continues.[6] No association with smoking has been observed. No association with head trauma has been observed for neuroepithelial tumors.

Biology

Primary brain tumors are morphologically heterogeneous, with respect to both the varied histological subtypes (intertumoral heterogeneity) and the appearances of the cells constituting a given tumor subtype (intratumoral heterogeneity). Genetic alterations that govern cellular proliferation, survival, and invasion drive the development and progression of primary brain tumors. Most of the alterations identified over the past several decades have been mapped to three common pathways: the mitogenic signaling pathways, the protein 53 (p53) pathway, and the retinoblastoma (RB) pathway. Although interconnected, mitogenic signaling regulates cell division, survival, and motility while the p53 and RB pathways regulate cell cycle and influence the balance between cellular proliferation, senescence and apoptosis.

Numerous mitogens and their cognate receptor tyrosine kinases (RTKs) are activated in gliomas, often due to genomic alterations that constitutively activate signaling with reduced reliance upon extracellular mitogens. For example, epidermal growth factor receptor (*EGFR*) gene amplification, a common EGFR activating mutation (*EGFRvIII*), and platelet-derived growth factor receptor α gene (*PDGFRA*) amplification are common genetic alterations in gliomas. Phosphoinositide 3′-kinase (PI3K) and mitogen-activated protein kinase (MAPK) are key effectors of mitogenic signaling. Aberrant mitogenic signaling can occur through activating genetic alterations in PI3K and MAPK, or through inactivating mutations in components that suppress their activities, namely the tumor suppressor genes phosphatase and tensin homolog (*PTEN*) and neurofibromatosis 1 (*NF1*). Inactivation of the p53 pathway occurs most frequently through alterations of the gene encoding p53 (*TP53*) or proteins that regulate p53 degradation (*CDKN2A/ARF*, *MDM2*, and *MDM4*). Likewise, inactivation of the RB pathway occurs most frequently through alterations of the gene encoding RB or kinases that regulate the phosphorylation status, and thus activity, of RB (*CDKN2A/ P16INK4A*, *CDKN2B* and *CDK4*). Mutations that inactivate the RB and p53 pathways render tumors particularly susceptible to mitogenic signaling, underscoring the interconnected nature of these three pathways in regulating aberrant cell proliferation.

Targeted therapies against discrete components of the three core glioma pathways have met with limited success thus far, in part due to the enrollment of patients with molecularly heterogeneous glioma subtypes under broad histological inclusion criteria. These limitations are currently being addressed more effectively by comprehensive analyses of the glioma genome to define molecularly distinct subtypes for enhanced diagnostic and prognostic precision.[7–10]

One of the most striking findings from comprehensive mutational analysis has been the identification of the somatic mutations in the isocitrate dehydrogenase 1 gene (*IDH1*) in secondary GBMs.[8] Subsequent analysis of GBM and the lower grade gliomas from which secondary GBM evolve identified *IDH1* and *IDH2* mutations in approximately 75% of all WHO grade 2 and 3 astrocytomas, oligodendrogliomas and grade 4 secondary GBMs. Conversely, *IDH* mutations were found in only 8% or less of primary GBMs and generally not found in pilocytic astrocytoma, ependymoma, medulloblastoma or other primary brain tumor types.[11–13] Interestingly, *IDH* mutations seem to be exclusively found in adults and not in pediatric patients with similar glioma pathologies. Mutations in *IDH1* and *IDH2* are mutually exclusive and the vast majority of *IDH* mutations (over 95%) occur in *IDH1*. *IDH* mutation is currently the most powerful diagnostic marker available for identifying diffuse gliomas in biopsy material and distinguishing pathologically identical primary and secondary GBM.[12,14] Also of great importance, *IDH* mutation confers a better prognosis among WHO grade 3 and 4 glioma subtypes.[8,12,13,15] Furthermore, patients with *IDH*-mutated GBMs have a better prognosis than patients with *IDH* wild-type anaplastic astrocytomas, indicating that in this instance IDH status can be more prognostic than current WHO histopathological criteria.[13,16]

IDH1 and IDH2 are NADP⁺-dependent enzymes that produce nicotinamide adenine dinucleotide phosphate (NADPH) during the catalytic conversion of isocitrate to α-ketoglutarate (α-KG). The mutations found in gliomas occur at the active substrate recognition sites of the two enzymes, arginine R132 of IDH1 and R172 of IDH2, and confer the gain of a novel function to use α-KG as substrate to produce extremely high levels of 2-hydroxyglutarate (2HG) and consume NADPH.[17] 2HG is a competitive inhibitor of multiple α-KG-dependent enzymes including dioxygenases that regulate histone and DNA methylation.[18] As a result, IDH mutation produces global alterations in DNA methylation and thus gene

expression.[19] These findings demonstrate that in addition to the diagnostic and prognostic value of identifying *IDH* mutation, a mechanistic understanding may also impact on the development of novel therapeutics.

Another important dividend of comprehensive and coordinated efforts to analyze the genome of gliomas has been the implementation of gene expression profiles to identify four robust subtypes of GBM: proneural, neural, classical, and mesenchymal.[9,10] Specific genetic alterations also help to differentiate the GBM subtypes: the proneural subtype is characterized by alterations of *PDGFRA* and *IDH1* mutation, the classical by *EGFR* amplification and mutation (*EGFRvIII*), and the mesenchymal by *NF1* and *PTEN* mutations. Patients with the proneural GBM subtype demonstrate the longest survival times.[9] More aggressive therapy, however, significantly reduces mortality in patients with neural, classical and mesenchymal GBM subtypes but not proneural GBM.[10]

The GBM molecular subtypes were named to reflect their resemblances to stages in neurogenesis and to place them in the context of cancer stem cell biology. The prevailing model of cellular heterogeneity and progression had been based upon the stochastic clonal expansion model, whereby any cell having acquired sufficient mutations for transformation constituted the origins of the tumor and source of daughter cells with equal tumorigenic potential. The acquisition of additional mutations in any of these daughter cells could then give rise to new clones of cells expanded by new and perhaps differing advantages in growth, invasion or survival in unique microenvironments.

The discovery of cells with stem-like properties in many tumor types, and in particular of those with neural stem cell properties in brain tumors, has led to a new paradigm called the cancer stem cell (CSC) model. The CSC hypothesis models intratumoral cellular heterogeneity according to a hierarchical organization of differentiation states and has important implications for cell growth and treatment resistance. Under the appropriate culture conditions, CSCs isolated from GBM express neural stem cell (NSC) proteins and upon division give rise to more CSCs (self-renewal) or to more differentiated neural cell types that express markers for astrocytes, oligodendrocytes, or neurons. Among the diverse glioma cell types, only a relatively small proportion of multipotent glioma stem cells (GSCs) are tumorigenic in orthotopic xenograft transplantation models. That is, GSCs have the unique capacity to initiate and passage disease in immunodeficient mice and to give rise to secondary tumors containing GSCs and the bulk of nontumorigenic glioma cells. Several surface markers have been used to enrich for GSCs, and CD133 has been most commonly used to study GSC properties. In addition to tumorigenicity, enhanced resistance to cytotoxic therapies and promotion of angiogenesis indicate the clinical relevance of therapeutically targeting GSCs.[20–22]

Tissue-specific stem cells are appealing candidates as cells of origin because they are maintained into adulthood and can accumulate genetic alterations through sustained self-renewing proliferation. Integration of the genomic profiles, or transcriptome, of molecularly distinct subgroups of ependymoma with those of regionally specific NSCs suggests that this may indeed be the case, with adult spinal NSCs and embryonic cerebral NSCs representing the cells of origin for spinal and cerebral ependymomas, respectively.[23]

The importance of cellular context for manifesting oncogenic mutations has recently been highlighted by mouse genetics to trace the lineages of cells with *TP53* and *NF1* mutation during the formation of glioma. Introduction of the mutations in cerebral NSCs drives aberrant growth in oligodendrocyte precursor cells (OPCs) only and not in other NSC-derived lineages or in NSCs themselves. The transcriptome of OPCs most closely resembles that of proneural GBMs, suggesting a unique cell of origin for this GBM subtype. These findings underscore the important relationships between specific combinations of mutations and susceptible cell types for manifesting particular brain tumor subtypes.

The short-term dividend of these and other recent discoveries is enhanced diagnostic criteria, prognostic accuracy, and rationale for selecting treatment modalities. Longer term and more substantial dividends may be realized by enhanced preclinical models of the full spectrum of primary brain tumor subtypes to target relevant molecular pathways and cell types.

Clinical features and natural history

The symptoms and signs of primary CNS neoplasms represent a combination of localized or focal CNS dysfunction (i.e. seizures, aphasia, hemiparesis) sometimes with superimposed diffuse cerebral dysfunction resulting from mass effect and elevated intracranial pressure. The majority of patients with CNS neoplasms have a good performance status at diagnosis. A large percentage of patients with low-grade gliomas present with partial seizures without any other evidence of neurological deficit. Even among high-grade glioma patients, 60% present with a Karnofsky performance status of 70% or better.[24]

Since the majority of adult gliomas are frontal, temporal, or parietal in origin, focal cerebral hemispheric symptoms predominate. Seizures are more common in low-grade (70–80%) than in high-grade gliomas (20–30%).[25] In the absence of elevated intracranial pressure, only 36% of patients with supratentorial gliomas complain of headache. The headaches tend to be nondescript except for the recurring, persistent, or progressive nature. Severe headaches occur when substantial mass effect and elevated intracranial pressure develop. The classic early morning headache is seen only infrequently.[26]

Given the anatomical distribution of gliomas, personality and cognitive changes are often part of the presenting symptomatology. Apathy and blunted affect are strikingly common, and often attributed to depression for months prior to the diagnosis of a CNS neoplasm. Impaired cognition is among the most common symptoms. This may arise from localized cerebral dysfunction, such as aphasia due to dominant temporal/frontal dysfunction, and neglect or denial of illness due to nondominant parietal dysfunction. Progressive subacute dementia-like presentations occur with gliomas invading the corpus callosum, deep frontal, or midline structures, such as the thalamus. Recognizing cognitive dysfunction and the degree to which it impacts on daily life may be difficult. Family

members are often aware of subtle cognitive symptoms and changes in personality based on their persistence and evolution more than on the severity of these symptoms. Routine bedside testing of cognitive abilities is relatively insensitive for these types of deficits, particularly in older adults for whom minor abnormalities on mental status testing might be dismissed. Neurological deficits that alter personality and cognitive functions are particularly important to recognize and explain when educating the patient and caregivers about the illness, in treatment planning, and in the development of long-term care plans. For many adults with primary CNS neoplasms, the decision-making process regarding medical care will become the responsibility of caregivers, as the patient's capacity to comprehend, analyze, judge, and make decisions is progressively impaired. Particularly in regard to end-of-life issues, the need for early discussion is highlighted in this patient population.[27]

The rate of evolution of a CNS neoplasm has a significant impact on the severity of symptoms. For example, a 4 cm glioblastoma with surrounding edema may produce life-threatening brain herniation, while a 4 cm low-grade astrocytoma located in the same region may produce only focal seizures and otherwise be asymptomatic. Impairments resulting from bilateral involvement of homologous regions of the cerebral hemispheres produce substantially greater functional disability than those resulting from unilateral involvement. This caveat holds irrespective of the nature of the underlying process (i.e. direct involvement by tumor, hydrocephalus, treatment-related toxicity, or coincidental CNS pathology unrelated to the neoplasm).

The natural history of primary CNS neoplasms is commonly viewed from the perspective of high-grade gliomas, as these are the most common and most predictable. However, this view of their natural history cannot be generalized to all types of gliomas. Many low-grade gliomas can be static clinically and radiographically for many years. This tendency for long periods of stable disease makes interpretation of reports on small numbers of patients over short intervals (<3–5 years) very difficult.

Gliomas are neoplasms that fail therapy because of inadequate local control. Leptomeningeal metastases are uncommon, though not rare. These are infrequently observed with gliomas of all histologies and grades, although more commonly among the higher-grade neoplasms. Systemic metastases are extremely rare. In the absence of unexplained spinal symptoms such as radiculopathy or myelopathy, staging of the neuraxis with magnetic resonance imaging (MRI) scanning and cerebrospinal fluid (CSF) cytological evaluation is not warranted. In effect, the clinical history and neurological examination serve as disease staging evaluations. The important exceptions are the medulloblastoma/primitive neuroectodermal tumor (PNET) and childhood type of ependymoma, which do have a higher incidence of subarachnoid dissemination. With improvement of local control, the incidence of leptomeningeal spread in high-grade gliomas will likely increase. The staging evaluation and treatment design for many gliomas may eventually come to resemble those currently used for medulloblastoma.

Table 58.2 Overall survival for various neuroepithelial neoplasms by histology.

Neoplasm	Median survival (years)	Percentage survival				References
		1 year	2 years	5 years	10 years	
Glioblastoma	1.2	68.9	27.2	9.8	–	Stupp, 2009[28]
		34.6	12.6	4.7	2.8	CBTRUS, 2011[2]
MGMT methylated	1.9	94.5	59.4	5.4	–	Stupp, 2009[28]
MGMT unmethylated	1	62.9	14.8	5.5	–	Stupp, 2009[28]
MG (grade 3)*	2.9	95	63	46	–	Levin,[†] 1990[29]
Astrocytoma	7.3	98	84	60	40	Leighton et al., 1997[30]
Anaplastic astrocytoma	1.7	60	43	31	22	CBTRUS, 2011[2]
Oligodendroglioma	>10	94	90	80	64	CBTRUS, 2011[2]
1p/19q codeleted	14.9	100	100	90	70	Fallon, 2004[31]
1p/19q not codeleted	4.7	100	95	40	20	Fallon, 2004[31]
Anaplastic oligodendroglioma	5	80	66	49	35	CBTRUS, 2011[2]
Mixed oligodendroglioma/astrocytoma	10.8	99	93	83	63	Leighton et al., 1997[30]
Ependymoma						
Childhood	1.7	85	40	15	–	Lyons and Kelly,[‡] 1991[32]
Adult	>10	94	89	79	63	CBTRUS, 2011[2]

* MG, malignant glioma including multiple histologies, predominantly astrocytic neoplasms.
[†] These studies utilize minimum performance status requirements for entry, that is, Karnofsky >50%.
[‡] Posterior fossa only.

Table 58.3 Influence of clinical and treatment factors on median survival of adults with malignant gliomas.

	Median survival	References
Age		
<45 years	24 months	Shapiro et al., 1989[24]
>65 years	6 months	
Karnofsky status		
90–100	20 months	Shapiro et al., 1989[24]
70–80	13 months	
50–60	7 months	
30–40	5 months	
Residual tumor following surgery (by CT scan)		
<1 cm²	21 months	Wood et al., 1988[203]
>4 cm²	11 months	
Postsurgical treatment		
Supportive care	3.5 months	Walker et al., 1978[204]
BCNU	4.6 months	
Radiation	9.0 months	
Radiation and BCNU	8.6 months	Walker et al., 1978[204]
	13.1 months	Shapiro et al., 1989[24]
Radiation and temozolomide	14.6 months	Stupp et al., 2005[28]

Reproduced from Moots,[27] with permission from Thieme.
BCNU, bis-chloroethylnitrosourea (carmustine); CT; computed tomography.

Pathological anatomy and neuroimaging

Overview of pathology in glioma diagnosis

It is the role of the neuropathologist to assign a diagnostic category and WHO grade to tumor biopsy specimens. Hematoxylin and eosin (H&E) staining is performed to assess nuclear size, shape and chromatin pattern, cytoplasmic area and borders, proliferative activity as revealed by mitotic figures, and brain infiltration pattern. In most cases, additional immunohistochemical stains are performed. Reactivity for glial fibrillary acidic protein (GFAP) or synaptophysin can reveal glial differentiation or neural differentiation, respectively, of neoplastic cells. Epithelial membrane antigen (EMA) shows specific reactivity patterns in various tumor entities, with diffuse cytoplasmic reactivity in meningiomas and dot-like staining in ependymomas. Neurofilament immunohistochemistry may reveal incorporation of neural processes into a tumor mass, a finding that indicates tumor infiltration into the brain parenchyma. A commonly used marker of cycling cells, Ki-67, is frequently used to determine the percentage of proliferating cells in a neoplasm. "Special stains" are nonimmunohistochemical studies that demonstrate cell and extracellular matrix components. These are used less often than immunohistochemical methods but can be useful. An example is the reticulin connective tissue stain, which may aid the diagnosis of pleomorphic xanthoastrocytoma (PXA) by demonstrating basement membrane material surrounding individual tumor cells.

Once a particular histological category has been assigned, a tumor grade is determined. Grading follows a standardized, four-tier system set forth in the WHO manual.[33] Grade 1 tumors demonstrate recurrent potential but can be cured by surgical excision alone because the tendency for infiltration is low. Grade 2 tumors, while demonstrating low proliferative rates, are usually infiltrative with indistinct surgical and radiographic margins; these tend to recur, and often progress with acquisition of increasingly malignant features. Grade 3 tumors are characterized by higher cellularity and "anaplastic" histological features including frequent mitotic figures and marked variation in nuclear size and shape. Grade 4 tumors generally show marked hypercellularity, more advanced anaplasia, a proliferative tumor vasculature, and necrosis. It must be emphasized that the prognostic impact of tumor grade varies widely from one neoplastic entity to another. For example, grade 3 diffuse astrocytomas will invariably progress to grade 4 lesions (glioblastoma) while grade 3 ependymomas may be cured by modern treatments. And while progression along the grading spectrum characterizes the natural history of diffuse astrocytic tumors, other glial and neuroepithelial neoplasms, for example pilocytic astrocytoma and ganglioglioma, do not usually advance in grade.

While in the majority of cases categorization and grading of tumors are straightforward, diagnostic difficulties are common. These arise as a result of either histological overlap between tumor entities and/or ill-defined grading criteria. A common source of diagnostic difficulty is the histological overlap between astrocytic tumors and oligodendroglial neoplasms. Oligodendrogliomas classically show round nuclei with cytoplasmic clearing ("cytoplasmic halos") but astrocytic neoplasms may also demonstrate cytoplasmic clearing in a significant portion of cells. When other features that might permit classification of a tumor as either astrocytic or oligodendroglial are lacking, the pathologist must use the "roundness" of tumor nuclei to categorize the neoplasm. This is not a straightforward determination and one often finds high interpathologist variability, with some making a diagnosis of oligodendroglioma, some using the term astrocytoma, and others calling the tumor an "oligoastrocytoma."

The impact of ill-defined grading criteria on tumor classification is best illustrated by the difficulty in distinguishing grade 2 diffuse from grade 3 anaplastic astrocytomas. The WHO criteria state that while a single mitosis identified in a small stereotactic biopsy specimen indicates proliferative activity suggestive of anaplasia, a single mitosis in larger resection specimens is not sufficient for a WHO grade 3 designation.[34] The reference does not provide additional detail as to the frequency of mitotic figures required for anaplasia. Pathologists are accustomed to enumerating the number of mitotic figures per high-power microscopic field for other tumor entities but this mitotic frequency criterion does not exist in the astrocytoma grading spectrum. Since the degree of mitotic activity sufficient for anaplasia is not well codified, cases with borderline features are common and the diagnostic decision is difficult.[35]

Overview of neuroimaging in gliomas

With a few exceptions, neuroepithelial neoplasms grow by infiltration along nerve fibers and along the microvasculature through the brain parenchyma. This leads to characteristic gross patterns of growth because of the involvement of fiber tracts (i.e. subinsular extension of a temporal glioma, subpial accumulations of tumor cells).[36,37] Changes in the affected neuropil may be very modest for low-grade neoplasms. The cellularity is modestly increased compared to normal white matter. Some edema, neuronal satellitosis, subpial accumulation of tumors cells, endothelial hyperplasia, microcalcifications, cystic changes, and occasionally perivascular inflammatory infiltrates are seen. In low-grade neoplasms, the blood–brain barrier is generally relatively well preserved. These features are apparent on computed tomography (CT) and magnetic resonance imaging (MRI) scanning, although for low-grade gliomas MRI is considerably more sensitive (Fig. 58.1). Typically there is a region of increased signal on T2-weighted MRI images, indicating increased tissue fluid or loss of myelin content, with relatively indistinct margins. Evidence of mass effect, demonstrated by displacement of adjacent structures (e.g. compression of sulci, ventricular displacement), is almost always present. Mass effect often helps to distinguish low-grade neoplasms from demyelinating and other nonneoplastic processes. Typically, contrast enhancement is absent, indicating preservation of the blood–brain barrier. If contrast enhancement is observed in an otherwise typical low-grade diffuse astrocytoma, the prognosis is worse. However, a few less common variants of low-grade astrocytoma, particularly the pilocytic astrocytoma, characteristically demonstrate contrast enhancement and yet maintain an excellent prognosis.

High-grade gliomas are much more cellular with more extensive edema and mass effect, in part related to impairment of the blood–brain barrier. Barrier disruption results from multiple factors, including inflammation within the tumor, release of vasoactive substances by tumor cells, endothelial hyperplasia, and neovascularity. The central core of the neoplasm is a region of high cellularity often with necrosis, surrounded by tumor with high cellularity and vascular hyperplasia infiltrating the adjacent neuropil. The brain adjacent to this densely packed core is infiltrated by tumor cells often over distances of many centimeters.[38,39]

Magnetic resonance imaging scanning of high-grade gliomas demonstrates extensive edema and mass effect, often with radiographic evidence of temporal or subfalcine

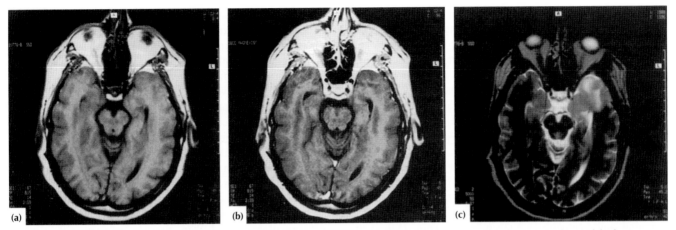

Figure 58.1 A 45-year-old right-handed male presented with episodes of confusion accompanied by guttural noises diagnosed as complex partial seizures. The precontrast T1-weighted MRI (a) demonstrates an indistinct fullness in the gyri of the anterior temporal lobe on the left. On postcontrast T1-weighted images (b), there is no contrast enhancement. T2-weighted images (c) reveal a poorly demarcated region of increased signal intensity that proved to be a low-grade astrocytoma.

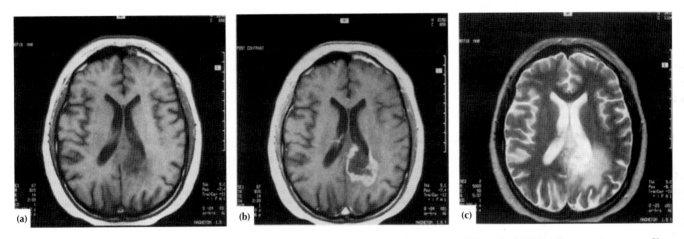

Figure 58.2 A 30-year-old male presented with incoordination of the right leg and headaches. The precontrast T1-weighted MRI (a) demonstrates an area of low signal intensity deep in the left parietal lobe. The postcontrast T1-weighted image (b) demonstrates peripheral enhancement. The T2-weighted images (c) reveal edema and infiltration by tumor without a sharp demarcation throughout the left parietal lobe as well as the corpus callosum. Pathologically, this neoplasm proved to be a glioblastoma.

herniation. The tumor core is typically well demonstrated after intravenous contrast as an outer region of intense enhancement with a poorly enhancing center. The extent of the invasive component is best depicted on T2-weighted views. Again, there is an increased T2 signal abnormality with margins that usually appear indistinct. Correlative pathology studies reveal that the T2 abnormality often approximates but does not perfectly demonstrate the true extent of the neoplasm with microscopic infiltration of tumor cells beyond the radiographically apparent margin (Fig. 58.2). The MRI fluid-attenuated inversion recovery (FLAIR) sequence provides a depiction similar to the T2 view but is sometimes easier to interpret because the CSF appears dark in the FLAIR sequence.

Despite remarkable advances in the ability to image the CNS, the information available from MRI scanning has important limitations with regard to assessment of most neuroepithelial tumors. The true extent of the tumor is not clearly defined. It is approximated by the T2-weighted abnormality more closely than by the region of contrast enhancement for most gliomas.[36,40] Changes in the T2-weighted and FLAIR images are multifactorial (i.e. edema, loss of myelin, gliosis, neoplastic infiltration) and often do not improve with treatment. In fact, these changes may worsen as a delayed result of radiation and some chemotherapies. Furthermore, both the degree of contrast enhancement and the extent of the T2-weighted abnormality may improve with escalation of corticosteroid dosage, and after bevacizumab.

These limitations are important to consider in relation to treatment planning for surgery and radiation therapy where extent of tumor involvement is a critical element in decision making. The limitations of MRI imaging for assessment of tumor response also have important implications that affect both the treatment decisions for individual patients (e.g. is radiographically stable disease while on chemotherapy in the months after radiation adequate justification for continuing maintenance chemotherapy?) and the design of clinical trials for gliomas, which typically assess tumor response based on the dimensions of the contrast-enhancing lesion.[41–46]

The MRI appearance of a CNS mass lesion can provide a strong impression that a lesion is a primary neoplasm but it does not provide diagnostic certainty to a degree sufficient to explain the prognosis or to develop treatment plans. Some enhancing lesions prove to be low-grade gliomas. Even multiple enhancing lesions that suggest metastatic disease occasionally prove to be multifocal high-grade gliomas. The distinction between high-grade glioma, CNS lymphoma, solitary metastasis, and abscess remains a challenge that has not been resolved by standard neuroimaging. The distinction between oligodendroglial and astrocytic neoplasms also remains very difficult. Positron emission tomography (PET) scanning and magnetic resonance spectroscopy (MRS) are additional tools that can help determine whether a lesion is neoplastic, and yet many of these difficulties are not settled by PET or MRS. To date, the need for a pathological diagnosis of a CNS neoplasm remains, and with the development of treatment strategies based on molecular characteristics, the need for a tissue diagnosis is increasing.

Two common situations in which treatment decisions are based solely on imaging are a brainstem lesion and an enhancing mass suspicious for high-grade glioma in an elderly or debilitated patient. Data on brainstem lesions in children provide some guidance in the former situation. In children with brainstem lesions who have the typical history and imaging features characteristic of a brainstem glioma, a diagnostic biopsy is generally not recommended. This is based on pathological studies showing that such lesions are astrocytoma, generally high grade, in 95% of cases. The risk of biopsy in these children is not warranted. In adults, brainstem gliomas are uncommon and thus there is a stronger rationale for biopsy but the risks remain substantial (see below).

In the situation of an older adult with advanced symptoms from an enhancing cerebral hemispheric mass, an invasive diagnostic procedure would often want to be avoided. Yet occasionally a process other than glioblastoma that might be more effectively treated, such as CNS lymphoma or abscess, will be missed for lack of a pathological diagnosis. In our experience, patients who are not well enough to undergo a biopsy either receive only palliative care with steroids or occasionally an abbreviated course of radiation.

Principles of glioma therapy

Surgery

Surgery for gliomas offers several important benefits. First is the ability to make an exact pathological diagnosis. A second benefit is the improvement of symptoms through reduction of mass effect. Removal of the mass is the quickest way to achieve symptomatic improvement. In some cases, this may be life-saving due to impending brain herniation. Surgical removal may improve seizure control and allow for lower doses of adjuvant corticosteroids.

Another benefit of surgery is the potential to change the natural history of a glioma. There is evidence in lower grade lesions

that complete surgical resection may be curative in selected patients. This is particularly true for grade 1 neoplasms such as pilocytic astrocytomas and gangliogliomas, as well as for certain grade 2 neoplasms such as pleomorphic xanthoastrocytomas. For higher grade neoplasms, emerging data suggest that improvements in overall survival and quality of survival are associated with more extensive resections, as long as new deficits are not created with surgery. Surgical resection of tumors also allows for smaller target areas for radiation therapy in some cases. Radiation may also be better tolerated with the associated reduction of mass effect after surgical removal.

A final benefit to surgical therapy for gliomas is the opportunity to use implantable therapies. This would include adjuvants such as carmustine wafers for high-grade gliomas, catheters for delivery of intrathecal chemotherapy, convection delivery of chemotherapy, or radiation sources for brachytherapy.

Surgical options include stereotactic biopsy, limited open biopsy, or open resection of lesions. Stereotactic biopsies offer advantages of limited exposure and shorter operating times but may be hindered by sample bias of the lesion and by the small but significant incidence of associated periprocedural hemorrhage. Open biopsy improves the accuracy of diagnosis due to larger samples but is associated with slightly higher risk. Open surgical resection provides the largest amount of tissue and gives the opportunity for relief from mass effect but carries higher risk due to the longer and more extensive nature of the procedure.

Decision making as to which patients are candidates for surgery and what type of surgery to perform is a complex process. Factors which must be accounted for include the patient's age, performance status, location of the lesion, associated symptoms, time course, and overall goals of therapy. Decisions are best made by a multidisciplinary team with input from neurosurgeons, medical oncologists, radiation oncologists, and neuroradiologists who are all experienced in the management of brain tumors. Risks and complications in the postoperative period include hemorrhage (either intraoperative or within the immediate postoperative period), seizures, leak of spinal fluid, creation of new neurological deficits, transient worsening of mass effect, obstruction or injury to venous sinuses, or arteries producing stroke or worsened mass effect, infection, obstruction of CSF pathways, cosmetic deformities, as well as usual risks of surgical procedures and anesthesia. Fortunately, with the adoption of advanced neuroanesthesia and microneurosurgical techniques, intraoperative mortality is an exceedingly rare event but major risks do remain with all procedures.

Craniotomy has been made much safer by the introduction of a variety of technical adjuncts. Chief among these are intraoperative navigation systems, which use infrared technology to correlate surface and deep brain anatomy with preloaded imaging studies. The accuracy of these systems allows for biopsy of lesions as small as 1–2 mm in size on a routine basis. These systems have also lessened the morbidity of cranial procedures by decreasing the size of necessary exposure and helping to define borders of lesions prior to resection. Other technical adjuncts include the use of intraoperative corticography for mapping out seizure foci, both before and after resection. Some cranial procedures are done with the patient only under intravenous sedation in a so-called "awake" craniotomy. These techniques are used when the surgeon needs to communicate with the patient during the procedure and are primarily helpful for localization of speech and motor function when an infiltrative lesion is located immediately adjacent to the two areas of brain eloquent for these functions. Intraoperative consultation with a neuropathologist for frozen section diagnosis is another important part of the surgical management of glioma patients. This can be a valuable guide to help intraoperative decision making about the extent of resection that is appropriate for a given diagnosis.

Postoperative imaging is recommended to assess the extent of resection for open cases and to determine accuracy of targeting for biopsy-only cases. It is important that this postoperative scan be done within 48 h after surgery as the breakdown of the blood–brain barrier is greatly accelerated after this time point and this will make determination of extent of resection difficult. Most clinicians favor waiting at least 14 days before initiating any form of radiotherapy to the operated field. An exception to this would be cases where stereotactic biopsy only has been done since there is a very small wound and healing issues are less important.

Radiation therapy

Radiation therapy is utilized in the treatment of most primary intracranial tumors either as definitive treatment or, more often, after maximal surgical resection. The goal of radiation is to eradicate tumor cells at the origin of the tumor or in the resection cavity. Additionally, a margin of brain tissue surrounding the tumor is included in the irradiation field due to the infiltrative behavior of gliomas. This margin varies depending on the histological subtype. Treatment is most often delivered with fractionated external beam photon irradiation over a course of 5–6 weeks.

For low-grade tumors that do not enhance, the target volume is often defined by T2 or FLAIR pulse sequence abnormalities. This volume is then expanded approximately 1–2 cm. For high-grade tumors, the T2 or FLAIR changes are contoured and expanded by 2 cm. After treatment of this area, additional boost irradiation is delivered to a smaller area consisting of the enhancing tumor with an additional 2 cm margin. The treatment planning process also includes the delineation of normal critical structures such as the optic nerves, optic chiasm, cochleae, and brainstem. Depending on the proximity of the tumor to these structures, the physician may choose treatment delivery with either three-dimensional (3D) conformal radiation or intensity modulated radiation therapy (IMRT) in order to achieve optimal normal tissue sparing without compromising tumor coverage.

Other options for radiotherapy delivery could include radiosurgery, stereotactic radiation therapy, or particle beam irradiation (i.e. protons). Radiosurgery and stereotactic radiation therapy are commonly used in the treatment of brain metastases but play a limited role in the treatment of gliomas. Charged particle irradiation with protons has been used, although there is not a clear advantage for most gliomas.

The side-effects of radiation treatment can be divided into those that occur during or directly after the course of radiation and those that are considered late sequelae. During the course of treatment, fatigue and worsening of pretreatment symptoms due to increased peritumoral edema are the major side-effects.

Long-term risks and complications of radiation are varied and depend on dose and location of treatment. One of the more serious complications is the development of radiation necrosis at the site of treatment that can occur months to years after treatment. Differentiating radionecrosis from tumor progression can be difficult both clinically and radiographically. Hearing loss is possible when cochlear tolerance is exceeded. The lens of the eye is very sensitive to radiation and patients should be counseled on the risk of cataract formation in tumors near the eye. Radiation-induced optic neuritis can manifest as focal visual loss, decreased acuity, or blindness. Patients are at increased risk for these sequelae with doses to the optic nerves and chiasm exceeding 5400 cGy. Treatment near the pituitary can lead to decreased hypothalamic and pituitary function.

Chemotherapy

Outcome measures assessed in phase 3 clinical trials are the strongest evidence-based indications for the use of chemotherapy as part of the initial treatment of gliomas. This information exists only for GBM, where chemotherapy modestly improves overall survival (OS), and for anaplastic oligodendroglioma in which chemotherapy increased progression-free survival (PFS) but not OS. Most recent trials have not shown a survival advantage with chemotherapy in anaplastic astrocytomas. In grade 2 gliomas, older trials have not demonstrated a benefit for the addition of chemotherapy. Ongoing trials are addressing whether chemotherapy combined with radiation is beneficial for grade 2 and 3 gliomas. Benefit has also been seen in a few rarer types of glioma such as the subependymal giant cell astrocytomas. Data for the use of chemotherapy in recurrent gliomas are weak but it is frequently used as salvage therapy given the limitations of surgery and radiation in this setting.

Other factors that impact chemotherapy decisions include age, performance status, expected survival, and the nature of symptoms. Older patients generally do not tolerate chemotherapy regimens as well as younger patients, and there are suggestions that older glioma patients have lower response rates. In the pivotal trials for glioblastoma, patients older than 70 years of age were excluded, and caution is advised when prescribing temozolomide for older patients.

With regard to performance status, many glioma trials use a Karnofsky performance status (KPS) of 70% or greater for eligibility. In general practice, a KPS of 60% is a very reasonable level at which to consider treatment. It would be uncommon to recommend chemotherapy as adjuvant therapy at diagnosis or for recurrent disease if the KPS is 50% or less. This guideline does not apply to all primary CNS neoplasms, particularly for CNS lymphomas, where aggressive therapy for a patient with low KPS can be very effective.

In certain cases chemotherapy can improve control of neurological symptoms. Improved seizure control is a quantifiable symptom for which multiple trials in low- and high-grade gliomas have demonstrated positive results. Yet it is uncommon for seizure control to improve sufficiently to allow discontinuation of anticonvulsants. Most focal neurological symptoms are not markedly improved by chemotherapy. Even an excellent tumor response to treatment will often leave a major neurological deficit unchanged or only modestly improved. Patients and families should understand that current therapies are not curative. The primary goals of treatment are delaying recurrence and improving survival. Symptom control is a valuable secondary goal, although the primary therapies for symptom relief remain surgery, corticosteroids, anticonvulsants, antidepressants, analgesics and others.[47]

Monitoring therapeutic efficacy is much more heavily weighted on neuroimaging (e.g. MRI) results than on symptomatic changes.[48] While MRI imaging is a more sensitive and more specific way to identify glioma response and progression than clinical assessment, it has many pitfalls. Radiation may cause transient worsening of contrast enhancement and edema (i.e. pseudoprogression), and steroid administration affects enhancement and edema. Maximal radiographic improvement may not occur until 3 months in glioblastomas and 6–12 months in low-grade gliomas. These issues have been highlighted by the difficulties that arise in interpreting MRI scans after treatment with bevacizumab. Expert attempts to standardize response criteria for clinical trials provide valuable insights for physicians treating glioma patients.[44,46]

Neuroepithelial neoplasms

Astrocytic neoplasms

Glioblastoma

Glioblastoma, or grade 4 astrocytoma, is a highly cellular, anaplastic neoplasm with frequent mitoses, vascular proliferation, and necrosis (Fig. 58.3). In most instances, glioblastoma is not difficult to diagnose histologically. There are a number of uncommon histological variants such as the small cell predominant glioblastoma and the gliosarcoma. These histological variants have a behavior and prognosis that are similar to the typical glioblastoma. The distinction from anaplastic oligodendroglioma may be difficult (see below). The distinction from some low-grade gliomas with unusually anaplastic or pleomorphic cytological features also can present a critical diagnostic challenge (see below).

Resections that accomplish removal of all enhancing tumor are described as "gross total resections." The term is an imprecise one and is often misleading to patients. This degree of resection can be accomplished in 40–60% of patients with high-grade gliomas. Resections that accomplish removal of 98% of enhancing tissue achieve an increase in median survival.[49] Even the most aggressive surgical resection cannot be considered treatment with curative potential.

The surgical mortality for resection of malignant gliomas (MG) is less than 3%. Transient worsening of neurological deficits is common. Persistent, functionally significant worsening is observed in about 20%.[50] A high incidence of venous thrombosis is also observed. This appears to result

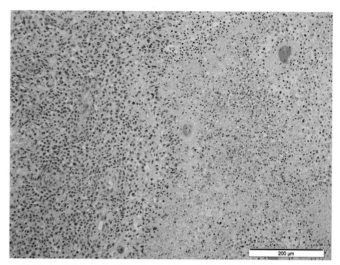
(a)

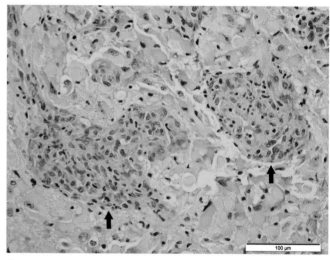
(b)

Figure 58.3 Glioblastoma. Glioblastomas are densely cellular with necrosis (a, *right half of field*; H&E, 200× original magnification) and/or vascular proliferation (b, *arrows*; H&E, 400× original magnification) characterized by multilayered blood vessels, often with a glomeruloid morphology.

from tumor-induced hypercoagulability. Treatment with anticoagulant therapy can be accomplished safely.[51]

Radiation therapy has the most significant impact on survival among all the treatment options for patients with gliomas. Compared with surgery and supportive care, the addition of fractionated radiation increased median survival for high-grade glioma patients three- to fourfold in multiple brain tumor support groups (BTSG) studies.[52] Current radiation therapy recommendations typically include fractionated doses to a total of 60.0 Gy over 6 weeks. With escalation of the dose to between 65 and 75 Gy, a modest decline in survival has been observed.[53]

The benefit of chemotherapy for glioblastoma and other high-grade gliomas was a highly debated issue for many years. The European Organization for Research and Treatment of Cancer (EORTC)/National Cancer Institute of Canada (NCIC) published the results of a large randomized phase 3 clinical trial in 2005 showing a statistically significant survival advantage using a treatment regimen consisting of 60 Gy of radiotherapy with concurrent daily temozolomide at 75 mg/m². After completion of the radiation therapy, monthly temozolomide was continued at 150–200 mg/m² on days 1–5 of a 28-day cycle for six cycles. The median survival in the experimental arm was 14.6 months, compared to 12.1 months with radiation treatment alone This study included patients with KPS ≥70 and age less than 70 years. After the publication of these data, temozolomide largely supplanted the nitrosoureas as the first choice of treatment for most gliomas. However, single-agent temozolomide does not have a substantially better response rate than bis-chloroethylnitrosourea (BCNU) or Lomustine (1- (2-chloroethyl)-3-cyclohexyl-1-nitrosourea; CCNU).[54] Single-agent BCNU, CCNU or the procarbazine, lomustine, and vincristine (PCV) regimen can be considered options for therapy at recurrence, although a trial of BCNU for recurrent glioma with MRI-based response assessment showed only a 10% response rate.[55] Bevacizumab has now relegated these regimens to third-line options (see below).

One important prognostic and predictive biomarker for GBM is the methylation status of the MGMT promoter. Epigenetic silencing of this gene reduces repair of alkylated DNA. Roughly 45% of GBMs have methylated MGMT promoters. In the EORTC/NCIC trial, methylation of the MGMT promoter was associated with a significantly prolonged progression-free survival and overall survival (median survival 21.7 months) after treatment with radiation and temozolomide compared to the unmethylated cohort of patients (median survival 12.2 months). Stratification by MGMT status has become the norm for GBM trials.[56,57]

The use of implantable BCNU-containing wafers (Gliadel®, Eisai) placed at the time of resection provides high-dose therapy for microscopic residual disease. There is minimal systemic distribution which avoids the usual hematological toxicities of BCNU. Implantation of BCNU wafers combined with radiation improves overall survival compared to radiation alone (13.1 versus 10.9 months).[58] Only a small percentage of patients, about 10% at our institution, receive these wafers due to anatomical and surgical constraints. There is an increased risk of seizures, cerebral edema, impaired wound healing, and intracranial infections following implantation. We proceed with radiation and temozolomide after BCNU wafers are implanted.[59]

The average time to recurrence for GBMs after treatment with radiation and temozolomide is 7 months. Re-resection can be considered at progression if there is significant mass effect causing seizures or other symptoms but there is no survival benefit to additional surgery.[60] Reirradiation or stereotactic radiosurgery can also be offered at the time of recurrence but this is controversial and should be recommended on a case-by-case basis. Salvage chemotherapy, usually with a regimen containing bevacizumab (Avastin®, Genentech/Roche), is the most common course of treatment at present. Measurement of disease response is obscured by the diminution of contrast enhancement that is seen after bevacizumab is given. In one large, noncomparative phase 2 trial, bevacizumab in combination with irinotecan resulted in an estimated

6-month progression-free survival (PFS) rate of 50.3%, a median overall survival of 8.9 months, and a response rate of 37.8%.[61] Bevacizumab as a single agent has also been shown to be an effective option for recurrent GBM, with a 6-month rate of progression-free survival of 35.1%.[62] Bevacizumab is well tolerated, improves symptoms caused by peritumoral edema, and allows for significant reduction or cessation of steroids.

Other drugs used in the treatment of recurrent GBM include nitrosoureas, cisplatin, carboplatin, procarbazine, irinotecan, and etoposide, although response rates are generally in the 5–20% range. Temozolomide has only limited activity in patients with recurrent glioblastomas, with a response rate of 5.4% and 6-month progression-free survival rate of 21%.[2] Alternative schedules of temozolomide, "dose dense" every other week or "metronomic" protracted daily dosing, have been reported to produce a higher response rate. Drugs that inhibit the EGFR, such as erlotinib and gefinitib, have been largely disappointing despite the frequency of EGFR vIII mutations in GBM.

Gliosarcoma

The 2007 WHO classification classifies primary gliosarcoma (PGS) as a distinct variant of GBM. Gliosarcomas represent approximately 1.8–2.8% of GBMs, and occur almost twice as frequently in men as in women. The symptoms at presentation and the age of presentation (sixth to seventh decade of life) are similar in GBM and PGS. These tumors are composed of two distinctly identifiable biphasic components: a grade 4 glial neoplasm which fulfills histological criteria for GBM, and a metaplastic mesenchymal component. There is no consensus about the morphology of the mesenchymal portion of these tumors, which may display fibroblastic, cartilaginous, osseous, muscle, or adipose features.[63] Secondary gliosarcoma (SGS) is a rare but distinct entity, whereby a primary GBM develops sarcomatoid features, usually after treatment with radiation and concurrent temozolomide. In one single-institution retrospective series of 30 patients, those who initially received concurrent and adjuvant temozolomide for GBM had much worse survival after developing SGS than those who did not receive temozolomide (4.3 and 10.5 months survival, respectively).[64]

Although classified as a GBM variant, PGS have several clinical features which suggest that these tumors may be a distinct entity. First, PGS is found exclusively supratentorially, with a predilection for the temporal and frontal lobes. Secondly, it has a much higher incidence of extracranial metastases when compared to GBM. The most common sites of metastases are the lung and liver, and this is thought to be through hematogenous spread. A well-documented phenomenon is the occurence of metastases which contain only sarcomatous elements.[65] CSF metastases are also well documented, and imaging of the entire neuraxis can be considered.[66] Finally, as molecular classification of these tumors became more refined, certain molecular differences between GBM and PGS became apparent. EGFR gene amplification is a common event in more than half of GBMs but occurs in fewer than 10% of gliosarcomas.[67] Gliosarcomas also seem to have more genetic stability, based on the decreased frequency of chromosomal imbalances. It is important to note that the gliomatous and sarcomatous elements often have identical mutations, including *p16* deletion, *PTEN* mutation, *CDK4* amplification, and p53 nuclear accumulation, further reinforcing the monoclonal origin of PGS.[67]

Four studies of PGS patients with matched GBM control groups revealed that survival for gliosarcoma is similar to that for GBM. The total number of PGS patients was small (66 PGS compared to over 3000 GBM patients) but there was no statistically significant difference in survival. Gross total resection should be the initial treatment goal. Postsurgical radiation therapy improves survival (10.6 months median survival with radiation versus 6.25 months without) but the data for chemotherapy in these tumors are limited. The authors recommend using the standard GBM chemotherapy regimen (i.e. low-dose temozolomide with radiation, followed by monthly full-dose temozolomide), given the aggressive nature of these tumors.

Anaplastic astrocytoma

Principles of surgery and radiation are similar to those for glioblastoma. The use of chemotherapy has been evaluated in trials specific to this grade. One report demonstrated a statistically significant improvement in outcome for patients receiving PCV as opposed to single-agent BCNU.[29] However, an attempt by the EORTC to reproduce this finding was negative.[68] Current trials are looking at whether temozolomide is more active. Many neurooncologists continue to favor including chemotherapy in the initial treatment of anaplastic astrocytoma. However, support from a large randomized trial that uses radiation only as the control arm is not available (Fig. 58.4).

Astrocytoma

The term "astrocytoma" is used by pathologists to refer grade 1 or 2 astrocytomas, which are often called low-grade astrocytomas. The older term, benign astrocytoma, is pathologically imprecise and clinically misleading. Its use should be avoided (Fig. 58.5).

Multiple series suggest that resection of typical low-grade astrocytoma is beneficial, although no randomized trials have been performed to address this question.[69,70] Fractionated radiation therapy produces an increase in PFS and clinical benefit such as improved seizure control at doses somewhat lower than those for high-grade gliomas (i.e. 45 Gy).[71] However, its impact on overall survival benefit is less clear.[30] Multiple randomized trials have shown equivalent overall survival for patients treated at diagnosis versus those treated when subsequent progression is observed radiographically, although the use of salvage therapies confounds the interpretation of these results.[72]

Analysis of these treatment options must also include consideration of long-term sequelae of cranial radiation in adults. While severe cognitive impairment has been associated with whole-brain and opposed parallel port delivery, modern radiation planning provides a lower risk of delayed neurotoxicity. For many patients the neuropsychological deficits are modest and difficult to separate from tumor-related phenomena.[73] The cognitive sequelae of cranial

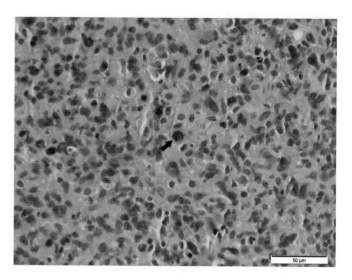

Figure 58.4 Anaplastic astrocytoma. Mitotic activity (*arrow*) distinguishes anaplastic astrocytoma from grade 2 diffuse astrocytoma. Anaplastic astrocytomas also demonstrate increased cellularity and greater variation in nuclear size and shape in comparison to grade 2 tumors. H&E, 600× original magnification.

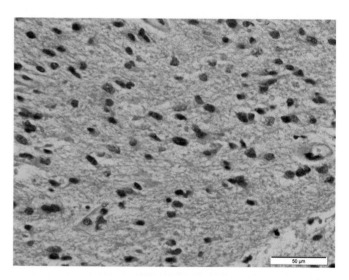

Figure 58.5 Diffuse astrocytoma. The nuclei of this moderately cellular tumor are ovoid to angular in shape and show mild pleomorphism. No significant mitotic activity is appreciated. H&E, 600× original magnification.

irradiation are much more apparent in children. However, since low-grade astrocytoma has a peak incidence in early to mid-adult life and a significant percentage of patients will be 5- and 10-year survivors, these long-term sequelae are important considerations.

To date, there is no defined role for chemotherapy in the initial management of low-grade astrocytoma. A randomized trial of radiotherapy versus radiotherapy plus CCNU for incompletely resected low-grade glioma by the Southwest Oncology Group (SWOG) showed equivalent median survival.[74] Current trials are comparing radiation with or without temozolomide for patients with poor prognostic factors such as age >40 years and large postoperative tumor volume.[75,76]

Important astrocytic variants

In addition to grading, certain histological and anatomical features distinguish subgroups of astrocytoma for which specific prognostic information or treatment recommendations can be described. These are: (i) pilocytic astrocytoma, (ii) pilomyxoid astrocytoma, (iii) optic pathway glioma, (iv) gemistocytic astrocytoma, (v) pleomorphic xanthoastrocytoma, (vi) subependymal giant cell astrocytoma, (vii) ganglion cell neoplasm (ganglioglioma/gangliocytoma), and (viii) dysembryoplastic neuroepithelial tumor. These are relatively rare tumors. Most of these have a predilection to occur in children and young adults. Aside from the gemistocytic and pilomyxoid astrocytomas, these are neoplasms that display a low potential for malignant progression. However, in all of these subtypes, progression to high-grade histological features and aggressive clinical behavior sometimes occurs. Additionally, diffuse infiltrating astrocytomas in adults will on rare occasions arise in the brainstem or spinal cord, and treatment of these neoplasms also deserves consideration.

Pilocytic and pilomyxoid astrocytoma

Pilocytic astrocytomas (PAs) demonstrate low-to-moderate cellularity and classically show a biphasic histological pattern. Bipolar, piloid ("hair-like") cells set in a dense, fibrillar background alternate with multipolar cells set in a loose, spongy stroma. Elongate, eosinophilic, corkscrew-shaped structures termed "Rosenthal fibers" are a frequent finding in dense tumor regions while globular aggregates of hyaline droplets termed "eosinophilic granular bodies" (EGBs) are more common in the spongy tumor regions. Clear cell differentiation may occur, resulting in tumor zones with an oligodendroglioma-like appearance. Pilocytic astrocytomas are highly vascular, often demonstrating vascular proliferation similar to that seen in glioblastoma. Mitotic figures are rare in this neoplasm (Fig. 58.6a).

In addition to the optic nerve and hypothalamus, predominantly pilocytic astrocytomas can arise in the thalamus, cerebellum, and less frequently in the cerebral hemispheres, the brainstem, and spinal cord. The majority are observed in children.

About 15% of PAs occur in patients with NF1. Biallelic inactivation of the *NF1* gene results in increased activity in the MAPK pathway. The *NF1* gene is intact in sporadic PAs but the MAPK pathway activity is enhanced in these tumors by other genetic changes, the most common of which are *BRAF* rearrangements or mutations. These are found in 70% of sporadic PAs in the posterior fossa.[77,78] Only 10% of sporadic PAs in the optic pathways and hypothalamus have *BRAF* rearrangements. These have *NOTCH2* upregulation and features of radial glia, suggesting an important biological distinction from cerebellar PAs.[79]

These tumors are remarkable for the presence of intense contrast enhancement on MRI, a feature not seen in the more common low-grade fibrillary astrocytoma. Unlike medulloblastoma, they are hypointense on diffusion weighted imaging.[80] Additionally, they are not highly infiltrative and total resection may be curative. Even subtotal resection may be followed by long progression-free intervals. The truly localized nature of these neoplasms makes them amenable to radiosurgery. Conventional fractionated radiation therapy (RT) will also control their growth, with a 5-year PFS of 69%. Better control is achieved in posterior fossa PAs than in supratentorial tumors.[81] As with optic gliomas (see below), chemotherapy with carboplatin, often combined with vincristine, has demonstrated efficacy with a 42% response rate.[82] Temozolomide has a somewhat lower response rate in optic pathway glioma (OPG)/PA with a 15% response rate and 38% stable diseases being observed in children on monthly cycles.[83] However, some patients do achieve durable control with a 3-year EFS of 57% in one small report.[84]

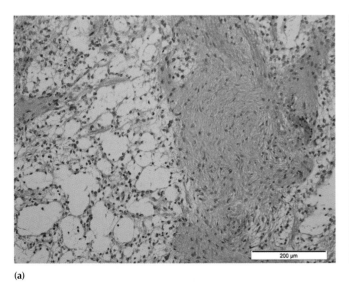

(a)

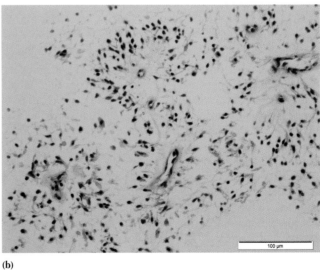

(b)

Figure 58.6 Pilocytic and pilomyxoid astrocytoma. (a) Pilocytic astrocytoma. Biphasic pattern of dense, process-rich areas with Rosenthal fibers (*right side of field*) and hypocellular areas with microcysts (*left side of field*). H&E, 200× original magnification. (b) Pilomyxoid astrocytoma. Monomorphous tumor cells in a myxoid matrix often show radial angiocentric arrangements. No Rosenthal fibers or eosinophilic granular bodies are seen. H&E, 400× original magnification.

Pilocytic astrocytomas occur in adults, although much more rarely. As in children, they often have a good prognosis after aggressive local therapy.[85] A prospective trial of supratentorial PAs yielded 95% 5-year OS and PFS.[86] A retrospective report of 30 adults with PA demonstrated good overall results with 5- and 10-year OS rates of 95% and 85% respectively, and PFS of 63% and 35%. Median PFS was 8.4 years. Although observation is a common practice following even a partial resection, adjuvant radiation was associated with a higher 5-year PFS in this report (91% versus 42%).[87] Recurrence after a relatively short duration has been reported in adults, a high percentage of whom have progression to anaplastic histological features.[88]

Pilomyxoid astrocytomas (PMAs) have been recently recognized as more aggressive astrocytomas that share histological features with pilocytic astrocytomas. These tumors are composed of bipolar tumor cells with piloid morphology very similar to those seen in the dense regions of pilocytic astrocytomas. Pilomyxoid astrocytomas, however, are mono-phasic neoplasms with a prominent myxoid tumor matrix. Rosenthal fibers and eosinophilic granular bodies are absent. The monomorphic tumor cells of this entity demonstrate unique rosette-like, radial angiocentric arrangements. Mitotic figures may be observed (Fig. 58.6b).

This tumor more commonly arises in young children with a mean age of less than 2 years at diagnosis but a few cases have been reported in adults. It most commonly arises in the hypothalamic region, which is also a common location for pilocytic astrocytoma. However, local recurrence is much more frequent after resection, subarachnoid dissemination is considerably more common (14%), and progression-free survival is much shorter than for pilocytic astrocytoma (26 versus 147 months), as is overall survival (60 versus 233 months).[89]

Pilomyxoid astrocytoma is considered a grade 2 astrocytoma in the WHO classification scheme. In certain cases, pathological features are intermediate between classic PA and PMA, making a clear distinction between the two impossible.[90]

Optic pathway glioma

Optic pathway gliomas (OPGs) are usually pilocytic astrocytomas and most are characterized as WHO grade 1. A small number of optic pathway tumors are more aggressive, including pilomyxoid astrocytomas in young children (see above) and glioblastoma in middle-aged adults. Approximately 25% of OPGs are confined to the optic nerve, while 75% arise or extend more posteriorly to involve the optic chiasm, optic tracts, or hypothalamus. Despite the low-grade histological appearance, they usually enhance prominently with gadolinium on MRI scanning. Twenty-five to thirty percent of patients with OPGs have neurofibromatosis type I (NF1). Sixty percent occur in children under 10 years of age, 20% occur between ages 10 and 20 years, 16% occur between 20 and 50 years, and 4% in patients greater than 50 years. The most common presentations are slowly evolving visual complaints, hypothalamic and/or endocrine dysfunction, and hydrocephalus. Hydrocephalus is associated with a poorer outcome, reflecting posterior extension of the tumor.

Optic pathway gliomas are the most common CNS neoplasm occurring in association with NF1. About 8–10% of NF1 patients will be found to harbor an optic glioma, and occasionally bilateral optic nerve gliomas arise in this setting. Among NF1 patients, almost all symptomatic OPGs are diagnosed by age 6 years. The diagnosis of a new OPG or progression of known OPG after this age is unusual. All children with NF1 should be screened with annual visual examinations. Those with abnormal visual exams, whether symptomatic or not, should have MRI scanning performed.

Optic pathway gliomas often show long progression-free intervals, measured in many years. Even when visual symptoms progress, the MRI findings are often unchanged. More remarkably, spontaneous regression has been reported in a small number of cases. Thus, many patients are observed with serial MRI scans until evidence of progression is documented.

The treatment of tumors that are limited to the prechiasmatic optic nerve is surgical if visual preservation is no longer a goal. In this circumstance, complete resection is usually curative. Ten-year progression-free survival is 95%. Extension into the optic chiasm or beyond to the hypothalamus removes any chance of surgical cure. Many of the anteriorly located OPGs do not eliminate functional vision and more conservative, function-sparing approaches are warranted. The attendant risk of progression with anatomical extension to structures that preclude curative surgery makes these management decisions very difficult.

Both radiation and chemotherapy have been used as more conservative, function-sparing approaches. Radiation therapy is effective at controlling tumor progression.[91,92] In a retrospective study of 50 patients, those with optic nerve tumors treated with radiation in the range of 42–54 Gy had a 72% PFS at 10 years. Those with chiasmal-hypothalamic tumors had a 68% PFS at 5 years.[93] IMRT and fractionated radiosurgery are now being used frequently in an effort to minimize delayed radiation injury to adjacent structures. Five-year PFS was 72% and OS 90% in a small series using fractionated stereotactic radiotherapy.[94]

Attempts to defer radiation in young children by initiating treatment with chemotherapy have demonstrated significant activity for carboplatin and vincristine.[95–98] In 59 children with newly diagnosed or recurrent OPGs treated with this combination, the response rate was 58% and 3-year PFS was 70%.[95] In a smaller trial of 15 patients, the 5-year PFS was 63%.[99] This approach can also be used in adults. Oral VP-16 produced a 36% response rate in a small cohort with recurrent chiasmatic-hypothalamic gliomas.[100]

Gemistocytic astrocytoma

Gemistocytes are astrocytes with a large round eosinophilic cytoplasm and eccentrically placed nuclei. While occasional gemistocytes may be seen in the more common diffuse astrocytoma and smaller gemistocytic-appearing cells may be useful in identifying some oligodendrogliomas, gemistocytes are a conspicuous component of the gemistocytic astrocytomas. A diagnosis of gemistocytic astrocytoma is rendered when gemistocytic cells with plump cytoplasm and displaced nuclei account for more than 20% of all tumor cells[101–103]

(Fig. 58.7). A fraction of greater than 20% gemistocytes is also considered by some to be a poor prognostic sign. These tumors lack mitoses and vascular proliferation and are considered grade 2 in the WHO classification.[102] Some authors diagnose tumors composed of >60% gemistocytes as "pure" gemistocytic astrocytoma, although these often include anaplastic features.

Sixty to eighty percent of gemistocytic astrocytomas have *p53* mutations, which is notably higher than in fibrillary astrocytomas. Loss of heterozygosity (LOH) on chromosomes 1p and 19 is not found in gemistocytic astrocytomas. These tumors have a low proliferation index with the gemistocytes appearing to be an inert, nonreplicating fraction. They accumulate due to abnormalities in *bcl-2*, resulting in reduced apoptotic death.[104] Perivascular lymphocytic infiltration or "cuffing" is common. They also contain large numbers of microglia. These cells and the gemistocytes themselves express major histocompatibility complex (MHC) class II.[105,106]

Gemistocytic astrocytomas are essentially all supratentorial in location and predominantly frontal. Median age of diagnosis is in the fourth decade. Age greater than 35 years was associated with a poorer prognosis.[107] Despite otherwise low-grade histological features and a low proliferative index, the median survival with treatment is approximately 2.5–3 years. A retrospective study of 48 patients with incompletely resected gemistocytic astrocytoma who received postoperative radiation reported a 5-year survival rate of only 30%. These results are more typical of anaplastic astrocytoma than low-grade astrocytoma, and many authors favor more aggressive therapy for these patients.[101]

Not all reports concur with the long-held view that gemistocytic astrocytomas have a worse prognosis.[108] In an analysis of 25 astrocytomas with >20% gemistocytes, those with no evidence of anaplasia in the background astrocytic components (*n* = 16) had median survivals of 158 months, similar to other grade 2 astrocytomas. Those with anaplasia had a median survival of only 25 months. These findings suggest that the degree of anaplasia is more important for prognosis than the presence of gemistocytes.[109,110]

Pleomorphic xanthoastrocytoma

Pleomorphic xanthoastrocytomas (PXAs) are usually encountered in the second decade of life, typically presenting with seizures or hemiparesis. Radiographically, the majority form a cyst with a tumor nodule. These tumors are well circumscribed, although extension into the leptomeninges is common. The neoplastic cells of this tumor entity are pleomorphic – they are highly variable in size and shape. Spindle-shaped cells, giant cells, and even multinucleated cells are observed as well as occasional xanthomatous cells containing intracellular lipid droplets. Immunohistochemical staining for GFAP demonstrates the glial nature of these cells. Tumor cell nuclei are bizarre in shape and intranuclear inclusions are frequent. Eosinophilic granular bodies (EGBs) can usually be identified. Perivascular and interstitial lymphocytes are often present (Fig. 58.8). While most PXAs lack mitoses and necrosis, and are considered to be grade 2 neoplasms,[111] a subset of these tumors shows significant mitotic activity (five or more mitoses per 10 high-power microscopic fields). These mitotically active tumors show a more aggressive clinical course and are termed "pleomorphic xanthoastrocytoma with anaplastic features."[112] Recent studies have highlighted the presence of neuronal differentiation in tumor elements such as dysmorphic ganglion cells. Adjacent cortical dysplasia is not uncommon. Thus, PXAs have become part of the growing number of "glioneuronal" tumors.[113] When necrosis and vascular proliferation are present, distinguishing anaplastic PXA from glioblastoma may be impossible. Recent genetic studies revealed that about 60% of grade 2 PXAs have V600E *BRAF* mutations, a potential therapeutic target.[114]

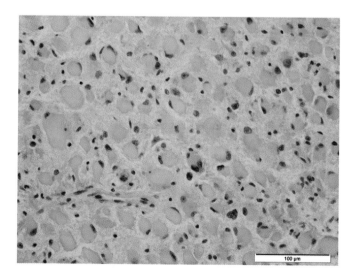

Figure 58.7 Gemistocytic astrocytoma. These astrocytomas are populated by gemistocytes with round eosinophilic cytoplasm and ovoid eccentric nuclei. H&E, 400× original magnification.

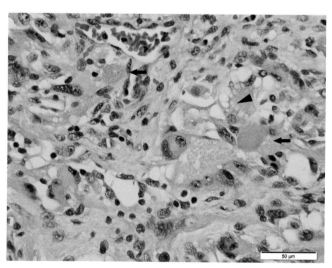

Figure 58.8 Pleomorphic xanthoastrocytoma. Pleomorphic xanthoastrocytomas show extreme variation in nuclear size, multinucleated cells (*center of image*), xanthomatous cells with intracellular lipid accumulation (*arrowhead*), and eosinophilic granular bodies (*arrows*). H&E, 600× original magnification.

For typical PXAs, surgical resection is the treatment of choice. In a review of 71 patients with a median age of 26 years, the PFS was 72% at 5 years and 61% at 10 years. The respective overall survival rates were 81% and 70%.[112] The outcome appears much worse in those who do not achieve a gross total resection, many of whom will recur within 1 year.[115] Approximately 15% underwent progressive anaplastic evolution. Optimal treatment for those with malignant degeneration has not been established but generally includes radiotherapy and often temozolomide.

Subependymal giant cell astrocytomas

Subependymal giant cell astrocytomas (SEGAs) are slow-growing, WHO grade 1 neoplasms associated with the tuberous sclerosis complex. Tuberous sclerosis is a relatively common autosomal dominant condition affecting one in 6000 people. Between 5% and 20% of patients with tuberous sclerosis will develop SEGAs during their lifetimes, typically during the first two decades. These tumors tend to arise from the head of the caudate nucleus near the foramen of Monro. SEGAs are circumscribed tumors composed of cells with astrocytic morphology that vary in shape from large and polygonal with abundant glassy cytoplasm to smaller and elongate. Nuclei vary in size and multinucleated cells are often seen (Fig. 58.9). Certain SEGAs have a potential for rapid growth, resulting in obstruction of the foramen of Monro or intratumoral hemorrhage.

Although these tumors are listed as astrocytic neoplasms under the latest WHO CNS tumor classification, there is controversy regarding the pure astrocytic nature of these tumors. Histologically, SEGAs have mixed glial-neuronal features by immunohistochemistry. They are formed by three dominant cell types: fibrillated spindle cells, gemistocytic-like cells, and giant pyramidal cells with a ganglioid appearance. In one recent study, the majority of these tumors stained positively for GFAP, neuron-specific enolase, synaptophysin, and neurofilaments.[116,117] Because of shared astrocytic and neuronal features, the term "subependymal giant cell tumor" is sometimes used to describe these lesions. While mitotic activity or necrosis may be observed, these features are not considered indicative of anaplastic progression.[118]

Currently, the standard of care is complete surgical resection, which can be curative. However, the deep location of SEGAs can render neurosurgical extirpation difficult, with significant perioperative risks. Radiation therapy is generally avoided, given the risks of secondary malignancy in patients already lacking one copy of a tumor suppressor gene. There is some evidence for long-term control with stereotactic radiosurgery in SEGAs, which reduces the risks of secondary tumors.[119]

As more information about the genetic aberrations of tuberous sclerosis has been discovered, molecular targets for treatment of SEGAs have been better defined. Over 85% of tuberous sclerosis patients harbor a mutation in one of the two tuberous sclerosis genes, *TSC1* (hamartin) or *TSC2* (tuberin). Deficiencies in either protein result in constitutive upregulation of the mammalian target of rapamycin complex 1 (mTOR) pathway, a serine/threonine protein kinase that helps regulate cell division and proliferation. Recent evidence

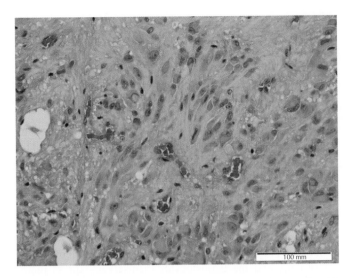

Figure 58.9 Subependymal giant cell astrocytoma (SEGA). Tumor cells with pleomorphic, eccentric nuclei, and distinct nucleoli palisade around a central vascular structure. H&E, 400× original magnification.

indicates that everolimus (RAD001, Novartis), a drug which inhibits mTOR, is an effective alternative to surgery. In a recent prospective study of young patients with SEGAs, everolimus administration resulted in a significant reduction in tumor burden. Seventy-five percent of patients had at least a 30% reduction in tumor volume over 6 months of treatment, with one-third of the patients demonstrating greater than 50% tumor shrinkage. Additionally, patients treated with everolimus had a clinically meaningful decrease in seizure frequency and hydrocephalus, resulting in improved quality of life.[120]

Ganglion cell neoplasms (gangliogliomas and gangliocytomas)

Ganglion cell tumors are composed of "dysplastic neurons" characterized by:

- loss of cytoarchitectural organization
- subcortical localization
- clustered appearance
- cytomegaly
- perimembranous aggregated Nissl substance
- presence of bi- or multinucleated neurons.[121]

At one end of the spectrum of ganglion cell neoplasms are gangliocytomas, which contain dysplastic mature neurons and a minimal, nonneoplastic glial component. At the other end are gangliogliomas, which contain a neuronal component that may be quite limited and a prominent, neoplastic glial population (Fig. 58.10). The neoplastic glial population shows substantial variability and may resemble fibrillary astrocytoma, oligodendroglioma, or pilocytic astrocytoma. Distinguishing ganglioglioma from a purely glial tumor (i.e. an astrocytoma) with entrapped neurons can be difficult, and these cases therefore present a diagnostic challenge for the neuropathologist. Other characteristic features include calcifications, perivascular lymphocytic infiltrates, Rosenthal fibers, EGBs, and vascular proliferation. Desmoplasia is common in tumors that involve the subarachnoid space.

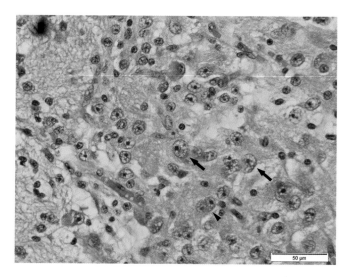

Figure 58.10 Ganglion cell tumor. Ganglioglioma. Dysplastic neurons in this image show a clustered appearance with nucleomegaly (*arrows*) and binucleate forms (*arrowhead*). H&E, 600× original magnification.

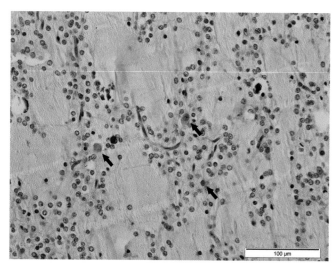

Figure 58.11 Dysembryoplastic neuroepethelial tumor. Oligodendroglial-like cells in columns and "floating" neurons (*arrows*) are set in a mucinous matrix. H&E, 400× original magnification.

Gangliogliomas are rare low-grade tumors that arise predominantly in the temporal and frontal lobes but can arise elsewhere. Most are well circumscribed. Cyst formation and calcification are common. The glial component of gangliogliomas may show anaplastic features such as high mitotic activity and necrosis; tumors with these features are considered "anaplastic gangliogliomas" and are assigned a WHO grade 3 status. Notably, cytological atypia within the astrocytic component does not portend the same poor prognosis that such features predict in pure astrocytomas. The appropriate treatment for gangliogliomas is complete resection. Additional therapy should be reserved for recurrent tumors, which are fortunately uncommon.[122,123]

Dysembryoplastic neuroepithelial tusmors

The dysembryoplastic neuroepithelial tumor (DNT) is an entity that also demonstrates ganglionic differentiation. It manifests a benign course and a high propensity to be mistaken for more aggressive glial neoplasms, particularly mixed oligoastrocytomas. DNTs are encountered in young adults with long-standing partial seizures, often present since childhood. The majority arise in the temporal lobes or, less commonly, the frontal lobes. Radiographic evidence of minor cranial bone deformation adjacent to the tumor is found in one-third of patients. DNTs involve and expand the cerebral cortex. They have a multinodular architecture, occasionally with microcyst formation.

Microscopic examination of DNTs reveals the seminal histological feature, the "specific glioneuronal element": parallel strands of small oligodendroglial-like cells in an alveolar or columnar pattern, lining axon bundles. Between these cell columns, "floating" neurons appear suspended in a mucinous matrix (Fig. 58.11). Further distinction between "simple" and "complex" DNTs is made based on the appearance of the adjacent oligodendroglial and astrocytic elements. In the complex variant of DNT, glial nodules of variable size are observed in association with the glioneuronal element. Neuronal elements

perpendicular to the cortical surface are surrounded by variable numbers of neoplastic oligodendroglia, producing the macroscopically nodular appearance. Surrounding areas of cortical dysplasia are common. Anaplasia, vascular proliferation, mitotic activity, and necrosis are not features of this neoplasm. However, in a small or poorly representative sample, the distinction from an oligodendroglioma or oligoastrocytoma may be impossible. The ganglionic elements are generally not cytologically bizarre, a feature that helps distinguish DNTs from gangliogliomas.[124,125]

Brainstem gliomas in adults

Brainstem gliomas in adults are rare. Histologically, most are astrocytic neoplasms and more often are low grade histologically than in children. Oligodendroglioma are rarer still in this location. Adult brainstem gliomas are sometimes located in the dorsal midbrain (tectal glioma) or laterally in the medulla, extend into the cerebellar peduncles or over multiple brainstem segments. This is in contrast to the central pontine location that is so typical of the childhood brainstem glioma. The clinical course in adults is often more indolent than that of the childhood brainstem glioma. This fact is critical to point out when discussing this type of tumor with adult patients because almost every source of information available to the patient about brainstem gliomas will describe the childhood version, which has an extremely poor prognosis.

Multiple retrospective series of adult brainstem gliomas have been published.[109,126–130] Age at diagnosis is typically in the mid-30s. A wide variety of presenting symptoms is reported but the most common are diplopia, facial weakness or numbness, ataxia, and limb weakness that sometimes is bilateral. The median duration of symptoms is 4 months but can be much longer. Prognosis is poorer if the time from symptom onset to diagnosis is less than 3 months. Other factors suggesting a poor prognosis include a Karnofsky score of ≤70, age greater than 40 years, tumor grade, and non-Caucasian ethnicity.

Magnetic resonance imaging reveals expansion of the affected region with hyperintensity on T2 and FLAIR sequences. Half are nonenhancing and appear diffusely infiltrative. Cystic components (12%), exophytic growth (12%), and hydrocephalus are occasional features. MR spectroscopy and fluordeoxyglucose (FDG) PET scanning have been used to support the diagnosis of a neoplasm but their reliability has not been rigorously established. Those tumors with a diffuse infiltrating picture that closely mimic the pediatric pontine glioma are generally not biopsied. In those with unusual imaging features a biopsy should be considered. In one series of 46 adult patients who underwent biopsy, the diagnoses included pilocytic astrocytoma (2), low grade astrocytoma (14), anaplastic astrocytoma/GBM (12), and three nondiagnostic biopsies.[131] More rarely, metastases, lymphoma, PNET, ependymoma, or other tumors will be discovered.

Observation with serial MRI scans every 6 months is a good option for those patients with very long-standing, slowly progressing symptoms. Radiation, fractionated over 6 weeks to 54 Gy, is the mainstay of therapy. Temozolomide added to radiation has not been beneficial in children and that observation holds in adults as well.

Radiographic responses to radiation are uncommon but at least 50% of patients will report clinical improvement. A significant number of patients will achieve stable symptoms for a few years and then slowly worsen without obvious MRI progression. The timing of initiation of salvage chemotherapy is a difficult decision, particularly in view of the meager efficacy of chemotherapy to date. Median survival in the largest reported series ($n = 101$ patients) was 85 months with 5- and 10-year overall survival rates of 58% and 41%. However, median survival in those with high-grade histology was approximately 1 year, while in the low-grade group it was almost 10 years.[132]

One subgroup of special note is that of nonenhancing gliomas of the tectal region. Tectal gliomas are often stable without treatment for many years. They tend to present with hydrocephalus due to obstruction of the cerebral aqueduct. Ventricular shunt placement or third ventriculostomy is often required but the neoplasm can be observed with serial MRI scans. There are some proponents of surgical resection of progressive neoplasms in this region. More commonly, progressive glial tumors in this region have been treated with radiation.[133]

Spinal cord gliomas in adults

Primary glial tumors arising in the spinal cord account for less than 5% of all gliomas. The incidence is about one per 100,000 person-years. The most common histologies are ependymoma and astrocytoma which will be considered together in this section. Oligodendrogliomas are exceedingly rare in the spinal cord. About half of the ependymomas arising in the region of the cauda equina/filum terminale display a distinctive histological pattern, termed myxopapillary, a feature that is essentially limited to ependymomas in this location. The relative frequency of the two common histologies varies by age, with astrocytomas of the spinal cord being more common in children while in adults ependymomas are more common. Over 90% of these gliomas are histologically low grade and

thus the symptomatology is commonly that of a slowly progressive myelopathy with symptoms present for many months, and not uncommonly over a year prior to diagnosis. Sensory symptoms tend to predominate early, followed by weakness. Sixty percent have only minor motor deficit at diagnosis. Modest localized back pain is a common early symptom.[134] Multiple ependymomas may occur, usually in the setting of neurofibromatosis.

The symptomatology also varies based on the level of involvement of the spinal cord. Astrocytomas most often arise in the cervical and upper thoracic region. Classic myelopathic features are seen. These include upper motor neuron findings in the legs, sometimes asymmetrical motor and sensory features such as in the Brown–Sequard syndrome, Lhermitte phenomenon, and occasionally superimposed radicular or lower motor neuron findings in the arms. Ependymomas are more equally divided between the cervical and lumbar regions although in patients older than 50 years, the thoracic region is commonly affected. Lumbar region ependymomas often arise from the filum terminale and are technically outside the spinal cord proper (i.e. extramedullary). They tend to produce cauda equina symptoms with radicular findings in the legs, such as dermatomal sensory loss, weakness with lower motor neuron signs (i.e. localized atrophy, fasciculation), absent reflexes, and also incontinence.

Magnetic resonance imaging is the best method of imaging for spinal tumors. Most ependymomas will enhance with gadolinium. A few low-grade astrocytomas will also enhance but many do not. As with intracranial astrocytomas, the high-grade spinal astrocytomas generally do enhance. Contiguous cysts or syringomyelia are seen in at least 30% of intraparenchymal spinal cord tumors. Evidence of subarachnoid seeding should be sought. It is unusually common in high-grade astrocytomas of the spinal cord, and is infrequent but not rare with ependymomas. The histological diagnosis of intramedullary spinal cord tumors can often be suspected from the patient's age, the location (e.g. lumbar versus other), and the MRI characteristics. Yet these features are not accurate enough to provide a certain diagnosis. CSF studies are rarely helpful in establishing the diagnosis of a spinal cord neoplasm but often serve to address other diagnostic concerns such as inflammatory or demyelinating lesions that can mimic neoplasms.

The diagnosis of a spinal cord neoplasm should be established by biopsy, generally performed through a dorsal midline myelotomy. The astrocytomas, while generally low grade, are infiltrative which often makes surgical resection impossible. Occasionally internal decompression/resection of the tumor and cyst decompression can be accomplished, yet the lack of an established plane around the tumor makes the likelihood of surgical injury to the spinal cord high. Pilocytic astrocytomas account for almost half of the spinal cord astrocytomas. They are generally not infiltrative and often are amenable to resection. Ependymomas tend to be very sharply demarcated. Even though they lack a true capsule, a plane of dissection can sometimes be established, allowing for complete resection and potentially a surgical cure.[135] Gross total resection is accomplished in 30–50% of the intramedullary spinal ependymomas and in a higher percentage of the extramedullary filum terminale ependymomas. Some reports indicate that major resections are associated with a worse outcome for infiltrative astrocytomas, especially if high grade. Selection bias likely plays a part in that finding, with more aggressive resections being attempted on high-grade infiltrative tumors but major neurological deficits after surgery might also contribute to a poor outcome.[136] Other reports suggest that major resection can be beneficial, with a radiographic gross total resection achieved in half of the grade 3 patients but rarely in grade 4 patients. However, 40% had a neurological decline postoperatively. A trend towards improved survival was observed in the grade 3 patients who achieved a radical resection versus those who did not (OS 78% versus 38% at 4 years).[137]

While symptomatic improvement is sometimes observed after surgery, patients with long-standing and functionally significant neurological deficits are not likely to improve. The goal of surgery with respect to neurological function is to prevent progression of deficits. Postoperatively, 10% of patients have a significant decline in functional neurological status, mainly judged by ability to walk. One-third of these patients will recover to baseline. However, lesser degrees of neurological deficit such as new paresthesias, incontinence, and pain are common. Resection of tumors in the upper cervical region or cervicomedullary junction can also lead to impairment of breathing. When high risks such as these are weighed against the potential for a curative resection, the decision is a very difficult one. Both the decision making and the procedure itself, if undertaken, should be done by a neurosurgeon with extensive experience in the resection of spinal neoplasms.[27,138–140]

Recommendations for treatment after surgery are based almost entirely on retrospective series and by inference on the treatment of intracranial gliomas. Patients who achieve a complete or near complete resection of a pilocytic astrocytoma or low-grade ependymoma should be followed with serial MRI scans, usually at 6-month intervals. At the time of progression, a second resection should be considered but radiation should also be offered at this point. This strategy would also be reasonable for a low-grade pilocytic astrocytoma that is not resectable if the symptoms are mild (i.e. pain only or paresthesias) and nonprogressive. Adult patients presenting with progressive symptoms from a low-grade astrocytoma or ependymoma, and for whom a substantial resection cannot be achieved, should receive radiation therapy. Long-term control can be achieved in most patients, although this cannot be considered curative therapy. Survival is better for those who received >35 Gy than those receiving <35 Gy (26 versus 9 months).[136] All high-grade astrocytomas (i.e. grades 3 and 4) should receive radiation.

There is no role for chemotherapy in the initial treatment plan for adult low-grade spinal gliomas. In the exceptional situation in which deferring radiation is essential for an adult with a progressive spinal cord astrocytoma, temozolomide can be tried initially. Temozolomide in typical monthly cycles was evaluated in 22 patients with recurrent spinal astrocytomas, all of whom had prior surgery and radiation. Radiographic partial response was observed in 18% and stable disease was achieved in 55%. Median time to progression was 14.5 months.[141] In children, a radiographic response will be achieved in 20–30%

with various regimens that generally have included alkylating agents.[142] By inference from intracranial tumors, some authors recommend chemotherapy, usually temozolomide, for high-grade astrocytomas of the spine.

There are very few data on chemotherapy for adult ependymomas. Multiagent regimens have been used in young children with intracranial ependymomas with the goal of deferring radiation, and responses are achieved in a significant minority. However, the biology of those childhood tumors and their clinical course are so different from those of adult spinal ependymoma that inferences regarding treatment are of little help. Recurrent intracranial ependymomas have generally appeared to respond more frequently to platinum-based therapy than to nitrosoureas and the combination of carboplatin and etoposide is frequently recommended. A retrospective review of 16 patients, predominantly adults, with progressive ependymomas found that the response rate achieved with platinum-based regimens exceeded that of nitrosourea-based regimens (67% versus 25%).[143]

Long-term outcome for adults with spinal cord gliomas varies on the basis of histology, age, duration of symptoms, and neurological function at diagnosis, and tumor location. Patients with low-grade astrocytoma have a much better 5-year survival rate than those with high-grade histology (70–90% versus 30%). In one large retrospective analysis of the SEER database, the 5-year overall survival for grade 1, 2, 3, and 4 spinal cord astrocytomas was 82%, 70%, 28%, and 14%, respectively.[144] Those with pilocytic astrocytoma do the best among this group, with a median survival of 98 months compared with 68 months for grade 2 and 15 months for grades 3 and 4 astrocytomas. Ten-year survival is much better for pilocytic compared with diffuse astrocytoma (78% versus 17%) but in both groups the PFS curves maintain an extended plateau well beyond 10 years.[136]

For intramedullary ependymomas, the 5- and 10-year survival rates are approximately 85% and 57%, respectively. For grade 1, 2, and 3 spinal cord ependymomas, the 5-year overall survival is predicted to be 92%, 97%, and 58%, respectively.[144] Complete resection of a filum terminale ependymoma is associated with a 5-year PFS of nearly 100%.[145,146] Young patients have longer survival than older patients. Symptom duration of greater than 6 months is a favorable indicator with a 5-year survival of 71% versus 42% for a shorter duration of symptoms. Patients with spinal cord astrocytomas and good neurological function pre- and postoperatively have a better 5-year overall survival than those with poor neurological function (73% versus 22%).[147] Similar results are reported for Karnofsky performance status. Upper cervical tumors tend to be the most disabling and the worst prognostically, while the extramedullary filum terminale tumors have a particularly good prognosis.

Oligodendroglial neoplasms

Since the late 1980s, the prognostic value of distinguishing low-grade (grade 2) and high-grade (grade 3) oligodendrogliomas has been confirmed.[148] Yet these neoplasms are not as predictable as their astrocytic counterparts, and within these two grades much more histological variation is observed than among different grades of astrocytoma. Attempts to characterize them on the basis of histological and gross morphological features demonstrate their wide variability.[149,150]

Oligodendrogliomas are composed of monomorphic cells with round nuclei and perinuclear halos, the latter feature representing a retraction artifact of fixation; these features recapitulate the appearance of nonneoplastic oligodendrocytes. An interlacing "chicken-wire" network of capillaries is usually observed and microcalcifications are common (Fig. 58.12). The neoplastic cells of oligodendroglioma are unique in their propensity to form "secondary structures" including perivascular aggregates, perineuronal aggregates, and subpial tumor "mounds." Tumor cells also display a tendency to cluster together, forming nodules evident at low magnification. Anaplastic features including high mitotic activity, vascular proliferation, necrosis, high cellularity, and marked cytological atypia may indicate progression to anaplastic oligodendroglioma (Fig. 58.13). Varying numbers of cells with astrocyte-like cytological features may be seen in oligodendrogliomas. Often termed "minigemistocytes," these cells show eccentric eosinophilic cytoplasm reminiscent of gemistocytic astrocytes but retain round oligodendroglial nuclei.

The observation that a high percentage of oligodendroglial neoplasms demonstrate LOH at loci on chromosomes 1p and 19q moved their classification strongly towards a molecular definition. Initially this observation was coupled with a high response rate to PCV chemotherapy, giving rise to its use as a predictive marker of chemoresponsiveness. Subsequently improved outcome with radiation was also reported in patients with codeletions of 1p and 19q. More recently, the impression is that this codeletion identifies gliomas with more indolent growth characteristics, giving it prognostic significance rather than a predictive value. After years without a clear biological basis, it is now known that in many tumors a translocation of 1p and 19q [t(1,19(q10;p10)] gives rise to a fusion gene that alters growth characteristics. Median survival for low-grade tumors with the translocation is 12 years versus 8 years for those without the translocation.[151] Tumors with only one of the two deletions do not appear prognostically favorable. Many new clinical trials are designed specifically with LOH 1p and 19q as an eligibility requirement or a stratification factor.

Oligoastrocytoma is the designation given to tumors with a mixed population of oligodendroglial cells with round nuclei and astrocytic cells with angular nuclei. Interobserver variability for diagnosing oligoastrocytoma is high. Oligoastrocytomas often exhibit LOH at 1p and 19q, further suggesting that these are best classified as an oligodendroglioma variant.[152] Treatment response data also support this view.[153–155]

Both pure oligodendroglioma and mixed oligoastrocytoma may evolve to a higher grade of anaplasia. Forty-five percent of grade 2 pure oligodendrogliomas recur as grade 3 or 4 neoplasms, and in almost half of these the histology found at recurrence is that of mixed oligoastrocytoma. For grade 2 oligoastrocytomas, 70% demonstrate grade 3 or 4 features at recurrence, many with predominantly astrocytic features including a high percentage that appear as glioblastoma.[156]

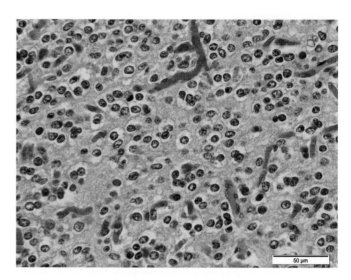

Figure 58.12 Oligodendroglioma. Tumor cells demonstrate round nuclei and perinuclear cytoplasmic clearing. They form "secondary structures" around neurons and blood vessels. A delicate vascular pattern is observed. H&E, 600× original magnification.

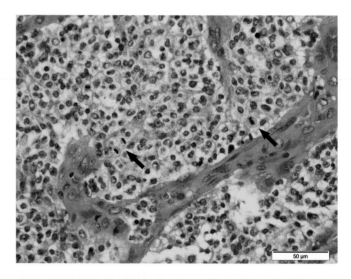

Figure 58.13 Anaplastic oligodendroglioma. Mitotic figures (*arrows*) and vascular proliferation are depicted. H&E, 600× original magnification.

Anaplastic oligodendroglioma may exhibit areas of classic oligodendroglioma with monomorphous nuclei and an interlacing delicate vascular pattern but features of malignancy are observed as well. Since vascular proliferation and mitotic activity appear to be of particular importance in predicting tumor behavior,[157] the diagnosis of anaplastic oligodendroglioma should require either the presence of conspicuous vascular proliferation and/or high mitotic activity.[158] Prognosis becomes significantly less favorable once six or more mitotic figures are identified in a count of 10 high-power fields, and for this reason some authors use this value as a cutoff point for assigning WHO grade 3 status to an oligodendroglioma.[159] Necrosis may be present as well and often shows a pseudopalisading morphology; this change, however, does not indicate progression to glioblastoma. Unlike anaplastic oligodendroglioma in which necrosis does not increase tumor grade from 3 to 4, anaplastic oligoastrocytomas with necrosis are termed "glioblastoma with oligodendroglial component" (GBM-O).[160]

Low-grade oligodendroglioma

Low-grade oligodendrogliomas are typically cerebral hemispheric nonenhancing masses. Rarely they arise in the cerebellum, brainstem, or spinal cord. They are the most indolent of the major forms of infiltrating glioma. Therapeutic recommendations derive from retrospective reports, a few small prospective trials, and a few large phase 3 trials that combine low-grade oligodendroglioma with low-grade astrocytoma.[72] Although pragmatic, this protocol design is unfortunate given the clear differences between oligodendroglioma and astrocytoma in important biological features and in natural history. However, relatively small patient numbers, follow-up requirements of 5–10 years and more, and similarities in treatment options foster this phase 3 trial design.

Tumor grade is the strongest predictor of outcome and most important guide for therapy at present, with more conservative approaches recommended for low-grade oligodendrogliomas, given their highly variable but often indolent natural history. Clinical variables including younger age, high performance status, and extent of resection are predictors of a better outcome. Those low-grade tumors with contrast enhancement on MRI do less well.[161] LOH on chromosomes 1p and 19q has become a major contributing factor in assessment of prognosis.

Most retrospective studies suggest that a survival benefit is obtained with surgical resection. Patients with a gross total resection demonstrate a greater than twofold increase in 10-year survival compared to subtotal resection (59% versus 23%). Extent of resection correlated with outcome in multiple large retrospective trials.[70,162,163]

Conventional fractionated radiation therapy appears beneficial, although its impact on survival is not entirely clear. Radiation doses of >50 Gy are associated with median survival about twice that of patients receiving less than 50 Gy (7.9 versus 4.5 years).[148] However, not all reports demonstrate a survival advantage associated with radiation therapy. Larger randomized trials that include a high percentage of astrocytomas have shown that upfront radiation improves PFS (5.3 years versus 3.4 years) but that overall survival is not affected.[72] Symptom control, specifically seizure control, is improved with radiation, although delayed neuropsychological sequelae are found in over half of patients when carefully tested over long intervals.[164]

Low-grade oligodendrogliomas do have relatively good response rates to alkylating agents. Initial reports utilizing nitrosourea-based regimens such as PCV demonstrate response or stable disease in a high percentage (90%) of patients with low-grade oligodendrogliomas.[165] Overall survival with PCV as initial treatment for low-grade oligodendroglioma at 5 and 10 years was 57% and 50% respectively in a report of 33 patients.[166] Another report demonstrated 5- and 10-year PFS of 75% and 46% in 36 patients treated with PCV.[167] These observations followed reports of high response rates (60–90%) achieved in anaplastic oligodendrogliomas with PCV (see below).

Recent reports have also demonstrated responses to temozolomide, and many favor its use over the nitrosoureas because of a better toxicity profile. A low-dose protracted temozolomide schedule (75 mg/m²; 7 weeks on/4 weeks off) resulted in 20% partial response (PR) and 75% stable disease (SD) at a median follow-up of 39 months.[168] Effective salvage chemotherapy for recurrent oligodendroglioma has also been described, particularly with combinations that include VP-16 and cisplatin or carboplatin, and with bevacizumab.[169–173]

In summary, the initial treatment of low-grade oligodendrogliomas should include resection aimed at removal of radiographically visible tumor or as much as is feasible while maintaining acceptable neurological function. Observation is often chosen for young patients (i.e. <40 years), especially if a major resection can be accomplished. Serial MRI scans at 4–6-month intervals and deferring other therapy until evidence of progression is a common approach. Many still consider fractionated radiation in doses of 45–54 Gy to be standard therapy. Chemotherapy is increasingly being considered an important alternative to radiation for initial management. The need for prospective randomized trials is evident.[174]

Anaplastic oligodendroglioma

Anaplastic oligodendroglioma generally presents as an enhancing cerebral hemispheric mass. The enhancement tends to be diffuse and patchy. A well-defined enhancing ring with a central core of lower signal is less commonly seen than with glioblastoma. As with other high-grade gliomas, the initial management must provide stabilization of neurological symptoms. Gross total resection should be performed whenever feasible.

Postoperative therapy is recommended with a strong consensus, although both radiation and chemotherapy have demonstrated long-term control in a high percentage of patients.[175,176] Over the past 20 years this has fostered a very interesting and informative series of large-scale trials comparing upfront chemotherapy and radiation.

In a large randomized trial comparing an intensive PCV regimen for four cycles followed by radiation (59 Gy) to radiation alone, the OS was nearly equal in the two groups (4.7 versus 4.9 years respectively). Progression-free survival was better in the combined therapy group than with RT alone: 2.6 versus 1.7 years. However, grade 3 and 4 toxicities were observed in 65% of the patients on chemotherapy, including one chemotherapy-related death.[177] Another randomized trial comparing RT followed by six cycles of standard PCV versus RT alone yielded very similar results, with significant improvement in PFS (23 versus 12 months) but no significant difference in OS (40 versus 30 months). However, 82% of the RT-only patients received chemotherapy at progression.[178] *MGMT* promoter methylation, *IDH1* mutations, and 1p/19q codeletion were prognostic of a better outcome irrespective of treatment.[179,180]

Given the remarkable chemosensitivity of these infiltrating, histologically high-grade gliomas, initial treatment with chemotherapy and deferred radiation has been under investigation. A phase 2 trial of monthly cycles of temozolomide without radiation in 40 patients with anaplastic oligodendroglioma (11) or anaplastic oligoastrocytoma (29) demonstrated

CR in 38%, PR in 15%, and SD in 23%. The 6-month PFS was 77% and the median PFS was 21 months.[181]

Another strategy has been to treat anaplastic oligodendroglioma patients demonstrating LOH 1p/19q with chemotherapy alone, and use combined modality therapy for those without the codeletion. A phase 2 trial of 48 anaplastic oligodendroglioma patients found that 75% had codeletion; in this group upfront temozolomide achieved a PFS of 28 months. In the 25% of patients lacking the codeletion, upfront temozolomide was followed by radiation and concurrent temozolomide. The PFS for this group was only 13.5 months.[182] A similar study of preradiation temozolomide, using a 7 day on/7 day off schedule for 6 months followed by concurrent RT plus temozolomide, yielded important response and progression data. Among 39 patients the CR was 6% and PR 26%. Progression prior to radiation occurred in 10%.[183]

Upfront chemotherapy with deferred radiation is an attractive strategy in older adult patients where the risk of radiation-related neurotoxicity is higher. In a study of 44 patients older than 70 years, initial therapy with temozolomide yielded PR in 32% and SD in 41%. Median PFS was 6.9 months and median OS was 12.4 months.[184] Patients with MGMT promoter methylation survived the longest, with an OS of 16 months.

Encouraged by high response rates seen in anaplastic oligodendroglial neoplasms, further intensification of chemotherapy has been investigated. A small phase 2 trial of myeloablative therapy using busulfan and thiotepa, enrolling patients who had an objective response to intensive PCV, reported that 15 of 20 (75%) patients achieved a response, and this group had a PFS and OS of >36 months. However, one treatment-related death occurred.[185] Long-term follow-up of 39 patients in a similar trial using I-PCV followed by high-dose thiotepa demonstrated a median PFS of 78 months. Median OS had not been reached but 46% of patients had relapsed at a median follow-up of 80 months.[186]

The treatment of recurrent anaplastic oligodendroglial tumors should be viewed as distinct from glioblastoma because of the better efficacy of salvage regimens. In addition to temozolomide and nitrosourea-based therapy, durable responses have been achieved with carboplatin, cisplatin plus etoposide, cytoxan, and more recently bevacizumab.[169–173]

Ependymoma

Ependymomas account for 2.1% of all primary brain tumors, regardless of age. In the pediatric population, these tumors are the third most common histology, representing 6.4% of tumors in the 0–14-year age group and 5% in the 15–19-year age group. Children more frequently have posterior fossa ependymomas, while supratentorial tumors are more common in adults. There is a slightly higher incidence in males (0.37 per 100,000 person-years) compared with females (0.33 per 100,000 person-years), and in Caucasians (0.38 per 100,000 person-years) compared with African-Americans (0.20 per 100,000 person-years). The revised 2007 WHO classification of brain tumors recognizes three grades of ependymoma: grade 1 (subependymoma and myxopapilllary ependymoma),

grade 2 (ependymoma), and grade 3 (anaplastic ependymoma). There are four histological variants of ependymoma: cellular, papillary, clear cell, and tanycytic.

Ependymomas are moderately cellular, well-circumscribed tumors composed of a monotonous population of ependymal cells with distinctive nuclear morphology and perivascular architecture. Tumor cell nuclei are monomorphous with an ovoid shape and fine, speckled chromatin. The nuclei stand apart from blood vessels, resulting in perivascular anuclear zones. Radially arranged tumor cells and perivascular anuclear zones together create "perivascular pseudorosettes," the most distinguishing histological feature of ependymoma (Fig. 58.14). True ependymal rosettes composed of columnar cells around a central lumen are occasionally seen. A minority are frankly anaplastic with mitotic figures, nuclear atypia, and vascular proliferation. The predictive value of the histological distinction between low-grade and anaplastic ependymoma is not as great as with other types of glioma.[187] Immunohistochemical staining of ependymomas is positive for GFAP and EMA, while neuronal markers are negative. GFAP immunohistochemistry highlights tumor cell processes in pseudorosettes. EMA immunohistochemistry demonstrates dot-like cytoplasmic staining and can be diagnostically useful.

Spinal cord ependymomas, which occur primarily in adults, are discussed in the "Spinal cord glioma in adults" section (see above). The majority of adult ependymomas are well-circumscribed masses arising in the spinal cord. The tendency for recurrence and dissemination of spinal ependymomas is so entirely different from that of childhood intracranial ependymomas that these represent distinct clinical entities.

Complete surgical resection is considered to be the standard of care for treatment of ependymomas. As with many brain tumors, gross total resection (GTR) results in superior survival compared to subtotal resection (STR). In the pediatric population, this is often difficult given the infratentorial location and local extension into the brainstem. In adults, complete surgical resection is more easily attainable, with 62% of patients

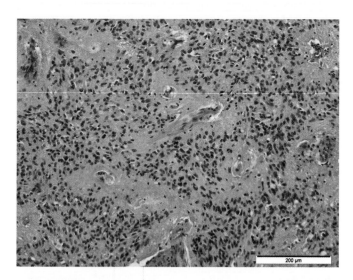

Figure 58.14 Ependymoma. "Perivascular pseudorosettes" (perivascular anuclear zones) are a histological hallmark of ependymomas. H&E, 200× original magnification.

achieving total resection.[188] Since resection is potentially curative, a second attempt at resection is often considered if substantial residual disease is apparent on postoperative scans or at the time of first recurrence. Emergency ventriculostomy may be indicated for rapidly progressive hydrocephalus from fourth ventricle tumors, and some patients will require permanent ventriculoperitoneal shunting once the tumor is removed. Preoperative MRI scanning of the entire neuraxis, and postoperative CSF analysis (if safely obtained), is recommended, as ependymomas have a higher likelihood of subarachnoid dissemination than astrocytic neoplasms, although less than medulloblastoma/PNET.

The role of postoperative radiation treatment in ependymomas is less clearly defined. In grade 3 (anaplastic) ependymomas, adjuvant radiation treatment is generally recommended, even after GTR, using fractionated radiation to a dose of 45–54 Gy to the tumor bed plus a margin. Focal radiation is also recommended for infratentorial grade 2 and some incompletely resected supratentorial grade 2 ependymomas. However, in lower grade supratentorial tumors, the role of radiation after GTR is not as well defined. Radiation does improve local control, yet with careful monitoring it can often be deferred until recurrence. With over 90% of recurrences being at the primary site, an attempt at re-resection is often recommended prior to irradiation. In children under the age of 3, radiation therapy is often deferred for multiagent chemotherapy due to the profound side-effects of radiation in young children.[189] Craniospinal radiation is limited to those patients, including adults, with evidence of subarachnoid dissemination.[32,190,191]

In general, ependymomas are considered to be chemotherapy-resistant tumors. Most of the data for chemotherapy are based on treatment of recurrent disease, rather than in the adjuvant setting. The efficacy of chemotherapy for childhood ependymoma is less than that observed with medulloblastoma. In young children treated with multiagent chemotherapy (cisplatin, VP-16, vincristine, and cyclophosphamide) following surgery, the response rate (CR + PR) was 48%.[189] However, cooperative group trials have not demonstrated a substantial impact of chemotherapy on survival.

There is a paucity of prospective trials in adults with ependymoma. A large number of chemotherapy agents have been used, usually in multiagent combinations. The best response rate (31–67%) is seen with regimens containing either cisplatin or carboplatin.[192] The nitrosoureas demonstrate lower response rates in the 25% range.[193] Nonplatinum-containing regimens with cyclophosphamide, vincristine, or etoposide are commonly used but response rates are only 11–13%. Although it showed little activity in platinum-resistant patients, temozolomide is in phase 2 testing in combination with lapatinib.[194] Agents targeting the ErbB2(her-2/neu), PDGFR-α, and α-v-β-3 integrin pathways are currently being investigated in ependymoma.[195]

The prognosis for patients with intracranial ependymoma varies with age. Children carry a higher likelihood of recurrence, most of which are local recurrences. About 10% of recurrences involve concurrent or isolated subarachnoid metastases. Metastases outside the neuraxis are exceedingly rare. Five-year PFS estimates for children are 50–70%.

Ten-year OS after gross total resection is 70% but with subtotal resection, only 33% of pediatric patients are alive. Adults fare better with 5- and 10-year OS rates of 86% and 81%, respectively.[196]

Anaplastic ependymomas

Ependymomas which exhibit hypercellularity, cellular and nuclear pleomorphism, frequent mitoses, pseudopalisading necrosis, and vascular proliferation on pathological examination are given the designation of WHO grade 3 anaplastic ependymomas, or "malignant ependymomas." Perivascular pseudorosettes can still be identified but the anuclear zones may be narrowed in comparison to usual ependymomas (Fig. 58.15).

Grade 3 tumors can arise through the malignant progression of grade 2 ependymomas. MRI of the spine and CSF analysis are essential parts of staging for these tumors, as the incidence of spinal cord seeding is 8–20%. Postoperative radiation treatment is considered the standard of care in grade 3 tumors. Anaplastic ependymomas have a much worse prognosis compared to lower grade ependymomas, with 5-year survival rates ranging from 10% to 47%.

Myxopapillary ependymomas

Myxopapillary ependymomas (MPEs) are slow-growing, grade 1 ependymomas, which represent the most common glioma arising in the conus-filum region. Most occur in adults. In children, these tumors are vanishingly rare, with only around 100 MPE patients reported in the literature. MPEs are intradural, extramedullary tumors. The tumor cells of MPE demonstrate a radial perivascular arrangement similar to usual ependymoma but are separated from the central blood vessel by a myxoid matrix. The myxoid matrix not only forms a "collar" separating the tumor cells from vessels but also extends into the tumor stroma in the form of intercellular microcysts. Clustering of cells around the tumor vasculature creates a papillary appearance. Mitotic activity is low (Fig. 58.16).

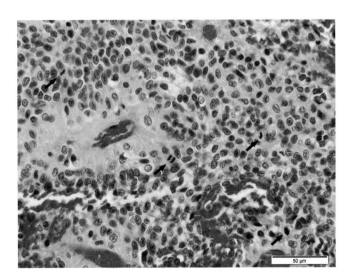

Figure 58.15 Anaplastic ependymoma. Mitotic figures (*arrows*) are present in high numbers in this tumor. Vascular proliferation and necrosis are often present as well. H&E, 600× original magnification.

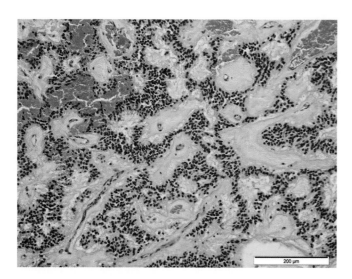

Figure 58.16 Myxopapillary ependymoma. A gray, myxoid matrix is interposed between blood vessels and radially arranged tumor cells. H&E, 200× original magnification.

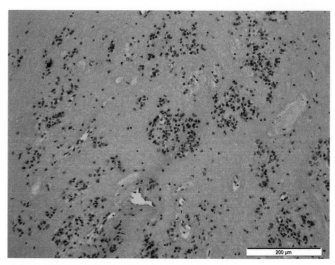

Figure 58.17 Subependymoma. Tumor cells form clusters in a dense, fibrillar stroma. H&E, 200× original magnification.

As with other ependymomas, the ability to achieve a GTR is the most important prognostic factor.[197] However, the location of MPEs renders GTR difficult. These tumors often present late with local extensions and attachment to the surrounding nerve roots and conus medullaris. In one of the largest surgical series, of 77 patients with MPE, recurrence rates were lowest after gross total resection of encapsulated tumors (10% recurrence) when compared with those removed in piecemeal (34%) or subtotally resected tumors (41%).[198] Adjuvant radiation treatment can be offered after subtotal resection or in the context of salvage therapy. In a recent large series of mainly adult patients with MPE, adjuvant high-dose RT (>50.4 Gy) was associated with a significant improvement in 5-year PFS.[199] There is no well-defined role for chemotherapy in MPEs.

The long-term survival for adult MPE patients is excellent, with 97% of patients alive at 10 years. Progression-free survival (62%) and local control (72%) at 10 years are also quite good.[200]

Subependymoma

Subependymomas are WHO grade 1 neoplasms that usually arise in the lateral and fourth ventricles. Ependymomas and subependymomas can usually be distinguished by imaging: ependymomas are generally periventricular, while subependymomas are entirely intraventricular. These tumors tend to be asymptomatic, unless they reach a size, usually in the 3–5 cm range, which results in CSF flow obstruction and hydrocephalus.[201] They are more common in males, usually presenting with symptoms in the fourth to sixth decades of life. These tumors are exceedingly rare: one study reported an incidence of 0.7% among 1000 patients with pathologically documented intracranial neoplasms.

Histological examination reveals a hypocellular neoplasm composed of clusters of nuclei with ependymal features (Fig. 58.17). Glial cell processes form a dense, fibrillar stroma that surrounds the clustered tumor cell nuclei. Small cysts are often observed within the stroma. A lobular tumor architecture may be appreciated on low magnification. Mitoses are uncommon and the MIB-1 labeling index is low.[202] Rare combined tumors with regions of ependymoma and subependymoma are encountered; these lesions are graded based on the ependymoma component. By MRI, these tumors are usually well-defined solid or mixed solid-cystic intraventricular masses with variable enhancement.

Complete surgical excision is the recommended treatment, which is more easily accomplished with supratentorial subependymomas than with their fourth ventricle counterparts. Potential injury to cranial nerves often limits the resectability of fourth ventricle tumors. Adjuvant radiation treatment is not recommended unless residual tumor is present. Radiation can also be used in the setting of unresectable lesions or in cases of progressive disease. There is no role for chemotherapy in subependymomas.

References

1. Louis DN, *et al*. The 2007 WHO classification of tumours of the central nervous system. Acta Neuropathol 2007; 114(2): 97–109.
2. Central Brain Tumor Registry of the United States. Statistical Report: Primary Brain and Central Nervous System Tumors Diagnosed in the United States in 2004–2007. www.cbtrus.org.
3. Porter KR, *et al*. Prevalence estimates for primary brain tumors in the United States by age, gender, behavior, and histology. Neuro Oncol 2010: 12(6): 520–7.
4. Wrensch M, *et al*. Familial and personal medical history of cancer and nervous system conditions among adults with glioma and controls. Am J Epidemiol 1997; 145(7): 581–93.
5. Bohnen N, Radhakrishnan K, O'Neill BP, Kurland LT. Descriptive and analytic epidemiology of brain tumors. In: Black P, Loeffler JS (eds) *Cancer of the Nervous System*. Cambridge: Blackwell Science, 1997. pp.1–22.
6. INTERPHONE Study Group. Brain tumour risk in relation to mobile telephone use: results of the INTERPHONE international case–control study. Int J Epidemiol 2010; 39(3): 675–94.
7. Cancer Genome Atlas Research Network, Comprehensive genomic characterization defines human glioblastoma genes and core pathways. Nature 2008; 455(7216): 1061–8.

8. Parsons DW, *et al.* An integrated genomic analysis of human glioblastoma multiforme. Science 2008; 321(5897): 1807–12.

9. Phillips HS, *et al.* Molecular subclasses of high-grade glioma predict prognosis, delineate a pattern of disease progression, and resemble stages in neurogenesis. Cancer Cell 2006; 9(3): 157–73.

10. Verhaak RG, *et al.* Integrated genomic analysis identifies clinically relevant subtypes of glioblastoma characterized by abnormalities in PDGFRA, IDH1, EGFR, and NF1. Cancer Cell 2010; 17(1): 98–110.

11. Hartmann C, *et al.* Type and frequency of IDH1 and IDH2 mutations are related to astrocytic and oligodendroglial differentiation and age: a study of 1,010 diffuse gliomas. Acta Neuropathol 2009; 118(4): 469–74.

12. Nobusawa S, *et al.* IDH1 mutations as molecular signature and predictive factor of secondary glioblastomas. Clin Cancer Res 2009; 15(19): 6002–7.

13. Yan H, *et al.* IDH1 and IDH2 mutations in gliomas. N Engl J Med 2009; 360(8): 765–73.

14. Capper D, *et al.* Application of mutant IDH1 antibody to differentiate diffuse glioma from nonneoplastic central nervous system lesions and therapy-induced changes. Am J Surg Pathol 2010; 34(8): 1199–204.

15. Weller M, *et al.* Molecular predictors of progression-free and overall survival in patients with newly diagnosed glioblastoma: a prospective translational study of the German Glioma Network. J Clin Oncol 2009; 27(34): 5743–50.

16. Hartmann C, *et al.* Patients with IDH1 wild type anaplastic astrocytomas exhibit worse prognosis than IDH1-mutated glioblastomas, and IDH1 mutation status accounts for the unfavorable prognostic effect of higher age: implications for classification of gliomas. Acta Neuropathol 2010; 120(6): 707–18.

17. Dang L, Jin S, Su SM. IDH mutations in glioma and acute myeloid leukemia. Trends Mol Med 2010; 16(9): 387–97.

18. Xu W, *et al.* Oncometabolite 2-hydroxyglutarate is a competitive inhibitor of alpha-ketoglutarate-dependent dioxygenases. Cancer Cell 2011; 19(1): 17–30.

19. Laffaire J, *et al.* Methylation profiling identifies 2 groups of gliomas according to their tumorigenesis. Neuro Oncol 2011; 13(1): 84–98.

20. Bao S, *et al.* Glioma stem cells promote radioresistance by preferential activation of the DNA damage response. Nature 2006; 444(7120): 756–60.

21. Bao S, *et al.* Stem cell-like glioma cells promote tumor angiogenesis through vascular endothelial growth factor. Cancer Res 2006; 66(16): 7843–8.

22. Liu G, *et al.* Analysis of gene expression and chemoresistance of CD133+ cancer stem cells in glioblastoma. Mol Cancer 2006; 5: 67.

23. Johnson RA, *et al.* Cross-species genomics matches driver mutations and cell compartments to model ependymoma. Nature 2010; 466(7306): 632–6.

24. Shapiro WR, *et al.* Randomized trial of three chemotherapy regimens and two radiotherapy regimens and two radiotherapy regimens in postoperative treatment of malignant glioma. Brain Tumor Cooperative Group Trial 8001. J Neurosurg 1989; 71(1): 1–9.

25. Moots PL, *et al.* The course of seizure disorders in patients with malignant gliomas. Arch Neurol 1995; 52(7): 717–24.

26. Forsyth PA, Posner JB. Headaches in patients with brain tumors: a study of 111 patients. Neurology 1993; 43(9): 1678–83.

27. Moots PL. Pitfalls in the management of patients with malignant gliomas. Semin Neurol 1998; 18(2): 257–65.

28. Stupp R, *et al.* Effects of radiotherapy with concomitant and adjuvant temozolomide versus radiotherapy alone on survival in glioblastoma in a randomised phase III study: 5-year analysis of the EORTC-NCIC trial. Lancet Oncol 2009; 10(5): 459–66.

29. Levin VA, *et al.* Superiority of post-radiotherapy adjuvant chemotherapy with CCNU, procarbazine, and vincristine (PCV) over BCNU for anaplastic gliomas: NCOG 6 G61 final report. Int J Radiat Oncol Biol Phys 1990; 18(2): 321–4.

30. Leighton C, *et al.* Supratentorial low-grade glioma in adults: an analysis of prognostic factors and timing of radiation. J Clin Oncol 1997; 15(4): 1294–301.

31. Fallon KB, *et al.* Prognostic value of 1p, 19q, 9p, 10q, and EGFR-FISH analyses in recurrent oligodendrogliomas. J Neuropathol Exp Neurol 2004; 63(4): 314–22.

32. Lyons MK, Kelly PJ. Posterior fossa ependymomas: report of 30 cases and review of the literature. Neurosurgery 1991; 28(5): 659–64; discussion 664–5.

33. Kleihues P, *et al.* WHO grading of tumours of the central nervous system. In: Louis DN, Ohgaki H, Wiestler OD, Cavenee WK (eds) *WHO Classification of Tumours of the Central Nervous System.* Lyon: IARC Press, 2007. p.10.

34. Kleihues P, *et al.* Anaplastic astrocytoma. In: Louis DN, Ohgaki H, Wiestler OD, Cavenee WK (eds) *WHO Classification of Tumours of the Central Nervous System.* Lyon: IARC Press, 2007. pp.30–2.

35. Jaros E, *et al.* Prognostic implications of p53 protein, epidermal growth factor receptor, and Ki-67 labelling in brain tumours. Br J Cancer 1992; 66(2): 373–85.

36. Daumas-Duport C, Scheithauer BW, Kelly PJ. A histologic and cytologic method for the spatial definition of gliomas. Mayo Clin Proc 1987; 62(6): 435–49.

37. Scherer HJ. The forms of glioma growth and their practical significance. Brain 1940; 63(1): 1–35.

38. Burger PC, *et al.* Computerized tomographic and pathologic studies of the untreated, quiescent, and recurrent glioblastoma multiforme. J Neurosurg 1983; 58(2): 159–69.

39. Burger PC, *et al.* Topographic anatomy and CT correlations in the untreated glioblastoma multiforme. J Neurosurg 1988; 68(5): 698–704.

40. Kelly PJ. Stereotactic histologic correlations of computed tomography- and magnetic resonance imaging-defined abnormalities in patients with glial neoplasms. Mayo Clin Proc 1987; 62(6): 450–9.

41. Friedman HS, *et al.* Criteria for termination of phase II chemotherapy for patients with progressive or recurrent brain tumor. Neurology 1989; 39(1): 62–6.

42. Macdonald DR, *et al.* Response criteria for phase II studies of supratentorial malignant glioma. J Clin Oncol 1990; 8(7): 1277–80.

43. Reardon DA, *et al.* Clinical trial end points for high-grade glioma: the evolving landscape. Neuro Oncol 2011; 13(3): 353–61.

44. Van den Bent MJ, *et al.* Response assessment in neuro-oncology (a report of the RANO group): assessment of outcome in trials of diffuse low-grade gliomas. Lancet Oncol; 2011; 12(6): 583–93.

45. Wen PY, Kesari S. Malignant gliomas in adults. N Engl J Med 2008; 359(5): 492–507.

46. Wen PY, *et al.* Updated response assessment criteria for high-grade gliomas: response assessment in neuro-oncology working group. J Clin Oncol 2010; 28(11): 1963–72.

47. Wen PY, *et al.* Medical management of patients with brain tumors. J Neurooncol 2006; 80(3): 313–32.

48. Galanis E, *et al.* Efficacy of neuroradiological imaging, neurological examination, and symptom status in follow-up assessment of patients with high-grade gliomas. J Neurosurg 2000; 93(2): 201–7.

49. Lacroix M, *et al.* A multivariate analysis of 416 patients with glioblastoma multiforme: prognosis, extent of resection, and survival. J Neurosurg 2001; 95(2): 190–8.

50. Fadul C, *et al.* Morbidity and mortality of craniotomy for excision of supratentorial gliomas. Neurology 1988; 38(9): 1374–9.

51. Norris LK, Grossman SA. Treatment of thromboembolic complications in patients with brain tumors. J Neurooncol 1994; 22(2): 127–37.

52. Shapiro WR. Therapy of adult malignant brain tumors: what have the clinical trials taught us? Semin Oncol 1986; 13(1): 38–45.

53. Buatti J, *et al.* Radiation therapy of pathologically confirmed newly diagnosed glioblastoma in adults. J Neurooncol 2008; 89(3): 313–37.

54. Yung WK, *et al.* A phase II study of temozolomide vs. procarbazine in patients with glioblastoma multiforme at first relapse. Br J Cancer 2000; 83(5): 588–93.

55. Brandes AA, *et al.* How effective is BCNU in recurrent glioblastoma in the modern era? A phase II trial. Neurology 2004; 63(7): 1281–4.

56. Hegi ME, *et al.* MGMT gene silencing and benefit from temozolomide in glioblastoma. N Engl J Med 2005; 352(10): 997–1003.

57. Weller M, *et al.* MGMT promoter methylation in malignant gliomas: ready for personalized medicine? Nat Rev Neurol 2010; 6(1): 39–51.

58. Westphal M, *et al.* A phase 3 trial of local chemotherapy with biodegradable carmustine (BCNU) wafers (Gliadel wafers) in patients with primary malignant glioma. Neuro Oncol 2003; 5(2): 79–88.

59. Bock HC, *et al.* First-line treatment of malignant glioma with carmustine implants followed by concomitant radiochemotherapy: a multicenter experience. Neurosurg Rev 2010; 33(4): 441–9.

60. Clarke JL, *et al.* Is surgery at progression a prognostic marker for improved 6-month progression-free survival or overall survival for patients with recurrent glioblastoma? Neuro Oncol 2011; 13(10): 1118–24.

61. Vredenburgh JJ, *et al.* Bevacizumab plus irinotecan in recurrent glioblastoma multiforme. J Clin Oncol 2007; 25(30): 4722–9.

62. Cloughesy TF, *et al.* A phase II, randomized, non-comparative clinical trial of the effect of bevacizumab (BV) alone or in combination with irinotecan (CPT) on 6-month progression free survival (PFS6) in recurrent, treatment-refractory glioblastoma (GBM). J Clin Oncol 2008; 26(Suppl): abstract 2010b.

63. Han SJ, *et al.* Primary gliosarcoma: key clinical and pathologic distinctions from glioblastoma with implications as a unique oncologic entity. J Neurooncol 2010; 96(3): 313–20.

64. Han SJ, *et al.* Secondary gliosarcoma after diagnosis of glioblastoma: clinical experience with 30 consecutive patients. J Neurosurg 2010; 112(5): 990–6.

65. Beaumont TL, *et al.* Gliosarcoma with multiple extracranial metastases: case report and review of the literature. J Neurooncol 2007; 83(1): 39–46.

66. Demirci S, *et al.* Multiple spinal metastases of cranial gliosarcoma: a case report and review of the literature. J Neurooncol 2008; 88(2): 199–204.

67. Actor B, *et al.* Comprehensive analysis of genomic alterations in gliosarcoma and its two tissue components. Genes Chromosomes Cancer 2002; 34(4): 416–27.

68. Hildebrand J, *et al.* Adjuvant dibromodulcitol and BCNU chemotherapy in anaplastic astrocytoma: results of a randomised European Organisation for Research and Treatment of Cancer phase III study (EORTC study 26882). Eur J Cancer 2008; 44(9): 1210–16.

69. Berger MS, *et al.* The effect of extent of resection on recurrence in patients with low grade cerebral hemisphere gliomas. Cancer 1994; 74(6): 1784–91.

70. McGirt MJ, *et al.* Extent of surgical resection is independently associated with survival in patients with hemispheric infiltrating low-grade gliomas. Neurosurgery 2008; 63(4): 700–7; author reply 707–8.

71. Karim AB, *et al.* A randomized trial on dose-response in radiation therapy of low-grade cerebral glioma: European Organization for Research and Treatment of Cancer (EORTC) Study 22844. Int J Radiat Oncol Biol Phys 1996; 36(3): 549–56.

72. Van den Bent MJ, *et al.* Long-term efficacy of early versus delayed radiotherapy for low-grade astrocytoma and oligodendroglioma in adults: the EORTC 22845 randomised trial. Lancet 2005; 366(9490): 985–90.

73. Taphoorn MJ, *et al.* Cognitive functions and quality of life in patients with low-grade gliomas: the impact of radiotherapy. Ann Neurol 1994; 36(1): 48–54.

74. Eyre HJ, *et al.* A randomized trial of radiotherapy versus radiotherapy plus CCNU for incompletely resected low-grade gliomas: a Southwest Oncology Group study. J Neurosurg 1993; 78(6): 909–14.

75. Daniels TB, *et al.* Validation of EORTC prognostic factors for adults with low-grade glioma: a report using intergroup 86-72-51. Int J Radiat Oncol Biol Phys 2011; 81(1): 218–24.

76. Pignatti F, *et al.* Prognostic factors for survival in adult patients with cerebral low-grade glioma. J Clin Oncol 2002; 20(8): 2076–84.

77. Yu J, *et al.* Alterations of BRAF and HIPK2 loci predominate in sporadic pilocytic astrocytoma. Neurology 2009; 73(19): 1526–31.

78. Pomeroy SL, Pathologic intracellular signaling in childhood pilocytic astrocytomas. Neurology 2009; 73(19): 1522–3.

79. Tchoghandjian A, *et al.* Pilocytic astrocytoma of the optic pathway: a tumour deriving from radial glia cells with a specific gene signature. Brain 2009; 132(Pt 6): 1523–35.

80. Komotar RJ, *et al.* Magnetic resonance imaging characteristics of pilomyxoid astrocytoma. Neurol Res 2008; 30(9): 945–51.

81. Mansur DB, *et al.* Radiation therapy for pilocytic astrocytomas of childhood. Int J Radiat Oncol Biol Phys 2011; 79(3): 829–34.

82. Moghrabi A, *et al.* Phase II study of carboplatin (CBDCA) in progressive low-grade gliomas. Neurosurg Focus 1998; 4(4): e3.

83. Gururangan S, *et al.* Temozolomide in children with progressive low-grade glioma. Neuro Oncol 2007; 9(2): 161–8.

84. Khaw SL, *et al.* Temozolomide in pediatric low-grade glioma. Pediatr Blood Cancer 2007; 49(6): 808–11.

85. Bell D, *et al.* Pilocytic astrocytoma of the adult – clinical features, radiological features and management. Br J Neurosurg 2004; 18(6): 613–16.

86. Brown PD, *et al.* Adult patients with supratentorial pilocytic astrocytomas: a prospective multicenter clinical trial. Int J Radiat Oncol Biol Phys 2004; 58(4): 1153–60.

87. Ishkanian A, *et al.* Upfront observation versus radiation for adult pilocytic astrocytoma. Cancer 2011; 117: 4070–9.

88. Ellis JA, *et al.* Rapid recurrence and malignant transformation of pilocytic astrocytoma in adult patients. J Neurooncol 2009; 95(3): 377–82.

89. Komotar RJ, *et al.* Pilocytic and pilomyxoid hypothalamic/chiasmatic astrocytomas. Neurosurgery 2004; 54(1): 72–9; discussion 79–80.

90. Johnson MW, *et al.* Spectrum of pilomyxoid astrocytomas: intermediate pilomyxoid tumors. Am J Surg Pathol 2010; 34(12): 1783–91.

91. Flickinger JC, Torres C, Deutsch M. Management of low-grade gliomas of the optic nerve and chiasm. Cancer 1988; 61(4): 635–42.

92. Wong JY, *et al.* Optic gliomas. A reanalysis of the University of California, San Francisco experience. Cancer 1987; 60(8): 1847–55.

93. Khafaga Y, *et al.* Optic gliomas: a retrospective analysis of 50 cases. Int J Radiat Oncol Biol Phys 2003; 56(3): 807–12.

94. Combs SE, *et al.* Fractionated stereotactic radiotherapy of optic pathway gliomas: tolerance and long-term outcome. Int J Radiat Oncol Biol Phys 2005; 62(3): 814–19.

95. Friedman HS, *et al.* Treatment of children with progressive or recurrent brain tumors with carboplatin or iproplatin: a Pediatric Oncology Group randomized phase II study. J Clin Oncol 1992; 10(2): 249–56.

96. Listernick R, *et al.* Optic pathway gliomas in children with neurofibromatosis 1: consensus statement from the NF1 Optic Pathway Glioma Task Force. Ann Neurol 1997; 41(2): 143–9.

97. Packer RJ, *et al.* Brainstem gliomas. Neurosurg Clin North Am 1992; 3(4): 863–79.

98. Packer RJ, *et al.* Treatment of chiasmatic/hypothalamic gliomas of childhood with chemotherapy: an update. Ann Neurol 1988; 23(1): 79–85.

99. Silva MM, *et al.* Optic pathway hypothalamic gliomas in children under three years of age: the role of chemotherapy. Pediatr Neurosurg 2000; 33(3): 151–8.

100. Chamberlain MC. Recurrent chiasmatic-hypothalamic glioma treated with oral etoposide. Arch Neurol 1995; 52(5): 509–13.

101. Krouwer HG, *et al.* Gemistocytic astrocytomas: a reappraisal. J Neurosurg 1991; 74(3): 399–406.

102. Tihan T, *et al.* Definition and diagnostic implications of gemistocytic astrocytomas: a pathological perspective. J Neurooncol 2006; 76(2): 175–83.

103. Von Deimling A, *et al.* Diffuse astrocytoma. In: Louis DN, Ohgaki H, Wiestler OD, Cavenee WK (eds) *WHO Classification of Tumours of the Central Nervous System.* Lyon: IARC Press, 2007. pp.25–9.

104. Watanabe K, *et al.* Role of gemistocytes in astrocytoma progression. Lab Invest 1997; 76(2): 277–84.

105. Geranmayeh F, *et al.* Microglia in gemistocytic astrocytomas. Neurosurgery 2007; 60(1): 159–66; discussion 166.

106. Kosel S, *et al.* Genotype-phenotype correlation in gemistocytic astrocytomas. Neurosurgery 2001; 48(1): 187–93; discussion 193–4.

107. Nowak-Sadzikowska J, *et al.* Postoperative irradiation of incompletely excised gemistocytic astrocytomas. Clinical outcome and prognostic factors. Strahlenther Onkol 2005; 181(4): 246–50.

108. Martins DC, et al. Gemistocytes in astrocytomas: are they a significant prognostic factor? J Neurooncol 2006; 80(1): 49–55.

109. Avninder S, et al. Gemistocytic astrocytomas: histomorphology, proliferative potential and genetic alterations – a study of 32 cases. J Neurooncol 2006; 78(2): 123–7.

110. Yang HJ, et al. The significance of gemistocytes in astrocytoma. Acta Neurochir (Wien) 2003; 145(12): 1097–103; discussion 1103.

111. Kepes JJ, et al. Pleomorphic xanthoastrocytoma: a distinctive meningocerebral glioma of young subjects with relatively favorable prognosis. A study of 12 cases. Cancer 1979; 44(5): 1839–52.

112. Giannini C, et al. Pleomorphic xanthoastrocytoma: what do we really know about it? Cancer 1999; 85(9): 2033–45.

113. Im SH, et al. Pleomorphic xanthoastrocytoma: a developmental glioneuronal tumor with prominent glioproliferative changes. J Neurooncol 2004; 66(1–2): 17–27.

114. Dias-Santagata D, et al. BRAF V600E mutations are common in pleomorphic xanthoastrocytoma: diagnostic and therapeutic implications. PLoS One 2011; 6(3): e17948.

115. Rao AA, et al. Pleomorphic xanthoastrocytoma in children and adolescents. Pediatr Blood Cancer 2010; 55(2): 290–4.

116. Buccoliero AM, et al. Subependymal giant cell astrocytoma (SEGA): is it an astrocytoma? Morphological, immunohistochemical and ultrastructural study. Neuropathology 2009; 29(1): 25–30.

117. Lopes MB, et al. Immunohistochemical characterization of subependymal giant cell astrocytomas. Acta Neuropathol 1996; 91(4): 368–75.

118. Shepherd CW, et al. Subependymal giant cell astrocytoma: a clinical, pathological, and flow cytometric study. Neurosurgery 1991; 28(6): 864–8.

119. Campen CJ, Porter BE. Subependymal giant cell astrocytoma (SEGA) treatment update. Curr Treat Options Neurol 2011; 13(4): 380–5.

120. Krueger DA, et al. Everolimus for subependymal giant-cell astrocytomas in tuberous sclerosis. N Engl J Med 2010; 363(19): 1801–11.

121. Becker AJ, et al. Ganglioglioma and gangliocytoma. In: Louis DN, Ohgaki H, Wiestler OD, Cavenee WK (eds) WHO Classification of Tumours of the Central Nervous System. Lyon: IARC Press, 2007. pp.103–5.

122. Hakim R, et al. Gangliogliomas in adults. Cancer 1997; 79(1): 127–31.

123. Hirose T, et al. Ganglioglioma: an ultrastructural and immunohistochemical study. Cancer 1997; 79(5): 989–1003.

124. Daumas-Duport C. Dysembryoplastic neuroepithelial tumours. Brain Pathol 1993; 3(3): 283–95.

125. Daumas-Duport C, et al. Dysembryoplastic neuroepithelial tumor: a surgically curable tumor of young patients with intractable partial seizures. Report of thirty-nine cases. Neurosurgery 1988; 23(5): 545–56.

126. Guillamo JS, et al. Brain stem gliomas. Curr Opin Neurol 2001; 14(6): 711–15.

127. Guillamo JS, et al. Brainstem gliomas in adults: prognostic factors and classification. Brain 2001; 124(Pt 12): 2528–39.

128. Kesari S, et al. Prognostic factors in adult brainstem gliomas: a multicenter, retrospective analysis of 101 cases. J Neurooncol 2008; 88(2): 175–83.

129. Laigle-Donadey F, et al. Brainstem gliomas in children and adults. Curr Opin Oncol 2008; 20(6): 662–7.

130. Salmaggi A, et al. Natural history and management of brainstem gliomas in adults. A retrospective Italian study. J Neurol 2008; 255(2): 171–7.

131. Rachinger W, et al. Serial stereotactic biopsy of brainstem lesions in adults improves diagnostic accuracy compared with MRI only. J Neurol Neurosurg Psychiatry 2009; 80(10): 1134–9.

132. Selvapandian S, et al. Brainstem glioma: comparative study of clinico-radiological presentation, pathology and outcome in children and adults. Acta Neurochir (Wien) 1999; 141(7): 721–6; discussion 726–7.

133. Yeh DD, et al. Management strategy for adult patients with dorsal midbrain gliomas. Neurosurgery 2002; 50(4): 735–8; discussion 738–40.

134. Shrivastava RK, et al. Intramedullary spinal cord tumors in patients older than 50 years of age: management and outcome analysis. J Neurosurg Spine 2005; 2(3): 249–55.

135. Kucia EJ, et al. Surgical technique and outcomes in the treatment of spinal cord ependymomas, part 1: intramedullary ependymomas. Neurosurgery 2011; 68(1 Suppl Operative): 57–63; discussion 63.

136. Minehan KJ, et al. Prognosis and treatment of spinal cord astrocytoma. Int J Radiat Oncol Biol Phys 2009; 73(3): 727–33.

137. McGirt MJ, et al. Extent of surgical resection of malignant astrocytomas of the spinal cord: outcome analysis of 35 patients. Neurosurgery 2008; 63(1): 55–60; discussion 60–1.

138. Jallo GI, et al. Intrinsic spinal cord tumor resection. Neurosurgery 2001; 49(5): 1124–8.

139. Parsa AT, et al. Spinal cord and intradural-extraparenchymal spinal tumors: current best care practices and strategies. J Neurooncol 2004; 69(1–3): 291–318.

140. Sandalcioglu IE, et al. Functional outcome after surgical treatment of intramedullary spinal cord tumors: experience with 78 patients. Spinal Cord 2005; 43(1): 34–41.

141. Chamberlain MC. Temozolomide for recurrent low-grade spinal cord gliomas in adults. Cancer 2008; 113(5): 1019–24.

142. Balmaceda C. Chemotherapy for intramedullary spinal cord tumors. J Neurooncol 2000; 47(3): 293–307.

143. Gornet MK, et al. Chemotherapy for advanced CNS ependymoma. J Neurooncol 1999; 45(1): 61–7.

144. Milano MT, et al. Primary spinal cord glioma: a Surveillance, Epidemiology, and End Results database study. J Neurooncol 2010; 98(1): 83–92.

145. Henson JW. Spinal cord gliomas. Curr Opin Neurol 2001; 14(6): 679–82.

146. Robinson CG, et al. Long-term survival and functional status of patients with low-grade astrocytoma of spinal cord. Int J Radiat Oncol Biol Phys 2005; 63(1): 91–100.

147. Lee HK, et al. The prognostic value of neurologic function in astrocytic spinal cord glioma. Neuro Oncol 2003; 5(3): 208–13.

148. Shaw EG, et al. Oligodendrogliomas: the Mayo Clinic experience. J Neurosurg 1992; 76(3): 428–34.

149. Daumas-Duport C, et al. Oligodendrogliomas. Part II: A new grading system based on morphological and imaging criteria. J Neurooncol 1997; 34(1): 61–78.

150. Daumas-Duport C, et al. Oligodendrogliomas. Part I: Patterns of growth, histological diagnosis, clinical and imaging correlations: a study of 153 cases. J Neurooncol 1997; 34(1): 37–59.

151. Jenkins RB, et al. A t(1;19)(q10;p10) mediates the combined deletions of 1p and 19q and predicts a better prognosis of patients with oligodendroglioma. Cancer Res 2006; 66(20): 9852–61.

152. Kraus JA, et al. Shared allelic losses on chromosomes 1p and 19q suggest a common origin of oligodendroglioma and oligoastrocytoma. J Neuropathol Exp Neurol 1995; 54(1): 91–5.

153. Glass J, et al. The treatment of oligodendrogliomas and mixed oligodendroglioma-astrocytomas with PCV chemotherapy. J Neurosurg 1992; 76(5): 741–5.

154. Kim L, et al. Procarbazine, lomustine, and vincristine (PCV) chemotherapy for grade III and grade IV oligoastrocytomas. J Neurosurg 1996; 85(4): 602–7.

155. Kyritsis AP, et al. The treatment of anaplastic oligodendrogliomas and mixed gliomas. Neurosurgery 1993; 32(3): 365–70; discussion 371.

156. Jaeckle KA, et al. Transformation of low grade glioma and correlation with outcome: an NCCTG database analysis. J Neurooncol 2011; 104(1): 253–9.

157. Giannini C, et al. Oligodendrogliomas: reproducibility and prognostic value of histologic diagnosis and grading. J Neuropathol Exp Neurol 2001; 60(3): 248–62.

158. Reifenberger G, et al. Anaplastic oligodendroglioma. In: Louis DN, Ohgaki H, Wiestler OD, Cavenee WK (eds) WHO Classification of Tumours of the Central Nervous System. Lyon: IARC Press, 2007. pp.60–2.

159. Burger PC, Scheithauer BW. Tumors of the Central Nervous System. AFIP Atlas of Tumor Pathology, Series 4. Washington DC: Armed Forces Institute of Pathology, 2007. pp.122–45.

160. Miller CR, et al. Significance of necrosis in grading of oligodendroglial neoplasms: a clinicopathologic and genetic study of newly diagnosed high-grade gliomas. J Clin Oncol 2006; 24(34): 5419–26.

161. Chaichana KL, *et al.* Prognostic significance of contrast-enhancing low-grade gliomas in adults and a review of the literature. Neurol Res 2009; 31(9): 931–9.

162. Schomas DA, *et al.* Intracranial low-grade gliomas in adults: 30-year experience with long-term follow-up at Mayo Clinic. Neuro Oncol 2009; 11(4): 437–45.

163. Smith JS, *et al.* Role of extent of resection in the long-term outcome of low-grade hemispheric gliomas. J Clin Oncol 2008; 26(8): 1338–45.

164. Douw L, *et al.* Cognitive and radiological effects of radiotherapy in patients with low-grade glioma: long-term follow-up. Lancet Neurol 2009; 8(9): 810–18.

165. Mason WP, *et al.* Low-grade oligodendroglioma responds to chemotherapy. Neurology 1996; 46(1): 203–7.

166. Lebrun C, *et al.* Treatment of newly diagnosed symptomatic pure low-grade oligodendrogliomas with PCV chemotherapy. Eur J Neurol 2007; 14(4): 391–8.

167. Iwadate Y, *et al.* Favorable long-term outcome of low-grade oligodendrogliomas irrespective of 1p/19q status when treated without radiotherapy. J Neurooncol 2011; 102(3): 443–9.

168. Kesari S, *et al.* Phase II study of protracted daily temozolomide for low-grade gliomas in adults. Clin Cancer Res 2009; 15(1): 330–7.

169. Brandes AA, *et al.* Carboplatin and teniposide as third-line chemotherapy in patients with recurrent oligodendroglioma or oligoastrocytoma: a phase II study. Ann Oncol 2003; 14(12): 1727–31.

170. Chamberlain MC, Johnston S. Bevacizumab for recurrent alkylator-refractory anaplastic oligodendroglioma. Cancer 2009; 115(8): 1734–43.

171. Peterson K, *et al.* Salvage chemotherapy for oligodendroglioma. J Neurosurg 1996; 85(4): 597–601.

172. Soffietti R, *et al.* Second-line treatment with carboplatin for recurrent or progressive oligodendroglial tumors after PCV (procarbazine, lomustine, and vincristine) chemotherapy: a phase II study. Cancer 2004; 100(4): 807–13.

173. Taillibert S, *et al.* Bevacizumab and irinotecan for recurrent oligodendroglial tumors. Neurology 2009; 72(18): 1601–6.

174. Levin VA. Controversies in the treatment of low-grade astrocytomas and oligodendrogliomas. Curr Opin Oncol 1996; 8(3): 175–7.

175. Cairncross G, *et al.* Chemotherapy for anaplastic oligodendroglioma. National Cancer Institute of Canada Clinical Trials Group. J Clin Oncol 1994; 12(10): 2013–21.

176. Cairncross JG, *et al.* Aggressive oligodendroglioma: a chemosensitive tumor. Neurosurgery 1992; 31(1): 78–82.

177. Cairncross JG, *et al.* Phase III trial of chemotherapy plus radiotherapy compared with radiotherapy alone for pure and mixed anaplastic oligodendroglioma: Intergroup Radiation Therapy Oncology Group Trial 9402. J Clin Oncol 2006; 24(18): 2707–14.

178. Van den Bent MJ, *et al.* Adjuvant procarbazine, lomustine, and vincristine improves progression-free survival but not overall survival in newly diagnosed anaplastic oligodendrogliomas and oligoastrocytomas: a randomized European Organisation for Research and Treatment of Cancer phase III trial. J Clin Oncol 2006; 24(18): 2715–22.

179. Van den Bent MJ, *et al.* IDH1 and IDH2 mutations are prognostic but not predictive for outcome in anaplastic oligodendroglial tumors: a report of the European Organization for Research and Treatment of Cancer Brain Tumor Group. Clin Cancer Res 2010; 16(5): 1597–604.

180. Van den Bent MJ, *et al.* MGMT promoter methylation is prognostic but not predictive for outcome to adjuvant PCV chemotherapy in anaplastic oligodendroglial tumors: a report from EORTC Brain Tumor Group Study 26951. J Clin Oncol 2009; 27(35): 5881–6.

181. Gan HK, *et al.* A phase II trial of primary temozolomide in patients with grade III oligodendroglial brain tumors. Neuro Oncol 2010; 12(5): 500–7.

182. Mikkelsen T, *et al.* Temozolomide single-agent chemotherapy for newly diagnosed anaplastic oligodendroglioma. J Neurooncol 2009; 92(1): 57–63.

183. Vogelbaum MA, *et al.* Phase II trial of preirradiation and concurrent temozolomide in patients with newly diagnosed anaplastic oligodendrogliomas and mixed anaplastic oligoastrocytomas: RTOG BR0131. Neuro Oncol 2009; 11(2): 167–75.

184. Ducray F, *et al.* Up-front temozolomide in elderly patients with anaplastic oligodendroglioma and oligoastrocytoma. J Neurooncol 2011; 101(3): 457–62.

185. Mohile NA, *et al.* A phase II study of intensified chemotherapy alone as initial treatment for newly diagnosed anaplastic oligodendroglioma: an interim analysis. J Neurooncol 2008; 89(2): 187–93.

186. Abrey LE, *et al.* High-dose chemotherapy with stem cell rescue as initial therapy for anaplastic oligodendroglioma: long-term follow-up. Neuro Oncol 2006; 8(2): 183–8.

187. Ross GW, Rubinstein LJ. Lack of histopathological correlation of malignant ependymomas with postoperative survival. J Neurosurg 1989; 70(1): 31–6.

188. Armstrong TS, *et al.* Clinical course of adult patients with ependymoma: results of the Adult Ependymoma Outcomes Project. Cancer 2011; 117(22): 5133–41.

189. Duffner PK, *et al.* Postoperative chemotherapy and delayed radiation in children less than three years of age with malignant brain tumors. N Engl J Med 1993; 328(24): 1725–31.

190. Shaw EG, *et al.* Postoperative radiotherapy of intracranial ependymoma in pediatric and adult patients. Int J Radiat Oncol Biol Phys 1987; 13(10): 1457–62.

191. Wallner KE, *et al.* Intracranial ependymomas: results of treatment with partial or whole brain irradiation without spinal irradiation. Int J Radiat Oncol Biol Phys 1986; 12(11): 1937–41.

192. Brandes AA, *et al.* A multicenter retrospective study of chemotherapy for recurrent intracranial ependymal tumors in adults by the Gruppo Italiano Cooperativo di Neuro-Oncologia. Cancer 2005; 104(1): 143–8.

193. Gilbert MR, *et al.* Ependymomas in adults. Curr Neurol Neurosci Rep 2010; 10(3): 240–7.

194. Chamberlain MC, Johnston SK. Temozolomide for recurrent intracranial supratentorial platinum-refractory ependymoma. Cancer 2009; 115(20): 4775–82.

195. Shonka NA. Targets for therapy in ependymoma. Target Oncol 2011; 6(3): 163–9.

196. Metellus P, *et al.* Adult intracranial WHO grade II ependymomas: long-term outcome and prognostic factor analysis in a series of 114 patients. Neuro Oncol 2010; 12(9): 976–84.

197. Kucia EJ, *et al.* Surgical technique and outcomes in the treatment of spinal cord ependymomas: part II: myxopapillary ependymoma. Neurosurgery 2011; 68(1 Suppl Operative): 90–4; discussion 94.

198. Sonneland PR, *et al.* Myxopapillary ependymoma. A clinicopathologic and immunocytochemical study of 77 cases. Cancer 1985; 56(4): 883–93.

199. Pica A, *et al.* The results of surgery, with or without radiotherapy, for primary spinal myxopapillary ependymoma: a retrospective study from the rare cancer network. Int J Radiat Oncol Biol Phys 2009; 74(4): 1114–20.

200. Akyurek S, *et al.* Spinal myxopapillary ependymoma outcomes in patients treated with surgery and radiotherapy at M.D. Anderson Cancer Center. J Neurooncol 2006; 80(2): 177–83.

201. Scheithauer BW. Symptomatic subependymoma. Report of 21 cases with review of the literature. J Neurosurg 1978; 49(5): 689–96.

202. Prayson RA, Suh JH. Subependymomas: clinicopathologic study of 14 tumors, including comparative MIB-1 immunohistochemical analysis with other ependymal neoplasms. Arch Pathol Lab Med 1999; 123(4): 306–9.

203. Wood JR *et al.* The prognostic importance of tumor size in malignant gliomas: a computer tomographic scan study by the Brain Tumor Cooperative Group. J Clin Oncol 1988; 6: 338–43.

204. Walker MD *et al.* Evaluation of BCNU and/or radiotherapy in the treatment of anaplastic gliomas. J Neurosurg 1978; 49: 333–43.

Section 10: Neurological Malignancies

59 Medulloblastoma in Adults

Paul L. Moots[1,3] **and Anna Marie Kenney**[2]

[1] Department of Medicine and Department of Neurology, [2] Departments of Neurological Surgery and Cell Biology,
Vanderbilt-Ingram Cancer Center, Vanderbilt University Medical Center, Nashville, TN, USA
[3] Tennessee Valley Healthcare Systems, Veterans Administration Medical Center, Nashville, TN, USA

Introduction

Medulloblastoma and other central nervous system (CNS) primitive neuroectodermal tumors (PNET) account for 25% of primary CNS neoplasms in the pediatric age range but only 1% of adult primary CNS neoplasms. The peak incidence is in the midportion of the first decade. The incidence declines rapidly after the mid-teens. Its occurrence is exceptionally rare after age 40 and there is not a second peak in incidence affecting older adults. Yet 10–20% of patients with medulloblastoma are above 16 years of age.[1,2]

Our understanding of the biology of medulloblastoma has advanced dramatically in recent years. This neoplasm evolves from progenitor cells in the primordium of the cerebellum, dorsal brainstem, or as yet unidentified precursors.[3,4] Analogous populations at other sites in the CNS likely give rise to other types of embryonal CNS neoplasms such as supratentorial PNETs. The association of medulloblastoma with genetic syndromes such as Turcot and Gorlin syndromes raised the suspicion that specific mutations were etiologic. Elegant studies on genetically engineered mice with mutations in pathways controlling proliferation and differentiation have established some of the critical alterations in the cellular developmental program that lead to neoplasia. Some of these alterations differ in adults compared with children.

There are also important clinical distinctions between childhood and later arising medulloblastoma. Histological differences, including a higher likelihood of desmoplastic medulloblastoma, are seen in adults. The risk of subarachnoid metastases appears highest in young children and somewhat lower in adults. Recurrences in the first 2 years are more common in children while late recurrences (e.g. >5–7 years) are more common in adults.

Treatment planning for adults has generally been inferred from results of randomized studies in children that have distinguished between patients at "standard risk" and those at "high risk" for recurrence when treated with craniospinal radiation alone. Clinical criteria defining high risk typically have included substantial residual disease at the primary site after resection and any evidence of metastases. The high-risk children have a substantial improvement in survival with the addition of chemotherapy. It is not clear whether that advantage is also obtained in adults. Chemotherapy has also become a component of therapy for standard-risk children, allowing a reduction of the craniospinal radiation dose and thus reducing delayed sequelae of radiation. Whether that strategy would be effective in adults is unknown.

Late effects of treatment are a major concern at any age. Although cognitive sequelae are not as severe in adults as in young children, they are still an important concern. Other late sequelae include endocrine dysfunction, fertility problems, vasculopathy, second cancers, premature aging, and in some adolescents linear growth may still be an important factor. Despite these important concerns, medulloblastoma is one of the few curable primary CNS neoplasms. This engenders an aggressive treatment approach and leads to a high long-term survivorship with many patients experiencing multiple treatment sequelae.

Biology and epidemiology

The incidence of medulloblastoma/PNET in children and teens is 0.51 per 100,000 person-years. In the 20–34-year age range, it is 0.15 per 100,000 and decreases by half in each of the subsequent two decades.[1,2]

A small percentage of medulloblastoma arises in patients with well-defined genetic predispositions to cancer. These include Turcot and Gorlin syndromes, and hereditary retinoblastoma. Taken together, these genetic causes account for perhaps 5% of cases. Remarkably, neurofibromatosis types 1 and 2, which are strongly associated with the development of astrocytoma and ependymoma respectively, are not associated with the development of medulloblastoma/PNET.

Textbook of Uncommon Cancer, Fourth Edition. Edited by Derek Raghavan, Charles D. Blanke, David H. Johnson, Paul L. Moots, Gregory H. Reaman, Peter G. Rose and Mikkael A. Sekeres.
© 2012 John Wiley & Sons, Inc. Published 2012 by John Wiley & Sons, Inc.

The developing brain has a relatively high susceptibility and/or propensity to undergo neoplastic transformation. Brain tumors are the most common solid tumor type in children but this includes many distinct subtypes. The brain has an extended period of histogenesis compared with other solid organs. The immaturity of the blood–brain barrier during fetal and early postnatal life may also be a contributing factor in the high relative incidence of brain tumors in children. The populations of neuroepithelial precursors that are vulnerable to carcinogenic effects vary in location and temporal sequence during brain development. It is likely that the various discrete populations of neuroprogenitor cells have at least partially distinct molecular mechanisms of neoplastic transformation, and differ in their susceptibility to various carcinogens. These factors may explain the important differences between medulloblastoma, CNS PNET, and the glial (i.e. astrocytic, oligodendroglial, and ependymal) neoplasms common in children. These differential susceptibilities are also reflected in the marked differences in the types of brain tumors arising in children compared with adults.[5]

Medulloblastomas can be divided into 4–6 genetically and histologically defined subgroups.[6,7] These subgroups identify specific patient groups and prognoses. Certain subgroups are marked by upregulation of expression of sonic hedgehog (Shh) or Wnt pathway targets, and others are marked by amplification or upregulation of c-myc ("Group C") or elevated expression of OTX2 and the presence of isochromosome 17q ("Group D"). Overall, Group C patients fare the worst. In adults, medulloblastomas generally fall into the Shh (60%), Wnt (15%), or Group D (25%) subgroups, with the Wnt group having the best overall survival and progression-free survival, followed by the Shh group.[8] Interestingly, comparisons between adult and pediatric Shh medulloblastomas reveal distinct differences in terms of gene expression and prognosis.[9] For example, infant Shh medulloblastomas showed high levels of extracellular matrix gene expression, whereas adult Shh medulloblastomas featured increased expression of synaptogenesis and tissue morphogenesis genes.

The cells of origin for Group C and Group D medulloblastomas are not known. Shh-associated medulloblastoma derives from neural precursors in the rhombic lip.[10] These cells, cerebellar granule neuron precursors (CGNPs), are destined to form the external granular layer (EGL) of the cerebellar cortex, where they will undergo a period of rapid, Shh-induced proliferation before migrating inward to form the internal granule layer of the cerebellum. The Shh ligand, secreted by Purkinje neurons, interacts with the 12-transmembrane domain receptor Patched (Ptc), which inhibits Smoothened, a 7-transmembrane pass protein with resemblance to G-protein coupled receptors. Shh interaction with Ptc relieves the inhibition of Smoothened, resulting in pathway activation and translocation to the nucleus of Gli family transcription factors, which activate target genes driving CGNP proliferation and inhibiting differentiation.[11–13]

Shh medulloblastomas can be modeled in mice by deletion of Ptc, a negative regulator of Shh signaling, or by activation of Smoothened, the positive transducer of the Shh signal. Typically, approximately 15% of mice heterozygous for Ptc will develop medulloblastomas by 1 year of age.[14] Tumor incidence can be increased by placing the $Ptc^{+/-}$ mice on a $p53^{-/-}$ background, irradiating $Ptc^{+/-}$ pups, or conditionally deleting Ptc from cerebellar granule neuron progenitors.[15–17] These animal models have a very strong resemblance to human medulloblastoma, and many of the genes that are implicated in Shh pathway-mediated medulloblastoma formation in mouse models are found to be abnormal in human Shh medulloblastoma. For example, both human and mouse Shh-associated medulloblastomas have upregulation of N-myc, which has been identified as a Shh transcriptional target during normal cerebellar development.[18] These tumors also have increased expression of the microRNA miR 17/92, an N-myc target, and amplification of the oncogenic transcription cofactor yes-associated protein (YAP), all of which have been shown to be regulated by Shh in primary CGNP cultures derived from the neonatal murine cerebellum and in the mouse EGL in vivo.[19–21]

Inhibitors of the hedgehog pathway have been developed and tested for use in medulloblastoma patients. For the most part, these inhibitors target Smoothened. Initial studies in $Ptc^{+/-}/p53^{-/-}$ mice indicated that such inhibitors (HhAntag) effectively blocked tumor growth and prolonged survival of treated mice.[22] However, follow-up studies showed that HhAntag treatment was detrimental to bone structure in young mice, an indicator that such Smoothened inhibitors might not be suitable for young patients.[23] More recently, great excitement was generated when a Smoothened inhibitor developed by Genentech (GDC-0449) was used to treat a 26-year-old patient with metastatic medulloblastoma whose tumors exhibited Ptc loss of heterozygosity or somatic mutation.[24] The patient experienced rapid regression of the tumors, although he ultimately succumbed to the disease. Analysis of the recurrent tumors identified a novel mutation in Smoothened rendering it resistant to the drug. Importantly, medulloblastoma-bearing mice treated with GDC-0449 developed resistance through mutation of the same amino acid, underscoring the high degree of conservation between mouse and human Shh medulloblastomas.[25]

A recent, elegant study by the Gilbertson group has demonstrated that in both mice and humans, Wnt medulloblastomas are likely to arise from the embryonic dorsal brainstem.[26] Patients with Wnt medulloblastomas have activating mutations in the Wnt pathway effector CTNNB1 (β-catenin). Moreover, medulloblastoma incidence is increased in patients with familial adenomatous polyposis coli (APC, Turcot syndrome), and mutations in APC and the Wnt antagonists AXIN1 and AXIN2 have also been reported in medulloblastomas.[27–30]

Wnt is a secreted ligand which binds to and activates a receptor termed Frizzled (Fz), which like Smoothened resembles a 7-transmembrane pass G-protein coupled receptor. Fz activation results in inactivation of the APC gene product, whose function is to promote the degradation of β-catenin. APC inhibition allows β-catenin to accumulate and translocate to the nucleus, where it interacts with a transcription factor partner, TCF, to activate target genes, including the myc oncogenes.[31,32] Consistent with this, Wnt medulloblastomas have high myc expression levels.[33] In the Gibson study, activating mutations in Ctnnb1 drove proliferation and accumulation of cells on the embryonic dorsal brainstem.

These lesions progressed to tumor formation when *Tp53* was deleted, and the resultant tumors had characteristics and expression profiles resembling those of human Wnt medulloblastomas. It is noteworthy that although loss of *p53* can increase medulloblastoma formation in mice, its use as a prognostic indicator in humans remains controversial. Indeed, recent studies have reported *p53* loss or mutation in Wnt medulloblastomas, which generally have a favorable prognosis.[34]

Primitive neuroectodermal tumors are a heterogeneous group of tumors that occur in the central nervous system and are composed of neuroepithelial-like cells. Supratentorial PNETs (s-PNET) occur in the cerebral hemispheres but very rarely in adults. Adult and pediatric s-PNETs resemble each other histopathologically, containing cells with a variety of differentiation patterns. However, at the genetic level, pediatric s-PNETs often feature *MYCC* or *MYCN* amplification, which was not observed in the limited number of adult s-PNET available for study, while TP53 mutations are found in adult s-PNET but not pediatric s-PNET.[35] However, analysis of a different group of adult s-PNETs revealed that MYCC amplifications could be detected in some specimens.[36] Adult s-PNETs are rare enough that it has been difficult to identify prognostic markers that might dictate the course of treatment or predict survival. One small study found a correlation between the presence of intratumoral calcification and improved survival but again, the sample size (12) makes it difficult to draw solid conclusions.[37]

Some of the important goals in the molecular understanding of neoplasia include the use of molecular markers as prognostic indicators, as criteria for stratification into different treatment groups, and as indicators of likely response to a particular therapy. However, the development of patient subgroup stratification based on molecular diagnosis for prognostic purposes and for targeted therapies in individual patients has lagged behind the knowledge base.[38] Today, criteria for risk stratification in medulloblastoma still rely almost entirely on the clinical features of residual disease after surgery and the presence or absence of metastases. However, the field is rapidly advancing and recently a very simple and practical method for using immunostaining to differentiate between the four genetic subclasses has been reported.[33] With widespread adoption of such methodologies, it may become possible to also tailor clinical trials to patients belonging to groups most likely to respond to novel molecularly targeted therapeutics.

Epidemiological studies of childhood brain tumors provide some very interesting suggestions about environmental factors. As with adult gliomas, exposures to nitroso compounds are associated with an increased relative risk. These may come from dietary sources, medications, and other chemical exposures. Exposure during gestation as well as in postnatal life may be important. Exposure to ionizing radiation also increases the risk of brain tumors, and again with a long latency. There is some evidence to suggest that exposures to pesticides during pregnancy or soon after birth or parental exposure to some pesticides are associated with an increased risk of childhood brain tumors. Tobacco use in adults has not been associated with brain tumor development. Epidemiological studies in children

of parents who smoke have given mixed results. Some studies indicate that paternal smoking is associated with an increased risk of brain tumors, while other studies have been negative. Exposure to common viral infections such as influenza, as well as exposure to SV-40 virus, has been associated with an increased risk in some studies. Remarkably, prenatal vitamin use has been associated with a decreased risk of childhood brain tumors, perhaps related to direct effects on CNS development analogous to the reduced risk of spinal dysraphism associated with folate use or due to antioxidant effects that limit prenatal exposure to potential carcinogens.

Clinical presentation

The most common presenting symptoms for adults with medulloblastoma are headaches (83%), nausea/vomiting (43%), gait imbalance (40%), and dizziness (23%). Cranial neuropathies including diplopia are less common. Presentations with spinal symptomatology such as back or radicular pain, or with signs of myelopathy due to subarachnoid "drop metastases," are uncommon in adults but when an apparently isolated intradural-extramedullary spinal lesion is found, medulloblastoma should be included in the differential diagnosis. The duration of symptoms prior to diagnosis is typically 2–3 months but can be more than 6 months.[39,40]

A few patients will present with a dramatic decline after a very short duration of symptoms. Intratumoral hemorrhage or obstruction of cerebrospinal fluid (CSF) flow through the cerebral aqueduct and fourth ventricle can lead to acute hydrocephalus and cerebellar herniation through the foramen magnum. This life-threatening complication requires emergency measures for neurological stabilization. Medical interventions such as high-dose corticosteroids (e.g. dexamethasone 40–100 mg IV bolus), mannitol, and hyperventilation may provide a few hours for definitive management. Intubation can sometimes precipitate such a decline. Definitive treatment of this neurological emergency is surgical decompression often accompanied by ventriculostomy.

Magnetic resonance imaging (MRI) scanning is currently the best method of assessment for the types of symptoms related to intracranial tumors (Figs 59.1, 59.2). This is particularly true for posterior fossa lesions because MRI scanning provides a much better image of the posterior fossa with fewer artifacts than does computed tomography (CT) scanning. Medulloblastoma is generally an intensely enhancing, relatively discrete mass in the cerebellar midline or hemisphere.[41] A lateral hemispheric location is more common in adults than in children (Fig. 59.3). Occasionally, the mass may appear to arise in the cerebellopontine angle or the middle cerebellar peduncle. In a small percentage, enhancement is absent or minimal. Due to high cellularity many medulloblastomas have an abnormal appearance on diffusion-weighted imaging, a finding that may help to distinguish them from cerebellar astrocytomas and ependymomas. Rarely, the mass appears cystic. Evidence of invasion of the floor of the fourth ventricle carries a poor prognosis in some adult medulloblastoma series. The scan should be carefully reviewed for evidence of subarachnoid or intraventricular subependymal spread, as well as for hydrocephalus.

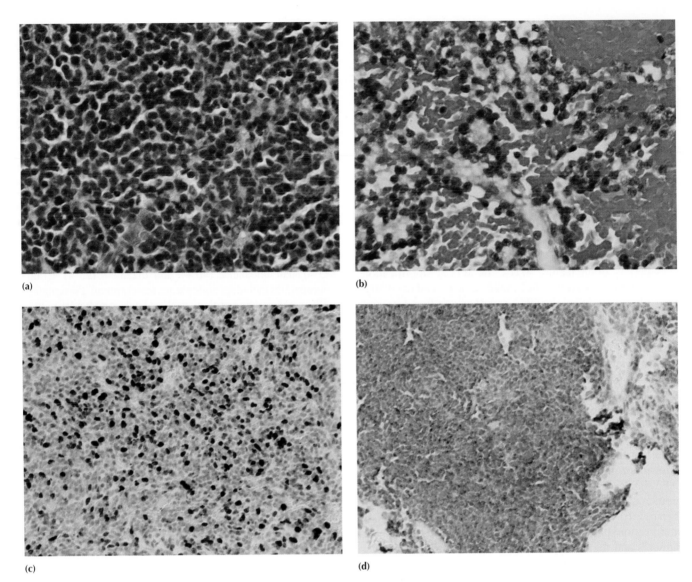

Figure 59.1 Medulloblastoma histopathology. (a,b) Hematoxylin and eosin staining of a medulloblastoma demonstrates a highly cellular lesion populated by cells with hyperchromatic nuclei and little cytoplasm. Apoptotic bodies, scattered mitotic figures, and rudimentary Homer–Wright rosette formation (b) were observed. Necrosis was not observed in this specimen. (c) The proliferative index as assessed by MIB-1 immunohistochemistry is very high. (d) Evidence for differentiation was identified in this case by immunohistochemical staining for the neuronal marker, synaptophysin. This medulloblastoma was resected from the 52-year-old man whose MRI is demonstrated in Fig. 59.2.

The differential diagnosis arising from the posterior fossa location and MRI characteristics includes ependymoma and cerebellar forms of astrocytoma such as pilocytic astrocytoma. The latter often but not always have a distinctive cystic appearance. Other types of glioma such as glioblastoma and anaplastic oligodendroglioma are exceedingly rare in this location. In the adult population, metastasis is an important part of the differential. The fact that most adult medulloblastomas present as solitary lesions, and the age being rarely over 40, tends to favor a primary neoplasm rather than a metastasis. A few other mass lesions arising in the posterior fossa, such as meningioma, choroid plexus papilloma, and acoustic schwannoma of the cerebellopontine angle, will on occasion have an atypical appearance that will be difficult to distinguish from medulloblastoma radiographically.

In children, the importance of identifying subarachnoid metastases is well established. Detailed staging of the neuraxis with MRI imaging of the entire spine and CSF cytology studies are warranted if medulloblastoma is suspected. There is an advantage to obtaining these studies prior to surgery when feasible. Postoperative artifacts, including meningeal enhancement at the operative site, meningeal enhancement more widely intracranially, spinal meningeal enhancement, and blood tracking along the spinal epidural space, may be difficult to distinguish from meningeal metastases. CSF cytology is also an important part of neuraxis staging but is often contraindicated until after surgical decompression.

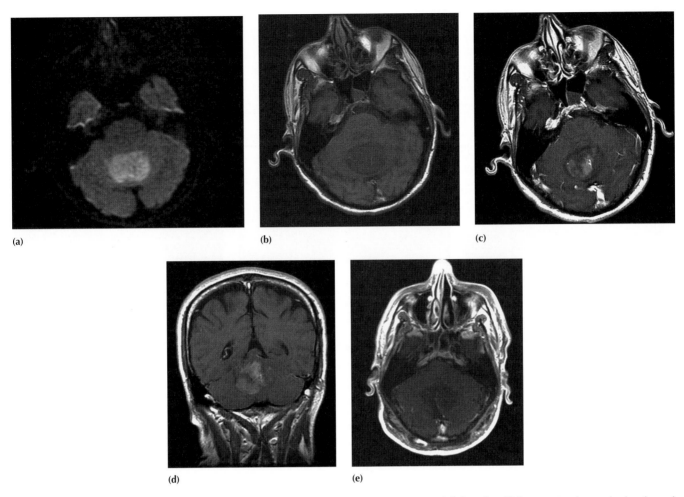

(a)

(b)

(c)

(d)

(e)

Figure 59.2 Magnetic resonance imaging of midline medulloblastoma in an adult. The patient is a 52-year-old man who presented with a 2-month history of gait ataxia and slurred speech. MRI diffusion-weighted images (a) reveal a diffusion abnormality suggestive of a highly cellular neoplasm, thus favoring medulloblastoma. Axial T1-weighted views obtained before gadolinium (b) and after gadolinium (c) reveal patchy enhancement. A coronal T1-weighted postgadolinium view (d) demonstrates the vermian location and extension superiorly. Hydrocephalus was not present. The 24 h postoperative axial T1-weighted postgadolinium image (e) demonstrates a complete resection of the mass. Blood products mixed with CSF give the fluid in the surgical cavity a slightly higher intensity than CSF. MRI imaging of the spine and CSF cytology were negative for dissemination.

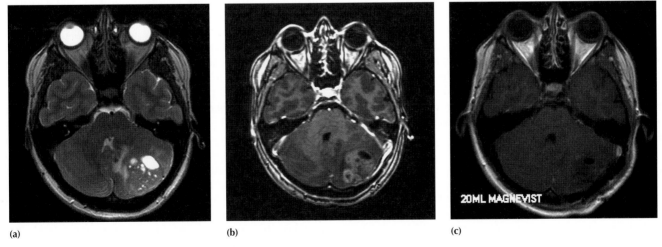

(a)

(b)

(c)

Figure 59.3 Magnetic resonance imaging of lateral cerebellar hemispheric medulloblastoma in an adult. The patient is a 27-year-old woman who presented with a 3-week history of nausea, vomiting, and headaches. The T2 (a) and T1 postgadolinium (b) images demonstrate a laterally placed cerebellar hemispheric mass, a characteristic location for adult medulloblastoma. The mass is relatively well demarcated and partially cystic. There is distortion of the fourth ventricle. At 24 h postoperatively (c) the T1 postgadolinium images reveal a complete resection. Subsequent MRI of the spine and CSF cytology were negative.

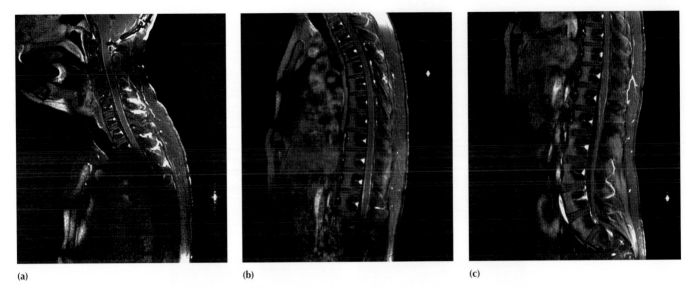

(a)   (b)   (c)

Figure 59.4 Recurrent medulloblastoma with leptomeningeal dissemination. This 30-year-old man presented with myelopathy and lumbar nerve root symptoms 6 months after resection of a large cell/anaplastic medulloblastoma. Staging at the time of diagnosis, including total spine MRI and CSF cytology, was negative. He received craniospinal proton irradiation which accounts for the unusual vertebral bone marrow appearance. He also received multiagent chemotherapy. This T1 postgadolinium cervical (a), thoracic (b), and lumbosacral (c) MRI demonstrates a diffuse thin coating of contrast enhancement throughout the spinal leptomeninges. CSF cytology was positive at this time.

It is widely held that neuraxis staging is also essential in adults with medulloblastoma/PNET.[42] The presence of subarachnoid metastases or positive CSF cytology at diagnosis is less common in adults (10–30%) than in children (Fig. 59.4). Many but not all adult studies identify subarachnoid metastases as a poor prognostic factor. The demonstration of subarachnoid metastases will alter the radiation planning, often including boosts to regions of bulky metastases. Chemotherapy decisions also are heavily influenced by staging results.

Hydrocephalus is another problem that contributes to the presenting symptomatology of headaches, nausea, and vomiting. About 25% of adults have hydrocephalus that requires placement of a ventriculoperitoneal (VP) shunt. Many neurosurgeons prefer to place a temporary ventriculostomy drain prior to or at the time of surgery. After resection of the tumor, CSF flow is often reestablished to an adequate degree. At that point, the ventriculostomy can be clamped and then removed after a period of observation. This avoids the need for a permanent VP shunt for some patients. Shunt malfunction, infection, and the relatively rare occurrence of tumor dissemination with peritoneal seeding via the shunt are considerations leading away from VP shunting when possible.[43]

Medulloblastoma in children

Advances in the treatment of childhood medulloblastoma have come from numerous randomized prospective trials dating back to the mid-1980s.[44–46] Fundamental conclusions derived from these trials include:
- risk stratification guides management
- the quality of radiation planning and delivery is important
- chemotherapy following radiation produces a substantial increase in 5-year event-free survival compared to radiation

alone (48% versus 0%) for children with high-risk characteristics
- for standard-risk patients a decrease in the craniospinal radiation dose is associated with a decline in event-free survival but the addition of chemotherapy allows lower craniospinal radiation.[47,48]

Risk stratification

Clinical variables have been the most important factors in risk stratification. Since the mid-1990s age, extent of resection, and the presence or absence of metastases have been the primary stratification factors.[49] Age less than 3 years is associated with a worse outcome than older patients, with a 5-year event-free survival of only 32%. This has in part been attributed to a higher percentage of M+ patients. The inclusion of young patients with atypical teratoid/rhabdoid tumor (AT/RT) in older trials may also have influenced the outcome results. Postoperative assessment of residual disease replaced the preoperative T stage for assessment of risk.[50] Now almost entirely based on MRI assessment, residual disease postoperatively of greater than 1–1.5 cm^2 carries a poor prognosis. Yet this criterion is somewhat arbitrary and among high-risk patients localized residual disease is not as strong a prognostic indicator as the presence of metastases (for M stage; Box 59.1). In children M+ is worse than M0 and this appears to hold over all ages (see Box 59.1). Based on these clinical criteria, children are categorized as standard risk (>3 years, no or minimal residual tumor, M0) or high risk (<3 years, >1–1.5 cm^2 residual tumor, M1–M4). When treated with radiation therapy alone, the respective 5-year event-free survival rates for these groups are approximately 65% and 0%.[44]

Some investigators now include certain histological subtypes as part of the risk stratification scheme. Of the four histological subtypes of medulloblastoma, the large cell/anaplastic subtype has a worse prognosis.[51] Since the pathological criteria used to diagnose this subtype are somewhat subjective, their use has not been as well embraced as the clinical characteristics mentioned above but are becoming more so in current trials. Conversely, a better prognosis has been associated with desmoplastic and nodular medulloblastoma. This is increasingly recognized in young children, although traditionally it has been considered more common in adults.[52] Important biological characteristics have been associated with particular histologies and are encouraging the move to a molecular-based risk stratification.

The blossoming molecular understanding of the origins of medulloblastoma has provided a wealth of biological attributes that appear useful in risk stratification. Tumors that overexpress N-myc appear to have a worse prognosis and often display large cell/anaplastic histological features. Medulloblastomas with activated Shh pathways have a better prognosis and a high percentage display desmoplastic or extensive nodular features. Other groups with separate prognostic results can be distinguished based on molecular genetic features. At present, these stratification schemes are being validated and it is expected that they will be incorporated into risk stratification for trials in the near future.[33,53–55]

One major step provided by the combined forces of molecular classification and histological assessment of posterior fossa embryonal neoplasms was recognition of the distinction between CNS atypical teratoid/rhabdoid tumor (AT/RT) and medulloblastoma. The histological appearance of AT/RT can be difficult to distinguish from medulloblastoma. The diagnosis is established by mutational analysis of the SMARCB1 gene (also called INI1).[56,57] AT/RT is predominantly found in children under 3 years of age, and in that age group comprises up to 20% of malignant CNS tumors. AT/RT has an extremely poor prognosis with a 15% 2-year survival for children less than 3 years of age. Older children have a somewhat better outcome.[58] Mutational analysis is becoming a standard part of the pathological evaluation of malignant CNS tumors in young children. Assessment of SMARCB1/INI1 expression can also be done by immunohistochemistry.[59] The exclusion of AT/RT from current medulloblastoma trials in the young age group may give the appearance of improved outcomes in current trials.

Recent results and current trials

Infants

The treatment of infants has been heavily oriented towards chemotherapy because of the severe neurocognitive and other adverse developmental effects of craniospinal radiation.[60,61] Intensive chemotherapy regimens, some including myeloablative therapy with stem cell support, have been investigated with the aim of deferring or avoiding radiation. This approach also provides some insights regarding the potential of neoadjuvant chemotherapy in older children and adults.

In infants the response rates and long-term efficacy of chemotherapy have been studied utilizing a variety of agents and combinations. The combination of cisplatin, cyclophosphamide, VP-16, and vincristine produced a response rate (complete response plus partial response [CR + PR]) of 48% with a 2-year event-free survival of 34%.[62] This multiagent combination has also been used as an intensive induction regimen prior to myeloablative chemotherapy with carboplatin, thiotepa and etoposide and autologous bone marrow rescue. More recently, high-dose methotrexate has been added to this induction regimen. This achieved a 5-year event-free survival (EFS) of 52% for all patients, 64% for those with gross total resection and 29% for those with residual tumor.[63] Seventy-one percent avoided radiation. Another infant study incorporating high-dose methotrexate as well as intrathecal methotrexate along with the multiagent combination demonstrated 5-year EFS for complete resection, residual tumor or metastatic disease of 82%, 50%, and 33% respectively.[64] Other approaches currently being investigated in young children include intensive systemic plus intrathecal chemotherapy, and systemic chemotherapy followed by focal radiation of the posterior fossa.[65]

Radiation therapy remains an efficacious salvage therapy for infants and young children who have recurrence after chemotherapy. A complete response to radiation therapy was achieved in six of 11 patients (55%) who progressed during chemotherapy.[66] High-dose chemotherapy with autologous bone marrow rescue may also serve as effective salvage therapy for these children.[67]

Recent trends in the treatment of very young children include the important separation of AT/RT from medulloblastoma mentioned above, the observation that desmoplastic/nodular medulloblastoma is not rare in this age group and appears to have a more favorable prognosis, and increasingly intensive therapy for the core group of high-risk infants. As diagnostic accuracy and better risk stratification evolve based on new pathological and molecular assessments, the validity of historical comparisons is reduced. There is some concern that apparent improvements in outcome may reflect changes in patient selection, and this will have to be carefully addressed in trial design and reporting.

Older children

The treatment of medulloblastoma in patients from mid-childhood through the early teen years forms the bulk of our knowledge about this neoplasm, and the core of information from which adult treatment strategies are inferred. Within this age range, a comparison of event-free survival rates for older children (i.e. 4–7 and 8–13 years) is not statistically different from that for teens (>14 years) in most trials. However, some studies focusing specifically on teenagers (age 10–20 years) demonstrate a positive linear relationship between age and time to relapse.[68] A longer time to relapse has also been observed in adults.

Standard treatment for these children includes a resection of the primary mass if feasible. Craniospinal radiation with boosts to the primary site and to areas of gross metastatic disease are used for all patients. Traditionally the entire posterior fossa is treated with 54–56 Gy. Conformal radiation to the tumor and surrounding tissue also appears to be effective and reduces the radiation dose to the cochlea.[69,70] Among high-risk patients the craniospinal dose is 36 Gy and the boost to the primary site and foci of gross metastatic disease is an additional 18 Gy. Most often this is done in daily fractions of 1.8–2.0 Gy. Other fractionation schedules, particularly twice daily "hyperfractionation," have been investigated based on the potential to reduce delayed radiation toxicity and to escalate the dose modestly. Another alternative that is gaining some support is proton therapy which is delivered with little penetration beyond the intended target, and may reduce marrow toxicity and second malignancies.[71] (See Fig. 59.4.) Neither of these would be considered standard therapy at present.

Radiation dosing for prevention of recurrence beyond the primary site (e.g. craniospinal dosing) has undergone careful scrutiny because of the concern for delayed neurocognitive, endocrine, and growth sequelae. Reduction of the craniospinal dose to 2.4 Gy was accompanied by an increase in early relapses.[47] Long-tem follow-up has shown that the difference is lost as time elapses. The addition of chemotherapy for standard-risk patients treated with reduced-dose craniospinal radiation does show good EFS and reduced radiation sequelae.[48]

For poor-risk patients postradiation chemotherapy with CCNU (lomustine) and vincristine, or CCNU, vincristine, and cisplatin demonstrated an improved outcome.[44,45] Packer et al. reported a 5-year event-free survival of 85% using the latter combination in a cohort of 63 high-risk patients, results that equaled the outcome for standard-risk patients.[72] Current trials for high-risk patients are investigating concurrent chemoradiation, for example with weekly carboplatin during radiation, followed by cycles of maintenance chemotherapy.

The use of neoadjuvant chemotherapy followed by craniospinal radiation in children with poor-risk medulloblastoma/PNET has been evaluated in prospective trials. Using a regimen derived from experience in infants, a major cytoreductive response was achieved in 60% of medulloblastoma/PNET patients using an intensive regimen of cisplatin, cyclophosphamide, etoposide, and vincristine prior to radiotherapy.[73] This regimen has been adapted to adults (see below). Others have made similar observations. A radiographically documented response rate of 43% was achieved in 30 patients using prera-

diation cyclophosphamide, cisplatin, and vincristine. The 2-year event-free survival was 40%.[74] In fact, numerous reports demonstrate favorable response rates with neoadjuvant regimens.[75–78] Yet some reports suggest that the delay in starting radiation may be detrimental.[79] Progression prior to radiation in neoadjuvant trials is typically in the range of 15–20%. Preradiation chemotherapy has seemed especially suited for adults where reduced tolerance to the myelosuppressive effects of chemotherapy following craniospinal radiation is particularly problematic. However, larger randomized pediatric trials using a neoadjuvant design have not shown improved long-term results.[80] These trials will be discussed further below.

Outcome for high-risk children, particularly M + patients, remains unsatisfactory with 5 years EFS often reported as less than 60%. Intensification of radiotherapy dosing has been incorporated in some programs. Risk-adapted radiotherapy dosing has been evaluated at St Jude using craniospinal doses of 23.4 Gy for average risk, 36 Gy for M0–1, and 39.6 Gy for M2–3. Added conformal dosing to the tumor bed totaled 55.8 Gy, and gross metastatic disease was treated locally to 50.4 Gy.[81] Intensification of radiation dosing using a hyperfractionated schedule has also been attempted following intensive multiagent chemotherapy, again with craniospinal dosing to 39 Gy for high-risk patients and 60 Gy to the primary site.[82] These risk-adapted radiotherapy approaches were incorporated into intensive multiagent chemotherapy schedules that were also risk adapted. In the St Jude program this included preradiation topotecan and postradiation dose-intensive cytoxan-based myeloablative chemotherapy with stem cell rescue. In the Milan trial preradiation chemotherapy was followed by CCNU and vincristine for 1 year for patients who achieved a complete response prior to radiation. Those who did not achieve a complete response received postradiation myeloablative chemotherapy using thiotepa with peripheral stem cell support. The 5-year PFS was 70% in the St Jude cohort and 72% in the Milan report.[82]

Sequelae of therapy

Toxicities related to craniospinal radiation have been a major consideration in the evolution of treatment strategies for medulloblastoma. The major delayed sequelae involve neurocognitive and other neurological problems, linear growth, endocrine complications, and second malignancies. Neurocognitive sequelae are heavily influenced by age at treatment, with young children suffering substantial reductions in IQ and school progress. Fundamental elements of attention, recall, speed of mental processing, and learning are impaired.[83,84] In reports of survivors of greater than 5 years, these problems exceed 40%.[85] Chemotherapy-related neuropathy is common but relatively mild in children. Late-onset hearing loss was self- or proxy-reported in 7% of children treated for medulloblastoma.[86] Audiological analysis yields higher numbers. Eight of nine medulloblastoma patients developed late-onset hearing loss in a retrospective report including many cancer types.[87] Regimens that include cisplatin and posterior fossa radiation cause the highest risk. This risk is reduced with regimens designed to spare radiation to, or limit cochlear exposure.[69,70,88] Other late-onset (>5 years post diagnosis) neurological disorders reported by medulloblastoma/PNET patients include seizures in 8%, coordination deficits in 4%, and motor deficits in 4%.[86]

Endocrine sequelae are primarily attributable to hypothalamic and pituitary dysfunction. Growth hormone deficiency is the most common and along with direct radiation effects on bone, tends to limit linear growth. Hypothyroidism, hypogonadism, and infertility are also relatively common.[89] Second neoplasms occurred in 11% of long-term pediatric CNS tumor survivors at 25 years, nonmelanotic skin cancers, meningiomas, and second CNS tumors being most common. The increasing recognition of syndromes with hereditary cancer predisposition is important in this regard, with Gorlin and Turcot syndromes being related to medulloblastoma.

Although neurocognitive issues are one of the most significant long-term sequelae and are largely related to craniospinal radiation, quality-of-life measures and long-term health status measures were lower in patients who received craniospinal radiation plus chemotherapy than in those who received only radiation. They had poorer health status by self-report. They also had more behavioral and emotional problems, and poorer quality of life by parent-report.[90] Quality-of-life issues including college graduation rate, marital status, and income are reduced in long-term survivors compared with siblings.[85]

Survival is also reduced in long-term survivors of medulloblastoma compared with the general population. Cumulative late mortality in 5-year survivors of pediatric brain tumors was 13% at 15 years and 26% at 30 years.[85] The highest rates were observed in medulloblastomas with a standardized mortality ratio of 17% at 30 years. The most common causes of death were recurrence (61%) and other medical causes (21%), including second neoplasms (9%), cardiac disease (3%), and pulmonary disease (3%).[85]

Medulloblastoma in adults

In adult medulloblastoma series the 5-year survival rates range from 48% to 84%, and 10-year rates from 40% to 56%.[39,40,42,91–99] The SEER database analyses of 5- and 10-year survival for patients >18 years of age are 64% and 50%, with a 10.6-year median survival.[100] Cumulative relative or age-adjusted survival rates are marginally better in children than adults at 5 years (62% versus 59%) but are significantly better for children at 10 years (57% versus 46%).[101]

Risk stratification

Currently stratification of risk for adults follows pediatric guidelines. The recommendations include postoperative MRI scanning within 48 h to assess the amount of residual disease at the operative site. MRI scanning of the total spine and CSF cytology should also be performed. These are typically done 2 weeks postoperatively in order to avoid postoperative artifacts such as epidural blood collections and transiently positive cytology respectively. Bone scans and bone marrow biopsy are not routinely done for staging unless specific symptoms or laboratory results raise concern for systemic dissemination. Patients with greater than $1.5\,cm^2$ residual disease or with metastases (M + neuraxis staging) have an unfavorable prognosis.[42] However, not all adult studies find these criteria to be significant prognostic factors.[98,99,102,103]

With postoperative imaging and neuraxis staging high-risk patients account for 43–72% in various adult medulloblastoma series. In a large retrospective analysis, Prados et al. found that 55% of adults were high risk, including 33% staged as M1–3. High-risk patients had a significantly worse prognosis than standard-risk patients, with 5-year PFS and OS in the two groups being 58% versus 38% and 81% versus 54% respectively.[42] Another large retrospective series including 253 patients classified 124 (57%) as standard risk and 95 (43%) as high risk, with 34 patients having insufficient data. The standard-risk group had a significantly better 5-year OS (77% versus 65%) and 10-year OS (62% versus 49%).[99] A prospective trial of 36 adult patients revealed a better outcome for standard-risk patients at a median follow-up of 3.7 years (5-year PFS of 76% versus 61%). However, reanalysis of this same cohort with a median follow-up of 7.6 years demonstrated that this difference was no longer significant[98,102] (also see below, Prospective adult trials).

Among high-risk adults, M + patients have a worse outcome than M0 patients, with a 5-year PFS of 75% versus 45%.[102] This finding is consistent with pediatric reports demonstrating that high-risk M + patients have a worse prognosis than high-risk patients with only residual local disease.[72] Here too, with a longer duration of follow-up, the difference in outcome between the M0 ($n = 23$) and M + ($n = 13$) adult groups was no longer statistically significant with 5-year PFS rates of 78% versus 61% respectively.[98]

Other clinical factors that have been significant predictors of outcome in adult medulloblastoma, albeit less consistently, include fourth ventricular involvement, brainstem involvement (T3b or T4 in the Chang system), postoperative performance status, and posterior fossa radiation dose of less than 50 Gy.[99,103]

Recent attempts at molecular risk stratification of medulloblastoma have included some important observations in adults, as previously discussed. Most notable is the strong association in transcriptional analysis with Shh pathway activation. The Shh type medulloblastoma accounts for 71% of adult medulloblastoma. Shh tumors are also highly represented in infant medulloblastoma. However, the adult and infant Shh tumors differ substantially in the expression of other gene families, with cellular development and synaptic formation-related genes being upregulated in adults and extracellular matrix genes upregulated in infants. The prognosis in infants is very good, while that of Shh adults is intermediate. Cytogenetic changes, particularly 10q deletions, are common in Shh tumors in both age groups but appear to confer an unfavorable prognosis only for adults.[6,9,104] About 7% of Wnt medulloblastoma are in young adults. This group has a favorable prognosis. Adult medulloblastomas rarely appear in the Group C category which carries a poor prognosis but represent 13% of the Group D patients with an outcome considered intermediate.[53,105,106]

Standard-risk adults

Treatment outcomes for adult medulloblastoma patients have been reported in many retrospective series but not all distinguish standard- and high-risk patients, the criteria used for assessment of risk are varied, and assignment of risk retrospectively is challenging.

Resection to the fullest extent possible followed by craniospinal radiation has been the cornerstone of therapy for standard-risk adults. Typically a craniospinal dose of 36 Gy is delivered in daily fractions of 1.8–2.0 Gy over about 4 weeks. The posterior fossa receives additional radiation to a total of 54 Gy, with lower doses being less effective.[107] Care must be taken to include the full extent of the neuraxis with special attention paid to the cribiform plate and the lateral and caudal projections of the spinal theca. Traditionally, the radiation port for the primary site is defined anatomically as the entire posterior fossa. Less commonly, the port is defined as the enhancing mass plus a 2 cm margin. The use of three-dimensional conformal planning or intensity-modulated radiation therapy (IMRT) appears to provide effective local control while sparing radiation to the temporal bones and cochlea.[69,70] This reduces the likelihood of cochlear and auditory nerve damage.

Most adults complete craniospinal radiation without interruption. However, radiation-related neutropenia was seen in 17% of adults.[42] Nadir white blood counts (WBCs) tend to be in the 2000–2500 m⁻³ range. In adults treated with nitrosourea-based chemotherapy following radiation, significant myelosuppression was observed in 33–45%, usually requiring dose reduction.

Most reports indicate that long-term outcomes for standard-risk adult patients are similar to those observed in children. Prados observed a 5-year PFS of 81% and OS of 58% in 21 standard-risk patients treated between 1975 and 1991.[42] In 14 standard-risk patients accrued between 1988 and 2011, Brandes et al. observed a 5-year PFS of 80% and OS of 80% when evaluated at a median follow-up of 7.6 years. However, late recurrences were common in this group.[98]

Reduction of the craniospinal dose in conjunction with adjuvant chemotherapy for standard-risk children is a strategy that has not been evaluated prospectively in adults. One large retrospective report found that a craniospinal radiation dose of less than 34 Gy yielded a significantly poorer outcome. Overall survival was not significantly different for patients who received greater than 34 Gy compared with those who received less than 34 Gy and also received chemotherapy.[99] Combined modality therapy is an attractive concept in that delayed radiation sequelae are radiation dose related. Yet the severity of the neurocognitive problems tends to be less in adults than seen in children. Additionally, the efficacy of chemotherapy is less well defined in adult medulloblastoma. Thus predictions about the relative risks and benefits of applying reduced craniospinal radiation dosing while adding chemotherapy for standard-risk adults are not directly inferable from pediatric results. Conventional radiation dosing without chemotherapy is the most common recommendation for standard-risk adults at present.[103]

High-risk adults

In series that report long-term outcome for high-risk adults the 5-year PFS ranges from 38% to 47% and 5-year OS from 54% to 65%, with M+ patients doing more poorly than M0 patients.[42,94,98,99]

Consideration of surgical goals in the setting of a suspected high-risk medulloblastoma patient presents some difficult issues. In addition to the need to establish a tissue diagnosis, patients with a large cerebellar mass extending to involve the cerebellar peduncle, floor of the fourth ventricle or deeper brainstem regions derive a benefit from judicious resection for the purpose of decompression. It is also likely that a long-term benefit might be obtained, based on the impression that a small volume of residual disease postoperatively appears to be more important than preoperative T stage with regard to long-term control. A more difficult scenario is the situation in which preoperative scanning provides evidence of extensive subarachnoid dissemination. Surgical decompression may still have a compelling rationale for a large posterior fossa mass in order to avoid acute neurological deterioration. However, the degree of local residual disease after resection is no longer the major determinant of risk stratification based on the evidence that M+ patients do worse than M0. In the exceptional situation that the diagnosis is established on CSF cytology, resection of the primary site may not be warranted if extensive meningeal seeding is apparent.

Radiation therapy for high-risk adults follows the same format as treatment for standard-risk patients but additional boosts to total 45 Gy are given to areas of obvious radiographically defined bulky disease, particularly in the spinal canal. A dilemma is encountered when leptomeningeal spread is so extensive that the entire spine or the whole brain would be considered the boost target. Full-dose boosts to large volumes in either region would add considerably to both the acute and delayed sequelae. A judicious attempt to boost the region(s) most severely affected radiographically, or the region that is most symptomatic, is recommended in this circumstance.

The timing of radiation has also been a subject of concern. Delays in starting or completing radiation because of upfront chemotherapy have been associated with poorer outcome in some pediatric studies. Progression prior to radiation, which is seen more often in M+ patients, occurs in 0–38% of patients, with most studies demonstrating about 15–20%.[74,76,77,108–110] Similar results have been found in adults. In the prospective trial by Brandes et al., progression on preradiation chemotherapy was 0%, while in the prospective Eastern Cooperative Oncology Group (ECOG) trial it was 25%.[98,111,112] Interruption during radiation, another concern raised in pediatric reports, was highlighted by Chan et al. who reported that adult medulloblastoma patients who required more than 48 days to complete craniospinal RT fared worse than those who completed radiation in less than 48 days.[94]

The addition of chemotherapy for high-risk adults is widely recommended by inference from the pediatric experience. This is supported by relatively high response rates to the same spectrum of agents used for pediatric patients.[93,95] However, among retrospective series of adult medulloblastoma, statistical analysis has not conclusively shown a survival benefit with chemotherapy.[97,99] Two prospective adult trials have been performed, although neither accrued sufficient numbers to answer the question as to the benefit of chemotherapy.[98,112] Despite these limitations, there have been advocates of preradiation chemotherapy, postradiation chemotherapy, and both. There has also been consideration of dose intensification, including high-dose chemotherapy with bone marrow reconstitution.

Preradiation chemotherapy has been used in adults in part to allow more intensive chemotherapy regimens than are feasible in the postradiation setting. In pediatric prospective high-risk trials, the response to preradiation platinum or cyclophosphamide-based chemotherapy ranges from 29% to 74%.[62,74,76,77,108,109] Response rates appear lower in M+ medulloblastoma. Upfront response data in adults are limited. Spreafico et al. observed a CR in three of five M1–3 patients after an intensive preradiation regimen including methotrexate, etoposide, cytoxan, and carboplatin. At completion of radiation the CR rate in this small group was 100%.[96] Greenberg et al. report on seven patients, six of whom were high risk, treated with preradiation cisplatin, etoposide, cyclophosphamide, and vincristine based on a Pediatric Oncology Group (POG) protocol. They observed three PR after two or three cycles of chemotherapy. These three patients achieved a CR after radiation.[95] In a prospective ECOG trial of 16 high-risk adults using a regimen of cisplatin, etoposide, cyclophosphamide, and vincristine, the objective response rate (OR) prior to the completion of chemotherapy was 19%, with six being inevaluable. The OR at the completion of radiation was 44%.[111,112]

Considering long-term outcomes with preradiation chemotherapy, three randomized phase 3 trials in high-risk pediatric patients using regimens containing platinum/cyclophosphamide followed by craniospinal radiation and maintenance chemotherapy have failed to show an improved PFS or OS. In two, CCG921 and HIT'91, the EFS was poorer in the preradiation group.[46,108] The third trial, POG 9031, showed no difference in EFS.[113,114] These results, coupled with some evidence for poorer efficacy when radiation is delayed or interrupted, have led to reduced enthusiasm for upfront chemotherapy in adults.

The best results to date for high-risk pediatric patients were achieved by Packer et al. using postradiation cisplatin, CCNU, and vincristine. In this trial, the 5-year PFS was 85%, with M0 patients faring much better than M+ patients.[72] Variations of this regimen are widely used in adults, although in a few small series the outcome for adults has not been as good. For example, in the report by Greenberg et al., 10 patients treated with the Packer protocol had a median survival of 36 months.[95] Increased hematological toxicities and more severe vincristine-related neuropathy are seen in adults than in children.

Prospective adult trials

In a prospective trial of adult medulloblastoma patients, Brandes et al. enrolled 36 patients over a 12-year period.[98,102] Twenty-two high-risk patients received preradiation chemotherapy, and those with metastatic disease ($n = 13$ or 60% M+) received additional postradiation chemotherapy. A MOPP-like regimen was used prior to 1995. Thereafter the combination of cisplatin, etoposide, and cyclophosphamide was used. Standard-risk patients received craniospinal RT (36 Gy) and a boost to the primary site to total 54.8 Gy. Preradiation response

data were not presented but no patients progressed during preradiation chemotherapy. At a median follow-up of 3.7 years, standard-risk patients had a 5-year PFS of 76% and OS of 89%. The high-risk patients had a 61% PFS and 69% OS at 5 years. M0 patients did significantly better than M+ patients with a 5-year PFS of 75% versus 45%.

Long-term follow-up data on this cohort revealed different findings, however. At a median follow-up of 7.6 years the 5-year PFS rates for the standard-risk and high-risk groups were 80% versus 69%. The 5-year OS was 80% versus 73%. Neither of these differences was significant. Late recurrence in the standard-risk group contributed to this loss of statistical significance. Neither M status (M0 versus M+) nor residual disease after surgery was significant in regard to outcome at the longer follow-up point. T stage (T3b/T4) had borderline significance for 5-year PFS: 82% versus 44%. Given the trends that are apparent, the number of patients may be too few to provide a firm conclusion.[98,103]

A prospective trial of moderately intensive multiagent preradiation chemotherapy followed by craniospinal radiation for high-risk adult patients was conducted by ECOG and the Southwest Oncology Group (SWOG) (ECOG 4397). Sixteen patients were enrolled over 7 years, giving an accrual rate of 2.5 patients per year, which is very similar to that achieved by Brandes et al. The chemotherapy regimen was modeled very closely after a protocol for high-risk pediatric patients used by Jennings et al.[73,111,112] Dosing in the pediatric trial was 30% greater for the cisplatin, etoposide, and cyclophosphamide arm, and four cycles were used instead of three. That pediatric cohort of 10 patients achieved a CR of 50% and an OR of 60% by the completion of radiation. The median PFS was 44 months. Median OS had not been reached at 48 months. In E4397 the OR observed at the completion of chemotherapy was 19% with six inevaluable, and the OR after radiation was 44%. PFS in E4397 was very similar to the pediatric group at 46.2 months. The difference in OR may in part be attributed to greater chemotherapy dose intensity in the pediatric group, although here too, the small number of patients precludes a firm conclusion.

The long-term efficacy achieved in E4397, a 5-year OS of 61%, is very similar to that in numerous high-risk pediatric trials and in the adult trial by Brandes et al.[98,102] The time to progression of 46.2 months and 5-year PFS of 36% are similar to those reported in high-risk patients and particularly M+ patients. This is obtained despite the impression that upfront and postradiation response rates were lower in the adults. If chemotherapy efficacy is less in adult medulloblastoma, reflecting inherently lower chemosensitivity or less dose-intense therapy, concern is raised about inferences drawn from pediatrics for the treatment of standard-risk adult medulloblastoma patients. The results achieved with lower craniospinal radiation dosing in conjunction with chemotherapy in pediatric standard-risk patients may not be achieved in adults.

One additional prospective trial under way involves adults and children with recurrent medulloblastoma utilizing a Shh pathway inhibitor, GDC-0449. This is an oral selective inhibitor of Smoothened. It blocks pathway activity even when Ptc mutations produce ligand-independent constitutive activity, and in mouse models of medulloblastoma causes tumor regression. Testing is under way in a variety of adult and pediatric solid tumors. Remarkable but transient responses have been reported in adult medulloblastoma.[24,115,116]

High-dose chemotherapy in adults

A small number of reports have focused on high-dose chemotherapy with autologous bone marrow or stem cell rescue in adults with recurrent medulloblastoma, based on pediatric findings that long-term survival is achieved for some patients.[117–119] Major toxicities and a relatively high mortality rate have limited enthusiasm for this approach. In a single-institution retrospective experience, Gill *et al.* compared outcomes for 13 adult patients who received conventional salvage chemotherapy with that of 10 patients who received high-dose thiotepa and carmustine followed by PBSC.[120] There were no long-term survivors in the conventional treatment group. Median time to progression was 1.25 years for the transplant group versus 0.58 years for the conventionally treated group. Four of 10 high-dose patients were progression free with a median follow-up of 2.9 years. Median survival for the high-dose group was 3.5 years versus 2.0 years for the conventional chemotherapy group. Despite the anticipated hematological toxicities, there were no treatment-related deaths.

Supratentorial primitive neuroectodermal tumor in adults

Supratentorial PNETs include a collection of rare neoplasms that share embryonal histological features with medulloblastoma (Fig. 59.5). They account for 2–3% of all pediatric CNS neoplasms, approximately one-tenth as common as medulloblastoma, and are extremely rare in adults. In some instances, the histological appearance of a PNET is indistinguishable from a medulloblastoma but the neoplasm is located outside the cerebellum. In other instances, the neoplasm may demonstrate distinctive histological features of differentiation such as ependymal rosettes, neural rosettes, or evidence of pineal differentiation. These various neoplasms, ependymoblastoma, cerebral neuroblastoma, pineoblastoma, and the otherwise undifferentiated s-PNET also share with medulloblastoma a relatively high risk of subarachnoid dissemination, and responsiveness to the same spectrum of chemotherapy agents as medulloblastoma, although not with the same efficacy. Pineoblastoma is often discussed separately from the remainder of the s-PNETs with most reports indicating a better response and prognosis (see Chapter 60). Recently supratentorial neoplasms with features of glioblastoma and elements of PNET have been described. These add a new component to the spectrum of overlapping or mixed neoplasms and their treatment is highly debated.[121]

As a group, the PNETs have a considerably shorter PFS and OS than medulloblastoma, and thus are considered high risk even if M- and in the setting of a gross total resection. Staging does help in formulating radiation treatment planning and provides important prognostic information, with patients who are

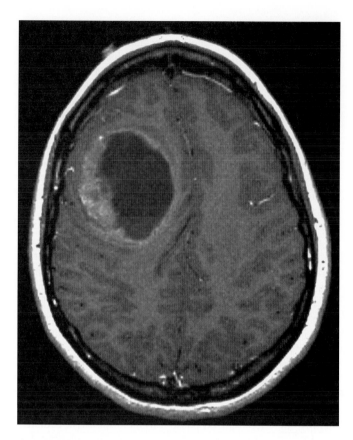

Figure 59.5 Magnetic resonance imaging in an adult with a supratentorial PNET. This 21-year-old woman presented with progressive headaches over a few weeks. The T1 postgadolinium image reveals an enhancing, relatively well-demarcated cystic or necrotic mass. There is a faint fluid–fluid level in the cavity suggestive of either blood products or proteinaceous debris. This proved to be a s-PNET without histological or immunohistochemical evidence of differentiation. Staging with spine MRI and CSF cytology was negative.

M+ at diagnosis having a worse prognosis. Treatment strategies have paralleled those developed for medulloblastoma. Intensification of chemotherapy and risk-adapted radiation and chemotherapy plans have evolved.

The response to chemotherapy appears to be less frequent than that observed for medulloblastoma. In infants, the OR of multiagent chemotherapy using cisplatin, etoposide, cyclophosphamide, and vincristine administered with the intention of deferring radiation was 29% for s-PNET, with a 2-year PFS of 19% and OS of 21%.[62] The response rate to the "8-in-1" regimen was 33% for s-PNET and 0% for pineoblastoma, with a 3-year PFS of 25%.[122,123]

Further intensification of therapy for sPNET has been a major theme in pediatric trials. In two related trials an intensive induction regimen including cisplatin, etoposide, cyclophosphamide, and vincristine, with high-dose methotrexate added in the second version, was used.[124] These trials enrolled 43 patients with a median age of 3.1 years. Eighty-eight percent of those with a subtotal resection had an objective response to the induction therapy. Thirty-two patients with a gross total resection or complete response to induction proceeded to consolidation with myeloablative therapy using carboplatin, thiotepa, and etoposide followed by autologous stem cell rescue.

The 5-year EFS and OS rates were 39% and 49% respectively for the entire group. Sixteen patients eventually received radiation, although often local rather than craniospinal. Twelve of 20 survivors never received any radiation.

A risk-adapted strategy similar to that used for medulloblastoma has been evaluated in older children with s-PNET.[125] Patients between 3 and 6 years of age with neuraxis staging demonstrating <1.5 cm^2 residual disease after surgery and M0, designated standard risk, received craniospinal RT to 23.4 Gy and a total of 55.8 Gy to the tumor bed. High-risk patients (>1.5 cm^2 residual disease or M+) received preradiation topotecan and craniospinal radiation to 36–39.6 Gy with a tumor dose of 55.8 Gy. All patients then received four cycles of high-dose nonmyeloablative chemotherapy including cisplatin, cyclophosphamide, and vincristine with autologous stem cell or bone marrow rescue after each cycle. Sixteen patients (median age 7.9 years) were treated: eight considered standard risk and eight high risk. Eleven were M0, one was M2 and four were M3. The 5-year EFS and OS rates for the entire group were 68% and 74%. Standard-risk patients had better 5-year EFS and OS than high-risk patients (EFS 75% versus 60%; OS 88% versus 58% respectively). As with medulloblastoma, it is suggested that a reduced craniospinal radiation dosing combined with intensive chemotherapy can be used to achieve good results in patients with relatively favorable initial staging.

These results point to the importance of intensified therapy for this group of highly refractory embryonal CNS neoplasms. Whether these therapies are feasible in adults is a difficult question. More conventional chemotherapy regimens when applied to young adults with s-PNET have not been as effective. In a retrospective comparison including children and young adults, outcomes were assessed for 11 nonpineal s-PNET patients, eight of whom were treated with craniospinal radiation followed by cisplatin, CCNU, and vincristine following the Packer regimen. The 5-year OS was 12%. Considered by age, the 5-year OS was 25% for five children aged 4–13 years and 0% for six adults aged 20–35 years.[126]

High-dose chemotherapy with stem cell rescue has been reported with some encouraging results in this relatively refractory population. In a study of 17 PNET patients, all but two of whom were pediatric (median age 3.6 years), s-PNETs (n = 7) did remarkably well, with five remaining disease free at a median of 8 years after treatment. Four of these received radiation following the chemotherapy.[127] However, pineoblastomas (n = 8) did extremely poorly. Another trial of high-dose chemotherapy and radiation for newly diagnosed pineoblastoma, including six children and six adults, achieved a median PFS of 62 months for nine patients.[128]

Sequelae of therapy in adults

The major sequelae of therapy include neurocognitive and other neurological sequelae, endocrinopathies, infertility, vasculopathy, early aging, hematological sequelae, and second malignancies. The spectrum of sequelae closely overlaps that seen in children for whom better documentation exists. The major differences are that linear growth is not an issue and the severity of neurocognitive sequelae, which is strongly related

to age at treatment, is less severe although still very important in adults.

In the absence of confounding factors such as hydrocephalus, most young adults who receive craniospinal radiation do not experience a severe decline in cognitive function. Many adult patients maintain the capacity to live independently, although complaints of poor memory, fatigue, and slow mental processing are common. This differs considerably from patients treated at younger ages for whom independent living, academic performance, job status, marriage, and driving status are all substantially reduced.[129] Detailed neuropsychological assessment of 10 adults who were disease free for greater than 3 years indicated a decline in overall IQ compared to predicted premorbid levels, with memory, verbal and nonverbal reasoning, and arithmetic scores reduced. Reading and spelling scores tend to be maintained.[130] Also notable in adults is the rarity of "cerebellar mutism" after posterior fossa craniotomies.[131,132]

The most common other neurological sequelae are neuropathy related to vincristine or cisplatin, and hearing loss. Neuropathy is common, and tends to be more severe and persistent in adults than in children. It is not rare to find vincristine omitted or stopped especially when used as weekly therapy concurrent with radiation following the Packer regimen. Cranial nerve palsies, various mononeuropathies, and autonomic neuropathy also occur occasionally with vincristine. When these arise a detailed workup is required to exclude leptomeningeal recurrence as the cause. Hearing loss relates to radiation and/or cisplatin.

Endocrinopathies are most commonly attributable to radiation-related hypothalamic injury, although direct injury to the thyroid gland and ovaries is important in contributing to delayed sequelae.[133] Endocrinopathies tend to become apparent a few years after treatment. Growth hormone deficiency is the most common problem in children, occurring in 40–80% of patients. This is followed in frequency by hypothyroidism (6–60%), adrenocorticotropic hormone or glucocorticoid deficiency (24%), and hypogonadism (25–50%).[134] Hypothyroidism and hypogonadism are the most common symptomatic endocrinopathies in adults. Hypothyroidism results from direct radiation exposure to the thyroid more often than from hypothalamic injury but lower craniospinal radiation doses do not reduce its occurrence. The possibility of ovarian damage from direct radiation exposure is an added concern in young women receiving craniospinal radiation. Reduced fertility, estimated at 23%, and early menopause were reported for young women who were postpubertal when treated with radiation to the abdomen or pelvis or alkylating chemotherapy for a variety of childhood cancers. These were not as common for females who were treated when prepubertal.[135]

Other direct craniospinal radiation-related injuries include reduced bone growth in children and osteopenia in adults, cardiac toxicity with decreased maximal cardiac index on exercise tests, and restrictive lung disease.[134] Evidence for cardiac and pulmonary injury comes from detailed testing but only infrequently are they major symptomatic concerns.[136]

The incidence of second malignancies in children treated for medulloblastoma is 5.4 times the expected rate.[137] These often arise many years after treatment. Meningiomas and gliomas are the most common. Adenocarcinomas of the colon, breast and lung, thyroid cancer, leukemia, myelodysplasia, and sarcomas have all been observed. Basal cell cancers in irradiated areas have been observed and raise concern for Gorlin syndrome.

Recommendations

Given the rarity of medulloblastoma and s-PNET in adults, we would encourage referral to a major medical center with a multidisciplinary neurooncology team experienced in the care of pediatric and adult medulloblastoma patients. Major resection of the primary tumor is the surgical goal for almost all medulloblastoma and PNET patients. All patients should have detailed staging of the nervous system including total spine MRI and CSF studies, including cytology.

The treatment of standard-risk medulloblastoma patients remains craniospinal radiation with standard craniospinal doses and a full dose to the posterior fossa. Fragmentary evidence suggests that lowering the craniospinal dose with the addition of chemotherapy can be done in adults with acceptable long-term results, although the comparative efficacy of chemotherapy in adults remains a question. For high-risk medulloblastoma and supratentorial PNET, conventional radiation followed by multiagent chemotherapy is recommended. Although the treatment data in adults are limited, the potential for cure in this young adult patient population contributes to a justifiable bias towards more aggressive therapy.

Prospective randomized trials in adults are not feasible. Despite the obstacles, expansion of pediatric medulloblastoma trials to include young adults, for example to age 30, would be a way to extend the information on their treatment and outcome. Integration of recent scientific advances into study design and treatment selection remains the best path to improved therapy and outcomes for these rare patients.

References

1. Central Brain Tumor Registry of the United States. *Statistical Report: Primary Brain Tumors in the United States 2004–2007*. Hinsdale, IL: Central Brain Tumor Registry of the United States, 2011.
2. Giordana MT, *et al.* Epidemiology of adult medulloblastoma. Int J Cancer 1999; 80: 689–92.
3. Eberhart CG. Even cancers want commitment: lineage identity and medulloblastoma formation. Cancer Cell 2008; 14: 105–7.
4. Gibson P, *et al.* Subtypes of medulloblastoma have distinct developmental origins. Nature 2010; 468: 1095–9.
5. Rubinstein LJ. The correlation of neoplastic vulnerability with central neuroepithelial cytogeny and glioma differentiation. J Neurooncol 1987; 5: 11–27.
6. Northcott PA, *et al.* Medulloblastoma comprises four distinct molecular variants. J Clin Oncol 2011; 29: 1408–14.
7. Cho YJ, *et al.* Integrative genomic analysis of medulloblastoma identifies a molecular subgroup that drives poor clinical outcome. J Clin Oncol 2011; 29: 1424–30.
8. Remke M, *et al.* Adult medulloblastoma comprises three major molecular variants. J Clin Oncol 2011; 29: 2717–23.
9. Northcott PA, *et al.* Pediatric and adult sonic hedgehog medulloblastomas are clinically and molecularly distinct. Acta Neuropathol 2011; 122: 231–40.
10. Eberhart CG. Even cancers want commitment: lineage identity and medulloblastoma formation. Cancer Cell 2008; 14: 105–7.
11. Wechsler-Reya RJ, Scott MP. Control of neuronal precursor proliferation in the cerebellum by sonic hedgehog. Neuron 1999; 22: 103–14.
12. Dahmane N, Ruiz I, Altaba A. Sonic hedgehog regulates the growth and patterning of the cerebellum. Development 1999; 126: 3089–4100.
13. Wallace VA. Purkinje-cell-derived Sonic hedgehog regulates granule neuron precursor cell proliferation in the developing mouse cerebellum. Curr Biol 1999; 9: 445–8.
14. Goodrich LV, Scott MP. Hedgehog and patched in neural development and disease. Neuron 1998; 21: 1243–57.
15. Pazzaglia S, *et al.* High incidence of medulloblastoma following X-ray irradiation of newborn Ptc1 heterozygous mice. Oncogene 2002; 21: 7580–4.
16. Wetmore C, Eberhart DE, Curran T. Loss of p53 but not ARF accelerates medulloblastoma in mice heterozygous for patched. Cancer Res 2001; 61: 513–16.
17. Yang ZJ, *et al.* Medulloblastoma can be initiated by deletion of Patched in lineage-restricted progenitors or stem cells. Cancer Cell 2008; 14: 135–45.
18. Kenney AM, Cole MD, Rowitch DH. Nmyc upregulation by sonic hedgehog signaling promotes proliferation in developing cerebellar granule neuron precursors. Development 2003; 130: 15–28.
19. Northcott PA, *et al.* The miR-17/92 polycistron is up-regulated in sonic hedgehog-driven medulloblastomas and induced by N-myc in sonic hedgehog-treated cerebellar neural precursors. Cancer Res 2009; 69: 3249–55.
20. Uziel T, *et al.* The miR-17~92 cluster collaborates with the Sonic Hedgehog pathway in medulloblastoma. Proc Natl Acad Sci USA 2009; 106: 2812–17.
21. Fernandez LA, *et al.* YAP-1 is amplified and up-regulated in hedgehog-associated medulloblastomas and mediates Sonic hedgehog-driven neural precursor proliferation. Genes Dev 2009; 23: 2729–41.
22. Romer JT, *et al.* Suppression of the Shh pathway using a small molecule inhibitor eliminates medulloblastoma in Ptc(+/-)p53(-/-) mice. Cancer Cell 2004; 6: 229–40.
23. Kimura H, Ng JM, Curran T. Transient inhibition of the Hedgehog pathway in young mice causes permanent defects in bone structure. Cancer Cell 2008; 13: 249–60.
24. Rudin CM, *et al.* Treatment of medulloblastoma with hedgehog pathway inhibitor GDC-0449. N Engl J Med 2009; 361: 1173–8.
25. Yauch RL, *et al.* Smoothened mutation confers resistance to a Hedgehog pathway inhibitor in medulloblastoma. Science 2009; 326: 572–4.
26. Gibson P, *et al.* Subtypes of medulloblastoma have distinct developmental origins. Nature 2010; 468: 1095–9.
27. Amlashi SF, Riffaud L, Brassier G, Morandi X. Nevoid basal cell carcinoma syndrome: relation with desmoplastic medulloblastoma in infancy. A population-based study and review of the literature. Cancer 2003; 98: 618–24.
28. Huang H, *et al.* APC mutations in sporadic medulloblastomas. Am J Pathol 2000; 156: 433–7.
29. Baeza N, Masuoka J, Kleihues P, Ohgaki H. AXIN1 mutations but not deletions in cerebellar medulloblastomas. Oncogene 2003; 22: 632–6.
30. Koch A, *et al.* Mutations of the Wnt antagonist AXIN2 (Conductin) result in TCF-dependent transcription in medulloblastomas. Int J Cancer 2007; 121: 284–91.
31. Willert K, Nusse R. Beta-catenin: a key mediator or Wnt signaling. Curr Opin Genet Dev 1998; 8: 95–102.
32. He TC, *et al.* Identification of c-MYC as a target of the APC pathway. Science 1998; 281: 1509–12.
33. Northcott PA, *et al.* Medulloblastoma comprises four distinct molecular variants. J Clin Oncol 2011; 29: 1408–14.
34. Lindsey JC, *et al.* TP53 mutations in favorable-risk Wnt-Wingless-subtype medulloblastomas. J Clin Oncol 2011; 29: e344–6.
35. Gessi M, *et al.* Supratentorial primitive neuroectodermal tumors of the central nervous system in adults: molecular and histopathologic analysis of 12 cases. Am J Surg Pathol 2011; 35: 573–82.

36. Behdad A, Perry A. Central nervous system primitive neuroectodermal tumors: a clinicopathologic and genetic study of 33 cases. Brain Pathol 2010; 20: 441–50.

37. Kim DG, et al. Supratentorial primitive neuroectodermal tumors in adults. J Neurooncol 2002; 60: 43–52.

38. Gilbertson RJ, Gajjar A. Molecular biology of medulloblastoma: will it ever make a difference to clinical management? J Neurooncol 2005; 75: 273–8.

39. Kunschner LJ, et al. Survival and recurrence factors in adult medulloblastoma: the MD Anderson Cancer Center experience from 1978 to 1998. Neuro Oncol 2001; 3: 167–73.

40. Peterson K, Walker, RW. Medulloblastoma/primitive neuroectodermal tumor in 45 adults. Neurology 1995; 45: 440–2.

41. Malheiros SM, et al. MRI of medulloblastoma in adults. Neuroradiology 2003; 45: 463–7.

42. Prados MD, et al. Medulloblastoma in adults. Int J Radiat Oncol Biol Phys 1995; 32: 1145–52.

43. Magtibay PM, et al. Unusual presentation of adult metastatic peritoneal medulloblastoma associated with a ventricular shunt: a case study and review of the literature. Neuro Oncol 2003; 5: 217–20.

44. Evans AE, et al. The treatment of medulloblastoma. Results of a prospective randomized trial of radiation therapy with and without CCNU, vincristine and prednisone. J Neurosurg 1990; 72: 572–82.

45. Tait DM, et al. Adjuvant chemotherapy for medulloblastoma: the first multi-centre control trial of the International Society of Pediatric Oncology (SIOP I). Eur J Cancer 1990; 26: 464–9.

46. Zeltzer PM, et al. Metastasis stage, adjuvant treatment and residual tumor are prognostic factors for medulloblastoma in children: conclusions from the Children's Cancer Group 921 randomized phase III trial. J Clin Oncol 1999; 17: 832–45.

47. Thomas PR, et al. Low-stage medulloblastoma: final analysis of a trial comparing standard-dose with reduced dose neuraxis radiation. J Clin Oncol 2000; 18: 3004–11.

48. Packer RJ, et al. Phase III study of craniospinal radiation followed by adjuvant chemotherapy for newly diagnosed average risk medulloblastoma. J Clin Oncol 2006; 24: 4202–8.

49. Packer RJ, Rood BR, MacDonald TJ. Medulloblastoma: present concepts of stratification into risk groups. Pediatr Neurosurg 2003; 39: 60–7.

50. Chang CH, Housepian EM, Herbert C. An operative staging system and megavoltage radiotherapeutic technique for cerebellar medulloblastoma. Radiology 1969; 93: 1351–9.

51. Eberhart CG, et al. Histopathologic grading of medulloblastomas: a Pediatric Oncology Group study. Cancer 2002; 94: 552–60.

52. Rutkowski S, et al. Survival and prognostic factors of early childhood medulloblastoma: an international meta-analysis. J Clin Oncol 2010; 28: 4961–8.

53. Ellison DW, et al. Definition of disease risk stratification groups in childhood medulloblastoma using combined clinical, pathologic, and molecular variables. J Clin Oncol 2011; 29: 1400–7.

54. Tamayo P, et al. predicting relapse in patients with medulloblastoma by integrating evidence from clinical and genomic features. J Clin Oncol 2011; 29: 1415–23.

55. Packer RJ. Risk stratification of medulloblastoma: a paradigm for future childhood brain tumor management strategies. Curr Neurol Neurosci Rep 2011; 11: 124–6.

56. Biegel JA, et al. Germline and acquired mutations of INI1 in atypical and rhabdoid tumors. Cancer Res 1999; 59: 74–9.

57. Hilden JM, et al. Central nervous system atypical teratoid/rhabdoid tumor: results of therapy in children enrolled in a registry. J Clin Oncol 2004; 22: 2877–84.

58. Tekautz TM, et al. Atypical teratoid/rhabdoid tumors (ATRT): improved survival in children 3 years of age and older with radiation and high-dose alkylator-based chemotherapy. J Clin Oncol 2005; 23: 1491–9.

59. Judkins AR, et al. Immunohistochemical analysis of hSNF5/INI1 in pediatric CNS neoplasms. Am J Surg Pathol 2004; 28: 644–50.

60. Kiltie AE, et al. Survival and late effects in medulloblastoma patients treated with craniospinal irradiation under three years old. Med Pediatr Oncol 1997; 28: 348–54.

61. Palmer SL, et al. Patterns of intellectual development among survivors of pediatric medulloblastoma: a longitudinal analysis. J Clin Oncol 2001; 19: 2302–8.

62. Duffner PK, et al. Postoperative chemotherapy and delayed radiation in children less than three years of age with malignant brain tumors. N Engl J Med 1993; 328: 1725–31.

63. Dhall G, et al. Outcome of children less than three years old at diagnosis with non-metastatic medulloblastoma treated with chemotherapy on the "Head Start" I and II protocols. Pediatr Blood Cancer 2008; 50: 1169–75.

64. Rutkowski S, et al. Treatment of early childhood medulloblastoma by postoperative chemotherapy alone. N Eng J Med 2005; 352: 978–86.

65. Rutkowski S, et al. Medulloblastoma in young children. Pediatr Blood Cancer 2010; 54: 635–7.

66. Gajjar A, et al. Medulloblastoma in very young children. Outcome of definitive craniospinal irradiation following incomplete response to chemotherapy. J Clin Oncol 1994; 12: 1212–16.

67. Dupuis-Girod S, et al. Will high dose chemotherapy followed by autologous bone marrow transplantation supplant craniospinal irradiation in young children treated for medulloblastoma? J Neurooncol 1996; 27: 87–98.

68. Tabori U, et al. Distinctive clinical course and pattern of relapse in adolescents with medulloblastoma. Int J Radiat Oncol Biol Phys 2006; 64: 402–7.

69. Merchant TE, et al. Multi-institution prospective trial of reduced-dose craniospinal radiation (23.4 Gy) followed by conformal posterior fossa (36 Gy) and primary site radiation (55.8 Gy) and dose-intensive chemotherapy for average-risk medulloblastoma. Int J Radiat Oncol Biol Phys 2008; 70: 782–7.

70. Breen SL, et al. A comparison of conventional, conformal and intensity-modulated coplanar radiotherapy plans for posterior fossa treatment. Br J Radiol 2004: 77(Suppl): 768–77.

71. Kirsch DG, Tarbell NJ. New technologies in radiation therapy for pediatric brain tumors: the rationale for proton radiation therapy. Pediatr Blood Cancer 2004; 42: 461–4.

72. Packer RJ, et al. Outcome for children with medulloblastoma treated with radiation and cisplatin, CCNU, and vincristine chemotherapy. J Neurosurg 1994; 81: 690–8.

73. Jennings MT, et al. Differential responsiveness among "high risk" pediatric brain tumors in a pilot study of dose-intensive induction chemotherapy. Pediatr Blood Cancer 2004; 43: 46–54.

74. Mosijczuk AD, et al. Preradiation chemotherapy in advanced medulloblastoma. A Pediatric Oncology Group pilot study. Cancer 1993; 72: 2755–62.

75. Kovnar EH, et al. Preirradiation cisplatin and etoposide in the treatment of high-risk medulloblastoma and other malignant embryonal tumors of the central nervous system. A phase II study. J Clin Oncol 1990; 8: 330–6.

76. Heideman RL, et al. Preirradiation chemotherapy with carboplatin and etoposide in newly diagnosed embryonal pediatric CNS tumors. J Clin Oncol 1995; 13: 2247–54.

77. Pendergass TW, et al. Eight drugs in one day chemotherapy for brain tumors: experience in 107 children and rationale for preradiation chemotherapy. J Clin Oncol 1987; 5: 1221–31.

78. Stewart CF, et al. Results of a phase II upfront window of pharmacologically guided topotecan in high-risk medulloblastoma and supratentorial primitive neuroectodermal tumor. J Clin Oncol 2004; 22: 3357–65.

79. Attard-Montalto S, et al. Is there a danger in delaying radiotherapy in childhood medulloblastoma? Br J Radiol 1993; 66: 807–13.

80. Bailey CC, et al. Prospective randomized trial of chemotherapy given before radiotherapy in childhood medulloblastoma. International Society of Paediatric Oncology (SIOP) and the (German) Society of Paediatric Oncology (GPO): SIOP II. Med Pediatr Oncol 1995; 25: 166–78.

81. Gajjar A, *et al*. Risk adapted craniospinal radiation followed by high-dose chemotherapy and stem-cell rescue in children with newly diagnosed medulloblastoma (St Jude Medulloblastoma-96): long-term results form a prospective, multicenter trial. Lancet Oncol 2006; 7: 813–20.

82. Gandola L, *et al*. Hyperfractionated accelerated radiotherapy in the Milan strategy for metastatic medulloblastoma. J Clin Oncol 2009; 27: 566–71.

83. Palmer SL, Reddick WE, Gajjar A. Understanding the cognitive impact on children who are treated for medulloblastoma. J Pediatr Psychol 2007; 32: 1040–9.

84. Edelstein K, *et al*. Early aging in adult survivors of childhood medulloblastoma: long-term neurocognitive, functional and physical outcomes. Neuro Oncol 2011; 13: 536–45.

85. Armstrong GT, *et al*. Long-term outcomes among adult survivors of childhood central nervous system malignancies in the Childhood Cancer Survivor Study. J Natl Cancer Inst 2009; 101: 946–58.

86. Packer RJ, *et al*. Long-term neurologic and neurosensory sequelae in adult survivors of a childhood brain tumor: childhood cancer survivor study. J Clin Oncol 2003; 21: 3255–61.

87. Kolinsky DC, *et al*. Late onset hearing loss: a significant complication of cancer survivors treated with cisplatin containing chemotherapy regimens. J Pediatr Hematol Oncol 2010; 32: 119–23.

88. Orgei E, *et al*. Hearing loss among survivors of childhood brain tumors treated with an irradiation sparing approach. Pediatr Blood Cancer 2012; 58(6): 953–8.

89. Gurney JG, *et al*. Endocrine and cardiovascular late effects among adult survivors of childhood brain tumors: Childhood Cancer Survivor Study. Cancer 2003; 97: 663–73.

90. Bull KS, *et al*. Reduction of health status 7 years after addition of chemotherapy to craniospinal radiation for medulloblastoma: a follow-up study in PNET3 trial survivors – on behalf of the CCLG (formerly UKCCSG). J Clin Oncol 2007; 25: 4239–45.

91. Bloom HJG, Bessell EM. Medulloblastoma in adults: a review of 47 patients treated between 1952 and 1981. Int J Radiat Oncol Biol Phys 1990; 18: 763–72.

92. Hazuka MB, DeBoise DA, Henderson RA, Kinzie JJ. Survival in adult patients treated for medulloblastoma. Cancer 1992; 69: 2143–8.

93. Galanis E, *et al*. Effective chemotherapy for advanced CNS embryonal tumors in adults. J Clin Oncol 1997; 15: 2939–44.

94. Chan AW, *et al*. Adult medulloblastoma: prognostic factors and patterns of relapse. Neurosurgery 2000; 47: 623–31.

95. Greenberg HS, Chamberlain MC, Glantz MJ, Wang PS. Adult medulloblastoma: multiagent chemotherapy. Neuro Oncol 2001; 3: 29–34.

96. Spreafico F, *et al*. Survival in adults treated for medulloblastoma using paediatric protocols. Eur J Cancer 2005; 41: 1304–10.

97. Herrlinger U, *et al*. Adult medulloblastoma: prognostic factors and response to therapy at diagnosis and at relapse. J Neurol 2005; 252: 291–9.

98. Brandes AA, *et al*. Long-term results of a prospective study on the treatment of medulloblastoma in adults. Cancer 2007; 110: 2035–41.

99. Padovani L, *et al*. Common strategy for adult and pediatric medulloblastoma: a multicenter series of 253 patients. Int J Radiat Oncol Biol Phys 2007; 68: 433–40.

100. Lai R. Survival of patients with adult medulloblastoma. Cancer 2008; 112: 1568–74.

101. Smoll NR. Relative survival of childhood and adult medulloblastomas and primitive neuroectodermal tumors. Cancer 2012; 118(5): 1313–22.

102. Brandes AA, *et al*. The treatment of adults with medulloblastoma: a prospective study. Int J Radiat Oncol Biol Phys 2003; 57: 755–61.

103. Brandes AA, *et al*. Adult neuroectodermal tumors of the posterior fossa (medulloblastoma) and of supratentorial sites (stPNET). Crit Rev Oncol Hematol 2009; 71: 165–79.

104. Korshunov A, *et al*. Adult and pediatric medulloblastomas are genetically distinct and require different algorithms for molecular risk stratification. J Clin Oncol 2010; 28: 3054–60.

105. Pfister SM, *et al*. Molecular diagnostics of CNS embryonal tumors. Acta Neuropathol 2010; 120: 553–66.

106. Eberhart CG. Molecular diagnostics in embryonal brain tumors. Brain Pathol 2011; 21: 96–104.

107. Moody AM, Norman AR, Tait D. Paediatric tumors in the adult population. The experience of the Royal Marsden Hospital 1974–1990. Med Pediatr Oncol 1996; 26: 153–9.

108. Kortman RD, *et al*. Postoperative neoadjuvant chemotherapy before radiotherapy as compared to immediate radiotherapy followed by maintenance chemotherapy in the treatment of medulloblastoma in childhood: results of the German prospective randomized trial HIT '91. Int J Radiat Oncol Biol Phys 2000; 46: 269–79.

109. Verlooy J, *et al*. Treatment of high risk medulloblastoma in children above the age of 3 years: A SFOP study. Eur J Cancer 2006; 42: 3004–14.

110. Strother D, *et al*. Feasibility of four consecutive high-dose chemotherapy cycles with stem cell rescue for patients with newly diagnosed medulloblastoma or supratentorial primitive neuroectodermal tumor after craniospinal radiation. J Clin Oncol 2001; 19: 2696–704.

111. Moots PL, *et al*. Toxicities associated with chemotherapy followed by craniospinal radiation for adults with poor-risk medulloblastoma/PNET and disseminated ependymoma: a preliminary report of ECOG 4397. ASCO Annual Meeting, New Orleans, June 2004.

112. Moots PL, *et al*. Preradiation chemotherapy for adult poor risk medulloblastoma, PNET and ependymoma: ECOG 4397. (Technical report available at ecog.org; manuscript in preparation 2012.)

113. Tarbell NJ, *et al*. Outcome for children with high stage medulloblastoma: results of the Pediatric Oncology Group 9031. Int J Radiat Oncol Biol Phys 2000; 48(Suppl 3): S179.

114. Miralbell R, *et al*. Radiotherapy in pediatric medulloblastoma. Quality assessment of Pediatric Oncology Group Trial 9031. Int J Radiat Oncol Biol Phys 2006; 64: 1325–30.

115. Gupta S, Takebe N, Lorusso P. Targeting the Hedgehog pathway in cancer. Ther Adv Med Oncol 2010; 2: 237–50.

116. Lorusso PM, *et al*. Pharmacokinetic dose-scheduling study of hedgehog pathway inhibitor vismodegib (GDC-0449) in patients with locally-advanced or metastatic solid tumors. Clin Cancer Res 2011; 17(17): 5774–82.

117. Dunkel IJ, *et al*. High-dose carboplatin, thiotepa and etoposide with autologous stem-cell rescue for patients with recurrent medulloblastoma. Children's Cancer Group. J Clin Oncol 1998; 16: 222–8.

118. Zia MI, *et al*. Possible benefits of high-dose chemotherapy and autologous stem cell transplantation for adults with recurrent medulloblastoma. Bone Marrow Transplant 2002; 30: 565–9.

119. Abrey LE, *et al*. High dose chemotherapy with autologous stem cell rescue in adults with malignant primary brain tumors. J Neurooncol 1999; 44: 147–53.

120. Gill P, *et al*. High-dose chemotherapy with autologous stem cell transplantation in adults with recurrent embryonal tumors of the central nervous system. Cancer 2008; 112: 1805–11.

121. Perry A, *et al*. Malignant gliomas with primitive neuro-ectodermal tumor-like components: a clinicopathologic and genetic study of 53 cases. Brain Pathol 2009; 19: 81–90.

122. Geyer JR, *et al*. Survival of infants with primitive neuroectodermal tumors or malignant ependymomas of the CNS treated with eight drugs in 1 day: a report from the Children's Cancer Group. J Clin Oncol 1994; 12: 1607–15.

123. Hong TS, *et al*. Patterns of treatment failure in infants who were treated on CCG-921: a phase III combined modality study. Pediatr Blood Cancer 2005; 45: 676–82.

124. Fangusaro J, *et al*. Intensive chemotherapy followed by consolidative myeloablative chemotherapy with autologous hematopoetic cell rescue (AuHCR) in young children with newly diagnosed supratentorial primitive neuroectodermal tumors (sPNETs): report of the Head Start I and II Experience. Pediatr Blood Cancer 2008; 50: 312–18.

125. Chintagumpala M, *et al*. A pilot study of risk-adapted radiotherapy and chemotherapy in patients with supratentorial PNET. Neuro Oncol 2009; 11: 33–40.

126. Biswas S, *et al*. Non-pineal supratentorial primitive neuroectodermal tumors (s PNET) in teenagers and young adults: time to reconsider cisplatin based chemotherapy after craniospinal irradiation? Pediatr Blood Cancer 2009; 52: 796–803.

127. Broniscer A, *et al*. High dose chemotherapy with autologous stem cell rescue in the treatment of patients with recurrent non-cerebellar primitive neuroectodermal tumors. Pediatr Blood Cancer 2004; 42: 261–7.

128. Gururangan S, *et al*. High-dose chemotherapy with autologous stem cell rescue in children and adults with newly diagnosed pineoblastomas. J Clin Oncol 2003; 21: 2187–91.

129. Edelstein K, *et al*. Early aging in adult survivors of childhood medulloblastoma: long-term neurocognitive, functional and physical outcomes. Neuro Oncol 2011; 13: 536–45.

130. Kramer J, *et al*. Neuropsychological sequelae of medulloblastoma in adults. Int J Radiat Oncol Biol Phys 1997; 38: 21–6.

131. Mariën P, *et al*. Posterior fossa syndrome in adults: a new case and comprehensive survey of the literature. Cortex 2011; July 22 [Epub ahead of print].

132. Frasanito P, Massimi L. Cerebellar mutism: review of the literature. Child Nerv Syst 2011; 27: 867–88.

133. Brandes AA, *et al*. Endocrine dysfunction in patients treated for brain tumors: incidence and guidelines for management. J Neurooncol 2000; 47: 85–92.

134. Fossati P, *et al*. Pediatric medulloblastoma: toxicity of current treatment and potential role for proton therapy. Cancer Treat Rev 2009; 35: 79–96.

135. Chiarelli AM, *et al*. Early menopause and infertility in females after treatment for childhood cancer diagnosed in 1964–1988 in Ontario, Canada. Am J Epidemiol 1999; 150: 245–54.

136. Endicott TJ, *et al*. Pulmonary sequelae after electron spinal irradiation. Radiother Oncol 2001; 60: 267–72.

137. Goldstein AM, Yuen J, Tucker MA. Second cancers after medulloblastoma: population-based results from the United States and Sweden. Cancer Causes Control 1997; 8: 865–71.

60 Pineal Parenchymal Tumors

Shota Tanaka,[1,3,4] Stephen W. Clark,[2] and Patrick Y. Wen[3,4]

[1] Stephen E. and Catherine Pappas Center for Neuro-Oncology, Massachusetts General Hospital, Boston, MA, USA

[2] Division of Neuro-Oncology, Department of Neurology, Vanderbilt-Ingram Cancer Center, Vanderbilt University Medical Center, Nashville, TN, USA

[3] Center for Neuro-Oncology, Dana-Farber Cancer Institute, Boston, MA, USA

[4] Harvard Medical School, Boston, MA, USA

Introduction

Pineal parenchymal tumors (PPTs) are rare rumors of the pineal gland in children and young adults. Given the deep narrow corridor to the pineal gland and the complexity of the surrounding vasculature, surgical treatment for pineal region tumors (PRTs) has always been challenging. Without the advantages of high-resolution imaging, operative microscope, sophisticated anesthesia, or chemotherapeutic agents that we enjoy today, a surgical resection used to carry a tremendously high risk of complications.[1] Oppenheim and Krause first reported removal of a PRT in 1913.[2] Dandy reported total resections of PRTs via interhemispheric transcallosal approach in 1921.[2–4] Subsequently, several surgical approaches were proposed. However, it was only after the operative microscope was introduced to neurosurgery that resection of PRTs could be performed with acceptable risks. Continued advances in diagnostic imaging such as computed tomography and magnetic resonance imaging have further simplified the detection of these tumors and enabled accurate preoperative planning. Moreover, the advent of stereotaxy, as well as the advances of adjuvant chemoradiotherapy, have contributed to improved treatment outcomes of PRTs and PPTs.

Among various kinds of tumors located in the pineal region, PPTs are derived from pineocytes, which secrete melatonin, serotonin, and other neurotransmitters, and account for 10–30% of PRTs.[5–9] According to the World Health Organization (WHO) classification of brain tumors, PPTs are divided into three categories determined by the degree of differentiation on histology: pineocytoma, pineal parenchymal tumor of intermediate differentiation (PPTID), and pineoblastoma.[10] Treatments and prognosis widely vary depending upon histology. This chapter will discuss the epidemiology, diagnosis, treatment, and prognosis of PPTs.

Epidemiology

Tumors in the pineal region are rare, affecting roughly 130 people per year in the United States.[11] The age-adjusted incidence rate is 0.04 per 100,000 person-years. They account for only 0.2% of all central nervous system (CNS) and spinal tumors; however, they account for 3% of CNS tumors in the pediatric population. Notably, they affect pediatric patients of all age groups, although the incidence is slightly higher among patients less than 4 years old and there tends to be a slight female predominance.

Among PRTs, germ cell tumors (GCTs) are the most common and account for 30–60% of all tumors [6,8,9,12] whereas PPTs account for 14–27%.[5,6] Other tumors include astrocytomas and, more rarely, meningiomas, ependymomas, choroid plexus papillomas, metastases, and lymphomas.[8] Among PPTs, pineocytoma and pineoblastoma account for 14–33% and 24–50%, respectively.[6,13–15] Age at presentation is variable for PPTs, with pineocytoma predominantly affecting adults (median age 38 years) whereas pineoblastoma most often affects a younger population (median age 18.5 years).[5,10,13,14,16–19] No gender preference is apparent.

Pathogenesis

The pathogenesis of PPTs is closely linked to the development of the pineal gland and the pineocyte, a cell with photosensory and neuroendocrine functions.[20] A pathological study of pineal glands from infants indicated a remarkable morphological and functional evolution of this endocrine organ in postnatal life.[21] Closely packed, dark, nucleated cells (type I) with occasional rosette formation and positivity for S-100 predominated in neonates, whereas loosely arranged, large, clear cells (type II) with strong positivity for neuron-specific enolase gradually increased in number with age.

Due to the rarity of these tumors, little is known about their cytogenetics. Of note, medulloblastoma, the second most common pediatric brain tumor after pilocytic astrocytoma,[11] occurs in the posterior fossa and is a counterpart to supratentorial primary neuroectodermal tumors (PNET), including pineoblastoma. It is known to harbor a deletion of chromosome 17p in less than 50% of cases.[22] Several small cytogenetic studies in

Textbook of Uncommon Cancer, Fourth Edition. Edited by Derek Raghavan, Charles D. Blanke, David H. Johnson, Paul L. Moots, Gregory H. Reaman, Peter G. Rose and Mikkael A. Sekeres.
© 2012 John Wiley & Sons, Inc. Published 2012 by John Wiley & Sons, Inc.

the literature have failed to identify any consistent changes in PPTs.[23–30] Except for structural aberrations of chromosome 1, which is seen in medulloblastoma, a review of the literature found no consistent chromosomal changes in pineoblastoma.[23] A comparative genomic hybridization of nine PPTs (three each for pineocytoma, PPTID, and pineoblastoma) demonstrated an average of zero chromosomal changes in pineocytoma, 5.3 in PPTID (3.3 gains, 2.0 losses), and 5.6 in pineoblastoma (2.3 gains, 3.3 losses).[30] The most frequent DNA copy number changes were gains of 12q (three cases), 4q, 5p, and 5q (four cases), as well as losses of 22 (4/6 cases), 9q, and 16q (4/6 cases). Based on this work, PPTIDs are cytogenetically more similar to pineoblastomas than to pineocytomas.

Further studies involving DNA microarray analysis and real-time polymerase chain reaction (PCR) have revealed differential gene expression in PPTs when compared to normal brain and the fetal pineal gland.[31] For example, puromycin-sensitive aminopeptidase (PSA) and teratocarcinoma-derived growth factor 3 (TDGF3) were upregulated in PPT and in medulloblastoma, and adenomatous polyposis coli was down-regulated only in PPT. PSA is expressed in cortical and cerebellar neurons of normal brain[32] and it codes for the most abundant aminopeptidase in the brain, which is involved in proteolytic events essential for cell growth.[33] TDGF3 is a member of the Cripto family, cell surface-associated molecules which are upregulated in a wide range of epithelial cancers,[34] and Cripto overexpression may play an early role in cancer progression.[35] Upregulated expression of chromosome 17 open reading frame 1A was seen in high-grade but not in low-grade PPT. This gene codes for a plasma membrane protein and is located in 17q12, where genetic alterations are common in medulloblastoma.[36] Another microarray study of two pineocytomas revealed that genes coding for enzymes of melatonin biosynthesis (*TPH* and *HIOMT*) and those related to phototransduction in the retina (*OPN4*, *RGS16*, and *CRB3*) were highly expressed in pineocytoma.[37]

The expression of these photosensory-related proteins in PPTs may provide a useful diagnostic tool for better characterizing the differentiation of these tumors. In addition, several genes (*PRAME*, *CD24*, *POU4F2*, and *HOXD13*) were more robustly expressed in high-grade than in low-grade PPTID, suggesting their potential utility in tumor grading.

Pathology

In the current WHO classification of brain tumors, PPTs are classified into three categories: pineocytoma, PPTID, and pineoblastoma.[10] One interesting retrospective study reported that the histological diagnosis of PPT was considered inappropriate in 10.6% of 281 patients with PRTs after central pathology review, which highlights the importance of appropriate surgical specimens and careful pathology review by experienced neuropathologists.[15] Typical pineocytoma is a well-differentiated, moderately cellular neoplasm composed of relatively small, uniform, mature pineocyte-like cells. It usually grows in sheets or ill-defined lobules, and often features pineocytomatous rosettes with nuclear-free spaces filled with a fine meshwork of cell processes. Mitotic figures are lacking in most cases. Immunohistochemistry is usually strongly positive for neuronal markers such as synaptophysin, neuron-specific enolase, and neurofilament protein, as well as neuroendocrine markers such as chromogranin A.[17,38] Photosensory differentiation is associated with immunoreactivity for retinal S-antigen and rhodopsin.[17,39,40] Pineocytoma corresponds histologically to WHO grade 1.

Pineoblastomas are composed of densely packed, small, poorly differentiated neuroectodermal cells, resembling other small cell or primitive neuroectodermal tumors (PNETs). The individual tumor cells have minimal cytoplasm and contain hyperchromatic irregular nuclei. Mitoses are frequent with variable amounts of necrosis. Pineocytomatous rosettes are not seen, but Homer–Wright rosettes may be seen similarly to medulloblastoma. Flexner–Wintersteiner rosettes seen in some cases are interpreted as evidence of photoreceptor differentiation. Immunohistochemistry of pineoblastoma resembles that of pineocytoma and it expresses neuronal and photosensory markers. Pineoblastoma corresponds histologically to WHO grade 4.

Pineal parenchymal tumors are considered to represent a spectrum of tumors composed of primitive parenchymal cells to well-differentiated pineocytes[20]; a fair percentage of PPTs fit neither pineocytoma nor pineoblastoma. Among such tumors, some consist of cells with histological features intermediate between typical pineocytomas and pineoblastomas and thus are called PPTs of intermediate differentiation. Others are the mixture of well-differentiated pineocyte-like cells and poorly differentiated pineoblastoma-like cells and thus are referred to as mixed pineocytoma/pineoblatomas, which account for approximately 10% of PPTs.[39] PPTID may correspond to WHO grade 2 or 3 but definite grading criteria have yet to be established.[20]

Although this classic classification has clinical advantages in selecting the appropriate therapeutic regimen for a given patient and estimating his/her prognosis, the histological distinction between these three types remains unclear and somewhat confusing from a practical standpoint, partially because the morphological criteria have not been well established and remain subjective.[18] Rather, PPTs are believed to exist along a continuum. In fact, a recent case report presented a pineoblastoma that had been transformed from a conservatively managed pineocytoma.[41] Thus, extensive efforts have been undertaken to try to differentiate the spectrum of PPTs more clearly. A mitotic index has been consistently suggested as a useful prognostic marker of PPTs in the literature[14,40,42,43]; immunopositivity of neurofilaments is also suggested as a potential marker enabling a clear distinction between different grades of PPTs.[14,18,43]

A large retrospective study of 66 PPTs in 12 institutions correlated the histological features with patient survival, and a new grading system was proposed using morphology, mitotic index, and neurofilaments on immunohistochemistry.[14] Using this grading system, pineocytoma (WHO grade 1) and pineoblastoma (WHO grade 4) fell into grade 1 and grade 4, respectively. PPTID was divided into the two grades: grade 2 consisting of transitional, lobulated, or diffuse PPT with strong immunostaining for neurofilaments and less than six mitoses, and grade 3 consisting of lobulated or diffuse PPT with either six or more mitoses or fewer than six mitoses but without immunostaining for neurofilaments. Grade 3 also includeed mixed pineocytoma-pineoblastoma. Prognostically, this grading system was useful, with an overall survival (OS) rate at 5 years approaching 90% for grade 1 tumors, 80% for grade 2 tumors, 40% for grade 3 tumors, and 10% for grade 4 tumors.

A challenge remains in discerning a pineocytoma from a normal pineal gland or pineal cyst.[44] Whereas pineocytoma generally forms sheets or extended lobules, the normal pineal gland has small lobules and well-formed fibrovascular septae. A pineal cyst typically has a three-layered pattern. This differentiation, however, is crucial as misdiagnosing pineal cyst as pineocytoma, for example, may lead to unnecessary therapy for nonneoplastic pineal lesion.[39]

Clinical presentation

It is not possible to differentiate PPTs from other PRTs or pineocytoma from pineoblastoma by symptoms and signs alone, although the interval between initial symptoms and diagnosis tends to be shorter for high-grade PPTs compared to low-grade.[45] Given their close association to the aqueduct, PPTs may cause obstructive hydrocephalus and patients may present with signs of increased intracranial pressure. These tumors may also cause cranial nerve deficits such as upward gaze palsy, convergence nystagmus, and near-light dissociation (Parinaud syndrome) by compressing the dorsal midbrain. No signs or symptoms are pathognomonic for PPTs. If they compress the cerebellum or the hypothalamus, patients present with ataxia or hormonal insufficiency. In one retrospective study of 30 patients with PPTs, common symptoms and signs included headache (73%), impaired vision (47%), nausea and vomiting (40%), impaired gait (37%), papilledema (60%), ataxia (50%), and upward gaze palsy (30%).[13] In rare cases, patients present with intratumoral hemorrhage.[19]

Diagnostic considerations

Lesions that arise in the pineal region are diverse and include not only PRTs but also metastasis, vascular lesions such as cavernomas, infectious lesions such as tuberculoma, and arachnoid cyst.[5–8] PRTs also represent a wide variety of tumors with significantly different natural histories, and thus accurate histological diagnosis is warranted to allow the proper choice of treatment modalities and regimens. As GCTs are the most common tumors in the pineal region,[6,8,9,12] sampling of GCT markers (β-human chorionic gonadotropin, α-fetoprotein, placental alkaline phosphatase) from serum and cerebrospinal fluid (CSF) should be obtained. Most commonly, CSF is obtained during the initial CSF diversion procedure, as lumbar puncture is contraindicated for patients presenting with signs of increased intracranial pressure. Cytology should also be checked as CSF seeding may be present at the time of presentation, especially in pineoblastoma and high-grade PPTID.[14,15,46,47] Spinal magnetic resonance imaging (MRI) s should be considered to evaluate for possible seeding.

It is difficult to discern the various types of PRTs solely on imaging. PPTs are generally hyperintense on T2-weighted images, whereas GCTs tend to be isointense to the gray matter; however, there is significant overlap in imaging characteristics among PRTs.[48] Among PPTs, signal intensity may be higher with pineocytoma than with pineoblastoma on fluid-attenuated inversion-recovery sequence, and pineocytoma is more likely to have a cystic component.[49] Whereas pineocytoma tends to enhance homogeneously, pineoblastoma and PPTIDs show a more heterogeneous pattern (Fig. 60.1).[50] Irregular borders with brain invasion are commonly demonstrated in high-grade PPTs such as pineoblastoma.[9]

With the increasing use of diagnostic imaging such as MRI, abnormality in the pineal region is now detected more

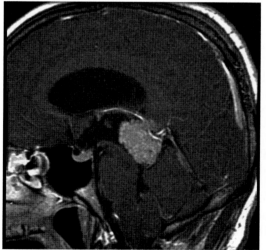
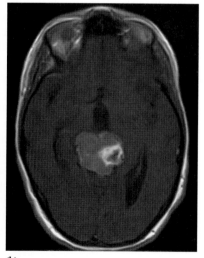
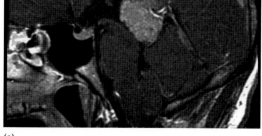

Figure 60.1 (a) A postcontrast sagittal T1 image of a pineoblastoma. (b) PPTID revealing its heterogeneous enhancement.

(a)

(b)

frequently. One area of concern is distinguishing radiographically a pineal cyst from a pineocytoma or pilocytic astrocytoma.[39] This is important clinically because the incidence of pineal cyst is not trivial, ranging from 1% to 4%, and thus a misdiagnosis can result in inappropriate therapy[51–53]; typically a pineal cyst has a very benign natural history.[52,54] Some authors advocate a thin <2 mm rim of enhancement and no nodularity as criteria to differentiate pineal cyst from neoplasm.[55,56]

Treatment

Surgery

Given the diversity in PRTs and the lack of tumor markers for PPTs, surgical treatment is warranted in virtually all cases to obtain a histological diagnosis. Two approaches are commonly taken for biopsies of PRTs. One is a stereotactic biopsy. Its diagnostic yield in the literature ranges from 92% to 100%.[5–7,57] However, in one retrospective study, 18 of 61 patients who had undergone a stereotactic biopsy went on to have resection and the correlation of the biopsy with the histological diagnosis was 89%.[6] This low rate of concordance may represent an issue with stereotactic biopsy for PRTs; they may have mixed histology within the same lesion (for example, mixed germ cell tumors and mixed pineocytoma/pineoblastoma). Furthermore, this histological discordance supports the importance of surgical resection in PRTs. Given the depth of the tumors and the complex surrounding vasculature such as the vein of Galen and internal cerebral veins, high rates of complications are often quoted by neurosurgeons associated with stereotactic biopsy in this location[58]; however, its morbidity and mortality rates are generally low in the literature.[5–7,59] For example, a large retrospective study of 370 stereotactic biopsies of PRTs reported a mortality rate of 1.3% and a persistent morbidity rate of 0.8%, which was not necessarily thought to be higher than those of stereotactic biopsy in general.[5]

Another approach is endoscopic biopsy via a transventricular approach.[60–62] Its biggest advantage is that it can simultaneously treat obstructive hydrocephalus with third ventriculostomy during one general anesthesia.[63] Furthermore, endoscopic third ventriculostomy can avoid ventriculoperitoneal shunts which are associated with the inherent risks of shunt infection and malfunction indefinitely. The diagnostic yield of endoscopic biopsy is generally high at 86.7–100%.[60–62] However, it has not gained popularity, probably because it can only be done safely by experienced neurosurgeons. Endoscopic surgery for PRTs is particularly difficult due to the long reach and possible need of a flexible endoscope.

The efficacy of radical resection for PPTs has been debated, especially with regard to high-grade PPTs. Aggressive debulking as opposed to biopsy can potentially restore CSF flow if a patient suffers from obstructive hydrocephalus secondary to the tumor, although obstructive hydrocephalus is generally handled successfully with CSF diversion procedures such as ventriculoperitoneal shunt and endoscopic third ventriculostomy. Complete resection is achievable for some benign PPTs such as pineocytoma, and constitutes optimal

management with excellent long-term recurrence-free survival.[13,64,65] A recent systematic review of the literature found a total of 166 patients with pineocytoma and reported 1- and 5-year progression-free survival (PFS) rates of 97% and 89% for the resection group and 90% and 75% for the biopsy group.[65] Notably, these rates were 100% and 100% for patients undergoing gross total resection (GTR) (61 patients, 42%). This favorable tumor control with GTR likely reflects upon the survival benefit of GTR as compared to subtotal resection (STR) or biopsy. The OS rates at 1 and 5 years were 91% and 84% for the GTR group (without radiotherapy) and 88% and 17% for the STR group (with radiotherapy), and the difference was statistically significant. It has to be mentioned that aggressive surgery in the pineal region carries the inherent risk of catastrophic postoperative neurological deterioration given the depth of the tumor and the surrounding vasculature. Its risks and benefits have to be seriously assessed and fully discussed with patients preoperatively. The reported surgical complication rates vary among the series (mortality 0–10%, morbidity 0–18%).[6,66–69]

Local anatomy has to be fully reviewed to determine the approach of choice for tumor resection. Specifically, the extent of a tumor (rostral-caudal, anterior, lateral), its relationship to the deep venous system (the vein of Galen, internal cerebral veins, veins of Rosenthal), the angle of tentorium, and the drainage of the sinuses (straight sinus, transverse sinus, superior sagittal sinus) will be discussed. An approach along the cerebellar tentorium is preferred in the majority of cases to obtain good access to the pineal region. It has two variations: supracerebellar-infratentorial approach and occipital-supratentorial approach. The caudal extension of the tumor may mandate a posterior interhemispheric transcallosal approach. Detailed discussion regarding surgical approaches is outside the scope of this chapter but is extensively outlined elsewhere.[2,6,66,70,71]

The benefits of aggressive tumor resection, on the other hand, are less clear for malignant tumors such as pineoblastoma,[72,73] although some studies argue for the survival benefit of GTR.[74,75] Given that GTR (residual <1–1.5 cm³) is a positive prognostic factor for medulloblastoma,[76–78] aggressive tumor resection may improve survival for patients with pineoblastoma as well, although the complicated local anatomy discussed earlier may result in high postoperative complication rates and degrade its survival benefit. PPTID is thought to be closer in behavior and prognosis to pineoblastoma than to pineocytoma, and thus it is generally treated similarly to pineoblastoma.

Radiotherapy

The rarity of pineocytoma precludes either a prospective study or a large-scale retrospective study regarding the efficacy of adjuvant radiotherapy.[79] In the previously mentioned comprehensive review of pineocytoma treatment, 66 patients (40%) underwent adjuvant treatment with either fractionated radiotherapy or stereotactic radiosurgery (SRS).[65] Adjuvant radiotherapy was not able to compensate for incomplete resection in that tumor control rates were clearly better with GTR than with STR combined with radiotherapy. Furthermore, adjuvant radiotherapy after STR did not significantly add to tumor control rates compared with STR alone, questioning a benefit of adjuvant radiotherapy after STR. However, postoperative radiotherapy to reduce local recurrence is generally recommended for pineocytomas that are subtotally resected or only biopsied.[4] If radiotherapy is delivered, localized fields should be used and cranial-spinal irradiation (CSI) should be reserved for patients with overt leptomeningeal spread. All previous studies evaluating SRS for pineocytoma are retrospective and contain small numbers of patients.[80-83] Thus, no definitive conclusion can be drawn regarding the indication of SRS for this benign tumor except as an initial treatment in cases of pineocytomas whereby GTR is deemed impossible or achievable only with unacceptable risk.[84]

Numerous studies have demonstrated the benefit of radio-therapy for pineoblastoma and PPTID, in both the pediatric[13] and adult[13,74,85] populations. High-grade PPT, especially pineo-blastoma, is prone to shed into the CSF (14–45% of cases[6,8,46]) and therefore CSI is warranted along with chemotherapy regardless of extent of surgical resection.[8] Typically, a dose of 30–36 Gy to the neuraxis followed by a boost to the primary site to 50–55 Gy is recommended.[4] Gross spinal metastases receive 45–50.4 Gy.[4,86] Localized radiotherapy almost inevitably fails in pineoblastoma. For example, SRS does not seem promising for pineoblastoma, in contrast to pineocytoma[83]; in one retrospective study, the local control rate was 85% at 5 years for pineocytoma whereas it was merely 30% at 2 years for pineoblastoma.[82]

Given the difficulty of microsurgery for PRTs and the risk of stereotactic biopsy for such deep-seated lesions, many patients are treated with radiotherapy without a histological diagnosis. In a review of the literature involving over 200 PRTs treated with radiotherapy, including nonbiopsied patients, patients with PPTs, patients with germinomas, and patients with nongerminomatous GCTs, response to radiotherapy varied widely, emphasizing the importance of histological confirmation.[87]

Chemotherapy

Treatment strategies for patients with supratentorial PNETs including pineoblastoma are derived from those employed in medulloblastoma and include chemotherapy and CSI. Interestingly, treatment results differ between the two despite the similarity of histological features, with pineoblastoma being less responsive than medulloblastoma.[73,88–91]

Patients with pineoblastomas have been put in the same group as patients with other supratentorial PNETs in the majority of studies mainly because of their rarity. However, pineoblastoma may respond to treatments differently than other supratentorial PNETs. In the Children's Cancer Group (CCG) study, patients with pineoblastomas responded to CSI and chemotherapy better than patients with other supratentorial PNETs.[72,90] Patients in this study were randomized to receive either vincristine, lomustine, and prednisone or the eight-drugs-in-one-day (8-in-1) regimen (methylprednisone,

vincristine, lomustine or carmustine, procarbazine, hydroxy-urea, cisplatin, cytarabine, and cyclophosphamide).

Chemotherapy for pineoblastoma varies significantly among institutions and groups, and the optimal regimen or timing of chemotherapy is yet to be determined.[15] The agents that have been used include carboplatin, carmustine, cisplatin, cyclophosphamide, cytarabine, etoposide, ifosfamide, hydroxyurea, lomustine, methotrexate, procarbazine, vinblastine, and vincristine.[15,72,85,92]

More intense chemotherapy regimens followed by autologous stem cell transplant have been explored. In one study of recurrent supratentorial PNETs, 17 patients were treated with high-dose chemotherapy (HDC) followed by autologous stem cell rescue (ASCR).[93] Conditioning consisted of carboplatin, thiotepa, and etoposide. Eight patients harbored pineoblastoma, and their 5-year event-free survival was significantly worse than that of patients with other supratentorial PNETs (0% versus 62.5%). This difference apparently stemmed from the fact that five patients with cortical PNETs remained alive disease free at a median of 8.3 years of follow-up. Given that surgery at relapse was found to be a favorable prognostic factor in that study, the difficulties of surgical debulking for recurrent pineoblastoma might be an important causal factor for its worse outcome. Of note in this study, two patients (11%) died of toxicity and six patients had a grade 3/4 nonhematological toxicity. Moreover, the patients uniformly required blood product transfusions and nine patients developed infections despite broad-spectrum antibiotic use. In the newly diagnosed setting, 12 pineoblastoma patients (six children and six adults) were treated with surgery, induction chemotherapy, and radiotherapy (all but two patients), followed by HDC (cyclophosphamide, melphalan or busulfan, and melphalan) and ASCR.[94] Nine patients were alive with no evidence of disease recurrence at a median of 62 months from diagnosis (range 28–125 months), including three patients with metastatic disease and two infants who did not receive any radiotherapy. The actuarial 4-year OS and PFS rates were 71% and 69%, respectively. HDC in addition to radiotherapy seems to be an effective treatment in selected patients with newly diagnosed pineoblastomas.

Treatment of pineoblastoma in infants presents a significant challenge.[95] The desire to avoid long-term complications associated with CSI in very young children has led to the pursuit of alternative approaches. Delaying radiotherapy by giving upfront chemotherapy in infants with pineoblastoma has been tried, with dismal results.[72,91,96] In the Pediatric Oncology Group study, 11 pineoblastoma patients all less than 3 years old received intensive chemotherapy with cyclophosphamide, vincristine, cisplatin, and etoposide without radiation, all of whom failed within 12 months after diagnosis.[96] The OS after diagnosis ranged from 4 months to 13 months. Similar results were reported in the CCG study, in which eight infants all less than 18 months were treated with the 8-in-1 chemotherapy without radiation.[72] All patients developed progressive disease 3–14 months (median 4 months) from the start of treatment. The median OS was merely 10 months. Thus, controversy remains regarding the optimal treatment strategy for infants with pineoblastomas.

Table 60.1 A historical comparison of overall survival and progression-free survival between pineocytoma, PPTID, and pineoblastoma.

Reference		Pineocytoma					PPTID					Pineoblastoma				
		Number of patients	Median OS	5-year OS rate	Median PFS	5-year PFS rate	Number of patients	Median OS	5-year OS rate	Median PFS	5-year PFS rate	Number of patients	Median OS	5-year OS rate	Median PFS	5-year PFS rate
Schild et al.[13]	1993	9	NA	67	NA	NA	6	NA	58*	NA	NA	15	NA	58*	NA	NA
Mena et al.[17]	1995	21	NR	NA	NA	NA	3	NA	NA	NA	NA	11	24	NA	NA	NA
Jakacki et al.[72]	1995	–	–	–	–	–	–	–	–	–	–	17	Dissem.: 30, No-dissem.: NR	61 (3-year)	NA	73 (3-year)
Chang et al.[46]	1995	–	–	–	–	–	–	–	–	–	–	10	NA	NA	NA	NA
Fauchon et al.[15]	2000	19	NR	91	NA	NA	GII: 27, GIII: 20	GII: NR, GIII: 38	GII: 74, GIII 39	NA	NA	18	16	10	NA	NA
Lutterbach et al.[85*]	2002	–	–	–	–	–	37	165	80	93	NA	64	77	51	46	NA
Gururangan et al.[94]	2003	–	–	–	–	–	–	–	–	–	–	12	NR	69 (4-year)	NR	71 (4-year)
Lee et al.[74*]	2005	–	–	–	–	–	–	–	–	–	–	34	25.7	NA	NA	NA
Hinkes et al.[92†]	2007	–	–	–	–	–	–	–	–	–	–	Age >3: 6, Age <3: 5	Age >3: 106, Age <3: 11	NA	Age >3: 95, Age <3: 7	NA
Clark et al.[64,65]	2010	166, 168§	NR	Resection: 76, Biopsy: 64	NR	Resection: 89, Biopsy: 75	–	–	–	–	–	–	–	–	–	–

Dissem, disseminated; GII, grade II; GIII, grade III; NA, not available; NR, not reached; OS, overall survival; PFS, progression-free survival.
* Adults only.
† Children only.
§ 166 for PFS analysis, 168 for OS analysis.

Prognosis

The prognosis of PPTs varies significantly depending upon the histological grades.[14] The survival data of patients with PPTs as found in the literature are summarized in Table 60.1. In a retrospective study of 76 patients, the 5-year OS rates were 91%, 74%, 39%, and 10% for pineocytoma, PPTID (grade 2), PPTID (grade 3), and pineoblastoma, respectively.[15]

Favorable outcomes have been achieved with surgery with or without radiotherapy in pineocytoma, with a 5-year OS rate ranging from 67% to 91%.[13,15,64,86] GTR is the most consistent favorable prognostic factor of OS. In a retrospective study of 168 patients with pineocytomas, the 5-year OS rate was 82% and 64% for the resection group and the biopsy group, respectively.[64] Moreover, STR could not achieve as good survival outcomes as GTR even with the support of radiotherapy.

Recent aggressive multimodality treatment strategies have achieved more promising results regarding the survival of patients with high-grade PPTs (pineoblastomas and PPTIDs) (see Table 60.1). In one series of patients with pineoblastoma or PPTID treated with various treatment modalities, the projected 1-, 3-, and 5-year OS rates were 88%, 78%, and 58%, respectively.[13] In a subanalysis of the aforementioned CCG randomized study of supratentorial PNETs, 17 pineoblastoma patients aged 18 months or older were treated with CSI and multiagent chemotherapy; the OS and PFS rates at 3 years were $73 \pm 12\%$ and $61 \pm 13\%$, respectively.[72] In contrast, survival of very young children with pineoblastomas remains dismal. In the same CCG study, all of eight infants aged less than 18 months treated with the 8-in-1 chemotherapy alone developed progressive disease at a median of 4 months, suggesting that age and/or the use of radiation are important determinants of survival.[72]

Malignant PPTs are rare among adult patients and they are generally treated with the pediatric protocols. In one small series, five adult patients with disseminated pineoblastoma had a median OS of 30 months despite multimodality treatments, whereas all of five patients with pineoblastoma without dissemination were alive after a median follow-up of 26 months.[46] In a multicenter, retrospective study of 101 adult patients with malignant PPTs, the median OS rates were 165 months and 77 months for patients with PPTID and those with pineoblastoma, respectively.[85] In a multivariate analysis, extent of disease (localized versus disseminated), histology (PPTID versus pineoblastoma), and residual disease after surgery and radiotherapy (no/minor versus major) were independent prognostic factors of OS.

Recommendations

Pineal parenchymal tumors are rare tumors arising in the pineal gland and represent a wide spectrum of tumors composed of well-differentiated pineocytes to primitive parenchymal cells. Therefore, accurate histological diagnosis is crucial for optimization of adjuvant treatments, which is usually obtained by surgery.

Pineocytoma is a slow-growing tumor and can potentially be curable with gross total resection. Given the difficulty of aggressive resection due to the depth of the lesion and the surrounding vital structures, surgery should preferably be performed by experienced neurosurgeons. Preoperatively, surgical planning has to be thoroughly done, and the risks and benefits of surgical resection have to be fully discussed with patients and their families. The efficacy of adjuvant radiotherapy has not been fully proven. If it is entertained for residual disease, it should be localized and should not cover the entire neuroaxis.

In contrast, pineoblastoma is a highly aggressive tumor mandating multimodality approaches with surgery, chemotherapy, and radiotherapy. It is not clear if the extent of resection makes a difference in treatment outcomes, although surgical debulking may alleviate mass effect and facilitate further treatment in some cases. Various chemotherapy regimens have been reported, with platinum agents being the mainstay; more recently, high-dose chemotherapy followed by autologous stem cell rescue has been vigorously explored and seems to achieve promising outcomes in carefully selected patients. Radiotherapy should be delivered to the brain and the whole spine regardless of extent of resection because of the propensity of dissemination. Treatment of very young children remains extremely challenging, with most cases rapidly progressing despite aggressive chemotherapy; this is likely related to the fact that radiotherapy is usually deferred for fear of its long-term adverse effect.

Pineal parenchymal tumor of intermediate differentiation is believed to behave more similarly to pineoblastoma than to pineocytoma, and thus is treated the same as pineoblastoma.

References

1. Donat JF, Okazaki H, Gomez MR, Reagan TJ, Baker HL, Laws ER. Pineal tumors. A 53-year experience. Arch Neurol 1978; 35(11): 736–40.
2. Winn R. *Youmans Neurological Surgery*. Philadelphia: Elsevier Saunders, 2011.
3. Sherman IJ, Kretzer RM, Tamargo RJ. Personal recollections of Walter E. Dandy and his brain team. J Neurosurg 2006; 105(3): 487–93.
4. Mehta MP, Chang SM, Guha A, Newton HB, Vogelbaum MA. *Principles and Practice of Neuro-oncology: A Multidisciplinary Approach*. New York: Demos Medical, 2010.
5. Regis J, Bouillot P, Rouby-Volot F, Figarella-Branger D, Dufour H, Peragut JC. Pineal region tumors and the role of stereotactic biopsy: review of the mortality, morbidity, and diagnostic rates in 370 cases. Neurosurgery 1996; 39(5): 907–12.
6. Konovalov AN, Pitskhelauri DI. Principles of treatment of the pineal region tumors. Surg Neurol 2003; 59(4): 250–68.
7. Kreth FW, Schätz CR, Pagenstecher A, Faist M, Volk B, Ostertag CB. Stereotactic management of lesions of the pineal region. Neurosurgery 1996; 39(2): 280–9; discussion 289–91.
8. Blakeley JO, Grossman SA. Management of pineal region tumors. Curr Treat Options Oncol 2006; 7(6): 505–16.
9. Parker JJ, Waziri A. Preoperative evaluation of pineal tumors. Neurosurg Clin North Am 2011; 22(3): 353–8.
10. Louis DN, Ohgaki H, Wiestler OD, *et al.* The 2007 WHO classification of tumours of the central nervous system. Acta Neuropathol 2007; 114(2): 97–109.
11. Central Brain Tumor registry of the United States. *Statistical Report: Primary Brain and Central Nervous System Tumors Diagnosed in the United States 2004–2007*. Washington, DC: Central Brain Tumor Registry of the United States, 2011.
12. Shibui S, Nomura K. Statistical analysis of pineal tumors based on the data of Brain Tumor Registry of Japan. Prog Neurol Surg 2009; 23: 1–11.

13. Schild SE, Scheithauer BW, Schomberg PJ, *et al.* Pineal parenchymal tumors. Clinical, pathologic and therapeutic aspects. Cancer 1993; 72(3): 870–80.

14. Jouvet A, Saint-Pierre G, Fauchon F, *et al.* Pineal parenchymal tumors: a correlation of histological features with prognosis in 66 cases. Brain Pathol 2000; 10(1): 49–60.

15. Fauchon F, Jouvet A, Paquis P, *et al.* Parenchymal pineal tumors: a clinicopathological study of 76 cases. Int J Radiat Oncol Biol Phys 2000; 46(4): 959–68.

16. Herrick MK, Rubinstein LJ. The cytological differentiating potential of pineal parenchymal neoplasms (true pinealomas). A clinicopathological study of 28 tumours. Brain 1979; 102(2): 289–320.

17. Mena H, Rushing EJ, Ribas JL, Delahunt B, McCarthy WF. Tumors of pineal parenchymal cells: a correlation of histological features, including nucleolar organizer regions, with survival in 35 cases. Hum Pathol 1995; 26(1): 20–30.

18. Yamane Y, Mena H, Nakazato Y. Immunohistochemical characterization of pineal parenchymal tumors using novel monoclonal antibodies to the pineal body. Neuropathology 2002; 22(2): 66–76.

19. Hoffman HJ, Yoshida M, Becker LE, Hendrick EB, Humphreys RP. Pineal region tumors in childhood. Experience at the Hospital for Sick Children, 1983. Pediatr Neurosurg 1994; 21(1): 91–103; discussion 104.

20. Louis DN, Ohgaki H, Wiestler OD, Cavenee WK. *WHO Classification of Tumors of the Central Nervous System.* Lyon: IARC Press, 2007. pp.121–7.

21. Min KW, Seo IS, Song J. Postnatal evolution of the human pineal gland. An immunohistochemical study. Lab Invest 1987; 57(6): 724–8.

22. Biegel JA, Janss AJ, Raffel C, *et al.* Prognostic significance of chromosome 17p deletions in childhood primitive neuroectodermal tumors (medulloblastomas) of the central nervous system. Clin Cancer Res 1997; 3(3): 473–8.

23. Brown AE, Leibundgut K, Niggli FK, Betts DR. Cytogenetics of pineoblastoma: four new cases and a literature review. Cancer Genet Cytogenet 2006; 170(2): 175–9.

24. Sawyer JR, Sammartino G, Husain M, Linskey ME. Constitutional t(16;22)(p13.3;q11.2 approximately 12) in a primitive neuroectodermal tumor of the pineal region. Cancer Genet Cytogenet 2003; 142(1): 73–6.

25. Roberts P, Chumas PD, Picton S, Bridges L, Livingstone JH, Sheridan E. A review of the cytogenetics of 58 pediatric brain tumors. Cancer Genet Cytogenet 2001; 131(1): 1–12.

26. Bigner SH, McLendon RE, Fuchs H, McKeever PE, Friedman HS. Chromosomal characteristics of childhood brain tumors. Cancer Genet Cytogenet 1997; 97(2): 125–34.

27. Sreekantaiah C, Jockin H, Brecher ML, Sandberg AA. Interstitial deletion of chromosome 11q in a pineoblastoma. Cancer Genet Cytogenet 1989; 39(1): 125–31.

28. Griffin CA, Hawkins AL, Packer RJ, Rorke LB, Emanuel BS. Chromosome abnormalities in pediatric brain tumors. Cancer Res 1988; 48(1): 175–80.

29. Li MH, Bouffet E, Hawkins CE, Squire JA, Huang A. Molecular genetics of supratentorial primitive neuroectodermal tumors and pineoblastoma. Neurosurg Focus 2005; 19(5): E3.

30. Rickert CH, Simon R, Bergmann M, Dockhorn-Dworniczak B, Paulus W. Comparative genomic hybridization in pineal parenchymal tumors. Genes Chromosomes Cancer 2001; 30(1): 99–104.

31. Champier J, Jouvet A, Rey C, Brun V, Bernard A, Fèvre-Montange M. Identification of differentially expressed genes in human pineal parenchymal tumors by microarray analysis. Acta Neuropathol 2005; 109(3): 306–13.

32. Tobler AR, Constam DB, Schmitt-Gräff A, Malipiero U, Schlapbach R, Fontana A. Cloning of the human puromycin-sensitive aminopeptidase and evidence for expression in neurons. J Neurochem 1997; 68(3): 889–97.

33. Constam DB, Tobler AR, Rensing-Ehl A, Kemler I, Hersh LB, Fontana A. Puromycin-sensitive aminopeptidase. Sequence analysis, expression, and functional characterization. J Biol Chem 1995; 270(45): 26931–9.

34. Shen MM. Decrypting the role of Cripto in tumorigenesis. J Clin Invest 2003; 112(4): 500–2.

35. Morkel M, Huelsken J, Wakamiya M, *et al.* Beta-catenin regulates Cripto- and Wnt3-dependent gene expression programs in mouse axis and mesoderm formation. Development 2003; 130(25): 6283–94.

36. Aldosari N, Rasheed BK, McLendon RE, Friedman HS, Bigner DD, Bigner SH. Characterization of chromosome 17 abnormalities in medulloblastomas. Acta Neuropathol 2000; 99(4): 345–51.

37. Fèvre-Montange M, Champier J, Szathmari A, *et al.* Microarray analysis reveals differential gene expression patterns in tumors of the pineal region. J Neuropathol Exp Neurol 2006; 65(7): 675–684.

38. Jouvet A, Fèvre-Montange M, Besançon R, *et al.* Structural and ultrastructural characteristics of human pineal gland, and pineal parenchymal tumors. Acta Neuropathol 1994; 88(4): 334–48.

39. Hirato J, Nakazato Y. Pathology of pineal region tumors. J Neurooncol 2001; 54(3): 239–49.

40. Numoto RT. Pineal parenchymal tumors: cell differentiation and prognosis. J Cancer Res Clin Oncol 1994; 120(11): 683–90.

41. Howard BM, Hofstetter C, Wagner PL, Muskin ET, Lavi E, Boockvar JA. Transformation of a low-grade pineal parenchymal tumour to secondary pineoblastoma. Neuropathol Appl Neurobiol 2009; 35(2): 214–17.

42. Fèvre-Montange M, Vasiljevic A, Frappaz D, *et al.* Utility of Ki67 immunostaining in the grading of pineal parenchymal tumours: a multicentre study. Neuropathol Appl Neurobiol 2012; 38(1): 87–94.

43. Arivazhagan A, Anandh B, Santosh V, Chandramouli BA. Pineal parenchymal tumors – utility of immunohistochemical markers in prognostication. Clin Neuropathol 2008; 27(5): 325–33.

44. Scheithauer BW. Pathobiology of the pineal gland with emphasis on parenchymal tumors. Brain Tumor Pathol 1999; 16(1): 1–9.

45. Borit A, Blackwood W, Mair WG. The separation of pineocytoma from pineoblastoma. Cancer 1980; 45(6): 1408–18.

46. Chang SM, Lillis-Hearne PK, Larson DA, Wara WM, Bollen AW, Prados MD. Pineoblastoma in adults. Neurosurgery 1995; 37(3): 383–90.

47. Dahiya S, Perry A. Pineal tumors. Adv Anat Pathol 2010; 17(6): 419–27.

48. Gaillard F, Jones J. Masses of the pineal region: clinical presentation and radiographic features. Postgrad Med J 2010; 86(1020): 597–607.

49. Korogi Y, Takahashi M, Ushio Y. MRI of pineal region tumors. J Neurooncol 2001; 54(3): 251–61.

50. Nakamura M, Saeki N, Iwadate Y, Sunami K, Osato K, Yamaura A. Neuroradiological characteristics of pineocytoma and pineoblastoma. Neuroradiology 2000; 42(7): 509–14.

51. Mamourian AC, Towfighi J. Pineal cysts: MR imaging. Am J Neuroradiol 1986; 7(6): 1081–6.

52. Al-Holou WN, Garton HJ, Muraszko KM, Ibrahim M, Maher CO. Prevalence of pineal cysts in children and young adults. Clinical article. J Neurosurg Pediatr 2009; 4(3): 230–6.

53. Al-Holou WN, Terman SW, Kilburg C, *et al.* Prevalence and natural history of pineal cysts in adults. J Neurosurg 2011; 115(6): 1106–14.

54. Al-Holou WN, Maher CO, Muraszko KM, Garton HJ. The natural history of pineal cysts in children and young adults. J Neurosurg Pediatr 2010; 5(2): 162–6.

55. Fakhran S, Escott EJ. Pineocytoma mimicking a pineal cyst on imaging: true diagnostic dilemma or a case of incomplete imaging? Am J Neuroradiol 2008; 29(1): 159–63.

56. Barboriak DP, Lee L, Provenzale JM. Serial MR imaging of pineal cysts: implications for natural history and follow-up. Am J Roentgenol 2001; 176(3): 737–43.

57. Dempsey PK, Kondziolka D, Lunsford LD. Stereotactic diagnosis and treatment of pineal region tumours and vascular malformations. Acta Neurochir (Wien) 1992; 116(1): 14–22.

58. Field M, Witham TF, Flickinger JC, Kondziolka D, Lunsford LD. Comprehensive assessment of hemorrhage risks and outcomes after stereotactic brain biopsy. J Neurosurg 2001; 94(4): 545–51.

59. Linggood RM, Chapman PH. Pineal tumors. J Neurooncol 1992; 12(1): 85–91.

60. Pople IK, Athanasiou TC, Sandeman DR, Coakham HB. The role of endoscopic biopsy and third ventriculostomy in the management of pineal region tumours. Br J Neurosurg 2001; 15(4): 305–11.

61. Morgenstern PF, Osbun N, Schwartz TH, Greenfield JP, Tsiouris AJ, Souweidane MM. Pineal region tumors: an optimal approach for simultaneous endoscopic third ventriculostomy and biopsy. Neurosurg Focus 2011; 30(4): E3.

62. Chernov MF, Kamikawa S, Yamane F, Ishihara S, Kubo O, Hori T. Neurofiberscopic biopsy of tumors of the pineal region and posterior third ventricle: indications, technique, complications, and results. Neurosurgery 2006; 59(2): 267–77.

63. Oi S, Shibata M, Tominaga J, et al. Efficacy of neuroendoscopic procedures in minimally invasive preferential management of pineal region tumors: a prospective study. J Neurosurg 2000; 93(2): 245–53.

64. Clark AJ, Sughrue ME, Ivan ME, et al. Factors influencing overall survival rates for patients with pineocytoma. J Neurooncol 2010; 100(2): 255–60.

65. Clark AJ, Ivan ME, Sughrue ME, et al. Tumor control after surgery and radiotherapy for pineocytoma. J Neurosurg 2010; 113(2): 319–24.

66. Bruce JN, Ogden AT. Surgical strategies for treating patients with pineal region tumors. J Neurooncol 2004; 69(1–3): 221–36.

67. Shin HJ, Cho BK, Jung HW, Wang KC. Pediatric pineal tumors: need for a direct surgical approach and complications of the occipital transtentorial approach. Childs Nerv Syst 1998; 14(4–5): 174–8.

68. Demetri GD, van Oosterom AT, Garrett CR, et al. Efficacy and safety of sunitinib in patients with advanced gastrointestinal stromal tumour after failure of imatinib: a randomised controlled trial. Lancet 2006; 368(9544): 1329–38.

69. Cuccia V, Rodríguez F, Palma F, Zuccaro G. Pinealoblastomas in children. Childs Nerv Syst 2006; 22(6): 577–85.

70. Mehta MP, Chang SM, Guha A, Newton HB, Vogelbaum MA. *Principles and Practice of Neuro-oncology: A Multidisciplinary Approach.* New York: Demos Medical, 2010.

71. Bernstein M, Berger M. *Neuro-oncology: The Essentials.* New York: Thieme Medical Publishers, 2008.

72. Jakacki RI, Zeltzer PM, Boyett JM, et al. Survival and prognostic factors following radiation and/or chemotherapy for primitive neuroectodermal tumors of the pineal region in infants and children: a report of the Childrens Cancer Group. J Clin Oncol 1995; 13(6): 1377–83.

73. Reddy AT, Janss AJ, Phillips PC, Weiss HL, Packer RJ. Outcome for children with supratentorial primitive neuroectodermal tumors treated with surgery, radiation, and chemotherapy. Cancer 2000; 88(9): 2189–93.

74. Lee JY, Wakabayashi T, Yoshida J. Management and survival of pineoblastoma: an analysis of 34 adults from the brain tumor registry of Japan. Neurol Med Chir (Tokyo) 2005; 45(3): 132–41.

75. Gilheeney SW, Saad A, Chi S, et al. Outcome of pediatric pineoblastoma after surgery, radiation and chemotherapy. J Neurooncol 2008; 89(1): 89–95.

76. Rutkowski S, von Hoff K, Emser A, et al. Survival and prognostic factors of early childhood medulloblastoma: an international meta-analysis. J Clin Oncol 2010; 28(33): 4961–8.

77. Jenkin D, Goddard K, Armstrong D, et al. Posterior fossa medulloblastoma in childhood: treatment results and a proposal for a new staging system. Int J Radiat Oncol Biol Phys 1990; 19(2): 265–74.

78. Chan AW, Tarbell NJ, Black PM, et al. Adult medulloblastoma: prognostic factors and patterns of relapse. Neurosurgery 2000; 47(3): 623–31.

79. Stoiber EM, Schaible B, Herfarth K, et al. Long term outcome of adolescent and adult patients with pineal parenchymal tumors treated with fractionated radiotherapy between 1982 and 2003 – a single institution's experience. Radiat Oncol 2010; 5: 122.

80. Kano H, Niranjan A, Kondziolka D, Flickinger JC, Lunsford D. Role of stereotactic radiosurgery in the management of pineal parenchymal tumors. Prog Neurol Surg 2009; 23: 44–58.

81. Reyns N, Hayashi M, Chinot O, et al. The role of Gamma Knife radiosurgery in the treatment of pineal parenchymal tumours. Acta Neurochir (Wien) 2006; 148(1): 5–11; discussion 11.

82. Mori Y, Kobayashi T, Hasegawa T, Yoshida K, Kida Y. Stereotactic radiosurgery for pineal and related tumors. Prog Neurol Surg 2009; 23: 106–18.

83. Kobayashi T, Kida Y, Mori Y. Stereotactic gamma radiosurgery for pineal and related tumors. J Neurooncol 2001; 54(3): 301–9.

84. Lekovic GP, Gonzalez LF, Shetter AG, et al. Role of Gamma Knife surgery in the management of pineal region tumors. Neurosurg Focus 2007; 23(6): E12.

85. Lutterbach J, Fauchon F, Schild SE, et al. Malignant pineal parenchymal tumors in adult patients: patterns of care and prognostic factors. Neurosurgery 2002; 51(1): 44–55.

86. Schild SE, Scheithauer BW, Haddock MG, et al. Histologically confirmed pineal tumors and other germ cell tumors of the brain. Cancer 1996; 78(12): 2564–71.

87. Fuller BG, Kapp DS, Cox R. Radiation therapy of pineal region tumors: 25 new cases and a review of 208 previously reported cases. Int J Radiat Oncol Biol Phys 1994; 28(1): 229–45.

88. Geyer JR, Zeltzer PM, Boyett JM, et al. Survival of infants with primitive neuroectodermal tumors or malignant ependymomas of the CNS treated with eight drugs in 1 day: a report from the Childrens Cancer Group. J Clin Oncol 1994; 12(8): 1607–15.

89. Mikaeloff Y, Raquin MA, Lellouch-Tubiana A, et al. Primitive cerebral neuroectodermal tumors excluding medulloblastomas: a retrospective study of 30 cases. Pediatr Neurosurg 1998; 29(4): 170–7.

90. Cohen BH, Zeltzer PM, Boyett JM, et al. Prognostic factors and treatment results for supratentorial primitive neuroectodermal tumors in children using radiation and chemotherapy: a Childrens Cancer Group randomized trial. J Clin Oncol 1995; 13(7): 1687–96.

91. Geyer JR, Sposto R, Jennings M, et al. Multiagent chemotherapy and deferred radiotherapy in infants with malignant brain tumors: a report from the Children's Cancer Group. J Clin Oncol 2005; 23(30): 7621–31.

92. Hinkes BG, von Hoff K, Deinlein F, et al. Childhood pineoblastoma: experiences from the prospective multicenter trials HIT-SKK87, HIT-SKK92 and HIT91. J Neurooncol 2007; 81(2): 217–23.

93. Broniscer A, Nicolaides TP, Dunkel IJ, et al. High-dose chemotherapy with autologous stem-cell rescue in the treatment of patients with recurrent non-cerebellar primitive neuroectodermal tumors. Pediatr Blood Cancer 2004; 42(3): 261–7.

94. Gururangan S, McLaughlin C, Quinn J, et al. High-dose chemotherapy with autologous stem-cell rescue in children and adults with newly diagnosed pineoblastomas. J Clin Oncol 2003; 21(11): 2187–91.

95. Jakacki RI. Pineal and nonpineal supratentorial primitive neuroectodermal tumors. Childs Nerv Syst 1999; 15(10): 586–91.

96. Duffner PK, Cohen ME, Sanford RA, et al. Lack of efficacy of postoperative chemotherapy and delayed radiation in very young children with pineoblastoma. Pediatric Oncology Group. Med Pediatr Oncol 1995; 25(1): 38–44.

61 Craniopharyngiomas

Gazanfar Rahmathulla,[1] John J. Park,[2] and Gene H. Barnett[1]

[1] Rose Ella Burkhardt Brain Tumor and Neuro-Oncology Center, Cleveland Clinic, Cleveland, OH, USA
[2] Texas Spine and Neurosurgery Center, Methodist Sugar Land Hospital, Sugar Land, TX, USA

Introduction

Craniopharyngiomas (CPs) are slow-growing, histologically benign, sellar, and suprasellar tumors whose location and adherence to surrounding critical structures often result in a malignant course of endocrinological, behavioral, and visual abnormalities leading ultimately to premature death. In 1904, Jakob Erdheim described this as a "hypophyseal duct tumor"[1] and subsequently Harvey Cushing coined the term "craniopharyngioma,"[2] thus establishing it as a distinctly separate tumor arising in the pituitary region. It has been postulated to arise from the hypophyseal duct or Rathke's pouch,[3] a theory that remains popular today.

Complete microsurgical resection is the traditional goal of treatment and may lead to cure.[4–6] However, due to the critical location and adherent nature of these lesions, such an aggressive approach can be fraught with hazards and lead to debilitating outcomes. In the 1950s operative mortality rates varied between 10% and 40%[7] but subsequent advances in neurosurgical techniques brought this down to between 0% and 10%.[8,9] The propensity of these tumors to recur following gross total resection can be as high as 57%, necessitating the use of alternative treatment modalities for tumor control. A multitude of therapeutic options has therefore been developed[10–14] to manage these lesions, and controversy still exists with regard to optimal therapy. In this chapter, we will review the nature of these rare tumors, consider various management options, discuss their use alone and in combination, and make recommendations regarding contemporary management.

Anatomy

Craniopharyngiomas are tumors of the sellar, suprasellar, and/or anterior third ventricle regions along the path of development of Rathke's pouch.[3,4,15] Most CPs arise near the infundibular stalk, in intimate connection to the hypothalamus and optic apparatus (Fig. 61.1), as well as the major arteries in the region such as the internal carotid arteries. While sellar tumors are supplied by small vessels arising from the adjacent dura of the cavernous sinus, suprasellar CPs are directly supplied by small branches of the arteries of the anterior diencephalon. These include the anterior cerebral artery, the anterior communicating artery, and the posterior communicating artery. They generally are not supplied by the posterior circulation (i.e. posterior cerebral arteries and vertebrobasilar distribution), a fact that has important surgical connotations.

Surgeons typically categorize CPs as sellar, prechiasmatic, and retrochiasmatic because of implications regarding surgical approach. Radiographically, about three-quarters of CPs are suprasellar, 20% are sellar and suprasellar, while only about 5% are entirely sellar in nature. They may also occur in the optic chiasm or third ventricle, and even in the nasopharynx, pineal regions, or sphenoid bone.[16]

Embryology and epidemiology

In the third to fourth weeks of gestation, the ectoderm of the stomodeum (roof of the oral cavity) invaginates toward the diencephalon to meet the downwardly projecting infundibular bud, thus forming the primitive craniopharyngeal duct. Rathke's pouch is then formed as the development of the sphenoid bone pinches off the invagination from the pharyngeal epithelium. The pouch then surrounds the infundibulum and subsequently goes on to form the adenohypophysis. It is believed by many that embryonic rests of cells that would otherwise be destined to become tooth buds or oral epithelium may be deposited during this development along the craniopharyngeal duct and are responsible for the development of CPs. CPs are true cystic tumors and should not be confused with Rathke's cleft cysts, although these may also have embryonic origins. Some adult tumors with squamous papillary pathology (see below) may arise by different mechanisms.[4,17]

Craniopharyngiomas may be diagnosed at any age, although there is a bimodal distribution (Fig. 61.2)[18] with peaks in childhood (5–14 years) and later years (50–74 years). The

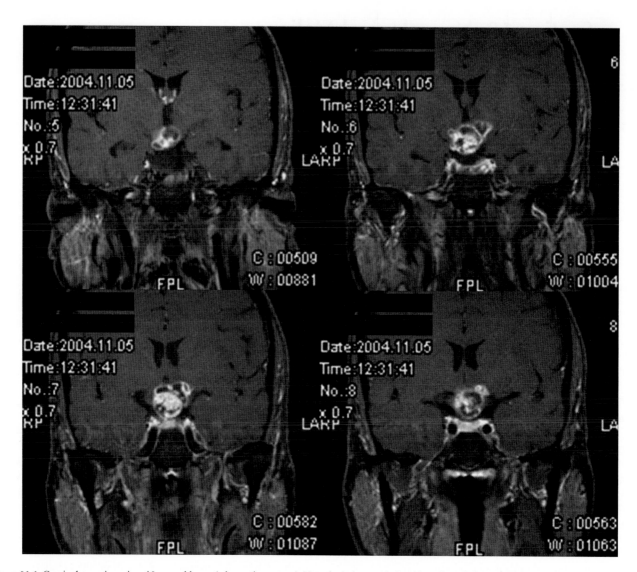

Figure 61.1 Craniopharyngioma in a 46-year-old man (adamantinomatous). Note the intimate relationship to hypothalamus and optic pathways.

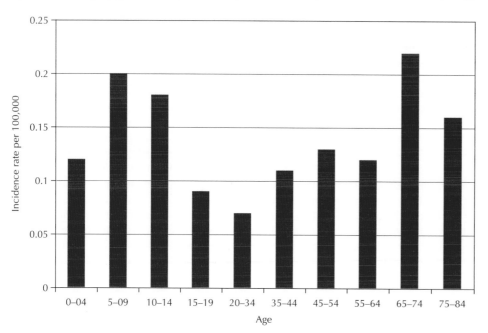

Figure 61.2 Age distribution of craniopharyngioma in 135 cases compiled by the Central Brain Tumor Registry of the United States (CBTRUS), 1990–1993. Reproduced with permission from Bunin et al.[18]

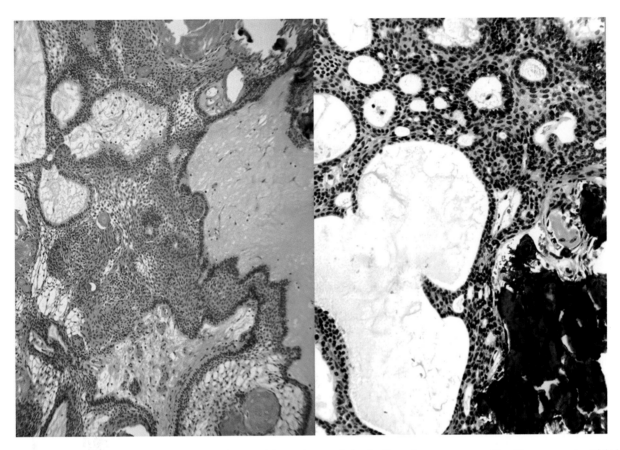

Figure 61.3 Histology of adamantinomatous craniopharyngioma. Left image shows typical palisading columnar squamous cells with spongy center. Right image shows flattened epithelium lining a cyst with calcification at bottom right.

overall incidence is about 0.5–2.5 per 100,000 person-years and is independent of gender or race, although there are some data suggesting male predominance in childhood[19] and an increased incidence in Japanese children. Approximately 338 cases of CP are expected to occur annually in the United States, with 96 occurring in children from 0 to 14 years of age. They constitute about 5–10% of all childhood tumors but less than 1% of adult intracranial tumors. Of parasellar tumors, they represent 50% in children and 20% in adults.

Although there have been a few reports of occurrences in siblings, there is no known genetic predisposition to CPs. Reports on the molecular characteristics of these tumors have been largely unrevealing to date but mutations in the *CTNNB1* gene that codes for β-catenin protein have been associated with adamantinomatous CPs.

Pathology

Craniopharyngiomas are typically composed of a combination of solid portions with a benign histology and cystic components to a greater or lesser degree.[4] Their size at diagnosis is variable, and it is not uncommon for tumors to be larger than 5 cm when discovered. They are World Health Organization (WHO) grade 1 tumors, indicating that they are potentially curable with complete surgical resection. The tumor elicits an intense glial reaction from the adjacent hypothalamus, optic pathways, and infundibulum and may be particularly adherent to these and

nearby vessels. These points of attachment often limit the role of surgery or contribute to postoperative morbidity.

Two distinct histopathologies are found – the adamantinomatous and the papillary varieties. The former is found in childhood CPs and in about half of adult-onset tumors, and is composed of ribbons and bands of palisaded, columnar, or polygonal epithelial cells around the periphery of these structures and internally more loosely arranged with spongy architecture. The cysts may be lined with flattened epithelium (Fig. 61.3). This pattern resembles the adamantinomatous pattern of tooth buds and leads to the initial postulates that the tumors are derived from Rathke's duct. "Wet" keratin, calcifications, and cholesterol deposits are also common. The cysts are laden with oily brown, cholesterol-rich fluid, and microscopic tumor projections into the adjacent brain occur frequently. The adamantinomatous tumor is usually separated from adjacent parenchyma by a gliotic reaction varying in thickness, hence creating a safe plane for a more complete surgical resection when present.[20–22]

The squamous papillary variety occurs almost exclusively in adults with a predilection for involving the third ventricle.[23] It is composed of sheets of squamous epithelium forming pseudopapillae and papillae resembling metaplastic respiratory epithelium (Fig. 61.4).[24,25] Cysts are typically lined with simple squamous epithelium and lack the machine oil quality. Calcifications are rare. These tumors may derive from cell rests attempting to differentiate into oral mucosa or from

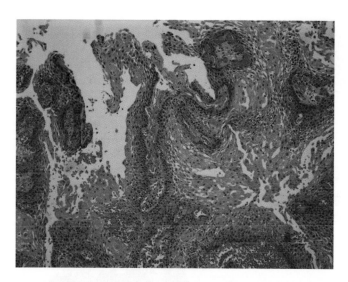

Figure 61.4 Histology of squamous papillary craniopharyngioma. The image shows solid epithelium in papillary architecture without stellate zones. They are solid, few small cysts with minimal dark oily fluid as compared to the adamantinomatous type.

squamous cells present in the adult sellar region. The absence of cysts and calcification in papillary tumors increases the likelihood of a gross total resection, although the risk of recurrence and response to radiotherapy (RT) remain the same following subtotal resections (STR).[26,27]

Labeling indices such as MIB-1 are typically <2% and of limited predictive value regarding behavior except when >7% where recurrence is considered likely. Spontaneous malignant transformation and metastases are said not to occur but seeding along biopsy or surgical tracts has been reported, as well as a report of distant leptomeningeal metastasis after surgical resection.[28] Radiation-induced conversion to squamous carcinoma has also been reported.[29]

Clinical presentation and diagnostic considerations

Presenting symptoms of CP are due to compression of the adjacent structures, namely the optic apparatus causing visual symptoms, the pituitary stalk and gland giving rise to endocrinological symptoms, hypothalamic compression causing behavioral disorders and when large and obstructing cerebrospinal fluid (CSF) outflow secondary to ventricular compression causes symptoms of raised intracranial pressure (ICP) such as headaches.[6,30]

Adults are more likely to present with symptoms of visual impairment or endocrinological abnormalities than children. Visual disturbances are particularly prevalent in adults, with findings indicating the pattern of growth of these tumors and commonly including bitemporal hemianopsia, homonymous hemianopsia, or unilateral and bilateral decreased acuity or blindness. Children usually tolerate gradual visual field changes and are not symptomatic until their vision is significantly compromised. In one series, formal visual field testing showed visual compromise in 74.5% of patients at the time of diagnosis. Visual impairment was particularly noted in

patients scheduled for transcranial surgery as opposed to those scheduled for transsphenoidal surgery (84.3 versus 42.9%). Papilledema is found in 29% of adults at presentation and in about 20% of children.[31]

Endocrinological symptoms are the presenting complaints in about 30% of adults, although testing may reveal hormonal abnormalities in 80–90% of individuals. Gonadal insufficiency causes loss of libido and reduced masculine hair growth in adult males and secondary dysmenorrhea in women. Hyperprolactinemia occurs in 20% of patients due to compression of the hypothalamus or pituitary stalk and the decrease in the normally inhibitory effect on pituitary prolactin release. Diabetes insipidus is seen in 9–17% of patients prior to surgery. Other endocrinological abnormalities include hypothyroidism and secondary adrenal insufficiency.

Hypothalamic disturbances can include central hyperphagia with obesity, disturbances of thirst, and alterations in sleep cycles but tend to affect adults less frequently than children. On the other hand, mental disturbance is more commonly seen in adults than in children, with more than 30% of patients older than 45 years of age suffering from dementia or intermittent confusion, apathy, depression, or psychomotor slowing. Increased intracranial pressure and obstructive hydrocephalus secondary to upward tumor growth into the third ventricle are seen more frequently in children than in adults. In one series, only 29% of adult patients had evidence of hydrocephalus at presentation, compared to over 50% in pediatric patients. In addition, headache (80% versus 30%), nausea or vomiting (60% versus 20%), and short stature (30% versus 15%) are more common in children than adults.[4] The combination of progressive visual disturbance with endocrinological disorder should suggest a possible lesion in the sellar or suprasellar region such as CP.

Imaging

Contemporary neuroimaging studies such as computed tomography (CT) and magnetic resonance imaging (MRI) have greatly facilitated the radiographic diagnosis of these lesions compared to the era limited to pneumoencephalography, angiograms, and skull x-rays where displacement of the ventricles and vessels, and suprasellar calcifications or sellar erosions, often suggested the diagnosis of CP. The radiographic hallmark of CP is an enhancing solid/cystic lesion in the sellar, suprasellar, and/or anterior third ventricle. Adamantinomatous lesions are typically mixed solid/cystic and calcified on CT scan, whereas papillary lesions are often isodense, solid, and rarely show calcifications. Almost all CPs enhance after administration of intravenous contrast[32] (Fig. 61.5). On MRI, the tumors are usually heterointense with cystic components varying in signal intensity on T1-weighted imaging. T2 and fluid-attenuated inversion recovery (FLAIR) images characteristically demonstrate high signal in the cysts, variable signal in the solid component, and high signal in the adjacent brain, which may indicate gliosis, edema from compression of the optic chiasm or tracts, tumor invasion, and irritation from leaking fluid[33] (Fig. 61.6). Magnetic resonance spectroscopy (MRS) demonstrates high lipid content in the cystic components.

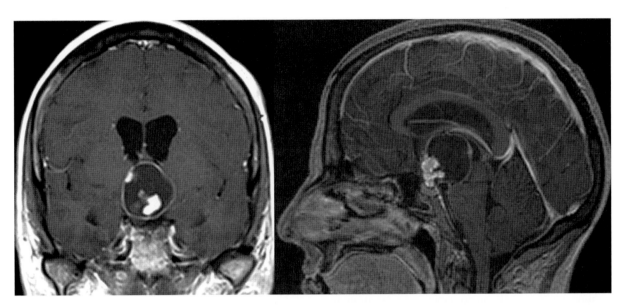

Figure 61.5 Magnetic resonance imaging scans. The left side reveals a coronal T1 contrast enhanced image and the right a sagittal contrast enhanced image with a large sellar suprasellar mixed cystic lesion containing a solid enhancing nodule within it. Suprasellar extension is noted to cause compression of the optic chiasm, and retrochiasmatic extension of the cystic component into the posterior fossa is noted to cause brainstem compression.

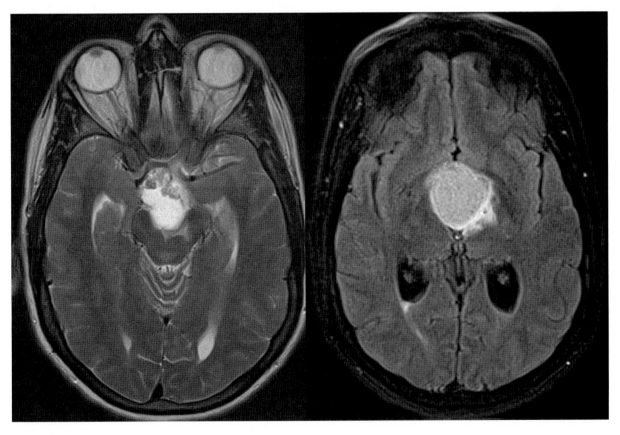

Figure 61.6 Axial T2 image on the left and FLAIR on the right revealing a hyperintense cystic lesion with a solid nodule within the cyst. The mass is compressing the adjacent optic apparatus anteriorly and the brainstem is deformed posteriorly.

These two imaging modalities complement each other, with CT providing information about the bony anatomy of the skull base and presence of calcifications, whereas the MRI provides three-dimensional (3D) information about the tumor in relation to the adjacent neuroanatomical structures such as the optic apparatus, pituitary gland, and diencephalic structures, essential to deciding the best approach in treating these tumors.

Table 61.1 Radiographic differential diagnosis of craniopharyngiomas.

Lesion	Distinguishing feature(s)
Rathke's cleft cyst	Does not enhance, no solid component, less heterogeneous
Pituitary adenoma	Confluent enhancement (unless hemorrhagic and cystic), sellar origin
Arachnoid cyst	Does not enhance, no calcifications
Epidermoid/dermoid cysts	Nonenhancing, low CT density, MRI diffusion changes
Pilocytic/infiltrating astrocytoma of chiasm or hypothalamus	Solid or microcystic, robust enhancement, not calcified, possible necrosis
Xanthoastrocytoma	Adolescent age group
Thrombosed aneurysm	MRI flow changes, blood products

CT, computed tomography; MRI, magnetic resonance imaging.

Box 61.1 Minimum preoperative neuroendocrine assessment.

- Detailed clinical history and examination including fluid intake and output
- Plasma and urine electrolytes and osmolality
- Serum urea and electrolytes
- Thyroid function tests (free T3, T4 and thyroid stimulating hormone)
- Morning cortisol (if patient is not on maintenance doses of steroids)
- Prolactin levels
- Insulin-like growth factor-1
- Follicle stimulating hormone/luteinizing hormone

Reproduced with permission from Hopper et al.[34]

Conventional CT or MR angiography may be used for preoperative planning and better visualization of the vasculature in relation to the tumor, showing displaced and/or encased vessels, but is usually of little benefit. The radiographic differential diagnosis is shown in Table 61.1.

Medical and endocrinological evaluation

In view of the clinical presentation, a complete evaluation prior to treatment consists of a neuroophthalmological, neuroendocrine workup along with neuropsychological evaluation in children and appropriate radiological imaging. These tests are not diagnostic of CP *per se* but when suggestive of a visual, pituitary, and/or hypothalamic dysfunction, they can help localize the lesion and direct preoperative management. The neuroophthalmological exam consists of visual field and acuity charting and a fundus examination to look for papilledema.

Neuroendocrine assessment is essential to identify baseline hormonal levels and the need for appropriate replacement during the course of the treatment (Box 61.1). The common endocrine abnormalities include evidence of one or more insufficiencies of the anterior pituitary (adenohypophyseal) products (adrenocorticotropic hormone, thyroid stimulating hormone, luteinizing hormone, follicle stimulating hormone, growth hormone/insulin-like growth factor-1) and/or mild overproduction of prolactin due to disruption of physiological infundibular inhibition of prolactin production (also known as the "stalk effect"). Patients may also exhibit diabetes insipidus due to posterior pituitary dysfunction and an inability to concentrate urine.

Neuropsychological evaluation, although not routinely required in adults, may be necessary in children who more often present with cognitive changes, psychomotor decline, and personality disturbances.

Neuroimaging with CT and MRI is essential to plan the best surgical approach and assess the ventricles for hydrocephalus, as well as to discuss the potential complications and differential diagnosis with the patient and family.

The impact on preoperative management is discussed below.

Treatment

Controversy continues over the best way to treat CPs. Various therapeutic strategies exist, which can be combined to create a multimodality approach individualized to each patient. Microsurgical resection continues to remain the mainstay of treatment with other adjuvant modalities combined to minimize recurrence and symptomatic progression following surgery. Aggressive and complete surgical resection would be ideal for achieving a complete cure but the benefits must be weighed against the potential for significant complications.

Pretreatment management

Prior to beginning therapy, a medical and endocrine evaluation as described in the previous section should be performed in order to address the spectrum of symptoms brought on by these lesions.[4,15] The potential for damage to the optic apparatus and the need to correct underlying hormonal deficiencies prior to and following surgery are essential components in the overall management of these patients. In cases where pituitary dysfunction is present, steroid administration will be required perioperatively for those undergoing surgery. Hydrocephalus may require shunting for cerebrospinal fluid diversion, although normalization of ventricular size is often seen following efficacious treatment of the tumor.

Surgery

The traditional management of these tumors is aggressive microsurgical resection. Numerous surgical approaches have been described for the resection of these lesions, detailed descriptions of which are beyond the scope of this chapter. Choice of an approach is dictated primarily by the location of the tumor.[35–37] The subfrontal approach (below the frontal lobes) is the most commonly employed and allows good visualization of both optic nerves and the internal carotid artery. The pterional (frontotemporal) approach provides a shorter trajectory to the parasellar space along the Sylvian fissure and lateral sphenoid wing. The subtemporal (below the temporal lobes) approach is rarely used for these lesions, and is

Table 61.2 Summary of results of conventional radiotherapy (CRT) on craniopharyngiomas.

Authors	Patients	Treatment	Median dose (Gy)	Tumor size (mL)	Follow-up (months)	Control (%)	Complications (%)
Regine[59]	58	CRT	56–62	NA	17 years	82 at 10 years	NA
Rajan[60]	173	CRT	50	NA	12	83 & 79 at 10 & 20 years	50
Hetelekidis[61a]	37	CRT	54	NA	49	86 at 10 years	60
Habrand[62a]	37	CRT	50	NA	NA	78 & 56.5 at 5 & 10 years	40
Merchant[38a]	15	CRT	54	NA	72	94 at 5 years	80
Moon[63]	50	CRT	54	12	12.8 years	96 & 91 at 5 & 10 years	15
Merchant[64a]	28	CRT	55	NA	36	90 at 3 years	NA

[a] series of adult patients treated with CRT not inclusive of any pediatric cases.

primarily for unilateral retrochiasmatic tumors. The transsphenoidal or endoscopic (via the nose) approaches are ideal for tumors confined to the sellar or suprasellar region or with a significant cystic component.[11]

Although the potential for cure is maximized by aggressive initial surgical resection, complete resection is not a guarantee for cure (so-called "false cures") and often cannot be attained without considerable morbidity. Overall surgical mortality ranges between 0% and 4% in recent large surgical series, with a notable rate of 16.7% in a series by Yasargil *et al.* where aggressive total resection (ATR) was performed in all patients.[35] Aggressive surgery also appears to increase the risk of serious morbidities including visual, other neurological, behavioral, and endocrinological (particularly diabetes insipidus).[38–40] Location may also contribute to the morbidity of ATR as lesions in the third ventricle may also have a mortality of about 17%.[41] Subtotal resection (STR) is often dictated by tumor adherence to vital neurovascular structures and the desire to minimize morbidity.[8] In this setting, ATRs are achieved in about 50–60% of cases by the transcranial routes.[42]

More minimally invasive approaches have become increasingly popular in an effort to reduce surgical discomfort, morbidity, and recovery time. These include "keyhole" approaches through eyebrow incisions,[43,44] endoscopic procedures for sellar[45] and even suprasellar lesions,[30–32] stereotactic or endoscopic placement of drainage or delivery catheters for the management of CP cysts[46] and stereotactic biopsy for the purposes of diagnosis and cyst drainage.[47,48] There is a growing trend of combining minimally invasive stereotactic surgical procedures with drug or radiation (interstitial, fractionated radiotherapy, stereotactic radiosurgery [SRS]) treatments for a multimodality approach of maintaining lesion control at minimum risk.[49]

Radiotherapy

Radiation for CPs is traditionally delivered via external fractionated delivery in total doses ranging from 50 to 60 Gy.[50,51] Such radiotherapy is rarely used alone for the treatment of these lesions[52] but is used most commonly after STR at the time of tumor recurrence,[53] with results that are typically superior to reoperation (Table 61.2). There appears to be no clear benefit in terms of local control or survival for using radiation after gross total resection; however, there is good evidence to support its use after STR, with 5- and 10-year survivals of about

70% and 65% respectively in one series.[54] Less clear is the timing of treatment after STR – empirically if incomplete or waiting until progression/recurrence. There appears to be no difference in survival between either of these approaches, so many advocate the latter delayed approach to minimize the risk of late radiation toxicities such as cognitive impairment, malignant transformation, or induction of benign[55] or malignant secondary tumors.[56] An advance in the external delivery of fractionated radiation is the use of stereotactic techniques – so-called stereotactic radiotherapy which allows more conformal delivery, limiting collateral damage to surrounding structures.

Even with control of the solid tumor by surgery or radiotherapy, growth of existing or development of new cysts can lead to progressive neurological dysfunction. Intracavitary use of radioactive solutions delivered using stereotactically directed catheters and, at times, subcutaneous Ommaya reservoirs appears to be an important tool in the management of tumor cysts.[57,58] Such therapeutic agents include phosphorus-32, yttrium-90, iridium-192, gold-198 colloid, and iodine-125.

Radiosurgery

More controversial than the issues pertaining to radiotherapy and CPs is the use of SRS in the management of new or recurrent CPs. SRS is a combined surgical/radiation oncology technique where high-dose radiation is delivered to a small volume in a single (or few) session(s) with the intention of ablating or inactivating the target, using the precision of image-guided stereotactic techniques to direct this energy, sparing nearby structures. There are certain radiobiological advantages of SRS over fractionated radiotherapy for benign lesions[65] but there is also concern about possible injury to the optic nerves and hypothalamus for certain CPs. Nonetheless, there is a blossoming literature (Table 61.3) supporting the use of SRS for newly diagnosed, incompletely resected, or recurrent tumors. SRS may be used alone or in combination with other techniques such as preoperative cyst aspiration (to reduce the size of the tumor) or interstitial radiotherapy (to better control cysts).[66–68] Some advocate using SRS only for sellar CPs.[69] Regardless, tumor doses should be at least 6 if not 9.5 Gy[68] with dose to the optic nerves and chiasm no more than 8–10 Gy (the less the better).[70,71] Risk of postoperative visual or endocrinological deficits is typically less than 4% with extended (12-year) tumor control of about 85% when adhering

Authors	Patients	Treatment	Marginal dose (Gy)	Follow-up (years)	Tumor control rate %	Complications
Prasad[67]	9	GKRS	13	NA	88	No data
Chung[72]	31	GKRS	12	3	87	2/31
Amendola[73]	14	GKRS	14	3.3	86	None
Ulfarsson[68]	21	GKRS	3–25	13.6	33	No data
Kobayashi[14]	98	GKRS	11	5.5	80	6

FSRT, fractionated stereotactic radiotherapy; GKRS, gamma knife radiosurgery.

Table 61.3 Reported results of gamma knife radiosurgery (GKRS) for craniopharyngiomas.

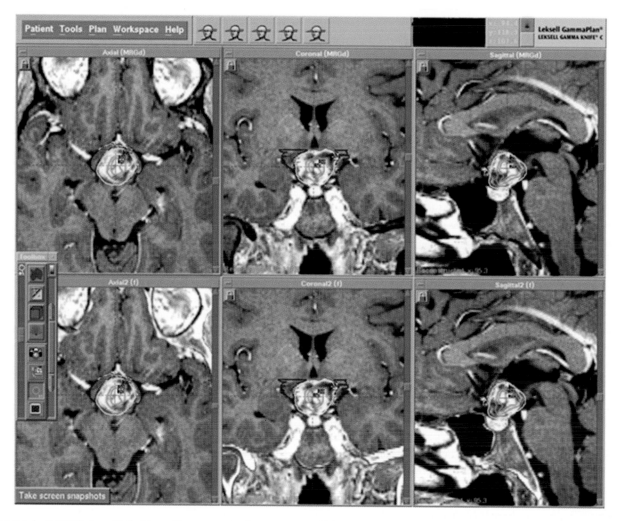

Figure 61.7 Leksell GKRS plan with the blue outline representing the optic nerves which are the organ at risk (to be protected from radiation) in the treatment plan. The red boundary outlines the tumor contour, with the 90% isodose line represented in green and the 55% isodose line in yellow.

to these parameters. Figure 61.7 shows the treatment plan of a patient treated with gamma-knife radiosurgery.

Chemotherapy

The principal use of chemotherapy for CPs is for control of tumoral cysts or for surgical/radiation failures of the lesion as a whole. Intratumoral bleomycin (typically intracystic delivery, 3 mg every other day) may help control otherwise intractable cyst expansion.[74] Extracavitary extravasation of the drug,

however, can cause blindness or even death, tempering enthusiasm for this approach.[75]

Systemic chemotherapy may be of benefit in some otherwise treatment-refractory cases of CP. Reported successes have been achieved with a combination of vincristine, carmustine (BCNU) and procarbazine, or doxorubicin and lomustine (CCNU)[76], and also with a cisplatin-based regimen.[77] The identification of estrogen receptors in some of these tumors has not yet translated into successful treatments exploiting this finding.[78]

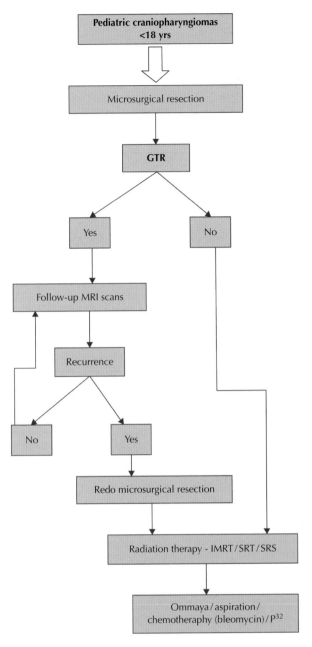

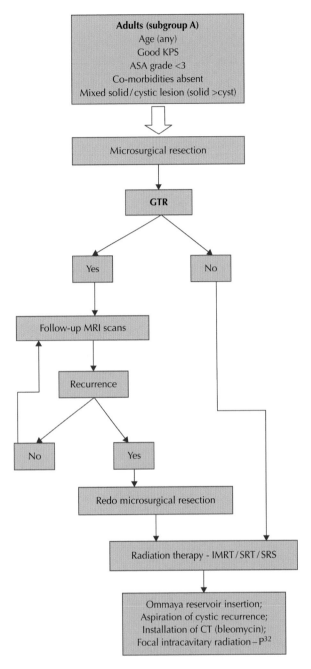

Figure 61.8 Algorithm for the management of pediatric patients (<18 years). The goal would be a GTR. If this is achieved, the child will subsequently require regular clinical follow-up and imaging at 3-month intervals for about a year and then at 6-month intervals for 2–3 years and then yearly. In recurrent disease appropriate treatment options should be chosen based on the age and tolerance to various therapies.

Figure 61.9 Algorithm for the management of adult patients with no comorbidities. GTR is the goal of surgery and if achieved, observation and MR imaging are performed at regular intervals. In case of a STR, radiation therapy is the treatment of choice if reoperation is not possible. Recurrent disease can be treated using aspiration if there is a cystic recurrence, Ommaya insertion or chemotherapy instillations into the cyst cavity are available options.

Recommendations

Because of the heterogeneous locations, histologies, and age populations, no single strategy is appropriate for all CPs. We have proposed a simple algorithm which outlines our approach to CPs in the pediatric (<18 years) and adult population (Figs 61.8–61.10). In the pediatric population (see Fig. 61.8), the goal would be to achieve a gross total resection (GTR) and to follow up with close observation clinically and with imaging every 3 months for about a year and then at 6-month intervals or

longer, depending on the interval since surgery. In adult patients without any significant comorbidity and with a good Karnofsky performance status (KPS), microsurgical resection with a goal of achieving a GTR would be the preferred treatment. If a GTR is achieved and postoperative imaging reveals no evidence of any residual component of tumor, the patients can be followed up with observation and imaging at regular intervals (see Fig. 61.9). In cases where a STR has been achieved, the patient is followed

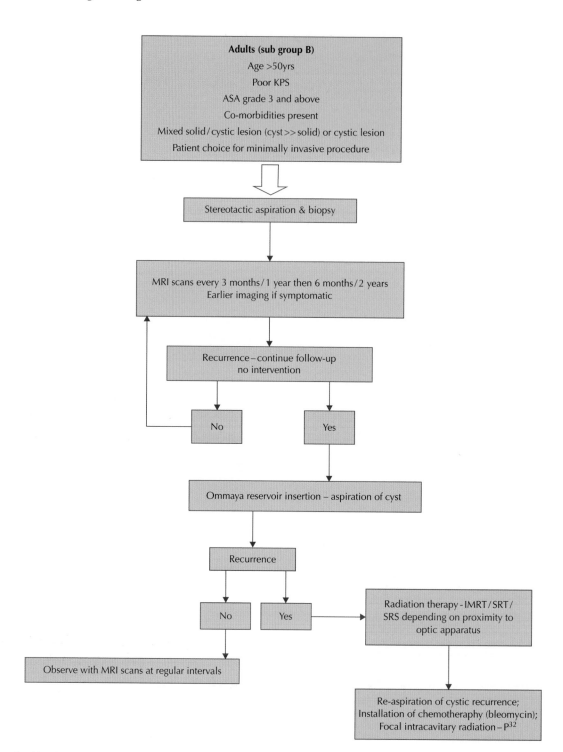

Figure 61.10 Algorithm for management of a subset of adult patients (subset B) with associated comorbidities or requiring minimally invasive therapeutic options.

up with imaging in 3–6 months and they receive adjuvant focal radiation therapy (intensity-modulated radiotherapy [IMRT], GKRS or SRS), depending on the size and proximity to the optic apparatus.

At our institute, in a selected subgroup of patients who may not be able to tolerate a craniotomy, have poor KPS or American Society of Anesthesiologists (ASA) physical status grading and elect to have an alternative approach, we use our minimally invasive paradigm. This includes using a combination of

procedures such as cyst aspiration, focal radiotherapy techniques (GKRS, SRS or IMRT), and Ommaya reservoir insertion. Our algorithm is described in Figure 61.10 and is based on our personal experience and outcomes. To date, we have treated 11 patients with one or all the above-mentioned procedures, and on long-term follow-up (1–10 years) have had good results without any procedural mortality or morbidity. Because of the small number of patients, inadequate data exist to formulate guidelines, so there are no level I or II data to create a generalized algorithm to treat craniopharyngiomas and every case has to be individualized in its approach, depending on the presenting variables.

Some generalities are probably valid, despite the lack of any level I evidence in this disorder. Patients with sellar lesions can be well managed with transsphenoidal microsurgery or endoscopic surgery, or high-precision SRS (such as with the GKRS, Elekta Medical Instruments, Stockholm, Sweden). Microsurgical resection (tempered with the fallback of STR if too adherent to critical structures) should be considered for suprasellar lesions, with or without endoscopic techniques. Third ventricular tumors, particularly if they show adjacent brain changes, may best be approached by a multimodality approach of stereotactic aspiration, high-precision SRS, and intracavitary treatment for progressive cysts. Radiotherapy should probably be reserved for progressive or progressive subtotally resected lesions. It is likely that the role of multimodality minimally invasive stereotactic techniques will become even more prevalent as patients demand lower risk, less invasive approaches to management of intracranial disease.

Prognosis

In a review by Bunin et al.[18] of the National Cancer Data Base (NCDB), of the 63,252 intracranial tumors operated on between 1985 to 1992, data on 285 CP patients was analyzed by them, with the overall 5-year survival rate being 80%. However, age was a significant negative prognostic factor with 5-year survivals of 99%, 79%, and 37% for individuals diagnosed at ages of less than 20, 20–64, and 65 years or older, respectively. Survival in children appears to have improved over time. In our series of adult patients treated with a minimally invasive approach (cyst drainage±Ommaya±SRS/IMRT), 5-year survival rates have reached 100% and do not mirror the results of the NCDB.

References

1. Erdheim J. Ueber hypophysengangsgeschwulste und hirncholesteratome. Akad Wiss Wien 1904; 113: 537–726.
2. Cushing H. Intracranial tumours. J Nervous Mental Dis 1932; 76: 539.
3. Mott FW, Barratt JOW. Three cases of tumour of the third ventricle. Arch Neurol London 1907; 1: 417.
4. Carmel P. Craniopharyngiomas. New York: McGraw-Hill, 1985.
5. Matson DD, Crigler JF Jr. Management of craniopharyngioma in childhood. J Neurosurg 1969; 30: 377–90.
6. Moore KD CW. Craniopharyngioma. New York: Thieme Medical Publishers, 2000.
7. Backlund EO. Treatment of craniopharyngiomas: the multimodality approach. Pediatr Neurosurg 1994; 21(Suppl 1): 82–9.
8. Fahlbusch R, Honegger J, Paulus W, Huk W, Buchfelder M. Surgical treatment of craniopharyngiomas: experience with 168 patients. J Neurosurg 1999; 90: 237–50.
9. Baskin DS, Wilson CB. Surgical management of craniopharyngiomas. A review of 74 cases. J Neurosurg 1986; 65: 22–7.
10. Barajas MA, Ramirez-Guzman G, Rodriguez-Vazquez C, et al. Multimodal management of craniopharyngiomas: neuroendoscopy, microsurgery, and radiosurgery. J Neurosurg 2002; 97: 607–9.
11. Cappabianca P, Cavallo LM, Colao A, et al. Endoscopic endonasal transsphenoidal approach: outcome analysis of 100 consecutive procedures. Minim Invasive Neurosurg 2002; 45: 193–200.
12. Coffey RJ, Lunsford LD. The role of stereotactic techniques in the management of craniopharyngiomas. Neurosurg Clin North Am 1990; 1: 161–72.
13. Scott RM, Hetelekidis S, Barnes PD, Goumnerova L, Tarbell NJ. Surgery, radiation, and combination therapy in the treatment of childhood craniopharyngioma – a 20-year experience. Pediatr Neurosurg 1994; 21 (Suppl 1): 75–81.
14. Kobayashi T, Kida Y, Mori Y, Hasegawa T. Long-term results of gamma knife surgery for the treatment of craniopharyngioma in 98 consecutive cases. J Neurosurg 2005; 103: 482–8.
15. Janzer R. Craniopharyngioma. Lyon, France: IARC Press, 2000.
16. Fujimoto Y, Matsushita H, Velasco O, Rosemberg S, Plese JP, Marino R Jr. Craniopharyngioma involving the infrasellar region: a case report and review of the literature. Pediatr Neurosurg 2002; 37: 210–16.
17. Gsponer J, de Tribolet N, Deruaz JP, et al. Diagnosis, treatment, and outcome of pituitary tumors and other abnormal intrasellar masses. Retrospective analysis of 353 patients. Medicine (Baltimore) 1999; 78: 236–69.
18. Bunin GR, Surawicz TS, Witman PA, Preston-Martin S, Davis F, Bruner JM. The descriptive epidemiology of craniopharyngioma. Neurosurg Focus 1997; 3: e1.
19. Stewart AM, Lennox EL, Sanders BM. Group characteristics of children with cerebral and spinal cord tumours. Br J Cancer 1973; 28: 568–74.
20. Kobayashi T, Kageyama N, Yoshida J, Shibuya N, Yonezawa T. Pathological and clinical basis of the indications for treatment of craniopharyngiomas. Neurol Med Chir (Tokyo) 1981; 21: 39–47.
21. Hoffman HJ. Craniopharyngiomas. Can J Neurol Sci 1985; 12: 348–52.
22. Sweet WH. Radical surgical treatment of craniopharyngioma. Clin Neurosurg 1976; 23: 52–79.
23. Crotty TB, Scheithauer BW, Young WF Jr, et al. Papillary craniopharyngioma: a clinicopathological study of 48 cases. J Neurosurg 1995; 83: 206–14.
24. Russell DS, Rubinstein LJ. Pathology of Tumours of the Nervous System. Baltimore, MD: Williams and Wilkins, 1977.
25. Miller D. Pathology of craniopharyngiomas: clinical import of pathological findings. Pediatr Neurosurg 1994; 21: 11–17.
26. Albright AL, Adelson PD, Pollack IF. Principles and Practice of Pediatric Neurosurgery. New York: Thieme Medical, 2007.
27. Weiner HL, Wisoff JH, Rosenberg ME, et al. Craniopharyngiomas: a clinicopathological analysis of factors predictive of recurrence and functional outcome. Neurosurgery 1994; 35: 1001–10; discussion 10–1.
28. Gupta K, Kuhn MJ, Shevlin DW, Wacaser LE. Metastatic craniopharyngioma. Am J Neuroradiol 1999; 20: 1059–60.
29. Kristopaitis T, Thomas C, Petruzzelli GJ, Lee JM. Malignant craniopharyngioma. Arch Pathol Lab Med 2000; 124: 1356–60.
30. Carmel PW. Tumours of the third ventricle. Acta Neurochir (Wien) 1985; 75: 136–46.
31. Kaye AH, Black PML. Operative Neurosurgery. Edinburgh: Churchill Livingstone, 2000.
32. FitzPatrick M, Tartaglino LM, Hollander MD, Zimmerman RA, Flanders AE. Imaging of sellar and parasellar pathology. Radiol Clin North Am 1999; 37: 101–21, x.
33. Saeki N, Uchino Y, Murai H, et al. MR imaging study of edema-like change along the optic tract in patients with pituitary region tumors. Am J Neuroradiol 2003; 24: 336–42.
34. Hopper N, Albanese A, Ghirardello S, Maghnie M. The pre-operative endocrine assessment of craniopharyngiomas. J Pediatr Endocrinol Metab 2006; 19(Suppl 1): 325–7.
35. Yasargil MG, Curcic M, Kis M, Siegenthaler G, Teddy PJ, Roth P. Total removal of craniopharyngiomas. Approaches and long-term results in 144 patients. J Neurosurg 1990; 73: 3–11.
36. Spaziante R, de Divitiis E, Irace C, Cappabianca P, Caputi F. Management of primary or recurring grossly cystic craniopharyngiomas by means of draining systems. Topic review and 6 case reports. Acta Neurochir (Wien) 1989; 97: 95–106.

37. Choux M, Lena G. Bases of surgical management of craniopharyngioma in children [proceedings]. Acta Neurochir (Wien) 1979; 28(Suppl): 348.

38. Merchant TE, Kiehna EN, Sanford RA, et al. Craniopharyngioma: the St. Jude Children's Research Hospital experience 1984–2001. Int J Radiat Oncol Biol Phys 2002; 53: 533–42.

39. Honegger J, Barocka A, Sadri B, Fahlbusch R. Neuropsychological results of craniopharyngioma surgery in adults: a prospective study. Surg Neurol 1998; 50: 19–28; discussion 9.

40. Honegger J, Buchfelder M, Fahlbusch R. Surgical treatment of craniopharyngiomas: endocrinological results. J Neurosurg 1999; 90: 251–7.

41. Behari S, Banerji D, Mishra A, Sharma S, Chhabra DK, Jain VK. Intrinsic third ventricular craniopharyngiomas: report on six cases and a review of the literature. Surg Neurol 2003; 60: 245–52; discussion 52–3.

42. Van Effenterre R, Boch AL. Craniopharyngioma in adults and children: a study of 122 surgical cases. J Neurosurg 2002; 97: 3–11.

43. Jho HD. Orbital roof craniotomy via an eyebrow incision: a simplified anterior skull base approach. Minim Invasive Neurosurg 1997; 40: 91–7.

44. Jho HD, Carrau RL. Endoscopic endonasal transsphenoidal surgery: experience with 50 patients. J Neurosurg 1997; 87: 44–51.

45. Laws ER Jr. Transsphenoidal microsurgery in the management of craniopharyngioma. J Neurosurg 1980; 52: 661–6.

46. Joki T, Oi S, Babapour B, et al. Neuroendoscopic placement of Ommaya reservoir into a cystic craniopharyngioma. Childs Nerv Syst 2002; 18: 629–33.

47. Gahbauer H, Sturm V, Schlegel W, et al. Combined use of stereotaxic CT and angiography for brain biopsies and stereotaxic irradiation. Am J Neuroradiol 1983; 4: 715–18.

48. Mundinger F, Ostertag CB, Birg W, Weigel K. Stereotactic treatment of brain lesions. Biopsy, interstitial radiotherapy (iridium-192 and iodine-125) and drainage procedures. Appl Neurophysiol 1980; 43: 198–204.

49. Nicolato A, Foroni R, Rosta L, Gerosa M, Bricolo A. Multimodality stereotactic approach to the treatment of cystic craniopharyngiomas. Minim Invasive Neurosurg 2004; 47: 32–40.

50. Jephcott CR, Sugden EM, Foord T. Radiotherapy for craniopharyngioma in children: a national audit. Clin Oncol (R Coll Radiol) 2003; 15: 10–13.

51. Gurkaynak M, Ozyar E, Zorlu F, Akyol FH, Atahan IL. Results of radiotherapy in craniopharyngiomas analysed by the linear quadratic model. Acta Oncol 1994; 33: 941–3.

52. Honegger J, Grabenbauer GG, Paulus W, Fahlbusch R. Regression of a large solid papillary craniopharyngioma following fractionated external radiotherapy. J Neurooncol 1999; 41: 261–6.

53. Jose CC, Rajan B, Ashley S, Marsh H, Brada M. Radiotherapy for the treatment of recurrent craniopharyngioma. Clin Oncol (R Coll Radiol) 1992; 4: 287–9.

54. Danoff BF, Cowchock FS, Kramer S. Childhood craniopharyngioma: survival, local control, endocrine and neurologic function following radiotherapy. Int J Radiat Oncol Biol Phys 1983; 9: 171–5.

55. Kano T, Zama A, Ono N, et al. [A juvenile case of radiation-induced meningioma two years after radiation for craniopharyngioma]. No Shinkei Geka 1994; 22: 367–70.

56. Ushio Y, Arita N, Yoshimine T, Nagatani M, Mogami H. Glioblastoma after radiotherapy for craniopharyngioma: case report. Neurosurgery 1987; 21: 33–8.

57. Yu X, Liu Z, Li S. Combined treatment with stereotactic intracavitary irradiation and gamma knife surgery for craniopharyngiomas. Stereotact Funct Neurosurg 2000; 75: 117–22.

58. Schefter JK, Allen G, Cmelak AJ, et al. The utility of external beam radiation and intracystic 32P radiation in the treatment of craniopharyngiomas. J Neurooncol 2002; 56: 69–78.

59. Regine WF, Mohiuddin M, Kramer S. Long-term results of pediatric and adult craniopharyngiomas treated with combined surgery and radiation. Radiother Oncol 1993; 27: 13–21.

60. Rajan B, Ashley S, Gorman C, et al. Craniopharyngioma – long-term results following limited surgery and radiotherapy. Radiother Oncol 1993; 26: 1–10.

61. Hetelekidis S, Barnes PD, Tao ML, et al. 20-year experience in childhood craniopharyngioma. Int J Radiat Oncol Biol Phys 1993; 27: 189–95.

62. Habrand JL, Saran F, Alapetite C, Noel G, El Boustany R, Grill J. Radiation therapy in the management of craniopharyngioma: current concepts and future developments. J Pediatr Endocrinol Metab 2006; 19(Suppl 1): 389–94.

63. Moon SH, Kim IH, Park SW, et al. Early adjuvant radiotherapy toward long-term survival and better quality of life for craniopharyngiomas – a study in a single institute. Childs Nerv Syst 2005; 21: 799–807.

64. Merchant TE. Craniopharyngioma radiotherapy: endocrine and cognitive effects. J Pediatr Endocrinol Metab 2006; 19(Suppl 1): 439–46.

65. Lunsford LD, Kondziolka D, Flickinger JC. Stereotactic radiosurgery for benign intracranial tumors. Clin Neurosurg 1993; 40: 475–97.

66. Suh JH, Barnett GH. Stereotactic radiosurgery for brain tumors in pediatric patients. Technol Cancer Res Treat 2003; 2: 141–6.

67. Prasad D, Steiner M, Steiner L. Gamma knife surgery for craniopharyngioma. Acta Neurochir (Wien) 1995; 134: 167–76.

68. Ulfarsson E, Lindquist C, Roberts M, et al. Gamma knife radiosurgery for craniopharyngiomas: long-term results in the first Swedish patients. J Neurosurg 2002; 97: 613–22.

69. Jackson AS, St George EJ, Hayward RJ, Plowman PN. Stereotactic radiosurgery. XVII: Recurrent intrasellar craniopharyngioma. Br J Neurosurg 2003; 17: 138–43.

70. Tishler RB, Loeffler JS, Lunsford LD, et al. Tolerance of cranial nerves of the cavernous sinus to radiosurgery. Int J Radiat Oncol Biol Phys 1993; 27: 215–21.

71. Hasegawa T, Kobayashi T, Kida Y. Tolerance of the optic apparatus in single-fraction irradiation using stereotactic radiosurgery: evaluation in 100 patients with craniopharyngioma. Neurosurgery 2010; 66: 688–94; discussion 694–5.

72. Chung WY, Pan DH, Shiau CY, Guo WY, Wang LW. Gamma knife radiosurgery for craniopharyngiomas. J Neurosurg 2000; 93(Suppl 3): 47–56.

73. Amendola BE, Wolf A, Coy SR, Amendola MA. Role of radiosurgery in craniopharyngiomas: a preliminary report. Med Pediatr Oncol 2003; 41: 123–7.

74. Savas A, Arasil E, Batay F, Selcuki M, Kanpolat Y. Intracavitary chemotherapy of polycystic craniopharyngioma with bleomycin. Acta Neurochir (Wien) 1999; 141: 547–8; discussion 549.

75. Savas A, Erdem A, Tun K, Kanpolat Y. Fatal toxic effect of bleomycin on brain tissue after intracystic chemotherapy for a craniopharyngioma: case report. Neurosurgery 2000; 46: 213–16; discussion 216–17.

76. Lippens RJ, Rotteveel JJ, Otten BJ, Merx H. Chemotherapy with Adriamycin (doxorubicin) and CCNU (lomustine) in four children with recurrent craniopharyngioma. Eur J Paediatr Neurol 1998; 2: 263–8.

77. Plowman PN, Besser GM, Shipley J, Summersgill B, Geddes J, Afshar F. Dramatic response of malignant craniopharyngioma to cisplatin-based chemotherapy. Should craniopharyngioma be considered as a suprasellar 'germ cell' tumour? Br J Neurosurg 2004; 18: 500–5.

78. Izumoto S, Suzuki T, Kinoshita M, et al. Immunohistochemical detection of female sex hormone receptors in craniopharyngiomas: correlation with clinical and histologic features. Surg Neurol 2005; 63: 520–5; discussion 5.

Section 10: Neurological Malignancies

62 Ophthalmic Cancers

Maria M. Choudhary[1] and Arun D. Singh[2]

[1] Department of Internal Medicine, [2] Department of Ophthalmic Oncology, Cole Eye Institute, Cleveland Clinic, Cleveland, OH, USA

Introduction

Primary ophthalmic tumors, although less common than metastases, arise from various ophthalmic and adnexal structures. In general, they can be anatomically classified as eyelid tumors, conjunctival/corneal tumors, uveal tumors, retinal tumors, and orbital/adnexal tumors (Table 62.1). Ophthalmic tumors, similar to neoplasia elsewhere, can be benign, premalignant, and malignant, presenting in both children (retinoblastoma) and adults (uveal melanoma). Symptomatology and clinical presentation vary depending upon the anatomic location of the tumor. In general, treatment options include surgery, radiation, and chemotherapy. In addition, specialized ophthalmic procedures such as thermotherapy and brachytherapy are used for localized lesions. In this chapter, we limit our discussion to general aspects of the most common types of ophthalmic cancers from each region: eyelid (sebaceous carcinoma), conjunctiva (squamous cell carcinoma [SCC]), uvea (melanoma), and retina (retinoblastoma).

Sebaceous carcinoma of the eyelid

Historical background

Current understanding of sebaceous carcinoma was initiated by a review by Straatsma in 1956, which established the origin of this neoplasm.[1] Historical developments are summarized elsewhere.[2] The terms sebaceous gland carcinoma, sebaceous cell carcinoma, and sebaceous carcinoma are interchangeably used in the literature.[3,4]

Anatomy

The tarsal plate of the eyelid offers structural support to the eyelid. It is a fibrous tissue, which contains meibomian glands within its substance. Meibomian glands are modified sebaceous glands contributing to the oil layer of the tear film. Zeis glands, which are also sebaceous in nature, are located closer to the eyelid margin in association with the eyelashes.

Biology and epidemiology

Sebaceous carcinoma can occur in a variety of sites but the ocular and orbital involvement accounts for about 75% of all cases. Overall, sebaceous carcinoma represents about 1% of all eyelid tumors with an incidence of 0.5 per million white population in the United States.[5] However, sebaceous carcinoma represents a greater proportion of eyelid tumors (28–33%) in the Asian population.[6,7]

The etiology of sebaceous carcinoma remains obscure. In a small minority of cases, genetic predisposition such as that seen in retinoblastoma and Muir–Torre syndrome may play a contributory role.[8–10] External beam radiotherapy, especially in children, is a known risk factor.[11] Immunosuppression as seen in acquired immunodeficiency syndrome (AIDS) may also be associated with sebaceous carcinoma.[12]

Histopathology

Four histopathological variants are known: lobular, comedocarcinoma, papillary, and mixed with variable amount of differentiation. The lobular pattern is most common, mimicking the structure of a normal sebaceous gland.[13] All variants contain lipids, which is readily demonstrated by oil red O stain. Immunohistochemically, the sebaceous carcinoma expresses human milk fat globule-1 and epithelial membrane antigen but not cytokeratins unlike squamous cell or basal cell carcinoma.[14]

Sebaceous carcinoma tends to spread locally to the lacrimal gland and to the draining (preauricular and submandibular) lymph nodes. The incidence of regional lymph node spread may be lower nowadays compared to the historic reports of 30%.[15–17] Distant hematogenous metastasis to the lung, liver, bone, and brain is also becoming uncommon.[17]

Table 62.1 Common ophthalmic tumors classified by anatomic layers.

Structure	Benign	Malignant
Eyelid	Papilloma	Basal cell carcinoma
	Nevus	Squamous cell carcinoma
	Hemangioma	Meibomian gland carcinoma
Conjunctiva/cornea	Nevus	Squamous cell carcinoma
Retina	Retinocytoma	Retinoblastoma
Uvea	Nevus	Uveal melanoma
	Hemangioma	Uveal metastasis
Orbital/adnexal	Dermoid cysts	Rhabdomyosarcoma
	Hemangioma	Lymphoma
	Lymphangioma	Orbital metastasis

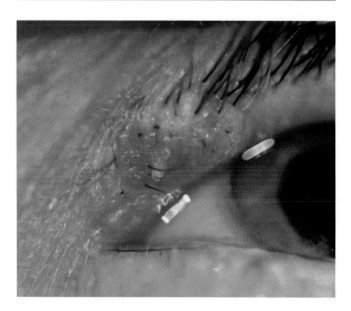

Figure 62.1 Photograph showing typical external appearance of a localized sebaceous carcinoma.

Clinical presentation and diagnostic considerations

Because of its rarity, sebaceous carcinoma is often misdiagnosed both clinically and histopathologically. It typically affects older females.[3] In the periocular region, the neoplasm arises from meibomian glands, Zeis glands, caruncle, conjunctiva, and eyebrows.[18] Sebaceous carcinoma can appear as a solitary nodule when arising from the Zeis glands or presents as diffuse thickening of the eyelid when arising from meibomian glands (Fig. 62.1). The upper eyelid (63%) is more often involved than the lower eyelid (27%) with involvement of both eyelids (5%) in a minority of cases.[2] The localized form is often misdiagnosed as chalazion and the diffuse form as blepharitis.[2]

A high index of suspicion is a must for early diagnosis. Excisional or incisional biopsy must include full thickness of the eyelid so that the tarsus can be examined histopathologically. Because of its tendency to show pagetoid spread along the conjunctival epithelium and have multicentric origin, biopsies from multiple sites, especially of the conjunctiva (mapping biopsy), may be necessary to establish the full extent of the disease.[19]

Treatment

Surgical excision with about 5 mm of clear margins is considered the standard of care.[20] Clear margins may be obtained either with frozen section control or Mohs technique with comparable results.[20] Mapping biopsy of the conjunctiva is also indicated to determine the extent of the disease.[19] Supplemental cryotherapy is advocated but its benefits remain to be established.[21] Topical mitomycin therapy is useful for treatment of conjunctival involvement.[22] Radiotherapy offers only palliative treatment and is recommended when a patient declines or is unfit for surgery.[20,23,24] Exenteration is performed for extensive orbital extension.[20,25] Sentinel lymph node biopsy offers the possibility of early detection of regional spread.[26]

Recommendations

Excision with mapping biopsy as outlined above is generally performed. In the presence of extensive orbital involvement, exenteration is recommended.

Prognosis

The prognosis with sebaceous carcinoma is rather poor because of delayed diagnosis, its tendency for multicentric origin, and the risk of regional/distant spread. Nevertheless, it appears that survival with sebaceous carcinoma may be improving as recent studies have indicated mortality rates of less than 10%.[15–17]

Conjunctival squamous cell carcinoma

Historical background

Squamous cell carcinoma (SCC) of the conjunctiva was described as early as 1860 by von Graefe.[27] He used the term "epithelioma" to describe gelatinous elevations of the conjunctiva typified by variable amounts of vascularity and keratinization. Although SCC of the conjunctiva is often considered a low-grade carcinoma, timely diagnosis and appropriate management are essential to prevent visual disability, disfigurement, and life-threatening invasive disease.[28]

Anatomy

The conjunctiva is a membranous lining composed of nonkeratinized squamous epithelium and columnar epithelium with a deeper substantia propria, which extends from the eyelid margin to the corneal limbus.[29] SCC is considered within the clinical spectrum of ocular surface squamous neoplasia (OSSN), which includes all epithelial tumors, whether dysplastic or carcinomatous, that affect the conjunctiva or the cornea.[29]

Biology and epidemiology

Although SCC of the conjunctiva is an uncommon ophthalmic tumor, it is the most common malignancy of the conjunctiva in the United States.[30] Incidence ranges from 0.03 to 2.8 per

100,000 person-years.[31,32] SCC is most commonly observed in older male Caucasians (mean age: 56 years).[29]

At the limbus, a transition from the columnar conjunctival epithelium of the fornices to the stratified squamous epithelium of the cornea occurs. This region is biologically akin to other transitional tissues such as the uterine cervix that are also prone to dysplasia.[32] Most squamous tumors originate from the interpalpebral limbus and involve both the conjunctiva and the cornea.

Ultraviolet-B (UV-B) light exposure has consistently emerged as a major etiological factor.[33] Chronic environmental exposure to wind, dust, petroleum, and cigarette smoke is also believed to be a significant risk factor. Human papillomavirus (subtypes 16 and 18) has also been associated with SCC but is probably not an independent cause of conjunctival neoplasia.[34] The mechanism of squamous transformation after UV-B radiation may be related to point mutations of the p53 tumor suppressor gene.[35] Patients with xeroderma pigmentosa have a much higher incidence and account for most SCC in young patients.[32] Systemic immunosuppression, as seen in AIDS, may increase the risk of developing OSSN by as much as 13-fold.[36]

Histopathology

SCC can be broadly divided into corneal/conjunctival intraepithelial neoplasia (CIN) and invasive SCC. Lesions that are confined to the epithelium are preferentially termed CIN.[32,37] Tumors that infiltrate the substantia propria are referred to as invasive SCC of the conjunctiva or cornea.[38] Within the heterogeneous category of CIN, dysplasia may range from mild (less than one-third thickness occupied by atypical cells) to severe (near full-thickness involvement). Full-thickness obliteration of normal cells without penetration of the basement membrane is referred to as carcinoma *in situ*.

The predominant cell type is the spindle variety, characterized by small elliptical cells without prominent nucleoli, a weakly basophilic cytoplasm, and frequent mitotic figures. The epidermoid variety with larger polyhedral cells is less frequent (5%).[33] Mucoepidermal carcinoma is a rare variant characterized by mucus-filled cysts and a greater propensity to local invasion.[39]

Clinical presentation and diagnostic considerations

Unilateral red eye and ocular irritation are the most common presenting symptoms, and diffuse tumors can often be misdiagnosed as chronic conjunctivitis. On examination, nodular thickening of the interpalpebral limbal conjunctiva with a gelatinous, papillomatous, or leukoplakic appearance is typically observed (Fig. 62.2).[40] The lesion may mimic or even coexist with benign conjunctival degenerations such as pingueculae and pterygia.[30]

Clinical differentiation of CIN from invasive SCC of the conjunctiva or cornea is unreliable.[41] Rose Bengal stain may be useful in delineating abnormalities of the mucin layer associated with OSSN. While features such as size and extensive involvement of the limbal circumference have been associated with invasive disease,[42] the diagnosis is ultimately histopathological and relies on careful evaluation for violation of the epithelial basement membrane. Nonsurgical ascertainment of OSSN may be enhanced with exfoliative or impression cytology but the ability to distinguish carcinoma *in situ* from minimally invasive SCC is limited.[40]

Treatment

Management is influenced primarily by the extent of the lesion. Surgical excision with 2–3 mm margins has been the preferred approach for OSSN involving less than 4 clock hours of limbal

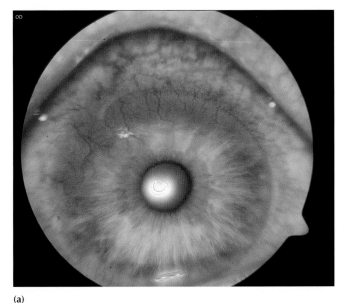

(a)

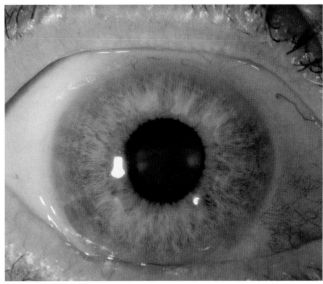

(b)

Figure 62.2 Slit-lamp photograph of the left eye. (a) Note nodular thickening and vascularization of the superior limbal conjunctiva with corneal extension. (b) After four cycles of topical mitomycin 0.04% therapy.

conjunctiva.[43] Alcohol epitheliectomy of any corneal component is generally followed by removal of the conjunctival component via lamellar scleral resection. Application of intraoperative supplemental cryotherapy (double freeze–thaw cycles) to conjunctival margins reduces the risk of tumor recurrence.[44] Mohs technique has also been described in the management of conjunctival SCC.[45] Surgical management is more complicated with larger lesions, where attempts at total surgical excision carry a risk of limbal stem cell depletion, corneal scarring, and visual loss. Extensive excisions for locally invasive disease can require limited or *en masse* removal of affected ocular and orbital tissues followed by reconstruction with conjunctival autografts, amniotic membrane grafts, or keratolimbal stem cell grafts.

Topical chemotherapy has been advocated both intraoperatively and postoperatively as an adjuvant for incomplete excision of large and diffuse primary or recurrent tumors.[46,47] More recently, topical therapy has been explored as an alternative to excision in selected cases.[48] It has also been reported to be effective as a neoadjuvant therapy.[49] While mitomycin-C (MCC) is the best studied of the chemotherapeutic agents, other topical agents including 5-fluorouracil[48] and interferon-$\alpha 2b$[50] have also been investigated.[51] Protocols for topical therapy typically involve temporary punctual occlusion followed by alternating weeks of 0.04% MCC drops four times daily and rest until resolution occurs.[47] A reversible chemical keratoconjunctivitis is common with all agents, although interferon-$\alpha 2b$ produces less epithelial toxicity *in vitro*.[52] Radiation is rarely indicated.[33]

Recommendations

In general, complete excision, where feasible, should be attempted. Supplemental cryotherapy is always performed. In patients with larger, diffuse, or recurrent involvement, incisional biopsy followed by topical MMC therapy is effective.[53]

Prognosis

Most CIN lesions do not progress to invasive SCC.[42] When conjunctival SCC does occur, it is rarely metastatic but the risk of regional and distant metastasis is much greater in the face of immunosuppression and HIV infection.[38] Recurrence occurs at rates between 16% and 52% in long-term studies and is predicted by larger lesion size, positive surgical margins, lack of supplemental cryotherapy, increased patient age (>60 years), and elevated proliferation index by Ki-67 immunostaining.[40,42,44] The histological type and severity of dysplasia or clinical appearance cannot predict the likelihood of recurrence. Currently, recurrence rates of 5–10% are expected with a median time to recurrence of about 18 months.[53] Annual follow-up is recommended. Intraocular (13%) or orbital (11%) involvement requiring enucleation or orbital exenteration is uncommon.[54] Fortunately, metastatic conjunctival SCC is extremely rare. The most important factor in cases resulting in visual loss or death is a delay in diagnosis.[33]

Uveal melanoma

Historical background

Until the 1980s, the optimal management for uveal melanomas, small, medium, or large, was debatable[55,56] because the majority of data were derived from retrospective studies based only on a small number of patients treated at a given center.[57,58] Moreover, the benefit of enucleation was being questioned.[59,60] In 1984, funded by the National Eye Institute (Bethesda, Maryland), Collaborative Ocular Melanoma Study (COMS) trials were designed. Over the last 20 years, a wealth of reliable data derived from COMS and other studies has offered clearer guidelines for the management of patients with uveal melanoma.

Anatomy

The uvea is the middle coat of the eyeball, with the sclera external to it and the retina being the innermost layer. The uvea extends anteriorly from the pupil to the optic disk posteriorly. The uvea is divided into three parts: iris, ciliary body, and choroid (from anterior to posterior). The uvea is a highly vascular layer with abundant melanocytes of neuroectodermal origin.

Biology and epidemiology

Uveal melanoma is the most common primary intraocular malignant tumor (85%).[61] Even so, melanomas of the ocular and adnexal structures comprise approximately 5% of all melanomas[62] whereas primary eyelid, conjunctival, and orbital melanomas are very rare.[62,63]

Uveal melanoma is a primary malignant tumor of the uvea arising from uveal melanocytes. On the basis of anatomical location, it is classified into three types: iris melanoma, ciliary body melanoma, and choroidal melanoma. Although uveal melanocytes and cutaneous melanocytes share common embryologic origin and some morphological properties, several significant differences exist between cutaneous and uveal melanomas in terms of the prognostic factors, site of distant metastasis, and response of metastatic disease to chemotherapy. Cell type, an important prognostic factor in uveal melanoma, is of minor significance in cutaneous melanoma.[64] Cutaneous melanoma tends to show nonvisceral metastasis involving skin, subcutaneous tissues, and distant lymph nodes more often than visceral involvement. In contrast, uveal melanoma predominantly metastasizes to liver. The chemotherapy regimen currently used in the treatment of metastatic cutaneous melanoma is ineffective against metastatic uveal melanoma.[65]

Incidence

The global incidence of uveal melanoma ranges from 5.3 to 10.9 cases per million.[66] The incidence of uveal melanoma in the United States and European countries is similar to that in Australia[67] and New Zealand,[68] where the population is exposed to a higher intensity of ultraviolet light. The overall mean incidence of uveal melanoma is 4.3 per million, with a higher rate in males (4.9 per million) as compared to females (3.7 per million).[61] Unlike trends for cutaneous melanoma, the incidence of uveal melanoma has remained stable in the United States for the last 50 years.[61,69]

Host factors

Among the host factors, race seems to be the most significant, as uveal melanoma is about 150 times more common in whites than in blacks.[63,70] Light skin color, blond hair, and blue eyes are specific host risk factors. Genetic factors such as family history and other syndromic associations, except oculo(dermal) melanocytosis, play only a minor role in predisposition to uveal melanoma.[66]

Environmental factors

The evidence with respect to the contributory role of sunlight exposure in the etiopathogenesis of uveal melanoma is at best weak and contradictory.[63,70] In addition, there is no consistent evidence indicating that a specific occupational exposure, ultraviolet light or a chemical agent is a risk factor for uveal melanoma.[63,70]

Histopathology

Uveal melanoma is composed of melanocytes with variable amounts of intrinsic vascularity. Areas of hemorrhage, necrosis, and lymphocytic infiltration are also observed. The tumors are composed of spindle cells, epithelioid cells, or most commonly a mixture of both types of cells (mixed cell type).[71]

Clinical presentation

Iris melanoma presents as a pigmented raised lesion. A ciliary body melanoma can cause blurred vision due to lenticular astigmatism. Loss of vision, flashing light sensation, and exudative retinal detachment are some of the common presentations of a choroidal melanoma. The diagnosis is essentially clinical based on indirect ophthalmoscopy, angiographic studies, and the ultrasonographic pattern (Fig. 62.3). The diagnostic accuracy with such techniques is 99% and therefore biopsy is performed only in very atypical cases.

Treatment

The treatment of uveal melanoma is surgical or radiation therapy. Visual acuity, potential for retaining vision, vision in the unaffected eye, tumor size and location, and patient preference are important factors when considering the treatment options.[72] For smaller tumors, surgical resection (iridectomy, cyclectomy, choroidectomy) is performed. Larger tumors and those associated with significant loss of vision or those that have no potential for maintaining vision are managed by enucleation. Medium-sized tumors can be treated with proton beam radiotherapy, brachytherapy (iodine-125, ruthenium-106), or enucleation. Smaller choroidal tumors are also amenable to transpupillary thermotherapy (TTT).

The COMS divided choroidal melanoma according to size into small, medium, and large tumors on the basis of the largest basal diameter (LBD) and height (Table 62.2).[73] COMS comprises two randomized trials, one each for medium[74] and large tumors,[75] and one observational study for small tumors.[76] The small choroidal melanoma observational study identified clinical features associated with time to tumor growth. The Kaplan–Meier estimate of the probability of growth was 11% and 31% by 1 and 5 years respectively.[76] It must be realized that about two-thirds of tumors did not show evidence of growth, even though these tumors were classified as small choroidal melanoma. Patients with medium choroidal melanoma were randomized to receive enucleation or iodine-125 brachytherapy.[74,77,78] The Kaplan–Meier estimates of 5-year all-cause and melanoma-related mortality rates were comparable for both treatment arms. Patients with a large choroidal melanoma were randomly assigned to enucleation with and without pre-enucleation radiation (20 Gy was delivered in five daily fractions).[75,79] The Kaplan–Meier estimates of 5-year all-cause mortality and melanoma-related mortality were comparable for both treatment arms.

Recommendations

Tumor size is the most significant factor that influences the treatment recommendation. In general, COMS guidelines are followed. Small-sized choroidal melanomas that are less than 4 mm in thickness may be treated by TTT.

Prognosis

The survival in patients with uveal melanoma is compromised due to the tendency of uveal melanoma to undergo hepatic metastasis. Among other factors, tumor size, tumor cell type, and presence of cytogenetic changes are significant prognostic factors.[64] The COMS data indicate approximate melanoma-related mortality at 5 years of 1%, 10%, and 25% for small, medium, and large choroidal melanoma respectively. Currently used screening protocols of annual chest x-rays and semi-annual liver function tests are not helpful, unless liver imaging studies are included.[80]

Prognostication of uveal melanoma based upon tumor cytogenetic and molecular assays has now become feasible.[81] Nonrandom karyotype abnormalities including loss of chromosome 3 (monosomy 3), loss of 6q, and gain of chromosome 8q are associated with increased risk of metastatic death.[82,83] Gene expression profiling can classify uveal melanoma into less aggressive class 1 tumors and class 2 tumors with a higher risk of metastasis.[84,85] Tumor samples may be obtained after enucleation or resection and even after fine needle aspiration biopsy.[86,87] The ultimate goal is to develop targeted adjuvant therapies for patients with high risk of metastasis.[88]

Metastatic uveal melanoma

The treatment of metastatic uveal melanoma has been dismissal so far.[89] Encouraging results have been reported with compassionate use of ipilimumab (human anticytotoxic

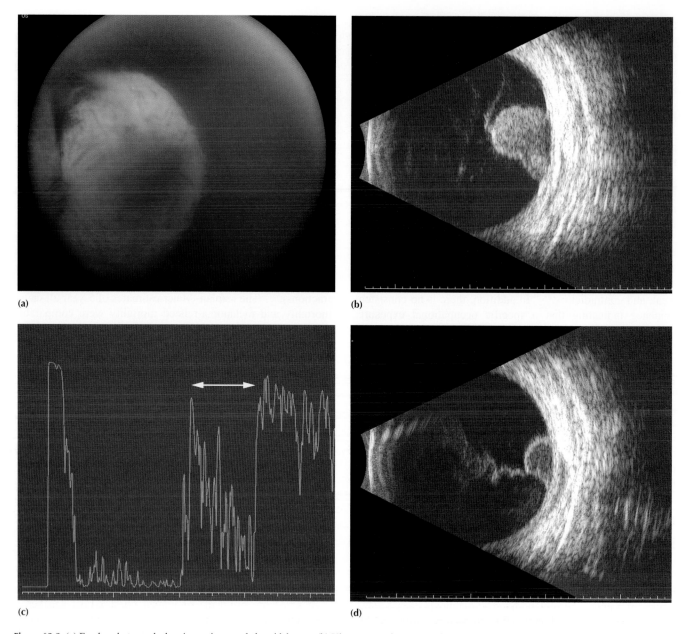

Figure 62.3 (a) Fundus photograph showing a pigmented choroidal mass. (b) Ultrasonography B- scan demonstrates a dome-shaped choroidal mass with retinal detachment. (c) On A-scan, the tumor has typical low internal reflectivity (*between arrows*). (d) Twelve months after treatment with iodine-125 plaque radiation; note regression of the tumor.

Table 62.2 Classification system and design of Collaborative Ocular Melanoma Trials.*

| Classification | Size (mm) | | Design | Treatment groups |
	Diameter	Height		
Nevus	<5.0	<1.0		
Small melanoma	5.0–16.0	1.0–2.5	Nonrandomized	Observation[†]
Medium melanoma	≤16.0	2.5–10.0	Randomized	Iodine-125 plaque radiotherapy Enucleation
Large melanoma	>16.0	>10.0	Randomized	Preenucleation radiotherapy Enucleation

* After November, 1990.
[†] Treatment offered initially or during follow-up based on the discretion of the patient and treating ophthalmologist.

T lymphocyte antigen- 4 monoclonal antibody) in a small number of patients who had failed or could not tolerate previous systemic or locoregional therapies.[90]

Retinoblastoma

Historical background

James Wardrop in 1809 was the first to recognize retinoblastoma as a specific entity and called it fungus haematodes. Enucleation with removal of a long stump of optic nerve as a treatment for retinoblastoma was recommended by von Graefe in 1884. Hilgartner first used external beam radiotherapy in 1903[91] and Kupfer used chemotherapy in 1953 for the treatment of retinoblastoma.[92] Reese and Ellsworth proposed a classification for retinoblastoma, which has guided treatment for the last 50 years.[93] More recently, there has been a move towards new classification of retinoblastoma which has better correlation with currently used methods of treatment.[94]

Anatomy

The retina is the innermost layer of the eyeball. It is a highly complex neural structure and embryologically represents a direct extension of the brain. Retinoblastoma arises from the as yet unidentified retinoblasts that transiently populate the pediatric retina.

Biology and epidemiology

Retinoblastoma is the most common primary intraocular malignant tumor in children with an incidence of 1 in 15,000 live births. The average annual incidence of retinoblastoma in the United States is 11.8 per million for children younger than 4 years.[95]

Retinoblastoma is a familial disorder with an autosomal-dominant inheritance. It can be classified in three different ways: familial or sporadic, bilateral or unilateral, and heritable or nonheritable. Approximately 10% of newly diagnosed retinoblastoma cases are familial and 90% are sporadic. All familial cases are due to an inherited germline mutation. All bilateral cases and about 15% of unilateral cases represent new onset of germline mutations.[96]

The human retinoblastoma susceptibility gene (RB1), a tumor suppressor gene, is located on chromosome 13 q14.[97] The mutations are distributed throughout the RB1 gene with no mutational hotspots. Retinoblastoma protein (pRB) arrests the cell cycle at the G1 restriction point by binding to E2F transcription factors. In the absence of both alleles of RB1, one due to the inactivating mutation and the other due to either a separate somatic mutation or chromosomal mechanisms, there is almost complete lack of pRB. In the absence of pRB, there is uncontrolled cell proliferation leading to retinoblastoma.[98]

Histopathology

Retinoblastoma growth patterns can be classified as one of four types: exophytic, endophytic, mixed, and diffuse infiltrating. Endophytic tumor grows toward the vitreous cavity and mimics endophthalmitis. Exophytic tumors tend to grow outwards, leading to retinal detachment. Diffuse infiltrating tumors lack localized tumor prominence and are usually misdiagnosed as uveitis. Histopathologically, retinoblastoma is a neuroblastic tumor with large basophilic nuclei and scanty cytoplasm. Necrosis, mitosis, and calcification are common features. Flexner–Wintersteiner rosettes are highly characteristic of retinoblastoma (Fig. 62.4).[99]

Clinical presentation and diagnostic considerations

Leukocoria (a white pupil) and strabismus are the most common presenting signs (see Fig. 62.4).[100] Other less common presentations include intraocular inflammation, discoloration of the iris due to neovascularization, hyphema (blood in the anterior chamber), and glaucoma. As children with a family history of retinoblastoma are screened prospectively by periodic indirect ophthalmoscopy, early retinoblastoma may be detected by screening examinations. Diagnosis is usually based on the ophthalmoscopic appearance of a white tumor with intrinsic calcifications demonstrated by ultrasonography or computed tomography (CT) scan. Intraocular biopsy in the setting of retinoblastoma is contraindicated because of concerns regarding seeding of malignant cells.[101]

Metastatic disease is rare at presentation so lumbar puncture with cerebrospinal fluid analysis, bone marrow aspiration, and bone scan are not performed on a routine basis.[102] However, these tests are indicated in children with advanced intraocular disease or who show evidence of extraocular disease at presentation. Retinocytoma or the so-called spontaneously regressed retinoblastoma is the benign equivalent of retinoblastoma.[103]

Treatment

In recent years, there has been a trend away from enucleation, with the increased use of alternative globe-conserving methods of treatment including laser photocoagulation, cryotherapy, TTT, plaque radiotherapy, external beam radiotherapy, and chemotherapy.[104] Laser photocoagulation and cryotherapy are used to treat very small tumors.[105] TTT is used for small tumors in conjunction with chemotherapy.[106] Plaque radiotherapy is highly effective in treating medium-sized tumors.[107] External beam radiation therapy was used for large and multiple tumors associated with vitreous seeding.[108] It is used less frequently nowadays due to concerns of inducing second malignant neoplasms (SMNs). Enucleation is still a valid primary therapeutic option for advanced unilateral retinoblastoma.

Since the 1990s, chemoreduction has been increasingly used for the management of retinoblastoma to avoid external beam radiotherapy or enucleation.[109] Chemotherapy is delivered intravenously to reduce the volume of intraocular retinoblastoma and also to make it amenable to focal therapy such as cryotherapy, thermotherapy, or brachytherapy. Six-cycle chemoreduction using three agents (vincristine, etoposide, and carboplatin) is generally prescribed.[110] On the basis of available (noncomparative series) data, it can be concluded that

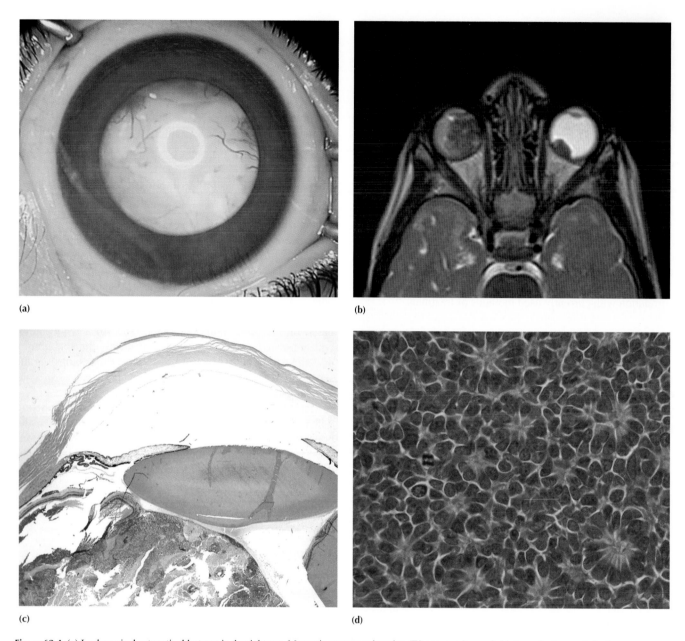

Figure 62.4 (a) Leukocoria due to retinoblastoma in the right eye. Magnetic resonance imaging (T2 sequence) revealed intraocular tumors in both eyes. (b) Calcification in the right eye is evident as black spaces within the tumor. Histopathology of the enucleated globe revealed partially necrotic tumor (c) with Flexner–Wintersteiner rosettes (d).

chemoreduction combined with adjuvant focal therapy offers about a 50–90% probability of avoiding enucleation or external beam radiotherapy, depending upon the severity of disease at initial presentation.[111] It must be realized that chemoreduction is not without its problems. Recurrence of the neoplasm while on chemotherapy has been observed.[112] Immediate complications related to transient bone marrow suppression requiring hospital admissions and intravenous antibiotics with consequent delay in examinations under anesthesia are frequent.[113] Risk of late complications such as drug-induced leukemia have not yet been excluded.

More recently, there has been a trend towards superselective delivery of chemotherapy (melphalan) via cannulation of the ophthalmic artery.[114,115] The aim of such an approach is to avoid systemic complications and to achieve higher drug levels within the vitreous cavity. Although the initial results are encouraging, such treatments should only be conducted within a framework of clinical trial in a specialized center.[116] There are several clinical trials that are being conducted by the Children's Oncology Group.[117]

Recommendations

The decision-making process for treatment of retinoblastoma is rather complex as several factors such as family history, status of the other eye, number, size, and location of tumors, and the visual potential are important considerations. In general, advanced unilateral disease is best managed by enucleation with continued monitoring of the uninvolved eye. Treatment of bilateral disease is initiated by chemotherapy (chemoreduction) with local therapy comprising cryotherapy, thermotherapy, or brachytherapy. External beam radiation therapy as an initial treatment for bilateral disease is generally not recommended.

Prognosis

Survival in patients with retinoblastoma is compromised by three independent diseases: metastatic retinoblastoma, trilateral retinoblastoma, and SMNs. Recent advances in the treatment of retinoblastoma have led to improved 5-year survival rates of greater than 90% in developed countries.[95] However, in underdeveloped countries, retinoblastoma is associated with a high mortality rate because it tends to present or is diagnosed at a much more advanced stage.

Metastasis in retinoblastoma usually occurs within 1 year of diagnosis of retinoblastoma and almost never after 5 years.[118] Involvement of the central nervous system and hematogenous spread are the most common sites of metastasis. Survival with metastatic retinoblastoma is generally limited to 6 months.[118,119] Several histopathological risk factors for metastasis have been identified, in the presence of which, chemotherapy is generally recommended.[120,121] In about 8% of cases with germline retinoblastoma, a primary intracranial tumor is observed (trilateral retinoblastoma).[122] The primary intracranial malignant tumor can be varied in its location and histopathological features. The majority of tumors are located in the pineal region but the tumors can also occur in the suprasellar and parasellar regions. The histopathological appearance is that of a pinealoblastoma or a primitive neuroectodermal tumor.[122,123]

In the United States, more patients die of SMNs than from their initial retinoblastoma.[124] SMNs typically occur in adolescence in children with germline mutations. Treatment with external beam radiotherapy enhances the risk for SMNs.[125] A variety of tumors are seen within the spectrum of SMNs but osteogenic sarcoma, soft tissue sarcomas, and cutaneous melanomas are most frequently observed.[126]

References

1. Straatsma BR. Meibomian gland tumors. AMA Arch Ophthalmol 1956; 56(1): 71–93.
2. Kass LG, Hornblass A. Sebaceous carcinoma of the ocular adnexa. Surv Ophthalmol 1989; 33(6): 477–90.
3. Shields JA, Demirci H, Marr BP, Eagle RC Jr, Shields CL. Sebaceous carcinoma of the ocular region: a review. Surv Ophthalmol 2005; 50(2): 103–22.
4. Loeffler KU. Eyelid adnexal tumors. In: Singh AD, Damato BE, Pe'er J, Murphree AL, Perry JD (eds) Clinical Ophthalmic Oncology. Philadelphia: Saunders-Elsevier, 2007. pp.94–8.
5. Margo CE, Mulla ZD. Malignant tumors of the eyelid: a population-based study of non-basal cell and non-squamous cell malignant neoplasms. Arch Ophthalmol 1998; 116(2): 195–8.
6. Ni C, Searl SS, Kuo PK, Chu FR, Chong CS, Albert DM. Sebaceous cell carcinomas of the ocular adnexa. Intl Ophthalmol Clin 1982; 22(1): 23–61.
7. Abdi U, Tyagi N, Maheshwari V, Gogi R, Tyagi SP. Tumours of eyelid: a clinicopathologic study. J Indian Med Assoc 1996; 94(11): 405–9, 416, 418.
8. Stockl FA, Dolmetsch AM, Codere F, Burnier MN Jr. Sebaceous carcinoma of the eyelid in an immunocompromised patient with Muir–Torre syndrome. Can J Ophthalmol 1995; 30(6): 324–6.
9. Rundle P, Shields JA, Shields CL, Eagle RC Jr, Singh AD. Sebaceous gland carcinoma of the eyelid seventeen years after irradiation for bilateral retinoblastoma. Eye (London) 1999; 13(Pt 1): 109–10.
10. Kivela T, Asko-Seljavaara S, Pihkala U, Hovi L, Heikkonen J. Sebaceous carcinoma of the eyelid associated with retinoblastoma. Ophthalmology 2001; 108(6): 1124–8.
11. Rumelt S, Hogan NR, Rubin PA, Jakobiec FA. Four-eyelid sebaceous cell carcinoma following irradiation. Arch Ophthalmol 1998; 116(12): 1670–2.
12. Yen MT, Tse DT. Sebaceous cell carcinoma of the eyelid and the human immunodeficiency virus. Ophthal Plast Reconstr Surg 2000; 16(3): 206–10.
13. Rao NA, Hidayat AA, McLean IW, Zimmerman LE. Sebaceous carcinomas of the ocular adnexa: a clinicopathologic study of 104 cases, with five-year follow-up data. Hum Pathol 1982; 13(2): 113–22.
14. Sinard JH. Immunohistochemical distinction of ocular sebaceous carcinoma from basal cell and squamous cell carcinoma. Arch Ophthalmol 1999; 117(6): 776–83.
15. Doxanas MT, Green WR. Sebaceous gland carcinoma. Review of 40 cases. Arch Ophthalmol 1984; 102(2): 245–9.
16. Muqit MM, Roberts F, Lee WR, Kemp E. Improved survival rates in sebaceous carcinoma of the eyelid. Eye (London) 2004; 18(1): 49–53.
17. Hornblass A, Lauer SA. Sebaceous carcinoma of the eyelids. Ophthalmology 2004; 111(12): 2149–50.
18. Boniuk M, Zimmerman LE. Sebaceous carcinoma of the eyelid, eyebrow, caruncle, and orbit. Trans Am Acad Ophthalmol Otolaryngol 1968; 72(4): 619–42.
19. Putterman AM. Conjunctival map biopsy to determine pagetoid spread. Am J Ophthalmol 1986; 102(1): 87–90.
20. Cook BE Jr, Bartley GB. Treatment options and future prospects for the management of eyelid malignancies: an evidence-based update. Ophthalmology 2001; 108(11): 2088–98.
21. Lisman RD, Jakobiec FA, Small P. Sebaceous carcinoma of the eyelids. The role of adjunctive cryotherapy in the management of conjunctival pagetoid spread. Ophthalmology 1989; 96(7): 1021–6.
22. Rosner M, Hadar I, Rosen N. Successful treatment with mitomycin C eye drops for conjunctival diffuse intraepithelial neoplasia with sebaceous features. Ophthal Plast Reconstr Surg 2003; 19(6): 477–9.
23. Nunery WR, Welsh MG, McCord CD Jr. Recurrence of sebaceous carcinoma of the eyelid after radiation therapy. Am J Ophthalmol 1983; 96(1): 10–15.
24. Yen MT, Tse DT, Wu X, Wolfson AH. Radiation therapy for local control of eyelid sebaceous cell carcinoma: report of two cases and review of the literature. Ophthal Plast Reconstr Surg 2000; 16(3): 211–15.
25. Callahan EF, Appert DL, Roenigk RK, Bartley GB. Sebaceous carcinoma of the eyelid: a review of 14 cases. Dermatol Surg 2004; 30(8): 1164–8.
26. Wilson MW, Fleming JC, Fleming RM, Haik BG. Sentinel node biopsy for orbital and ocular adnexal tumors. Ophthal Plast Reconstr Surg 2001; 17(5): 338–44.
27. Duke-Elder S, Leigh A. Diseases of the outer eye. In: Duke-Elder S (ed) Systems of Ophthalmology, vol 7. St Louis, MO: CV Mosby, 1985.
28. Pe'er J, Frucht-Pery J. Ocular surface squamous neoplasia. In: Singh AD, Damato BE, Pe'er J, Murphree AL, Perry JD (eds) Clinical Ophthalmic Oncology. Philadelphia: Saunders-Elsevier, 2007. pp.136–40.
29. Spencer W. Conjunctiva. In: Spencer W (ed) Ophthalmic Pathology: An Atlas and Textbook. Philadelphia: WB Saunders, 1996.

30. Grossniklaus HE, Green WR, Luckenbach M, Chan CC. Conjunctival lesions in adults. A clinical and histopathologic review. Cornea 1987; 6(2): 78–116.

31. Sun EC, Fears TR, Goedert JJ. Epidemiology of squamous cell conjunctival cancer. Cancer Epidemiol Biomarkers Prevent 1997; 6(2): 73–7.

32. Pizzarello LD, Jakobiec FA. Bowen's disease of the conjunctiva: a misnomer. In: Jakobiec FA (ed) *Ocular and Adnexal Tumors*. Birmingham, AL: Aesculapius, 1978. pp.553–71.

33. Lee GA, Hirst LW. Ocular surface squamous neoplasia. Surv Ophthalmol 1995; 39(6): 429–50.

34. McDonnell JM, McDonnell PJ, Sun YY. Human papillomavirus DNA in tissues and ocular surface swabs of patients with conjunctival epithelial neoplasia. Invest Ophthalmol Vis Sci 1992; 33(1): 184–9.

35. Brash DE, Ziegler A, Jonason AS, Simon JA, Kunala S, Leffell DJ. Sunlight and sunburn in human skin cancer: p53, apoptosis, and tumor promotion. J Investig Dermatol Symp Proc 1996; 1(2): 136–42.

36. Kestelyn P. Ocular problems in AIDS. Int Ophthalmol 1990; 14(3): 165–72.

37. Waring GO 3 rd, Roth AM, Ekins MB. Clinical and pathologic description of 17 cases of corneal intraepithelial neoplasia. Am J Ophthalmol 1984; 97(5): 547–59.

38. Shields CL, Shields JA. Tumors of the conjunctiva and cornea. Surv Ophthalmol 2004; 49(1): 3–24.

39. Rao NA, Font RL. Mucoepidermoid carcinoma of the conjunctiva: a clinicopathologic study of five cases. Cancer 1976; 38(4): 1699–709.

40. McKelvie PA, Daniell M, McNab A, Loughnan M, Santamaria JD. Squamous cell carcinoma of the conjunctiva: a series of 26 cases. Br J Ophthalmol 2002; 86(2): 168–73.

41. Lee GA, Hirst LW. Retrospective study of ocular surface squamous neoplasia. Aust N Z J Ophthalmol 1997; 25(4): 269–76.

42. Erie JC, Campbell RJ, Liesegang TJ. Conjunctival and corneal intraepithelial and invasive neoplasia. Ophthalmology 1986; 93(2): 176–83.

43. Shields JA, Shields CL, de Potter P. Surgical management of conjunctival tumors. The 1994 Lynn B. McMahan Lecture. Arch Ophthalmol 1997; 115(6): 808–15.

44. Fraunfelder FT, Wingfield D. Management of intraepithelial conjunctival tumors and squamous cell carcinomas. Am J Ophthalmol 1983; 95(3): 359–63.

45. Buus DR, Tse DT, Folberg R, Buuns DR. Microscopically controlled excision of conjunctival squamous cell carcinoma. Am J Ophthalmol 1994; 117(1): 97–102.

46. Frucht-Pery J, Sugar J, Baum J, et al. Mitomycin C treatment for conjunctival-corneal intraepithelial neoplasia: a multicenter experience. Ophthalmology 1997; 104(12): 2085–93.

47. Frucht-Pery J, Rozenman Y, Pe'er J. Topical mitomycin-C for partially excised conjunctival squamous cell carcinoma. Ophthalmology 2002; 109(3): 548–52.

48. Yeatts RP, Ford JG, Stanton CA, Reed JW. Topical 5-fluorouracil in treating epithelial neoplasia of the conjunctiva and cornea. Ophthalmology 1995; 102(9): 1338–44.

49. Singh AD, Jacques R, Rundle PA, Rennie IG, Mudhar HS, Slater D. Neoadjuvant topical mitomycin C chemotherapy for conjunctival and corneal intraepithelial neoplasia. Eye (London) 2006; 20(9): 1092–4.

50. Vann RR, Karp CL. Perilesional and topical interferon alfa-2b for conjunctival and corneal neoplasia. Ophthalmology 1999; 106(1): 91–7.

51. Sepulveda R, Pe'er J, Midena E, Seregard S, Dua HS, Singh AD. Topical chemotherapy for ocular surface squamous neoplasia: current status. Br J Ophthalmol 2010; 94(5): 532–5.

52. Smith M, Trousdale MD, Rao NA, Robin JB. Lack of toxicity of a topical recombinant interferon alpha. Cornea 1989; 8(1): 58–61.

53. Singh AD. Excision and cryosurgery of conjunctival malignant epithelial tumours. Eye (London) 2003; 17(2): 125–6.

54. Glasson WJ, Hirst LW, Axelsen RA, Moon M. Invasive squamous cell carcinoma of the conjunctiva. Arch Ophthalmol 1994; 112(10): 1342–5.

55. Schachat AP. Management of uveal melanoma: a continuing dilemma. Collaborative Ocular Melanoma Study Group. Cancer 1994; 74(11): 3073–5.

56. Fine SL. No one knows the preferred management for choroidal melanoma. Am J Ophthalmol 1996; 122(1): 106–8.

57. Markowitz JA, Hawkins BS, Diener-West M, Schachat AP. A review of mortality from choroidal melanoma. I. Quality of published reports, 1966 through 1988. Arch Ophthalmol 1992; 110(2): 239–44.

58. Diener-West M, Hawkins BS, Markowitz JA, Schachat AP. A review of mortality from choroidal melanoma. II. A meta-analysis of 5-year mortality rates following enucleation, 1966 through 1988. Arch Ophthalmol 1992; 110(2): 245–50.

59. Zimmerman LE, McLean IW, Foster WD. Does enucleation of the eye containing a malignant melanoma prevent or accelerate the dissemination of tumour cells? Br J Ophthalmol 1978; 62(6): 420–5.

60. Singh AD, Rennie IG, Kivela T, Seregard S, Grossniklaus H. The Zimmerman–McLean–Foster hypothesis: 25 years later. Br J Ophthalmol 2004; 88(7): 962–7.

61. Singh AD, Topham A. Incidence of uveal melanoma in the United States: 1973–1997. Ophthalmology 2003; 110(5): 956–61.

62. Chang AE, Karnell LH, Menck HR. The National Cancer Data Base report on cutaneous and noncutaneous melanoma: a summary of 84,836 cases from the past decade. The American College of Surgeons Commission on Cancer and the American Cancer Society. Cancer 1998; 83(8): 1664–78.

63. Singh AD, Bergman L, Seregard S. Uveal melanoma: epidemiologic aspects. Ophthalmol Clin North Am 2005; 18(1): 75–84, viii.

64. Singh AD, Shields CL, Shields JA. Prognostic factors in uveal melanoma. Melanoma Res 2001; 11(3): 255–63.

65. Singh AD, Borden EC. Metastatic uveal melanoma. Ophthalmol Clin North Am 2005; 18(1): 143–50, ix.

66. Vajdic CM, Kricker A, Giblin M, et al. Incidence of ocular melanoma in Australia from 1990 to 1998. Int J Cancer 2003; 105(1): 117–22.

67. Michalova K, Clemett R, Dempster A, Evans J, Allardyce RA. Iris melanomas: are they more frequent in New Zealand? Br J Ophthalmol 2001; 85(1): 4–5.

68. Strickland D, Lee JA. Melanomas of eye: stability of rates. Am J Epidemiol 1981; 113(6): 700–2.

69. Egan KM, Seddon JM, Glynn RJ, Gragoudas ES, Albert DM. Epidemiologic aspects of uveal melanoma. Surv Ophthalmol 1988; 32(4): 239–51.

70. Singh AD, Damato B, Howard P, Harbour JW. Uveal melanoma: genetic aspects. Ophthalmol Clin North Am 2005; 18(1): 85–97, viii.

71. Collaborative Ocular Melanoma Study. Histopathologic characteristics of uveal melanomas in eyes enucleated from the Collaborative Ocular Melanoma Study. COMS Report No. 6. Am J Ophthalmol 1998; 125(6): 745–66.

72. Damato BE. Management of patients with uveal melanoma. In: Singh AD, Damato BE, Pe'er J, Murphree AL, Perry JD (eds) *Clinical Ophthalmic Oncology*. Philadelphia: Saunders-Elsevier, 2007. pp.226–31.

73. Collaborative Ocular Melanoma Study. *Manual of Procedures: accession no. PBS 179693*. Springfield, VA: National Technical Information Service, 1995.

74. Diener-West M, Earle JD, Fine SL, et al. The COMS randomized trial of iodine 125 brachytherapy for choroidal melanoma, III: initial mortality findings. COMS Report No. 18. Arch Ophthalmol 2001; 119(7): 969–82.

75. Collaborative Ocular Melanoma Study. The Collaborative Ocular Melanoma Study (COMS) randomized trial of pre-enucleation radiation of large choroidal melanoma II: initial mortality findings. COMS Report No. 10. Am J Ophthalmol 1998; 125(6): 779–96.

76. Collaborative Ocular Melanoma Study. Mortality in patients with small choroidal melanoma. The Collaborative Ocular Melanoma Study Group. COMS Report No. 4. Arch Ophthalmol 1997; 115(7): 886–93.

77. Melia BM, Abramson DH, Albert DM, et al. Collaborative Ocular Melanoma Study (COMS) randomized trial of I-125 brachytherapy for

medium choroidal melanoma. I. Visual acuity after 3 years. COMS Report No. 16. Ophthalmology 2001; 108(2): 348–66.

78. Diener-West M, Earle JD, Fine SL, *et al.* The COMS randomized trial of iodine 125 brachytherapy for choroidal melanoma, II: characteristics of patients enrolled and not enrolled. COMS Report No. 17. Arch Ophthalmol 2001; 119(7): 951–65.

79. Collaborative Ocular Melanoma Study. The Collaborative Ocular Melanoma Study (COMS) randomized trial of pre-enucleation radiation of large choroidal melanoma III: local complications and observations following enucleation COMS Report No. 11. Am J Ophthalmol 1998; 126(3): 362–72.

80. Diener-West M, Reynolds SM, Agugliaro DJ, *et al.* Screening for metastasis from choroidal melanoma: the Collaborative Ocular Melanoma Study Group. COMS Report No. 23. J Clin Oncol 2004; 22(12): 2438–44.

81. Turell ME, Saunthararajah Y, Triozzi PL, Tubbs RR, Crabb JW, Singh AD. Recent advances in prognostication for uveal melanoma. Int Ophthalmol 2011; Winter: 45–8.

82. Prescher G, Bornfeld N, Hirche H, Horsthemke B, Jockel KH, Becher R. Prognostic implications of monosomy 3 in uveal melanoma. Lancet 1996; 347(9010): 1222–5.

83. Patel KA, Edmondson ND, Talbot F, Parsons MA, Rennie IG, Sisley K. Prediction of prognosis in patients with uveal melanoma using fluorescence in situ hybridisation. Br J Ophthalmol 2001; 85(12): 1440–4.

84. Tschentscher F, Husing J, Holter T, *et al.* Tumor classification based on gene expression profiling shows that uveal melanomas with and without monosomy 3 represent two distinct entities. Cancer Res 2003; 63(10): 2578–84.

85. Onken MD, Worley LA, Tuscan MD, Harbour JW. An accurate, clinically feasible multi-gene expression assay for predicting metastasis in uveal melanoma. J Mol Diagn 2010; 12(4): 461–8.

86. Midena E, Bonaldi L, Parrozzani R, Tebaldi E, Boccassini B, Vujosevic S. In vivo detection of monosomy 3 in eyes with medium-sized uveal melanoma using transscleral fine needle aspiration biopsy. Eur J Ophthalmol 2006; 16(3): 422–5.

87. Damato B, Duke C, Coupland SE, *et al.* Cytogenetics of uveal melanoma: a 7-year clinical experience. Ophthalmology 2007; 114(10): 1925–31.

88. http://clinicaltrials.gov/ct2/show/NCT01100528?term=uveal+melanoma+dacarbazine&rank=1, No. 3095, 2010.

89. Augsburger JJ, Correa ZM, Shaikh AH. Effectiveness of treatments for metastatic uveal melanoma. Am J Ophthalmol 2009; 148(1): 119–27.

90. Danielli R, Ridolfi R, Chiarion-Sileni V, *et al.* Ipilimumab in pretreated patients with metastatic uveal melanoma: safety and clinical efficacy. Cancer Immunol Immunother 2012; 61(1): 41–8.

91. Albert DM. Historic review of retinoblastoma. Ophthalmology 1987; 94(6): 654–62.

92. Kupfer C. Retinoblastoma treated with intravenous nitrogen mustard. Am J Ophthalmol 1953; 36(12): 1721–3.

93. Reese AB. *Tumors of the Eye.* New York: Harper and Row, 1976.

94. Murphree AL. Intraocular retinoblastoma: the case for a new group classification. Ophthalmol Clin North Am 2005; 18(1): 41–53, viii.

95. Broaddus E, Topham A, Singh AD. Incidence of retinoblastoma in the USA: 1975–2004. Br J Ophthalmol 2009; 93(1): 21–3.

96. Gallie BL, Dunn JM, Chan HS, Hamel PA, Phillips RA. The genetics of retinoblastoma. Relevance to the patient. Pediatr Clin North Am 1991; 38(2): 299–315.

97. Friend SH, Bernards R, Rogelj S, *et al.* A human DNA segment with properties of the gene that predisposes to retinoblastoma and osteosarcoma. Nature 1986; 323(6089): 643–6.

98. Gallie BL, Dunn JM, Hamel PA, Muncaster M, Cohen BL, Phillips RA. How do retinoblastoma tumours form? Eye (London) 1992; 6(Pt 2): 226–31.

99. Sang DN, Albert DM. Retinoblastoma: clinical and histopathologic features. Hum Pathol 1982; 13(2): 133–47.

100. Abramson DH, Frank CM, Susman M, Whalen MP, Dunkel IJ, Boyd NW 3rd. Presenting signs of retinoblastoma. J Pediatr 1998; 132(3 Pt 1): 505–8.

101. Shields CL, Honavar S, Shields JA, Demirci H, Meadows AT. Vitrectomy in eyes with unsuspected retinoblastoma. Ophthalmology 2000; 107(12): 2250–5.

102. Pratt CB, Crom DB, Howarth C. The use of chemotherapy for extraocular retinoblastoma. Med Pediatr Oncol 1985; 13(6): 330–3.

103. Singh AD, Santos CM, Shields CL, Shields JA, Eagle RC Jr. Observations on 17 patients with retinocytoma. Arch Ophthalmol 2000; 118(2): 199–205.

104. Murphree AL. Local therapy, brachytherapy, and enucleation. In: Singh AD, Damato BE, Pe'er J, Murphree AL, Perry JD (eds) *Clinical Ophthalmic Oncology.* Philadelphia: Saunders-Elsevier, 2007. pp.454–61.

105. Shields JA, Parsons H, Shields CL, Giblin ME. The role of cryotherapy in the management of retinoblastoma. Am J Ophthalmol 1989; 108(3): 260–4.

106. Journee-de Korver HG, Midena E, Singh AD. Infrared thermotherapy: from laboratory to clinic. Ophthalmol Clin North Am 2005; 18(1): 99–110, viii–ix.

107. Shields JA, Shields CL, de Potter P, Hernandez JC, Brady LW. Plaque radiotherapy for residual or recurrent retinoblastoma in 91 cases. J Pediatr Ophthalmol Strabismus 1994; 31(4): 242–5.

108. Hernandez JC, Brady LW, Shields JA, *et al.* External beam radiation for retinoblastoma: results, patterns of failure, and a proposal for treatment guidelines. Int J Radiat Oncol Biol Phys 1996; 35(1): 125–32.

109. Ferris FL 3rd, Chew EY. A new era for the treatment of retinoblastoma. Arch Ophthalmol 1996; 114(11): 1412.

110. Chan HS, Gallie BL, Munier FL, Beck Popovic M. Chemotherapy for retinoblastoma. Ophthalmol Clin North Am 2005; 18(1): 55–63, viii.

111. Shields CL, Honavar SG, Meadows AT, *et al.* Chemoreduction plus focal therapy for retinoblastoma: factors predictive of need for treatment with external beam radiotherapy or enucleation. Am J Ophthalmol 2002; 133(5): 657–64.

112. Scott IU, Murray TG, Toledano S, O'Brien JM. New retinoblastoma tumors in children undergoing systemic chemotherapy. Arch Ophthalmol 1998; 116(12): 1685–6.

113. Benz MS, Scott IU, Murray TG, Kramer D, Toledano S. Complications of systemic chemotherapy as treatment of retinoblastoma. Arch Ophthalmol 2000; 118(4): 577–8.

114. Yamane T, Kaneko A, Mohri M. The technique of ophthalmic arterial infusion therapy for patients with intraocular retinoblastoma. Int J Clin Oncol 2004; 9(2): 69–73.

115. Abramson DH. Super selective ophthalmic artery delivery of chemotherapy for intraocular retinoblastoma: 'chemosurgery'. The first Stallard lecture. Br J Ophthalmol 2010; 94(4): 396–9.

116. Shields CL, Shields JA. Intra-arterial chemotherapy for retinoblastoma: the beginning of a long journey. Clin Exper Ophthalmol 2010; 38(6): 638–43.

117. Meadows AT, Chintagumpala M, Dunkel IJ, Friedman D, Stoner JA, Villablanca JG. Children's Oncology Group (COG) trials for retinoblastoma. In: Singh AD, Damato BE, Pe'er J, Murphree AL, Perry JD (eds) *Clinical Ophthalmic Oncology.* Philadelphia: Saunders-Elsevier, 2007. pp. 491–5.

118. Kopelman JE, McLean IW, Rosenberg SH. Multivariate analysis of risk factors for metastasis in retinoblastoma treated by enucleation. Ophthalmology 1987; 94(4): 371–7.

119. MacKay CJ, Abramson DH, Ellsworth RM. Metastatic patterns of retinoblastoma. Arch Ophthalmol 1984; 102(3): 391–6.

120. Honavar SG, Singh AD, Shields CL, *et al.* Postenucleation adjuvant therapy in high-risk retinoblastoma. Arch Ophthalmol 2002; 120(7): 923–31.

121. Singh AD, Shields CL, Shields JA. Prognostic factors in retinoblastoma. J Pediatr Ophthalmol Strabismus 2000; 37(3): 134–41.

122. Singh AD, Shields CL, Shields JA. New insights into trilateral retinoblastoma. Cancer 1999; 86(1): 3–5.

123. Kivela T. Trilateral retinoblastoma: a meta-analysis of hereditary retino-blastoma associated with primary ectopic intracranial retinoblastoma. J Clin Oncol 1999; 17(6): 1829–37.

124. Eng C, Li FP, Abramson DH, *et al*. Mortality from second tumors among long-term survivors of retinoblastoma. J Nat Cancer Inst 1993; 85(14): 1121–8.

125. Abramson DH, Frank CM. Second nonocular tumors in survivors of bilateral retinoblastoma: a possible age effect on radiation-related risk. Ophthalmology 1998; 105(4): 573–9; discussion 579–80.

126. Kleinerman RA, Tucker MA, Tarone RE, *et al*. Risk of new cancers after radiotherapy in long-term survivors of retinoblastoma: an extended follow-up. J Clin Oncol 2005; 23(10): 2272–9.

63 Introduction to Rare Cancers of Childhood

Alberto S. Pappo[1] and Gregory H. Reaman[2]

[1] Division of Solid Tumors, St Jude Children's Research Hospital, Memphis, TN, USA
[2] Division of Oncology, Children's National Medical Center, Washington, DC, USA

Childhood cancer in itself is a rare disease since only 12,400 children under the age of 20 years are diagnosed with cancer each year in the United States.[1] Furthermore, the Rare Disease Act of 2002 (http://history.nih.gov/research/downloads/PL107-280.pdf) defines a rare disease as one that affects populations smaller than 200,000 persons in the United States. Thus the definition of a rare cancer in the pediatric population poses significant challenges.

Investigators from the Italian Cooperative Project on Rare Pediatric Tumors (TREP) defined a pediatric rare tumor as one that has an incidence of less than 2 per million population per year and is not the subject of specific clinical trials.[2] Unfortunately, this definition would exclude the two most common histological subtypes of rare cancers seen in children, melanoma and thyroid carcinoma, both having an incidence rate that exceed 5 per million per year (http://seer.cancer.gov/csr/1975_2008/results_merged/sect_29_childhood_cancer_iccc.pdf). The German Society of Pediatric Oncology and Hematology (GPOH) has opted to consider rare pediatric cancers as those tumors that are not registered within a specific pediatric GPOH study.[3] In the experience of German investigators, such tumors account for about 5.4% of all registered malignancies in patients less than 20 years of age and this number would translate into 50 children and adolescents with rare tumors per year who would be eligible for treatment.[3] The Children's Oncology Group (COG) has opted to use a broader and more descriptive definition of a rare cancer in children and has included the subset of tumors listed in the International Classification of Childhood Cancer subgroup XI of the Surveillance, Epidemiology, and End Results (SEER) section of the National Cancer Institute database.[1] This group of tumors includes adrenocortical carcinoma, nasopharyngeal carcinoma, malignant melanoma, nonmelanoma skin cancers, and other nonspecified carcinomas and accounts for about 9% of all childhood tumors (Fig. 63.1). About 75% of the tumors selected for study by the infrequent tumor subcommittee of the COG Rare Tumor Committee affect patients between 15 and 19 years of age, making their study extremely challenging.[6] Although the incidence rates for cancer in this age group are twice those reported in younger patients, clinical trial participation is one-fourth of the corresponding rates seen in younger patients.[4] Similarly, survival rates for 15–19 year olds have lagged behind when compared to the excellent outcomes seen in younger patients.[5]

When the Pediatric Oncology Group and the Children's Cancer Group merged in 2000, a unique opportunity to study rare cancers in North America emerged and in 2002, the Children's Oncology Group created the Rare Tumor Committee, composed of the infrequent tumor subcommittee, the liver tumor subcommittee, the germ cell tumor subcommittee, and more recently the retinoblastoma subcommittee. The main purpose of the infrequent tumor subcommittee was to facilitate the study of rare childhood cancers by fostering interdisciplinary multicenter collaborations. To better define the prevalence of these tumors in the pediatric population, the infrequent tumor subcommittee encouraged investigators to participate in the COG registry, a tool available to all member institutions which captures all new cases of childhood cancer referred to COG participating centers. As shown in Figure 63.2, based on information from the SEER database from 2002 to 2007, the expected number of registrations on the SEER registry for patients with rare cancers under the age of 20 years would have been 9756. However, only 686 (7%) cases were recorded in the COG registry,[6] a figure similar to what had been previously reported by both groups prior to the merger.[7] Interestingly, patients with the two most common "infrequent tumors," melanoma and thyroid carcinoma, had the lowest registration rates (about 5%) whereas other infrequent cancers such as adrenocortical and nasopharyngeal carcinoma had significantly higher registration rates.[6]

Our experience is similar to that of other investigators and confirms that registration rates for infrequent cancers are age and histology dependent.[8] These differences might be explained by the fact that younger patients afflicted with rare cancers such as adrenocortical carcinoma are often referred to centers with clinical expertise in the multimodal management of these patients. For younger patients with "adult-type cancers" such as nasopharyngeal carcinoma, referral to centers with multidisciplinary management teams is essential for successful treatment. In contrast, thyroid carcinoma and cutaneous melanoma are primarily surgical diseases and therapy can often be delivered by providers located outside a pediatric center. Furthermore, physicians in such centers may be eager to retain these patients and are likely unaware of the research opportunities offered by the pediatric cooperative groups.

Availability of paired normal and tumor tissue is vital for advancing research. Recent examples in pediatric rare cancers include the identification of a unique germline *p53* R337h mutation in Brazilian cases of pediatric adrenocortical carcinoma,[9] the presence of germline inactivating mutations of the RNase endonuclease *DICER1* in cases of familial pleuropulmonary blastoma,[10] and the presence of germline mutations in the succinate dehydrogenase complex II in subsets of patients with pediatric gastrointestinal stromal tumors.[11] Interestingly, the information generated from tumors and

patients in the examples cited above was derived from registries that were not linked to a national cooperative group. In this respect, Bleyer has published that available banked tumor tissue in the adolescent and young adult population is underrepresented and that this fact could hinder the research efforts in this patient population.[12] In the experience of the COG, the rate of tumor banking for infrequent cancers over a 5-year period was poor; only 56 samples out of 517 frozen specimens submitted to an open COG banking protocol were from patients with infrequent tumors.[6] Thus, if we take into consideration the low registration rates in the COG registry and the poor participation rates in the current COG banking protocol, we can expect that only about 1% of all pediatric and adolescents with rare cancers will have tissue banked for future research studies.

Clinical trial participation amongst adolescents and young adults with infrequent cancers is suboptimal[6,7] and the limited number of patients does not allow the conduct of prospective randomized trials. For this reason, investigators of various cooperative groups have undertaken different approaches to formulate diagnostic and treatment recommendations for these diseases. The COG partnered with the Eastern Cooperative Oncology Group and the Southwest Oncology Group and opened two randomized studies for the treatment of pediatric melanoma (age ≥10 years) but over a 4-year period, only four patients with melanoma were enrolled in these trials. In addition, the COG has developed two single-arm trials for the treatment of pediatric nasopharyngeal carcinoma and adrenocortical carcinoma but initial enrollment rates for these trials were disappointing.[6] The COG is currently in the process of publishing literature reviews summarizing diagnostic and treatment strategies for various rare pediatric cancers including pleuropulmonary blastoma, melanoma, and colorectal carcinoma.

The German cooperative group GPOH has opted to register all patients with solid tumors that do not fall into any GPOH prospective therapeutic trial and after the development of the registry and uniform therapeutic strategies, overall registration rates increased almost ten-fold in some diseases such as granulosa

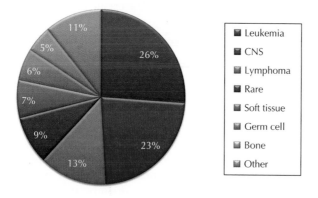

Figure 63.1 Percentage distribution of cancers in patients 0–19 years of age using the International Classification of Childhood Cancer, SEER 2004–2008.

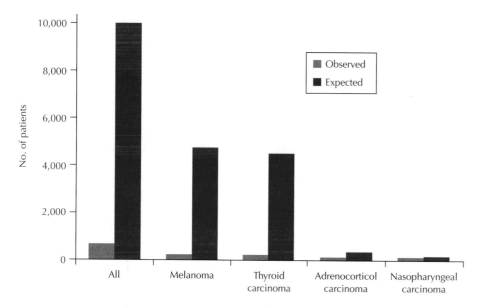

Figure 63.2 Observed versus expected numbers of rare cancers registered in the COG registry 2002–2007. Reproduced from Pappo *et al.*[6] with permission from The American Society of Clinical Oncology.

and Sertoli Leydig cell tumors. Other diseases that have been registered in their initiative include melanoma, epithelial tumors of the salivary glands, and gastrointestinal carcinomas.[3,13] The Italian TREP project has developed guidelines for treatment of specific diseases and has published reviews of various rare tumors that have been registered in the Italian network.[14–16]

It is clear that increased participation in registries and cooperative group initiatives is needed in order to move the field forward. The COG is currently exploring a new initiative called the Childhood Cancer Research Network in hopes of positively impacting registration rates of various pediatric cancers, including rare cancers. Additionally, we need to actively explore different mechanisms for reimbursement to institutions that actively participate in banking and therapeutic trials and expand our international collaborative opportunities in order to improve accrual to therapeutic trials and biology studies.

In the following chapters the reader will find a description of the salient clinical features and treatment options for children with various rare cancers.

References

1. Ries LAG, Smith MA, Gurney JG, et al. Cancer Incidence and Survival among Children and Adolescents: United States SEER Program 1975–1995. Pub No 99-4649. Bethesda, MD: National Cancer Institute, SEER Program, 1999.

2. Ferrari A, Bisogno G, de Salvo GL, et al. The challenge of very rare tumours in childhood: the Italian TREP project. Eur J Cancer 2007; 43: 654–9.

3. Brecht IB, Graf N, Schweinitz D, et al. Networking for children and adolescents with very rare tumors: foundation of the GPOH Pediatric Rare Tumor Group. Klin Padiatr 2009; 221: 181–5.

4. Bleyer A, Budd T, Montello M. Adolescents and young adults with cancer: the scope of the problem and criticality of clinical trials. Cancer 2006; 107: 1645–55.

5. Bleyer WA. Cancer in older adolescents and young adults: epidemiology, diagnosis, treatment, survival, and importance of clinical trials. Med Pediatr Oncol 2002; 38: 1–10.

6. Pappo AS, Krailo M, Chen Z, et al. Infrequent Tumor Initiative of the Children's Oncology Group: initial lessons learned and their impact on future plans. J Clin Oncol 2010; 28: 5011–16.

7. Liu L, Krailo M, Reaman GH, et al. Childhood cancer patients' access to cooperative group cancer programs: a population-based study. Cancer 2003; 97: 1339–45.

8. Ferrari A, Montello M, Budd T, et al. The challenges of clinical trials for adolescents and young adults with cancer. Pediatr Blood Cancer 2008; 50: 1101–4.

9. DiGiammarino EL, Lee AS, Cadwell C, et al. A novel mechanism of tumorigenesis involving pH-dependent destabilization of a mutant p53 tetramer. Nat Struct Biol 2002; 9:12–16.

10. Hill DA, Ivanovich J, Priest JR, et al. DICER1 mutations in familial pleuropulmonary blastoma. Science 2009; 325: 965.

11. Janeway KA, Kim SY, Lodish M, et al. Defects in succinate dehydrogenase in gastrointestinal stromal tumors lacking KIT and PDGFRA mutations. Proc Natl Acad Sci USA 2011; 108: 314–18.

12. Bleyer A, Barr R, Hayes-Lattin B, et al. The distinctive biology of cancer in adolescents and young adults. Nat Rev Cancer 2008; 8: 288–98.

13. Schneider DT, Brecht IB. Care for rare cancers: improved care requires improved communication. Klin Padiatr 2010; 222: 124–6.

14. Carretto E, Inserra A, Ferrari A, et al. Epithelial thymic tumours in paediatric age: a report from the TREP project. Orphanet J Rare Dis 2011; 6: 28.

15. Cecchetto G, Ferrari A, Bernini G, et al. Sex cord stromal tumors of the ovary in children: a clinicopathological report from the Italian TREP project. Pediatr Blood Cancer 2011; 56: 1062–7.

16. Dall'igna P, Cecchetto G, Bisogno G, et al. Pancreatic tumors in children and adolescents: the Italian TREP project experience. Pediatr Blood Cancer 2010; 54: 675–80.

64 Uncommon Tumors of the Gastrointestinal Tract in Children

Alberto S. Pappo[1] and Wayne L. Furman[2]

[1] Division of Solid Tumors, [2] Department of Oncology, St Jude Children's Research Hospital, Memphis, TN, USA

Introduction

In 2010, there were approximately 274,000 cases of cancer of the digestive system in the United States and the most common histologies were carcinomas of the colon, rectum, and pancreas.[1] The median age at diagnosis of these malignancies is approximately 70 years (http://seer.cancer.gov/statfacts/index.html). Adenocarcinomas account for the majority of gastrointestinal malignancies in adults and the remaining tumor types include carcinoid-neuroendocrine carcinoma, hepatocellular carcinoma, squamous cell carcinoma of the esophagus, malignant lymphoma, leiomyosarcoma, and malignant gastrointestinal stromal tumors (GISTs). With the exception of malignant lymphoma, the overwhelming majority of these neoplasms are diagnosed in individuals over the age of 40 years.

Gastrointestinal malignancies are rare in children (Table 64.1). Review of the Surveillance, Epidemiology and End Results (SEER) database from 2004 to 2008 identified 616 gastrointestinal malignancies in children under the age of 20 years. The most common sites and histologies are given in Table 64.2. Based on these figures, the most common epithelial malignancies of the gastrointestinal tract in children appear to be carcinoid tumors and colorectal carcinoma and most occur in older children.

Carcinoid tumors

Carcinoid tumors are neuroendocrine tumors that vary in their clinical behavior depending on their hormone production and site of origin. They can occur in lung,[6] bronchi,[7] and thymus[8,9] as well as the gastrointestinal tract,[10–12] pancreas,[13] and liver.[6,14,15] These tumors arise from enterochromaffin cells and most contain membrane-bound secretory granules which contain a variety of vasoactive peptides, the most common of which is serotonin.[16] Release of these vasoactive peptides into the systemic circulation produces symptoms referred to as the carcinoid syndrome.[16–21] Symptoms include episodic diarrhea and flushing, usually with a feeling of warmth, and can include bronchial constriction, peripheral vasomotor symptoms, and cyanosis.[16,17] These tumors can secrete a variety of biologically active substances besides serotonin, including histamine, somatostatin, growth hormone, calcitonin, gastrin, prostaglandins, dopamine, vasoactive intestinal peptide, and corticotropin, and symptoms vary with the type of vasoactive peptides secreted.[16,17] The preoperative diagnosis of carcinoid tumors is often based on urinary elevation of 5-hydroxyindoleacetic acid (5-HIAA), a serotonin metabolite.[16] Plasma levels of chromogranin A may also be a useful tumor marker.[22]

Although much of our discussion will apply to carcinoid tumors in any site, we will limit our discussion here to tumors arising in the abdominal cavity in children. Carcinoid tumors are more common in females, often occur in the appendix in pediatric series[18,23–30] and occur in 1–1.42 children per million younger than 15 years.[24] In adults they are most often found in the small intestine (45%).[16] A carcinoid tumor is found incidentally in approximately 1 in 2–300 appendectomies.[17] With rare exceptions,[31] these tumors are small (<2 cm[32]), and in children rarely produce the carcinoid syndrome,[18,24,29,33,34] although one series reports a single 8-year-old male with a 4 mm tumor who presented with the carcinoid syndrome in addition to abdominal pain and fever.[35] Generally appendiceal carcinoids require only simple surgical resection unless there is evidence of metastases or the tumor is greater than 2 cm.[36,37] In these larger tumors or if there is evidence of metastases, right hemicolectomy is sometimes recommended,[11,17,37–39] although in children this may not be necessary.[29,32]

The appropriate diagnostic evaluation depends on the primary tumor site.[40] Recommendations for initial staging include computed tomography (CT) of chest, abdomen, and pelvis, Technethium 99-bone scan as well as 24-h urine for 5-HIAA[35] and plasma chromogranin A.[22,41] In cases where CT imaging is unclear, magnetic resonance imaging (MRI) may be helpful.[42] Since a majority of carcinoid tumors express somatostatin receptors, octreotide scans are also often used.[43–46]

Textbook of Uncommon Cancer, Fourth Edition. Edited by Derek Raghavan, Charles D. Blanke, David H. Johnson, Paul L. Moots, Gregory H. Reaman, Peter G. Rose and Mikkael A. Sekeres.
© 2012 John Wiley & Sons, Inc. Published 2012 by John Wiley & Sons, Inc.

The treatment of choice is complete surgical resection, when possible.[10,16,21,38,40–42,47] There is no known effective therapy for unresectable metastatic tumors. When resection is not possible, chemoembolization or radiofrequency ablation have been used to palliate symptoms and improve survival.[48–50] For patients with metastatic disease, the choices are less clear-cut. If patients have carcinoid syndrome, treatment with octreotide and its analogs often improves the symptoms and has resulted in significant clinical responses in some patients.[51–53] The addition of interferon-α to octreotide confers extra benefit to some patients, especially those resistant to octreotide alone.[42,54,55] Most carcinoid tumors are resistant to cytotoxic chemotherapy, although some responses have been seen with 5-fluorouracil (5-FU) and streptozotocin or doxorubicin.[42] More recently, encouraging results have been seen with sunitinib[56] and everolimus with octreotide long-acting release (LAR).[57]

Table 64.1 Pediatric series of gastrointestinal tumors.

Author	No. of patients	Lymphoma	Colorectal	Carcinoid	Other
Ladd[2]	58	30	6	2	20
Bethel[3]	55	41	3	9	2
Skinner[4]	39	22	4	1	12
Hameed[5]	57	47	7		3

Colorectal carcinoma

Although colorectal carcinoma (CRC) is the third most common cancer in adults,[58] it is very rare in children and adolescents. Our knowledge of CRC in pediatrics is based on a handful of case series and case reports.[59–78] Apart from one small clinical trial,[62] there has been a lack of prospective clinical studies in this age group. These publications have suggested that compared to adults with CRC, there is a higher frequency of mucinous histology and more advanced stage disease at diagnosis. We will summarize the available data on the epidemiology, biology, risk factors, presenting features, prognosis, and treatment of CRC in children and adolescents.

Epidemiology

In the United States every year, approximately 150,000 cases of CRC are diagnosed with more than 90% occurring in patients older than 50 years of age[58] (Fig. 64.1),[79] although it has been reported in a child as young as 9 months of age.[80] However, fewer than 100 cases are diagnosed each year in children, adolescents and young adults (see Fig. 64.1 insert).[77] CRC accounts for 2.1% of malignancies in the 15–29-year age group[79] (Fig. 64.2).[79] At St Jude Children's Research Hospital, where more than 20,000 children and adolescents with cancer have been seen since March 1962, CRC has been diagnosed in only 77 children ≤20 years of age.[59]

Table 64.2 Digestive system malignancies by age, SEER 2004–2008.

	00 years	01–04 years	05–09 years	10–14 years	15–19 years
	Count	Count	Count	Count	Count
Digestive system	105	192	52	71	196
Esophagus	0	0	^	0	0
Stomach	0	^	^	^	19
Small intestine	0	0	0	^	^
Colon and rectum	^	^	0	13	87
Colon excluding rectum	^	^	0	13	68
Cecum	^	0	0	0	9
Appendix	0	0	0	7	15
Ascending colon	0	0	0	0	9
Hepatic flexure	0	0	0	^	^
Transverse colon	0	0	0	^	6
Splenic flexure	^	0	0	^	5
Descending colon	0	0	0	0	^
Sigmoid colon	0	^	0	^	13
Large intestine, not otherwise specified	0	0	0	0	^
Rectum and rectosigmoid junction	0	0	0	0	19
Rectosigmoid junction	0	0	0	0	^
Rectum	0	0	0	0	16
Anus, anal canal and anorectum	0	^	0	0	^
Liver and intrahepatic bile duct	67	124	28	29	52
Liver	67	124	28	28	52
Intrahepatic bile duct	0	0	0	^	0
Gallbladder	0	0	0	^	0
Other biliary	0	^	0	0	^
Pancreas	0	^	^	^	15
Retroperitoneum	34	57	18	16	11
Peritoneum, omentum and mesentery	^	^	^	^	^
Other digestive organs	^	0	0	0	^

^, fewer than five cases.

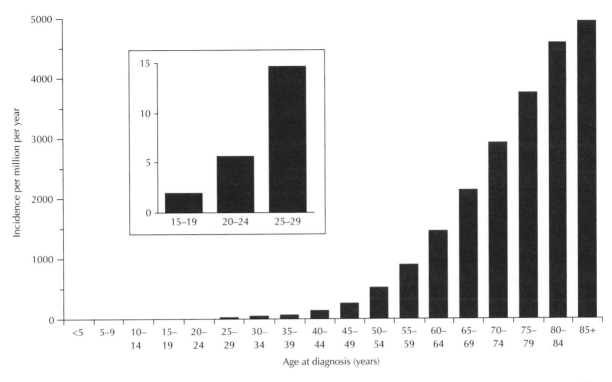

Figure 64.1 Incidence of colorectal cancer by age group in the period 1975–2000, based on the national SEER data. Reproduced from Bleyer *et al.*[79]

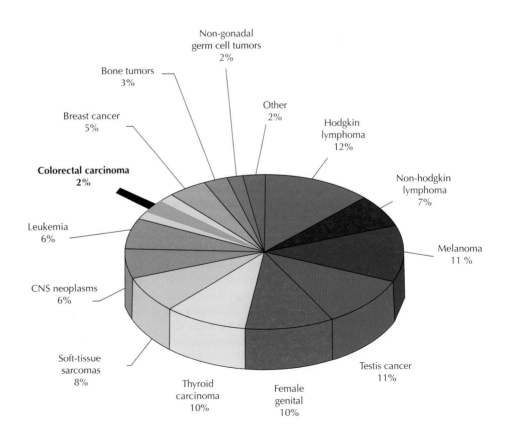

Figure 64.2 Cancer subtypes in the 15–29 year age group. Reproduced from Bleyer *et al.*[79]

Risk factors

In adults, CRC is more common in developed countries. Although the cause of this disparity is not well understood, dietary differences have been suggested as a major factor. Other factors reported to be associated with an increased incidence of CRC in adults include obesity,[81] a high-calorie diet, high consumption and/or overcooking of red meat,[82] excess alcohol consumption,[83,84] sedentary lifestyle,[85] and cigarette smoking.[86] However, the disparate incidence in developed and undeveloped countries is more likely to reflect complex interactions among multiple factors, including genetics, lifestyle, and environment, as well as diet.[87] Most of these factors are unlikely to exert a major effect in children. Although case series offer clues about the biological nature of CRC in patients less than 20 years of age, definitive conclusions cannot be drawn from the small numbers of patients studied.

Most CRC in adults arise from stepwise changes that occur in preexisting adenomas. In 1990 Fearon and Vogelstein put forth a model for the development of CRC, based on observations of genetic mutations in samples of colonic adenomas and carcinomas. They suggested that these colonic lesions progressed from epithelial hyperplasia to adenomas to invasive carcinomas.[88,89] Adenomatous polyps are thought to require more than 5 years of growth before becoming clinically significant, and the progression from adenoma to carcinoma is thought to occur over about 10 years.[90] Although this model seems to hold true in most adult CRC,[90–92] it may not apply to childhood cases of this disease. There are several factors that argue for a different pathogenesis in children: CRC has been seen in children as young as 9 months[80]; premalignant adenomas are rarely seen in proximity to sporadic CRC in children; and CRC in children tends to be of mucinous histology.[77] Children with familial polypoid syndromes of the gastrointestinal tract such as the familial adenomatous polyposis (FAP) syndromes are an exception in which Fearon and Vogelstein's model may hold true.[88,89] In children with FAP, CRC occurs at younger ages, due to inherited genetic susceptibilities that result in accelerated progression of adenomas and malignant transformation.[93–95]

About 20–30% of adult CRC patients will have a significant family history, defined as a first- or second-degree relative with CRC; however, only about 5% have a well-defined inherited genetic syndrome.[96] The most common of these (3–5% of all patients) is hereditary nonpolyposis CRC (HNPCC) or Lynch syndrome; the second most common (~1%) is FAP or Gardner syndrome.[97] The remainder are syndromes involving hamartomatous polyps, such as Peutz–Jeghers syndrome and familial juvenile polyposis.[98] For the majority of these cases the specific genes remain to be characterized.[99] The incidence of these well-defined genetic syndromes in children with CRC cannot be clearly determined from available pediatric series.[59–61,64,65,69–72,74,75,77,94,95,100] Other predisposing risk factors for CRC in children include inflammatory bowel disease,[101,102] prior radiation exposure,[103] and certain hereditary conditions.

Familial adenomatous polyposis is inherited as a dominant trait with 90% penetrance and may be associated with the appearance of multiple cancers by the age of 37 years.[104,105]

Early diagnosis and total colectomy eliminate the risk of development of CRC for these patients. Because nearly every patient with FAP will eventually develop CRC if left untreated, the standard of care is prophylactic colectomy. However, the optimal timing of colectomy in children with FAP is unknown.[93,95] Colonic polyps appear at a median age of 16 years[106] but have been seen in children as young as 5 years.[107] The majority of children with FAP who developed CRC had a severe polyposis phenotype (more than 1000 colonic polyps).[108]

Other syndromes associated with colorectal carcinoma in young people include Turcot syndrome,[109] for which the frequent mutation of the adenomatous polyposis coli gene has been found,[110] Oldfield syndrome,[111] and Gardner syndrome.[112] There may be an association of neurofibromatosis and polyposis coli,[113] and one individual with multiple adenomatous polyps and multiple colonic carcinomas had a constitutional deletion of the p53 gene, also in association with neurofibromatosis.[113]

Clinical features

Most large series suggest that children tend to present with late-stage disease and mucinous histology and that they have a relatively poor outcome.[59–62,64,65,69–72,75,77,78,94] However, a recent review of data from the SEER program suggests that these findings may reflect reporting bias.[79] Early signs of colorectal carcinoma are difficult to distinguish from more common and benign causes of abdominal complaints in children. The presenting complaints are often vague and nonspecific and include abdominal pain, weight loss, change in bowel habits, anemia, and bleeding.[59,77,114] In a recent review of 77 children with CRC who presented to St Jude Children's Research Hospital, patients had experienced symptoms for a median of 3 months and most were anemic.[59] All the presenting complaints are so common in pediatric care that the possible diagnosis of CRC may be overlooked, whereas in an older adult these same complaints would prompt a colonoscopy. This delay in considering a diagnosis of CRC may be partially responsible for many children presenting with advanced-stage disease. As in most other pediatric series (summarized in Saab and Furman[77]), 66 of 77 patients (86%) at St Jude presented with advanced-stage disease, 48(62%) had mucinous histology, 33 (43%) had >10% signet ring cells, and the 10-year event-free survival estimate overall was only 17.7%±5.1%.[59] All these parameters are "worse" than those reported in adults with CRC.[58,115] However, while vigilance for pediatric CRC remains important, adult-type screening exams (e.g. colonoscopy, routine fecal occult blood testing, and sigmoidoscopy) are not likely to be cost-effective and will generally identify many false positives in the absence of known risk factors.

In the St Jude review,[59] the median duration from the onset of symptoms to diagnosis was 3 months (range 1 day to 18 months). This wide range of time to diagnosis was evident in almost all reviews of CRC in children,[77] with the duration of symptoms before diagnosis ranging from 1 day to 6 years and a median duration of several months. This may be due to the rarity of CRC in children and the fact that multiple benign pediatric abdominal conditions present with similar symptoms and are much more common. This delay in diagnosis has

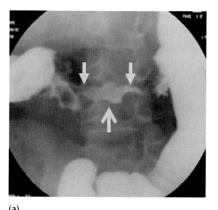
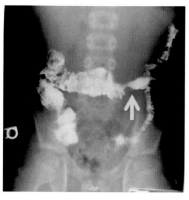
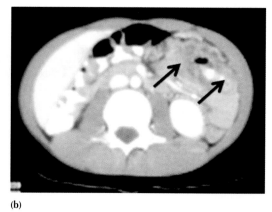

(a)　　　　　　　　　　　　　　　　　　　　　　　　　　　　　　(b)

Figure 64.3 (a) Barium enema of a 14 year old with colorectal carcinoma, showing an apple-core lesion in the transverse colon (*arrows*). (b) CT scan of the abdomen in the same patient, showing circumferential thickening of the colonic wall (*arrows*). Courtesy of Dr Sue Kaste, St Jude Children's Research Hospital, Memphis, TN, USA.

also been presumed to be one reason why children with CRC present at more advanced disease stages than adults. However, in the review from St Jude,[59] a comparison between patients whose time to diagnosis was less than 2 months (20 patients) and those whose diagnosis occurred after 2–6 months (12 patients) from the onset of symptoms revealed that those with a longer time to diagnosis tended to have a lower stage of disease ($p = 0.063$) and better estimates of event-free survival ($p < 0.001$) and overall survival ($p = 0.014$). These data suggest that the longer time to diagnosis may be a result of differences in tumor biology rather than simply a delay in recognizing the symptoms.[116]

Children and adolescents with CRC also often present with acute abdominal conditions such as acute obstruction, perforation, or severe pain mimicking appendicitis. In adults, intestinal obstruction is the presenting symptom in 15–20%.[117] In some pediatric reports, acute presentations, including intestinal obstruction and acute pain mimicking appendicitis, account for close to 50% of presentations.[61,64,67–70] This high frequency has been partially blamed on the fact that symptoms are often missed in children until the tumor is large enough to cause an acute abdominal presentation. Another explanation could be more aggressive tumor biology in children, leading to rapidly advanced local disease and acute symptomatology.

Diagnosis and staging

Once the diagnosis is suspected, evaluation often includes abdominal x-rays, barium enema, CT of abdomen and pelvis, and MRI if CT is inadequate. Typically these studies will reveal obstruction, narrowing of the colonic lumen, or an abdominal mass (Fig. 64.3). Depending on the situation, either colonoscopy with excision of a polyp or actual biopsy with excision of the mass would be the next step. Histopathological examination of tissue is required for diagnosis (Fig. 64.4). The procedure used to obtain tissue is best determined in consultation with surgical colleagues and depends on the patient's clinical situation. Decisions about how tissue is to be obtained should take into account that surgery is the most important component of effective therapy.

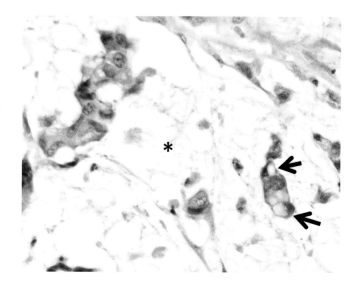

Figure 64.4 Histological section of colorectal carcinoma of the mucinous subtype. Copious mucinous material (*asterisk*) and signet cells (*arrowhead*) in the tumor. Courtesy of Dr Jesse Jenkins, St Jude Children's Research Hospital, Memphis, TN, USA.

Once the diagnosis has been established, evaluation for distant metastatic disease should be completed, including a CT of the chest. Positron emission tomography (PET)-CT may be considered for selected patients but is not routinely indicated.[118] At this point, the utility of fluorodeoxyglucose PET (FDG-PET) scans is unclear. This method appears to be less useful in detecting lesions of mucinous histology.[119] Because mucinous lesions appear to predominate in children, FDG-PET scans may be less helpful in these patients.

Other tests to consider include a total colonoscopy to identify other synchronous lesions or polyps, complete blood count, blood chemistry panel with liver enzymes, and typically a serum carcinoembryonic antigen (CEA) level. Although this antigen is useful in adults[120] to monitor disease and predict recurrence or progression, it is less likely to be useful in most pediatric cases. In a study by Rao *et al.*,[63] CEA levels in nine of 23 pediatric patients did not correspond with either residual disease or disease progression. In a follow-up study, the same group concluded that CEA is not an effective marker for monitoring most children with CRC.[121] Staging guidelines for adult patients should be applied to children with CRC. Currently the American Joint Commission on Cancer (AJCC) guidelines[122] is the most widely used staging system.

Treatment

Because there is only one prospective clinical trial for CRC in children and young adults,[62] treatment recommendations must be adapted from adult experience. Complete surgical resection is the treatment of choice and cure is usually not possible if this is not achieved. The surgical approach should follow guidelines established for the treatment of adults with comparative extents of disease.[118] The basic surgical principles are an *en bloc* resection of the tumor with any organs or structures attached to the tumor, including the major vascular pedicle supplying the tumor along with its lymphatics. At least a 5 cm margin of normal bowel should be obtained on either side of the tumor to minimize the possibility of an anastomotic recurrence.[123,124] Adequate lymph node resection is imperative. The number of lymph nodes examined by the pathologist is prognostic of survival,[125] and therefore a minimum of 12 negative lymph nodes should be examined to define node-negative disease.[118] If the diagnosis was not made preoperatively and CRC is found in a patient being urgently explored for an acute abdomen, the surgeon should convert the procedure to a standard colon cancer resection with excision of draining lymphatics. Unfortunately for many children, adolescents and young adults, CRC is rarely considered in the initial differential diagnosis and therefore the initial surgical approach is often inadequate. In those cases, reexploration of the abdomen, with the goals of bowel resection with adequate margins and adequate lymph node sampling, should be done at a center experienced in this type of surgery.

Because of the rarity of CRC in children, few pediatric oncologists will have any substantial experience with this disease. Consultation with medical oncologists experienced in evaluating adults with colorectal carcinoma is essential. The treatment for children should be adapted from current adult treatment recommendations. Five-year overall survival for stage I disease, treated with surgery alone is at least 90%.[58] For stage II disease, in general the benefit of adjuvant chemotherapy is still being studied. Currently, adjuvant chemotherapy does not appear to improve survival by more than 5%.[118,126,127] Careful observation is a reasonable recommendation for most adults who have no evidence of disease after resection. However, adjuvant therapy may be recommended for those with any poor prognostic features, such as poorly differentiated histology, perforation, T4 lesion, peritumoral lymphovascular involvement, or inadequate lymph node sampling.[118,126] Unfortunately, many pediatric patients with CRC present with one or more of the poor prognostic features. For example, in the largest available pediatric series, the eight children with stage II disease had only a 37.5% ± 15% 10-year event-free survival (EFS) estimate,[59] although 5-year disease-free survival is 60–80%+ in most adult studies.[126]

The best option for children with CRC is participation in a clinical trial, although this opportunity is rarely available. The relative prevalence of one or more negative prognostic factors at diagnosis and young age by definition suggests that adjuvant chemotherapy be strongly considered (and carefully discussed by the oncologist with the family) for most children with stage II disease. For stage III or IV disease, chemotherapy has demonstrated a clear survival benefit in adults[118,128] and children should be treated in a similar fashion. Although the FOLFOX regimen[129,130] or one of its derivatives, such as modified FOLFOX-6,[131] is the current regimen of choice,[128] chemotherapy for advanced-stage disease is under active investigation and changing rapidly. Addition of the targeted agents bevacizumab,[132,133] cetuximab,[134] and panitumumab[135–137] to standard chemotherapy regimens has shown benefit in selected patient groups. There is accumulating evidence that some patients who present with stage IV disease can be cured, if complete surgical resection can eventually be attained.[138] In considering options for a pediatric patient with advanced-stage disease, one should carefully review the current medical literature and consult with an adult oncologist experienced in treating CRC before recommending a specific regimen.

Gastrointestinal stromal tumors

Gastrointestinal stromal tumors (GIST) are the most common gastrointestinal mesenchymal neoplasm of adults,[139] with an estimated incidence of 6.8 cases per million.[140] The median age at diagnosis is 60 years and tumors most commonly arise in the stomach (60%) and small bowel (25%).[140] Pathologically, the majority of GIST are characterized by spindle cell histology.[141] The risk of metastasis has been correlated with the mitotic rate, size, and anatomical location of the tumor (Table 64.3).

Approximately 90% of adult GIST have activating mutations of the KIT or PDGFR protooncogenes and the use of selective receptor tyrosine kinase inhibitors such as imatinib and sunitinib have proven to be very effective in the treatment of a disease that was considered to be chemoresistant.[140,143–145] GISTs rarely occur in pediatric patients. The exact number of pediatric GISTs in the United States is not known. In one series from St Jude Children's Research Hospital, GIST accounted for 2% of all pediatric nonrhabdomyosarcoma

Table 64.3 Prognosis of adult GIST based on 1684 patients.

Group	Tumor parameters: size (cm), mitotic rate per 50 HPF	Patient with progression/ malignant potential (%) gastric, small intestine
1	≤2 ≤5	0 very low, 0 very low
2	>2 ≤5	1.9 low, 4.3 low
3a	>5 ≤10	3.6 low, 24 intermediate
3b	>10 ≤5	12 intermediate, 52 high
4	≤2 >5	0 low, 50 high
5	>2 ≤5 >5	16 intermediate, 73 high
6a	>5 ≤10 >5	55 high, 85 high
6b	>10 >5	86 high, 90 high

HPF, high-power field.
Reprinted from Miettinen and Lasota[142] with permission from Archives of Pathology & Laboratory Medicine. Copyright 2006. College of American Pathologists.

soft tissue sarcomas seen at that institution and in one series from Memorial Sloan-Kettering Hospital, the authors estimated that about 1.5–2% of all GISTs seen at their center occurred in the pediatric population.[146,147] A report from the UK National Registry of Childhood Tumours reported an annual incidence rate of 0.02 per million in children under 14 years of age[148] and estimates from the SEER population database suggest that the expected incidence of GIST in patients under 19 years of age in the United States is approximately 0.08 per million.

Predisposing conditions

Gastrointestinal stromal tumors can occur sporadically or in association with four genetic syndromes: familial GIST,[149] neurofibromatosis type 1,[150] Carney triad,[151] and Carney–Stratakis syndrome.[152] Pediatric GIST has been linked to the latter two syndromes which are described below.

Carney triad was first described in 1977[153,154] and is characterized by the occurrence of GIST, extraadrenal paraganglioma, and pulmonary chondroma. In a series of 104 patients, the mean age at diagnosis was 22 years and 88% of the patients were female.[154] The most common site of GIST in these patients was the stomach and within this location, the antrum was most often involved. In addition, multifocality and nodal metastases were frequently reported (29%). Over 80% of GISTs in this patient population were of epithelioid histology and in this series the clinical behavior of the tumor did not correlate with the risk classification system described in Table 64.3. Metastases were documented in nearly 49 patients (47%) yet the median survival time for all patients was 26.5 years and the estimated 10- and 40-year survival rates were 100% and 73% respectively. None of the tumors analyzed had KIT, PDGFR, succinate dehydrogenase (SDH) B, C, or D coding sequence alterations.[154]

The Carney–Stratakis syndrome, first described in 2002, is characterized by the presence of paragangliomas and GIST.[155] Unlike the Carney triad, this dyad has an autosomal dominant pattern of inheritance with incomplete penetrance and is characterized by the presence of germline mutations of the SDH subunits B, C, and D.[156] Patients with this syndrome have an average age at presentation of 23 years. GISTs in these patients are more commonly located in the stomach and tend to be multifocal.[157]

Clinical presentation

Several reviews and case series have summarized the clinical presentation and outcome of pediatric patients with GIST[148,158,159] and these differences are highlighted in Table 64.4.[159] Briefly, the median age at presentation for pediatric GIST is approximately 13 years. Females are more commonly affected than males and the majority of pediatric GISTs (85%) arise within the stomach. The most common presenting symptom is anemia secondary to gastrointestinal bleeding. Tumors are multifocal in up to 70% of cases and lymph node metastases are commonly reported, a feature that explains the large number of incomplete tumor resections and high incidence of local recurrences reported in the literature. Tumor size has been

Table 64.4 Clinical and pathological features of pediatric versus adult GIST.

Characteristic	Pediatric	Adult
Median age	13	60
Sex predominance	Female	Equal male and female
Location/extent of disease	Stomach Multifocal Lymph nodes	Stomach
Histology	Epithelioid or mixed	Spindle
KIT/PDGFR mutations	Rare	Common
Inherited predisposition	Common	Rare
Natural history/ outcome	Slow growth Indolent Multiple locoregional recurrences Poor response to tyrosine kinase inhibitors	Highly responsive to tyrosine kinase inhibitors

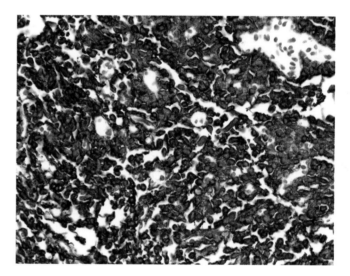

Figure 64.5 Pediatric GIST showing intense c-KIT immunostaining (40×). Courtesy of Dr Armita Bahrami, St Jude Children's Research Hospital, Memphis, TN, USA.

reported to vary greatly, with a median size of about 6 cm, and the proposed criteria for assessing prognosis in adult GIST (see Table 64.3) do not appear to predict the clinical outcome or behavior of these tumors in pediatric patients. Most tumors have an epithelioid or mixed epithelioid and spindle cell component. Two patients have been reported to have had prior malignancies (osteosarcoma and neuroblastoma) and about 10% of patients had a documented diagnosis of Carney triad or Carney–Stratakis syndrome.

Biology

Only about 15% of pediatric GIST have KIT or PDGFR mutations, thus limiting the clinical usefulness of tyrosine kinase inhibitor therapy in these patients.[158] Despite the lack of KIT mutations, KIT is expressed and activated in pediatric GIST (Fig. 64.5).[160]

The incidence of *BRAF* V600E mutations in this population is not known but in adults this variant is detected in up to 13% of wild-type GIST.[161] Because new therapies such as vemurafenib are now available for BRAF mutated tumors,[162] one could argue that GISTs that lack KIT and PDGFR mutations should also be screened for the presence of BRAF mutations. As mentioned previously, inactivating germline mutations of SDHB, C, and D predispose to the development of GIST and about 12% of patients with sporadic wild-type GIST occurring in the absence of a personal or family history of paraganglioma have germline mutations in one of the SDH genes.[163] Furthermore, all pediatric wild-type GISTs and several adult wild-type GISTs lack enzymatic activity and protein expression of SDH in the absence of mutations in the SDHB, C or D genes, suggesting that dysregulation of this pathway may play a pivotal role in the pathogenesis of this subset of GIST.[163] Recent studies have also demonstrated that there is strong insulin-like growth factor (IGF)-1R expression in adult and pediatric wild-type GISTs, implicating this pathway as a potential therapeutic alternative for these patients.[164]

Management guidelines

To date, there are no published guidelines summarizing the diagnostic workup and treatment of pediatric GIST. Figure 64.6 summarizes suggested guidelines for diagnosis and treatment of pediatric GIST. Initial assessment should include a thorough medical history to identify potential predisposing conditions such as the Carney triad or Carney–Stratakis syndrome. Initial laboratory workup should include a complete blood count (CBC) (anemia is the most common presenting finding), serum chemistries, chest x-ray (to look for chondromas) and CT scan of abdomen and pelvis. The routine use of PET scans is not recommended.

Since 10–15% of pediatric GIST patients will have activating mutations of KIT and PDGFR and will therefore respond to targeted therapies,[165] tumor tissue should be sent for this analysis. SDHB immunocytochemistry in formalin-fixed and paraffin-embedded tissue should be performed in wild-type tumors. Absent SDHB expression correlates well with the presence of SDHB, C, and D germline mutations and should prompt investigators to conduct testing and screening for these syndromes.[166]

Since most pediatric GIST (80%) arise in the stomach, the diagnostic use of upper gastrointestinal imaging and endoscopy is important in establishing the diagnosis. GISTs are often intramural so biopsies must be deep enough to obtain a representative tissue sample.

The traditional view that surgery is the mainstay of therapy for adult GIST needs to be evaluated carefully in pediatric wild-type GISTs since these tumors have an indolent course and a high recurrence rate. The recurrences often occur as small nodules in the peritoneum and some can be remote from

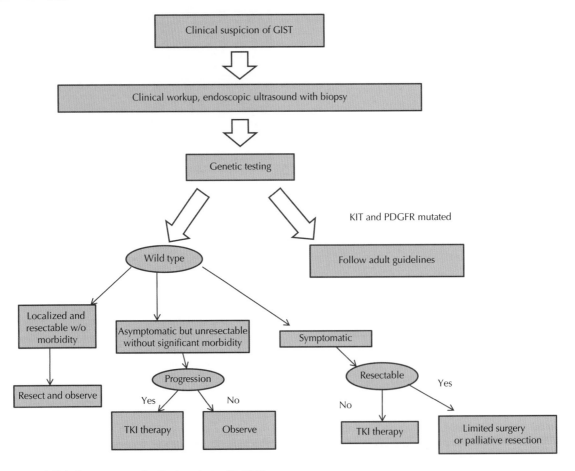

Figure 64.6 Proposed clinical management of pediatric patients with GIST.

the primary site.[146] These data support the use of conservative surgical approaches such as wedge resection of the involved stomach with preservation of gastric tissue.

If the tumor has KIT or PDGFR mutations, treatment should follow the guidelines published by the National Comprehensive cancer Network (www.nccn.org). For children and adolescents with wild-type tumors, surgical resection if feasible can be followed by careful observation (Fig 64.6). If a patient is asymptomatic and has a large unresectable tumor or metastatic disease, careful observation appears warranted since these tumors have an indolent course and respond poorly to targeted therapies. However, if the tumor progresses or causes symptoms, a trial of tyrosine kinase inhibitors appears warranted. Responses to imatinib in pediatric GIST have been suboptimal, with one partial response (PR) and three stable disease (SD) in 10 patients.[158] In vitro data demonstrate that the IC50 for sunitinib in wild-type KIT is 10 times lower than that of imatinib[146] and clinical studies have shown a higher clinical benefit rate in adult patients with wild-type GIST.[167,168] In pediatric patients, antitumor activity has been reported, with one of seven patients achieving a partial response and five achieving stable disease.[169]

Future plans to study pediatric gastrointestinal stromal tumor

To further study pediatric GIST, 10 clinicians from seven academic institutions in the United States and one in Australia have developed the Consortium for Pediatric and wildtype GIST Research (CPGR) (www.pediatricgist.cancer.gov/Source/CPGR/CPGR.aspx). This consortium organizes a biannual clinic that brings physicians who have the most experience treating and studying GIST together with children and adults who have wild-type GIST. Since its inception in 2008, 80 patients have attended and 36% of these were pediatric patients.

Tumors of the pancreas

Primary neoplasms of the pancreas are rare in children. Based on information from the UK National Registry of Childhood Tumours, the estimated annual incidence of pancreatic tumors in children 15 years of age or younger is 0.1 per million population.[206] The SEER database registered 69 patients under 20 years of age with pancreatic tumors between 1976 and 2006 with an estimated age-adjusted annual incidence of 0.19 per million.[170] Neoplasms of the pancreas are classified histogenetically into exocrine and endocrine tumors. Those arising from the exocrine pancreas include the ductal and acinar cell tumors. Islet cell tumors comprise the endocrine neoplasms of the pancreas. Two tumor types of importance in the pediatric age group, pancreatoblastoma and solid pseudopapillary tumor, have been classified with the exocrine pancreatic neoplasms, though both may contain minor populations of tumor cells with neuroendocrine features by electron microscopy and/or immunohistochemistry as an implication of their primordial or dysontogenetic nature.

The histological diagnosis of pediatric pancreatic tumors in six series comprising 201 patients is given in Table 64.5.

Ductal type adenocarcinoma is extremely rare in patients under 40 years of age but it is the most common primary malignancy of the pancreas in older adults, accounting for 85% of all cases. When this malignancy occurs in younger patients, it often affects those who are 15–19 years of age.[173] In one review, only 20 of 71 tumors pancreatic tumors in patients under 40 years of age who were reported in the literature could be categorized as ductal adenocarcinomas.[177]

Acinar cell carcinoma is another malignant exocrine neoplasm of the pancreas and accounts for 1% of all pancreatic tumors.[178] This tumor type has been recognized in children although, like ductal adenocarcinomas, most cases have been diagnosed in adults. There is a variant, the mixed acinar-endocrine carcinoma of the pancreas. The importance of these

Table 64.5 Series of pediatric patients with pancreatic tumors.

Author	No. of pts	Solid pseudopapillary tumor	Pancreatoblastoma	Carcinoma	Other
Shorter[171]	17	7	5	1	Endocrine 2 PNET 2
Dall'Igna[172]	21	12	4	2	Endocrine 3
Perez[173]	58	10	10	11	Endocrine 19 Sarcomas 5 Unknown 3
Park[174]	32	19	2	4	Endocrine 2 Lymphoma 3 PNET 1 Hemangioendothelioma 1
Yu[175]	18	4	0	6	Endocrine 5 Sarcoma 1 Adenoma 2
*Ellerkamp[176]	55	38	5	12	0
Total	201	90	26	36	49

* Includes exocrine tumors only.
PNET, primitive neuroectodermal tumor.

tumors is the overlapping pathological similarity in some cases to pancreatoblastomas and solid pseudopapillary tumors that occur in young children and adolescents/young adults, respectively.

Pancreatoblastoma is an embryonal tumor of the pancreas that arises from multipotential cells and recapitulates the normal embryology of the pancreas. The term pancreatoblastoma was first coined by Horie in 1977.[179] This malignancy is rare, with only 153 cases reported in the literature from 1966 to 2003.[180] In a series for the Kiel Pediatric Tumor Registry, pancreatoblastoma accounted for only 0.01% of the 22,783 malignancies registered.[180] Furthermore, from 1973 to 2004, the SEER database registered only 10 cases[173] and the UK National Registry of Childhood Tumours recorded only 11 cases over a 30-year period.[170] More recently, the Italian Rare Tumor Group (TREP) recorded 4 cases over an 8-year period.[181] Because of the rarity of this disease, national groups across Europe (Italy, France, United Kingdom, Poland, and Germany) interested in rare cancers have joined forces and developed an international working group called EXPeRT (European Cooperative Study Group for Pediatric Rare Tumors). The first publication of this group identified 20 cases of pancreatoblastoma from 2000 to 2009.[181]

This neoplasm was first described in 1959 by Frantz. The tumor has a distinct organoid structure with squamoid corpuscles and is surrounded by acinar arrangements and divided into lobules.[179] This tumor occurs almost exclusively in children with a median age at diagnosis of 5 years; 78% of cases occur within the first 10 years of life.[180] The tumor affects males more commonly and preferentially involves the head of the pancreas (Fig. 64.7).[180,182] Pancreatoblastoma has been reported in association with the Beckwith–Wiedemann syndrome[183–186] and familial adenomatous polyposis.[187] Approximately 153 cases of pancreatoblastoma[180] had been reported through 1997.[146,148] Cytogenetic analysis revealed two translocations, t(13;22)(q10;q10) and t(13;13)(q10;q10), in a 4-year-old boy and analysis of one cell line from a 14 year old showed complex cytogenetic changes most often affecting chromosomes 1, 2, 3, 6, 7, 8, 12, 13, 14, 16, 19, 20, 21, 22, and X. Comparative genomic hybridization (CGH) detected amplification in chromosomes 1p, 6p, 7q, 8q, 17q, 21q, and X, and increased copy number in regions of chromosomes 2p, 2q, 3p, 4p, 4q, 9q, 13, 14q, and 20.[188,189] IGF-2 overexpression has been documented within small undifferentiated cells as well as maternal allele-specific loss of heterozygosity (LOH) at 11p15.5[190] Aberrant expression of β-catenin in the squamoid corpuscles and occasional mutations of the gene with concomitant overexpression of cyclin D1 have also been reported and these findings may be important in the morphogenesis of the squamoid corpuscles which are characteristic of pancreatoblastoma.[191]

The majority of patients present with an asymptomatic incidentally detected abdominal mass. Presenting symptoms may include weight loss, vomiting, and obstructive jaundice and patients usually present with advanced-stage disease which is either locally extensive or metastatic.[180,181,192] About 17–35% present with metastases, most commonly involving the liver.[180] Nodal metastases affecting portal and splenic areas and lung can also be present. Serum α-fetoprotein level may be elevated

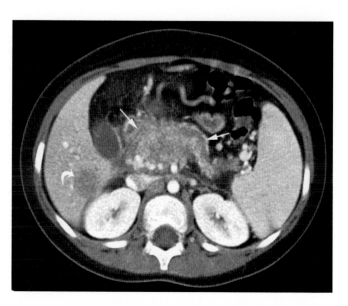

Figure 64.7 Axial contrast-enhanced CT image through the upper abdomen demonstrates a pancreatoblastoma (*straight arrows*) involving the pancreatic head, neck, and proximal body. One of the hepatic metastatic deposits is shown (*curved arrow*). Courtesy of Dr Jamie Coleman, St Jude Children's Research Hospital, Memphis, TN, USA.

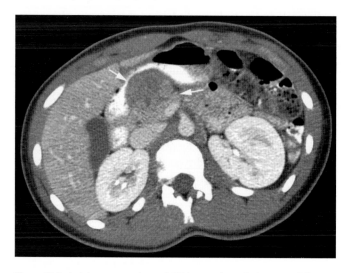

Figure 64.8 Axial contrast-enhanced CT images through the upper abdomen demonstrate a solid well-defined mass arising from the pancreatic head compatible with a solid papillary epithelial neoplasm of the pancreas. Courtesy of Dr Jamie Coleman, St Jude Children's Research Hospital, Memphis, TN, USA.

in up to 75% of patients; in one series, the median value was 658 IU/mL.[180,181] Surgery is the mainstay of therapy and surgical procedures such as pancreatoduodenectomy can achieve complete surgical resection in the majority of patients.[181] For patients with unresectable or metastatic tumors, chemotherapy has proven very active and in one series, over 70% of patients experienced a response. The most active agents include cisplatin, doxorubicin, cyclophosphamide and etoposide but the use of a cisplatin-doxorubin (PLADO) regimen is recommended.[181] Since these tumors are chemosensitive, current therapies should incorporate upfront chemotherapy followed by delayed, optimally planned surgical resection. The role of adjuvant chemotherapy and radiotherapy has not been well established. In one series, the 5-year event-free survival and overall survival rates were 58% and 79% respectively.[181] Tumor respectability, response to chemotherapy, and absence of metastases are associated with improved outcome.[180,181]

Solid pseudopapillary tumor of the pancreas or Frantz tumor (Fig. 64.8) is a rare and distinctive neoplasm of the pancreas which accounts for 1–2% of pancreatic tumors in adults but for the majority of cases of pancreatic tumors in children (see Table 64.5).[193] This tumor almost exclusively affects women (M:F ratio of 1:8 to 1:9) with a mean age at presentation of 22 years.[194] About 20% of patients are between the ages of 1 and 18 years.[194] Grossly, the tumors are cystic and hemorrhagic with focal areas of solid grayish white tissue. Microscopically, the tumor has uniform growth and is characterized by solid, pseudopapillary, or hemorrhagic pseudocystic structures in varying proportions. The presence of solid sheets of uniform vacuolated-to-eosinophilic tumor cells and discohesive, pseudopapillary profiles of cells is the principal microscopic finding. The solid areas may have a trabecular perithelial appearance, whereas other foci have pseudoglandular features with hyaline-myxoid stroma. The tumor cells are usually positive for vimentin, α1-antitrypsin, neuron-specific enolase, and α1-antichymoptrypsin.[193] The tumor most often involves the pancreatic head and tail and rarely invades the retroperitneum or mesentery.[193] In a series of 25 Taiwanese patients, solid pseudopapillary tumors uniformly expressed and harbored CTNNB1 gene mutations, suggesting that the Wnt pathway is critical for the development of this rare disease.[195]

The clinical presentation is nonspecific and about one-third of the patients are asymptomatic. When symptoms are present, abdominal pain is the predominant finding.[193] Other symptoms such as fever, jaundice, and weight loss are seen in less than 5% of patients.[193,194]

Surgery is the mainstay of therapy. In a series of 553 patients treated surgically, local resections or enucleations without the use of extensive surgeries were performed in one-third of the patients. In another series, distal pancreatectomy could be safely performed in 31% of 315 patients and pancreatoduodenectomy was done in 25% of the patients.[193] Chemotherapy has been used in isolated reports suggesting that ifosfamide, cisplatin, etoposide,[196] gemcitabine,[197] and vincristine[198] have clinical activity against the disease. Other therapeutic strategies such as transarterial chemoembolization, radiation, and radiofrequency ablation have also been reported.[193] Outcome for patients with this disease is excellent, with estimated 1–, 3–, and 5-year survival rates of 99.4%, 97.5%, and 96.9% respectively.

Islet cell neoplasms include adenomas and carcinomas whose pathological discriminants from each other are not sharply defined in all cases. These tumors constitute a larger proportion of all pancreatic neoplasms in children in comparison to the adult experience. The possibility of multiple endocrine neoplasia type 1 should be considered in children who present with a nonislet cell tumor.[199] Most insulinomas are adenomas and require only surgical resection. Most gastrin-producing islet cell tumors of the Zollinger–Ellison syndrome are carcinomas with regional lymph node and/or liver metastases at diagnosis.[200]

For cases in which surgical cure cannot be accomplished, medical management may be appropriate. Somatostatin analogs and interferon control symptoms in up to 75% of patients and cause disease stabilization in about 50% of patients.[201] Chemotherapy with streptozotocin in combination with fluorouracil or doxorubicin can produce responses that last about 9 months in up to 40% of patients with pancreatic neuroendocrine tumors.[202] More recently, when compared to patients who were treated with best supportive care, the administration of sunitinib or everolimus was associated with improvements in progression-free survival rates of about 6 months in patients with advanced neuroendocrine tumors of the pancreas.[203,204]

The use of peptide receptor radionuclide therapy with the somatostatin-based radiopeptide (90) yttrium-labeled 1,4,7,10-tetraazacyclododecane-1,4,7,10-tetraacetic acid ([90] Y-DOTA]-TOC) also appears promising and has been reported to produce responses in about one-third of patients with neuroendocrine tumors.[205]

References

1. Jemal A, Siegel R, Xu J, *et al.* Cancer statistics, 2010. CA Cancer J Clin 2010; 60: 277–300.
2. Ladd AP, Grosfeld JL. Gastrointestinal tumors in children and adolescents. Semin Pediatr Surg 2006; 15: 37–47.
3. Bethel CA, Bhattacharyya N, Hutchinson C, *et al.* Alimentary tract malignancies in children. J Pediatr Surg 1997; 32: 1004–8; discussion 1008–9.
4. Skinner MA, Plumley DA, Grosfeld JL, *et al.* Gastrointestinal tumors in children: an analysis of 39 cases. Ann Surg Oncol 1994; 1: 283–9.
5. Hameed R, Parkes S, Davies P, *et al.* Paediatric malignant tumours of the gastrointestinal tract in the West Midlands, UK, 1957–2000: a large population based survey. Pediatr Blood Cancer 2004; 43: 257–60.
6. Broaddus RR, Herzog CE, Hicks MJ. Neuroendocrine tumors (carcinoid and neuroendocrine carcinoma) presenting at extra-appendiceal sites in childhood and adolescence. Arch Pathol Lab Med 2003; 127: 1200–3.
7. Moraes TJ, Langer JC, Forte V, *et al.* Pediatric pulmonary carcinoid: a case report and review of the literature. Pediatr Pulmonol 2003; 35: 318–22.
8. Dusmet ME, McKneally MF. Pulmonary and thymic carcinoid tumors. World J Surg 1996; 20: 189–95.
9. Luh SP, Kuo C, Liu WS, *et al.* Carcinoid tumor of the thymus: a clinicopathologic report of two cases with a review of the literature. Int Surg 2005; 90: 270–4.
10. Pasieka JL. Carcinoid tumors. Surg Clin North Am 2009; 89: 1123–37.
11. Sarvida ME, O'Dorisio MS. Neuroendocrine tumors in children and young adults: rare or not so rare. Endocrinol Metab Clin North Am 2011; 40: 65–80, vii.
12. La Ferla G, Baxter RA, Tavadia HB, *et al.* Multiple colonic carcinoid tumours in a child. Br J Surg 1984; 71: 843.
13. Kelemen D, Horvath OP, Juhasz Z, *et al.* Pancreatic carcinoid in childhood. Eur J Pediatr Surg 2009; 19: 268–9.
14. Foley DS, Sunil I, Debski R, *et al.* Primary hepatic carcinoid tumor in children. J Pediatr Surg 2008; 43: e25–8.
15. Modlin IM, Lye KD, Kidd M. A 5-decade analysis of 13,715 carcinoid tumors. Cancer 2003; 97: 934–59.
16. Pinchot SN, Holen K, Sippel RS, *et al.* Carcinoid tumors. Oncologist 2008; 13: 1255–69.
17. Doherty GM. Neuroendocrine (carcinoid) tumors and the carcinoid syndrome. In: De Vita V, Lawrence T, Rosenberg S. *Cancer Principles and Practice of Oncology*, 9th edn. Philadelphia: Lippincott, 2011. pp. 1503–1515.
18. Spunt SL, Pratt CB, Rao BN, *et al.* Childhood carcinoid tumors: the St Jude Children's Research Hospital experience. J Pediatr Surg 2000; 35: 1282–6.

19. Yang K, Ulich T, Cheng L, *et al.* The neuroendocrine products of intestinal carcinoids. An immunoperoxidase study of 35 carcinoid tumors stained for serotonin and eight polypeptide hormones. Cancer 1983; 51: 1918–26.

20. King MD, Young DG, Hann IM, *et al.* Carcinoid syndrome: an unusual cause of diarrhoea. Arch Dis Child 1985; 60: 269–71.

21. Kulke MH, Mayer RJ. Carcinoid tumors. N Engl J Med 1999; 340: 858–68.

22. Campana D, Nori F, Piscitelli L, *et al.* Chromogranin A: is it a useful marker of neuroendocrine tumors? J Clin Oncol 2007; 25: 1967–73.

23. Neves GR, Chapchap P, Sredni ST, *et al.* Childhood carcinoid tumors: description of a case series in a Brazilian cancer center. Sao Paulo Med J 2006; 124: 21–5.

24. Parkes SE, Muir KR, al Sheyyab M, *et al.* Carcinoid tumours of the appendix in children 1957–1986: incidence, treatment and outcome. Br J Surg 1993; 80: 502–4.

25. Andersson A, Bergdahl L. Carcinoid tumors of the appendix in children. A report of 25 cases. Acta Chir Scand 1977; 143: 173–5.

26. Moertel CG, Hanley JA. Combination chemotherapy trials in metastatic carcinoid tumor and the malignant carcinoid syndrome. Cancer Clin Trials 1979; 2: 327–34.

27. Svendsen LB, Bulow S. Carcinoid tumours of the appendix in young patients. Acta Chir Scand 1980; 146: 137–9.

28. Pelizzo G, La Riccia A, Bouvier R, *et al.* Carcinoid tumors of the appendix in children. Pediatr Surg Int 2001; 17: 399–402.

29. Dall'Igna P, Ferrari A, Luzzatto C, *et al.* Carcinoid tumor of the appendix in childhood: the experience of two Italian institutions. J Pediatr Gastroenterol Nutr 2005; 40: 216–19.

30. Field JL, Adamson LF, Stoeckle HE. Review of carcinoids in children. Functioning carcinoid in a 15-year-old male. Pediatrics 1962; 29: 953–60.

31. Volpe A, Willert J, Ihnken K, *et al.* Metastatic appendiceal carcinoid tumor in a child. Med Pediatr Oncol 2000; 34: 218–20.

32. Corpron CA, Black CT, Herzog CE, *et al.* A half century of experience with carcinoid tumors in children. Am J Surg 1995; 170: 606–8.

33. Moertel CL, Weiland LH, Telander RL. Carcinoid tumor of the appendix in the first two decades of life. J Pediatr Surg 1990; 25: 1073–5.

34. Doede T, Foss HD, Waldschmidt J. Carcinoid tumors of the appendix in children – epidemiology, clinical aspects and procedure. Eur J Pediatr Surg 2000; 10: 372–7.

35. Hatzipantelis E, Panagopoulou P, Sidi-Fragandrea V, *et al.* Carcinoid tumors of the appendix in children: experience from a tertiary center in northern Greece. J Pediatr Gastroenterol Nutr 2010; 51: 622–5.

36. Assadi M, Kubiak R, Kaiser G. Appendiceal carcinoid tumors in children: does size matter? Med Pediatr Oncol 2002; 38: 65–6.

37. Moertel CG, Dockerty MB, Judd ES. Carcinoid tumors of the vermiform appendix. Cancer 1968; 21: 270–8.

38. Boudreaux JP, Putty B, Frey DJ, *et al.* Surgical treatment of advanced-stage carcinoid tumors: lessons learned. Ann Surg 2005; 241: 839–45; discussion 845–6.

39. Moertel CG, Weiland LH, Nagorney DM, *et al.* Carcinoid tumor of the appendix: treatment and prognosis. N Engl J Med 1987; 317: 1699–701.

40. NCCN Clinical Practice Guidelines in Oncology. *NCCN Guidelines: Neuroendocrine Tumors.* Fort Washington, PA: National Comprehensive Cancer Network,.2011.

41. Schmidt C, Bloomston M, Shah MH. Well-differentiated neuroendocrine tumors: a review covering basic principles to loco-regional and targeted therapies. Oncogene 2011; 30: 1497–505.

42. Kulke MH. Clinical presentation and management of carcinoid tumors. Hermatol Oncol Clin North Am 2007; 21: 433–55; vii–viii.

43. Lebtahi R, Cadiot G, Delahaye N, *et al.* Detection of bone metastases in patients with endocrine gastroenteropancreatic tumors: bone scintigraphy compared with somatostatin receptor scintigraphy. J Nucl Med 1999; 40: 1602–8.

44. Ganim RB, Norton JA. Recent advances in carcinoid pathogenesis, diagnosis and management. Surg Oncol 2000; 9: 173–9.

45. Oberg K, Eriksson B. Nuclear medicine in the detection, staging and treatment of gastrointestinal carcinoid tumours. Best Pract Res Clin Endocrinol Metab 2005; 19: 265–76.

46. Lamberts SW, Bakker WH, Reubi JC, *et al.* Somatostatin-receptor imaging in the localization of endocrine tumors. N Engl J Med 1990; 323: 1246–9.

47. Chan JA, Kulke MH. New treatment options for patients with advanced neuroendocrine tumors. Curr Treat Options Oncol 2011; 12: 136–48.

48. Bloomston M, Al-Saif O, Klemanski D, *et al.* Hepatic artery chemoembolization in 122 patients with metastatic carcinoid tumor: lessons learned. J Gastrointest Surg 2007; 11: 264–71.

49. Ahrar K, Gupta S. Hepatic artery embolization for hepatocellular carcinoma: technique, patient selection, and outcomes. Surg Oncol Clin North Am 2003; 12: 105–26.

50. Gupta S, Yao JC, Ahrar K, *et al.* Hepatic artery embolization and chemoembolization for treatment of patients with metastatic carcinoid tumors: the M.D. Anderson experience. Cancer J 2003; 9: 261–7.

51. Leong WL, Pasieka JL. Regression of metastatic carcinoid tumors with octreotide therapy: two case reports and a review of the literature. J Surg Oncol 2002; 79: 180–7.

52. O'Toole D, Ducreux M, Bommelaer G, *et al.* Treatment of carcinoid syndrome: a prospective crossover evaluation of lanreotide versus octreotide in terms of efficacy, patient acceptability, and tolerance. Cancer 2000; 88: 770–6.

53. Rubin J, Ajani J, Schirmer W, *et al.* Octreotide acetate long-acting formulation versus open-label subcutaneous octreotide acetate in malignant carcinoid syndrome. J Clin Oncol 1999; 17: 600–6.

54. Frank M, Klose KJ, Wied M, *et al.* Combination therapy with octreotide and alpha-interferon: effect on tumor growth in metastatic endocrine gastroenteropancreatic tumors. Am J Gastroenterol 1999; 94: 1381–7.

55. Pape UF, Wiedenmann B. Adding interferon-alpha to octreotide slows tumour progression compared with octreotide alone but evidence is lacking for improved survival in people with disseminated midgut carcinoid tumours. Cancer Treat Rev 2003; 29: 565–9.

56. Kulke MH, Lenz HJ, Meropol NJ, *et al.* Activity of sunitinib in patients with advanced neuroendocrine tumors. J Clin Oncol 2008; 26: 3403–10.

57. Yao JC, Phan AT, Chang DZ, *et al.* Efficacy of RAD001 (everolimus) and octreotide LAR in advanced low- to intermediate-grade neuroendocrine tumors: results of a phase II study. J Clin Oncol 2008; 26: 4311–18.

58. American Cancer Society. Colorectal Cancer Facts & Figures 2011–2013, www.cancer.org/acs/groups/content/@epidemiologysurveilance/documents/document/acspc–028323.pdf. Atlanta, GA: American Cancer Society, 2011.

59. Hill DA, Furman WL, Billups CA, *et al.* Colorectal carcinoma in childhood and adolescence: a clinicopathologic review. J Clin Oncol 2007; 25: 5808–14.

60. Ferrari A, Rognone A, Casanova M, *et al.* Colorectal carcinoma in children and adolescents: the experience of the Istituto Nazionale Tumori of Milan, Italy. Pediatr Blood Cancer 2008; 50: 588–93.

61. La Quaglia MP, Heller G, Filippa DA, *et al.* Prognostic factors and outcome in patients 21 years and under with colorectal carcinoma. J Pediatr Surg 1992; 27: 1085–9; discussion 1089–90.

62. Pratt CB, Rao BN, Merchant TE, *et al.* Treatment of colorectal carcinoma in adolescents and young adults with surgery, 5-fluorouracil/leucovorin/interferon-alpha 2a and radiation therapy. Med Pediatr Oncol 1999; 32: 459–60.

63. Rao BN, Pratt CB, Fleming ID, *et al.* Colon carcinoma in children and adolescents. A review of 30 cases. Cancer 1985; 55: 1322–6.

64. Andersson A, Bergdahl L. Carcinoma of the colon in children: a report of six new cases and a review of the literature. J Pediatr Surg 1976; 11: 967–71.

65. Middelkamp JN, Haffner H. Carcinoma of the colon in children. Pediatrics 1963; 32: 558–71.

66. Chabalko JJ, Fraumeni JF Jr. Colorectal cancer in children: epidemiologic aspects. Dis Colon Rectum 1975; 18: 1–3.

67. Lamego CM, Torloni H. Colorectal adenocarcinoma in childhood and adolescent. Report of 11 cases and review of the literature. Pediatr Radiol 1989; 19: 504–8.

68. Brown RA, Rode H, Millar AJ, *et al.* Colorectal carcinoma in children. J Pediatr Surg 1992; 27: 919–21.

69. Karnak I, Ciftci AO, Senocak ME, *et al.* Colorectal carcinoma in children. J Pediatr Surg 1999; 34: 1499–504.

70. Radhakrishnan CN, Bruce J. Colorectal cancers in children without any predisposing factors. A report of eight cases and review of the literature. Eur J Pediatr Surg 2003; 13: 66–8.

71. Chantada GL, Perelli VB, Lombardi MG, *et al.* Colorectal carcinoma in children, adolescents, and young adults. J Pediatr Hematol Oncol 2005; 27: 39–41.

72. Taguchi T, Suita S, Hirata Y, *et al.* Carcinoma of the colon in children: a case report and review of 41 Japanese cases. J Pediatr Gastroenterol Nutr 1991; 12: 394–9.

73. Bhatia MS, Chandna S, Shah R, *et al.* Colorectal carcinoma in Indian children. Indian Pediatr 2000; 37: 1353–8.

74. Vastyan AM, Walker J, Pinter AB, *et al.* Colorectal carcinoma in children and adolescents – a report of seven cases. Eur J Pediatr Surg 2001; 11: 338–41.

75. Sharma AK, Gupta CR. Colorectal cancer in children: case report and review of literature. Trop Gastroenterol 2001; 22: 36–9.

76. Sharma MS, Kumar S, Agarwal N. Childhood colorectal carcinoma: a case series. Afr J Paediatr Surg 2009; 6: 65–7.

77. Saab R, Furman WL. Epidemiology and management options for colorectal cancer in children. Paediatr Drugs 2008; 10: 177–92.

78. Sultan I, Rodriguez-Galindo C, El-Taani H, *et al.* Distinct features of colorectal cancer in children and adolescents: a population-based study of 159 cases. Cancer 2010; 116: 758–65.

79. Spunt SLF, Furman WL, La Quaglia M, *et al.* Colon and rectal cancer. In: Bleyer A, O'Leary M, Barr R, Ries L (eds) *Cancer Epidemiology in Older Adolescents and Young Adults 15 to 29 Years of Age, Including SEER Incidence and Survival: 1975–2000.* NIH Pub. No. 06–5767. Bethesda, MD: National Cancer Institute, 2006. pp.123–33.

80. Kern WH, White WC. Adenocarcinoma of the colon in a 9-month-old infant; report of a case. Cancer 1958; 11: 855–7.

81. Donohoe CL, Pidgeon GP, Lysaght J, *et al.* Obesity and gastrointestinal cancer. Br J Surg 2010; 97: 628–42.

82. Skjelbred CF, Saebo M, Hjartaker A, *et al.* Meat, vegetables and genetic polymorphisms and the risk of colorectal carcinomas and adenomas. BMC Cancer 2007; 7: 228.

83. Anderson JC, Alpern Z, Sethi G, *et al.* Prevalence and risk of colorectal neoplasia in consumers of alcohol in a screening population. Am J Gastroenterol 2005; 100: 2049–55.

84. Wu AH, Henderson BE. Alcohol and tobacco use: risk factors for colorectal adenoma and carcinoma? J Nat Cancer Inst 1995; 87: 239–40.

85. Boutron-Ruault MC, Senesse P, Meance S, *et al.* Energy intake, body mass index, physical activity, and the colorectal adenoma-carcinoma sequence. Nutr Cancer 2001; 39: 50–7.

86. Leufkens AM, van Duijnhoven FJ, Siersema PD, *et al.* Cigarette smoking and colorectal cancer risk in the European Prospective Investigation into Cancer and Nutrition study. Clin Gastroenterol Hepatol 2011; 9: 137–44.

87. Potter JD. Colorectal cancer: molecules and populations. J Nat Cancer Inst 1999; 91: 916–32.

88. Fearon ER, Vogelstein B. A genetic model for colorectal tumorigenesis. Cell 1990; 61: 759–67.

89. Vogelstein B, Fearon ER, Hamilton SR, *et al.* Genetic alterations during colorectal-tumor development. N Engl J Med 1988; 319: 525–32.

90. Cappell MS. Pathophysiology, clinical presentation, and management of colon cancer. Gastroenterol Clin North Am 2008; 37: 1–24, v.

91. Winawer SJ, Zauber AG, Ho MN, *et al.* Prevention of colorectal cancer by colonoscopic polypectomy. The National Polyp Study Workgroup. N Engl J Med 1993; 329: 1977–81.

92. Winawer SJ, Zauber AG, O'Brien MJ, *et al.* Randomized comparison of surveillance intervals after colonoscopic removal of newly diagnosed adenomatous polyps. The National Polyp Study Workgroup. N Engl J Med 1993; 328: 901–6.

93. Alkhouri N, Franciosi JP, Mamula P. Familial adenomatous polyposis in children and adolescents. J Pediatr Gastroenterol Nutr 2010; 51: 727–32.

94. Durno C, Aronson M, Bapat B, *et al.* Family history and molecular features of children, adolescents, and young adults with colorectal carcinoma. Gut 2005; 54: 1146–50.

95. Durno CA, Gallinger S. Genetic predisposition to colorectal cancer: new pieces in the pediatric puzzle. J Pediatr Gastroenterol Nutr 2006; 43: 5–15.

96. Gatalica Z, Torlakovic E. Pathology of the hereditary colorectal carcinoma. Fam Cancer 2008; 7: 15–26.

97. De la Chapelle A. Genetic predisposition to colorectal cancer. Nature reviews. Cancer 2004; 4: 769–80.

98. Rowley PT. Inherited susceptibility to colorectal cancer. Annu Rev Med 2005; 56: 539–54.

99. Grady WM. Genetic testing for high-risk colon cancer patients. Gastroenterology 2003; 124: 1574–94.

100. Datta RV, La Quaglia MP, Paty PB. Genetic and phenotypic correlates of colorectal cancer in young patients. N Engl J Med 2000; 342: 137–8.

101. Kayton ML. Cancer and pediatric inflammatory bowel disease. Semin Pediatr Surg 2007; 16: 205–13.

102. Eaden J. Review article: Colorectal carcinoma and inflammatory bowel disease. Aliment Pharmacol Ther 2004; 20(Suppl 4): 24–30.

103. O'Connor TW, Rombeau JL, Levine HS, *et al.* Late development of colorectal cancer subsequent to pelvic irradiation. Dis Colon Rectum 1979; 22: 123–8.

104. Houlston RS, Murday V, Harocopos C, *et al.* Screening and genetic counselling for relatives of patients with colorectal cancer in a family cancer clinic. BMJ 1990; 301: 366–8.

105. Dean PA. Hereditary intestinal polyposis syndromes. Rev Gastroenterol Mex 1996; 61: 100–11.

106. Corredor J, Wambach J, Barnard J. Gastrointestinal polyps in children: advances in molecular genetics, diagnosis, and management. J Pediatr 2001; 138: 621–8.

107. Distante S, Nasioulas S, Somers GR, *et al.* Familial adenomatous polyposis in a 5 year old child: a clinical, pathological, and molecular genetic study. J Med Genet 1996; 33: 157–60.

108. Church JM, McGannon E, Burke C, *et al.* Teenagers with familial adenomatous polyposis: what is their risk for colorectal cancer? Dis Colon Rectum 2002; 45: 887–9.

109. Turcot J, Despres JP, St Pierre F. Malignant tumors of the central nervous system associated with familial polyposis of the colon: report of two cases. Dis Colon Rectum 1959; 2: 465–8.

110. Hamilton SR, Liu B, Parsons RE, *et al.* The molecular basis of Turcot's syndrome. N Engl J Med 1995; 332: 839–47.

111. Oldfield MC. The association of familial polyposis of the colon with multiple sebaceous cysts. Br J Surg 1954; 41: 534–41.

112. Gardner EJ. Follow-up study of a family group exhibiting dominant inheritance for a syndrome including intestinal polyps, osteomas, fibromas and epidermal cysts. Am J Hum Genet 1962; 14: 376–90.

113. Pratt CB, Jane JA. Multiple colorectal carcinomas, polyposis coli, and neurofibromatosis, followed by multiple glioblastoma multiforme. J Nat Cancer Inst 1991; 83: 880–1.

114. Pizzo PA, Poplack DG. *Principles and Practice of Pediatric Oncology,* 6th edn. Philadelphia: Wolters Kluwer/Lippincott Williams and Wilkins Health, 2011.

115. Consorti F, Lorenzotti A, Midiri G, *et al.* Prognostic significance of mucinous carcinoma of colon and rectum: a prospective case-control study. J Surg Oncol 2000; 73: 70–4.

116. Tricoli JV, Seibel NL, Blair DG, *et al.* Unique characteristics of adolescent and young adult acute lymphoblastic leukemia, breast cancer, and colon cancer. J Nat Cancer Inst 2011; 103: 628–35.

117. Lee YM, Law WL, Chu KW, *et al.* Emergency surgery for obstructing colorectal cancers: a comparison between right-sided and left-sided lesions. J Am Coll Surg 2001; 192: 719–25.

118. NCCN Clinical Practice Guidelines in Oncology. *Colon Cancer.* Fort Washington, PA: National Comprehensive Cancer Network, 2011.

119. Berger KL, Nicholson SA, Dehdashti F, *et al.* FDG PET evaluation of mucinous neoplasms: correlation of FDG uptake with histopathologic features. Am J Roentgenol 2000; 174: 1005–8.

120. Goldstein MJ, Mitchell EP. Carcinoembryonic antigen in the staging and follow-up of patients with colorectal cancer. Cancer Invest 2005; 23: 338–51.

121. Angel CA, Pratt CB, Rao BN, et al. Carcinoembryonic antigen and carbohydrate 19-9 antigen as markers for colorectal carcinoma in children and adolescents. Cancer 1992; 69: 1487–91.

122. Edge SB, Byrd DR, Compton CC, et al. (eds). *AJCC Cancer Staging Manual*, 7th edn. New York: Springer, 2010.

123. Rodriguez-Bigas MA, Hoff PM, Crane CH. Carcinoma of the colon and rectum. In: Kuff DW, Bast RC Jr, Hait WN, et al. (eds) *Cancer Medicine 7*. London: BC Decker Inc, 2006.

124. Nelson H, Petrelli N, Carlin A, et al. Guidelines 2000 for colon and rectal cancer surgery. J Natl Cancer Inst 2001; 93: 583–96.

125. Gunderson LL, Jessup JM, Sargent DJ, et al. Revised TN categorization for colon cancer based on national survival outcomes data. J Clin Oncol 2010; 28: 264–71.

126. Benson AB 3rd, Schrag D, Somerfield MR, et al. American Society of Clinical Oncology recommendations on adjuvant chemotherapy for stage II colon cancer. J Clin Oncol 2004; 22: 3408–19.

127. Figueredo A, Charette ML, Maroun J, et al. Adjuvant therapy for stage II colon cancer: a systematic review from the Cancer Care Ontario Program in Evidence-Based Care's gastrointestinal cancer disease site group. J Clin Oncol 2004; 22: 3395–407.

128. Saltz LB. Adjuvant therapy for colon cancer. Surg Oncol Clin North Am 2010; 19: 819–27.

129. Andre T, Boni C, Mounedji-Boudiaf L, et al. Oxaliplatin, fluorouracil, and leucovorin as adjuvant treatment for colon cancer. N Engl J Med 2004; 350: 2343–51.

130. Andre T, Boni C, Navarro M, et al. Improved overall survival with oxaliplatin, fluorouracil, and leucovorin as adjuvant treatment in stage II or III colon cancer in the MOSAIC trial. J Clin Oncol 2009; 27: 3109–16.

131. Tournigand C, Andre T, Achille E, et al. FOLFIRI followed by FOLFOX6 or the reverse sequence in advanced colorectal cancer: a randomized GERCOR study. J Clin Oncol 2004; 22: 229–37.

132. Hurwitz H, Fehrenbacher L, Novotny W, et al. Bevacizumab plus irinotecan, fluorouracil, and leucovorin for metastatic colorectal cancer. N Engl J Med 2004; 350: 2335–42.

133. Hurwitz HI, Yi J, Ince W, et al. The clinical benefit of bevacizumab in metastatic colorectal cancer is independent of K-ras mutation status: analysis of a phase III study of bevacizumab with chemotherapy in previously untreated metastatic colorectal cancer. Oncologist 2009; 14: 22–8.

134. Cunningham D, Humblet Y, Siena S, et al. Cetuximab monotherapy and cetuximab plus irinotecan in irinotecan-refractory metastatic colorectal cancer. N Engl J Med 2004; 351: 337–45.

135. Addeo R, Caraglia M, Cerbone D, et al. Panitumumab: a new frontier of target therapy for the treatment of metastatic colorectal cancer. Expert Rev Anticancer Ther 2010; 10: 499–505.

136. Giusti RM, Shastri KA, Cohen MH, et al. FDA drug approval summary: panitumumab (Vectibix). Oncologist 2007; 12: 577–83.

137. Van Cutsem E, Peeters M, Siena S, et al. Open-label phase III trial of panitumumab plus best supportive care compared with best supportive care alone in patients with chemotherapy-refractory metastatic colorectal cancer. J Clin Oncol 2007; 25: 1658–64.

138. VanderMeer TJ, Callery MP, Meyers WC. The approach to the patient with single and multiple liver metastases, pulmonary metastases, and intra-abdominal metastases from colorectal carcinoma. Hematol Oncol Clin North Am 1997; 11: 759–77.

139. Perez EA, Livingstone AS, Franceschi D, et al. Current incidence and outcomes of gastrointestinal mesenchymal tumors including gastrointestinal stromal tumors. J Am Coll Surg 2006; 202: 623–9.

140. Corless CL, Fletcher JA, Heinrich MC. Biology of gastrointestinal stromal tumors. J Clin Oncol 2004; 22: 3813–25.

141. Blay JY, Bonvalot S, Casali P, et al. Consensus meeting for the management of gastrointestinal stromal tumors. Report of the GIST Consensus Conference of 20–21 March 2004, under the auspices of ESMO. Ann Oncol 2005; 16: 566–78.

142. Miettinen M, Lasota J. Gastrointestinal stromal tumors: review on morphology, molecular pathology, prognosis, and differential diagnosis. Arch Pathol Lab Med 2006; 130: 1466–78.

143. Demetri GD, von Mehren M, Blanke CD, et al. Efficacy and safety of imatinib mesylate in advanced gastrointestinal stromal tumors. N Engl J Med 2002; 347: 472–80.

144. DeMatteo RP, Heinrich MC, El-Rifai WM, et al. Clinical management of gastrointestinal stromal tumors: before and after STI-571. Hum Pathol 2002; 33: 466–77.

145. DeMatteo RP, Lewis JJ, Leung D, et al. Two hundred gastrointestinal stromal tumors: recurrence patterns and prognostic factors for survival. Ann Surg 2000; 231: 51–8.

146. Agaram NP, La Quaglia MP, Ustun B, et al. Molecular characterization of pediatric gastrointestinal stromal tumors. Clin Cancer Res 2008; 14: 3204–15.

147. Cypriano MS, Jenkins JJ, Pappo AS, et al. Pediatric gastrointestinal stromal tumors and leiomyosarcoma. Cancer 2004; 101: 39–50.

148. Benesch M, Wardelmann E, Ferrari A, et al. Gastrointestinal stromal tumors (GIST) in children and adolescents: a comprehensive review of the current literature. Pediatr Blood Cancer 2009; 53: 1171–9.

149. Li FP, Fletcher JA, Heinrich MC, et al. Familial gastrointestinal stromal tumor syndrome: phenotypic and molecular features in a kindred. J Clin Oncol 2005; 23: 2735–43.

150. Miettinen M, Fetsch JF, Sobin LH, et al. Gastrointestinal stromal tumors in patients with neurofibromatosis 1: a clinicopathologic and molecular genetic study of 45 cases. Am J Surg Pathol 2006; 30: 90–6.

151. Matyakhina L, Bei TA, McWhinney SR, et al. Genetics of Carney triad: recurrent losses at chromosome 1 but lack of germline mutations in genes associated with paragangliomas and gastrointestinal stromal tumors. J Clin Endocrinol Metab 2007; 92: 2938–43.

152. Pasini B, McWhinney SR, Bei T, et al. Clinical and molecular genetics of patients with the Carney–Stratakis syndrome and germline mutations of the genes coding for the succinate dehydrogenase subunits SDHB, SDHC, and SDHD. Eur J Hum Genet 2008; 16: 79–88.

153. Carney JA, Sheps SG, Go VL, et al. The triad of gastric leiomyosarcoma, functioning extra-adrenal paraganglioma and pulmonary chondroma. N Engl J Med 1977; 296: 1517–18.

154. Zhang L, Smyrk TC, Young WF Jr, et al. Gastric stromal tumors in Carney triad are different clinically, pathologically, and behaviorally from sporadic gastric gastrointestinal stromal tumors: findings in 104 cases. Am J Surg Pathol 2010; 34: 53–64.

155. Carney JA, Stratakis CA. Familial paraganglioma and gastric stromal sarcoma: a new syndrome distinct from the Carney triad. Am J Med Genet 2002; 108: 132–9.

156. McWhinney SR, Pasini B, Stratakis CA. Familial gastrointestinal stromal tumors and germ-line mutations. N Engl J Med 2007; 357: 1054–6.

157. Carney JA, Stratakis CA. Familial paraganglioma and gastric stromal sarcoma: a new syndrome distinct from the Carney triad. Am J Med Genet 2002; 108: 132–9.

158. Pappo AS, Janeway KA. Pediatric gastrointestinal stromal tumors. Hematol Oncol Clin North Am 2009; 23: 15–34, vii.

159. Benesch M, Leuschner I, Wardelmann E, et al. Gastrointestinal stromal tumours in children and young adults: a clinicopathologic series with long-term follow-up from the database of the Cooperative Weichteilsarkom Studiengruppe (CWS). Eur J Cancer 2011; 47: 1692–8.

160. Janeway KA, Liegl B, Harlow A, et al. Pediatric KIT wild-type and platelet-derived growth factor receptor alpha-wild-type gastrointestinal stromal tumors share KIT activation but not mechanisms of genetic progression with adult gastrointestinal stromal tumors. Cancer Res 2007; 67: 9084–8.

161. Hostein I, Faur N, Primois C, et al. BRAF mutation status in gastrointestinal stromal tumors. Am J Clin Pathol 2010; 133: 141–8.

162. Chapman PB, Hauschild A, Robert C, et al. Improved survival with vemurafenib in melanoma with BRAF V600E mutation. N Engl J Med 2011; 364: 2507–16.

163. Janeway KA, Kim SY, Lodish M, *et al.* Defects in succinate dehydrogenase in gastrointestinal stromal tumors lacking KIT and PDGFRA mutations. Proc Natl Acad Sci USA 2011; 108: 314–18.

164. Belinsky MG, Rink L, Cai KQ, *et al.* The insulin-like growth factor system as a potential therapeutic target in gastrointestinal stromal tumors. Cell Cycle 2008; 7: 2949–55.

165. Demetri GD. Targeting the molecular pathophysiology of gastrointestinal stromal tumors with imatinib. Mechanisms, successes, and challenges to rational drug development. Hematol Oncol Clin North Am 2002; 16: 1115–24.

166. Pasini B, Stratakis CA. SDH mutations in tumorigenesis and inherited endocrine tumours: lesson from the phaeochromocytoma-paraganglioma syndromes. J Intern Med 2009; 266: 19–42.

167. Heinrich MC, Corless CL, Demetri GD, *et al.* Kinase mutations and imatinib response in patients with metastatic gastrointestinal stromal tumor. J Clin Oncol 2003; 21: 4342–9.

168. Heinrich MC, Maki RG, Corless CL, *et al.* Primary and secondary kinase genotypes correlate with the biological and clinical activity of sunitinib in imatinib-resistant gastrointestinal stromal tumor. J Clin Oncol 2008; 26: 5352–9.

169. Janeway KA, Albritton KH, van den Abbeele AD, *et al.* Sunitinib treatment in pediatric patients with advanced GIST following failure of imatinib. Pediatr Blood Cancer 2009; 52: 767–71.

170. Brennan B. Pediatric pancreatic tumors: the orphan looking for a home. Pediatr Blood Cancer 2010; 54: 659–60.

171. Shorter NA, Glick RD, Klimstra DS, *et al.* Malignant pancreatic tumors in childhood and adolescence: the Memorial Sloan-Kettering experience, 1967 to present. J Pediatr Surg 2002; 37: 887–92.

172. Dall'Igna P, Cecchetto G, Bisogno G, *et al.* Pancreatic tumors in children and adolescents: the Italian TREP project experience. Pediatr Blood Cancer 2010; 54: 675–80.

173. Perez EA, Gutierrez JC, Koniaris LG, *et al.* Malignant pancreatic tumors: incidence and outcome in 58 pediatric patients. J Pediatr Surg 2009; 44: 197–203.

174. Park M, Koh KN, Kim BE, *et al.* Pancreatic neoplasms in childhood and adolescence. J Pediatr Hematol Oncol 2011; 33: 295–300.

175. Yu DC, Kozakewich HP, Perez-Atayde AR, *et al.* Childhood pancreatic tumors: a single institution experience. J Pediatr Surg 2009; 44: 2267–72.

176. Ellerkamp V, Warmann SW, Vorwerk P, *et al.* Exocrine pancreatic tumors in childhood in Germany. Pediatr Blood Cancer 2012; 58: 366–71.

177. Luttges J, Stigge C, Pacena M, *et al.* Rare ductal adenocarcinoma of the pancreas in patients younger than age 40 years. Cancer 2004; 100: 173–82.

178. Holen KD, Klimstra DS, Hummer A, *et al.* Clinical characteristics and outcomes from an institutional series of acinar cell carcinoma of the pancreas and related tumors. J Clin Oncol 2002; 20: 4673–8.

179. Horie A, Yano Y, Kotoo Y, *et al.* Morphogenesis of pancreatoblastoma, infantile carcinoma of the pancreas: report of two cases. Cancer 1977; 39: 247–54.

180. Dhebri AR, Connor S, Campbell F, *et al.* Diagnosis, treatment and outcome of pancreatoblastoma. Pancreatology 2004; 4: 441–51; discussion 452–3.

181. Bien E, Godzinski J, Dall'Igna P, *et al.* Pancreatoblastoma: a report from the European Cooperative Study Group for Paediatric Rare Tumours (EXPeRT). Eur J Cancer 2011; 47: 2347–52.

182. Levey JM, Banner BF. Adult pancreatoblastoma: a case report and review of the literature. Am J Gastroenterol 1996; 91: 1841–4.

183. Drut R, Jones MC. Congenital pancreatoblastoma in Beckwith–Wiedemann syndrome: an emerging association. Pediatr Pathol 1988; 8: 331–9.

184. Koh TH, Cooper JE, Newman CL, *et al.* Pancreatoblastoma in a neonate with Wiedemann–Beckwith syndrome. Eur J Pediatr 1986; 145: 435–8.

185. Sorrentino S, Conte M, Nozza P, *et al.* Simultaneous occurrence of pancreatoblastoma and neuroblastoma in a newborn with Beckwith–Wiedemann syndrome. J Pediatr Hematol Oncol 2010; 32: e207–9.

186. Muguerza R, Rodriguez A, Formigo E, *et al.* Pancreatoblastoma associated with incomplete Beckwith–Wiedemann syndrome: case report and review of the literature. J Pediatr Surg 2005; 40: 1341–4.

187. Abraham SC, Wu TT, Klimstra DS, *et al.* Distinctive molecular genetic alterations in sporadic and familial adenomatous polyposis-associated pancreatoblastomas: frequent alterations in the APC/beta-catenin pathway and chromosome 11p. Am J Pathol 2001; 159: 1619–27.

188. Wiley J, Posekany K, Riley R, *et al.* Cytogenetic and flow cytometric analysis of a pancreatoblastoma. Cancer Genet Cytogenet 1995; 79: 115–18.

189. Barenboim-Stapleton L, Yang X, Tsokos M, *et al.* Pediatric pancreatoblastoma: histopathologic and cytogenetic characterization of tumor and derived cell line. Cancer Genet Cytogenet 2005; 157: 109–17.

190. Kerr NJ, Chun YH, Yun K, *et al.* Pancreatoblastoma is associated with chromosome 11p loss of heterozygosity and IGF2 overexpression. Med Pediatr Oncol 2002; 39: 52–4.

191. Tanaka Y, Kato K, Notohara K, *et al.* Significance of aberrant (cytoplasmic/nuclear) expression of beta-catenin in pancreatoblastoma. J Pathol 2003; 199: 185–90.

192. Klimstra DS, Wenig BM, Adair CF, *et al.* Pancreatoblastoma. A clinicopathologic study and review of the literature. Am J Surg Pathol 1995; 19: 1371–89.

193. Yu PF, Hu ZH, Wang XB, *et al.* Solid pseudopapillary tumor of the pancreas: a review of 553 cases in Chinese literature. World J Gastroenterol 2010; 16: 1209–14.

194. Papavramidis T, Papavramidis S. Solid pseudopapillary tumors of the pancreas: review of 718 patients reported in English literature. J Am Coll Surg 2005; 200: 965–72.

195. Huang SC, Ng KF, Yeh TS, *et al.* Clinicopathological analysis of beta-catenin and Axin-1 in solid pseudopapillary neoplasms of the pancreas. Ann Surgical Oncol 2011; Jul 19 [Epub ahead of print].

196. Rebhandl W, Felberbauer FX, Puig S, *et al.* Solid-pseudopapillary tumor of the pancreas (Frantz tumor) in children: report of four cases and review of the literature. J Surg Oncol 2001; 76: 289–96.

197. Kanter J, Wilson DB, Strasberg S. Downsizing to resectability of a large solid and cystic papillary tumor of the pancreas by single-agent chemotherapy. J Pediatr Surg 2009; 44: e23–5.

198. Hah JO, Park WK, Lee NH, *et al.* Preoperative chemotherapy and intraoperative radiofrequency ablation for unresectable solid pseudopapillary tumor of the pancreas. J Pediatr Hematol Oncol 2007; 29: 851–3.

199. Tonelli F, Giudici F, Fratini G, *et al.* Pancreatic endocrine tumors in multiple endocrine neoplasia type 1 syndrome: review of literature. Endocr Pract 2011; 17: 33–40.

200. Wilson SD. Zollinger–Ellison syndrome in children: a 25-year follow-up. Surgery 1991; 110: 696–702; discussion 702–3.

201. Modlin IM, Moss SF, Oberg K, *et al.* Gastrointestinal neuroendocrine (carcinoid) tumours: current diagnosis and management. Med J Aust 2010; 193: 46–52.

202. Kouvaraki MA, Ajani JA, Hoff P, *et al.* Fluorouracil, doxorubicin, and streptozocin in the treatment of patients with locally advanced and metastatic pancreatic endocrine carcinomas. J Clin Oncol 2004; 22: 4762–71.

203. Raymond E, Dahan L, Raoul JL, *et al.* Sunitinib malate for the treatment of pancreatic neuroendocrine tumors. N Engl J Med 2011; 364: 501–13.

204. Yao JC, Shah MH, Ito T, *et al.* Everolimus for advanced pancreatic neuroendocrine tumors. N Engl J Med 2011; 364: 514–23.

205. Imhof A, Brunner P, Marincek N, *et al.* Response, survival, and long-term toxicity after therapy with the radiolabeled somatostatin analogue [90Y-DOTA]-TOC in metastasized neuroendocrine cancers. J Clin Oncol 2011; 29: 2416–23.

206. Brennan B. Pediatric pancreatic tumors: The orphan looking for a home. Pediatr Blood Cancer 2010: 54: 659–660.

65 Rare Pediatric Malignancies of the Head and Neck

Cynthia E. Herzog,[1] Michael E. Kupferman,[2] Winston Huh,[1] and Anita Mahajan[3]

[1] Division of Pediatrics, [2] Department of Head and Neck Surgery, [3] Department of Radiation Oncology, The University of Texas MD Anderson Cancer Center, Houston, TX, USA

Introduction

Head and neck tumors account for about 12% of malignancies in patients under age 19 according to data from the Surveillance, Epidemiology, and End Results (SEER) database.[1] Some of these tumors are more commonly occurring pediatric cancers that occur in nonhead and neck sites as well: lymphoma (27%) and bone and soft tissue sarcomas (14%). Others are specific to the head and neck region: thyroid tumors (21%) and retinoblastoma (16%). The remaining 22% are accounted for by a number of rare tumors, including salivary gland tumors (4%) and nasopharyngeal carcinoma (1%).

Treatment of pediatric head and neck tumors requires a multidisciplinary approach, which can include surgery, pediatric oncology, radiation oncology, ophthalmology, oral surgeons, and dentists. Special consideration needs to be given to the fact that structures are still growing and developing in these patients and late effects can occur long after treatment is given. This chapter will address salivary gland tumors and nasopharyngeal carcinoma, which are true malignancies. In addition, giant cell tumors of the jaw, which can be locally aggressive, will be addressed.

Salivary gland tumors

Tumors of the salivary glands represent approximately 1% of cancers in the US population, and present in either the major (parotid and submandibular) or minor (oral cavity, paranasal sinuses, larynx, oropharynx, trachea) salivary glands. Data in the pediatric population are limited, as the majority of studies on salivary gland malignancies have not provided subgroup analysis in minor salivary gland tumors in children and few reports in the literature are available.

Epidemiology

In the pediatric population, salivary gland malignancies account for 10% of all pediatric head and neck cancers. Only 5% of all salivary gland tumors occur in children and, unique to this age group, the majority (45–55%) of these are epithelial malignancies.[2–7] Large population-based studies of salivary gland tumors, both benign and malignant, have found approximately 0.4–1 tumor per 100,000 population per year, of which 15–25% are localized to the minor salivary glands.[6,8,9] The percentage of these tumors that are malignant varies by report, and ranges from 40% to 80%.[6,9] These tumors encompass a wide variety of histologies and their diversity confounds issues related to surgical management and the roles of adjuvant therapies.[10] Population studies have demonstrated that only 5% of minor salivary gland tumors occur in children, approximately half of which are malignant.

Pathology and biology

Mucoepidermoid carcinoma (MEC) is the most common pathology seen in the major salivary glands (45%), followed by acinic cell carcinoma (26%) and adenoid cystic carcinoma (15%). The majority of these are low- or intermediate-grade tumors (78%), while high-grade histologies are associated with adverse prognosis. In the minor salivary glands, the distribution of tumor histologies favors mucoepidermoid carcinoma (60%), with adenoid cystic carcinoma (25%) and adenocarcinoma (10%) comprising the remaining histologies. The presence of perineural invasion is associated with adverse prognosis and indicates the need for adjuvant treatments.

Clinical presentation and patterns of spread

The majority of patients present in the adolescent years with a neck mass, either in the parotid region or at the submandibular gland. Cranial nerve or sensorimotor symptoms can occur in 10–15% of patients and are a barometer for an aggressive malignancy, as they often indicate perineural spread of tumor. Metastatic lymphadenopathy is rarely seen at presentation

Textbook of Uncommon Cancer, Fourth Edition. Edited by Derek Raghavan, Charles D. Blanke, David H. Johnson, Paul L. Moots, Gregory H. Reaman, Peter G. Rose and Mikkael A. Sekeres.

(<10%). Frequently, the clinical signs and symptoms are present for 6–12 months until evaluation is sought.

By stage at presentation, small tumors predominate, with 70–75% of tumors presenting as either T1 (≤2 cm) or T2 (>2 cm and <4 cm) lesions; uncommonly, these tumors can involve local bony structures when they arise in the major salivary glands. However, this is not the case with minor salivary gland tumors, which can invade local structures when present in the sinonasal tract. Nodal metastasis can occur in up to 40% of patients, with the majority metastasizing from the parotid gland.

Evaluation

A careful history and physical examination will greatly aid in the initial evaluation of a patient and development of a differential diagnosis. Dedicated imaging using either computed axial tomography (CT) or magnetic resonance imaging (MRI) is important to determine extent, invasiveness of disease and potential nodal involvement. Each imaging modality has its own distinct advantages. CT scans are preferable when evaluating for bony erosion or involvement of the skull base, while MRI scans typically have advantages with evaluating soft tissue definition and intracranial involvement. Any imaging study should include the full length of the neck in order to fully evaluate for any suspicious lymph nodes that may require biopsy. Metabolic imaging, such as 18 F-fluorodeoxyglucose positron emission tomography (FDG PET), can provide additional information regarding evaluation of abnormal metabolic activity of a primary mass and assessing for lymph node involvement. However, FDG PET has limitations in terms of determining metabolic activity in lesions less than 1 cm and sometimes differentiating inflammatory conditions from malignant diseases.

If there is difficulty in differentiating between a benign or malignant diagnosis, then fine needle aspiration (FNA) can be used to obtain material for histological diagnosis. While less invasive, there is a greater risk for a nondiagnostic biopsy with FNA compared to core needle or open biopsy techniques. If there is little question that a mass is malignant, then a core needle or open biopsy technique is generally recommended in order to obtain sufficient material for additional studies, such as immunohistochemical panels or cytogenetic studies.

Differential diagnosis

The differential diagnosis of pediatric head and neck masses can be divided into four general categories: congenital lesions, inflammatory/infection-related lesions, other benign lesions, and malignant neoplasms. Fortunately, most pediatric head and neck masses are benign in nature. Age of the patient at presentation and anatomical location of the primary tumor will aid in refining the differential diagnosis. Congenital lesions such as thyroglossal duct cysts would be less likely to be part of the differential for parotid gland masses because these lesions tend to occur in the anterior triangle region of the neck. The entire list of potential nonmalignant diagnoses is quite large and an extensive review would be beyond the scope of this chapter.

With regard to other malignancies to consider, rhabdomyosarcoma is the most common soft tissue sarcoma encountered in the head and neck in children, and a parameningeal rhabdomyosarcoma of the masticator space can mimic the presentation of a parotid gland tumor.[1] Other malignancies to consider include synovial sarcoma, malignant peripheral nerve sheath tumor, lymphoma, osteosarcoma, thyroid carcinoma, and metastatic lesions from malignancies such as neuroblastoma.[11–14] Desmoid fibromatosis and Langerhans cell histiocytosis are nonmalignant disorders that should also be considered since they often require aggressive treatment.

Treatment

For cancers of the major and minor salivary glands, surgical resection has been the primary treatment modality. For the majority of parotid tumors, this generally entails a superficial parotidectomy with preservation of the facial nerve. For larger or deep lobe tumors, a total parotidectomy may be necessary. The decision to resect the facial nerve is fraught with cosmetic, functional, and psychological implications that will affect the child for life, and thus a frank discussion of this issue must be undertaken in the preoperative setting. Reconstructive surgery at the time of primary resection is preferable, particularly for management of anticipated facial nerve resection.

Nodal dissection should be performed for high-grade histologies, large tumors, and when nodal metastasis are present. For submandibular gland cancers, a comprehensive resection of levels I–III should be performed with complete resection of the submandibular gland and the primary nodes. For minor salivary gland cancers, surgical resection may necessitate skull base resection or transoral resection, depending on the primary tumor site. More details of these techniques can be found in other texts. While complete oncological resection remains the primary goal, functional and cosmetic issues should be considered in choosing the optimal surgical approach.

Locoregional therapy should be intensified among patients with high-grade lesions, positive surgical margins, and invasive features, as they are at risk for not only recurrence but also unfavorable prognosis. While combined chemotherapy and radiotherapy is recommended for squamous histologies in the postoperative setting, this aggressive strategy has received little attention for treatment of salivary malignancies, especially in pediatric patients. The use of traditional cytotoxic chemotherapy has been mainly reserved for patients with progressive, metastatic disease. Unfortunately, evaluating the results of many of these studies is difficult since the patient cohorts tend to be small in number with mixed histological diagnoses and with variable prior history of medical treatment. The reported response rates for a variety of single chemotherapy agent studies have been quite poor. The most common studied chemotherapy combination has been cisplatin, doxorubicin, and cyclophosphamide (CAP regimen). Response rates of 25–50% have been reported but the CAP regimen has been associated with significant toxicities.[15,16]

With the advent of newer molecular-targeted agents, there is interest in determining the genetic profiles of salivary gland malignancies. For example, overexpression of c-kit has been observed in a significant number of adenoid cystic carcinomas. Also, epidermal growth factor receptor (EGFR) overexpression has been reported for MEC and adenoid cystic carcinomas.[17–19] Unfortunately, however, no objective responses have been observed in clinical trials using imatinib, gefitinib, cetuximab, lapatinib, and bortezomib.[10,15–28] Thus greater understanding of the molecular pathways involved is required to determine which pathways are critical for tumor development and therefore suitable as candidates for targeted therapy. It remains to be seen whether this approach would benefit pediatric patients.

The role of radiotherapy has evolved over time as conformal techniques have improved. Radiotherapy is reserved for patients with adverse histological features or recurrent disease.[21,29,30] The radiation field is dependent upon the location of tumor, invasive features, and presence of nodal disease.

Prognosis

Outcomes for pediatric patients with major salivary gland malignancies have generally been excellent, with 5-year disease-free survival of 80–94%.[20–23]

Treatment-related sequelae from the management of salivary gland cancers can be profound in the pediatric population. Delayed side-effects include permanent xerostomia, facial paralysis, craniofacial growth dysmorphism, visual impairment, osteoradionecrosis, and cosmetic deformity. Despite the favorable prognosis of salivary gland tumors in the pediatric population, there is a significant risk of developing secondary radiation-associated neoplasms in these patients.[31]

Long-term morbidities are in line with those typically seen in adult patients, namely facial nerve dysfunction, xerostomia, and dental caries. For adult survivors of pediatric malignancies, most morbidity is primarily associated with systemic therapy and cranial irradiation, although midface irradiation in children less than 10 years old is associated with midface hypoplasia and ocular abnormalities. Based upon these data, we conclude that intensification of local therapy for salivary gland cancers in the pediatric population is associated with few late side-effects but should be carefully considered in therapeutic decision making. However, these results should not alter the current guidelines of the Institute of Medicine (IOM), which recommends intensive monitoring of irradiated pediatric patients.[32]

Individualized monitoring can be established for those who received surgery alone, as they would be categorized as low risk in the IOM guidelines. Particular to salivary gland cancers, recurrences beyond 5 years were common, with the locoregional recurrences presenting at a median of 8 years after treatment.

Nasopharygeal carcinoma

Nasopharyngeal cancer (NPC) (see Chapter 8) is a rare primary cancer that represents only 1% of all childhood malignancies. NPC is challenging to treat and generally requires carefully planned interdisciplinary care to obtain optimal results. Much of the treatment for pediatric NPC is extrapolated from adult studies where larger numbers of patients are available.

Epidemiology

Nasopharyngeal carcinoma appears to have a multifactorial etiology which varies with genetic, environmental, and viral factors. There is a strong geographic/genetic predilection with high rates noted in South East Asian, Inuit, and North African populations. The incidence is 15–20 cases per 10^5 person-years in endemic areas in comparison to less than one case per 10^5 person-years in most other parts of the world. Environmental risk factors include cigarette smoke, occupational exposures to formaldehyde, and wood dust.[33] In adults, 70% of all primary nasopharyngeal tumors are NPC and the incidence appears to have a bimodal age distribution, in the fourth and sixth decades. There is a strong correlation with Epstein–Barr virus (EBV) exposure and the diagnosis of NPC, particularly in endemic areas. Nasopharyngeal carcinoma has been associated with specific HLA types and other genetic factors may play a role, especially in low-incidence populations.

In endemic areas, the incidence of NPC is low in the pediatric population but in other populations a substantial proportion of NPC cases occur in the pediatric age group, primarily in adolescents. It is diagnosed worldwide at a rate of 1–1.5 cases per 10^6 person-years but in endemic cases, the incidence can be up to 8–25 cases per 10^5 person-years. NPC is diagnosed in 35–50% of all primary nasopharyngeal tumors. It occurs in males twice as often as in females and is more common in blacks in the United States. In the pediatric population most NPC tumors are World Health Organization (WHO) type 3 (undifferentiated, also known as lymphoepithelioma).[34] EBV has been found in almost all cases of undifferentiated, nonkeratinizing NPC.[35]

Pathology

The WHO initially described three different histological subgroups of NPC: type 1 (squamous cell), type 2 (nonkeratinizing), and type 3 (undifferentiated). In 2005, a new classification was proposed: keratinizing squamous cell carcinoma, nonkeratinizing carcinoma (differentiated and undifferentiated), and basaloid squamous cell carcinoma.[36] Nonkeratinizing tumors are most frequently diagnosed: 99% in endemic areas, 75% in the United States. Keratinizing tumors constitute only 1% of NPC tumors in Hong Kong in contrast to 25% in the United States. Basaloid squamous cell carcinoma is very rare but may have a lower clinical aggressiveness in comparison to other subtypes of NPC.

Biology

Epstein–Barr virus has been found in almost all cases of undifferentiated, nonkeratinizing NPC.[35] EBV transformation of epithelial cells results in a type 2 latent infection, in which the genes for EBV encoded small nuclear RNAs (EBERs), EBV nuclear antigen 1 (EBNA1), and latent membrane protein 1 and 2 (LMP1 and LMP2) are transcribed. This differs from the type 3 latent infection seen with B lymphocytes, in which additional genes, including those for EBNA2 and EBNA3, are also transcribed.[37]

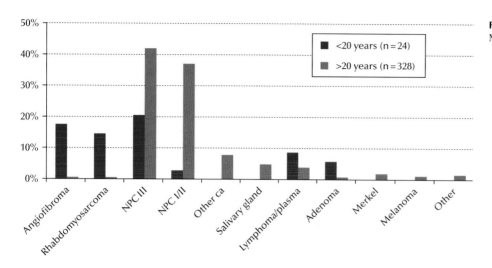

Figure 65.1 Nasopharyngeal tumors seen at MDA from 2000 to 2010.

Legend for figure:
- <20 years (n = 24)
- >20 years (n = 328)

Chart categories: Angiofibroma, Rhabdomyosarcoma, NPC III, NPC I/II, Other ca, Salivary gland, Lymphoma/plasma, Adenoma, Merkel, Melanoma, Other

Pattern of spread

The nasopharynx is an open area defined anteriorly by the choanae of the nasal cavity, inferiorly by the upper surface of the soft palate, superiorly and posteriorly by the skull base and cervical vertebrae 1 and 2. The lateral walls incorporate the eustachian tube orifices which are defined by the torus tubarius and the fossa of Rosenmuller. The majority of NPCs arise from the lateral walls around the fossa of Rosenmuller. NPCs grow anteriorly into the nasal cavity, posteriorly and superiorly to the skull base, sphenoid sinus, prevertebral space, and clivus. The foramen lacerum and foramen ovale are paths of direct extension into the cavernous sinus and middle cranial fossa. The rich lymphatic drainage allows early spread to draining lymph nodes. Cervical lymphadenopathy is present in over 85% of patients. The jugulodigastric nodes are most commonly involved. Bilateral neck node involvement is found in 50% of patients.[38] Hematogenous spread is reported in 3% of patients at diagnosis but is noted in up to 50% of cases over the course of their disease.

Clinical presentation

Most pediatric patients present with advanced locoregional disease manifesting as cervical lymphadenopathy. Other findings are epistaxis, hearing loss, nasal congestion, pain, and cranial nerve deficits.[39] Many patients present with multiple symptoms. In most cases the lactate dehydrogenase level is elevated but this finding is nonspecific. The diagnosis is established from a biopsy of the nasopharynx or cervical lymph nodes.

Evaluation

All patients presenting with a painless enlarging neck mass should undergo a thorough clinical evaluation of the head and neck area. A CT scan and MRI of the nasopharynx, skull base, paranasal sinuses, and cervical areas should be obtained to determine the extent of locoregional disease. To determine the origin and extent of disease, a fiberoptic nasopharygoscopy should be attempted with a biopsy to establish the diagnosis.

A full staging workup can include chest x-ray, bone scan, CT scans of the chest and abdomen, or PET scan. This evaluation should be tailored to the patient's symptoms and laboratory evaluation. Monitoring EBV titers may be useful in evaluating disease status.

Differential diagnosis

In the United States the differential diagnosis for nasopharyngeal tumors in children is quite extensive, with NPC being a less common diagnosis. Other tumors that occur in the nasopharynx include angiofibroma, rhabdomyosarcoma, lymphoma, adenoma, salivary gland tumors, and others. Figure 65.1 shows the distribution of diagnosis in patients presenting with nasopharyngeal tumors at a single institution over 10 years, comparing children to adults.

Treatment

Multimodality therapy is required for the management of NPC. Radiation therapy has been the mainstay of treatment for NPC, and for patients with limited local disease, good overall survival rates can be accomplished with this modality alone. Because most patients present with advanced stages, surgery is usually limited to establishment of the diagnosis. As supported by prospective randomized trial and more recent metaanalysis, chemotherapy has improved local control and overall survival when used in a neoadjuvant and adjuvant fashion in adults.[40–42] A review of published randomized trials in adults of radiotherapy alone verses radiotherapy in combination with chemotherapy reports consistent survival benefit for concurrent radiation and chemotherapy.[34,43] The benefit of neoadjuvant or adjuvant chemotherapy is less consistently seen but it does appear to decrease locoregional and distant failure. There are a number of reports on the addition of chemotherapy to high-dose radiotherapy in children with advanced-stage disease but the rarity of NPC has limited randomized trials in the pediatric population. The Pediatric Oncology Group and St Jude studies support the use of chemotherapy with radiotherapy as primary treatment of NPC.[44]

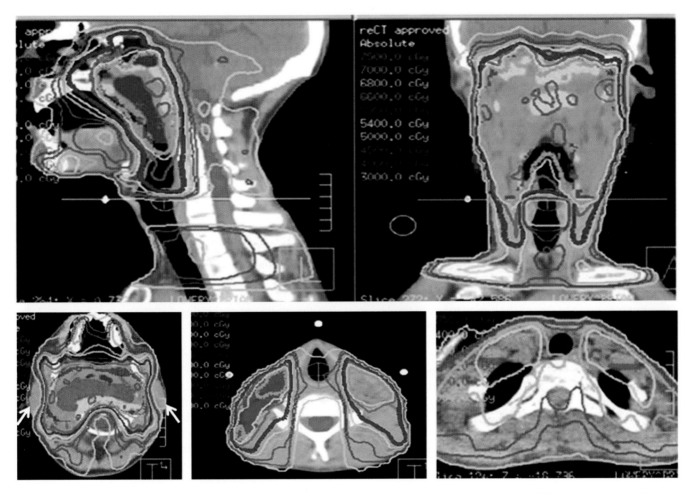

Figure 65.2 Radiotherapy dosimetry using IMRT for a patient with NPC. A concomitant boost technique was used to deliver 70 Gy to the primary site, 56 Gy to the high-risk lymph nodes and 50 Gy to the supraclavicular lymph nodes.

Radiotherapy planning is complex since the area of concern extends from the skull base to the supraclavicular fossae in order to incorporate all the areas at risk from primary tumor involvement and lymphatic dissemination. MRI/CT-based planning is critical to identify normal and target regions. Radiation dose to the parotid glands, oral mucosa, mandible, brainstem, spinal cord, temporal lobes, pituitary gland, hypothalamus, cochlea, optic nerves, optic chiasm, retina, and lens should be monitored and lowered as much as possible. Typical radiotherapy doses range from 50 Gy for subclinical sites of involvement to 70 Gy for gross sites of disease, given in 1.8–2 Gy daily fractions 5 days a week. Various fractionation schemes and planning techniques such as concurrent boosts or simultaneous integrated boosts have been incorporated for practical reasons with no adverse or beneficial effect on tumor control.

Advanced radiotherapy techniques such as intensity modulated radiotherapy (IMRT), arc therapy, tomotherapy, image guidance, and proton therapy may allow sparing of normal tissues and decrease radiation-associated morbidity.[45–47] An example of an 18-year-old patient with undifferentiated NPC with positive lymphadenopathy treated with IMRT and a simultaneous boost technique is shown in Figure 65.2. Note

the reduction of dose to the parotid glands as annotated by the white arrows.

Even with the improvements in survival seen after the addition of chemotherapy to standard high-dose radiotherapy, a large number of patients with advanced-stage NPC will relapse and/or develop distant metastatic disease. In addition, toxicities secondary to high-dose radiation in patients with NPC include, but are not limited to, mucositis, chronic xerostomia, hypopituitarism, significant hearing loss, and occasional cases of temporal lobe necrosis and osteoradionecrosis.[48] This has led to efforts to develop less toxic, more effective therapies by targeting EBV which is associated with almost all cases of pediatric NPC.

The use of EBV-CTL adoptive immunotherapy for the treatment of NPC has been reported by several groups. This therapy appears to be safe and can be associated with significant antitumor activity.[49]

Prognosis

Survival rates for adult NPC have steadily increased over the past 60 years. Recent studies report 5-year overall survival rates of 75% in comparison to 35% in 1940–60 and 55–60% in

1970–90.[47,50] Local control continues to be quite good at 80% at 5 years. There continue to be local failures and distant metastases which require additional monitoring and intervention as needed.

For children in particular, the irradiation of normal tissues may be associated with many significant morbidities including ototoxicity, vision loss, cataract formation, temporal lobe necrosis, brainstem injury, neuroendocrine insufficiencies with associated growth retardation, trismus, xerostomia, dental problems, malocclusion, and secondary neoplasms. These issues should be monitored and timely interventions should be planned in order to minimize the impact on quality of life. The addition of chemotherapy can impact toxicities such as hearing loss further.

Central giant cell lesions

In 1953, Jaffe used the term giant cell reparative granuloma of jawbones for what he considered a local reparative reaction.[51] This term was meant to convey the benign nature of this lesion and to distinguish it from malignant giant cell tumor of long bones. Chuong et al. recognized that some of these jaw tumors had an aggressive course but that the aggressive tumors could not be distinguished histologically from more benign tumors and suggested the term central giant cell lesion (CGCL).[52]

Epidemiology

The etiology of CGCL is unknown. De Lange et al. reported an analysis of CGCL in the Dutch population which found that CGCL occurred more commonly in the mandible (67%), in females (56%) and in younger patients, with a peak in males at age 10–14 years and in females at age 15–19 years.[53] These findings are in agreement with other reports.[54,55] However, aggressive lesions were seen less commonly in the Danish population than has been reported by others.[54,55] This likely reflects the fact that other reports are not population based but are patient series, with a likely referral bias toward more aggressive lesions.

Pathology

The diagnosis is confirmed by means of incisional biopsy. Histological features are spindle-shaped stromal cells, the presence of giant cells is not very abundant, with irregular distribution that is often seen focally around areas of hemorrhage.[52,55]

Biology

The behavior of this tumor is variable, ranging from indolent to locally aggressive. Chuong et al. analysed samples from 17 patients with CGCL in 1986 in an attempt to identify histological factors that could distinguish between aggressive and nonaggressive.[52] Aggressive lesions were characterized clinically by pain, rapid growth, root resorption, cortical perforation, and high recurrence rate. There was no histological difference between the two types but the patients with aggressive tumors were younger and had larger tumors. The term central giant cell lesion, with clinical classification as aggressive or nonaggressive, was then proposed for these tumors. Rare cases of true malignancy have been reported.[56]

Clinical presentation and patterns of spread

Most present with painless swelling of the jaw that is often noted on routine dental x-rays. A small number have pain or neuresthenia. Bone destruction, with loosening and displacement of teeth and malocclusion, is common. CGCL does not metastasize but can be locally aggressive.

Evaluation

Serial CT scans can be used but concerns over exposure of the patient to radiation and expense limit the frequency of radiological examination by this method. In addition, it is difficult to position the patient so as to reproduce exactly the same sections through the same structures every time, compromising the ability to make direct comparisons between serial examinations.

Differential diagnosis

Routine serum analysis of calcium, phosphate, and parathyroid hormone levels should be obtained to distinguish these lesions from the "brown tumors" that can occur with primary or secondary hyperparathyroidism. Cherubism must be considered, especially in the case of bilateral disease. Although CGCL has been reported in Noonan syndrome and neurofibromatosis type 1, the incidence is very low and may be coincidental.[55]

Treatment

Surgery

Standard therapy is surgery, with curettage being the most common. The management of aggressive subtypes requires wide surgical resection with margins of 5 mm or more, and this compounds the morbidity of what is already a deforming condition. However, due to the location, en bloc resection can be associated with significant morbidity, triggering attempts to identify effective alternative therapies.

Nonsurgical adjunctive therapies could potentially minimize surgically induced damage to vital structures in proximity to the tumors, including growth centers, permanent teeth, nerves, joints, and the skeletal structures which support the esthetic contours of the face. Ideally one would seek to devise a totally nonsurgical modality for definitive treatment of these tumors, thereby avoiding iatrogenic damage altogether.

Intralesional steroids

The use of intralesional injections of steroids for CGCL was first reported by Jacoway et al. in 1988.[57] Since then there have been several case reports and small series which were reviewed by de Lange et al.[55] Most reported use of triamcinolone 10 mg/mL mixed 1:1 with 0.5% marcaine or lidocaine, with 2–6 mL given weekly for 6 weeks. Complete or considerable remission was noted in all 12 patients and only one patient required additional treatment with surgery. A larger series of 21 patients was reported by Nogueira et al., using triamcinolone hexacetonide 20 mg/mL mixed 1:1 with 2% lidocaine/1:200,000 epinephrine, with 1 mL/1 cm of tumor given twice weekly for 6 weeks.[58] No response was seen in two patients, four had a moderate response and 15 a good response. In the aggressive type no response was seen in two, moderate response in three and good response in five versus one moderate response and 10 good responses in nonaggressive tumors. It is unclear whether the lower response rate seen by Nogueira et al. was due to inclusion of aggressive lesions, which appear to have a lower response rate, or to the use of an alternative steroid.

Bone remodeling and healing of the lesion have been shown after intralesional steroid. This treatment is relatively simple and inexpensive but should be used with caution in patients in whom the use of steroids may be problematic, such as immunocompromised patients or those with diabetes or peptic ulcer disease.

Calcitonin

The use of human calcitonin was first reported by Harris in 1993; then when human calcitonin was no longer available, the use of salmon calcitonin was reported by Pogrel et al.[59,60] Both subcutaneous and intranasal calcitonin have been used. A review by de Lange et al. in 2007 indicates variable response.[55] There is only one double-blind, placebo-controlled trial of calcitonin.[61] This study compared placebo to intranasal salmon calcitonin at 200 IU/day for 3 months, then all patients were continued on calcitonin for a year. There was no difference seen in size after 3 months, or after 15 months. Continued regression of tumor was seen after treatment was discontinued.

Interferon

In 1999, Kaban et al. reported a case of a patient with CGCL treated with interferon after disease recurrence following two prior surgical resections and progression on calcitonin.[62] The experience with 26 patients with aggressive CGCL treated with interferon following enucleation of the tumor has subsequently been reported by Kaban et al.[63] Patients were treated for a mean of 8.0 ± 3.1 months with interferon-α at 3 million units/m^2 given subcutaneously daily. Sixteen patients had been off therapy for at least 2 years with no evidence of recurrence. Six were without evidence of recurrence less than 2 years off therapy and four were still on therapy

Busaidy et al. also reported their experience in five patients using interferon in an attempt to avoid surgery.[64] Subsequently 14 patients have been treated (unpublished data). Five patients have required no surgical intervention, three patients 3–5 years after interferon and another two patients 9–12 months after interferon. Six patients had conservative surgery in addition to interferon. One patient was noncompliant and had progressive disease requiring surgical resection. Two patients were lost to follow-up.

Prognosis

Recurrence after surgical treatment ranges from 11% to 49%,[55] with higher rates, up to 72%, when only aggressive lesions are considered.[52] The recurrence rate in aggressive tumors may be decreased with chemotherapy but information on the best treatment and proof of effectiveness are lacking.

Conclusion

Tumors of the head and neck are relatively rare in the pediatric population, with approximately 12% of pediatric malignancies occurring in the head and neck region. Salivary gland tumors, nasopharyngeal carcinoma, and central giant cell lesions are rare head and neck tumors in the pediatric population. Treatment of these tumors requires a multidisciplinary approach that usually includes surgery, pediatric oncology, and radiation oncology, and in some cases may involve other disciplines such as ophthalmology, oral surgery, and dentistry. Better understanding of the biology of these rare diseases is needed for more effective treatment interventions.

References

1. Albright JT, Topham AK, Reilly JS. Pediatric head and neck malignancies: US incidence and trends over 2 decades. Arch Otolaryngol Head Neck Surg 2002; 128(6): 655–9.
2. Hicks J, Flaitz C. Mucoepidermoid carcinoma of salivary glands in children and adolescents: assessment of proliferation markers. Oral Oncol 2000; 36(5): 454–60.
3. Luna MA, Batsakis JG, el-Naggar AK. Salivary gland tumors in children. Ann Otol Rhinol Laryngol 1991; 100(10): 869–71.
4. Shikhani AH, Johns ME. Tumors of the major salivary glands in children. Head Neck Surg 1988; 10(4): 257–63.
5. Tian Z, Li L, Wang L, Hu Y, Li J. Salivary gland neoplasms in oral and maxillofacial regions: a 23–year retrospective study of 6982 cases in an eastern Chinese population. Int J Oral Maxillofac Surg 2010; 39(3): 235–42.
6. Eveson JW, Cawson RA. Salivary gland tumours. A review of 2410 cases with particular reference to histological types, site, age and sex distribution. J Pathol 1985; 146(1): 51–8.
7. Lopes MA, Santos GC, Kowalski LP. Multivariate survival analysis of 128 cases of oral cavity minor salivary gland carcinomas. Head Neck 1998; 20(8): 699–706.
8. Buchner A, Merrell PW, Carpenter WM. Relative frequency of intra-oral minor salivary gland tumors: a study of 380 cases from northern California and comparison to reports from other parts of the world. J Oral Pathol Med 2007; 36(4): 207–14.
9. Spiro RH. Salivary neoplasms: overview of a 35-year experience with 2,807 patients. Head Neck Surg 1986; 8(3): 177–84.
10. Lack EE, Upton MP. Histopathologic review of salivary gland tumors in childhood. Arch Otolaryngol Head Neck Surg 1988; 114(8): 898–906.
11. Alam K, Khan R, Jain A, et al. The value of fine-needle aspiration cytology in the evaluation of pediatric head and neck tumors. Int J Pediatr Otorhinolaryngol 2009; 73(7): 923–7.
12. Anne S, Teot LA, Mandell DL. Fine needle aspiration biopsy: role in diagnosis of pediatric head and neck masses. Int J Pediatr Otorhinolaryngol 2008; 72(10): 1547–53.
13. Torsiglieri AJ Jr, Tom LW, Ross AJ 3rd, Wetmore RF, Handler SD, Potsic WP. Pediatric neck masses: guidelines for evaluation. Int J Pediatr Otorhinolaryngol 1988; 16(3): 199–210.
14. Huh WW, Fitzgerald N, Mahajan A, Sturgis EM, Beverly Raney R, Anderson PM. Pediatric sarcomas and related tumors of the head and neck. Cancer Treat Rev 2011; 37(6): 431–9.
15. Dreyfuss AI, Clark JR, Fallon BG, Posner MR, Norris CM Jr, Miller D. Cyclophosphamide, doxorubicin, and cisplatin combination chemotherapy for advanced carcinomas of salivary gland origin. Cancer 15 1987; 60(12): 2869–72.

16. Licitra L, Cavina R, Grandi C, *et al.* Cisplatin, doxorubicin and cyclophosphamide in advanced salivary gland carcinoma. A phase II trial of 22 patients. Ann Oncol 1996; 7(6): 640–2.

17. Holst VA, Marshall CE, Moskaluk CA, Frierson HF Jr. KIT protein expression and analysis of c-kit gene mutation in adenoid cystic carcinoma. Mod Pathol 1999; 12(10): 956–60.

18. Jeng YM, Lin CY, Hsu HC. Expression of the c-kit protein is associated with certain subtypes of salivary gland carcinoma. Cancer Lett 2000; 154(1): 107–11.

19. Laurie SA, Licitra L. Systemic therapy in the palliative management of advanced salivary gland cancers. J Clin Oncol 2006; 24(17): 2673–8.

20. Kupferman ME, de la Garza GO, Santillan AA, *et al.* Outcomes of pediatric patients with malignancies of the major salivary glands. Ann Surg Oncol 2010; 17(12): 3301–7.

21. Guzzo M, Ferrari A, Marcon I, *et al.* Salivary gland neoplasms in children: the experience of the Istituto Nazionale Tumori of Milan. Pediatr Blood Cancer 2006; 47(6): 806–10.

22. Bentz BG, Hughes CA, Ludemann JP, Maddalozzo J. Masses of the salivary gland region in children. Arch Otolaryngol Head Neck Surg 2000; 126(12): 1435–9.

23. Shapiro NL, Bhattacharyya N. Clinical characteristics and survival for major salivary gland malignancies in children. Otolaryngol Head Neck Surg 2006; 134(4): 631–4.

24. Agulnik M, Cohen EW, Cohen RB, *et al.* Phase II study of lapatinib in recurrent or metastatic epidermal growth factor receptor and/or erbB2 expressing adenoid cystic carcinoma and non adenoid cystic carcinoma malignant tumors of the salivary glands. J Clin Oncol 2007; 25(25): 3978–84.

25. Locati LD, Bossi P, Perrone F, *et al.* Cetuximab in recurrent and/or metastatic salivary gland carcinomas: a phase II study. Oral Oncol 2009; 45(7): 574–8.

26. Hotte SJ, Winquist EW, Lamont E, *et al.* Imatinib mesylate in patients with adenoid cystic cancers of the salivary glands expressing c-kit: a Princess Margaret Hospital phase II consortium study. J Clin Oncol 2005; 23(3): 585–90.

27. Pfeffer MR, Talmi Y, Catane R, Symon Z, Yosepovitch A, Levitt M. A phase II study of imatinib for advanced adenoid cystic carcinoma of head and neck salivary glands. Oral Oncol 2007; 43(1): 33–6.

28. Laurie SA, Ho AL, Fury MG, Sherman E, Pfister DG. Systemic therapy in the management of metastatic or locally recurrent adenoid cystic carcinoma of the salivary glands: a systematic review. Lancet Oncol 2010; 12(8): 815–24.

29. Conley J, Tinsley PP Jr. Treatment and prognosis of mucoepidermoid carcinoma in the pediatric age group. Arch Otolaryngol 1985; 111(5): 322–4.

30. Chong GC, Beahrs OH, Chen ML, Hayles AB. Management of parotid gland tumors in infants and children. Mayo Clin Proc 1975; 50(5): 279–83.

31. Callender DL, Frankenthaler RA, Luna MA, Lee SS, Goepfert H. Salivary gland neoplasms in children. Arch Otolaryngol Head Neck Surg 1992; 118(5): 472–6.

32. Hewitt M, Weiner SL, Simone JV. *Childhood cancer survivorship: improving care and quality of life.* Washington DC: National Academies Press, 2003.

33. Yu MC, Yuan JM. Epidemiology of nasopharyngeal carcinoma. Semin Cancer Biol 2002; 12(6): 421–9.

34. Ma BB, Chan AT. Recent perspectives in the role of chemotherapy in the management of advanced nasopharyngeal carcinoma. Cancer 2005; 103(1): 22–31.

35. Niedobitek G. Epstein–Barr virus infection in the pathogenesis of nasopharyngeal carcinoma. Mol Pathol 2000; 53(5): 248–54.

36. Chan JKC, Pilch BZ, Kuo TT, Wenig BM, Lee AWM. Tumours of the nasopharynx. In: Barnes L, Eveson JW, Reichart P, Sidransky D (eds) *Pathology and Genetics of Head and Neck Tumours*, vol 9, 3rd edn. Lyon: IARC Press, 2005. pp.85–97.

37. Raab-Traub N. Epstein–Barr virus in the pathogenesis of NPC. Semin Cancer Biol 2002; 12(6): 431–41.

38. Lindberg R. Distribution of cervical lymph node metastases from squamous cell carcinoma of the upper respiratory and digestive tracts. Cancer 1972; 29(6): 1446–9.

39. Skinner DW, van Hasselt CA, Tsao SY. Nasopharyngeal carcinoma: modes of presentation. Ann Otol Rhinol Laryngol 1991; 100(7): 544–51.

40. Al-Sarraf M, LeBlanc M, Giri PG, *et al.* Chemoradiotherapy versus radiotherapy in patients with advanced nasopharyngeal cancer: phase III randomized Intergroup study 0099. J Clin Oncol 1998; 16(4): 1310–17.

41. Baujat B, Audry H, Bourhis J, *et al.* Chemotherapy in locally advanced nasopharyngeal carcinoma: an individual patient data meta-analysis of eight randomized trials and 1753 patients. Int J Radiat Oncol Biol Phys 2006; 64(1): 47–56.

42. Zhang L, Zhao C, Ghimire B, *et al.* The role of concurrent chemoradiotherapy in the treatment of locoregionally advanced nasopharyngeal carcinoma among endemic population: a meta-analysis of the phase III randomized trials. BMC Cancer 2010; 10: 558.

43. Agulnik M, Siu LL. State-of-the-art management of nasopharyngeal carcinoma: current and future directions. Br J Cancer 2005; 92(5): 799–806.

44. Rodriguez-Galindo C, Wofford M, Castleberry RP, *et al.* Preradiation chemotherapy with methotrexate, cisplatin, 5-fluorouracil, and leucovorin for pediatric nasopharyngeal carcinoma. Cancer 2005; 103(4): 850–7.

45. Wolden SL, Chen WC, Pfister DG, Kraus DH, Berry SL, Zelefsky MJ. Intensity-modulated radiation therapy (IMRT) for nasopharynx cancer: update of the Memorial Sloan-Kettering experience. Int J Radiat Oncol Biol Phys 2006; 64(1): 57–62.

46. Widesott L, Pierelli A, Fiorino C, *et al.* Intensity-modulated proton therapy versus helical tomotherapy in nasopharynx cancer: planning comparison and NTCP evaluation. Int J Radiat Oncol Biol Phys 2008; 72(2): 589–96.

47. Xiao WW, Huang SM, Han F, *et al.* Local control, survival, and late toxicities of locally advanced nasopharyngeal carcinoma treated by simultaneous modulated accelerated radiotherapy combined with cisplatin concurrent chemotherapy: long-term results of a phase 2 study. Cancer 2011; 117(9): 1874–83.

48. Kam MK, Teo PM, Chau RM, *et al.* Treatment of nasopharyngeal carcinoma with intensity-modulated radiotherapy: the Hong Kong experience. Int J Radiat Oncol Biol Phys 2004; 60(5): 1440–50.

49. Louis CU, Straathof K, Bollard CM, *et al.* Adoptive transfer of EBV-specific T cells results in sustained clinical responses in patients with locoregional nasopharyngeal carcinoma. J Immunother 2010; 33(9): 983–90.

50. Zhang L, Zhao C, Ghimire B, *et al.* The role of concurrent chemoradiotherapy in the treatment of locoregionally advanced nasopharyngeal carcinoma among endemic population: a meta-analysis of the phase III randomized trials. BMC Cancer 2010; 10: 558.

51. Jaffe HL. Giant-cell reparative granuloma, traumatic bone cyst, and fibrous (fibro-osseous) dysplasia of the jawbones. Oral Surg Oral Med Oral Pathol 1953; 6(1): 159–75.

52. Chuong R, Kaban LB, Kozakewich H, Perez-Atayde A. Central giant cell lesions of the jaws: a clinicopathologic study. J Oral Maxillofac Surg 1986; 44(9): 708–13.

53. De Lange J, van den Akker HP, Klip H. Incidence and disease-free survival after surgical therapy of central giant cell granulomas of the jaw in The Netherlands: 1990–1995. Head Neck 2004; 26(9): 792–5.

54. Whitaker SB, Waldron CA. Central giant cell lesions of the jaws. A clinical, radiologic, and histopathologic study. Oral Surg Oral Med Oral Pathol 1993; 75(2): 199–208.

55. De Lange J, van den Akker HP, van den Berg H. Central giant cell granuloma of the jaw: a review of the literature with emphasis on therapy options. Oral Surg Oral Med Oral Pathol Oral Radiol Endod 2007; 104(5): 603–15.

56. Mintz GA, Abrams AM, Carlsen GD, Melrose RJ, Fister HW. Primary malignant giant cell tumor of the mandible. Report of a case and review of the literature. Oral Surg Oral Med Oral Pathol 1981; 51(2): 164–71.

57. Jacoway J, Howell F, Terry B. Central giant cell granuloma: an alternative to surgical therapy. Oral Surg Oral Med Oral Pathol 1988; 66(5): 572.

58. Nogueira RL, Teixeira RC, Cavalcante RB, Ribeiro RA, Rabenhosrt SH. Intralesional injection of triamcinolone hexacetonide as an alternative treatment for central giant-cell granuloma in 21 cases. Int J Oral Maxillofac Surg 2010; 39(12): 1204–10.

59. Harris M. Central giant cell granulomas of the jaws regress with calcitonin therapy. Br J Oral Maxillofac Surg 1993; 31(2): 89–94.

60. Pogrel MA, Regezi JA, Harris ST, Goldring SR. Calcitonin treatment for central giant cell granulomas of the mandible: report of two cases. J Oral Maxillofac Surg 1999; 57(7): 848–53.

61. De Lange J, van den Akker HP, Veldhuijzen van Zanten GO, Engelshove HA, van den Berg H, Klip H. Calcitonin therapy in central giant cell granuloma of the jaw: a randomized double-blind placebo-controlled study. Int J Oral Maxillofac Surg 2006; 35(9): 791–5.

62. Kaban LB, Mulliken JB, Ezekowitz RA, Ebb D, Smith PS, Folkman J. Antiangiogenic therapy of a recurrent giant cell tumor of the mandible with interferon alfa-2a. Pediatrics 1999; 103(6 Pt 1): 1145–9.

63. Kaban LB, Troulis MJ, Wilkinson MS, Ebb D, Dodson TB. Adjuvant antiangiogenic therapy for giant cell tumors of the jaws. J Oral Maxillofac Surg 2007; 65(10): 2018–24; discussion 2024.

64. Busaidy K, Wong M, Herzog C, Flaitz C, Marchena J, Eftekhari F. Alpha interferon in the management of central giant cell granuloma: early experiences. J Oral Maxillofac Surg 2002; 2(5): 86–7.

66 Uncommon Pediatric Tumors of the Thorax

Yoav H. Messinger,[1] Kris Ann P. Schultz,[1] and Louis P. Dehner[2]

[1] Department of Pediatric Hematology/Oncology, Children's Hospitals and Clinics of Minnesota, Minneapolis, MN, USA
[2] Lauren V. Ackerman Department of Surgical Pathology, Barnes-Jewish Hospital; Department of Pathology and Immunology, St Louis Children's Hospital, Washington University Medical Center, St Louis, MO, USA

Introduction

Although common in the adult population, primary pulmonary malignancies in the age group less than 20 years at diagnosis are quite rare.[1,2] The most common malignant pulmonary neoplasms in children are, in fact, metastases from other primary tumors, primarily sarcomas[3] (Fig. 66.1). The purpose of this chapter is to discuss a group of neoplasms of diverse pathological type, which have in common their origin from intrathoracic organs or structures or the chest wall, and have been described in children. Most of these neoplasms are malignant, including lymphomas and neuroblastic tumors, although the clinical behavior is dependent upon the specific tumor type and the pathological stage. Several of the tumor types are diagnosed almost exclusively in children, especially the pleuropulmonary blastoma (PPB), which is the most common primary malignancy of the lung in children.[4]

The epidemiology of primary pulmonary neoplasms in children is not well documented when compared to the established associations of carcinomas and mesotheliomas with environmental factors such as tobacco smoke and asbestos exposure in adults. Children with primary or secondary immunodeficiency syndromes and neurofibromatosis occasionally develop pulmonary or mediastinal neoplasms of hematopoietic and/or sarcomatous nature.[5] Infants with tuberous sclerosis complex develop cardiac rhabdomyoma(s) which is arguably a hamartoma with its capacity for spontaneous regression rather than a neoplasm.[6] A unique syndrome resulting in predisposition to PPBs is recognized and the genetic basis has been elucidated.[7,8] Other than these few associations and relationships, epidemiological factors in children have yet to be elucidated.

Presenting symptoms of an intrathoracic tumor in a child are generally the consequence of the direct mass effect or airway obstruction. In some cases, the mass may have been detected in utero by ultrasonography. Cough, dyspnea, chest pain, fever, superior vena cava syndrome, and pneumothorax are some of the more common clinical manifestations.

A minority of neoplasms are associated with digital clubbing as seen in intrathoracic lymphomas,[9] spinal cord compression with limb weakness or bowel/bladder dysfunction seen in neurogenic or vertebral malignancies,[10] or autoimmune phenomena seen in mediastinal hematolymphoid malignancies or thymic neoplasms.

Because most pulmonary neoplasms present as a mass, the tumor is often initially recognized in a standard chest radiograph in a child with suspected respiratory tract infection or pneumothorax.[11] If the tumor is asymptomatic, the identification of a mass may be entirely incidental, which is the experience in some cases of inflammatory myofibroblastic tumor (IMT).[12] Some metastatic lesions to the lung and PPB may have a combination of cysts in the lung and a pneumothorax. For instance, both primary pleuropulmonary synovial sarcoma and metastatic synovial sarcoma present in the latter fashion.[13] Diffuse reticulonodular infiltrates in the parenchyma with or without mediastinal adenopathy, or a mass(es) in an immunosuppressed child should alert one to the possibility of a hematolymphoid disorder, Epstein–Barr virus (EBV)-associated smooth muscle neoplasm, or an infectious process.[14] A similar presentation is seen in children with Langerhans cell histiocytosis or juvenile xanthogranuloma with lung involvement.

Computed tomography (CT) allows for more exact localization of the lesion(s) and improves the sensitivity for metastatic disease.[15] Magnetic resonance imaging (MRI) provides additional refinements about tissue densities, an opportunity for multiple views, and clear images of the vertebral column and neural foramina. Unfortunately, it is not as satisfactory in identifying intrapulmonary lesions, and may have limited use for diagnosis and follow-up of PPB, for example. Recently, positron emission tomography (PET)/CT scans have provided an additional tool to follow aggressive, highly metabolically active tumors such as the solid PPB or lymphoma. Ultrasonography, fluoroscopy, and angiography can also be of diagnostic value on rare occasions.

Textbook of Uncommon Cancer, Fourth Edition. Edited by Derek Raghavan, Charles D. Blanke, David H. Johnson, Paul L. Moots, Gregory H. Reaman, Peter G. Rose and Mikkael A. Sekeres.
© 2012 John Wiley & Sons, Inc. Published 2012 by John Wiley & Sons, Inc.

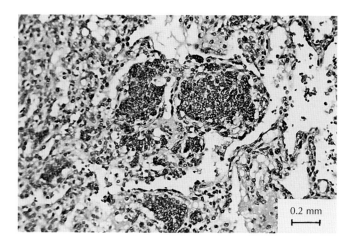

Figure 66.1 Wilm's tumor metastatic to the lung showing nodules of neoplastic blastoma in the interstitium. H&E, ×200.

Histological diagnosis is necessary for nearly all intrathoracic solid tumors, regardless of the presumed site of origin, with the exception of hematolymphoid malignancies diagnosed in the blood or bone marrow. Flexible, fiberoptic bronchoscopy with biopsy is sometimes carried out before definitive surgery. Communication among the various physicians involved in the diagnosis and management is essential for comprehensive preoperative planning.

Since pediatric cancer protocols often require risk assignment according to various morphological and biological characteristics of the neoplasm, it is necessary, if possible, to obtain sufficient diagnostic tissue for complete evaluation. The particular type of biopsy must be weighed in light of potential complications but in most cases an open biopsy is preferred, if not complete resection in the case of a well-circumscribed mass. If a biopsy is performed, sufficient tissue should be obtained for the purposes of an intraoperative frozen section to insure the presence of diagnostic tissue. Some tissue should be set aside for flow cytometry in the case of a suspected hematolymphoid malignancy as well as lesional tissue that was not subjected to the unavoidable artifacts of frozen section.

Mediastinum

The mediastinum is divided into anterior, middle, and posterior compartments, each of which has several specific tumor types associated with it. There are also differences in the frequency and tumor types between children and adults. Overall, 60–65% of mediastinal masses in children are benign (including teratomas, ganglioneuromas, and vascular malformations) and the remainder are malignant (35–40%).[16–20]

Hematolymphoid malignancies, both Hodgkin and non-Hodgkin lymphoma, present in the anterior mediastinum of children, either in the thymus or lymph nodes. Nodular sclerosis Hodgkin, T lymphoblastic and large B cell lymphomas (Fig. 66.2a,b) account for the majority of lymphoid malignancies presenting in the mediastinum of children (75% or more of cases).

Thymic-based tumors other than the lymphoproliferative malignancies are notably uncommon in children.[21] Only 1–2% of mediastinal tumors in children arise from the epithelial

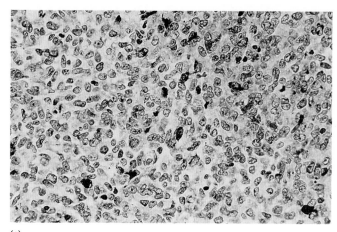

(a)

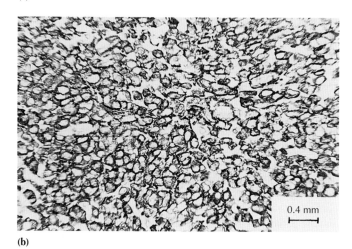

(b)

Figure 66.2 Lymphoblastic lymphoma presenting as an enlarging anterior mediastinal mass in a 16-year-old male. A mediastinal biopsy showing an infiltrate of malignant thymic lymphoblasts with convoluted and nonconvoluted nuclei (a). An immunoperoxidase stain for CD99 or 013, the antibody to the *MIC2* gene product showing a uniform membrane reaction (b). The tumor cells were also immunopositive for CD45RO. H&E, ×400; immunoperoxidase, ×400.

component of the thymus that defines a thymoma (see Chapter 20).[17,21,22] Only 32 cases of thymoma in children were identified in a recent literature review.[23] The median age was 11.5 years with a range from 1 to 16 years. Myasthenia gravis was the most common paraneoplastic syndrome in 13% of cases, followed by immune deficiency and hypoplastic anemia (Good syndrome). Lymphocyte-rich thymomas (types B1 and B2) can be mistaken for a lymphoma since the epithelial cells are relatively inconspicuous in the background whereas epithelial-predominant thymoma (type B3) must be differentiated from thymic carcinoma.[23–25] Like adults, thymoma staging is based on the Masaoka-Koga staging system (Table 66.1). Encapsulation, invasion through the capsule and involvement of surrounding sites (pericardium, pleura) are the pathological findings of prognostic importance (Table 66.1). Flow cytometry in cases of thymoma has a similar pattern to T cell lymphoblastic lymphoma (double positive CD4+ CD8+, CD1a+, TdT+). The only difference is variable surface CD3 (sCD3) expression versus forward scatter of thymocytes from thymoma

Table 66.1 Masaoka–Koga staging system.

Stage	Definition
I	Grossly and microscopically completely encapsulated tumor
IIa	Microscopic transcapsular invasion
IIb	Macroscopic invasion into thymic or surrounding fatty tissue, or grossly adherent to but not breaking through mediastinal pleura or pericardium
III	Macroscopic invasion into neighboring organ (i.e. pericardium, great vessel or lung)
IVa	Pleural or pericardial metastases
IVb	Lymphogenous or hematogenous metastasis

Reproduced with permission from Koga.[32]

compared to a well-defined, coherent single population without variability of CD3 expression in T cell lymphoblastic lymphoma/leukemia.[26] The demonstration of a dispersed population of cytokeratin-positive epithelial cells readily differentiates a lymphocyte-rich thymoma from T cell lymphoblastic lymphomas. Stage of disease and histological type of thymoma are the major determinants of prognosis.[27–31]

The management of a thymoma is not age dependent since the behavior of these tumors is consistent regardless of age. However, there is a suggestion that thymomas in male children 10 years old or less at diagnosis have a poorer outcome than thymomas in females over 10 years of age.[23] Surgical resection should be attempted in those cases with localized disease.[23,33] The prognosis for stage I and II tumors is excellent with near 100% survival.[34] Resectable stage III disease is treated with surgical resection with postoperative radiation; unresectable stage III tumor requires chemotherapy with or without radiation therapy and if possible debulking surgery.[35] Stage IVa thymoma (pleural dissemination) should be treated with surgery when possible and chemotherapy; there is doubt whether radiation is helpful.[35] Stage IVb is treated with chemotherapy. Chemotherapy regimens for thymoma include platinum in various combinations with etoposide, doxorubicin, epirubicine, vincristine, cyclophosphamide, and prednisone.[36]

Recent data on activated pathways in thymic tumors have led to investigation of targeted therapy, with a poor response to epidermal growth factor receptor (EGFR) inhibitors due to the rarity of EGFR mutations and for the same reason to imatinib as KIT mutations are uncommon. The new targeted agents anti-IGF-1R antibody and the CDK inhibitor (PHA-848,125AC) are in clinical trials and may be more promising.[37]

Thymic carcinoma, unlike thymoma, is a neoplasm whose histopathological features are those of a malignant epithelial tumor, often resembling a moderately differentiated squamous cell carcinoma. For every thymic carcinoma in a child, there are 10–15 thymomas in the same age group. In adults they comprise 10–25% of thymic tumors.[27] In contrast to thymic carcinomas, thymomas are organotypic tumors (i.e. their morphology is unique to the thymus and not found in tumors of other organs, and they exhibit functional features of a normal thymus, i.e. the generation of immature T cells by the neoplastic epithelium). Thymic carcinomas are nonorganotypic tumors in that they have similar pathological features to neoplasms in the lung and salivary gland, as two examples. These tumors do not

have the capacity to promote the maturation of intratumorous immature T cells like the thymoma.[38]

There is a correlation between the pathological type of thymic carcinoma and outcome. For instance, thymic squamous cell carcinoma, confined to the thymus, can have a 10-year survival rate up to 65%. Well-differentiated neuroendocrine tumors (typical and atypical carcinoids) of the thymus may have 5-year survival rates of less than 50%.[39] The highly aggressive carcinoma with the t(15;19) involving the fusion gene *BRD4-NUT* and also termed "NUT midline carcinoma" is seen in adolescents and young adults.[40] Histologically, this neoplasm often resembles a poorly differentiated squamous cell carcinoma and has a poor prognosis.[38] Lymphoepithelioma-like carcinoma of the thymus is seen in children and one of our cases in a 14-year-old male was EBER (EBV) positive. These tumors are usually nonresectable, with advanced stage at presentation, and the outcome with surgery and chemotherapy with/without radiation is unfavorable.

There are three reviews of thymic carcinoma in children with a total of 20 cases.[41–43] These tumors usually present in late childhood or early adolescence and have a male predilection.[42,43] Histopathological subtypes in two studies have included lymphoepithelioma-like carcinoma (eight cases), poorly differentiated carcinoma (five cases), small cell (two cases), squamous cell carcinoma (two cases) and carcinoma with neuroendocrine differentiation (one case).[41,43] Paraneoplastic syndromes have been reported in eight (28%) of 29 cases and have included hypertrophic osteopathy, systemic lupus erythematosus, polymyositis, and nephrotic syndrome.[41,43,44] Most thymic carcinomas in children are advanced stage at presentation and with metastatic spread to multiple sites including the lungs, liver, lymph nodes, and bone. Complete resection is possible in only a minority of cases but a biopsy is indicated to exclude a hematolymphoid malignancy.

Chemotherapy with regimens that include cisplatin, doxorubicin, cyclophosphamide and/or other agents was given to almost all with a few exceptions.[41–43] Local radiation therapy has limited value with a poor response in most cases accounting for the 70% death rate. Virtually the only long-term survivors are those patients whose tumor had been completely resected and without evidence of metastasis. This poor outcome may reflect the high proportion of lymphoepithelioma-like carcinomas in children; these tumors have a similarly poor outcome in adults.[45]

There has been recent interest in the evaluation of new targeted agents such as tyrosine kinase inhibitors in the management of thymic carcinoma. Caution regarding the applicability of results in adults with thymic squamous cell carcinoma is warranted since the latter is uncommon in children.[38] Even though EGFR is strongly expressed in 35% of thymic carcinomas, disappointing activity was documented in two clinical phase 2 studies using the EGFR inhibitors erlotinib and gefitinib.[46,47] Interestingly, c-kit (CD117) is highly expressed in most thymic squamous cell and basaloid carcinomas. However, imatinib activity is restricted to those tumors with c-kit mutations which are only found in 5–10% of cases, so this agent has limited potential for activity.[38] The multi-kinase inhibitor sunitinib may be a more attractive agent since it is active in the presence of both mutated and wild-type c-kit; it has shown preliminary activity in four patients with squamous cell (three cases) and undifferentiated thymic carcinomas (one case).[48] Though these data are promising, caution is again appropriate in the application of these results to children in whom these pathological subtypes are less common. It is important to verify that the putative target is expressed in any thymic carcinoma in a child.

Thymolipoma is a benign, generally slow-growing mediastinal mass composed of lobules of mature adipose tissue and thymic tissue consisting of epithelial cells, lymphocytes, and Hassall's bodies and rarely a hemangioma-like pattern.[49] Thymolipoma may be associated with hyperthyroidism or myasthenia gravis. Resection is the treatment of choice.[50] Like thymoma, this tumor is also seen in children.

Thymic cyst presents as either a multilocular structure or as a single cyst which is lined by thymic epithelium and thymocytes. The multilocular thymic cyst in a child is reported in association with HIV-acquired immunodeficiency syndrome. Hodgkin lymphoma, Langerhans cell histiocytosis, germinoma, teratoma, and thymoma may present as a thymic cyst; these neoplasms are often initially identified in the microscopic examination.[51–54]

Germ cell neoplasms (GCN), although uncommon, account for nearly 10–20% of mediastinal masses in children. The mediastinum is the second most common extragonadal site for such neoplasms, exceeded only by the sacrococcygeal region.[55] These tumors occur almost exclusively in the anterior mediastinum, where they comprise almost 25% of all masses in this compartment.[56] Overall, approximately 5–6% of all GCNs in children present in the anterior mediastinum.[56] Most GCNs of the anterior mediastinum (75–80% of cases) are mature teratomas, whose cystic or mixed cystic and solid areas are composed of mature tissues of ectodermal, endodermal, and mesodermal types.[57,58] Unlike GCNs in adults (with the characteristic chromosomal gain of 12q) imbalances in chromosome 1, deletions of 4q and 6q and gains of 20q are the cytogenetic aberrations in these tumors in children.[59] Teratomas in the fetal period may be associated with hydrops fetalis. Takayasu *et al.* described a case of fetal teratoma complicated by hydrops fetalis managed by fetal aspiration of cyst fluid and successful resection after birth.[60]

The remaining GCNs of the mediastinum are malignant as defined by one or more of the following histopathological patterns: germinoma (seminoma), embryonal carcinoma, yolk sac tumor (endodermal sinus tumor), choriocarcinoma, immature teratoma, and nongerminal sarcomas.[58] These neoplasms often have residual teratomatous elements in addition to the malignant components. In females, yolk sac tumor is often the only malignant element, whereas in males, mixed malignant patterns are commonly seen.[61] It is also the fact that malignant GCNs of the mediastinum occur overwhelmingly in males between the ages of 12 and 35 years.[55,62] There is an increased risk for mediastinal GCNs in Klinefelter syndrome.[63,64] Serum α-fetoprotein and/or human chorionic gonadotropin are invariably elevated at diagnosis. Since the mediastinum is a potential site for metastases from a testicular GCN, the possibility of an occult primary tumor in the testis should not be overlooked in the clinical evaluation.[65]

Germinoma (seminoma) is the most common subtype of malignant GCN of the mediastinum; 10% of cases are diagnosed between the ages of 10 and 19 years.[66] These tumors may be cystic and have a prominent lymphocytic component that may resemble Hodgkin lymphoma, thymoma, or diffuse large B cell lymphoma. Complete resection is the treatment of choice and the prognosis correlates with extent of disease. Other malignant patterns include yolk sac tumor (endodermal sinus tumor) and choriocarcinoma.[67,68] Mixed histological patterns of malignant GCNs occur in the mediastinum with combinations of embryonal carcinoma, teratoma (often immature), and yolk sac tumor. Immature teratoma behaves in a malignant fashion when diagnosed in an adolescent or young adult, in contrast to the benign behavior of a similar-appearing tumor in an infant or young child (Fig. 66.3). Nongerminal malignancies in the form of angiosarcoma, rhabdomyosarcoma or granulocytic sarcoma are a rare but well-documented phenomenon in mediastinal GCNs (Fig. 66.4).[69] Some of the hematological malignancies have been demonstrated to arise from germ cells rather than host hematopoietic cells.[70–73]

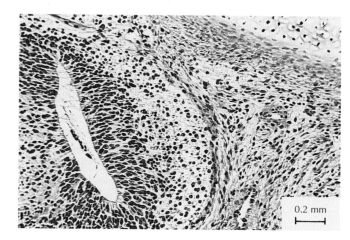

Figure 66.3 Immature teratoma of the anterior mediastinum, showing an embryonic or primitive-appearing neural canal with palisading neuroblast-like cells. Fibrous stroma and cartilage are also present. H&E, ×200.

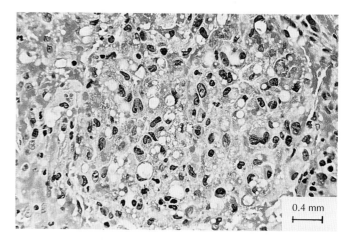

Figure 66.4 Epithelioid angiosarcoma arising in a malignant mixed germ cell neoplasm of the anterior mediastinum in a 15-year-old male. The signet ring-like cells are the malignant endothelial cells. H&E, ×400.

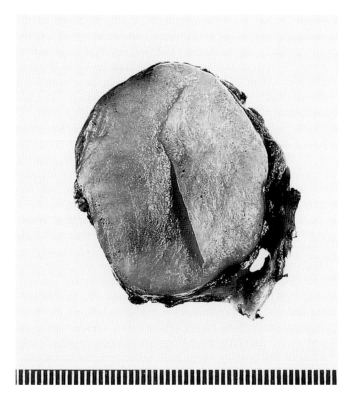

Figure 66.5 Composite ganglioneuroblastoma (nodular stroma-rich ganglioneuroblastoma) of the posterior mediastinum in a 1-year-old female. The circumscribed grayish-tan mass represents the stroma-rich ganglioneuromatous component surrounded by hemorrhagic tissue containing the neuroblasts.

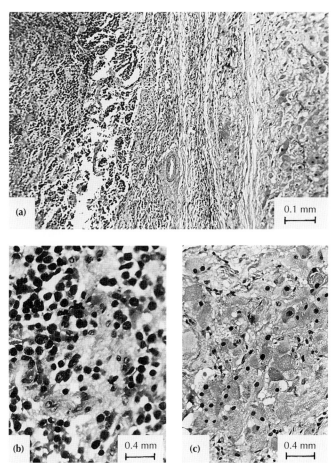

Figure 66.6 Composite ganglioneuroblastoma (nodular stroma-rich ganglioneuroblastoma), showing a sharp plane of fibrous tissue separating the ganglioneuromatous from the neuroblastomatous component (a). Poorly differentiated neuroblastoma (b) and ganglioneuroma (c) are seen at higher magnification. H&E, ×100, ×400, ×400.

Several studies have confirmed poorer outcomes for patients with mediastinal GCNs when compared to their gonadal morphological counterparts. Complete surgical resection and cisplatin-based chemotherapy have yielded the best results in the management of these tumors. If complete resection is feasible, it should be attempted to include a margin of resection with contiguous nonvital structures such as the thymus. When the tumor is unresectable, the diagnosis should be confirmed with a biopsy that may reveal only necrosis or a less than representative sample of the tumor as a whole since these tumors are often heterogeneous. The biopsy may only have mature teratoma. The treatment decision will then require the incorporation of clinical findings and tumor markers. Those children with advanced disease may experience a variable disease-free interval after platinum-based regimens.[61]

In children with initially unresectable tumors, chemotherapy may reduce the tumor volume so that a complete resection becomes more feasible.[61] One study has compared the use of combination chemotherapy including cisplatin, bleomycin, and etoposide to the use of carboplatin, bleomycin, and etoposide; carboplatin-based regimens was not only less toxic but also more effective than the cisplatin-based regimens.[74] The Children's Cancer Group and Pediatric Oncology Group study 8882 evaluated response rate and survival using etoposide and bleomycin with platinum randomized to high or low dose. Mediastinal GCNs were analyzed for clinical and operative findings, and the results emphasized the need for aggressive

surgical resection either before or after chemotherapy.[61] Kesler *et al.* studied the pathological features of postchemotherapy specimens and found that tumor necrosis and teratoma were predictors of survival, and that those with persistent nonteratomatous GCN or sarcomatous degeneration warranted additional surgery.[75] Refractory GCNs may be successfully treated with cycles of paclitaxel and ifosfamide alternating with carboplatin and etoposide with stem cell support.[76] Kesler also studied 431 patients with testicular nonseminomas with lung or mediastinal metastases who were treated with chemotherapy followed by surgical resection. A total of 640 surgical procedures were performed in 431 patients with a survival close to 70% after average follow-up of 5.6 years. These authors suggested that an aggressive postchemotherapy surgical approach to resect any residual teratoma in the lung or mediastinum is reasonable.[77]

Neurogenic neoplasms are those soft tissue tumors that arise from sympathetic-parasympathetic ganglion peripheral nerves. These tumors have a predilection for the posterior mediastinum where 90% or more of cases originate in the chest (Figs 66.5, 66.6). Approximately 25% of all mediastinal masses in children are neurogenic, compared to 15–20% in adults.[20,78,79] In children,

10–25% of all neuroblastic tumors present in the thorax and specifically in the posterior mediastinum.[80] Virtually all neurogenic tumors of the mediastinum in children under 2 years of age are either poorly differentiated neuroblastomas (NB) or intermixed ganglioneuroblastomas (GNB); these neoplasms tend to be low stage (stages I and II, 50–90% of cases) and have favorable histology and biological markers whereas the older children have higher stage disease, a trend comparable to nonthoracic NBs. Into later childhood and adolescence, a neurogenic tumor is more likely to be a ganglioneuroma, schwannoma or neurofibroma. A cautionary note about the ganglioneuroma in children is the presence, usually focally, of intermixed GNB but in most cases, the management and favorable prognosis are unlikely to be altered in a significant manner.

Localized or locoregional ganglioneuroma and intermixed GNB have excellent outcomes with overall survival of 98%, whereas GNB will be treated according to the status of the neuroblastic nodule: stage, favorable versus unfavorable histology, *MYCN* amplification, 11q aberration, and ploidy.[81] Surgical management of neurogenic tumors of the mediastinum in children is influenced by the size of tumor; smaller neurogenic tumors can usually be resected thoracoscopically and larger tumor via thoracotomy.[82] Complete resection is unnecessary to effect a favorable outcome.[83]

Paraganglioma arises from the sympathetic and parasympathetic ganglia; the sympathetic paraganglioma is histogenetically related to the adrenal pheochromocytoma. Approximately 15–20% of the latter two neoplasms present in the first two decades of life. Only 1–2% of all mediastinal masses, regardless of the specific age group, are paragangliomas and most arise in the posterior mediastinum, with a few in the anterior and middle mediastinum. The importance of the paraganglioma in children is the distinct likelihood of its occurrence in the setting of a familial genetic disorder. Some syndromes are manifested by a pheochromocytoma only (MEN 2A and MEN 2B with *RET* mutations, 10q11.2; NFI with *NFI* mutations 17q11.2) or pheochromocytoma and/or paraganglioma (von Hippel–Lindau with mutations, 3p26-p25; Carney triad; Carney–Stratakis syndrome, mutations *SDHB* 1p36.1p35, *SDHD*, 11q23, *SDHC*).[84–86] Paragangliomas arising in the posterior mediastinum, whether in a child or adult, metastasize in 50–70% of cases.[87] Long-term follow-up is usually necessary since metastatic disease can occur long after the initial resection of the primary tumor. If the paraganglioma is functional, paroxysmal hypertension must be anticipated and controlled preoperatively with α-adrenergic and, if necessary, β-adrenergic blockade but serious intraoperative hypertension may still occur.[88] Surgical excision is the treatment of choice.[88,89]

Thymic neuroendocrine tumor (NET) or thymic carcinoid is uncommon in any age group but the incidence is increasing, for reasons that are not entirely clear.[90] A NET arising in the thymus accounts for 2–4% of mediastinal masses without regard to a specific age group but in the first two decades of life, it comprises less than 1% of tumors in this site. There are individual case reports of NETs and examples in children and adolescents in various case series.[91–96] This highly aggressive neoplasm has a propensity to metastasize and can be associated with Cushing syndrome and multiple endocrine neoplasia

(MEN) 1.[97,98] If possible, complete *en bloc* resection of the tumor, usually with the pericardium, pleura and sometimes the great vessels, is the treatment of choice, resulting in improved survival.[90,99] Tumor size and stage (localized, regional, distant), grade and extent of surgical resection have been correlated with survival.[90,100] Chemotherapy and radiotherapy have not been shown to be effective in any age group with a NET.[90,99] However, some benefit from imatinib mesylate has been reported in those thymic NETs with c-kit (CD117) overexpression.[101] The targeted agent sunitinib malate, an oral tyrosine kinase inhibitor, had very limited activity in NETs in a recently reported phase 2 study.[102] However, combined sunitinib and octreotide did significantly decrease the size of a thymic NET in one patient, allowing eventual complete surgical resection.[103] Overall, the outcome for thymic NETs is poor with only 20–25% long-term survival.[90]

The other neurogenic neoplasms are those that arise from the peripheral nerves in the form of neurofibromas and schwannomas; it is important to note that the stroma of a ganglioneuroma has microscopic features resembling both of the latter two neoplasms. Both neurofibromas and schwannomas are found in the paravertebral-paraspinal location, in addition to the lateral and anterior chest wall. Other neoplasms included under the broad rubric of neurogenic tumors with an origin in the mediastinum are melanotic neuroectodermal tumor of infancy, granular cell tumor, myxopapillary ependymoma and malignant peripheral nerve sheath tumor.[104–106]

Soft tissue neoplasms of virtually all types have been diagnosed in the thoracic space and may present as an organ-based tumor in the thymus, lung, heart or in the nonorgan soft tissues. Several examples of *lipoblastoma* have been reported in young children in the anterior mediastinum.[107] *Cystic hygroma*, a lymphatic malformation of infancy, occurs as an isolated mass-like lesion but more often as a diffuse infiltrative process with involvement of the neck and axilla. *Rhabdomyosarcoma*, as a *de novo* neoplasm or less often as a nongerminal sarcoma in a mediastinal teratoma, is the most common primary sarcoma of the mediastinum in children. Another distinctive pathological setting is the solid PPB with its often predominant rhabdomyosarcomatous component. In fact, most rhabdomyosarcoma arising in the thoracic cavity in children less than 5 years of age are probably examples of PPB. Exclusive of that clinicopathological context, most rhabdomyosarcomas in the chest are the embryonal rhabdomyosarcoma subtype. Mediastinal paraspinal rhabdomyosarcoma should be differentiated from neuroblastoma and Ewing sarcoma- primitive neuroectodermal tumor. Complete resection, if possible, is recommended for rhabdomyosarcoma in the thoracic space but preoperative adjuvant therapy may be required before a challenging resection is possible. There is one older report from the Intergroup Rhabdomyosarcoma Study on the results and outcome of 10 children with mediastinal rhabdomyosarcoma (RMS).[108] A later study from the same group evaluated truncal rhabdomyosarcomas, 10 of which were in the paraspinal region, and after chemotherapy and radiation therapy, seven patients were without evidence of disease 3–7 years after diagnosis.[109] Recent reports from the Children's Oncology Group (COG) and the European Cooperative Soft Tissue Sarcoma trial (CWS) group have included thorax and mediastinum in the trunk, and no specific data are available regarding the outcome of primary rhabdomyosarcoma in these sites. A report from the Societé Internationale d'Oncologie Pédiatrique (SIOP) does include eight of 146 (5.5%) primary thoracic metastatic RMS but specific outcome is not included.[110]

Malignant peripheral nerve sheath tumor, another sarcoma presenting in the mediastinum, typically arises in the setting of a child with neurofibromatosis type 1 whose plexiform neurofibroma of the middle or posterior mediastinum has undergone malignant transformation. Ewing sarcoma-primitive neuroectodermal tumor, synovial sarcoma, hemangiopericytoma, malignant rhabdoid tumor, chondrosarcoma, myxoid liposarcoma, alveolar soft part sarcoma, epithelioid sarcoma, solitary fibrous tumor, and angiosarcoma are other tumor types that have been reported in the mediastinum of children.[111–120]

Heart, pericardium, great vessels

Primary neoplasms of the heart, pericardium, and great vessels constitute a rare group of tumors in children and adults with a reported frequency in autopsy of only 0.001–0.03%.[121] These tumors are almost exclusively mesenchymal in derivation, with a few exceptions such as the pericardial teratoma.

Myxoma is the most common primary tumor of the heart in adults, accounting for 80% of all cases, usually in the left atrium and sporadic in occurrence. Less than 8% of all cardiac myxomas present before the age of 20 years.[122] Myxomas on the right side of the heart, on a valve or multifocal in a child should raise the distinct possibility of the Carney complex; this syndrome is present in 7–10% of all cases of cardiac myxomas.[123] Rhabdomyoma and fibroma together represent 60–70% of primary cardiac tumors in children. Rhabdomyomas account for 60–85% of congenital cardiac tumors and at least 50% of all primary tumors of the heart in children.[124] Primary cardiac neoplasms in children are pathologically benign in 85–90% of cases but that does not diminish the fact that these tumors may cause death and even sudden death secondary to a lethal arrhythmia.[125]

Rhabdomyoma of the heart is arguably a hamartoma rather than a true neoplasm. These tumors are often detected prenatally by fetal echocardiography and MRI.[124] The clinical presentation varies from an asymptomatic incidental finding to fetal hydrops, potentially fatal arrhythmias, inflow and/or outflow tract obstruction, cardiac failure, valve dysfunction and systemic or pulmonary embolism.[122,124] The presence of multiple tumors diagnosed by echocardiography (and sometimes MRI) is mostly compatible with rhabdomyoma, in contrast to cardiac fibroma which is usually a solitary mass.[122] It is estimated that 50–80% of cardiac rhabdomyoma are a manifestation of tuberous sclerosis complex (TSC), with mutations of the *TSC1* or *TSC2* gene.[6,124,125] There is rapid growth of rhabdomyoma in the second trimester with stabilization after 32 weeks' gestation. Fetal hydrops, fetal dysrhythmia, and large tumor size ≥20–40 mm are predictive of neonatal morbidity.[6,124] Spontaneous regression is reported in a majority of cases, usually completed before 4 years of age.[122,124,126] Surgical resection may be necessary in some cases when there is obstruction to blood flow or a refractory arrhythmia.[122,127] The clinical outcome is favorable in most cases (80–90%).[6,124] The typical gross presentation is that of multiple lobulated masses arising from the ventricular wall, atrioventricular valves or interventricular septum. These masses are composed of large rounded cells with abundant clear cytoplasm.[128]

Fibroma, like the cardiac rhabdomyoma, often presents in the prenatal or neonatal period and early infancy but is also diagnosed into adolescence.[129] Arrhythmia, heart failure, cyanosis, syncope, chest pain or sudden death are the various clinical presentations but one-third of cases may be asymptomatic.[122] Approximately 3% of patients with the Gorlin–Goltz syndrome, an autosomal dominant disorder, have cardiac fibromas in addition to multiple basal cell carcinoma, odontogenic keratocysts, and skeletal anomalies.[130,131] Unlike the rhabdomyoma, the fibroma is usually a solitary mass which arises in the interventricular septum or as a large intracavitary circumferential mass involving the septum and free wall of the left ventricle (Fig. 66.7). Multiple fibromas of the heart may be found in neonates with congenital generalized

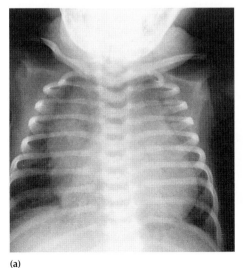

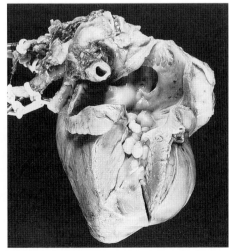

Figure 66.7 Cardiac fibroma in a neonate who presented with tachypnea and cyanosis while feeding. A chest x-ray showed marked cardiomegaly (a). The infant died at 16 days of age. At autopsy, the heart weighed 54 g (normal = 21 ± 5 g) and the left ventricle and cavity had been replaced by a grayish-white myocardial mass (b).

(a)

(b)

myofibromatosis. A uniform proliferation of spindle cells, arranged in broad fascicles, replaces the myocardium. Necrosis and dystrophic calcifications are other microscopic features. The fibroma is thought to be an equivalent neoplasm pathologically to infantile myofibromatosis of the soft tissues. Mass effect on the inflow or outflow tract, or coronary flow may require debulking surgery although the fibroma can remain dormant for years and the potential for spontaneous regression is limited. The fibroma is the most commonly resected heart tumor in children, usually before 1 year of age in 30–35% of cases, and is the second most common tumor found at autopsy in children.[130] If a surgical resection cannot be accomplished, cardiac transplantation may be necessary.[122,124,132]

Inflammatory myofibroblastic tumor (IMT) is also reported in the heart in children of all ages.[133] This tumor arises from the endocardium, including the valve leaflets, or may extend from the lung to the heart.[134] Multifocal tumors are known to occur. Surgical resection or cardiac transplantation is required as the clinical circumstances may dictate. It is generally acknowledged that the IMT is a neoplasm.[135] The calcifying fibrous pseudotumor of the myocardium is probably not related to the IMT.

Histiocytoid or oncocytic cardiomyopathy (cardiac hamartoma), an enigmatic tumefactive lesion(s), presents with potentially life-threatening arrhythmias or sudden death in infants and young children, less than 2 years of age.[136] Multifocal yellowish nodules are present in the subendocardium, myocardium, and even the heart valves. These lesions are composed of pale-staining polygonal cells arranged in cohesive aggregates, often situated beneath the endocardium (Fig. 66.8). The cytoplasm has an eosinophilic to granular appearance. This nonneoplastic disorder affecting cardiac myocytes is now thought to represent a type of mitochondriopathy with point mutations in the mitochondrial cytochrome B gene.[137] Noncompaction of the left ventricular myocardium may be an associated finding. In infants with intractable arrhythmias, treatment includes surgical resection or

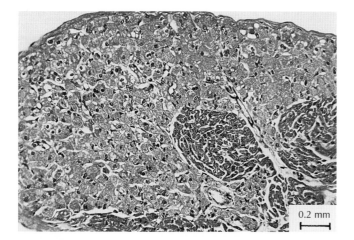

Figure 66.8 Histiocytoid (oncocytic) cardiomyopathy in an infant who died suddenly without an apparent cause of death. Multiple yellowish nodules were present throughout the heart and were composed of uniform polygonal cells resembling granular cells. H&E, ×200.

cryoablation of the multiple small nodules, and survival is about 80%.[130]

Lipoblastoma has been reported in the heart of a child.[138] Hemangiomas may be based in the endocardium or are intramuscular, and in neonates are usually in the right atrium. Most cases are not associated with extracardiac hemangiomas or diffuse neonatal hemangiomatosis.[139]

Primary sarcoma of the heart is exceedingly rare and may have been erroneously reported as sarcoma but is actually an IMT, especially if associated with long-term survival.[130] Various types of sarcomas have been described including undifferentiated sarcoma, angiosarcoma, rhabdomyosarcoma, and osteosarcoma. Most patients are dead within 13 months.[130] A primary alveolar soft part sarcoma of the heart correlated with the presence of the ASPL-TFE3 fusion transcript has been reported in an 11-year-old girl.[140] In another case, we have seen synovial sarcoma of the heart in a 14-year-old boy. Sarcomas of the aorta and pulmonary artery in children are even less common than those arising in the heart.[141,142] These tumors are neoplasms that are often difficult to classify, arising from subintimal fibroblasts.

Teratoma of the pericardium is the most common primary neoplasm in this site in childhood.[142] These tumors usually present in infancy, with cardiorespiratory distress and an enlarged cardiac silhouette, or can be detected prenatally.[143,144] Those tumors with a prenatal and/or perinatal presentation may require prenatal pericardiocentesis or laser ablation of the vascular supply to the mass. The mortality in the perinatal cases exceeds 40%.[143] A glistening cystic mass attached to the adventitia of the aorta with the tumor positioned on the right side of the heart is the gross appearance of the tumor. These multicystic, glistening tumors are composed of mature and occasionally immature teratomatous elements. Immature somatic elements in these tumors do not alter the excellent prognosis with successful surgical resection. Malignant mesothelioma rarely occurs in the pericardium of children.[124]

The single most common category of cardiac neoplasms in the pediatric age group is represented by those malignancies with secondary or metastatic involvement of the heart. Approximately 75% of all cardiac neoplasms in children are examples of leukemic or lymphomatous infiltrates or metastases from various types of bone and soft tissue sarcomas and Wilms tumor.[128,142] Lymphoblastic leukemia-lymphoma seems to have a particular predilection for cardiac involvement.

Lung and airways

The overwhelming majority of pulmonary and airway neoplasms in children are metastatic or secondary tumors, with Hodgkin lymphoma, Wilms tumor, and osteosarcoma as the most common examples.[4] These are parenchymal-based tumors. There are several examples of tumefactive and neoplastic lesions which are based in the airway with symptoms often related to obstruction.

Tracheobronchial papillomas-papillomatosis is an HPV-driven proliferation (HPV-6 and HPV-11) of upper and lower airway mucosa. The infection is typically transmitted vertically from mother to infant through the birth canal. The lesions are initially discovered on the larynx with subsequent contiguous spread to the trachea and bronchi with a conversion of respiratory to squamous mucosa in a minority of cases. Tracheobronchial papillomatosis on the basis of HPV-11 can rarely transform to squamous cell carcinoma.

Tracheal and bronchial tumors presenting as an endophytic mass are restricted principally to a group of epithelial neoplasms arising from the submucosal glands and several types of mesenchymal-stromal tumors.[145,146]

Bronchial carcinoid (low-grade neuroendocrine tumor) is the most common primary airway epithelial malignancy in childhood.[1,2] Approximately 10% of cases are diagnosed in the first two decades of life, between 3 and 19 years of age.[147,148] The obstructing nature of these tumors is manifested by wheezing, treatment-resistant pneumonitis, and atelectasis.[149] Fiberoptic bronchoscopy with biopsy has a high diagnostic yield, but there is a risk of bleeding.[150] Because of the prominent vascular component, endoscopic removal of these lesions can be hazardous and currently is generally not recommended.[145,151] Complete surgical resection is the treatment and current management includes parenchymal sparing procedures (e.g. sublobar and bronchoplastic resections).[150] Of the 25 pediatric cases reported in the literature, five (20%) had local recurrence, with subsequent death in three patients several years after the initial diagnosis.[145,152,153] Choroidal metastases have been described in one case.[153] These subepithelial neoplasms have a firm texture and project into the lumen of the airway. The apparent circumscription from the luminal perspective can be misleading since the tumor often infiltrates around and through the bronchial cartilage and into the adjacent lung parenchyma. Uniform, polygonal tumor cells are arranged in trabecular, insular and ribbon-like profiles. Mitotic activity to any degree separates the typical from the atypical carcinoid; the latter tumor is more clinically aggressive in contrast to more common typical carcinoid. Metaplastic bone is an uncommon feature.

Bronchial carcinoid has been shown to be radioresponsive. Atypical carcinoid (which carries a worse prognosis) responds to combinations of cisplatin and etoposide, and even early-stage atypical carcinoid seems to benefit from postoperative chemoradiotherapy.[154–156] The carcinoid syndrome is rarely encountered with bronchial carcinoids.[157,158]

Mucoepidermoid carcinoma and adenoid cystic carcinoma may present in the trachea, as well as more commonly in the bronchus.[159,160] Like the bronchial carcinoid, the presenting symptoms are those of airway obstruction. These tumors typically arise from the mucous glands in the main stem bronchus or in the proximal or lobar bronchus as an endobronchial polypoid growth that is covered by normal respiratory epithelium. Bronchial lavage and brushing are seldom diagnostic, and forceps biopsy must be performed with the same admonition about bleeding.[145,161,162] It has been suggested that *mucoepidermoid carcinoma* of the bronchus may be as prevalent in children as the bronchial carcinoid.[163] Most mucoepidermoid carcinomas of the bronchus are low-grade neoplasms with an excellent outcome, and even the high-grade tumors do not necessarily behave in an aggressive fashion (Fig. 66.9).[145,153,161,164,165] Though most low-grade mucoepidermoid carcinomas are

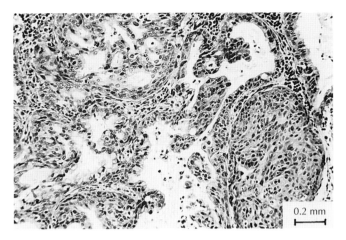

Figure 66.9 Mucoepidermoid carcinoma of the bronchus in a 10-year-old male who presented with wheezing and shortness of breath. Solid nests of low-grade squamous epithelium and glands and cysts lined by well-differentiated mucin epithelium are the features of this low-grade neoplasm. H&E, ×200.

readily identified pathologically, the high-grade tumor may be difficult to distinguish from standard squamous cell carcinomas or NUT-midline carcinoma. Treatment consists of complete resection, with preservation of parenchyma whenever possible. Sleeve resection of the affected segment of bronchus has been performed with success in children and adults alike.[166]

Adenoid cystic carcinoma is the least common of the so-called bronchial adenomas in children.[163,167] This tumor presents as often in the trachea as in the bronchus. Cough and postobstructive pneumonia are the most common clinical manifestations. In adults this tumor may be associated with history of smoking.[168] Complete resection is accomplished more often when this tumor presents in the trachea where infiltration is more limited than in the bronchus. Small cylindroid nests of uniform tumor cells both expand and infiltrate throughout the background and often demonstrate perineural invasion which explains the high rate of local recurrence. This tumor metastases not only to lymph nodes but also to the lungs and rarely liver or brain.[168] Pleomorphic adenoma, malignant myoepithelioma, and acinic cell carcinoma are other rare examples of salivary gland analog tumors in the bronchus.[169]

Sarcomas of the respiratory tree include rhabdomyosarcoma of the larynx[170,171] or bronchus,[172] leiomyosarcoma, and fibrosarcoma.[173–176] The latter two neoplasms with a congenital or neonatal presentation have been collectively designated as *congenital peribronchial myofibroblastic tumor* in the World Health Organization (WHO) classification.[177] These tumors may be associated with nonimmune fetal hydrops. Bronchial fibrosarcomas in children are generally low-grade neoplasms with a favorable outcome after resection.[175,178]

Inflammatory myofibroblastic tumor may present as an obstructing endotracheal or endobronchial mass.[179] This tumor, like its pulmonary counterpart, is a spindle cell proliferation with a background of lymphocytes and plasma cells. The recommended treatment for IMT is complete surgical resection since incomplete resection may be associated with recurrence, as in the case of IMT of the lung.[180] Laser ablation is an excellent alternative treatment in those cases with difficult surgical options.[145] Radiation therapy, immunomodulatory therapy, steroids, and combination of chemotherapeutic agents have been used in recurrent cases.[145] Another possibly related lesion is the *fibrous histiocytoma*, which may have some microscopic features in common with the IMT but is composed of mononuclear cells with occasional giant cells (Fig. 66.10). Although the fibrous histiocytoma is regarded in the pathological sense as a benign tumor, it may recur locally on multiple occasions, just as the IMT does in a minority of cases.[181,182] The differentiation of an endobronchial fibrous histiocytoma from juvenile xanthogranuloma has proven to be problematic in some cases.

Pleuropulmonary blastoma (PPB) is the most common primary malignancy of pulmonary parenchyma in childhood.[4] It is the pulmonary analog of the more familiar dysontogenetic embryonal tumors of childhood such as nephroblastoma

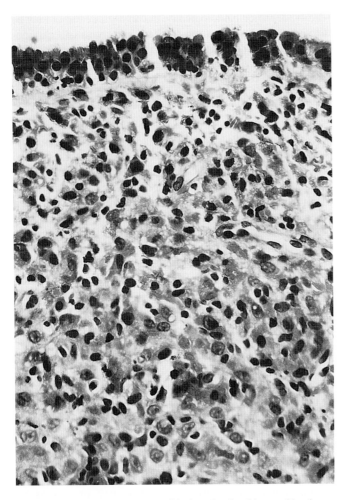

Figure 66.10 Fibrous histiocytoma of the bronchus in a 16-year-old male who presented with shortness of breath. The tumor is composed predominantly of mononuclear cells with some spindle cells in the background. These tumors may be locally aggressive, as in this case, with multiple local recurrences.

(Wilms tumor), neuroblastoma, hepatoblastoma, and others. This tumor is thought to arise from primitive pleuropulmonary mesenchyme which may explain its occurrence in peripheral lung parenchyma as well as the visceral or parietal pleura. From its original description of 11 cases as an entity in 1988, the International PPB Registry (IPPBR) has enrolled more than 340 cases.

Like the other more common early childhood malignancies, PPB is diagnosed in the first 3–5 years of life. During this period, the PPB transforms into a solid high-grade multipatterned sarcoma (type III PPB) from an initial purely cystic lesion (type I PPB) whose clinical and imaging features are often interpreted as a congenital cystic adenomatoid or pulmonary airway malformation (CCAM-CPAM). Pathological progression is recognized by sarcomatous overgrowth with partial obliteration of the epithelial lined cysts (type II) and the emergence of a solid neoplasm (type III), which often fills the entire thoracic cavity and extends into the mediastinum in some cases. The pathological progression through the three types occurs from birth (even prenatally) to approximately age 72 months, at which age 97% of PPBs have been diagnosed (Fig. 66.11). There are critical therapeutic and prognostic implications that correlate with the pathological type. Most PPBs are unifocal in the affected lobe but approximately 12% of cases are multifocal and/or bilateral, cystic lesions with one or two affected adjacent lobes. The median age at diagnosis of the type I PPB is 10 months and for type III 41 months.

An air-filled multilocular peripheral cyst measuring 2 cm or less (the cysts are rarely fluid filled) is the typical appearance of the type I PPB (Fig. 66.12). At the extreme, the cyst may occupy the entire hemithorax. The cyst may be exophytic (on stalks), pleural or replace most or all of a lobe. Multifocal and/ or bilateral cysts should suggest the possibility of type I PPB rather than CCAM-CPAM.[183] At surgery, the multicystic structure is located at the periphery of the lung in the visceral subpleura rather than within the lung parenchyma as in the case of CCAM-CPAM.

A partially solid and cystic lesion is the appearance of type II PPB; the solid component is often appreciated in the imaging studies.[183] Unlike purely cystic PPB, which is often resected in a more limited fashion as a presumed CCAM-CPAM, type II PPB is usually resected as a lobectomy. A solid lobar-based mass is the presentation of type III PPB (Fig. 66.13). Adhesions between the mass and the chest wall and apparent replacement of the entire lung are some of the challenges offered by solid PPB. These tumors are often soft and friable on the basis of extensive hemorrhage and necrosis, which may convey the impression of a cystic mass. Tumor contamination of the thoracic cavity may be present in those cases with gross invasion beyond the lung. An unfavorable operative situation may lend itself to a biopsy only and later surgery after chemotherapy.

The interrelationship of type I PPB to the more complex types II and III PPB was suggested initially in the pathological features with the overlap between type II and the purely cystic type I PPB and the exclusively solid type III PPB

Figure 66.11 Age-type histograms.
(a) Age at presentation of type I PPB. (b) Age at presentation of type II PPB. (c) Age at presentation of type III PPB.
* Type II patients diagnosed at ages 222, 236, and 431 not included in this data.

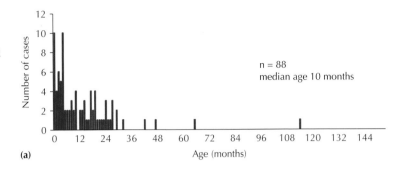

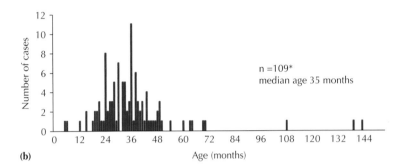

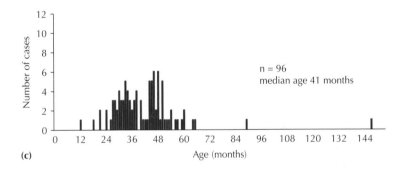

whose histological features overlapped with the solid foci of type II PPB. The delicate cystic structures of type I PPB with its population of primitive small cells with or without rhabdomyoblastic differentiation and nodules of fetal cartilage are the features in common with the residual cystic areas of type II PPB (Fig. 66.14). Obliterations and absence of any cystic foci by a complex sarcoma with embryonal rhabdomyosarcoma, high-grade spindle cell sarcoma, scattered large, bizarre-appearing anaplastic cells, and nodules of sarcomatous cartilage are features of type III PPB. All four basic patterns are not necessarily represented or represented equally in any one type III PPB. Across this morphological spectrum, the median ages at diagnosis for types I, II, and III PPB are 10, 35, and 41 months, respectively (see Fig. 66.11). Later age at diagnosis is correlated with pathological progression and an increasing tendency to metastasize with a decreasing likelihood of cure.

Approximately 27% of PPBs are presently diagnosed as type I lesions. It is uncertain whether every case of PPB begins

as a type I lesion since it is not known what proportions of types II and III PPBs are preceded by a purely cystic lesion. One child is known who had a normal chest CT (done for unrelated reasons) prior to diagnosis of type III PPB 41 months later. Among 228 types II and III PPB cases collected to date, most had no prior radiographic evaluation (chest CT is the most sensitive test). However, there are cases in the literature and in the PPB registry whose clinical course began in infancy with a "history of a congenital lung cyst" diagnosed as a CCAM-CPAM which upon re-review was found to be a cystic PPB; these children later presented with a type II or type III PPB (see Figs 66.12, 66.13).

The recognition of the type I PPB with regressive or involutional microscopic features (type Ir) by Hill and associates has suggested that the fate of all cystic PPBs is not inevitable progression to a type II or type III PPB.[184] These multilocular cysts with the architecture of the type I PPB lack the subepithelial primitive small cell population and have a hyalinized interstitium. Type Ir PPB has been observed primarily in older relatives

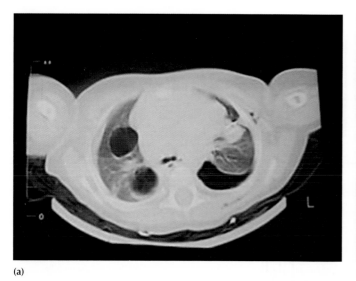
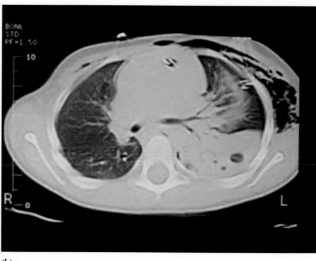

(a)   (b)

Figure 66.12 CT images of type I and type II PPB developing in the same patient 39 months later. (a) Bilateral, multifocal type I PPB with pneumothorax. Cysts were extensively distributed in both lungs. Cysts were resected on two occasions, because of pneumothorax and infection, respectively. (b) Type II PPB in the left lung 39 months after initial type I resection. The patient is alive more than 10 years later.

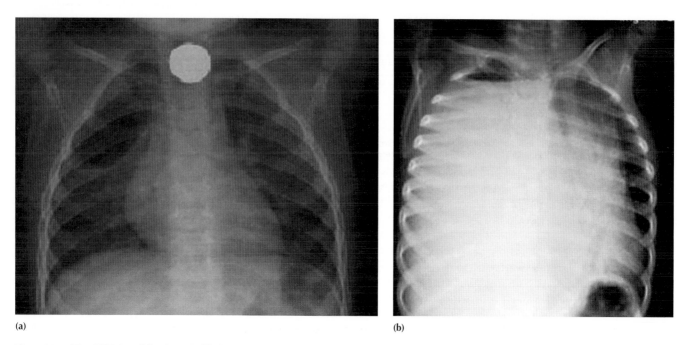

(a)   (b)

Figure 66.13 Type II PPB evolving from air-filled cystic lesion. (a) Chest radiograph obtained because of coin ingestion. Right upper chest cystic lesion not appreciated. (b) The same patient 6 months later with a large cystic/solid tumor with pleural effusion.

of PPB patients and has been discovered during adolescence and into young adulthood. Like type I PPB in the infant, the type Ir lesion may present with a spontaneous pneumothorax. These same regressive features in the type Ir PPB are also observed in type I lesions in infants and may account for the focal present of small primitive cells and rhabdomyoblasts; this feature must be addressed by extensive tissue sampling of these filmy multicystic lesions regardless of the patient's age. Unresected presumed type Ir PPBs in older relatives of PPB patients have minimal potential to progress to a type II or III lesions. Among 91 type I PPBs in the IPPBR, the oldest

age at which type I PPB has been diagnosed is 114 months. Unusually late progression of known cysts is extremely uncommon; one case has been reported of a radiographically documented lung cyst at age 53 months which developed into type II PPB at age 90 months.[185] Asymptomatic lung cysts discovered in a PPB family member after the age of 6 years (after the age at which >95% type II and III are diagnosed) are likely type Ir lesions; though resection may be considered it is not mandatory. The regressed or involved cystic PPB illustrates that the process of pathological progression is not an inevitable event which is a lesson shared with neuroblastoma

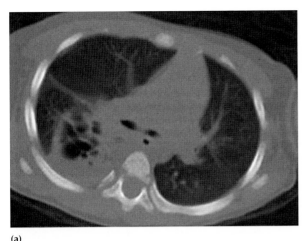
(a)

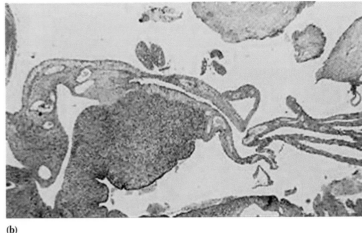
(b)

Figure 66.14 Type II PPB. (a) Axial CT image of solid tumor encroaching upon residual air-filled cystic spaces. Thirty months earlier, a large right lower lobe cyst was apparent on an abdominal flat plate radiograph obtained for abdominal pain (*not shown*). This cyst was not appreciated. (b) Sarcomatous overgrowth of cyst septa (different patient from (a)).

in situ in the adrenal and involuted nephrogenic rests in the kidney.

As noted earlier, approximately 12% of patients may have more than one lesion and the lesions are not necessarily synchronous or coincidental in terms of their pathological features. For instance, a patient with type II or III PPB may have type I and/or a type Ir lesion elsewhere in other lobes of the lung. Type I PPB in one lung has been accompanied by a contralateral type II PPB. There is no understanding of the unsynchronized behavior of cysts.

Most cases of type I PPB are first recognized in the microscopic example of a "congenital lung cyst." If a cystic PPB is suspected, complete cyst resection is recommended; this may involve removal of an exophytic stalk-based cyst complex, "cystectomy" of a large bleb-like pleural surface cyst or lobectomy for cyst(s) which replace most or all of one lobe of a lung. It has been noted that the remaining lung and other unaffected lobes readily expand even when completely atelectatic before resection. A large cyst or tension pneumothorax may compress cysts in surrounding atelectatic lung; therefore, it is recommended to perform an early postoperative CT scan that may reveal residual cysts. If residual contiguous cysts are identified after resection, they should be excised or if not, monitored carefully with follow-up imaging. In some children, cysts may be found in more than one ipsilateral or contralateral lobe, making complete resection impractical; it is recommended that the pathological diagnosis should be based on resection of one or more of the larger cysts.

Complete surgical resection is recommended either primarily or following neoadjuvant chemotherapy for suspected type II and III PPB. Because these neoplasms are often quite large, a preoperative biopsy may be the initial step. However, when primary resection is attempted, the procedure is usually more manageable than predicted based on the radiographic extent of disease. In those cases in which mechanical ventilation has been unable to sustain respiratory adequacy, resection should be attempted. Two to four courses of neoadjuvant chemotherapy may lead to reduction in tumor volume

of 30–90%. Local control with re-resection should be attempted approximately 10–14 weeks after diagnosis because tumors have been demonstrated to recrudesce thereafter. Chemotherapy alone cannot be expected to produce complete disease eradication.

At surgery, the type II or III tumor may appear completely encapsulated (Fig. 66.15) or conversely highly necrotic and friable with a tendency to fragment and rupture, requiring piecemeal removal. The prognostic importance of intrathoracic spillage has not been evaluated rigorously. Typically, type II and III PPBs overtake one or two lobes with sparing of residual lung. Intrathoracic spread may involve direct invasion of pleural surfaces including the mediastinum or more distant pleural studding. Ribs and intercostal muscles are only rarely invaded but invasion of diaphragmatic muscle does occur; focal resection of the diaphragm with fabric graft has been done. Examples of type III PPB arising from the parietal pleura may completely spare the lung. Occasionally, so extensive is the involvement of lung and both pleural surfaces that an extrapleural pneumonectomy is required; in several cases the procedure has been well tolerated and associated with long-term disease-free status. Regional lymph node metastases are uncommon.

To date, no prospective treatment trial for PPB has been done and therefore experience with chemotherapy is largely retrospective. One retrospective study of 38 patients with type I PPB suggested that adjuvant chemotherapy may improve outcome.[186] Among 38 patients, 20 had surgery alone; eight (40%) recurred as type II or III PPBs and five of the eight were dead of tumor. The remaining 18 had a resection and adjuvant chemotherapy; one (5%) of these 18 had a recurrence as a type III PPB and went on to die. Some of the 38 cases occurred before wide recognition of type I PPB and had been considered a CCAM-CPAM at the time; the diagnosis of type I PPB was made retrospectively. Therefore postresection surveillance was limited. The outcome for patients with well-documented type I PPBs who are closely followed for recurrence cannot be predicted from this study. If physicians select adjuvant

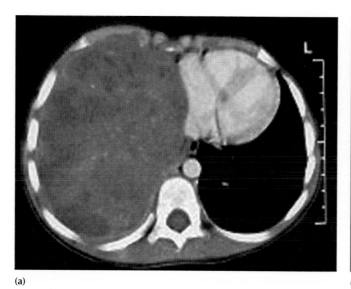
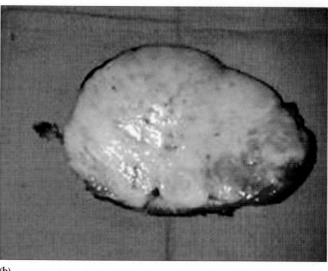

(a)   (b)

Figure 66.15 Type III PPB. (a) Axial chest CT image of large right hemithoracic mass. (b) Cut section of encapsulated solid PPB resected prior to chemotherapy. This child developed bifrontal cerebral metastases 12 months following chest PPB diagnosis. Chest disease did not recur. The child is alive 10 years from chest diagnosis.

chemotherapy for type I PPB, the recommendation of the IPPBR suggests approximately 10 months of vincristine, actinomycin-D, and cyclophosphamide (VAC).

Combined multimodal therapy including surgery and aggressive chemotherapy regimens is necessary in cases of type II and III PPB. Neoadjuvant chemotherapy may be chosen for large neoplasms in order to reduce tumor volume and facilitate surgical resection. Primary resection may be selected in those cases with tumor seemingly localized to a lobe. However, neither approach has been evaluated in a prospective manner for its prognostic effect. In either case, the goal is complete surgical resection in addition to a reduction in the frequency of local recurrence and metastatic spread. It is the impression from the IPPBR experience that long-term disease-free status is attained almost exclusively in those cases treated with the combination of surgery and chemotherapy. In order to achieve this goal, second- and even third-look surgeries should be considered in order to maintain complete resection status based upon the local tumor response as monitored by chest CT scans.

Historically, chemotherapy regimens for types II and III PPBs have typically been based on other childhood sarcoma regimens with a vincristine (V), actinomycin-D (A), and cyclophosphamide (C) regimen (VAC) or VA with ifosfamide (I) (VAI) or four-drug combinations such as doxorubicin (Do) added to VAC (VACDo) or to VAI (VAIDo). IVADo is a four-drug regimen in which the four agents are used together in early courses.[187] Multidrug regimens such as carboplatinum (C), epirubicin (E), VAI, and etoposide (E) (CEVAIE) have been used but are not currently recommended. As noted above, neoadjuvant therapies with tumor volume reductions of 30–90% have demonstrated in a convincing fashion that chemotherapy is active for solid PPB. However, the optimum regimen, its duration and timing vis-à-vis surgical resection have not been the subject of any concerted retrospective or prospective study.

The role of radiation therapy in PPB has not been established in any systematic manner. Several reports suggest that radiation

is effective for PPB but these reports are limited by the fact that the diagnosis of PPB had not been confirmed.[188,189] An earlier report from the IPPBR suggested that radiation therapy is not associated with any improvement in patient survival.[190] In 2011, the IPPBR confirmed this lack of improvement in survival; we have compared the survival in 44 children with PPB receiving radiation as part of the primary treatment with surgery and chemotherapy to 130 patients who were treated with surgery and chemotherapy without radiation therapy. The overall survival was 63% in the former group and 64% in the latter patients ($p = 0.69$, log rank test) (unpublished observation, YHM). It is suggested that the role of radiation therapy is limited to those cases with measurable residual disease after local control by second- or even third-look surgery, for brain metastasis or local recurrence in the chest. Dosage appropriate for high-grade sarcoma (44 Gy or above) by external beam radiation therapy is probably required as suggested in one report.[188] Thoracic recurrences of PPB tend to occur within 36 months of diagnosis. For type I PPB recurring as type II or III after surgery alone, the therapy should be the same as for *de novo* type II or III PPB with an equivalent prognosis. Therapy for recurrence of type II and III PPB is not standardized as yet. Some children have survived after recurrence(s) with multimodal therapy which may include radiation therapy and high-dose chemotherapy with autologous stem cell rescue.

Types II and III PPB can and do metastasize whereas it has not been observed in type I PPB which has not recurred as a type II or III PPB. The most common site for metastasis is the brain with life-table estimates of 11% in the case of type II PPB and 55% in type III PPBs.[191] Most metastasis to the brain occurs within 36 months of imaging detection of the primary tumor and is *independent* of disease status in the chest; 50% of cerebral metastases occur in the absence of detectable disease in the chest. Seizures and symptoms of increased intracranial pressure are the clinical manifestations of brain metastasis. Multiple synchronous and metachronous metastases are known to occur.

Cerebral metastasis has been observed within 6 weeks of normal surveillance brain imaging as an indication of the rapid growth of a metastasis to the brain. Therapy must be prompt; stereotactic radiosurgery followed by focal conformal radiotherapy would be a minimum for therapy although some children have had additional chemotherapy, including stem cell therapy. From among approximately 50 children with cerebral metastasis in the IPPBR, perhaps 10–20% have been cured with satisfactory neurodevelopmental function. Only one case has been observed in which the leptomeninges were the apparent first site of central nervous system metastasis but the cerebrospinal fluid (CSF) cytology was negative. "Drop" metastases along the spinal cord may be a late complication of cerebral disease; CSF cytology may or may not reveal disease even in such late complications of central nervous system disease. Other metastatic sites include intrathoracic "drop" metastasis along pleural surfaces and more rarely liver and bone metastasis. The latter has rarely been identified at the time of initial presentation. Bone marrow metastasis is distinctly unusual and routine surveillance at diagnosis or thereafter is not necessary unless a small biopsy only demonstrates rhabdomyosarcoma, in which case there is some uncertainty whether the particular tumor is a pure rhabdomyosarcoma or not. Lung parenchymal metastasis is rare; one must recognize that PPB is not infrequently multifocal or bilateral when considering this possibility of pulmonary parenchymal metastasis.

The prognosis of PPB is correlated with the pathological type as a reflection of the increasingly aggressive nature of this neoplasm from a purely cystic to a solid. Based on the IPPBR retrospective series of over 300 cases with non-standardized treatment from many institutions, the long-term survival for type I PPB is generally greater than 90% and for types II and III it is in the range of 45–60% (Fig. 66.16).

In approximately one-third of PPB cases, a highly distinctive familial tumor and dysplasia syndrome (OMIM #601200) affects the patient and/or family.[7] Heterozygous germline mutations in *DICER1* underlie this syndrome, as first reported by Hill and associates.[8] A recent report from our group showed that 36 of 68 (53%) children with PPB have heterozygous germline loss-of-function mutations in *DICER1*.[192] *DICER1* is an endoribonuclease producing mature small RNA molecules (miRNA) with critical messenger RNA regulating activity. Penetrance is quite low and the syndrome is highly pleiotropic.

The phenotype of the familial syndrome is not yet fully elucidated but the most frequent manifestations of the syndrome affecting children with PPB or their relatives include cystic nephroma (CN),[193] multinodular hyperplasia of the thyroid[194] and ovarian sex cord stromal cell tumors, especially Sertoli–Leydig cell tumor (SLCT).[194,195] In addition to CN and SLCT, other highly distinctive diseases occurring with PPB and/or *DICER1* mutation are nasal chondromesenchymal hamartoma,[196] ciliary body medulloepithelioma,[197] embryonal rhabdomyosarcoma (ERMS) of uterine cervix,[198,199] and pituitary blastoma.[200,201] Other childhood neoplasms have been seen including Wilms tumor, ERMS of the bladder and medulloblastoma.[202] Single examples of synovial sarcoma and other soft tissue sarcomas, primary cerebral sarcoma, and cerebral medulloepithelioma have been observed. Also single examples of pulmonary sequestration, transposition of the great vessels, and seminoma have been observed in *DICER1* mutation carriers but may be coincidental.[199,202] Pleuropulmonary blastoma, CN, and bladder ERMS are mainly seen in children less than 6 years of age whereas the nasal and ocular tumors are diagnosed by age 10 years. Ovarian tumors have occurred between the ages of 2 and 35 years. Cervical ERMS is concentrated in teenage years.[198] Thyroid disease, which may include differentiated thyroid carcinoma, occurs from ages 5 to 35+ years,

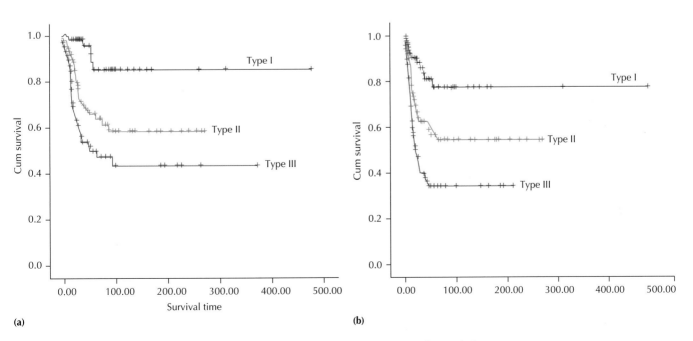

(a)   **(b)**

Figure 66.16 Kaplan–Meier curves types I, II, III. (a) PPB event-free survival. (b) PPB recurrence-free survival.

typically in the teens. There is no apparent increase in any adult-onset neoplasm associated with this syndrome but an ongoing National Cancer Institute study may clarify this further.

Fetal lung interstitial tumor (FLIT) presents as a solid mass prenatally and up to 3 months of age, and may cause fetal hydrops.[203,204] A spongy, lobar-based lesion is composed of irregular airspace-like structures with microcystic features and immature interstitial cells within expanded septa. In contrast to the type I PPB, FLIT is a solid though spongy lesion. A case of FLIT was reported with trisomy 8, suggesting that this lesion is a variant of type I PPB.[205]

Various types of *sarcomas*, presumably as primary neoplasms in the lung, have been reported in children as single case studies in most instances. Rhabdomyosarcoma of the lung parenchyma without a known primary site elsewhere has been seen rarely in children.[108] Other examples of pulmonary rhabdomyosarcoma have been reported in association with CCAM-CPAM but it is generally thought that many if not most of these cases are cystic PPBs.[206,207]

Fibrosarcoma, leiomyosarcoma, malignant fibrous histiocytoma, epithelioid hemangioendothelioma, and synovial sarcoma of the lung are other sarcomas seen in the first two decades of life.[176,178,208–211] Many pulmonary fibrosarcomas present in early childhood and not infrequently in the neonatal period; these tumors together with the so-called congenital leiomyosarcoma are collectively designated as congenital peribronchial myofibroblastic tumors (Fig. 66.17).[177,212] Moran and associates reported their experience with 18 cases of pulmonary leiomyosarcoma; two patients in this series were 5 and 17 years at diagnosis.[213] Both benign and malignant smooth muscle neoplasms have been documented in several visceral sites, including the lung, in children with HIV-AIDS or who have been organ transplant recipients.[214] Epstein–Barr virus has been implicated in the pathogenesis of those smooth muscle neoplasms in the immunosuppressed setting.[14,215,216] High pathological grade is correlated with a poor prognosis. At least nine cases of pulmonary *Kaposi sarcoma* have been reported in immunosuppressed children.[217,218]

Synovial sarcoma is recognized as a primary pleuropulmonary neoplasm.[13] It presents as a pleural-based tumor with symptoms such as chest pain or cough although it can rarely present with pneumothorax. Pathologically, it is a cystic/bullous lesion with only subtle evidence of a malignant spindle cell proliferation with or without an epithelial component. The diagnosis can be confirmed and corroborated by immunohistochemistry (vimentin, cytokeratin, epithelial membrane antigen, CD99, and bcl-2 positive) and the t(X;18)(p11.2;q11.2) translocation by fluorescence *in situ* hybridization (FISH). We have seen examples of cystic synovial sarcomas of the lung in older children and adolescents with the question of cystic PPB. Metastatic synovial sarcoma to the lung is more common than its primary counterpart.

Hemangiopericytoma has been observed rarely; the outcome was fatal in those cases despite surgery and chemotherapy.[219,220] *Malignant fibrous histiocytoma* has been reported in the lung of children.[221,222] *Epithelioid hemangioendothelioma (intravascular bronchioloalveolar tumor)* is a low-grade angiosarcoma which is reported in older children and adolescents as multiple, often bilateral nodules; these tumors in the lung are usually metastases from a primary vascular neoplasm in the liver.[223,224] Both Ewing sarcoma-primitive neuroectodermal tumor and desmoplastic small round cell tumor have been reported in the lung.[225,226]

Bronchogenic carcinoma of the common adult types is extremely rare in children, as noted in the few available epidemiological studies.[227,228] The term bronchogenic carcinoma that has been used to include both small cell and nonsmall cell lung cancers (commonly squamous cell, large cell, and adenocarcinoma) has been replaced in the most recent WHO classification guidelines by each tumor type individually.[229]

Carcinomas in all anatomical sites comprise 2% or less of all malignant neoplasms in children. Hancock and associates, in their review of primary pediatric malignant neoplasms of the lung, reported that approximately 17% of tumors were bronchogenic carcinomas.[2] The three major types, squamous cell carcinoma, adenocarcinoma, and small cell undifferentiated carcinoma, have been described in older children and adolescents.[230–235] The pathological features and natural history of these tumor types are seemingly comparable to the same tumors in adults (Fig. 66.18). Some selected problems that may arise in the pathological diagnosis of these tumors include the differentiation of mucoepidermoid carcinoma and tracheobronchial papillomatosis from squamous cell carcinoma,[236] and avoiding the misinterpretation of a bronchial carcinoid or a lymphoproliferative process as a small cell undifferentiated carcinoma. Adenocarcinoma is proportionately more common in adolescents and young adults than the other major subtypes of bronchogenic carcinoma.[4,237–239] The acinar and bronchioloalveolar carcinomas are documented in later childhood and adolescence. Several examples of bronchioloalveolar carcinoma or atypical goblet cell hyperplasia arising in CCAM-CPAM would suggest more than a coincidental relationship.[240–242]

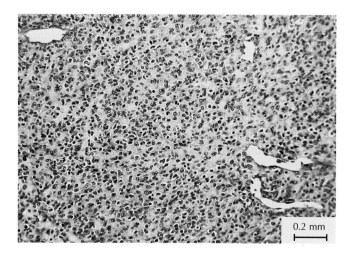

0.2 mm

Figure 66.17 Congenital fibrosarcoma of the lung, showing a cellular neoplasm with focal cleft-like vascular spaces resembling a hemangiopericytoma. Despite the large size, cellularity, and mitotic activity of these neoplasm presenting in the neonatal period, the prognosis is excellent upon successful resection. H&E, ×200.

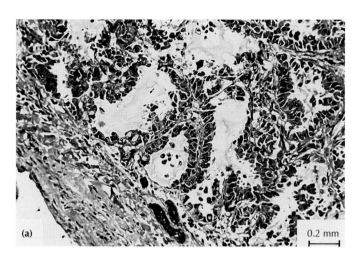

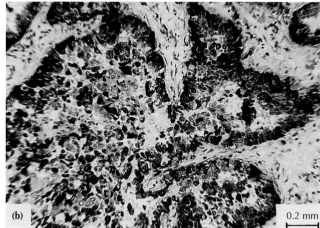

Figure 66.18 Bronchioloalveolar carcinoma in a 15-year-old male who presented with acute respiratory distress and lung infiltrates, who expired before a diagnosis was established. An adenocarcinoma with the characteristic growth of neoplastic columnar cells along airspaces was seen on microscopic examination (a). The tumor cells were strongly immunopositive for carcinoembryonic antigen (b). H&E, ×200; immunoperoxidase, ×200.

A thorough staging with mediastinoscopy should be done in the young patient with a bronchogenic carcinoma, as in an adult with the same tumor. The decision about surgery is predicated on the extent of disease. A consultation with a medical oncologist is appropriate since the therapeutic options are basically the same without regard to age. Several molecular targets, including p53 mutations, EGFR mutations with subsequent dysregulation of the ras/raf kinase pathway and k-ras mutations, have lead to the development of new targeted therapy approaches.[235] Tumors should be resected primarily whenever possible, followed by chemotherapy, irradiation and targeted therapy, usually applied according to the TMN staging and the molecular signature. Primary pulmonary adenocarcinomas were found in young patients with other nonlung pediatric cancers; three out of six whose tumors were tested had common EGFR and *KRAS* mutations, in three they preceded the administration of cytotoxic chemotherapy.[243] Though all eight were alive at a short follow-up,[243] the outcome of advanced adenocarcinoma in children is believed to be very poor.[4,237–239]

Fetal pulmonary adenocarcinoma (pulmonary endodermal tumor resembling fetal lung) is a type of well-differentiated adenocarcinoma whose complex glandular pattern resembles the pseudoglandular stage of lung development.[244] The majority of these tumors present in adults but they are also encountered in late childhood and adolescence.[245,246] Elongated tubular rounded glands with or without papillary enfoldings with minimal interstitium are the principal microscopic features (Fig. 66.19). Solid formations of tumor cells have a morular appearance. The columnar cells have abundant glycogen-rich clear cytoplasm and nuclei with low- to intermediate-grade cytological abnormalities. Lobectomy is the treatment of choice and the prognosis is favorable in the absence of high-grade cytological abnormalities in the epithelial component or a sarcomatous stroma. Koss and associates have proposed a histogenetic relationship between fetal pulmonary adenocarcinoma, PPB, and classic pulmonary blastoma.[247]

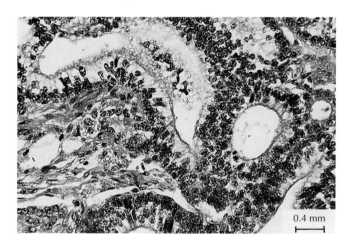

Figure 66.19 Fetal pulmonary adenocarcinoma in a 14-year-old female, showing the characteristic tubular glands lined by stratified columnar cells with clear atypical cytoplasm. H&E, ×400.

Pulmonary blastoma is a malignant neoplasm with a biphasic pattern of primitive-appearing tubuloglandular profiles in a stroma composed of immature cells.[248] Various lines of differentiation have been reported in these tumors, including cartilage and even yolk sac tumor. A review of 63 cases over a 15-year period yielded only three cases in individuals less than 20 years old (16, 17, 19 years old).[249] This tumor occurs almost exclusively in adults which made it a poor candidate as a neoplasm related to the other dysontogenetic tumors of childhood.

Inflammatory myofibroblastic tumor is one of the more common primary neoplasms of lung in children and adolescents, which typically presents as a solitary mass. A minority of children may have symptoms and signs of an inflammatory process, which is mediated by cytokines produced by the tumor. Multifocal tumors in separate sites are known to occur in less than 5% of cases.[250] The neoplastic nature of the IMT has been supported by the observation that a substantial

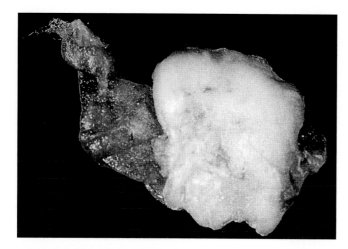

Figure 66.20 Inflammatory myofibroblastic tumor resected from the right lower lobe of a 4-year-old female. A well-circumscribed mass measuring 1.5 cm has a faintly nodular, pale tannish-white surface with small yellowish puncta of calcification. Courtesy of Stanley B. Smith.

proportion of cases have a translocation in the anaplastic lymphoma kinase (ALK) receptor tyrosine kinase locus region at 2p23.[251–253] Dystrophic calcification may or may not be identified in the gross examination of these firm, well-circumscribed tumors with a tan nodular surface (Fig. 66.20). Spindle cells, lymphocytes, plasma cells, and foci of dense fibrosis are the basic microscopic features (Fig. 66.21). The spindle cells have the ultrastructure and immunophenotype of myofibroblasts (Fig. 66.22). A lobectomy is curative in most cases. A minority of IMTs may behave aggressively with extension into the chest wall that may be accompanied by an alteration in the microscopic features to a more overtly sarcomatous appearance with necrosis and anaplasia (Fig. 66.23).[221,254]

Chest wall, diaphragm, and pleura

Primary malignant lesions of the chest wall, diaphragm, and pleura, although uncommon in children, are well documented.[255–257] Pinto and associates have reviewed the topic of pleural tumors in childhood.[12] Thoracic wall lesions in children and thoracic tumors have been reviewed by several authors.[214,258,259] Ewing sarcoma-primitive neuroectodermal tumor (EWS-PNET) is the most common primary malignant tumor of the chest wall.[260] Another similar neoplasm in terms of its pathological features and immunophenotype is the *desmoplastic small round cell tumor* (DSRCT) which has been reported as a pleural-based tumor and in the lung.[261–263] Both the EWS-PNET and DSRCT have translocations involving the *EWS* gene on 22q12 but different fusion partners.[264] These aggressive neoplasms have been treated with resection, radiotherapy, and adjuvant chemotherapy including vincristine, actinomycin-D, cyclophosphamide, doxorubicin, ifosfamide, and etoposide.[260,265,266] Chemotherapy prior to surgery has resulted in improved survival and better local control of EWS-PNET.[265,266] Surgery with wide uninvolved margins provides for the best survival but in the case of an intrathoracic

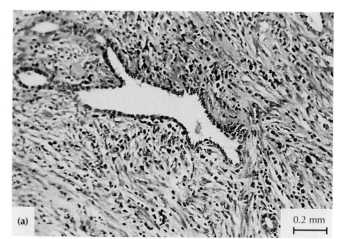

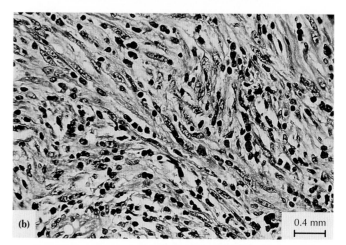

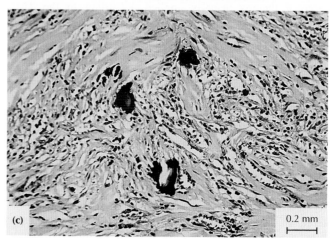

Figure 66.21 Inflammatory myofibroblastic tumor, showing three characteristic microscopic patterns in a tumor resected from the lung of a 4-year-old female. An entrapped airspace surrounded by dense fibroinflammatory tissue (a), spindle cells intermixed with plasma cells and lymphocytes (b), and foci of calcification in a dense hypocellular collagen (c) are the histological features. H&E, ×200, ×400, ×200.

tumor, this can be difficult to achieve in some cases.[266] Event-free survival (EFS) at 5 years is approximately 60% for EWS-PNET which is comparable to the outcome in other primary

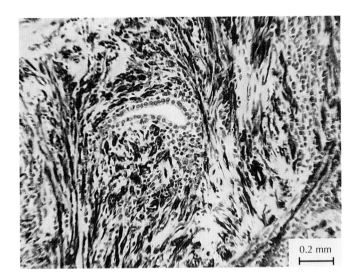

Figure 66.22 Inflammatory myofibroblastic tumor, showing immunoreactivity for smooth muscle actin in the spindle cell component. Immunoperoxidase, ×200.

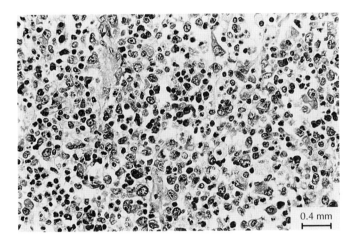

Figure 66.23 Inflammatory myofibroblastic tumor of the lung presenting in a 14-year-old female. In addition to the typical spindle cell pattern in the lung mass, a portion of the tumor had grown into the pleural space and chest wall whose histological appearance was a mixed cellular infiltrate with atypical round cells with the immunophenotype of histiocytes rather than myofibroblasts (see Fig. 66.20). H&E, ×400.

sites.[265] Hemithorax radiation has improved EFS to 63% at 7 years[267] and ifosfamide and etoposide improved the outcome.[265] Those children with metastatic disease at diagnosis have a poor prognosis.[260]

Chest wall *rhabdomyosarcoma* is the second most common primary chest wall malignancy in children.[258,266] Hayes-Jordan *et al.* reviewed the Intergroup Rhabdomyosarcoma Study experience with 130 patients treated on IRS studies I–IV.[268] There was a median age of 9 years at diagnosis (range 0–20 years). Alveolar rhabdomyosarcoma was reported in 37% of cases and almost 40% had group IV disease at diagnosis. Progressive improvement in failure-free survival (FFS) and overall survival (OS) was achieved from IRS study I to IRS study IV. Metastatic disease at diagnosis had a

profoundly deleterious effect on outcome (7% with metastasis, 61% without). The 5-year FFS and OS rates for patients with group I, II, III, and IV disease were not statistically different. Histological subtype (alveolar or undifferentiated versus embryonal or spindle cell) or size had no effect on FFS or OS in nonmetastatic disease. Moreover, complete surgical resection of the tumor either before or after induction chemotherapy did not alter the outcome; most patients with positive microscopic margins received radiation therapy. If the surgeon expresses confidence that negative margins can be obtained "upfront," then primary surgical resection should be attempted; otherwise the recommendation is biopsy only followed by chemotherapy and later surgical resection.[268] The most significant factors resulting in improved outcome over the four sequential studies (IRS-I to IRS-IV) were enhancements in chemotherapy and radiation. No improvement in the treatment of metastatic disease was achieved over the several decades, and the outcome remains extremely poor.[268]

Other rare malignant chest wall or pleural tumors in children include extraskeletal myxoid chondrosarcoma,[269] hemangiopericytoma,[266,270] and malignant mesothelioma.[271] Though thoracic lymphoma usually presents as a mediastinal mass, it can occur on the thoracic wall as an isolated soft tissue mass or by direct mediastinal or parenchymal extension.[258]

References

1. Cohen MC, Kaschula RO. Primary pulmonary tumors in childhood: a review of 31 years' experience and the literature. Pediatr Pulmonol 1992; 14(4): 222–32.
2. Hancock BJ, Di Lorenzo M, Youssef S, Yazbeck S, Marcotte JE, Collin PP. Childhood primary pulmonary neoplasms. J Pediatr Surg 1993; 28(9): 1133–6.
3. Abel RM, Brown J, Moreland B, Parikh D. Pulmonary metastasectomy for pediatric solid tumors. Pediatr Surg Int 2004; 20(8): 630–2.
4. Dishop MK, Kuruvilla S. Primary and metastatic lung tumors in the pediatric population: a review and 25-year experience at a large children's hospital. Arch Pathol Lab Med 2008; 132(7): 1079–103.
5. Balarezo FS, Joshi VV. Proliferative and neoplastic disorders in children with acquired immunodeficiency syndrome. Adv Anat Pathol 2002; 9(6): 360–70.
6. Chao AS, Chao A, Wang TH, et al. Outcome of antenatally diagnosed cardiac rhabdomyoma: case series and a meta-analysis. Ultrasound Obstet Gynecol 2008; 31(3): 289–95.
7. Priest JR, Watterson J, Strong L, et al. Pleuropulmonary blastoma: a marker for familial disease. J Pediatr 1996; 128(2): 220–4.
8. Hill DA, Ivanovich J, Priest JR, et al. DICER1 mutations in familial pleuropulmonary blastoma. Science 2009; 325(5943): 965.
9. Staalman CR, Umans U. Hypertrophic osteoarthropathy in childhood malignancy. Med Pediatr Oncol 1993; 21(9): 676–9.
10. Baten M, Vannucci RC. Intraspinal metastatic disease in childhood cancer. J Pediatr 1977; 90(2): 207–12.
11. Cohen MD. *Imaging of Children with Cancer*. St Louis: Mosby Year Book, 1982.
12. Pinto A, Machin GA, Trevenen CL. Respiratory tract and serosal tumors. In: Parham DR (ed) *Pediatric Neoplasia: Morphology and Biology*. Philadelphia: Lippincott-Raven, 1996. pp. 423–47.
13. Cummings NM, Desai S, Thway K, et al. Cystic primary pulmonary synovial sarcoma presenting as recurrent pneumothorax: report of 4 cases. Am J Surg Pathol 2010; 34(8): 1176–9.

14. Jenson HB, Leach CT, McClain KL, *et al*. Benign and malignant smooth muscle tumors containing Epstein–Barr virus in children with AIDS. Leuk Lymphoma 1997; 27(3–4): 303–14.

15. Rosenfield NS, Keller MS, Markowitz RI, Touloukian R, Seashore J. CT differentiation of benign and malignant lung nodules in children. J Pediatr Surg 1992; 27(4): 459–61.

16. Simpson I, Campbell PE. Mediastinal masses in childhood: a review from a paediatric pathologist's point of view. Prog Pediatr Surg 1991; 27: 92–126.

17. Takeda S, Miyoshi S, Akashi A, *et al*. Clinical spectrum of primary mediastinal tumors: a comparison of adult and pediatric populations at a single Japanese institution. J Surg Oncol 2003; 83(1): 24–30.

18. Tansel T, Onursal E, Dayloglu E, *et al*. Childhood mediastinal masses in infants and children. Turk J Pediatr 2006; 48(1): 8–12.

19. Temes R, Allen N, Chavez T, Crowell R, Key C, Wernly J. Primary mediastinal malignancies in children: report of 22 patients and comparison to 197 adults. Oncologist 2000; 5(3): 179–84.

20. Wright CD. Mediastinal tumors and cysts in the pediatric population. Thorac Surg Clin 2009; 19(1): 47–61, vi.

21. Spigland N, di Lorenzo M, Youssef S, Russo P, Brandt M. Malignant thymoma in children: a 20-year review. J Pediatr Surg 1990; 25(11): 1143–6.

22. Dhall G, Ginsburg HB, Bodenstein L, *et al*. Thymoma in children: report of two cases and review of literature. J Pediatr Hematol Oncol 2004; 26(10): 681–5.

23. Liang X, Lovell MA, Capocelli KE, *et al*. Thymoma in children: report of 2 cases and review of the literature. Pediatr Dev Pathol 2010; 13(3): 202–8.

24. Ocal T, Turken A, Ciftci AO, Senocak ME, Tanyel FC, Buyukpamukcu N. Thymic enlargement in childhood. Turk J Pediatr 2000; 42(4): 298–303.

25. Rice HE, Flake AW, Hori T, Galy A, Verhoogen RH. Massive thymic hyperplasia: characterization of a rare mediastinal mass. J Pediatr Surg 1994; 29(12): 1561–4.

26. Gorczyca W, Tugulea S, Liu Z, Li X, Wong JY, Weisberger J. Flow cytometry in the diagnosis of mediastinal tumors with emphasis on differentiating thymocytes from precursor T-lymphoblastic lymphoma/leukemia. Leuk Lymphoma 2004; 45(3): 529–38.

27. Chalabreysse L, Roy P, Cordier JF, Loire R, Gamondes JP, Thivolet-Bejui F. Correlation of the WHO schema for the classification of thymic epithelial neoplasms with prognosis: a retrospective study of 90 tumors. Am J Surg Pathol 2002; 26(12): 1605–11.

28. Chen G, Marx A, Chen WH, *et al*. New WHO histologic classification predicts prognosis of thymic epithelial tumors: a clinicopathologic study of 200 thymoma cases from China. Cancer 2002; 95(2): 420–9.

29. Myojin M, Choi NC, Wright CD, *et al*. Stage III thymoma: pattern of failure after surgery and postoperative radiotherapy and its implication for future study. Int J Radiat Oncol Biol Phys 2000; 46(4): 927–33.

30. Okumura M, Ohta M, Tateyama H, *et al*. The World Health Organization histologic classification system reflects the oncologic behavior of thymoma: a clinical study of 273 patients. Cancer 2002; 94(3): 624–32.

31. Suster S, Moran CA. Thymoma classification: current status and future trends. Am J Clin Pathol 2006; 125(4): 542–54.

32. Koga K, Matsuno Y, Noguchi M, *et al*. A review of 79 thymomas: modification of staging system and reappraisal of conventional division into invasive and non-invasive thymoma. Pathol Int 1994; 44(5): 359–67.

33. Casey EM, Kiel PJ, Loehrer PJ Sr. Clinical management of thymoma patients. Hematol Oncol Clin North Am 2008; 22(3): 457–73.

34. Detterbeck FC, Parsons AM. Management of stage I and II thymoma. Thorac Surg Clin 2011; 21(1): 59–67, vi–vii.

35. Fujii Y. Published guidelines for management of thymoma. Thorac Surg Clin 2011; 21(1): 125–9, viii.

36. RaA, Giaccone G. Chemotherapy for thymic tumors: induction, consolidation, palliation. Thorac Surg Clin 2011; 21(1): 107–114, viii.

37. Girard N. Targeted therapies for thymic malignancies. Thorac Surg Clin 2011; 21(1): 115–123, viii.

38. Marx A, Rieker R, Toker A, Langer F, Strobel P. Thymic carcinoma: is it a separate entity? From molecular to clinical evidence. Thorac Surg Clin 2011; 21(1): 25–31, v–vi.

39. Cardillo G, Treggiari S, Paul MA, *et al*. Primary neuroendocrine tumours of the thymus: a clinicopathologic and prognostic study in 19 patients. Eur J Cardiothorac Surg 2010; 37(4): 814–18.

40. French CA. Pathogenesis of NUT midline carcinoma. Annu Rev Pathol 2012; 7: 247–65.

41. Carretto E, Inserra A, Ferrari A, *et al*. Epithelial thymic tumours in paediatric age: a report from the TREP project. Orphanet J Rare Dis 2011; 6: 28.

42. Stachowicz-Stencel T, Bien E, Balcerska A, *et al*. Thymic carcinoma in children: a report from the Polish Pediatric Rare Tumors Study. Pediatr Blood Cancer 2010; 54(7): 916–20.

43. Yaris N, Nas Y, Cobanoglu U, Yavuz MN. Thymic carcinoma in children. Pediatr Blood Cancer 2006; 47(2): 224–7.

44. Kilis-Pstrusinska K, Medynska A, Zwolinska D, Dobaczewski G. Lymphoepithelioma-like thymic carcinoma in a 16-year-old boy with nephrotic syndrome – a case report. Pediatr Nephrol 2008; 23(6): 1001–3.

45. Hartmann CA, Roth C, Minck C, Niedobitek G. Thymic carcinoma. Report of five cases and review of the literature. J Cancer Res Clin Oncol 1990; 116(1): 69–82.

46. Christodoulou C, Murray S, Dahabreh J, *et al*. Response of malignant thymoma to erlotinib. Ann Oncol 2008; 19(7): 1361–2.

47. Kurup A, Burns M, Dropcho S, *et al*. Phase II study of gefitinib treatment in advanced thymic malignancies. J Clin Oncol 2005; 23(16S): 7068.

48. Strobel P, Bargou R, Wolff A, *et al*. Sunitinib in metastatic thymic carcinomas: laboratory findings and initial clinical experience. Br J Cancer 2010; 103(2): 196–200.

49. Moran CA, Rosado-de-Christenson M, Suster S. Thymolipoma: clinicopathologic review of 33 cases. Modern Pathol 1995; 8(7): 741–4.

50. Kitano Y, Yokomori K, Ohkura M, Kataoka T, Narita M, Takemura T. Giant thymolipoma in a child. J Pediatr Surg 1993; 28(12): 1622–5.

51. Bouziri A, Khaldi A, Louati H, Menif K, Khayati A, Ben Jaballah N. Respiratory failure revealing a multilocular thymic cyst in an infant. Ann Thorac Surg 2010; 90(1): 305–8.

52. Kontny HU, Sleasman JW, Kingma DW, *et al*. Multilocular thymic cysts in children with human immunodeficiency virus infection: clinical and pathologic aspects. J Pediatr 1997; 131(2): 264–70.

53. Rakheja D, Weinberg AG. Multilocular thymic cyst associated with mature mediastinal teratoma: a report of 2 cases. Arch Pathol Lab Med 2004; 128(2): 227–8.

54. Wakely P Jr, Suster S. Langerhans' cell histiocytosis of the thymus associated with multilocular thymic cyst. Hum Pathol 2000; 31(12): 1532–5.

55. Moran CA, Suster S. Primary germ cell tumors of the mediastinum: I. Analysis of 322 cases with special emphasis on teratomatous lesions and a proposal for histopathologic classification and clinical staging. Cancer 1997; 80(4): 681–90.

56. Mullen B, Richardson JD. Primary anterior mediastinal tumors in children and adults. Ann Thorac Surg 1986; 42(3): 338–45.

57. Dulmet EM, Macchiarini P, Suc B, Verley JM. Germ cell tumors of the mediastinum. A 30-year experience. Cancer 1993; 72(6): 1894–901.

58. Rosado-de-Christenson ML, Templeton PA, Moran CA. From the archives of the AFIP. Mediastinal germ cell tumors: radiologic and pathologic correlation. Radiographics 1992; 12(5): 1013–30.

59. Schneider DT, Schuster AE, Fritsch MK, *et al*. Genetic analysis of childhood germ cell tumors with comparative genomic hybridization. Klin Padiatr 2001; 213(4): 204–11.

60. Takayasu H, Kitano Y, Kuroda T, *et al*. Successful management of a large fetal mediastinal teratoma complicated by hydrops fetalis. J Pediatr Surg 2010; 45(12): e21–4.

61. Billmire D, Vinocur C, Rescorla F, *et al*. Malignant mediastinal germ cell tumors: an Intergroup study. J Pediatr Surg 2001; 36(1): 18–24.

62. Gooneratne S, Keh P, Sreekanth S, Recant W, Talerman A. Anterior mediastinal endodermal sinus (yolk sac) tumor in a female infant. Cancer 1985; 56(6): 1430–3.

63. Nichols CR, Heerema NA, Palmer C, Loehrer PJ Sr, Williams SD, Einhorn LH. Klinefelter's syndrome associated with mediastinal germ cell neoplasms. J Clin Oncol 1987; 5(8): 1290–4.

64. Zon R, Orazi A, Neiman RS, Nichols CR. Benign hematologic neoplasm associated with mediastinal mature teratoma in a patient with Klinefelter's syndrome: a case report. Med Pediatr Oncol 1994; 23(4): 376–9.

65. Dehner LP. Germ cell tumors of the mediastinum. Semin Diagn Pathol 1990; 7(4): 266–84.

66. Moran CA, Suster S, Przygodzki RM, Koss MN. Primary germ cell tumors of the mediastinum: II. Mediastinal seminomas – a clinicopathologic and immunohistochemical study of 120 cases. Cancer 1997; 80(4): 691–8.

67. Moran CA, Suster S. Primary mediastinal choriocarcinomas: a clinicopathologic and immunohistochemical study of eight cases. Am J Surg Pathol 1997; 21(9): 1007–12.

68. Moran CA, Suster S, Koss MN. Primary germ cell tumors of the mediastinum: III. Yolk sac tumor, embryonal carcinoma, choriocarcinoma, and combined nonteratomatous germ cell tumors of the mediastinum – a clinicopathologic and immunohistochemical study of 64 cases. Cancer 1997; 80(4): 699–707.

69. Suster S, Moran CA, Koss MN. Rhabdomyosarcomas of the anterior mediastinum: report of four cases unassociated with germ cell, teratomatous, or thymic carcinomatous components. Hum Pathol 1994; 25(4): 349–56.

70. Chaganti RS, Ladanyi M, Samaniego F, et al. Leukemic differentiation of a mediastinal germ cell tumor. Genes Chromosomes Cancer 1989; 1(1): 83–7.

71. Domingo A, Romagosa V, Callis M, Vivancos P, Guionnet N, Soler J. Mediastinal germ cell tumor and acute megakaryoblastic leukemia. Ann Intern Med 1989; 111(6): 539.

72. Lee KC. Hematopoietic precursor cells within the yolk sac tumor component are the source of secondary hematopoietic malignancies in patients with mediastinal germ cell tumors. Cancer 1994; 73(5): 1535–6.

73. Orazi A, Neiman RS, Ulbright TM, Heerema NA, John K, Nichols CR. Hematopoietic precursor cells within the yolk sac tumor component are the source of secondary hematopoietic malignancies in patients with mediastinal germ cell tumors. Cancer 1993; 71(12): 3873–81.

74. Mann JR, Raafat F, Robinson K, et al. UKCCSG's germ cell tumour (GCT) studies: improving outcome for children with malignant extracranial non-gonadal tumours – carboplatin, etoposide, and bleomycin are effective and less toxic than previous regimens. United Kingdom Children's Cancer Study Group. Med Pediatr Oncol 1998; 30(4): 217–27.

75. Kesler KA, Rieger KM, Ganjoo KN, et al. Primary mediastinal nonseminomatous germ cell tumors: the influence of postchemotherapy pathology on long-term survival after surgery. J Thorac Cardiovasc Surg 1999; 118(4): 692–700.

76. Feldman DR, Sheinfeld J, Bajorin DF, et al. TI-CE high-dose chemotherapy for patients with previously treated germ cell tumors: results and prognostic factor analysis. J Clin Oncol 2010; 28(10): 1706–13.

77. Kesler KA, Kruter LE, Perkins SM, et al. Survival after resection for metastatic testicular nonseminomatous germ cell cancer to the lung or mediastinum. Ann Thorac Surg 2011; 91(4): 1085–93; discussion 1093.

78. King RM, Telander RL, Smithson WA, Banks PM, Han MT. Primary mediastinal tumors in children. J Pediatr Surg 1982; 17(5): 512–20.

79. Macchiarini P, Ostertag H. Uncommon primary mediastinal tumours. Lancet Oncol 2004; 5(2): 107–18.

80. Demir HA, Yalcin B, Buyukpamukcu N, et al. Thoracic neuroblastic tumors in childhood. Pediatr Blood Cancer 2010; 54(7): 885–9.

81. Cohn SL, Pearson AD, London WB, et al. The International Neuroblastoma Risk Group (INRG) classification system: an INRG Task Force report. J Clin Oncol 2009; 27(2): 289–97.

82. Fraga JC, Aydogdu B, Aufieri R, et al. Surgical treatment for pediatric mediastinal neurogenic tumors. Ann Thorac Surg 2010; 90(2): 413–18.

83. De Bernardi B, Gambini C, Haupt R, et al. Retrospective study of childhood ganglioneuroma. J Clin Oncol 2008; 26(10): 1710–16.

84. Almeida MQ, Stratakis CA. Solid tumors associated with multiple endocrine neoplasias. Cancer Genet Cytogenet 2010; 203(1): 30–6.

85. Musil Z, Puchmajerova A, Krepelova A, et al. Paraganglioma in a 13-year-old girl: a novel SDHB gene mutation in the family? Cancer Genet Cytogenet 2010; 197(2): 189–92.

86. Waguespack SG, Rich T, Grubbs E, et al. A current review of the etiology, diagnosis, and treatment of pediatric pheochromocytoma and paraganglioma. J Clin Endocrinol Metab 2010; 95(5): 2023–37.

87. Ayala-Ramirez M, Feng L, Johnson MM, et al. Clinical risk factors for malignancy and overall survival in patients with pheochromocytomas and sympathetic paragangliomas: primary tumor size and primary tumor location as prognostic indicators. J Clin Endocrinol Metab 2011; 96(3): 717–25.

88. Singh J, Rana SS, Sharma R, Ghai B, Puri GD. A rare cause of hypertension in children: intrathoracic pheochromocytoma. Pediatr Surg Int 2008; 24(7): 865–7.

89. Spector JA, Willis DN, Ginsburg HB. Paraganglioma (pheochromocytoma) of the posterior mediastinum: a case report and review of the literature. J Pediatr Surg 2003; 38(7): 1114–16.

90. Gaur P, Leary C, Yao JC. Thymic neuroendocrine tumors: a SEER database analysis of 160 patients. Ann Surg 2010; 251(6): 1117–21.

91. Brown LR, Aughenbaugh GL, Wick MR, Baker BA, Salassa RM. Roentgenologic diagnosis of primary corticotropin-producing carcinoid tumors of the mediastinum. Radiology 1982; 142(1): 143–8.

92. Gartner LA, Voorhess ML. Adrenocorticotropic hormone-producing thymic carcinoid in a teenager. Cancer 1993; 71(1): 106–11.

93. Lin KL, Chen CY, Hsu HH, Kao PF, Huang MJ, Wang HS. Ectopic ACTH syndrome due to thymic carcinoid tumor in a girl. J Pediatr Endocrinol Metab 1999; 12(4): 573–8.

94. McCaughey ES, Walker V, Rolles CJ, Scheurmier NI, Hale AC, Rees LH. Ectopic ACTH production by a thymic carcinoid tumour. Eur J Pediatr 1987; 146(6): 590–1.

95. Salyer WR, Salyer DC, Eggleston JC. Carcinoid tumors of the thymus. Cancer 1976; 37(2): 958–73.

96. Wick MR, Carney JA, Bernatz PE, Brown LR. Primary mediastinal carcinoid tumors. Am J Surg Pathol 1982; 6(3): 195–205.

97. McEvoy MP, Rich BS, New M, Tang LH, La Quaglia MP. Thymic carcinoid presenting with Cushing's syndrome in a 17-year-old boy: a case report and review of the literature. J Clin Oncol 2011; 29(25): e716–18.

98. Teh BT, Zedenius J, Kytola S, et al. Thymic carcinoids in multiple endocrine neoplasia type 1. Ann Surg 1998; 228(1): 99–105.

99. Dusmet ME, McKneally MF. Pulmonary and thymic carcinoid tumors. World J Surg 1996; 20(2): 189–95.

100. Moran CA, Suster S. Neuroendocrine carcinomas (carcinoid tumor) of the thymus. A clinicopathologic analysis of 80 cases. Am J Clin Pathol 2000; 114(1): 100–10.

101. Hamada S, Masago K, Mio T, Hirota S, Mishima M. Good clinical response to imatinib mesylate in atypical thymic carcinoid with KIT overexpression. J Clin Oncol 2011; 29(1): e9–10.

102. Kulke MH, Lenz HJ, Meropol NJ, et al. Activity of sunitinib in patients with advanced neuroendocrine tumors. J Clin Oncol 2008; 26(20): 3403–10.

103. Dham A, Truskinovsky AM, Dudek AZ. Thymic carcinoid responds to neoadjuvant therapy with sunitinib and octreotide: a case report. J Thorac Oncol 2008; 3(1): 94–7.

104. Estrozi B, Queiroga E, Bacchi CE, et al. Myxopapillary ependymoma of the posterior mediastinum. Ann Diagn Pathol 2006; 10(5): 283–7.

105. Kruse-Losler B, Gaertner C, Burger H, Seper L, Joos U, Kleinheinz J. Melanotic neuroectodermal tumor of infancy: systematic review of the literature and presentation of a case. Oral Surg Oral Med Oral Pathol Oral Radiol Endod 2006; 102(2): 204–16.

106. Machida E, Haniuda M, Eguchi T, et al. Granular cell tumor of the mediastinum. Intern Med 2003; 42(2): 178–81.

107. Salem R, Zohd M, Njim L, et al. Lipoblastoma: a rare lesion in the differential diagnosis of childhood mediastinal tumors. J Pediatr Surg 2011; 46(5): e21–3.

108. Crist WM, Raney RB Jr, Newton W, Lawrence W Jr, Tefft M, Foulkes MA. Intrathoracic soft tissue sarcomas in children. Cancer 1982; 50(3): 598–604.

109. Wharam MD, Hanfelt JJ, Tefft MC, et al. Radiation therapy for rhabdomyosarcoma: local failure risk for Clinical Group III patients on

Intergroup Rhabdomyosarcoma Study II. Int J Radiat Oncol Biol Phys 1997; 38(4): 797–804.

110. McDowell HP, Foot AB, Ellershaw C, Machin D, Giraud C, Bergeron C. Outcomes in paediatric metastatic rhabdomyosarcoma: results of the International Society of Paediatric Oncology (SIOP) study MMT-98. Eur J Cancer 2010; 46(9): 1588–95.

111. D'Abrera VS, Burfitt-Williams W. A melanotic neuroectodermal neoplasm of the posterior mediastinum. J Pathol 1973; 111(3): 165–72.

112. Flieder DB, Moran CA, Suster S. Primary alveolar soft-part sarcoma of the mediastinum: a clinicopathological and immunohistochemical study of two cases. Histopathology 1997; 31(5): 469–73.

113. Gross E, Rao BN, Pappo A, et al. Epithelioid sarcoma in children. J Pediatr Surg 1996; 31(12): 1663–65.

114. Khoddami M, Squire J, Zielenska M, Thorner P. Melanotic neuroectodermal tumor of infancy: a molecular genetic study. Pediatr Dev Pathol 1998; 1(4): 295–9.

115. Klimstra DS, Moran CA, Perino G, Koss MN, Rosai J. Liposarcoma of the anterior mediastinum and thymus. A clinicopathologic study of 28 cases. Am J Surg Pathol 1995; 19(7): 782–91.

116. Mack TM. Sarcomas and other malignancies of soft tissue, retroperitoneum, peritoneum, pleura, heart, mediastinum, and spleen. Cancer 1995; 75(1 Suppl): 211–44.

117. Mikkilineni RS, Bhat S, Cheng AW, Prevosti LG. Liposarcoma of the posterior mediastinum in a child. Chest 1994; 106(4): 1288–9.

118. Schmidt D, Harms D, Burdach S. Malignant peripheral neuroectodermal tumours of childhood and adolescence. Virchows Arch A Pathol Anat Histopathol 1985; 406(3): 351–65.

119. Suster S, Moran CA. Malignant cartilaginous tumors of the mediastinum: clinicopathological study of six cases presenting as extraskeletal soft tissue masses. Hum Pathol 1997; 28(5): 588–94.

120. Suster S, Moran CA, Koss MN. Epithelioid hemangioendothelioma of the anterior mediastinum. Clinicopathologic, immunohistochemical, and ultrastructural analysis of 12 cases. Am J Surg Pathol 1994; 18(9): 871–81.

121. Lam KY, Dickens P, Chan AC. Tumors of the heart. A 20-year experience with a review of 12,485 consecutive autopsies. Arch Pathol Lab Med 1993; 117(10): 1027–31.

122. Bruce CJ. Cardiac tumours: diagnosis and management. Heart 2011; 97(2): 151–60.

123. Jain D, Maleszewski JJ, Halushka MK. Benign cardiac tumors and tumorlike conditions. Ann Diagn Pathol 2010; 14(3): 215–30.

124. Yinon Y, Chitayat D, Blaser S, et al. Fetal cardiac tumors: a single-center experience of 40 cases. Prenat Diagn 2010; 30(10): 941–9.

125. Beghetti M, Gow RM, Haney I, Mawson J, Williams WG, Freedom RM. Pediatric primary benign cardiac tumors: a 15-year review. Am Heart J 1997; 134(6): 1107–14.

126. Smythe JF, Dyck JD, Smallhorn JF, Freedom RM. Natural history of cardiac rhabdomyoma in infancy and childhood. Am J Cardiol 1990; 66(17): 1247–9.

127. Takach TJ, Reul GJ, Ott DA, Cooley DA. Primary cardiac tumors in infants and children: immediate and long-term operative results. Ann Thorac Surg 1996; 62(2): 559–64.

128. Burke AP, Virmani R. Cardiac rhabdomyoma: a clinicopathologic study. Modern Pathol 1991; 4(1): 70–4.

129. De Montpreville VT, Serraf A, Aznag H, Nashashibi N, Planche C, Dulmet E. Fibroma and inflammatory myofibroblastic tumor of the heart. Ann Diagn Pathol 2001; 5(6): 335–42.

130. Burke A, Virmani R. Pediatric heart tumors. Cardiovasc Pathol 2008; 17(4): 193–8.

131. Boutet N, Bignon YJ, Drouin-Garraud V, et al. Spectrum of PTCH1 mutations in French patients with Gorlin syndrome. J Invest Dermatol 2003; 121(3): 478–81.

132. Michler RE, Goldstein DJ. Treatment of cardiac tumors by orthotopic cardiac transplantation. Semin Oncol 1997; 24(5): 534–9.

133. Burke A, Li L, Kling E, Kutys R, Virmani R, Miettinen M. Cardiac inflammatory myofibroblastic tumor: a "benign" neoplasm that result in syncope, myocardial infarction, and sudden death. Am J Surg Pathol 2007; 31(7): 1115–22.

134. Corneli G, Alifano M, Forti Parri S, Lacava N, Boaron M. Invasive inflammatory pseudo-tumor involving the lung and the mediastinum. Thorac Cardiovasc Surg 2001; 49(2): 124–6.

135. Miller DV, Tazelaar HD. Cardiovascular pseudoneoplasms. Arch Pathol Lab Med 2010; 134(3): 362–8.

136. Shehata BM, Patterson K, Thomas JE, Scala-Barnett D, Dasu S, Robinson HB. Histiocytoid cardiomyopathy: three new cases and a review of the literature. Pediatr Dev Pathol 1998; 1(1): 56–69.

137. Vallance HD, Jeven G, Wallace DC, Brown MD. A case of sporadic infantile histiocytoid cardiomyopathy caused by the A8344G (MERRF) mitochondrial DNA mutation. Pediatr Cardiol 2004; 25(5): 538–40.

138. Dishop MK, O'Connor WN, Abraham S, Cottrill CM. Primary cardiac lipoblastoma. Pediatr Dev Pathol 2001; 4(3): 276–80.

139. Isaacs H Jr. Fetal and neonatal cardiac tumors. Pediatr Cardiol 2004; 25(3): 252–73.

140. Luo J, Melnick S, Rossi A, Burke RP, Pfeifer JD, Dehner LP. Primary cardiac alveolar soft part sarcoma. A report of the first observed case with molecular diagnostics corroboration. Pediatr Dev Pathol 2008; 11(2): 142–7.

141. Burke AP, Cowan D, Virmani R. Primary sarcomas of the heart. Cancer 1992; 69(2): 387–95.

142. Chan HS, Sonley MJ, Moes CA, Daneman A, Smith CR, Martin DJ. Primary and secondary tumors of childhood involving the heart, pericardium, and great vessels. A report of 75 cases and review of the literature. Cancer 1985; 56(4): 825–36.

143. MacKenzie S, Loken S, Kalia N, et al. Intrapericardial teratoma in the perinatal period. Case report and review of the literature. J Pediatr Surg 2005; 40(12): e13–18.

144. Tollens M, Grab D, Lang D, Hess J, Oberhoffer R. Pericardial teratoma: prenatal diagnosis and course. Fetal Diagn Ther 2003; 18(6): 432–6.

145. Al-Qahtani AR, di Lorenzo M, Yazbeck S. Endobronchial tumors in children: institutional experience and literature review. J Pediatr Surg 2003; 38(5): 733–6.

146. Mathisen DJ. Tracheal tumors. Chest Surg Clin North Am 1996; 6(4): 875–98.

147. Moraes TJ, Langer JC, Forte V, Shayan K, Sweezey N. Pediatric pulmonary carcinoid: a case report and review of the literature. Pediatr Pulmonol 2003; 35(4): 318–22.

148. Wang LT, Wilkins EW Jr, Bode HH. Bronchial carcinoid tumors in pediatric patients. Chest 1993; 103(5): 1426–8.

149. Hulka GF, Rothschild MA, Warner BW, Bove KE. Carcinoid tumor of the trachea in a pediatric patient. Otolaryngol Head Neck Surg 1996; 114(6): 822–5.

150. Machuca TN, Cardoso PF, Camargo SM, et al. Surgical treatment of bronchial carcinoid tumors: a single-center experience. Lung Cancer 2010; 70(2): 158–62.

151. Schreurs AJ, Westermann CJ, van den Bosch JM, Vanderschueren RG, Brutel de la Riviere A, Knaepen PJ. A twenty-five-year follow-up of ninety-three resected typical carcinoid tumors of the lung. J Thorac Cardiovasc Surg 1992; 104(5): 1470–5.

152. Andrassy RJ, Feldtman RW, Stanford W. Bronchial carcinoid tumors in children and adolescents. J Pediatr Surg 1977; 12(4): 513–17.

153. Lack EE, Harris GB, Eraklis AJ, Vawter GF. Primary bronchial tumors in childhood. A clinicopathologic study of six cases. Cancer 1983; 51(3): 492–7.

154. Kaplan B, Stevens CW, Allen P, Liao Z, Komaki R. Outcomes and patterns of failure in bronchial carcinoid tumors. Int J Radiat Oncol Biol Phys 2003; 55(1): 125–31.

155. Musi M, Carbone RG, Bertocchi C, et al. Bronchial carcinoid tumours: a study on clinicopathological features and role of octreotide scintigraphy. Lung Cancer 1998; 22(2): 97–102.

156. Chakravarthy A, Abrams RA. Radiation therapy in the management of patients with malignant carcinoid tumors. Cancer 1995; 75(6): 1386–90.

157. Doppman JL, Nieman L, Miller DL, et al. Ectopic adrenocorticotropic hormone syndrome: localization studies in 28 patients. Radiology 1989; 172(1): 115–24.

158. Davila DG, Dunn WF, Tazelaar HD, Pairolero PC. Bronchial carcinoid tumors. Mayo Clin Proc 1993; 68(8): 795–803.

159. Bellah RD, Mahboubi S, Berdon WE. Malignant endobronchial lesions of adolescence. Pediatr Radiol 1992; 22(8): 563–7.

160. Hause DW, Harvey JC. Endobronchial carcinoid and mucoepidermoid carcinoma in children. J Surg Oncol 1991; 46(4): 270–2.

161. Granata C, Battistini E, Toma P, et al. Mucoepidermoid carcinoma of the bronchus: a case report and review of the literature. Pediatr Pulmonol 1997; 23(3): 226–32.

162. Torres AM, Ryckman FC. Childhood tracheobronchial mucoepidermoid carcinoma: a case report and review of the literature. J Pediatr Surg 1988; 23(4): 367–70.

163. Roby BB, Drehner D, Sidman JD. Pediatric tracheal and endobronchial tumors: an institutional experience. Arch Otolaryngol Head Neck Surg 2011; 137(9): 925–9.

164. Giusti RJ, Flores RM. Mucoepidermoid carcinoma of the bronchus presenting with a negative chest X-ray and normal pulmonary function in two teenagers: two case reports and review of the literature. Pediatr Pulmonol 2004; 37(1): 81–4.

165. Seo IS, Warren J, Mirkin LD, Weisman SJ, Grosfeld JL. Mucoepidermoid carcinoma of the bronchus in a 4-year-old child. A high-grade variant with lymph node metastasis. Cancer 1984; 53(7): 1600–4.

166. Gaissert HA, Mathisen DJ, Grillo HC, Vacanti JP, Wain JC. Tracheobronchial sleeve resection in children and adolescents. J Pediatr Surg 1994; 29(2): 192–7; discussion 197–8.

167. Ahel V, Zubovic I, Rozmanic V. Bronchial adenoid cystic carcinoma with saccular bronchiectasis as a cause of recurrent pneumonia in children. Pediatr Pulmonol 1992; 12(4): 260–2.

168. Molina JR, Aubry MC, Lewis JE, et al. Primary salivary gland-type lung cancer: spectrum of clinical presentation, histopathologic and prognostic factors. Cancer 2007; 110(10): 2253–9.

169. Sabaratnam RM, Anunathan R, Govender D. Acinic cell carcinoma: an unusual cause of bronchial obstruction in a child. Pediatr Dev Pathol 2004; 7(5): 521–6.

170. Diehn KW, Hyams VJ, Harris AE. Rhabdomyosarcoma of the larynx: a case report and review of the literature. Laryngoscope 1984; 94(2 Pt 1): 201–5.

171. Doddo JM, Wieneke KF, Rosman PM. Laryngeal rhabdomyosarcoma. Case report and literature review. Cancer 1987; 59(5): 1012–18.

172. Fallon G, Schiller M, Kilman JW. Primary rhabdomyosarcoma of the bronchus. Ann Thorac Surg 1971; 12(6): 650–4.

173. Lai DS, Lue KH, Su JM, Chang H. Primary bronchopulmonary leiomyosarcoma of the left main bronchus in a child presenting with wheezing and atelectasis of the left lung. Pediatr Pulmonol 2002; 33(4): 318–21.

174. Ferrari A, Collini P, Casanova M, Meazza C, Podda M, Mazza EA. Response to chemotherapy in a child with primary bronchopulmonary leiomyosarcoma. Med Pediatr Oncol 2002; 39(1): 55–7.

175. Garnett JD, Cook CB. Primary bronchopulmonary fibrosarcoma of the trachea in a child. South Med J 1993; 86(11): 1283–5.

176. Kunst PW, Sutedja G, Golding RP, Risse E, Kardos G, Postmus PE. Unusual pulmonary lesions: case 1. A juvenile bronchopulmonary fibrosarcoma. J Clin Oncol 2002; 20(11): 2745–51.

177. Travis WD. Congenital peribronchial myofibroblastic tumour. In: Travis WD, et al. (eds) Pathology and Genetics of the Lung, Pleura, Thymus and Heart. World Health Classification of Tumors. Lyon: IARC Press, 2004. pp.102–3.

178. Pettinato G, Manivel JC, Saldana MJ, Peyser J, Dehner LP. Primary bronchopulmonary fibrosarcoma of childhood and adolescence: reassessment of a low-grade malignancy. Clinicopathologic study of five cases and review of the literature. Hum Pathol 1989; 20(5): 463–71.

179. Dewar AL, Connett GJ. Inflammatory pseudotumor of the trachea in a ten-month-old infant. Pediatr Pulmonol 1997; 23(4): 307–9.

180. Cerfolio RJ, Allen MS, Nascimento AG, et al. Inflammatory pseudotumors of the lung. Ann Thorac Surg 1999; 67(4): 933–6.

181. Sculerati N, Mittal KR, Greco MA, Ambrosino MM. Fibrous histiocytoma of the trachea: management of a rare cause of upper airway obstruction. Int J Pediatr Otorhinolaryngol 1990; 19(3): 295–301.

182. Tagge E, Yunis E, Chopyk J, Wiener E. Obstructing endobronchial fibrous histiocytoma: potential for lung salvage. J Pediatr Surg 1991; 26(9): 1067–9.

183. Priest JR, Williams GM, Hill DA, Dehner LP, Jaffe A. Pulmonary cysts in early childhood and the risk of malignancy. Pediatr Pulmonol 2009; 44(1): 14–30.

184. Hill DA, Jarzembowski JA, Priest JR, Williams G, Schoettler P, Dehner LP. Type I pleuropulmonary blastoma: pathology and biology study of 51 cases from the International Pleuropulmonary Blastoma Registry. Am J Surg Pathol 2008; 32(2): 282–95.

185. Dosios T, Stinios J, Nicolaides P, Spyrakos S, Androulakakis E, Constantopoulos A. Pleuropulmonary blastoma in childhood. A malignant degeneration of pulmonary cysts. Pediatr Surg Int 2004; 20(11–12): 863–5.

186. Priest JR, Hill DA, Williams GM, et al. Type I pleuropulmonary blastoma: a report from the International Pleuropulmonary Blastoma Registry. J Clin Oncol 2006; 24(27): 4492–8.

187. Bisogno G, Ferrari A, Bergeron C, et al. The IVADo regimen – a pilot study with ifosfamide, vincristine, actinomycin D, and doxorubicin in children with metastatic soft tissue sarcoma: a pilot study of behalf of the European Pediatric Soft Tissue Sarcoma Study Group. Cancer 2005; 103(8): 1719–24.

188. Indolfi P, Bisogno G, Casale F, et al. Prognostic factors in pleuropulmonary blastoma. Pediatr Blood Cancer 2007; 48(3): 318–23.

189. Kamenova B, Braverman AS, Axiotis CA, Sohn C, Goff DJ. Complete remission of an unrectable pleuropulmonary blastoma in an adult after radiation therapy. Am J Clin Oncol 2006; 29(6): 641–2.

190. Priest JR, McDermott MB, Bhatia S, Watterson J, Manivel JC, Dehner LP. Pleuropulmonary blastoma: a clinicopathologic study of 50 cases. Cancer 1997; 80(1): 147–61.

191. Priest JR, Magnuson J, Williams GM, et al. Cerebral metastasis and other central nervous system complications of pleuropulmonary blastoma. Pediatr Blood Cancer 2007; 49(3): 266–73.

192. Hill DA, Wang JD, Schoettler P, et al. Germline DICER1 mutations are common in both hereditary and presumed sporadic pleuropulmonary blastoma [Abstract]. Lab Invest 2010; 90: 311.

193. Boman F, Hill DA, Williams GM, et al. Familial association of pleuropulmonary blastoma with cystic nephroma and other renal tumors: a report from the International Pleuropulmonary Blastoma Registry. J Pediatr 2006; 149(6): 850–4.

194. Rio Frio T, Bahubeshi A, Kanellopoulou C, et al. DICER1 mutations in familial multinodular goiter with and without ovarian Sertoli–Leydig cell tumors. JAMA 2011; 305(1): 68–77.

195. Schultz KA, Pacheco MC, Yang J, et al. Ovarian sex cord-stromal tumors, pleuropulmonary blastoma and DICER1 mutations: a report from the International Pleuropulmonary Blastoma Registry. Gynecol Oncol 2011; 122(2): 246–50.

196. Priest JR, Williams GM, Mize WA, Dehner LP, McDermott MB. Nasal chondromesenchymal hamartoma in children with pleuropulmonary blastoma – a report from the International Pleuropulmonary Blastoma Registry Registry. Int J Pediatr Otorhinolaryngol 2010; 74(11): 1240–4.

197. Priest JR, Williams GM, Manera R, et al. Ciliary body medulloepithelioma: four cases associated with pleuropulmonary blastoma – a report from the International Pleuropulmonary Blastoma Registry. Br J Ophthalmol 2011; 95(7): 1001–5.

198. Dehner LP, Hill DA, Jarzembowski J, Williams G, Wikenheiser-Brokamp KA, Messinger Y. Pleuropulmonary blastoma (PPB): a clinicopathologic report of 342 cases from the International PPB Registry (IPPBR). USACP 2012 Annual Meeting, Vancouver.

199. Foulkes WD, Bahubeshi A, Hamel N, et al. Extending the phenotypes associated with DICER1 mutations. Hum Mutat 2011; 32(12): 1381–4.

200. Scheithauer BW, Horvath E, Abel TW, et al. Pituitary blastoma: a unique embryonal tumor. Pituitary 2011; Jul 30 [Epub ahead of print].

201. Wildi-Runge S, Bahubeshi A, Carret AS, et al. New phenotype in the familial DICER1 tumor syndrome: pituitary blastoma presenting at age 9 months [Abstract]. Endocr Rev 2011; 32(03): 1–777.

202. Slade I, Bacchelli C, Davies H, *et al*. DICER1 syndrome: clarifying the diagnosis, clinical features and management implications of a pleiotropic tumour predisposition syndrome. J Med Genet 2011; 48(4): 273–8.

203. Dishop MK, McKay EM, Kreiger PA, *et al*. Fetal lung interstitial tumor (FLIT): a proposed newly recognized lung tumor of infancy to be differentiated from cystic pleuropulmonary blastoma and other developmental pulmonary lesions. Am J Surg Pathol 2010; 34(12): 1762–72.

204. Lazar DA, Cass DL, Dishop MK, *et al*. Fetal lung interstitial tumor: a cause of late gestation fetal hydrops. J Pediatr Surg 2011; 46(6): 1263–6.

205. De Chadarevian JP, Liu J, Pezanowski D, *et al*. Diagnosis of "fetal lung interstitial tumor" requires a FISH negative for trisomies 8 and 2. Am J Surg Pathol 2011; 35(7): 1085; author reply 1086–7.

206. Ozcan C, Celik A, Ural Z, Veral A, Kandiloglu G, Balik E. Primary pulmonary rhabdomyosarcoma arising within cystic adenomatoid malformation: a case report and review of the literature. J Pediatr Surg 2001; 36(7): 1062–5.

207. Pai S, Eng HL, Lee SY, *et al*. Correction: Pleuropulmonary blastoma, not rhabdomyosarcoma in a congenital lung cyst. Pediatr Blood Cancer 2007; 48(3): 370–1.

208. Guccion JG, Rosen SH. Bronchopulmonary leiomyosarcoma and fibrosarcoma. A study of 32 cases and review of the literature. Cancer 1972; 30(3): 836–47.

209. Beluffi G, Bertolotti P, Mietta A, Manara G, Luisetti M. Primary leiomyosarcoma of the lung in a girl. Pediatr Radiol 1986; 16(3): 240–4.

210. Spillane AJ, A'Hern R, Judson IR, Fisher C, Thomas JM. Synovial sarcoma: a clinicopathologic, staging, and prognostic assessment. J Clin Oncol 2000; 18(22): 3794–803.

211. Etienne-Mastroianni B, Falchero L, Chalabreysse L, *et al*. Primary sarcomas of the lung: a clinicopathologic study of 12 cases. Lung Cancer 2002; 38(3): 283–9.

212. McGinnis M, Jacobs G, el-Naggar A, Redline RW. Congenital peribronchial myofibroblastic tumor (so-called "congenital leiomyosarcoma"). A distinct neonatal lung lesion associated with nonimmune hydrops fetalis. Modern Pathol 1993; 6(4): 487–92.

213. Moran CA, Suster S, Abbondanzo SL, Koss MN. Primary leiomyosarcomas of the lung: a clinicopathologic and immunohistochemical study of 18 cases. Modern Pathol 1997; 10(2): 121–8.

214. Van Hoeven KH, Factor SM, Kress Y, Woodruff JM. Visceral myogenic tumors. A manifestation of HIV infection in children. Am J Surg Pathol 1993; 17(11): 1176–81.

215. Cheuk W, Li PC, Chan JK. Epstein–Barr virus-associated smooth muscle tumour: a distinctive mesenchymal tumour of immunocompromised individuals. Pathology 2002; 34(3): 245–9.

216. Monforte-Munoz H, Kapoor N, Saavedra JA. Epstein–Barr virus-associated leiomyomatosis and posttransplant lymphoproliferative disorder in a child with severe combined immunodeficiency: case report and review of the literature. Pediatr Dev Pathol 2003; 6(5): 449–57.

217. Marais BJ, Pienaar J, Gie RP. Kaposi sarcoma with upper airway obstruction and bilateral chylothoraces. Pediatr Infect Dis J 2003; 22(10): 926–8.

218. Theron S, Andronikou S, George R, *et al*. Non-infective pulmonary disease in HIV-positive children. Pediatr Radiol 2009; 39(6): 555–64.

219. Van Damme H, Dekoster G, Creemers E, Hermans G, Limet R. Primary pulmonary hemangiopericytoma: early local recurrence after perioperative rupture of the giant tumor mass (two cases). Surgery 1990; 108(1): 105–9.

220. Daghfous J, Beji M, Kanoun N, Labbene N, Kilani T. [Primary pulmonary hemangiopericytoma in a child]. Rev Mal Respir 1993; 10(1): 46–8.

221. Nistal M, Jimenez-Heffernan JA, Hardisson D, Viguer JM, Bueno J, Garcia-Miguel P. Malignant fibrous histiocytoma of the lung in a child. An unusual neoplasm that can mimic inflammatory pseudotumour. Eur J Pediatr 1997; 156(2): 107–9.

222. Shah SJ, Craver RD, Yu LC. Primary malignant fibrous histiocytoma of the lung in a child: a case report and review of literature. Pediatr Hematol Oncol 1996; 13(6): 531–8.

223. Buggage RR, Soudi N, Olson JL, Busseniers AE. Epithelioid hemangioendothelioma of the lung: pleural effusion cytology, ultrastructure, and brief literature review. Diagn Cytopathol 1995; 13(1): 54–60.

224. Roepke JE, Heifetz SA. Pathological case of the month. Epithelioid hemangioendothelioma (intravascular bronchioloalveolar tumor) of the lung. Arch Pediatr Adolesc Med 1997; 151(3): 317–19.

225. Morton RL, Eid NS, Coventry S, Raj A. Clinicopathologic conference: a large pulmonary cavitary lesion in a 2-year-old boy. J Pediatr 2004; 144(1): 107–11.

226. Syed S, Haque AK, Hawkins HK, Sorensen PH, Cowan DF. Desmoplastic small round cell tumor of the lung. Arch Pathol Lab Med 2002; 126(10): 1226–8.

227. Al-Sheyyab M, Muir KR, Cameron AH, *et al*. Malignant epithelial tumours in children: incidence and aetiology. Med Pediatr Oncol 1993; 21(6): 421–8.

228. Stiller CA. International variations in the incidence of childhood carcinomas. Cancer Epidemiol Biomarkers Prev 1994; 3(4): 305–10.

229. Travis WD, *et al*. (eds). *Pathology and Genetics of Tumours of the Lung, Pleura, Thymus and Heart*. Lyon: IARC Press, 2004.

230. Asamura H, Nakayama H, Kondo H, *et al*. AFP-producing squamous cell carcinoma of the lung in an adolescent. Jpn J Clin Oncol 1996; 26(2): 103–6.

231. Curcio LD, Cohen JS, Grannis FW Jr, Paz IB, Chilcote R, Weiss LM. Primary lymphoepithelioma-like carcinoma of the lung in a child. Report of an Epstein–Barr virus-related neoplasm. Chest 1997; 111(1): 250–1.

232. Kojima R, Mizuguchi M, Bessho F, *et al*. Pulmonary carcinoma associated with hamartoma in an 11-year-old boy. Am J Pediatr Hematol Oncol 1993; 15(4): 439–42.

233. Icard P, Regnard JF, de Napoli S, Rojas-Miranda A, Dartevelle P, Levasseur P. Primary lung cancer in young patients: a study of 82 surgically treated patients. Ann Thorac Surg 1992; 54(1): 99–103.

234. Kim HS, Lee JJ, Cho AR, Kim DH, Choi CW. Squamous cell carcinoma of the lung in an autistic child who has never smoked. J Pediatr Hematol Oncol 2011; 33(5): e216–19.

235. Ackert U, Haffner D, Classen CF. Non-small cell lung carcinoma in an adolescent manifested by acute paraplegia due to spinal metastases: a case report. J Med Case Rep 2011; 5(1): 486.

236. Zawadzka-Glos L, Jakubowska A, Chmielik M, Bielicka A, Brzewski M. Lower airway papillomatosis in children. Int J Pediatr Otorhinolaryngol 2003; 67(10): 1117–21.

237. Hartman GE, Shochat SJ. Primary pulmonary neoplasms of childhood: a review. Ann Thorac Surg 1983; 36(1): 108–19.

238. Lal DR, Clark I, Shalkow J, *et al*. Primary epithelial lung malignancies in the pediatric population. Pediatr Blood Cancer 2005; 45(5): 683–6.

239. Yu DC, Grabowski MJ, Kozakewich HP, *et al*. Primary lung tumors in children and adolescents: a 90-year experience. J Pediatr Surg 2010; 45(6): 1090–5.

240. Granata C, Gambini C, Balducci T, *et al*. Bronchioloalveolar carcinoma arising in congenital cystic adenomatoid malformation in a child: a case report and review on malignancies originating in congenital cystic adenomatoid malformation. Pediatr Pulmonol 1998; 25(1): 62–6.

241. MacSweeney F, Papagiannopoulos K, Goldstraw P, Sheppard MN, Corrin B, Nicholson AG. An assessment of the expanded classification of congenital cystic adenomatoid malformations and their relationship to malignant transformation. Am J Surg Pathol 2003; 27(8): 1139–46.

242. Stacher E, Ullmann R, Halbwedl I, *et al*. Atypical goblet cell hyperplasia in congenital cystic adenomatoid malformation as a possible preneoplasia for pulmonary adenocarcinoma in childhood: a genetic analysis. Hum Pathol 2004; 35(5): 565–70.

243. Kayton ML, He M, Zakowski MF, *et al*. Primary lung adenocarcinomas in children and adolescents treated for pediatric malignancies. J Thorac Oncol 2010; 5(11): 1764–71.

244. Nakatani Y, Kitamura H, Inayama Y, *et al*. Pulmonary adenocarcinomas of the fetal lung type: a clinicopathologic study indicating differences in histology, epidemiology, and natural history of low-grade and high-grade forms. Am J Surg Pathol 1998; 22(4): 399–411.

245. Singh SP, Besner GE, Schauer GM. Pulmonary endodermal tumor resembling fetal lung: report of a case in a 14-year-old girl. Pediatr Pathol Lab Med 1997; 17(6): 951–8.

246. DiFurio MJ, Auerbach A, Kaplan KJ. Well-differentiated fetal adenocarcinoma: rare tumor in the pediatric population. Pediatr Dev Pathol 2003; 6(6): 564–7.

247. Koss MN, Hochholzer L, O'Leary T. Pulmonary blastomas. Cancer 1991; 67(9): 2368–81.

248. Weissferdt A, Moran CA. Malignant biphasic tumors of the lungs. Adv Anat Pathol 2011; 18(3): 179–89.

249. Van Loo S, Boeykens E, Stappaerts I, Rutsaert R. Classic biphasic pulmonary blastoma: a case report and review of the literature. Lung Cancer 2011; 73(2): 127–32.

250. Crespo C, Navarro M, Gonzalez I, Lorente MF, Gonzalez R, Mayol MJ. Intracranial and mediastinal inflammatory myofibroblastic tumour. Pediatr Radiol 2001; 31(8): 600–2.

251. Chun YS, Wang L, Nascimento AG, Moir CR, Rodeberg DA. Pediatric inflammatory myofibroblastic tumor: anaplastic lymphoma kinase (ALK) expression and prognosis. Pediatr Blood Cancer 2005; 45(6): 796–801.

252. Debelenko LV, Arthur DC, Pack SD, Helman LJ, Schrump DS, Tsokos M. Identification of CARS-ALK fusion in primary and metastatic lesions of an inflammatory myofibroblastic tumor. Lab Invest 2003; 83(9): 1255–65.

253. Dehner LP. Inflammatory myofibroblastic tumor: the continued definition of one type of so-called inflammatory pseudotumor. Am J Surg Pathol 2004; 28(12): 1652–4.

254. Morotti RA, Legman MD, Kerkar N, Pawel BR, Sanger WG, Coffin CM. Pediatric inflammatory myofibroblastic tumor with late metastasis to the lung: case report and review of the literature. Pediatr Dev Pathol 2005; 8(2): 224–9.

255. Saenz NC, Ghavimi F, Gerald W, Gollamudi S, LaQuaglia MP. Chest wall rhabdomyosarcoma. Cancer 1997; 80(8): 1513–17.

256. Raney RB Jr, Ragab AH, Ruymann FB, et al. Soft-tissue sarcoma of the trunk in childhood. Results of the intergroup rhabdomyosarcoma study. Cancer 1982; 49(12): 2612–16.

257. Gonzalez-Crussi F, Wolfson SL, Misugi K, Nakajima T. Peripheral neuroectodermal tumors of the chest wall in childhood. Cancer 1984; 54(11): 2519–27.

258. Garcia-Pena P, Barber I. Pathology of the thoracic wall: congenital and acquired. Pediatr Radiol 2010; 40(6): 859–68.

259. Wong KS, Hung IJ, Wang CR, Lien R. Thoracic wall lesions in children. Pediatr Pulmonol 2004; 37(3): 257–63.

260. Shamberger RC, Tarbell NJ, Perez-Atayde AR, Grier HE. Malignant small round cell tumor (Ewing's-PNET) of the chest wall in children. J Pediatr Surg 1994; 29(2): 179–84; discussion 184–5.

261. Ostoros G, Orosz Z, Kovacs G, Soltesz I. Desmoplastic small round cell tumour of the pleura: a case report with unusual follow-up. Lung Cancer 2002; 36(3): 333–6.

262. Parkash V, Gerald WL, Parma A, Miettinen M, Rosai J. Desmoplastic small round cell tumor of the pleura. Am J Surg Pathol 1995; 19(6): 659–65.

263. Muramatsu T, Shimamura M, Furuichi M, Nishii T, Takeshita S, Shiono M. Desmoplastic small round cell tumor of the lung. Ann Thorac Surg 2010; 90(6): e86–7.

264. Romeo S, dei Tos AP. Soft tissue tumors associated with EWSR1 translocation. Virchows Arch 2010; 456(2): 219–34.

265. Shamberger RC, La Quaglia MP, Krailo MD, et al. Ewing sarcoma of the rib: results of an Intergroup study with analysis of outcome by timing of resection. J Thorac Cardiovasc Surg 2000; 119(6): 1154–61.

266. Van Den Berg H, van Rijn RR, Merks JH. Management of tumors of the chest wall in childhood: a review. J Pediatr Hematol Oncol 2008; 30(3): 214–21.

267. Schuck A, Ahrens S, Konarzewska A, et al. Hemithorax irradiation for Ewing tumors of the chest wall. Int J Radiat Oncol Biol Phys 2002; 54(3): 830–8.

268. Hayes–Jordan A, Stoner JA, Anderson JR, et al. The impact of surgical excision in chest wall rhabdomyosarcoma: a report from the Children's Oncology Group. J Pediatr Surg 2008; 43(5): 831–6.

269. Hachitanda Y, Tsuneyoshi M, Daimaru Y, et al. Extraskeletal myxoid chondrosarcoma in young children. Cancer 1988; 61(12): 2521–6.

270. Raafat F, Cameron AH, Mann JR, Stevens MC, Spooner D. Recurrent hemangiopericytoma of the chest wall: report of a case in a 5-year-old boy. Pediatr Pathol 1994; 14(1): 19–25.

271. Vanneuville G, Escande G, Dechelotte P, et al. Malignant pleural tumor in a child mimicking a mesothelioma. Eur J Pediatr Surg 1993; 3(6): 362–5.

67 Uncommon Adrenal Tumors in Children and Adolescents

Raul C. Ribeiro,[1,3] **Carlos Rodriguez-Galindo,**[4] **Emilia M. Pinto,**[2,3] **Gerard P. Zambetti,**[2] **and Bonald C. Figueiredo**[5]

[1] Department of Oncology, [2] Department of Biochemistry, [3] International Outreach Program, St Jude Children's Research Hospital, Memphis, TN, USA
[4] Department of Pediatric Oncology, Dana-Farber Cancer Institute; Harvard Medical School, Boston, MA, USA
[5] Pelé Pequeno Príncipe Research Institute, Faculdades Pequeno Príncipe, Curitiba, PR, Brazil

Adrenocortical tumors

Introduction

The first case of childhood adrenocortical tumor (ACT) was reported in 1865.[1] Cushing described the classic features of hypercortisolism in 1912 but the role of adrenal tumors in this syndrome was not well understood until 1934.[2]

Childhood ACT has peculiar clinical and biological features unlike those observed in other pediatric carcinomas. The incidence of most childhood carcinomas increases with age, whereas 65% of ACTs occur in children younger than 5 years.[3,4] In fact, this age distribution resembles that of tumors of embryonic origin. In this chapter, we summarize the clinical and biological characteristics of and treatment outcome in children with ACTs.

Epidemiology

Only about 0.2% of all cases of childhood malignancies are ACTs. The frequency of ACT is 0.4 per million during the first 4 years of life, and it decreases to 0.1 per million during the subsequent 10 years. It then rises to 0.2 per million during the late teen years and reaches another peak during the fourth decade of life. This pattern is consistent with the concept that pediatric ACTs comprise at least two distinct disease groups. From the United States Surveillance, Epidemiology, and End Results (SEER) program data, it is estimated that there are 19–20 new cases of adrenocortical carcinoma per year in the United States in children and adolescents.[5] The estimates do not include cases of adrenocortical carcinoma that are misdiagnosed as adenomas and therefore are not reported. If it is assumed that one-third of all ACTs are adenomas, 25–30 cases of ACTs are estimated to occur annually in patients under the age of 20 in the United States. The incidence of ACT differs worldwide across geographic regions. The incidence per million in children less than 14 years of age ranges from 0.1 in Hong Kong and Mumbai to 0.4 in Los Angeles to 3.4 in southern Brazil.[5–9]

There is overwhelming evidence of a clustering of pediatric ACT in southern Brazil, with 375 cases reported over a 39-year span[10,11] (Table 67.1). In the United States, in contrast, only 79 cases have been reported to the SEER program in about 30 years.[5] Similarly, a report from Eurocare that included population-based cancer registries of 20 European countries (1983–1994) revealed that only 65 of 25,457 cases of pediatric solid malignancy (0.26%) were ACTs.[7] Moreover, there is compelling evidence that the germline *TP53* R337H mutation explains the high incidence of pediatric adrenocortical carcinoma in southern Brazil and is involved in its tumorigenesis.[12,13] First, constitutional *TP53* mutations, in general, increase the predisposition to pediatric ACT.[14] Second, laboratory findings that strongly implicate the *TP53* R337H substitution in adrenal tumorigenesis include the loss of heterozygosity (LOH) with retention of the mutant allele in tumor cells, the accumulation of the R337H protein in the nucleus,[12] and the folding and other properties of the missense R337H protein *in vitro*.[13] The penetrance of ACT has been estimated at about 10% in a large cohort of carriers of the *TP53* R337H from families known to have children with ACT.[15] Other genetic changes found with variable frequency in children with the *TP53* R337H and ACT, including amplification of the 9q34 chromosomal region (detected in eight of nine tumor samples from children with ACT in Curitiba, Brazil),[16] an increased copy number of the steroidogenic factor 1 (*SF-1*) gene in eight of the cases with 9q34 amplification,[17] germline missense mutation in the inhibin α-subunit gene,[18] and other yet to be determined factors, may contribute to adrenal cell transformation.[19,20]

Pathogenesis

The adrenal cortex arises from the coelomic mesoderm during approximately the fourth to sixth weeks of development.

Table 67.1 Comparison of cases of ACTs registered in select hospitals in the Brazilian states of São Paulo, Paraná, and Bahia versus cases in the United States and Europe.

Institution	State	Period	Number of patients	Age (years)	*TP53* R337H tested/positive (%)
HCACC[11]	São Paulo	1978–2003	56	<21	NA
SCSP[11]	São Paulo	1985–2004	17	<14	NA
CIDB[31]	São Paulo	1980–2004	78	<18	20/20 (100)
IC[11]	São Paulo	1977–2002	46	<13	NA
HCFMSP[11]	São Paulo	1982–2003	27	<16	21/27 (78)
HCC[10]	Paraná	1966–2003	124	<13	61/65 (93.8)
HCFMRP[32]	São Paulo	1985–2003	21	<12	12/16 (75)
ONCO/HSR[33]	Bahia	1981–2004	6	<12	0/5 (0)
SEER[5]	USA	1973–2007	79	<20	NA
Eurocare[7]	Europe	1983–1994	65	<15	NA

CIDB, Centro Infantil Domingos Boldrini, Universidade de Campinas; HCACC, Hospital do Cancer AC Camargo; HCC, Hospital de Clínicas de Curitiba, Universidade Federal do Paraná; HCFMRP, Hospital das Clínicas da Faculdade de Medicina de Ribeirão Preto; HCFMSP, Hospital das Clínicas da Faculdade de Medicina da Universidade de São Paulo; IC, Instituto da Criança da Universidade de São Paulo; ONCO/HSR, Sociedade de Oncologia da Bahia Ltda/Hospital São Rafael; SCSP, Santa Casa de São Paulo; SEER, Surveillance Epidemiology and End Results; NA, not available. Modified from Pianovski *et al.*[34] with permission from John Wiley & Sons, Inc.

Table 67.2 Constitutional genetic abnormalities associated with adrenocortical tumors (ACT).

Condition	Tumor types	Observations
Li–Fraumeni syndrome and other germline *TP53* mutations	Adenomas, carcinomas	4% of all tumors in Li–Fraumeni syndrome are pediatric ACT
Beckwith–Wiedemann syndrome	Adenomas, carcinomas	ACT is the second most common tumor (approx. 15% of children with this syndrome have ACT)
Hemihypertrophy	Adenomas, carcinomas	20% of these tumors are ACT
Congenital adrenal hyperplasia	Adenoma, carcinoma (very rare)	Testicular tumors of heterotopic adrenal cortical tissue
Carney complex	Primary pigmented nodular adrenocortical disease (PPNAD)	PPNAD occurs in approx. 25% of patients; common in children
Multiple endocrine neoplasia type I	Nodules, adenomas, carcinomas	Median age of patients with carcinomas is 40 years

Modified from Ribeiro and Figueiredo[35] with permission from Elsevier.

These mesothelial cells proliferate between the dorsal mesentery and the developing gonad, delineating two histologically distinct components: an outer zone from which the "adult cortex" originates and a more central zone called the *fetal cortex*. The latter is the largest portion of the adrenal cortex at birth. It begins to undergo apoptosis by the last intrauterine month and disappears toward the end of the first year of life.[21,22] The fetal cortex is responsible for 90% of the mother's production of dehydroepiandrosterone (DHEA) and its sulfated derivative (DHEA-S).[23]

Predisposing constitutional genetic factors have been found in the majority of children and adolescents with ACT (Table 67.2). Li and Fraumeni observed a remarkably high frequency of ACT (four cases, or 10%) among 44 malignancies in children from families in which diverse cancers segregated in an autosomal-dominant pattern.[24,25] In addition to childhood sarcoma and premenopausal breast cancer, members of these families were at increased risk for other malignancies, including leukemia, brain tumors, osteosarcomas, and adrenocortical carcinomas.[26] Other possible tumors associated with this syndrome include melanoma, carcinomas of the lung, pancreas, stomach,[27] and prostate, and gonadal germ cell tumors.[25,28] In 1990, Malkin *et al.*[28] screened five of these families and found germline mutations clustered in exon 7 of the *TP53* gene

in all the five. It is now well recognized that most of the constitutional genetic abnormalities in young children with ACT are the germline mutations in various exons of *TP53*. In fact, it is likely that about 70% of young children with ACT have constitutional *TP53* mutations. For example, Varley *et al.*[14] found germline *TP53* mutations in nine of 14 cases of pediatric ACT selected without reference to the family's history of cancer. These observations support the recommendation that cases of ACT in children and adolescents should be screened for germline *TP53* mutations.[29,30]

Beckwith–Wiedemann syndrome (BWS) is also a rare genetic disorder with a higher than expected incidence of ACT. It includes congenital umbilical hernia, macroglossia, and gigantism[36] but a wide phenotypic expression has been noted. Genetic linkage analysis has provided evidence that familial BWS is associated with regulatory abnormalities at the chromosome 11p15 region.[37,38] The genes for insulin-like growth factor-2 (IGF-II) and H19 have been mapped to this site. Adjacent genes have been shown to be paternally imprinted and maternally expressed.[39] They appear to be important regulators of fetal adrenal growth and tumorigenesis.[40–42] The loss of imprinting of these genes may cause their overexpression, thereby leading to oncogenesis.[43] Other abnormalities involving both chromosomes 11 and 17, such

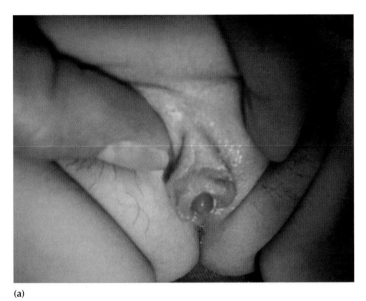

(a)

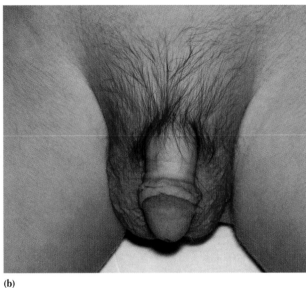

(b)

Figure 67.1 Clinical signs of adrenocortical tumors. (a) Precocious pseudopuberty (clitoromegaly) in a girl with adrenocortical carcinoma. (b) Precocious pseudopuberty in a boy with adrenocortical carcinoma. Panel (b) is reproduced from Ribeiro *et al.*[74] with kind permission from Springer Science+Business Media.

as LOH,[20,4] translocations,[45] and mutations,[46,47] have been reported.

Congenital hemihypertrophy, an unusual entity associated with an asymmetrical overgrowth of a whole side or part of the body, has consistently been associated with several benign and malignant neoplasias, including ACT.[48–52] Chronic stimulation of the adrenal gland by adrenocorticotropic hormone (ACTH) is thought to contribute to tumorigenesis.[53,54] However, ACTs are described only rarely in patients with congenital adrenal hyperplasia[55–57] and the role of 21-hydroxylase in the pathogenesis of adrenal masses has been challenged.[58] Carney complex and multiple endocrine neoplasia (MEN) 1[59–64] are reviewed elsewhere in this chapter.

The relationship between environmental factors and ACT is difficult to prove. Mann *et al.*[65] reported the case of a child with ACT whose mother ingested hydroxyprogesterone hexanoate during pregnancy to prevent miscarriage. Hornstein *et al.*[66] described a case of adrenocortical carcinoma in a child with fetal alcohol syndrome; however, the child also had hemihypertrophy and a familial history of cancer. Dedov and Norets[67] administered [^{75}Se]selenomethionine to rats on days 11–13 of the gestation period. They found that prenatal exposure to the radionuclide was associated with the development of ACTs along with other endocrine and nonendocrine tumors in their offspring. The origin of the *TP53* R337H mutation in southern Brazil, once thought to have environmental causes, has been shown to be due to a founder effect.[68]

Clinical features

Among 254 children enrolled in the International Pediatric Adrenocortical Tumor Registry (IPACTR),[4] the median age at diagnosis of ACT was 3.2 years. Fewer than 15% of patients were 13 years or older at diagnosis. The incidence was higher among girls, with the overall female:male ratio being 1.6:1;

Table 67.3 Signs and symptoms of adrenocortical tumors in 58 children.

Feature	n	%
Pubic hair	53	91
Hypertrophy		84
Clitoris	36	62
Penis	13	22
Acne	42	72
Deep voice	32	55
Hypertension	32	55
Facial hair	29	50
Facial hyperemia	28	48
Palpable tumor	28	48
Weight gain	22	38
Hirsutism	21	36
Moon face	19	33
Accelerated growth velocity	17	29
Centripetal fat distribution	14	24
Buffalo hump of the neck	11	19
Seizures	7	12

Reproduced with permission from Sandrini *et al.*[73] Copyright 1997, The Endocrine Society.

however, the ratio ranged from 1.7:1 in the 0–3-year-old group to 6.2:1 in adolescents (≥13 years). Although the reason for this prevalence in females is not understood, there is evidence of gender-specific physiological changes in the adrenal glands.[69,70] Signs and symptoms of virilization were the most common presenting clinical manifestation (>80% of patients) (Fig. 67.1).[71–74] Clinical manifestations of ACT can be present at birth.[75] An acute abdomen due to spontaneous tumor rupture is rarely the presenting clinical manifestation of ACT.[76]

In a detailed review of the presenting features of 58 cases of childhood ACT[73] (Table 67.3), features of virilization included pubic hair, facial acne, clitoromegaly, voice change, facial hair, hirsutism, muscle hypertrophy, growth acceleration, and increase in penis size (see Fig. 67.1). Virilization was observed either alone (virilizing tumors, 40% of patients) or accompanied by clinical manifestations of the overproduction of other adrenal cortical hormones, including glucocorticoids, androgens, aldosterone, or estrogens (mixed type, 45%). About 10% of patients showed no clinical evidence of an endocrine syndrome at presentation (nonfunctional tumors). Finally, overproduction of glucocorticoids alone (Cushing syndrome) was evident in only 3% of patients. Interestingly, patients with an excess of glucocorticoid did not show striae. Primary hyperaldosteronism (Conn syndrome)[77] and pure feminization occur very rarely.[78–80] None of the patients in the registry manifested either syndrome. The most common presenting clinical manifestations of hyperaldosteronism include headache, weakness of

proximal muscle groups, polyuria, tachycardia with or without palpitation, hypocalcemia, and hypertension. The most frequent sign of feminization is gynecomastia.

Tumor size varied widely among children for whom this information was available in the IPACTR. The tumor weight was more than 200 g in 83 of 182 cases.[4] There was no predominant tumor laterality. Bilateral tumors have been occasionally reported.[81,82] Ectopic ACT, which occurs very rarely, has been described in the spinal canal[83,84] and intrathoracic cavity.[85] Ectopic adrenal cortical tissue is commonly detected retroperitoneally in the celiac plexus, kidney, genitalia, broad ligaments, epididymis, and spermatic cord,[86] and any of these can be a potential site for the development of ACT. Other relevant clinical presenting features of 58 cases of childhood ACT included elevated blood pressure in 55% of the patients,

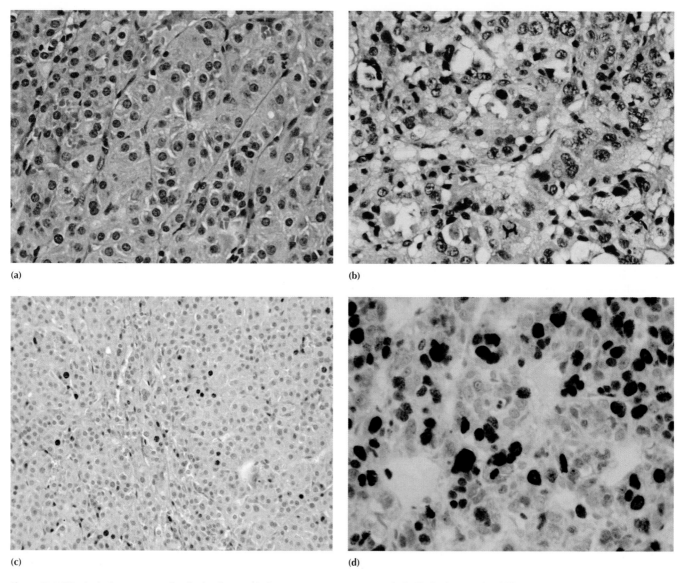

(a)

(b)

(c)

(d)

Figure 67.2 Histological appearance of pediatric adrenocortical tumors. (a) Adenoma is composed of compact cells arranged in nests and cords. There was no cytological atypia, necrosis, or increased mitotic activity. Occasional bi- and multinucleated cells can be present. H&E, 400×. (b) Carcinoma is composed of cells that have eosinophilic cytoplasm and enlarged and pleomorphic nuclei with prominent nucleoli. Mitotic figures are frequently present (*arrowhead*). H&E, 400×. (c) Proliferative index in adenoma and (d) carcinoma assessed by nuclear expression of Ki-67 antigen, 400×.

12% of whom had hypertensive crisis (associated with seizures in one patient). Hypertension was common in patients with glucocorticoid-secreting tumors (Cushing or mixed type); it also occurred in half of the patients with signs of virilization only and in three patients with nonfunctioning tumors. Treatment of hypertension in patients with ACT can be challenging. Fatalities due to hypertensive crisis have been reported.[73] In general, patients have responded well to captopril, although in some cases it has been necessary to add other drugs, such as ketoconazole.[87]

Children and adolescents with functional ACT are subject to growth disturbances.[88] Pure androgen and estrogen excess most often results in increased growth velocity and premature epiphyseal closure. In the Curitiba series, the height and weight of children with ACT often exceeded the 50th percentile at diagnosis. Patients with a greater than expected height for age included not only those with the virilizing form of ACT but also those with the mixed form. Bone age was advanced more than 1 year in 68% of the patients. Markers of growth and development have consistently remained within the normal range in long-term survivors.[89] True precocious puberty is rarely noted.

In many instances, the increased somatic growth of these children, their generally healthy appearance, and the lack of a palpable abdominal mass diverted pediatricians from the possibility of a malignancy. To avoid delaying the diagnosis of ACT, any child less than 4 years with pubarche should be considered to have ACT until proven otherwise. In addition, the presence of acne in an infant can be considered pathognomonic of an adrenocortical lesion. Finally, because Cushing syndrome is very rare in children, it should be considered highly indicative of ACT in children younger than 10 years.[90]

Diagnosis

The diagnosis of ACT is made on the basis of the gross and histological appearance of tissue obtained surgically. The pathological classification of pediatric ACT is troublesome. Even an experienced pathologist can find it difficult to differentiate pediatric adenoma from carcinoma (Fig. 67.2).[91] Weiss *et al.*[92,93] and Hough *et al.*[94] formulated classification systems on the basis of macroscopic, microscopic, and clinical features present at diagnosis. Bugg *et al.*[95] used modified criteria of Weiss *et al.*[92,93] to analyze a large series of pediatric ACT. In this study, the adrenal tumors were divided into three groups: adrenocortical adenomas, high-grade carcinomas, and low-grade carcinomas. High-grade carcinoma and tumor weight were the most reliable predictors of outcome. However, histological criteria that predict outcome in adult adrenocortical tumors are not reliable in pediatric ACT.

Because about 80% of pediatric ACTs secrete one or more adrenal cortex hormones, careful preoperative laboratory evaluation is critical for early and long-term management.[96] Routine laboratory evaluation for suspected ACT includes measurement of plasma cortisol, DHEA-S, testosterone, androstenedione, 17-hydroxyprogesterone, aldosterone, renin activity, deoxycorticosterone (DOC), and other 17-deoxysteroid precursors. This comprehensive panel of tests not only contributes to the diagnosis but also provides useful markers for the detection of tumor recurrence. In our experience, a dexamethasone suppression test has rarely been necessary. Elevated glucocorticoid and androgen levels are strong indications of adrenal tumor.

Several imaging modalities are used to corroborate the diagnosis of ACT and provide critical information for disease extent and surgical planning.[97] Because incidentaloma is not found in children, it is not necessary to use imaging in an attempt to separate incidentalomas from carcinomas. Computed tomography (CT), sonography, magnetic resonance imaging (MRI), and positron emission tomography (PET) scanning are most commonly used in cases with a presumptive diagnosis of ACT. At St Jude Children's Research Hospital, the use of MRI has steadily increased over the past few years. This modality has several advantages over CT, including the absence of ionizing radiation, the capability of imaging multiple planes, and improved tissue contrast differentiation. On CT imaging, ACT is usually well demarcated with an enhancing peripheral capsule. Large tumors usually have a central area of stellate appearance caused by hemorrhage, necrosis, and fibrosis. This stellate zone is hyperintense on T2-weighted and short-inversion recovery (STIR) MR images. Calcifications are common. Because ACT is metabolically active, fluorodeoxyglucose (FDG)-PET imaging is increasingly used in patients with ACT (Fig. 67.3).[98–100] C-metomidate (MTO), a marker of sustained 11-β-hydroxylase activity, has been investigated as an alternative PET tracer for adrenocortical imaging. The clinical indications of PET with this new tracer are still evolving.[101] Although FDG/MTO-PET is unlikely to add information to that obtained with CT or MRI of the primary tumor and its regional extension, it can reveal distant metastases that are not readily detected on CT or MRI. PET imaging can also detect tumor recurrence in areas that may be missed on routine follow-up imaging and tumor invasion of the inferior vena cava[102] (Fig. 67.4). Newer imaging modalities are being developed and may improve our ability to maintain the efficacy of the existent modalities and decrease patients' exposure to ionizing irradiation.[103]

Currently, our recommendation is that, in addition to sonography, all patients who have a suspected adrenal tumor should be examined by CT and MRI. Because the liver and lungs are the most common sites of metastasis at the time of diagnosis, CT scans of the chest and MRI of abdomen are recommended for all patients with newly diagnosed ACT. The skeleton and central nervous system are involved in a few cases. Technetium bone scans are typically obtained in the initial evaluation of children with ACT. Imaging of the central nervous system is not routinely performed at presentation.

Treatment

Surgery

Surgery is the single most important procedure in the successful treatment of ACT. It is performed by a transabdominal approach, usually using an ipsilateral subcostal incision, which may be modified to a chevron or bilateral subcostal incision.

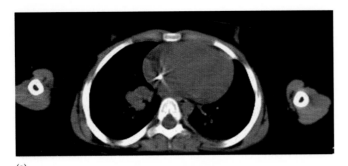

(a)

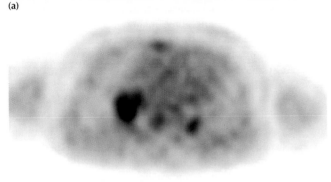

(b)

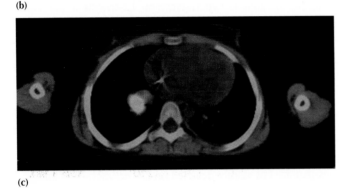

(c)

Figure 67.3 A 4-year-old girl with pulmonary metastatic adrenocortical carcinoma. (a) CT scan shows abnormal soft tissue in the right and left lower lobes. (b) Corresponding FDG-PET image shows increased accumulation of FDG within the lesions shown on the CT scan, consistent with metastatic tumor. (c) Fusion of CT and PET images in upper panels.

En bloc resection, which may include the kidney, portions of the pancreas and/or liver, or other adjacent structures, may be necessary in rare cases of large, locally invasive tumors. A thoracoabdominal incision is indicated in rare cases. The role of regional lymph node dissection in pediatric ACT has not been evaluated but it has been advocated because patients with large tumors commonly experience local relapse. An ipsilateral modified node dissection is performed, extending from the renal vein to the level of bifurcation of the common iliac vessel. If there are contralateral clinically enlarged lymph nodes, they should be removed as well. Surgical resection of recurrent local and distant disease is also important. In the latter case, multiple surgical resections may be necessary to render patients free of disease.[104] This aggressive approach is associated with prolonged survival, particularly when combined with chemotherapy.[105,106] Because of tumor friability, rupture of the capsule and tumor spillage are frequent (occurring in approximately 20% of cases during the initial

procedure and in 43% after local recurrence).[73] Infiltration of the vena cava may make radical surgery difficult in some cases, although successful complete resection of the tumor thrombus has been reported with cardiopulmonary bypass.[107,108]

Surgery requires careful and precise perioperative planning. All patients with a glucocortical-secreting tumor are assumed to have suppression of the contralateral adrenal gland, and therefore steroid replacement therapy is given. Special attention to electrolyte balance, hypertension, surgical wound care, and infectious complications is imperative.

Chemotherapy

The role of chemotherapy in the management of childhood ACT has not been established. Mitotane (1,1-dichloro-2-(*o*-chlorophenyl)-2-(*p*-chlorophenyl)ethane, or *o, p*′-DDD), an insecticide derivative that produces adrenocortical necrosis, has been used extensively in adults with ACT[109,110] but its efficacy in children is not known. Mitotane has been used to treat advanced metastatic ACT, given prior to surgery in cases of inoperable tumors or after surgery in patients at high risk for relapse (adjuvant chemotherapy), combined with other agents, and used to control symptoms associated with increased production of adrenal hormones. Objective responses to mitotane are obtained in 15–60% of treated adult patients.[111] The wide variation in response rates may, in part, reflect the pharmacokinetics of mitotane. There has been evidence of greater tumor response when the plasma concentration of mitotane is above 14 mg/L.[112] The most important common toxicities of mitotane are nausea, vomiting, diarrhea, and abdominal pain. Less frequent reactions include somnolence, lethargy, ataxic gait, depression, and vertigo. Of interest, prepubertal patients can develop gynecomastia or thelarche. Another shortcoming of mitotane treatment is that it significantly alters steroid hormone metabolism, so that blood and urine steroid measurements cannot be used as markers of tumor relapse. Mitotane should be considered an experimental agent in the treatment of children with ACT. Other chemotherapeutic agents, including 5-fluorouracil, etoposide, cisplatin, carboplatin, cyclophosphamide, doxorubicin, gemcitabine, and streptozocin, have been used alone or in combination to treat ACT, with varied results.[113–115]

There has been no formal trial of conventional chemotherapy agents in pediatric ACT but the available case reports and the experience of the IPACTR suggest that a subset of pediatric ACT is sensitive to chemotherapy. Emerging treatment approaches have been described and can potentially be utilized in pediatric adrenocortical tumors.[116–119] The role of radiotherapy in treatment of ACT is controversial but its use has been advocated by some investigators.[120–122] Because children with ACT usually carry a germline *TP53* mutation, the use of radiotherapy in these patients has to be carefully considered.[123,124] The adjuvant combination used most often in pediatrics consists of cisplatin and doxorubicin with or without etoposide given with mitotane.

Outcome

In the IPACTR series, of the 254 patients with known outcomes, 97 (38.2%) died and 157 (61.8%) were alive at a median follow-up of 2 years and 5 months (range 5 days to 22 years).[4]

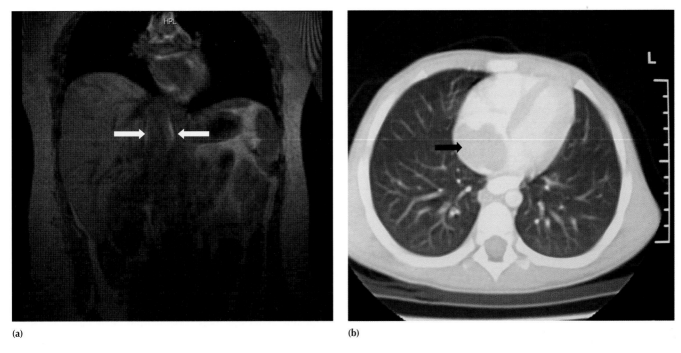

(a)   (b)

Figure 67.4 (a) Vena cava involvement by intraluminal extension of adrenocortical tumor. (b) Axial magnetic resonance image of a large intraatrial tumor thrombus.

Table 67.4 Staging of adrenocortical tumors in children (Children's Oncology Group).

Stage	Definition
I	Completely resected, small tumors (<100 g and <200 cm³) with normal postoperative hormone levels
II	Completely resected, large tumors (≥100 g or ≥200 cm³) with normal postoperative hormone levels
III	Unresectable, gross or microscopic residual disease Tumor spillage Patients with stage I and II tumors whose hormone levels fail to normalize after surgery Patients with retroperitoneal lymph node involvement
IV	Presence of distant metastases

The survival rate in this study is similar to that reported by others.[125] Five patients died of causes unrelated to tumor progression (two died of infection, one of hypertensive complications, one of massive hemorrhage during surgery, and one of an unspecified complication). The 5-year event-free survival (EFS) and overall survival estimates were 54.2% (95% confidence interval [CI] 48.2–60.2%) and 54.7% (95% CI 48.7–60.7%), respectively.

Prognostic factors

Complete tumor resection is the single most important prognostic indicator. Patients who have residual disease after surgery have a dismal prognosis. Of 57 patients in the IPACTR who had distant or local, gross or microscopic residual disease after surgery, only eight have remained free of disease. Conversely, the long-term survival rate is around 75% for children with completely resected tumors. Among the latter, tumor size has prognostic value. Registry data showed that among 192 such patients, those with tumors weighing more

than 200 g had an EFS estimate of 39%, compared with 87% for those with smaller tumors. Tumor size has been consistently associated with prognosis in several studies of ACT.[126,127] Children whose tumors produce excess glucocorticoid appear to have a worse prognosis than those who have pure virilizing manifestations.

Classification schemes or disease staging systems to guide therapy for pediatric ACT are still evolving. A modification of the staging system of Sandrini and colleagues[73] including tumor volume and resectability has been adapted for use in the Children's Oncology Group treatment protocol (Table 67.4). Note that in this set of disease staging criteria, histology is not considered a variable due to the well-known difficulties in distinguishing independent histological parameters in pediatric ACT. It is likely that prognostic factor analysis can be further refined by adding other predictive factors.[128–130] For example, rupture of the tumor pseudocapsule during surgery and invasion of the vena cava were associated with poor prognosis even among patients whose tumors were completely resected but these variables are yet to be prospectively analyzed. Moreover, some histological tumor features, such as vascular or capsular invasion, extensive necrosis, and marked mitotic activity, were independently associated with prognosis in a 2003 study.[126]

St Jude International Pediatric Adrenocortical Tumor Registry

Because of its rarity, the pathogenesis, natural history, and best practices in pediatric ACT remain largely unknown. The International Pediatric Adrenocortical Tumor Registry (IPACTR, www.ipactr.org) was created by St Jude Children's Research Hospital investigators in 1990 to collect clinical and laboratory features, treatment practices, and outcome data for children with ACT. Moreover, a translational research program was developed to investigate the disease pathogenesis and test drug efficacy in ACT preclinical models. As previously noted, 50–70% of children with ACT carry *de novo*, inherited, or somatic *TP53* mutations. Family members of children who inherited *TP53* mutations are also at an increased risk for malignancy, although the risk appears to vary depending on the type of mutation. It is possible that tissue-specific factors interact with mutated p53 in promoting tumorigenesis. Moreover, it has become increasingly evident that common polymorphisms of selected genes might modulate the oncogenic potential of p53[131] (Fig. 67.5).

Therefore, the study of pediatric ACT provides unique opportunities to identify cell pathways implicated in tumorigenesis in general. However, there are major challenges to

studying rare tumors. First, a large number of cases is necessary for meaningful clinical and laboratory studies. Second, specific uniform treatment protocols are required for survival and prognostic factor analysis. Third, for carriers of constitutional mutations, long-term follow-up of affected children and updated information on their relatives' history of cancer are required. Finally, availability of genomic material is essential for genotype-phenotype correlative analysis.

Rare tumor registries such as the IPACTR can overcome many of the challenges associated with low patient numbers, variable treatment management, and lack of follow-up information and blood and tumor samples for translational research. Since 1990, 321 children with ACT have been enrolled on the IPACTR study. The clinical and ancillary laboratory data for the first 254 patients registered have been reported.[4] Since this report, an additional 67 children and adolescents with ACT and two relatives (breast cancer and renal cell carcinoma) from the United States and other countries (Argentina, Brazil, Colombia, England, Greece, Honduras, Spain, and United Arab Emirates) have been enrolled.[132] Li–Fraumeni syndrome was observed in nine cases (13.4%). To date, the *TP53* status has been determined in 50 pediatric ACT cases. Tumor tissue DNA was available in 45 ACT cases. The wild-type *TP53* sequence was observed in 13 cases (28.8%). In the remaining 32 (71.2%), *TP53* mutations were noted. Somatic *TP53* mutations were observed in four cases, all of them in heterozygous state, and germline *TP53* mutations in 24 cases. Of the 15 germline mutations cases in which patient and parental blood DNA was available for study, 10 cases were inherited and five were "*de novo*" *TP53* mutations. In nine germline *TP53* cases, blood from parents was not accessed to define inheritance. There were 24 different *TP53* mutations observed in our cohort, and only three were reported more than once (Arg337His, Arg175His, and Arg273Cys). These mutations occurred through the *TP53* gene and no hot spot site was evident (Fig. 67.6). Two mutations, *TP53*

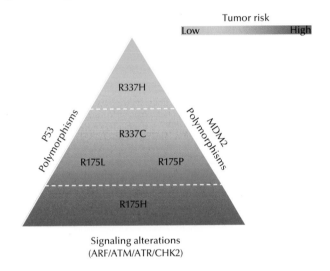

Figure 67.5 Different *TP53* mutations have shown a spectrum of activity (p53 gradient effect). Alterations in components of the p53 cellular pathway, including *TP53* and MDM2 polymorphisms, might modulate the oncogenic potential of p53 and influence tumor susceptibility. Reproduced with permission from Zambetti.[131]

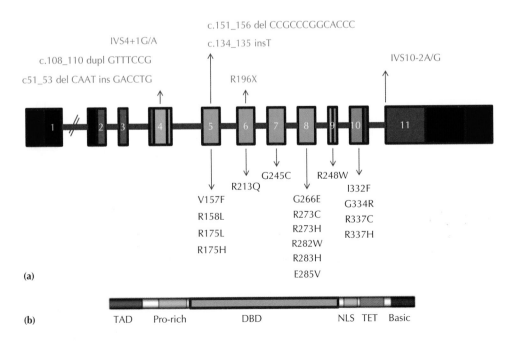

Figure 67.6 *TP53* mutations observed in childhood adrenocortical tumors registered through the International Pediatric Adrenocortical Tumor Registry. (a) *TP53* mutations were detected within and outside the DNA binding domain. Most mutations represent single nucleotide substitutions (*black*), although nonsense and complex mutations were also observed (*red*). (b) The schematic outlines the coding region of *TP53* spanning exons 1 to 11 (colors represent functional domains). Reproduced from Pinto.[132] Reprinted by permission of SAGE Publications.

Ile332Phe and Gly334Arg, both located in the tetramerization domain of p53, have not been previously reported.

Children's Oncology Group Adrenocortical Tumor Trial

Cooperative, multiinstitutional efforts have been pivotal in the advancement of pediatric oncology during the past several decades. Rare pediatric tumors, however, have remained research orphans and children with these rare malignancies have yet to benefit from group initiatives. In 2002, the Children's Oncology Group (COG) created the rare tumor committee, which currently integrates subcommittees on liver tumors, germ cell tumors, retinoblastoma, and infrequent tumors. The main objectives of the infrequent tumor subcommittee were to create an organizational framework to facilitate the study of these infrequent malignancies and to develop registries, biospecimen banks, and clinical trials. Building from the experience of the IPACTR, the COG rare tumor committee sought to encourage registration of all pediatric rare cancers into the COG research registry. Based on the estimates from the SEER database, 71% of the expected cases of adrenocortical carcinoma were registered, which compares very favorably with other pediatric rare tumors such as melanoma (14%) and retinoblastoma (38%). While these data are very encouraging, they continue to highlight the obstacles in the development of clinical research in very rare cancers.[133]

Initial efforts were followed by the development of the ARAR0332 protocol (Treatment of Adrenocortical Tumors with Surgery plus Lymph Node Dissection and Multiagent Chemotherapy), a collaboration between the COG and Brazilian institutions. This protocol investigates three main clinical questions:
• the efficacy of surgery alone for stage I tumors (disease stage system, see Table 67.4)
• the role of retroperitoneal lymph node resection in reducing local recurrence of stage II tumors
• the impact of mitotane and cisplatin-based chemotherapy for unresectable and metastatic disease (Table 67.5).
The ARAR0332 protocol opened in August 2006 in the North American institutions and in June 2008 in the two institutions in southern Brazil. Sixty patients had been enrolled as of July 2011. Importantly, more than one-third of the patients enrolled are from the ACT cluster area in southern Brazil, which highlights the importance of collaborative studies for pediatric ACT and will allow gathering a significant amount of data on the clinical characteristics, treatment, and outcomes for children with ACT and will increase our knowledge of its biology and epidemiology. Initiatives that coordinate efforts in pediatric ACT are clearly needed. It is only through the development of international collaborative projects that we can further our knowledge of the epidemiology and biology of this neoplasm.

Acknowledgments

This work was supported in part by grants P30 CA-21765 and PO1 CA-20180 from the National Cancer Institute and by the American Lebanese Syrian Associated Charities (ALSAC). We thank David Galloway for expert review of the manuscript.

References

1. Pitman. General melasma and short hair over the entire body of a child of three years, with conversion of the left supra-renal capsule into a large malignant tumor; the external organs of generation resembling that of adult life. Lancet 1865; 1: 175.
2. Walters W, Wilder R, Kepler E. The suprarenal cortical syndrome with presentation of ten cases. Ann Surg 1934; 100: 670.
3. Ribeiro RC, Sandrini Neto RS, Schell MJ, Lacerda L, Sambaio GA, Cat I. Adrenocortical carcinoma in children: a study of 40 cases. J Clin Oncol 1990; 8(1): 67–74.
4. Michalkiewicz E, Sandrini R, Figueiredo B, et al. Clinical and outcome characteristics of children with adrenocortical tumors: a report from the International Pediatric Adrenocortical Tumor Registry. J Clin Oncol 2004; 22(5): 838–45.
5. Surveillance, Epidemiology, and End Results (SEER) Program (www.seer.cancer.gov) SEER*Stat Database: Incidence – SEER 9 Regs Research Data, Nov 2009 Sub (1973–2007)<Single Ages to 85+, Katrina/Rita Population Adjustment>– Linked To County Attributes – Total U.S., 1969–2007 Counties, National Cancer Institute, DCCPS, Surveillance Research Program, Cancer Statistics Branch, released April 2010, based on the November 2010 submission.
6. Drut R, Hernandez A, Pollono D. Incidence of childhood cancer in La Plata, Argentina, 1977–1987. Int J Cancer 1990; 45(6): 1045–7.
7. Gatta G, Capocaccia R, Stiller C, Kaatsch P, Berrino F, Terenziani M. Childhood cancer survival trends in Europe: a EUROCARE Working Group study. J Clin Oncol 2005; 23(16): 3742–51.
8. Gatta G, Zigon G, Capocaccia R, et al. Survival of European children and young adults with cancer diagnosed 1995–2002. Eur J Cancer 2009; 45(6): 992–1005.
9. Stiller CA. International patterns of cancer incidence in adolescents. Cancer Treat Rev 2007; 33(7): 631–45.
10. Pereira RM, Michalkiewicz E, Sandrini F, et al. Childhood adrenocortical tumors. Arq Bras Endocrinol Metabol 2004; 48(5): 651–8.
11. Latronico AC, Mendonca BB. Adrenocortical tumors – new perspectives. Arq Bras Endocrinol Metabol 2004; 48(5): 642–6.
12. Ribeiro RC, Sandrini F, Figueiredo B, et al. An inherited p53 mutation that contributes in a tissue-specific manner to pediatric adrenal cortical carcinoma. Proc Natl Acad Sci USA 2001; 98(16): 9330–5.
13. DiGiammarino EL, Lee AS, Cadwell C, et al. A novel mechanism of tumorigenesis involving pH-dependent destabilization of a mutant p53 tetramer. Nat Struct Biol 2002; 9(1): 12–16.
14. Varley JM, McGown G, Thorncroft M, et al. Are there low–penetrance TP53 Alleles? evidence from childhood adrenocortical tumors. Am J Hum Genet 1999; 65(4): 995–1006.

Table 67.5 Treatment on the Children's Oncology Group ARAR0332 protocol.

Stage	Treatment
Stage I	Surgery alone
Stage II	Surgery
	RPLN dissection
Stage III	Mitotane
	CDDP/ETO/DOX
	Surgery + RPLN dissection
Stage IV	Mitotane
	CDDP/ETO/DOX
	Surgery + RPLN dissection

CDDP, cisplatin; DOX, doxorubicin; ETO, etoposide; RPLN, retroperitoneal lymph node.

15. Figueiredo BC, Sandrini R, Zambetti GP, *et al*. Penetrance of adrenocortical tumours associated with the germline TP53 R337H mutation. J Med Genet 2006; 43(1): 91–96.

16. Figueiredo BC, Stratakis CA, Sandrini R, *et al*. Comparative genomic hybridization analysis of adrenocortical tumors of childhood. J Clin Endocrinol Metab 1999; 84(3): 1116–21.

17. Figueiredo BC, Cavalli LR, Pianovski MA, *et al*. Amplification of the steroidogenic factor 1 gene in childhood adrenocortical tumors. J Clin Endocrinol Metab 2005; 90(2): 615–19.

18. Longui CA, Lemos-Marini SH, Figueiredo B, *et al*. Inhibin alpha-subunit (INHA) gene and locus changes in paediatric adrenocortical tumours from TP53 R337H mutation heterozygote carriers. J Med Genet 2004; 41(5): 354–9.

19. West AN, Neale GA, Pounds S, *et al*. Gene expression profiling of childhood adrenocortical tumors. Cancer Res 2007; 67(2): 600–8.

20. Ragazzon B, Assie G, Bertherat J. Transcriptome analysis of adrenocortical cancers: from molecular classification to the identification of new treatments. Endocr Relat Cancer 2011; 18(2): R15–R27.

21. Kempna P, Fluck CE. Adrenal gland development and defects. Best Pract Res Clin Endocrinol Metab 2008; 22(1): 77–93.

22. Lalli E. Adrenal cortex ontogenesis. Best Pract Res Clin Endocrinol Metab 2010; 24(6): 853–64.

23. Malendowicz LK. 100th anniversary of the discovery of the human adrenal fetal zone by Stella Starkel and Leslaw Wegrzynowski: how far have we come? Folia Histochem Cytobiol 2010; 48(4): 491–506.

24. Li FP, Fraumeni JF Jr. Rhabdomyosarcoma in children: epidemiologic study and identification of a familial cancer syndrome. J Natl Cancer Inst 1969; 43(6): 1365–73.

25. Li FP, Fraumeni JF Jr. Prospective study of a family cancer syndrome. JAMA 1982; 247(19): 2692–4.

26. Malkin D. Li–Fraumeni syndrome. Genes Cancer 2011; 2(4): 475–84.

27. Masciari S, Dewanwala A, Stoffel EM, *et al*. Gastric cancer in individuals with Li–Fraumeni syndrome. Genet Med 2011; 13(7): 651–7.

28. Malkin D, Li FP, Strong LC, *et al*. Germ line p53 mutations in a familial syndrome of breast cancer, sarcomas, and other neoplasms. Science 1990; 250(4985): 1233–8.

29. Villani A, Tabori U, Schiffman J, *et al*. Biochemical and imaging surveillance in germline TP53 mutation carriers with Li–Fraumeni syndrome: a prospective observational study. Lancet Oncol 2011; 12(6): 559–67.

30. Tinat J, Bougeard G, Baert-Desurmont S, *et al*. 2009 version of the Chompret criteria for Li Fraumeni syndrome. J Clin Oncol 2009; 27(26): e108–e109.

31. Hirose PF, Capellanno AM, Oliveira A, *et al*. Adrenocortical tumors in children: the Brazilian experience in a single institution. J Clin Oncol 2005; 23: A8506.

32. Sandrini F, Villani DP, Tucci S, Moreira AC, de Castro M, Elias LL. Inheritance of R337H p53 gene mutation in children with sporadic adrenocortical tumor. Horm Metab Res 2005; 37(4): 231–5.

33. Barreto JHS, Dórea MDF, Mendonça N. Carcinoma do córtex adrenal na infância. Arq Bras Endocrinol Metabol 2001; 45: S383.

34. Pianovski MA, Maluf EM, de Carvalho DS, *et al*. Mortality rate of adrenocortical tumors in children under 15 years of age in Curitiba, Brazil. Pediatr Blood Cancer 2006; 47(1): 56–60.

35. Ribeiro RC, Figueiredo B. Childhood adrenocortical tumours. Eur J Cancer 2004; 40(8): 1117–26.

36. Choufani S, Shuman C, Weksberg R. Beckwith–Wiedemann syndrome. Am J Med Genet C Semin Med Genet 2010; 154C(3): 343–54.

37. Koufos A, Grundy P, Morgan K, *et al*. Familial Wiedemann–Beckwith syndrome and a second Wilms tumor locus both map to 11p15.5. Am J Hum Genet 1989; 44: 711.

38. Ping AJ, Reeve AE, Law DJ, *et al*. Genetic linkage of Beckwith–Wiedemann syndrome to 11p15. Am J Hum Genet 1989; 44: 720.

39. Nativio R, Sparago A, Ito Y, Weksberg R, Riccio A, Murrell A. Disruption of genomic neighbourhood at the imprinted IGF2-H19 locus in Beckwith–Wiedemann syndrome and Silver–Russell syndrome. Hum Mol Genet 2011; 20(7): 1363–74.

40. Liu J, Kahri AI, Heikkila P, Ilvesmaki V, Voutilainen R. H19 and insulin-like growth factor-II gene expression in adrenal tumors and cultured adrenal cells. J Clin Endocrinol Metab 1995; 80(2): 492–6.

41. Mesiano S, Mellon SH, Jaffe RB. Mitogenic action, regulation, and localization of insulin-like growth factors in the human fetal adrenal gland. J Clin Endocrinol Metab 1993; 76(4): 968–76.

42. Wilkin F, Gagne N, Paquette J, Oligny LL, Deal C. Pediatric adrenocortical tumors: molecular events leading to insulin-like growth factor II gene overexpression. J Clin Endocrinol Metab 2000; 85(5): 2048–56.

43. Sparago A, Russo S, Cerrato F, *et al*. Mechanisms causing imprinting defects in familial Beckwith–Wiedemann syndrome with Wilms' tumour. Hum Mol Genet 2007; 16(3): 254–64.

44. Yano T, Linehan M, Anglard P, *et al*. Genetic changes in human adrenocortical carcinomas. J Natl Cancer Inst 1989; 81: 518.

45. Limon J, Clin PD, Gaeta J, Sandberg AA. Translocation t(4; 11)(q35; p13) in an adrenocortical carcinoma. Cancer Genet Cytogenet 1987; 28: 343.

46. Henry I, Jeanpierre M, Couillin P, *et al*. Molecular definition of the 11p15.5 region involved in Beckwith–Wiedemann syndrome and probably in predisposition to adrenocortical carcinoma. Hum Genet 1989; 81(3): 273–7.

47. Herrmann ME, Rydstedt LL, Talpos GB, Ratner S, Wolman SR, Lalley PA. Chromosomal aberrations in two adrenocortical tumors, one with a rearrangement at 11p15. Cancer Genet Cytogenet 1994; 75(2): 111–16.

48. Benson RF, Vulliamy DG, Taubman JO. Congenital hemihypertrophy and malignancy. Lancet 1963; 1: 468–9.

49. Fraumeni JF Jr, Miller RW. Adrenocortical neoplasms with hemihypertrophy, brain tumors, and other disorders. J Pediatr 1967; 70(1): 129–38.

50. Muller S, Gadner H, Weber B, Vogel M, Riehm H. Wilms' tumor and adrenocortical carcinoma with hemihypertrophy and hamartomas. Eur J Pediatr 1978; 127: 219–26.

51. Tank ES, Kay R. Neoplasms associated with hemihypertrophy, Beckwith–Wiedemann syndrome and aniridia. J Urol 1980; 124: 266.

52. Clericuzio CL, Martin RA. Diagnostic criteria and tumor screening for individuals with isolated hemihyperplasia. Genet Med 2009; 11(3): 220–2.

53. Van Seters AP, van Aalderen W, Moolenaar AJ, Gorsiro MC, van Roon F, Backer ET. Adrenocortical tumour in untreated congenital adrenocortical hyperplasia associated with inadequate ACTH suppressibility. Clin Endocrinol (Oxf) 1981; 14(4): 325–34.

54. Shinohara N, Sakashita S, Terasawa K, Nakanishi S, Koyanagi T. [Adrenocortical adenoma associated with congenital adrenal hyperplasia]. Nippon Hinyokika Gakkai Zasshi 1986; 77(9): 1519–23.

55. Varan A, Unal S, Ruacan S, Vidinlisan S. Adrenocortical carcinoma associated with adrenogenital syndrome in a child. Med Pediatr Oncol 2000; 35(1): 88–90.

56. Daeschner GL. Adrenal cortical adenoma arising in a girl with congenital adrenogenital syndrome. Pediatrics 1965; 36: 140.

57. Pang S, Becker D, Cotelingam J, *et al*. Adrenocortical tumor in a patient with congenital adrenal hyperplasia due to 21-hydroxylase deficiency. Pediatrics 1981; 68: 242.

58. Barzon L, Maffei P, Sonino N, *et al*. The role of 21-hydroxylase in the pathogenesis of adrenal masses: review of the literature and focus on our own experience. J Endocrinol Invest 2007; 30(7): 615–23.

59. Carney JA, Hruska LS, Beauchamp GD, Gordon H. Dominant inheritance of the complex of myxomas, spotty pigmentation, and endocrine overactivity. Mayo Clin Proc 1986; 61(3): 165–72.

60. Stratakis CA, Carney JA, Lin JP, *et al*. Carney complex, a familial multiple neoplasia and lentiginosis syndrome. Analysis of 11 kindreds and linkage to the short arm of chromosome 2. J Clin Invest 1996; 97(3): 699–705.

61. Almeida MQ, Stratakis CA. Solid tumors associated with multiple endocrine neoplasias. Cancer Genet Cytogenet 2010; 203(1): 30–6.

62. Libe R, Horvath A, Vezzosi D, *et al*. Frequent phosphodiesterase 11A gene (PDE11A) defects in patients with Carney complex (CNC) caused by PRKAR1A mutations: PDE11A may contribute to adrenal and testicular tumors in CNC as a modifier of the phenotype. J Clin Endocrinol Metab 2011; 96(1): E208–E214.

63. Chandrasekharappa SC, Guru SC, Manickam P, *et al.* Positional cloning of the gene for multiple endocrine neoplasia type 1. Science 1997; 276(5311): 404–7.

64. Schaefer S, Shipotko M, Meyer S, *et al.* Natural course of small adrenal lesions in multiple endocrine neoplasia type 1: an endoscopic ultrasound imaging study. Eur J Endocrinol 2008; 158(5): 699–704.

65. Mann JR, Cameron AH, Gornall P, Rayner PH, Shah KJ. Transplacental carcinogenesis (adrenocortical carcinoma) associated with hydroxyprogesterone hexanoate. Lancet 1983; 2: 580.

66. Hornstein L, Crowe C, Gruppo R. Adrenal carcinoma in child with history of fetal alcohol syndrome [letter]. Lancet 1977; 2(8051): 1292–3.

67. Dedov VI, Norets TA. State of the endocrine system in the progeny of female rats treated with 75Se-selenomethionine. Radiobiologiia 1982; 22(3): 409–12.

68. Pinto EM, Billerbeck AE, Villares MC, Domenice S, Mendonca BB, Latronico AC. Founder effect for the highly prevalent R337H mutation of tumor suppressor p53 in Brazilian patients with adrenocortical tumors. Arq Bras Endocrinol Metabol 2004; 48(5): 647–50.

69. Nowak D, Goralczyk K, Zurada A, Gielecki J. Morphometrical analysis of the human suprarenal gland between the 4th and 7th months of gestation. Ann Anat 2007; 189(6): 575–82.

70. Bielohuby M, Herbach N, Wanke R, *et al.* Growth analysis of the mouse adrenal gland from weaning to adulthood: time- and gender-dependent alterations of cell size and number in the cortical compartment. Am J Physiol Endocrinol Metab 2007; 293(1): E139–E146.

71. Lee PDK, Winter RJ, Green OC. Virilizing adenocortical tumors in childhood. Eight cases and a review of the literature. Pediatrics 1985; 76: 437–44.

72. Lack EE, Mulvihill JJ, Travis WD, Kozakewich HP. Adrenal cortical neoplasms in the pediatric and adolescent age group. Clinicopathologic study of 30 cases with emphasis on epidemiological and prognostic factors. Pathol Annu 1992; 27(Pt 1): 1–53.

73. Sandrini R, Ribeiro RC, DeLacerda L. Childhood adrenocortical tumors. J Clin Endocrinol Metab 1997; 82(7): 2027–31.

74. Ribeiro RC, Rodriguez-Galindo C, Zambetti GP. Childhood adrenocortical carcinoma. In: Schwab M (ed) *Encyclopedia of Cancer.* Berlin: Springer, 2009. pp.635–9.

75. Artigas JL, Niclewicz ED, Padua GS, Ribas DB, Athayde SL. Congenital adrenal cortical carcinoma. J Pediatr Surg 1976; 11(2): 247–52.

76. Leung LY, Leung WY, Chan KF, Fan TW, Chung KW, Chan CH. Ruptured adrenocortical carcinoma as a cause of paediatric acute abdomen. Pediatr Surg Int 2002; 18(8): 730–2.

77. Dinleyici EC, Dogruel N, Acikalin MF, Tokar B, Oztelcan B, Ilhan H. An additional child case of an aldosterone-producing adenoma with an atypical presentation of peripheral paralysis due to hypokalemia. J Endocrinol Invest 2007; 30(10): 870–2.

78. Halmi KA, Lascari AD. Conversion of virilization to feminization in a young girl with adrenal cortical carcinoma. Cancer 1971; 27: 931–5.

79. Itami RM, Admundson GM, Kaplan SA, *et al.* Prepubertal gynecomastia caused by an adrenal tumor. Am J Dis Child 1982; 136: 584–6.

80. Leditschke JF, Arden F. Feminizing adrenal adenoma in a five-year-old boy. Aust Paediatr J 1974; 10(4): 217–21.

81. Ranew RB, Meadows AT, d'Angio GJ. Adrenocortical carcinoma in children: experience at the Children's Hospital of Philadelphia, 1961–1980. In: Humphrey GB, Grindey GB, Dehner LP, Acton RT, Pysher TJ (eds) *Adrenal and Endocrine Tumors in Children.* Boston: Martinus Nijhoff Publishers, 1983. pp.303–5.

82. Loridan L, Senior B. Cushing's syndrome in infancy. J Pediatr 1969; 75(3): 349–59.

83. Kepes JJ, O'Boynick P, Jones S, Baum D, McMillan J, Adams ME. Adrenal cortical adenoma in the spinal canal of an 8-year-old girl. Am J Surg Pathol 1990; 14(5): 481–4.

84. Rodriguez FJ, Scheithauer BW, Erickson LA, Jenkins RB, Giannini C. Ectopic low-grade adrenocortical carcinoma in the spinal region: immunohistochemical and molecular cytogenetic study of a pediatric case. Am J Surg Pathol 2009; 33(1): 142–8.

85. Medeiros LJ, Anasti J, Gardner KL, Pass HI, Nieman LK. Virilizing adrenal cortical neoplasm arising ectopically in the thorax. J Clin Endocrinol Metab 1992; 75(6): 1522–5.

86. Page DL, DeLellis RA, Hough AJ. Embryology and postnatal development. In: Page DL, DeLellis RA, Hough AJ (eds) *Tumors of the Adrenal.* Washington, DC: Armed Forces Institute of Pathology, 1986. pp.25–35.

87. Veytsman I, Nieman L, Fojo T. Management of endocrine manifestations and the use of mitotane as a chemotherapeutic agent for adrenocortical carcinoma. J Clin Oncol 2009; 27(27): 4619–29.

88. Hauffa BP, Roll C, Muhlenberg R, Havers W. Growth in children with adrenocortical tumors. Klin Padiatr 1991; 203(2): 83–7.

89. Schmit-Lobe MC, DeLacerda L, Ribeiro RC, Kohara SK, Sandrini R. Patterns of growth and development in 26 children operated for adrenocortical carcinoma (ACC) and disease-free for more than one year. Pediatr Res 1990; 38, 622.

90. Gilbert MG, Cleveland WW. Cushing's syndrome in infancy. Pediatrics 1970; 46: 217–29.

91. Dehner LP, Hill DA. Adrenal cortical neoplasms in children: why so many carcinomas and yet so many survivors? Pediatr Dev Pathol 2009; 12(4): 284–91.

92. Weiss LM, Medeiros LJ, Vickery AL Jr. Pathologic features of prognostic significance in adrenocortical carcinoma. Am J Surg Pathol 1989; 13(3): 202–6.

93. Weiss LM. Comparative study of 43 metastasizing and nonmetastasizing adrenocortical tumors. Am J Surg Pathol 1984; 8: 163–9.

94. Hough AJ, Hollifield JW, Page DL, Hartmann WH. Prognostic factors in adrenal cortical tumors: a mathematical analysis of clinical and morphologic data. Am J Clin Pathol 1979; 72: 390–9.

95. Bugg MF, Ribeiro RC, Roberson PK, *et al.* Correlation of pathologic features with clinical outcome in pediatric adrenocortical neoplasia. A study of a Brazilian population. Brazilian Group for Treatment of Childhood Adrenocortical Tumors. Am J Clin Pathol 1994; 101(5): 625–9.

96. Shen WT, Lee J, Kebebew E, Clark OH, Duh QY. Selective use of steroid replacement after adrenalectomy: lessons from 331 consecutive cases. Arch Surg 2006; 141(8): 771–4.

97. Blake MA, Cronin CG, Boland GW. Adrenal imaging. Am J Roentgenol 2010; 194(6): 1450–60.

98. Ahmed M, Al Sugair A, Alarifi A, Almahfouz A. Al Sobhi S. Whole-body positron emission tomographic scanning in patients with adrenal cortical carcinoma: comparison with conventional imaging procedures, Clin Nucl Med 2003; 28(6): 494–7.

99. Wong KK, Arabi M, Zerizer I, Al-Nahhas A, Rubello D, Gross MD. Role of positron emission tomography/computed tomography in adrenal and neuroendocrine tumors: fluorodeoxyglucose and nonfluorodeoxyglucose tracers. Nucl Med Commun 2011; 32(9): 764–81.

100. Mackie GC, Shulkin BL, Ribeiro RC, *et al.* Use of [18 F]fluorodeoxyglucose positron emission tomography in evaluating locally recurrent and metastatic adrenocortical carcinoma. J Clin Endocrinol Metab 2006; 91(7): 2665–71.

101. Minn H, Salonen A, Friberg J, *et al.* Imaging of adrenal incidentalomas with PET using (11)C-metomidate and (18)F-FDG. J Nucl Med 2004; 45(6): 972–9.

102. Cheng MF, Wu YW, Tzen KY, Yen RF. F-18 FDG PET/CT illustrating tumor invasion in the IVC from adrenocortical carcinoma. Clin Nucl Med 2007; 32(11): 891–2.

103. Sauter AW, Wehrl HF, Kolb A, Judenhofer MS, Pichler BJ. Combined PET/MRI: one step further in multimodality imaging. Trends Mol Med 2010; 16(11): 508–15.

104. Kemp CD, Ripley RT, Mathur A, *et al.* Pulmonary resection for metastatic adrenocortical carcinoma: the National Cancer Institute experience. Ann Thorac Surg 2011; 92(4): 1195–200.

105. Arai H, Rino Y, Yamanaka S, *et al.* Successful treatment of adrenocortical carcinoma with pulmonary metastasis in a child: report of a case. Surg Today 2008; 38(10): 965–9.

106. Hermsen IG, Gelderblom H, Kievit J, Romijn JA, Haak HR. Extremely long survival in six patients despite recurrent and metastatic adrenal carcinoma. Eur J Endocrinol 2008; 158(6): 911–19.

107. Godine LB, Berdon WE, Brasch RC, Leonidas JC. Adrenocortical carcinoma with extension into inferior vena cava and right atrium: report of 3 cases in children. Pediatr Radiol 1990; 20(3): 166–8; discussion 169.

108. Chesson JP, Theodorescu D. Adrenal tumor with caval extension – case report and review of the literature. Scand J Urol Nephrol 2002; 36(1): 71–3.

109. Terzolo M, Angeli A, Fassnacht M, et al. Adjuvant mitotane treatment for adrenocortical carcinoma. N Engl J Med 2007; 356(23): 2372–80.

110. Schteingart DE. Adjuvant mitotane therapy of adrenal cancer – use and controversy. N Engl J Med 2007; 356(23): 2415–18.

111. Icard P, Goudet P, Charpenay C, et al. Adrenocortical carcinomas: surgical trends and results of a 253-patient series from the French Association of Endocrine Surgeons study group. World J Surg 2001; 25(7): 891–7.

112. Baudin E, Pellegriti G, Bonnay M, et al. Impact of monitoring plasma 1,1-dichlorodiphenildichloroethane (o,p'DDD) levels on the treatment of patients with adrenocortical carcinoma. Cancer 2001; 92(6): 1385–92.

113. Berruti A, Terzolo M, Pia A, Angeli A, Dogliotti L. Mitotane associated with etoposide, doxorubicin, and cisplatin in the treatment of advanced adrenocortical carcinoma. Italian Group for the Study of Adrenal Cancer. Cancer 1998; 83(10): 2194–200.

114. Khan TS, Imam H, Juhlin C, et al. Streptozocin and o,p'DDD in the treatment of adrenocortical cancer patients: long-term survival in its adjuvant use. Ann Oncol 2000; 11(10): 1281–7.

115. Sperone P, Ferrero A, Daffara F, et al. Gemcitabine plus metronomic 5-fluorouracil or capecitabine as a second-/third-line chemotherapy in advanced adrenocortical carcinoma: a multicenter phase II study. Endocr Relat Cancer 2010; 17(2): 445–53.

116. Fassnacht M, Libe R, Kroiss M, Allolio B. Adrenocortical carcinoma: a clinician's update. Nat Rev Endocrinol 2011; 7(6): 323–35.

117. Tacon LJ, Prichard RS, Soon PS, Robinson BG, Clifton-Bligh RJ, Sidhu SB. Current and emerging therapies for advanced adrenocortical carcinoma. Oncologist 2011; 16(1): 36–48.

118. Spiegel AM, Libutti SK. Future diagnostic and therapeutic trends in endocrine cancers. Semin Oncol 2010; 37(6): 691–5.

119. Haluska P, Worden F, Olmos D, et al. Safety, tolerability, and pharmacokinetics of the anti-IGF-1R monoclonal antibody figitumumab in patients with refractory adrenocortical carcinoma. Cancer Chemother Pharmacol 2010; 65(4): 765–73.

120. Sabolch A, Feng M, Griffith K, Hammer G, Doherty G, Ben-Josef E. Adjuvant and definitive radiotherapy for adrenocortical carcinoma. Int J Radiat Oncol Biol Phys 2011; 80(5): 1477–84.

121. Hermsen IG, Groenen YE, Dercksen MW, Theuws J, Haak HR. Response to radiation therapy in adrenocortical carcinoma. J Endocrinol Invest 2010; 33(10): 712–14.

122. Polat B, Fassnacht M, Pfreundner L, et al. Radiotherapy in adrenocortical carcinoma. Cancer 2009; 115(13): 2816–23.

123. Ferrarini A, Auteri-Kaczmarek A, Pica A, et al. Early occurrence of lung adenocarcinoma and breast cancer after radiotherapy of a chest wall sarcoma in a patient with a de novo germline mutation in TP53. Fam Cancer 2011; 10(2): 187–92.

124. Salmon A, Amikam D, Sodha N, et al. Rapid development of post-radiotherapy sarcoma and breast cancer in a patient with a novel germline 'de-novo' TP53 mutation. Clin Oncol (R Coll Radiol) 2007; 19(7): 490–3.

125. Chudler RM, Kay R. Adrenocortical carcinoma in children. Urol Clin North Am 1989; 16(3): 469–79.

126. Wieneke JA, Thompson LD, Heffess CS. Adrenal cortical neoplasms in the pediatric population: a clinicopathologic and immunophenotypic analysis of 83 patients. Am J Surg Pathol 2003; 27(7): 867–81.

127. Michalkiewicz EL, Sandrini R, Bugg MF, et al. Clinical characteristics of small functioning adrenocortical tumors in children. Med Pediatr Oncol 1997; 28(3): 175–8.

128. El Wakil A, Doghman M, Latre De Late P, Zambetti GP, Figueiredo BC, Lalli E. Genetics and genomics of childhood adrenocortical tumors. Mol Cell Endocrinol 2011; 336(1–2): 169–73.

129. Mateo EC, Lorea CF, Duarte AA, et al. A study of adrenocortical tumors in children and adolescents by a comparative genomic hybridization technique. Cancer Genet 2011; 204(6): 298–308.

130. Leal LF, Mermejo LM, Ramalho LZ, et al. Wnt/beta-catenin pathway deregulation in childhood adrenocortical tumors. J Clin Endocrinol Metab 2011; 96(10): 3106–14.

131. Zambetti GP. The p53 mutation "gradient effect" and its clinical implications. J Cell Physiol 2007; 213(2): 370–3.

132. Pinto EM, Ribeiro RC, Figueiredo BC, Zambetti GP. TP53-associated pediatric malignancies. Genes Cancer 2011; 2(4): 485–90.

133. Pappo AS, Krailo M, Chen Z, Rodriguez-Galindo C, Reaman G. Infrequent tumor initiative of the Children's Oncology Group: initial lessons learned and their impact on future plans. J Clin Oncol 2010; 28(33): 5011–16.

68 Uncommon Pediatric Genitourinary Tumors

Barbara Bambach,[1] Hans G. Pohl,[2] and Jeffrey S. Dome[3]

[1] Department of Pediatrics, Roswell Park Cancer Institute; Department of Pediatrics, State University of New York at Buffalo, NY, USA
[2] Division of Urology, [3] Division of Oncology, Children's National Medical Center; George Washington University School of Medicine, Washington, DC, USA

Introduction

Pediatric genitourinary tumors account for approximately 10% of malignancies up to age 19 years.[1] The most common of these are Wilms tumor of the kidney, gonadal germ cell tumors, and rhabdomyosarcoma of the testicular adnexa, vagina, uterus, bladder, and prostate. This chapter focuses on the less common pediatric genitourinary tumors. For the purposes of this review, the genitourinary tumors are divided by the site of origin: the kidney, the female reproductive system (cervix, vagina, uterus, and ovary), and the male reproductive system (penis, prostate, and testes).

The kidney

Renal cell carcinoma

Pediatric renal cell carcinoma (RCC) (see Chapter 1) is the second most common renal malignancy in children and adolescents. Whereas Wilms tumor is the most common kidney cancer up to age 14 years, RCC becomes more common in the 15–19-year age group.[1] The median age at presentation in pediatric series is 9–10 years, with an equal ratio of boys to girls.[2–4] The clinical presenting features are pain (30–40%), gross hematuria (30–40%), and abdominal mass (20–25%). Nonspecific complaints such as fever, weight loss, and lethargy are seen in 15–40% of children.[2,3]

The biology of pediatric RCC is distinct from its adult counterpart. Whereas the vast majority of adult RCCs have clear cell histology, pediatric RCC has other histological types. Historically, most pediatric RCCs were reported to have clear cells with papillary architecture.[5] After translocation renal cell carcinoma was described and recognized as a distinct entity by the World Health Organization (WHO) in 2004, it became apparent that a significant proportion, if not the majority, of pediatric RCCs are the translocation subtype (Fig. 68.1).[6–8] Translocation RCC is associated with translocations involving genes that encode members of the microophthalmia (MiTF) family of transcription factors. The most commonly involved gene is *TFE3* on chromosome Xp11, which can fuse to several partners including *ASPL* (17q25), *PRCC* (1q21), *PSF* (1p34), *NonO* (Xq12), and *CLTC* (17q23).[9] A less common subtype of translocation RCC involves a fusion of the untranslated *alpha* gene (11q12) to the *TFEB* gene (6p21).[10,11] Among adults and children with translocation RCC, age ≥25 years, lymph node involvement, Fuhrman grade, and presence of distant metastatic disease were associated with poor survival.[12] In pure pediatric series, however, local lymph node involvement was not associated with unfavorable outcome, even among patients who did not receive adjuvant therapy.[7] Interestingly, 15% of translocation RCCs occur in individuals who were previously treated with chemotherapy for a variety of malignancies (Wilms tumor, acute myeloid leukemia, neuroblastoma) and nonmalignant conditions (lupus erythematosus).[13] A separate entity of oncocytoid RCC following neuroblastoma has been described that is distinct from translocation RCC and represents its own category in the WHO classification.[14] Other types of RCC described in children and teenagers include the papillary, chromophobe, sarcomatoid, and collecting duct subtypes. The common clear cell subtype seen in adults has also been described but is distinctly uncommon in children.

The most common sites of metastasis for pediatric RCC are the lymph nodes, lungs, bone, and brain. Modern studies of pediatric RCC use the American Joint Committee on Cancer (TNM) staging system but the historical literature reported results based on the modified Robson classification. Using this system, approximately 60% of pediatric patients present with advanced stage (III or IV) disease (Table 68.1).[15] As with adult RCC, survival is stage dependent (see Table 68.1).

Tumor resection is the mainstay of therapy for pediatric RCC. Most patients are presumed to have Wilms tumor and undergo radical nephrectomy and lymph node sampling according to Wilms tumor surgical guidelines. Many patients

Textbook of Uncommon Cancer, Fourth Edition. Edited by Derek Raghavan, Charles D. Blanke, David H. Johnson, Paul L. Moots, Gregory H. Reaman, Peter G. Rose and Mikkael A. Sekeres.
© 2012 John Wiley & Sons, Inc. Published 2012 by John Wiley & Sons, Inc.

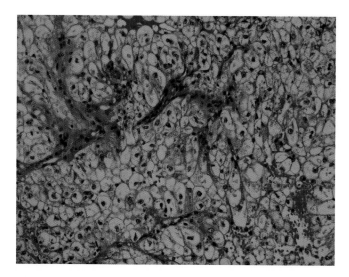

Figure 68.1 Translocation renal cell carcinoma. Solid nests of large cells with abundant clear cytoplasm, rounded nuclei, and prominent nucleoli. H&E, 400×. Courtesy of D. Ashley Hill.

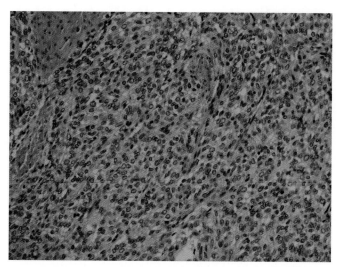

Figure 68.2 Clear cell sarcoma of the kidney, classic pattern. Nests of pale-stained tumor cells are separated by a delicate but distinct network of fine vascular septa. Nuclei are vesicular, with poorly stained chromatin and inconspicuous nucleoli. H&E, 200×. Courtesy of D. Ashley Hill.

Table 68.1 Frequency and outcome for pediatric RCC by modified Robson stage.

Stage	I	II	III	IV
No. of patients (%)	79 (32.5)	26 (10.7)	66 (27.1)	72 (29.6)
% surviving	92.4	84.6	72.7	13.9

with localized disease (including those with local lymph node involvement) have fared well without adjuvant therapy. The Children's Oncology Group (COG) AREN0321 study is prospectively testing the hypothesis that adjuvant therapy is not needed for localized pediatric RCC. Patients with metastatic disease have a poor prognosis. Although successes with high-dose interleukin-2 have been reported,[16] it is recognized in that nonclear cell renal cell carcinomas do not respond well to immunotherapy.[17] The authors do not consider immunotherapy to be first-line treatment for pediatric RCC. Reports of responses to tyrosine kinase inhibitors and therapies directed against vascular endothelial growth factor (VEGF) (sunitinib, sorafenib, ramucirumab) in translocation and other nonclear cell RCC have been published recently.[18,19] Responses to gemcitabine/doxorubicin alternating with gemcitabine/oxaliplatin have also been observed.[7]

Clear cell sarcoma of the kidney

Clear cell sarcoma of the kidney (CCSK) is the second most common renal malignancy in children under 15 years of age. Unlike pediatric RCC, which affects older children, CCSK has an age distribution similar to Wilms tumor, with a mean age at presentation of 3 years.[20] CCSK is indistinguishable from Wilms tumor on clinical presentation (abdominal mass, pain, and hematuria) and imaging studies, so the diagnosis is usually unexpected.[21] The classic morphological pattern of clear cell sarcoma is defined by nests or cords of cells containing abundant extracellular matrix giving the clear cell appearance

(Fig. 68.2). The nests of cells are separated by a network of capillary vascular arcades that are often surrounded by more spindled septal cells. Several variant patterns of CCSK can invite confusion with other pediatric renal tumors.[20]

The genetic etiology of CCSK is poorly understood. Most cases of CCSK have normal karyotypes, though a recurrent t(10;17) translocation has been identified.[22–24] Other recurrent abnormalities detected by either conventional karyotyping or comparative genomic hybridization (CGH) include chromosome 14q deletion and 1q gain.[24–26] Gene expression studies of CCSK have revealed frequent upregulation of neural markers with activation of the sonic hedgehog and phosphoinositide-3-kinase/Akt pathways.[27] Among the upregulated members of the Akt signaling pathway is the epidermal growth factor receptor (*EGFR*) gene. Most CCSKs exhibit EGFR protein staining by immunohistochemistry. *EGFR* gene amplification, somatic *EGFR* mutations, and mutations of *PTEN*, a negative regulator of the Akt pathway, have been reported. Immunostaining studies also demonstrated frequent overexpression of c-kit.[28] Loss of imprinting (LOI) studies found a high rate of LOI at *IGF-2*.[25] The overexpression of insulin-like growth factor (IGF)-2 and EGFR indicates that these proteins may represent novel therapeutic targets for CCSK.

Although CCSK has been called the "bone metastasizing renal tumor of childhood," distant metastatic spread at the time of diagnosis is uncommon, affecting only 4–5% of patients.[20,29] When CCSK does spread, the most common sites are the bone, lung, and liver. Spread to regional lymph nodes is present at diagnosis in about 30% of patients.[20] Relapse-free and overall survival (OS) estimates for patients with CCSK have improved markedly over time. The addition of doxorubicin to vincristine/dactinomycin-based chemotherapy regimens was one of the key factors associated with improved outcome.[20,29] The fourth National Wilms Tumor Study demonstrated improved relapse-free survival (RFS) in patients treated with a 14–16-month chemotherapy regimen with vincristine, dactinomycin, doxorubicin, and flank radiation (8-year RFS, 87.8%) compared to a 6-month regimen (8-year RFS, 60.6%, $p = 0.08$). However, overall survival rates were similar for the long (8-year OS, 87.5%) and short (8-year OS, 85.9%) duration of therapy.[30] The fifth National Wilms Tumor Study evaluated a new regimen consisting of vincristine, doxorubicin, cyclophosphamide, etoposide, and flank radiation given over a 6-month period. With this approach, 5-year event-free survival was 100% (stage I), 87% (stage II), 74% (stage III), and 36% (stage IV).[31]

On older studies, the bones and lungs were the most common sites of recurrence[29,30] but now the brain is the most common site.[31–33] The explanation for this change in natural history is unclear but it suggests that the brain is a sanctuary site for CCSK cells that is relatively protected from chemotherapy. Although CCSK was previously associated with late recurrences, with modern treatment regimens the vast majority of recurrences occur within 3 years of diagnosis.[31]

Rhabdoid tumor of the kidney

Approximately 2% of renal neoplasms in children are malignant rhabdoid tumor of the kidney (RTK).[34] RTK was originally thought to be a rhabdomyosarcomatoid variant of Wilms tumor but lack of myoblastic differentiation and morphological linkage to Wilms tumor led to its classification as a separate entity (Fig. 68.3).[35] The median age of diagnosis is 13 months; 75% of cases occur before age 3 years and 90% occur before age 4 years.[34] Common features at clinical presentation include fever, hypertension, gross or microscopic hematuria, and irritability (pain is difficult to assess in infants).[36] Hypercalcemia has been described in up to 26% of patients, a sign that distinguishes RTK from Wilms tumor.[36]

Although first described in the kidney, rhabdoid tumors can arise at many sites, including the brain (termed "atypicalteratoid/rhabdoid tumor"), liver, and soft tissues throughout the body. There has been debate in the pathology literature whether extrarenal rhabdoid tumors represent the same entity as RTK versus another tumor type with "rhabdoid features."[37,38] The discovery of deletions and mutations of the *SMARCB1* gene on chromosome 22q (also referred to as *INI1*, *BAF47*, and *hSNF5*) in the vast majority of renal and extrarenal rhabdoid tumors has clarified that rhabdoid tumor is indeed a distinct entity.[39–41] The description of patients with both renal and brain rhabdoid tumors and germline *SMARCB1* mutations bolstered the premise that rhabdoid tumors at different sites share a common pathogenesis.[42,43] *SMARCB1* encodes a member of the SWI/SNF chromatin remodeling complex, which regulates transcription by controlling access of transcription machinery to gene promoters.[44] The precise genes involved in the development of rhabdoid tumor remain to be elucidated but several lines of evidence indicate that these tumors have altered expression of members of the p16$^{\text{INK4A}}$/CyclinD1/E2F pathway, which regulates the cell cycle.[45–47]

Rhabdoid tumor of the kidney is one of the most aggressive pediatric malignancies. These tumors may metastasize to the lung, abdomen, liver, brain, bone, or lymph nodes. Current treatment regimens include vincristine, cyclophosphamide

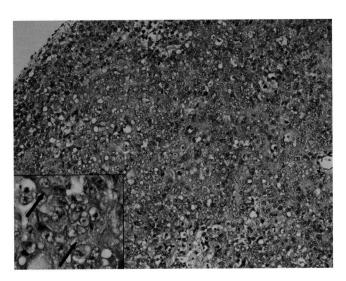

Figure 68.3 Malignant rhabdoid tumor of the kidney. Sheets of undifferentiated cells with large nuclei and prominent nucleoli. Apoptotic cells and necrosis are common. Occasional cells in this field show paranuclear eosinophilic inclusions termed rhabdoid cells (*inset*). H&E, 200×; 400× inset. Courtesy of D. Ashley Hill.

and/or ifosfamide, doxorubicin, carboplatin, and etoposide, as well as radiation therapy. Despite the use of multiagent treatment regimens, the overall survival rate for RTK has remained stubbornly low at around 20%.[48,49] Lower stage (stage I and II) disease and older age at diagnosis have been associated with more favorable outcome.[48] Some investigators have recommended high-dose therapy with stem cell rescue for rhabdoid tumors[50] but it is not clear whether this provides a benefit because survivors with advanced-stage disease have also been reported without stem cell transplant.[51,52]

Congenital mesoblastic nephroma

Congenital mesoblastic nephroma (CMN) is a rare tumor that accounts for about 3% of pediatric renal tumors.[53] The median age at presentation is 2.2 months and it is the most common renal neoplasm in the first 2 months of infancy.[53,54] Common presenting signs and symptoms include abdominal mass, hypertension, and hematuria.[53]

There are two main histological subtypes of CMN: classic (or conventional) and cellular (or atypical), based on the degree of cellularity and mitotic activity (Fig. 68.4).[55,56] A third variant has features of both subtypes in which the two histological patterns coexist. Cellular CMN is histologically similar to infantile fibrosarcoma (IFS) and both have the same chromosome translocation, t(12;15)(p13;q25), which results in a fusion of the *ETV6* gene on chromosome 12 with the *NTRK3* gene on chromosome 15.[57–59] The *ETV6 (TEL)* gene is also implicated in the t(12;21)(p13;q22) of pediatric precursor B cell acute lymphoblastic leukemia, and encodes a transcription factor with a helix-loop-helix protein dimerization domain. NTRK3 is a receptor tyrosine kinase. The chimeric ETV6-NTRK3 protein is postulated to have constitutively active tyrosine kinase growth pathway signaling.[60]

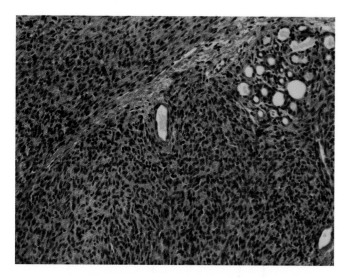

Figure 68.4 Congenital mesoblastic nephroma. Cellular spindle cell neoplasm composed of cells with bland ovoid to spindled nuclei, indistinct nucleoli, and poorly defined cell borders. A characteristic feature is the infiltration of normal kidney at the edges of the tumor; tumor infiltrating renal tubules is shown in upper right. H&E, 400×. Courtesy of D. Ashley Hill.

Outcomes for patients with CMN are generally excellent when treated with nephrectomy only, with overall survival rates of 95%.[53] Rare cases of recurrence and metastasis have been reported, with spread to the lung and brain.[61,62] The few tumors that recur are almost exclusively the cellular variant. It remains to be established whether patients with stage III cellular CMN benefit from adjuvant chemotherapy. In a series published by the German Pediatric Oncology Group (GPOH), two of five patients with stage III cellular CMN developed recurrent disease, whereas only one of the remaining 45 patients had recurrence.[63] Similar to the experience with IFS, studies of cellular CMN have shown that these tumors respond to regimens based on various combinations of vincristine, dactinomycin, doxorubicin, and cyclophosphamide.[63,64]

Metanephric adenoma, metanephric stromal tumor, and metanephric adenofibroma

Metanephric tumors comprise a spectrum of benign renal tumors that include a purely epithelial lesion (metanephric adenoma), a purely stromal lesion (metanephric stromal tumor), and a mixed stromal-epithelial lesion (metanephric adenofibroma).[65] Metanephric adenomas can occur in childhood but typically occur in the fifth to sixth decades of life. They are often discovered incidentally but can present with pain and hematuria. About 10% of patients have polycythemia, which resolves once the tumor is resected. The tumors are benign and do not require adjuvant therapy. Metanephric stromal tumor (MST) presents at a median age of 13 months (range, newborn to 13 years). The lesion resembles the spindle cell stroma of classic congenital mesoblastic nephroma but is a distinct entity.[66] No cases of recurrence have been described but three cases were associated with vascular abnormalities such as aneurysms and angiodysplasia.[66] Metanephric adenofibroma

(MAF), previously called nephrogenic adenofibroma,[67] has a median age of 30 months (range, 5 months to 36 years).[68] MAF has been subclassified into a usual type, MAF with mitoses, MAF in the setting of Wilms tumor, and MAF in the setting of papillary renal cell carcinoma. Regardless of the subtype, patients with MAF uniformly do well.[68]

Renal medullary carcinoma

Renal medullary carcinoma (RMC) is a highly aggressive malignant tumor that occurs in adolescent and young adult patients with sickle cell trait or hemoglobin SC disease.[69] Interestingly, only two cases have been described in patients homozygous for sickle cell disease (hemoglobin SS).[70] Mean age of presentation is 19 years, with a range from 5 to 40 years and a male:female ratio of 2:1.[70] There is no single pathognomonic genetic abnormality seen in RMC but *BCR-ABL* translocations or *ABL* gene amplication have been described in rare cases, as have *ALK* gene rearrangements.[70–72] Absence of SMARCB1/INI1/hSNF5/BAF47 staining by immunohistochemistry has been observed in RMC, suggesting that rhabdoid tumor of the kidney and RMC may have a common pathogenesis.[73]

Patients with RMC almost always present with metastatic disease and have fatal outcomes.[69,70] Transient responses have been observed after treatment with methotrexate/vinblastine/doxorubicin/cisplatin (MVAC) or platinum/gemcitabine/taxane.[70,74–77] A patient with RMC was shown to have a complete tumor response after treatment with the proteosome inhibitor bortezomib.[78]

The female reproductive tract

Cervix (see Chapter 40)

Cervical carcinoma

Cervical cancer rates in adolescents are exceedingly low; the Surveillance, Epidemiology, and End Results (SEER) database shows an incidence of 0.1 cases per 100,000 in girls aged 15–19 years of age from 1990 to 2006.[79] However, human papillomavirus (HPV) infection, the cause of cervical cancer, is extremely common in adolescents, with infection rates higher than any other age group. More than 50% of sexually active adolescents develop anogenital HPV infections.[80] Seventy-four percent of all new HPV infections occur in the 15–24-year age group, accounting for 9.2 million infected adolescents or young adults.[81] The Centers for Disease Control and Prevention (CDC) estimates that 80% of women who reach age 50 years will have had a genital HPV infection.[81] More than 100 species of HPV are identified, with approximately 40 of them occurring in the anogenital area. Fifteen are "high risk" for development of cervical cancer. HPV-16 and HPV-18 cause 70% of all cervical cancer and precancerous lesions.[81] HPV-6 and HPV-11 are "low risk" and are responsible for benign disease such as genital warts and most cases of cervical intraepithelial neoplasia (CIN) 1.[81]

Although frank cervical cancer is very rare in adolescents, abnormal cytology is more prevalent. The Bethesda System for cervical cytology is the current classification used for reporting Pap results in the United States. This system classifies changes as squamous intraepithelial lesions (SIL) or atypical squamous cells (ASC), replacing WHO categories of CIN for cytology.[82] ASC of undetermined significance (ASCUS) is thought to be relatively benign, although "ASC, cannot rule out high grade" (ASC-H) has a greater prediction for more serious lesions.[82] Cervical biopsy samples obtained from colposcopy still use the WHO classification of CIN 1, 2, or 3. CIN 1 is considered benign but CIN 3 is precancerous, with 30–70% progressing to cancer.[82] CIN 2 prognosis is somewhat uncertain. It may be difficult for pathologists to identify reliably[80,82] and many pathologists will group this as CIN 2/3. Some studies have shown that the majority of CIN 2 lesions in adolescents regress over time, although there may be age differences in this regression rate.[82]

Screening of young women has not changed rates of cervical cancer in women less than 30 years old.[80] Therefore, screening recommendations have been revised such that cervical screening should start at age 21 years, with no caveats regarding the age of first sexual activity.[80] There is no place for HPV testing in adolescents due to its high prevalence. Guidelines for triaging abnormal cytology results in adolescents have recently been updated to minimize surgical intervention, which can result in increased risk of preterm delivery and low birthweight.[80]

The US Food and Drug Administration (FDA) has approved twp vaccines for prevention of HPV infection and hence cervical cancer. One is a quadrivalent vaccine (HPV-4) with serotypes HPV-6, -11, -16, and -18 (Gardasil, Merck). The other is bivalent (HPV-2) with serotypes -16 and -18 (Cervarix, GlaxoSmithKline). Efficacy studies have shown that among women naïve to HPV serotypes in the vaccine, efficacy rates were close to 100%, though efficacy appears less for subjects not vaccine type naïve.[83–85] Knowing that adolescents have high rates of HPV infection and that the vaccine trials suggest better efficacy in those who are HPV naïve, targeting younger girls for vaccination seems to maximize the benefits. In the United States, the Advisory Committee for Immunization Practices (ACIP) recommends three doses of either the bivalent or quadrivalent HPV vaccine for girls aged 11–12 years, though it can be started as early as 9 years.[86] Either vaccine is recommended for prevention of cervical cancers and precancers, although only the quadrivalent vaccine is recommended for protection against genital warts, vulvar, and vaginal cancers.

Sarcoma botryoides (embryonal rhabdomyosarcoma)

Sarcoma botryoides, a subtype of embryonal rhabdomyosaroma, is most typically seen in the vagina of infants but rare cases arising from the cervix in girls less than 18 years old have been reported.[87,88] These patients are typically treated with regimens used for rhabdomyosarcoma, with surgery, vincristine and dactinomycin-based chemotherapy, and radiation therapy for locally advanced disease. The prognosis is excellent. Recently, an association between cervical rhabdomyosarcoma, the rare pediatric lung cancer pleuropulmonary blastoma, and Sertoli–Leydig cell tumor has been reported. One patient had a documented DICER1 gene mutation, which is associated with the pleuropulmonary blastoma family tumor and dysplasia syndrome.[89]

Vagina and uterus

Alveolar soft part sarcoma

Alveolar soft part sarcoma (ASPS) is usually located in the extremities, pelvis, head, and neck in children.[90] However, a handful of these tumors have been reported arising from the vagina or uterus.[91–95] Most patients presented with menometrorrhagia. Cytogenetically, there is an unbalanced translocation, der(17)t(X;17)(p11;q25), which results in a fusion of the ASPL gene on chromosome 17 to the TFE3 gene on chromosome X.[96] Patients described in the literature with uterine disease had hysterectomies with or without bilateral salpingo-oophorectomy.[95] No adjuvant therapy was given and no recurrences or metastatic disease were seen, with an average follow-up of 46 months (range 9–78 months). Four of five patients with vaginal ASPS received radiation therapy ranging from 4500 to 8200 cGy, and one patient received chemotherapy with cisplatin and cyclophosphamide.[92] Three patients were alive and free of disease 3–17 years from diagnosis and the status of the other two patients was unknown.

The usual metastatic sites are lungs, brain, and bone. ASPS of the uterus and vagina seems to have a better prognosis than ASPS arising outside the female genital tract. However, this may be due to the relatively short follow-up period reported, as approximately one-third of reported recurrences have been 10 years or more after diagnosis. ASPS is resistant to most conventional chemotherapy agents and the role of radiation therapy is debated. Recent reports suggest that the tyrosine kinase inhibitor sunitinib and antiangiogenesis agent bevacizumab have efficacy in ASPS.[97–99]

Endodermal sinus tumor

Although this germ cell tumor usually arises in the ovary, there have been reports of vaginal endodermal sinus tumors, primarily in children less than 2 years old.[100–105] The typical presentation is vaginal bleeding. On physical examination, polypoid tumors extending into the vaginal lumen may be found. Clinically, vaginal endodermal sinus tumors may be misdiagnosed as botryoid rhabdomyosarcoma. On the basis of the success of chemotherapy regimens for germ cell tumors at other sites, current therapy consists of cisplatin, bleomycin and etoposide, or vinblastine. Chemotherapy should be used as upfront therapy prior to consideration of exenterative surgery or radiation therapy.

Ovary

Juvenile granulosa cell tumor

Juvenile granulosa cell tumor (JGCT) is a rare cause of gonadotropin-releasing hormone (GnRH)-independent sexual precocity in girls. Rare reports of androgenic JGCT also exist with virilization.[106] The juvenile form accounts for 5% of all granulosa cell tumors, and comprises 90% of all prepubertal sex cord tumors.[107] Inhibin and müllerian inhibiting substance may be useful tumor markers.[108,109] Stage is the most important prognostic factor.[106,110] The majority are stage I (International Federation of Gynecology and Obstetrics [FIGO] classification) at diagnosis and have 90% survival[106,111,112] whereas stages II and III have historically been almost uniformly fatal.[113] At laparotomy, the contralateral ovary and fallopian tube should be inspected along with the intraabdominal organs and peritoneal surfaces. Pelvic washings should be performed, and pelvic and paraaortic lymph node sampling done for complete primary surgical staging.[114,115] Unilateral oophorectomy for stage IA is sufficient because of the low rate of bilateral disease and favorable prognosis. Chemotherapy is advocated for patients with advanced or recurrent disease.[113,116–120] Cisplatin-based chemotherapy has generally been used, similar to regimens for germ cell tumors.[116,117] Recurrences are generally within 3 years but some later recurrences have been reported.[121]

Small cell carcinoma with hypercalcemia

The average age of presentation for this tumor is 23 years, with a reported range of 14 months to 44 years.[122,123] Symptoms are nonspecific, such as abdominal pain and swelling. Small cell carcinomas of the ovary are almost always unilateral. Hypercalcemia is reported in two-thirds of patients,[124] although only 2.5% have symptoms of hypercalcemia.[125] The mechanism of the hypercalcemia is not understood entirely but parathyroid hormone-related protein (PTHrP) may be produced by the tumor.[126] Serum calcium can be used as a tumor marker postoperatively. Small cell carcinomas are very aggressive tumors with only 30% survival in stage IA patients[124]; most patients die within 6 months of diagnosis.[122] Pediatric data are limited to mostly case reports or small series. Most authors recommend intensive adjuvant chemotherapy.[123,127] Distelmaier et al. have recommended therapy with cisplatin, ifosfamide, and doxorubicin for six cycles followed by high-dose chemotherapy with carboplatin and etoposide.[123] Others have suggested other chemotherapy regimens without high-dose therapy.[125,128,129]

No consensus exists in the literature regarding surgical approach for these patients. Some argue that due to the aggressiveness of this tumor, even low-stage disease should have aggressive surgery with bilateral salpingo-oophorectomy, hysterectomy, pelvic, and paraaortic node sampling.[130] Others argue that since the majority of these tumors are unilateral, if the uterus and opposite ovary appear normal, only unilateral salpingo-oophorectomy is needed.[124,131]

Metastatic tumors to the ovary

There is very little literature on this phenomenon in children. The largest report describes 14 cases.[132] The majority of these cases were diagnosed at autopsy, although five were symptomatic premortem and were initially misdiagnosed as primary ovarian tumors. The most common tumor metastatic to the ovary was neuroblastoma, with autopsy specimens frequently showing an ovary diffusely replaced by tumor. This must be differentiated from primary neuroblastoma of the ovary, of which there were five reported cases (presumably arising from teratoma).[132] The next most common tumor metastatic to the ovary was rhabdomyosarcoma.[132,133] Other tumors that have been reported to spread to the ovary include Ewing sarcoma, retinoblastoma, medulloblastoma, desmoplastic small round cell tumor, and Wilms tumor.[132–134] There are very rare reports

of colorectal carcinoma and gastric carcinoma metastatic to the ovary in adolescents.[132] This is seen more frequently in adults.

Leukemia and lymphoma

Ovarian involvement occurs frequently in acute lymphoblastic leukemia (ALL) at the end-stages of disease or at autopsy. An ovarian mass may also rarely be the initial manifestation of recurrent ALL.[135,136] In a series of patients with ALL relapse in the ovary, nine patients had bilateral disease and 13 had unilateral disease, although the contralateral ovary was not always biopsied.[135] In this series, approximately 20% had positive cerebrospinal fluid (CSF) cytology, and 20% had bone marrow relapse. Most of the cases occurred late, often more than 36 months after the initial diagnosis. Abdominal pain was the most frequent presenting symptom, and the majority of evaluable cases had palpable abdominal masses. Patients with ALL involving the ovary are treated with systemic chemotherapy, similar to the management of patients with extramedullary relapse at other sites. Although the numbers are small, there appears to be no obvious advantage for salpingo-oophorectomy. The role of radiation therapy is unclear. One-third of the patients were reported in continuous complete remission with a median follow-up of 42 months.[135]

The ovary has been reported as the initial presenting site of newly diagnosed lymphoma in children, though only a few tumors have been reported to arise from the ovary primarily.[137–139] Patients have presented with abdominal or back pain, swelling of the lower extremity, B symptoms, irregular vaginal bleeding, ascites, and pleural effusions. In a large retrospective study including adult and pediatric ovarian lymphomas, the major histologies seen were small noncleaved Burkitt type and diffuse large cell.[140]

Primary ovarian sarcoma

Less than 3% of all ovarian tumors are sarcomas.[141] They may arise from teratomas, malignant mixed mesodermal tumors, or Sertoli–Leydig cell tumors.[142,143] Many different histologies have been reported, including rhabdomyosarcoma, stromal cell sarcoma, fibrosarcoma, and leiomyosarcoma. Surgical therapy is the primary treatment modality for these tumors, including bilateral salpingo-oophorectomy and hysterectomy.[141] For the majority of the histologies, the benefit of adjuvant chemotherapy or radiotherapy is unknown, and the prognosis is poor.[141–145] Survival is excellent, however, for low-grade stromal sarcoma, even when there is spread beyond the ovary.[141]

The male reproductive system

Penis

Malignancies of the penis have rarely been reported in children. Squamous cell carcinoma of the penis occurs in the sixth and seventh decades of life, although there have been five cases reported in children less than 15 years of age.[146,147] It is postulated that poor hygiene in males with intact foreskin increases the risk for penile cancer, since squamous cell carcinoma is almost unheard of in circumcised men.[148–150] Lesions are found on the glans penis, coronal sulcus, or inner preputial skin. The treatment is entirely surgical, with low-stage disease (<1 cm) being amenable to cure with either laser therapy or Mohs micrographic therapy.[151]

While rhabdomyosarcoma is one of the more frequent neoplasms in children, its origin in the penis is uncommon. Six pediatric patients were reported in the literature.[152–157] These cancers have presented as dorsal penopubic masses, with the exception of one that was ventral and associated with priapism. Therapy includes surgery and/or radiation as well as traditional chemotherapy for rhabdomyosarcoma, and is dependent on the stage of the disease, as with rhabdomyosarcomas originating elsewhere.

Prostate

Adenocarcinoma of the prostate is a very rare tumor in men less than 35 years, with 14 reports in children less than 18 years, the youngest being 20 months old.[158–161] Children usually present with urinary retention and hematuria and tend to have a large tumor burden at diagnosis. The pediatric patient invariably has a poorly differentiated, aggressive tumor with negative tumor markers of prostatic acid phosphatase (PAP) and prostate-specific antigen (PSA).[160,161] These tumors metastasize to regional and distant lymph nodes and lungs. Bony metastases usually develop late and are osteolytic, unlike those in adults.[159,161] The majority of pediatric patients described have had advanced disease at diagnosis not amenable to radical surgery, and have responded poorly to radiation and hormonal therapy. Chemotherapy may be of some benefit (unlike in adults), including vincristine, doxorubicin, and ifosfamide.[158] However, most patients die within 1 year.

Testes

One percent of childhood malignancies are testicular tumors, which occur in one in 1,000,000 Caucasian Americans.[162] In general, testicular neoplasms that occur in prepubertal boys differ in incidence, histological distribution, and prognosis from those occurring in postpubertal males. Testicular tumors are ten times more frequent in postpubertal males than in boys younger than 12 years old, with a reported incidence of 5.4 per 100,000 in adults compared with 0.5 per 100,000 in children.[163] Seminoma, embryonal carcinoma and choriocarcinoma, the more commonly encountered malignant germ cell tumors in adults, are not reported in prepubertal testis tumors. Conversely, 98% of malignant germ cell tumors in prepubertal testes are pure yolk sac histology, with the remaining cases identified as gonadoblastomas and the rare malignant stromal cell tumors, Sertoli cell tumors, and mixed stromal cell tumors.[150] When yolk sac histology is identified in postpubertal testis tumors, it is usually present as a component of a histologically mixed tumor along with teratoma, embryonal carcinoma, and syncytiotrophoblasts.[164]

Based on large national testicular tumor registries, textbooks and literature surveys, yolk sac tumor has been reported as the most common primary testis tumor in prepubertal males. In the American Academy for Pediatrics Prepubertal Testis Tumor Registry (AAP PTTR), yolk sac tumors represent 62% of 398 tumors. Similarly, in the Armed Forces Institute of Pathology Adolescent Testis Tumor Registry (AFIP ATTR), yolk sac tumor was the predominant cell type in prepubertal patients. In sharp contrast, the pooled data of four major pediatric hospitals reflect a very different experience, with benign lesions representing 74% of all tumors, the most common being teratomas (48%) and epidermoid cysts (14%). The most likely explanation for this discrepancy is the tendency to underreport benign lesions to tumor registries.

All solid tumors of the testes should be approached through an inguinal excision with a high inguinal orchiectomy for suspected malignancy. However, the predominance of benign lesions among prepubertal testis tumors strongly supports the evolving changes in the standard approach. Testis-sparing enucleation of benign tumors is rapidly becoming the standard of care for prepubertal teratomas, epidermoid cysts, and other benign tumors.

When faced with a prepubertal boy presenting with a nontender testicular mass, sonography and measurement of serum α-fetoprotein (AFP) can help determine which tumors may be amenable to a testis-sparing approach. Teratoma, epidermoid cyst, cystic granulosa cell tumor, cystic dysplasia, and simple cysts can all usually be differentiated by sonography from more solid-appearing prepubertal testis tumors such as yolk sac tumors and most gonadal stromal cell tumors. Preoperative AFP levels further differentiate yolk sac tumors from other tumors preoperatively since at least 93% of yolk sac tumors stain positively for this marker and are associated with elevated serum levels. In the United Kingdom Children's Cancer Group Study, serum AFP was elevated in all 64 patients with yolk sac tumor in whom it was measured. In contrast, teratomas and other benign tumors do not exhibit such staining and are associated with normal serum AFP levels. Therefore, when an intratesticular mass is discovered preoperatively in a prepubertal boy with a normal serum AFP level, one can exclude yolk sac tumor preoperatively with almost absolute certainty, particularly if the mass has cystic features on sonography.

Gonadoblastoma

This rare tumor is seen in patients with gonadal dysgenesis and a Y-chromosome cell line. The majority of patients are phenotypic girls with various degrees of virilization. The remainder are phenotypic boys with hypospadias and cryptorchidism. These tumors are usually benign but do have significant potential for malignant transformation, often to dysgerminoma, and should thus have prophylactic gonadectomy. Scully reported the largest review,[165] in which 57% had 46XY, 30% had 45X/46XY, one patient had 45X, and the remainder had other mosaicisms. One-third of these tumors are bilateral at diagnosis.[166] Histologically, three distinct elements are seen: large germ cells similar to seminoma, sex cord nongerminal elements (Sertoli or granulosa), and mesenchymal or stromal elements (Leydig cells). Calcifications may be seen. One-half will have an overgrowth of the germ cell component, and 10% of these will metastasize.[165] This entity has been described in the newborn period in a patient with dysgenetic testes,[167] emphasizing the importance of early diagnosis and prophylactic gonadectomy.

Seminoma

While this is the most common testicular tumor in adults, it is rarely seen in prepubertal boys.[168] Recommended therapy is the same as for adults: orchiectomy for stage I, orchiectomy plus chemotherapy or radiation for stage II, and preoperative chemotherapy followed by surgery, radiation, and additional chemotherapy for stage III.[169] Chemotherapy is with cisplatin and bleomycin. *In situ* seminoma of the testes has been seen in young males who are infertile as well as in dysgenetic gonads.[170]

Sertoli cell tumor (see Chapter 5)

Less than 1% of testicular tumors are Sertoli cell tumors, and 15% of these occur in children.[166] These usually present as a painless testicular mass. The most common associated endocrine disorder is gynecomastia. There has also been an association with Peutz–Jeghers syndrome.[171,172] The majority of these are benign but malignant variants have been reported in children, one of which metastasized.[173] Treatment is inguinal orchiectomy but retroperitoneal extension must be excluded. Retroperitoneal lymphadenectomy is indicated for Sertoli cell tumors with malignant features (e.g. metastasis, retroperitoneal extension).[174] A variant of Sertoli cell tumor, large cell calcifying Sertoli cell tumor of the testis, is often bilateral, and occurs more frequently with endocrine disturbances such as gynecomastia secondary to estrogen elevation.[175] These tumors have been reported in association with cardiac myxoma, as well as endocrine disorders, including adrenocortical hyperplasia, pituitary adenoma, and sexual precocity. Treatment is similar to that of other Sertoli cell tumors.

Metastatic disease to the testes

Neuroblastoma and Wilms tumor metastases to the testes have been described in patients with widely disseminated disease.[176,177] Up to 4% of patients with neuroblastoma have been found to have testicular metastases.[178] These patients usually present with an adrenal primary and metastatic disease to the retroperitoneal nodes, bone, and bone marrow. The testicular involvement is usually discovered at autopsy.[176] Wilms tumor metastases have been reported in two cases.[177,179] One patient had involvement of all the veins throughout the testis and spermatic cord, suggesting retrograde venous extension, without other systemic metastasis. The second patient had multiple metastases after orchiectomy and died within a year.

Leukemia and lymphoma

Historically, 20% of boys with ALL were found to have testicular disease grossly at diagnosis,[180] although this is now estimated to be 5% because of improved early diagnosis. If routine testicular biopsies are performed, the incidence of testicular leukemia may be as high as 35%.[180] Patients usually have painless testicular swelling, which may be unilateral or bilateral. Patients at highest risk for testicular disease at diagnosis as well as testicular relapse are those with T-cell lymphoblastic leukemia and higher lymphoblast counts at diagnosis. Since isolated testicular relapses can lead to systemic relapse, therapy involves irradiation of both testes (18–24 Gy) plus subsequent chemotherapy.[181] Routine testicular biopsy in the absence of clinical findings at diagnosis or at the conclusion of maintenance therapy is not indicated.

Overt infiltration of the testes with non-Hodgkin lymphoma (NHL) has been described either at diagnosis or relapse.[182,183] Most reported series are of adult patients, with relatively few pediatric patients described. In a review of the St Jude experience, Kellie *et al.* found 5% of all boys with NHL, and 7% of those with advanced-stage disease had testicular involvement.[184] Six of nine patients had disease at diagnosis and presented with painless testicular enlargement. In two, the disease was bilateral. Four patients had diffuse undifferentiated non-Burkitt lymphoma and one patient had lymphoblastic lymphoma. All six patients responded to induction therapy with a clinical complete response; four of these patients remained disease free for 2.9–8.3 years. Two of these patients received radiation to the testes (2250–2400 cGy), and one patient had an orchiectomy. In a study by the French Society of Pediatric Oncology, 5.3% (30/742) of boys with small noncleaved B cell lymphoma had testicular involvement and were treated without radiation. Five patients underwent diagnostic orchiectomy, the remainder did not. Twenty-eight patients achieved complete remission and 26 patients were alive without progressive disease with a median follow-up of 6.5 years.[185]

Juvenile granulosa cell tumor of the testis

There are 24 cases reviewed in the literature:[186] 14 in the newborn period, nine between the ages of 1 and 6 months, and one at 21 months. These tumors usually present as enlargement of the scrotal testis without endocrine abnormalities. Five patients had ambiguous genitalia or abnormal karyotype. All 12 patients for whom follow-up is known were well 6 months to 7 years after unilateral orchiectomy. The tumors can be reliably differentiated from yolk sac tumors based on positive histological staining for inhibin-α and negative staining for AFP. Shukla *et al.* have successfully demonstrated that these tumors can be managed by enucleation with preservation of the testis.[187]

Epidermoid cyst

Although these occur most frequently in adults, pediatric cases have been reported.[188–190] They usually present as painless nodules or cysts, and clinically mimic germ cell tumors. Thus, they are usually not diagnosed prior to surgery. The absence of testicular intraepithelial neoplasia distinguishes them from teratoma. Typically, these tumors have a benign course, and testis-sparing excisions have been performed with no reports of local recurrences.[188,191]

References

1. Howlader N NA, Krapcho M, Neyman N, *et al.* SEER Cancer Statistics Review, 1975–2008. 2011; http://seer.cancer.gov/csr/1975_2008/
2. Castellanos RD, Aron BS, Evans AT. Renal adenocarcinoma in children: incidence, therapy and prognosis. J Urol 1974; 111: 534–7.
3. Indolfi P, Terenziani M, Casale F, *et al.* Renal cell carcinoma in children: a clinicopathologic study. J Clin Oncol 2003; 21(3): 530–5.
4. Selle B, Furtwangler R, Graf N, Kaatsch P, Bruder E, Leuschner I. Population-based study of renal cell carcinoma in children in Germany, 1980–2005: more frequently localized tumors and underlying disorders compared with adult counterparts. Cancer 2006; 107(12): 2906–14.

5. Lack EE, Cassady JR, Sallan SE. Renal cell carcinoma in childhood and adolescence: a clinical and pathological study of 17 cases. J Urol 1985; 133: 822–8.

6. Bruder E, Passera O, Harms D, et al. Morphologic and molecular characterization of renal cell carcinoma in children and young adults. Am J Surg Pathol 2004; 28(9): 1117–32.

7. Geller JI, Argani P, Adeniran A, et al. Translocation renal cell carcinoma: lack of negative impact due to lymph node spread. Cancer 2008; 112(7): 1607–16.

8. Ramphal R, Pappo A, Zielenska M, Grant R, Ngan BY. Pediatric renal cell carcinoma: clinical, pathologic, and molecular abnormalities associated with the members of the mit transcription factor family. Am J Clin Pathol 2006; 126(3): 349–64.

9. Argani P, Ladanyi M. Translocation carcinomas of the kidney. Clin Lab Med 2005; 25(2): 363–78.

10. Argani P, Hawkins A, Griffin CA, et al. A distinctive pediatric renal neoplasm characterized by epithelioid morphology, basement membrane production, focal HMB45 immunoreactivity, and t(6;11)(p21.1;q12) chromosome translocation. Am J Pathol 2001; 158(6): 2089–96.

11. Davis IJ, His BL, Arroyo JD, et al. Cloning of a novel alpha-TFEB fusion in renal tumors harboring the t(6;11)(p21;q12) chromosome translocation. Proc Natl Acad Sci USA 2003(100): 6051–6.

12. Malouf GG, Camparo P, Molinie V, et al. Transcription factor E3 and transcription factor EB renal cell carcinomas: clinical features, biological behavior and prognostic factors. J Urol 2011; 185(1): 24–9.

13. Argani P, Lae M, Ballard ET, et al. Translocation carcinomas of the kidney after chemotherapy in childhood. J Clin Oncol 2006; 24(10): 1529–34.

14. Medeiros LJ, Palmedo G, Krigman HR, Kovacs G, Beckwith JB. Oncocytoid renal cell carcinoma after neuroblastoma: a report of four cases of a distinct clinicopathologic entity. Am J Surg Pathol 1999; 23(7): 772–80.

15. Geller JI, Dome JS. Local lymph node involvement does not predict poor outcome in pediatric renal cell carcinoma. Cancer 2004; 101(7): 1575–83.

16. MacArthur CA, Isaacs H Jr, Miller JH, Ozkaynak F. Pediatric renal cell carcinoma: a complete response to recombinant interleukin-2 in a child with metastatic disease at diagnosis. Med Pediatr Oncol 1994; 23(4): 365–71.

17. Upton MP, Parker RA, Youmans A, McDermott DF, Atkins MB. Histologic predictors of renal cell carcinoma response to interleukin-2-based therapy. J Immunother 2005; 28(5): 488–95.

18. Malouf GG, Camparo P, Oudard S, et al. Targeted agents in metastatic Xp11 translocation/TFE3 gene fusion renal cell carcinoma (RCC): a report from the Juvenile RCC Network. Ann Oncol 2010; 21(9): 1834–8.

19. Choueiri TK, Lim ZD, Hirsch MS, et al. Vascular endothelial growth factor-targeted therapy for the treatment of adult metastatic Xp11.2 translocation renal cell carcinoma. Cancer 2010; 116(22): 5219–25.

20. Argani P, Perlman EJ, Breslow NE, et al. Clear cell sarcoma of the kidney: a review of 351 cases from the National Wilms Tumor Study Group Pathology Center. Am J Surg Pathol 2000; 24(1): 4–18.

21. Sotelo-Avila C, Gonzalez-Crussi F, Sadowinski S, Gooch WM III, Pena R. Clear cell sarcoma of the kidney: a clinicopathologic study of 21 patients with long-term follow-up evaluation. Hum Pathol 1985; 16(12): 1219–30.

22. Punnett HH, Halligan GE, Zaeri N, Karmazin N. Translocation 10;17 in clear cell sarcoma of the kidney. A first report. Cancer Genet Cytogenet 1989; 41(1): 123–8.

23. Rakheja D, Weinberg AG, Tomlinson GE, Partridge K, Schneider NR. Translocation (10;17)(q22;p13): a recurring translocation in clear cell sarcoma of kidney. Cancer Genet Cytogenet 2004; 154(2): 175–9.

24. Brownlee NA, Perkins LA, Stewart W, et al. Recurring translocation (10;17) and deletion (14q) in clear cell sarcoma of the kidney. Arch Pathol Lab Med 2007; 131(3): 446–51.

25. Schuster AE, Schneider DT, Fritsch MK, Grundy P, Perlman EJ. Genetic and genetic expression analyses of clear cell sarcoma of the kidney. Lab Invest 2003; 83(9): 1293–9.

26. Barnard M, Bayani J, Grant R, Zielenska M, Squire J, Thorner P. Comparative genomic hybridization analysis of clear cell sarcoma of the kidney. Med Pediatr Oncol 2000; 34(2): 113–16.

27. Cutcliffe C, Kersey D, Huang CC, Zeng Y, Walterhouse D, Perlman EJ. Clear cell sarcoma of the kidney: up-regulation of neural markers with activation of the sonic hedgehog and Akt pathways. Clin Cancer Res 2005; 11(22): 7986–94.

28. Jones C, Rodriguez-Pinilla M, Lambros M, et al. c-KIT overexpression, without gene amplification and mutation, in paediatric renal tumours. J Clin Pathol 2007; 60(11): 1226–31.

29. Green DM, Breslow NE, Beckwith JB, Moksness J, Finklestein JZ, d'Angio GJ. Treatment of children with clear-cell sarcoma of the kidney: a report from the National Wilms' Tumor Study Group. J Clin Oncol 1994; 12(10): 2132–7.

30. Seibel NL, Li S, Breslow NE, et al. Effect of duration of treatment on treatment outcome for patients with clear-cell sarcoma of the kidney: a report from the National Wilms' Tumor Study Group. J Clin Oncol 2004; 22(3): 468–73.

31. Seibel NL, Sun J, Anderson JR, et al. Outcome of clear cell sarcoma of the kidney (CCSK) treated on the National Wilms Tumor Study-5 (NWTS). Proc Am Soc Clin Oncol 2006; 24(18 S): 502 S.

32. Radulescu VC, Gerrard M, Moertel C, et al. Treatment of recurrent clear cell sarcoma of the kidney with brain metastasis. Pediatr Blood Cancer 2008; 50(2): 206–9.

33. Furtwangler R, Reignhard H, Beier R, et al. Clear-cell sarcoma (CCSK) of the kidney-results of the SIOP 93-01/GPOH trial. Pediatr Blood Cancer 2005; 45(4): 423.

34. Weeks DA, Beckwith JB, Mierau GW, Luckey DW. Rhabdoid tumor of kidney. A report of 111 cases from the National Wilms' Tumor Study Pathology Center. Am J Surg Pathol 1989; 13(6): 439–58.

35. Haas JE, Palmer NF, Weinberg AG, Beckwith JB. Ultrastructure of malignant rhabdoid tumor of the kidney. A distinctive renal tumor of children. Hum Pathol 1981; 12(7): 646–57.

36. Amar AM, Tomlinson G, Green DM, Breslow NE, de Alarcon PA. Clinical presentation of rhabdoid tumors of the kidney. J Pediatr Hematol Oncol 2001; 23: 105–8.

37. Weeks DA, Beckwith JB, Mierau GW. Rhabdoid tumor. An entity or a phenotype? Arch Pathol Lab Med 1989; 113(2): 113–14.

38. Wick MR, Ritter JH, Dehner LP. Malignant rhabdoid tumors: a clinicopathologic review and conceptual discussion. Semin Diagn Pathol 1995; 12(3): 233–48.

39. Versteege I, Sevenet N, Lange J, et al. Truncating mutations of hSNF5/INI1 in aggressive paediatric cancer. Nature 1998; 394(6689): 203–6.

40. Biegel JA, Zhou JY, Rorke LB, Stenstrom C, Wainwright LM, Fogelgren B. Germ-line and acquired mutations of INI1 in atypical teratoid and rhabdoid tumors. Cancer Res 1999; 59(1): 74–9.

41. Eaton KW, Tooke LS, Wainwright LM, Judkins AR, Biegel JA. Spectrum of SMARCB1/INI1 mutations in familial and sporadic rhabdoid tumors. Pediatr Blood Cancer 2010; 56(1): 7–15.

42. Biegel JA, Fogelgren B, Wainwright LM, Zhou JY, Bevan H, Rorke LB. Germline INI1 mutation in a patient with a central nervous system atypical teratoid tumor and renal rhabdoid tumor. Genes Chromosomes Cancer 2000; 28: 31–7.

43. Savla J, Chen TTY, Schneider NR, Timmons CF, Delattre O, Tomlinson GE. Mutations of the hSNF5/INI1 gene in renal rhabdoid tumors with second primary brain tumors. J Natl Cancer Inst 2000; 92: 648–50.

44. Roberts CW, Biegel JA. The role of SMARCB1/INI1 in development of rhabdoid tumor. Cancer Biol Ther 2009; 8(5): 412–16.

45. Betz BL, Strobeck MW, Reisman DN, Knudsen ES, Weissman BE. Re-expression of hSNF5/INI1/BAF47 in pediatric tumor cells leads to G1 arrest associated with induction of p16ink4a and activation of RB. Oncogene 2002; 21(34): 5193–203.

46. Tsikitis M, Zhang Z, Edelman W, Zagzag D, Kalpana GV. Genetic ablation of Cyclin D1 abrogates genesis of rhabdoid tumors resulting from Ini1 loss. Proc Natl Acad Sci USA 2005; 102(34): 12129–34.

47. Isakoff MS, Sansam CG, Tamayo P, et al. Inactivation of the Snf5 tumor suppressor stimulates cell cycle progression and cooperates with p53 loss in oncogenic transformation. Proc Natl Acad Sci USA 2005; 102(49): 17745–50.

48. Tomlinson GE, Breslow NE, Dome J, *et al.* Rhabdoid tumor of the kidney in the National Wilms' Tumor Study: age at diagnosis as a prognostic factor. J Clin Oncol 2005; 23(30): 7641–5.

49. Van den Heuvel-Eibrink MM, van Tinteren H, Rehorst H, *et al.* Malignant rhabdoid tumours of the kidney (MRTKs), registered on recent SIOP protocols from 1993 to 2005: a report of the SIOP renal tumour study group. Pediatr Blood Cancer 2011; 56(5): 733–7.

50. Madigan CE, Armenian SH, Malogolowkin MH, Mascarenhas L. Extracranial malignant rhabdoid tumors in childhood: the Childrens Hospital Los Angeles experience. Cancer 2007; 110(9): 2061–6.

51. Waldron PE, Rodgers BM, Kelly MD, Womer RB. Successful treatment of a patient with stage IV rhabdoid tumor of the kidney: case report and review. J Pediatr Hematol Oncol 1999; 21(1): 53–7.

52. Wagner L, Hill DA, Fuller C, *et al.* Treatment of metastatic rhabdoid tumor of the kidney. J Pediatr Hematol Oncol 2002; 24(5): 385–8.

53. Howell CG, Othersen HB, Kiviat NE, Norkool P, Beckwith JB, d'Angio GJ. Therapy and outcome in 51 children with mesoblastic nephroma: a report of the National Wilms' Tumor Study. J Pediatr Surg 1982; 17: 826–31.

54. Van den Heuvel-Eibrink MM, Grundy P, Graf N, *et al.* Characteristics and survival of 750 children diagnosed with a renal tumor in the first seven months of life: a collaborative study by the SIOP/GPOH/SFOP, NWTSG, and UKCCSG Wilms tumor study groups. Pediatr Blood Cancer 2008; 50(6): 1130–4.

55. Joshi VV, Kasznica J, Walters TR. Atypical mesoblastic nephroma. Pathologic characterization of a potentially aggressive variant of conventional congenital mesoblastic nephroma. Arch Pathol Lab Med 1986; 110(2): 100–6.

56. Pettinato G, Manivel JC, Wick MR, Dehner LP. Classical and cellular (atypical) congenital mesoblastic nephroma: a clinicopathologic, ultrastructural, immunohistochemical, and flow cytometric study. Hum Pathol 1989; 20(7): 682–90.

57. Knezevich SR, Garnett MJ, Pysher TJ, Beckwith JB, Grundy PE, Sorensen PH. ETV6-NTRK3 gene fusions and trisomy 11 establish a histogenetic link between mesoblastic nephroma and congenital fibrosarcoma. Cancer Res 1998; 58(22): 5046–8.

58. Knezevich SR, McFadden DE, Tao W, Lim JF, Sorensen PH. A novel ETV6-NTRK3 gene fusion in congenital fibrosarcoma. Nature Genet 1998; 18(2): 184–7.

59. Rubin BP, Chen CJ, Morgan TW, *et al.* Congenital mesoblastic nephroma t(12;15) is associated with ETV6-NTRK3 gene fusion: cytogenetic and molecular relationship to congenital (infantile) fibrosarcoma. Am J Pathol 1998; 153(5): 1451–8.

60. Wai DH, Knezevich SR, Lucas T, Jansen B, Kay RJ, Sorensen PH. The ETV6-NTRK3 gene fusion encodes a chimeric protein tyrosine kinase that transforms NIH3T3 cells. Oncogene 2000; 19(7): 906–15.

61. Steinfeld AD, Crowley CA, O'Shea PA, Tefft M. Recurrent and metastatic mesoblastic nephroma in infancy. J Clin Oncol 1984; 2: 956–60.

62. Heidelberger KP, Ritchey ML, Dauser RC, McKeever PE, Beckwith JB. Congenital mesoblastic nephroma metastatic to the brain. Cancer 1993; 72(8): 2499–502.

63. Furtwaengler R, Reinhard H, Leuschner I, *et al.* Mesoblastic nephroma – a report from the Gesellschaft fur Padiatrische Onkologie und Hamatologie (GPOH). Cancer 2006; 106(10): 2275–83.

64. Loeb DM, Hill DA, Dome JS. Complete response of recurrent cellular congenital mesoblastic nephroma to chemotherapy. J Pediatr Hematol Oncol 2002; 24(6): 478–81.

65. Argani P. Metanephric neoplasms: the hyperdifferentiated, benign end of the Wilms tumor spectrum? Clin Lab Med 2005; 25(2): 379–92.

66. Argani P, Beckwith JB. Metanephric stromal tumor: report of 31 cases of a distinctive pediatric renal neoplasm. Am J Surg Pathol 2000; 24(7): 917–26.

67. Hennigar RA, Beckwith JB. Nephrogenic adenofibroma. A novel kidney tumor of young people. Am J Surg Pathol 1992; 16(4): 325–34.

68. Arroyo MR, Green DM, Perlman EJ, Beckwith JB, Argani P. The spectrum of metanephric adenofibroma and related lesions: clinicopathologic study of 25 cases from the National Wilms Tumor Study Group Pathology Center. Am J Surg Pathol 2001; 25(4): 433–44.

69. Davis CJ Jr, Mostofi FK, Sesterhenn IA. Renal medullary carcinoma. The seventh sickle cell nephropathy. Am J Surg Pathol 1995; 19(1): 1–11.

70. Simpson L, He X, Pins M, *et al.* Renal medullary carcinoma and ABL gene amplification. J Urol 2005; 173(6): 1883–8.

71. Stahlschmidt J, Cullinane C, Roberts P, Picton SV. Renal medullary carcinoma: prolonged remission with chemotherapy, immunohistochemical characterisation and evidence of bcr/abl rearrangement. Med Pediatr Oncol 1999; 33(6): 551–7.

72. Marino-Enriquez A, Ou WB, Weldon CB, Fletcher JA, Perez-Atayde AR. ALK rearrangement in sickle cell trait-associated renal medullary carcinoma. Genes Chromosomes Cancer 2011; 50(3): 146–53.

73. Cheng JX, Tretiakova M, Gong C, Mandal S, Krausz T, Taxy JB. Renal medullary carcinoma: rhabdoid features and the absence of INI1 expression as markers of aggressive behavior. Mod Pathol 2008; 21(6): 647–52.

74. Pirich LM, Chou P, Walterhouse DO. Prolonged survival of a patient with sickle cell trait and metastatic renal medullary carcinoma. J Pediatr Hematol Oncol 1999; 21(1): 67–9.

75. Strouse JJ, Spevak M, Mack AK, Arceci RJ, Small D, Loeb DM. Significant responses to platinum-based chemotherapy in renal medullary carcinoma. Pediatr Blood Cancer 2005; 44(4): 407–11.

76. Walsh A, Kelly DR, Vaid YN, Hilliard LM, Friedman GK. Complete response to carboplatin, gemcitabine, and paclitaxel in a patient with advanced metastatic renal medullary carcinoma. Pediatr Blood Cancer 2010; 55(6): 1217–20.

77. Bell MD. Response to paclitaxel, gemcitabine, and cisplatin in renal medullary carcinoma. Pediatr Blood Cancer 2006; 47(2): 228.

78. Ronnen EA, Kondagunta GV, Motzer RJ. Medullary renal cell carcinoma and response to therapy with bortezomib. J Clin Oncol 2006; 24(9): e14.

79. Watson M, Saralya M, Ahmed F, *et al.* Using population-based cancer registry data to assess the burden of human papillomavirus-associated cancers in the United States: overview of methods. Cancer 2008; 113(Suppl 10): 2841–5.

80. Moscicki AB. Human papillomavirus disease and vaccines in adolescents. Adolesc Med 2010; 21: 347–63.

81. Hager WDM. Human papilloma virus infection and prevention in the adolescent population. J Pediatr Adolesc Gynecol 2009; 22(4): 197–204.

82. Widdice LE, Moscicki AB. Updated guidelines for Papanicolau tests, colposcopy, and human papillomavirus testing in adolescents. J Adolesc Health 2008; 43: S41–S51.

83. FUTURE II Study Group. Quadrivalent vaccine against human papillomavirus to prevent high-grade cervical lesions. N Engl J Med 2007; 356: 1915–27.

84. Ault KA, FUTURE II Study Group. Effect of prophylactic human papillomavirus L1 virus-like particle vaccine on risk of cervical intraepithelial neoplasia grade 2, grade 3, and adenocarcinoma in situ: a combined analysis of four randomized clinical trials. Lancet 2007; 369: 1861–8.

85. Garland SM, Hernandez-Avila M, Wheeler CM, *et al.* Quadrivalent vaccine against human papillomavirus to prevent anogenital diseases. N Engl J Med 2007; 356: 1928–43.

86. Centers for Disease Control and Prevention. Vaccine recommendations for HPV2 and HPV4. Morb Mortal Wkly Rep 2010; 59(20): 626–9.

87. Daya DA SR. Sarcoma botryoides of the uterine cervix in young women: a clinicopathological study of 13 cases. Gynecol Oncol 1988; 29: 290–304.

88. Arndt CA, Donaldson SS, Anderson JR, *et al.* What constitutes optimal therapy for patients with rhabdomyosarcoma of the female genital tract? Cancer 2001; 91(12): 2454–68.

89. Dehner LP, Jarzembowski JA, Hill DA. Embryonal rhabdomyosarcoma of the uterine cervix: a report of 14 cases and a discussion of its unusual clinicopathological associations. Mod Pathol 2011; Dec 9 [Epub ahead of print].

90. Kayton ML, Meyers P, Wexler LH, Gerald WL, La Quaglia MP. Clinical presentation, treatment, and outcome of alveolar soft part sarcoma in children, adolescents, and young adults. J Pediatr Surg 2006; 41(1): 187–93.

91. Kasai K, Yoshida Y, Okumara M. Alveolar soft part sarcoma of the vagina: clinical features and morphology. Gynecol Oncol 1980; 9: 227.

92. Chapman GW, Benda J, Williams T. Alveolar soft-part sarcoma of the vagina. Gynecol Oncol 1984; 18: 125.

93. O'Toole RV, Tuttle SE, Lucas JG, Sharma HM. Alveolar soft part sarcoma of the vagina: an immunochemical and electron microscopic study. Int J Gynecol Pathol 1985; 4: 258–65.

94. Carinelli SG, Giudici MN, Brioschi D, Cefis F. Alveolar soft part sarcoma of the vagina. Tumori 1990; 76: 77–80.

95. Nielsen GP, Oliva E, Young RH, Rosenberg AE, Dickersin GR, Scully RE. Alveolar soft-part sarcoma of the female genital tract: a report of nine cases and review of the literature. Int J Gynecol Pathol 1995; 14: 283–92.

96. Folpe AL, Deyrup AT. Alveolar soft part sarcoma: a review and update. J Clin Pathol 2006; 59(11): 1127–32.

97. Stacchiotti S, Negri T, Zaffaroni N, et al. Sunitinib in advanced alveolar soft part sarcoma: evidence of a direct antitumor effect. Ann Oncol 2011; 22(7): 1682–90.

98. Banihani M, Al Mansara A. Spontaneous regression in alveolar soft part sarcoma: case report and literature review. World J Surg Oncol 2009; 7: 53.

99. Schultheis B, Kummer G, Tannapfel A, Strumberg D. Successful sequential antiangiogenic therapy for alveolar soft part sarcoma – a case report. Int J Clin Pharmacol Ther 2010; 48(7): 468–9.

100. SenGupta SK, Murthy DP, Martin WM, Klufio C. A rare case of endodermal sinus tumor of the vagina in an infant. Aust N Z J Obstet Gynecol 1991; 31(4): 381–2.

101. Young RH, Scully RE. Endodermal sinus tumor of the vagina. A report of nine cases and review of the literature. Gynecol Oncol 1984; 18: 380–92.

102. Kohorn EL, McIntosh S, Lytton B, Knowlton AH, Merino M. Case reports: endodermal sinus tumour of the infant vagina. Gynecol Oncol 1985; 20: 196–203.

103. Andersen WA, Sabio H, Durso N, Mills SE, Levien M, Underwood PB Jr. Endodermal sinus tumour of the vagina: the role of primary chemotherapy. Cancer 1985; 56: 1025–7.

104. Collins HS, Burke TW, Heller PB, Olson TA, Woodward JE, Park RC. Endodermal sinus tumour of the infant vagina treated exclusively by chemotherapy. Obstet Gynecol 1989; 73: 507–9.

105. Gangopadhyay M, Raha K, Sinha SK, De A, Bera P, Pati S. Endodermal sinus tumor of the vagina in children: a report of two cases. Indian J Pathol Microbiol 2009; 52(3): 403–4.

106. Nomelini RS, Micheletti AM, Adad SJ, Murta EF. Androgenic juvenile granulosa cell tumor of the ovary with cystic presentation: a case report. Eur J Gynecol Oncol 2007; 28(3): 236–8.

107. Silverman LA, Gitelman SE. Immunoreactive inhibin, mullerian inhibitory substance, and activin as biochemical markers for juvenile granulosa cell tumors. J Pediatr 1996; 129(6): 918–21.

108. Lappöhn RE, Burger HG, Bouma J, Bangah M, Krans M, de Bruijn HW. Inhibin as a marker for granulosa cell tumors. N Engl J Med 1989; 321: 790–3.

109. Gustafson ML, Lee MM, Scully RE, et al. Müllerian inhibiting substance as a marker for sex-cord tumor. N Engl J Med 1992; 326: 466–71.

110. Schneider DT, Calaminus G, Wessalowski R. Therapy of advanced ovarian juvenile granulosa cell tumors. Klin Pediatr 2002; 214(4): 173–8.

111. Calaminus G, Wessalowski R, Harms D, Gobel U. Juvenile granulosa cell tumors of the ovary in children and adolescents: results from 33 patients registered in a prospective cooperative study. Gynecol Oncol 1997; 65(3): 447–52.

112. Stuart CE, Dawson LM. Update on granulosa cell tumors of the ovary. Curr Opin Obstet Gynecol 2003; 15(1): 33–7.

113. Powell JL, Johnson NA, Bailey CI, Otis CN. Management of advanced juvenile granulosa cell tumor of the ovary. Gynecol Oncol 1993; 48(1): 119–23.

114. Kaur H, Bagga R, Saha SC, et al. Juvenile granulosa cell tumor of the ovary presenting with pleural effusion and ascites. Int J Clin Oncol 2009; 14: 78–81.

115. Abu-Rustum NR, Restivo A, Ivy J. Retroperitoneal nodal metastasis in primary and recurrent granulosa cell tumors of the ovary. Gynecol Oncol 2006; 103: 31–4.

116. Cecchetto G, Ferrari A, Bernini G, et al. Sex-cord stromal tumors of the ovary in children: a clinicopathological report from the italian TREP project. Pediatr Blood Cancer 2010; 56: 1062–7.

117. Powell JL, Otis CN. Case report: management of advanced juvenile granulosa cell tumor of the ovary. Gynecol Oncol 1997; 64(2): 282–4.

118. Colombo N, Sessa C, Landoni F, Sartori E, Pecorelli S, Mangioni C. Cisplatin, vinblastine and bleomycin combination chemotherapy in metastatic granulosa cell tumor of the ovary. Obstet Gynecol 1986; 67(2): 265–8.

119. Vassal G, Flamont F, Gailand JM. Juvenile granulosa cell tumor of the ovary in children: a clinical study of 15 cases. J Clin Oncol 1988; 6(6): 990–5.

120. Wessalowski R, Spaar HJ, Pape H. Successful liver treatment of a juvenile granulosa cell tumor in a 4-year-old child by regional deep hyperthermia, systemic chemotherapy, and irradiation. Gynecol Oncol 1995; 57(3): 417–22.

121. Frausto SD, Geisler JP, Fletcher MS. Late recurrence of juvenile granulosa cell tumor of the ovary. Am J Obstet Gynecol 2004; 191: 366–7.

122. Benrubi GI, Pitel P, Lammert N. Small cell carcinoma of the ovary with hypercalcemia responsive to sequencing chemotherapy. South Med J 1993; 86(2): 247–8.

123. Distelmaier F, Calaminus G, Harms D, et al. Ovarian small cell carcinoma of the hypercalcemic type in children and adolescents: a prognostically unfavorable but curable disease. Cancer 2006; 107(9): 2298–306.

124. Scully RE. Small cell carcinoma of hypercalcemic type. Int J Gynecol Pathol 1993; 12: 148–52.

125. Dykgraaf RH, de Jong D, van Veen M, Ewing-Graham PC, Helmerhorst TJM, van der Burg ME. Clinical management of ovarian small-cell carcinoma of the hypercalcemic type. Int J Gynecol Cancer 2009; 19(3): 348–53.

126. Baeyens L, Amat S, Vanden Houte K, Vanhoutte P, L'Hermite M. Small cell carcinoma of the ovary successfully treated with radiotherapy only after surgery: case report. Eur J Gynecol Oncol 2008; 29(5): 535–7.

127. Harrison ML, Hoskins P, du Bois A, et al. Small cell of the ovary, hypercalcemic type – analysis of combined experience and recommendation for management. A GCIG study. Gynecol Oncol 2006; 100(2): 233–8.

128. Senekjian EK, Weiser PA, Talerman A, Herbst AL. Vinblastine, cisplatin, cyclophosphamide, bleomycin, doxorubicin, and etoposide in the treatment of small cell carcinoma of the ovary. Cancer 1989; 64: 1183–7.

129. Rana S, Warren BK, Yamada SD. Stage IIIC small cell carcinoma of the ovary: survival with conservative surgery and chemotherapy. Obstet Gynecol 2004; 103: 1120–3.

130. Reed WC. Small cell carcinoma of the ovary with hypercalcemia: report of a case of survival without recurrence 5 years after surgery and chemotherapy. Gynecol Oncol 1995; 199: 5452–5.

131. McAfee JL, McCoy RD. Uterine and ovarian conservation in advanced small cell carcinoma of the ovary. Obstet Gynecol 1998; 91(5 Pt 2): 846–8.

132. Young RH, Kozakewich HP, Scully RE. Metastatic ovarian tumors in children: a report of 14 cases and review of the literature. Int J Gynecol Pathol 1993; 12: 8–19.

133. Moore JG, Schifrin BS, Erez S. Ovarian tumors in infancy, childhood and adolescence. Am J Obstet Gynecol 1967; 99: 913–22.

134. Paterson E. Distant metastases from medulloblastoma of the cerebellum. Brain 1961; 84: 301–9.

135. Pais RC, Kim TH, Zwiren GT, Ragab AH. Ovarian tumors in relapsing acute lymphoblastic leukemia: a review of 23 cases. J Pediatr Surg 1991; 26(1): 70–4.

136. Kim JW, Cho MK, Kim CH, et al. Ovarian and multiple lymph nodes recurrence of acute lymphoblastic leukemia: a case report and review of literature. Pediatr Surg Int 2008; 24(11): 1269–73.

137. Chong AL, Ngan BY, Weitzman S, Abla O. Anaplastic large cell lymphoma of the ovary in a pediatric patient. J Pediatr Hematol Oncol 2009; 31(9): 702–4.

138. Koksal Y, Caliskan U, Ucar C, Reisli I. A case of primary ovarian lymphoma in a child with high levels of CA125 and CA19-9. J Pediatr Hematol Oncol 2005; 27(11): 594–5.

139. Monterroso V, Jaffe ES, Merino MJ, Medeiros LJ. Malignant lymphomas involving the ovary. A clinicopathologic analysis of 39 cases. Am J Surg Pathol 1993; 17(2): 154–70.

140. Paladugu RR, Bearman RM, Rappaport H. Malignant lymphoma with primary manifestation in the gonad: a clinicopathologic study of 38 patients. Cancer 1980; 45: 561–71.

141. Shakfeh SM, Woodruff JD. Primary ovarian sarcomas: report of 46 cases and review of the literature. Obstet Gynecol Surv 1987; 42(6): 331–49.

142. Kefeli M, Kandemir B, Akpolat I, Yildirim A, Kokcu A. Rhabdomyosarcoma arising in a mature cystic teratoma with contralateral serous carcinoma: case report and review of the literature. Int J Gynecol Pathol 2009; 28: 372–5.

143. Cribbs RK, Shehata BM, Ricketts RR. Primary ovarian rhabdomyosarcoma in children. Pediatr Surg Int 2008; 24: 593–5.

144. Taskm S, Taskm EA, Uzum N, Ataoglu O, Ortac F. Primary ovarian leiomyosarcoma: a review of the clinical and immunohistochemical features of the rare tumor. Obstet Gynecol Surv 2007; 62(7): 480–6.

145. Arslan OS, Sumer C, Cihangiroglu G, Kanat-Pektas M, Gungor T. A rare tumor of the female genital tract: primary ovarian leiomyosarcoma. Arch Gynecol Obstet 2011; 283(Suppl 1): S83–5.

146. Hemal AK, Kumar R, Wadhwa SN. Carcinoma penis in a young boy. A case report. Indian J Cancer 1996; 33(2): 108–10.

147. Narasimharao KL, Chatterjee H, Veliath AJ. Penile carcinoma in the first decade of life. Br J Urol 1985; 57: 358.

148. Schelhammer PF, Jordan GH, Schlossberg SM. Tumors of the penis. In: Walsh PC, Retik AB, Stamey TA, Vaughan ED Jr (eds) *Campbell's Urology*. Philadelphia: WB Saunders, 1992. pp.1269–76.

149. Persky L. Epidemiology of cancer of the penis. Cancer Res 1977; 60: 97–109.

150. Bissada NK, Morcos RR, el-Senoussi M. Post circumcision carcinoma of the penis (clinical aspects). J Urol 1986; 135: 283–5.

151. Mohs FE, Snow SN, Larson PO. Mohs micrographic surgery for penile tumors. Urol Clin North Am 1992; 19(2): 291–304.

152. Dalkin B, Zaontz MR. Rhabdomyosarcoma of the penis in children. J Urol 1989; 141: 908–9.

153. Maresch R, Chiari H. Harnorgare mannliche Geschlechtsorgane Das Sarkom des Glides. In: Henke F, Lubarsch O (eds) *Handbuch der Speziellen Pathologischen Anatomic und Histologic*. Berlin: Springer-Verlag, 1931. p.369.

154. Ramos JZ, Pack GT. Primary embryonal rhabdomyosarcoma of the penis in a 2-year-old child. J Urol 1966; 96: 928–32.

155. Puhl H. Zur Kenntnis der Sarkome der Harnrohre (Mitteilungeines Falles von Myosarkom). Z Urol 1929; 23: 583.

156. Castellanos-Yodo U. Rhabdomyosarcoma primario del pene (relate de un cas). Arch Cuba Cancerol 1955; 14: 348.

157. Pak K, Sakaguchi N, Takayama H, Tomoyoshi T. Rhabdomyosarcoma of the penis. J Urol 1986; 136: 438–9.

158. Sandhu DPS, Munson KW, Benghiat A, Hopper IP. Natural history and prognosis of prostate carcinoma in adolescents and men under 35 years of age. Br J Urol 1992; 69: 525–9.

159. Shimada H, Misugi K, Sasaki Y, Iizuka A, Nishihira H. Carcinoma of the prostate in childhood and adolescence: report of a case and review of the literature. Cancer 1980; 46: 2534–42.

160. Briet S, Tremeaux JC, Piard F. Adenocarcinoma of the prostate in adolescents and young adults. Apropos of a case in a 20-year-old man. J Urol 1986; 92: 565–8.

161. Chiu CL, Weber DL. Prostatic carcinoma in young adults. JAMA 1974; 4: 724–6.

162. Connolly JA, Gearhart JP. Management of yolk sac tumors in children. Urol Clin North Am 1993; 20(1): 7–14.

163. Brosman SA. Testicular tumors in prepubertal children. Urology 1979; 13(6): 581–8.

164. Mostofi FK. Proceedings: Testicular tumors. Epidemiologic, etiologic, and pathologic features. Cancer 1973; 32(5): 1186–201.

165. Scully R. Gonadoblastoma: a review of 74 cases. Cancer 1970; 25: 1340.

166. Coppes MJ, Rackley R, Kay R. Primary testicular and paratesticular tumors in childhood. Med Pediatr Oncol 1994; 22: 329–40.

167. Hung W, Randolph JG, Chandra R, Belman AB. Gonadoblastoma in dysgenetic testis causing male pseudohermaphroditism in newborn. Urology 1981; 17: 584–7.

168. Viprakasit D, Navarro C, Guarin UK, Garnes HA. Seminoma in children. Urology 1977; 9: 568–70.

169. Albers P, Albrecht W, Algaba F, *et al.* EAU guidelines on testicular cancer: 2011 update. Eur Urol 2011; 60(2): 304–19.

170. Dehner L. Gonadal and extragonadal germ cell neoplasia of childhood. Hum Pathol 1983; 14: 493–511.

171. Dubois RS, Hoffman WH, Krishnan TH, *et al.* Feminizing sex-cord tumor with annular tubules in a boy with Peutz–Jeghers syndrome. J Pediatr 1982; 101: 568–71.

172. Cantú JM, Rivera H, Ocampo-Campos R, *et al.* Peutz–Jeghers syndrome with feminizing Sertoli cell tumor. Cancer 1980; 46: 223–8.

173. Sharma S, Seam RK, Kapoor HL. Malignant Sertoli cell tumor of the testis in a child. J Surg Oncol 1990; 44: 129–31.

174. Henley JD, Young RH, Ulbright TM. Malignant sertoli cell tumors of the testis: a study of 13 examples of a neoplasm frequently misinterpreted as seminoma. Am J Surg Pathol 2002; 26(5): 541–50.

175. Proppe K, Scully RE. Large-cell calcifying Sertoli cell tumor of the testis. Am J Clin Pathol 1980; 74: 607–19.

176. Kushner BH, Vogel R, Hajdu SI, Helson L. Metastatic neuroblastoma and testicular involvement. Cancer 1985; 56: 1730–2.

177. Sauter E, Schorin MA, Farr GH Jr, Falterman KW, Arensman RM. Wilms' tumor with metastasis to the left testis. Am Surg 1990; 56: 260–2.

178. Cortez JC, Kaplan GW. Gonadal stromal tumors, gonadoblastomas, epidermoid cysts, and secondary tumors of the testis in children. Urol Clin North Am 1993; 20(1): 15–26.

179. Trobs RB, Friedrich T, Lotz I, Bennek J. Wilms' tumour metastasis to the testis: long-term survival. Pediatr Surg Int 2002; 18(5–6): 541–2.

180. Gutjhar P, Humpl T. Testicular lymphoblastic leukemia/lymphoma. World J Urol 1995; 13: 230–2.

181. Finkelstein JZ, Miller DR, Feusner J, *et al.* Treatment of overt isolated testicular relapse in children on therapy for acute lymphoblastic leukemia – a report from the Children's Cancer Group. Cancer 1994; 73: 219–23.

182. Jaffe N, Buell D, Cassady JR, Traggis D, Weinstein H. Role of staging in childhood non-Hodgkin's lymphoma. Cancer Treat Res 1977; 61: 1001–7.

183. Al-Attar A, Pritchard J, Al-Saleem T, Al-Naimi M, Alash N, Attra A. Intensive chemotherapy for non-localized Burkitt's lymphoma. Arch Dis Child 1986; 61: 1013–19.

184. Kellie SJ, Pul CH, Murphy SB. Childhood non-Hodgkin's lymphoma involving the testis: clinical features and treatment outcome. J Clin Oncol 1989; 7(8): 1066–70.

185. Dalle JH, Mechinaud F, Michon J, *et al.* Testicular disease in childhood B-cell non-Hodgkin's lymphoma: the French Society of Pediatric Oncology experience. J Clin Oncol 2001; 19(9): 2397–403.

186. Groisman GM, Dische MR, Fine EM, Unger PD. Juvenile granulosa cell tumor of the testis: a comparative immunohistochemical study with normal infantile gonads. Pediatr Pathol 1993; 13: 389–400.

187. Shukla AR, Huff DS, Canning DA, *et al.* Juvenile granulosa cell tumor of the testis: contemporary clinical management and pathological diagnosis. J Urol 2004; 171(5): 1900–2.

188. Dieckmann KP, Loy V. Epidermoid cyst of the testis: a review of clinical and histogenetic considerations. Br J Urol 1994; 73(4): 436–41.

189. Malek RS, Rosen JS, Farrow GM. Epidermoid cyst of the testis: a critical analysis. Br J Urol 1986; 58: 55–9.

190. Price EB Jr. Epidermoid cysts of the testis: a clinical and pathologic analysis of 69 cases from the testicular tumor registry. J Urol 1969; 102: 708–13.

191. Ross JH, Kay R, Elder J. Testis sparing surgery for pediatric epidermoid cysts of the testis. J Urol 1993; 149(2): 353–6.

69 Uncommon Pediatric Brain Tumors

Robert C. Castellino,[1] Matthew Schniederjan,[2] and Tobey J. MacDonald[1]

[1] Pediatric Neuro-Oncology Program, Aflac Cancer Center and Blood Disorders Service, Children's Healthcare of Atlanta; Emory University School of Medicine, Emory Children's Center, Atlanta, GA, USA
[2] Department of Pathology, Children's Healthcare of Atlanta, Atlanta, GA, USA

Introduction

Brain tumors are the most common solid cancers of childhood. The subject of this chapter is those tumors which have been typically classified as "other" or that remain "unclassified" due to the relative rarity of each tumor type.

Angiocentric glioma

Clinical presentation

This entity was first described in 2005 and fewer than 40 cases have been documented, although the clinical and pathological findings are distinct and consistent enough to warrant recent inclusion into the World Health Organization (WHO) nomenclature. Along with ganglioglioma and dysembryoplastic neuroepithelial tumor, angiocentric glioma is a low-grade tumor strongly associated with long-standing, drug-resistant epilepsy. Only a small fraction (7%) have presented solely with headaches or visual disturbances and no seizures. Depending on location, some patients have also presented with focal deficits. The mean duration of symptoms prior to surgery is approximately 7 years.[1] Males and females are equally affected, with onset of seizures occurring typically in childhood or adolescence, but seizures may occur later, accounting for the broad age range at diagnosis (2–70 years, mean 16 years).[2–5]

Neuroimaging of angiocentric glioma shows a solitary, superficial, cortical area of T2/fluid-attenuated inversion recovery (FLAIR) hyperintensity that usually does not enhance with contrast administration. T1-weighted sequences may show a thin rim of cortical hyperintensity.[2,3] All reported cases have been supratentorial, except one case from the midbrain.[6] There is no obvious predilection for any specific lobe, as there is for temporal lobe in ganglioglioma.

Histopathology

The cells of this tumor are intermingled with brain parenchyma in an infiltrative pattern. Other areas may exhibit a more solid growth pattern but the lesion lacks the pushing border of many other low-grade neoplasms. Individual cells and fascicles stream through the affected area and orient around small and large blood vessels, radially, longitudinally, or concentrically. The radial arrays of tumor cells resemble the perivascular pseudorosettes in ependymomas and astroblastomas. Similar arrangements may be formed along the subpial surface, with the bipolar tumor cells either parallel or perpendicular to the pia. The tumor cells are uniform and mostly bipolar with cigar-shaped nuclei and thick glial cytoplasmic processes. A small nucleolus may be apparent. Some cells contain an eosinophilic structure within the cytoplasm that corresponds to microlumens seen by electron microscopy.[5] Glial fibrillary acidic protein (GFAP) is generally positive but can be variable or weak. Cytoplasmic microlumens appear as solid, round, or irregular points of reactivity on epithelial membrane antigen (EMA) staining. EMA also labels membranes and cytoplasm in an inconsistent manner. Proliferation rates, as measured by staining with a specific monoclonal antibody, called MIB1, against the protein Ki-67, in angiocentric glioma are generally very low, around 1–2%.[2]

Treatment and outcome

The vast majority of reported cases have maintained an indolent course, with documented long-term survival in all except for one case in which the onset of seizures was during adulthood and the patient subsequently died of progressive disease.[1] Most patients are cured of their epilepsy after removal of the tumor, unless it is subtotally resected. Although a small number of cases have received postoperative radiotherapy, because of the excellent results with gross total resection and the benign nature of this disease, postoperative radiotherapy or chemotherapy does not appear to be warranted.

Astroblastoma

Clinical presentation

This entity was first described by Bailey and Bucy in 1930 and to date, fewer than 100 reports have been described in the literature, many as single cases.[7] The precise definition and histogenesis of this tumor remain undecided. Astroblastoma is generally a neoplasm of childhood and early adulthood, with a mean age of 17 years from 51 patients in five series, although the distribution extends well into adulthood, up to 58 years.[8–12] Females account for most of the reported cases, with a ratio around 3:1. No familial predisposition or other disease associations have been described. Clinical symptoms depend on tumor location, size, and mass effect. Headache, focal deficits, nausea and vomiting, visual disturbances, and seizures are the most common presenting symptoms.

Magnetic resonance imaging (MRI) and computed tomography (CT) studies most often reveal a supratentorial mass that is calcified, well circumscribed, and heterogeneously enhancing.[12] The vast majority of cases have been in the cerebral hemispheres but rare examples have arisen elsewhere. An identifying feature of astroblastoma on postcontrast T1-weighted images is a "bubbly" appearance created by multiple intratumoral cysts.[12] The extent of surrounding edema is highly variable.

Histopathology

The exact histological criteria defining this entity are not universally agreed upon. The unifying feature of astroblastoma is perivascular pseudorosettes similar to those of ependymoma but with broad column-like foot processes extending out from the vessel surface. The perivascular cells in astroblastoma are distinct with well-defined cell borders, whereas the fibrillar processes in ependymoma overlap and obscure the intercellular borders. The stout bands of cytoplasm terminate in an uneven layer of nuclei that have little or no cytoplasm on their outer aspect. The other central features of astroblastoma are circumscription and vascular hyalinization. Histologically malignant features in astroblastoma include elevated mitotic rates, vascular proliferation, nuclear atypia and loss of architecture; however, the boundary between malignant and low-grade astroblastoma is not distinct and its refinement will require more experience with these lesions. Astroblastomas react with antibodies to S-100 protein, GFAP, and vimentin, although each may be only focal. Dot- and ring-like EMA reactivity, such as that seen in ependymomas, is not present in astroblastomas.

Treatment and outcome

The prognosis and optimal management for astroblastoma have yet to be established. Two general categories of histological aggressiveness are recognized: well differentiated and malignant. Gross total resection (GTR) is likely important for long-term progression-free survival for either histological type and is generally feasible in the majority of patients, even when very large, given the peripheral location and well-circumscribed nature of these tumors.[10,13] Subtotally resected tumors will typically be treated with postoperative irradiation, although clear evidence for radiation efficacy has yet to be established. In a metaanalysis of 116 patients, 5-year progression-free survival (PFS) in those who underwent GTR was 83% compared to 55% in those undergoing subtotal resection and postoperative radiotherapy, even after controlling for histological grade.[13] This analysis also demonstrated that 5-year PFS was not significantly different between those who underwent GTR alone (94%) and those who underwent GTR and radiation (73%).[13] In the recurrent setting of well-differentiated lesions, re-resection is advocated followed by radiotherapy.

Occasionally this tumor can behave aggressively, with short survival times observed, and because the natural course of this disease remains unclear, some will opt for radiotherapy after resection in all cases regardless of histological appearance and degree of resection. Although adjuvant chemotherapy with agents such as temozolomide has been employed in malignant-appearing tumors, no definitive results with chemotherapy are available.[10]

Atypical teratoid/rhabdoid tumor

Clinical presentation

Atypical teratoid/rhabdoid tumor (AT/RT) is a rare, highly malignant tumor that occurs in children and adults but has a predilection for infants under the age of 3 years. Rhabdoid tumors were first described as occurring in the kidney as a variant of Wilms tumor with poor prognosis.[14] Subsequent case reports identified rhabdoid tumors outside the kidney in soft tissues[15] and in the central nervous system (CNS).[16] CNS AT/RT was recognized as a distinct tumor type in 1996[17] and in 2000 was classified by the WHO as a grade IV neoplasm of the CNS.[18] AT/RTs also occur in the setting of the "familial rhabdoid tumor predisposition syndrome."[19] Rhabdoid tumor predisposition syndrome is a consequence of germline mutation in the *SMARCB1* (*INI1/hSNF5*) tumor suppressor gene on chromosome 22q11.2, causing a nonfunctioning allele. Patients bearing this germline mutation are prone to tumor formation when a somatic "second hit" occurs at the *SMARCB1* locus.

Studies from single institutions report prevalence for AT/RT tumors of 0.9–1.3% of all childhood brain tumors.[20,21] A population-based study recently published by the Austrian Brain Tumor Registry covering the period from 1996 to 2006 reports an age-standardized incidence rate of AT/RT of 1.38 per 1,000,000 person-years in children up to the age of 15.[22] However, in children under the age of 3, AT/RT was as common as supratentorial primitive neuroectodermal tumor (PNET) or medulloblastoma (17.3%, 16%, and 13.3%, respectively). Furthermore, 50% of AT/RT were misdiagnosed initially, which corresponded with a inferior 5-year overall survival (66.7% versus 15% 5-year overall survival of patients diagnosed initially versus those tumors reclassified as AT/RT).[22]

To date, only 31 cases of AT/RT in adults between the ages of 18 and 45 years old have been published.[23–27] In contrast with children in whom most AT/RTs arise in the ventricles or posterior fossa, most adult AT/RTs are found in the cerebral hemispheres. Adults with AT/RT have been considered to have a better overall survival, ranging from 1 to 30 months after diagnosis in the 11 cases with molecular and/or genetic verification of AT/RT by sequencing for loss or mutation of *SMARCB1*, fluorescent *in situ* hybridization (FISH) for *SMARCB1*, and/or immunohistochemistry (IHC) for absent INI1 staining.[23] It is unclear whether this may be due to the greater amenability to resection of cerebral AT/RTs in adults, more widespread use of radiation therapy in adults, or biological differences between AT/RT tumors in adults and children.

Since 50% of AT/RTs in children are located in the posterior fossa, they often present with symptoms that include early-morning headache, vomiting, lethargy, and ataxia. AT/RTs located above the tentorium, along the meninges, or along the spinal canal can present with other symptoms, including seizures, paraplegia, progressive neuropathy, or cranial nerve palsies. Median age at diagnosis is 24 months. Approximately 30% of patients are older than 3 years old at diagnosis.[28,29] Some studies have also noted a slight predominance of males diagnosed with AT/RT.[29,30]

Atypical teratoid/rhabdoid tumor may occur anywhere in the brain, with an approximately equal distribution between supratentorial and infratentorial compartments.[30–32] Cases occasionally arise within the spinal cord, probably at a rate consistent with the relative volume of the cord to the brain.[33] On MRI, AT/RT is generally circumscribed, with heterogeneous contrast enhancement and signal intensity, usually secondary to areas of hemorrhage and necrosis. Leptomeningeal spread is a common radiological finding, being present in approximately a fifth to a quarter of cases at diagnosis.[31]

Histopathology

Histological heterogeneity is characteristic of AT/RT, with neuroectodermal, mesenchymal, and, rarely, epithelial differentiation being evident. The neuroectodermal component can closely mimic medulloblastoma. Most AT/RTs are composed of sheets of pleomorphic cells that typically have large nuclei with open chromatin and prominent nucleoli, and a small to moderate amount of lightly eosinophilic cytoplasm. Most cases contain foci of cells with prominent cytoplasmic vacuoles. Many cases have at least focal rhabdoid morphology with eccentric smooth pink cytoplasmic inclusions that indent the nucleus.[17,34] These cytoplasmic inclusions are composed of whorled aggregates of intermediate filaments.[35] However, the presence of rhabdoid inclusions is not required for the diagnosis of AT/RT.

Atypical teratoid/rhabdoid tumor has a characteristically heterogeneous immunophenotype. Focal membranous and cytoplasmic staining for EMA is one of the most consistent features, with foci of smooth muscle actin (SMA), vimentin, cytokeratin, GFAP, synaptophysin, and neurofilament reactivity. Unlike other CNS neoplasms, AT/RTs demonstrate remarkable uniformity in genetic alterations of the *SMARCB1* locus

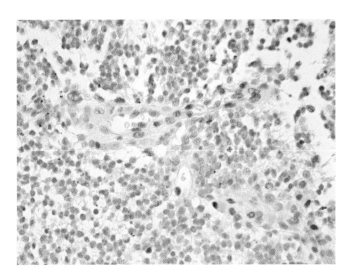

Figure 69.1 Atypical teratoid/rhabdoid tumor. Immunohistochemistry demonstrates loss of INI1 expression in tumor cells while native endothelial cells retain staining (brown) for INI1.

on chromosome 22q11.2.[36,37] Reported alterations include homo- and heterozygous deletions, loss of heterozygosity, and mutations of *SMARCB1*, especially in exons 5 or 9.[38,39] Since loss of expression or function of INI1 is thought to be a key molecular event in the formation of AT/RT, demonstration of its loss or mutation is a reliable way to diagnose AT/RT in patients who present with an embryonal brain tumor (Fig. 69.1). Use of FISH along with genomic sequencing permits identification of more than 75% of AT/RTs.[39,40] While there are embryonal brain tumors that exhibit histology consistent with AT/RT but positive immunohistochemical staining for the *SMARCB1* protein, INI1, these are considered even more rare and are thought to represent only 2% of all AT/RTs.[41] Choroid plexus carcinoma and CNS-PNET have previously been reported to lack INI1 reactivity. In one small series antisera to the tight junction protein claudin-6 reacted with seven of seven AT/RTs and no PNETs, offering an alternative to INI1/BAF47, although larger series are needed.[42]

Treatment and outcome

Atypical teratoid/rhabdoid tumor is an aggressive tumor that carries a poor overall prognosis. Published studies report a median survival from 8 to 17 months from diagnosis, despite treatment that includes maximal surgical resection, combination chemotherapy, with or without craniospinal irradiation. A recent study of 36 patients with AR/RT reported an 11% event-free and 17% overall survival of children under the age of 3, who comprised 71% of the study participants.[32] Two factors that have repeatedly been associated with a poor outcome are age less than 3 at diagnosis and presence of metastatic disease.[17,32] Conversely, maximal surgical resection has been strongly associated with increased survival.[30]

The role of conventional versus high-dose chemotherapy (HDC) with autologous stem cell rescue remains controversial. At least two published studies report a greater than 50% survival when patients with an AT/RT were treated with a carboplatin-thiotepa-based HDC regimen.[30,43] However, another study using a modified rhabdomyosarcoma-type IRS-III regimen along with intrathecal chemotherapy and either focal or craniospinal irradiation reports a 64% survival with a median follow-up of 1.7 years.[44] Also controversial are the role and timing of radiotherapy. Some clinicians consider radiotherapy as crucial to treatment of AT/RT[45] while others prefer to defer use of irradiation due to its potentially devastating side-effects on cognition when used in young children.[46] Data from St Jude Children's Hospital lend support to the early use of irradiation for AT/RT.[32] Overall, newer treatment regimens have improved the prognosis for survival from AT/RT and have led to a long-term cure in a minority of patients.[44]

Medulloepithelioma

Clinical presentation

As with other embryonal tumors, medulloepithelioma occurs most often in young children, typically between 6 months and 5 years of age, with an even distribution between females and males.[47] This rare PNET, which was first described by Bailey and Cushing in 1926, may arise anywhere in the neuraxis, and even peripherally in the orbit[48] and pelvis.[49] On imaging, medulloepitheliomas are noncontrast enhancing, hypo- to isointense on T1-weighted MRI, and hyperintense on T2.[48] They tend to be well circumscribed and only slightly heterogeneous. Symptoms and signs are related to the specific location of the tumor.

Histopathology

Medulloepithelioma is characterized by a "back-to-back" proliferation of tubular structures composed of pseudostratified columnar epithelium that resembles the primitive/embryonic neural tube (Fig. 69.2). These structures are also reminiscent of

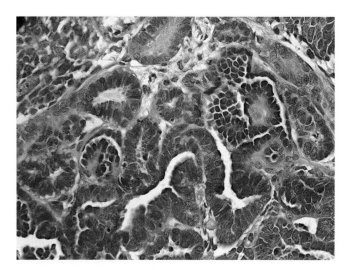

Figure 69.2 Medulloepithelioma. Hematoxylin and eosin staining reveals typical glandular structures in medulloepithelioma that resemble the embryonic neural tube.

the malignant glands of well-differentiated adenocarcinoma and, like that lesion, the columnar cells of medulloepithelioma rest on a shared basement membrane. Although tubules dominate the histological picture of this lesion, areas of undifferentiated proliferation are also seen. Tumor cells often lack significant pleomorphism and have a high nuclear to cytoplasmic ratio, with large, regular, elliptical nuclei that contain coarse, open chromatin and prominent, often multiple nucleoli. Mitoses are abundant. Medulloepitheliomas may show divergent differentiation into glial, neural, and mesenchymal lineages.[47,50–52] Care must be taken in the face of nonneuroepithelial differentiation that the lesion in question is not actually an immature teratoma. Reticulin staining and immunostaining for type IV collagen emphasize the shared basement membrane of tumor epithelium, as does periodic acid-Schiff (PAS) staining. Typical neuroepithelial markers, such as S-100, synaptophysin, and GFAP, are not expressed in the epithelial cells of medulloepithelioma, although they may be seen in nonepithelial areas.

Treatment and outcome

Unlike other PNETs, medulloepitheliomas have a dismal prognosis, with a reported median survival of 5 months and to date, only three of the 36 cases reported in the literature have documented survival longer than 5 years following treatment. In all three cases, patients underwent gross total surgical resection and had no evidence of tumor dissemination, including negative cerebrospinal fluid (CSF) cytology for malignant cells. In one of the three cases, craniospinal irradiation and multiagent systemic chemotherapy, similar to that administered for other cerebral PNETs, were employed while in another case only local stereotactic radiotherapy to 20 Gy was administered with equally good results.[53,54] For reasons that are not known, intraorbital medulloepithelioma appears to have an excellent prognosis, having relatively good long-term survival following simple enucleation.

Embryonal tumor with abundant neuropil and true rosettes

Clinical presentation

Embryonal tumor with abundant neuropil and true rosettes (ETANTR) was first described by Eberhart et al. in 2000, with fewer than 50 cases reported to date.[55–60] ETANTR occurs in young children, with a mean age of about 2 years, ranging up to 4 years, with a female predominance of around 2:1.[55] The most common MRI appearance is an heterogeneously enhancing, well-circumscribed, solid mass that arises within the supratentorial and infratentorial compartments.[55]

Histopathology

The histological appearance consists of islands of embryonal tumor cells in a sea of neuropil-like matrix, forming luminal or "ependymoblastic" rosettes (Fig. 69.3). The ependymoblastic rosettes appear in both the hypo- and hypercellular areas, and

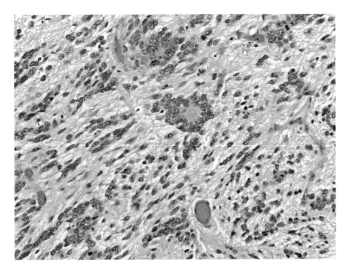

Figure 69.3 Embryonal tumor with abundant neuropil and true rosettes. Although hematoxylin and eosin staining demonstrates relatively low cellularity compared to other CNS malignancies, ETANTR is a highly aggressive embryonal tumor.

are formed of pseudostratified, elongated tumor cells arranged radially around a well-defined, round to slit-like lumen. Sometimes the lumen is rudimentary and contains small amounts of granular material. Similar to nodular medulloblastomas, ETANTR tumor cells show varying levels of differentiation, from embryonal within the areas of cellularity to neurocytic, and even occasionally ganglionic, within the hypocellular areas. Although the undifferentiated cells within the clusters generally fail to stain for neuronal or glial markers, NeuN, synaptophysin, and neurofilament staining can be strong within the more differentiated cells of the neuropil-like areas. GFAP stains scattered, entrapped astrocytes and the occasional tumor cell.

Treatment and outcome

The projected survival in patients with ETANTR is typically less than 1 year from diagnosis, although clinical outcome has been accurately documented in only seven cases to date, all aged less than 3 years and all without evidence of leptomeningeal dissemination at diagnosis. In six patients with subtotal surgical resection and aggressive adjuvant therapy with radiation and/or chemotherapy, only one was reported alive without disease 34 months after diagnosis following multiple resections and high-dose chemotherapy.[59] Of the 46 cases reported to date, the longest reported survival was 42 months.[61]

Pineoblastoma

Clinical presentation

Tumors that encompass the parenchyma of the pineal gland are rare entities, constituting less than 1% of primary CNS neoplasms and less than a third of pineal region tumors.[62,63] Pineoblastomas are primarily identified in childhood and early adulthood. Prevalence is the same in males and females. Pineal

parenchymal tumors can present with symptoms of acute obstructive hydrocephalus or Parinaud syndrome, an upward gaze paralysis with retraction nystagmus due to compression of the tectum. Rarely, it can present with spontaneous hemorrhage.[64]

Rarely, pineoblastoma can present in the context of germline mutation of the *RB1* gene. It is well known that tissues in the pineal gland and retina are developmentally related. Retinal and pineal photosensory cells are both derived from diverticles of the third ventricle of the diencephalon.[65] When pineoblastoma is identified synchronously with bilateral retinoblastoma, it is termed "trilateral retinoblastoma" and is associated with a significantly worse prognosis than those with a diagnosis of retinoblastoma alone.[66] Pineoblastoma has also rarely been reported in patients with a diagnosis of familial adenomatous polyposis.[67]

Histopathology

Pineoblastomas closely resemble other PNETs and consist of sheets of small and poorly differentiated embryonal cells, frequently with necrosis, numerous mitoses, and vascular proliferation. Some cases may have large angular cells with prominent nucleoli and other features of anaplasia, the significance of which is unknown. Both luminal (Flexner–Wintersteiner)[67] and fibrillary (Homer Wright)[68] rosettes sometimes appear. Pineoblastoma may also coexist with lower grade elements. Some pathologists have observed skeletal muscle, cartilage, and melanotic epithelia within pineoblastomas. These cases resemble similar lesions of the retina and are called pineal anlage tumors.[69,70] Endodermal structures in such a lesion are grounds for a diagnosis of immature teratoma. Although pineoblastomas are morphologically identical to PNETs in other locations, such as medulloblastoma or nonpineal supratentorial PNET (sPNET), and similarly have a tendency for CSF dissemination, they behave differently. In fact, pineoblastoma is distinguished from other PNETs more by its location than any morphological or immunohistochemical findings.

Treatment and outcome

Overall, age at diagnosis is a major factor in the outcome of treatment for pineoblastoma, with an abysmal progression-free (PFS) and overall survival (OS) in children age 3 and under at diagnosis. This is likely due to the decision of most oncologists to avoid radiation therapy in children less than 3 years old in order to avoid the substantial deleterious effects of ionizing radiation on the developing brain. The overall strategy in these patients has been to use chemotherapy until children are old and stable enough to receive radiation. Unfortunately, pineoblastoma carries a uniformly fatal prognosis in children under the age of 3 irrespective of whether they are treated with conventional or high-dose chemotherapy.

The best results to date come from the Head Start I and II trials where investigators reported a 5-year PFS of 15% in children with pineoblastoma versus 48% in children with nonpineal sPNET.[71] Interestingly, children over 3 years old with pineoblastoma tend to fare better than those with sPNET.

The best results reported to date come from the SIOP/UKCCSG PNET3 study in which children were treated with combination chemotherapy followed by craniospinal irradiation (CSI) and a boost to the primary site. The 5-year PFS was 92.9% for pineal tumors and 40.7% for nonpineal sPNETs. However, OS did not differ between the two groups. In the US, investigators of the CCG-99701 study, in which children older than 3 years received CSI with a primary site boost, daily carboplatin, and weekly vincristine, followed by six cycles of chemotherapy, report a 3-year PFS of 76% for pineoblastoma patients and 49% for patients diagnosed with a nonpineal sPNET.[71]

Choroid plexus carcinoma

Clinical presentation

Tumors of the choroid plexus constitute less than 0.5% of all primary CNS tumors. However, in children under the age of 2, they account for 12% of CNS tumors. Up to 20% of tumors of the choroid plexus are choroid plexus carcinomas and 70% of all choroid plexus carcinomas present in children under the age of 2.[72-74] The median age for all choroid plexus tumors was reported as 3.5 years with males and females equally represented in one extensive review.[75] Unlike lower WHO grade choroid plexus papillomas, which have a high cure rate after complete resection, choroid plexus carcinomas carry a dismal prognosis.[76] The most common presentation of choroid plexus carcinoma is with obstructive hydrocephalus due to intraventricular growth of the lesion. The most common location for a choroid plexus carcinoma is in the lateral ventricles.[75] Neuroimaging of choroid plexus neoplasms shows a solid, well-circumscribed, contrast-enhancing mass that is sometimes internally cystic. Choroid plexus carcinomas also tend to disseminate in the CSF.

Choroid plexus carcinomas have been noted to occur in the context of Li–Fraumeni syndrome, some with confirmed germline *TP53* mutations.[77,78] Although choroid plexus carcinoma is not particularly common among Li–Fraumeni-related cancers, it has been suggested that germline mutations of the *TP53* gene are common in children with choroid plexus carcinoma.

Histopathology

Choroid plexus carcinomas are proliferative, disorganized, and malignant. One study used four or more of the following criteria to diagnose a choroid plexus carcinoma: mitoses >5/10 high-power field (HPF), hypercellularity, necrosis, loss of papillary architecture, and pleomorphism.[79] Choroid plexus carcinomas usually develop *de novo* but can develop from a preexisting lower-grade choroid plexus papilloma. Choroid plexus carcinomas usually express cytokeratins and lack expression for prealbumin (transthyretin) and S-100, which are normally expressed in lower grade papillomas.[80,81] MIB1 staining measures 14% in most choroid plexus carcinomas.[82] Other markers of adenocarcinoma, such as BerEP4, TTF1, and CDX2, should be negative in choroid plexus carcinomas.[83]

Treatment and outcome

The primary treatment approach for a choroid plexus carcinoma is surgical resection, frequently along with chemotherapy. Extent of resection is one of the most important prognostic factors.[73,84] Historically, choroid plexus carcinomas have been reported to have a 5-year OS rate of around 30–35%, although long-term cures have been achieved after complete resection.[85] Due to the invasive nature and vascularity which can prevent gross total resection, some authors have suggested a two-stage surgical approach with an initial biopsy followed by neoadjuvant chemotherapy and definitive surgery. A retrospective analysis of 12 patients at the Hospital for Sick Children who failed an initial attempt at gross total resection reports that 11 of 12 were able to undergo a greater than 95% resection following four cycles of chemotherapy with ifosfamide, carboplatin, and etoposide (ICE). A median total of seven additional cycles of ICE chemotherapy was administered after second-look surgery. Eight patients survived at a median follow-up of 6.9 years. Interestingly, none received treatment with ionizing radiation but six of eight experienced significant neurocognitive and sensory deficits following treatment.[74]

Radiation therapy also seems to have benefit but its role in the treatment of choroid plexus carcinoma remains unclear.[86] A recent retrospective study analyzed the effects of radiotherapy in 56 patients diagnosed with choroid plexus carcinoma.[87] The median age of patients in the study was 2.7 years. The OS and PFS survival rates for the entire cohort were 59.5% and 37.2%, respectively. Gross total resection and CSI were the two factors that positively affected PFS. In fact, the 5-year PFS for patients who received CSI was 44.2% versus a PFS of 15.3% in those who only received involved field radiation.[87]

Desmoplastic infantile ganglioglioma/astrocytoma

Clinical presentation

Desmoplastic infantile ganglioglioma/astrocytoma (DAI/DIG) primarily presents in infants, with a mean and median age at presentation of 6 months[88,89] although more than 15 cases that presented later in childhood have been reported.[90,91] The male to female ratio is 1.5:1. Most patients who present beyond 6 months are male.[92] Infants classically present with a bulging fontanelle, increased head circumference, and stupor. MRI of the brain shows a large heterogeneous and partially cystic mass compressing a cerebral hemisphere and abutting the dura (Fig. 69.4). DAI/DIGs described to date have only been found above the tentorium. MRI reveals a superficial, contrast-enhancing, T1-isointense solid area and a central, cystic T2-hyperintense region. Imaging may also demonstrate edema, calcification, and bone remodeling.[93]

Histopathology

Most DAI/DIGs show two patterns of growth within the same lesion. The solid component of the mass near the skull consists of astroglia dispersed in a background of wavy dense collagen fibrils and spindle-shaped fibroblasts in a storiform pattern.[89]

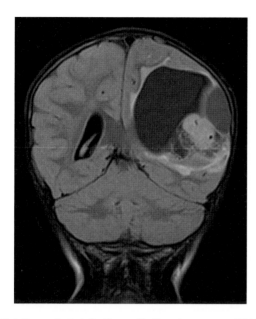

Figure 69.4 Desmoplastic infantile ganglioglioma/astrocytoma. FLAIR magnetic resonance imaging captures the typical imaging features of DIG: large, superficial, heterogeneous and cystic.

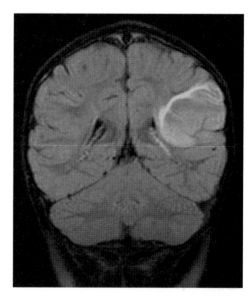

Figure 69.5 Dysembryoplastic neuroepithelial tumor. FLAIR magnetic resonance imaging demonstrates how DNET tends to expand the cortical ribbon without exerting significant mass effect.

The ratio of tumor cells to collagen can vary widely, even within the same tumor, with areas of sclerosis and hypocellularity in some portions of the tumor. Neurons, which are the sole difference between DAI and DIG, may be found in this component, most often as small polygonal cells with little obvious neuronal differentiation and less often as overt ganglion cells. Collagen fibrils are intimately deposited between tumor cells and can be clearly displayed by reticulin staining. An immature or embryonal component is usually present focally, composed of small basophilic cells with scant cytoplasm and little morphological differentiation. This component lacks a dense collagen background and occasionally contains mitoses and necrosis that are worrisome for but not indicative of a more aggressive neoplasm. These hypercellular areas do not have clear prognostic significance.[160,161]

Although DAI/DIGs are typically well circumscribed, they frequently invade surroundings tissues along perivascular spaces. Staining for GFAP helps to expose subtle astrocytes embedded in a desmoplastic background. Because H&E staining may also fail to show clear neuronal differentiation, staining for synaptophysin can reveal neoplastic neurons. MIB1 labeling is generally seen in 5% or fewer tumor nuclei. Instances of aggressive DAI/DIG with high MIB1 rates and metastases have been reported.[160,161]

Treatment and outcome

Gross total resection is the treatment of choice for DAI/DIG. When achievable, GTR is the only required treatment. Re-resection should be attempted in cases of tumor recurrence. According to published literature, only 56% of patients are able to experience GTR. Nevertheless, one group has reported spontaneous regression in two infants who only had subtotal resection of their tumors. The main obstacles to complete resection are deep location of tumors, bilateral tumor extension, and significant tumor-associated vasculature. To date, only 11 patients have been treated with chemotherapy and 12 with radiotherapy for DAI/DIGs that were not amenable to surgical resection, with mixed results overall.[94] However, patients with gross total and incomplete tumor resection can both expect long-term cure.

Dysembryoplastic neuroepithelial tumor

Clinical presentation

Dysembryoplastic neuroepithelial tumor (DNET) is a low-grade tumor that is strongly associated with intractable partial seizures. It was first identified in temporal lobe specimens removed for seizure control.[95] Most patients present with a long history of refractory epilepsy beginning in childhood but can have onset well into adulthood. DNETs are classically supratentorial, located within the mesial cortex of the temporal lobe. However, they can be located in other areas of cortex and ventricles, in the cerebellum, or the brainstem.[96–99] On MRI, DNETs expand the cortex without mass effect or edema (Fig. 69.5). Multiple small cystic or pseudocystic structures may be present. T1-weighted MRI shows hypo- or isointensity, while T2-weighted images are hyperintense. DNETs do not usually enhance with contrast. CT examination often shows evidence of tumor-associated calcification.[100]

Histopathology

The pathognomonic lesion of DNET is the specific glioneuronal element, an arrangement of axons clustered in columns perpendicular to the cortical surface and flanked by oligodendroglia-like cells and microcystic pools of acidic mucopolysaccharide material. The microcysts occasionally contain "floating neurons," a unique characteristic of DNET.[95] The specific glioneuronal element also contains "glial nodules" that project a multinodular appearance. Microvascular proliferation, necrosis, rare mitoses, and nuclear atypia can all be seen but have no impact on tumor prognosis.[101] The vascular proliferation can form glomeruloid structures or long arcing rims of redundant vessels. Some reports have identified findings consistent with cortical dysplasia in brain adjacent to lesions of DNET.[102,103] Immunohistochemical analysis of DNET reveals oligodendroglia-like cells that stain positively for S-100 but are only sporadically positive for synaptophysin, neurofilament, and class III β-tubulin.[104] One study reports that 70% of DNETs stain positively for the antiapoptotic proteins BCL-2 and BCL-X.[105] MIB1 may be the most useful antibody in distinguishing DNET, with a rate below 1% in most cases.[106]

Treatment and outcome

Gross total resection is the treatment of choice for DNET. Published series have reported that three-quarters of those treated with surgery achieve control of epilepsy. Tumor recurrence after partial or total resection is rare. Total resection may give a more favorable long-term outcome. Postoperative malignant transformation has been reported to be very rare, with only three cases described in the literature. In two cases, adjuvant treatment consisted of radiation and chemotherapy, whereas in one patient there was no adjuvant treatment. Treatment with chemotherapy and/or ionizing radiation does not seem to affect tumor progression or recurrence.[107]

Myxopapillary ependymoma

Clinical presentation

Myxopapillary ependymomas have a preferential localization to the region of the cauda equina, where they often arise from the filum terminale (Fig. 69.6). Rarely, they occur in other CNS locations and can also present as sacrococcygeal tumors involving subcutaneous soft tissue. Myxopapillary ependymomas occur in young adults (mean age 36 years) and in males more than females. Tumors generally grow as circumscribed, sausage-shaped masses extending down from the cauda equina and filling the intradural sac. They present clinically with low back pain and lower extremity symptoms, including sensory changes and motor deficits. Back stiffness and bladder dysfunction may also be observed at presentation. Almost all children present with lumbar, sacral, or radicular pain.[108]

Histopathology

Histologically, these tumors are commonly not papillary but have a microcystic appearance with numerous pools of mucinous material among a monomorphic population of fibrillar glial cells and thickly hyalinized blood vessels. True to their name, myxopapillary ependymomas may be composed of fibrillar cuboidal-to-columnar cells surrounding a central vessel and connective tissue stroma, giving a distinctly papil-

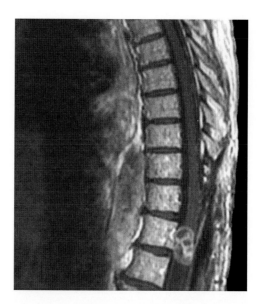

Figure 69.6 Myxopapillary ependymoma. A representative T2-weighted magnetic resonance image shows the usual location of myxopapillary ependymomas at the L1-L2 level of the conus medullaris.

lary architecture. One reliable but not always seen feature is the presence of a rim of hyaline or mucin surrounding the central blood vessel and separating it from the circumferential ependymal tumor cells. The resulting distinctive histology of myxopapillary ependymoma comes from this pattern of degenerative, myxoid change and the production of mucin by tumor cells. Occasionally, the hyaline deposition around blood vessels almost completely replaces the original lesion, leaving little recognizable as myxopapillary ependymoma. Like more typical ependymomas, the myxopapillary type is positive for GFAP, S-100 protein, vimentin, and CD99. No histological criteria for predicting metastatic or locally aggressive behavior of these lesions exist.

Treatment and outcome

Because of the rarity of this tumor, therapeutic guidelines have not been established. Although metastases from such lesions are reported,[109–112] the prognosis for patients with these tumors is generally quite good following complete resection. The overall survival is approximately 94%.[108] For this reason, myxopapillary ependymomas are designated as WHO grade I. Children, however, appear to have a clinically more aggressive course, with a much higher rate of local recurrence and dissemination within the neuraxis compared to that observed in adults (64% versus 32%).[108] GTR is associated with favorable outcome in both adults and children, although recurrence rates of 10–20% have been reported even after GTR.[108] The majority of cases not involving the conus medullaris or cauda equina are amenable to complete resection but only about 10% of the cases involving the conus can be completely removed.[113] In children, about 8–12% of the cases will have conus involvement and in these children, disease-free progression has been reported to be as low as 20%.[108] There is no proven benefit of radiotherapy or chemotherapy following complete resection in children; however, subtotally resected tumors are generally treated with local, whole spine, or craniospinal irradiation. Locally recurrent tumors may be re-resected without further therapy if there is no residual or disseminated disease. Postoperative neurological impairment, notably bladder dysfunction, may be seen in up to 25% of patients, especially those with unencapsulated tumors, and may be irreversible. Other postoperative complications such as tethered cord and paraplegia may also be observed.[113]

Pilomyxoid astrocytoma

Clinical presentation

Pilomyxoid astrocytomas (PMA), which are distinct from pilocytic astrocytomas (PAs), are most common in the first 3 years of life, with a mean age of 18 months at diagnosis (versus mean age of 58 months for PA). Like PAs, PMAs occur in progressively lower frequencies as age increases.[114] Rare examples have been described in adults.[115,116] Most cases are centered in the chiasmatic/hypothalamic area but pilomyxoid astrocytoma can be found anywhere in the neuraxis. Several cases from the spinal cord have been described.[116,117] Symptoms are typically related to increased intracranial pressure, including failure to thrive, developmental delay, altered consciousness, vomiting, feeding difficulties, and generalized weakness. Focal deficits related to vision or hypothalamic function may also be observed. In infants, enlarged head circumference or bulging fontanelle may be observed. Neuroimaging is similar between pilocytic and pilomyxoid astrocytomas.[118]

Histopathology

This tumor is architecturally monomorphic, lacking the densely fibrillar element and biphasic appearance of classic pilocytic astrocytoma, instead demonstrating a loose myxoid pattern throughout. Although classic pilocytic astrocytoma can be monomorphically myxoid, pilomyxoid astrocytoma has a distinctive perivascular orientation of tumor cells, similar to the perivascular pseudorosettes of ependymomas (Fig. 69.7). Rosenthal fibers are lacking but rare eosinophilic granular bodies (EGBs) are allowable.[119] Infiltration of surrounding tissue is limited but reported to exceed that of classic pilocytic astrocytoma.[120] For a diagnosis of pilomyxoid astrocytoma, the vast majority of the tumor should show typical pilomyxoid features.

Treatment and outcome

Compared to pilocytic astrocytomas, pilomyxoid lesions are more aggressive, having an increased local recurrence rate (50% versus 76%, respectively) and higher CSF dissemination rate. Currently, there are no specific treatment guidelines for PMA and most are treated identically to classic PAs with conventional chemotherapy regimens for low-grade gliomas (e.g. carboplatin and vincristine). Similar to metastatic PA, disseminated PMA may be treated with focal or craniospinal irradiation. Initial reports suggested that PMAs have a lower

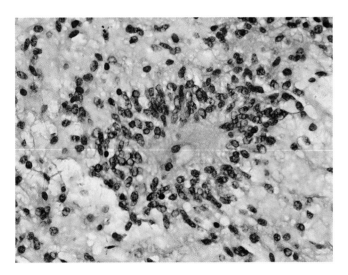

Figure 69.7 Pilomyxoid astrocytoma. Hematoxylin and eosin staining reveals perivascular orientation of tumor cells amid a uniformally myxoid background.

rate of survival compared to PAs,[119] even when controlling for the effect of location and age.[114,121]

Primary melanocytic neoplasms

Melanocytic lesions in the CNS arise in the meninges from meningeal melanocytes. Primary CNS melanocytic neoplasms are unusual and account for less than 1% of all primary intracranial tumors. Tumors can be grouped into three categories: melanocytosis, melanocytoma, and primary CNS melanoma.

Congenital melanocytosis (neurocutaneous melanosis)

Clinical presentation

Melanocytosis occurs almost exclusively in the context of an inherited phakomatosis, neurocutaneous melanosis, a syndrome with giant or multiple large hairy congenital nevi with diffuse meningeal melanocytosis or melanomatosis.[122] During normal embryonic development, melanoblasts migrate from the neural crest along the leptomeninges and eventually to the skin. Aberrant migration may lead to the deposition of melanocytes along the leptomeninges, resulting in neurocutaneous melanosis. Even controlled proliferation of benign melanocytes along the leptomeninges can result in symptoms of increased intracranial pressure.[123] Neurocutaneous melanosis is usually diagnosed before the age of 2. Patients present with large hairy nevi and can either be asymptomatic or exhibit variably severe, progressive neurological symptoms such as hydrocephalus, seizures, ataxia, or cranial nerve deficits. In two prospective cohort studies, approximately 7% of children with large congenital melanocytic nevi developed neurocutaneous melanosis. No patients in the cohort developed cutaneous melanoma. The 5-year cumulative risk of developing malignant melanoma was 2.3% and for neurocutaneous melanoma was 2.5%.[123] There is no gender or racial predilection.[122,124] Brain MRI reveals meningeal thickening with bright homogeneous enhancement and adjacent T2 hyperintensity due to edema.

Histopathology

Melanocytosis is characterized by a monotonous population of cells that can be spindled, oval, or polygonal.[122] Tumor cells fill and expand the subarachnoid space and track down the cortical perivascular spaces. This should not be misidentified as true parenchymal invasion. Nuclear atypia, mitoses, necrosis, large or multiple nucleoli and invasion of neuropil all suggest malignant transformation. Pigment deposition is variable from scant to extremely heavy with numerous melanophages.

Treatment and outcome

Even in patients with benign CNS melanocytosis, the outlook is grim, with a median survival of less than 3 years from presentation. Chemotherapy and radiation fail to significantly alter the course of disease.[124]

Melanocytoma

Clinical presentation

Melanocytomas present at a median age of 56, although the range of ages is wide.[125] There are more cases reported in females than males. Melanocytomas present with symptoms similar to those of meningioma. When pigmented, melanocytomas are identifiable on MRI by their singularly bright T1 hyperintensity and T2 hypointensity.[126] Lesions are usually found in the posterior fossa, brainstem, or spinal cord, since most meningeal melanocytes can be identified in these same locations.

Histopathology

Melanocytomas are derived from leptomeningeal melanocytes.[127] Melanocytomas contain mildly spindled cells with oval to elongate grooved nuclei arranged into small sheets and variably dense clusters. A minority of melanocytomas exhibit epithelioid features.[125] Clusters of cells can mimic the appearance of meningothelial whorls. Nuclear atypia, mitoses, necrosis, large or multiple nucleoli and invasion of neuropil all suggest malignant transformation; although ≤1/10 Hpf mitotic figures are allowed.[125]

Treatment and outcome

Although few cases exist in the literature, survival without recurrence for melanocytomas is typical, even following incomplete resection.[125] However, these tumors can recur locally and should be followed closely after surgical resection.

Melanoma

Clinical presentation

Primary CNS melanoma is a rare and aggressive tumor that accounts for 1% of all cases of melanoma. Age and anatomical distribution of CNS melanomas mirror that of melanocytomas.

Histopathology

Primary CNS melanoma resembles cutaneous melanoma. Melanomas exhibit more anaplastic nuclei, have a higher cell density than melanocytoma, and often demonstrate tissue invasion and necrosis. With occult noncutaneous primary sites, it can be difficult to prove that a CNS lesion is not metastatic from a cutaneous lesion. Immunohistochemistry in primary CNS melanocytic lesions follows that of extracranial cases, with immunoreactivity for S-100, HMB-45, tyrosinase (MART-1), and microphthalmia transcription factor (MITF).

Treatment and outcome

Primary CNS melanomas tend to be aggressive and frequently fatal, regardless of their clinical management.[125]

Pleomorphic xanthoastrocytoma

Clinical presentation

Pleomorphic xanthoastrocytoma (PXA) is an uncommon low-grade glial neoplasm primarily affecting children and young adults. PXA is most common in the first three decades of life but 40% of cases occur after the age of 25 years.[128] Males and females are equally affected. Most present with a long-term history of intractable seizures. Fifty percent of PXAs arise within the temporal lobe; another 40% occur elsewhere in the cerebral hemispheres. The tumor maintains a superficial cortical position, often abutting and extending into the leptomeninges. Around 8% of PXAs arise within the cerebellum.[129] MRI shows a circumscribed tumor that is isointense to gray matter on T1-weighted sequences, mildly hyperintense on T2, and intensely contrast enhancing.[130] The pattern of contrast enhancement is typically heterogeneous within the solid tumor. Most contain cystic areas that form the "cyst with mural nodule" configuration.

Histopathology

Pleomorphic xanthoastrocytoma can be described as a circumscribed astrocytoma with pleomorphic large cells and multinucleate giant cells on a background of tumor cells that tend to be elongated and arranged in fascicles. Evidence of vascular proliferation and calcification is uncommon. Increased mitoses (>5/10 HPF) or necrosis are each sufficient to warrant a diagnosis of "pleomorphic xanthoastrocytoma with anaplastic features," which is associated with an increased rate of recurrence.[128]

Dense cellularity and pleomorphism typical of PXA should bring ganglioglioma, glioblastoma (GBM), giant cell glioblastoma (gcGBM), gliosarcoma, and pleomorphic sarcoma into the differential diagnosis. The presence of eosinophilic granular bodies and compact architecture should also introduce pilocytic astrocytoma into the differential diagnosis.[131] PXA overlaps with ganglioglioma in location, age distribution, clinical presentation, and imaging features. Both tumors have similar architecture, reticulin background, protein aggregates, and perivascular lymphocytes. As in ganglioglioma and pilocytic astrocytoma, most PXAs contain varying forms of protein aggregates. Reticulin staining marks the basal lamina that surrounds individual cells in PXA and distinguishes it from the giant cell pattern of glioblastoma.

The immunophenotype of PXA generally follows expectations for an astrocytic neoplasm, with diffuse positivity for

S-100 and GFAP. Most PXAs stain negatively for the neuronal markers synaptophysin, neurofilament, and microtubule-associated protein 2 (MAP2).[132] Class III β-tubulin immunopositivity is seen in most PXAs.[133] MIB1/Ki-67 labeling indices are generally below 3%. The hallmarks of PXA that are not seen in giant cell glioblastoma include a fascicular architecture, EGBs, and extensive intercellular reticulin deposition. TP53 is expressed diffusely in the majority of giant cell glioblastomas and only focally in a minority of PXA. Neuronal markers, except class III β-tubulin, are also more restricted to PXA.[134] A recent study identified BRAF V600E mutations in 12 of 20 (60%) PXAs and increased expression of phospho-ERK was detected in all PXAs independent of the BRAF mutation status. BRAF V600E mutations were identified in only two of 71 (2.8%) GBMs, including one of nine (11.1%) gcGBMs.[131]

Treatment and outcome

The principal treatment for PXA is surgical resection followed by close monitoring with MRI. Overall survival is 80% at 5 years and 70% at 10 years. However, the recurrence rate following surgery is 30% at 5 years and 40% at 10 years. But, many cases in the literature also received radiation and chemotherapy in varying doses and regimens. One group identified extent of surgical resection as the single most important factor in progression-free survival, with atypical mitoses and ≥5 mitoses/10 HPF also significantly correlated in a univariate analysis.[128] Overall survival was not associated with totality of resection but mitotic index of ≥5 mitoses/10 Hpf correlated with deaths, as did necrosis and atypical mitoses to a lesser extent.[128] Recurrent lesions or tumors that demonstrate anaplastic features at primary resection are treated with radiation[135] and chemotherapeutic protocols[128,136] that are also used to treat anaplastic astrocytoma and glioblastoma.

Rosette-forming glioneuronal tumor (of the fourth ventricle)

Clinical presentation

This entity is named for the location in which all cases of it had originally occurred, until it was found elsewhere, specifically the chiasm, spinal cord, and cerebellum.[137–139] Although fewer than 50 cases have been reported, most of those have occurred within the second to fourth decades of life with no significant sex predilection. Headache and ataxia, along with other symptoms of increased intracranial pressure, are common in rosette-forming glioneuronal tumor (RGNT) due to obstruction of the cerebral aqueduct, and are seen in about half of reported cases. However, the onset of symptoms is slow, often lasting for months before the mass lesion is discovered. MRI typically shows a solid and partially cystic circumscribed midline mass that is hyperintense on T2 sequences and hypointense on T1. Administration of contrast material shows at least focal nodular enhancement in most cases.[140] Calcification is present in about half of reported cases.

Histopathology

Although distinct, RGNT shares some features with DNET and may represent a category of extracortical DNET. The major cellular component is monotonous with small, round, hyperchromatic nuclei and scant fibrillar cytoplasm. These cells line areas of granular fibrillarity that form columns, perivascular pseudorosettes, and small fibrillar rosettes in a background of myxoid material. Like pilocytic astrocytomas and DNET, the cells can also grow in sheets of oligodendroglia-like cells and form mucinous microcysts with "floating neurons." Immunohistochemistry shows synaptophysin reactivity around vessels and within rosettes and diffuse GFAP staining among more piloid astroglial cells. A MIB1 proliferation index should be below 2–3%.

Treatment and outcome

In keeping with the histologically low-grade appearance of this lesion, RGNT has been treated primarily by surgical resection. Many patients with RGNT have had lasting neurological deficits after treatment but this may reflect attempts at aggressive surgical resection in and around the fourth ventricle.[141] Almost all RGNTs do not recur following complete resection but there is a low rate of progression following subtotal resection or biopsy alone. In one report, only one case out of 35 (2.9%) with follow-up recurred 10 years after surgery.[142] Reports of stable unresected satellite lesions following 2-year follow-up suggest that biopsy alone to confirm the diagnosis or limited resection to alleviate symptoms may be all that is indicated for the treatment of these tumors.[141] Postoperative morbidity most commonly reported has been ataxia and cranial nerve palsies in up to 20% of patients. Thus, care should be taken in limiting resection of these benign tumors to avoid morbidity. Radiation and chemotherapy have no proven benefit.

Subependymal giant cell astrocytoma

Clinical presentation

Few primary CNS neoplasms originate in a more stereotyped clinical setting than the subependymal giant cell astrocytoma (SEGA). The vast majority of SEGAs are thought to occur in the context of tuberous sclerosis[143] but because of variable penetrance, many SEGA patients will not show clinically apparent signs of the syndrome (facial angiofibromas, cortical tubers, intractable seizures, subungual fibromas, "ash-leaf spots" and shagreen patches) until later, if at all.[144,145] The age at tumor diagnosis extends from congenital[146] to 75 years[147] but most cases present in the first two decades. Males and females are affected at similar rates. Almost all SEGAs occur in the lateral or third ventricles, with a large majority of those centered near the foramina of Monro (Fig. 69.8). Because of the proximity to this conduit of CSF flow, some patients will present with signs and symptoms of CSF obstruction, but onset of seizures may also precipitate the discovery of SEGA. CT shows a partially calcified nodule on the medial wall of the lateral ventricle that is T1 isointense and T2 hyperintense by

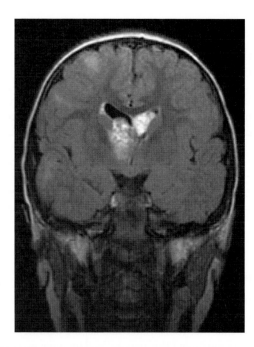

Figure 69.8 Subependymal giant cell astrocytoma. Magnetic resonance imaging of a SEGA in a typical location in the lateral ventricles, centered near the foramen of Monro.

MR.[148] Contrast material intensely enhances the lesion. Other findings may include smaller subependymal nodules ("candle gutterings"), cortical tubers and curvilinear white matter abnormalities.[149]

Histopathology

Sheet-like growth of large polygonal cells is seen in most cases of SEGA. The cells are large with eccentric, smooth, eosinophilic cytoplasm and one or two neuron-like nuclei with open chromatin and prominent central nucleoli. Although SEGA contains rather large cells, truly giant cells are an uncommon component. Microcalcifications are common and can occasionally overshadow the tumor cells but are not present in a minority of cases.[150] Mitoses and necrosis have been described in cases with benign courses, suggesting that they are not worrisome observations.[151]

Most SEGAs express both glial and neuronal antigens, with varying mixtures of GFAP, S-100, neurofilament, class III β-tubulin, synaptophysin, neuron-specific enolase, and MAP2 in most examples.[150,152] This biphenotypic profile, supported by ultrastructural evidence, has led to a gradual, though incomplete, reclassification of this tumor as glioneuronal in nature.[150] The other tumors seen in the tuberous sclerosis complex, such as renal angiomyolipoma and cardiac rhabdomyoma, react with the monoclonal antibody HMB45 but this characteristic is not seen in SEGA.[144,153]

Treatment and outcome

Treatment consists of gross total resection in symptomatic cases, or when a lesion progresses during surveillance.[154] Rates of growth following complete resection are low, making

surgery a successful and permanent therapeutic modality. Resected cases, however, are only seen in less than 10–20% of tuberous sclerosis (TS) patients.[143,155] For inoperable tumors or those displaying continued growth, treatment with conformal or gamma-knife irradiation may be warranted. More recently, administration of an inhibitor of the mammalian target of rapamycin (mTOR), the primary growth-promoting pathway perturbed in TS, has been shown to be efficacious. Rapamycin and rapamycin analogs such as everolimus that inhibit mTOR have been reported to cause regression in up to 70% of SEGA tumors and may offer a lower risk alternative to surgical intervention and irradiation.[156–158] Medical treatment with mTOR inhibitors may also lower the seizure burden and treat other TS-associated lesions; however, therapy with mTOR inhibitors carries additional risks of immunosuppression and hypercholesterolemia, and may need to be given chronically.[159] The full benefits and risks of this treatment have yet to be determined.

References

1. Mott RT, Ellis TL, Geisinger KR. Angiocentric glioma: a case report and review of the literature. Diagn Cytopathol 2010; 38: 452–6.
2. Lellouch-Tubiana A, Boddaert N, Bourgeois M, *et al.* Angiocentric neuroepithelial tumor (ANET): a new epilepsy-related clinicopathological entity with distinctive MRI. Brain Pathol 2005; 15: 281–6.
3. Preusser M, Hoischen A, Novak K, *et al.* Angiocentric glioma: report of clinico-pathologic and genetic findings in 8 cases. Am J Surg Pathol 2007; 31: 1709–18.
4. Shakur SF, McGirt MJ, Johnson MW, *et al.* Angiocentric glioma: a case series. J Neurosurg Pediatr 2009; 3: 197–202.
5. Wang M, Tihan T, Rojiani AM, *et al.* Monomorphous angiocentric glioma: a distinctive epileptogenic neoplasm with features of infiltrating astrocytoma and ependymoma. J Neuropathol Exp Neurol 2005; 64: 875–81.
6. Covington DB, Rosenblum MK, Brathwaite CD, Sandberg DI. Angiocentric glioma-like tumor of the midbrain. Pediatr Neurosurg 2009; 45: 429–33.
7. Bailey P, Bucy PC. Astroblastomas of the brain. Acta Psychiatr Neurol 1930; 5: 439–61.
8. Thiessen B, Finlay J, Kulkarni R, Rosenblum MK. Astroblastoma: does histology predict biologic behavior? J Neurooncol 1998; 40: 59–65.
9. Bonnin JM, Rubinstein LJ. Astroblastomas: a pathological study of 23 tumors, with a postoperative follow-up in 13 patients. Neurosurgery 1989; 25: 6–13.
10. Brat DJ, Hirose Y, Cohen KJ, Feuerstein BG, Burger PC. Astroblastoma: clinicopathologic features and chromosomal abnormalities defined by comparative genomic hybridization. Brain Pathol 2000; 10: 342–52.
11. Salvati M, d'Elia A, Brogna C, *et al.* Cerebral astroblastoma: analysis of six cases and critical review of treatment options. J Neurooncol 2009; 93: 369–78.
12. Bell JW, Osborn AG, Salzman KL, Blaser SI, Jones BV, Chin SS. Neuroradiologic characteristics of astroblastoma. Neuroradiology 2007; 49: 203–9.
13. Sughrue ME, Choi J, Rutkowski MJ, *et al.* Clinical features and postsurgical outcome of patients with astroblastoma. J Clin Neurosci 2011; 18: 750–4.
14. Beckwith JB, Palmer NF. Histopathology and prognosis of Wilms tumors: results from the First National Wilms' Tumor Study. Cancer 1978; 41: 1937–48.
15. Lynch HT, Shurin SB, Dahms BB, Izant RJ Jr, Lynch J, Danes BS. Paravertebral malignant rhabdoid tumor in infancy. In vitro studies of a familial tumor. Cancer 1983; 52: 290–6.

16. Bonnin JM, Rubinstein LJ, Palmer NF, Beckwith JB. The association of embryonal tumors originating in the kidney and in the brain. A report of seven cases. Cancer 1984; 54: 2137–46.

17. Rorke LB, Packer RJ, Biegel JA. Central nervous system atypical teratoid/rhabdoid tumors of infancy and childhood: definition of an entity. J Neurosurg 1996; 85: 56–65.

18. Fritz A, Percy C, Jack A, et al. International Classification of Diseases for Oncology, 3rd edn. Geneva: World Health Organization, 2000.

19. Sevenet N, Sheridan E, Amram D, Schneider P, Handgretinger R, Delattre O. Constitutional mutations of the hSNF5/INI1 gene predispose to a variety of cancers. Am J Hum Genet 1999; 65: 1342–8.

20. Rickert CH, Paulus W. Epidemiology of central nervous system tumors in childhood and adolescence based on the new WHO classification. Childs Nerv Syst 2001; 17: 503–11.

21. Kaderali Z, Lamberti-Pasculli M, Rutka JT. The changing epidemiology of paediatric brain tumours: a review from the Hospital for Sick Children. Childs Nerv Syst 2009; 25: 787–93.

22. Woehrer A, Slavc I, Waldhoer T, et al. Incidence of atypical teratoid/rhabdoid tumors in children: a population-based study by the Austrian Brain Tumor Registry, 1996–2006. Cancer 2010; 116: 5725–32.

23. Samaras V, Stamatelli A, Samaras E, et al. Atypical teratoid/rhabdoid tumor of the central nervous system in an 18-year-old patient. Clin Neuropathol 2009; 28: 1–10.

24. Ingold B, Moschopulos M, Hutter G, et al. Abdominal seeding of an atypical teratoid/rhabdoid tumor of the pineal gland along a ventriculo-peritoneal shunt catheter. Acta Neuropathol 2006; 111: 56–9.

25. Arita K, Sugiyama K, Sano T, Oka H. Atypical teratoid/rhabdoid tumour in sella turcica in an adult. Acta Neurochir (Wien) 2008; 150: 491–5; discussion 496.

26. Takei H, Adesina AM, Mehta V, Powell SZ, Langford LA. Atypical teratoid/rhabdoid tumor of the pineal region in an adult. J Neurosurg 2010; 113: 374–9.

27. Takahashi K, Nishihara H, Katoh M, et al. A case of atypical teratoid/rhabdoid tumor in an adult, with long survival. Brain Tumor Pathol 2011; 28: 71–6.

28. Cohn RD, Frank Y, Stanek AE, Kalina P. Malignant rhabdoid tumor of the brain and kidney in a child: clinical and pathologic features. Pediatr Neurol 1995; 13: 65–8.

29. Athale UH, Duckworth J, Odame I, Barr R. Childhood atypical teratoid rhabdoid tumor of the central nervous system: a meta-analysis of observational studies. J Pediatr Hematol Oncol 2009; 31: 651–63.

30. Hilden JM, Meerbaum S, Burger P, et al. Central nervous system atypical teratoid/rhabdoid tumor: results of therapy in children enrolled in a registry. J Clin Oncol 2004; 22: 2877–84.

31. Meyers SP, Khademian ZP, Biegel JA, Chuang SH, Korones DN, Zimmerman RA. Primary intracranial atypical teratoid/rhabdoid tumors of infancy and childhood: MRI features and patient outcomes. Am J Neuroradiol 2006; 27: 962–71.

32. Tekautz TM, Fuller CE, Blaney S, et al. Atypical teratoid/rhabdoid tumors (ATRT): improved survival in children 3 years of age and older with radiation therapy and high-dose alkylator-based chemotherapy. J Clin Oncol 2005; 23: 1491–9.

33. Warmuth-Metz M, Bison B, Dannemann-Stern E, Kortmann R, Rutkowski S, Pietsch T. CT and MR imaging in atypical teratoid/rhabdoid tumors of the central nervous system. Neuroradiology 2008; 50: 447–52.

34. Rorke LB, Packer R, Biegel J. Central nervous system atypical teratoid/rhabdoid tumors of infancy and childhood. J Neurooncol 1995; 24: 21–8.

35. Inenaga C, Toyoshima Y, Mori H, Nishiyama K, Tanaka R, Takahashi H. A fourth ventricle atypical teratoid/rhabdoid tumor in an infant. Brain Tumor Pathol 2003; 20: 47–52.

36. Roberts CW, Biegel JA. The role of SMARCB1/INI1 in development of rhabdoid tumor. Cancer Biol Ther 2009; 8: 412–16.

37. Versteege I, Sevenet N, Lange J, et al. Truncating mutations of hSNF5/INI1 in aggressive paediatric cancer. Nature 1998; 394: 203–6.

38. Biegel JA, Tan L, Zhang F, Wainwright L, Russo P, Rorke LB. Alterations of the hSNF5/INI1 gene in central nervous system atypical teratoid/

rhabdoid tumors and renal and extrarenal rhabdoid tumors. Clin Cancer Res 2002; 8: 3461–7.

39. Jackson EM, Sievert AJ, Gai X, et al. Genomic analysis using high-density single nucleotide polymorphism-based oligonucleotide arrays and multiplex ligation-dependent probe amplification provides a comprehensive analysis of INI1/SMARCB1 in malignant rhabdoid tumors. Clin Cancer Res 2009; 15: 1923–30.

40. Jalali GR, Vorstman JA, Errami A, et al. Detailed analysis of 22q11.2 with a high density MLPA probe set. Hum Mutat 2008; 29: 433–40.

41. Fruhwald MC, Hasselblatt M, Wirth S, et al. Non-linkage of familial rhabdoid tumors to SMARCB1 implies a second locus for the rhabdoid tumor predisposition syndrome. Pediatr Blood Cancer 2006; 47: 273–8.

42. Birks DK, Kleinschmidt-DeMasters BK, Donson AM, et al. Claudin 6 is a positive marker for atypical teratoid/rhabdoid tumors. Brain Pathol 2010; 20: 140–50.

43. Gardner SL, Asgharzadeh S, Green A, Horn B, McCowage G, Finlay J. Intensive induction chemotherapy followed by high dose chemotherapy with autologous hematopoietic progenitor cell rescue in young children newly diagnosed with central nervous system atypical teratoid rhabdoid tumors. Pediatr Blood Cancer 2008; 51: 235–40.

44. Chi SN, Zimmerman MA, Yao X, et al. Intensive multimodality treatment for children with newly diagnosed CNS atypical teratoid rhabdoid tumor. J Clin Oncol 2009; 27: 385–9.

45. Chen YW, Wong TT, Ho DM, et al. Impact of radiotherapy for pediatric CNS atypical teratoid/rhabdoid tumor (single institute experience). Int J Radiat Oncol Biol Phys 2006; 64: 1038–43.

46. Radcliffe J, Bunin GR, Sutton LN, Goldwein JW, Phillips PC. Cognitive deficits in long-term survivors of childhood medulloblastoma and other noncortical tumors: age-dependent effects of whole brain radiation. Int J Dev Neurosci 1994; 12: 327–34.

47. Molloy PT, Yachnis AT, Rorke LB, et al. Central nervous system medulloepithelioma: a series of eight cases including two arising in the pons. J Neurosurg 1996; 84: 430–6.

48. Viswanathan S, Mukul D, Qureshi S, Ramadwar M, Arora B, Kane SV. Orbital medulloepitheliomas – with extensive local invasion and metastasis: a series of three cases with review of literature. Int J Pediatr Otorhinolaryngol 2008; 72: 971–5.

49. Bruggers CS, Welsh CT, Boyer RS, Byrne JL, Pysher TJ. Successful therapy in a child with a congenital peripheral medulloepithelioma and disruption of hindquarter development. J Pediatr Hematol Oncol 1999; 21: 161–4.

50. Auer RN, Becker LE. Cerebral medulloepithelioma with bone, cartilage, and striated muscle. Light microscopic and immunohistochemical study. J Neuropathol Exp Neurol 1983; 42: 256–67.

51. Scheithauer BW, Rubinstein LJ. Cerebral medulloepithelioma. Report of a case with multiple divergent neuroepithelial differentiation. Childs Brain 1979; 5: 62–71.

52. Deck JH. Cerebral medulloepithelioma with maturation into ependymal cells and ganglion cells. J Neuropathol Exp Neurol 1969; 28: 442–54.

53. Moftakhar P, Fan X, Hurvitz CH, Black KL, Danielpour M. Long-term survival in a child with a central nervous system medulloepithelioma. J Neurosurg Pediatr 2008; 2: 339–45.

54. Matsumoto M, Horiuchi K, Sato T, et al. Cerebral medulloepithelioma with long survival. Neurol Med Chir (Tokyo) 2007; 47: 428–33.

55. Gessi M, Giangaspero F, Lauriola L, et al. Embryonal tumors with abundant neuropil and true rosettes: a distinctive CNS primitive neuroectodermal tumor. Am J Surg Pathol 2009; 33: 211–17.

56. Eberhart CG, Brat DJ, Cohen KJ, Burger PC. Pediatric neuroblastic brain tumors containing abundant neuropil and true rosettes. Pediatr Dev Pathol 2000; 3: 346–52.

57. Dunham C, Sugo E, Tobias V, Wills E, Perry A. Embryonal tumor with abundant neuropil and true rosettes (ETANTR): report of a case with prominent neurocytic differentiation. J Neurooncol 2007; 84: 91–8.

58. Pfister S, Remke M, Castoldi M, et al. Novel genomic amplification targeting the microRNA cluster at 19q13.42 in a pediatric embryonal tumor with abundant neuropil and true rosettes. Acta Neuropathol 2009; 117: 457–64.

59. La Spina M, Pizzolitto S, Skrap M, *et al*. Embryonal tumor with abundant neuropil and true rosettes. A new entity or only variations of a parent neoplasms (PNETs)? This is the dilemma. J Neurooncol 2006; 78: 317–20.

60. Fuller C, Fouladi M, Gajjar A, Dalton J, Sanford RA, Helton KJ. Chromosome 17 abnormalities in pediatric neuroblastic tumor with abundant neuropil and true rosettes. Am J Clin Pathol 2006; 126: 277–83.

61. Manjila S, Ray A, Hu Y, Cai DX, Cohen ML, Cohen AR. Embryonal tumors with abundant neuropil and true rosettes: 2 illustrative cases and a review of the literature. Neurosurg Focus 2011; 30: E2.

62. Jouvet A, Saint-Pierre G, Fauchon F, *et al*. Pineal parenchymal tumors: a correlation of histological features with prognosis in 66 cases. Brain Pathol 2000; 10: 49–60.

63. Cho BK, Wang KC, Nam DH, *et al*. Pineal tumors: experience with 48 cases over 10 years. Childs Nerv Syst 1998; 14: 53–8.

64. Schild SE, Scheithauer BW, Schomberg PJ, *et al*. Pineal parenchymal tumors. Clinical, pathologic, and therapeutic aspects. Cancer 1993; 72: 870–80.

65. Vigh B, Rohlich P, Gorcs T, *et al*. The pineal organ as a folded retina: immunocytochemical localization of opsins. Biol Cell 1998; 90: 653–9.

66. Bader JL, Meadows AT, Zimmerman LE, *et al*. Bilateral retinoblastoma with ectopic intracranial retinoblastoma: trilateral retinoblastoma. Cancer Genet Cytogenet 1982; 5: 203–13.

67. Ikeda J, Sawamura Y, van Meir EG. Pineoblastoma presenting in familial adenomatous polyposis (FAP): random association, FAP variant or Turcot syndrome? Br J Neurosurg 1998; 12: 576–8.

68. Borit A, Blackwood W, Mair WG. The separation of pineocytoma from pineoblastoma. Cancer 1980; 45: 1408–18.

69. McGrogan G, Rivel J, Vital C, Guerin J. A pineal tumour with features of "pineal anlage tumour". Acta Neurochir (Wien) 1992; 117: 73–7.

70. Schmidbauer M, Budka H, Pilz P. Neuroepithelial and ectomesenchymal differentiation in a primitive pineal tumor ("pineal anlage tumor"). Clin Neuropathol 1989; 8: 7–10.

71. Dhall G, Khatua S, Finlay JL. Pineal region tumors in children. Curr Opin Neurol 2010; 23: 576–82.

72. Berger C, Thiesse P, Lellouch-Tubiana A, Kalifa C, Pierre-Kahn A, Bouffet E. Choroid plexus carcinomas in childhood: clinical features and prognostic factors. Neurosurgery 1998; 42: 470–5.

73. McEvoy AW, Harding BN, Phipps KP, *et al*. Management of choroid plexus tumours in children: 20 years experience at a single neurosurgical centre. Pediatr Neurosurg 2000; 32: 192–9.

74. Lafay-Cousin L, Mabbott DJ, Halliday W, *et al*. Use of ifosfamide, carboplatin, and etoposide chemotherapy in choroid plexus carcinoma. J Neurosurg Pediatr 2010; 5: 615–21.

75. Wolff JE, Sajedi M, Brant R, Coppes MJ, Egeler RM. Choroid plexus tumours. Br J Cancer 2002; 87: 1086–91.

76. Gupta N. Choroid plexus tumors in children. Neurosurg Clin North Am 2003; 14: 621–31.

77. Krutilkova V, Trkova M, Fleitz J, *et al*. Identification of five new families strengthens the link between childhood choroid plexus carcinoma and germline TP53 mutations. Eur J Cancer 2005; 41: 1597–603.

78. Dickens DS, Dothage JA, Heideman RL, Ballard ET, Jubinsky PT. Successful treatment of an unresectable choroid plexus carcinoma in a patient with Li–Fraumeni syndrome. J Pediatr Hematol Oncol 2005; 27: 46–9.

79. Jeibmann A, Hasselblatt M, Gerss J, *et al*. Prognostic implications of atypical histologic features in choroid plexus papilloma. J Neuropathol Exp Neurol 2006; 65: 1069–73.

80. Matsushima T, Inoue T, Takeshita I, Fukui M, Iwaki T, Kitamoto T. Choroid plexus papillomas: an immunohistochemical study with particular reference to the coexpression of prealbumin. Neurosurgery 1988; 23: 384–9.

81. Paulus W, Janisch W. Clinicopathologic correlations in epithelial choroid plexus neoplasms: a study of 52 cases. Acta Neuropathol 1990; 80: 635–41.

82. Vajtai I, Varga Z, Aguzzi A. MIB-1 immunoreactivity reveals different labelling in low-grade and in malignant epithelial neoplasms of the choroid plexus. Histopathology 1996; 29: 147–51.

83. Gottschalk J, Jautzke G, Paulus W, Goebel S, Cervos-Navarro J. The use of immunomorphology to differentiate choroid plexus tumors from metastatic carcinomas. Cancer 1993; 72: 1343–9.

84. Fitzpatrick LK, Aronson LJ, Cohen KJ. Is there a requirement for adjuvant therapy for choroid plexus carcinoma that has been completely resected? J Neurooncol 2002; 57: 123–6.

85. Packer RJ, Perilongo G, Johnson D, *et al*. Choroid plexus carcinoma of childhood. Cancer 1992; 69: 580–5.

86. Mazloom A, Wolff JE, Paulino AC. The impact of radiotherapy fields in the treatment of patients with choroid plexus carcinoma. Int J Radiat Oncol Biol Phys 2010; 78(1): 79–84.

87. Mazloom A, Wolff JE, Paulino AC. The impact of radiotherapy fields in the treatment of patients with choroid plexus carcinoma. Int J Radiat Oncol Biol Phys 2010; 78: 79–84.

88. VandenBerg SR. Desmoplastic infantile ganglioglioma and desmoplastic cerebral astrocytoma of infancy. Brain Pathol 1993; 3: 275–81.

89. VandenBerg SR, May EE, Rubinstein LJ, *et al*. Desmoplastic supratentorial neuroepithelial tumors of infancy with divergent differentiation potential ("desmoplastic infantile gangliogliomas"). Report on 11 cases of a distinctive embryonal tumor with favorable prognosis. J Neurosurg 1987; 66: 58–71.

90. Qaddoumi I, Ceppa EP, Mansour A, Sughayer MA, Tihan T. Desmoplastic noninfantile ganglioglioma: report of a case. Pediatr Dev Pathol 2006; 9: 462–7.

91. Per H, Kontas O, Kumandas S, Kurtsoy A. A report of a desmoplastic non-infantile ganglioglioma in a 6-year-old boy with review of the literature. Neurosurg Rev 2009; 32: 369–74; discussion 374.

92. Pommepuy I, Delage-Corre M, Moreau JJ, Labrousse F. A report of a desmoplastic ganglioglioma in a 12-year-old girl with review of the literature. J Neurooncol 2006; 76: 271–5.

93. Trehan G, Bruge H, Vinchon M, *et al*. MR imaging in the diagnosis of desmoplastic infantile tumor: retrospective study of six cases. Am J Neuroradiol 2004; 25: 1028–33.

94. Gelabert-Gonzalez M, Serramito-Garcia R, Arcos-Algaba A. Desmoplastic infantile and non-infantile ganglioglioma. Review of the literature. Neurosurg Rev 2010; 34: 151–8.

95. Daumas-Duport C, Scheithauer BW, Chodkiewicz JP, Laws ER Jr, Vedrenne C. Dysembryoplastic neuroepithelial tumor: a surgically curable tumor of young patients with intractable partial seizures. Report of thirty-nine cases. Neurosurgery 1988; 23: 545–56.

96. Baisden BL, Brat DJ, Melhem ER, Rosenblum MK, King AP, Burger PC. Dysembryoplastic neuroepithelial tumor-like neoplasm of the septum pellucidum: a lesion often misdiagnosed as glioma: report of 10 cases. Am J Surg Pathol 2001; 25: 494–9.

97. Altinors N, Calisaneller T, Gulsen S, Ozen O, Onguru O. Intraventricular dysembryoplastic neuroepithelial tumor: case report. Neurosurgery 2007; 61: E1332–3; discussion E1333.

98. Kuchelmeister K, Demirel T, Schlorer E, Bergmann M, Gullotta F. Dysembryoplastic neuroepithelial tumour of the cerebellum. Acta Neuropathol 1995; 89: 385–90.

99. Fujimoto K, Ohnishi H, Tsujimoto M, Hoshida T, Nakazato Y. Dysembryoplastic neuroepithelial tumor of the cerebellum and brainstem. Case report. J Neurosurg 2000; 93: 487–9.

100. Stanescu Cosson R, Varlet P, Beuvon F, *et al*. Dysembryoplastic neuroepithelial tumors: CT, MR findings and imaging follow-up: a study of 53 cases. J Neuroradiol 2001; 28: 230–40.

101. Daumas-Duport C. Dysembryoplastic neuroepithelial tumours. Brain Pathol 1993; 3: 283–95.

102. Daumas-Duport C, Varlet P, Bacha S, Beuvon F, Cervera-Pierot P, Chodkiewicz JP. Dysembryoplastic neuroepithelial tumors: nonspecific histological forms – a study of 40 cases. J Neurooncol 1999; 41: 267–80.

103. Takahashi A, Hong SC, Seo DW, Hong SB, Lee M, Suh YL. Frequent association of cortical dysplasia in dysembryoplastic neuroepithelial tumor treated by epilepsy surgery. Surg Neurol 2005; 64: 419–27.

104. Hirose T, Scheithauer BW, Lopes MB, VandenBerg SR. Dysembryoplastic neuroeptihelial tumor (DNT): an immunohistochemical and ultrastructural study. J Neuropathol Exp Neurol 1994; 53: 184–95.

105. Prayson RA. Bcl-2, bcl-x, and bax expression in dysembryoplastic neuroepithelial tumors. Clin Neuropathol 2000; 19: 57–62.

106. Prayson RA, Morris HH, Estes ML, Comair YG. Dysembryoplastic neuroepithelial tumor: a clinicopathologic and immunohistochemical study of 11 tumors including MIB1 immunoreactivity. Clin Neuropathol 1996; 15: 47–53.

107. Preuss M, Nestler U, Zuhlke CJ, Kuchelmeister K, Neubauer BA, Jodicke A. Progressive biological behavior of a dysembryoplastic neuroepithelial tumor. Pediatr Neurosurg 2010; 46: 294–8.

108. Bagley CA, Wilson S, Kothbauer KF, Bookland MJ, Epstein F, Jallo GI. Long term outcomes following surgical resection of myxopapillary ependymomas. Neurosurg Rev 2009; 32: 321–34; discussion 334.

109. Davis C, Barnard RO. Malignant behavior of myxopapillary ependymoma. Report of three cases. J Neurosurg 1985; 62: 925–9.

110. Jatana KR, Jacob A, Slone HW, Ray-Chaudhury A, Welling DB. Spinal myxopapillary ependymoma metastatic to bilateral internal auditory canals. Ann Otol Rhinol Laryngol 2008; 117: 98–102.

111. Mridha AR, Sharma MC, Sarkar C, et al. Myxopapillary ependymoma of lumbosacral region with metastasis to both cerebellopontine angles: report of a rare case. Childs Nerv Syst 2007; 23: 1209–13.

112. Woesler B, Moskopp D, Kuchelmeister K, Schul C, Wassmann H. Intracranial metastasis of a spinal myxopapillary ependymoma. A case report. Neurosurg Rev 1998; 21: 62–5.

113. Sakai Y, Matsuyama Y, Katayama Y, et al. Spinal myxopapillary ependymoma: neurological deterioration in patients treated with surgery. Spine 2009; 34: 1619–24.

114. Komotar RJ, Mocco J, Carson BS, et al. Pilomyxoid astrocytoma: a review. Med Gen Med 2004; 6: 42.

115. Omura T, Nawashiro H, Osada H, Shima K, Tsuda H, Shinsuke A. Pilomyxoid astrocytoma of the fourth ventricle in an adult. Acta Neurochir (Wien) 2008; 150: 1203–6; discussion 1206.

116. Sajadi A, Janzer RC, Lu TL, Duff JM. Pilomyxoid astrocytoma of the spinal cord in an adult. Acta Neurochir (Wien) 2008; 150: 729–31.

117. Komotar RJ, Carson BS, Rao C, Chaffee S, Goldthwaite PT, Tihan T. Pilomyxoid astrocytoma of the spinal cord: report of three cases. Neurosurgery 2005; 56: 191.

118. Linscott LL, Osborn AG, Blaser S, et al. Pilomyxoid astrocytoma: expanding the imaging spectrum. Am J Neuroradiol 2008; 29: 1861–6.

119. Tihan T, Fisher PG, Kepner JL, et al. Pediatric astrocytomas with monomorphous pilomyxoid features and a less favorable outcome. J Neuropathol Exp Neurol 1999; 58: 1061–8.

120. Fernandez C, Figarella-Branger D, Girard N, et al. Pilocytic astrocytomas in children: prognostic factors – a retrospective study of 80 cases. Neurosurgery 2003; 53: 544–53; discussion 554–5.

121. Komotar RJ, Burger PC, Carson BS, et al. Pilocytic and pilomyxoid hypothalamic/chiasmatic astrocytomas. Neurosurgery 2004; 54: 72–9; discussion 79–80.

122. Kadonaga JN, Frieden IJ. Neurocutaneous melanosis: definition and review of the literature. J Am Acad Dermatol 1991; 24: 747–55.

123. Slutsky JB, Barr JM, Femia AN, Marghoob AA. Large congenital melanocytic nevi: associated risks and management considerations. Semin Cutan Med Surg 2010; 29: 79–84.

124. Pavlidou E, Hagel C, Papavasilliou A, Giouroukos S, Panteliadis C. Neurocutaneous melanosis: report of three cases and up-to-date review. J Child Neurol 2008; 23: 1382–91.

125. Brat DJ, Giannini C, Scheithauer BW, Burger PC. Primary melanocytic neoplasms of the central nervous systems. Am J Surg Pathol 1999; 23: 745–54.

126. Ahluwalia S, Ashkan K, Casey AT. Meningeal melanocytoma: clinical features and review of the literature. Br J Neurosurg 2003; 17: 347–51.

127. Limas C, Tio FO. Meningeal melanocytoma ("melanotic meningioma"). Its melanocytic origin as revealed by electron microscopy. Cancer 1972; 30: 1286–94.

128. Giannini C, Scheithauer BW, Burger PC, et al. Pleomorphic xanthoastrocytoma: what do we really know about it? Cancer 1999; 85: 2033–45.

129. Hamlat A, Le Strat A, Guegan Y, Ben-Hassel M, Saikali S. Cerebellar pleomorphic xanthoastrocytoma: case report and literature review. Surg Neurol 2007; 68: 89–94; discussion 95.

130. Tien RD, Cardenas CA, Rajagopalan S. Pleomorphic xanthoastrocytoma of the brain: MR findings in six patients. Am J Roentgenol 1992; 159: 1287–90.

131. Dias-Santagata D, Lam Q, Vernovsky K, et al. BRAF V600E mutations are common in pleomorphic xanthoastrocytoma: diagnostic and therapeutic implications. PLoS One 2011; 6: e17948.

132. Giannini C, Scheithauer BW, Lopes MB, Hirose T, Kros JM, VandenBerg SR. Immunophenotype of pleomorphic xanthoastrocytoma. Am J Surg Pathol 2002; 26: 479–85.

133. Katsetos CD, del Valle L, Geddes JF, et al. Aberrant localization of the neuronal class III beta-tubulin in astrocytomas. Arch Pathol Lab Med 2001; 125: 613–24.

134. Martinez-Diaz H, Kleinschmidt-DeMasters BK, Powell SZ, Yachnis AT. Giant cell glioblastoma and pleomorphic xanthoastrocytoma show different immunohistochemical profiles for neuronal antigens and p53 but share reactivity for class III beta-tubulin. Arch Pathol Lab Med 2003; 127: 1187–91.

135. Koga T, Morita A, Maruyama K, et al. Long-term control of disseminated pleomorphic xanthoastrocytoma with anaplastic features by means of stereotactic irradiation. Neuro Oncol 2009; 11: 446–51.

136. Chang HT, Latorre JG, Hahn S, Dubowy R, Schelper RL. Pediatric cerebellar pleomorphic xanthoastrocytoma with anaplastic features: a case of long-term survival after multimodality therapy. Childs Nerv Syst 2006; 22: 609–13.

137. Scheithauer BW, Silva AI, Ketterling RP, Pula JH, Lininger JF, Krinock MJ. Rosette-forming glioneuronal tumor: report of a chiasmal-optic nerve example in neurofibromatosis type 1: special pathology report. Neurosurgery 2009; 64: E771–2; discussion E772.

138. Anan M, Inoue R, Ishii K, et al. A rosette-forming glioneuronal tumor of the spinal cord: the first case of a rosette-forming glioneuronal tumor originating from the spinal cord. Hum Pathol 2009; 40: 898–901.

139. Shah MN, Leonard JR, Perry A. Rosette-forming glioneuronal tumors of the posterior fossa. J Neurosurg Pediatr 2010; 5: 98–103.

140. Komori T, Scheithauer BW, Hirose T. A rosette-forming glioneuronal tumor of the fourth ventricle: infratentorial form of dysembryoplastic neuroepithelial tumor? Am J Surg Pathol 2002; 26: 582–91.

141. Marhold F, Preusser M, Dietrich W, Prayer D, Czech T. Clinicoradiological features of rosette-forming glioneuronal tumor (RGNT) of the fourth ventricle: report of four cases and literature review. J Neurooncol 2008; 90: 301–8.

142. Solis OE, Mehta RI, Lai A, et al. Rosette-forming glioneuronal tumor: a pineal region case with IDH1 and IDH2 mutation analyses and literature review of 43 cases. J Neurooncol 2011; 102: 477–84.

143. Shepherd CW, Scheithauer BW, Gomez MR, Altermatt HJ, Katzmann JA. Subependymal giant cell astrocytoma: a clinical, pathological, and flow cytometric study. Neurosurgery 1991; 28: 864–8.

144. Gyure KA, Prayson RA. Subependymal giant cell astrocytoma: a clinicopathologic study with HMB45 and MIB-1 immunohistochemical analysis. Mod Pathol 1997; 10: 313–17.

145. Sharma M, Ralte A, Arora R, Santosh V, Shankar SK, Sarkar C. Subependymal giant cell astrocytoma: a clinicopathological study of 23 cases with special emphasis on proliferative markers and expression of p53 and retinoblastoma gene proteins. Pathology 2004; 36: 139–44.

146. Hussain N, Curran A, Pilling D, et al. Congenital subependymal giant cell astrocytoma diagnosed on fetal MRI. Arch Dis Child 2006; 91: 520.

147. Takei H, Adesina AM, Powell SZ. Solitary subependymal giant cell astrocytoma incidentally found at autopsy in an elderly woman without tuberous sclerosis complex. Neuropathology 2009; 29: 181–6.

148. Inoue Y, Nemoto Y, Murata R, et al. CT and MR imaging of cerebral tuberous sclerosis. Brain Dev 1998; 20: 209–21.

149. Iwasaki S, Nakagawa H, Kichikawa K, et al. MR and CT of tuberous sclerosis: linear abnormalities in the cerebral white matter. Am J Neuroradiol 1990; 11: 1029–34.

150. Buccoliero AM, Franchi A, Castiglione F, et al. Subependymal giant cell astrocytoma (SEGA): is it an astrocytoma? Morphological, immunohistochemical and ultrastructural study. Neuropathology 2009; 29: 25–30.

151. Chow CW, Klug GL, Lewis EA. Subependymal giant-cell astrocytoma in children. An unusual discrepancy between histological and clinical features. J Neurosurg 1988; 68: 880–3.

152. Lopes MB, Altermatt HJ, Scheithauer BW, Shepherd CW, VandenBerg SR. Immunohistochemical characterization of subependymal giant cell astrocytomas. Acta Neuropathol 1996; 91: 368–75.

153. Sharma MC, Ralte AM, Gaekwad S, Santosh V, Shankar SK, Sarkar C. Subependymal giant cell astrocytoma – a clinicopathological study of 23 cases with special emphasis on histogenesis. Pathol Oncol Res 2004; 10: 219–24.

154. Clarke MJ, Foy AB, Wetjen N, Raffel C. Imaging characteristics and growth of subependymal giant cell astrocytomas. Neurosurg Focus 2006; 20: E5.

155. Goh S, Butler W, Thiele EA. Subependymal giant cell tumors in tuberous sclerosis complex. Neurology 2004; 63: 1457–61.

156. Franz DN, Leonard J, Tudor C, *et al.* Rapamycin causes regression of astrocytomas in tuberous sclerosis complex. Ann Neurol 2006; 59: 490–8.

157. Koenig MK, Butler IJ, Northrup H. Regression of subependymal giant cell astrocytoma with rapamycin in tuberous sclerosis complex. J Child Neurol 2008; 23: 1238–9.

158. Krueger DA, Care MM, Holland K, *et al.* Everolimus for subependymal giant-cell astrocytomas in tuberous sclerosis. N Engl J Med 2010; 363: 1801–11.

159. Campen CJ, Porter BE. Subependymal giant cell astrocytoma (SEGA) treatment update. Curr Treat Options Neurol 2011; 13: 380–5.

160. De Munnynck K, *et al.* Desmoplastic infantile ganglioglioma: a potentially malignant tumor? Am J Surg Pathol 2002; 26: 1515–22.

161. Darwish B, *et al.* Desmoplastic infantile ganglioglioma/astrocytoma with cerebrospinal metastasis. J Clin Neurosci 2007; 14: 498–501.

70 Malignant Tumors of the Skin and Subcutaneous Tissue in Children

Alberto S. Pappo[1] and Carlos Rodriguez-Galindo[2]

[1] Division of Solid Tumors, St Jude Children's Research Hospital, Memphis, TN, USA
[2] Department of Pediatric Oncology, Dana-Farber Cancer Institute; Harvard Medical School, Boston, MA, USA

Introduction

Malignant tumors of the skin and subcutaneous tissue are rare in childhood. Only about 1% of skin tumors in children are malignant.[1–4] In a review of 36,207 pediatric dermatology patients seen at a large treatment center over 20 years, 53 tumor diagnoses (36 primary and 17 metastatic) were malignant; the most common histologies included rhabdomyosarcoma, 25%; lymphomas, 19%; basal cell carcinoma, 13%; leukemia, 13%; neuroblastoma, 10%; malignant melanoma, 6%; squamous cell carcinoma, 6%; unclassified sarcomas, 4%; epithelioid schwannoma, 2%; and ependymoma, 2%.[5] In another review, leukemia (38%), histiocytosis (20%), neuroblastoma (17%), rhabdoid tumor (11%), and rhabdomyosarcoma (6%) were the most common malignancies associated with cutaneous metastases in neonates.[6]

In this chapter we review some of the most relevant primary and metastatic tumors of the skin and subcutaneous tissues.

Melanoma

Pediatric melanoma is rare and accounts for about 3% of cancers in patients under 20 years of age but comprises 7% of cancer cases in patients between 15 and 19 years of age (Fig. 70.1).[7] In the pediatric age group, melanoma is more common in females but males predominate after the age of 40 years.[8] The incidence of pediatric melanoma has increased at a rate of 1.5% per year from 1975 through 2008 (http://seer.cancer.gov/csr/1975_2008/results_merged/sect_29_childhood_cancer_iccc.pdf). The incidence of melanoma increases with age and over 90% of pediatric cases occur in patients older than 10 years of age; 74% are seen in 15–19 year olds.[8]

Risk factors

Risk factors associated with the development of melanoma in adults have also been documented in children and include light skin, tendency to freckle, and increased number of melanocytic nevi.[9] In addition, subsets of pediatric patients have unique predisposing factors.

- Xeroderma pigmentosum (XP),[10] an autosomal recessive disorder characterized by extreme photosensitivity to ultraviolet radiation and caused by mutations of the nucleotide excision repair complementation groups. Patients with XP have a 2000-fold increased risk of developing melanoma at a median age of 22 years.[11]
- Survivors of hereditary retinoblastoma,[12] regardless of whether they were irradiated or not, have a 30-fold increased risk of developing melanoma.[12]
- Werner syndrome.[13]
- Congenital melanoma.[14]
- Giant congenital melanocytic nevi (Fig. 70.2).[15] These patients have about a 5% lifetime risk of developing melanoma; larger size and numerous satellite nevi increase the risk.[15]
- Neurocutaneous melanosis[16] is a rare disorder characterized by large or multiple congenital nevi in association with meningeal melanoma or melanosis.[16] The risk of developing neurocutaneous melanosis in patients with large congenital nevi ranges from 2.5% to 12%.[16] About one-fourth of asymptomatic patients with large congenital nevi have radiographic evidence of central nervous system melanosis but these patients rarely develop symptomatic disease.[16]
- Immunosupression as a result of immunodeficiencies or following solid organ or bone marrow transplantation is associated with an increased of melanoma.[17–19] Childhood cancer survivors are also at increased risk of developing melanoma.[20]
- Genetic and environmental factors including the use of tanning beds.[21,22]

Clinical manifestations

Pediatric melanoma has a similar clinical presentation to adult melanoma but delays in diagnosis are seen in up to 60% of patients.[23,24] Initial signs and symptoms may include bleeding, ulceration, increasing mole size, itching, and a palpable

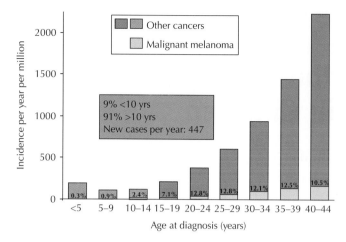

Figure 70.1 Incidence of malignant melanoma relative to all cancer. SEER, 1975–2000.

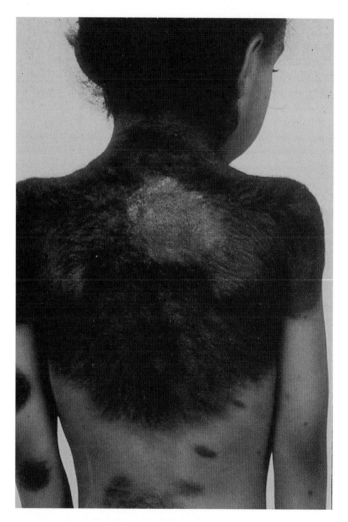

Figure 70.2 Giant congenital melanocytic nevi.

mass.[25] A review of two large series of pediatric melanoma comprising over 4400 patients reveals that female sex predominates in this patient population and over 90% are white.[26,27] Although the majority of patients present with localized disease, younger patients (<10 years) are more likely to present with advanced-stage disease, head and neck primaries, and nodular melanomas.[26,27]

Diagnosis and work-up

Establishing the diagnosis of pediatric melanoma can be challenging. In a study by Wechsler,[28] amongst eight experienced dermatopathologists who reviewed 85 childhood melanoma cases, it was demonstrated that complete agreement with the diagnosis was accomplished in only 39% of the cases and in a study by Leman, eight of 13 cases of melanoma in patients under 15 years of age were reclassified as unusual nevi.[29] Emerging terms such as tumors of unknown metastatic potential (MELTUMPS) and atypical spitz nevus are often confusing[30] and the terminology may affect the decisions of the treating clinician who ultimately has to make a therapeutic recommendation. In one publication of 57 MELTUMPS, only 50% of the participants were able to diagnose clinically favorable lesions as benign and 73% with unfavorable behavior as malignant.[31] New molecular tests such as comparative genomic hybridization[32] and fluorescent *in situ* hybridization (FISH) may aid in the classification of these controversial melanocytic lesions. For example, four-color FISH probes for *RREB1n* (6p25), *MYB* (6q23), *CCND1* (11q13), and *CEP6* (6p11.1-q11) may help identify lesions at risk for metastases.[33] *BRAF* V600E and *HRAS* mutations have also been reported in pediatric melanomas and atypical melanocytic lesions.[33]

Staging

Guidelines for staging pediatric melanoma have not been developed so most clinicians use the adult American Joint Commission on Cancer (AJCC) classification of melanoma to stage and assign therapy to these patients (Fig. 70.3). In the new AJCC system, patients are stratified into four different groups and those with localized tumors are subsequently stratified into two stages (I and II) based on primary tumor thickness, presence or absence of ulceration, and mitotic rate. Stage III patients have nodal disease and stage IV patients have distant metastases. Pediatric patients, particularly those with atypical melanocytic lesions, appear to have a higher rate of nodal disease although this feature may not affect clinical outcome.[34–38] In one large series, stage was predictive of clinical outcome (Fig. 70.4). The routine use of computed tomography (CT) to detect metastatic disease in children with melanoma has not been studied well but one publication suggests that thick primary lesions have an increased incidence of clinically unsuspected metastases.[25]

Treatment

The 5-year melanoma-specific survival for children with melanoma is 93.5%.[26] Surgical resection is the mainstay of therapy for pediatric melanoma. Current surgical guidelines recommend the following margins of resection: 0.5 cm for melanoma *in situ*, 1.0 cm for melanoma thickness under 1 mm, 1–2 cm for melanoma thickness of 1.01–2 mm, and 2 cm for tumor thickness greater than 2 mm (www.nccn.org/professionals/

American Joint Committee on Cancer

Melanoma of the Skin Staging
7th EDITION

Definitions

Primary Tumor (T)

TX   Primary tumor cannot be assessed (for example, curettaged or severely regressed melanoma)

T0   No evidence of primary tumor

Tis   Melanoma in situ

T1   Melanomas 1.0 mm or less in thickness

T2   Melanomas 1.01–2.0 mm

T3   Melanomas 2.01–4.0 mm

T4   Melanomas more than 4.0 mm

NOTE: a and b subcategories of T are assigned based on ulceration and number of mitoses per mm^2, as shown below:

T CLASSIFICATION	THICKNESS (mm)	ULCERATION STATUS/MITOSES
T1	≤1.0	a: w/o ulceration and mitosis <1/mm^2 b: with ulceration or mitoses ≥1/mm^2
T2	1.01–2.0	a: w/o ulceration b: with ulceration
T3	2.01–4.0	a: w/o ulceration b: with ulceration
T4	>4.0	a: w/o ulceration b: with ulceration

Regional Lymph Nodes (N)

NX   Patients in whom the regional nodes cannot be assessed (for example, previously removed for another reason)

N0   No regional metastases detected

N1-3   Regional metastases based upon the number of metastatic nodes and presence or absence of intralymphatic metastases (in transit or satellite metastases)

NOTE: N1–3 and a–c subcategories assigned as shown below:

N CLASSIFICATION	NO. OF METASTATIC NODES	NODAL METASTATIC MASS
N1	1 node	a: micrometastasis[1] b: macrometastasis[2]
N2	2–3 nodes	a: micrometastasis[1] b: macrometastasis[2] c: in transit met(s)/satellite(s) *without* metastatic nodes
N3	4 or more metastatic nodes, or matted nodes, or in transit met(s)/satellite(s) with metastatic node(s)	

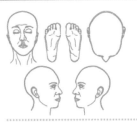

Distant Metastatis (M)

M0   No detectable evidence of distant metastases

M1a   Metastases to skin, subcutaneous, or distant lymph nodes

M1b   Metastases to lung

M1c   Metastases to all other visceral sites or distant metastases to any site combined with an elevated serum LDH

NOTE: Serum LDH is incorporated into the M category as shown below:

M CLASSIFICATION	SITE	SERUM LDH
M1a	Distant skin, subcutaneous, or nodal mets	Normal
M1b	Lung metastases	Normal
M1c	All other visceral metastases	Normal
	Any distant metastasis	Elevated

ANATOMIC STAGE/PROGNOSTIC GROUPS

Clinical Staging[3]				Pathologic Staging[4]			
Stage 0	Tis	N0	M0	0	Tis	N0	M0
Stage IA	T1a	N0	M0	IA	T1a	N0	M0
Stage IB	T1b	N0	M0	IB	T1b	N0	M0
	T2a	N0	M0		T2a	N0	M0
Stage IIA	T2b	N0	M0	IIA	T2b	N0	M0
	T3a	N0	M0		T3a	N0	M0
Stage IIB	T3b	N0	M0	IIB	T3b	N0	M0
	T4a	N0	M0		T4a	N0	M0
Stage IIC	T4b	N0	M0	IIC	T4b	N0	M0
Stage III	Any T	≥ N1	M0	IIIA	T1-4a	N1a	M0
					T1-4a	N2a	M0
				IIIB	T1-4b	N1a	M0
					T1-4b	N2a	M0
					T1-4a	N1b	M0
					T1-4a	N2b	M0
					T1-4a	N2c	M0
				IIIC	T1-4b	N1b	M0
					T1-4b	N2b	M0
					T1-4b	N2c	M0
					Any T	N3	M0
Stage IV	Any T	Any N	M1	IV	Any T	Any N	M1

Financial support for AJCC
7th Edition Staging Posters
provided by the American Cancer Society

Notes

[1] Micrometastases are diagnosed after sentinel lymph node biopsy and completion lymphadenectomy (if performed).

[2] Macrometastases are defined as clinically detectable nodal metastases confirmed by therapeutic lymphadenectomy or when nodal metastasis exhibits gross extracapsular extension.

[3] Clinical staging includes microstaging of the primary melanoma and clinical/radiologic evaluation for metastases. By convention, it should be used after complete excision of the primary melanoma with clinical assessment for regional and distant metastases.

[4] Pathologic staging includes microstaging of the primary melanoma and pathologic information about the regional lymph nodes after partial or complete lymphadenectomy. Pathologic Stage 0 or Stage IA patients are the exception; they do not require pathologic evaluation of their lymph nodes.

Figure 70.3 AJCC classification of melanoma. Reproduced from Edge *et al.*[121] Used with the permission of the American Joint Committee on Cancer (AJCC), Chicago, Illinois. The original source for this material is the AJCC Cancer Staging Manual, Seventh Edition (2010) published by Springer Science and Business Media LLC, www.springer.com

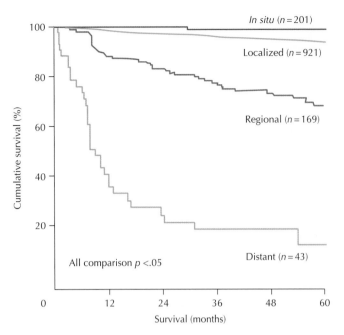

In situ (n = 201)

Localized (n = 921)

Regional (n = 169)

All comparison p < .05

Distant (n = 43)

Figure 70.4 Survival of childhood melanoma by stage. Data from Lange *et al.*[27] Reprinted with permission. © 2008 American Society of Clinical Oncology. All rights reserved.

Table 70.1 Primary soft tissue sarcomas of the skin and subcutaneous tissues.

Cell of origin	Neoplasm
Vascular	Kaposi sarcoma
	Angiosarcoma
	Epithelioid hemangioendothelioma
	Endovascular papillary angioendothelioma
	Retiform hemangioendothelioma
	Malignant glomus tumor
Fibrous	Dermatofibrosarcoma protuberans
	Angiomatoid fibrous histiocytoma
	Infantile myofibromatosis
	Atypical fibroxanthoma
	Dermatofibroma
	Plexiform fibrohistiocytic tumor
Smooth muscle	Superficial leiomyosarcoma
	Superficial leiomyoma
	Hamartoma
	Angiolipoleiomyoma
Nerve sheath	Cutaneous malignant peripheral nerve sheath tumor
Neural crest	Clear cell sarcoma
Neuroectodermal	Primary superficial Ewing sarcoma
Adipose	Superficial liposarcoma
Unknown	Epithelioid sarcoma

physician_gls/pdf/melanoma.pdf). Patients with thin lesions (≤1 mm) and ulceration, mitotic rate >1 mm^2, young age, and all lesions >1 mm with or without adverse features such as increased mitotic rate, ulceration, and lymphovascular invasion should undergo sentinel node sampling.[39] If the sentinel node is positive, patients should be offered a complete lymph node dissection although this procedure may not ultimately affect overall survival.[40] Patients with high-risk primary cutaneous melanoma, especially with regional lymph node involvement, should be offered the option to receive adjuvant interferon-α2b, a therapy that is well tolerated in children.[39,41,42] Limited numbers of pediatric patients with metastatic melanoma have been treated with dacarbazine (DTIC) and interleukin-2[43,44] and newer therapies such as ipilimumab and the *BRAF* inhibitor vemurafenib have not been well studied and developed to date in the pediatric population.[45,46]

Malignant epithelial tumors of the skin

Both basal cell and squamous cell carcinoma are rare in children. In a series of over 36,000 dermatology patients seen at a large center in Mexico City, only 53 malignant cutaneous tumors were identified and of these, only 25% were either squamous cell or basal cell carcinomas.[5] Table 70.1 shows some of the most common skin and subcutaneous tumors. Basal cell carcinomas are rare in pediatrics and usually arise within the context of predisposing conditions such as xeroderma pigmentosum[11] and Gorlin syndrome, an entity characterized by germline *PTCH1* mutations and an increased risk for developing various tumors including basal cell carcinoma, rhabdomyosarcoma, medulloblastoma, fibrosarcoma, mengioma, and ovarian fibromas.[47] These patients have increased rates of ionizing radiation-induced chromosomal aberrations[48] and can therefore benefit

from therapies that avoid local radiation therapy. One such therapy, GDC-0449 (vismodegib),[49] a potent small molecule inhibitor of the Hedgehog pathway, has proven effective in the treatment of patients with medulloblastoma and advanced-stage basal cell carcinoma.[49–51] Nevus sebaceous is one of the few nongenetic lesions associated with basal cell carcinoma in childhood but this is a rare occurrence as only eight cases have been reported.[52]

Squamous cell carcinoma (SCC) of the skin is rare in children and the majority of cases have been described in children with xeroderma pigmentosum.[11,53] Other causes include chronic poorly healed scars, immunosuppression, interferon-γ receptor 2 deficiency, dystrophic epidermolysis bullosa, and systemic sclerosis or pansclerotic morphea.[54–57] As with adults, location and size of the tumor affect treatment selection. The lesions are most frequently surgically excised. Other treatments include radiation, chemotherapy, Mohs micrographic surgery (MMS), and photodynamic therapy. Prognosis depends on size and depth of the tumor and seems to mirror that in adults, with early lesions readily curable and more advanced lesions being less responsive to treatment.

Histiocytoses

Histiocytoses are a heterogeneous group of disorders characterized by the proliferation and accumulation of reactive or neoplastic histiocytes. Based on the cell of origin and the clinical and biological behavior, histiocytoses are grouped into three classes; skin involvement is a known characteristic in all the histiocytic proliferations (see Table 70.2).

Class I: Langerhans cell histiocytosis

Langerhans cell histiocytosis (LCH) is a disease caused by clonal proliferation of Langerhans cells that share phenotypic

Table 70.2 Histiocytic disorders with skin involvement.

Class	Disease
I	Langerhans cell histiocytosis
	Self-healing reticulohistiocytosis of Hashimoto–Pritzker
II	Juvenile xanthogranuloma
	Rosai–Dorfman disease
	Hemophagocytic lymphohistiocytosis
	Multicentric reticulohistiocytosis
	Sea-blue histiocytic syndrome
	Necrobiotic xanthogranuloma
	Xanthoma disseminatum
III	Malignant histiocytosis

characteristics with the primary antigen-presenting cells of the epidermis. Molecular analyses of mouse models and human LCH samples suggest that LCH's cell of origin may not be the epidermal LC itself but a myeloid-derived precursor. Advanced genomic technologies have revealed the presence of activating, somatic *BRAF* mutations in the majority of specimens. Together, these observations have produced a new picture of LCH as a myeloid neoplasm.[58]

Langerhans cell histiocytosis is characterized by a spectrum of varying degrees of organ involvement and dysfunction. Patients may present with limited disease or with multisystem involvement. Treatment of LCH is risk adapted; patients with single lesions may respond well to local treatment, whereas patients with multisystem disease and risk-organ involvement (hematopoietic, liver, spleen) require more intensive therapy. While survival for patients without organ dysfunction is excellent, mortality rates for patients with organ dysfunction may reach 30–40%. For patients with low-risk disease, while cure is almost universal, disease reactivation rates are in excess of 30%.[59]

Langerhans cell histiocytosis can affect many different organs, including the skeleton, skin, lymph nodes, liver, lungs, spleen, and the hematopoietic and central nervous systems. The skin may be involved in LCH either as single-organ involvement or as part of multisystem disease, and up to 50% of patients will present initially with a rash.[60] Any part of the skin can be affected, including the nails. Scalp involvement is very common, and more typical of infants, followed by flexural areas in neck, axillae and, very characteristically, the genitourinary (diaper) area. It presents as diffuse and widespread tender scaly erythematous patches that may become petechial and exhibit small erosions with serous crusts. On the trunk, the rash tends to be more maculopapular and scaly, resembling guttate psoriasis or pityriasis rosea. The genitalia are very typically affected in older women.[60]

Isolated skin LCH has a good prognosis in general, with approximately 50% regression within a few months. However, LCH reactivation in the skin or progression to the disseminated, sometimes fatal form can also occur. Close observation for a prolonged period is mandatory, especially in newborns and infants, since up to 60% progress to multisystem disease, usually with risk-organ involvement.[61–63] In the pediatric age group, skin involvement is particularly typical of newborns and infants; cutaneous LCH is the most common initial

manifestation in both single-system (92%) and multisystem (86%) disease.[62] In this age group, a close distinction from the self-healing reticulohistiocytosis of Hashimoto–Pritzker is key. This self-limited form of LCH generally starts in the neonatal period with eruption of nodular lesions that resemble those of healing chicken pox and that affect any body part, including palms and soles. These lesions resolve over weeks, although new lesions may appear while old lesions regress. It is not often possible to distinguish which cases will regress spontaneously based on clinical or histopathological features.[61,63,64] However, infants with severe multisystem involvement usually have the more acute cutaneous form, with papulosquamous eruption in scalp, flexural areas, and trunk. LCH presenting as blueberry muffin baby has also been reported.[65]

Treatment of cutaneous LCH needs to be considerd in the context of the age of the patient and the degree of involvement of other organs. Surgical excision for isolated nodules may be occasionally indicated but mutilating surgery is never warranted. Topical steroids can be beneficial as first-line therapy, particularly for erythematous lesions, but recurrence after therapy is common. In severe skin disease, topical nitrogen mustard, topical tacrolimus or psoralen with ultraviolet (PUVA) photochemotherapy may be effective. Mild systemic chemotherapy such as prednisone and vinblastine is recommended in widespread disease but more intensive therapy may be required in cases of multisystem involvement.[59]

Class II: benign non-Langerhans cell histiocytoses

The cell of origin of this group of diseases is the monocyte/macrophage, a cell of diverse differentiation potential. Several disorders are included, and most of them have preferential skin involvement (see Table 70.2).

Juvenile xanthogranuloma (JXG) is the most common histiocytic disease; it appears usually in infancy or early childhood (median age 5–12 months) and usually regresses spontaneously.[66–68] Classically, patients develop a solitary small reddish-yellow firm papule with a surface telangiectasia, but multiple lesions may develop and systemic involvement, including CNS, liver/spleen, lung, eye, and muscle, has been reported. The eye is the most common extracutaneous site, and all children with JXG should have proper ophthalmological evaluation.[67] Two-thirds of patients develop solitary skin lesions; these lesions present as a small (<1 cm) firm nodule, usually during the first years of life (median age 2 years), and with predilection for head and neck.[66] In approximately 16% of patients, JXG may present as a solitary subcutaneous nodule or deep soft tissue mass; in this form lesions may be larger, up to 3 or 4 cm, and patients are diagnosed earlier in life (median age 3 months).[66,68] Multiple skin lesions are present in less than 10% of patients; this form usually presents during infancy, with numerous firm nodules that decrease or resolve over the years. A minority of patients (<5%) present with skin and visceral involvement (liver, lungs, spleen, kidneys, and brain); this systemic form is almost exclusive to the neonatal period and a fatal outcome is common.[66,68]

The pathology of JXG is characterized by dense, poorly defined infiltrates of small histiocytes with foreign body giant cells (Touton giant cells), and foam cells in the papillary and reticular dermis. Extension into the subcutaneous tissue, fascia, and peripheral muscle occurs in up to 38% of cases.[66,67] The characteristic histiocytes are clearly distinguishable from Langerhans cells by positivity for CD68, factor XIIIa, and vimentin. In general, no treatment is needed for JXG limited to the skin but systemic therapy may be required for JXG with visceral involvement, although it is considered a chemoresistant disease.

Sinus histiocytosis with massive lymphadenopathy (Rosai–Dorfman disease) is a reactive histiocytosis, generally benign, self-limited, and confined mainly to cervical lymph nodes. It usually affects young adults, who present with painless bilateral cervical lymphadenopathies usually with elevated erythrocyte sedimentation rate (ESR) and polyclonal gammopathy. Up to 40% of affected individuals have extranodal disease, and the skin is the most common site, followed by bone, salivary gland, CNS, and genitourinary, respiratory, and gastrointestinal systems. Isolated skin involvement is rare but well described.[67] Cutaneous lesions are yellow, sometimes erythematous papules or nodules, up to 4 cm in diameter, and spontaneous regression is commonly seen. The pathology of Rosai–Dorfman disease is defined by a characteristic expansion of the lymph node sinuses by large foamy histiocytes admixed with plasma cells. Fibrosis of the capsule and lymphocytophagocytosis (emperipolesis) are prominent. Typical cutaneous lesions include a dense upper dermal histiocyte infiltration with scattered multinucleated giant cells (Touton cells). These pathological histiocytes are negative for CD1a but positive for XIIIa.[67] There is no treatment with well-documented efficacy in Rosai–Dorfman disease, and close observation is usually recommended but steroids or LCH-type therapy may be indicated in cases of disease progression or involvement of critical structures.

Hemophagocytic lymphohistiocytosis (HLH) is a rare, life-threatening, rapidly progressive histiocytosis characterized by a benign proliferation of activated macrophages induced by T cell activation causing an uncontrolled phagocytic syndrome. This phenomenon may occur secondary to infections at any age or, most typically, during infancy in children with constitutional defects in NK lytic function. Skin rashes consisting of nonspecific, transient, generalized, maculopapular eruptions are present in up to 65% of patients. Erythroderma and purpuric macules/papules are also reported; isolated skin involvement does not occur. Treatment of HLH includes systemic chemotherapy for cytoreduction coupled with immunomodulation, with consolidation with allogeneic hematopoietic stem cell transplantation for patients with constitutional HLH.[67]

Much less frequent class II histiocytoses with skin involvement but with very rare occurrence in children are multicentric reticulohistiocytosis, sea-blue histiocytic syndrome, necrobiotic xanthogranuloma, and xanthoma disseminatum (see Table 70.2; reviewed in Newman *et al.*[67]).

Class III: malignant histiocytosis

Malignant histiocytosis is a very rare, life-threatening disease characterized by widespread neoplastic proliferation of histiocytic cells involving liver, spleen, lymph nodes, and bone marrow. It presents usually with painful lymphadenopathies, hepatosplenomegaly, fever, and night sweats.[67] In up to 50% of patients, extranodal extension is seen, mostly affecting skin, bone, and gastrointestinal tract. Skin involvement is present in 10–15% of cases, with single or multiple paponodular lesions, ranging from skin-colored to violaceous. Lesions can occur anywhere but predilection for extremities, especially lower legs and buttocks, is seen. Pathology shows deep dermal and subcutaneous infiltrate of atypical histiocytes around adnexal structures and blood vessels; emperipolesis is also common. Treatment of malignant histiocytosis is not well defined but management using the general guidelines of treatment of anaplastic large cell lymphomas is usually recommended. Recently, the use of alemtuzumab has been reported to be effective.[69]

Primary soft tissue sarcomas of the skin and the subcutaneous tissue

Primary sarcomas of the skin are extremely rare, representing <1% of malignant solid tumors in the adults, and even less in children (see Table 70.1).[70]

Kaposi sarcoma

Kaposi sarcoma (KS), an angioproliferative disorder, is the most common cutaneous soft tissue sarcoma in population-based studies, accounting for more than 70% of all cutaneous malignancies, with a higher incidence in males in all age groups.[70] There are four main types of KS: classic KS, which typically occurs among elderly Mediterranean men or Ashkenazi Jews; epidemic or HIV-associated KS; endemic KS, which presents in individuals of Central African countries; and transplantation-related KS. All four types have been associated with infection with human herpesvirus (HHV)-8, also known as KS-associated herpesvirus (KSHV).[71–73] The KSHV does not cause a very ubiquitous infection, and major variations in geographical prevalence occur. KSHV is very common in sub-Saharan Africa with seropositivity rates >50%, moderately prevalent in Mediterranean countries (20–30%), and less prevalent in Europe, the US, and Australia (<10%). Prevalence is most elevated in homosexual men.

Kaposi sarcoma is characterized by the development of purplish or dark macules, plaques, and cutaneous nodules that may ulcerate and bleed easily. In the classic form, these lesions can remain unchanged for months to years, although they can also grow rapidly and disseminate in weeks to months.[71–73] In children, KS is mostly limited to the epidemic form in countries with high prevalence of HIV/AIDS and, much less frequently, the transplantation-associated form. While cutaneous lesions are observed in >90% of adults with KS, cutaneous KS is less common in children with or without HIV infection. KS in young children with the epidemic form predominantly involves the lymph nodes, which is an atypical presentation in adults that has been associated with HHV-8 seroconversion.[74]

Effective antiretroviral therapy is key in the management of the epidemic form of KS, through immune reconstitution and control of HIV viremia, and it has also been shown to prevent the development of KS. Mild worsening may be seen with initiation of antiretroviral therapy due to the immune reactivation inflammatory syndrome. KS is not considered to be a curable tumor but durable remissions can be achieved. Indications to initiate treatment for KS include rapidly progressive disease, visceral disease, and bulky cutaneous disease. Different local treatments have been shown to be effective, including radiotherapy, cryotherapy, and intralesional injection of neoplastics. Systemic therapy is indicated for bulky and rapidly progressing disease. Regimens that include combinations of vincristine, bleomycin, doxorubicin, etoposide, and paclitaxel have proved to be effective.[72–74] Liposomal doxorubicin is currently the agent of choice; pegylated liposomes preferentially accumulate in highly vascularized KS lesions, and randomized trials have shown single-agent liposomal doxorubicin to be superior to a regimen combining vincristine, bleomycin, and doxorubicin.[72,73] Also, the preferential infection of endothelial cells and secondary production of vascular endothelial growth factor (VEGF) provide a strong rationale for the use of antiangiogenic agents. Targeting mTOR using rapamycin has been found to be effective in posttransplant KS and is currently being used to prevent and treat this disease.[72,73]

Dermatofibrosarcoma protuberans

Dermatofibrosarcoma protuberans (DFSP) is a rare cutaneous tumor of low-grade malignancy that typically manifests as a nodular mass on the trunk or proximal extremities and is characterized by an infiltrative growth pattern, a high rate of recurrence after simple excision, and a low potential for metastasis.[71,75] DFSP is the second most common cutaneous sarcoma, representing 18% of cutaneous sarcomas in population-based studies.[70] Incidence rates rise exponentially until 20 years of age to peak in the fourth and fifth decades, and subsequently decline. There appears to be a higher incidence in females across the age spectrum, and progesterone receptor expression may contribute to the rapid growth during pregnancy.[70] Ultrastructural and immunohistochemical data suggest that DFSP is of fibroblastic origin. In >90% of cases, DFSP featured t(17;22)(q22;q13) or a supernumerary ring chromosome composed of hybrid material derived from t(17;22). This results in fusion of *PDGF* gene on chromosome 22 with the *collagen 1 alpha 1 (COL1A1)* gene on chromosome 17 and constitutive production of COL1A1-PDGF-β fusion protein that is postranslationally processed to form functional PDGF-β.[71,75]

Dermatofibrosarcoma protuberans occurs most commonly in individuals aged 20–50 years, most frequently on the trunk (50–60%), proximal extremities (20–30%), and head and neck (10–15%).[75] The lesions appear as indurated pink, violet red, or flesh-colored plaques, and the surrounding skin may display telangiectasia. DFSP has a very indolent course, with a lengthy interval (months to years) preceding the onset of symptoms. Lesions typically are fixed to the dermis but not to deeper lying tissue, and typically do not exhibit a nodular/protuberant growth pattern until late in their course.[75–77] Some cases feature flat or depressed atrophic plaques that may remain nonprotuberant for many years.[77] Pathology is defined by the presence of large, bland spindle cell tumors of irregularly interwoven fascicles often in a storiform pattern, extending to deep dermis and fat with finger-like projections that can be difficult to distinguish from dermal fibroblasts. These lesions have a unique immunohistochemistry pattern, with positivity to CD34 and factor XIIIa and negativity for S-100, which helps differentiate them from factor XIIIa-negative dermatofibroma and S-100-positive neurofibroma. The low-grade, classic form of DFSP constitutes approximately 85–90% of cases; the remaining patients present with a fibrosarcomatous high-grade variant (FS-DFSP) with higher risk of local and distant metastases.[75]

The extent of tumor and degree of fixation to underlying tissue are generally assessed by physical examination; however, magnetic resonance imaging (MRI) may be useful for determining deep tumor invasion. Standard surgical excision is associated with local recurrence rates of 30–50%. Mohs micrographic surgery is the mainstay of treatment; mapping of tumors using this method has shown that tumors often exhibit tentacle-like extensions that are clinically unapparent and may extend beyond the clinically evident tumor by as much as 3 cm.[71,75,78] If conventional surgery is used, very wide margins (>3 cm) should be attempted. Adjuvant RT may benefit patients who have undergone resection whose specimens showed close margins.[75] The constitutive activation of platelet-derived growth factor (PDGF) typical of DFSP provides a strong rationale for the use of imatinib in the rare patients with metastatic disease, and in patients with inoperable presentations or with recurrent or extensive disease. In those cases, the use of imatinib in the neoadjuvant setting may help reduce the tumor burden, possibly allowing a more conservative surgical procedure.[75,79]

The clinical diagnosis of DFSP in childhood remains difficult, as it often resembles a vascular birthmark; the diagnosis of DFSP is uncommon in children younger than 16 and is usually established later, typically in the third or fourth decades of life.[76] Congenital cases of DFSP are also well described; however, a delay in diagnosis of congenital cases by several years is common.[76]

Angiomatoid (malignant) fibrous histiocytoma

Angiomatoid (malignant) fibrous histiocytoma (AMFH) was originally regarded as a variant of malignant fibrous histiocytoma, based on the presence of metastases in a proportion of cases. However, subsequent investigations have proven the generally indolent behavior of this neoplasm, with metastases in less than 5% of cases, usually in the regional lymph nodes.[80] AMFH is the third most common cutaneous neoplasm, accounting for 5% of the cases in population-based studies.[70] It typically occurs in children and young adults, usually in subcutis or deep dermis and presents as a solitary mass, most commonly in the extremities. Clinically it may resemble hematoma, hemangioma, or a benign cyst. It may be associated with systemic manifestations such as fever, weight loss and anemia, probably due to cytokine production by the tumor, as the systemic findings resolve shortly after surgery.[80,81]

Histology is very distinctive, with a dense fibrous capsule and a surrounding lymphocytic infiltrate that may closely mimic metastatic disease involving a lymph node; this chronic inflammatory infiltrate is generally most prominent around the periphery of the tumor. Blood-filled cystic spaces for which this tumor is named are common but not universal. AMFH has a unique immunophenotype, with positivity to desmin, epithelial membrane antigen, CD68, and CD99.[80,81] Myogenin and MyoD1 are always negative, which is an important element in the differential diagnosis of desmin-positive tumors in children. Despite their name, AMFHs do not express endothelial markers. AMFH is defined genetically by the translocation of the *ATF1* gene on 12q13 with either *FUS* (or *TLS*) on 16p11 or *EWSR1* on 22q12. There is no correlation between type of fusion and clinicopathological features.[81] Importantly, the *AFT1/EWSR1* translocation is identical to the one found in clear cell sarcoma (see below).

Treatment of AMFH is surgical and there is no role for systemic chemotherapy except for the rare cases of extranodal metastatic disease.

Cutaneous and subcutaneous leiomyosarcoma (superficial leiomyosarcoma)

Primary superficial leiomyosarcoma (LMS) is a rare indolent smooth cell neoplasm, accounting for less than 3% of all cutaneous soft tissue sarcomas.[70,82] Two groups of superficial LMS are described: cutaneous (arising in dermis, with or without extension into the subcutis, from the arrector pili or genital dartoic muscle) and subcutaneous (arising in the subcutis, from the smooth muscle wall of blood vessels).[71] Superficial LMS presents as indurated, erythematous, slow-growing single or clustered nodules, and often exhibits local discoloration, ranging from red, dark blue, black to whitish. The subcutaneous type presents as a palpable mass that may resemble lipoma, cyst or neurofibroma.[71] Superficial LMS has been described at all ages, from infants to the elderly, but highest frequency is in the middle age group.[71,82,83] It usually presents as solitary or grouped nodules in the hair-bearing surfaces of the extremities, particularly the lower extremities.[71,82] Treatment is mainly surgical, although local recurrence rates are in the range of 30–50% in both the cutaneous and subcutaneous forms. For this reason, wide local excisions, with 3–5 cm margins, or Mohs micrographic surgery are recommended.[82] While distant metastases are rare in the cutaneous form, and often limited to the regional lymph nodes, up to 40% of subcutaneous LMS metastasize.[82]

Angiosarcoma and other vascular neoplasms

Angiosarcoma

Angiosarcoma is a very aggressive, malignant endothelial cell tumor of vascular or lymphatic origin, accounting for approximately 2–5% of all cutaneous sarcomas.[70,84] It may occur at any age but its incidence is higher in the elderly, and its occurrence in children is extremely rare. Angiosarcoma is classified into five types: cutaneous, lymphedema associated, radiation induced, primary breast, and soft tissue.[84,85] Cutaneous angiosarcoma typically presents in elderly white men and preferentially involves the scalp. It can resemble a bruise, is typically multifocal and can be mistaken for a simple benign lesion, leading to delayed diagnosis. With increasing tumor size, tissue infiltration, edema, tumor fungation, ulceration, and hemorrhage can develop.[84] Lymphedema-associated cutaneous angiosarcoma (Stewart–Treves syndrome) has been described secondary to a variety of mechanisms, but most cases occur after mastectomy.[85] Radiation-induced cutaneous angiosarcoma usually occurs after long intervals, and it usually presents as diffuse infiltrative plaques or papulonodules, with ulceration.[85] Treatment is based on radical surgery, with the use of chemotherapy (taxanes or combinations of ifosfamide/doxorubicin) in cases of unresectable, recurrent, or metastatic disease.[84]

Pediatric angiosarcoma typically presents as soft tissue or visceral disease, although up to 30% of cases may occur in superficial locations in the head and neck.[86] True cutaneous angiosarcoma is extremely rare in children but appears to have some distinctive features. Tumors appear to predominate in lower extremities, with female predominance and presence of preexisting conditions such as congenital hemihypertrophy, Aicardi syndrome, congenital lymphedema, and congenital hemangioma treated with radiotherapy (RT).[87]

Epithelioid hemangioendothelioma

Epithelioid hemangioendothelioma (EHE) is considered to be a low-grade angiosarcoma; it usually appears as a solitary, slightly painful soft tissue tumor. It may occur at any age but is rare during childhood. At least half the cases are closely associated with a vessel, usually a vein, and in some cases, the occlusion of the vessel accounts for most of the symptoms, such as edema or thrombophlebitis. Treatment includes wide excision and clinical evaluation of lymph nodes. There are also forms of epithelioid angiosarcoma that may be confused with EHE.[85]

Endovascular papillary angioendothelioma (Dabska tumor)

This is a rare variant of low-grade angiosarcoma, initially described in the head and neck and extremities of six children ranging from 4 months to 15 years. Treatment consists of wide excision and regional lymphadenectomy if the nodes are clinically involved.[85]

Retiform hemangioendothelioma

A distinctive variant of low-grade angiosarcoma of the skin, preferentially involving the upper and lower extremities. It has been described in all age groups, and clinically presents as slow-growing exophytic masses or plaque-like dermal and subcutaneous nodules. It has a very low metastatic potential, and treatment is surgical, although local recurrences are common.[85]

Malignant glomus tumor

The majority of glomus tumors are small, benign neoplasms that occur in the dermis or subcutis of the extremities. However, occasional glomus tumors may show more aggressive clinical behavior, and the name glomangiosarcoma is commonly used. Atypical and malignant glomus tumors are exceptionally rare; lesions are larger and deeper than conventional glomus tumor and metastases may occur. Pathology may show sarcomatous areas intermingled with areas of benign glomus tumor.[85,88] This entity is extremely rare in children but cases have been described.[88]

Other cutaneous neoplasms with a significant vascular component include multinucleate cell angiohistiocytoma, angiofibroma, angioleiomyoma, angiolipoma, angiolipoleiomyoma, and angiomyxoma.[85]

Epithelioid sarcoma

Epithelioid sarcoma (ES) is a very rare soft tissue sarcoma, accounting for <1% of all soft tissue sarcomas.[89] Its histogenesis is unknown but it appears to be a mesenchymal tumor with predominant epithelial differentiation, showing reactivity for both epithelial and mesenchymal markers, such as cytokeratin, epithelial membrane antigen, vimentin, and CD34.[90] Unlike most soft tissue sarcomas, it characteristically spreads via lymphatics to noncontiguous areas of skin, deep soft tissue, fascia, and bone. Two types of epithelioid sarcoma are recognized: classic and proximal. In its conventional or classic form, it is usually a solitary or multifocal tumor involving the dermis, subcutis, or deeper soft tissues in the distal extremities of young adults, and is frequently associated with ulceration of the overlying skin. The classic-type ES is rare in children and older individuals. The proximal type has a more axial distribution (mediastinum, pelvis, perineum, trunk), with more deep-seated locations and more aggressive clinical behavior from the outset, and occurs predominantly in adults.

Histologically, the proximal or axial type is differentiated from the classic type by the presence of larger epithelioid cells, with vesicular nuclei and prominent nucleoli and atypia, and presence of rhabdoid features. Inactivation of *SMARCB1/INI1* in 22q11 (and corresponding absent INI1 staining) has been described in the proximal but not classic type, thus including this variant of epithelioid sarcoma in the rhabdoid family of tumors.

Epithelioid sarcoma is an aggressive neoplasm and local recurrence is the rule. It recurs persistently, often with successive lesions appearing more proximally, and eventually metastasizes.[90] Wide, total surgical excision with clear margins is needed. Metastases affecting the lymph nodes are common and sentinel node biopsies may be indicated in the diagnostic workup.

Clear cell sarcoma of tendons and aponeuroses

Clear cell sarcoma (CCS) is a rare sarcoma also referred to as malignant melanoma of the soft parts and thought to derive from neural crest cells. There is evidence of melanocyte differentiation by immunohistochemical, ultrastructural, and genomic profiling studies. Genetically it is characterized by the presence of a t(12;22)(q13;q12) that results in the *AFT1/EWSR1* fusion.[91] CCS has a predilection for the distal extremities of adolescents and young adults, especially the lower limbs, and a high propensity for regional or distant metastases. Histologically, the lesion is usually found to be infiltrating into tendons and aponeuroses. In accordance with the slow-growing behavior of this neoplasm, mitotic features are rare. The clear cell appearance is due to accumulation of glycogen. Immunohistochemistry is significant for expression of antigens associated with melanin synthesis such as HMB-45, Melan-A, and S-100, which make it indistinguishable from malignant melanoma. Treatment is mainly surgical and radical resections are usually indicated. Chemotherapy and radiation therapy usually have a very limited role. Sentinel node biopsies are also helpful for staging and for guiding the extent of surgery.[91,92]

Primary superficial Ewing sarcoma

Cutaneous and subcutaneous Ewing sarcoma is a rare but well-described entity with unique clinical features.[93–95] It typically develops in the hypodermis (and less frequently in the dermis) of adolescents and young adults (median age 17 years) and has a strong female predominance. Different from classic Ewing sarcoma, superficial Ewing sarcoma appears to have a predilection for the extremities (up to 60% of cases), followed by head and neck areas (20%).[93] It is histologically and molecularly indistinguishable from classic Ewing sarcoma. When treated following the standard guidelines of Ewing sarcoma, with chemotherapy and aggressive local control, the outcome of superficial Ewing sarcoma is excellent, with long-term survival rates in excess of 90%. Patients treated with surgery only have high local and distant recurrence rates.[93–95]

Infantile myofibromatosis

Infantile myofibromatosis (IM) is a rare fibrous tumor of infancy that can be solitary or multiple. Familial cases in siblings and successive generations have been described. Three types of IM are recognized: solitary IM, characterized by a single lesion affecting mainly skin or muscle of the head, neck, or trunk, and less frequently extremities, accounting for approximately 75% of the cases; multifocal IM without visceral involvement; and multifocal IM with visceral involvement or generalized (multicentric lesions arising not only in skin and muscle but also in bone, lung, heart, and gastrointestinal tract). While the solitary form is more common in males, the multifocal forms are more frequent in females. IM is almost exclusive to infants and children: 88% of cases are diagnosed before 2 years and 60% are noted at birth or shortly thereafter. Approximately 50% of the solitary and 90% of multifocal cases are congenital.[96,97]

Infantile myofibromatosis lesions appear as grossly well-demarcated, painless and nontender, 0.5–7 cm rubbery firm to hard subcutaneous nodules or masses covered by normal skin. Primary skin lesions may resemble hemangioma because of its prominent vascularity. Microscopically they form well-circumscribed nodules with biphasic features, with peripheral zone of spindle-shaped cells arranged in interweaving bundles or a whorled disposition (smooth muscle-like fascicles), and a central portion with rounder cells with perivascular disposition, extending from dermis to the subcutaneous tissue. Necrosis or a hemangiopericytoma-like pattern is often found in the center of the tumor nodules. Positive immunostaining for muscle actin, vimentin and desmin, and negative staining for S-100, strongly suggest the myofibroblastic origin of the spindle cells.[96,97]

Forms without visceral involvement have an excellent outcome, with spontaneous regression common, particularly in the multifocal forms, within 1–2 years. Surgery may be indicated for solitary lesions when excision is possible but radical surgeries should not be attempted. Patients with visceral involvement may have more severe disease, particularly those with gastrointestinal or cardiopulmonary compromise, and fatal outcomes have been described. Chemotherapy may promote tumor regression in those cases; combinations of vinblastine and methotrexate, or more intense sarcoma regimens have proven to be effective.[96–98]

Cutaneous malignant peripheral nerve sheath tumor

Cutaneous malignant peripheral nerve sheath tumor (cMPNST) is a very rare cutaneous sarcoma that may arise in patients with and without neurofibromatosis (NF)-1. It has the capacity for repeated local recurrence but appears to be associated with a lower propensity for metastasis. cMPNST may present at any age and anywhere on the body, although it appears to be more common in head, neck, and upper trunk. A plexiform variant of cMPNST that presents in infancy and childhood as either a congenital or acquired tumor also conforms to this pattern of local aggressive growth and a low propensity for metastases.[71]

Atypical fibroxanthoma

Atypical fibroxanthoma is a malignant fibrohohistiocytic neoplasm that most commonly arises on sun-damaged skin of elderly individuals, tends to recur locally, and has low potential for metastasis, less than that of its deeper soft tissue counterpart, the malignant fibrous histiocytoma. Atypical fibroxanthoma may also arise on nonexposed sites in younger individuals, typically after irradiation, and in children with xeroderma pigmentosum. It commonly presents as a nodule, often ulcerated, on markedly sun-damaged or irradiated skin of head and neck. Treatment is surgical; wide margins are typically required. Mohs micrographic surgery is also recommended.[71]

Cutaneous and subcutaneous leiomyoma

Solitary and multiple piloleiomyomas arise from the arrectores pilorum muscles, and solitary genital leiomyomas arise from the mamillary, vulvar, or dartoic muscles. The most common type of presentation is multiple piloleiomyomas that appear as grouped, linear or dermatomal arrangements of firm, red to brown intradermal nodules, which are fixed to the skin but not to deeper tissues. Extremities are most frequently involved, particularly in extensor surfaces, followed by trunk and face/neck. Pain may be induced by cold, emotions, touch, trauma or pressure, and it is believed to be secondary to pressure on nerve fibers within the tumor or contraction of muscle fibers. Patients with mutiple leiomyomas may also develop uterine leiomyomas and, rarely, leiomyosarcoma. In cases of multiple lesions, the clinical course is gradual progression, with no spontaneous regressions.

Treatment depends on number of lesions and the presence or absence of symptoms. Surgery with skin grafting may be indicated but frequent recurrences may occur, particularly in patients with multiple lesions. This entity is extremely rare in children.[82]

Smooth muscle hamartoma

Smooth muscle hamartoma is a rare benign proliferation of smooth muscle that may present in two forms. In the *congenital form*, lesions typically occur in the trunk and proximal extremities, may contain dark, long or thick hair, and have variable pigmentation. The degree of hypertrichosis, pigmentation, and induration may change with time. Enlargement with the growth of the child may also occur. Transient piloerection or elevation of a lesion induced by rubbing, referred to as the pseudo-Darier sign, is often seen. Pathology characteristically shows discrete, hyperplastic smooth muscle bundles within the reticular dermis; these bundles may extend into the subcutaneous tissue or may be associated with hair follicles in up to 40% of cases.[82] In the *adolescent or Becker nevus form*, hamartomas with hyperpigmentation and hypertrichosis occur usually on the shoulder of adolescent males. The differential diagnosis of smooth muscle hamartoma is with solitary mastocytoma, café-au-lait spot, and congenital pigmented hairy nevocellular nevus.[82]

Other cutaneous and subcutaneous mesenchymal neoplasms that are extremely rare in children include superficial liposarcoma, cutaneous angiolipoleiomyoma, dermatofibroma, plexiform fibrohistiocytic tumor, soft tissue giant cell tumor, and cutaneous malignant rhabdoid tumor.[80,82]

Metastatic tumors to the skin and subcutaneous tissues

Many pediatric malignancies are known to metastasize to the skin and subcutaneous tissues. In fact, it is estimated that approximately 50% of malignant cutaneous tumors in children are metastatic.[99] The most common solid malignancies which metastasize to the skin are neuroblastoma and sarcomas.[99,100] Approximately one-third of neonatal and 3% of all neuroblastoma cases present with cutaneous metastases. The typical lesions are firm, blue to purple papules and nodules with a blueberry muffin appearance. Catecholamine release may cause nodules to develop blanching with surrounding erythema when stroked.[100] The most common sarcoma causing skin metastases is rhabdomyosarcoma, particularly the alveolar subtype,[99,100] and skin involvement is also a common presentation in neonatal rhabdomyosarcoma.[101] Osteosarcoma also appears to have a predilection for skin metastases;[102,103] in those situations, the differential diagnosis with soft tissue giant cell tumor is important. Finally, neonatal and infantile malignant rhabdoid tumor has also been reported to metastasize to the skin.[104]

Blueberry muffin baby

Blueberry muffin baby is a descriptive term of purpuric lesions reflective of extramedullary hematopoiesis. The clinical lesions most commonly result from intrauterine infections, such as rubella and cytomegalovirus (CMV), and less commonly from malignancy and hematological disorders. The phenotypic designation blueberry muffin baby was first used in the 1960s to describe the characteristic appearance of neonates affected by congenital rubella. The multiple, dark to purple papules and nodules result from viral-induced dermal extramedullary hematopoiesis.[65] However, over the past 40 years, other causes of blueberry muffin baby have been reported in association with a variety of intrauterine congenital infections (toxoplasma, CMV, rubella, herpesvirus), hematological disorders (hereditary spherocytosis, hemolytic anemia, twin–twin transfusion syndrome), autoimmune conditions (neonatal lupus), and proliferative diseases (congenital leukemia, Langerhans cell histiocytosis, metastatic neuroblastoma, rhabdomyosarcoma, choriocarcinoma or malignant rhabdoid tumor). Most lesions display the characteristic histological features observed in skin metastases, with dermal-situated nodules.[65,105]

Primary cutaneous lymphomas

The World Health Organization-European Organization for Research and Treatment of Cancer (WHO-EORTC) classification of primary cutaneous lymphomas is summarized in Table 70.3.[106] Cutaneous T cell lymphoma is the most common cutaneous lymphoma, and includes mycosis fungoides, Sezary syndrome, cutaneous CD30[+] T cell lymphoproliferative disorders, and primary cutaneous peripheral T cell lymphoma. Cutaneous B cell lymphomas are very rare and almost exclusive to adults. Primary cutaneous lymphomas are of rare occurrence in children – only 5% occur in patients <20 years of age.[107] Most cases correspond to primary cutaneous T cell lynphoma but other unusual cutaneous lymphomas have also been described.

Cutaneous T cell and NK cell lymphomas

Mycosis fungoides
Mycosis fungoides is the most common cutaneous lymphoma, accounting for 50% of all primary cutaneous lymphomas in adults. It is characterized by a proliferation of small- to medium-sized T lymphocytes with cerebriform nuclei, and it typically affects older adults, who present with patches (generally in sun-protected areas) that progress over the years to form plaques and tumors.[106,108] In later stages of the disease, lymph nodes and visceral organs may become involved. The neoplastic cells have a mature CD4[+] T cell phenotype and clonal T cell receptor gene rearrangements are present. Local treatment alone is usually indicated for patients with disease limited to the skin, including phototherapy, topical application of nitrogen mustard, or radiotherapy; systemic multiagent chemotherapy is used only in case of extracutaneous involvement. Prognosis is usually excellent and depends on the stage, type and extent of the skin lesions; 10-year disease-specific survival rates range from 98% for patients with limited patch disease to less than 20% for patients with nodal involvement.[106] Mycosis fungoides is rare but well described in children and adolescents, and its clinical course does not seem to differ from the indolent course described in adults.[106,109]

Primary cutaneous CD30[+] lymphoproliferative disease
This entity includes primary cutaneous anaplastic large cell lymphoma (C-ALCL), lymphomatoid papulosis (LyP), and borderline cases. It is now generally accepted that C-ALCL and LyP form a spectrum of diseases, and that histological criteria alone are often insufficient to differentiate between these two ends of the spectrum. The clinical appearance and course are used as decisive criteria for the definite diagnosis and choice of treatment.

Primary cutaneous anaplastic large cell lymphoma
Primary C-ALCL is defined by the presence of large cells with anaplastic, pleomorphic, or immunoblastic cytomorphology and expression of the CD30 antigen. It presents mainly in adults with a male to female ratio of 2–3:1. Most patients present with solitary or localized nodules or tumors, often with ulceration. Multifocal lesions are present in 20% of the cases.

Table 70.3 WHO-EORTC classification of cutaneous lymphomas.

Category	Neoplasm
Cutaneous T cell and NK cell lymphomas	Mycosis fungoides
	Sezary syndrome
	Adult T cell leukemia/lymphoma
	Primary cutaneous CD30[+] lymphoproliferative disorders:
	– Primary cutaneous anaplastic large cell lymphoma
	– Lymphomatoid papulosis
	Subcutaneous panniculitis-like T cell lymphoma
	Extranodal NK/T cell lymphoma, nasal type
	Primary cutaneous peripheral T cell lymphoma:
	– Primary cutaneous epidermotropic CD8[+] T cell lymphoma
	– Cutaneous ϒ/∂ T cell lymphoma
	– Primary cutaneous CD4[+] small/medium-sized pleomorphic T cell lymphoma
Cutaneous B cell lymphomas	Primary cutaneous marginal zone B cell lymphoma
	Primary cutaneous follicle center lymphoma
	Primary cutaneous diffuse large B cell lymphoma, leg type
	Primary cutaneous diffuse large B cell lymphoma, other
Precursor hematological neoplasm	CD4[+]/CD56[+] hematodermic neoplasm (blastic NK cell lymphoma)

Source: Willemze et al.[106]

Skin lesions may show partial or complete spontaneous regression, as in LyP (see below). These lymphomas frequently relapse in the skin; extracutaneous dissemination occurs in approximately 10% of patients and mainly involves lymph nodes. Immunophenotypically, the neoplastic cells generally show an activated CD4+ T cell phenotype. Most cases show clonal rearrangement of T cell receptor genes. The t(2;5) (p23;35) translocation and its variants, which are a characteristic feature of systemic ALCL, is not or very rarely found in C-ALCL. Treatment is usually with surgical excision or radiation therapy. If multiple lesions are present, good results have been obtained with low-dose methotrexate. In cases of disease progression or extracutaneous involvement, ALCL-type therapy is indicated. In general, the prognosis is excellent, with long-term disease-free survival in excess of 80%.[106,107]

Lymphomatoid papulosis

Lymphomatoid papulosis is defined as a chronic, recurrent, self-healing papulonecrotic or papulonodular skin disease with histological features suggestive of a CD30+ malignant lymphoma. It typically presents in the fourth or fifth decades, with a slight male predominance, but pediatric cases are well described. Lesions appear as papular or papulonecrotic small nodules at different stages of development, predominantly on trunk and limbs. Duration may vary from several months to more than 40 years. Pathology is characterized by clusters of large CD30+ cells intermingled with a variable proportion of inflammatory cells; however, findings may vary with the age of the lesion. Similar to C-ALCL, the neoplastic lesions have clonally rearranged T cell receptor genes and absence of the t(2;5)(p23;35) translocation. Prognosis is excellent as most lesions resolve spontaneously.[107] Low-dose oral methotrexate is the most effective therapy to suppress the occurrence of new lesions.[106]

Nasal-type NK/T cell lymphoma

Extranodal nasal-type NK/T cell lymphoma is included as a separate CD56+ entity in the WHO-EORTC classification of cutaneous lymphomas. It is relatively common in Asian countries and also well described in Central and South America, but very infrequent in Europe and North America. Most cases originate from nasopharynx or tonsils; the disease is usually localized but up to one-third of patients may have B symptoms. Frequent angioinvasion and necrosis, association with Epstein–Barr virus (EBV), predilection for young males, and propensity for skin involvement are characteristic features. Nasal-type NK/T cell lymphoma is highly sensitive to radiation therapy but relatively resistant to chemotherapy.[106,110]

Other cutaneous T cell lymphomas

Cutaneous peripheral T cell lymphoma represents a heterogeneous group that includes all T cell neoplasms that do not fit into any other subtypes. It is very rare in pediatrics but up to 15% of nonanaplastic peripheral T cell lymphoma in children may have cutaneous involvement.[109,111]

Subcutaneous panniculitis-like T cell lymphoma is characterized by the presence of primary subcutaneous infiltrates of T cells and macrophages, predominantly affecting the legs, and often with an associated hemophagocytic syndrome. In the absence of extracutaneous involvement and hemophagocytosis, the clinical course may be rather indolent.[106,109]

Cutaneous B cell lymphoma

Cutaneous B cell lymphoma is much less frequent, accounting for less than 30% of primary cutaneous lymphomas in adults.[108] It includes three entities: marginal zone B cell lymphoma, follicle center lymphoma, and diffuse large B cell lymphoma, all of them extremely rare in children.[108,109,112,113]

CD4/CD56 hematodermic neoplasms

CD4/CD56 hematodermic neoplasm (formerly known as blastic NK cell lymphoma) is a recently recognized entity characterized by blastoid tumor cells expressing CD4 and CD56; it has high incidence of skin involvement and harbors the risk of leukemia dissemination. Although originally thought to be a NK neoplasm, recent studies suggest that it derives from a plasmacytoid dendritic cell.[106,114] Common B cell, T cell, NK, and myelomonocytic lineage markers are negative. Median age is 65 years, and patients usually present with solitary lesions that spread to multiple with time. Involvement of lymph nodes and bone marrow occurs in 10–20% of the cases. This entity has been described in childhood, although its true incidence and clinical behavior in this age group are not yet well known.[115]

Secondary skin involvement by hematological malignancies

Leukemia cutis is a general term used for cutaneous manifestations of leukemia; lesions result from infiltration of skin by neoplastic leukocytes or their precursors. Leukemia cutis can be seen in both congenital and childhood leukemias, including acute and chronic lymphoblastic leukemia (ALL, CLL), acute and chronic myelocytic leukemia (AML, CML). In general, the presence of leukemia cutis tends to be associated with a high tumor burden and a poor prognosis.[100] The frequency of leukemia cutis is 25–30% in congenital leukemia (where it can present with the typical appearance of blueberry muffin syndrome), 10–15% in AML, and only about 1–2% in ALL. Clinically lesions of leukemia cutis are highly variable, ranging from erythematous to violaceous papules, nodules, and/or plaques, and their clinical appearance is not specific to a particular type of leukemia.[100,116]

Lymphoma cutis is relatively rare in children with lymphoma. The incidence of skin involvement in lymphoblastic lymphoma is around 10%[116] but it can be as high as 26% in children with anaplastic large cell lymphoma (ALCL).[117] In ALCL, the skin is the most common extranodal site, and cutaneous involvement has an independent adverse prognostic factor.[117]

Myeloid sarcoma is an extramedullary tumor mass composed of immature cells of the myeloid series, which occurs in the setting of AML or myelodysplastic syndrome (MDS). Although myeloid sarcoma may occur at any age, it is most common in patients under 15 years. Primary myelosarcomas have a predilection for the skin but other organs can be affected, including the orbit, skeleton, and genitourinary or gastrointestinal tracts.[118,119] The incidence of myeloid sarcoma in the course of AML has been reported to be 3–5%, and may often precede the diagnosis of overt AML.[118,119] Skin infiltration is the most frequent localization associated with a myelomonocytic differentiation.[119] With proper AML therapy, outcome is comparable to children with overt AML.[119]

Cutaneous mastocytosis

The skin is the organ most frequently involved in mastocytosis. Cutaneous mastocytosis tends to appear early in life, and it is often accompanied by symptoms of mast cell activation such as flushing, pruritus, urtication, abdominal pain, nausea, vomiting, diarrhea, bone pain, vascular instability, headache, and neuropsychiatric problems. Three types of skin involvement are recognized: nodular, maculopapular, and diffuse cutaneous mastocytosis. Bullous lesions can occur in all forms and are related to the lesional mast cell load. *Nodular cutaneous mastocytosis* accounts for approximately 10–15% of the cases and always presents early in life, typically within the first 3 months. Lesions are also called mastocytomas, are either solitary or few in number and present as plaques or nodules, more frequently on the extremities. They are usually sharply defined, with an orange/yellow color, and when rubbed show the Darier sign (urtication and an axon flare). *Maculopapular cutaneous mastocytosis* is the most common form, accounting for more than 80% of the cases. It is characterized by generalized eruption of macules, papules, and plaques in random distribution, including mucous membranes but sparing palms and soles. Pruritus, dermographism, and Darier sign are additional features of these eruptions. Infants present with a papular variant that tends to involute before puberty; older children and adolescents present with urticaria pigmentosa, with large numbers and disseminated disease, also sparing palms and soles, persisting into adulthood. The least common form is *diffuse cutaneous mastocytosis*, which usually presents as erythroderma involving almost the entire skin. Darier sign is pronounced and often associated with hemorrhage and blister formation. Due to widespread and heavy mast cell load, these children have flushing, hypotension, shock, and diarrhea.[120]

References

1. Hamm H, Hoger P. Skin tumors in childhood. Dtsch Arztebl Int 2011; 108: 347–53.
2. Knight PJ, Reiner CB. Superficial lumps in children: what, when, and why? Pediatrics 1983; 72: 147–53.
3. Hamm H, Hoger PH. Skin tumors in childhood. Deutsch Arzteblatt Int 2011; 108: 347–53.
4. Knight PJ, Reiner CB. Superficial lumps in children: what, when, and why? Pediatrics 1983; 72: 147–53.
5. De la Luz Orozco-Covarrubias M, Tamayo-Sanchez L, Duran-McKinster C, Ridaura C, Ruiz-Maldonado R. Malignant cutaneous tumors in children. Twenty years of experience at a large pediatric hospital. J Am Acad Dermatol 1994; 30: 243–9.
6. Isaacs H Jr. Cutaneous metastases in neonates: a review. Pediatr Dermatol 2011; 28: 85–93.
7. Ries L, Gurney J, Tamra T, Young J, Bunin G. Cancer incidence and survival among children and adolescents: United States SEER Program 1975–1995. SEER Program NIH Pub 99–4649. Bethesda, MD: National Cancer Institute, 1999.
8. Bleyer A, Barr R, Ries LA. Cancer epidemiology in older adolescents and young adults 15 to 29 years of age including SEER incidence and survival: 1975–2000. Bethesda, MD: National Cancer Institute, 2006.
9. Youl P, Aitken J, Hayward N, et al. Melanoma in adolescents: a case–control study of risk factors in Queensland, Australia. Int J Cancer 2002; 98: 92–8.
10. Kraemer KH, DiGiovanna JJ, Moshell AN, Tarone RE, Peck GL. Prevention of skin cancer in xeroderma pigmentosum with the use of oral isotretinoin. N Engl J Med 1988; 318: 1633–7.
11. Bradford PT, Goldstein AM, Tamura D, et al. Cancer and neurologic degeneration in xeroderma pigmentosum: long term follow-up characterises the role of DNA repair. J Med Genet 2011; 48: 168–76.
12. Kleinerman RA, Tucker MA, Tarone RE, et al. Risk of new cancers after radiotherapy in long-term survivors of retinoblastoma: an extended follow-up. J Clin Oncol 2005; 23: 2272–9.
13. Muftuoglu M, Oshima J, von Kobbe C, Cheng WH, Leistritz DF, Bohr VA. The clinical characteristics of Werner syndrome: molecular and biochemical diagnosis. Hum Genet 2008; 124: 369–77.
14. Alexander A, Samlowski WE, Grossman D, et al. Metastatic melanoma in pregnancy: risk of transplacental metastases in the infant. J Clin Oncol 2003; 21: 2179–86.
15. Hale EK, Stein J, Ben-Porat L, et al. Association of melanoma and neurocutaneous melanocytosis with large congenital melanocytic naevi – results from the NYU-LCMN registry. Br J Dermatol 2005; 152: 512–17.
16. Makkar HS, Frieden IJ. Neurocutaneous melanosis. Semin Cutan Med Surg 2004; 23: 138–44.
17. Ceballos PI, Ruiz-Maldonado R, Mihm MC Jr. Melanoma in children. N Engl J Med 1995; 332: 656–62.
18. Curtis RE, Rowlings PA, Deeg HJ, et al. Solid cancers after bone marrow transplantation. N Engl J Med 1997; 336: 897–904.
19. Euvrard S, Kanitakis J, Claudy A. Skin cancers after organ transplantation. N Engl J Med 2003; 348: 1681–91.
20. Friedman DL, Whitton J, Leisenring W, et al. Subsequent neoplasms in 5-year survivors of childhood cancer: the Childhood Cancer Survivor Study. J Natl Cancer Inst 2010; 102: 1083–95.
21. Lazovich D, Vogel RI, Berwick M, Weinstock MA, Anderson KE, Warshaw EM. Indoor tanning and risk of melanoma: a case–control study in a highly exposed population. Cancer Epidemiol Biomarkers Prev 2010; 19: 1557–68.
22. Pappo AS. Melanoma in children and adolescents. Eur J Cancer 2003; 39: 2651–61.
23. Saenz NC, Saenz-Badillos J, Busam K, LaQuaglia MP, Corbally M, Brady MS. Childhood melanoma survival. Cancer 1999; 85: 750–4.
24. Melnik MK, Urdaneta LF, Al-Jurf AS, Foucar E, Jochimsen PR, Soper RT. Malignant melanoma in childhood and adolescence. Am Surg 1986; 52: 142–7.
25. Kaste SC, Pappo AS, Jenkins JJ 3rd, Pratt CB. Malignant melanoma in children: imaging spectrum. Pediatr Radiol 1996; 26: 800–5.
26. Strouse JJ, Fears TR, Tucker MA, Wayne AS. Pediatric melanoma: risk factor and survival analysis of the surveillance, epidemiology and end results database. J Clin Oncol 2005; 23: 4735–41.
27. Lange JR, Palis BE, Chang DC, Soong SJ, Balch CM. Melanoma in children and teenagers: an analysis of patients from the National Cancer Data Base. J Clin Oncol 2007; 25: 1363–8.
28. Wechsler J, Bastuji-Garin S, Spatz A, et al. Reliability of the histopathologic diagnosis of malignant melanoma in childhood. Arch Dermatol 2002; 138: 625–8.
29. Leman JA, Evans A, Mooi W, MacKie RM. Outcomes and pathological review of a cohort of children with melanoma. Br J Dermatol 2005; 152: 1321–3.
30. Mones JM, Ackerman AB. "Atypical" Spitz's nevus, "malignant" Spitz's nevus, and "metastasizing" Spitz's nevus: a critique in historical perspective of three concepts flawed fatally. Am J Dermatopathol 2004; 26: 310–33.
31. Cerroni L, Barnhill R, Elder D, et al. Melanocytic tumors of uncertain malignant potential: results of a tutorial held at the XXIX Symposium of

the International Society of Dermatopathology in Graz, October 2008. Am J Surg Pathol 2010; 34: 314–26.

32. Bastian BC, LeBoit PE, Hamm H, Brocker EB, Pinkel D. Chromosomal gains and losses in primary cutaneous melanomas detected by comparative genomic hybridization. Cancer Res 1998; 58: 2170–5.

33. Massi D, Cesinaro AM, Tomasini C, et al. Atypical Spitzoid melanocytic tumors: a morphological, mutational, and FISH analysis. J Am Acad Dermatol 2011; 64: 919–35.

34. Lohmann CM, Coit DG, Brady MS, Berwick M, Busam KJ. Sentinel lymph node biopsy in patients with diagnostically controversial spitzoid melanocytic tumors. Am J Surg Pathol 2002; 26: 47–55.

35. Berk DR, LaBuz E, Dadras SS, Johnson DL, Swetter SM. Melanoma and melanocytic tumors of uncertain malignant potential in children, adolescents and young adults – the Stanford experience 1995–2008. Pediatr Dermatol 2010; 27: 244–54.

36. Su LD, Fullen DR, Sondak VK, Johnson TM, Lowe L. Sentinel lymph node biopsy for patients with problematic spitzoid melanocytic lesions: a report on 18 patients. Cancer 2003; 97: 499–507.

37. Busam KJ, Murali R, Pulitzer M, et al. Atypical spitzoid melanocytic tumors with positive sentinel lymph nodes in children and teenagers, and comparison with histologically unambiguous and lethal melanomas. Am J Surg Pathol 2009; 33: 1386–95.

38. Moore-Olufemi S, Herzog C, Warneke C, et al. Outcomes in pediatric melanoma: comparing prepubertal to adolescent pediatric patients. Ann Surg 2011; 253: 1211–15.

39. Shah NC, Gerstle JT, Stuart M, Winter C, Pappo A. Use of sentinel lymph node biopsy and high-dose interferon in pediatric patients with high-risk melanoma: the Hospital for Sick Children experience. J Pediatr Hematol Oncol 2006; 28: 496–500.

40. Morton DL, Thompson JF, Cochran AJ, et al. Sentinel-node biopsy or nodal observation in melanoma. N Engl J Med 2006; 355: 1307–17.

41. Navid F, Furman WL, Fleming M, et al. The feasibility of adjuvant interferon alpha-2b in children with high-risk melanoma. Cancer 2005; 103: 780–7.

42. Chao MM, Schwartz JL, Wechsler DS, Thornburg CD, Griffith KA, Williams JA. High-risk surgically resected pediatric melanoma and adjuvant interferon therapy. Pediatr Blood Cancer 2005; 44: 441–8.

43. Ribeiro RC, Rill D, Roberson PK, et al. Continuous infusion of interleukin-2 in children with refractory malignancies. Cancer 1993; 72: 623–8.

44. Bauer M, Reaman GH, Hank JA, et al. A phase II trial of human recombinant interleukin-2 administered as a 4-day continuous infusion for children with refractory neuroblastoma, non-Hodgkin's lymphoma, sarcoma, renal cell carcinoma, and malignant melanoma. A Childrens Cancer Group study. Cancer 1995; 75: 2959–65.

45. Flaherty KT, Puzanov I, Kim KB, et al. Inhibition of mutated, activated BRAF in metastatic melanoma. N Engl J Med 2010; 363: 809–19.

46. Hodi FS, O'Day SJ, McDermott DF, et al. Improved survival with ipilimumab in patients with metastatic melanoma. N Engl J Med 2010; 363: 711–23.

47. Gerstenblith MR, Goldstein AM, Tucker MA. Hereditary genodermatoses with cancer predisposition. Hematol Oncol Clin North Am 2010; 24: 885–906.

48. Leonard JM, Ye H, Wetmore C, Karnitz LM. Sonic Hedgehog signaling impairs ionizing radiation-induced checkpoint activation and induces genomic instability. J Cell Biol 2008; 183: 385–91.

49. Dierks C. GDC-0449 – targeting the hedgehog signaling pathway. Recent Results Cancer Res 2010; 184: 235–8.

50. Rudin CM, Hann CL, Laterra J, et al. Treatment of medulloblastoma with hedgehog pathway inhibitor GDC-0449. N Engl J Med 2009; 361: 1173–8.

51. Von Hoff DD, LoRusso PM, Rudin CM, et al. Inhibition of the hedgehog pathway in advanced basal-cell carcinoma. N Engl J Med 2009; 361: 1164–72.

52. Altaykan A, Ersoy-Evans S, Erkin G, Ozkaya O. Basal cell carcinoma arising in nevus sebaceous during childhood. Pediatr Dermatol 2008; 25: 616–19.

53. Kraemer KH, Slor H. Xeroderma pigmentosum. Clin Dermatol 1985; 3: 33–69.

54. Jensen P, Hansen S, Moller B, et al. Skin cancer in kidney and heart transplant recipients and different long-term immunosuppressive therapy regimens. J Am Acad Dermatol 1999; 40: 177–86.

55. Horn HM, Tidman MJ. The clinical spectrum of dystrophic epidermolysis bullosa. Br J Dermatol 2002; 146: 267–74.

56. Toyoda H, Ido M, Nakanishi K, et al. Multiple cutaneous squamous cell carcinomas in a patient with interferon gamma receptor 2 (IFN gamma R2) deficiency. J Med Genet 2010; 47: 631–4.

57. Wollina U, Buslau M, Weyers W. Squamous cell carcinoma in pansclerotic morphea of childhood. Pediatr Dermatol 2002; 19: 151–4.

58. Badalian-Very G, Vergilio JA, Degar BA, Rodriguez-Galindo C, Rollins BJ. Recent advances in the understanding of Langerhans cell histiocytosis. Br J Haematol 2012; 156(2): 163–72.

59. Abla O, Egeler RM, Weitzman S. Langerhans cell histiocytosis: current concepts and treatments. Cancer Treat Rev 2010; 36: 354–9.

60. Munn S. Langerhans cell histiocytosis of the skin. Hematol Oncol Clin North Am 1998; 12: 269–86.

61. Lau L, Krafchik B, Trebo MM, Weitzman S. Cutaneous Langerhans cell histiocytosis in children under one year. Pediatr Blood Cancer 2006; 46: 66–71.

62. Minkov M, Prosch H, Steiner M, et al. Langerhans cell histiocytosis in neonates. Pediatr Blood Cancer 2005; 45: 802–7.

63. Stein SL, Haut PR, Mancini AJ. Langerhans cell histiocytosis presenting in the neonatal period: a retrospective case series. Arch Pediatr Adolesc Med 2001; 155: 778–83.

64. Battistella M, Teillac DH, Brousse N, de Prost Y, Bodemer C. Neonatal and early infantile cutaneous Langerhans cell histiocytosis: comparison of self-regressive and non-self regressive forms. Arch Dermatol 2010; 146: 149–56.

65. Shaffer MP, Walling HW, Stone MS. Langerhans cell histiocytosis presenting as blueberry muffin baby. J Am Acad Dermatol 2005; 53: S143–6.

66. Dehner L. Juvenile xanthogranulomas in the first two decades of life: a clinicopathologic study of 174 cases with cutaneous and extracutaneous manifestations. Am J Surg Pathol 2003; 27: 579–93.

67. Newman B, Hu W, Nigro K, Gilliam AC. Aggressive histiocytic disorders that can involve the skin. J Am Acad Dermatol 2007; 56: 302–16.

68. Janssen D. Juvenile xanthogranuloma in childhood and adolescence: a clinicopathologic study of 129 patients from the Kiel pediatric tumor registry. Am J Surg Pathol 2005; 29: 21–8.

69. Shukla N, Kobos R, Renaud T, et al. Successful treatment of refractory metastatic histiocytic sarcoma with alemtuzumab. Cancer 2011; Dec 13 [Epub ahead of print].

70. Rouhani P, Fletcher CDM, Devesa SS, Toro JR. Cutaneous soft tissue sarcoma incidence patterns in the U.S. Cancer 2008; 113: 616–27.

71. Guillen DR, Cockerell CJ. Cutaneous and subcutaneous sarcomas. Clin Dermatol 2001; 19: 262–8.

72. Uldrick T, Whitby D. Update on KSHV epidemiology, Kaposi sarcoma pathogenesis, and treatment of Kaposi sarcoma. Cancer Lett 2011; 305: 150–62.

73. Mesri EA, Cesarman E, Boshoff C. Kaposi's sarcoma and its associated herpesvirus. Nat Rev Cancer 2010; 10: 707–19.

74. Gantt S, Kakuru A, Wald A, et al. Clinical presentation and outcome of epidemic Kaposi sarcoma in Ugandan children. Pediatr Blood Cancer 2010; 54: 670–4.

75. McArthur G. Dermatofibrosarcoma protuberans: recent clinical progress. Ann Surg Oncol 2007; 14: 2876–86.

76. Checketts SR, Hamilton TK, Baughman RD. Congenital and childhood dermatofibrosarcoma protuberans: a case report and review of the literature. J Am Acad Dermatol 2000; 42: 907–13.

77. Martin L, Combemale P, Dupin M, et al. The atrophic variant of dermatofibrosarcoma protuberans in childhood: a report of six cases. Br J Dermatol 1998; 139: 719–25.

78. Paradisi A, Abeni D, Rusciani A, et al. Dermatofibrosarcoma protuberans: wide local excision vs. Mohs micrographic surgery. Cancer Treat Rev 2008; 34: 728–36.

79. Gooskens SLM, Oranje AP, van Adrichem LNA, *et al*. Imatinib mesylate for children with dermatofibrosarcoma protuberans (DFSP). Pediatr Blood Cancer 2010; 55: 369–73.

80. Billings SD, Folpe AL. Cutaneous and subcutaneous fibrohistiocytic tumors of intermediate malignancy: an update. Am J Dermatol 2004; 26: 141–55.

81. Thway K. Angiomatoid fibrous histiocytoma: a review with recent genetic findings. Arch Pathol Lab Med 2008; 132: 273–7.

82. Holst VA, Junkins-Hopkins JM, Elenitsas R. Cutaneous smooth muscle neoplasms: clinical features, histologic findings, and treatment options. J Am Acad Dermatol 2002; 46: 477–90.

83. Blaise G, Nikkels AF, Quatresooz P, *et al*. Childhood cutaneous leiomyosarcoma. Pediatr Dermatol 2009; 26: 477–9.

84. Young RJ, Brown NJ, Reed MW, Hughes D, Woll PJ. Angiosarcoma. Lancet Oncol 2010; 11: 983–91.

85. Requena L, Sangueza OP. Cutaneous vascular proliferations. Part III. Malignant neoplasms, other cutaneous neoplasms with significant vascular component, and disorders erroneously considered as vascular neoplasms. J Am Acad Dermatol 1998; 38: 143–75.

86. Ayadi L, Khabir A. Pediatric angiosarcoma of soft tissue: a rare clinicopathologic entity. Arch Pathol Lab Med 2010; 134: 481–5.

87. Deyrup A, Miettinen M, North P, *et al*. Pediatric cutaneous angiosarcomas: a clinicopathologic study of 10 cases. Am J Surg Pathol 2011; 35: 70–5.

88. Folpe A, Fanburg-Smith J, Miettinen M, Weiss S. Atypical and malignant glomus tumor: analysis of 52 cases, with a proposal for the reclassification of glomus tumors Am J Surg Pathol 2001; 25: 1–12.

89. Ferrari A, Sultan I, Huang TT, *et al*. Soft tissue sarcoma across the age spectrum: a population-based study from the Surveillance Epidemiology and End Results database. Pediatr Blood Cancer 2011; 57: 943–9.

90. Armah HB, Parwani AV. Epithelioid sarcoma. Arch Pathol Lab Med 2009; 133: 814–19.

91. Dim DC, Cooley LD, Miranda RN. Clear cell sarcoma of tendons and aponeuroses: a review. Arch Pathol Lab Med 2007; 131: 152–6.

92. Hantschke M, Mentzel T, Rutten A, *et al*. Cutaneous cell sarcoma: a clinicopathologic, immunohistochemical, and molecular analysis of 12 cases emphasizing its distinction from dermal melanoma. Am J Surg Pathol 2010; 34: 216–22.

93. Delaplace M, Lhommet C, de Pinieux G, Vergier B, de Muret A, Machet L. Primary cutaneous Ewing's sarcoma: a systematic review focused on treatment and outcome. Br J Dermatol 2011; Nov 19 [Epub ahead of print].

94. Machado I, Llombart B, Calabuig-Fariñas S, Llombart-Bosch A. Superficial Ewing's sarcoma family of tumors: a clinicopathological study with differential diagnoses. J Cutan Pathol 2011; 38: 636–43.

95. Terrier-Lacombe MJ, Guillou L, Chibon F, *et al*. Superficial primitive Ewing's sarcoma: a clinicopathologic and molecular cytogenetic analysis of 14 cases. Mod Pathol 2008; 22: 87–94.

96. Chung EB, Enzinger FM. Infantile myofibromatosis. Cancer 1981; 48: 1807–18.

97. Larralde M, Hoffner MV, Boggio P, Abad ME, Luna PC, Correa N. Infantile myofibromatosis: report of nine patients. Pediatr Dermatol 2010; 27: 29–33.

98. Levine E, Fréneaux P, Schleiermacher G, *et al*. Risk-adapted therapy for infantile myofibromatosis in children. Pediatr Blood Cancer 2011; Oct 28 [Epub ahead of print].

99. Wesche WA, Khare VK, Chesney TM, Jenkins JJ. Non-hematopoietic cutaneous metastases in children and adolescents: thirty years experience at St. Jude Children's Research Hospital. J Cutan Pathol 2000; 27: 485–92.

100. Wright T. Cutaneous manifestations of malignancy. Curr Opin Pediatr 2011; 23: 407–11.

101. Rodriguez-Galindo C, Hill DA, Onyekwere O, *et al*. Neonatal alveolar rhabdomyosarcoma with skin and brain metastases. Cancer 2001; 92: 1613–20.

102. Collier DAH, Busam K, Salob S. Cutaneous metastasis of osteosarcoma. J Am Acad Dermatol 2003; 49: 757–60.

103. Larsen S, Davis DMR, Comfere NI, Folpe AL, Sciallis GF. Osteosarcoma of the skin. Int J Dermatol 2010; 49: 532–40.

104. Hsueh C, Kuo T. Congenital malignant rhabdoid tumor presenting as a cutaneous nodule: report of 2 cases with review of the literature. Arch Pathol Lab Med 1998; 122: 1099–102.

105. Isaacs H. Cutaneous metastases in neonates: a review. Pediatr Dermatol 2011; 28: 85–93.

106. Willemze R, Jaffe ES, Burg Gn, *et al*. WHO-EORTC classification for cutaneous lymphomas. Blood 2005; 105: 3768–85.

107. Yu JB, Blitzblau RC, Decker RH, Housman DM, Wilson LD. Analysis of primary CD30+ cutaneous lymphoproliferative disease and survival from the Surveillance, Epidemiology, and End Results database. J Clin Oncol 2008; 26: 1483–8.

108. Bradford PT, Devesa SS, Anderson WF, Toro JR. Cutaneous lymphoma incidence patterns in the United States: a population-based study of 3884 cases. Blood 2009; 113: 5064–73.

109. Fink-Puches R, Chott A, Ardigó M, *et al*. The spectrum of cutaneous lymphomas in patients less than 20 years of age. Pediatr Dermatol 2004; 21: 525–33.

110. Li YX, Fang H, Liu QF, *et al*. Clinical features and treatment outcome of nasal-type NK/T-cell lymphoma of Waldeyer ring. Blood 2008; 112: 3057–64.

111. Hutchison RE, Laver JH, Chang M, *et al*. Non-anaplastic peripheral t-cell lymphoma in childhood and adolescence: a Children's Oncology Group study. Pediatr Blood Cancer 2008; 51: 29–33.

112. Boccara O, Laloum-Grynberg E, Jeudy Gr, *et al*. Cutaneous B-cell lymphoblastic lymphoma in children: a rare diagnosis. J Am Acad Dermatol 2012; 66(1): 51–7.

113. Sharon V, Mecca PS, Steinherz PG, Trippett TM, Myskowski PL. Two pediatric cases of primary cutaneous B-cell lymphoma and review of the literature. Pediatr Dermatolo 2009; 26: 34–9.

114. Assaf C, Gellrich S, Whittaker S, *et al*. CD56-positive haematological neoplasms of the skin: a multicentre study of the Cutaneous Lymphoma Project Group of the European Organisation for Research and Treatment of Cancer. J Clin Pathol 2007; 60: 981–9.

115. Ruggiero A, Maurizi P, Larocca L, Arlotta A, Riccardi R. Childhood CD4+/CD56+ hematodermic neoplasm: case report and review of the literature. Haematologica 2006; 91: ECR48.

116. Millot F, Robert A, Bertrand Y, *et al*. Cutaneous involvement in children with acute lymphoblastic leukemia or lymphoblastic lymphoma. Pediatrics 1997; 100: 60–4.

117. Le Deley MC, Reiter A, Williams D, *et al*. Prognostic factors in childhood anaplastic large cell lymphoma: results of a large European intergroup study. Blood 2008; 111: 1560–6.

118. Breccia M, Mandelli F, Petti MC, *et al*. Clinico-pathological characteristics of myeloid sarcoma at diagnosis and during follow-up: report of 12 cases from a single institution. Leukemia Res 2004; 28: 1165–9.

119. Reinhardt D, Creutzig U. Isolated myelosarcoma in children – update and review. Leukemia Lymphoma 2002; 43: 565–74.

120. Wolff K, Komar M, Petzelbauer P. Clinical and histopathological aspects of cutaneous mastocytosis. Leukemia Res 2001; 25: 519–28.

121. Edge SB, Byrd DR, Compton CC, (eds). *AJCC Cancer Staging Manual*, 7th edn. New York, NY: Springer, 2010.

Index

Textbook of Uncommon Cancer, Fourth Edition. Edited by Derek Raghavan, Charles D. Blanke, David H. Johnson, Paul L. Moots, Gregory H. Reaman, Peter G. Rose and Mikkael A. Sekeres.
© 2012 John Wiley & Sons, Inc. Published 2012 by John Wiley & Sons, Inc.

esophagus 382–3
lung *see* pulmonary large cell neuroendocrine
  carcinoma
laryngectomy 126–7
larynx
  anatomy 119, *120*
  function-sparing treatment 126–7
  tumors 119–29
    clinical presentation 119
    epithelial 120, 121–3
    imaging 119–20
    mesenchymal 124–5
    neuroendocrine 125–6
    pathological subtypes 121–6
    salivary gland-derived 123–4
    staging 119, **121, 122**
    submucosal 119, 120
    treatment 126–9
"leiomyoblastoma" 557
leiomyoma
  benign metastasizing (BML) 557
  cutaneous/subcutaneous pediatric 952
  esophagus *380*, 380–1
  urethra 37
  uterus 550, 551, **551**
    variants mimicking cancer 557
leiomyomatosis
  disseminated peritoneal 557
  intravenous 557
  and renal cell carcinoma syndrome,
    hereditary 557
leiomyosarcoma (LMS)
  bile duct 432
  bladder 32
  cervix 580
  colon and rectum 458
  cutaneous/subcutaneous 675
    pediatric 950
  esophagus 381
  gallbladder 428
  liver 433
  lung 305, *305*
    children 892
    epidemiology 303
    immunohistochemistry 305, **305**
    prognosis 313–14
    treatment 314–15
  oral cavity *105*, 105–6
  prostate 55–6, *56*
  renal 13
  respiratory tree, children 885
  small bowel 446
  subcutaneous 675
  superficial 675
    pediatric 950
  uterus 550–3
    benign mesenchymal tumors mimicking 557
    chemotherapy 548, **548, 549**, 552–3
    pathology *550*, 550–1, **551,** *551*
    radiotherapy 548, 552
  vulva 593
lenalidomide
  5q- syndrome 613
  myeloproliferative neoplasms 652, **653**
lepidic predominant adenocarcinoma (LPA),
  lung 355, 360
leptomeningeal melanomatosis, primary 709
  neuroimaging 710–11, *711*
leptomeninges
  choroid plexus tumors 759, 762, *762*
  glioma metastases 770
  primary CNS lymphoma 748, 749
letrozole
  endometrial carcinoma 544, **544**

male breast cancer 237, 238
Letterer–Siwe disease 108
leucovorin, urachal cancer 31
leukemia
  acute 601–7, **602**
  B cell 617–19
  bilineal *606*, 606–7
  biphenotypic 606
  cutis, children 954
  myeloproliferative neoplasm-associated 601–5
  ovarian involvement 920
  prostatic involvement 65, 66
  stem cell 606–7
  testicular involvement 922
  see also specific types
leukemia/lymphoma-related factor (LRF), prostate
  cancer 66
leukocoria, retinoblastoma 841, *842*
leukocyte alkaline phosphatase (LAP) score 603,
  603, 654
leukoencephalopathy, treatment-related, primary
  CNS lymphoma 753
leuprolide acetate, stromal ovarian tumors 510, **511**
Leydig cells 81
  hyperplasia 81
Leydig cell tumors (LCT)
  ovary 516
  testis 81–3
    management 82–3, **83**
    pathology 81–2, *82*
lichen sclerosus, vulvar 587
Li–Fraumeni syndrome
  adrenocortical tumors 173, **173**, 904, **904**, 910
  choroid plexus tumors 760, 932
  paratesticular rhabdomyosarcoma 88
  phyllodes tumor of breast 243–4, 246
  uterine leiomyosarcoma 550
light chain, serum free 628
linitis plastica, bladder adenocarcinoma 28
lipid cell tumors *see* steroid cell tumors
lipoblastoma
  heart 884
  mediastinum 882
liposarcoma
  breast 249
  esophagus 381
  renal 13
  skin 675–6
liver
  anatomy *423*
  fibrolamellar carcinoma 432–3
  lymphoma 434
  mesenchymal tumors 433–4
  metastatic tumors *see* hepatic metastases
  neuroendocrine tumors 434
  tumors 432–4
liver flukes, bile duct tumors 429
liver transplantation
  bile duct tumors 430
  fibrolamellar carcinoma 432–3
  hepatoblastoma 434
  metastatic gastrointestinal stromal tumors 476
  neuroendocrine tumors 434
LNH-84 protocol, T cell lymphoblastic
  lymphoma 660–1
lobular carcinoma, male breast 235
lomustine *see* CCNU
loss of heterozygosity (LOH)
  adrenocortical carcinoma 173, 174
  chordomas 723
  embryonal rhabdomyosarcoma 596
  malignant mesothelioma 319
  meningioma 736
  oligodendrogliomas 786, 787, 788

parathyroid carcinoma 203
salivary gland adenoid cystic carcinoma 102
thymoma 281
LP cells 622, *622*
lung
  atypical adenomatous hyperplasia (AAH) 356
  benign lesions, imitating sarcoma 312
  congenital cystic adenomatoid malformation
    (CCAM-CPAM) 886
  inflammatory pseudotumors 312
  lymphangioleiomatosis 312
  transplantation, bronchioloalveolar
    carcinoma 359
  tumors *see* pulmonary tumors
Lung Cancer Study Group (LCSG) 358
luteinizing hormone (LH) receptors, adrenocortical
  carcinoma 174
lymphangioleiomatosis, pulmonary 312
lymphedema-associated angiosarcoma 673–4, 950
lymph node dissection
  cervical cancer 567, 583
  cervical melanoma 581–2
  colorectal carcinoids 455
  endometrial cancer 541–2
  endometrial stromal sarcoma 554
  fallopian tube cancer 535
  gastrointestinal stromal tumors 470
  medullary thyroid carcinoma 190, 191
  pediatric adrenocortical tumors 908
  pediatric colorectal carcinoma 856
  stromal ovarian tumors 509
  testicular Leydig cell tumors 83
  uterine leiomyosarcoma 551
  vulvar cancer 588–9, 591
  see also axillary lymph node dissection; neck
    dissection; retroperitoneal lymph node
    dissection; sentinel lymph node biopsy
lymph node involvement (LNI)
  adenoid cystic carcinoma of breast 221
  anorectal melanoma 695, 696
  borderline tumors of ovary 499, 503
  esthesioneuroblastoma 158–9
  fallopian tube cancer 533–4
  gastric lymphoma 402
  laryngeal cancer 128
  male breast cancer 235, 237
  malignant mesothelioma of tunica vaginalis 87
  medullary thyroid carcinoma 190
  metaplastic breast carcinoma 215
  nasopharyngeal carcinoma 137, 141
  renal Xp11 translocation neoplasms 6, 915
  small bowel adenocarcinoma 445
  vulvar cancer 588, 589
lymphoblastic lymphoma, T cell (T-LBL) 659–61
lymphocytes
  breast lobulitis 227
  Langerhans cell histiocytosis 716
  nasopharyngeal carcinoma 135, *135*, 136
  thymic development 280
  thymoma 281, 283, *283*
  thymus 281, 282
"lymphoepithelial carcinomas," nasopharynx 136
lymphoepithelial lesions, breast lymphoma 226, 227
lymphoepithelioma
  bladder 29
  nasopharynx 135, 139, 140
lymphoepithelioma-like carcinoma (LELC)
  cervix 571
  esophagus 384
  skin 671
  stomach 403, *403*
  thymus (LETC) 286, *286*
    molecular biology 287
    pediatric patients 879